Schizophrenia

For Teresa
and Georgina, Colette, Eleanor and Phineas
SRH

For Leslie and Collin
DRW

Schizophrenia

Edited by

Steven R. Hirsch
MD FRCP FRCPsych
*Professor of Psychiatry Emeritus, Division of Neuroscience
and Psychological Medicine, Imperial College Faculty of
Medicine, and Director of Teaching Governance,
West London Mental Health NHS Trust
London, UK*

Daniel R. Weinberger
MD
*Chief, Clinical Brain Disorders Branch
Intramural Research Program
National Institute of Mental Health
Bethesda
MD 20982, USA*

SECOND EDITION

Blackwell
Publishing

First published 1995
Reprinted 1996, 1997
Second edition 2003

Library of Congress Cataloging-in-Publication Data
Schizophrenia/edited by Steven R. Hirsch, Daniel R. Weinberger. —2nd ed.
p.; cm.
Includes bibliographical references and index.
ISBN 0-632-06388-2 (hardback)
1. Schizophrenia.
[DNLM: 1. Schizophrenia. WM 203 S33721 2003] I. Hirsch, Steven R. II. Weinberger, Daniel R. (Daniel Roy)
RC 514.S33413   2003
616.89′82—dc21   2002151908

ISBN 0-632-06388-2

A catalogue record for this title is available from the British Library

Set in 9/12 Sabon by SNP Best-set Typesetter Ltd., Hong Kong
Printed and bound in Great Britain at the Bath Press, Bath

Commissioning Editor: Stuart Taylor
Managing Editor: Rupal Malde
Editorial Assistant: Geraldine Jeffers
Production Editor: Lindsey Williams
Production Controller: Chris Downs

For further information on Blackwell Science, visit our website:
www.blackwellpublishing.com

Contents

Contributors, vii

Foreword by Nancy C. Andreasen, xi

Preface to the Second Edition, xiii

Preface to the First Edition, xv

Part 1: Descriptive Aspects

1 Concepts and classification of schizophrenia, 3
   J.K. Wing & N. Agrawal
2 Descriptive psychopathology, 15
   J. Cutting
3 The symptoms of schizophrenia, 25
   R.L.M. Fuller, S.K. Schultz & N.C. Andreasen
4 Child and adolescent onset schizophrenia, 34
   C. Hollis
5 Atypical psychotic disorders, 54
   C.B. Pull, J.M. Cloos & N.V. Murthy
6 Late-onset schizophrenia, 68
   R. Howard & D.V. Jeste
7 The schizophrenia spectrum personality disorders, 80
   K. O'Flynn, J. Gruzelier, A. Bergman & L.J. Siever
8 Course and outcome of schizophrenia, 101
   H. Häfner & W. an der Heiden
9 Depression and schizophrenia, 142
   S.G. Siris & C. Bench
10 Neurocognitive deficits in schizophrenia, 168
   T.E. Goldberg, A. David & J.M. Gold

Part 2: Biological Aspects

11 The secondary schizophrenias, 187
   T.M. Hyde & S.W. Lewis
12 The epidemiological horizon, 203
   A. Jablensky
13 Risk factors for schizophrenia: from conception to birth, 232
   J.J. McGrath & R.M. Murray
14 Genetics and schizophrenia, 251
   B. Riley, P. Asherson & P. McGuffin
15 Intermediate phenotypes in genetic studies of schizophrenia, 277
   M.F. Egan, M. Leboyer & D.R. Weinberger
16 Electrophysiology, 298
   D.F. Salisbury, S. Krljes & R.W. McCarley

17 Neuropathology of schizophrenia, 310
   P.J. Harrison & D.A. Lewis
18 Schizophrenia as a neurodevelopmental disorder, 326
   D.R. Weinberger & S. Marenco
19 The neurochemistry of schizophrenia, 349
   B. Moghaddam & J.H. Krystal
20 Dopamine transmission in the schizophrenic brain, 365
   M. Laruelle
21 Animal models of schizophrenia, 388
   B.K. Lipska & D.R. Weinberger
22 Brain imaging in schizophrenia, 403
   P. Liddle & C. Pantelis

Part 3: Physical Treatments

23 The neuroscience and clinical psychopharmacology of first- and second-generation antipsychotic drugs, 421
   J.L. Waddington, S. Kapur & G.J. Remington
24 Acute pharmacological treatment of schizophrenia, 442
   S. Miyamoto, T.S. Stroup, G.E. Duncan, A. Aoba & J.A. Lieberman
25 Maintenance treatment, 474
   S.R. Marder & D.A. Wirshing
26 Treatment-resistant schizophrenia, 489
   T.R.E. Barnes, P. Buckley & S.C. Schulz
27 Electroconvulsive therapy and schizophrenia, 517
   H.A. Sackeim
28 Neuroleptic-induced acute extrapyramidal syndromes and tardive dyskinesia, 552
   V.S. Mattay & D.E. Casey
29 Non-neurological side-effects of antipsychotic drugs, 573
   D.C. Goff & R.I. Shader

Part 4: Psychosocial Aspects

30 Schizophrenia and violence, 591
   P.J. Taylor & S.E. Estroff
31 Schizophrenia and psychosocial stresses, 613
   P.E. Bebbington & E. Kuipers
32 Psychiatric rehabilitation, 637
   T.K.J. Craig, R.P. Liberman, M. Browne, M.J. Robertson & D. O'Flynn
33 Psychological treatments for schizophrenia, 657
   B.V. Martindale, K.T. Mueser, E. Kuipers, T. Sensky & L. Green
34 Mental health services, 688
   M. Muijen, F. Holloway & H. Goldman

CONTENTS

35 Psychosis and recovery: some patients' perspectives, 701
P. Chadwick, R. Lundin, G. Brown, A. McPartlin,
C. Brookman & J. Antoniou

36 Economics of the treatment of schizophrenia, 713
S.M. Essock, L.K. Frisman & N.H. Covell

Index, 725

Contributors

N. Agrawal MB BS MD MSc MRCPsych
Specialist Registrar and Honorary Clinical Research Fellow, Department of Psychological Medicine, Imperial College School of Medicine, Chelsea & Westminster Hospital, London SW10 9NG, UK

N.C. Andreasen MD PhD
Andrew H. Woods Chair of Psychiatry, Roy J. and Lucille A. Carver College of Medicine, The University of Iowa, IA, USA; Director, The MIND Institute, Adjunct Professor of Psychiatry and Neurology, The University of New Mexico, NM, USA

J. Antoniou
Patient contributor

A. Aoba MD PhD
Professor, Department of Neuropsychiatry, St Marianna University School of Medicine, Japan

P.J. Asherson MRCPsych PhD
Senior Lecturer in Molecular Psychiatry, MRC Social Developmental Genetic Psychiatry Centre, Institute of Psychiatry, De Crespigny Park, London SE5 8AF, UK

T.R.E. Barnes MD FRCPsych DSc
Professor of Clinical Psychiatry, Department of Psychological Medicine, Imperial College Faculty of Medicine, London W6 8RP, UK

P.E. Bebbington PhD FRCP FRCPsych
Professor of Social and Community Psychiatry, University College London, London, UK

C. Bench PhD
Senior Lecturer in Clinical Psychiatry, Division of Neuroscience and Psychological Medicine, Faculty of Medicine, Imperial College of Science, Technology and Medicine, London W6 8RP, UK

A. Bergman PhD
Department of Psychology, St John's University, Jamaica, NY 11439, USA

C. Brookman
Patient contributor

G. Brown (alias)
Patient contributor

M. Browne MA
Department of Psychology, University of Nebraska – Lincoln, Lincoln, NE, USA

P.F. Buckley MD
Professor and Chairman, Department of Psychiatry, Medical College of Georgia, Augusta, GA 30912, USA

D.E. Casey MD
Associate Director of Research, VISN 20 MIRECC, Mental Illness Research, Education and Clinical Center, Portland VA Medical Center; Professor of Psychiatry and Neurology, Oregon Health and Science University, Portland, OR, USA

P.K. Chadwick
Lecturer in Psychology, Birkbeck College Faculty of Continuing Education, University of London, London, UK

J.M. Cloos MD
Centre Hospitalier de Luxembourg, 1210 Luxembourg

N.H. Covell PhD
Research Associate, Connecticut Department of Mental Health and Addiction Services (DMHAS), Hartford; Department of Psychology, University of Connecticut, Storrs, CT, USA

T.K.J. Craig MB BS PhD FRCPsych
Professor, Division of Psychological Medicine, Guy's, King's and St Thomas' School of Medicine, St Thomas's Hospital, London SE1 7EH, UK

J. Cutting MD FRCP FRCPsych MPhil
Consultant Psychiatrist, Honorary Senior Lecturer, Institute of Psychiatry, London, UK

A. David
Section of Cognitive Neuropsychiatry, Institute of Psychiatry and GKT School of Medicine, London SE5 8AF, UK

G.E. Duncan PhD
Associate Professor, Department of Psychiatry, University of North Carolina at Chapel Hill School of Medicine, Chapel Hill, NC, USA

M. Egan MD
Staff Clinician and Principal Investigator, Clinical Brain Disorders Branch, National Institute of Mental Health, Bethesda, MD 20814-9692, USA

S.M. Essock PhD
Professor and Director of the Division of Health Services Research, Department of Psychiatry, Mount Sinai School of Medicine of New York University, New York; Evaluation Director, Veterans Affairs New York Healthcare System, Mental Illness Research, Education, and Clinical Center (MIRECC), Bronx, NY, USA

S.E. Estroff
Professor, Department of Social Medicine, Adjunct Professor in Anthropology and Psychiatry, University of North Carolina at Chapel Hill, Chapel Hill, NC, USA

L.K. Frisman PhD
Director of Research, Connecticut Department of Mental Health and Addiction Services (DMHAS), Hartford; Research Professor, Department of Psychology, University of Connecticut, Storrs, CT, USA

R.L.M. Fuller PhD
Postdoctoral Research Fellow, Maryland Psychiatric Research Center, University of Maryland School of Medicine, Baltimore, MD, USA

D. Goff MD
Director, Schizophrenia Program, Massachusetts General Hospital, Harvard Medical School, Cambridge, MA, USA

J.M. Gold PhD
Associate Professor, Maryland Psychiatric Research Center, University of Maryland School of Medicine, Baltimore, MD, USA

T.E. Goldberg PhD
Chief, Unit on Experimental Neuropsychology, Clinical Brain Disorders Branch, IRP, NIMH, Bethesda, MD 20892, USA

H. Goldman
Professor of Psychiatry, University of Maryland School of Medicine, Baltimore, MD 21201, USA

L. Green MA MB BS MRCPsych MSc
Specialist Registrar in General Adult Psychiatry, The Gordon Hospital, London SW1V 2RH, UK

J. Gruzelier
Department of Cognitive Neuroscience and Behaviour, Imperial College School of Medicine, London W6 8RP, UK

H. Häfner MD PhD Dres.h.c. Professor em. of Psychiatry
Professor of Psychiatry, Head, Schizophrenia Research Unit, Central Institute of Mental Health, D-68159 Mannheim, Germany

P.J. Harrison
Professor of Psychiatry, University of Oxford, Oxford, UK

W. an der Heiden DIPL.-PSYCH PhD
Deputy Head, Schizophrenia Research Unit, Central Institute of Mental Health, D-68159 Mannheim, Germany

C. Hollis BSc PhD DCH MRCPsych
Professor of Child and Adolescent Psychiatry, University of Nottingham, Queen's Medical Centre, Nottingham NG7 2UH, UK

F. Holloway FRCPsych
Consultant Psychiatrist and Clinical Director, Croydon Integrated Adult Mental Health Service, Bethlem Royal Hospital, Beckenham, Kent BR3 3BX, UK

R. Howard MD
Professor of Old Age Psychiatry and Psychopathology, Institute of Psychiatry, De Crespigny Park, London SE5 8AF, UK

T.M. Hyde MD PhD
Neuropathology Section, Clinical Brain Disorders Branch, National Institute of Mental Health, Intramural Research Program, National Institutes of Health, Bethesda, MD 20892, USA

A. Jablensky MD DMSc FRCPsych
Professor of Psychiatry, School of Psychiatry and Clinical Neuroscience, University of Western Australia, Australia

D.V. Jeste MD
Estelle and Edgar Levi Chair in Aging, Professor of Psychiatry and Neurosciences, Chief, Division of Geriatric Psychiatry, University of California; VA San Diego Healthcare System, San Diego, CA, USA

S. Kapur MD PhD FRCP(C)
Research Chair in Schizophrenia and Neuroscience, Clarke Division of CAMH, University of Toronto, Toronto M5T 1R8, Canada

S. Krljes MSc
Department of Psychiatry, Faculty of Medicine, Imperial College, London, UK

J.H. Krystal MD
Professor of Psychiatry, Yale University School of Medicine, New Haven, CT, USA

E. Kuipers BSc MSc PhD FBPsS
Professor of Clinical Psychology, Department of Psychology, Institute of Psychiatry, De Crespigny Park, London SE5 8AF, UK

M. Laruelle MD
Associate Professor of Psychiatry and Radiology, Columbia University College of Physicians and Surgeons, New York State Psychiatric Institute, New York, NY 10032, USA

M. Leboyer
Hôpital Albert Chenevier, Service de Psychiatrie Adulte, 94000 Créteil, France

D.A. Lewis MD
Professor, Departments of Psychiatry and Neuroscience, Director, Center for the Neuroscience of Mental Disorders, University of Pittsburgh, Pittsburgh, PA, USA

S.W. Lewis MD FRCPsych
Professor of Adult Psychiatry, School of Psychiatry and Behavioural Sciences, University of Manchester, Manchester M23 9LT, UK

R.P. Liberman MD
Professor, UCLA Department of Psychiatry and Biobehavioral Sciences; Director, UCLA Psych REHAB Program, 300 UCLA Medical Plaza, Los Angeles, CA 90095, USA

P. Liddle BM BCh PhD MRCPsych
Professor of Psychiatry, University of Nottingham, Queen's Medical Centre, Nottingham NG7 2UH, UK

J.A. Lieberman MD
Thad and Alice Eure Distinguished Professor of Psychiatry, Vice-Chairman, Department of Psychiatry, Professor of Psychiatry, Pharmacology and Radiology, University of North Carolina School of Medicine, NC, USA

B.K. Lipska PhD
Chief, Unit on Animal Models, Clinical Brain Disorders Branch, NIMH, Bethesda, MD 20892, USA

R. Lundin
Patient contributor

R.W. McCarley MD
Professor and Director, Laboratory of Neuroscience, and Chair, Harvard Department of Psychiatry, Deputy Chief of Staff/Mental Health Services, VA Boston Healthcare System, Brockton, MA 02301, USA

J.J. McGrath MB BS FRANZCP
Queensland Centre for Schizophrenia Research, University of Queensland, The Park Centre for Mental Health, Wacol, Q4076, Australia

P. McGuffin MB PhD FRCP FRCPsych
Director and Professor of Psychiatric Genetics, MRC Social Genetic and Developmental Psychiatry (SGDP) Research Centre, Institute of Psychiatry, De Crespigny Park, London SE5 8AF, UK

A. McPartlin
Patient contributor

S.R. Marder MD
Professor and Vice Chair, Department of Psychiatry and Biobehavioral Sciences, David Geffen School of Medicine at UCLA; Director, Department of Veterans Affairs VISN 22 Mental Illness Research, Education, and Clinical Center, Los Angeles, CA, USA

S. Marenco MD
Senior Staff Fellow, NIMH, Clinical Brain Disorders Branch, Bethesda, MD 20892, USA

B.V. Martindale MB BS MRCP FRCPsych
Consultant Psychiatrist in Psychotherapy and Honorary Senior Lecturer, Imperial College School of Medicine, West London Mental Health Trust, Southall, Middlesex UB1 3EU, UK

V.S. Mattay MD
Chief, Unit on Clinical Neuroimaging, Clinical Brain Disorders Branch, NIMH, NIH, Bethesda, MD 20892, USA

S. Miyamoto MD PhD
Instructor, Department of Neuropsychiatry, St Marianna University School of Medicine, Japan

B. Moghaddam PhD
Professor of Psychiatry and Neurobiology, Yale University School of Medicine, New Haven, CT, USA

K.T. Mueser PhD
Licensed Clinical Psychologist, Professor, Department of Psychiatry and Community and Family Medicine, Dartmouth Medical School, New Hampshire–Dartmouth Psychiatric Research Center, Concord, NH 03301, USA

M. Muijen
Chief Executive, Sainsbury Centre for Mental Health, London SE1 1LB, UK

R.M. Murray MD DSc FRCP FRCPsych
Institute of Psychiatry, De Crespigny Park, London SE5 8AF, UK

N.V. Murthy DPM MSc MRCPsych
Specialist Registrar, West London Mental Health NHS Trust, Southall, Middlesex UB1 3HS, UK

D. O'Flynn MB BS MRCPsych
Consultant Psychiatrist, Rehabilitation Services, Lambeth Hospital, South London; Maudsley NHS Trust, London SW9 9NT, UK

K. O'Flynn MD
Fellow, Department of Psychiatry, Mount Sinai School of Medicine, New York, NY 10029, USA

C. Pantelis MB BS MRCPsych FRANZCP
Associate Professor and Head, Cognitive Neuropsychiatry Research and Academic Unit, Department of Psychiatry, The University of Melbourne, Australia; Co-ordinator, Applied Schizophrenia Division, Mental Health Research Institute, Principal Fellow, Centre for Neuroscience, The University of Melbourne, Australia

C.B. Pull MD MA
Professor of Psychiatry, Chairman of the Department of Neurosciences, Centre Hospitalier de Luxembourg, 1210 Luxembourg

G.J. Remington MD PhD FRCP(C)
Professor of Psychiatry, Clarke Division of CAMH, University of Toronto, Toronto M5T 1R8, Canada

B. Riley PhD
Director of Molecular Genetics, Assistant Professor, Departments of Psychiatry and Human Genetics, Virginia Institute of Psychiatric and Behavioral Genetics, Virginia Commonwealth University, Richmond, VA, USA

M.J. Robertson MS
Research Associate, UCLA Neuropsychiatric Institute; Administrator and Director of Training, UCLA Psych REHAB Program, 300 UCLA Medical Plaza, Los Angeles, CA 90095, USA

H.A. Sackeim PhD
Chief, Department of Biological Psychiatry, New York State Psychiatric Institute, NY, USA; Professor, Departments of Psychiatry and Radiology, College of Physicians and Surgeons of Columbia University, NY, USA

CONTRIBUTORS

D.F. Salisbury PhD
Assistant Professor, Harvard Medical School, Boston, MA; Cognitive Neuroscience Laboratory, McLean Hospital, Belmont, MA, USA; Laboratory of Neuroscience, Boston Veterans Affairs Healthcare System, Brockton Division, Brockton, MA, USA

S.K. Schultz MD
Associate Professor of Psychiatry, University of Iowa College of Medicine, Iowa City, IA, USA

S.C. Schulz MD
Professor and Head, Department of Psychiatry, Medical School, University of Minnesota, MN, USA

T. Sensky BSc PhD MB BS FRCPsych
Reader in Psychological Medicine, Imperial College of Science, Technology and Medicine, West Middlesex University Hospital, Isleworth, Middlesex TW7 6AF, UK

R.I. Shader MD
Professor of Pharmacology and Experimental Therapeutics, Program Director for Graduate Education, Professor of Psychiatry, Tufts University School of Medicine and Sackler School of Graduate Biomedical Sciences, Boston, MA 02111, USA

L.J. Siever MD
Professor of Psychiatry, Department of Psychiatry, Mount Sinai School of Medicine, New York, NY 10029, USA

S.G. Siris MD
Professor of Psychiatry, Albert Einstein College of Medicine; Director, Division of Continuing Psychiatric Services for Schizophrenia and Related Conditions, The Zucker-Hillside Hospital, Long Island Jewish Medical Center, Long Island, NY, USA

T.S. Stroup MD MPH
Associate Professor, Department of Psychiatry, University of North Carolina at Chapel Hill School of Medicine, Chapel Hill, NC 27599-7160, USA

P.J. Taylor MB BS MRCP FRCPsych
Department of Forensic Psychiatry, Institute of Psychiatry, London SE5 8AF, UK; Honorary Consultant Forensic Psychiatrist, Broadmoor Hospital, Crowthorne RG45 7EG, UK

J.L. Waddington PhD DSc
Professor of Neuroscience, Department of Clinical Pharmacology, Royal College of Surgeons in Ireland, Dublin 2, Ireland

D.R. Weinberger MD
Chief, Clinical Brain Disorders Branch, Intramural Research Program, National Institute of Mental Health, Bethesda, MD 20892, USA

J.K. Wing CBE MD
Retired

D.A. Wirshing MD
Associate Professor of Psychiatry, Department of Psychiatry and Biobehavioral Sciences, David Geffen School of Medicine at UCLA; Staff Psychiatrist, VA Greater Los Angeles Health Care System, Los Angeles, CA, USA

Foreword

For much of the past century, schizophrenia was the 'poor stepchild' of psychiatry. Its prognosis and outcome were thought to be nearly hopeless. Its mechanisms seemed inexplicable. Many of the people who suffered from it were hidden away in state hospitals devoted to the long-term care of the chronically mentally ill or mentally retarded. Particularly in the USA, most of the best and brightest psychiatrists avoided evaluating and treating people with schizophrenia, because they were perceived to be inaccessible to 'state-of-the-art' therapies such as psychoanalysis. Fortunately, British and other European colleagues were wiser, developing structured imaging tools such as the Present State Examination and conducting classic studies such as the International Pilot Study of Schizophrenia.

However, during the past several decades, the status of schizophrenia has gradually changed. Now, at the beginning of the twenty-first century, schizophrenia has in some respects become the poster child of psychiatry. Recent films such as *A Beautiful Mind* or *Shine* have captured the imagination and compassion of the general public, creating a much-needed sympathy for, and curiosity about, severe psychotic mental illnesses. The outcome of schizophrenia and related psychotic disorders is no longer considered to be hopeless. The discovery of chlorpromazine in 1952, and the more recent development of second-generation neuroleptics, has shown psychotic symptoms can be substantially reduced, and that, perhaps, even negative symptoms may be ameliorated. Neuroimaging tools have opened up the brain to scientific investigation. Scientists can now conduct *in vivo* studies of brain anatomy, physiology and chemistry using techniques such as structural magnetic resonance, positron emission tomography, functional magnetic resonance and magnetic resonance spectroscopy. The classic tools of epidemiology and genetic and family studies have now been complemented with the modern methods of molecular genetics, functional genomics and proteomics. Pessimism has changed to guarded optimism, and aversion has changed to hopeful curiosity. This new era of affirmation and hopefulness in the twenty-first century was launched in the year 2000, when Arvid Carlsson received the Nobel Prize for his studies on dopamine and Paul Greengard received the Nobel Prize for his work on signal transduction. Furthermore, Eric Kandel, a psychiatrist, was also honoured for his work on the mechanisms of learning and memory. The work of all of these men clearly indicates that the study of schizophrenia rests on a solid scientific foundation.

This second edition of the single best book on schizophrenia, edited by Steven Hirsch and Daniel Weinberger, therefore appears at a propitious time in history. It is particularly appropriate that its editors bring together the best of both American and European psychiatry, a fact that is reflected by the international cast of scientists who have contributed to this book. It provides a comprehensive and up-to-date summary of all aspects of schizophrenia, ranging from clinical description to mechanisms and treatment. This book will provide a useful roadmap for all students, both young and old, who are preparing to set forth on the exciting journey of understanding the causes of schizophrenia during the twenty-first century and seeking better ways both to treat and ultimately to prevent it.

Nancy C. Andreasen MD PhD

Preface to the Second Edition

Considerable advances in the understanding and progress of treatment of schizophrenia are reflected in this totally revised and updated second edition. In many respects, the field of schizophrenia research has changed dramatically since the first edition of this book. There are now several genes that appear to be valid susceptibility factors for illness, and these discoveries will very probably lead to a new understanding of causation and to new targets for therapeutic intervention. Likewise, new pharmacological treatments have emerged since the first edition, and much more clinical experience with the so-called 'atypical antipsychotics' has been acquired. The brain biology of schizophrenia has also matured considerably, with replicable molecular changes in the brain that implicate specific processes in synaptic function, and with much more sophisticated neuroimaging paradigms revealing patterns of abnormalities in specific functional neuronal networks. With these many recent developments in hand, the second edition of *Schizophrenia* is essentially a new work.

New topics include Chapter 35, written by patients who give their perspective of schizophrenia; Chapter 30 on the economics of schizophrenia and its treatment; Chapter 4 on schizophrenia in childhood; and Chapters 15 and 16 on the biology of genetic susceptibility and the electrophysiology of schizophrenia respectively. Several chapters have new authors and have been completely rewritten, including Chapter 8 on the course and outcome, Chapter 17 on the neuropathology of schizophrenia, Chapter 19 on the neurochemistry, Chapter 20 on the dopamine theory and Chapter 21 on animal neuropharmacology and prediction of clinical response. The section on physical treatments of schizophrenia has been reorganized and rewritten with new authors, including Chapter 24 on acute treatment, Chapter 25 on maintenance medication and relapse prevention and Chapter 26 on treatment-resistant schizophrenia. Chapter 1, on the concept and classification of schizophrenia, has been revised to include discussion of the differences between ICD-10 and DSM-IV-TR. This chapter links in with Chapter 5 (atypical psychotic disorders) to cover most of the diagnostic groups, but the chapter on schizoaffective disorders in the first edition has not been included because there has been very little research in that area.

Readers are referred to Chapter 7 of the first edition for discussion of schizoaffective disorders. Similarly, Chapter 17, the new chapter on the neuropathology of schizophrenia, focuses mainly on recent developments and should be read in conjunction with Chapter 15 of the first edition (Falkai and Bogerts) to comprehensively cover findings in that field. This can also be said of Chapter 19 on the neurochemistry of schizophrenia, which should be read in conjunction with Chapter 19 of the first edition (Owen and Simpson) to cover all the previous research findings, some of which are relevant but less topical today. Developments concerning the dopamine theory have been considerable and Chapter 20 focuses on these, leaving previous findings and a review of older theories to Chapter 20 of the first edition. Likewise, readers wanting a full historical perspective on animal neuropharmacology should refer to Chapter 21 of the first edition, after consulting new developments in the current edition. Part 4 on psychosocial aspects has similarly been completely revised and made more comprehensive by the addition of new authors and the inclusion of subjects not considered in the first edition.

We worked with the authors to try to reduce unnecessary redundancy where it does not add to our understanding of the subject, and to cross-reference between chapters and provide a very thorough index to enable the reader to use this volume as a resource text. Thus, we have endeavoured to provide a comprehensive account and revision of current-day knowledge of our understanding of the causes of schizophrenia, with its biological, social and psychological elements, the clinical manifestations of the condition with its various routes to management and treatment including physical treatments, psychological therapies and the organization of community services. Some of the limitations in these approaches are reflected in the chapter written by patients who give their own critical accounts of their experience. However, our perspective about the textbook is little changed from the view we expressed in the Preface to the First Edition.

Steven R. Hirsch
Daniel R. Weinberger

Preface to the First Edition

Schizophrenia has been a controversial topic since the term was first proposed by Eugen Bleuler to describe a uniquely human syndrome of profoundly disturbed behaviour. In the years following Bleuler's original work the controversies have continued at least as vigorously, but their content has changed. The debate is no longer about the nature of intra-psychic mechanisms, or whether schizophrenia really exists, or whether it is an illness as opposed to a life choice, or whether it is an important public health concern. Indeed, a recent editorial in *Nature* reified the current status of schizophrenia in the biomedical research establishment by declaring, 'Schizophrenia is arguably the worst disease affecting mankind, even AIDS not excepted' (*Nature* Editorial, 1988). In the United States alone it is estimated to cost over $40 billion each year in economic terms: the price that is paid by affected individuals and their families is inestimable.

The debate has shifted away from the view that schizophrenia is caused by a fault in the infant–mother psychological relationship. This had gained the status of orthodoxy during the late/middle part of this century and has been radically revised. Early parenting as a aetiologic factor never stood up to scientific scrutiny (Hirsch & Leff, 1975). The evidence that schizophrenia is associated with objective changes in the anatomy and function of the brain and has a genetic predisposition is incorporated in a major revision of the concept of schizophrenia encompassed in this book.

Schizophrenia has assumed an increasingly important place in neuroscience and molecular biological research programs around the world. Provocative evidence has suggested that aberrations of complex molecular processes responsible for the development of the human brain may be responsible for this illness. The possibility of finding a specific genetic defect that may participate in the liability to develop this disease has never seemed brighter. At the same time, the pharmaceutical industry has revitalized the search for effective new medical treatments. Where it was believed for almost three decades that all antipsychotic drugs were equally effective, it has now been shown that this is not the case. Moreover, it is clear that more effective drugs can be developed which are safer and have fewer side effects.

This textbook of schizophrenia represents a major shift of thinking influenced by the recent changes in our understanding of the brain, the developments in methodology which have influenced scientifically informed notions of our clinical practice, and the changes in our culture which have led to new concepts of management and treatment and a new understanding of the factors which are likely to affect relapse.

While we have asked the authors to make their chapters up to date and comprehensive, we have also worked with them to maintain a 'textbook' orientation so that students and researchers from other disciplines, as well as clinical and research specialists in the field, may be intelligibly informed about schizophrenia.

Promising as some of the basic science may seem, schizophrenia is still a disease whose diagnosis depends on clinical acumen and careful assessment. Therefore all the traditional subject areas are covered. This includes a series of chapters that discuss current issues in the phenomenological characterization of the illness, from its history to the ongoing debate about clinical subtypes, modifying factors, spectrum disorders, and the very nature and prognostic implications of the fundamental symptoms. The increased recognition of the importance of neuropsychological deficits in the chronic disability and outcome of this illness is highlighted by several contributors.

The series of chapters focused around the theme of aetiological factors emphasizes the dramatic shift in thinking on the medical aspects of schizophrenia. The application of new methods for studying the brain during life and at post-mortem examination has provided compelling data that subtle abnormalities are associated with the illness. The precise nature of the fundamental pathological process is unknown, and many uncertainties about it need to be answered. Is brain development disturbed in a characteristic way? Is there a common aetiology, or can schizophrenia arise from a myriad of causes, any of which affect a final common path of brain disturbance? Could the developmental abnormality result solely from environmental causes, or is a genetic factor essential? What is the correspondence between pathological changes and clinical manifestations? Does everyone with the pathological change manifest the illness, or is it possible to have the defect but compensate for it? What makes decompensation happen? What factors encourage clinical recovery?

The application of recombinant DNA technology involves a new language in asking the old question of how and what genetic factors play a role in the illness. While it is widely believed that a simple Mendelian genetic defect does not account for schizophrenia, what does it take in genetic terms? How many genes could be involved in liability? Are the genes likely to be recognizable as having anything to do with the phenotype as we have traditionally perceived it? What should relatives of a patient be advised about genetic risk? The straightforward dopamine hypothesis that had guided most researchers for the seventies and eighties has become much more sophisticated and enlightened. It is still important in understanding how the illness is treated, but it clearly has much less explanatory power than it seemed to have in the past. Is dopamine really involved in schizophrenia, or is it simply a way of modulating symptoms by affecting neurotransmission in a relatively unimportant but peripherally connected brain system? Can the illness be treated with drugs that do not touch the dopamine system?

Intensive, insight oriented psychotherapy on an individual basis is no longer used to treat patients with schizophrenia. Indeed, controlled outcome studies indicate that doing so is potentially harmful. However, more rationally based cognitive behavioural methods have shown real gains in symptom control and are becoming increasingly important in modern management. There is solid evidence that therapy aimed at altering the family environment significantly reduces the risk of relapse. The value of community rather than hospital based treatment is a modern trend, but the evidence from carefully controlled research leaves many questions unanswered: yet, a consensus is beginning to emerge on several of the basic issues.

We have invited leading experts to review established knowledge of the major fields of study in schizophrenia. This in-evitably leads us to include new topical areas of interest including homelessness, the risk of violence and the relationship of depression to schizophrenia, as well as brain imaging studies and the treatment of refractory states which would not have appeared in texts a decade ago. The result is a radical revision of our concepts and understanding which we believe justifies the effort of our authors whom we gratefully thank for their contribution.

Steven R. Hirsch
Daniel R. Weinberger

References

Editorial. (1988) Where next with psychiatric illness? *Nature*, 336, 95–96.

Hirsch, S.R. & Leff, J. (1975) *Abnormalities in Parents of Schizophrenics: Review of the Literature and an Investigation of Communication Defects and Deviances*. Maudsley Monograph Services, No. 22 (Oxford University Press).

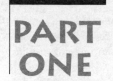

PART ONE

Descriptive Aspects

1 Concepts and classification of schizophrenia

J.K. Wing and N. Agrawal

Early concepts, 3
    Griesinger, 3
    Kraepelin, 4
    Bleuler, 4
The phenomena of schizophrenia, 5
    Positive symptoms, 5
    Negative symptoms, 6
    The concept of autism, 6
The concept of disease, 7
    Disease as entity or as deviation from normal
        functioning, 7
    Hierarchy in psychiatric disorders, 7
    Other types of theory, 8
Empirical approaches to the classification of
    schizophrenia, 8

Testing clinical concepts, 8
From concepts to classification, 9
Standards for symptom definition and
    combination, 9
Modern classifications of schizophrenia and their
    limitations, 9
ICD-10 and DSM-IV concepts of schizophrenia and
    related disorders, 10
    Diagnostic criteria for schizophrenia, 10
    Course and subtypes of schizophrenia, 11
    Diagnostic criteria for related
        psychotic disorders, 11
Conclusions, 12
References, 12

Each account of the concept of 'schizophrenia' reaches into the past from a viewpoint in a contemporary present. Berrios and Hauser (1988) commented that such accounts were unhistorical because we still lived in a Kraepelinian world. That was fair comment at the time and could be applied to many emerging disciplines whose concepts became temporarily stuck. It is also true that most people who have been concerned with such concepts over a professional lifetime find that the accumulation of new knowledge requires them to take a critical look back along several progressively different sightlines. This chapter is limited to the past two centuries, but a comment by John Locke over 300 years ago illustrates the confusion arising from terms used to describe severe deviations from mental health.

> Locke was 'astonished at the Obstinacy of a worthy man, who yields not to the Evidence of reason, though laid before him as clear as Day-light . . . I shall be pardoned for calling it by so harsh a name as *Madness*, when it is considered that opposition to Reason deserves that Name and is really Madness; and there is scarce a man so free from it, but that if he should always on all occasions argue or do as in some cases he constantly does, would not be thought fitter for *Bedlam*, than for Civil Conversation. I do not here mean when he is under the power of an unruly Passion, but in the calm steady course of his Life.' (Locke 1959)

Locke carefully distinguished 'madness' in the sense of unreasonableness, which was as common in his time as in ours, and the effects of being overpowered by 'an unruly passion', which was rare. His terminology is upside down to current readers but his distinction is clear and surprisingly modern.

Nevertheless, Michel Foucault would have none of it. To him, madness was always a form of opposition to 'established' reason. He thought that the way people react to it was a function of the historical epoch in which they lived (Foucault 1967). Such issues have not gone away, but one of the strongest tendencies in modern psychiatry is towards accepting Locke's basic differentiation between 'unreasonableness', which is common, and illness, which is rare. The international acceptance of specified definitions for mental disorders, with 'schizophrenia' as perhaps the outstanding example, may, however, have created an undue confidence in the durability of the global concepts. It is less likely that definitions of the constituent 'symptoms', about which people understandably complain and which are the most obvious and accessible phenomena, will change much in the foreseeable future. However, there is a gradual acceptance that standardized definitions of symptoms, plus new means of investigating brain functions, might eventually lead to the combination, break-up or abandonment of some current disease concepts, schizophrenia conceivably among them.

Even to the sceptical eye of the present authors, there has been sufficient advance in knowledge during the past decade to make another retrospective worthwhile, both for its own sake and because of the possible implications for future development.

Early concepts

Griesinger

There has been no time since attempts at classification began when controversy about the nature of 'schizophrenia' was absent. However, there have been periods when a sort of orthodoxy was accepted. One of these was based on Griesinger's teaching that only what we would now call affective and schizoaffective disorders constituted a 'primary' disease process (Griesinger 1861). What we now call chronic schizophrenic impairments could develop secondarily, but only after earlier affective episodes. Griesinger eventually came to agree that there could be a primary psychosis, even in the absence of these preliminaries, and thus 'abandoned the classification system of mental disorders hitherto traditional for him and his time' (Janzarik 1987). Thirty years of confusion about the relationships between a multiplicity of syndromes followed.

Kraepelin

It was not until the publication of the fifth edition of Kraepelin's textbook (1896/1987) that a firm line of demarcation was drawn between dementia praecox and affective psychosis and a sort of consensus again achieved. Both Griesinger's and Kraepelin's concepts were couched in terms of 'disease entities', following the lines of successful developments in medicine at that time. The discovery of the anatomical and physiological concomitants of clinically identified syndromes, often with a 'natural' history and a pathology, and sometimes with what appeared to be a single causal agent such as the tubercle bacillus or the cholera vibrio, proved irresistible to the neuropsychiatrists who were also carving more specific syndromes out of the global concepts of dementia, delirium and insanity that preceded them. Because cause was unknown, although variously postulated, classification depended largely on the course and outcome of groups of symptoms.

Kraepelin introduced a simple distinction between conditions characterized by mental deterioration such as the catatonia and hebephrenia of his contemporary Kahlbaum (1874/1973), which with paranoid deterioration became subdivisions of the disease, and more periodic forms of mania and melancholia, such as the *folie circulaire* of Falret (1854). His follow-up data suggested a mental state profile recognizable at the time of presentation and a 'generally regular and progressive' course. The chief symptoms were auditory and tactile hallucinations, delusions, thought disorder, incoherence, blunted affect, negativism, stereotypies and lack of insight. The phenomena were expressed as psychological rather than physical abnormalities, with catatonic symptoms, for example, being described in terms of disorders of the will. Paranoia was regarded as a separate disorder, characterized by incorrigible delusions often circumscribed in topic, a general absence of hallucinations, and a chronic but non-deteriorating course. Kraepelin also adopted Kahlbaum's model – general paralysis of the insane – as his prototype for a disease based on unity of cause, course and outcome. The nature of the disease was obscure although probably related to 'a tangible morbid process in the brain'.

A sympathetic and illuminating account of the development of Kraepelin's ideas up to 1913 has been provided by Berrios and Hauser (1988). They point out that his concept was neither as simple nor as rigid as is generally assumed and that it continued to develop. Indeed, Kraepelin (1920) eventually came to agree that dementia praecox and manic-depressive psychosis could coexist and, thus, that a unitary psychosis could not be ruled out.

Bleuler

The term 'schizophrenia' stems from Eugen Bleuler (1911/1950), who acknowledged in his preface his indebtedness to Kraepelin for 'grouping and description of the separate symptoms' and to Freud, whose ideas Bleuler used to 'advance and enlarge the concepts of psychopathology'. He retained the separation from manic-depressive psychosis while pointing out that affective symptoms could coexist. His concept was based on an assumption that the manifold external clinical manifestations masked an inner clinical unity that 'clearly marked [them] off from other types of disease'. Moreover, he argued that 'each case nevertheless reveals some significant residual symptoms common to all'. The end results were identical, 'not quantitatively but qualitatively'.

Bleuler's primary symptom was cognitive: a form of 'thought disorder', loosening of the associations. It provided links to Kraepelin's 'dementia' and to the biological origins of the disease, but also, through 'psychic complexes', to disorders of affectivity, ambivalence, autism, attention and will. These essential symptoms could be observed in every case. Catatonia, delusions, hallucinations and behavioural problems he regarded as accessory psychological reactions, not caused by the biological process or processes.

A substantial subgroup was designated 'simple schizophrenia', in which no accessory symptoms (the most easy to recognize) need be present. Diem (1903/1987), who worked with Bleuler, gave a description of two cases that he thought were caused by simple dementing forms of dementia praecox. Both were apparently normal as children, but as young men they began inexplicably to lose volition and purpose, ending as vagrants. Delusions and hallucinations were absent. Although no early developmental history was provided, these two people certainly became severely impaired in psychological and personal functioning and fitted Bleuler's severe version of simple schizophrenia. Bleuler's own examples are less easy to recognize. Among the lower classes, they 'vegetate as day labourers, peddlars, even as servants'. At higher levels, 'the most common type is the wife . . . , who is unbearable, constantly scolding, nagging, always making demands but never recognizing duties'. Beyond this 'simple' form of the disease, the largest subgroup was labelled 'latent schizophrenia': 'irritable, odd, moody, withdrawn or exaggeratedly punctual people'. Bleuler thought it 'not necessary to give a detailed description' of the manifestations in this group but there is a clear merger with subsequent concepts of schizoid and schizotypal personality (e.g. Kendler 1985).

This is in contrast to Kraepelin, whose account even of the 'mild' form of the course sounds severe. Thus, although Bleuler separated those with the disease from those without, the concept was in effect dimensional. Although accepting much of Kraepelin's formulation, Bleuler substantially widened the concept, while continuing to describe his concept as a disease entity. The simple and latent forms, whose vaguely defined primary symptoms could be elaborated through 'psychic complexes', were thus able to carry the weight, power and putative severity of a widely recognized diagnosis. Under the influence of contrasting types of theory – one psychoanalytical, the other biological – Bleuler's least differentiated subgroups came to exert an undue influence on the way that the diagnosis of schizophrenia was made and used in the USA and USSR during the 1970s (Wing 1978, chapter 6).

The phenomena of schizophrenia

Many attempts have been made to carry forward, refine or break up the syndromes described by the two conceptual giants. One motive was to improve earlier formulations of the fundamental characteristics that might underlie all the others. Berze (1914/1987), for example, drew on Griesinger's 'lowered mental energy' to postulate a basic factor, described in terms of a primary insufficiency of mental activity. This negative factor was responsible for the secondary positive phenomena as in Bleuler's theory, but without the psychic complexes. The mechanism was similar to that in Jackson's (1869/1932) theory of a hierarchy of levels of functional organization in the nervous system. A (negative) loss of function higher up can result in a (positive) disturbance of functions lower down. Gruhle (1929) pointed to the difficulty of applying such explanations to the phenomena of schizophrenia. He also made the unexceptionable, but rarely heeded, comment that some experiences and behaviours in schizophrenia cannot easily be fitted into either category. Gruhle distinguished between sets of primary negative and primary positive features, each specifiable descriptively.

Thus, issues connected with theories of 'negative' and 'positive' abnormalities have been hotly debated since at least the time of Griesinger. A more recent attempt to examine the relationships between symptoms in long-term schizophrenia used a profile of four measures:
1 flatness of affect;
2 poverty of quantity and/or content of speech;
3 incoherence of speech; and
4 specific types of coherently expressed delusions and hallucinations.
Affective flattening was particularly associated with poverty of speech, less so with incoherence and least with coherently expressed delusions. There was no evidence that the three types of speech abnormality were mutually exclusive categories (Wing 1961).

In a study comparing three hospitals with different social environments, poverty of content and quantity of speech were classified together with social withdrawal, flat affect, slowness, underactivity and low motivation as a 'negative' syndrome. Incoherence of speech was included with delusions, hallucinations, overactivity and socially embarrassing behaviour as a 'positive' syndrome (Wing & Brown 1961).

Crow (1985) gave added point to the descriptive separation by suggesting that different neural mechanisms might underlie the two syndromes, which he designated types I and II. Whether there are two, three or more syndromes has continued to be strongly debated, but now with fresh impetus to validate such clinical constructions by demonstrating biological differences. Crow has subsequently suggested that the 'first-rank symptoms' provide clues to the process of separation of the two hemispheres of the brain 'that is the species-defining characteristic of the brain of *Homo Sapiens*' (Crow 1998).

Positive symptoms

In the preface to the second edition, published in 1919, of his book on general psychopathology, Karl Jaspers wrote:
> We trail around with us a great number of vague generalities. I have tried to clarify them as far as possible. But the deep intentions, which sometimes find expression through them, should not simply be set aside and let fall because full clarification has not been attained . . . .

Jaspers did indeed provide illumination at both levels (1946/1963). In order to clarify the key problem of delusion formation he discriminated between phenomena that can be understood in terms of some antecedent factor such as social beliefs or abnormal affects (overvalued and delusion-like ideas), and those that are based on irreducible experiences, not comprehensible in such terms. 'There is an immediate intrusive knowledge of the meaning and it is this which is itself the delusional experience.' In the examples he quotes, Jaspers makes it clear that such experiences are direct and sudden in onset, and not congruent with affect.

He and Kurt Schneider kept up a regular correspondence during the years 1921–55 (Janzarik 1984). Schneider (1959, 1976) composed a list of experiences that could, in practice, be used to differentiate schizophrenia from manic-depressive psychosis with reasonable reliability. His 'first-rank' symptoms included:
• thoughts experienced as spoken aloud, or echoed, or removed, or broadcast or alien;
• voices heard commenting on the patient's thoughts or making references in the third person;
• experiencing bodily functions, movements, emotions or will as under the control of some external force or agency;
• delusional atmosphere; and
• delusional perception.

Any of these experiences could be elaborated according to the personal preoccupations of the individual concerned, including those that were socially shared. Schneider did not suggest that the first-rank symptoms carried any special theoretical or prognostic significance but did think (correctly: World Health Organization 1973) that most clinicians would make a diagnosis of schizophrenia if they were present in the absence of evident brain disease.

This still left a small group of seemingly inexplicable delusions that did not fit Schneider's primary criteria. For example, Kraepelin had regarded paranoia as a separate category. In 1918, Kretschmer (1966/1974) published a monograph on a group of disorders characterized by delusions that developed following a specific stress occurring to someone with a sensitive personality. These conditions could become chronic but were not accompanied by deterioration. Other, usually monothematic delusional disorders have been separated from schizophrenia. For example, a single delusion that other people think the individual smells, or that some part of the anatomy is distorted or missing, in the absence of any apparent basis in affective, or any other, disorder. One such symptom can ruin the sufferer's whole life. Acute delusional or hallucinatory states of brief duration, with no subsequent development of schizophrenic symptoms, were classified by French psychiatrists as *bouffées délirantes*, following Magnan (1893). This rich vein of clinical description facilitated subsequent attempts to operationalize the concepts.

Negative symptoms

Another line of development followed the ideas of Kahlbaum (1874/1973), who had been the first to describe both hebephrenia and catatonia, and of Kraepelin, who included catatonia as a form of dementia praecox. Bleuler gave a detailed description of catatonic signs but regarded them as 'accessory' phenomena and tended to interpret them in psychoanalytical terms.

Fisher (1983) noted that, 'prior to 1900, when neurological and psychiatric syndromes were being delineated, the symptoms of psychomotor retardation, slowness, apathy and lack of spontaneity were universally regarded as manifestations of abulia'. Much of the literature was concerned with the most severe state, akinetic mutism. Kleist (1960) and Leonhard (1957; Fish 1958) delineated narrow clinical syndromes intended to serve as indicators of equally specific brain abnormalities, but were unable to convince sceptics who pointed to the lack of evidence of specific pathology.

More recently, there has been a recrudescence of interest in motor disorders associated with psychological abnormalities. Rogers (1992) has reviewed the history of the concept of catatonia and its long-standing separation from extrapyramidal neurological disorders (dyskinesias and parkinsonism). He pointed to the occurrence of both kinds of symptom in schizophrenia, affective disorders, obsessive–compulsive disorder and mental handicap.

The motor phenomena observed in schizophrenia before the advent of psychotropic medication included reduced and increased speech and behaviours, abnormalities of non-verbal means of communication, symptoms such as negativism, ambitendence, forced grasping, echopraxia and echolalia, opposition, automatic obedience, mannerisms, posturing and stereotypies. This list is taken from the tenth edition of the Present State Examination (PSE) (WHO 1999). Some of these phenomena, such as automatic obedience, forced grasping and negativism, can be interpreted as disturbances of volition. Extrapyramidal and catatonic signs were highly correlated in a sample of patients with schizophrenia examined by McKenna *et al.* (1991). More specifically, there were 'independent associations between tardive dyskinesia and "positive" catatonic phenomena (i.e. those distinguished by the presence of an abnormality), and between parkinsonism and "negative" catatonic phenomena (i.e. those featuring the absence or diminution of a normal function)'.

The concept of autism

Bleuler (1919) regarded autism as one of the fundamental features of schizophrenia. He described it as an *active* withdrawal from contact with reality in order to live in an inner world of fantasy. Gruhle (1929) pointed out that it was just as likely to be forced on the patient by the cognitive disorder. Kanner (1943) recognized, in a flash of genius, a syndrome worth separating from the then amorphous mass of 'subnormality' and 'psychosis' in children. His observations were precise and brilliant, but at the same time he adopted the much less exact term 'autism' to describe it, thus linking it to Bleuler's concept. Within a year, Asperger (1944/1991) independently described a behaviour pattern he called 'autistic psychopathy', now referred to as Asperger's syndrome. Both Kanner's and Asperger's syndromes had in common a range of disorders of development present from birth or early childhood (Wing 1981, 2000; Tantam 1988; Frith & Frith 1991; Gillberg 2002). The results of an epidemiological study in south-east London (Wing & Gould 1979) showed typical examples of each syndrome, but identified many more children who shared features of both, or who met some but not all the diagnostic criteria for either. The authors developed the hypothesis of an autistic spectrum, characterized by a triad of impairments affecting the development of social interaction, communication and imagination, associated with a narrow repetitive pattern of activities.

The chief feature of the triad was social impairment, which could be manifested in several ways. Three groups were particularly evident.

1 Aloofness and indifference to others, e.g. avoiding social contact except for simple needs or to obtain pleasure from physical stimulation such as tickling. Those in this group tended to be the most disabled because of intellectual, behavioural and language impairments.

2 Passive acceptance of approaches from others but little or no spontaneous social interaction.

3 Initiating contacts in an odd one-sided way, unaffected by the reaction of the person approached. Those in this group tended to have less global impairment but behaviour was markedly abnormal.

The borders between groups are not neatly differentiated and can change over time; for example, some children change from aloofness to passivity, or to active but odd participation, as they grow up. Psychological examination has suggested that affected children and adults have an inborn difficulty that limits their understanding of other people's thoughts and feelings (Frith 1989). This lack is one part of a more general and fundamental problem shared by all those with the spectrum, which limits the attribution of meaning to experiences (Wing 1982; Frith 1989; Frith & Happé 1994). This hypothesis comes closer to Gruhle's view that autism is a consequence of cognitive disorder rather than of an 'active withdrawal' as suggested by Bleuler, and is in striking contrast to Jasper's description of the intrusion of abnormal meaning in the primary delusions of schizophrenia.

The diagnosis of autistic spectrum disorders in adults depends on characteristics of early development that are rarely considered by psychiatrists when taking histories from adult patients. For some diagnostic categories used in adult psychiatry, the ICD-10 criteria overlap with those in the autistic spectrum. For example, the criteria for schizoid and schizotypal personality disorders are closely similar to those for Asperger's syndrome as defined in ICD-10 and DSM-IV. Sula Wolff (1995) followed up children with 'schizoid personality disorder' and came to consider that they were better placed in the autistic spectrum, representing the most able individuals who fit Asperger's descriptions.

Many of the features of catatonia, as recently described by Joseph (1992), Bush *et al.* (1996) and by Rogers (1992), are identical to those found in autistic spectrum disorders, especially in younger and more severely disabled children. Follow-up into adult life has shown that a small proportion of those with autistic disorders, at any level of ability, have marked exacerbation of catatonic features in adolescence or early adult life. Some become severely incapacitated as a result (Wing & Shah 2000).

The narrow repetitive range of activities characteristic of autistic spectrum disorders can be mistaken for obsessive–compulsive disorder but the more common misdiagnosis is that of schizophrenia, although the diagnostic criteria for the latter are substantially different from those of autism. Such mistakes tend to be based on a misinterpretation of the social aloofness and passivity, or the odd speech and ideas that are found in people with active but odd social interaction. There is no evidence that medications, whether 'typical' or 'atypical', have a useful effect on the core symptoms of autism, although their tranquillizing effects are sometimes useful. The 'management' of autistic spectrum disorders depends on the provision of an appropriately structured environment, with well-programmed activities that encourage the use of any potential skills.

The concept of disease

Disease as entity or as deviation from normal functioning

Kendell (1987) has pointed out that none of the four types of psychosis – schizophrenic, affective, good prognosis acute and chronic paranoid – discussed above has been clearly demonstrated to be a disease entity. Does it matter? Kraepelin and Bleuler thought it did. But even so well 'validated' a disease as tuberculosis cannot be said to be an 'entity' in the sense that everyone with the bacillus in the bloodstream has the same (or any) symptoms, let alone the same course or outcome.

Cohen (1961) argued that the concept of disease that 'still dominates our textbook descriptions, as illustrated by the so-called classical pictures of typhoid fever, influenza, disseminated sclerosis and the rest, is little more helpful in diagnosis than would be a composite portrait of a football team in revealing whether any one individual is a member'.

Throughout medicine, but particularly during the past 50 years, rigid disease categories have been replaced by more useful concepts that are constantly evolving in the light of the experimental evidence. As disease concepts evolve in the light of the successes and failures of hypothesis testing, it becomes obvious that some diseases previously thought to be 'entities' are actually linked and that the fundamental processes involve deviations or blockages in the functioning of normal homeostatic cycles. Hypertension, diabetes and coronary heart disease are obvious examples, but so, increasingly, are most well-known diseases. Different defining formulae that use the same name have to fight against each other for survival. Which is more successful at any one time depends on the weight of evidence its protagonists can provide.

The evidence must also include the epidemiology of schizophrenia: the genetics, age and sex distribution, excess of births in the winter months and the possibility that the course and even the incidence varies both geographically and over time.

Hierarchy in psychiatric disorders

Some sense can be made of the relationships between psychiatric disorders if dimensional as well as categorical concepts are borne in mind. Both are useful so long as it is recognized that it is essential to move easily between them. The ancient hierarchies divided mental faculties into conative, cognitive and affective. If brain function is profoundly impaired, there can be no or only negligible function of will. Movement, thought and emotion will then be absent or distorted.

It is possible that each of the three faculties can be impaired independently of the others and that the conventional hierarchical system of diagnosis would have more than just practical use if based on three or four dimensions (the extra one representing motor functions). Positive and negative aspects would then be represented at every level.

At the moment, in practice, diagnoses tend to be made as follows:
• At the top are disorders such as dementia, which, at least in the early stages, can be associated with any other type of problem. For example, 'schizophrenic symptoms' occurring in the course of Huntington's disease or temporal lobe epilepsy or severe learning disability tend to be discounted for the purpose of diagnosis.
• Similarly, disorders in the autistic spectrum, if diagnosed on the developmental history and the spectrum, should not be given a primary diagnosis of schizophrenia.

• In general, schizophrenic symptoms, in the absence of 'organic' disorder, take precedence in diagnosis and for treatment over bipolar psychoses if both are present.

• Affective psychoses in turn take precedence over unipolar depression and the anxiety that is so commonly associated with all the above disorders.

• Symptoms such as fatigue, worry and muscular tension are regarded as non-specific.

The hierarchy is generally non-reflexive, i.e. each disorder tends to manifest the symptoms of those lower down (Foulds 1965; Sturt 1981) but not those of disorders higher up. By the same token, *all* disorders can be seen in cross-section as well as longitudinally, manifesting a complex of symptoms, some negative and some positive, and many 'non-specific' for the 'diagnosis'. Both perspectives are legitimate for different purposes (Wing 1978, chapter 3; 1991).

Other types of theory

A review of the history of concepts of schizophrenia would not be complete without a reference to theories of 'not-schizophrenia', although these tend to be logically self-destructive. Most are variants of those by Goffman (1961), Laing and Esterson (1964), Scheff (1966) and Szasz (1971), which have been dealt with elsewhere (Wing 1978, chapter 5).

This is far from saying that there are no other components to the aetiology of schizophrenia than those that involve purely biological elements. In fact, from the time of Kraepelin, concepts of disordered attention or arousal have suggested that environmental events may influence symptoms for better or worse. Certainly, some sufferers have learned for themselves how to cope with symptoms without losing control, and many carers have found, without help from professionals, how to provide an optimal environment (Creer & Wing 1974; Wing 1975). Interactive biosocial theories that suggest how environmental over- and understimulation may act to improve or exacerbate the positive and negative impairments (Wing 1978) cannot be taken seriously by those who reject any deviation from a purely biological approach. Thus, an absolute biologism is as limiting and ultimately sterile as an absolute rejection of biology.

The value of cognitive–behaviour therapy for the enhancement, in some cases, of the effects of the new medications during recovery from an attack of schizophrenia, and the acquisition of a degree of control over symptoms during convalescence and between attacks, is not only a success of the past decade but a pointer to the future. Tools for assessing claims of efficacy for such treatment methods are available, and must be applied according to strict rules by disinterested investigators.

Excluding clinical concepts that cannot be expressed clearly and numerically does not mean they are clinically valueless. Some may in time prove to be significant, but they have to wait until someone with the clinical intuition of Alzheimer, Asperger, Kanner or Kurt Schneider clarifies them.

Some critics of formulations such as schizophrenia (e.g. Bentall *et al.* 1988) have suggested that there is no need to do more than study symptoms, pointing to evidence that symptom-based therapies can provide relief and greater autonomy to sufferers and their families. It has yet to be demonstrated how far control of one symptom will generalize to others, how long relief lasts and what proportion of sufferers can benefit. A more specific disadvantage is that concentrating on single symptoms, instead of – rather than as well as – syndromes, may divert attention from the *clinical context* of the symptoms, with a resulting detriment to problems that are multifaceted and interconnected.

Empirical approaches to the classification of schizophrenia

Many of the clinical concepts of schizophrenia summarized so far, selected from a range that could be broadened to include dozens more authors, have been unsatisfactory in several ways:

• their symptomatic and syndromic components overlap but are not identical;

• they cannot be stated in precisely reproducible terms;

• the weights given to individual symptoms when formulating a diagnosis are not specified but left to clinical interpretation;

• other criteria, such as course, are of uncertain value for classification; and

• until recently there has been little convincing evidence for specific pathologies or physical causes in the large majority of cases.

Testing clinical concepts

New syndromes can be derived from symptom lists by the application of statistical techniques. There is a long line of such studies, many of them initiated in the 1950s and 1960s in order to overcome the unreliability then being demonstrated in day-to-day clinical diagnosis (e.g. Lorr 1966). They were successful in achieving reasonable reliability, but the usefulness of the statistical syndromes was not demonstrated, except in the sense that the factors often looked very similar to the diagnoses they tried to leave behind.

Kendell (1989) addressed the problem in a more practical way. He suggested utilizing statistical methods to refine syndromes, which could then be tested against outcome and used to generate or test biological hypotheses. His own studies (Kendell & Brockington 1980) did not demonstrate a point of statistical discontinuity between schizophrenic and affective psychoses. This could be due in part to fluctuation over time; cross-sections cannot display the clinical picture that eventually emerges. In addition, the hierarchies that run through psychiatric classification ensuring that disorders higher up, such as dementia, schizophrenia and bipolar disorder, which tend to be co-morbid with symptoms of disorders lower down, must also be considered. A high proportion of people with schizophrenia in the International Pilot Study of Schizophrenia (WHO 1973) would have been classified by the PSE computer program known as CATEGO as having affective disorders if symptoms discriminating for schizophrenia had been left out (Wing et al. 1974). Moreover, some at least of the affective symptoms so common in acute schizophrenia must be reactive to the stress of the primary experiences.

From concepts to classification

The clinical concepts, especially those of Kraepelin and Bleuler, can be recognized as early attempts to classify schizophrenia, but there were differences in their approach to defining schizophrenia as an entity. While Kraepelin emphasized the value of onset and course as well as descriptions in diagnosis and classification of schizophrenia, Bleuler and Schneider preferred a cross-sectional approach based on patients' current mental state, emphasizing fundamental and characteristic distinguishing symptoms. Recent recognizable international classification systems such as DSM and ICD have attempted syntheses of these concepts to foster international consensus.

Early DSM and ICD classifications (such as DSM-II and ICD-8) included a very broad definition of psychosis based on severity of social and personal dysfunction, thereby allowing for considerable overlap with personality disorders. This, in addition to the prevalent influence of the psychoanalytic movement in the USA, led to significant differences in the interpretation of diagnostic guidelines and definitions of concepts of psychosis and schizophrenia. These differences were clearly reflected in studies such as the US–UK study (Kendell et al. 1971), which displayed the range of concepts of schizophrenia from a broad one in the USA to a very narrow one in Europe.

One obvious line of development, therefore, has been to try to provide comprehensive, accurate and technically specifiable means of describing and classifying the component concepts (phenomena) in order to allow more meaningful comparisons between clinicians, academic schools, research laboratories and public health statistics.

Standards for symptom definition and combination

In the case of schizophrenia, the first essential is to provide differential definitions of the symptoms and signs, based as far as possible on deviations from normal psychological functioning. The descriptions of Jaspers and Kurt Schneider are well suited to such an exercise. These descriptions influenced attempts of clinical standardization in the form of development of definitions and structured interviews and diagnostic criteria such as the PSE (Wing & Brown 1970), Schedule for Affective Disorders and Schizophrenia (SADS) (Endicott & Spitzer 1978) and Research Diagnostic Criteria (RDC) (Spitzer et al. 1975). The 10th edition of PSE (now with other materials called Schedule for Clinical Assessment in Neuropsychiatry (SCAN); Wing et al. 1998, WHO 1999) is a more recent attempt of clinical standardization, as is the Diagnostic Interview for Social and Communication Disorders (DISCO) for social and communication disorders (Leekam et al. 2002; Wing et al. 2002). The definitions of symptoms and the algorithms for standardized diagnosis they provide make it possible to undertake more reliable and comparable clinical studies and more specific tests of biological functioning. These developments influenced further revisions of ICD and DSM concepts and classifications of schizophrenia. The American diagnostic classification (DSM) in the next revision of DSM-III and -IIIR made the concept of schizophrenia one of the narrowest, whereas the concept in ICD-9 remained very broad. However, in their most recent revisions, DSM-IV and ICD-10 have tried to bridge these differences by bringing the criteria closer.

Modern classifications of schizophrenia and their limitations

ICD-10 and DSM-IV provide the criteria for diagnosing schizophrenia and other psychotic disorders. At best, they can only be considered an 'arbitrary but well informed consensus on the definition of schizophrenia aimed at reliable communication' (Andreasen & Carpenter 1993). These reflect our current understanding of the concept of schizophrenia.

These diagnostic concepts must be considered provisional constructs intended to fulfil the need for international communication and research. Therefore, a need for constant revision based on epidemiological, pathophysiological, aetiological validation and evaluation of emerging neurosciences and genetic data cannot be denied. This must be an ongoing process. These classification systems currently use descriptive diagnostic criteria based on the intensity and duration of systems. They are operationalized to a variable extent (more in DSM-IV than in ICD-10) with explicit exclusion and inclusion criteria.

The conditions recognized by applying the criteria laid down in DSM-III, and its successors DSM-IIIR and DSM-IV (American Psychiatric Association 1993), and also in ICD-10 (WHO 1993), are not described as diseases but as disorders. The rules for schizophrenia laid down in the Diagnostic Criteria for Research in subchapter F20 of ICD-10 are far from describing a disease concept. They list most of the symptoms described by Kraepelin but do not include a long-term course or a particular outcome, or refer to a pathology or a cause. The distinction from bipolar disorder if both are present is limited to a clinical judgement as to which type of symptom occurs first. Schizophrenia in ICD-10 is not a disease but a disorder. The introduction explains that this terminology is adopted:

so as to avoid even greater problems inherent in the use of terms such as 'disease' and 'illness'. 'Disorder' is not an exact term, but it is used here to imply the existence of a clinically recognizable set of symptoms or behaviour that in most cases is associated with distress and with interference with functions.

An article in the Schizophrenia Bulletin illustrated the position clearly (Flaum & Andreason 1991). The authors listed DSM-IIIR and ICD-10 criteria, and three further versions then under consideration for DSM-IV. It is unlikely that a disease concept will change its nature by choosing two of one kind of item and three of another, rather than three of the first kind and two of the second. In fact, in the version eventually adopted (DSM-IV), the chief distinctions from ICD-10 (the requirement for a 6-month course and deterioration in social functioning) remain. Nevertheless, the coding system for DSM-IV is still mapped to that of ICD-9. However, both sets of criteria should be applied, using standardized instruments such as SCAN/PSE10 and the Composite International Diagnostic Interview (CIDI) (Robins *et al*. 1988) in research and public health projects, in order to foster international comparisons and comparisons with locally favoured alternatives.

ICD-10 and DSM-IV concepts of schizophrenia and related disorders

Although attempts have been made to bridge the gap between ICD-10 and DSM-IV and move them closer, significant differences still persist concerning the definition, duration and subtypes of schizophrenia and the nomenclature of various other psychotic disorders classified with schizophrenia. ICD-10 classifies schizotypal disorder, persistent delusional disorder, acute and transient psychotic disorders, induced delusional disorder and schizoaffective disorders together with schizophrenia (Table 1.1). DSM-IV does not include the category of schizotypal disorders with psychotic disorders but classifies it along with cluster A personality disorders (see Chapter 7).

Induced delusional disorder in ICD-10 is called shared psychotic disorder in DSM-IV; persistent delusional disorder in ICD-10 is called delusional disorder in DSM-IV (Table 1.2). The major difference is in the category of acute and transient psychotic disorder of ICD-10, which overlaps with brief psychotic disorder and schizophreniform disorder of DSM-IV.

The other major difference is in the classification of psychotic illness secondary to substance misuse and to general medical conditions, which are classified together with schizophrenia in DSM-IV but are classified with disorder due to psychoactive substance misuse (F10–F19) and organic mental disorder (F00–F09), respectively, in ICD-10.

ICD-10 avoids criteria based on social and occupational

dysfunction for the diagnosis of schizophrenia on the basis that it is difficult to equate these criteria between different cultures. This is a major inclusion criterion in DSM-IV that is essential for the diagnosis of schizophrenia.

Diagnostic criteria for schizophrenia

ICD-10 requires either one of the Schneiderian first-rank symptoms, or bizarre delusions, or two or more symptoms including persistent hallucinations, thought disorder, catatonic behaviour, negative symptoms or significant and persistent behavioural change. These features are required to be present for a 1-month duration or longer. ICD-10 recognizes that there may be a prodromal phase associated with schizophrenia, but as a prodrome typical of and specific to schizophrenia could not be described reliably it is not included in the diagnostic criteria. The 1-month duration of schizophrenia according to ICD-10 does not include the prodromal phase (Table 1.3).

ICD-10 requires exclusion of substance use or organic brain disease if they may be causing features of schizophrenia. As described earlier, the presence of the schizophrenia-like symptoms caused by either organic brain disease or substance use are classified along with organic mental disorder and substance misuse disorders, respectively, in ICD-10, not with schizophrenia.

DSM-IV requires, for the diagnosis of schizophrenia, 1 month's duration of characteristic symptoms with at least two of the symptoms of delusions, hallucinations, disorganized speech, grossly disorganized catatonic behaviour or negative symptoms (Table 1.4). However, only one of these is required if delusions are bizarre or third-person auditory hallucination or running commentary are present. This criterion brings the DSM-IV diagnosis of schizophrenia closer to that of ICD-10. In

Table 1.2 Brief outline of DSM-IV classification of schizophrenia and other psychotic disorders.

295.x	Schizophrenia
295.4	Schizophreniform disorder
295.7	Schizoaffective disorder
297.1	Delusional disorder
298.8	Brief psychotic disorder
297.3	Shared psychotic disorder
293.x	Psychotic disorder due to (specify medical condition):
.81	with delusions
.82	with hallucinations
293.x	Substance-induced psychotic disorders:
.xx	onset during intoxication
.xx	onset during withdrawal
297.1	Delusional disorder
298.8	Brief psychotic disorder
297.3	Shared psychotic disorder
298.9	Psychotic disorder NOS

NOS, not otherwise specified.

Table 1.1 Brief outline of ICD-10 classification of schizophrenia and other psychotic disorders.

F20	Schizophrenia
F21	Schizotypal disorder
F22	Persistent delusional disorder
F23	Acute and transient psychotic disorders
F24	Induced delusional disorders
F25	Schizoaffective disorder
F28	Other non-organic psychotic disorders
F29	Unspecified non-organic psychosis

Table 1.3 ICD-10 diagnostic criteria for schizophrenia.

Characteristic symptoms
At least one of:
   Thought echo, thought insertion/withdrawal/broadcast
   Passivity, delusional perception
   Third person auditory hallucination, running commentary
   Persistent bizarre delusions
or two or more of:
   Persistent hallucinations
   Thought disorder
   Catatonic behaviour
   Negative symptoms
   Significant behaviour change

Duration
More than 1 month

Exclusion criteria
Mood disorders, schizoaffective disorder
Overt brain disease
Drug intoxication or withdrawal

Table 1.4 DSM-IV diagnostic criteria for schizophrenia.

Characteristic symptoms
At least one of:
   Bizarre delusions
   Third person auditory hallucinations
   Running commentary
or two or more of:
   Delusions
   Hallucinations
   Disorganized speech
   Grossly disorganized behaviour
   Negative symptoms

Duration
1 month of characteristic symptoms
With 6 months of social/occupational dysfunction

Exclusion criteria
Schizoaffective or mood disorders
Direct consequence of substance use or general medical condition
Pervasive developmental disorders

addition to this criterion, DSM-IV requires a total duration of at least 6 months, including 1 month of active symptoms and social and occupational disfunction during this time. This criterion is significantly different from ICD-10 as the duration required is only 1 month in ICD-10 and social and occupational dysfunction is not required at all. DSM-IV recognizes the prodrome of schizophrenia and the duration of prodrome is included in the total 6-month duration required for its diagnosis. Specific exclusion criteria are similar to those of ICD-10, including those of schizoaffective and mood disorders and exclusion of disorders secondary to general medical condition and substance misuse. In the DSM-IV, schizophrenia-like illness secondary to a general medical condition or substance misuse is classified in the chapter on schizophrenia and related psychotic disorders. This is in contrast with ICD-10, as described above, and avoids hierarchical assumptions.

Course and subtypes of schizophrenia

Both ICD-10 and DSM-IV provide broadly similar classifications of longitudinal course. The subtypes of schizophrenia included in both ICD-10 and DSM-IV are paranoid, catatonic, undifferentiated and residual schizophrenia. Hebephrenic schizophrenia is called disorganized type in DSM-IV. The requirement for the subtypes is similar in both classification systems, although they are more clearly operationalized in DSM-IV.

Common subtypes in ICD-10 and DSM-IV

- Paranoid
- Catatonic
- Hebephrenic (disorganized in DSM-IV)

- Residual
- Undifferentiated

Additional subtypes in ICD-10

- Simple
- Postschizophrenic depression

ICD-10 also includes subcategories of simple schizophrenia and postschizophrenic depression as subtypes of schizophrenia. ICD-10 clarifies retention of simple schizophrenia as a subtype of schizophrenia, with the requirement of certain described features for at least 2 years because of its continued use in some countries and because of the uncertainty about its nature, which will require additional information for resolution. Diagnosis of postpsychotic depression requires a clear diagnosis of schizophrenia within the past 12 months with the presence of some features of schizophrenia and predominant depressive symptoms, which meet a threshold of depressive episode, for 2 weeks.

In addition to a categorical description of schizophrenia subtypes, DSM-IV offers a dimensional alternative in its Appendix B:
- psychotic dimension;
- disorganized dimension; and
- negative dimension.

ICD-10 does not give a description of any dimensions yet as these are difficult to define.

Diagnostic criteria for related psychotic disorders

Schizotypal disorder in ICD-10 is classified in the 'Schizophrenia and other psychotic disorders' section as this disorder is described as possessing many of the characteristic features of schizophrenia without its obvious delusions and hallucinations. The diagnosis requires the presence of more than three of the characteristic features without meeting the criteria for schizophrenia itself. In contrast, DSM-IV classifies the condition with the cluster A personality disorders, such as schizoid and paranoid.

Persistent delusional disorder of ICD-10 and delusional disorder of DSM-IV have similar diagnostic criteria except for differences in the duration of illness required, which is 3 months in ICD-10 and only 1 month in DSM-IV. Both classifications define this condition by the presence of a non-bizarre persistent delusion or set of related delusions. DSM-IV, in addition, specifies seven subtypes of this condition.

Any disorder of acute onset with typical schizophrenic features or other psychotic features lasting for more than 1 day to less than 1 month is classified in DSM-IV as brief psychotic disorder. This disorder is associated with a return to the premorbid level of functioning with good prognosis and may or may not be associated with marked stressors. This condition in ICD-10 is classed as acute and transient psychotic disorder. If the disorder persists for more than 1 month with schizophrenia-like symptoms, it is classified as schizophrenia in ICD-10, whereas in DSM-IV it will be classed as schizophreniform disorder. It will only be reclassified as schizophrenia if it lasts for more than 6 months. If the acute and transient psychosis has features of schizophrenia and has non-bizarre delusions, DSM-IV will class it as delusional disorder after 1 month whereas ICD-10 will class it as persistent delusional disorder only after a 3-month duration.

Schizoaffective disorder is diagnosed according to ICD-10 when both definite affective symptoms and schizophrenic symptoms are prominent simultaneously or within a few days of each other within the same episode of illness. In addition, DSM-IV requires the presence of typical schizophrenic features for at least 2 weeks along with the presence of prominent mood features. A substantial proportion of the illness should be characterized by the presence of mood features. Both classifications subdivide the disorder into manic or bipolar type and depressive type.

Induced delusional disorder is a rare disorder defined in ICD-10 as a condition in which two or more people share the same delusion or delusional system, support each other in this belief and have an unusually close relationship. The dominant person usually develops the illness first and induces the delusion later in the passive person. The DSM-IV diagnostic criteria for this illness are the same, although the disorder is called shared psychotic disorder.

Both ICD-10 and DSM-IV, while providing the basis for an effective communication between the professionals and a basis for research, also confer the disadvantages of creating an impression of discrete entities by imposing a framework on what are in fact complex and overlapping phenomena. These classification systems are complex, difficult to follow in day-to-day practice and the criteria are constantly revised; consequently, the research based on these systems becomes rapidly obsolete and difficult to apply in a clinical setting. Nevertheless, it is very hard to imagine working in a complex field such as schizophrenia and related psychotic disorders and not having a reasonable level of shared understanding of modern widely used concepts and definitions.

Conclusions

This review began with 'unitary psychosis'. Has this ceased to exist because there is no code for it in ICD-10 or DSM-IV? Should those who regard basic schizophrenic phenomena as symptoms of dysfunctions in the central nervous system classify them under F06.2 (organic schizophrenia-like disorder) or F20 (schizophrenia)? Another problem of the same order concerns the significance of the difference between G93.3 (postviral fatigue syndrome) and F48, which includes fatigue syndrome.

Being able to pose these questions does not demonstrate the futility of providing standardized definitions for international use. The examples do not inspire confidence but the effort to provide reference criteria is essential. It does demonstrate that, whether called 'diseases' or 'disorders', we are dealing with constantly changing concepts. That is not all. The same is true of 'syndromes' and of 'symptoms'. They, too, are concepts that must compete with each other. The more precisely they, and the predictions that follow from them, are stated, the more easily they can be refuted if they are wrong. It may pay, in the short term, to be vague; however, a greater distraction from the search for knowledge is that some protagonists, even when using an impeccably sceptical approach in their scientific work, tend to use the terminology of 'disease entities' and seem to want to believe that the Snark or the Boojum really exist. Others react against each such provocation and waste their time and wit in polemic.

Such arguments are inevitable and will continue. However, looking back from this new vantage point, it is still possible to discern a pattern amid the noise.

References

American Psychiatric Association (1993) *Diagnostic and Statistical Manual of Mental Disorders*, 4th edn. APA, Washington, DC.

Andreasen, N.C. & Carpenter, W.T. (1993) Diagnosis and classification of schizophrenia. *Schizophrenia Bulletin* **19**, 199–211.

Asperger, H. (1944/1991) Autistic psychopathy in childhood. In: *Autism and Asperger Syndrome*. Cambridge University Press, Cambridge. Translated and annotated by U. Frith, from: Die 'Autistischen Psychopathen' im Kindesalter. *Archiv für Psychiatrie und Nervenkrankheiten* **117**, 76–136.

Bentall, R.P., Jackson, H.F. & Pilgrim, D. (1988) Abandoning the concept of schizophrenia. *British Journal of Psychology* **27**, 303–324.

Berrios, G.E. & Hauser, R. (1988) The early development of Kraepelin's ideas on classification: a conceptual history. *Psychological Medicine* **18**, 813–821.

Berze, J. (1914/1987) Primary insufficiency of mental activity. In: *The Clinical Roots of the Schizophrenia Concept* (eds J. Cutting &

M. Shepherd), pp. 51–58. Translated from Chapter 4 of *Die primäre Insuffizienz der psychischen Aktivität*. Deuticke, Leipzig.

Bleuler, E. (1911/1950) Dementia praecox or the group of schizophrenias. New York: International Universities Press. Translated by J. Zinkin from Dementia Praecox oder der Gruppe der Schizophrenien. In: *Handbuch der Geisteskrankheiten* (ed. G. Aschaffenburg). Deuticke, Leipzig.

Bleuler, E. (1919) *Das Autistisch-Indisziplinierte Denken in der Medizin und Seine Überwindung*. Springer, Berlin.

Bush, G., Fink, M., Petrides, G. *et al.* (1996) Catatonia. I. Rating scale and standardised examination. *Acta Psychiatrica Scandinavica* 93, 129–136.

Cohen, H. (1961) The evolution of the concept of disease. In: *Concepts of Medicine* (ed. B. Lush), pp. 159–169. Pergamon, Oxford.

Creer, C. & Wing, J.K. (1974) *Schizophrenia at Home*. National Schizophrenia Fellowship, London. [Reprinted with a new preface, 1988.]

Crow, T.J. (1985) The two syndrome concept: origns and current status. *Schizophrenia Bulletin* 11, 471–486.

Crow, T.J. (1998) Nuclear schizophrenic symptoms as a window on the relationship between thought and speech. *Schizophrenia Research* 28, 127–141.

Diem, O. (1903/1987) The simple dementing form of dementia praecox. In: *The Clinical Roots of the Schizophrenia Concept* (eds J. Cutting & M. Shepherd), pp. 25–34. Translated from Die einfach demente Form der Dementia Praecox. *Archiv für Psychiatrie und Nervenkrankheiten* 37, 81–87.

Endicott, J. & Spitzer, R.L. (1978) A diagnostic interview: the Schedule for Affective Disorders and Schizophrenia. *Archives of General Psychiatry* 35, 837–844.

Falret, J. (1854) *Leçons Cliniques de Médicine Mentale*. Baillière, Paris.

Fish, F.J. (1958) Leonhard's classification of schizophrenia. *Journal of Mental Science* 104, 103.

Fisher, C.M. (1983) Abulia minor versus agitated behavior. *Clinical Neurosurgery* 31, 9–31.

Flaum, M. & Andreason, N.C. (1991) Diagnostic criteria for schizophrenia and related disorders: options for DSM-IV. *Schizophrenia Bulletin* 17, 143–156.

Foucault, M. (1967) *Madness and Civilisation*. Tavistock, London.

Foulds, G.A. (1965) *Personality and Personal Illness*. Tavistock, London.

Frith, C.D. & Frith, U. (1991) Elective affinities in schizophrenia and childhood autism. In: *Social Psychiatry. Theory, Methodology and Practice* (ed. P.E. Bebbington), pp. 65–88. Transaction, New Brunswick.

Frith, U. (1989) *Autism: Explaining the Enigma*. Blackwell, Oxford.

Frith, U. & Happé, F. (1994) Autism: beyond theory of mind. *Cognition* 50, 115–132.

Gillberg, C. (2002) *A Guide to Asperger Syndrome*. Cambridge University Press, Cambridge.

Goffman, E. (1961) Asylums. *Essays on the Social Situation of Mental Patients and Other Inmates*. Penguin, Harmonsworth.

Griesinger, W. (1861) *Die Pathologie und Therapie der Psychischen Krankheiten*. Krabbe, Stuttgart.

Gruhle, H.W. (1929) Psychologie der Schizophrenie. In: *Psychologie der Schizophrenie* (eds J. Berze & H.W. Gruhle). Springer, Berlin.

Jackson, J.H. (1869/1932) Certain points in the study and classification of diseases of the nervous system. Reprinted in: *Selected Writings of John Hughlings Jackson*, Vol. 2. (ed. J. Taylor). Hodder and Stoughton, London.

Janzarik, W. (1984) Jaspers, Kurt Schneider und die Heidelberger Psychopathologie. *Nervenarzt* 55, 18–24.

Janzarik, W. (1987) The concept of schizophrenia: history and problems. In: *Search for the Causes of Schizophrenia* (eds H. Häfner, W.F. Gattaz & W. Janzarik). Springer-Verlag, Heidelberg.

Jaspers, K. (1946/1963) *General Psychopathology*. Manchester University Press, Manchester. Translated by J. Hoenig & M. Hamilton from *Allgemeine Psychopathologie*. Springer Verlag, Heidelberg.

Joseph, A.B. (1992) Catatonia. In: *Movement Disorders in Neurology and Neuropsychiatry* (eds A.B. Joseph & R.R. Young), pp. 335–342. Blackwell Scientific, Boston.

Kahlbaum, K. (1874/1973) *Catatonia*. Johns Hopkins University Press, Baltimore. Translated by Y. Levij & T. Priden from *Die Katatonie oder das Spannungs-Irresein*. Hirschwald, Berlin.

Kanner, L. (1943) Autistic disturbances of affective contact. *Nervous Child* 2, 217–250.

Kendell, R.E. (1987) Diagnosis and classification of functional psychoses. *British Medical Bulletin* 43, 499–513.

Kendell, R.E. (1989) Clinical validity. *Psychological Medicine* 19, 45–55.

Kendell, R.E. & Brockington, I.F. (1980) The identification of disease entities and the relationship between schizophrenic and affective psychoses. *British Journal of Psychiatry* 137, 324–331.

Kendell, R.E., Cooper, J.E., Gourlay, A.J. *et al.* (1971) Diagnostic criteria of American and British psychiatrists. *Archives of General Psychiatry* 25 (2), 123–130.

Kendler, K.S. (1985) Diagnostic approaches to schizotypal personality disorder: a historical perspective. *Schizophrenia Bulletin* 11, 538–553.

Kleist, K. (1960) Schizophrenic symptoms and cerebral pathology. *Journal of Mental Science* 106, 246–255.

Kraepelin, E. (1896/1987) Dementia praecox. In: *The Clinical Roots of the Schizophrenia Syndrome* (eds J. Cutting & M. Shepherd), pp. 15–24. Cambridge University Press, Cambridge. Translated from *Lehrbuch der Psychiatrie*, 5th edn, pp. 426–441. Barth, Leipzig.

Kraepelin, E. (1920) Die Erscheinungsformen des Irreseins. *Zeitschrift für Neurologie und Psychiatrie* 62, 1–29.

Kretschmer, E. (1966/1974) The sensitive delusion of reference. In: *Themes and Variations in European Psychiatry* (eds S.R. Hirsch & M. Shepherd). Wright, Bristol. Translated from *Der sensitiver Beziehungswahn*. Springer, Heidelberg.

Laing, R.D. & Esterson, A. (1964) *Sanity: Madness and the Family*. Tavistock, London.

Leekam, S.R., Libby, S.J., Wing, L. *et al.* (2002) The diagnostic interview for social and communication disorders. Algorithms for ICD 10 childhood autism and autistic spectrum disorders. *Journal of Child Psychology and Psychiatry* 43, 325–327.

Leonhard, K. (1957) *Aufteilung der Endogenen Psychosen*. Akademie Verlag, Berlin.

Locke, J. (1959) *Essay Concerning Human Understanding*, Vol. 1, 2nd edn (ed. A.C. Fraser). Dover, New York.

Lorr, M. (1966) *Explorations in Typing Psychotics*. Pergamon, London.

McKenna, P.J., Lund, C.E., Mortimer, A.M. & Biggins, C.A. (1991) Motor, volitional and behavioural disorders in schizophrenia. II. The 'conflict of paradigms' hypothesis. *British Journal of Psychiatry* 158, 328–336.

Magnan, V. (1893) *Leçons Cliniques Sur les Maladies Mentales*. Battaille, Paris.

Robins, L.N., Wing, J., Wittchen, H.U. *et al.* (1988) The Composite International Diagnostic Interview: an epidemiological instrument suitable for use in conjunction with different diagnostic systems and in different cultures. *Archives of General Psychiatry* 45, 1069–1077.

Rogers, D. (1992) *Motor Disorder in Psychiatry: Towards a Neurological Psychiatry*. Wiley, New York.

Scheff, T.J. (1966) *Being Mentally Ill*. Aldine, Chicago.

Schneider, K. (1959) *Clinical Psychopathology*. Translated by M.W. Hamilton. Grune & Stratton, New York.

Schneider, K. (1976) *Klinische Psychopathologie*, 11th edn. Thieme, Stuttgart.

Spitzer, R.L., Endicott, J. & Robins, E. (1975) *Research Diagnostic Criteria: Rationale and Reliability*. Hodder and Stoughton, London.

Sturt, E. (1981) Hierarchical patterns in the distribution of psychiatric symptoms. *Psychological Medicine* **11**, 783–794.

Szasz, T. (1971) *The Manufacture of Madness*. Routledge, London.

Tantam, D. (1988) Asperger's syndrome. *Journal of Child Psychology and Psychiatry* **29**, 245–255.

Wing, J.K. (1961) A simple and reliable subclassification of chronic schizophrenia. *Journal of Mental Science* **107**, 862–875.

Wing, J.K., ed. (1975) *Schizophrenia from Within*. National Schizophrenia Fellowship, London.

Wing, J.K. (1978) *Reasoning About Madness*. Oxford University Press, London.

Wing, J.K. (1991) Social psychiatry. In: *Social Psychiatry: Theory, Methodology and Practice* (ed. P.E. Bebbington), pp. 3–22. Transaction, New Brunswick.

Wing, J.K. & Brown, G.W. (1961) Social treatment of chronic schizophrenia: a comparative survey of three mental hospitals. *Journal of Mental Science* **107**, 847–861.

Wing, J.K. & Brown, G.W. (1970). *Institutionalism and Schizophrenia*. Cambridge University Press, London.

Wing, J.K., Cooper, J.E. & Sartorius, N. (1974) *The Description and Classification of Psychiatric Symptoms: an Instruction Manual for the PSE and CATEGO System*. Cambridge University Press, London.

Wing, J.K., Sartorius, N. & Üstün, T.B. (1998) *Diagnosis and Clinical Measurement in Psychiatry: the SCAN System*. Cambridge University Press, Cambridge.

Wing, L. (1981) Asperger's syndrome. *Psychological Medicine* **11**, 115–129.

Wing, L. (1982) Development of concepts, classification and relationship to mental retardation. In: *Psychoses of Uncertain Aetiology* (eds J.K. Wing & L.G. Wing), pp. 185–190. Cambridge University Press, Cambridge.

Wing, L. (2000) Past and future research on Asperger Syndrome. In: *Asperger Syndrome* (eds A. Klin, F. Volkmar & S. Sparrow). Guildford Press, New York.

Wing, L. & Gould, J. (1979) Severe impairments of social interaction and associated abnormalities in children: epidemiology and classification. *Journal of Autism and Developmental Disorder* **9**, 11–29.

Wing, L. & Shah, A. (2000) Catatonia in autistic spectrum disorders. *British Journal of Psychiatry* **176**, 357–362.

Wing, L., Leekam, S.R., Libby, S.J. *et al.* (2002) The diagnostic interview for social and communication disorders. *Journal of Child Psychology and Psychiatry* **43**, 307–325.

Wolff, S. (1995) *Loners: The Life Path of Unusual Children*. Routledge, London.

World Health Organization (1973) *The International Pilot Study of Schizophrenia*. WHO, Geneva.

World Health Organization (1993) *The ICD-10 Classification of Mental and Behavioural Disorders: Diagnostic Criteria for Research*. WHO, Geneva.

World Health Organization (1999) *Schedules for Clinical Assessment in Neuropsychiatry*. World Health Organization, Geneva.

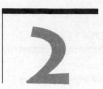

Descriptive psychopathology

J. Cutting

Introduction, 15
Hallucinations and other abnormal
    experiences, 15
    Definitions and classification, 15
    Incidence and variety in schizophrenia, 16
Delusions, 17
    Definitions and classification, 17
    Incidence and variety in schizophrenia, 17
Catatonia, 18
    Definition and classification, 18
    Incidence and variety in schizophrenia, 19
Thought disorder, 19
    Definitions and classification, 19

Incidence and variety in schizophrenia, 20
Disturbance of emotion, 21
    Definitions and classification, 21
    Incidence and variety in schizophrenia, 21
Psychological deficit, 22
    Attentional impairment, 22
    Intellectual decline, 22
    Memory failures, 22
    Perceptual impoverishment, 22
    Lack of will, 22
Clustering of phenomena/symptoms, 22
Explanatory theories, 23
References, 23

Introduction

In schizophrenia the apparatus of the mind disintegrates, severely and pervasively. It does so, moreover, in such a fashion that an experienced clinician can distinguish the condition from all other psychiatric disorders by the pattern of what is left after the mayhem. What we encounter in an individual suffering from schizophrenia are two sets of features: (i) the absence of certain functions or aspects of the mind which should be present in a normal individual – sometimes called 'negative symptoms'; and (ii) the presence of certain phenomena which are not present in a normal individual, and which probably represent a response of the healthy part of the schizophrenic's mind to the absent functions – sometimes called 'positive symptoms'. Some schizophrenics display only the latter, some only the former, but most display a combination of both.

For practical purposes the descriptive psychopathology of schizophrenia can be treated in three sections:

1 purely positive symptoms – *hallucinations and other abnormal experiences*, *delusions* and *catatonia*;

2 traditional psychopathological groupings containing positive and negative symptoms – *thought disorder* and *disturbances of emotions*; and

3 what used to be referred to as *psychological deficit*, purely negative symptoms – *impaired attention*, *intelligence*, *memory*, *perception* and *will*.

Neither the positive symptoms (or phenomena) nor the negative symptoms (or signs, because strictly speaking they are things we observe rather than what a patient complains about) exhaust the entire gamut of a schizophrenic's subjective experience or entirely account for all the possible behaviour. The condition has such a pervasive effect on the mind that all aspects are affected, including, for example, an individual's sense of time and appreciation of space. Moreover, schizophrenics may engage in bizarre behaviour which cannot be explained in terms of the categories of negative symptoms listed above. (see also Chapter 3.)

Hallucinations and other abnormal experiences

Definitions and classification

There are four categories of experience within this group of phenomena: anomalous experiences, illusions, hallucinations and pseudohallucinations.

Anomalous experiences, or distortions of a real perceptual experience, are those where a real perception of an object (i.e. the object actually perceived is really there) does not accord with its normal quality. Its colour may be different from usual, its shape may be strange, its size may be smaller or larger than realistically possible or it may be altered in a very subtle way – less or more familiar, less or more distant (or louder or softer in the auditory modality), less or more real or even less or more accentuated relative to the rest of the perceptual environment. None of these experiences is a hallucination, illusion or pseudohallucination (see below) because a real object is there, it is recognized as such, but it is merely registered as different from hitherto. Some of the experiences have attracted a specific label, e.g. *déjà vu* for an increase in familiarity, derealization for a loss of the sense of reality and micropsia if the perceived object looks smaller than normal.

Illusions are false perceptual experiences where an object that really exists 'out there' is completely misrecognized as an entirely different class of object, e.g. a moving curtain for a burglar or a rubber band for a snake. It is not an anomalous experience, because it is not a qualitative alteration in the perception of a correctly recognized object, but rather the complete misrecognition of something – the new 'something' looking exactly like a real example of what it would in fact look like. Illusions are mentioned here for completeness, but are not specific or indicative of schizophrenia.

A hallucination is a perception of something when in fact nothing exists in the perceptual field, a perception without an object, in short.

15

Table 2.1 Subtypes of hallucinations.

Modality
Visual
Auditory
Olfactory
Gustatory
Tactile, somatic, kinaesthetic

Timing with respect to sleep
Hypnagogic: just before falling asleep
Hypnopompic: on just waking up

Precipitation by sensory stimulus
Synaesthetic: precipitation by sensation in a different modality from
  hallucination (e.g. voice after seeing flashing light)
Functional (or reflex): precipitation by sensation in same modality (e.g.
  voice after hearing dripping tap. NB This is not an illusion because
  the dripping tap and the voice are *both* heard)

Content
e.g. Musical
Autoscopic
  Of self
Lilliputian
  Smaller than realistic
Teichopsia
  Geometrical shapes, particularly of battlements
  Characteristic of migraine

Table 2.2 Examples of anomalous experiences in schizophrenia.

Colour
'Colours meant a lot to me . . . stood out, not meant a lot, especially
traffic lights.'

'All bright colours were ones that frightened me most – orange and
red.'

Faces/people
'All I could see were people in a car and they looked like ghosts. They
looked different, like statues or monuments, dead, as if cremated.'

'The right side [in his left field] of my mother's and sister's faces went
completely black. When I looked in the mirror the right half of my own
face [really the left half as it was a mirror image] also looked black.'

Environment
'I couldn't recognize any of my surroundings – people, places. I could
recognize certain things. I could recognize qualities of a place, of
surfaces. It was the organization of things which was different.'

'It was like being in one of my paintings [patient was an art student]. I
used to go out and see the houses with fascination. I would stare out of
the window for hours.'

A pseudohallucination is variously defined in the psycho-pathological literature. One school of thought (Hare 1973) considers it to be a hallucination with preserved insight. In other words, I might perceive an elephant in front of me (when none actually exists), and at the same time be aware of the falseness of my perceptual experience, i.e. I know that no elephant is there even though I see it. Another school of thought (Jaspers 1913) regards it as a hallucination, but one where the hallucinated object lacks the reality of a perception of the same object if it were really there – less vivid, less 'real', etc. This latter school of thought is perhaps a more philosophically correct perspective, because the distinction between a hallucination and a pseudo-hallucination may be more one of degree, as a careful analysis of most hallucinations (Merleau-Ponty 1962) will reveal that the apparent object is rarely experienced as 'realistically' as the comparable real object.

Hallucinations themselves are further divided into various types, according to modality, timing with respect to sleep, their occasional precipitation by a sensory stimulus and their content (Table 2.1). There are numerous causes of hallucinations besides schizophrenia (Cutting 1996).

Incidence and variety in schizophrenia

The incidence of all types of anomalous experiences in schizo-phrenia is about 50% (Cutting & Dunne 1989), and of all types of hallucinations about 50%. Visual hallucinations occur in 15% of all subjects, auditory in 50% of all subjects and tactile in 5% of all subjects (Cutting 1990).

The pattern of the anomalous experiences is very varied. Some examples are shown in Table 2.2. Colours and faces are often the focus of the anomalous experience, but there may be a complete alteration in the quality of the entire environment. This understandably induces a feeling of perplexity in the sufferer, and constitutes what is called delusional mood, because the experiences later solidify as beliefs about what was going on then, e.g. people looking at me in a funny way, etc. The anomalous experiences usually occur at the onset of an episode, and are often forgotten or become delusionally elaborated by the time the patient is interviewed.

The pattern of the hallucinations, on the other hand, is quite specific. The most common hallucination is a voice – not just any auditory hallucination, but a voice. Moreover, this voice has certain characteristics that make it even more specific for the condition: it is usually heard in a grammatical form that is different from how we experience our own thoughts (e.g. instead of 'I wonder what I'm going to have for supper tonight', the voice says, '*he* is wondering what to have for supper') and the sex of the voice (male or female) is nearly always identified, but the owner of the voice is usually not someone who is known to the subject. Added to all this is the fact that schizophrenic voices diminish if there is meaningful conversation going on around, and intensify if there is no background auditory noise or if the background noise is devoid of meaning (Margo *et al.* 1981). Moreover, schizophrenics with voices do not differ from schizophrenics without voices on measures of auditory acuity

(Collicutt & Hemsley 1981) or imagery (Starker & Jolin 1982). Typical examples of schizophrenic voices are: 'He's getting things the wrong way' (presumably referring to how he thought about himself), 'You're not going to smoke the cigarette the way you want to but the way we want you to.'

Schneider (1958) was so impressed with the regular occurrence of such 'voices' in schizophrenic patients that he elevated three types to the rank of first-rank symptoms of the condition:
1 voices speaking thoughts aloud;
2 voices arguing (two or more hallucinatory voices discussing the person in the third person); and
3 voices commenting on the subject's actions.

Other characteristics of the 'voices' are that they may be experienced outside the head, but they are usually poorly localized, and some patients do not distinguish them completely from their thoughts, i.e. they fulfil certain criteria for a pseudohallucination.

Finally, consider this example of ethological research: Green and Preston (1981) applied a throat microphone to one hallucinating schizophrenic, by means of which they picked up the following conversation (supporting the view that 'voices' are subvocalizations of real thoughts experienced by a subject rather than incorrect perceptual accounts of auditory stimuli in their environment). *Voice*, 'Mind your own business darling; I don't want him [referring to the experimenter] to know what I was doing.' When the experimenter asked the subject what was going on, he replied 'See that, I spoke to ask her [the owner of the voice] what she was doing, and she said, mind your own business.'

The pattern of a schizophrenic's visual hallucinations is less well established. Although infrequent, visual hallucinations do occur in a substantial minority of schizophrenics (Guttmann & Maclay 1937; Feinberg 1962; Cutting 1996). They appear to be of things which do not actually exist in the real world, or of part-objects, e.g. leg on a bedroom wall, 'a big animal like an octopus', 'something like a mouse running across the floor', 'mirages of a desert' or 'rat tail coming out of own anus'.

Illusions, in general, are rare, as are pseudohallucinations (barring the problem of establishing the strict phenomenological status of schizophrenic 'voices'). Olfactory (Rubert *et al.* 1961) and gustatory (De Morsier 1938) hallucinations are also rare. Somatic hallucinations are less rare (Cutting 1990).

Delusions

Definitions and classification

Various definitions of delusion exist (Schmidt 1940). Possibly the three best ones are Jaspers' (1913), that of the DSM-IIIR (American Psychiatric Association 1987) and Spitzer's (1990).

Jaspers' definition proposed three criteria: (i) it is a belief held with extraordinary conviction, with an incomparable subjective certainty; (ii) there is an imperviousness to other experiences

and to compelling counterargument; and (iii) the content is impossible.

That in DSM-IIIR is:
A false personal belief based on incorrect inference about external reality and firmly sustained in spite of what almost everyone else believes and in spite of what constitutes incontrovertible and obvious proof or evidence to the contrary. The belief is not one ordinarily accepted by other members of the person's culture or sub-culture (i.e. it is not an article of religious faith). When a false belief involves an extreme value judgement, it is regarded as a delusion only when the judgement is so extreme as to defy credibility.

Spitzer defines delusion as follows:
X's statement is a delusion if it concerns the world, and is not an analytic statement (i.e. a linguistic tautology), and it is held with a subjective certainty only appropriate for statements about the mind.

The main differences between these definitions are Jaspers' emphasis on the inappropriate conviction, DSM-IIIR's mapping of the social context in which the delusion has to be placed, and Spitzer's restriction to a concern with the world (rather than self, body or mind). Given the complexity of the topic, all three definitions should be taken into account for their respective insights.

Delusions are currently classified according to four independent principles:
1 degree of inexplicability, e.g. primary;
2 nature of subverted mental function, e.g. delusional perception;
3 nosological significance, i.e. the extent to which the delusional state has been accorded independent status from the three major psychoses, e.g. sensitive delusion of reference; and
4 thematic content, e.g. jealousy.

These four classificatory systems are summarized in Table 2.3, along with a fifth system (Cutting 1996) which groups the themes in a more logical way.

Incidence and variety in schizophrenia

Delusions occur at some stage of the condition in more than 90% of schizophrenics.

Concerning the various types of delusions categorized in Table 2.3, some are more common than others and some have been elevated to the status of diagnostic criteria for schizophrenia.

Jaspers (1913) believed that primary delusions were pathognomonic of schizophrenia. In addition to the three properties that he believed belonged to any delusion – conviction, imperviousness to other experiences and impossibility of content – primary delusions possessed the further properties of 'ununderstandability', 'being unmediated by thought' and 'involvement of the whole personality' (Walker 1991).

Schneider (1958) was unhappy with this general formulation because of the practical problems of establishing whether a delusion fulfilled these latter three criteria. Only in the case of delusional perception, according to Schneider, could the

Table 2.3 Classification of delusions.

According to degree of inexplicability
Primary, pure, true
Secondary, delusion-like ideas
Overvalued idea

According to subverted mental function
Delusional perception
Delusional notion
Delusional memory
Delusional awareness
Delusional atmosphere/mood

According to degree of independent nosological status, e.g.
Paranoia
Delusional loving (de Clérambault's syndrome)
Monosymptomatic hypochondriacal psychosis

According to thematic content (traditional), e.g.
Lycanthropy (transformation into an animal)
Jealousy
Grandiosity
Influence/control

According to thematic content (logical, comprehensive, mutually exclusive)
Concerning the world
  Altered identity/class of things, e.g. Capgras' syndrome
  Altered quality, e.g. spouse unfaithful
  Altered chronicle of events, e.g. world going to blow up
  Altered evaluation, e.g. persecutory
  Altered self-reference, e.g. reference
  Nihilism, e.g. spouse dead
Concerning the mind
  Altered boundaries, e.g. thought broadcasting
  Altered function, e.g. cannot think
  Altered autonomy, e.g. thought insertion
Concerning the self
  Altered identity, e.g. X=Napoleon
  Altered ability, e.g. X is spiritual healer
  Altered autonomy, e.g. someone taken X over
  Altered evaluation, e.g. guilt
Concerning the body
  Altered structure, e.g. no brain
  Altered function, e.g. bowels do not work
  Altered autonomy, e.g. X's sensations are not X's

Table 2.4 Characteristic schizophrenic delusions.

Delusional perception	Normal perception has private and illogical meaning
Thought withdrawal	Thoughts cease and are simultaneously experienced as removed by external force
Thought insertion	Thoughts have a quality of not being own and are ascribed to external agency
Thought broadcasting	Thoughts escape into outside world where they are experienced by others
Made feelings	Feelings do not seem to be own, but are attributable to external force
Made impulses	Drive or impulse seems to be alien and external
Made volitional acts	Actions and movements felt to be under outside control
Somatic passivity	Experience of bodily sensations imposed by external agency
Bizarre delusions	e.g. parents exist in another time and place
Multiple delusions	e.g. nurses are Japanese, mirrors reflect the wrong way, haloperidol is made from shark's pancreas
Widespread delusions	e.g. husband acted in a sexually indiscrete way at a party, earthquake happening, grandson seriously ill

psychiatrist be sure that 'some abnormal significance . . . were attached . . . without any comprehensible rational or emotional justification'. This, according to Schneider, was because a two-stage process was involved: a normal perception and then an 'irrational and emotionally incomprehensible . . . delusional course'.

As well as delusional perception, Schneider also elevated certain delusional themes to the status of first-rank symptoms – the common denominator of which is a loss of autonomy or boundaries in the spheres of body, self or mind. These are usually regarded as seven in number (Table 2.4). More recent formulations (e.g. Research Diagnostic Criteria (RDC); Carpenter *et al.* 1973; Spitzer *et al.* 1975; DSM-IIIR) recognize the fact that deluded schizophrenics *may not have* such first-rank symptoms but manics *may have* them, and give the following categories of delusion equal diagnostic significance – bizarre, multiple or widespread (involving more than one area of life). Of the themes listed in Table 2.3, the most diagnosis-specific in schizophrenia, relative to manics and psychotic depressives (all diagnosed by non-delusional criteria), were (McGilchrist & Cutting 1995; Cutting 1996) altered bodily structure, altered bodily autonomy, altered boundaries of mind, altered autonomy of mind and altered identity of the world.

Catatonia

Definition and classification

Catatonia refers to a set of complex movements, postures and actions whose common denominator is their involuntariness (Table 2.5). Not all involuntary movements fall within the

Table 2.5 Catatonic phenomena.

Stupor	Virtual absence of movement and speech in the presence of full consciousness
Catalepsy	Maintenance of unusual postures for long periods of time and no sense of discomfort, often accompanied by waxy flexibility (external manipulation of limb as though made of wax)
Automatism	Automatic obedience to commands, regardless of consequence
Mannerisms	Peculiar social habits, e.g. style of dress, handshake, writing or speech, at variance with social setting
Stereotypies	Repetitive movements of a single part of the body, divorced from mainstream of bodily activities
Posturing and grimacing	Peculiar positions of body (posturing) or face (grimacing) inappropriate to mainstream activity and social situation
Negativism	Behaviour which is consistently in opposition to social and apparent individual demands of a situation
Echopraxia	Automatic repetition of visually perceived actions of others

category of catatonia; tics, chorea, dyskinesia, athetosis and ballismus are involuntary but not catatonic. It is partly convention and partly complexity that allocates certain movements or postures to the category. They are a heterogeneous bunch, ranging from a peculiar way of holding the head (posturing) to the entire annihilation of free will (as in negativism).

Incidence and variety in schizophrenia

According to the International Pilot Study of Schizophrenia (World Health Organization 1973), 7% of 811 schizophrenics exhibited one or other phenomenon. Other estimates (Morrison 1973; Guggenheim & Barbigian 1974) also gave a figure of between 5% and 10%. According to Abrams and Taylor (1976), mannerisms are the most common, followed, in descending order of frequency, by stereotypies, stupor, negativism, automatism and echopraxia.

Mannerisms, stereotype, negativism, catalepsy, automatism and posturing or grimacing are most specifically linked with schizophrenia. Stupor is more commonly linked with depressive psychosis or brainstem lesions (Johnson 1984; Barnes *et al.* 1986). Echopraxia is also seen in cases with frontal lobe lesions (Lhermitte *et al.* 1986). Abrams and Taylor (1976) claimed that all varieties of catatonia could occur in mania, but this is not my experience.

There is evidence that catatonic phenomena have diminished in frequency since Kraepelin's turn-of-the-century estimate of 20% in his series of patients with dementia praecox. There is also evidence that they are more common in schizophrenics from developing countries (World Health Organization 1973).

Table 2.6 Components of thought disorder.

Disorder of content, i.e. delusion including delusions about the autonomy of a subject's own thought processes, e.g. thought insertion

Disorder of form, i.e. formal thought disorder
Disorder of the mechanisms of thinking as characterized descriptively (intrinsic thinking disturbance, dyslogia)
    Concrete thinking
    Loosening of associations
    Overinclusion
    Illogicality
Disorder of language and speech
    Derailment, tangentiality, knight's move thinking
    Neologisms
    Poverty of speech (alogia)
    Poverty of content of speech
    Incoherence
    Pressure of speech
    Flight of ideas
    Retarded speech, mutism

Nowadays, there is a tendency to lump catatonic phenomena with other involuntary movements such as tics, dyskinesia and chorea, and to deny them special status in schizophrenics (Rogers 1985).

Thought disorder

Definitions and classification

The term thought disorder covers a variety of positive *and* negative symptoms of schizophrenia, and is largely a misnomer because much of what is traditionally referred to as thought disorder is a disorder of spoken language.

The various components are set out in Table 2.6. The first distinction, identified by Schilder (1920), is between *disordered content* and *disordered form*. The former is synonymous with delusion. The latter comprises two categories (Andreasen 1982a; Cutting & Murphy 1988); (i) an intrinsic disturbance of thinking itself; and (ii) disordered language and speech.

The intrinsic disturbance of thinking includes such inferred and hypothetical descriptive notions as concrete thinking, overinclusion, illogicality and loosening of associations.

Concrete thinking is a tendency to select one aspect of a thing or concept, usually a physical quality or a personal association, at the expense of its overall meaning. It is traditionally tested by proverb interpretation, a concrete response being one which fails to take proper account of the metaphorical nature of proverbs.

Overinclusion is the tendency to include false or irrelevant items in a concept or category, in other words, to inappropriately widen the boundaries of a concept or category. It is sometimes assessed in the course of an object-sorting task, an overinclusive response being one which incorporates too many or inappropriate items within a category.

Illogicality is a tendency to offer bizarre explanations for things and events, explanations which not only grossly contravene the laws of logic, but also the 'way of the world'. It is traditionally tested by inviting a subject to complete a syllogism (e.g. if all alligators are reptiles, and some reptiles are green, then are all alligators green? True or false?)

Loosening of associations is sometimes used as a synonym for derailment (see below), in which case it refers to a disorder in the form of spoken speech. In the present context it carries the meaning of a disordered conceptual structure, as illustrated by the reply of a schizophrenic subject to one of the questions in the similarities subscale of the Wechsler Adult Intelligence Scale: in what way are an orange and a banana alike? They are Nature's produce! This is not wrong, just loose. Note that the traditional tests for these thinking disorders are not good at discriminating schizophrenics from normal subjects, with significant numbers of the latter overlapping with the former.

Disordered language and speech are usually held to contain the following main varieties. First, there is *derailment* or tangentiality or knight's move thinking – a failure to conform to the social rules of conversation and the needs of a listener by picking up on personal or idiosyncratic aspects of a word or phrase and not sticking to the overall theme of the discourse. Next there is *neologism*, the creation of new words, subsuming an allied phenomenon, word approximations or paraphasia, where recognized words are given a new meaning. Then there is *poverty of speech*, which is a grossly reduced output of speech, and *poverty of content of speech* where, despite an adequate fluency, the number of ideas expressed is substantially reduced. *Incoherence* refers to a breakdown in the grammatical structure of what is expressed, sometimes to such an extent that the speech resembles aphasia – hence schizophasia or 'word salad'. *Pressure of speech* is a speeding-up of the flow of speech; *flight of ideas* is a combination of pressure of speech and derailment; and *retardation*, of which *mutism* is an extreme form, is self-explanatory.

Two alternative classifications are in use, one theoretical (Chaika 1990) and one practical (Andreasen 1979a). Chaika proposes four levels in the breakdown of language, each responsible for some of the traditional clinical varieties. Level 1, the subtlest disorder, affects the richness of expression of ideas, of which poverty of content of speech is an example. At level 2, there is an internal lack of coherence in the construction of sentences, illustrated by derailment. By level 3, the conventionally agreed shared meanings of words is dispensed with, hence neologisms. Finally, at level 4, even the conventional rules of grammar disappear, and the utterance becomes an unintelligible jumble – incoherence.

Some items of thought disorder are regarded as positive symptoms of schizophrenia, e.g. derailment and illogicality; others are regarded as negative symptoms, e.g. poverty of speech. Several schedules for the assessment of the various types exist and the most useful of these are reviewed in Cutting (1994).

Incidence and variety in schizophrenia

Andreasen's (1979a) study on the incidence of 18 varieties of thought disorder in schizophrenics and manics still provides the best picture of its incidence and specificity in schizophrenia. Cutting and Murphy (1988) studied the incidence of four types of intrinsic thinking disturbance, and had neurotic controls, not manics.

In Andreasen's study, derailment (56%) was the most common variety in schizophrenia, but did not significantly distinguish this group from manics, whereas poverty of content of speech (40% schizophrenics, 19% manics) did discriminate the two diagnostic groups. Pressure of speech (27% schizophrenics, 72% manics) was another significant discriminator. Neologisms (2% schizophrenics) were rare.

Cutting and Murphy found that a loosening of associations (based on impaired ability to appreciate conceptual similarities)

Table 2.7 Examples of thought disorder in schizophrenia.

Derailment
'Mum loves God. She always compares me with God.
I want to know if there are any eggs in my ovaries.'

'They were frightening me about wishes and when I was 20 I blew out a candle and I was frightened of my mother.'

Incoherence
'That is when God pardoned the GP at 9.30 this morning, the catching of an instant philosophically speaking into time that only occurs at both at death turkeys in the freezer.'

'To do to ask is at the behest of my parents which seems a fairly inappropriate reason to me.'

Neologisms/word approximations

'Oumana'	God's love beyond me
'Cytic'	Extrasensory perception
'I froze people out'	Made them older
'Medetary'	Smoked cannabis because it was good for him
'Criton'	Something which expresses sexual identity
'Psycasm'	Like a Lucky Strike cigarette

Poverty of content of speech
'I asked for pudding. I wanted to get a pudding. I accepted the pudding. I brought the pudding to the room. I ate the pudding. I am an affair of certain self-fermenting proteins catalysing their own growth. I am certainly not going to accept a continuous adjustment of internal to external relations.'

'I need to see the appropriateness of today.'

Illogicality
'I went through the colour black in quite an easy task.'

'In my mind the kissing and cuddling in 1960 makes it rain in 1980.'

'I want to have a haircut because there's no oxygen on the ward.'

occurred in 5% of schizophrenics; overinclusion (based on the number of category inclusions of items ranging from appropriate to inappropriate) occurred in 25% of schizophrenics; concrete thinking (rated as concreteness in proverb interpretation) occurred in none of 20 schizophrenics; and illogicality (false conclusions in syllogisms) occurred in 10% of schizophrenics. All figures refer to the proportion of subjects falling outside of 2 SD from the control mean.

Examples of the main varieties encountered in schizophrenia are shown in Table 2.7. Four of the five examples given – loosening of associations, incoherence, poverty of content of speech and illogicality – are the only varieties of thought disorder considered to have diagnostic specificity in DSM-IIIR.

Disturbance of emotion

Definitions and classification

Emotion is a general term covering *feelings* ('individual unique and radical commotions of the psyche'; Jaspers 1913), *affect* ('a momentary and complex emotional process of great intensity with conspicuous bodily accompaniment and sequelae'; Jaspers 1913) and *mood* ('states of feeling or frames of mind that come about with prolonged emotion'; Jaspers 1913). Philosophers such as Jaspers and Wittgenstein (1980) emphasize the fact that emotion is an experience. Other philosophers (e.g. Ryle 1949) and behaviourist psychologists (e.g. Izard & Buechler 1980) emphasize the *motivational* aspect of emotion.

Feelings, affect, mood and motivation all have their psychopathological counterparts (Table 2.8), and examples from all four categories can be encountered in schizophrenia. Only one type – inappropriate affect – is generally held to be a positive symptom of schizophrenia, whereas several – blunting (or flattening) of affect, anhedonia (loss of feeling) and apathy (loss of motivation) – are regarded as negative symptoms.

Incidence and variety in schizophrenia

Anhedonia (loss of feeling) is sometimes divided into social, e.g. loss of pleasure from being with friends, and physical, e.g. loss of pleasure from seeing a beautiful sunset, being massaged, drinking, etc. It can be rated using a questionnaire (Chapman *et al.* 1980) or at interview (Harrow *et al.* 1977). Using the questionnaire of Chapman *et al.*, Watson *et al.* (1979) found that 45% of 312 schizophrenics fell outside the 90th percentile of alcoholic controls, although Cook and Simukonda (1981), who used the same questionnaire, found that only 34% of 52 schizophrenics fell outside 1 SD of nurses; social anhedonia accounted for most of this. Schuck *et al.* (1984) also found that physical anhedonia was no more prevalent in schizophrenics than in depressives. Harrow *et al.* (1977) found that only chronic, not acute, schizophrenics were significantly anhedonic.

Intensification of feelings is reported at the onset of schizo-

Table 2.8 Disturbances of emotion.

Normal aspects	Main psychopathological varieties
Feeling	Loss of feeling – anhedonia
	Heightened feeling
Affect	Inappropriate affect
	Flattened, blunting of, affect
Mood	Depression
	Elation
	Anxiety
Motivation	Apathy

phrenia, but there are no adequate studies of the topic. A patient of McGhie and Chapman (1961), for example, recalled:

> You have no idea what it's like doctor. You would have to experience it yourself. When you feel yourself going into a sort of coma you get really scared. It's like waiting on a landing craft going into D-Day. You tremble and panic. It's like no other fear on earth.

Inappropriate affect or parathymia is the display of an emotion considered inappropriate to the situation. It is usually an outburst of empty giggling and occurs in about 20% of acutely ill schizophrenics (Andreasen 1979b).

Flattening of affect or blunted affect can be observed in about 50% of acute (Andreasen 1979b) or chronic schizophrenics (McCreadie 1982). According to Andreasen, it is a composite rating by an observer of the following elements, in descending order of weighted significance: paucity of expressive gestures (57%); unchanging facial expression (53%); lack of vocal inflection (53%); decreased spontaneous movement (37%); poor eye contact (37%); affective non-responsivity (30%); slowed speech (17%); and increased latency of response (10%).

Depression is a non-specific accompaniment of schizophrenia. It is much more frequent in acute schizophrenia (70% – neurotic depression in CATEGO (Wing *et al.* 1974) – Knights & Hirsch 1981) than expected, although probably not much higher in chronic schizophrenia (clinical depression (10%) Barnes *et al.* 1989) than in the normal population. The relationship between depression and schizophrenia is more complicated than these bare figures indicate. There is the diagnostic dilemma to consider: do you exclude patients with 'first-rank symptoms of schizophrenia' from the category of depressive psychosis even if they fulfil all other criteria for this? According to Hirsch (1982), depression and schizophrenia both arise from a 'shared pathophysiological mechanism', and depression is 'revealed' as an integral part of schizophrenia in so far as it does not become obvious until after the acute phase has subsided, although the symptoms of depression are indeed most prevalent in the acute phase if systematically rated (Knights & Hirsch 1981). According to Crow (1986), who revives Griesinger's (1845) unitary psychosis theory, depression and schizophrenia are only far ends of the same spectrum. According to Galdi (1983), depression is increased by the use of neuroleptics. According to McGlashan and Carpenter (1976), remitted schizophrenics experience more depression as part of a recovery of insight into what they have been through.

Elation is also a non-specific accompaniment of schizophrenia, but may complicate the diagnostic issue in the same way as depression, as discussed above.

Anxiety is particularly marked at the outset, but is pathologically absent in the chronic stages.

Apathy is the most troublesome negative symptom of all (at least for carers of the sufferer). Although regarded as the psychopathological counterpart of the motivational component of emotion, it is, in my view, better regarded as a manifestation of impaired will in the condition, and will be discussed below. Its mention here is justified because most psychologists and many psychiatrists regard motivation as an aspect of emotion.

Psychological deficit

The terms dementia praecox, deterioration, defect state and pseudodementia have all been applied to the combination of impaired attention, apparent decline in intelligence, failures in memory, perceptual impoverishment and lack of will. The individual components are also referred to as psychological deficits or negative symptoms.

Attentional impairment

There is a large body of literature demonstrating that attention, particularly maintenance of attention, is impaired in schizophrenia (e.g. Asarnow & MacCrimmon 1978; Van den Bosch 1982). The various components of attention – maintenance, selectivity, span, shifting of focus – are not equally affected, and the brunt is borne by maintenance, shifting, span and selectivity in that order of severity.

Intellectual decline

Numerous studies have shown a decline in formally measured intelligence from a prepsychotic state to psychosis (Rappaport & Webb 1950) and, further, from acute to chronic psychosis (Trapp & James 1937). The intellectual decline affects all subtests of the Wechsler Adult Intelligence Scale, but particularly the performance subtests, and particularly digit symbol and picture arrangement (Cutting 1990). There is growing evidence, and some controversy, that schizophrenics have a particular profile of intellectual decline, relative to Alzheimer's disease (see Chapter 10).

Memory failures

Although amnesia is traditionally regarded as a symptom of organic psychosis and should not, according to this view, be prominent in a functional psychosis such as schizophrenia, there is increasing evidence that chronic schizophrenics do have a pervasive disturbance of memory. McKenna *et al.* (1990) demonstrated that the memory impairment in chronic schizophrenics was equivalent to a group of patients with definite brain injury (see Chapter 10).

Perceptual impoverishment

Schizophrenics turn away from the outside world and become preoccupied with their own subjective state (Sass 1992), and it is difficult to assess the patency of the actual perceptual processes. There is ample evidence that their perception of the world differs qualitatively from that of a normal person (Cutting 1990); this, in consequence, leads to an impoverishment in their appreciation of the outside world.

Lack of will

Chronic schizophrenics suffer from a profound apathy, sometimes known as abulia, and this stems from a fundamental deficiency in the mainspring of their life. Kraepelin (1913/1919) considered this their essential psychological problem. Unfortunately, the term 'will' has fallen into disuse for most of this century and there have been no experimental studies to assess the significance of Kraepelin's views.

Clustering of phenomena/symptoms

There is no shortage of attempts to classify the above psychopathological features of schizophrenia.

Bleuler (1911/1950) proposed a distinction between 'fundamental symptoms', those which were virtually pathognomonic, and 'accessory symptoms', those which occurred in other conditions as well. The former comprised disturbances of association and affectivity, ambivalence and autism. The latter included delusions, alterations in personality, speech and writing disorders and catatonia.

Schneider (1958) proposed a distinction between first-rank symptoms (see Table 2.4) and other symptoms, regarding the former as atheoretical diagnostic aids.

Andreasen (1982b) and Crow (1980) adapted Jackson's formulation of positive and negative symptoms as applied to neurological disorders to schizophrenia, and this has proved, in my view, one of the most useful classifications of phenomena. Andreasen recognizes five categories of negative symptoms: affective flattening, attentional impairment, alogia (poverty of speech), avolition (apathy) and anhedonia (asociality). Hallucinations, delusions, bizarre behaviour and certain instances of thought disorder (derailment, flight of ideas, illogicality) are the positive symptoms.

Liddle (1987) identified three statistical clusters of symptoms, calling them the psychomotor poverty syndrome (poverty of speech, flattened affect and decreased spontaneous movement), the disorganization syndrome (formal thought disorder and inappropriate affect) and the reality distortion syndrome (delusions and hallucinations).

Huber *et al.* (1980) divided symptoms into 'characteristic schizophrenic deficiency' types and 'non-characteristic'. The former included what he called '*coanaesthetic* symptoms', body hallucinations and the latter such complaints as 'reduced capacity for adaptation'.

All such classifications can be criticized on the grounds of either reliability or validity, and their usefulness will almost certainly be undermined or corroborated by neurobiological advances over the next decade or so.

Explanatory theories

Explanatory theories for schizophrenic phenomena abound (Cutting 1985). It may be that all these are so closely attached to a psychological theory of the mind that subsequent generations, who eschew that particular theory, will have to grasp the schizophrenic experience afresh. The best modern account is actually given in a book that relates schizophrenia to the artistic history of the last century – *Madness and Modernism* (Sass 1992) – emphasizing that the 'descriptive' psychopathology of schizophrenia is still a powerful source of information for all those interested in the workings of the mind in 'normals', as well as for those endeavouring to understand the nature and cause of schizophrenia.

References

Abrams, R. & Taylor, M.A. (1976) Catatonia. *Archives of General Psychiatry* 33, 579–581.

American Psychiatric Association (1987) *Diagnostic and Statistical Manual of Mental Disorders*, 3rd edn. American Psychiatric Association, Washington DC.

Andreasen, N.C. (1979a) Thought, language and communication disorders. *Archives of General Psychiatry* 36, 1315–1330.

Andreasen, N.C. (1979b) Affective flattening and the criteria for schizophrenia. *American Journal of Psychiatry* 136, 944–947.

Andreasen, N.C. (1982a) Should the term 'thought disorder' be revised? *Comprehensive Psychiatry* 23, 291–299.

Andreasen, N.C. (1982b) Negative symptoms in schizophrenia. *Archives of General Psychiatry* 39, 784–788.

Asarnow, R.F. & MacCrimmon, D.J. (1978) Residual performance deficit in clinically remitted schizophrenics: a marker of schizophrenia? *Journal of Abnormal Psychology* 87, 597–608.

Barnes, M.P., Saunders, M., Walls, T.J., Saunders, I. & Kirk, C.A. (1986) The syndrome of Karl Ludwig Kahlbaum. *Journal of Neurology, Neurosurgery and Psychiatry* 49, 991–996.

Barnes, T.R.E., Curson, D.A., Liddle, P.F. & Patel, M. (1989) The nature and prevalence of depression in chronic schizophrenic in-patients. *British Journal of Psychiatry* 154, 486–491.

Bleuler, E. (1911/1950) *Dementia Praecox*. International University Press, New York. Translated by J. Zinkin, from *Dementia Praecox oder die Gruppe der Schizophrenien*. Deuticke, Leipzig.

Carpenter, W.T., Strauss, J.S. & Bartko, J.J. (1973) Flexible system for the diagnosis of schizophrenia. *Science* 182, 1275–1278.

Chaika, E. (1990) *Understanding Psychotic Speech: Beyond Freud and Chomsky*. Charles C. Thomas, Springfield.

Chapman, L.J., Chapman, J.P. & Raulin, M.L. (1980) Scales for physical and social anhedonia. *Journal of Abnormal Psychology* 85, 374–382.

Collicutt, J.R. & Hemsley, D.R. (1981) A psychophysical investigation of auditory functioning in schizophrenia. *British Journal of Social and Clinical Psychology* 20, 199–204.

Cook, M. & Simukonda, F. (1981) Anhedonia and schizophrenia. *British Journal of Psychiatry* 139, 523–525.

Crow, T.J. (1980) Molecular pathology of schizophrenia: more than one disease process? *British Medical Journal* i, 66–68.

Crow, T.J. (1986) The continuum of psychosis and its implications for the structure of the gene. *British Journal of Psychiatry* 149, 419–429.

Cutting, J. (1985) *The Psychology of Schizophrenia*. Churchill Livingstone, Edinburgh.

Cutting, J. (1990) *The Right Cerebral Hemisphere and Psychiatric Disorders*. Oxford University Press, Oxford.

Cutting, J. (1994) The assessment of thought disorder. In: *Assessment of Psychosis: A Practical Handbook* (eds T. Barnes & H. Nelson), pp. 41–50. Farrand Press, London.

Cutting, J. (1996) *Two Worlds, Two Minds, Two Hemispheres: A Reinterpretation of Psychopathology*. Oxford University Press, Oxford.

Cutting, J. & Dunne, F. (1989) Subjective experience of schizophrenia. *Schizophrenia Bulletin* 15, 217–231.

Cutting J. & Murphy, D. (1988) Schizophrenia thought disorder. *British Journal of Psychiatry* 152, 310–319.

De Morsier, G. (1938) Les hallucinations. *Revue d'Oto'neuro-ophthalmologie* 16, 241–252.

Feinberg, I. (1962) A comparison of the visual hallucinations in schizophrenia with those induced by mescaline and LSD-25. In: *Hallucinations* (ed. L.J. West), pp. 64–76. Grune & Stratton, New York.

Galdi, J. (1983) The causality of depression in schizophrenia. *British Journal of Psychiatry* 142, 621–625.

Green, P. & Preston, M. (1981) Reinforcement of vocal correlates of auditory hallucinations by auditory feedback. *British Journal of Psychiatry* 139, 204–208.

Griesinger, W. (1845) *Mental Pathology and Therapeutics*. New Sydenham Society, London. Translated (1867) from *Die Pathologie und Therapie der Psychischen Krankheiten*. Krabbe, Stuttgart.

Guggenheim, F.G. & Barbigian, H.M. (1974) Catatonic schizophrenia: epidemiology and clinical course. *Journal of Nervous and Mental Diseases* 158, 291–305.

Guttmann, E. & Maclay, W.S. (1937) Clinical observations on schizophrenic drawings. *British Journal of Medical Psychology* 16, 184–205.

Hare, E.H. (1973) A short note on pseudohallucinations. *British Journal of Psychiatry* 122, 469–476.

Harrow, M., Grinker, R.R., Holzman, P.S. & Kayton, L. (1977) Anhedonia and schizophrenia. *American Journal of Psychiatry* 134, 794–797.

Hirsch, S.R. (1982) Depression 'revealed' in schizophrenia. *British Journal of Psychiatry* 140, 421–424.

Huber, G., Gross, G., Schuttler, R. & Linz, M. (1980) Longitudinal studies of schizophrenic patients. *Schizophrenia Bulletin* 6, 592–605.

Izard, C.E. & Buechler, S. (1980) Aspects of consciousness and personality in terms of differential emotions theory. In: *Emotion; Theory, Research and Experience* (eds R. Plutchik & H. Kellerman), Vol. 1, pp. 165–187. Academic Press, New York.

Jaspers, K. (1913/1963) *General Psychopathology*. Manchester

University Press, Manchester. Translated by J. Hoenig & M.W. Hamilton from *Allgemeine Psychopathologie*. Springer Verlag, Berlin.

Johnson, J. (1984) Stupor and akinetic mutism. In: *Contemporary Neurology* (ed. M.J.G. Harrison), pp. 96–102. Butterworths, London.

Knights, A. & Hirsch, S.R. (1981) 'Revealed' depression and drug treatment of schizophrenia. *Archives of General Psychiatry* 38, 806–811.

Kraepelin, E. (1913/1919) *Psychiatrie*, 8th edn, Vol. 3, Part 2. Churchill Livingstone, Edinburgh. Translated by R.M. Barclay as *Dementia Praecox and Paraphrenia*.

Lhermitte, F., Pillon, B. & Serdaru, M. (1986) Human autonomy and the frontal lobes. I. Imitation and utilization behaviour, a neuropsychological study of 75 patients. *Annals of Neurology* 19, 326–334.

Liddle, P.F. (1987) Schizophrenic syndromes, cognitive performance and neurological dysfunction. *Psychological Medicine* 17, 49–57.

McCreadie, R.G. (1982) The Nithsdale schizophrenia survey. I. Psychiatric and social handicaps. *British Journal of Psychiatry* 140, 582–586.

McGhie, A. & Chapman, J. (1961) Disorders of attention and perception in early schizophrenia. *British Journal of Medical Psychology* 34, 103–115.

McGilchrist, I. & Cutting, J. (1995) Somatic delusions in schizophrenia and the affective psychoses. *British Journal of Psychiatry* 167, 350–361.

McGlashan, T.H. & Carpenter, W.T. (1976) Postpsychotic depression in schizophrenia. *Archives of General Psychiatry* 33, 231–239.

McKenna, P.J., Tamlyn, D., Lund, C.E. *et al.* (1990) Amnesic syndrome in schizophrenia. *Psychological Medicine* 20, 967–972.

Margo, A., Hemsley, D.R. & Slade, P.D. (1981) The effects of varying auditory input on schizophrenic hallucinations. *British Journal of Psychiatry* 139, 122–127.

Merleau-Ponty, M. (1962) *Phenomenology of Perception*. Routledge & Kegal Paul, London.

Morrison, J.R. (1973) Catatonia: retarded and excited types. *Archives of General Psychiatry* 28, 39–41.

Rappaport, S.R. & Webb, W.B. (1950) An attempt to study intellectual deterioration by premorbid and psychotic testing. *Journal of Consulting Psychology* 14, 95–98.

Rogers, D. (1985) The motor disorders of severe psychiatric illness: a conflict of paradigms. *British Journal of Psychiatry* 147, 221–232.

Rubert, S.L., Hollender, M.H. & Mehrhof, E.G. (1961) Olfactory hallucinations. *Archives of General Psychiatry* 5, 313–318.

Ryle, G. (1949) *The Concept of Mind*. Penguin, Harmondsworth.

Sass, L.A. (1992) *Madness and Modernism*. Basic Books, New York.

Schilder, P. (1920) On the development of thoughts. In: *Organisation and Pathology of Thought* (ed. D. Rappaport), pp. 497–518. Columbia University Press, New York. Translated by Rappaport, D. (1951).

Schmidt, G. (1940) A review of the German literature on delusion between 1914 and 1939. In: *The Clinical Roots of the Schizophrenia Concept* (eds J. Cutting & M. Shepherd), pp. 104–134. Cambridge University Press, Cambridge. Translated by H. Marshall (1987) from Der Wahn in deutschsprachigen Schriftum der letzten 24 Jahre (1914–1939). *Zentrulblatt für die gesamte Neurologie und Psychiatrie* 97, 113–143.

Schneider, K. (1958) *Clinical Psychopathology*. Translated by M.W. Hamilton (1959). Grune & Stratton, New York.

Schuck, J., Leventhal, D., Rothstein, H. & Irizarry, V. (1984) Physical anhedonia and schizophrenia. *Journal of Abnormal Psychology* 93, 342–344.

Spitzer, M. (1990) On defining delusions. *Comprehensive Psychiatry* 31, 377–397.

Spitzer, R.L., Endicott, J. & Robins, E. (1975) *Research Diagnostic Criteria*. New York State Psychiatric Institute, New York.

Starker, S. & Jolin, A. (1982) Imagery and hallucinations in schizophrenic patients. *Journal of Nervous and Mental Diseases* 170, 448–451.

Trapp, C.E. & James, E.B. (1937) Comparative intelligence ratings on the four types of dementia praecox. *Journal of Nervous and Mental Diseases* 86, 399–404.

Van den Bosch, R.J. (1982) *Attentional Correlates of Schizophrenia and Related Disorders*. Lisse, Swets & Zeitlinger.

Walker, C. (1991) Delusion: What did Jaspers really say? *British Journal of Psychiatry* 159, (Suppl. 14), 94–103.

Watson, C.G., Jacobs, L. & Kucala, T. (1979) A note on the pathology of anhedonia. *Journal of Clinical Psychology* 35, 740–743.

Wing, J.K., Cooper, J.E. & Sartorius, N. (1974) *Measurement and Classification of Psychiatric Symptoms*. Cambridge University Press, Cambridge.

Wittgenstein, L. (1980) *Remarks on the Philosophy of Psychology*. Basil Blackwell, Oxford.

World Health Organization (1973) *Report of the International Pilot Study of Schizophrenia*, Vol. 1. World Health Organization, Geneva.

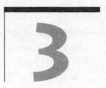

3 | The symptoms of schizophrenia

R.L.M. Fuller, S.K. Schultz and N.C. Andreasen

History of positive and negative symptoms, 25
Models of schizophrenia, 26
  Categorical models, 26
  Dimensional models, 27
  Unitary models, 27
Course of positive and negative symptoms, 28
  Stability of positive and negative symptoms, 28
  Prognostic significance of positive and negative symptoms, 28

Neurobiological correlates, 29
  Neuroimaging studies, 29
  Neuropsychology and cognitive impairment, 30
  Genetic studies, 30
  Response to treatment, 30
Conclusions, 30
References, 30

Schizophrenia is characterized by a multiplicity of symptoms arising from almost all domains of mental function, e.g. language, emotion, reasoning, motor activity and perception. These symptoms vary between patients, creating very diverse symptom profiles. The symptoms can include experiencing false perceptions (hallucinations), having false beliefs of control or danger (delusions), expressing disorganized speech and behaviour (positive formal thought disorder, bizarre behaviour), having impaired goal-directed behaviour (avolition), exhibiting blunted affect, being unable to find pleasure in activities or in the company of others (anhedonia/asociality), poverty of speech and thought (alogia) and impaired attention. The symptoms are often divided into positive and negative. Positive symptoms reflect an excess or distortion of normal function (e.g. hallucinations and delusions), while negative symptoms reflect a diminution or loss of normal function (e.g. flattening of affect and poverty of speech). (See also Chapter 2.)

History of positive and negative symptoms

The nineteenth century English physicians John Russell Reynolds and John Hughlings Jackson first used the terms 'positive' and 'negative'. Reynolds (1858, 1861) discussed positive and negative symptoms within the context of epilepsy in a descriptive and theoretical way. Jackson (1931) suggested that they should be understood in terms of inhibitory processes. (The temporal relationship of these publications is misleading because Jackson was Reynolds' contemporary, but his works were published posthumously.)

> Disease is said to 'cause' the symptoms of insanity. I submit that disease only produces negative mental symptoms, answering to the dissolution, and that all elaborate positive mental symptoms (illusions, hallucinations, delusions, and extravagant conduct) are the outcome of activity of nervous elements untouched by any pathological process; that they arise during activity on the lower level of evolution remaining.

Jackson (1931) believed that the florid positive symptoms were a release phenomenon, occurring when underlying brain processes become disinhibited as a result of a pathological insult to a higher level of brain functioning, while negative symptoms represented a more generalized loss of functions.

While many of the pioneers of psychiatric phenomenology recognized the importance of negative symptoms, they did not use this term. For example, Emil Kraepelin wrote extensively about avolition and affective flattening as central and defining features of 'dementia praecox'.

> There are apparently two principal groups of disorders that characterize the malady. On the one hand we observe a weakening of those emotional activities which permanently form the mainsprings of volition. . . . Mental activity and instinct for occupation become mute. The result of this highly morbid process is emotional dullness, failure of mental activities, loss of mastery over volition, of endeavour, and ability for independent action. . . . The second group of disorders consists in the *loss of the inner unity* of activities of intellect, emotion, and volition in themselves and among one another. . . . The near connection between thinking and feeling, between deliberation and emotional activity on the one hand, and practical work on the other is more or less lost. Emotions do not correspond to ideas. The patient laughs and weeps without recognizable cause, without any relation to their circumstances and their experiences, smile as they narrate a tale of their attempted suicide. (Kraepelin 1919, pp. 74–75)

Eugen Bleuler (1911/1950) spoke of the 'group of schizophrenias', but argued that a single defining feature was present in all people suffering from the illness. This feature, a disturbance in the ability to formulate coherent thought and language (often referred to as 'thought disorder' or 'loose associations'), was the most important of the 'fundamental symptoms'. Bleuler considered these 'fundamental symptoms' to be present in all patients: loss of continuity of associations, loss of affective responsiveness, loss of attention, loss of volition, ambivalence and autism. Bleuler held that these symptoms reflect underlying abnormalities in basic cognitive and emotive processes, while he relegated hallucinations and delusions to the status of 'accessory' or secondary symptoms.

Certain symptoms of schizophrenia are present in every case and in every period of the illness even though, as with every other disease symptom, they must have attained a certain degree of intensity before they can be recognized with any certainty. . . . Besides the specific permanent or fundamental symptoms, we can find a host of other, more accessory manifestations such as delusions, hallucinations, or catatonic symptoms. . . . As far as we know, the fundamental symptoms are characteristic of schizophrenia, while the accessory symptoms may also appear in other types of illness. (Bleuler 1911/1950, p. 13)

Kurt Schneider (1959) changed the focus of schizophrenia symptomatology with his assertion that the fundamental symptoms of schizophrenia reflect an inability to define the boundaries between self and non-self, resulting in experiences such as voices conversing or commenting, delusions of control or passivity, and thought withdrawal or insertion. He posited that these easily identifiable florid positive symptoms, which he called 'first rank symptoms', were the defining characteristics of schizophrenia (Schneider 1959). The clinical definition of schizophrenia shifted at this point to an emphasis on these positive or Schneiderian first-rank symptoms. A series of diagnostic tools were developed, such as the Present State Examination (Wing 1970), the Schedule for Affective Disorders and Schizophrenia (Endicott & Spitzer 1978), Research Diagnostic Criteria (Spitzer et al. 1978) and the DSM-III (American Psychiatric Association 1980), which defined schizophrenia according to a narrow band of positive symptoms.

However, clinical realties relatively quickly led to a corrective return to Bleulerian and Kraepelinian ideas, reintroduced as an emphasis on the importance of negative symptoms as central to the concept of schizophrenia. With this realization came three types of explanatory models attempting to account for the heterogeneity of the symptom profile in schizophrenia. These models include categorical, dimensional and unitary approaches to schizophrenia. Each model will be described in detail below.

Models of schizophrenia

Categorical models

Interest in negative symptoms re-emerged in the 1970s, as exemplified by Strauss and Carpenter (1974) and Andreasen (1979a,b,c). The turning point came perhaps from the works of Crow who, in 1980, proposed a new typology for schizophrenia, which integrated clinical presentation, pathophysiology and treatment response in a single model (Crow 1980; Crow et al. 1981). Patients with type I schizophrenia presented clinically with positive symptoms such as delusions and hallucinations; Crow posited that the underlying pathophysiological mechanism for this subtype was a biochemical imbalance, such as an excess of dopamine D_2 receptors. Therefore, he hypothe-

sized that the resulting clinical manifestations would be more likely to respond favourably to antipsychotic medication, to be characterized by exacerbations and remissions, and to have a more favourable outcome. Conversely, patients with type II schizophrenia, presenting with symptoms such as affective flattening and poverty of speech, were said to be manifestating an underlying structural/anatomical abnormality reflected by ventricular enlargement and cortical atrophy in neuroimaging studies. These symptoms therefore would tend to be poorly responsive to somatic treatment, follow a chronic course, and predict poor outcome.

Crow's original model did not specify which of the various descriptors of type I vs. type II should be used in studies designed to disconfirm or verify the hypothesized dichotomy; that is, clinical presentation, pathophysiology or treatment response. Therefore the model was difficult to test. Andreasen developed two detailed standardized rating scales, the Scale for the Assessment of Negative Symptoms (SANS) (Andreasen 1983) and the Scale for the Assessment of Positive Symptoms (SAPS) (Andreasen 1984), for reliably assessing symptoms and exploring other aspects of the relationships between positive symptoms, negative symptoms and cognitive, psychosocial and neurobiological correlates of schizophrenia. One result from validation studies of these scales was Andreasen's proposal of three subtypes of patients with schizophrenia: negative, positive and mixed (Andreasen & Olsen 1982). Both Crow (1980) and Andreasen et al. (1982) proposed that the negative symptoms of schizophrenia were indicators of a single 'subtype'.

Dividing patients into mutually exclusive subgroups is firmly rooted in the 'disease model' in medicine. Symptomatology is the measure used to identify a category, and at this point the categories are referred to as 'syndromes' (literally, a running together), because they constitute an identifiable clinical pattern that makes sense in the context of observed relationships of the symptoms. Once a specific pathophysiology or aetiology is identified, syndromes are elevated to the status of recognized diseases. In the 'categorical approach' it is assumed that the subtypes identified will differ from one another (and that this will eventually be discovered and documented) in terms of their pathophysiological mechanisms or aetiology, which may be reflected in differing responses to treatment, course of morbidity and underlying neurobiology.

The typology of schizophrenia proposed by Crow was inherently categorical, with subjects classified as either type I or II. The expansion of this conceptualization by Andreasen to include a mixed type was also categorical. The research produced from the categorical approach was prolific throughout the 1980s, but eventually the need for a new type of explanatory model arose. Dividing patients into mutually exclusive groups based on positive and negative symptoms was eventually abandoned, for several reasons. First, most patients were of a 'mixed' subtype, and many fewer were purely 'positive' or 'negative' (Andreasen 1985). Secondly, longitudinal studies revealed that the symptoms of patients varied over time (Breier et al. 1987; Marneros et al. 1991).

One of the most difficult problems in the investigation and assessment of negative symptoms in schizophrenia involves the recognition that their measurement may be confounded by a variety of other factors. The four most commonly implicated factors are:

1 neuroleptic side-effects, such as akinesia;

2 depression, which has been reported to be present in schizophrenia in the early course of the illness (Knights & Hirsch 1981; Wassink et al. 1999), not to decrease in severity as the psychotic symptoms abate with medication (Knights & Hirsch 1981) and to be frequent during the residual phase (Siris 1991);

3 a response to positive symptoms, for example avoiding social interactions because of paranoia; and

4 environmental understimulation resulting from chronic institutionalization (Carpenter et al. 1985).

Carpenter and his group have been most active in their attempts to disentangle 'primary' and 'secondary' negative symptoms (Carpenter & Kirkpatrick 1988). Carpenter defines primary, or 'deficit', symptoms as enduring core-negative symptoms of schizophrenia such as anhedonia and blunted affect. The secondary symptoms, however, are those negative symptoms that may be considered consequential to other symptoms or treatment of schizophrenia. Carpenter's deficit symptoms include flattened affect, anhedonia, poverty of speech, curbing of interest and decrease in curiosity, lack of sense of purpose and diminished social drive. By definition, these symptoms must not be fully accounted for by depression, anxiety, medication effects or environmental deprivation. The non-deficit syndrome is defined by an absence of these deficit symptoms with the presence of any other schizophrenia symptoms, such as disorganized thought or hallucinations.

Dimensional models

A more recent strategy for addressing the heterogeneity of the phenotype in schizophrenia is the dimensional approach. While 'categories' traditionally arise from disease models, 'dimensions' are often derived from the study of normal psychology; therefore, students of dimensional approaches have shown less concern about identifying brain–behaviour relationships. Dimensions define groups of symptoms that co-occur, but the co-occurrence is noted through statistical techniques such as factor analysis. While categories classify individuals, dimensions classify symptoms. Therefore, dimensions can overlap within a given individual and be additive.

Bilder et al. (1985) identified three distinct clusters of symptoms using correlative analysis of symptom ratings and neuropsychological data, providing the first validating evidence for the distinction between symptom dimensions.

1 The disorganization cluster included alogia, attentional impairment, positive formal thought disorder and bizarre behaviour.

2 The blunted affect and volition cluster included affective flattening, avolition/apathy and anhedonia.

3 The florid psychotic cluster included delusions, hallucinations and 'breadth of psychosis'.

Impaired neuropsychological performance was strongly association with the disorganized symptoms and, to a lesser extent, was associated with the blunted affect symptoms but was not associated with the psychotic symptoms. Andreasen and Grove (1986) replicated this finding in the second study, validating this distinction of three symptom dimensions, and subsequently many others have had similar findings (Kulhara et al. 1986; Liddle 1987a,b; Arndt et al. 1991; Gur et al. 1991; Brown & White 1992; Minas et al. 1992; Miller et al. 1993). Arndt et al. (1995) found that the negative symptoms, unlike the psychotic or disorganized symptoms, are stable over time. Liddle (1987b) used factor analysis to examine the relationship between symptoms in a group of patients with schizophrenia and began using the often cited dimension names of 'disorganization', 'psychomotor poverty' and 'reality distortion'. He also provided further validating evidence for these dimensions with imaging data (Liddle et al. 1992; see Chapter 22 for further discussion).

Later studies have further validated the finding that the negative and disorganized dimensions are associated with impairments in cognitive functioning (Liddle 1987a,b; Liddle & Morris 1991). O'Leary et al. (2000) further specified the nature of the impairment by investigating a large sample (134) of patients with schizophrenia. Negative symptoms were related to generalized brain dysfunction, the disorganized symptoms were related to verbal processing abnormalities and the psychotic symptoms showed no relationship to cognitive impairment.

One potential drawback of the dimensional approach is its disregard for the boundaries of the classical disease model which searches for the underlying construct of an illness. A comparable approach would be to search for the principal basis of a feature existing both in schizophrenia and other diseases, e.g. hallucinations, as they are found in schizophrenia, mania and epilepsy. The consequence of many investigations has been to treat dimensions as categories, resulting in attempts to localize specific symptoms.

Unitary models

A newer alternative, the unitary model, draws from the tradition of Bleuler (1911/1950), who attempted to identify what he considered to be the single fundamental abnormality in schizophrenia. Bleuler defined the fundamental symptoms of schizophrenia as those caused by a 'loosening of associations', which were present in all patients, tended to occur only in schizophrenia and therefore were pathognomonic of the illness. Thus, the unitary model stresses that there is a single unifying construct which explains the heterogeneity of the phenotype of schizophrenia. This model proposes that schizophrenia has one fundamental problem in a basic cognitive process.

One recent unitary model suggests that the fundamental deficit is a disruption of the fluid co-ordination of mental activity, called 'cognitive dysmetria' (Andreasen et al. 1996, 1998, 1999; Andreasen 1997, 1999). Synchrony refers to the normal fluid processing of information required during thought and speech, and 'dysmetria of thought' (Schmahmann 1991) or 'cognitive dysmetria' conveys its disturbance. This disruption would manifest itself in cognition, emotion and behaviour. Thus, the phenotype is defined by a unitary cognitive abnormality (cognitive dysmetria), which leads to the varied symptoms experienced by patients. This abnormality, not the symptoms, should be used to define the phenotype of the illness.

According to this unitary model, schizophrenia is a neurodevelopmental and cognitive disorder with an aetiology reflecting the interaction of genetics and environment and a pathophysiology consisting of the resultant abnormalities of brain development (which continues into early adulthood). Similar to the 'multiple hit' model of cancer, the unitary model suggests that the development of schizophrenia results from multiple aetiological factors leading to a shared pathophysiology and neurobiology in all people with schizophrenia. These complications in brain development from conception to early adulthood lead to disruptions in anatomic and functional connectivity, resulting in neural 'misconnections' expressed as 'cognitive dysmetria' and ultimately manifested as symptoms such as flattened affect, avolition, disorganized thought, hallucinations or delusions.

Several other theories have also attempted to explain the symptoms of schizophrenia via impairment in a single underlying cognitive process. These are the theories of willed action (Frith 1992), working memory (Goldman-Rakic 1994) and information processing and attention (Braff 1993).

Frith proposed that the general mechanism underlying the symptoms in schizophrenia is a disorder of consciousness or self-awareness, impairing one's ability to think with 'metarepresentations' (higher order abstract concepts which are representations of mental states) (Frith 1992). The impairment in self-awareness is the basis for three features of schizophrenia.
1 A disorder of willed action which leads to an inability to generate spontaneous or willed acts, resulting in poverty of action, perseveration or inappropriate action.
2 A disorder in self-monitoring. An inability to monitor willed intentions may lead to delusions of control, auditory hallucinations or thought insertion.
3 A disorder in monitoring the intentions of others, which leads to delusions of reference or paranoid delusions.

Goldman-Rakic (1994) suggested that another cognitive operation, working memory, may be disrupted in schizophrenia, leading to behavioural disorganization and certain positive and negative symptoms. Working memory is defined as a memory system in which items are held 'on-line' while needed and then discarded after use. There is evidence that the prefrontal cortex is involved in the organization and processing of this transitory memory system. Dysfunction in one or more components of working memory could result in the diverse symptoms of schizophrenia. Alogia would result from impaired information retrieval. The inability to hold a concept in mind may lead to thought disorder. A failure to reference internal or external stimuli against established memories may lead to misrepresenta-

tions of causality, resulting in delusions and hallucinations. Thus, the prefrontal cortex and its circuitry may be disrupted in schizophrenia, leading to impairments in working memory which surface as some of the positive symptoms and negative symptoms.

Braff (1993) hypothesized that patients with schizophrenia may have a fundamental deficit in information processing and attention. Patients are unsuccessful in allocating attentional resources to relevant tasks while inhibiting attention towards irrelevant stimuli. Subjectively, they may report trouble 'focusing' and feeling overwhelmed by external stimuli. On a wide variety of experimental paradigms to assess information processing and attention (such as prepulse inhibition, P50 gating, ocular motor function, continuous performance task and event-related potentials), patients with schizophrenia are less able to process information rapidly and efficiently, particularly in the context of distractions, high processing loads and multiple tasks.

Course of positive and negative symptoms

The symptoms of schizophrenia are important both clinically and theoretically. There is great interest in identifying the course and characteristics of the symptoms in schizophrenia to determine the differential nature of prognosis and outcome.

Stability of positive and negative symptoms

In his original model, Crow predicted that the negative syndrome would be stable, as it was hypothesized to reflect structural brain damage (Crow 1980; Crow et al. 1981). Studies have generally shown that negative symptoms are more stable than positive symptoms and are the least likely to improve over the course of the illness (Pfohl & Winokur 1982; Pogue-Geile & Harrow 1985; Johnstone et al. 1986; Lindenmayer et al. 1986; Addington & Addington 1991; Andreasen et al. 1991; Hull et al. 1997). In a longitudinal study of symptoms, Arndt et al. (1995) found that the negative symptoms were already prominent at the time of the patients' first episode and remained relatively stable throughout the 2 years in which the patients were followed. The positive symptoms of disorganization and psychoticism were found to be prominent at intake and declined over the course of the follow-up period (Arndt et al. 1995).

Prognostic significance of positive and negative symptoms (see also Chapter 8)

Early investigators attempted to distinguish those symptoms that were more likely to predict a good vs. a poor outcome in patients suffering from acute psychosis (Stephens 1978; Vaillant 1978). Yet, despite the sometimes severe distress associated with the psychotic symptoms, it is the negative symptoms which are most closely linked to prognosis. Patients who previously were deemed 'recovered' upon remission from hallucinations and delusions remained unemployed or socially isolated. Many studies have shown that the level of negative symptoms is related to a poor level of psychosocial functioning (Roff & Knight 1978; Johnstone *et al*. 1979; Knight *et al*. 1979; Kolakowska *et al*. 1985; Pogue-Geile & Harrow 1985; Biehl *et al*. 1986; Keefe *et al*. 1987; Munk-Jorgensen & Mortensen 1989; Breier *et al*. 1991; Fenton & McGlashan 1992). However, some studies found that a high level of positive symptoms also correlates with poor functioning (Pogue-Geile & Harrow 1984; Keefe *et al*. 1987; Breier *et al*. 1991).

Some retrospective studies have suggested an association between a longer duration of untreated initial psychosis and poor outcome in schizophrenia (Lo & Lo 1977; Inoue *et al*. 1986; Fenton & McGlashan 1987; Waddington *et al*. 1995; Scully *et al*. 1997; Wyatt *et al*. 1997). However, others have failed to confirm this relationship (Barnes *et al*. 2000; Craig *et al*. 2000; Ho *et al*. 2000). For example, Ho *et al*. demonstrated no relationship between poor outcome and duration of untreated initial psychosis in a longitudinal study of consistently well-characterized patients which controlled for other prognosticators of schizophrenia such as gender, age of illness onset and premorbid functioning.

Neurobiological correlates

Postmortem and neuroimaging studies have provided evidence of structural and physiological abnormalities in the brains of patients with schizophrenia. Studies using neuroimaging techniques, studies investigating cognitive impairment, genetic investigations and studies of response to treatment have made advancements in identifying the correlates of the neurobiology and symptoms of schizophrenia.

Neuroimaging studies

Neuroimaging has been used to investigate neuroanatomy and neurofunctioning in schizophrenia. Computerized tomography (CT) permitted the first systematic investigations of brain structure in schizophrenia, providing an opportunity to investigate relationships between symptomotology and structure. In this first phase of neuroimaging, investigators attempted to validate the positive and negative subtypes. Enlarged ventricles were associated with more severe negative symptoms as well as more cognitive impairment and greater impairment in premorbid functioning (Johnstone *et al*. 1976; Weinberger *et al*. 1980; Andreasen *et al*. 1982).

Further advancement of technology has provided magnetic resonance imaging (MRI), which allows for high levels of contrast between grey and white matter and cerebrospinal fluid through superior resolution capabilities. Functional neuroimaging allows for the exploration of relationships between symptomatology and dysfunction of specific brain regions. Earlier work used single photon emission computerized tomography (SPECT), while more recent studies utilized positron emission tomography (PET), both of which measure cerebral blood flow. Another method, functional magnetic resonance imaging (fMRI), uses the paramagnetic effects of deoxyhaemoglobin to measure regional blood flow and metabolic activity.

During the second phase of neuroimaging, investigators attempted to identify areas of impaired performance linked with the symptom dimensions in schizophrenia. Liddle *et al*. examined the three symptom clusters (reality distortion, disorganized symptoms and psychomotor poverty), finding increased cerebral blood flow present in left mesiotemporal structures in patients with hallucinations and delusions as well as increased flow in the right anterior cingulate cortex, left superior temporal gyrus and dorsomedial thalamus. In contrast, a relative decrease in blood flow was observed in the left prefrontal and parietal cortex among patients exhibiting the negative symptom of psychomotor poverty (see Chapter 22; Friston *et al*. 1992; Liddle *et al*. 1992). A number of imaging studies have linked hypofrontality of the frontal lobe with increased negative symptoms in patients with schizophrenia (Volkow *et al*. 1987; Andreasen *et al*. 1992, 1994; Wolkin *et al*. 1992; Schroeder *et al*. 1995). Other work using PET imaging to assess cerebral blood flow in relation to negative symptom measures was completed by Tamminga *et al*. (1992), similarly demonstrating decreased cerebral metabolism in frontal and parietal cortex as well as thalamic areas associated with the severity of negative symptoms.

Several studies have indicated that the temporal lobe volume is reduced in people with schizophrenia (Dewan *et al*. 1983; Cohen *et al*. 1989; Barta *et al*. 1997; Buchsbaum *et al*. 1997). Others have found reduced activation in the right temporal lobe (Jernigan *et al*. 1985; Post *et al*. 1987). Some have suggested that there may be more regionally specific abnormalities in areas such as the superior temporal gyrus or planum temporale which correlate with the presence of hallucinations, positive formal thought disorder or reality distortion (Barta *et al*. 1990; Shenton *et al*. 1992; Nelson *et al*. 1998; Portas *et al*. 1998).

Imaging technologies continue to reinforce the fact that clearly measurable abnormalities exist in schizophrenia. Imaging research has now shifted from single region models to circuit models. Advances in neuroimaging may help researchers to address the many intriguing questions that remain regarding the abnormalities of these circuits. For example, studies are being carried out to examine whether the differences seen in schizophrenia reflect anatomical or functional circuits misconnected through abnormal brain development, neuronal loss or other regressive changes, an epiphenomenon of treatment, or pathological sequelae of long-term illness. There is a growing consensus from research in first-episode never-medicated patients that fundamental differences exist in brain structure and function that antedate treatment and chronicity effects (Chapter 22).

Neuropsychology and cognitive impairment

There have been reports of cognitive impairment in schizophrenia since the illness was first described by Kraepelin (1919) and Bleuler (1911/1950). A remarkably consistent pattern emerges; cognitive impairment is associated with negative (Andreasen & Olsen 1982; Cornblatt *et al.* 1985; Gaebel *et al.* 1987; Keilp *et al.* 1988; Braff 1989; Andreasen *et al.* 1990; Merriam *et al.* 1990) and disorganized symptoms (Bilder *et al.* 1985; Frith *et al.* 1991), but is not associated with psychotic symptoms (Bilder *et al.* 1985; Cuesta & Peralta 1995; O'Leary *et al.* 2000). Further validating evidence exists. Negative symptoms have been found to be associated with impaired conceptual thinking, object naming and long-term memory (Liddle 1987a,b), a slowing of mental activity (Liddle & Morris 1991) and poor performance on tests of verbal learning and memory, verbal fluency, visual memory and visual–motor sequencing (O'Leary *et al.* 2000). Disorganized symptoms are associated with poor performance on tests of concentration, immediate recall and list learning (Liddle 1987a,b), an inability to inhibit inappropriate responses (Liddle & Morris 1991), lower verbal IQ and poor concept attainment (see Chapter 10; O'Leary *et al.* 2000).

Genetic studies

It has been recognized for many decades that schizophrenia aggregates among relatives of schizophrenic patients to a greater degree than in the general population. However, very little information exists on the correlation of genetics and the symptoms of schizophrenia. It has been proposed that the negative dimension of schizophrenia may represent a genetic subtype of the illness. In support of this hypothesis, some studies (Kay *et al.* 1986; McGuffin & Owen 1991), but not all (Pearlson *et al.* 1985; Alda *et al.* 1991), showed that first-degree relatives of patients with schizophrenia and high levels of negative symptoms have a higher morbid risk than the relatives of patients with schizophrenia and predominantly positive symptoms. Patients with a family history of schizophrenia are reported to have more treatment-resistant negative symptoms, which are related to poor psychosocial functioning, than those patients with no family history (Malaspina *et al.* 2000). Moreover, a reanalysis of previously published twin studies showed that negative symptoms in one twin predicts a higher concordance rate (Dworkin *et al.* 1988).

Kendler *et al.* (2000) attempted to provide evidence for linkage between families with schizophrenia-related disorders and chromosomal regions based on major symptoms of the illness. They found that families with positive evidence for linkage on the genomic region 8p (D8S283–D8S552) were likely to include probands with symptom profiles of thought disorder, affective deterioration, chronic course, poor outcome and minimal depressive symptoms.

Population-based association studies typically use the psychiatric diagnosis, i.e. the symptoms, as the phenotypic expression of illness. However, it is possible to use biological traits correlated with the illness as other indicators of phenotypic expression. For example, a specific pathological indicator such as the p50 auditory sensory gating deficit in schizophrenia may be used to identify susceptibility loci (Freedman 1998). Other examples include impaired prepulse inhibition, impaired habituation to the startle reflex, as well as eye-tracking and eye-blinking abnormalities. Such approaches may identify useful phenotypes for schizophrenia that are not based solely on diagnostic categories. Strategies like these are continuing to evolve at a rapid pace, each offering the potential for new insights into the genetic factors involved in the expression of schizophrenia (see Chapters 14 and 15).

Response to treatment

Medication is effective in reducing both positive and, to some extent, negative symptoms, but this is covered in detail in other chapters (see Chapters 8, 10 and 24–26).

Conclusions

The last two or three decades have been a rich era for the conceptualization and study of the role of symptoms in schizophrenia. The concepts of symptom dimensions have been carefully investigated, providing knowledge of cognitive impairment, structural and functional neuroanatomy and genetic bases for schizophrenia. The new horizon involves investigating the construct of an underlying cognitive dysfunction (e.g. cognitive dysmetria, working memory, a disturbance in consciousness, impaired information processing) that contributes to all the symptoms, both positive and negative.

References

Addington, J. & Addington, D. (1991) Positive and negative symptoms of schizophrenia: their course and relationship over time. *Schizophrenia Research* **5**, 51–59.

Alda, M., Zvolsky, P. & Dvorakova, M. (1991) Study of chronic schizophrenics with positive and negative family histories of psychosis. *Acta Psychiatrica Scandinavica* **83**, 334–337.

American Psychiatric Association (1980) *Diagnostic and Statistical Manual of Mental Disorders (DSM-III)*, 3rd edn. American Psychiatric Association, Washington DC.

Andreasen, N.C. (1979a) Affective flattening and the criteria for schizophrenia. *American Journal of Psychiatry* **136**, 944–947.

Andreasen, N.C. (1979b) Thought, language, and communication disorders. I. Clinical assessment, definition of terms, and evaluation of their reliability. *Archives of General Psychiatry* **36**, 1315–1321.

Andreasen, N.C. (1979c) Thought, language, and communication disorders. II. Diagnostic significance. *Archives of General Psychiatry* **36**, 1325–1330.

Andreasen, N.C. (1983) *The Scale for the Assessment of Negative Symptoms (SANS)*. University of Iowa, Iowa City, IA.

Andreasen, N.C. (1984) *The Scale for the Assessment of Positive Symptoms (SAPS)*. University of Iowa, Iowa City, IA.

Andreasen, N.C. (1985) Positive vs. negative schizophrenia: a critical evaluation. *Schizophrenia Bulletin* **11**, 380–389.

Andreasen, N.C. (1997) Linking mind and brain in the study of mental illnesses: a project for a scientific psychopathology. *Science* **275**, 1586–1593.

Andreasen, N.C. (1999) A unitary model of schizophrenia: Bleuler's 'fragmented phrene' as schizencephaly. *Archives of General Psychiatry* **56**, 781–787.

Andreasen, N.C. & Grove, W.M. (1986) Evaluation of positive and negative symptoms in schizophrenia. *Psychiatrie and Psychobiologie* **1**, 108–121.

Andreasen, N.C. & Olsen, S. (1982) Negative versus positive schizophrenia: definition and validation. *Archives of General Psychiatry* **39**, 789–794.

Andreasen, N.C., Olsen, S.A., Smith, M.R., Dennert, J.W. & Smith, M.R. (1982) Ventricular enlargement in schizophrenia: definition and prevalence. *American Journal of Psychiatry* **139**, 297–302.

Andreasen, N.C., Ehrhardt, J.C., Swayze, V.W. II *et al.* (1990) Magnetic resonance imaging of the brain in schizophrenia: the pathophysiologic significance of structural abnormalities. *Archives of General Psychiatry* **47**, 35–44.

Andreasen, N.C., Flaum, M., Arndt, S. *et al.* (1991) Positive and negative symptoms: assessment and validity. *Negative Versus Positive Schizophrenia* (eds A. Marneros, N.C. Andreasen & M.T. Tsuang), pp. 28–51. Springer-Verlag Berlin, Heidelberg.

Andreasen, N.C., Rezai, K., Alliger, R. *et al.* (1992) Hypofrontality in neuroleptic-naive and in patients with chronic schizophrenia: assessment with xenon-133 single-photon emission computed tomography and the Tower of London. *Archives of General Psychiatry* **49**, 943–958.

Andreasen, N.C., Flashman, L., Flaum, M. *et al.* (1994) Regional brain abnormalities in schizophrenia measured with magnetic resonance imaging. *Journal of the American Medical Association* **272**, 1763–1769.

Andreasen, N.C., O'Leary, D.S., Cizadlo, T. *et al.* (1996) Schizophrenia and cognitive dysmetria: a positron-emission tomography study of dysfunctional prefrontal–thalamic–cerebellar circuitry. *Procedures of the National Academy of Sciences of the USA* **93**, 9985–9990.

Andreasen, N.C., Paradiso, S. & O'Leary, D.S. (1998) 'Cognitive dysmetria' as an integrative theory of schizophrenia: a dysfunction in cortical–subcortical–cerebellar circuitry? *Schizophrenia Bulletin* **24** (2), 203–218.

Andreasen, N.C., Nopoulos, P., O'Leary, D.S. *et al.* (1999) Defining the phenotype of schizophrenia: cognitive dysmetria and its neural mechanisms. *Biological Psychiatry* **46**, 908–920.

Arndt, S., Alliger, R.J. & Andreasen, N.C. (1991) The distinction of positive and negative symptoms: the failure of a two-dimensional model. *British Journal of Psychiatry* **158**, 317–322.

Arndt, S., Andreasen, N.C., Flaum, M., Miller, D. & Nopoulos, P. (1995) A longitudinal study of symptom dimensions in schizophrenia: prediction and patterns of change. *Archives of General Psychiatry* **52** (5), 352–360.

Barnes, T.R., Hutton, S.B., Chapman, M.J. *et al.* (2000) West London first-episode study of schizophrenia: clinical correlates of duration of untreated psychosis. *British Journal of Psychiatry* **177** (3), 207–211.

Barta, P.E., Pearlson, G.D. & Powers, R.E. (1990) Auditory hallucinations and smaller superior temporal gyrus volume in schizophrenia. *American Journal of Psychiatry* **147**, 1457–1462.

Barta, P.E., Powers, R.E., Aylward, E.H. *et al.* (1997) Quantitative MRI volume changes in late onset schizophrenia and Alzheimer's disease compared to normal controls. *Psychiatry Research* **68**, 65–75.

Biehl, H., Maurer, K. & Schubart, C. (1986) Prediction of outcome and utilization of medical services in a prospective study of first onset schizophrenics: results of a prospective 5-year follow-up study. *European Archives of Psychiatry and Neurological Sciences* **236**, 139–147.

Bilder, R.M., Mukherjee, S. & Rieder, R.O. (1985) Symptomatic and neuropsychological components of defect states. *Schizophrenia Bulletin* **11**, 409–491.

Bleuler, E. (1911/1950) *Dementia Praecox or the Group of Schizophrenias.* Translated by J. Zinkin. International Universities Press, New York.

Braff, D.L. (1989) Sensory input deficits and negative symptoms in schizophrenic patients. *American Journal of Psychiatry* **146**, 1006–1011.

Braff, D.L. (1993) Information processing and attention dysfunctions in schizophrenia. *Schizophrenia Bulletin* **19**, 233–259.

Breier, A., Wolkowitz, O.M., Doran, A.R. *et al.* (1987) Neuroleptic responsivity of negative and positive symptoms in schizophrenia. *American Journal of Psychiatry* **144** (12), 1549–1555.

Breier, A., Schreiber, J. & Dyer, J. (1991) National Institute of Mental Health longitudinal study of chronic schizophrenia: prognosis and predictors of outcome. *Archives of General Psychiatry* **48**, 239–246.

Brown, K. & White, T. (1992) Syndromes of chronic schizophrenia and some clinical correlates. *British Journal of Psychiatry* **161**, 317–322.

Buchsbaum, M.S., Yang, S., Hazlett, E. *et al.* (1997) Ventricular volume and asymmetry in schizotypal personality disorder and schizophrenia assessed with magnetic resonance imaging. *Schizophrenia Research* **27**, 45–53.

Carpenter, W.T. & Kirkpatrick, B. (1988) The heterogeneity of the long-term course of schizophrenia. *Schizophrenia Bulletin* **14**, 645–659.

Carpenter, W.T., Strauss, J.S. & Bartko, J.J. (1985) On the heterogeneity of schizophrenia. In: *Controversies in Schizophrenia* (ed. M. Alpert), pp. 25–37. Guildford Press, New York.

Cohen, M.B., Lake, R.R., Graham, L.S. *et al.* (1989) Quantitative iodine-123 IMP imaging of brain perfusion in schizophrenia. *Journal of Nuclear Medicine* **30** (10), 1616–1620.

Cornblatt, B.A., Lenzenweger, M.F. & Dworkin, R.H. (1985) Positive and negative schizophrenic symptoms: attention and information processing. *Schizophrenia Bulletin* **11**, 397–407.

Craig, T.J., Bromet Fennig, E.J., Tanenberg-Karant, S., Lavelle, M. & Galambos, J. (2000) Is there an association between duration of untreated psychosis and 24-month clinical outcome in a first-admission series? *American Journal of Psychiatry* **157**, 60–66.

Crow, T.J. (1980) Molecular pathology of schizophrenia: more than one disease process? *British Medical Journal* **280**, 66–68.

Crow, T.J., Corsellis, J.A.N., Cross, A.J. *et al.* (1981) The search for changes underlying the type II syndrome. In: *Biological Psychiatry* (eds C. Perris, G. Struwe & B. Jansson), pp. 727–731. Elsevier North-Holland Biomedical Press, Amsterdam,

Cuesta, M. & Peralta, V. (1995) Cognitive disorders in the positive, negative and disordered syndromes of schizophrenia. *Psychiatry Research* **58**, 227–235.

Dewan, M.J., Pandurangi, A.K., Lee, S.H. *et al.* (1983) Central brain morphology in chronic schizophrenic patients: a controlled CT study. *Biological Psychiatry* **18** (10), 1133–1140.

Dworkin, R.H., Lenzenweger, M.F. & Moldin, S.O. (1988) A multidimensional approach to the genetics of schizophrenia. *American Journal of Psychiatry* **145**, 1077–1083.

Endicott, J. & Spitzer, R.L. (1978) A diagnostic interview: the Schedule for Affective Disorders and Schizophrenia (SADS). *Archives of General Psychiatry* **35**, 837–844.

Fenton, W.S. & McGlashan, T.H. (1987) Sustained remission in drug-free schizophrenic patients. *American Journal of Psychiatry* **144**, 1306–1309.

Fenton, W.S. & McGlashan, T.H. (1992) Testing systems for assessment of negative symptoms in schizophrenia. *Archives of General Psychiatry* **49**, 179–184.

Freedman, R. (1998) Basic and clinical approaches to the genetics of deficits in schizophrenia. *Biological Psychiatry* **43** (Suppl. 8), 3.

Friston, K.J., Liddle, P.F., Frith, C.D., Hirsch, S.R. & Frackowiak, R.S. (1992) The left medial temporal region and schizophrenia: a PET study. *Brain* **115** (2), 367–382.

Frith, C.D. (1992) *The Cognitive Neuropsychology of Schizophrenia.* Lawrence Erlbaum, East Sussex.

Frith, C.D., Friston, K., Liddle, P.F. & Frackowiak, R.S. (1991) Willed action and the prefrontal cortex in man: a study with PET. *Proceedings of the Royal Society of London* **244**, 241–246.

Gaebel, W., Ulrich, G. & Frick, K. (1987) Visuomotor performance of schizophrenic patients and normal controls in a picture viewing task. *Biological Psychiatry* **22** (10), 1227–1237.

Goldman-Rakic, P.S. (1994) Working memory dysfunction in schizophrenia. *Journal of Neuropsychiatry and Clinical Neuroscience* **64**, 348–357.

Gur, R.E., Mozley, D., Resnick, S.M. *et al.* (1991) Relations among clinical scales in schizophrenia. *American Journal of Psychiatry* **148**, 472–478.

Ho, B.-C., Andreasen, N.C., Flaum, M., Nopoulos, P. & Miller, D. (2000) Untreated initial psychosis: its relation to quality of life and symptom remission in first-episode schizophrenia. *American Journal of Psychiatry* **157**, 808–815.

Hull, J.W., Smith, T.E., Anthony, D.T. *et al.* (1997) Patterns of symptom change: a longitudinal analysis. *Schizophrenia Research* **24**, 17–18.

Inoue, K., Nakajima, T. & Kato, N. (1986) A longitudinal study of schizophrenia in adolescence. I. The 1- to 3-year outcome. *Japanese Journal of Psychiatry and Neurology* **40**, 143–151.

Jackson, J.H. (1931) *Selected Writings.* Hodder and Stoughton, London.

Jernigan, T.L., Sargent, T. III, Pfefferbaum, A., Kusubov, N. & Stahl, S.M. (1985) 18Fluorodeoxyglucose PET in schizophrenia. *Psychiatry Research* **16** (4), 317–329.

Johnstone, E.C., Crow, T.J., Frith, C.D., Husband, J. & Kreel, L. (1976) Cerebral ventricular size and cognitive impairment in chronic schizophrenia. *Lancet* **2**, 924–926.

Johnstone, E., Frith, C. & Gold, A. (1979) The outcome of severe acute schizophrenic illnesses after 1 year. *British Journal of Psychiatry* **134**, 28–33.

Johnstone, E.C., Owens, D.G.C. & Frith, C.D. (1986) The relative stability of positive and negative features in chronic schizophrenia. *British Journal of Psychiatry* **150**, 60–64.

Kay, S.R., Opler, L.A. & Fiszbein, A. (1986) Significance of positive and negative symptoms in chronic schizophrenia. *British Journal of Psychiatry* **149**, 439–448.

Keefe, R., Mohs, R. & Losonczy, M. (1987) Characteristics of very poor outcome schizophrenia. *American Journal of Psychiatry* **144**, 889–895.

Keilp, J.G., Sweeney, J.A., Jacobsen, P. *et al.* (1988) Cognitive impairment in schizophrenia: specific regions to ventricular size and negative symptomatology. *Biological Psychiatry* **24**, 47–55.

Kendler, K., Myers, J., O'Neill, A. *et al.* (2000) Clinical features of schizophrenia and linkage to chromosomes 5q, 6p, 8p, and 10p in the Irish study of high-density schizophrenia families. *American Journal of Psychiatry* **157** (3), 402–408.

Knight, R.A., Roff, J.D., Barnet, J. & Moss, J.L. (1979) Concurrent and predictive validity of thought disorder and affectivity: a 22-year follow-up of acute schizophrenia. *Journal of Abnormal Psychology* **88**, 1–12.

Knights, A. & Hirsch, S.R. (1981) 'Revealed' depression and drug treatment for schizophrenia. *Archives of General Psychiatry* **38**, 806–811.

Kolakowska, T., Williams, A.O. & Ardern, M. (1985) Schizophrenia with good and poor outcome. I. Early clinical features, response to neuroleptics and signs of organic dysfunction. *British Journal of Psychiatry* **146**, 229–239.

Kraepelin, E. (1919) *Dementia Praecox and Paraphrenia.* Translated by R.M. Barkley. E. & S. Livingstone, Edinburgh.

Kulhara, P., Kota, S.K. & Joseph, S. (1986) Positive and negative subtypes of schizophrenia: a study from India. *Acta Psychiatrica Scandinavica* **74**, 353–359.

Liddle, P. (1987a) Schizophrenia symptoms, cognitive performance and neurological dysfunction. *Psychological Medicine* **17**, 49–57.

Liddle, P. (1987b) The symptoms of chronic schizophrenia: a re-examination of the positive–negative dichotomy. *British Journal of Psychiatry* **151**, 145–151.

Liddle, P. & Morris, D. (1991) Schizophrenic syndromes and frontal lobe performance. *British Journal of Psychiatry* **158**, 340–345.

Liddle, P., Friston, K.J. & Frith, C.D. (1992) Cerebral blood flow and mental processes in schizophrenia. *Journal of the Royal Society of Medicine* **85**, 224–226.

Lindenmayer, J.P., Kay, S.R. & Friedman, C. (1986) Negative and positive schizophrenic syndromes after the acute phase: a prospective follow-up. *Comprehensive Psychiatry* **27**, 276–286.

Lo, W.H. & Lo, T. (1977) A 10-year follow-up study of Chinese schizophrenics in Hong Kong. *British Journal of Psychiatry* **131**, 63–66.

McGuffin, P. & Owen, M. (1991) The molecular genetics of schizophrenia: an overview and forward view. *European Archives of Psychiatry and Clinical Neuroscience* **240**, 169–173.

Malaspina, D., Goetz, R.R., Yale, S. *et al.* (2000) Relation of familial schizophrenia to negative symptoms but not to the deficit syndrome. *American Journal of Psychiatry* **157**, 994–1003.

Marneros, A., Deister, A. & Rohde, A. (1991) Stability of diagnoses in affective, schizoaffective and schizophrenic disorders: cross-sectional versus longitudinal diagnosis. *European Archives of Psychiatry and Clinical Neuroscience* **241**, 1870–1192.

Merriam, A.E., Kay, S.R. & Opler, L.A. (1990) Neurological signs and the positive–negative dimension in schizophrenia. *Biological Psychiatry* **28**, 181–192.

Miller, D.D., Arndt, S.V. & Andreasen, N.C. (1993) Alogia, attentional impairment, and inappropriate affect: their status in the dimensions of schizophrenia. *Comprehensive Psychiatry* **34**, 221–226.

Minas, I.H., Stuart, G.W., Klimidis, S. *et al.* (1992) Positive and negative symptoms in the psychoses: multidimensional scaling of SAPS and SANS items. *Schizophrenia Research* **8**, 143–156.

Munk-Jorgensen, P. & Mortensen, P.B. (1989) Schizophrenia: a 13-year follow-up – diagnostic and psychopathological aspects. *Acta Psychiatrica Scandinavica* **79**, 391–399.

Nelson, M.D., Saykin, A.J., Flashman, L.A. & Riordan, H.J. (1998) Hippocampal reduction in schizophrenia as assessed by magnetic resonance imaging: a meta-analytic study. *Archives of General Psychiatry* **55** (5), 433–440.

O'Leary, D., Flaum, M., Kesler, M. *et al.* (2000) Cognitive correlates of the negative, disorganized, and psychotic symptom dimensions of schizophrenia. *Journal of Neuropsychiatry and Clinical Neurosciences* **12**, 4–15.

Pearlson, G.D., Garbacz, D.J. & Moberg, P.J. (1985) Symptomatic, familial, perinatal, and social correlates of computerized axial tomography (CAT) changes in schizophrenics and bipolars. *Journal of Nervous and Mental Disorders* **173**, 42–50.

Pfohl, B. & Winokur, G. (1982) The evolution of symptoms in institutionalized hebephrenic/catatonic schizophrenics. *British Journal of Psychiatry* **141**, 567–572.

Pogue-Geile, M.F. & Harrow, M. (1984) Negative and positive symptoms in schizophrenia and depression: a follow up. *Schizophrenia Bulletin* **10**, 371–387.

Pogue-Geile, M.F. & Harrow, M. (1985) Negative symptoms in schizophrenia: their longitudinal course and prognostic importance. *Schizophrenia Bulletin* **11**, 427–439.

Portas, C.M., Goldstein, J.M., Shenton, M.E. *et al.* (1998) Volumetric evaluation of the thalamus in schizophrenic male patients using MRI. *Biological Psychiatry* **43** (9), 649–659.

Post, R.M., DeLisi, L.E., Holcomb, H.H. *et al.* (1987) Glucose utilization in the temporal cortex of affectively ill patients: positron emission tomography. *Biological Psychiatry* **22** (5), 545–553.

Reynolds, J. (1858) On the pathology of convulsions, with special reference to those of children. *Liverpool Medico-chirurgie Journal* **2**, 1–14.

Reynolds, J. (1861) *Epilepsy: its Symptoms, Treatment and Relation to Other Chronic Convulsive Diseases*, Vol. 2. John Churchill, London.

Roff, J.D. & Knight, R. (1978) A schizophrenia checklist: reliability without stability, concurrent without predictive validity. *Psychological Report* **43**, 791–794.

Schmahmann, J. (1991) An emerging concept: the cerebellar contribution to higher function. *Archives of Neurology* **48**, 1178–1187.

Schneider, K. (1959) *Clinical Psychopathology*. Translated by M.W. Hamilton. Grune & Stratton, New York.

Schroeder, J., Buchsbaum, M.S., Siegel, B.V., Geider, F.J. & Niethammer, R. (1995) Structural and functional correlates of subsyndromes in chronic schizophrenia. *Psychopathology* **28**, 38–45.

Scully, P.J., Coakley, G., Kinsella, A. & Waddington, J.L. (1997) Psychopathology, executive (frontal) and general cognitive impairment in relation to duration of initially untreated versus subsequently treated psychosis in chronic schizophrenia. *Psychological Medicine* **27**, 1303–1310.

Shenton, M., Kikinis, R. & Jolesz, F. (1992) Abnormalities of the left temporal lobe and thought disorder in schizophrenia: a quantitative magnetic resonance imaging study. *New England Journal of Medicine* **327**, 604–612.

Siris, S.G. (1991) Diagnosis of secondary depression in schizophrenia: implications for DSM-IV. *Schizophrenia Bulletin* **17**, 75–98.

Spitzer, R., Endicott, J. & Robins, E. (1978) *Research Diagnostic Criteria (RDC) for a Selected Group of Functional Disorders, Biometrics Research*, 3rd edn. New York State Psychiatric Institute, New York.

Stephens, J.H. (1978) Long-term prognosis and follow-up in schizophrenia. *Schizophrenia Bulletin* **4**, 25–47.

Strauss, J. & Carpenter, W.T. (1974) Characteristic symptoms and outcome in schizophrenia. *Archives of General Psychiatry* **30**, 429–434.

Tamminga, C.A., Thaker, G.K., Buchanan, R.W. *et al.* (1992) Limbic-system abnormalities identified in schizophrenia using positron emission tomography with fluorodeoxyglucose and neocortical alternations with deficit syndrome. *Archives of General Psychiatry* **49**, 522–530.

Vaillant, G. (1978) A 10-year followup of remitting schizophrenics. *Schizophrenia Bulletin* **4**, 78–85.

Volkow, N.D., Wolf, A.P., Van Gelder, P. *et al.* (1987) Phenomenological correlates of metabolic activity in 18 patients with chronic schizophrenia. *American Journal of Psychiatry* **144** (2), 151–158.

Waddington, J.L., Youssef, H.A. & Kinsella, A. (1995) Sequential cross-sectional and 10-year prospective study of severe negative symptoms in relation to duration of initially untreated psychosis in chronic schizophrenia. *Psychological Medicine* **25**, 849–857.

Wassink, T., Flaum, M., Nopolous, P. & Andreasen, N. (1999) Prevalence of depressive symptoms early in the course of schizophrenia. *American Journal of Psychiatry* **156**, 315–316.

Weinberger, D.R., Bigelow, L.B., Kleinman, J.E. *et al.* (1980) Cerebral ventricular enlargement in chronic schizophrenia: an association with poor response to treatment. *Archives of General Psychiatry* **37**, 11–13.

Wing, J.K. (1970) A standard form of psychiatric Present State Examinations (PSE): a method for standardizing the classification of symptoms. In: *Psychiatric Epidemiology* (eds E.H. Hare & J.K. Wing). Oxford University Press, London.

Wolkin, A., Sanfilipo, M., Wolf, A.P. *et al.* (1992) Negative symptoms and hypofrontality in chronic schizophrenia. *Archives of General Psychiatry* **49** (12), 959–965.

Wyatt, R.J., Green, M.F. & Tuma, A.H. (1997) Long-term morbidity associated with delayed treatment of first admission schizophrenic patients: a re-analysis of the Camarillo State Hospital data. *Psychological Medicine* **27**, 261–268.

4

Child and adolescent onset schizophrenia

C. Hollis

History, 34
  Evolution of the concept of schizophrenia in
    childhood and adolescence, 34
Clinical features, 35
  Clinical phases of schizophrenia, 35
  Symptom dimensions, 36
Diagnosis and differential diagnosis, 37
  Diagnostic validity, 37
  Developmental issues in assessment of
    children, 37
  Differential diagnosis, 38
Epidemiology, 40
  Incidence and prevalence, 40
  Sex ratio, 40
Aetiology and risk factors, 40
  Pregnancy and birth complications, 40
  Puberty, 40
  Psychosocial risks, 41
Neurobiology of schizophrenia, 41
  Neurodevelopmental models of
    schizophrenia, 41
  Neuropathology, 42
  Structural brain abnormalities, 42
  Progressive brain changes, 42
  Functional brain imaging, 43

Implications for neurodevelopmental models of
    schizophrenia, 43
Genetics, 44
  Genetic risk and early onset schizophrenia, 44
  Cytogenetic abnormalities, 44
Neuropsychology, 44
  Pattern of cognitive deficits, 44
  Executive functions and onset of
    schizophrenia, 45
  Course of cognitive deficits, 45
Course and outcome, 46
  Short-term course, 46
  Long-term outcome, 46
  Mortality, 46
  Prognosis, 46
Treatment approaches, 47
  General principles, 47
  Primary prevention and early detection, 47
  Pharmacological treatments, 47
  Psychosocial and family interventions, 48
  Cognitive–behaviour therapy, 48
  Cognitive remediation, 48
  Organization of treatment services, 48
Conclusions, 49
References, 49

Schizophrenia is one of the most devastating psychiatric disorders to affect children and adolescents. Although extremely rare before the age of 10, the incidence of schizophrenia rises steadily through adolescence to reach its peak in early adult life. An accumulating body of evidence now supports the view that schizophrenia in childhood and adolescence shows continuity with the adult form of the disorder at the levels of symptoms, clinical course and underlying neurobiology. Like other disorders of presumed multifactorial origin (e.g. juvenile rheumatoid arthritis and diabetes), the early onset form of schizophrenia appears to lie at the extreme end of a continuum of disease severity and genetic liability.

This chapter focuses on the similarities and differences, from both a clinical and neurobiological perspective, between child and adolescent onset schizophrenia and the adult form of the disorder. Special attention will be given to the following topics. First, the historical development of the concept of schizophrenia in children and adolescents. Secondly, the clinical issues relating to the recognition, differential diagnosis and management of child and adolescent onset schizophrenia. Thirdly, the evidence from clinical and neurobiological studies for continuity between the childhood and adult onset forms of the disorder. Fourthly, the possible mechanisms and timing of events in brain development that may be responsible for the onset of schizophrenia in children and adolescents.

History

Evolution of the concept of schizophrenia in childhood and adolescence

Both Kraepelin and Bleuler believed that schizophrenia presented in a similar form, albeit more rarely, during childhood and adolescence. Kraepelin (1919) found that 3.5% of cases of dementia praecox began before the age of 10, with a further 2.7% arising between the ages of 10 and 15. Kraepelin also remarked that these childhood onset cases frequently had an insidious onset. Bleuler (1911/1950) suggested that about 5% of cases of schizophrenia had their onset prior to age 15. De Sanctis (1906) described a group of young children who exhibited catatonia, stereotopies, negativism, echolalia and emotional bluntening. De Sanctis viewed this condition as an early onset form of Kraepelin's dementia praecox, and coined the term 'dementia praecoccissima'. The twentieth century saw a shifting debate about how best to categorize schizophrenia in childhood. The expansion and contraction of the concept of schizophrenia in childhood closely mirrored a similar debate concerning the boundaries of the adult form of the disorder. It also echoed the debate about how best to conceptualize and define depression in childhood, with the idea of age-specific symptomatology (developmental heterotypy) competing with the idea of applying unmodified adult diagnostic criteria to children (developmental homotypy).

During the first third of the twentieth century the views of Kraepelin, Bleuler and De Sanctis held sway. During this period, schizophrenia in children and adults was seen as essentially the same disorder with a broadly similar clinical presentation. In the 1930s, however, coinciding with the emergence of child psychiatry as a separate discipline, an alternative 'unitary' view of childhood psychoses was proposed which conflated the present day concepts of autism, schizophrenia, schizotypal and borderline personality disorder (Potter 1933; Fish & Rivito 1979). This broad definition of 'childhood schizophrenia' dominated the second third of the twentieth century. From the mid-1930s until the 1970s the concepts of autism and childhood schizophrenia were synonymous, with autism and other developmental disorders viewed as early manifestations of adult schizophrenia. This perspective was endorsed by DSM-II and ICD-8 which grouped all childhood onset psychoses, including autism, under a separate category of 'childhood schizophrenia'.

The 'unitary' view of childhood psychoses was challenged in the 1970s, following the landmark studies of Kolvin (1971) and Rutter (1972) who demonstrated that autism and childhood onset schizophrenia could be distinguished in terms of age at onset, phenomenology and family history. This led to the differentiation of adult-type schizophrenia with childhood onset from autism. Hence, in the last third of the twentieth century, the pendulum swung back to the view that schizophrenia in children and adolescents should be defined using unmodified adult diagnostic criteria (developmental homotypy). This view was endorsed by DSM-III (American Psychiatric Association 1980) and ICD-9 (World Health Organization 1978), and has been maintained in DSM-IV (American Psychiatric Association 1994) and ICD-10 (World Health Organization 1992), with the removal of the separate category of 'childhood schizophrenia' and the application of the same diagnostic criteria at all ages.

Clinical features

Clinical phases of schizophrenia

Premorbid social and developmental impairments

Child and adolescent onset schizophrenia is characterized by poor premorbid functioning and early developmental delays (Alaghband-Rad et al. 1995; Hollis 1995). Similar developmental and social impairments in childhood have been reported in adult onset schizophrenia using population-based cohorts free from referral biases (Done et al. 1994; Jones et al. 1994; Jones & Done 1997; Malmberg et al. 1998). While age of onset comparisons are plagued by methodological difficulties, premorbid developmental impairments appear to be more common and severe in the child and adolescent onset forms of the disorder. Hollis (1995) in a retrospective case–control chart study of 61 cases of child and adolescent onset schizophrenia (aged 7–17) reported significant impairments in language development (23%),

motor development (31%) and social development (36%). Developmental impairments were most common in cases with onset of schizophrenia before age 13 years. Hence, a history of premorbid impairments appears to be most common in the very earliest onset cases. Nicholson et al. (2000) reported significant premorbid speech/language, motor and social impairments in 50% of childhood onset patients with onset of psychosis before the age of 12 years. In comparison, language and motor developmental delays are reported in only about 10% of individuals destined to develop schizophrenia in adult life (Jones et al. 1994). A consistent characteristic in the premorbid phenotype is impaired sociability. In child and adolescent onset schizophrenia, about one-third of cases have significant difficulties in social development affecting the ability to make and keep friends (Hollis 1995). Similar, but less frequent difficulties with premorbid sociability have been noted in representative population samples of adult schizophrenia (Malmberg et al. 1998). Interestingly, the Hollis study (1995) indicated that some cases would have met diagnostic criteria for Asperger syndrome, schizotypal personality disorder or atypical autism prior to the onset of psychosis. In the National Institute of Mental Health (NIMH) study of childhood onset schizophrenia, 34% of cases demonstrated transient symptoms of pervasive developmental disorder during the premorbid period (Alaghband-Rad et al. 1995).

Premorbid IQ appears to be lower in child and adolescent onset schizophrenia than in the adult form of the disorder. The mean premorbid IQ lies in the mid to low 80s, 10–15 IQ points lower than in most adult studies (R. Asarnow et al. 1994; Spencer & Campbell 1994; Alaghband-Rad et al. 1995). In the Maudsley study (Hollis 1999) one-third of child and adolescent onset cases had an IQ below 70 (mild learning disability range). One interpretation of these findings is that a subgroup of adolescent schizophrenic cases has abnormal premorbid development with the rest developing normally. In fact, careful analysis shows that there is no abnormal developmental subgroup – this is simply an artefact of using rather crude categorical measures of premorbid development. Continuous IQ measures show that the whole distribution of IQ is shifted down compared with both adolescent affective psychoses and adult schizophrenia.

These findings are consistent with the view that premorbid impairments are manifestations of a genetic/developmental liability to schizophrenia. It seems clear that the premorbid phenotype does not just represent non-specific psychiatric disturbance. Subtle problems of language, attention and social relationships are typical while, in contrast, conduct problems are rare. However, premorbid social and behavioural difficulties are not specific to schizophrenia. Premorbid deficits also occur in adolescent affective psychoses, at a lower rate than in schizophrenia but higher than in non-psychotic psychiatric controls (van Os et al. 1997; Sigurdsson et al. 1999).

Significance of premorbid impairments: a risk factor or precursor of psychosis?

Premorbid impairments could lie on a causal pathway for psychosis or, alternatively, they could be markers of an underlying neuropatholgical process, such as aberrant neural connectivity which may be the cause of both premorbid social impairment and psychosis. Causality is clearly implicit in ideas of primary prevention and the risk estimates provided by population-based epidemiological studies of prepsychotic impairments (Done *et al.* 1994; Jones *et al.* 1994; Malmberg *et al.* 1998). Frith (1994) speculated on the possible cognitive mechanisms that might link deficits in social cognition or 'theory of mind' in a causal pathway to both positive and negative psychotic symptoms. If these characteristics are causally related then modifying the 'primary' cognitive or social deficits should reduce the risk of psychosis. Alternatively, cognitive and social deficits, although often present, may not be necessary in the pathogenesis. The fact that individuals can develop schizophrenia without obvious premorbid impairments supports this view. In these circumstances, an intervention aimed at the neurobiological level (e.g. antipsychotic medication) may be necessary. Only a high-risk longitudinal intervention study can adequately address the issue of causality, and this would clearly require an intervention that had benefits for the majority of individuals with the premorbid phenotype who would not develop psychosis.

Prodromal phase

While some individuals show relatively stable patterns of subtle social and neurocognitive impairments, those who develop schizophrenia typically enter a prodromal phase characterized by a gradual but marked decline in social and academic functioning which precedes the onset of active psychotic symptoms. An insidious deterioration prior to onset of psychosis is typical of the presentation of schizophrenia in children and adolescents (Werry *et al.* 1994). In the Maudsley study of adolescent psychoses (Hollis 1999) a pattern of insidious onset was found more often in cases of schizophrenia than in affective psychoses. Non-specific behavioural changes including social withdrawal, declining school performance, uncharacteristic and odd behaviour began, on average, over 1 year before the onset of positive psychotic symptoms. In retrospect, it was often apparent that non-specific behavioural changes were frequently early negative symptoms, which in turn had their onset well before positive symptoms such as hallucinations and delusions.

Hence, early recognition of disorder can be very difficult, as premorbid cognitive and social impairments gradually shade into prodromal symptoms before the onset of active psychotic symptoms (Hafner & Nowotny 1995). Prodromal symptoms can include odd ideas, eccentric interests, changes in affect, unusual experiences and bizarre perceptual experiences. While these are also characteristic features of schizotypal personality disorder, in a schizophrenic prodrome there is usually progression to more severe dysfunction.

Psychotic symptoms

Child and adolescent onset schizophrenia is characterized by more prominent negative symptoms (e.g. flattened or inappropriate affect and bizarre manneristic behaviour), disorganized behaviour, hallucinations in different modalities and relatively fewer well-formed systematized or persecutory delusions than adult schizophrenia (Garralda 1984; Asarnow & Ben-Meir 1988; Green *et al.* 1992; Werry *et al.* 1994). Taking the DSM-IIIR subtypes of schizophrenia, Beratis *et al.* (1994) found that the disorganized and undifferentiated subtypes were predominantly of adolescent onset while the paranoid subtype was most frequently first diagnosed in adult life. While all subtypes can occur in adolescence, there is a relative predominance of the disorganized subtype which in earlier systems of classification would have been described as hebephrenia.

Symptom dimensions

While many studies in adult onset patients have shown evidence of at least three separate dimensions of psychopathology (negative symptoms, positive symptoms and disorganization; see Chapter 3), very few studies have examined symptom dimensions in child and adolescent onset patients. The existing evidence points to a similar pattern of symptom dimensions across the age range (Maziade *et al.* 1996; Hollis 1999). The main difference is the larger proportion of overall symptom variance explained by the negative symptom dimension in child and adolescent onset patients (Hollis 1999). Symptom dimensions in these younger patients show some expected associations with diagnostic categories: negative symptoms are specifically associated with schizophrenia and dimensions of mania and depression with affective psychoses. In contrast, the dimensions of disorganization and positive psychotic symptoms show less clear-cut associations with any specific diagnostic category. This lack of diagnostic specificity confirms that positive symptoms should not be regarded as pathognomonic of schizophrenia. In terms of prognosis, the dimensions of disorganization and negative symptoms predict a poor adult outcome while affective symptoms predict a more benign course and outcome, and positive symptoms (hallucinations–delusions and passivity–thought interference) have less prognostic value. Two other findings from the Maudsley study (Hollis 1999) are of particular interest. First, the negative symptom dimension was associated with premorbid developmental impairments, which suggests possible developmental and neurobiological continuity between these domains. Secondly, negative symptoms were associated with an increased familial risk of schizophrenia. Taken together these findings suggest that negative symptoms may be the most direct expression of a genetic and developmental risk for schizophrenia. These findings also lend support to the Bleulerian view that the fundamental features of schizophrenia are negative symptoms and cognitive deficits.

Diagnosis and differential diagnosis

Diagnostic validity

There is now compelling evidence that schizophrenia can be identified using unmodified adult criteria in children as young as 7 years of age (Green *et al.* 1984; Russell *et al.* 1989; Werry 1992). However, simply finding that some children fulfil adult diagnostic criteria for schizophrenia tells us nothing about whether the diagnosis is valid for this age group. In the absence of a biological diagnostic test, demonstrating diagnostic validity requires evidence that these early onset cases more closely resemble adult onset schizophrenia than other disorders in terms of clinical course, treatment response, family history and neurobiological correlates.

There are dangers of slavishly applying unmodified adult diagnostic criteria to children and adolescents. First, if a degree of age-dependent symptom variation exists in schizophrenia then applying unmodified adult criteria may result in some 'true' cases being missed (false-negative diagnoses). Secondly, some presentations of schizophrenia in early life could simply be phenocopies of adult schizophrenia (false-positive diagnoses) with a separate aetiology and clinical course. Hence, two issues need to be addressed. First, what is the validity of adult diagnostic criteria for schizophrenia when applied in childhood and adolescence? Secondly, are there partial syndromes or developmental variants of schizophrenia in childhood and adolescence that should be included as part of a broader schizophrenic spectrum?

Good evidence for the validity of the diagnosis of schizophrenia in childhood and adolescence comes from the recent Maudsley Child and Adolescent Psychosis Follow-up Study (Hollis 2000). The study was based on 110 cases of child and adolescent onset psychoses (mean age of onset 14.2 years, range 10–17 years) presenting as a consecutive series to the Maudsley Hospital from 1973 to 1991 (we refer to this subsequently as 'the Maudsley study'). The study used a 'catch-up' longitudinal design in which DSM-IIIR diagnoses were retrospectively applied to adolescent first-episode case notes and 85% (93/110) of the original cohort were then reassessed on average 11 years after their first admission. Of the 93 cases followed up, 51 had a baseline diagnosis of schizophrenia while 42 had a non-schizophrenic psychosis (bipolar, schizoaffective or atypical psychosis). The key findings with respect to diagnostic validity were as follows:

1 A DSM-IIIR diagnosis of schizophrenia in childhood and adolescence predicted a significantly poorer adult outcome compared with other non-schizophrenic psychosis.

2 The diagnosis of schizophrenia showed a high level of stability, with 80% having the same diagnosis recorded at adult follow-up.

These findings support the predictive validity of the DSM-IIIR diagnosis of schizophrenia in childhood and adolescence, and are likely to be equally applicable to DSM-IV criteria. The level of diagnostic stability for child and adolescent onset schizophrenia (using DSM-IIIR criteria) was very similar to that described in follow-up studies of adult first-episode schizophrenia.

However, there remains the issue of resolving the status of 'partial syndromes' that share some diagnostic features, or prodromal symptoms, of schizophrenia but do not meet full DSM-IV (American Psychiatric Association 1994) or ICD-10 (World Health Organization 1992) diagnostic criteria. For example, in the USA the term 'multidimensionally impaired' (MDI) (Jacobsen & Rapoport 1998; Kumra *et al.* 1998c) has been coined to describe children who have multiple early impairments in cognitive and social functioning and then develop transient psychotic symptoms in late childhood and early adolescence. A higher than expected rate of schizophrenia among first-degree relatives suggests that MDI children may lie on the schizophrenia spectrum, but longer follow-up studies are needed to tell if these cases progress to more typical schizophrenic presentations (Kumra *et al.* 1998c). At present, cases with partial or contiguous syndromes, such as the MDI syndrome or schizotypal personality disorder, require careful clinical follow-up to determine if they will develop schizophrenia. The question of how best to treat these presentations in clinical practice (e.g. whether they should be given low-dose antipsychotics) remains an important but unresolved question.

Developmental issues in assessment of children

The cognitive level of the child influences their ability to understand and express complex psychotic symptoms such as passivity phenomena, thought alienation and hallucinations. In younger children careful distinctions have to be made between developmental immaturity and psychopathology. For example, distinguishing true hallucinations from other subjective phenomena such as dreams may be difficult for young children.

Table 4.1 Differential diagnosis of schizophrenia in childhood and adolescence.

Psychoses	Affective psychoses (bipolar/major depressive disorder)
	Schizoaffective disorder
	Atypical psychosis
Developmental disorders	Autism spectrum disorders (Asperger syndrome)
	Developmental language disorder
	Schizotypal personality disorder
	'Multidimensionally impaired' disorder
Organic conditions	Drug-related psychosis (amphetamines, ecstasy, LSD, PCP)
	Complex partial seizures (temporal lobe epilepsy)
	Wilson's disease
	Metachromatic leucodystrophy

LSD, lysergic acid diethylamide; PCP, phencyclidine.

Developmental maturation can also affect the localization of hallucinations in space. Internal localization of hallucinations is more common in younger children and makes these experiences more difficult to differentiate subjectively from inner speech or thoughts (Garralda 1984). Formal thought disorder may also appear very similar to the pattern of illogical thinking and loose associations seen in children with immature language development. Negative symptoms can appear very similar to non-psychotic language and social impairments and can also be easily confused with anhedonia and depression.

Differential diagnosis

Psychotic symptoms in children and adolescents are diagnostically non-specific, occurring in a wide range of functional psychiatric, neurodevelopmental and organic brain disorders. The differential diagnosis of schizophrenia in childhood and adolescence is summarized in Table 4.1. A summary of physical investigations in children and adolescents with suspected schizophrenia is listed in Table 4.2.

Affective, schizoaffective and 'atypical' psychoses

The high rate of positive psychotic symptoms found in adolescent onset major depression and mania can lead to diagnostic confusion (Joyce 1984). Affective psychoses are most likely to be misdiagnosed as schizophrenia if a rigid Schneiderian concept of schizophrenia is applied with its emphasis on first-rank symptoms. Because significant affective symptoms also occur in about one-third of first-episode patients with schizophrenia, it may be impossible to make a definitive diagnosis on the basis of a single cross-sectional assessment. In DSM-IV the distinction between schizophrenia, schizoaffective disorder and affective psychoses is determined by the relative predominance and temporal overlap of psychotic symptoms (hallucinations and delusions) and affective symptoms (elevated or depressed mood). Given the difficulty in applying these rules with any precision, there is a need to identify other features to distinguish between schizophrenia and affective psychoses. Irrespective of the presence of affective symptoms, the most discriminating symptoms of schizophrenia are an insidious onset and the presence of negative symptoms (Hollis 1999). Similarly, complete remission from a first psychotic episode within 6 months of onset is the best predictor of a diagnosis of affective psychosis (Hollis 1999). Schizoaffective and atypical psychoses are unsatisfactory diagnostic categories with low predictive validity and little longitudinal stability (Hollis 2000).

Autistic spectrum and developmental language disorders

Kolvin (1971), in a landmark study, clearly distinguished the symptoms and correlates of core autism with onset before age 3 from adult-type schizophrenia beginning in late childhood and early adolescence. However, some children on the autistic spectrum (usually with atypical autism or Asperger syndrome) have social and cognitive impairments that overlap closely with the premorbid phenotype described in schizophrenia. Furthermore, children on the autistic spectrum may also develop psychotic symptoms in adolescence (Volkmar & Cohen 1991). Towbin *et al.* (1993) have labelled another group of children who seem to belong within the autistic spectrum as having 'multiplex developmental disorder'. An increased risk for psychosis has also been noted in developmental language disorders (Rutter & Mawhood 1991). While some children on the autistic spectrum can show a clear progression into classic schizophrenia, others show a more episodic pattern of psychotic symptoms without the progressive decline in social functioning and negative symptoms characteristic of child and adolescent onset schizophrenia.

Often it is only possible to distinguish between schizophrenia and disorders on the autistic spectrum by taking a careful developmental history that details the age of onset and pattern of autistic impairments in communication, social reciprocity and interests/behaviours. According to DSM-IV, schizophrenia

Table 4.2 Physical investigations in child and adolescent onset psychoses.

Investigation	Target disorder
Urine drug screen	Drug-related psychosis (amphetamines, ecstasy, cocaine, LSD and other psychoactive compounds)
EEG	Complex partial seizures/TLE
MRI brain scan	Ventricular enlargement, structural brain anomalies (e.g. cavum septum pellucidum)
	Enlarged caudate (typical antipsychotics)
	Demyelination (metachromatic leucodystrophy)
	Hypodense basal ganglia (Wilson's disease)
Serum copper and caeruloplasmin	Wilson's disease
Urinary copper	
Arylsulphatase A (white blood cell)	Metachromatic leucodystrophy
Karyotype/cytogenetics (FISH)	Sex chromosome aneuploidies, velocardiofacial syndrome (22q11 microdeletion)

FISH, fluorescence *in situ* hybridization; MRI, magnetic resonance imaging; TLE, temporal lobe apilepsy.

cannot be diagnosed in a child with autism/pervasive developmental disorder (PDD) unless hallucinations/delusions are present for at least 1 month. DSM-IV does not rank the active phase symptoms of thought disorder, disorganization or negative symptoms as sufficient to make a diagnosis of schizophrenia in the presence of autism. In contrast, ICD-10 does not include evidence of autism/PDD as an exclusion criteria for the diagnosis of schizophrenia.

'Multidimensionally impaired syndrome' and schizotypal personality disorder

'Multidimensionally impaired syndrome' (MDI) is a term coined to describe children who have brief transient psychotic symptoms, emotional lability, poor interpersonal skills, normal social skills and multiple deficits in information processing (Gordon et al. 1994). The diagnostic status of this group remains to be resolved. Short-term follow-up suggests that they do not develop full-blown schizophrenic psychosis. However, they have an increased risk of schizophrenia-spectrum disorders among first-degree relatives and the neurobiological findings (e.g. brain morphology) are similar to those in childhood onset schizophrenia (Kumra et al. 1998c). This group may possibly represent a genetically high-risk phenotype for schizophrenia rather than a prodromal state.

Children with schizotypal personality disorder (SPD) lie on a phenotypic continuum with schizophrenia and have similar cognitive and social impairments and are prone to magical thinking, mood disturbances and non-psychotic perceptual disturbances. Distinction from the prodromal phase of schizophrenia is particularly difficult when there is a history of social and academic decline without clear-cut or persisting psychotic symptoms. It has been reported that negative symptoms and attention in SPD improve with a low dose of risperidone (0.25–2.0 mg) (Rossi et al. 1997).

Epilepsy

Psychotic symptoms can occur in temporal and frontal lobe partial seizures. A careful history is usually sufficient to reveal an aura followed by clouding of consciousness and the sudden onset of brief ictal psychotic phenomena often accompanied by anxiety, fear, derealization or depersonalization. However, longer lasting psychoses associated with epilepsy can occur in clear consciousness during postictal or interictal periods (Sachdev 1998). In epileptic psychoses, hallucinations, disorganized behaviour and persecutory delusions predominate, while negative symptoms are rare. Children with complex partial seizures also have increased illogical thinking and use fewer linguistic-cohesive devices which can resemble formal thought disorder (Caplan et al. 1992). A positron emission tomography (PET) study has shown hypoperfusion in the frontal, temporal and basal ganglia in psychotic patients with epilepsy compared with non-psychotic epileptic patients (Gallhofer et al. 1985).

Epilepsy and schizophrenia may co-occur in the same individual, so that the diagnoses are not mutually exclusive. The onset of epilepsy almost always precedes psychosis unless seizures are secondary to antipsychotic medication. In a long-term follow-up of 100 children with temporal lobe epilepsy, 10% developed schizophrenia in adult life (Lindsay et al. 1979).

An EEG should be performed if a seizure disorder is considered in the differential diagnosis or arises as a side-effect of antipsychotic treatment. Ambulatory EEG monitoring and telemetry with event recording may be required if the diagnosis remains in doubt.

Neurodegenerative disorders

Rare neurodegenerative disorders occurring in late childhood and adolescence can mimic schizophrenia. The most important examples are Wilson's disease (hepatolenticular degeneration) and metachromatic leucodystrophy. These disorders usually involve significant extrapyramidal symptoms (e.g. tremor, dystonia and bradykinesia) or other motor abnormalities (e.g. unsteady gait) and a progressive loss of skills (dementia) that can aid the distinction from schizophrenia. Suspicion of a neurodegenerative disorder is one of the clearest indications for brain magnetic resonance imaging (MRI) in child and adolescent onset psychoses. Children and adolescents with schizophrenia show relative grey matter reduction with white matter sparing. In contrast, metachromatic leucodystrophy is characterized by frontal and occipital white matter destruction and demyelination. In Wilson's disease hypodense areas are seen in the basal ganglia, together with cortical atrophy and ventricular dilatation. The pathognomonic Kayser–Fleischer ring in Wilson's disease begins as a greenish-brown crescent-shaped deposit in the cornea above the pupil (this is most easily seen during slit lamp examination). In Wilson's disease there is increased urinary copper excretion, and reduced serum copper and serum caeruloplasmin levels. The biochemical marker for metachromatic leucodystrophy is reduced arylsulphatase-A (ASA) activity in white blood cells. This enzyme deficiency results in a deposition of excess sulphatides in many tissues including the central nervous system.

Drug psychoses

Recreational drug use is increasingly common among young people, so the co-occurrence of drug use and psychosis is to be expected. What is less certain is the nature of any causal connection. Psychotic symptoms can occur as a direct pharmacological effect of intoxication with stimulants (amphetamines, ecstasy and cocaine), hallucinogens (lysergic acid diethylamide 'LSD', psilocybin 'magic mushrooms' and mescaline) and cannabis (Poole & Brabbins 1996). The psychotic symptoms associated with drug intoxication are usually short-lived and resolve within a few days of abstinence from the drug. These drugs can have surprisingly long half-lives, with cannaboids still measurable up to 6 weeks after a single dose. Psychotic symptoms in the form of 'flashbacks' can also occur after cessation from chronic cannabis and LSD abuse. These phenomena are similar to alcoholic hallucinosis and typically involve transient vivid auditory hallucinations occurring in clear consciousness.

It is often assumed that there is a simple causal relationship between drug use and psychosis, with any evidence of drug use excluding the diagnosis of a functional psychosis. However, drug use can also be a consequence of psychosis with patients using drugs to 'treat' their symptoms in the early stages of a psychotic relapse. Overall, there is very little evidence to invoke a separate entity of 'drug-induced' psychosis in cases where psychotic symptoms arise during intoxication but then persist after the drug is withdrawn (Poole & Brabbins 1996). Patients whose so-called 'drug-induced' psychoses last for more than 6 months appear to have more clear-cut schizophrenic symptoms, a greater familial risk for psychosis and greater premorbid dysfunction (Tsuang et al. 1982). DSM-IV takes the sensible position that a functional psychosis should not be excluded unless there is compelling evidence that symptoms are entirely a result of drug use.

Other investigations

Whether any physical investigations should be viewed as 'routine' is debatable. However, it is usual to obtain a full blood count and biochemistry including liver and thyroid function and a drug screen (urine or hair analysis). The high yield of cytogenetic abnormalities reported in childhood onset schizophrenia (Kumra et al. 1998d; Nicholson et al. 1999) suggests the value of cytogenetic testing including karyotyping for sex chromosome aneuploidies and fluorescent in situ hybridization (FISH) for chromosome 22q11 deletions (velocardiofacial syndrome). The evidence of progressive structural brain changes (Rapoport et al. 1999) indicates the value of obtaining a baseline and annual follow-up brain MRI scans, although this is not a diagnostic test.

Epidemiology

Incidence and prevalence

Good population-based incidence figures for child and adolescent onset schizophrenia are notably lacking. What data do exist describe broader categories of psychosis, with diagnoses made without the benefit of standardized assessments. Gillberg et al. (1986) calculated age-specific prevalence for all psychoses (including schizophrenia, schizophreniform, affective psychosis, atypical psychosis and drug psychoses) in the age range 13–18 years using case-register data from Goteborg, Sweden. Of the cases, 41% had a diagnosis of schizophrenia. At age 13 years, the prevalence for all psychoses was 0.9/10 000, showing a steady increase during adolescence and reaching a prevalence of 17.6/10 000 at age 18 years.

Sex ratio

Males are over-represented in many clinical studies of childhood onset schizophrenia (Russell et al. 1989; Green et al. 1992; Russell 1994; Spencer & Campbell 1994). However, other studies of predominantly adolescent onset schizophrenia have described an equal sex ratio (Gordon et al. 1994; Werry et al. 1994; Hollis 2000). The interpretation of these studies is complicated by the possibility of referral biases to clinical centres. In an epidemiological study of first admissions for schizophrenia and paranoia in children and adolescents there was an equal sex ratio for patients under the age of 15 (Galdos et al. 1993; Lewine 1994). The finding of an equal sex distribution with adolescent onset is intriguing as it differs from the consistent male predominance (ratio 2:1) reported in incident samples of early adult onset schizophrenia (Castle & Murray 1991). Clearly, future studies require population-based incident samples free from potential referral biases.

Aetiology and risk factors

Pregnancy and birth complications

Pregnancy and birth complications (PBCs) have been implicated as a risk factor in schizophrenia (see Chapter 13). In a meta-analysis of 20 case–control studies, subjects who developed schizophrenia were more than twice as likely to have been exposed to PBCs as controls (Geddes & Lawrie 1995). However, the findings from two other large case–control studies suggest that the link between schizophrenia and PBCs may be much weaker than previously assumed (Kendall et al. 2000). In one case–control study of childhood onset schizophrenia, Matsumoto et al. (1999) reported an odds ratio of 3.5 for PBCs, suggesting a greater risk in very early onset cases. However, in the NIMH study of childhood onset schizophrenia, PBCs were no more common in cases than in sibling controls (Nicholson et al. 1999). Even if there is a significant association, it remains unclear whether there is any causal connection between PBCs and schizophrenia. There is a strong argument that PBCs are consequences rather than causes of abnormal neurodevelopment (Goodman 1988). This view is supported by the finding that schizophrenics have smaller head size at birth than controls (McGrath & Murray 1995), which is likely to be a consequence of either defects in genetic control of neurodevelopment or earlier environmental factors, such as viral exposure.

Puberty

The close temporal association between the onset of puberty and a marked increase in the incidence of schizophrenia suggests that biological (or social) events around puberty may be related to the expression of psychotic symptoms. Galdos et al. (1993) reported an association between the timing of menarche and onset of psychosis in girls. However, this finding has not been supported by subsequent studies. Frazier *et al.* (1997) found no relationship between the onset of psychosis and indices of puberty in cases recruited to the NIMH study of childhood onset schizophrenia. For both boys and girls the timing of pubertal events were similar for cases and controls.

Psychosocial risks

One possible explanation for an atypically early onset of schizophrenia could be differential exposure to psychosocial adversity, such as higher levels of parental hostility and criticism ('high EE'). High levels of expressed emotion (EE) among relatives of adult schizophrenics has been shown to be a predictor of psychotic relapse and poor outcome (Leff & Vaughn 1985). Although the role of high EE in precipitating the onset of schizophrenia has not been established, it is theoretically plausible that high EE might act to 'bring forward' the onset of the disorder in a vulnerable individual. Goldstein (1987) reported that parental EE measures of criticism and overinvolvement taken during adolescence were associated with an increased risk of schizophrenia spectrum disorders in young adulthood. However, a causal link is not proven, and the association may reflect either an expression of some common underlying trait or a parental response to premorbid disturbance in the preschizophrenic adolescent. Similarly, high EE in the parents of schizophrenic patients may be a reaction to the illness rather than a cause. There is no evidence that the parents of childhood onset patients show higher levels of EE than do parents of adult onset patients – in fact the reverse may be true. J.R. Asarnow *et al.* (1994) used the Five Minute Speech Sample to measure parental EE and found that childhood onset schizophrenics were no more likely to have 'high EE' parents than normal controls. Overall, there seems little evidence to suggest that the onset of schizophrenia in childhood can be explained by exposure to higher levels of parental criticism and hostility than that experienced by adult onset patients. Indeed, it appears that, on average, the parents of childhood onset schizophrenics generally express *lower* levels of criticism and hostility than parents of adult onset patients because of a greater tendency to attribute their childrens' behaviour to an illness which is beyond their control (Hooley 1987).

Neurobiology of schizophrenia

Neurodevelopmental models of schizophrenia

Over the last decade the concept of schizophrenia as a neurodevelopmental disorder has taken a strong hold, although 'neurodevelopmental' is often used with a wide range of meanings. It is possible to distinguish 'early' and 'late' neurodevelopmental models, with a third 'risk' model incorporating ideas from developmental psychopathology (Hollis & Taylor 1997).

The 'early' neurodevelopmental model emerged from the ideas of Fish (1957) who proposed that the neuropathology in schizophrenia was of perinatal origin. The 'early' neurodevelopmental model views the primary cause of schizophrenia as a static 'lesion' occurring during fetal brain development (Murray & Lewis 1987; Weinberger 1987). The putative 'lesion' could be of either neurogenetic or environmental origin (e.g. virus infection or fetal hypoxia). Two main lines of evidence support the 'early' neurodevelopmental model. First, there is an absence of gliosis in the postmortem brains of schizophrenic patients, which suggests a neurodevelopmental rather than a neurodegenerative pathology (see Chapter 17). Secondly, a more indirect line of evidence includes the association of schizophrenia with premorbid social and cognitive impairments (Foerster *et al.* 1991; Done *et al.* 1994; Jones *et al.* 1994), pregnancy and birth complications (Lewis & Murray 1987; McNeil 1995) and minor physical anomalies (Gualtieri *et al.* 1982; Guy *et al.* 1983). According to this 'early' model, during childhood the 'lesion' is relatively silent giving rise only to subtle behavioural symptoms (premorbid social and cognitive impairments). However, in adolescence, or early adult life, the 'lesion' interacts with the process of *normal* brain maturation (e.g. myelination of corticolimbic circuits and/or synaptic pruning and remodelling) to manifest itself in the form of psychotic symptoms.

There are several weaknesses in the 'early' neurodevelopmental model. First, it fails to provide a satisfactory account of the long latency between the putative perinatal damage/lesion and the typical onset of symptoms in late adolescence or early adult life. Secondly, an early neurodevelopmental insult on its own cannot account for the finding of increased extracerebral (sulcal) cerebrospinal fluid (CSF) space in schizophrenia. Diffuse loss of brain tissue limited to the pre- or perinatal periods would result in enlargement of the lateral ventricles but not increased extracerebral CSF space (Woods 1998).

The 'late' neurodevelopmental model, first proposed by Feinberg (1983, 1997), argues that the key neuropathological events in schizophrenia occur as a result of *abnormal* brain development during adolescence. The current formulation of the 'late' neurodevelopmental model proposes that *excessive* synaptic and/or dentritic elimination occurs during adolescence producing aberrant neural connectivity and psychotic symptoms (Woods 1998; McGlashen & Hoffman 2000). This 'late' model characterizes schizophrenia as a *progressive* late onset neurodevelopmental disorder in contrast to the 'early' model that proposes a *static* lesion during the perinatal period. The 'late' model predicts that progressive structural brain changes and cognitive decline will be seen in adolescence around the onset of psychosis. The excessive synaptic pruning during adolescence proposed in the 'late' model is simply an amplification of the normal process of neuronal remodelling with progressive pruning and elimination of synapses that begins in early childhood and extends through late adolescence (Huttenlocher 1979; Purves & Lichtmen 1980). These major regressive changes in adolescence with remodelling of neural connections are likely to be under genetic control with synaptic elimination in schizophrenia representing an extreme of normal variation (Feinberg 1983). In the 'late' model, premorbid abnormalities in early childhood are viewed as non-specific risk factors rather than early manifestations of an underlying schizophrenic neuropathology.

Both the 'early' and 'late' models suppose that there is a direct and specific expression of the eventual brain pathology as schizophrenic disorder. A third viewpoint, the 'risk' model, proposes that early and/or late brain pathology acts as a risk factor rather than a sufficient cause so that its effects can only be understood in the light of an individual's exposure to other risk and protective factors (Hollis & Taylor 1997). This latter formulation provides a probabilistic model of the onset of schizophrenia in which aberrant brain development is expressed as neurocognitive impairments that interact with the environment to produce psychotic symptoms. The following sections examine how well current neurobiological research evidence supports these competing neurodevelopmental models of schizophrenia (for further discussion of these theories see Chapters 13 and 15).

Neuropathology

In the postmortem brains of schizophrenic patients there is an absence of gliosis which is the necessary hallmark of neurodegeneration (Roberts *et al.* 1986). The prominent neuropathology in schizophrenia is not the classic form involving neuronal cell death, but instead a loss or reduction in dendritic spines and synapses which are the elements of neural connectivity (Garey *et al.* 1998; Glantz & Lewis 2000). As a result, the brain in schizophrenia is characterized by increased neuronal density, decreased intraneuronal space and reduced overall brain volume. Furthermore, the decrease in dentritic spine density appears to be both region and disease specific. A reduction in dendritic spine density has been reported on pyramidal cells in layer III of the temporal cortex (Garey *et al.* 1998) and the dorsolateral prefrontal cortex (Glantz & Lewis 2000) but not on pyramidal cells in the visual cortex of schizophrenic patients (Glantz & Lewis 2000). These findings are compatible with the hypothesis of reduced cortical and/or thalamic excitatory glutaminergic inputs to the dorsolateral prefrontal cortex in schizophrenia (see Chapter 17 for other perspectives on neuropathology).

Structural brain abnormalities

Neuroimaging and postmortem studies have shown that the brain as a whole and the frontal and temporal cortices in particular are smaller than in normal subjects (Andreasen *et al.* 1990; Nopoulos *et al.* 1995). Brain volume reductions in schizophrenia are specific to grey matter (Gur *et al.* 2000a) which supports neuropathological findings of increased neuronal density and reduced intraneuronal neurophil rather than neuronal loss (Selemon *et al.* 1995).

Across a range of neuroimaging studies, the volume of the hippocampus and amygdala is reduced bilaterally by 4.5–10% (Nelson *et al.* 1998; Gur *et al.* 2000a). Prefrontal grey matter volume is reduced by about 10% (Gur *et al.* 2000b). Enlargement of the third and lateral ventricles is a consistent finding,

with ventricular volume increased by about 40% bilaterally (Lawrie & Abukmeil 1998). Ventricular enlargement is associated with neuropsychological impairment and negative symptoms (Vita *et al.* 1991). Studies of the basal ganglia have produced more inconsistent results, possibly as a function of the increase in basal ganglia volume associated with the use of traditional antipsychotics. Interestingly, when patients are switched to the atypical antipsychotic clozapine there is a reduction of basal ganglia volume (Chakos *et al.* 1995).

The brain changes reported in child and adolescent onset schizophrenia appear to be very similar to those described in adult onset schizophrenia, supporting the idea of an underlying neurobiological continuity. In the NIMH study of childhood onset schizophrenia (onset less than 12 years of age), subjects had smaller brains than normal subjects, with larger lateral ventricles and reduced prefrontal lobe volume (Jacobsen & Rapoport 1998). Similar to findings from adult studies, reduced total cerebral volume is associated with negative symptoms (Alaghband-Rad *et al.* 1997). The midsagittal thalamic area is decreased while the midsagittal area of the corpus callosum is increased (Giedd *et al.* 1996), suggesting that the reduction in total cerebral volume in childhood onset schizophrenia is brought about by a relative reduction in grey matter with sparing of white matter. Childhood onset patients have a higher rate of developmental brain abnormalities than controls, including an increased frequency of an enlarged cavum septum pelucidum (Nopoulos *et al.* 1998). Abnormalities of the cerebellum have also been found including reduced volume of the vermis, midsagittal area and inferior posterior lobe (Jacobsen *et al.* 1997a).

Progressive brain changes

Two different types of progressive brain change have been described in schizophrenia. First, treatment with traditional antipsychotics appears to cause progressive enlargement of the basal ganglia, with these structures returning to their original size when patients are transferred to the atypical antipsychotic clozapine (Frazier *et al.* 1996). Secondly, there is evidence of progressive volume reductions in the temporal and frontal lobes during the first 2–3 years after the onset of schizophrenia (Gur *et al.* 1998). In the NIMH study of childhood onset schizophrenia, longitudinal repeated MRI scans through adolescence have revealed a progressive increase in ventricular volume and progressive decrease in cortical volume with frontal (11% decrease) and temporal lobes (7% decrease) disproportionately affected (Rapoport *et al.* 1997, 1999). Both patients and controls showed progressive reductions in frontal and parietal lobe volumes, with schizophrenic subjects showing a relatively greater loss of temporal lobe volume than controls (Jacobsen *et al.* 1998). The reduction seen in temporal lobe structures may occur rather later in the illness course than the reduction in frontal lobe and midsagittal thalamic structures. Progressive changes appear to be time limited to adolescence with the rate of volume reduction in frontal and temporal structures declining as subjects reach adult life.

Because progressive brain changes have been described *after* the onset of psychosis, it is possible that they are a consequence of neurotoxic effects of psychosis or, possibly, antipsychotic medication. Evidence that progressive brain changes precede the onset of psychosis is very limited. Pantelis *et al.* (2000) have provided a preliminary report of brain MRI findings in high-risk subjects scanned before and after the transition into psychosis. For those subjects who developed psychosis there were longitudinal volume reductions in the medial temporal region (hippocampus, entorhinal cortex, inferior frontal and fusiform gyrus). There were no significant longitudinal changes in cases that remained non-psychotic. These are potentially important findings which, if replicated, would provide strong support for the idea that excessive developmental reductions in temporal lobe volume have a key role in the onset of psychosis.

Functional brain imaging

The emergence of functional brain imaging technology has provided a unique opportunity to link symptoms and cognitive deficits in schizophrenia to underlying brain activity. Liddle *et al.* (1992) studied the relationship between symptom dimensions (negative, positive and disorganization) in adult schizophrenic subjects and regional cerebral blood flow (rCBF) using PET. Negative symptoms (e.g. affective blunting, avolition and alogia) were associated with reduced rCBF in the dorsolateral prefrontal cortex (DLPFC). Disorganization (e.g. formal thought disorder and bizarre behaviour) was associated with reduced rCBF in the right ventrolateral prefrontal cortex and increased rCBF in the anterior cingulate. Positive symptoms (e.g. hallucinations and delusions) were associated with increased rCBF in the left medial temporal lobe, and reduced rCBF in the posterior cingulate and left lateral temporal lobe. The most consistent association in the literature, across a variety of imaging methods, has been between negative symptoms and reduced frontal activity.

However, a simple description of 'hypofrontality' in schizophrenia does not capture the complex pattern of changes involving interconnected frontal areas and changes across time. In a PET study in childhood onset schizophrenia using the Continuous Performance Test (CPT), Jacobsen *et al.* (1997b) reported reduced activation compared with healthy controls in the mid and superior frontal gyrus, and increased activation in the inferior frontal, supramarginal gyrus and insula. The finding of hypofrontality in schizophrenia is a dynamic state-related phenomenon with evidence of remission of hypofrontality in asymptomatic patients (Spence *et al.* 1998). Localizationist models based on focal cerebral dysfunction in schizophrenia have tended to give way to more dynamic models of cerebral 'disconnectivity' based on dysfunctional neural networks or systems. Models of cerebral connectivity view normal higher brain function as depending on the integrated activity of widely distributed neurocognitive networks, rather than the activity of discrete brain areas in isolation (Bullmore *et al.* 1997). In normal individuals, the functional anatomy of a verbal fluency task (generation of words beginning with a given letter) can be examined using PET and has consistently shown activation of the left DLPFC and reciprocal deactivation of the superior temporal gyrus (STG). A number of investigators have reported a failure of normal STG deactivation (disconnectivity) in schizophrenic patients during a verbal fluency task (Friston *et al.* 1995; Dolan *et al.* 1996). However, left DLPFC–STG disconnectivity appears to be a state-related marker of psychosis as it is not found in asymptomatic schizophrenic patients (Dye *et al.* 1999; Spence *et al.* 2000) and may possibly be associated with active auditory hallucinations (Spence *et al.* 2000). In contrast, schizophrenic patients in remission do show reduced connectivity between the left DLPFC and anterior cingulate cortex relative to normal controls (Spence *et al.* 2000).

In summary, models of cerebral disconnectivity fit well with both neuropathological and functional neuroimaging data. What is becoming clear is that functional disconnectivity may both identify state-related changes associated with current symptomatology as well as more stable trait-related markers of neurocognitive vulnerability to psychosis.

Magnetic resonance spectroscopy: abnormal neuronal metabolism

Magnetic resonance spectroscopy (MRS) is an imaging technique that can be used to extract *in vivo* information on dynamic biochemical processes at a neuronal level. Proton (^{1}H) MRS focuses on changes in the neuronal marker *N*-acetylaspartate (NAA). Studies in adult schizophrenic patients have shown reductions in NAA in the hippocampal area and DLPFC. Similar reductions in NAA ratios specific to the hippocampus and DLPFC (Bertolino *et al.* 1998) and frontal grey matter (Thomas *et al.* 1998) have been reported in childhood onset schizophrenia, suggesting neuronal damage or malfunction in these regions.

Pettegrew *et al.* (1991) used phosphorus-31 (^{31}P) MRS in first-episode non-medicated schizophrenics and found reduced phosphomonoester (PME) resonance and increased phosphodiester (PDE) resonance in the prefrontal cortex. This result is compatible with reduced synthesis and increased breakdown of connective processes in the prefrontal cortex. A similar finding of reduced PME and increased PDE resonance has been reported in autistic adults, although they showed increased prefrontal metabolic activity, which was not seen in schizophrenic subjects (Pettegrew *et al.* 1991). It is possible that excessive synaptic elimination is not specific to schizophrenia, but its timing, location and extent may have crucial implications for the development of executive functions, and the risk of psychosis, in late childhood and adolescence.

Implications for neurodevelopmental models of schizophrenia

Taken together, the neuropathological and brain imaging findings provide considerable support for the idea of progressive neurodevelopmental changes in schizophrenia including excessive synaptic elimination resulting in aberrant neural connectivity. The 'early' neurodevelopmental model involving a static pre- or perinatal brain insult fails to account for the progressive nature of brain volume reductions in adolescence, and the fact that reduced brain volume is not accompanied by reduced intracranial volume. While early random events in fetal neurodevelopment (e.g. hypoxia, viruses) may affect baseline synaptic density, genetically determined excessive synaptic elimination as proposed by the 'late' neurodevelopmental model may be the neurobiological process underlying disorders in the schizophrenia spectrum (McGlashen & Hoffman 2000). What is unclear is whether excessive synaptic elimination in the prefrontal cortex (and possibly other brain regions) is a sufficient cause for psychosis to occur or whether it simply provides a vulnerable neurocognitive substrate that must interact with environmental stressors (e.g. cognitive or social demands) to produce psychotic symptoms.

Genetics

Genetic risk and early onset schizophrenia

If there is a continuum of transmitted liability for schizophrenia then, as with other disorders of presumed multifactorial origin, early onset cases of schizophrenia should be associated with a greater genetic loading (Childs & Scriver 1986). Pulver et al. (1990) found an increased morbid risk of schizophrenia in relatives of male probands under the age of 17. Meanwhile, Sham et al. (1994) found an increased morbid risk in females under age 21 compared with males or later onset females. While both of these studies suggest an inverse relationship between age at onset and transmitted liability, albeit with different gender-specific effects and age cut-offs, it would be dangerous to simply extrapolate these age trends to a younger childhood onset population. Unfortunately, there is a dearth of genetic studies of childhood onset schizophrenia that have used adequate methodology. In the only major twin study of childhood onset schizophrenia, Kallman and Roth (1956) reported an uncorrected MZ concordance rate of 88.2% and a DZ concordance rate of 22.9%. Adult onset schizophrenia clustered in the families of childhood onset probands, providing support for a similar genetic aetiology. Data from family studies suggest that child and adolescent onset schizophrenia carries a greater familial risk of psychosis than adult onset schizophrenia. In the Maudsley study, Hollis (1999) found that 20% of child and adolescent onset schizophrenia cases had at least one first-degree relative with schizophrenia, and 50% had a first-degree relative with psychosis. These rates are somewhat higher than those reported by Sham et al. (1994) for adult schizophrenic probands (13% of adult probands had a first-degree relative with schizophrenia and 23% had a first-degree relative with any psychosis). Data from the Maudsley study (Hollis 1999) also show that the presence of negative symptoms in the proband predicts a family history of schizophrenia. This provides further support for the idea that negative symptoms may represent the genetically transmitted phenotype in schizophrenia (Tsuang 1993).

Cytogenetic abnormalities

The association between schizophrenia and chromosomal deletions offers another possible clue to the location of candidate genes. The velocardiofacial syndrome (VCFS) microdeletion on chromosome 22q11 is associated with learning difficulties, short stature, palate abnormalities, cardiac anomalies and parkinsonism. VCFS has also been associated with schizophrenia, occurring at a rate of 2% compared with 0.02% in the normal population (Karayiorgou et al. 1995). VCFS appears to be associated with an earlier age of onset of schizophrenia in adults (Bassett et al. 1999). In the NIMH study of childhood onset schizophrenia, five cases out of 47 (10.6%) had previously undetected cytogenetic abnormalities (Nicholson et al. 1999). These included 3/47 (6.3%) with VCFS, one with Turner syndrome (deletion of a long arm of one X chromosome) and one with a balanced translocation of chromosomes 1 and 7. One study has reported an association, found only in males, between childhood onset schizophrenia and an excess of CAG/CTG trinucleotide expansions (Burgess et al. 1998). These findings point to possibly greater genetic heterogeneity in child and adolescent onset forms of schizophrenia.

Neuropsychology

Pattern of cognitive deficits

There is growing awareness that cognitive deficits in schizophrenia represent a core feature of the disorder and cannot simply be dismissed as secondary consequences of psychotic symptoms (Breier 1999). The degree of cognitive impairment is greater in child and adolescent onset than in adult onset patients. A consistent finding in child and adolescent onset patients is a mean IQ of between 80 and 85 (1 SD below the population mean), with about one-third of cases having an IQ below 70 (Jacobsen & Rapoport 1998; Hollis 1999). This represents a mean IQ score about 10 points lower than the mean IQ in adult schizophrenia. These findings raise several important questions. First, are the cognitive deficits specific or generalized: are some aspects of cognitive functioning affected more than others? Secondly, which deficits precede the onset of psychosis and could be causal, and which are consequences of psychosis? Thirdly, is the pattern of deficits specific to schizophrenia or shared with other developmental and psychotic disorders? Fourthly, are cognitive impairments progressive or static after the onset of psychosis?

Recent research (R. Asarnow et al. 1994, 1995) suggests that children with schizophrenia have specific difficulties with cognitive tasks that make demands on short-term working memory and selective and sustained attention and speed of processing.

These deficits are similar to the deficits reported in adult schizophrenia (Nuechterlain & Dawson 1984; Saykin et al. 1994). Deficits of attention, short-term and recent long-term memory have also been reported in adolescents with schizophrenia (Friedman et al. 1996). In contrast, well-established 'overlearned' rote language and simple perceptual skills are unimpaired in child and adolescent onset schizophrenia. Asarnow et al. (1991, 1995) have shown that children with schizophrenia have impairments on the span of apprehension task (a target stimulus has to be identified from an array of other figures when displayed for 50 ms). Performance on the task deteriorates markedly when increasing demands are made on information processing capacity (e.g. increasing the number of letters in the display from three to 10). Furthermore, event-related potentials on the span of apprehension task in both children and adults with schizophrenia, compared with age-matched controls, show less negative endogenous activity measured between 100 and 300 ms after the stimulus. Similar findings of reduced event-related potentials have been found during the CPT in both childhood and adult onset schizophrenia (Strandburg et al. 1999). These findings indicate a deficit in the allocation of attentional resources to a stimulus (Strandburg et al. 1994; Asarnow et al. 1995). As with adults, children and adolescents with schizophrenia show high basal autonomic activity and less autonomic responsivity than controls (Gordon et al. 1994), with attenuated increases in skin conductance following the presentation of neutral sounds (Zahn et al. 1997). Childhood onset patients, like adults, show increased reaction times with a loss of ipsimodal advantage compared with healthy controls (Zahn et al. 1998). Abnormalities in smooth pursuit eye movements (SPEM) have also been found in adolescent schizophrenics (mean age 14.5), which suggests continuity with the finding of abnormal SPEM in adult schizophrenics (Iacono & Koenig 1983). Children with schizophrenia also show similar impairments to adult patients on tests of frontal lobe executive function such as the Wisconsin Card Sorting Test (WCST; R. Asarnow et al. 1994).

In summary, while basic sensorimotor skills, associative memory and simple language abilities tend to be preserved in children with schizophrenia, deficits are most marked on tasks which require focused and sustained attention, flexible switching of cognitive set, high information processing speed and suppression of prepotent responses (Asarnow et al. 1995). Similar deficits affecting attention, memory and motor skills have been found in children genetically at 'high risk' for schizophrenia (Erlenmeyer-Kimling et al. 2000) and non-psychotic relatives of schizophrenic probands (Park et al. 1995). This adds further weight to the argument that cognitive deficits cannot be simply dismissed as non-specific consequences of schizophrenic symptoms, but rather are likely to be indicators of underlying genetic and neurobiological risk.

Executive functions and onset of schizophrenia

A diverse array of cognitive processes has been integrated under the cognitive domain of 'executive functions' which are presumed to be mediated by the prefrontal cortical system. Executive function skills are necessary to generate and execute goal-directed behaviour, especially in novel situations. Goal-orientated actions require that information in the form of plans and expectations are held 'on-line' in working memory and flexibly changed in response to feedback. Much of social behaviour and social development would appear to depend on these capacities as they involve integration of multiple sources of information, appreciation of others' mental states, inhibition of inappropriate prepotent responses and rapid shifting of attention.

Any cognitive theory of schizophrenia needs to explain the timing of onset which usually occurs during adolescence or early adulthood. Deficits in executive function and social cognition could be the developmental abnormality that predisposes to schizophrenia as executive function deficits impinge on social skills that usually emerge in early adolescence. This period is associated with a rapid growth in abstract analytical skills, together with the development of the sophisticated social and communication abilities that underlie successful social relationships. It is during this period of development (approximately age 8–15 years) that preschizophrenic social impairments become most apparent (Done et al. 1994) and there is also a relative decline in cognitive abilities in preschizophrenic subjects (Jones et al. 1994).

According to this 'risk' model of executive function deficit, the onset of psychosis depends on the interaction between social and cognitive capacities and the demands of the environment. During adolescence, increasing academic and social demands may act as stressors on a 'high-risk' subject, pushing them over the threshold for psychosis. The greater the premorbid impairment, the earlier the age that a critical liability threshold will be passed and symptoms emerge. This model predicts that similar executive function deficits are found in non-psychotic genetically 'high-risk' relatives. However, executive function deficits are probably not a primary cause of schizophrenia given that they also occur in other neurodevelopmental disorders including autism (Ozonoff et al. 1991; Hughes & Russell 1993) and attention deficit hyperactivity disorder (ADHD) (Welsh et al. 1991; Pennington et al. 1993; Karatekin & Asarnow 1998).

Course of cognitive deficits

Kraepelin's term 'dementia praecox' implied a progressive cognitive decline as part of the disease process. Jones et al. (1994) described how academic performance becomes progressively more deviant during adolescence in those individuals destined to develop schizophrenia in adult life. There is also some tentative evidence for a decline in IQ following the onset of psychosis in childhood onset schizophrenia. In the NIMH study (Alaghband-Rad et al. 1995), the mean postpsychotic IQ was 83.7 (SD 17.3) compared with a mean prepsychotic IQ of 87.7 (SD 25.4). Although a decline in IQ during the early phase of psychosis has been reported in adults with schizophrenia (Bilder *et al.* 1992), in the NIHM study the decline was in both raw and scaled IQ scores and continued for up to 24–48 months after onset (Jacobsen & Rapoport 1998). There was no evidence for a decline in postpsychotic IQ raw scores repeated after 2 years, although scaled (age-adjusted) IQ scores did still decline (Bedwell *et al.* 1999). Russell *et al.* (1997) found a small non-significant IQ decline, of only 2–3 points, in a 20-year longitudinal follow-up study of IQ in schizophrenia (about one-third of these cases had first onset of psychosis in adolescence).

In summary, when raw scores, rather than scaled scores, are analysed, there is little evidence for an absolute loss in cognitive ability in the early postpsychotic phase of schizophrenia. If a true decline does occur it is during, or before, the transition to psychosis. The small drop in IQ after the onset of psychosis could possibly be caused by the effect of psychotic symptoms on performance. Overall, the evidence points more to a premature arrest, or slowing, of normal cognitive development in child and adolescent onset schizophrenia rather than to a dementia.

Course and outcome

Short-term course

Child and adolescent onset schizophrenia characteristically runs a chronic course, with only a small minority of cases making a full symptomatic recovery from the first psychotic episode. In the Maudsley study of child and adolescent onset psychoses (Hollis 2000), only 12% of schizophrenic cases were in full remission at discharge, compared with 50% of cases with affective psychoses. The short-term outcome for schizophrenia presenting in early life appears to be worse than that of first-episode adult patients (Robinson *et al.* 1999). If full recovery does occur then it is most likely within the first 3 months of onset of psychosis. In the Maudsley study, those adolescent onset patients who were still psychotic after 6 months had only a 15% chance of achieving full remission, while over half of all patients who made a full recovery had active psychotic symptoms for less than 3 months (Hollis 1999). The clinical implication is that the early course over the first 6 months is the best predictor of remission and that longer observation over 6 months adds relatively little new information.

Long-term outcome

A number of long-term follow-up studies of child and adolescent onset schizophrenia all describe a typically chronic unremitting long-term course with severely impaired functioning in adult life (Eggers 1978; Werry *et al.* 1991; Schmidt *et al.* 1995; Eggers & Bunk 1997; Hollis 2000). Several common themes emerge from these studies. First, the generally poor outcome of early onset schizophrenia conceals considerable heterogeneity. About one-fifth of patients in most studies have a good outcome with only mild impairment, while at the other extreme about one-third of patients are severely impaired requiring intensive social and psychiatric support. Hence, for an individual patient diagnosis alone is a relatively crude prognostic indicator. Secondly, after the first few years of illness there is little evidence of further progressive decline. This suggests that in the first 10–15 years of illness, at least, the course is relatively stable, although further progression may occur later in life. Thirdly, child and adolescent onset schizophrenia has a worse outcome than either adolescent onset affective psychoses or adult onset schizophrenia. This suggests that outcome and clinical severity are related to both diagnosis and the age at onset. Fourthly, social functioning, in particular the ability to form friendships and love relationships, appears to be very impaired in early onset schizophrenia. Taken together, these findings confirm that schizophrenia presenting in childhood and adolescence lies at the extreme end of a continuum of phenotypic severity.

Mortality

The risk of premature death is increased in child and adolescent onset psychoses. In the Maudsley study (Hollis 1999), there were nine deaths out of the 106 cases followed up (8.5%). The standardized mortality ratio (SMR) was 1250 (95% CI 170–5500), which represents a 12-fold increase in the risk of death compared with an age- and sex-matched general UK population over the same period. Of the nine deaths in the cohort, seven were male and seven had a diagnosis of schizophrenia. Three subjects suffered violent deaths, two died from self-poisoning, and three had unexpected deaths resulting from previously undetected physical causes (cardiomyopathy and status epilepticus) which were possibly associated with high-dose antipsychotic medication.

The death rate in child and adolescent onset schizophrenia and other psychoses appears to be significantly higher than in the adult form of the disorder. In adults, the 'all cause' SMR for schizophrenia has been reported as 157 (95% CI 153–160) (Harris & Barraclough 1997). In a Norwegian study of adolescent psychiatric inpatients, Kjelsberg (2000) reported an SMR for psychosis of 390 in males and 1130 in females.

Prognosis

The predictors of poor outcome in adolescent onset affective psychoses include premorbid social and cognitive impairments (Werry & McClellan 1992; Hollis 1999), a prolonged first psychotic episode (Schmidt *et al.* 1995), extended duration of untreated psychosis (Hollis 1999) and the presence of negative symptoms (Hollis 1999). Premorbid functioning and negative symptoms at onset provide better prediction of long-term outcome than categorical diagnosis (Hollis 1999). This finding suggests that premorbid social and cognitive impairments and negative symptoms lie at the core of a valid clinical concept of schizophrenia.

Treatment approaches

General principles

While antipsychotic drugs remain the cornerstone of treatment in child and adolescent onset schizophrenia, all young patients with schizophrenia require a multimodal treatment package that includes pharmacotherapy, family and individual counselling, education about the illness and provision to meet social and educational needs (Clark & Lewis 1998).

Primary prevention and early detection

In theory at least, the onset of schizophrenia could be prevented if an intervention reduced the premorbid 'risk' status. However, the difficulty with the premorbid phenotype as currently conceived (subtle social and developmental impairments) is its extremely low specificity and positive predictive value for schizophrenia in the general population, assuming that these premorbid features are a causal risk factor (Erlenmeyer-Kimling et al. 2000). Future refinement of the premorbid phenotype is likely to include genetic and neurocognitive markers in order to achieve acceptable sensitivity and specificity. At present, primary prevention remains on the distant horizon.

In contrast to primary prevention, the aims of early detection are to identify the onset of deterioration in vulnerable individuals with a high predictive validity. Predictive power increases markedly in adolescence around the onset of the prodrome (Davidson et al. 1999). Recent work has attempted to identify 'high-risk' or early prodromal states with the aim of intervening to prevent the active phase of schizophrenia (McGrorry & Sing 1995; Yung et al. 1996). However, only about one-fifth of these 'high-risk' cases go on to develop frank psychosis and it has proved impossible to distinguish these 'high-risk' cases from others who remain non-psychotic. Clearly, interventions directed at 'high-risk' or prodromal states need to benefit the whole population at risk, the majority of whom will not develop schizophrenia. A pragmatic stance would be to monitor children and adolescents with a strong family history and/or suggestive prodromal symptoms to ensure prompt treatment of psychosis.

Strong claims have been made that early recognition and treatment of psychotic symptoms in schizophrenia improves outcome. The association between a long duration of untreated psychosis (DUP) and poor long-term outcome in schizophrenia (Loebel et al. 1992; Wyatt 1995; Birchwood et al. 1997) supports this view. A similar association has been found in child and adolescent onset psychoses (Hollis 1999). While the association between DUP and poor outcome seems secure, the causal connection is far less certain. DUP is also associated with insidious onset and negative symptoms which could confound links with poor outcome. While there are good a priori clinical reasons for the early treatment of symptoms to relieve distress and prevent secondary impairments, as yet it remains unproven whether early intervention actually alters the long-term course of schizophrenia.

Pharmacological treatments

Because of the very small number of trials of antipsychotics conducted with child and adolescent patients, it is necessary to extrapolate most evidence on drug efficacy from studies in adults. This seems a reasonable approach given that schizophrenia is essentially the same disorder whether it has onset in childhood or adult life. However, age-specific factors such as the greater risk of extrapyramidal side-effects (EPSs) and treatment resistance to traditional antipsychotics in younger patients (Kumra et al. 1998b) should also influence drug choice.

The typical antipsychotic haloperidol has been shown to be superior to placebo in two double-blind controlled trials of children and adolescents with schizophrenia (Pool et al. 1976; Spencer & Campbell 1994). It is estimated that about 70% of patients show good or partial response to antipsychotic treatment, although this may take 6–8 weeks to be apparent (Clark & Lewis 1998). The main drawbacks concerning the use of high-potency typical antipsychotics such as haloperidol in children and adolescents is the high risk of EPSs (produced by D_2 blockade of the nigrostriatal pathway), tardive dyskinesia and the lack of effect against negative symptoms and cognitive impairment. Treatment with typical antipsychotics is also associated with enlargement of the caudate nucleus which can be reversed with clozapine (Frazier et al. 1996). Clozapine (the prototypic atypical) has been shown to be superior to haloperidol in a double-blind trial of 21 cases of childhood onset schizophrenia (Kumra et al. 1996). Large open clinical trials of clozapine confirm its effectiveness in child and adolescent onset schizophrenia (Siefen & Remschmidt 1986; Remschmidt et al. 1994). Similar, although less marked, benefits of olanzepine over typical antipsychotics in childhood onset schizophrenia have been reported (Kumra et al. 1998a).

Drawing this evidence together, a strong case can be made for the first-line use of atypicals in child and adolescent schizophrenia (clozapine is only licensed in the UK for treatment-resistant schizophrenia). Treatment resistance in child and adolescent patients should be defined as follows:

1 non-response with at least two conventional antipsychotics (from different chemical classes) each used for at least 4–6 weeks; and/or

2 significant adverse effects with conventional antipsychotics. While atypicals reduce the risk of EPSs, they can produce other troublesome side-effects (usually dose-related) including weight gain (olanzapine), sedation, hypersalivation and seizures (clozapine). The risk of blood dyscrasias on clozapine is effectively managed by mandatory routine blood monitoring. However, knowledge about potential adverse reactions with the newest atypicals is very limited in child and adolescent patients. A further consideration is the cost of newer atypicals compared with traditional antipsychotics. In the UK, a 1-month supply of haloperidol costs less than £2, compared with £100–120 for the newer atypicals and £200 for clozapine. Although economic studies of cost-effectiveness have suggested that the costs of the atypicals are recouped in reduced inpatient stays and indirect

social costs (Aitchison & Kerwin 1997), the availability of these drugs, particularly in developing countries, may well be limited because of their high cost. In the late 1990s, the use of atypical antipsychotics by UK child psychiatrists was still low. Over a 2-year period, only 10% of child and adolescent psychiatrists who prescribed antipsychotics in the Trent Health Region had used an atypical drug (Slaveska *et al.* 1998).

Currently, there is no clear consensus about the choice of antipsychotics in children and adolescents with schizophrenia. Some authorities suggest starting with a trial of a traditional antipsychotic (e.g. haloperidol) with substitution of an atypical if the traditional antipsychotic is either not tolerated or ineffective after 6–8 weeks (Clark & Lewis 1998). However, clinical trial evidence suggests that clozapine is the most effective antipsychotic in child and adolescent onset schizophrenia, although its use is restricted to treatment-resistant cases.

A very powerful case can be made for using atypicals such as olanzapine, quetiapine or risperidone as a first-line treatment, given that child and adolescent onset schizophrenia is characterized by negative symptoms, cognitive impairments, sensitivity to EPSs and relative resistance to traditional antipsychotics.

Psychosocial and family interventions

The rationale for psychosocial family interventions follows from the association between high EE and the risk of relapse in schizophrenia (Leff & Vaughn 1985; Dixon & Lehman 1995). The overall aim is to prevent relapse (secondary prevention) and improve the patient's level of functioning by modifying the family atmosphere. Lam (1991) conducted a systematic review of published trials of psychoeducation and more intensive family interventions in schizophrenia and drew the following conclusions. First, education packages on their own increase knowledge about the illness but do not reduce the risk of relapse. Secondly, more intensive family intervention studies with high EE relatives have shown a reduction in relapse rates linked to a lowering of EE. Thirdly, family interventions tend to be costly and time-consuming with most clinical trials employing highly skilled research teams. Whether these interventions can be transferred into routine clinical practice is uncertain. Fourthly, interventions have focused on the reduction of EE in 'high-risk' families. Whether low EE families would also benefit from these interventions is less clear. This is particularly relevant to the families of children and adolescents with schizophrenia as, on average, these parents express *lower* levels of criticism and hostility than parents of adult onset patients (J.R. Asarnow *et al.* 1994). Hence, routine family interventions aiming to reduce high EE may be well-intentioned but misguided in their focus.

Cognitive–behaviour therapy

In adult patients, cognitive therapy has been used to reduce the impact of treatment-resistant positive symptoms (Tarrier *et al.* 1993). Cognitive–behaviour therapy (CBT) has been shown to be effective in treating negative as well as positive symptoms in schizophrenia resistant to standard antipsychotic drugs, with efficacy sustained over 9 months of follow-up (Sensky *et al.* 2000; see Chapter 33). Whether CBT is equally effective with younger patients, or those with predominant negative symptoms, remains to be established.

Cognitive remediation

Cognitive remediation is a relatively new psychological treatment which aims to arrest or reverse the cognitive impairments in attention, concentration and working memory seen in schizophrenia (Hayes & McGrath 2000; Wykes *et al.* 2000). The results of an early controlled trial in adults are promising, with gains found in the areas of memory and social functioning (Wykes *et al.* 2000). The relatively greater severity of cognitive impairments in child and adolescent patients suggests that early remediation strategies may be particularly important in these younger patients. Helpful advice can also be offered to parents, teachers and professionals, such as breaking down information and tasks into small manageable parts to reduce demands on working memory and speed of processing.

Organization of treatment services

It is a paradox that patients with very early onset schizophrenia have the most severe form of the disorder yet they often receive inadequate and poorly co-ordinated services. One reason for this state of affairs may be that the core responsibility for schizophrenia is seen to lie within adult psychiatric services. In the UK, community-based child and adolescent mental health services (CAMHS) provide the first-line assessment and care for child and young adolescent psychoses, with only about half of these cases referred to specialist inpatient units (Slaveska *et al.* 1998). While inpatient admission is often unnecessary, generic CAMHS services are usually not well placed to provide a comprehensive assessment and treatment service for very early onset psychoses. First, the very low population prevalence of psychosis reduces the predictive value of diagnosis outside specialist centres. Secondly, community-based services often lack familiarity with newer therapies for psychoses including atypical antipsychotics.

One possible model would be to establish specialist regional very early onset psychosis teams serving a population of about 5 million, akin to specialist cancer centres. These expert teams would be primarily outpatient-based but with access to inpatient facilities if required. Hence, the focus would be quite different from the more traditional general purpose adolescent inpatient unit. The teams could offer early diagnostic assessments for children and younger adolescents with suspected psychotic disorders and set up treatment plans in collaboration with more local child and adult psychiatric services. Ideally, these teams would be linked to a university academic centre with an interest in psychosis research and treatment evaluation.

Conclusions

The last decade has seen a dramatic growth in our understanding of the clinical course and neurobiological correlates of schizophrenia presenting in childhood and adolescence. It is now clear that adult-based diagnostic criteria have validity in this age group and the disorder has clinical and neurobiological continuity with schizophrenia in adults. Child and adolescent onset schizophrenia is a severe variant of the adult disorder associated with greater premorbid impairment, a higher familial risk, more severe clinical course and poorer outcome. The poor outcome of children and adolescents with schizophrenia has highlighted the need to target early and effective treatments and develop specialist services for this high-risk group. The last decade has witnessed the introduction of new atypical antipsychotics with improved side-effect profiles and efficacy, and these drugs are likely to replace the traditional antipsychotics as first-line drug therapy for child and adolescent onset schizophrenia.

However, a fundamental understanding of the underlying genetic and neurobiological basis of schizophrenia is still to be achieved. The finding of a progressive reduction in brain volume in very early onset patients and reduced synaptic density in the prefrontal cortex suggests the possibility that excessive synaptic elimination during adolescence may underlie the aetiology of schizophrenia. While significant advances in the next decade are likely to flow from technical developments in molecular genetics and neuroimaging, advance is limited by the defining diagnostic paradigm of schizophrenia. It is widely recognized that the clinical syndrome of schizophrenia contains considerable aetiological and clinical heterogeneity. Therefore, the challenge will be to identify the genetic, neurobiological and cognitive basis of this heterogeneity. Real advance in the field will depend on a more sophisticated understanding of the interplay between genetics, neurodevelopment and environment. This will involve identifying the molecular genetic basis of neurocognitive susceptibility traits for schizophrenia. The developmental mechanisms that translate neurocognitive risks into disorder will need to be understood. Unravelling neurocognitive and clinical heterogeneity should lead to improvements in our ability to deliver individually targeted treatments, as well as the ability to identify 'at risk' children and adolescents in order to prevent the onset of psychosis.

References

Aitchison, K.J. & Kerwin, R.W. (1997) The cost effectiveness of clozapine. *British Journal of Psychiatry* 171, 125–130.

Alaghband-Rad, J., McKenna, K., Gordon, C.T. *et al.* (1995) Childhood onset schizophrenia: the severity of premorbid course. *Journal of the American Academy of Child and Adolescent Psychiatry* 34, 1273–1283.

Alaghband-Rad, J., Hamburger, S.D., Giedd, J., Frazier, J.A. & Rapoport, J.L. (1997) Childhood onset schizophrenia: biological markers in relation to clinical characteristics. *American Journal of Psychiatry* 154, 64–68.

American Psychiatric Association (1980) *Diagnostic and Statistical Manual of Mental Disorders*, 3rd edn. American Psychiatric Association, Washington, DC.

American Psychiatric Association (1994) *Diagnostic and Statistical Manual of Mental Disorders*, 4th edn. American Psychiatric Association, Washington, DC.

Andreasen, N., Ehrhardt, J.C., Swazye, V.W. *et al.* (1990) Magnetic resonance imaging of the brain in schizophrenia. *Archives of General Psychiatry* 47, 35–44.

Asarnow, J.R. & Ben-Meir, S. (1988) Children with schizophrenia spectrum and depressive disorders: a comparative study of premorbid adjustment, onset pattern and severity of impairment. *Journal of Child Psychology and Psychiatry* 29, 477–488.

Asarnow, J.R., Thompson, M.C., Hamilton, E.B., Goldstein, M.J. & Guthrie, D. (1994) Family expressed emotion, childhood onset depression, and childhood onset schizophrenic spectrum disorders: is expressed emotion a non-specific correlate of psychopathology or a specific risk factor for depression? *Journal of Abnormal Psychology* 22, 129–146.

Asarnow, R., Granholm, E. & Sherman, T. (1991) Span of apprehension in schizophrenia. In: *Handbook of Schizophrenia*, Vol. 5. *Neuropsychology, Psychophysiology and Information Processing* (eds S.R. Steinhauer, J.H. Gruzelier & J. Zubin), pp. 335–370. Elsevier, Amsterdam.

Asarnow, R., Asamen, J., Granholm, E. *et al.* (1994) Cognitive/neuropsychological studies of children with schizophrenic disorder. *Schizophrenia Bulletin* 20, 647–669.

Asarnow, R., Brown, W. & Stranberg, R. (1995) Children with schizophrenic disorder: neurobehavioural studies. *European Archives of Psychiatry and Clinical Neuroscience* 245, 70–79.

Bassett, A.S., Chow, E., Scutt, L., Hodkinson, K. & Weksberg, R. (1999) Psychiatric phenotype of a genetic subtype of schizophrenia [Abstract]. *Schizophrenia Research* 36, 87.

Bedwell, J.S., Keller, B., Smith, A.K. *et al.* (1999) Why does postpsychotic IQ decline in childhood onset schizophrenia? *American Journal of Psychiatry* 156, 1996–1997.

Beratis, S., Gabriel, J. & Hoidas, S. (1994) Age at onset in subtypes of schizophrenic disorders. *Schizophrenia Bulletin* 20, 287–296.

Bertolino, A., Kumra, S., Callicott, J.H. *et al.* (1998) Common pattern of cortical pathology in childhood onset and adult onset schizophrenia as identified by proton magnetic resonance spectroscopic imaging. *American Journal of Psychiatry* 155, 1376–1383.

Bilder, R.M., Lipschutz-Broch, L., Reiter, G. *et al.* (1992) Intellectual deficits in first-episode schizophrenia: evidence for progressive deterioration. *Schizophrenia Bulletin* 18, 437–448.

Birchwood, M., McGorry, P. & Jackson, H. (1997) Early intervention in schizophrenia. *British Journal of Psychiatry* 170, 2–5.

Bleuler, E. (1911/1950) Dementia praecox. In: *The Group of Schizophrenias*. Translated by J. Zinkin. International Universities Press, New York.

Breier, A. (1999) Cognitive deficit in schizophrenia and its neurochemical basis. *British Journal of Psychiatry* 174 (Suppl. 37), 16–18.

Bullmore, E.T., O'Connell, P., Frangou, S. & Murray, R.M. (1997) Schizophrenia as a developmental disorder or neural network integrity: the dysplastic net hypothesis. In: *Neurodevelopment and Adult Psychopathology* (eds M.S. Keshervan & R.M. Murray), pp. 253–266. Cambridge University Press, Cambridge.

Burgess, C.E., Lindblad, K., Sidransky, E. *et al.* (1998) Large CAG/CTG repeats are associated with childhood onset schizophrenia. *Molecular Psychiatry* 3, 321–327.

Caplan, R., Guthrie, D., Shields, W.D. & Mori, L. (1992) Formal thought disorder in paediatric complex partial seizure disorder. *Journal of Child Psychology and Psychiatry* 33, 1399–1412.

Castle, D. & Murray, R. (1991) The neurodevelopmental basis of sex differences in schizophrenia. *Psychological Medicine* 21, 565–575.

Chakos, M.H., Lieberman, J.A., Alvir, J. *et al.* (1995) Caudate nuclei volumes in schizophrenic patients treated with typical antipsychotics or clozapine. *Lancet* 345, 456–457.

Childs, B. & Scriver, C.R. (1986) Age at onset and causes of disease. *Perspectives in Biology and Medicine* 29, 437–460.

Clark, A. & Lewis, S. (1998) Treatment of schizophrenia in childhood and adolescence. *Journal of Child Psychology and Psychiatry* 39, 1071–1081.

Davidson, M., Reichenberg, M.A., Rabinowitz, J. *et al.* (1999) Behavioral and intellectual markers for schizophrenia in apparently healthy male adolescents. *American Journal of Psychiatry* 156, 1328–1335.

De Sanctis, S. (1906) On some varieties of dementia praecox. In: *Rivista Sperimentale de Freniatria e Medicina Legale Delle Alienazioni Mentale* (ed. J.G. Howell), pp. 141–165. Translated by M.L. Osbourn. Brunner Mazel, New York.

Dixon, L.B. & Lehman, A.F. (1995) Family interventions for schizophrenia. *Schizophrenia Bulletin* 21, 631–643.

Dolan, R.J., Fletcher, P., Frith, C.D. *et al.* (1996) Dopaminergic modulation of impaired cognitive activation in the anterior cingulate cortex in schizophrenia. *Nature* 378, 180–182.

Done, J.D., Crow, T.J., Johnstone, E. & Sacker, A. (1994) Child-hood antecedents of schizophrenia and affective illness: social adjustment at ages 7 and 11. *British Medical Journal* 309, 699–703.

Dye, S.M., Spence, S.A., Bench, C.J. *et al.* (1999) No evidence for left superior temporal dysfunction in asymptomatic schizophrenia and bipolar disorder: PET study of verbal fluency. *British Journal of Psychiatry* 175, 367–374.

Eggers, C. (1978) Course and prognosis in childhood schizophrenia. *Journal of Autism and Childhood Schizophrenia* 8, 21–36.

Eggers, C. & Bunk, D. (1997) The long-term course of childhood onset schizophrenia: a 42-year follow-up. *Schizophrenia Bulletin* 23, 105–117.

Erlenmeyer-Kimling, L., Rock, D., Roberts, S.A. *et al.* (2000) Attention, memory and motor skills as childhood predictors of schizophrenia-related psychoses: the New York High Risk Project. *Archives of General Psychiatry* 157, 1416–1422.

Feinberg, I. (1983) Schizophrenia: caused by a fault in programmed synaptic elimination during adolescence. *Journal of Psychiatric Research* 17, 319–344.

Feinberg, I. (1997) Schizophrenia as an emergent disorder of late brain maturation. In: *Neuorodevelopment and Adult Psychopathology* (eds M.S. Keshervan & R.M. Murray), pp. 237–252. Cambridge University Press, Cambridge.

Fish, B. (1957) The detection of schizophrenia in infancy. *Journal of Nervous and Mental Diseases* 125, 1–24.

Fish, B. & Rivito, E.R. (1979) Psychoses of childhood. In: *Basic Handbook of Child Psychiatry*, Vol. 2 (ed. J.D. Noshpitz), pp. 249–304. Basic Books, New York.

Foerster, A., Lewis, S., Owen, M. & Murray, R.M. (1991) Pre-morbid adjustment and personality in psychosis. *British Journal of Psychiatry* 158, 171–176.

Frazier, J.A., Giedd, J.N., Kaysen, D. *et al.* (1996) Childhood onset schizophrenia: brain magnetic resonance imaging rescan after 2 years of clozapine maintenance. *American Journal of Psychiatry* 153, 564–566.

Frazier, J.A., Alaghband-Rad, J., Jacobsen, L. *et al.* (1997) Pubertal development and the onset of psychosis in childhood onset schizophrenia. *Psychiatry Research* 70, 1–7.

Friedman, L., Finding, R.L., Buch, J. *et al.* (1996) Structural MRI and neuropsychological assessments in adolescent patients with either schizophrenia or affective disorders. *Schizophrenia Research* 18, 189–190.

Friston, K.J., Herold, S., Fletcher, P. *et al.* (1995) Abnormal fronto-temporal interactions in schizophrenia. In: *Biology of Schizophrenia and Affective Diseases* (ed. S.J. Watson), pp. 449–481. Raven, New York.

Frith, C.D. (1994) Theory of mind in schizophrenia. In: *The Neuropsychology of Schizophrenia* (eds A. David & J.S. Cutting), pp. 147–161. Lawrence Erlbaum, Hove.

Galdos, P.M., van Os, J. & Murray, R. (1993) Puberty and the onset of psychosis. *Schizophrenia Research* 10, 7–14.

Gallhofer, B., Trimble, M.R., Frackowiak, R., Gibbs, J. & Jones, T. (1985) A study of cerebral blood flow and metabolism in epileptic psychosis using positron emission tomography and oxygen. *Journal of Neurology, Neurosurgery and Psychiatry* 48, 201–206.

Garey, L.J., Ong, W.Y., Patel, T.S. *et al.* (1998) Reduced dendritic spine density on cerebral cortical pyramidal neurons in schizophrenia. *Journal of Neurology, Neurosurgery and Psychiatry* 65 (4), 446–453.

Garralda, M.E. (1984) Hallucinations in children with conduct and emotional disorders. I. The clinical phenomena. *Psychological Medicine* 14, 589–596.

Geddes, J.R. & Lawrie, S.M. (1995) Obstetric complications and schizophrenia: a meta-analysis. *British Journal of Psychiatry* 167, 786–793.

Giedd, J.N., Castellanos, F.X., Rajapaske, J.C. *et al.* (1996) Quantitative analysis of grey matter volumes in childhood onset schizophrenia and attention deficit/hyperactivity disorder. *Society for Neuroscience Abstracts* 22, 1166.

Gillberg, C., Wahlstrom, J., Forsman, A., Hellgren, L. & Gillberg, J.C. (1986) Teenage psychoses: epidemiology, classification and reduced optimality in the pre-, peri- and neonatal periods. *Journal of Child Psychology and Psychiatry* 27, 87–98.

Glantz, L.A. & Lewis, D.A. (2000) Decreased dendritic spine density on prefrontal cortical pyramidal neurones in schizophrenia. *Archives of General Psychiatry* 57, 65–73.

Goldstein, M.J. (1987) The UCLA High Risk Project. *Schizophrenia Bulletin* 13, 505–514.

Goodman, R. (1988) Are complications of pregnancy and birth causes of schizophrenia? *Developmental Medicine and Child Neurology* 30, 391–406.

Gordon, C.T., Frazier, J.A., McKenna, K. *et al.* (1994) Childhood onset schizophrenia: a NIMH study in progress. *Schizophrenia Bulletin* 20, 697–712.

Green, W., Campbell, M., Hardesty, A. *et al.* (1984) A comparison of schizophrenic and autistic children. *Journal of the American Academy of Child Psychiatry* 23, 399–409.

Green, W., Padron-Gayol, M., Hardesty, A. & Bassiri, M. (1992) Schizophrenia with childhood onset: a phenomenological study of 38 cases. *Journal of the American Academy of Child and Adolescent Psychiatry* 31, 968–976.

Gualtieri, C.T., Adams, A. & Chen, C.D. (1982) Minor physical abnormalities in alcoholic and schizophrenic adults and hyperactive and autistic children. *American Journal of Psychiatry* 139, 640–643.

Gur, R.E., Cowell, P., Turetsky, B.I. *et al.* (1998) A follow-up magnetic resonance imaging study of schizophrenia: relationship of neuroanatomical changes to clinical and neurobehavioural measures. *Archives of General Psychiatry* 55, 145–152.

Gur, R.E., Turetsky, B.I., Cowell, P. *et al.* (2000a) Temporolimbic volume reductions in schizophrenia. *Archives of General Psychiatry* 57, 769–775.

Gur, R.E., Cowell, P., Latshaw, A. *et al.* (2000b) Reduced dorsal and orbital prefrontal gray matter volumes in schizophrenia. *Archives of General Psychiatry* 57, 761–768.

Guy, J.D., Majorski, L.V., Wallace, C.J. & Guy, M.P. (1983) The incidence of minor physical anomalies in adult schizophrenics. *Schizophrenia Bulletin* 9, 571–582.

Hafner, H. & Nowotny, B. (1995) Epidemiology of early onset schizophrenia. *European Archives of Psychiatry and Clinical Neuroscience* 245, 80–92.

Harris, E.C. & Barraclough, B. (1997) Excess mortality of mental disorder. *British Journal of Psychiatry* 173, 11–53.

Hayes, R.L. & McGrath, J.J. (2000) Cognitive rehabilitation for people with schizophrenia and related conditions: a systemic review and meta-analysis [Abstract]. *Schizophrenia Research* 41, 221–222.

Hollis, C. (1995) Child and adolescent (juvenile onset) schizophrenia: a case–control study of premorbid developmental impairments. *British Journal of Psychiatry* 166, 489–495.

Hollis, C. (1999) *A study of the course and adult outcomes of child and adolescent onset psychoses*. PhD thesis, University of London.

Hollis, C. (2000) The adult outcomes of child and adolescent onset schizophrenia: diagnostic stability and predictive validity. *American Journal of Psychiatry* 157, 1652–1659.

Hollis, C. & Taylor, E. (1997) Schizophrenia: a critique from the developmental psychopathology perspective. In: *Neuorodevelopment and Adult Psychopathology* (eds M.S. Keshervan & R.M. Murray), pp. 213–233. Cambridge University Press, Cambridge.

Hooley, J.M. (1987) The nature and origins of expressed emotion. In: *Understanding Major Mental Disorder: the Contribution of Family Interaction Research* (eds K. Hahlweg & M.J. Goldstein), pp. 176–194. Family Process, New York.

Hughes, C. & Russell, J. (1993) Autistic children's difficulty with mental disengagement with an object: its implications for theories of autism. *Developmental Psychology* 29, 498–510.

Huttenlocher, P.R. (1979) Synaptic density in human prefrontal cortex: developmental changes and effects of aging. *Brain Research* 163, 195–205.

Iacono, W.G. & Koenig, W.G.R. (1983) Features that distinguish smooth pursuit eye tracking performance in schizophrenic, affective disordered and normal individuals. *Journal of Abnormal Psychology* 92, 29–41.

Jacobsen, L. & Rapoport, J. (1998) Research update: childhood onset schizophrenia – implications for clinical and neurobiological research. *Journal of Child Psychology and Psychiatry* 39, 101–113.

Jacobsen, L., Giedd, J.N., Berquin, P.C. *et al.* (1997a) Quantitative morphology of the cerebellum and fourth ventricle in childhood onset schizophrenia. *American Journal of Psychiatry* 154, 1663–1669.

Jacobsen, L., Hamburger, S.D., Van Horn, J.D. *et al.* (1997b) Cerebral glucose metabolism in childhood onset schizophrenia. *Psychiatry Research* 75, 131–144.

Jacobsen, L., Giedd, J.N., Castellanos, F.X. *et al.* (1998) Progressive reductions in temporal lobe structures in childhood onset schizophrenia. *American Journal of Psychiatry* 155, 678–685.

Jones, P. & Done, J. (1997) From birth to onset: a developmental perspective of schizophrenia in two national birth cohorts. In: *Neuorodevelopment and Adult Psychopathology* (eds M.S. Keshervan & R.M. Murray), pp. 119–136. Cambridge University Press, Cambridge.

Jones, P., Rogers, B., Murray, R. & Marmot, M. (1994) Child development risk factors for adult schizophrenia in the British 1946 birth cohort. *Lancet* 344, 1398–1402.

Joyce, P.R. (1984) Age of onset in bipolar affective disorder and misdiagnosis of schizophrenia. *Psychological Medicine* 14, 145–149.

Kallman, F.J. & Roth, B. (1956) Genetic aspects of preadolescent schizophrenia. *American Journal of Psychiatry* 112, 599–606.

Karatekin, C. & Asarnow, R.F. (1998) Working memory in childhood onset schizophrenia and attention deficit/hyperactivity disorder. *Psychiatry Research* 80, 165–176.

Karayiorgou, M., Morris, M.A., Morrow, B. *et al.* (1995) Schizophrenia susceptibility associated with interstitial deletions of chromosome 22q11. *Proceedings of the National Academy of Sciences of the USA* 92, 7612–7616.

Kendall, R.E., McInneny, K., Juszczak, E. & Bain, M. (2000) Obstetric complications and schizophrenia: two case–control studies based on structured obstetric records. *British Journal of Psychiatry* 176, 516–522.

Kjelsberg, E. (2000) Adolescent psychiatric in-patients: a high risk group for premature death. *British Journal of Psychiatry* 176, 121–125.

Kolvin, I. (1971) Studies in the childhood psychoses. I. Diagnostic criteria and classification. *British Journal of Psychiatry* 118, 381–384.

Kraepelin, E. (1919) *Dementia Praecox*. Translated by R. Barclay. Livingstone, Edinburgh.

Kumra, S., Frazier, J.A., Jacobsen, L.K. *et al.* (1996) Childhood onset schizophrenia: a double blind clozapine–haloperidol comparison. *Archives of General Psychiatry* 53, 1090–1097.

Kumra, S., Jacobsen, L.K., Lenane, M. *et al.* (1998a) Childhood onset schizophrenia: an open-label study of olanzapine in adolescents. *Journal of the American Academy of Child and Adolescent Psychiatry* 37, 360–363.

Kumra, S., Jacobsen, L.K., Lenane, M. *et al.* (1998b) Case series: spectrum of neuroleptic-induced movement disorders and extrapyramidal side-effects in childhood onset schizophrenia. *Journal of the American Academy of Child and Adolescent Psychiatry* 37, 221–227.

Kumra, S., Jacobsen, L.K., Lenane, M. *et al.* (1998c) 'Multidimensionally impaired disorder': is it a variant of very early onset schizophrenia? *Journal of the American Academy of Child and Adolescent Psychiatry* 37, 91–99.

Kumra, S., Wiggs, E., Krasnewich, D. *et al.* (1998d) Brief report: association of sex chromosome anomalies with childhood onset psychotic disorders. *Journal of the American Academy of Child and Adolescent Psychiatry* 37, 292–296.

Lam, D.H. (1991) Psychosocial family intervention in schizophrenia: a review of empirical studies. *Psychological Medicine* 21, 423–441.

Lawrie, S.M. & Abukmeil, S.S. (1998) Brain abnormalities in schizophrenia: a systematic and quantitative review of volumetric magnetic resonance imaging studies. *British Journal of Psychiatry* 172, 110–120.

Leff, J. & Vaughn, C. (1985) *Expressed Emotion in Families: its Significance for Mental Illness*. Guilford Press, London.

Lewine, R.R.J. (1994) Comments on 'Puberty and the onset of psychosis' by P.M. Galdos *et al. Schizophrenia Research* 13, 81–83.

Lewis, S.W. & Murray, R.M. (1987) Obstetric complications, neurodevelopmental deviance and risk of schizophrenia. *Journal of Psychiatric Research* 21, 414–421.

Liddle, P., Friston, K.J., Frith, C.D. *et al.* (1992) Patterns of cerebral blood flow in schizophrenia. *British Journal of Psychiatry* 160, 179–186.

Lindsay, J., Ounsted, C. & Richards, P. (1979) Long-term outcome of children with temporal lobe seizures. II. Marriage, parenthood and sexual indifference. *Developmental Medicine and Child Neurology* 21, 433–440.

Loebel, A.D., Lieberman, J.A., Alvir, J.M.N. *et al.* (1992) Duration of psychosis and outcome in first episode schizophrenia. *American Journal of Psychiatry* **149**, 1183–1188.

McGlashen, T.H. & Hoffman, R.E. (2000) Schizophrenia as a disorder of developmentally reduced synaptic connectivity. *Archives of General Psychiatry* **57**, 637–648.

McGrath, J. & Murray, R. (1995) Risk factors for schizophrenia: from conception to birth. In: *Schizophrenia* (eds S.R. Hirsch & D.R. Weinberger), pp. 187–205. Blackwell Science, Oxford.

McGrory, P. & Sing, B. (1995) Schizophrenia: risk and possibility. In: *Handbook of Studies on Preventative Psychiatry* (eds B. Raphael & G. Burrows), pp. 491–514. Elsvier Science, Amsterdam.

McNeil, T.F. (1995) Perinatal risk factors and schizophrenia: selective review and methodological concerns. *Epidemiology Review* **17**, 107–112.

Malmberg, A., Lewis, G., David, A. & Allebeck, P. (1998) Premorbid adjustment and personality in people with schizophrenia. *British Journal of Psychiatry* **172**, 308–313.

Matsumoto, H., Takei, N., Saito, H., Kachi, K. & Mori, N. (1999) Childhood onset schizophrenia and obstetric complications: a case–control study. *Schizophrenia Research* **38**, 93–99.

Maziade, M., Bouchard, S., Gingras, N. *et al.* (1996) Long-term stability of diagnosis and symptom dimensions in a systematic sample of patients with onset of schizophrenia in childhood and early adolescence. II. Positive/negative distinction and childhood predictors of adult outcome. *British Journal of Psychiatry* **169**, 371–378.

Murray, R.M. & Lewis, S.W. (1987) Is schizophrenia a neurodevelopmental disorder? *British Medical Journal* **295**, 681–682.

Nelson, M.D., Saykin, A.J., Flashman, L.A. & Riodan, H.J. (1998) Hippocampal volume reduction in schizophrenia assessed by magnetic resonance imaging: a meta-analytic study. *Archives of General Psychiatry* **55**, 433–440.

Nicholson, R.M., Giedd, J.N., Lenane, M. *et al.* (1999) Clinical and neurobiological correlates of cytogenetic abnormalities in childhood onset schizophrenia. *American Journal of Psychiatry* **156**, 1575–1579.

Nicholson, R.M., Lenane, M., Singaracharlu, S. *et al.* (2000) Premorbid speech and language impairments in childhood onset schizophrenia: association with risk factors. *Schizophrenia Research* **41**, 55.

Nopoulos, P., Torres, I., Flaum, M. *et al.* (1995) Brain morphology in first-episode schizophrenia. *American Journal of Psychiatry* **152**, 1721–1723.

Nopoulos, P.C., Giedd, J.N., Andreasen, N.C. & Rapoport, J.L. (1998) Frequency and severity of enlarged septi pellucidi in childhood onset schizophrenia. *American Journal of Psychiatry* **155**, 1074–1079.

Nuechterlain, K.H. & Dawson, M.E. (1984) Information processing and attentional functioning in the developmental course of schizophrenic disorders. *Schizophrenia Bulletin* **10**, 160–203.

van Os, J., Jones, P., Lewis, G. *et al.* (1997) Developmental precursors of affective illness in a general population birth cohort. *Archives of General Psychiatry* **54**, 625–631.

Ozonoff, S., Pennington, B.F. & Rogers, S.J. (1991) Executive function deficits in high-functioning autistic individuals: relationship to theory of mind. *Journal of Child Psychology and Psychiatry* **32**, 1081–1105.

Pantelis, C., Velakoulis, D., Suchling, P. *et al.* (2000) Left medial temporal volume reduction occurs during transition from high-risk to first-episode psychosis. *Schizophrenia Research* **41**, 35.

Park, S., Holzman, P.S. & Goldman-Rakic, P.S. (1995) Spatial working memory deficits in the relatives of schizophrenic patients. *Archives of General Psychiatry* **52**, 821–828.

Pennington, B.F., Groisser, D. & Welsh, M.C. (1993) Contrasting deficits in attention deficit hyperactivity disorder versus reading disability. *Developmental Psychology* **29**, 511–523.

Pettegrew, J.W., Keshavan, M.S., Panchalingam, K. *et al.* (1991) Alterations in brain high energy phosphate and membrane phospholipid metabolism in first episode, drug naive schizophrenics: a pilot study of the dorsal prefrontal cortex by *in vivo* phosphorous-31 nuclear magnetic resonance spectroscopy. *Archives of General Psychiatry* **48**, 563–568.

Pool, D., Bloom, W., Miekle, D.H., Roniger, J.J. & Gallant, D.M. (1976) A controlled trial of loxapine in 75 adolescent schizophrenic patients. *Current Therapeutic Research* **19**, 99–104.

Poole, R. & Brabbins, C. (1996) Drug-induced psychosis. *British Journal of Psychiatry* **168**, 135–138.

Potter, H.W. (1933) Schizophrenia in children. *American Journal of Psychiatry* **12**, 1253–1270.

Pulver, A., Brown, C.H., Wolyniec, P. *et al.* (1990) Schizophrenia: age at onset, gender and familial risk. *Acta Psychiatrica Scandinavica* **82**, 344–351.

Purves, D.L. & Lichtmen, J.W. (1980) Elimination of synapses in the developing nervous system. *Science* **210**, 153–157.

Rapoport, J.L., Giedd, J., Kumra, S. *et al.* (1997) Childhood onset schizophrenia: progressive ventricular change during adolescence. *Archives of General Psychiatry* **54**, 897–903.

Rapoport, J.L., Giedd, J., Blumenthal, J. *et al.* (1999) Progressive cortical change during adolescence in childhood onset schizophrenia: a longitudinal magnetic resonance imaging study. *Archives of General Psychiatry* **56**, 649–654.

Remschmidt, H., Schultz, E. & Martin, M. (1994) An open trial of clozapine with thirty-six adolescents with schizophrenia. *Journal of Child and Adolescent Psychopharmacology* **4**, 31–41.

Roberts, G.W., Colter, N., Lofthouse, R. *et al.* (1986) Gliosis in schizophrenia: a survey. *Biological Psychiatry* **21**, 1043–1050.

Robinson, D., Woerner, M.G., Alvir, J.M. *et al.* (1999) Predictors of relapse following a first episode of schizophrenia or schizoaffective disorder. *Archives of General Psychiatry* **56**, 241–247.

Rossi, A., Mancini, F., Stratta, P. *et al.* (1997) Risperidone, negative symptoms and cognitive deficit in schizophrenia: an open study. *Acta Psychiatrica Scandinavica* **95**, 40–43.

Russell, A.J., Monro, J.C., Jones, P.B., Hemsley, D.R. & Murray, R.M. (1997) Schizophrenia and the myth of intellectual decline. *American Journal of Psychiatry* **154**, 635–639.

Russell, A.T. (1994) The clinical presentation of childhood onset schizophrenia. *Schizophrenia Bulletin* **20**, 631–646.

Russell, A.T., Bott, L. & Sammons, C. (1989) The phenomena of schizophrenia occurring in childhood. *Journal of the American Academy of Child and Adolescent Psychiatry* **28**, 399–407.

Rutter, M. (1972) Childhood schizophrenia reconsidered. *Journal of Autism and Childhood Schizophrenia* **2**, 315–407.

Rutter, M. & Mawhood, L. (1991) The long-term psychosocial sequelae of specific developmental disorders of speech and language. In: *Biological Risk Factors for Psychosocial Disorders* (eds M. Rutter & P. Casaer), pp. 233–259. Cambridge University Press, Cambridge.

Sachdev, P. (1998) Schizophrenia-like psychosis and epilepsy: the status of the association. *American Journal of Psychiatry* **155**, 325–336.

Saykin, A.J., Shtasel, D.L., Gur, R.E. *et al.* (1994) Neuropsychological deficits in neuroleptic-naive patients with first episode schizophrenia. *Archives of General Psychiatry* **512**, 124–131.

Schmidt, M., Blanz, B., Dippe, A., Koppe, T. & Lay, B. (1995) Course of patients diagnosed as having schizophrenia during first episode occurring under age 18 years. *European Archives of Psychiatry and Clinical Neuroscience* **245**, 93–100.

Selemon, L.D., Rajkowska, G. & Goldman-Rakic, P.S. (1995) Abnormally high neuronal density in the schizophrenic cortex: a morphometric analysis of prefrontal area 9 and occipital area 17. *Archives of General Psychiatry* **52**, 805–818.

Sensky, T., Turkington, D., Kingdon, D. *et al.* (2000) A randomized controlled trial of cognitive–behavioral therapy for persistent symptoms in schizophrenia resistant to medication. *Archives of General Psychiatry* **57**, 165–172.

Sham, P.C., Jones, P.B., Russell, A. *et al.* (1994) Age at onset, sex, and familial psychiatric morbidity in schizophrenia. Report from the Camberwell Collaborative Psychosis Study. *British Journal of Psychiatry* **165**, 466–473.

Siefen, G. & Remschmidt, H. (1986) Behandlungsergebnisse mit Clozapin bei schizophrenen Jungendlichen. *Zeitschrift fur Kinder- und Jungendpsychiatrie* **14**, 245–257.

Sigurdsson, E., Fombonne, E., Sayal, K. & Checkley, S. (1999) Neurodevelopmental antecedents of early onset bipolar affective disorder. *British Journal of Psychiatry* **174**, 121–127.

Slaveska, K., Hollis. C.P. & Bramble, D. (1998) The use of antipsychotics by the child and adolescent psychiatrists of Trent region. *Psychiatric Bulletin* **22**, 685–687.

Spence, S.A., Hirsch, S.R., Brooks, D.J. *et al.* (1998) Prefrontal cortex activity in people with schizophrenia and control subjects: evidence from positron emission tomography for remission of 'hypofrontality' with recovery from acute schizophrenia. *British Journal of Psychiatry* **172**, 316–323. [Published erratum appears in *British Journal of Psychiatry* 1998; **172**, 543.]

Spence, S.A., Liddle, P.F., Stefan, M.D. *et al.* (2000) Functional anatomy of verbal fluency in people with schizophrenia and those at genetic risk: focal dysfunction and distributed disconnectivity reappraised. *British Journal of Psychiatry* **176**, 52–60.

Spencer, E.K. & Campbell, M. (1994) Children with schizophrenia: diagnosis, phenomenology and pharmacotherapy. *Schizophrenia Bulletin* **20**, 713–725.

Strandburg, R.J., Marsh, J.T., Brown, W.S., Asarnow, R.F. & Guthrie, D. (1994) Information processing deficits across childhood and adult onset schizophrenia. *Schizophrenia Bulletin* **20**, 685–696.

Strandburg, R.J., Marsh, J.T., Brown. W.S. *et al.* (1999) Continuous-processing ERPS in adult schizophrenia: continuity with childhood onset schizophrenia. *Biological Psychiatry* **45**, 1356–1369.

Tarrier, N., Beckett, R., Harwood, S. *et al.* (1993) A trial of two cognitive behavioural methods of treating drug resistant residual symptoms in schizophrenic patients. I. Outcome. *British Journal of Psychiatry* **162**, 524–532.

Thomas, M.A., Ke, Y., Levitt, J. *et al.* (1998) Preliminary study of frontal lobe ^{1}H MR spectroscopy in childhood onset schizophrenia. *Journal of Magnetic Resonance Imaging* **8**, 841–846.

Towbin, K.R., Dykens, E.M., Pearson, G.S. & Cohen, D.J. (1993) Conceptualising 'borderline syndrome of childhood' and 'childhood schizophrenia' as a developmental disorder. *Journal of the American Academy of Child and Adolescent Psychiatry* **32**, 775–782.

Tsuang, M.T. (1993) Genotypes, phenotypes and the brain: a search for connections in schizophrenia. *British Journal of Psychiatry* **163**, 299–307.

Tsuang, M.T., Simpson, J.C. & Kronfold, Z. (1982) Subtypes of drug abuse with psychosis. *Archives of General Psychiatry* **39**, 141–147.

Vita, A., Dieci, M., Giobbio, G.M. *et al.* (1991) CT scan abnormalities and outcome of chronic schizophrenia. *American Journal of Psychiatry* **148**, 1577–1579.

Volkmar, F.R. & Cohen, D.J. (1991) Comorbid association of autism and schizophrenia. *American Journal of Psychiatry* **148**, 1705–1707.

Weinberger, D.R. (1987) Implications of normal brain development for the pathogenesis of schizophrenia. *Archives of General Psychiatry* **44**, 660–669.

Welsh, M.C., Pennington, B.F. & Groisser, D.B. (1991) A normative-developmental study of executive function: a window on pre-frontal function in children? *Developmental Neuropsychology* **7**, 131–139.

Werry, J.S. (1992) Child and adolescent (early onset) schizophrenia: a review in light of DSM-IIIR. *Journal of Autism and Developmental Disorders* **22**, 601–624.

Werry, J.S. & McClellan, J.M. (1992) Predicting outcome in child and adolescent (early onset) schizophrenia and bipolar disorder. *Journal of the American Academy of Child and Adolescent Psychiatry* **31**, 147–150.

Werry, J.S., McClellan, J.M. & Chard, L. (1991) Childhood and adolescent schizophrenia, bipolar and schizoaffective disorders: a clinical and outcome study. *Journal of the American Academy of Child and Adolescent Psychiatry* **30**, 457–465.

Werry, J.S., McClellan, J.M., Andrews, L. & Ham, M. (1994) Clinical features and outcome of child and adolescent schizophrenia. *Schizophrenia Bulletin* **20**, 619–630.

Woods, B.T. (1998) Is schizophrenia a progressive neurodevelopmental disorder? Toward a unitary pathogeneic mechanism. *American Journal of Psychiatry* **155**, 1661–1670.

World Health Organization (1978) *International Classification of Diseases*, 9th edn (ICD-9). World Health Organization, Geneva.

World Health Organization (1992) *The ICD-10 Classification of Mental and Behavioural Disorders: Diagnostic Criteria for Research*. World Health Organization, Geneva.

Wyatt, R.J. (1995) Early intervention in schizophrenia: can the course be altered? *Biological Psychiatry* **38**, 1–3.

Wykes, T., Reeder, C., Williams, C. *et al.* (2000) Cognitive remediation: predictors of success and durability of improvements [Abstract]. *Schizophrenia Research* **41**, 221.

Yung, A.R., McGorry, P.D., McFarlane, C.A. *et al.* (1996) Monitoring and care of young people at incipient risk of psychosis. *Schizophrenia Bulletin* **22**, 283–303.

Zahn, T.P., Jacobson, L.K., Gordon, C.T. *et al.* (1997) Autonomic nervous system markers of pathophysiology in childhood onset schizophrenia. *Archives of General Psychiatry* **54**, 904–912.

Zahn, T.P., Jacobson, L.K., Gordon, C.T. *et al.* (1998) Attention deficits in childhood onset schizophrenia: reaction time studies. *Journal of Abnormal Psychology* **107**, 97–108.

5 Atypical psychotic disorders

C.B. Pull, J.M. Cloos and N.V. Murthy

Historical background, 54
Transient psychotic disorders, 54
  Bouffées délirantes, 55
  Psychogenic or reactive psychoses, 55
  Schizophreniform psychoses, 55
  Cycloid psychoses, 56
  Culture-specific psychoses, 56
Persistent psychotic or delusional disorders, 56
  Paranoia and paranoid disorders, 56
  Paraphrenia, 57
  Chronic delusional states of French nosology, 58
  Delusional jealousy, 59
  Folie à deux, 59
  Capgras syndrome or *illusion des sosies*, 59
  Erotomania, 59
  Cotard syndrome, 60
  Kretschmer's *sensitiver Beziehungswahn*, 60

Schizotypal (personality) disorder, 60
Atypical psychotic disorders in DSM-IV, 60
  Delusional disorder, 61
  Brief reactive psychosis and brief psychotic disorder, 61
  Schizophreniform disorder, 61
  Schizoaffective disorder, 62
  Shared psychotic disorder, 62
  Schizotypal personality disorder, 62
Atypical psychotic disorders in ICD-10, 62
  Persistent delusional disorder, 62
  Acute and transient psychotic disorders, 63
  Induced delusional disorder, 64
  Schizoaffective disorders, 64
  Schizotypal disorder, 64
Conclusions, 64
References, 64

Atypical psychotic disorders designate psychotic conditions that cannot be easily classified as either schizophrenia or a mood disorder with psychotic features. They form a heterogeneous and poorly understood collection of disorders that are regarded as probably unrelated to schizophrenia and affective disorder, but on which surprisingly little empirical research has been carried out up to now. The terminology used to designate the individual disorders in this group as well as the proportion of patients that are regarded as having one of these disorders varies from country to country.

Atypical psychotic disorders can conveniently be divided according to their typical duration into a group of chronic persistent delusional disorders and a group of acute and transient psychotic disorders.

Schizoaffective disorder is described in a separate chapter and will not be detailed again here.

Historical background

In the successive editions of his *Textbook of Psychiatry* Kraepelin gradually evolved a system of classification to which all subsequent systems have paid tribute. In describing those conditions known today as functional psychoses, Kraepelin leaned heavily on clinical course and prognosis. In the sixth edition of his textbook, Kraepelin (1899) distinguished three classes of psychoses: manic-depressive psychoses, dementia praecox and paranoia. In the eighth edition, Kraepelin (1909–15) introduced the concept of the paraphrenias that are separated from the paranoid form of dementia praecox.

Kraepelin described dementia praecox as a single disease progressing towards 'psychic enfeeblement' (*psychische Schwäche*) and presenting three forms: hebephrenia, catatonia and dementia paranoides. Paranoia was characterized by systematized delusions, without hallucinations and accompanied by perfect presentation of clear and orderly thinking. Paraphrenia shared many of the characteristics of paranoia and schizophrenia. The main difference from paranoia was that in paraphrenia the delusions were accompanied by prominent hallucinations, and the main difference from schizophrenia was that paraphrenia did not progress to a dementia-like state.

Although Kraepelin's nosology was gradually to establish its position, several aspects of his classification have been either neglected or opposed, to varying degrees, depending on national schools of psychiatry. This has led to either an extension or a narrowing of the concept of dementia praecox, and consequently of schizophrenia. In Britain and in the USA, terms such as paranoia and paraphrenia were rarely used in practice, and psychoses that were not organic were classified, up to a recent past, as either schizophrenic or affective (Kendell 1993). The French, Scandinavian and German schools of psychiatry have, on the contrary, excluded from schizophrenia different types of acute and transient psychoses as well as a number of chronic delusional disorders (for a further discussion see Chapter 1).

Transient psychotic disorders

A considerable number of labels have been proposed to designate transient psychotic disorders which are regarded as neither schizophrenic nor affective. Although the different eponyms seem to refer to the same group of patients, systematic clinical information that would give rise to concepts that can be clearly defined and separated from each other is not yet available. The incidence of these disorders seems to be more frequent in developing countries than in other parts of the world (Sartorius *et al.* 1986).

Prominent concepts in this field are the *bouffées délirantes* of the French, the 'reactive' or 'psychogenic' psychoses and the 'schizophreniform' psychoses of the Scandinavian and the 'cycloid psychoses' of the German tradition, as well as a number of so-called culture-bound psychoses.

Bouffées délirantes

The concept of *bouffée délirante polymorphe des dégénérés* was introduced by Magnan and Legrain (1895), at the end of the nineteenth century, as part of a complex classification of the delusional states of degeneracy. The classical description of *bouffée délirante*, as given by Magnan's pupil Legrain (1886), rests on the following criteria:

1 sudden onset, 'like a bolt from the blue';
2 polymorphous delusions and hallucinations of any kind;
3 clouded consciousness associated with emotional instability;
4 absence of physical signs, i.e. the disorder is not caused by any organic mental disorder;
5 rapid return to the premorbid level of functioning; and
6 relapses may occur, but individual episodes are separated by symptom-free intervals.

Whereas Magnan and Legrain stated that *bouffées délirantes* occur without any identifiable precipitating factor, the current consensus holds that there is a variant of the disorder occasioned by psychological stressors.

Using the results of a national enquiry, the present author (Pull *et al.* 1987) has developed explicit diagnostic inclusion and exclusion criteria for both genuine or Magnan type as well as for stress-related *bouffée délirante*. The striking outcome of this enquiry is that the concept of *bouffée délirante*, as used by present-day French psychiatrists, has not changed in 100 years, with the exception that the theory of degeneracy is no longer used.

In the past, the disorder was diagnosed by French psychiatrists nearly three times as frequently as acute schizophrenia (Pichot & Debray 1971). According to Pichot (1990), empirical studies indicate that when stringent diagnostic criteria are applied, the disorder is not commonly reported among new cases. However, the concept of *bouffée délirante polymorphe* remains popular in France, as proven by a recent study in which nearly one-third of acute admissions were diagnosed with this disorder (Ferrey & Zebdi 1999).

Psychogenic or reactive psychoses

The concept of psychogenic or reactive psychosis has been developed in Scandinavia. The first comprehensive survey of the concept of psychogenic psychosis is to be found in a monograph by the Danish psychiatrist Wimmer (1916). According to Wimmer, psychogenic psychoses are clinically independent of schizophrenia and manic-depressive psychosis, usually develop in a predisposed individual, are caused by psychosocial factors (which also determine the content and form of the disorder), have a great tendency to recover and seem never to end in deterioration.

The prognostic validity of psychogenic psychosis has been investigated by Faergeman (1963), who made a follow-up study of Wimmer's cases. Of the 113 original cases of psychogenic psychosis, 66 were confirmed by Faergeman, whereas one-third were rediagnosed as suffering from schizophrenia.

According to Strömgren (1974, 1989), 65% of psychogenic psychoses are emotional reactions, 15% are disorders of consciousness and 20% are paranoid types. The results of a dual mating study suggest that reactive psychoses do not contribute liability factors to the development of schizophrenia or manic-depressive psychosis and that major psychoses do not contribute liability factors to reactive psychosis (Gottesman & Bertelsen 1989).

Pitta and Blay (1997) investigated the concepts of reactive psychoses as they are classified in standardized diagnostic systems by retrospectively applying criteria from DSM-IIIR, DSM-IV, ICD-10 and Present State Examination (PSE) diagnostic systems on 26 cases of reactive psychosis and psychosis not otherwise specified, to evaluate their agreement with those obtained using ICD-9. They found that case-note diagnoses obtained using DSM-IIIR, DSM-IV, ICD-10 criteria and the PSE-CATEGO program show a low level of agreement with ICD-9 diagnoses and although DSM-IIIR provides criteria for brief reactive psychosis, and DSM-IV and ICD-10 provide such criteria for brief or acute psychotic disorder, these bear little relationship to the original concept of the disorder.

Schizophreniform psychoses

The concept of schizophreniform psychosis was described in Norway by Langfeldt (1939). Langfeldt differentiated between two groups of psychoses usually diagnosed as schizophrenia: a group with poor prognosis, labelled 'genuine' or 'process' schizophrenia, and a group with good prognosis, labelled 'schizophreniform' psychosis.

The following factors were considered by Langfeldt to be correlated with good prognosis: a well-adjusted premorbid personality, the presence of identifiable precipitating factors, sudden onset, the presence among an otherwise schizophrenic symptomatology of disturbance of mood, clouding of consciousness and the absence of blunted affect.

A great deal of research (Garmezy 1968; Brockington *et al.* 1978) has been focused on an objective separation between 'process' schizophrenia and 'schizophreniform' psychosis, but there is no decisive evidence that two types are of a qualitatively different nature. Two studies reclassified Langfeldt's 100 cases of schizophreniform psychoses according to ICD-9 and DSM-III (Bergem *et al.* 1990), and DSM-IIIR, respectively (Guldberg *et al.* 1991), and concluded that most of the 'schizophreniform psychoses' turned out to be affective disorders with psychotic features.

Cycloid psychoses

The term 'cycloid psychoses' was coined by Leonhard (1957) to denominate endogenous psychotic syndromes characterized by a sudden onset, an admixture of symptoms belonging to the affective disorders and of symptoms belonging to schizophrenia and phasic course. Leonhard subdivided the cycloid psychoses into three forms: motility psychoses, confusional psychoses and anxiety–blissfulness psychoses.

The concept has been operationalized by Perris (1974) as follows: cycloid psychoses are psychotic episodes of sudden onset, mostly unrelated to stress, with good immediate outcome but with a high risk of recurrence, characterized by mood swings (from depression to elation) and at least two of the following:

1 various degrees of perplexity or confusion;
2 delusions (of reference, influence or persecution) and/or hallucinations not syntonic with mood;
3 motility disturbances (hypo- or hyperkinesia);
4 occasional episodes of ecstasy; and
5 states of overwhelming anxiety (pananxiety).

Findings of several empirical investigations (Cutting *et al.* 1978; Brockington *et al.* 1982; Maj 1990) suggest that cycloid psychoses meeting Perris' criteria represent a relatively consistent pattern of disorder with regard to onset, symptomatology, recurrence, outcome, response to treatment and family history.

The disorder appears to be a distinct nosological entity that differs from both schizophrenia and schizoaffective disorder. Cycloid psychoses predominate in severe postpartum psychiatric disorders (Lanczik *et al.* 1990; Pfuhlmann *et al.* 1998) and seem to constitute a substantial part of psychotic disorders among women (Lindvall *et al.* 1990). Disturbance of fetal brain maturation during the first trimester of gestation caused by maternal respiratory infection via live virus or disturbed maternal immune responses may be involved in the aetiology of cycloid psychoses, because the disorder is significantly associated with first-trimester maternal gestation respiratory infections (Stöber *et al.* 1997). Ventricular abnormalities in patients with cycloid psychoses were found in one study (Franzek *et al.* 1996), while another study showed no significant differences in brain images between normal controls and patients with cycloid psychoses, in contrast to patients with schizophrenia, who showed enlarged ventricles (Hoffler *et al.* 1997). Strik *et al.* (1997) found higher than normal P300 amplitudes in cycloid psychosis compared to normal controls. There were no differences in topographies and latencies. This finding is specific to cycloid psychosis and was explained by a generalized cerebral hyperarousal. Finally, Sigmund and Mundt (1999), using an integrative phenomenological methodology, showed that positive symptoms in cycloid psychosis are different from those of the core schizophrenia. They found absence of abnormalities of: (i) emotional expression and affect; (ii) thought; and (iii) movement impulses and sequences among patients with cycloid psychoses compared with those with schizophrenia.

Culture-specific psychoses

Disorders such as latah, amok, koro, windigo and a variety of other possibly culture-specific disorders share two principal features:

1 they are not easily accommodated by the categories in established and internationally used psychiatric classifications; and
2 they were first described in, and subsequently closely or exclusively associated with, a particular population or cultural area.

These disorders have also been referred to as culture-bound or culture-reactive, and as ethnic or exotic psychoses. Some are rare, some may be comparatively common, and the status of most is controversial. For example, classification of amok remains unsolved and has different criteria in modern psychiatric diagnostic systems when compared with the original Malay understanding of the term (Kon 1994; Hatta 1996). However, many researchers argue that culture-specific psychoses differ only in degree from disorders already included in existing classifications. As suggested by the tentative assignment of culture-specific disorders to categories in the ICD-10 (World Health Organization 1993), it would appear that most of these disorders are not even related to any identified psychosis, but rather to varying personality disorders, somatoform disorders, dissociative disorders or that they represent acute reactions to stress.

A list of culture-specific disorders and the codes suggested in ICD-10 for classifying them is given in Table 5.1.

Persistent psychotic or delusional disorders

The number and nature of persistent psychotic or delusional disorders that are regarded as neither schizophrenic nor affective varies greatly from country to country. Prominent in this field are the concepts of paranoia and paraphrenia, the *délires chroniques* of the French tradition, as well as a variety of other concepts, either included in the preceding or separated from them, such as delusional jealousy, *folie à deux*, Capgras syndrome, erotomania, Cotard syndrome, Kretschmer *sensitiver Beziehungswahn* and the more recent category of schizotypal disorder.

Paranoia and paranoid disorders

In the times before Kraepelin, the term paranoia was applied to a number of quite different disorders. In the eighth edition of his textbook, Kraepelin (1909–15) restricted the term to a group of psychoses characterized by the development of a permanent and unshakeable delusional system without hallucinations, accompanied by clear and orderly thinking, willing and acting. Kraepelin described different subtypes of paranoia, depending on the content of the delusions (persecutory, grandiose or jealous).

Since Kraepelin, the independence of paranoia from affective disorder and schizophrenia has been the object of much debate.

Table 5.1 Culture-bound syndromes and suggested ICD-10 codes.

Local term	ICD-10	Suggested code
Amok	F68.8	Other specified disorders of adult personality and behaviour
Dhat, dhatu, jiryan, shen-k'uei, shen-kui	F48.8 F45.34	Other specified neurotic disorders Somatoform autonomic dysfunction of the genitourinary system
Koro, jinjin bemar, suk yeong, suo-yang	F48.8 F45.34	Other specified neurotic disorders Somatoform autonomic dysfunction of the genitourinary system
Latah	F48.8 F44.88	Other specified neurotic disorders Other specified dissociative disorders
Nerfiza, nerves, nevra, nervios	F32.11 F48.0 F45.1	Moderate depressive episode with somatic syndrome Neurasthenia Undifferentiated somatoform disorder
Pa-leng, frigophobia	F40.2	Specific phobias
Pibloktoq, Arctic hysteria	F44.7 F44.88	Mixed dissociative disorders Other specified dissociative disorders
Susto, espanto	F45.1 F48.8	Undifferentiated somatoform disorder Other specified neurotic disorders
Taijin kyofusho, shinkeishitsu, anthropophobia	F40.1 F40.8	Social phobias Other phobic anxiety disorders
Ufufuyane, saka	F44.3 F44.7	Trance and possession disorders Mixed dissociative disorders
Uqamairineq	F44.88 F47.4	Other specified dissociative disorders Narcolepsy and cataplexy
Windigo	F68.8	Other specified disorders of adult personality and behaviour

In his 1980 literature review, Kendler concluded that the available data did not suggest that paranoia is a subtype of affective illness and that 'the bulk of the evidence suggests that paranoia and schizophrenia are distinct syndromes'.

The term 'paranoid disorders', which embraces paranoia, paraphrenia and a number of other delusional syndromes, has been the object of much controversy, in particular because the adjective 'paranoid' has had multiple different meanings over time and in different languages. In its original German meaning, it refers to all delusions relating to the subject. In the English-speaking community, it has been restricted by and large to designate persecutory delusions (Kendell 1993). In France, the term 'paranoïde' is used exclusively to differentiate a particular form of schizophrenia, i.e. paranoid schizophrenia (Pichot 1990). In current nomenclatures, the term 'delusional disorder' has been adopted for this group of disorders (Schmidt-Degenhard 1998; Schanda 2000).

Evidence supporting the independence of paranoia from schizophrenia comes primarily from family history studies (Kendler *et al*. 1981, 1985) and from course and outcome

studies (Opjordsmoen & Retterstol 1987; Schanda & Gariel 1988). However, a case–control epidemiological family study has demonstrated significant familial relationship between non-schizophrenic non-affective psychoses (schizoaffective disorder, schizophreniform disorder, delusional disorder and atypical psychosis) and schizophrenia and schizotypal disorder (Kendler *et al*. 1993).

Paraphrenia

The concept of paraphrenia was introduced by Kraepelin in the later editions of his textbook. Kraepelin described four types of paraphrenia: systematic, expansive, confabulatory and fantastic. For Kraepelin, paraphrenias could be distinguished from dementia praecox by the absence of deterioration despite a protracted course, and from paranoia because they were accompanied by prominent auditory hallucinations.

The independence of paraphrenia from schizophrenia has been questioned early on and, although the term has been part of most classifications up to a recent past, paraphrenia has been generally subsumed under schizophrenia. It appears that some psychiatrists recognize paraphrenia as a viable diagnostic entity, but label it 'atypical psychosis', 'schizoaffective disorder' or 'delusional disorder' for lack of a better diagnostic category in current diagnostic systems (Ravindran *et al.* 1999).

'Late paraphrenia' was defined by Roth (1955) as a well-organized system of paranoid delusions, with or without auditory hallucinations, existing in the setting of a well-presented personality and affective response. Paranoid psychoses with onset in late life appear to be rather heterogeneous (Almeida *et al.* 1995) and strongly associated with cognitive impairment (Forsell & Henderson 1998). Whether or not late paraphrenia should be considered a separate, although clinically not homogeneous, entity (Holden 1987) or a late-onset form of schizophrenia (Grahame 1984) continues to be debated up to the present (Howard *et al.* 1993); however, the high degree of similarity between patients with late paraphrenia provides a strong argument for the retention of the diagnosis as a clinical entity (Howard *et al.* 1994).

Chronic delusional states of French nosology

French psychiatrists traditionally separate from paranoid schizophrenia an important proportion of cases labelled *délires chroniques* (chronic delusional states). Chronic delusional states are subdivided into three broad categories:
1 chronic interpretative psychosis (also known as systematized or paranoiac psychosis);
2 chronic hallucinatory psychosis;
3 chronic imaginative (or paraphrenic or fantastic) psychosis.

Chronic interpretative psychosis

Chronic interpretative psychosis is subdivided into intellectual and emotional delusional states, according to the content of the delusional system and to whether or not the delusions are 'polarized' around a single theme.

In intellectual delusional states, the delusions spread progressively to contaminate all areas of mental activity. The original description of the disorder was provided by Sérieux and Capgras (1909). The disorder is defined by the authors as a chronic systematized psychosis, feeding on delusional interpretations and characterized by false reasoning originating in the misinterpretation of otherwise correctly perceived facts. The other essential features listed by Sérieux and Capgras are:
1 the complexity and coherence of the delusions;
2 the absence of prominent hallucinations;
3 unimpaired intellectual functioning;
4 progressive spreading of the delusional system; and
5 chronic course.
As described in current standard French textbooks, the disorder is essentially the same as that described in other nomenclatures by the term 'paranoia'.

In emotional delusional states, the delusional premise does not spread beyond the theme and person(s) involved in the original system. The disorder has been described by Sérieux and Capgras (1909) as a chronic systematized psychosis, in which a single, relentless and patently pathological thought subdues and dominates all other mental activity. The most commonly described variants are: (i) the vindictive delusional states of litigious persons, social reformers, religious fanatics or secretive inventors; and (ii) delusional jealousy and erotomania.

Emotional delusional states have been particularly well described by de Clérambault (in a series of papers collected in 1942), according to whom these disorders are characterized by a central delusional premise: 'I am the victim of an injustice', in the case of vindictive delusional states; 'he (she) is unfaithful to me', in delusional jealousy; and 'he (she) loves me', in erotomania.

A theoretical diagram of the traditional French classification of chronic interpretative psychosis (Pichot 1990) is presented in Table 5.2.

Chronic hallucinatory psychosis

Chronic hallucinatory psychosis was first described by Ballet (1911) as a disorder characterized by:

Table 5.2 Theoretical diagram of the traditional French classification of chronic delusional states. (From Pichot 1990.)

Class	Genus	Species	Variants
Chronic interpretative psychosis	Intellectual delusional states (not encapsulated)	Interpretative delusional states	
		Hypersensitive delusional states	Paranoia of spinsters and governesses Paranoia of immigrants or of culture shock
	Emotional delusional states (encapsulated)	Vindictive delusional states	Litigious paranoia Paranoia of social reformers and religious fanatics Paranoia of secretive inventors
		Sentimental delusional states	Conjugal paranoia Erotic paranoia (erotomania)

1 persistent hallucinatory activity;
2 delusions, most frequently of persecution; and
3 clear sensorium, unimpaired speech, appropriate behaviour and intact higher intellectual functions.

In addition to the preceding features, current explicit diagnostic criteria (Pull *et al.* 1987) emphasize the absence of schizophrenic thought disorder, onset in middle or late adult life, and relatively good psychosocial adjustment.

Chronic imaginative psychosis

Chronic imaginative psychosis was originally described by Dupré and Logre (1911). The disorder is characterized by paralogical magical thinking, fantastic and grandiose delusions, the predominance of confabulatory delusional mechanisms and good contact with reality contrasting with the extravagance of the delusions. The diagnosis is rarely made by French psychiatrists in the present day.

Delusional jealousy

Also called pathological jealousy, morbid jealousy or Othello syndrome, this disorder is characterized by an abnormal belief that one's sexual partner is unfaithful. According to Gelder *et al.* (1989), the condition is not uncommon in psychiatric practice and most full-time clinicians probably see one or two cases a year. As indicated by the result of surveys of subjects with delusional jealousy (Langfeldt 1961; Shepherd 1961; Mowat 1966; Vauhkonen 1968; Mullen & Maack 1985), the disorder is more frequent in men than women and may be present in demented patients (Breitner & Anderson 1994; Tsai *et al.* 1997). The prognosis depends on a number of factors, including the nature of any underlying psychiatric disorder and the patient's premorbid personality, and there is a risk that the patient may become violent to his or her partner or supposed rival. Delusional jealousy therefore continues to be an important subject for forensic psychiatry (Leong *et al.* 1994; Silva *et al.* 1998).

Folie à deux

Folie à deux was first described by Lasègue and Falret (1877), as a disorder in which the delusions held by a sick person are induced in, or shared by, a healthy person. The disorder, which may involve more than two people, typically develops in persons who are isolated from other people. Usually, the healthy partner(s) will lose the delusional beliefs when the relationship with the primary person is interrupted. The concept of *folie à deux*, which is listed apart in other nomenclatures, is not considered an independent disorder in traditional French nosology, but is subsumed under the category of interpretative delusional states. Modern nomenclatures also use the terms 'shared psychotic disorder' (DSM-IV) or 'induced delusional disorder' (ICD-10).

Capgras syndrome or *illusion des sosies*

Illusion des sosies was described by Capgras and Reboul-Lachaux (1923) as a delusional disorder in which the patient, usually a woman, is convinced that a particular person in her life, such as her husband or another person who is quite familiar and well known to her, has been replaced by a double (*sosie*), i.e. a look-alike impostor. Although originally described in France, the syndrome has received more attention in other countries (Sims & Reddie 1976) than in France, where the concept is hardly used at all. More than a dozen varieties of delusional misidentification have been reported in the psychiatric and neurological literature (Anderson & Williams 1994; de Pauw 1994a; Weinstein 1994; Ellis *et al.* 1996).

Capgras syndrome appears in both men and women over a wide age range and in a variety of illness states. In particular, the syndrome is associated with schizophrenia in more than half the cases (Berson 1983; Odom-White *et al.* 1995). Traditionally, the disorder was considered to have its origins in psychodynamic conflicts (de Pauw 1994b; Debruille & Stip 1996), but more recently another hypothesis, resulting from the observation of a high percentage of organic disorders associated with the syndrome, proposes a neuroanatomical and neuropsychological model for the delusion, involving the right hemisphere (Ellis 1994; Signer 1994). In a recent review of the phenomenology and cognitive neuropsychological origins of the Capgras syndrome, the authors report neuroimaging evidence suggesting right hemisphere abnormalities, particularly in the frontal and temporal regions. Neuropsychological research, reporting impairments in facial processing (a right hemisphere function), provides empirical support for these findings (Edelstyn & Oyebode 1999).

Erotomania

Also called de Clérambault syndrome outside of France, erotomania represents one of the emotional delusional states (*délires passionnels*) described by de Clérambault. The subject, usually a woman, is unshakably but unjustifiably convinced that another person, usually a man of higher social status or famous as a public figure, is infatuated with her. She finds 'proof' of his love for her everywhere, e.g. in casual remarks or in the way he dresses. In the beginning, the patient is quite confident that her 'lover' will eventually be able to come out of hiding, and tries to convince him with letters, phone calls or gifts. In the later stages of the disorder, the patient may become resentful, abusive, spiteful and even aggressive.

Recent reports suggest that erotomania is an aetiologically heterogeneous syndrome, which may be seen in a variety of mental disorders, most commonly in schizophrenia (Sims & White 1973; Jordan & Howe 1980; Ellis & Mellsop 1985). The presence of erotomania has also been noted in other conditions, including depression (Raskin & Sullivan 1974; Staner 1991), bipolar disorder (Remington & Book 1984; Signer & Swinson

1987; Signer 1991a) and organic mental disorder (Signer & Cummings 1987).

De Clérambault's original description of erotomania as a syndrome of pathological emotions that follow an orderly evolution differs from Kraeplin's views on erotomania, who placed the disorder among the paranoias (Signer 1991b). The term has undergone a number of reformulations in recent times and is now included in contemporary definitions as a specific form of delusional disorder ('erotomanic type'), characterized by delusional beliefs of being loved. This restrictive modern definition has been questioned by professionals involved in the research on 'stalking', a form of human behaviour characterized by obsessional following and harassing of a specific individual which now constitutes a criminal offence in most English-speaking nations, and in which erotomania often plays an important part (Mullen et al. 2000).

Cotard syndrome

Under the name *délire de négation*, Cotard (1880, 1882) described patients who complained of having lost not only their possessions and social status, but also their hearts, blood, intestines or brains. Currently, the term is often confined to the belief of being dead, which is conceptually too restrictive (Berrios & Luque 1995a). It has become rarer in recent years, at least in its complete form, probably because the underlying disorder responds to pharmacotherapy before the psychopathological manifestations of the syndrome develop. The syndrome is usually associated with severe forms of depression and chronic forms of the syndrome may occur in organic mental disorders.

A review of 100 cases of Cotard syndrome reported since 1880 found differences between younger and older subjects, the latter showing more organic disorder, auditory hallucinations and delusions of non-existence (Berrios & Luque 1995b). The cases were classified into a 'type I' group, being closer to the delusional than the affective disorders, and a mixed 'type II' group showing anxiety, depression and auditory hallucinations (Berrios & Luque 1995b). Some support exists that right hemisphere dysfunction, such as perceptual impairment and abnormal perceptual experience as well as an incorrect interpretation of these, contributes to the development of the syndrome, thus showing similarities to the neuropsychological origins of Capgras syndrome (Young et al. 1994; Gerrans 2000).

Kretschmer's *sensitiver Beziehungswahn*

In a monograph published in 1918, Kretschmer described a type of paranoia which developed in sensitive personalities when a precipitating event, termed key experience (*Schlüsselerlebnis*), occurred at the correct time in the person's life. According to Kretschmer, the prognosis was good. In particular, patients with the disorder did not develop schizophrenia. According to Pichot (1983), Kretschmer's description was to have a major impact on psychiatric thinking. By setting forth that a particular delu-

sional state could be 'understood', Kretschmer 'opened the path to the dissolution of process endogeny and the establishment of the psychogenic conception of the psychoses'.

Schizotypal (personality) disorder
(see also Chapter 7)

The term schizotypal was introduced to modern psychiatric nosology largely as the result of family studies in schizophrenia (Kety et al. 1978; Kendler et al. 1981). The disorder is more common among family members of individuals with schizophrenia and is part of the genetic 'spectrum' of disorders associated with schizophrenia. Schizotypal disorder is characterized by eccentric behaviour and anomalies of thinking and affect which resemble those seen in schizophrenia, and has been demonstrated to have phenomenological, biological, treatment and outcome characteristics similar to those of schizophrenia, although no definite and characteristic schizophrenic anomalies have occurred at any stage and no single feature is invariably present. Patients with schizotypal disorder show cognitive impairment as in schizophrenia, but the impairment appears to be more focal and involves mainly working memory, verbal learning and sustained attention rather than generalized intellectual deficits. Temporal lobe volume is reduced, as in schizophrenic patients, but the frontal lobe functions seem to be intact, thus preventing the more severe cognitive and social deteriorations seen in schizophrenia. A better capacity for compensatory buffering in lateral and subcortical brain regions may also explain the lower susceptibility of schizotypal patients to psychotic symptoms (Kirrane & Siever 2000).

The disorder is sometimes difficult to differentiate either from simple schizophrenia or from schizoid or paranoid personality disorders. It runs a chronic course with fluctuations of intensity. There is no definite onset and the evolution and course resemble those of a personality disorder. Schizotypal disorder is therefore listed among the personality disorders in DSM-IV, while ICD-10 places it under the atypical psychotic disorders.

Atypical psychotic disorders in DSM-IV
(for a further dicussion of classification issues and a comparison of DSM-IV and ICD-10 see Chapter 1)

In DSM-IV of the American Psychiatric Association (1994), atypical psychotic disorders (as defined here) are described under the heading 'Schizophrenia and Other Psychotic Disorders'. DSM-IV lists five major disorders in this section:
1 delusional disorder;
2 brief psychotic disorder;
3 schizophreniform disorder;
4 schizoaffective disorder;
5 induced or shared psychotic disorder (*folie à deux*).
Schizotypal disorder is listed among the personality disorders.

Table 5.3 DSM-IV classification of non-organic atypical psychotic disorders.

295.40	Schizophreniform disorder
	Specify if:
	    without good prognostic features
	    with good prognostic features

295.70	Schizoaffective disorder
	Specify type:
	    bipolar
	    depressive

297.1	Delusional disorder
	Specify type:
	    erotomanic, grandiose
	    jealous, persecutory
	    somatic, mixed, unspecified

298.8	Brief psychotic disorder
	Specify type:
	    with marked stressor(s) (brief reactive)
	    without marked stressor(s)
	    with postpartum onset

297.3	Shared psychotic disorder (*folie à deux*)
298.9	Psychotic disorder not otherwise specified

The DSM-IV classification of atypical psychotic disorders is presented in Table 5.3. Important changes have been made in the nomenclature and description of 'atypical' psychotic disorders from DSM-III (American Psychiatric Association 1981) to DSM-IIIR (American Psychiatric Association 1987; Kendler *et al.* 1989), and again from DSM-IIIR to DSM-IV (American Psychiatric Association 1994).

Delusional disorder

According to the DSM, current evidence from demographic, family and follow-up studies suggests that delusional disorder is probably distinct from both schizophrenia and mood disorders. In the three recent editions of the classification, the essential feature of the disorder is the presence of one or more persistent delusions that are not caused by any other mental disorder, such as schizophrenia, schizophreniform disorder, a mood disorder, an organic factor or the direct effects of a substance. Apart from the impact of the delusion(s) or its ramifications, functioning is not markedly impaired and behaviour is not obviously odd or bizarre.

The term 'paranoid', which was used in DSM-III to designate this type of disorder, has been changed to 'delusional' disorder in DSM-IIIR and DSM-IV. While the diagnosis of paranoid disorder could only be applied to people with delusions of persecution or jealousy, the inclusion criteria for delusional disorder are much broader in that they require only the presence of one or more 'non-bizarre' (non-schizophrenic) delusions, without further specification.

Two other important changes that were made in the criteria for delusional disorder in DSM-IIIR have been retained in DSM-IV. First, the minimum duration of the disorder has been increased from 1 week to 1 month and, secondly, persistent tactile and olfactory hallucinations are no longer excluded if related to the delusional theme (whereas auditory or visual hallucinations may not be present for more than a few hours).

Delusional disorder can be subdivided according to the predominant delusional theme in erotomanic type, grandiose type, jealous type, persecutory type, somatic type, mixed type (when delusions characteristic of more than one type are present but no one theme predominates) or unspecified type.

Although the prevalence is low, the disorder is not rare. Age of onset is usually middle or late adulthood; the older age being associated with the persecutory type, the younger with the somatic type (Yamada *et al.* 1998). The course is variable. Familial transmission is suspected and comorbid mood disorders may be present (Manschreck 1996). Cases seem to respond equally well to treatment whatever the specific delusional content and, when adequately treated, the prognosis is reasonably good (Munro & Mok 1995).

Campana *et al.* (1998) studied eye-tracking abnormalities in patients with delusional disorder and compared them with normal controls. They found abnormalities in smooth pursuit eye movements, which they concluded indicates a cerebral dysfunction similar to those detected in patients with schizophrenia.

Brief reactive psychosis and brief psychotic disorder

In DSM-III, the essential feature of brief reactive psychosis is the sudden onset of psychotic symptoms shortly after a recognizable psychosocial stressor, persisting for no more than 2 weeks, and with a full return to the premorbid level of functioning. In DSM-IIIR, the maximum duration of the disorder has been increased from 2 to 4 weeks, and there is acknowledgement that the stressors may be cumulative.

In DSM-IV, brief reactive disorder is listed as a subtype of a new category labelled brief psychotic disorder. The disorder is subdivided into three subtypes: with marked stressor(s), corresponding to the definition of brief reactive psychosis; without marked stressor(s); and with postpartum onset.

Schizophreniform disorder

The essential features of this disorder are identical to those of schizophrenia, with the exception that the duration is less than 6 months (but at least 1 month). Two subtypes may be specified, according to the presence or absence of 'good prognostic features' such as rapid onset, confusion or perplexity, good premorbid functioning and absence of blunted or flat affect.

There is little support for 'schizophreniform disorder' as a distinct diagnostic entity and a subtype of schizophrenia or affective illness. The clinical utility of the diagnosis is limited because it identifies a heterogeneous group of patients with new-onset schizophrenia, schizoaffective disorder and atypical affective disorder and only a small subgroup with a remitting non-affective psychosis, and a substantial number of patients are being rediagnosed during follow-up as schizophrenic. A review suggests that patients meeting criteria for schizophreniform disorder should instead be diagnosed as having 'psychotic disorder not otherwise specified' until additional clinical information (e.g. course of illness) becomes available (Strakowski 1994). Furthermore, the recent demonstration of impaired antioxidant defence and higher plasma lipid peroxides in unmedicated schizophreniform disorder than in normal controls was similar to the findings in unmedicated patients with first-episode schizophrenia (Mahadik *et al.* 1998). In addition, significantly higher soluble interleukin 2 receptor (sIL-2R) levels than normal controls were found in the sera of patients with both schizophrenia and schizophreniform disorder, thus implicating similar immunological mechanisms in both (Gaughran *et al.* 1998).

Schizoaffective disorder

The definition of schizoaffective disorder has been modified from DSM-III to DSM-IIIR, and again from DSM-IIIR to DSM-IV. In DSM-IV, the diagnosis is given to individuals who have had an uninterrupted period of illness during which, at some time, there was a major depressive episode or manic episode concurrent with symptoms of schizophrenia. During the same period of illness, there must have been delusions and hallucinations for at least 2 weeks in the absence of prominent mood symptoms. In addition, symptoms meeting criteria for a mood episode must be present for a substantial portion of the total duration of the illness.

Shared psychotic disorder

The DSM-IV definition of shared delusional disorder corresponds to the original description of *folie à deux* given by Lasègue and Falret (1877). A critical review of 61 case reports from 1942 to 1943 reveals that:
1 males and females were affected with equal frequency;
2 prevalence was equal in younger and older patients;
3 the majority of shared psychoses (90.2%) were equally distributed among married couples, siblings and parent–child dyads;
4 comorbid dementia, depression and mental retardation were common;
5 hallucinations were common; and
6 the majority of dyads (67.3%) were socially isolated.
The article concludes that shared psychotic disorder probably occurs in premorbidly disposed individuals in the context of social isolation that is shared with a psychotic person (Silveira & Seeman 1995).

Schizotypal personality disorder

In DSM-III, DSM-IIIR and DSM-IV, schizotypal disorder is listed among the personality disorders.

Atypical psychotic disorders in ICD-10

In ICD-10 (WHO 1992; Sartorius *et al.* 1993), atypical psychotic disorders (as defined here) are subdivided into five groups:
1 persistent delusional disorders;
2 acute and transient psychotic disorders;
3 induced delusional disorder;
4 schizoaffective disorder;
5 schizotypal disorder.
The ICD-10 classification of atypical psychotic disorders is presented in Table 5.4.

Persistent delusional disorder

The group of persistent delusional disorders includes a variety of disorders in which long-standing delusions constitute the only, or the most conspicuous, clinical characteristic, and which can-

Table 5.4 ICD-10 classification of non-organic atypical psychotic disorders.

F21	Schizotypal disorder	
F22	Persistent delusional disorders	
	F22.0	Delusional disorder (the following types may be specified if desired: persecutory, litiginous, self-referential, grandiose, hypochondriacal, jealous, erotomanic
	F22.8	Other persistent delusional disorders
	F22.9	Persistent delusional disorder, unspecified
F23	Acute and transient psychotic disorders	
	F23.0	Acute polymorphic psychotic disorder without symptoms of schizophrenia
	F23.1	Acute polymorphic psychotic disorder with symptoms of schizophrenia
	F23.2	Acute schizophrenia-like psychotic disorder
	F23.3	Other acute predominantly delusional psychotic disorder
	F23.8	Other acute and transient psychotic disorders
	F23.9	Acute and transient psychotic disorders, unspecified
	A fifth character may be used to identify the presence or absence of associated acute stress:	
	F23.x0	Without associated acute stress
	F23.x1	With associated acute stress
F24	Induced delusional disorder	
F25	Schizoaffective disorders	
	F25.0	Schizoaffective disorder, manic type
	F25.1	Schizoaffective disorder, depressed type
	F25.2	Schizoaffective disorder, mixed type
	F25.8	Other schizoaffective disorders
	F25.9	Schizoaffective disorder, unspecified
F28	Other non-organic psychotic disorders	
F29	Unspecified non-organic psychosis	

not be classified as organic, schizophrenic or affective. They are probably heterogeneous and have uncertain relationships to schizophrenia. The relative importance of genetic factors, personality characteristics and life circumstances in their genesis is uncertain and probably variable.

The category is subdivided into delusional disorder, other persistent delusional disorder and unspecified persistent delusional disorder.

Delusional disorder is characterized by the development of either a single delusion or a set of related delusions other than those listed as typically schizophrenic. The delusions are highly variable in content, the most common examples being persecutory, grandiose, hypochondriacal, jealous or erotic. They must be present for at least 3 months; they are usually persistent and sometimes lifelong. Persistent hallucinations in any modality must not be present and the general criteria of schizophrenia must not be fulfilled. Depressive symptoms may be present intermittently, provided that the delusions persist at times when there is no disturbance of mood. The following subtypes may be specified: persecutory, litigious, self-referential, grandiose, hypochondriacal or somatic, jealous and erotomanic.

The diagnostic criteria for research that are posed in ICD-10 for delusional disorder are presented in Table 5.5.

The category 'other persistent delusional disorders' should be used to classify disorders in which delusions are accompanied by persistent hallucinatory voices or by schizophrenic symptoms that are insufficient to meet the criteria for schizophrenia.

Table 5.5 Delusional disorder: ICD-10 diagnostic criteria for research.

A   A delusion or set of related delusions, other than those listed as typically schizophrenic (i.e. other than completely impossible or culturally inappropriate), must be present. The most common examples are persecutory, grandiose, hypochondriacal, jealous or erotic delusions

B   The delusion(s) in the first criterion must be present for at least 3 months

C   The general criteria for schizophrenia are not fulfilled

D   There must be no persistent hallucinations in any modality (but there may be transitory or occasional auditory hallucinations that are not in the third person or giving a running commentary)

E   Depressive symptoms (or even a depressive episode) may be present intermittently, provided that the delusions persist at times when there is no disturbance of mood

F   Most commonly used exclusion criteria. There must be no evidence of primary or secondary organic mental disorder, or of a psychotic disorder as a result of psychoactive substance use

Specification for possible subtypes. The following types may be specified if desired: persecutory, litiginous, self-referential, grandiose, hypochondriacal (somatic), jealous, erotomanic

Acute and transient psychotic disorders

ICD-10 explicitly recognizes that systematic clinical information that should provide definite guidance on the classification of acute and transient psychotic disorders is not yet available, and the limited data and clinical tradition that must therefore be used instead do not give rise to concepts that can be clearly defined and separated from each other.

The general diagnostic criteria for research that are proposed in ICD-10 for the group of acute and transient psychotic disorders are presented in Table 5.6.

To classify the disorders in this group, ICD-10 uses a diagnostic sequence that reflects the order of priority given to selected key features. Acute and transient psychotic disorders are subdivided according to whether the onset is acute (within a period of 2 weeks or less) or abrupt (within 48 h or less), whether the typical syndrome is polymorphic or typical of schizophrenia, and whether or not it is associated with acute stress. None of the disorders in the group meets the criteria for manic or depressive episodes, although emotional changes may be prominent from time to time. The disorders are also defined by the absence of

Table 5.6 Acute and transient psychotic disorders: ICD-10 diagnostic criteria for research.

G1   There is acute onset of delusions, hallucinations, incomprehensible or incoherent speech, or any combination of these. The interval between the first appearance of any psychotic symptoms and the presentation of the fully developed disorder should not exceed 2 weeks

G2   If transient states of perplexity, misidentification or impairment of attention and concentration are present, they do not fulfil the criteria for organically caused clouding of consciousness

G3   The disorder does not meet the symptomatic criteria for manic episode, depressive episode or recurrent depressive disorder

G4   There is insufficient evidence of recent psychoactive substance use to fulfil the criteria for intoxication, harmful use, dependence or withdrawal states. The continued moderate and largely unchanged use of alcohol or drugs in amounts or with the frequency to which the individual is accustomed does not necessarily rule out the use of this category; this must be decided by clinical judgement and the requirements of the research project in question

G5   Most commonly used exclusion clause. There must be no organic mental disorder or serious metabolic disturbances affecting the central nervous system (this does not include childbirth)

A fifth character should be used to specify whether the acute onset of the disorder is associated with acute stress (occurring 2 weeks or less before evidence of first psychotic symptoms)

For research purposes it is recommended that change of the disorder from a non-psychotic to a clearly psychotic state is further specified as either abrupt (onset within 48 h) or acute (onset in more than 48 h but less than 2 weeks)

organic causation and should not be diagnosed in the presence of obvious intoxication by a psychoactive substance.

The syndrome called 'polymorphic' is defined as a rapidly changing and variable state in which hallucinations, delusions, perceptual disturbances and emotional turmoil with intense feelings of happiness and ecstasy or anxiety and irritability are obvious but markedly variable, changing from day to day or even from hour to hour.

The most appropriate duration of acute and transient psychotic disorders is specified with regard to the duration of symptoms required for a diagnosis of schizophrenia and persistent delusional disorders. In ICD-10, the diagnosis of schizophrenia depends upon the presence of typical schizophrenic symptoms that persist for at least 1 month. When schizophrenic symptoms are consistently present during an acute psychotic disorder, the diagnosis should be changed to schizophrenia if the schizophrenic symptoms persist for more than 1 month. For patients with psychotic, but non-schizophrenic, symptoms that persist beyond 1 month, there is no need to change the diagnosis until the duration requirement of delusional disorder is reached (3 months).

Fifty-one patients with ICD-10 acute and transient psychotic disorder were followed up by a Danish team (Jorgensen *et al*. 1996). According to DSM-IV criteria these patients were classified into three diagnostic categories: schizophreniform disorder (41%), brief psychotic disorder (33%) and psychotic disorder not otherwise classified (25%). After a 1-year follow-up, the authors found that 52% of the patients had diagnostic stability. The rest had their diagnosis changed to either affective disorder (28%) or schizophrenia (15%). Demographic, social and clinical data could not differentiate between patients who changed their diagnosis and those who did not. Patients with an unchanged diagnosis continued to functioned fairly well throughout the year psychosocially, but brief psychotic episodes with an acute onset may also be an early manifestation of severe mental disorder (Jorgensen *et al*. 1997).

Induced delusional disorder

The ICD-10 definition of induced delusional disorder corresponds to the original description by Lasègue and Falret (1877).

Schizoaffective disorders

According to ICD-10, schizoaffective disorders are episodic disorders in which both affective and schizophrenic symptoms are prominent within the same episode of illness, and concurrently for at least part of the episode. The diagnosis rests upon an approximate equilibrium between the number, severity and duration of schizophrenic and affective symptoms. The disorder is subdivided into manic, depressive and mixed types. Two further subtypes may be specified according to the longitudinal development of the disorder, i.e. to whether or not schizophrenic symptoms persist beyond the duration of affective symptoms.

Table 5.7 Schizotypal disorder: ICD-10 diagnostic criteria for research.

A   The subject must have manifested at least four of the following over a period of at least 2 years, either continuously or repeatedly:
   1   Inappropriate or constricted affect, with the individual appearing cold and aloof
   2   Behaviour or appearance that is odd, eccentric or peculiar
   3   Poor rapport with others and a tendency to social withdrawal
   4   Odd beliefs or magical thinking, influencing behaviour and inconsistent with subcultural norms
   5   Suspiciousness or paranoid ideas
   6   Ruminations without inner resistance, often with dysmorphophobic, sexual or aggressive contents
   7   Unusual perceptual experiences, including somatosensory (bodily) or other illusions, depersonalization or derealization
   8   Vague, circumstantial, metaphoric, overelaborate or often stereotyped thinking, manifested by odd speech or in other ways, without gross incoherence
   9   Occasional transient quasipsychotic episodes with intense illusions, auditory or other hallucinations and delusion-like ideas, usually occurring without external provocation

B   The subject must never have met the criteria for schizophrenia

Schizotypal disorder

In ICD-10, schizotypal disorder is listed together with schizophrenia and delusional disorders. The diagnostic criteria for research that are proposed in ICD-10 for schizotypal disorder are presented in Table 5.7.

Conclusions

Atypical psychotic disorders represent a heterogeneous and poorly understood group of disorders. The nomenclature of these disorders is as uncertain as their nosological status. Little empirical evidence has been available up to now, and the limited data and clinical tradition used instead to define these disorders have generated concepts that remain controversial. However, there seems to be considerable international consensus as to which of these disorders should be classified, at least provisionally, apart from schizophrenia and the mood disorders. It is hoped that the specified atypical psychotic disorders that have been included in recent classification systems will lead to widespread critical appraisal of their usefulness and to increasingly rigorous empirical investigations into their true clinical value.

References

Almeida, O.P., Howard, R.J., Levy, R., *et al*. (1995) Clinical and cognitive diversity of psychotic states arising in late life (late paraphrenia). *Psychological Medicine* 25, 699–714.

American Psychiatric Association (1981) *Diagnostic and Statistical Manual of Mental Disorder (DSM-III)*, 3rd edn. American Psychiatric Association, Washington, DC.

American Psychiatric Association (1987) *Diagnostic and Statistical Manuel of Mental Disorder (DSM-IIIR)*, revised 3rd edn. American Psychiatric Association, Washington, DC.

American Psychiatric Association (1994) *Diagnostic and Statistical Manuel of Mental Disorder (DSM-IV)*, 4th edn. American Psychiatric Association, Washington, DC.

Anderson, D.N. & Williams, E. (1994) The delusion of inanimate doubles. *Psychopathology* 27, 220–225.

Ballet, G. (1911) La psychose hallucinatoire chronique. *Encéphale* 11, 401–411.

Bergem, A.M., Dahl, A.A., Guldberg, C.A. & Hansen, H. (1990) Langfeldt's schizophreniform psychoses fifty years later. *British Journal of Psychiatry* 157, 351–354.

Berrios, G.E. & Luque, R. (1995a) Cotard's delusion or syndrome? A conceptual history. *Comprehensive Psychiatry* 36, 218–223.

Berrios, G.E. & Luque, R. (1995b) Cotard's syndrome: analysis of 100 cases. *Acta Psychiatrica Scandinavica* 91, 185–188.

Berson, R.J. (1983) Capgras' syndrome. *American Journal of Psychiatry* 140, 969–978.

Breitner, B.C.C. & Anderson, D.N. (1994) The organic and psychological antecedents of delusional jealousy in old age. *International Journal of Geriatric Psychiatry* 9, 703–707.

Brockington, I.F., Kendell, R.E. & Leff, J.P. (1978) Definitions of schizophrenia: concordance and prediction of outcome. *Psychological Medicine* 8, 387–398.

Brockington, I.F., Perris, C., Kendell, R.E., Hillier, V.E. & Wainwright, S. (1982) The course and outcome of cycloid psychosis. *Psychological Medicine* 12, 97–105.

Campana, A., Gambini, O. & Scarone, S. (1998) Delusional disorder and eye tracking dysfunction: preliminary evidence of biological and clinical heterogeneity. *Schizophrenia Research* 30, 51–58.

Capgras, J. & Reboul-Lachaux, J. (1923) L'illusion des 'sosies' dans un délire systématisé chronique. *Annales Médico-Psychologiques* 81, 186–193.

de Clérambault, G. (1942) *Oeuvre Psychiatrique*, Presses Universitaires de France, Paris.

Cotard, J. (1880) Du délire hypochondriaque dans une forme grave de la mélancolie anxieuse. *Annales Médico-Psychologiques* 38, 168–174.

Cotard, J. (1882) Du délire des négations. *Archives de Neurologie* 11, 152–170; and 12, 282–296.

Cutting, J.C., Clarke, A.W. & Mann, A.H. (1978) Cycloid psychosis: an investigation of the diagnostic concept. *Psychological Medicine* 8, 637–648.

Debruille, J.B. & Stip, E. (1996) Capgras syndrome: evolution of hypotheses. *Canadian Journal of Psychiatry* 41, 181–187.

Dupré, E. & Logre, L. (1911) Les délires d'imagination: mythomanie délirante. *Encéphale* 10, 209–232.

Edelstyn, N.M. & Oyebode, F. (1999) A review of the phenomenology and cognitive neuropsychological origins of the Capgras' syndrome. *International Journal of Geriatric Psychiatry* 14, 48–59.

Ellis, H.D. (1994) The role of the right hemisphere in the Capgras delusion. *Psychopathology* 27, 177–185.

Ellis, H.D., Quayle, A.H., de Pauw, K.W., et al. (1996) Delusional misidentification of inanimate objects: a literature review and neuropsychological analysis of cognitive deficits in two cases. *Cognitive Neuropsychiatry* 1, 27–40.

Ellis, P. & Mellsop, G. (1985) De Clérambault's syndrome: a nosological entity? *British Journal of Psychiatry* 146, 90–95.

Faergeman, P.M. (1963) *Psychogenic Psychoses: A Description and Follow-Up of Psychoses Following Psychological Stress*. Butterworths, London.

Ferrey, G. & Zebdi, S. (1999) Evolution et pronostic des troubles psychotiques aigus (bouffée délirante polymorphe). *Encéphale* 25, 26–32.

Forsell, Y. & Henderson, A.S. (1998) Epidemiology of paranoid symptoms in an elderly population. *British Journal of Psychiatry* 172, 429–432.

Franzek, E., Becker, T., Hofmann, E. et al. (1996) Is computerized tomography ventricular abnormality related to cycloid psychosis? *Biological Psychiatry* 40, 1255–1266.

Garmezy, N. (1968) Process and reactive schizophrenia: some conceptions and issues. In: *The Role and Methodology of Classification in Psychiatry and Psychopathology* (eds M.M. Katz, J.O. Cole & W.E. Barton), pp. 419–430. Government Printing Office, Washington, DC.

Gaughran, F., O'Neil, E., Cole, M., et al. (1998) Increased soluble interleukin 2 receptor levels in schizophrenia. *Schizophrenia Research* 29, 263–267.

Gelder, M., Gath, D. & Mayou, R. (1989) Paranoid symptoms and paranoid syndromes. *Oxford Textbook of Psychiatry*, 2nd edn, pp. 324–344. Oxford University Press, Oxford.

Gerrans, P. (2000) Refining the explanation of Cotard's delusion. *Mind and Language* 15, 111–122.

Gottesman, I. & Bertelsen, A. (1989) Dual mating studies in psychiatry: offspring of inpatients with examples from reactive (psychogenic) psychoses. *International Review of Psychiatry* 1, 287–295.

Grahame, P.S. (1984) Schizophrenia in old age (late paraphrenia). *British Journal of Psychiatry* 145, 493–495.

Guldberg, C.A., Dahl, A.A., Hansen, H. & Bergem, A.M. (1991) Were Langfeldt's schizophreniform psychoses really affective? *Psychopathology* 24, 270–276.

Hatta, S.M. (1996) A Malay crosscultural worldview and forensic review of amok. *Australian and New Zealand Journal of Psychiatry* 30, 505–510.

Hoffler, J., Braunig, P., Kruger, S. & Ludvik, M. (1997) Morphology according to cranial computed tomography of first episode cycloid psychosis and its long-term course differences compared to schizophrenia. *Acta Psychiatrica Scandinavica* 96, 184–187.

Holden, N.L. (1987) Late paraphrenia or the paraphrenias? A descriptive study with a 10-year follow-up. *British Journal of Psychiatry* 150, 635–639.

Howard, R., Casde, D., Wessely, S. & Murray, R. (1993) A comparative study of 470 cases of early-onset and late-onset schizophrenia. *British Journal of Psychiatry* 163, 352–357.

Howard, R., Almeida, O. & Levy, R. (1994) Phenomenology, demography and diagnosis in late paraphrenia. *Psychological Medicine* 24, 397–410.

Jordan, H.W. & Howe, G. (1980) De Clérambault syndrome (erotomania): a review and case presentation. *Journal of the National Medical Association* 72, 979–985.

Jorgensen, P., Bennedsen, B., Christensen, J. & Hyllested, A. (1996) Acute and transient psychotic disorder: comorbidity with personality disorder. *Acta Psychiatrica Scandinavica* 94, 460–464.

Jorgensen, P., Bennedsen, B., Christensen, J. & Hyllested, A. (1997) Acute and transient psychotic disorder: a 1-year follow-up study. *Acta Psychiatrica Scandinavica* 96, 150–154.

Kendell, R.E. (1993) Paranoid disorders. In: *Companion to Psychiatric Studies* (eds R.E. Kendell & A.K. Zealley), pp. 459–471. Churchill Livingstone, Edinburgh.

Kendler, K.S., McGuire, M., Gruenberg, A.M., et al. (1993) The Roscommon Family Study. II. The risk of non-schizophrenic non-affective psychoses in relatives. *Archives of General Psychiatry* 50, 645–652.

Kendler, S.K. (1980) The nosologic validity of paranoia (simple delusional disorder): a review. *Archives of General Psychiatry* 37, 699–706.

Kendler, S.K., Gruenberg, A.M. & Strauss, J.S. (1981) An independent analysis of the Copenhagen sample of the Danish Adoption Study of schizophrenia. *Archives of General Psychiatry* 38, 985–987.

Kendler, S.K., Masterson, C.C. & Davis, K.L. (1985) Psychiatric illness in first-degree relatives of patients with paranoid psychosis, schizophrenia and medical illness. *British Journal of Psychiatry* 147, 524–531.

Kendler, S.K., Spitzer, R.L. & Williams, J.B.W. (1989) Psychotic disorders in DSM-IIIR. *American Journal of Psychiatry* 146, 953–962.

Kety, S.S., Rosenthal, D., Wender, P.H., Schulsinger, F. & Jacobson, B. (1978) The biologic and adoptive families of adopted individuals who became schizophrenic: prevalence of mental illness and other characteristics. In: *The Nature of Schizophrenia* (ed. L.D. Wynne). John Wiley & Sons, New York.

Kirrane, R.M. & Siever, L.J. (2000) New perspectives on schizotypal personality disorder. *Current Psychiatry Reports* 2, 62–66.

Kon, Y. (1994) Amok. *British Journal of Psychiatry* 165, 685–689.

Kraepelin, E. (1899) *Psychiatrie: Ein Lehrbuch Fur Studierende und Aerzte*, 6th edn. Barth, Leipzig.

Kraepelin, E. (1909–15) *Psychiatrie. Ein Lehrbuch Fur Studierende und Aerzte*, 8th edn. Barth, Leipzig.

Kretschmer, E. (1918) *Der Sensitive Beziehungswahn*. Springer-Verlag, Berlin.

Lanczik, M., Fritze, J. & Beckmann, H. (1990) Puerperal and cycloid psychoses: results of a retrospective study. *Psychopathology* 23, 220–227.

Langfeldt, G. (1939) *The Schizophreniform States*. Munsksgaard, Copenhagen/Oxford University Press, Oxford.

Langfeldt, G. (1961) The erotic jealousy syndrome: a clinical study. *Acta Psychiatrica Scandinavica Supplement* 151.

Lasègue, C. & Falret, J. (1877) La folie à deux ou folie communiquée. *Annales Médico-Psychologiques* 18, 321.

Legrain, M. (1886) *Du Délire Chez les Dégénérés*. Deshaye et Lecrosoier, Paris.

Leong, G.B., Silva, J.A., Garza-Trevino, E.S. *et al.* (1994) The dangerousness of persons with the Othello syndrome. *Journal of Forensic Sciences* 39, 1445–1454.

Leonhard, K. (1957) *Aufteilung der Endogenen Psychosen*. Akademie Verlag, Berlin.

Lindvall, M., Hagnell, O. & Ohman, R. (1990) Epidemiology of cycloid psychosis. *Psychopathology* 23, 228–232.

Magnan, V. & Legrain, M. (1895) *Les Dégénérés (Etat Mental et Syndromes Episodiques)*. Rueff et Cie, Paris.

Mahadik, S.P., Mukherjee, S., Scheffer, R., Correnti, E.F. & Mahadik, J.S. (1998) Elevated plasma lipid peroxides at the onset of nonaffective psychosis. *Biological Psychiatry* 43, 674–679.

Maj, M. (1990) Cycloid psychotic disorder: validation of the concept by means of a follow-up and a family study. *Psychopathology* 23, 196–204.

Manschreck, T.C. (1996) Delusional disorder: the recognition and management of paranoia. *Journal of Clinical Psychiatry* 57 (Suppl. 3), 32–38.

Mowat, R.R. (1966) *Morbid Jealousy and Murder*. Tavistock, London.

Mullen, P.E. & Maack, L.H. (1985) Jealousy, pathological jealousy and aggression. In: *Aggression and Dangerousness* (eds D.P. Farington & J. Gunn), pp. 103–126. Wiley, Chicester.

Mullen, P.E., Pathé, M. & Purcell, R. (2000) *Stalkers and Their Victims*. Cambridge University Press, Cambridge.

Munro, A. & Mok, H. (1995) An overview of treatment in paranoia/delusional disorder. *Canadian Journal of Psychiatry* 40, 616–622.

Odom-White, A., de Leon, J., Stanilla, J. *et al.* (1995) Misidentification syndromes in schizophrenia: case reviews with implications for classification and prevalence. *Australian and New Zealand Journal of Psychiatry* 29, 63–68.

Opjordsmoen, S. & Retterstol, N. (1987) Hypochondriacal delusions in paranoid psychoses: course and outcome compared with other types of delusions. *Psychopathology* 20, 272–284.

de Pauw, K.W. (1994a) Delusional misidentification: a plea for an agreed terminology and classification. *Psychopathology* 27, 123–129.

de Pauw, K.W. (1994b) Psychodynamic approaches to the Capgras delusion: a critical historical review. *Psychopathology* 27, 154–160.

Perris, C. (1974) A study of cycloid psychoses. *Acta Psychiatrica Scandinavica Supplement* 253.

Pfuhlmann, B., Stöber, G., Franzek, E. & Beckmann, H. (1998) Cycloid psychoses predominate in severe postpartum psychiatric disorders. *Journal of Affective Disorders* 50, 125–134.

Pichot, P. (1983) *A Century of Psychiatry*. Roger Dacosta, Paris.

Pichot, P. (1990) The diagnosis and classification of mental disorders in the French-speaking countries: background, current values and comparison with other classifications. In: *Sources and Traditions of Classification in Psychiatry* (eds N. Sartorius, A. Jablensky, D.A. Regier *et al.*), pp. 7–58. Hofgrete & Huber, Toronto.

Pichot, P. & Debray, H. (1971) *Hospitalisation Psychiatrique: Statistique Descriptive*. Sandoz Editions, Paris.

Pitta, J.C.N. & Blay, S.L. (1997) Psychogenic (reactive) and hysterical psychoses: a cross-system reliability study. *Acta Psychiatrica Scandinavica* 95, 112–118.

Pull, C.B., Pull, M.C. & Pichot, P. (1987) Des critères empiriques francais pour les psychoses. III. Algorithmes et arbre de décision. *Encéphale* 13, 59–66.

Raskin, D.E. & Sullivan, K.E. (1974) Erotomania. *American Journal of Psychiatry* 131, 1033–1035.

Ravindran, A.V., Yatham, L.N. & Munro, A. (1999) Paraphrenia redefined. *Canadian Journal of Psychiatry* 44, 133–137.

Remington, G. & Book, H. (1984) Case report of de Clérambault syndrome, bipolar affective disorder, and response to lithium. *American Journal of Psychiatry* 141, 1285–1287.

Roth, M. (1955) The natural history of mental disorder in old age. *Journal of Mental Science* 101, 281–301.

Sartorius, N., Jablenski, A., Korten, A. *et al.* (1986) Early manifestations and first contact incidence of schizophrenia in different cultures: a preliminary report on the initial evaluation phase of the WHO Collaborative Study on Determinants of Outcome of Severe Mental Disorders. *Psychological Medicine* 16, 909–928.

Sartorius, N., Kaelber, C.T. Cooper, J.E. *et al.* (1993) Progress toward achieving a common language in psychiatry: results from the field trial of the Clinical Guidelines accompanying the WHO Classification of Mental and Behavioural Disorders in ICD-10. *Archives of General Psychiatry* 50, 115–124.

Schanda, H. (2000) Paranoia and dysphoria: historical developments, current concepts. *Psychopathology* 33, 204–208.

Schanda, H. & Gabriel, E. (1988) Position of affective symptomatology in the course of delusional psychoses. *Psychopathology* 21, 1–11.

Schmidt-Degenhard, M. (1998) The history and psychopathology of paranoia. *Fortschritte der Neurologie-Psychiatrie* 66, 313–325.

Sérieux, P. & Capgras, J. (1909) *Les Folies Raisonnantes: le Délire d'Interprétation*. Felix Arcan, Paris.

Shepherd, M. (1961) Morbid jealousy: some clinical and social aspects of a psychiatric symptom. *Journal of Mental Science* **107**, 687–753.

Sigmund, D. & Mundt, C. (1999) The cycloid type and its differentiation from core schizophrenia: a phenomenological approach. *Comprehensive Psychiatry* **40**, 4–18.

Signer, S.F. (1991a) 'Les psychoses passionnelles' reconsidered: a review of de Clérambault's cases and syndrome with respect to mood disorders. *Journal of Psychiatry and Neuroscience* **16**, 81–90.

Signer, S.F. (1991b) Erotomania. *American Journal of Psychiatry* **148**, 1276.

Signer, S.F. (1994) Localization and lateralization in the delusion of substitution. *Psychopathology* **27**, 168–176.

Signer, S.F. & Cummings, J.L. (1987) De Clérambault's syndrome in organic affective disorder: two cases. *British Journal of Psychiatry* **151**, 404–407.

Signer, S.F. & Swinson, R.P. (1987) Two cases of erotomania (de Clérambault's syndrome) in bipolar affective disorder. *British Journal of Psychiatry* **151**, 853–855.

Silva, J.A., Ferrari, M.M., Leong, G.B. & Penny, G. (1998) The dangerousness of persons with delusional jealousy. *Journal of the American Academy of Psychiatry and the Law* **26**, 607–623.

Silveira, J.M. & Seeman, M.V. (1995) Shared psychotic disorder: a critical review of the literature. *Canadian Journal of Psychiatry* **40**, 389–395.

Sims, A. & Reddie, M. (1976) The de Clérambault and Capgras history. *British Journal of Psychiatry* **129**, 95–96.

Sims, A. & White, A. (1973) Coexistence of Capgras and de Clérambault's syndromes: a case history. *British Journal of Psychiatry* **123**, 635–637.

Staner, L. (1991) Sleep, dexamethasone suppression test, and response to somatic therapies in an atypical affective state presenting as erotomania: a case report. *European Psychiatry* **6**, 269–271.

Stöber, G., Kocher, I., Franzek, E. & Beckmann, H. (1997) First trimester maternal gestation infection and cycloid psychosis. *Acta Psychiatrica Scandinavica* **96**, 319–324.

Strakowski, S.M. (1994) Diagnostic validity of schizophreniform disorder. *American Journal of Psychiatry* **151**, 815–824.

Strik, W.K., Fallgatter, A.J., Stöber, G., Franzek, E. & Beckmann, H. (1997) Specific P300 features in cycloid psychosis. *Acta Psychiatrica Scandinavica* **95**, 67–72.

Strömgren, E. (1974) Psychogenic psychoses. In: *Themes and Variations in European Psychiatry* (eds S.R. Hirsch & M. Shepherd), pp. 97–117. Wright & Sons, Bristol.

Strömgren, E. (1989) The development of the concept of reactive psychoses. *British Journal of Psychiatry* **154**, 47–50.

Tsai, S.-J., Hwang, J.-P., Yang, C.-H. & Liu, K.-M. (1997) Delusional jealousy in dementia. *Journal of Clinical Psychiatry* **58**, 492–494.

Vauhkonen, K. (1968) On the pathogenesis of morbid jealousy. *Acta Psychiatrica Scandinavica Supplement* **202**, 1–261.

Weinstein, E.A. (1994) The classification of delusional misidentification syndromes. *Psychopathology* **27**, 130–135.

Wimmer, A. (1916) Psykogene Sindssygdomsformer. *Sct. Hans Mental Hospital 1816–1916*, Jubilee Publication, pp. 85–216. Gad, Copenhagen.

World Health Organization (1992) *The ICD-10 Classification of Mental and Behavioural Disorders: Clinical Descriptions and Diagnostic Guidelines.* World Health Organization, Geneva.

World Health Organization (1993) *The ICD-10 Classification of Mental and Behavioural Disorders: Diagnostic Criteria for Research.* World Health Organization, Geneva.

Yamada, N., Nakajima, S. & Noguchi, T. (1998) Age at onset of delusional disorder is dependent on the delusional theme. *Acta Psychiatrica Scandinavica* **97**, 122–124.

Young, A.W., Leafhead, K.M. & Szulecka, T.K. (1994) The Capgras and Cotard delusions. *Psychopathology* **27**, 226–231.

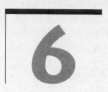

Late-onset schizophrenia

R. Howard and D. V. Jeste

Historical development, 68
   The European use of late paraphrenia, 68
   Current diagnosis of patients within ICD-10 and
     DSM-IV, 69
   Terminology and classification for the future, 70
Clinical features, 70
   Schizophrenic symptoms, 70
   Delusions, 70
   Affective symptoms, 70
   Cognitive deficits, 71
Aetiology, 71
   Genetic factors, 71

Brain abnormalities seen with imaging, 72
Gender, 73
Sensory deficits, 73
Premorbid personality and other factors, 74
Management/treatment, 74
   Establishing a therapeutic relationship, 75
   Rehousing, 75
   Cognitive and behavioural interventions, 75
   Antipsychotic medication, 75
Conclusions, 77
Acknowledgements, 77
References, 77

This chapter considers what has historically been a contentious area. Schizophrenia is generally regarded as an illness with onset in early adult life, yet cases of an illness that shows only minor phenotypical differences can arise for the first time in middle age and late life. Psychiatrists initially squabbled over whether or not such cases really existed. Once it was established that they did, researchers then disagreed about how they might relate to more 'typical' schizophrenia and what to call them. It may be difficult to understand the current view of these psychoses without some consideration of the historical development of the concepts and diagnoses involved.

Historical development

Both Kraepelin (1913) and Bleuler (1911) observed that there was a relatively small group of patients with schizophrenia who had an illness onset in late middle or old age and who, on clinical grounds, closely resembled those who had an onset in early adult life. Utilizing a very narrow conception of dementia praecox and specifically excluding cases of paraphrenia, Kraepelin (1913) reported that only 5.6% of 1054 patients had an onset after the age of 40 years. If the age of onset was set at 60 years or greater, only 0.2% of patients could be included.

Manfred Bleuler (1943) carried out the first specific and systematic examination of late-onset patients and defined late schizophrenia as follows:
1 onset after the age of 40;
2 symptomatology that does not differ from that of schizophrenia occurring early in life (or, if it does differ, it should not do so in a clear or radical way); and
3 it should not be possible to attribute the illness to a neuropathological disorder because of the presence of an amnestic syndrome or associated signs of organic brain disease.
Bleuler found that between 15% and 17% of two large series of schizophrenia patients had an onset after the age of 40. Of such late-onset cases, only 4% had become ill for the first time after the age of 60. Later authors confirmed that while onset of

schizophrenia after the age of 40 was unusual, onset after 60 should be considered even more rare. From 264 elderly schizophrenia patients admitted in Edinburgh in 1957, only seven had an illness that had begun after the age of 60 (Fish 1958). Using very broad criteria for the diagnosis of schizophrenia (including schizoaffective, paraphrenic and other non-organic non-affective psychoses) and studying 470 first contacts with the Camberwell Register, Howard *et al.* (1993) found 29% of cases to have been over 44 years at onset. Based on a literature review, Harris and Jeste (1988) noted that 23% of all schizophrenia inpatients reportedly had onset of their illness after age 40. There seemed to be a progressive decline in the number of patients with onset in later years.

Kraepelin and E. Bleuler both considered late-onset cases to have much in common with more typically early-onset schizophrenia and this view was supported by M. Bleuler's report (1943) of only very mild phenomenological variance from early-onset cases. However, his 126 late-onset cases were symptomatically milder, had less affective flattening and were less likely to have formal thought disorder than patients with a younger onset. Fish (1960) reported that the clinical picture presented by 23 patients with onset after 40 years did not differ importantly from patients who were younger at onset, but he believed that with increasing age at onset schizophrenia took on a more 'paraphrenic' form.

The European use of late paraphrenia

The notion of paraphrenia as a distinct diagnostic entity had been discredited by Mayer's follow-up of Kraepelin's 78 original cases. At least 40% of these patients had developed clear signs of dementia praecox within a few years and only 36% could still be classified as paraphrenic. Many of the paraphrenic patients had positive family histories of schizophrenia and the presenting clinical picture of those patients who remained 'true' paraphrenics did not differ from those who were later to develop signs of schizophrenia. Roth and Morrisey (1952) resurrected both the terminology and the controversy with their choice of the term 'late paraphrenia' to describe patients who they believed had schizophrenia, but with an onset delayed until after the age of 55 or 60 years. The term was intended to be descriptive: to distinguish the illness from the chronic schizophrenia patients seen in psychiatric institutions at the time and to emphasize the clinical similarities with the illness described by Kraepelin. Choice of the term was perhaps unfortunate because two particular points of misconception often seem to arise in relation to it and it is vital to set these straight. Late paraphrenia was never intended to mean the same thing as paraphrenia and Kraepelin certainly did not emphasize late age of onset as a feature of the illness. Kay and Roth (1961) studied a group of 39 female and three male patients diagnosed with late paraphrenia in Graylingwell Hospital between 1951 and 1955. All but six of these cases were followed up for 5 years. The case records of 48 female and nine male late paraphrenia patients admitted to a hospital in Stockholm between 1931 and 1940 were also collected and these cases were followed up till death or until 1956. Over 40% of the Graylingwell late paraphrenia patients were living alone, compared with 12% of affective disorder patients and 16% of those with organic psychoses who were of comparable ages. Late paraphrenia patients were also socially isolated. Although the frequency of visual impairment at presentation (15%) was no higher than that in comparison groups with other diagnoses, some impairment of hearing was present in 40% of late paraphrenic patients and this was considered severe in 15%. Deafness was only present in 7% of affective disorder patients. Focal cerebral disease was identified in only 8% of late paraphrenic patients at presentation. Primary delusions, feelings of mental or physical influence and hallucinations were all prominent and the prognosis for recovery was judged to be poor. From a detailed analysis of 1250 first admissions to a hospital in Gothenburg, Sjoegren (1964) identified 202 elderly individuals who conformed to the French concept of paraphrenia (Magnan 1893): well-organized and persistent paranoid delusions with hallucinations occurring in clear consciousness. Sjoegren argued cogently that, together with constitutional factors, ageing itself produced effects (feelings of isolation and loneliness, social and economic insecurity and heightened vulnerability) which contributed to the development of paranoid reactions.

Post (1966) collected a sample of 93 patients to whom he gave the non-controversial and self-explanatory label 'persistent persecutory states' and made a point of including cases regardless of coexisting organic brain change. Within this broad category he recognized three clinical subtypes: a schizophrenic syndrome (34 of 93 patients), a schizophreniform syndrome (37 patients) and a paranoid hallucinosis group (22 patients). Post regarded those patients with the schizophrenic syndrome as having a delayed form of the illness with only partial expression. Post's patients were treated with phenothiazines and he was able to demonstrate that the condition was responsive to antipsychotic medication. Success or failure of treatment was related to the adequacy of phenothiazine treatment and its long-term maintenance.

From a series of 45 female and two male late paraphrenic patients (identified using the same criteria as Kay & Roth's) admitted to St Francis' Hospital in Hayward's Heath between 1958 and 1964, Herbert and Jacobson (1967) confirmed many of Kay and Roth's (1961) observations. In addition, these investigators found an unexpectedly high prevalence of schizophrenia among the mothers (4.4%) and siblings (13.3%) of their patients.

Current diagnosis of patients within ICD-10 and DSM-IV

Diagnostic guidelines published by authoritative organizations such as the World Health Organization (WHO) or the American Psychiatric Association (APA) reflect the views of many contemporary clinicians who were consulted at the draft and field trial stages. Inclusion or exclusion of a particular diagnosis in published diagnostic schemes thus reflects the current credence given to the nosological validity of that diagnosis plus an indication of its general usefulness in clinical practice.

Late paraphrenia, included within ICD-9, has not survived as a separate codeable diagnosis into ICD-10. There are three possible diagnostic categories available for the accommodation of patients previously diagnosed as late paraphrenic: schizophrenia, delusional disorder and other persistent delusional disorders. It seems likely that most cases will be coded under schizophrenia (F20.0) (Quintal et al. 1991; Howard et al. 1994a), although the category of delusional disorder (F22.0) is suggested as a replacement for 'paraphrenia (late)' in the diagnostic guidelines. Distinction between cases of schizophrenia and delusional disorder within ICD-10 is very much dependent on the quality of auditory hallucinations experienced by patients and is subject to some unhelpful ageism. The guidelines for delusional disorder (F22.0) in ICD-10 state that: 'clear and persistent auditory hallucinations (voices) . . . are incompatible with this diagnosis'. Rather confusingly, the guidelines for a diagnosis of delusional disorder suggest that: 'occasional or transitory auditory hallucinations, particularly in elderly patients, do not rule out this diagnosis, provided that they are not typically schizophrenic and form only a small part of the overall clinical picture'. To add further to diagnostic dilemma, the guidelines also include the suggestion that: 'disorders in which delusions are accompanied by persistent hallucinatory voices or by schizophrenic symptoms that are insufficient to meet criteria for schizophrenia' should be coded under the category of other persistent delusional disorders (F22.8). Because the majority of late paraphrenic patients who hear distinct hallucinatory voices also have a rich variety of schizophrenic core symptoms, very few will be diagnosed as having other persistent delusional disorders.

The inclusion within DSM-IIIR (American Psychiatric Association 1987) of a separate category of late-onset schizophrenia for cases with an illness onset after the age of 44 years seems largely to have been a reaction to the unsatisfactory and arbitrary upper age limit for onset that had been included for DSM-III (American Psychiatric Association 1980) for a diagnosis of schizophrenia. DSM-IV (American Psychiatric Association 1994) contains no separate category for late-onset schizophrenia and this presumably reflects the current general North American view that there is a direct continuity between cases of schizophrenia whatever their age at onset.

Terminology and classification for the future

The important questions now are: have ICD-10 and DSM-IV been fair to abandon any facility for coding late-onset within schizophrenia, and do we need diagnostic categories that distinguish the functional psychoses with onset in later life from schizophrenia? These questions provided the spur to establish an international consensus on diagnosis and terminology (Howard *et al*. 2000), which may form the basis for consideration of these patients within future revisions of DSM and ICD. When the late-onset schizophrenia international consensus group met in 1998, it agreed that the available evidence from the areas of epidemiology, phenomenology and pathophysiology supported heterogeneity within schizophrenia with increasing age at onset up to the age of 60 years. Schizophrenia-like psychosis with onset after the age of 60 years (i.e. what some psychiatrists used to call late paraphrenia) was considered to be distinct from schizophrenia. The consensus group recommended that schizophrenia with onset between 40 and 59 years be termed late-onset schizophrenia and that chronic psychosis with onset after 60 years should be called very-late-onset schizophrenia-like psychosis (VLOSLP). The latter term is long-winded and unmemorable but at least is unambiguous and had the unprecedented support of both European and North American geriatric psychiatrists. There was no consensus regarding the exact age cut-offs of 40 and 60 years for defining late-onset schizophrenia and VLOSLP, and these were considered provisional until further research established evidence-based cut-points. From this point in this chapter the term late paraphrenia will be used only for patients already described as such in the literature.

Clinical features

Schizophrenic symptoms

Although Bleuler (1943) believed that it was not possible to separate early- and late-onset patients on clinical grounds, he acknowledged that a later onset was accompanied by less affective flattening and a more benign course. Formal thought disorder is seen in only about 5% of cases of DSM-IIIR late-onset schizophrenia (Pearlson *et al*. 1989) and could not be elicited from any of 101 late paraphrenic patients (Howard *et al*. 1994a). The first-rank symptoms of Schneider are seen, but may be somewhat less prevalent in later onset cases. Thought-insertion, block and withdrawal seem to be particularly uncommon (Grahame 1984; Pearlson *et al*. 1989; Howard *et al*. 1994b) and negative symptoms are less severe (Almeida *et al*. 1995a). In a multicentre study of late-onset schizophrenia, Jeste

et al. (1988) found that delusions, particularly of persecution, and auditory hallucinations were prominent in these patients. Late-onset schizophrenia typically resembled the paranoid subtype of early-onset schizophrenia. Other subtypes of schizophrenia, including catatonic and disorganized types, were very rare in old age. In studies at San Diego, Jeste *et al*. (1997) and Palmer *et al*. (2001) compared similarly aged patients with middle-age- and early-onset schizophrenia. The clinical symptoms were rated on the various scales used: Brief Psychiatric Rating Scale (BPRS), Scale for the Assessment of Positive Symptoms (SAPS), and Scale for the Assessment of Negative Symptoms (SANS) (Overall & Gorham 1962). The severity of positive symptoms was similar in the two groups, and both groups had significantly more positive symptoms, including thought disorder, than did normal subjects. Early-onset schizophrenia patients had more severe negative symptoms, including affective blunting, alogia, avolition and inattention, than did middle-age-onset schizophrenia patients. However, although middle-age-onset schizophrenia patients had less severe negative symptoms than early-onset schizophrenia patients, they still had consistently worse negative symptoms than normal subjects. These results suggest that middle-age-onset schizophrenia patients do have thought disorder and negative symptoms. It is worth noting that, by definition, patients with paranoid subtype lack a prominence of negative symptoms, and most patients with middle-age-onset schizophrenia have a paranoid type of schizophrenia (Andreasen 1982; Andreasen & Olsen 1982).

Delusions

Persecutory delusions usually dominate the presentation although, in a series of 101 late paraphrenic patients, delusions of reference (76%), control (25%), grandiose ability (12%) and of a hypochondriacal nature (11%) were also present (Howard *et al*. 1994a). Partition delusions are found in about two-thirds of cases and refer to the belief that people, animals, materials or radiation can pass through a structure that would normally constitute a barrier to such passage. This barrier is generally the door, ceiling, walls or floor of a patient's home and the source of intrusion is frequently a neighbouring residence (Herbert & Jacobson 1967; Pearlson *et al*. 1989; Howard & Levy 1992).

Affective symptoms

The coexistence of affective features in late-onset schizophrenia is well recognized clinically but there have been no controlled studies comparing such features in early- and late-onset cases. Atypical, schizoaffective and cycloid psychoses are all characterized by affective features, tend to arise later in life and affect women more than men (Cutting *et al*. 1978; Levitt & Tsuang 1988). Among late paraphrenic patients, Post (1966) reported depressive admixtures in 60% of cases, while Holden (1987) considered that 10 of his 24 'functional' late paraphrenic patients had affective or schizoaffective disorders. These patients also had a better outcome in terms both of institutionalization and 10-year survival compared with paranoid patients. Such observations have led to the suggestion that some later onset schizophrenic or late paraphrenic patients may have variants of primary affective disorder (Murray *et al*. 1992).

Cognitive deficits

Attempts to identify and characterize the patterns of cognitive impairment associated with these conditions began with Hopkins and Roth (1953), who administered the vocabulary subtest from the Wechsler–Bellevue Scale, a shortened form of Raven's Progressive Matrices, and a general test of orientation and information, to patients with a variety of diagnoses. Twelve late paraphrenic patients performed as well as a group of elderly depressive patients and better than patients with dementia on all three tests.

Naguib and Levy (1987) evaluated 43 late paraphrenic patients (having already excluded subjects with a diagnosable dementia) with the Mental Test Score (MTS), Digit Copying Test (DCT) and the Digit Symbol Substitution Test. Patients performed less well than age-matched controls on both the MTS and DCT.

Miller *et al*. (1991) have published neuropsychological data on patients with what they term 'late life psychosis'. These patients performed less well than age-matched controls on the Mini-Mental State Examination (MMSE), the Wechsler Adult Intelligence Scale–Revised, the Wisconsin Card Sorting Test, Logical Memory and Visual Reproduction subtests from the Wechsler Memory Scale, a test of verbal fluency and the Warrington Recognition Memory Test. However, patients were not well matched with controls for educational attainment and premorbid intelligence and some of the patients clearly had affective psychoses and dementia syndromes (Miller *et al*. 1992), so it is probably not fair to equate them with late paraphrenia or late-onset schizophrenia patients.

Almeida *et al*. (1995a) carried out a detailed neuropsychological examination of 40 patients with late paraphrenia in south London. Using cluster analysis of the results he identified two groups of patients. The first was a 'functional' group characterized by impairment restricted to executive functions, in particular a computerized test assessing extra- and intradimensional attention set shift ability and a test of planning. Such patients had a high prevalence and severity of positive psychotic symptoms and lower scores on a scale of neurological abnormalities. A second 'organic' group of late paraphrenic patients showed widespread impairment of cognitive functions together with a lower frequency of positive psychotic symptoms and a high prevalence of abnormalities on neurological examination (Almeida *et al*. 1995b).

Heaton *et al*. (1994, 2001) assessed cognitive performance with an expanded version of the Halstead–Reitan test battery in over 200 subjects. Overall, late-onset schizophrenia was similar to early-onset schizophrenia in terms of the pattern of neuropsychological impairment (Heaton *et al*. 1994). The neuropsychological deficit scores (corrected for age, gender and education) were similar among the schizophrenia groups and different from (intermediate between) those in the normal subjects and Alzheimer's disease patients. There was a dissociation in terms of learning and retaining information. The schizophrenia patients had mild to moderate impairment on learning but normal retention of information, whereas the patients with Alzheimer's disease were markedly impaired on both. Although the overall pattern of normal neuropsychological functioning for late- and early-onset schizophrenia groups was similar, there were some differences between late- and early-onset schizophrenia; these were in terms of learning and abstraction/flexibility of thinking, with the late-onset schizophrenia group being less impaired on these measures. Schizophrenia patients classified as having a normal learning and memory pattern had an older age of onset than patients with abnormal learning and memory profiles (Paulsen *et al*. 1995). Also, age of onset of schizophrenia was positively associated with total recall across learning trials and negatively associated with evidence of retrieval problems.

Paulsen *et al*. (1996) characterized the integrity of semantic memory in both late- and early-onset schizophrenia patients and found that the organization of semantic memory was almost normal in the late-onset schizophrenia patients, whereas it was significantly impaired in the early-onset schizophrenia patients.

Aetiology

Genetic factors

Reviewing the literature of family history in schizophrenia, Gottesman and Shields (1982) reported that the overall risk of schizophrenia in the relatives of an affected proband was about 10%, compared with a risk of around 1% for the general population. Kendler *et al*. (1987) concluded that there was no consistent relationship between age at onset and familial risk for schizophrenia, but data from patients with an onset in old age were not included in this analysis. The literature on familiality in late-onset schizophrenia and related psychoses of late life is sparse and inconclusive, partly because of variations in illness definition and age at onset, but principally because of the difficulties inherent in conducting family studies in patients who often have only a small number of surviving first-degree relatives. The results of the few studies specifically of late-onset psychoses, reviewed by Castle and Howard (1992), suggest a trend for increasing age at onset of psychosis to be associated with reduced risk of schizophrenia in first-degree relatives. Thus, studies involving subjects with illness onset after the age of 40 or 45 years have reported rates of schizophrenia in relatives of between 4.4% and 19.4% (Bleuler 1943; Huber *et al*. 1975; Pearlson *et al*. 1989), while those with onsets delayed to 50 or 60 years have yielded rates of between 1.0% and 7.3% (Funding 1961; Post 1966; Herbert & Jacobson 1967). More recently, studies of patients with psychosis onset after the age of 50 (Brodaty *et al*. 1999) and 60 years (Howard *et al*. 1997) reported no increase in the prevalence of schizophrenia among relatives of patients and those of healthy comparison subjects. In a controlled family study involving data from 269 first-degree relatives of patients with onset after 60 years and 272 relatives of healthy elderly subjects, the estimated lifetime risk for schizophrenia with an onset range of 15–90 years was 2.3% for the relatives of patients and 2.2% for the relatives of controls (Howard *et al.* 1997). In another study comparing patients with middle-age- with early-onset schizophrenia, there was no significant group difference in the proportion of first-degree relatives with schizophrenia (Jeste *et al.* 1997). Both the groups of schizophrenia patients had a significantly greater likelihood of having a first-degree relative with schizophrenia than normal subjects.

Brain abnormalities seen with imaging

Exclusion from computerized tomography (CT) studies of patients with obvious neurological signs or a history of stroke, alcohol abuse or dementia has shown that structural abnormalities other than large ventricles in patients with late paraphrenia are probably no more common than in healthy elderly controls. Despite adhering to such exclusions, Flint *et al.* (1991) found unsuspected cerebral infarction on the scans of five out of 16 of their late paraphrenic patients. Most of these infarcts were subcortical or frontal and they were more likely to occur in patients who had delusions but no hallucinations. The results of this study need to be interpreted with some caution, because only 16 of a collected sample of patients had actually undergone CT scanning and it is possible that these represented the more 'organic' cases, or at least those that were thought most likely to have some underlying structural abnormality.

The superiority of magnetic resonance imaging (MRI) over CT, both in terms of grey/white matter resolution and visualization of deep white matter, is established. The results of MRI studies of changes in periventricular and deep white matter in patients with paranoid psychosis, however, must be viewed with some caution because few have assessed abnormalities in white matter in any kind of standardized manner and appropriate control populations, matched for cerebrovascular risk factors, are rarely used. Miller *et al.* (1989, 1991, 1992) have reported the results of structural MRI investigations in patients with what they termed 'late life psychosis'. They have reported that 42% of non-demented patients with an onset of psychosis after the age of 45 (mean age at scanning 60.1 years) had white matter abnormalities on MRI, compared with only 8% of a healthy age-matched control group. The appearance of large patchy white matter lesions (WMLs) was six times more likely in the temporal lobe and four times more common in the frontal lobes of patients than controls (Miller *et al.* 1991). These authors hypothesized that, although insufficient to give rise to focal neurological signs, WMLs might produce dysfunction in the overlying frontal and temporal cortex and that this could contribute to psychotic symptomatology. They acknowledged that because WMLs in the occipital lobes could also be implicated, it might not be pos-

sible to pinpoint an isolated anatomical white matter lesion that predisposed to psychosis. When comparisons were made between the patients who had structural brain abnormalities on MRI (10) with those who did not (7), there were no significant differences in age, educational level, IQ or performance on a wide battery of neuropsychological tests. Measurements of ventricle–brain ratio (VBR) indicated a non-significant increase in patients (10.6%) compared with controls (8.8%). The DSM-IIIR (American Psychiatric Association 1987) diagnoses of the 24 patients at entry to this study were schizophrenic disorder (late-onset type) (10), delusional disorder (7), schizophreniform psychosis (2) and psychosis not otherwise specified (5), but at least 12 were shown to have organic cerebral conditions. Studies by Howard *et al.* (1995) of white matter signal hyperintensities among patients with late paraphrenia, from whom the authors have tried to exclude organic cases, have suggested that they may be no more common in such patients than in healthy community-living elderly controls.

Pearlson *et al.* (1993) have reported the results of a volumetric MRI study of late-onset schizophrenia patients based on a sample of 11 individuals with an illness onset after the age of 55 years. Third ventricle volume was significantly greater in late-onset schizophrenia patients than in an age-matched control group. VBR estimations were greater among the late-onset schizophrenia patients (mean 9.0) than controls (mean 7.1), but this difference did not reach statistical significance.

Howard *et al.* (1994b) have reported the results of volumetric MRI studies, based on the scans of 47 patients with late paraphrenia, 31 of whom satisfied ICD-10 criteria for a diagnosis of schizophrenia and 16 for delusional disorder. While total brain volume was not reduced in the patients compared with 35 elderly community-living controls, lateral and third ventricle volumes were increased. Measurements of the frontal lobes, hippocampus, parahippocampus, thalamus and basal ganglia structures failed to demonstrate further differences between patient and control subjects.

Symonds *et al.* (1997) found no significant differences among age-comparable late-onset schizophrenia, early-onset schizophrenia and normal control groups in terms of clinically relevant structural brain abnormalities such as strokes, tumours, cysts or other lesions that are obvious to a clinical neuroradiologist reporting on the MRI (Breitner *et al.* 1990). We believe that if there is a patient with a relevantly located stroke or brain tumour who develops new-onset psychosis, the diagnosis should be psychosis not otherwise specified or psychosis secondary to a general medical condition, rather than labelling it late-onset schizophrenia with stroke or tumour.

Corey-Bloom *et al.* (1995) performed a computerized quantitative analysis of grey matter, white matter and fluid volumes in different regions of the brain in a subset of the subjects (Jernigan *et al.* 1990, 1991). Comparing the three groups, late-onset schizophrenia, early-onset schizophrenia and normal controls ($n = 16$, 14 and 28, respectively), similar in age (all over 45), gender and education, the only significant differences in MRI measures were in ventricular and thalamic volumes. There were no significant differences between late- and early-onset schizophrenia groups in terms of non-specific structural brain abnormalities: ventricular enlargement and white matter hyperintensities. The ventricles were significantly larger in late-onset schizophrenia patients than in normal subjects, with early-onset schizophrenia being intermediate. The late-onset schizophrenia patients had a significantly larger thalamus than early-onset schizophrenia patients, with normal subjects being intermediate. (The difference in ventricular volume between early-onset schizophrenia and normal subjects, or in thalamic volume between either schizophrenia group and normal subjects was not significant, probably because of small sample sizes.) The functions of the thalamus include filtering stimuli, sensory gating and focusing attention (Sherman & Koch 1990), all of which are impaired in schizophrenia. Several studies have found a reduced neuronal number or density in the dorsomedial nucleus of thalamus in early-onset schizophrenia (Treff & Hempel 1958; Pakkenberg 1990, 1992). Andreasen et al. (1990, 1994) found a reduced thalamic volume on MRI, primarily on the right, and Buchsbaum et al. (1996) reported a reduced metabolic rate on positron emission tomography (PET), primarily in the right posterior and left anterior portions of the thalamus in neuroleptic-naive patients with schizophrenia. All of these investigations were restricted to early-onset schizophrenia patients. Hence, the preliminary finding of a larger thalamus in late-onset schizophrenia, if replicated, may have relevance to the differential age of onset of schizophrenia.

Gender

The female preponderance of individuals who have an onset of schizophrenia or a schizophrenia-like psychosis in middle or old age is a consistent finding. Among late-onset schizophrenia patients (onset after 40–50 years) females have been reported to constitute 66% (Bleuler 1943), 72% (Klages 1961), 82% (Gabriel 1978), 85% (Marneros & Deister 1984) and 87% (Pearlson et al. 1989) of patients. In studies of patients with an illness onset at 60 years or greater, the female preponderance is even greater: 75% (Sternberg 1972), 86% (Howard et al. 1994a), 88% (Kay & Roth 1961) and 91% (Herbert & Jacobson 1967).

Two recent reports have indicated the presence of a subgroup of female schizophrenia patients with later illness onset who typically do not have a positive family history of schizophrenia (Shimizu & Kurachi 1989; Gorwood et al. 1995). Typically, later illness onset, particularly in females, is associated with a milder symptom profile and better outcome, better premorbid social adjustment and a lower prevalence of structural brain abnormalities than in (mostly male) patients with early illness onset. This has led to the suggestion that sex differences in schizophrenia may reflect different psychiatric disorders. Lewine (1981) proposed two competing theories to account for age of onset and gender differences – the timing model and the subtype model. According to the timing model, men and women have the same form of schizophrenia but the age at onset of illness is different. There may be an earlier onset for men or a delayed onset for women because of biological and/or psychosocial gender differences. In this model, the age of onset would account for most of the gender differences. According to the subtype model, there are two distinct forms of schizophrenia: 'male' schizophrenia and 'female' schizophrenia. Castle and Murray (1991) have suggested that early-onset, typically male schizophrenia is essentially a heritable neurodevelopmental disorder, while late-onset schizophrenia in females may have aetiologically more in common with affective psychosis than with the illness seen in males.

In contrast, Lindamer et al. (2002) believe that the gender differences are better explained by Lewine's timing model. The less severe symptoms and more favourable course of schizophrenia seen in women might be related to the delayed onset of illness (for most disorders, the later the onset, the longer the period for normal premorbid functioning and the better the prognosis.) Because the evidence to support gender differences in heritability, neuropsychological impairment, structural brain abnormalities and treatment response is inconclusive, the hypothesis that there are two subtypes of schizophrenia based on gender is weakened. Given the lack of consistent evidence for important psychosocial factors in the age at onset differential, biological factors gain more credence as possible mediators of the timing effect. As a potential way of explaining gender differences in the distribution of age at onset in this 'timing' model, several lines of evidence suggest that oestrogen could act as one important neuroendocrine mediator to delay and/or protect against the illness.

Seeman has long proposed an important role for sex hormones, especially oestrogen, in the development of schizophrenia (Seeman 1981, 1999; Seeman & Lang 1990). It is hypothesized that those women with a genetic predisposition to schizophrenia are afforded protection between puberty and menopause from oestrogen, therefore delaying the onset of the illness (Riecher-Rossler et al. 1994; Lindamer et al. 2000). Direct evidence to support this hypothesis is so far lacking.

Sensory deficits

Deafness has been experimentally and clinically associated with the development of paranoid symptoms. Deficits of moderate to severe degree affect 40% of patients with late paraphrenia (Kay & Roth 1961; Herbert & Jacobson 1967) and are more prevalent than in elderly depressed patients or normal controls (Post 1966; Naguib & Levy 1987). Deafness associated with late-life psychosis is more usually conductive than degenerative (Cooper et al. 1974) and is generally of early onset, long duration, bilateral and profound (Cooper 1976; Cooper & Curry 1976). Corbin and Eastwood (1986) suggested that deafness may reinforce a pre-existing tendency to social isolation, withdrawal and suspiciousness. Further, auditory hallucinations are the psychopathological phenomena most consistently associated with deafness (Keshavan et al. 1992). There are several reports of improvement in psychotic symptoms after the fitting of a hearing aid (Eastwood et al. 1981; Khan et al. 1988; Almeida et al.

1993), although it has to be said that clinical practice suggests that this is not usually the case. Visual impairment, most commonly a consequence of cataract or macular degeneration, is also more common in elderly paranoid psychosis patients than those with affective disorder and there is a higher coincidence of visual and hearing impairment in paranoid than affective patients (Cooper & Curry 1976). An association between visual impairment and the presence of visual hallucinations (Howard et al. 1994a) echoes Keshavan's findings with deafness.

Somewhat different results were observed in a study by Prager and Jeste (1993). The authors conducted a case–control study involving a comparison of schizophrenic patients (early- and late-onset schizophrenia) with mood disorder patients and normal control subjects in terms of visual and auditory impairment. The results showed that all the psychiatric groups were similar to normal controls on uncorrected vision or hearing, but were significantly more impaired on corrected sensory function (i.e. with eyeglasses or hearing aids). These results suggest that the association between sensory impairment and late-life psychosis may be, at least in part, a result of insufficient correction of sensory deficits in older schizophrenia patients compared with normal controls. This could reflect a difficulty for these patients to access optimal health care, especially for the treatment of sensory impairment. In other words, the sensory deficits per se do not seem to predispose to late-onset schizophrenia but, rather, the sensory deficits remain largely uncorrected in older patients with schizophrenia. Alternatively, the causes for sensory deficits might be such that in this group the deficits are not correctable.

Premorbid personality and other factors

Premorbid personality in patients with late and mid-life paranoid psychoses and the quality of premorbid relationships within families and with friends were assessed retrospectively by Kay et al. (1976). This study is an important one because, through use of structured patient and informant interviews, it represented a first effort to overcome some of the problems inherent in any retrospective attempt at defining premorbid personality. From a consecutive series of first admissions to a psychiatric hospital, the authors selected 54 cases of paranoid and 57 of affective psychosis over the age of 50. Patients and close relatives or friends were independently given a semistructured clinical interview, designed to cover a wide range of paranoid traits. The paranoid patients were rated more highly, both by themselves and informants, on items that suggested that they had greater difficulty in establishing and maintaining satisfactory relationships premorbidly. They had also been significantly more shy, reserved, touchy and suspicious and less able to display sympathy or emotion. Through principal component analysis of the results, the authors derived a 'prepsychotic schizoid personality factor' consisting of unsociability, reticence, suspiciousness and hostility.

Retterstol (1966) has argued that because personality deviations in paranoid patients are recognizable at a very early age, factors in the childhood and adolescence of patients are impor-

tant in determining a predisposition to paranoid psychosis later in life. Key experiences in the later development of paranoid psychoses are proposed to be those that provoke feelings of insecurity or that damage the self-image of an individual whose personality is already overtly sensitive. Gurian et al. (1992) have also provided evidence for the importance of childhood experiences in the development of paranoid psychosis in late life. Among nine Israeli patients with delusional disorder, these authors found a high prevalence of 'war refugees'. These were individuals who had survived the Armenian or Nazi holocausts or been forced to leave their native country. The authors proposed an association between the presence of extremely life-threatening experiences in childhood, a failure to produce progeny and the development of paranoid delusional symptoms in late life in response to a stressful situation such as widowhood. Just how early the threatening experience needs to be is not clear. Cervantes et al. (1989) found the risk of developing a paranoid psychosis to be doubled in immigrants from Mexico and Central America who were escaping war or political unrest, compared with those who had moved for economic reasons. Thus, the period during which a personality may be rendered sensitive to the later development of paranoid psychosis by exposure to trauma is presumably not limited to early childhood.

Exactly how important abnormalities in personality functioning are in the aetiology and onset of late-life paranoid psychoses is unclear. While there is evidence linking social trauma in childhood or early adult life to the later development of psychosis, it is perhaps more plausible to view the abnormal premorbid personality as an early marker of impending psychosis rather than to regard the psychosis as an indication of earlier personality dysfunction.

In a small study, Lohr et al. (1997) found that middle-age-onset schizophrenia patients, similar to early-onset schizophrenia patients, had a greater number of minor physical anomalies than normal subjects and patients with Alzheimer's disease. This is an interesting finding because, as is generally accepted for early-onset schizophrenia patients, it suggests aberrations in the neurodevelopment of middle-age-onset schizophrenia patients.

According to the neurodevelopmental model (Weinberger 1987), the brain lesions putatively related to the pathogenesis of schizophrenia are of developmental origin and are not progressive or degenerative in nature. Studies by Jeste et al. (1997) suggest that the neurodevelopmental model also applies to late-onset schizophrenia. Differences in severity and specific locations or nature of these 'lesions' may account for a delay in the onset of schizophrenia. Wong et al. (1984) suggest that the later age of onset and a better prognosis for schizophrenia in women may relate to a later peak and a delayed regression of dopaminergic activity.

Management/treatment

There is limited published research addressing the treatment of late-onset schizophrenia. The available studies are generally characterized by small sample sizes and are often case reports or case series rather than well-controlled double-blind studies. Because the number of reports in late-onset schizophrenia is limited, we also include studies related to other psychotic disorders (e.g. early-onset schizophrenia, delusional disorder) in late life. Studies related to these other disorders may be applicable to patients with late-onset schizophrenia.

Establishing a therapeutic relationship

Although these patients are often described as hostile and their relationships with neighbours, primary care physicians and the local police may be affected by their psychotic symptoms by the time psychiatric referral is considered, the authors' experience is that they are often extremely lonely. Without entering into any kind of collusion, it is always possible to at least take the time to listen to the patient's account of his or her persecution and not difficult to express sympathy for the distress he or she is experiencing. Sometimes a brief admission to hospital or the establishment of regular community psychiatric nurse (CPN) visits can be rendered acceptable as an attempt to 'get to the bottom' of whatever is going on. Once a relationship of trust and support has been established, patients will often accept medication and visits from members of the psychiatric team. Use of compulsory admission powers should be reserved until all else has failed. Relatives and friends should be advised to encourage the patient to reserve discussion of such complaints to the time when the CPN visits if this is possible. However, there is no single strategy which is best for all patients. For most patients, interventions delivered to their own homes (CPN or volunteer visits, home helps and meals-on-wheels) seem to be most acceptable; although some will respond well to the activities and company provided by a day hospital or centre, some may decline to attend. The potential role of psychological treatments in the management of psychotic symptoms in younger patients is becoming clearer, but older psychotic patients are not routinely considered for these, which is unfortunate and unfair (Aguera-Ortiz & Reneses-Prieto 1999).

Rehousing

Because these patients may have highly restricted and encapsulated delusional systems, their complaints about neighbours or the home environment are sometimes taken at face value by social services staff. Hence, by the time of first psychiatric referral, a patient might have been rehoused at least once in the preceding months. As a general rule, even if it results in a brief reduction of complaints from the patient, provision of new accommodation is followed within a few weeks by a re-emergence of symptoms. The obvious distress this causes is sufficient reason always to advise patients and social workers against such moves unless they are being considered for non-delusional reasons or following successful treatment of psychosis.

Cognitive and behavioural interventions

Cognitive–behaviour therapy and social skills training have been found to be useful in younger adults with schizophrenia. Preliminary studies with older patients, including some with late-onset illness, suggest that age-appropriate combined cognitive behavioural–social skills training interventions may help to improve psychopathology and everyday functioning in older patients too (McQuaid et al. 2001; Granholm et al. 2002).

Antipsychotic medication

In general, neuroleptic or antipsychotic medications are the most effective symptomatic treatment for early- and late-onset chronic schizophrenia as these drugs improve both the acute symptoms and prevent relapses (Jeste et al. 1993). However, alterations in pharmacokinetics and pharmacodynamics complicate pharmacotherapy in older patients. In comparison to younger patients, geriatric patients show an increased variability of response and an increased sensitivity to medications (Salzman 1990).

Rabins et al. (1984) found no, or only a partial, response to neuroleptics in 43% of schizophrenic patients with an onset after 44 years, while Pearlson et al. (1989) reported that 54% of their patients fell into this category. In reports of patients with late paraphrenia, the comparable rates range from 49% (Post 1966) to 75% (Kay & Roth 1961). The general conclusion from such studies is that while drugs relieve some target symptoms, the overall treatment response to medication is modest.

It would be useful to know which illness parameters are associated with poor response to medication. Pearlson et al. (1989) found a poor response to neuroleptics to be associated with the presence of thought disorder and with schizoid premorbid personality traits. The presence of first-rank symptoms, family history of schizophrenia and gender had no effect on treatment response. In a late paraphrenic patient group, Holden (1987) found auditory hallucinations and affective features to predict a favourable response. However, this may simply reflect a better natural history in such patients.

Among a group of 64 late paraphrenic patients prescribed neuroleptic medication for at least 3 months, 42.2% showed no response, 31.3% a partial response and 26.6% a full response to treatment (Howard & Levy 1992). Compliance with medication, receiving depot rather than oral medication, and use of a community psychiatric nurse if the patient was an outpatient all had a positive effect on treatment response. Patients prescribed depot medication received on average a lower daily dose in chlorpromazine equivalents than those prescribed oral medication.

Rockwell et al. (1994) studied middle-aged and elderly patients with late-onset psychosis with somatic delusions (e.g. a delusional belief that the person has some physical defect, disorder or disease) with a mean age of 63. The delusional patients showed poor compliance with psychiatric treatment recommendations and rarely benefited from short-term psychopharmacological (mainly neuroleptic) intervention.

Dosage

In four North American clinical centres, the mean daily dosage prescribed to late-onset schizophrenia patients was several times lower than that in a group of young patients with schizophrenia (Jeste & Zisook 1988). Moreover, Jeste *et al.* (1997) found that the mean daily dosage of antipsychotics used in patients with late-onset schizophrenia was significantly smaller than that prescribed to age-comparable patients with early-onset schizophrenia.

Tardive dyskinesia

There is a serious risk associated with long-term use of typical neuroleptics. Patients may develop tardive dyskinesia (TD), a movement disorder characterized by involuntary, irregular or repetitive abnormal movements. In one study (Saltz *et al.* 1991) of elderly patients, ranging in age from 55 to 99 years, the incidence of TD was 31% after 43 weeks of cumulative neuroleptic treatment. Jeste *et al.* (1999b) reported the cumulative incidence of dyskinetic movements in elderly patients to be 29% following 12 months of typical neuroleptic use. This cumulative annual incidence of TD in older adults is five to six times that reported in younger adults. Higher dosage and longer duration of neuroleptic treatment, as well as other factors including alcohol dependence and subtle movement disorder at baseline, were found to increase the risk of TD in the older patient population (Jeste *et al.* 1995).

Novel antipsychotic medications

Because of its relatively weak blockade of striatal dopamine D_2-receptors, low-dose clozapine seemed a promising drug for the treatment of elderly psychotic patients who have individual sensitivity to extrapyramidal symptoms caused by typical neuroleptics. However, clozapine has anticholinergic, hypotensive and sedating effects and has been shown to impair memory function and, despite a few early positive case reports, has not found favour with those who regularly prescribe for older patients. Risperidone is a benzisoxazole derivative with strong binding affinity for serotonin $5-HT_2$-receptors, dopamine D_2-receptors and α_1- and α_2-adrenergic and histamine H_1-receptors. Of all the atypical antipsychotics, clinical experience with risperidone in the older patient group has so far been most extensive. Early reports with this drug suggested that activity at $5-HT_2$-receptors appeared to be important in the treatment of complex visual hallucinations, which had been traditionally regarded as treatment-resistant. Risperidone has efficacy in the treatment of hallucinations and delusions in elderly patients at low doses (typically, 0.5–2 mg/day). Jeste *et al.* (1999a) compared the 9-month cumulative incidence of TD with risperidone to that with haloperidol in older patients. Sixty-one patients on risperidone were matched with 61 patients from a larger sample of patients who received haloperidol in terms of age, diagnosis and length of pre-enrolment neuroleptic intake. The median daily dose of each medication was 1 mg. Results suggested that, over this 9-month period, risperidone was associated with a fivefold lower cumulative incidence of TD than haloperidol in a high-risk group of older patients. Risperidone should be prescribed to patients with late-onset schizophrenia at considerably lower dosage than those recommended for younger adults. The initial doses of risperidone should be between 0.25 and 0.5 mg/day, with increases not to exceed 0.5 mg/day. Maximum dosage in patients with schizophrenia should remain at 3 mg/day or less. The risk of extrapyramidal symptoms, postural hypotension and somnolence increases with higher dosage.

Olanzapine has a similar receptor-binding profile to clozapine but does not appear to cause the anticholinergic problems seen with the earlier agent. A starting dosage of 2.5–5 mg/day is generally well tolerated and can be increased to 10 or even 15 mg/day if no adverse events appear. Although data on the incidence of TD in elderly patients treated with olanzapine have not yet been reported, preliminary evidence indicates a low risk for extrapyramidal symptoms in this population and the risk of TD in young olanzapine-treated adults appears to be low (Tollefson *et al.* 1997). Anecdotal evidence suggests that olanzapine is less likely to cause extrapyramidal symptoms but more likely to produce sedation and weight gain.

Quetiapine, a newer atypical antipsychotic, also has a low risk of extrapyramidal symptoms, and probably of TD. It may cause sedation and postural hypotension at higher dosage. The recommended starting dosage is 25–50 mg/day, and the maintenance dosage range in older patients is 100–200 mg/day.

At this time, there is very little published information on ziprasidone in elderly patients with schizophrenia.

Comparative trials of different atypical antipsychotics are needed in older schizophrenia patients.

Guidelines for prescribing

There is no real evidence that any particular drug is more effective in this group of patients. The choice of drug for each individual patient should thus be based on considerations of concomitant physical illness and other treatments received, together with the specific side-effect profile of the drug (Tran-Johnson *et al.* 1994). Treatment should usually be commenced at a low dosage of an oral preparation and it is easy to argue that this should be one of the atypical agents because of the reduced risk of early and delayed emergent motor side-effects. Patients who do not respond to oral treatment (whether because of poor compliance or genuine treatment resistance) can be treated with depot. Successful treatment of patients with depot can often be at very modest dosage. For example, the mean dosage of prescribed depot in Howard and Levy's (1992) study was 14.4 mg flupenthixol decanoate or 9 mg fluphenazine decanoate every fortnight. Over the next few years we can expect to see the development of depot preparations of the atypical antipsychotics. Indeed, trials of depot risperidone are in progress at the time of writing. If these trials prove successful, we have little doubt that this will represent the optimal way of delivering antipsychotic treatment to at least some of these patients.

Conclusions

The history of schizophrenia and schizophrenia-like psychoses that have onset in later life is a long one, but it is only in the last three decades that any real attempts have been made to study patients with these conditions and understand how they might relate to psychoses which arise earlier in the life cycle. The aetiological roles of premorbid personality functioning, degenerative and genetic factors are still not fully elucidated, although most recent brain imaging studies indicate that gross degenerative changes are not present. If compliance with neuroleptic medication can be established and maintained, and supplemented by psychosocial therapy, the prognosis for symptomatic and functional improvement can be favourable.

Acknowledgements

This work was supported, in part, by the National Institute of Mental Health grants MH43695, MH49671 and MH19934 and by the Department of Veterans Affairs.

References

Aguera-Ortiz, L. & Reneses-Prieto, B. (1999) *The Place of Non-Biological Treatments*. In: *Late-Onset Schizophrenia* (eds R. Howard, P.V. Rabins & D.J. Castle), pp. 233–261. Wrightson Biomedical, Petersfield.

Almeida, O., Forstl, H., Howard, R. & David, A.S. (1993) Unilateral auditory hallucinations. *British Journal of Psychiatry* 162, 262–264.

Almeida, O.P., Howard, R.J., Levy, R. & David, A.S. (1995a) Psychotic states arising in late life (late paraphrenia): psychopathology and nosolgy. *British Journal of Psychiatry* 165, 205–214.

Almeida, O.P., Howard, R.J., Levy, R. *et al.* (1995b) Clinical and cognitive diversity of psychotic states arising in late life (late paraphrenia). *Psychological Medicine* 25, 699–714.

American Psychiatric Association (1980) *Diagnostic and Statistical Manual of Mental Disorders*, 3rd edn. American Psychiatric Press, Washington, DC.

American Psychiatric Association (1987) *Diagnostic and Statistical Manual of Mental Disorders–Revised*, 3rd edn. American Psychiatric Press, Washington, DC.

American Psychiatric Association (1994) *Diagnostic and Statistical Manual of Mental Disorders*, 4th edn. American Psychiatric Press, Washington, DC.

Andreasen, N.C. (1982) Negative symptoms in schizophrenia: definition and reliability. *Archives of General Psychiatry* 39, 784–788.

Andreasen, N.C. & Olsen, S. (1982) Negative vs. positive schizophrenia: definition and validation. *Archives of General Psychiatry* 39, 789–794.

Andreasen, N.C., Ehrhardt, J.C., Swayze, V.W. *et al.* (1990) Magnetic resonance imaging of the brain in schizophrenia. *Archives of General Psychiatry* 47, 35–44.

Andreasen, N.C., Arndt, S., Swayze, V.W. *et al.* (1994) Thalamic abnormalities in schizophrenia visualized through magnetic resonance image averaging. *Science* 266, 294–298.

Bleuler, E.P. (1911) *Dementia Praecox or the Group of Schizophrenias*. Deuticke, Leipzig.

Bleuler, M. (1943) Die spatschizophrenen krankheitsbilder. *Fortschritte der Neurologie Psychiatrie* 15, 259–290.

Breitner, J., Husain, M., Figiel, G., Krishnan, K. & Boyko, O. (1990) Cerebral white matter disease in late-onset psychosis. *Biological Psychiatry* 28, 266–274.

Brodaty, H., Sachdev, P., Rose, N., Rylands, K. & Prenter, L. (1999) Schizophrenia with onset after age 50 years. 1. Phenomenology and risk factors. *British Journal of Psychiatry* 175, 410–415.

Buchsbaum, M.S., Someya, T., Teng, C.Y. *et al.* (1996) PET and MRI of the thalamus in never-medicated patients with schizophrenia. *American Journal of Psychiatry* 153, 191–199.

Castle, D.J. & Howard, R. (1992) What do we know about the aetiology of late-onset schizophrenia. *European Psychiatry* 7, 99–108.

Castle, D.J. & Murray, R.M. (1991) The neurodevelopmental basis of sex differences in schizophrenia. *Psychological Medicine* 21, 565–575.

Cervantes, R.C., Salgado-Snyder, V.N. & Padilla, A.M. (1989) Post-traumatic stress in immigrants from Central American and Mexico. *Hospital Community Psychiatry* 40, 615–619.

Cooper, A.F. (1976) Deafness and psychiatric illness. *British Journal of Psychiatry* 129, 216–226.

Cooper, A.F. & Curry, A.R. (1976) The pathology of deafness in the paranoid and affective psychoses of later life. *Journal of Psychosomatic Research* 20, 97–105.

Cooper, A.F., Curry, A.R., Kay, D.W.K., Garside, R.F. & Roth, M. (1974) Hearing loss in paranoid and affective psychoses of the elderly. *Lancet* 2, 851–854.

Corbin, S.L. & Eastwood, M.R. (1986) Sensory deficits and mental disorders of old age: causal or coincidental associations? *Psychological Medicine* 16, 251–256.

Corey-Bloom, J., Jernigan, T., Archibald, S., Harris, M.J. & Jeste, D.V. (1995) Quantitative magnetic resonance imaging of the brain in late-life schizophrenia. *American Journal of Psychiatry* 152, 447–449.

Cutting, J.C., Clare, A.W. & Mann, A.H. (1978) Cycloid psychosi: investigation of the diagnostic concept. *Psychological Medicine* 8, 637–648.

Eastwood, R., Corbin, S. & Reed, M. (1981) Hearing impairment and paraphrenia. *Journal of Otolaryngology* 10, 306–308.

Fish, F. (1958) A clinical investigation of chronic schizophrenia. *British Journal of Psychiatry* 104, 34–54.

Fish, F. (1960) Senile schizophrenia. *Journal of Mental Science* 106, 938–946.

Flint, A.J., Rifat, S.I. & Eastwood, M.R. (1991) Late-onset paranoia: distinct from paraphrenia? *International Journal of Geriatric Psychiatry* 6, 103–109.

Funding, T. (1961) Genetics of paranoid psychosis of later life. *Acta Psychiatrica Scandinavica* 37, 267–282.

Gabriel, E. (1978) *Die Langfristige Entwicklung der Spatschizophrenien*. Karger, Basel.

Gorwood, P., Leboyer, M., Jay, M., Payan, C. & Feingold, J. (1995) Gender and age at onset in schizophrenia: impact of family history. *American Journal of Psychiatry* 152, 208–212.

Gottesman, I.I. & Shields, J. (1982) *Schizophrenia: the Epigenetic Puzzle.* Cambridge University Press, Cambridge.

Grahame, P.S. (1984) Schizophrenia in old age (late paraphrenia). *British Journal of Psychiatry* **145**, 493–495.

Granholm, E., McQuaid, J.R., McClure, F.S., Pedrelli, P. & Jeste, D.V. (2002) A randomized controlled pilot study of cognitive behavioral social skills training for older patients with schizophrenia. *Schizophrenia Research* **53**, 167–169.

Gurian, B.S., Wexler, D. & Baker, E.H. (1992) Late-life paranoia: possible association with early trauma and infertility. *International Journal of Geriatric Psychiatry* **7**, 277–284.

Harris, M.J. & Jeste, D.V. (1988) Late-onset schizophrenia: an overview. *Schizophrenia Bulletin* **14**, 39–55.

Heaton, R., Paulsen, J., McAdams, L.A. *et al.* (1994) Neuropsychological deficits in schizophrenia: relationship to age, chronicity and dementia. *Archives of General Psychiatry* **51**, 469–476.

Heaton, R.K., Gladsjo, J.A., Palmer, B. *et al.* (2001) The stability and course of neuropsychological deficits in schizophrenia. *Archives of General Psychiatry* **58**, 24–32.

Herbert, M.E. & Jacobson, S. (1967) Late paraphrenia. *British Journal of Psychiatry* **113**, 461–469.

Holden, N.L. (1987) Late paraphrenia or the paraphrenias: a descriptive study with a 10-year follow-up. *British Journal of Psychiatry* **150**, 635–639.

Hopkins, B. & Roth, M. (1953) Psychological test performance in patients over sixty. II. Paraphrenia, arteriosclerotic psychosis and acute confusion. *Journal of Mental Science* **99**, 451–463.

Howard, R. & Levy, R. (1992) Which factors affect treatment response in late paraphrenia? *International Journal of Geriatric Psychiatry* **7**, 667–672.

Howard, R., Castle, D., Wessely, S. & Murray, R.M. (1993) A comparative study of 470 cases of early and late-onset schizophrenia. *British Journal of Psychiatry* **163**, 352–357.

Howard, R., Almeida, O. & Levy, R. (1994a) Phenomenology, demography and diagnosis in late paraphrenia. *Psychological Medicine* **24**, 397–410.

Howard, R.J., Almeida, O., Levy, R., Graves, P. & Graves, M. (1994b) Quantitative magnetic resonance imaging volume try distinguishes delusional disorder from late-onset schizophrenia. *British Journal of Psychiatry* **165**, 474–480.

Howard, R., Cox, T., Almeida, O. *et al.* (1995) White matter signal hyperintensities in the brains of patients with late paraphrenia and the normal community-living elderly. *Biological Psychiatry* **38**, 86–91.

Howard, R., Graham, C., Sham, P. *et al.* (1997) A controlled family study of late-onset non-affective psychosis (late paraphrenia). *British Journal of Psychiatry* **170**, 511–514.

Howard, R., Rabins, P.V., Seeman, M.V. & Jeste, D.V. and the International Late-Onset Schizophrenia Group (2000) Late-onset schizophrenia and very-late-onset schizophrenia-like psychois: an international consensus. *American Journal of Psychiatry* **157**, 172–178.

Huber, G., Gross, G. & Schuttler, R. (1975) Spat schizophrenie. *Archiv Fur Psychiatrie und Nervenkrankheiten* **22**, 53–66.

Jernigan, T.L., Press, G.A. & Hesselink, J.R. (1990) Methods for measuring brain morphologic features on magnetic resonance images: validation and normal aging. *Archives of Neurology* **47**, 27–32.

Jernigan, T.L., Zisook, S., Heaton, R.K. *et al.* (1991) Magnetic resonance imaging abnormalities in lenticular nuclei and cerebral cortex in schizophrenia. *Archives of General Psychiatry* **48**, 881–890.

Jeste, D.V. & Zisook, S. (1988) Preface to psychosis and depression in the elderly. *Psychiatric Clinics of North America* **11**, xiii–xv.

Jeste, D.V., Harris, M.J., Pearlson, G.D. *et al.* (1988) Late-onset schizophrenia: studying clinical validity. *Psychiatric Clinics of North America* **11**, 1–14.

Jeste, D.V., Lacro, J.P., Gilbert, P.L., Kline, J. & Kline, N. (1993) Treatment of late-life schizophrenia with neuroleptics. *Schizophrenia Bulletin* **19** (4), 817–830.

Jeste, D.V., Caligiuri, M.P., Paulsen, J.S. *et al.* (1995) Risk of tardive dyskinesia in older patients: a prospective longitudinal study of 266 patients. *Archives of General Psychiatry* **52**, 756–765.

Jeste, D.V., Symonds, L.L., Harris, M.J. *et al.* (1997) Non-dementia non-praecox dementia praecox? Late-onset schizophrenia. *American Journal of Geriatric Psychiatry* **5**, 302–317.

Jeste, D.V., Lacro, J.P., Palmer, B. *et al.* (1999a) Incidence of tardive dyskinesia in early stages of neuroleptic treatment for older patients. *American Journal of Psychiatry* **156**, 309–311.

Jeste, D.V., Lacro, J.P., Palmer, B.W. *et al.* (1999b) Incidence of tardive dyskinesia in early stages of low-dose treatment with typical neuroleptics in older patients. *American Journal of Psychiatry* **156**, 309–311.

Kay, D.W.K. & Roth, M. (1961) Environmental and hereditary factors in the schizophrenias of old age ('late paraphrenia') and their bearing on the general problem of causation in schizophrenia. *Journal of Mental Science* **107**, 649–686.

Kay, D.W.K., Cooper, A.F., Garside, R.F. & Roth, M. (1976) The differentiation of paranoid from affective psychoses by patients' premorbid characteristics. *British Journal of Psychiatry* **129**, 207–215.

Kendler, K.S., Tsuang, M.T. & Hays, P. (1987) Age at onset in schizophrenia: a familial perspective. *Archives of General Psychiatry* **44**, 881–890.

Keshavan, M.S., David, A.S., Steingard, S. & Lishman, W.A. (1992) Musical hallucinations: a review and synthesis. *Neuropsychiatry, Neuropsychology and Behavioural Neurology* **5**, 211–223.

Khan, A.M., Clark, T. & Oyebode, F. (1988) Unilateral auditory hallucinations. *British Journal of Psychiatry* **152**, 297–298.

Klages, W. (1961) *Die Spatschizophrenie.* Enke, Stuttgart.

Kraepelin, E. (1913) *Psychiatrie, Ein Lehrbuch Fur Studierende und Artze.* Barth, Leipzig.

Levitt, J.J. & Tsuang, M.T. (1988) The heterogeneity of schizoaffective disorder: implications for treatment. *American Journal of Psychiatry* **145**, 926–936.

Lewine, R. (1981) Sex differences in schizophrenia: timing or subtype? *Psychological Bulletin* **90**, 432–444.

Lindamer, L.A., Harris, M.J., Gladsjo, J.A. *et al.* (2000) Gender and schizophrenia. In: *Sex Hormones, Aging, and Mental Disorders* (ed. M. Morrison), pp. 223–239. National Institute of Mental Health, Washington, DC.

Lindamer, L.A., Dunn, L.B. & Jeste, D.V. (2002) Gender and age of onset in schizophrenia: Lewine's hypothesis revisited. In: *Women's Health and Psychiatry* (eds K. Pearson & S.S. Rosenbaum). Lippincott Williams & Wilkins, New York.

Lohr, J.B., Alder, M., Flynn, K., Harris, M.J. & McAdams, L.A. (1997) Minor physical anomalies in older patients with late-onset schizophrenia, early-onset schizophrenia, depression, and Alzheimer's disease. *American Journal of Geriatric Psychiatry* **5**, 318–323.

McQuaid, J.R., Granholm, E., Roepke, S. *et al.* (2000) Development of an integrated cognitive–behavioral, social skills training intervention for older patients with schizophrenia. *Journal of Psychotherapy Research and Practice* **9**, 149–156.

Magnan, V. (1893) *Lecons Cliniques Sur les Maladies Mentales.* Bureaux de Progres Medical, Paris.

Marneros, A. & Deister, A. (1984) The psychopathology of 'late schizophrenia'. *Psychopathology* **17**, 264–174.

Miller, B.L., Lesser, I.M., Boone, K. *et al.* (1989) Brain white-matter lesions and psychosis. *British Journal of Psychiatry* 155, 73–78.

Miller, B.L., Lesser, I.M., Boone, K.B. *et al.* (1991) Brain lesions and cognitive function in late-life psychosis. *British Journal of Psychiatry* 158, 76–82.

Miller, B.L., Lesser, I.M., Mena, I. *et al.* (1992) Regional cerebral blood flow in late-life-onset psychosis. *Neuropsychiatry, Neuropsychology and Behavioural Neurology* 5, 132–137.

Murray, R.M., O'Callaghan, E., Castle, D.J. & Lewis, S.W. (1992) A neurodevelopmental approach to the classification of schizophrenia. *Schizophrenia Bulletin* 18, 319–332.

Naguib, M. & Levy, R. (1987) Late paraphrenia. neuropsychological impairment and structural brain abnormalities on computed tomography. *International Journal of Geriatric Psychiatry* 2, 83–90.

Overall, J.E. & Gorham, D.R. (1962) The Brief Psychiatric Rating Scale. *Psychological Reports* 10, 799–812.

Pakkenberg, B. (1990) Pronounced reduction of total neuron number in mediodorsal thalamic nucleus and nucleus accumbens in schizophrenia. *Archives of General Psychiatry* 47, 1023–1028.

Pakkenberg, B. (1992) The volume of the mediodorsal thalamic nucleus in treated and untreated schizophrenics. *Schizophrenia Research* 7, 95–100.

Palmer, B.W., McClure, F. & Jeste, D.V. (2001) Schizophrenia in late-life: findings challenge traditional concepts. *Harvard Review of Psychiatry* 9, 51–58.

Paulsen, J.S., Heaton, R.K., Sadek, J.R. *et al.* (1995) The nature of learning and memory impairments in schizophrenia. *Journal of the International Neuropsychological Society* 1, 88–99.

Paulsen, J.S., Romero, R., Chan, A. *et al.* (1996) Impairment of the semantic network in schizophrenia. *Psychiatry Research* 63, 109–121.

Pearlson, G.D., Kreger, L., Rabins, R.V. *et al.* (1989) A chart review study of late-onset and early-onset schizophrenia. *American Journal of Psychiatry* 146, 1568–1574.

Pearlson, G.D., Tune, L.E., Wong, D.F. *et al.* (1993) Quantitative D_2 dopamine receptor PET and structural MRI changes in late onset schizophrenia. *Schizophrenia Bulletin* 19, 783–795.

Post, F. (1966) *Persistent Persecutory States of the Elderly*. Pergamon Press, London.

Prager, S. & Jeste, D.V. (1993) Sensory impairment in late-life schizophrenia. *Schizophrenia Bulletin* 19, 755–772.

Quintal, M., Day-Cody, D. & Levy, R. (1991) Late paraphrenia and ICD-10. *International Journal of Geriatric Psychiatry* 6, 111–116.

Rabins, P., Pauker, S. & Thomas, J. (1984) Can schizophrenia begin after age 44? *Comprehensive Psychiatry* 25, 290–293.

Retterstol, N. (1966) *Paranoid and Paranoiac Psychoses: A Personal Follow-Up Investigation with Special Reference to Aetiological, Clinical and Prognostic Aspects*. Thomas Springfield. Oslo Universitetsforlaget.

Riecher-Rossler, A., Hafner, H., Stumbalum, M., Maurer, K. & Schmidt, R. (1994) Can estradiol modulate schizophrenic symptomatology? *Schizophrenia Bulletin* 20, 203–213.

Rockwell, E., Krull, A.J., Dimsdale, J. & Jeste, D.V. (1994) Late-onset psychosis with somatic delusions. *Psychosomatics* 35, 66–72.

Roth, M. & Morrisey, J.D. (1952) Problems in the diagnosis and classification of mental disorders in old age. *Journal of Mental Science* 98, 68–80.

Saltz, B.L., Woerner, M.G., Kane, J.M. *et al.* (1991) Prospective study of tardive dyskinesia incidence in the elderly. *Journal of the American Medical Association* 266, 2402–2406.

Salzman, C. (1990) Principles of psychopharmacology. In: *Verwoerdt's Clinical Geropsychiatry* (ed. D. Bienenfeld), pp. 235–249. Williams & Wilkins, Baltimore, MD.

Seeman, M.V. (1981) Gender and the onset of schizophrenia: neurohumoral influences. *Psychiatric Journal of the University of Ottawa* 6, 136–138.

Seeman, M.V. (1999) Oestrogens and psychosis. In: *Late Onset Schizophrenia* (eds. R. Howard, P.V. Rabins & D.J. Castle), pp. 165–180. Biomedical Publishing, Wrightson, Philadelphia.

Seeman, M.V. & Lang, M. (1990) The role of estrogens in schizophrenia gender differences. *Schizophrenia Bulletin* 16, 185–194.

Sherman, S.M. & Koch, C. (1990) Thalamus. In: *The Synaptic Organization of the Brain*, 3rd end (eds. G.M. Shepherd), pp. 246–278. Oxford University Press, New York.

Shimizu, A. & Kurachi, M. (1989) Do women without a family history of schizophrenia have a later onset of schizophrenia? *Japanese Journal of Psychiatry and Neurology* 43, 133–136.

Sjoegren, H. (1964) Paraphrenic, melancholic and psychoneurotic states in the pre-senile and senile periods of life. *Acta Psychiatrica Scandinavica Supplement* 176.

Sternberg, E. (1972) Neuere forschungsergebnisse bei spatschizophrenen psychosen. *Fortschritte der Neurologie Psychiatrie* 40, 631–646.

Symonds, L.L., Olichney, J.M., Jernigan, T.L. *et al.* (1997) Lack of clinically significant structural abnormalities in MRIs of older patients with schizophrenia and related psychoses. *Journal of Neuropsychiatry and Clinical Neuroscience* 9, 251–258.

Tollefson, G.D., Beasley, C.M., Tamura, R.N., Tran, P.V. & Potvin, J.H. (1997) Blind, controlled, long-term study of the comparative incidence of treatment-emerged tardive diskinesia with olanzapine or haloperidol. *American Journal of Psychiatry* 154, 1248–1254.

Tran-Johnson, T.K., Harris, M.J. & Jeste, D.V. (1994) Pharmacological treatment of schizophrenia and delusional disorders of late life. In: *Principles and Practices of Geriatric Psychiatry* (eds J.R.M. Copeland, M.T. Abou-Saleh & D.G. Blazer), pp. 685–692. John Wiley, New York.

Treff, W.M. & Hempel, K.J. (1958) Die Zelldichte bei Schizophrenen und klinisch Gesunden. *Journal für Hirnforschung* 4, 314–369.

Weinberger, D.R. (1987) Implications of normal brain development for the pathogenesis of schizophrenia. *Archives of General Psychiatry* 44, 660–669.

Wong, D.F., Wagner, H.N. Jr, Dannals, R.F. *et al.* (1984) Effects of age on dopamine and serotonin receptors measured by positron emission tomography in the living human brain. *Science* 226, 1393–1396.

7

The schizophrenia spectrum personality disorders

K. O'Flynn, J. Gruzelier, A. Bergman and L.J. Siever

Phenomenology, 80
  Psychometric assessment, 82
Spectrum personality disorders in premorbid clinical
    profiles of schizophrenic patients, 82
Genetics, 84
Psychophysiology, 84
  Prepulse inhibition, 84
  P50 suppression, 85
  Habituation, 85
  N100 and P300 evoked potentials, 86
  Eye movements, 86
Information processing and cognitive
    function, 86
  Visual processing, 86

Frontal and executive functions, 87
  Continuous performance test, 87
  Thought disorder and disinhibition, 88
  Memory, 88
  Lateralization, 89
Neurochemistry, 89
Imaging studies, 90
  Structural imaging, 90
  Functional imaging, 91
Treatment studies, 91
Outcome, 92
Integration of pathophysiology, 92
Conclusions, 93
References, 94

European phenomenologically orientated psychiatrists such as Kraeplin and Bleuler were among the first to observe that there may be gradations of schizophrenia-related disorders, with relatives of schizophrenic patients displaying mild psychotic-like symptoms and asociality similar but less severe than the signs and symptoms observed in chronic schizophrenia (Kraeplin 1919/1971; Bleuler 1950). More recently, the adoption studies of Kety *et al.* (1975) described the clinical profiles of probands and relatives with diagnoses of 'borderline schizophrenia' or 'latent schizophrenia'. These case histories were reviewed and the features identified provided the basis for the diagnosis 'schizotypal personality disorder' (SPD) which was included for the first time in DSM-III (Table 7.1; American Psychiatric Association 1980).

SPD is part of the 'odd' cluster of the personality disorders. Analogous to symptoms of chronic schizophrenia, the features of SPD may be viewed as psychotic-like (ideas of reference, magical thinking, suspiciousness) and deficit-related symptoms (social isolation, inadequate rapport). SPD represents the first personality disorder defined in part by its genetic relationship to schizophrenia and is the prototype of the schizophrenia-related personality disorders in the schizophrenia spectrum.

Studies of the phenomenology, genetics, biology, cognition, outcome and treatment response of SPD have consistently supported a close relationship of SPD to schizophrenia. Schizotypal patients do not, by definition, suffer from chronic psychosis, they have not been exposed to long-term medication, are usually not on current medication and are generally free from the effects of multiple hospital admissions or long-term institutionalization. These patients are therefore spared the multiple artefacts that potentially confound research in schizophrenia. Study of SPD patients may afford an opportunity to disentangle

the factors which interact to determine the schizophrenic process. In this chapter, we present an up to date perspective on research in this relatively novel and expanding area.

Phenomenology

Diagnostic criteria for schizotypal personality disorder or schizotypal disorder consist of attenuated psychotic-like symptoms such as ideas of reference and cognitive–perceptual distortions, as well as deficit-like symptoms of constricted affect, social isolation and related criteria reflecting eccentric appearance and speech. The ideas of reference of schizotypal personality disorder, while not held with the conviction characteristic of the chronic schizophrenic, are often persistent and disturbing to the patient. Schizotypal individuals may feel that others are staring at them or talking about them when they enter a bus or attend a social occasion. They often entertain unusual beliefs that are outside the social norms of their culture, sometimes in a superstitious or religious context and other times in an idiosyncratic fashion. For example, they may manifest 'magical thinking' such as the belief that one's thoughts anticipate tragic events such as accidental deaths. Illusions and other perceptual experiences are common, particularly in situations where information is ambiguous, such as in a darkened room, or in an altered state, such as drowsiness or fatigue. Schizotypal individuals may be socially isolated and have few friends in whom they confide and to whom they feel close in an enduring way. Their affect may be constricted, and they may be difficult to engage interpersonally. Rapport with others may be severely lacking. At other times, they may smile inappropriately and react emotionally in a way that appears incongruent with the content of

Table 7.1 DSM-IV diagnostic criteria for schizotypal personality disorder (American Psychiatric Association 1994).

A A pervasive pattern of social and interpersonal deficits marked by acute discomfort with, and reduced capacity for, close relationships as well as by cognitive or perceptual distortions and eccentricities of behaviour, beginning by early adulthood and present in a variety of contexts, as indicated by five (or more) of the following:

1 Ideas of reference (excluding delusions of reference)
2 Odd beliefs or magical thinking that influences behaviour and is inconsistent with subcultural norms (e.g. superstitiousness, belief in clairvoyance, telepathy or 'sixth sense'; in children or adolescents, bizarre fantasies or preoccupations)
3 Unusual perceptual experiences, including bodily illusions
4 Odd thinking and speech (e.g. vague, circumstantial, metaphorical, overelaborate, or stereotyped)
5 Suspiciousness or paranoid ideation
6 Inappropriate or constricted affect
7 Behaviour or appearance that is odd, eccentric or peculiar
8 Lack of close fiends or confidants other than first-degree relatives
9 Excessive social anxiety that does not diminish with familiarity and tends to he associated with paranoid fears rather than negative judgements about self

B Does not occur exclusively during the course of Schizophrenia, a Mood Disorder With Psychotic Features, another Psychotic Disorder, or a Pervasive Developmental Disorder

Note: If criteria are met prior to the onset of schizophrenia, add 'premorbid', e.g. 'schizotypal personality disorder (premorbid)'.

their speech context. They tend to be suspicious and guarded, attributing negative or persecutory intents to others. Their behaviour and appearance may also appear odd with idiosyncratic movements, expressions, mannerisms and style of dress. Their speech may also be unusual and may be concrete and impoverished or extraordinarily elaborate with frequent non-sequiturs.

The diagnostic criteria for paranoid personality disorder emphasize suspicious and mistrustful traits; distortions in cognition and perception may not be present. Thus, persons with this disorder have an expectancy of malevolent intent and behaviour on the part of others. They constantly question the loyalty of friends and close colleagues and see hidden threatening meanings that tend to justify their preconceptions. Because of their fear of the ill-will of others, they are reluctant to confide in them and are often volatile in response to perceived slights.

In contrast, schizoid personality disorder is grounded in the core traits of asociality and lack of enjoyment of interpersonal engagement. The schizoid person, like the schizotypal individual, may have no close friends or confidants, although people with schizoid personality disorder do not necessarily have the cognitive–perceptual distortions that are criteria for schizotypal personality disorder. The schizoid individual appears to prefer being alone and does not evidence desire for, or pleasure from, close relationships, whether friendly or intimate. Such individu-

als often appear indifferent to criticism and praise, and share with the schizotypal individual an aloof detached constricted appearance.

Schizotypal, schizoid and paranoid disorders are highly over-lapping in clinical samples (Kalus *et al.* 1996). Schizoid personality is least common in the clinical setting, perhaps because these individuals are stably isolated and thus do not experience the dysphoria, disruption of relationships and work function, along with the more eccentric appearance associated with the cognitive peculiarities of schizotypal and paranoid personality disorders. Paranoid and schizotypal personality disorders are highly overlapping in most clinical studies (Kalus *et al.* 1996), which is not surprising given the overlap between the criteria. However, it is not clear whether there is perhaps a group of individuals with paranoid personality disorder distinct from individuals meeting criteria for schizotypal personality disorder, who may be more closely related to delusional disorder or, in some cases, to the histrionic and dramatic spectrum of personality disorders. Further uncertainty involves the role of affect; in one study up to 40% of SPD patients had experienced episodes of major depression, a comorbidity also found in paranoid personality disorder (Bernstein *et al.* 1996; Siever *et al.* 1996).

The generally high comorbidity of these disorders and close relationship of their criteria raise the question of whether they are defining distinct disorders or are actually gradations of severity along the schizophrenia spectrum. According to the latter conception, schizoid personality disorder would represent one end of the continuum, at the other end of which is schizo-phrenia, with schizotypal personality disorder located between the two. Obviously, as one moves towards the more schizoid end of the spectrum, the relationship to schizophrenia is less strong and specific. However, from an aetiological point of view, heterogeneity might be found throughout the spectrum, because a variety of pathophysiological processes may lead to a final outcome of chronic schizophrenia.

There is also an overlap between schizophrenia spectrum personality disorders and borderline and avoidant personality disorders. However, the overlap with borderline personality disorder has been diminished as the criteria for each have become refined (Kavoussi & Siever 1992). The psychotic-like symptoms of borderline personality disorder are viewed as transient and often dissociative, in contrast to those of schizotypal personality disorder, which are more persistent and pervasive, and are accompanied by affective instability. Conceptually, avoidant personality disordered individuals yearn for social relationships but require an unusually strong degree of acceptance before engaging in them because of their anxiety, while schizoid and schizotypal individuals do not actively want or seek these relationships. However, in practice these distinctions are difficult to make. Schizotypal and schizotoid individuals may acknowledge a wistfulness for relationships and experience the limitations of their isolation. Furthermore, avoidant individuals may at times appear aloof and distant, and on neuropsychological testing show cognitive impairment (Cohen *et al.* 1996) that may not be clearly distinct in character from the neuropsychological abnormalities observed in the schizophrenia spectrum disorders.

Some of the symptoms characterizing these personality disorders have also been studied in non-clinical samples, who may be at the furthest end of the schizophrenia spectrum continuum. This line of research has focused on applying psychometric procedures to a normal population in order to detect individuals with an increased liability for schizophrenia. This psychometric high-risk strategy, which is used to identify hypothetically psychosis-prone individuals, is based on Meehl's conception of 'schizotaxia' reflecting an underlying schizophrenia genotype (Meehl 1962). Meehl hypothesized that individuals with schizotaxia who possess the genetic predisposition for schizophrenia but do not manifest the disorder will usually display some evidence of deviant psychological functioning, labelled 'schizotypy'. Meehl described a set of signs and symptoms that he believed were evident in those non-psychotic schizotypic individuals which he believed were based on a neurointegrative deficit termed 'schizotaxia'.

Psychometric assessment

Since Meehl's original description of schizotypic individuals, many self-report instruments have been developed to measure schizotypy in primarily non-clinical populations (Chapman *et al.* 1976, 1978; Eckblad & Chapman 1983; Claridge & Broks 1984; Venables *et al.* 1990; Raine 1991; Mason *et al.* 1997). When used as a high-risk methodology, this approach is a useful complement to the traditional genetic high-risk strategy because it should result in a more representative sample of future schizophrenics, given that only about 5–10% of schizophrenics have a schizophrenic parent (Chapman & Chapman 1985). Furthermore, the benefits of studying non-clinical populations include accessibility to larger numbers of subjects, elimination of potential confounds such as medication and institutionalization, and additional insight into the boundaries of the disorder, while the targeting of adult subjects instead of children shortens the period of follow-up.

The plethora of self-report scales differ in a number of ways, including item construction, conceptual bias and theoretical assumptions. Despite the wide range of techniques and conceptual frameworks evident in the various schizotypy scales, there are a number of findings that are relevant for the study of schizophrenia and schizophrenia spectrum personality disorders. When compared with schizophrenic patients, there is consistent evidence that non-clinical samples identified through these self-report inventories show similar, although often less severe, deficits in a number of areas such as neuropsychological, cognitive and psychophysiological functioning (Raine *et al.* 1995). These findings support the hypothesis that mild expression of schizotypy is genetically and clinically related to schizophrenia.

Another relevant contribution to the psychometric high-risk paradigm has been the number of studies investigating the factor structure underlying schizotypy. Despite the fact that these studies differed in terms of the specific scales used, some compatible

findings have emerged. The most consistent factor to emerge from these studies is that of 'positive' schizotypy, which consists of psychotic-like cognitive and perceptual experiences (Muntaner *et al.* 1988; Bentall *et al.* 1989; Hewitt & Claridge 1989; Raine & Allbutt 1989; Venables *et al.* 1990; Kendler & Hewitt 1992; Gruzelier 1996). Another factor comprises items reflecting 'negative', interpersonal or deficit-like characteristics (Muntaner *et al.* 1988; Bentall *et al.* 1989; Kendler & Hewitt 1992). Some studies have also found a third factor, which can be described as cognitive disorganization (Bentall *et al.* 1989), while others report a third factor of non-conformity (Muntaner *et al.* 1988; Bentall *et al.* 1989; Raine & Allbutt 1989; Kendler & Hewitt 1992), or a mixture of these features combined with activation (Gruzelier 1996; Gruzelier & Doig 1996). These factors have been based on data primarily gathered from non-clinical populations. However, the structure of these three factors has been replicated using non-psychotic outpatients (Battaglia *et al.* 1997) and parallels suggested with positive, negative and thought-disordered factors frequently found in studies of schizophrenia (Gruzelier 1999a). Furthermore, in a study of twins, Kendler *et al.* (1991) found two independent dimensions (positive and negative) of both clinically rated and self-rated schizotypy. These findings indicated that both positive and negative dimensions of both clinically rated and self-rated schizotypy correlated more highly in monozygotic twins than in dizygotic twins. A later paper focused solely on self-report scales of schizotypy and found three distinct factors (positive trait schizotypy, non-conformity and social schizotypy), all of which were influenced by genetic factors (Kendler & Hewitt 1992). These results suggest that genetic factors are important in all these areas of schizotypy.

While much of the research investigating the aetiology, pathophysiology and treatment of schizophrenia involves studies with schizophrenic patients, the concept of a schizophrenia spectrum has stimulated interest in studying both clinical and non-clinical schizotypic subjects. The results of studies utilizing self-report psychometric inventories of schizotypy confirm the importance and relevance of this research for the study of schizophrenia and schizophrenia spectrum personality disorders. In particular, it seems that the positive and negative factors of schizotypy may provide an important area to explore, as it has been suggested that positive and negative symptoms along the schizophrenia spectrum may be associated with distinct pathophysiologies (Siever 1991).

Spectrum personality disorders in premorbid clinical profiles of schizophrenic patients

Interest in the premorbid personality of schizophrenic patients is well established in the psychiatric literature. Both Kraepelin (1919/1971) and Bleuler (1950) observed that a proportion of schizophrenic patients displayed abnormal behaviour long before the onset of adult psychosis. Kretschmer's (1921) description of schizoid personality included solitariness, cold affect and eccentricity. Other descriptions have often included suspiciousness, rigidity and unusual speech (Foerster *et al.* 1991a). Given the recent interest in viewing schizophrenia spectrum personality disorders as milder schizophrenia-related disorders, the study of premorbid personality characteristics in schizophrenia may help to clarify the relationship between schizophrenia spectrum personality disorders and schizophrenia.

A variety of methodologies have been used to investigate the characteristics of adult psychiatric patients before the onset of an illness. These include follow-back studies of adult schizophrenic patients looking at previous school records (Watt 1978) or child guidance centre records, follow-up studies of children who have attended child guidance clinics (Robins 1966), and prospective high-risk studies following children who are presumably at high risk for schizophrenia, usually based on the genetic risk (Parnas & Jorgensen 1989). The majority of these studies did not involve the assessment of schizophrenia spectrum personality disorders as premorbid features of schizophrenia. However, some recent retrospective and high-risk studies have used assessments of personality features based on both patient reports and interviews with relatives (Squires-Wheeler *et al.* 1988; Foerster *et al.* 1991a,b; Peralta *et al.* 1991).

Many of the early retrospective and follow-back studies found that preschizophrenic boys were shy and withdrawn (Bower *et al.* 1960; Warnken & Seiss 1965; Barthell & Holmes 1968). One investigation of the school records of male and female schizophrenic patients indicated that preschizophrenic males were described as emotionally unstable and disagreeable beginning in grade seven which corresponds to early adolescence (Watt 1978). Preschizophrenic females, on the other hand, were described as emotionally unstable and introverted. Another study utilized information in the case notes of adult male schizophrenic patients who had attended a child guidance centre as children. The findings indicated that the diagnoses of these boys tended to consist of mixed emotional and conduct disorders. Similarly, a retrospective analysis from a birth cohort study found that children developing schizophrenia as adults were characterized by anxiety, depression, social withdrawal, aversive behaviour and poor motor control as well as cognitive underachievements, particularly in verbal abilities (Crow *et al.* 1995). In terms of follow-up studies, most have found that preschizophrenic boys were both aggressive and withdrawn (Michael *et al.* 1957; O'Neal & Robins 1958). However, those who were predominantly withdrawn seemed to have the poorest adult outcome (Ricks & Berry 1970; Roff *et al.* 1976).

A more efficient way of prospectively following preschizophrenic individuals is to identify children who are at increased genetic risk for developing schizophrenia as adults. All the studies that have compared high-risk children with normal controls have found significant behavioural differences. Some investigators have found high-risk children to have poor affective control, cognitive disturbance, social withdrawal, irritability and maladaptive behaviour (Glish *et al.* 1982; Parnas *et al.* 1982;

Olin & Mednick 1996). Attentional deficits potentiated by anhedonia were found in the New York High-Risk study (Freedman *et al.* 1998). There is also evidence that those high-risk subjects who develop predominantly negative-symptom schizophrenia will present with different premorbid behaviours than those subjects who develop predominantly positive-symptom schizophrenia (Cannon *et al.* 1990). This study reported that premorbid teacher ratings of predominantly negative-symptom schizophrenic patients consisted of more negative-type behaviours (passivity, lack of spontaneity, social unresponsiveness and isolation), while the predominantly positive schizophrenic patients were rated with more positive-type premorbid behaviours (overactivity, irritability, distractibility and aggression). One study compared the school reports of adults with schizotypal personality disorder with those suffering from schizophrenia (Olin *et al.* 1997). It was found that schizotypal personality was preceded by childhood behaviour that was disruptive and hyperexcitable, whereas schizophrenia was preceded by hypersensitivity to criticism (see also Huber 1997).

While the above studies clearly indicate that preschizophrenic and high-risk children demonstrate deviant behaviours compared with normal controls, some questions remain about the specificity of behavioural deviance to schizophrenia and whether these behaviours can be identified as schizophrenia spectrum personality disorders or traits. Studies that have compared the behaviours of high-risk children with psychiatric controls have found few, if any, behavioural differences (El-Guebaly *et al.* 1978; Weintraub & Neal 1984). Squires-Wheeler *et al.* (1988, 1989, 1992) investigated the rate of schizotypal personality traits in the New York High-Risk Project. Rates of schizotypal personality traits did not differ between the offspring of schizophrenic parents and the offspring of affective disorder parents (Squires-Wheeler *et al.* 1988, 1989). Furthermore, a subgroup of the offspring of affective disorder parents may be distinguished by transformation of schizotypal features to depression and/or anxiety (Squires-Wheeler *et al.* 1992). Taken together, these results do not provide conclusive evidence as to the specificity of schizotypal personality traits to schizophrenia in high-risk populations. Similarly, there is only limited support for the specificity of schizotypal traits in the premorbid personalities of schizophrenic patients vs. patients with affective psychosis (Foerster *et al.* 1991b).

Diagnostic specificity aside, it is clear that before the onset of illness a significant proportion of schizophrenic adults exhibit deviant characteristics including schizoid and schizotypal traits (Fish 1986; Hogg *et al.* 1990; Foerster *et al.* 1991b; Peralta *et al.* 1991). Furthermore, some investigators have found that premorbid personality traits are associated with specific dimensions of schizophrenic symptomatology (Jorgensen & Parnas 1990). For instance, there is evidence to support a relationship between premorbid schizoid personality disorder and negative symptoms in schizophrenic patients (Jorgensen & Parnas 1990; Peralta *et al.* 1991). These results are consistent with the hypothesis that the 'primary' genetic susceptibility to schizophrenia is manifested as deficit-like or negative traits (Siever 1991).

While findings of premorbid schizoid and schizotypal personality traits in schizophrenic patients lend support to the notion of a schizophrenia spectrum, it must also be noted that not all schizophrenic patients evidence abnormal personality traits before the onset of schizophrenia. In fact, one study found that a normal personality was the most frequent premorbid characterization of the schizophrenic sample (44%; Peralta *et al.* 1991). Another report indicated that 42% of the sample had no premorbid diagnosis based on the schedule for interviewing DSM-III personality disorders (SIDP), although when the Million Multiaxial Clinical Inventory (MMCI-I) was used, 70% of the same sample had at least one personality disorder diagnosis (Hogg *et al.* 1990). Once again, the heterogeneous nature of schizophrenia seems apparent.

In conclusion, it seems likely that a subgroup of schizophrenic patients can be characterized by premorbid personality disorders that are clearly related to schizophrenia. However, the relationship between abnormal personality traits and later schizophrenia is not clear. It may be that the presence of schizophrenia spectrum personality disorders is indicative of a higher morbidity for the development of schizophrenia, or that these personality disorders are part of the extended phenotype of schizophrenia. Furthermore, it is not clear whether a schizophrenia spectrum personality disorder is a necessary transitional stage occurring before the development of schizophrenia, which would indicate that all schizophrenic patients have a premorbid personality disturbance. Research investigating schizophrenia spectrum personality disorders in a variety of populations, including the premorbid personalities of schizophrenic patients, non-affected relatives of schizophrenic patients and clinically referred personality disordered patients, may help to answer some of the questions regarding the role of early personality disturbances in the development of schizophrenia.

Genetics

Adoption and family studies have provided strong evidence for a genetic relationship between schizophrenia and SPD (Kendler *et al.* 1981, 1993a, 1994; Frangos *et al.* 1985; Kendler 1985, 1988; Gershon *et al.* 1988; Maier *et al.* 1993). There is an increased incidence of SPD among the relatives of schizophrenic probands compared with the relatives of control subjects (Kendler *et al.* 1981, 1993b; Baron *et al.* 1982; Gunderson *et al.* 1983). An increased incidence of SPD has been reported in relatives of schizotypal probands, supporting a genetic basis for this personality disorder. An increase of schizophrenia-related disorders (Siever *et al.* 1990b) and of schizophrenia itself (Schulz *et al.* 1986; Battaglia *et al.* 1995) has been reported in the families of patients with SPD. The likelihood of having a schizophrenic relative is comparable for probands diagnosed with either SPD or schizophrenia (6.9% vs. 6.5%), further supporting common genetic substrates for the two disorders (Kendler *et al.* 1993a).

A further subject of investigation is the heritability of the factor structure of schizotypy. Certain SPD features suggest a closer genetic relationship to schizophrenia than others (Webb & Levinson 1993; Ingraham & Kety 2000). For example, an analysis of the Provincial sample of the Danish Adoption Study found suspiciousness, flat or spotty affectivity and reclusive withdrawn behaviour most frequent among the nonschizophrenic biological relatives of schizophrenic adoptees and each feature was significantly more common than among the biological relatives of controls. Psychotic-like symptoms, on the other hand, were not more prevalent among the biological relatives of schizophrenic adoptees than controls (Ingraham & Kety 2000). Several family studies have observed that, in contrast to positive psychotic-like SPD symptoms, the deficit-like SPD traits, primarily reflecting social and cognitive deficits, better characterized the relatives of schizophrenic probands compared with those of normal controls or other comparison groups (Gunderson *et al.* 1983; Kendler 1985; Torgersen *et al.* 1993; Webb & Levinson 1993; Maier *et al.* 1994). A study of twins from a nonclinical population (Kendler *et al.* 1991) found that positive and negative symptoms associated with SPD represent two relatively independent strongly heritable dimensions. However, only negative symptoms were related to other characteristics also associated with schizophrenia (Grove *et al.* 1991). These symptoms appear to underlie the core pathology across the spectrum, possibly reflecting a common neurodevelopmental abnormality.

It has been questioned whether there is a phenomenological difference between SPD patients who are relatives of schizophrenics and those who are identified clinically (Raine & Lencz 1995). For example, clinical patients may have more prominent psychotic-like symptoms. This may lead to an overlap in diagnosis between patients with borderline personality disorder and SPD patients where positive symptomatology is the prominent feature. This overlap was found to be considerable when DSM-III diagnostic criteria were used. An attempt to differentiate the psychotic-like symptoms of borderline personality disorder as transient, often dissociative and associated with periods of affective symptoms, as opposed to those of SPD which are more persistent and independent of affective symptoms, has been incorporated into DSM-IV (American Psychiatric Association 1994). As diagnostic criteria are refined, we are moving towards a more homogeneous SPD group, which will render interpretation of studies more meaningful. Studies involving populations from family, clinical and community sources may further clarify the underlying dimensions of schizotypy.

Psychophysiology (see also Chapter 16, which pertains to adults and patients with schizophrenia *per se*)

Prepulse inhibition

Dysfunctions at very early stages of sensory gating and information processing have been putatively associated with clinical features such as perceptual aberrations, hallucinations and

SCHIZOPHRENIA SPECTRUM PERSONALITY DISORDERS

distraction, which have been considered as potential precursors of sensory overload, cognitive fragmentation and disorganization. Among psychophysiological measures one approach has involved the startle reflex with the prepulse inhibition (PPI) paradigm. PPI refers to the inhibitory effect of a weak auditory prestimulus on the acoustic startle blink reflex to a loud noise. At short lead intervals this has the effect of markedly attenuating or 'gating' the amplitude of the startle response and facilitating its latency (Braff et al. 1991). Disruption of PPI occurs with agonists of dopamine and serotonin and with glutamate/N-methyl-D-aspartate (NMDA) antagonists (Swerdlow & Geyer 1998). Neurodevelopmental studies have shown that PPI is reduced by rearing rats in isolation, an effect which may be reversed by typical and atypical antipsychotic drugs. Furthermore, in rats with neonatal neurotoxic lesions of the hippocampus PPI is impaired after puberty, suggesting that early developmental lesions of the hippocampus create a vulnerability to hormonal influences on neuronal circuits that accompany puberty (Lipska et al. 1995).

Applications to the schizophrenia spectrum have shown that PPI is diminished in schizophrenia (Braff et al. 1991; Grillon et al. 1992; Bolino et al. 1994) and in schizotypal patients with positive and negative symptoms (Cadenhead et al. 1993). At the same time there have been disconfirmatory reports in both schizophrenia (Dawson et al. 1993) and in both positive and negative dimensions of schizotypy measured with the Chapman scales of perceptual aberration/magical ideation and anhedonia (Cadenhead et al. 1996). More subtle individual differences than simple positive–negative syndromes may assist with syndrome correlates. Swerdlow et al. (1995) reported an association with low Minnesota Multiphasic Personality Inventory (MMPI) hysteria scores, i.e. low scores on somatic anxiety, lassitude, social naivety and inhibited aggression, features in keeping with an activated syndrome (Gruzelier 1999a, 2002; Gruzelier et al. 2002).

The acoustic startle reflex is thought to involve inhibitory influences from descending frontolimbic circuitry elucidated in animals with pharmacological studies showing modulation by the hippocampal and medial prefrontal cortices and the basolateral amygdala. Accordingly, top-down modulatory influences may be important to control experimentally, as shown in recent-onset relatively asymptomatic schizophrenic patients (Dawson et al. 1993). Whereas PPI was normal in the conventional passive attention paradigm, there was a deficit in conditions where attention was required to the prepulse. Indeed, in schizophrenia higher level cognitive deficits have been associated with PPI attenuation and these include thought disorder, Wisconsin Card Sorting Test (WCST) performance, distractability on the Continuous Performance Test (CPT) and lateralized inattention on the Posner task (Karper et al. 1996). At the same time, Swerdlow et al. (1995) found no association in schizotypal individuals with cognitive tasks measuring disinhibition while Cadenhead et al. (1996) found no association with lower level processes including habituation of startle, visual backward masking and reaction time.

P50 suppression

Another measure of sensory gating involves a two-stimulus (S1, S2) evoked potential paradigm where normally the positive-going potential at 50 ms (P50) to the second stimulus (S2) is attenuated. A gating deficit at short interstimulus intervals is measured by a reduced ratio or difference between the two positive-going response amplitudes (P50s) at around 50 ms. This is typically interpreted as a failure to inhibit the response to the second stimulus, referred to as the P50 suppression anomaly. Neural underpinning is thought to involve desensitization of the alpha-7 nicotinic receptor (Griffith et al. 1998), which is modulated at the CA3 hippocampal level (Flach et al. 1996) and is linked with the same gene locus as schizophrenia (Freedman et al. 1997).

P50 suppression has been found deficient in many schizophrenic patients, their first-degree relatives and in SPD patients, as defined in Table 7.1 (Siegel et al. 1984; Waldo et al. 1991; Clementz et al. 1998; Cadenhead et al. 2000). Whereas symptom relations and the putative link with perceptual abnormalities have proved elusive in schizophrenia, a psychometric study in the normal population has found the unreality dimension to characterize those with abnormal P50 suppression (Croft et al. 2001). This relation was found not with P50 suppression per se but was caused by an attenuated amplitude to the first stimulus (S1), as well as to a failure of habituation of S2 amplitude, indicating the need for a closer look at the nature of the S1–S2 effect.

From a study of parents who carry the genetic inheritance, Freedman et al. concluded that the gating deficit may predispose to schizophrenia but that additional hippocampal pathology was necessary for the psychosis to develop (Harris et al. 1996). They found that while parents shared attentional deficits with patients, verbal learning deficits were only found in patients. Furthermore, in a sibling study, while schizophrenic and non-schizophrenic siblings shared the P50 gating deficit, hippocampal volumes, which correlated with IQ, were reduced only in those siblings with schizophrenia (Waldo et al. 1994). However, as will be shown below, short-term verbal learning deficits are not uncommon in schizotypes.

Habituation

Abnormalities in the response to novel stimuli and in the habituation of the response with stimulus repetition have also contributed to evidence of early stage anomalies of processing in schizophrenia and schizotypy. Habituation is a prerequisite for flexibility in selective attention and the redistribution of processing resources while the orienting response indexes the focusing of attention and a call for processing resources.

The more extensive examination of habituation in the schizophrenia spectrum has concerned electrophysiological approaches involving autonomic recording, electrodermal orienting activity in particular. A variety of abnormalities has been demonstrated, varying from over- to under-responsivity. In schizotypy, while a similar range of anomalies has been represented, irregular patterns of orientating and habituation are the most common and may coincide with cognitive disorganization (Gruzelier & Raine 1994; Raine et al. 1997). Interest in habituation deficits has extended to the P50 (Croft et al. 2001) and to habituation of the startle reflex (Bolino et al. 1992; Braff et al. 1992). In both cases, delayed habituation has been found to correlate with P50 and PPI deficits, as outlined in previous sections, suggesting shared central mechanisms (Schwarzkopf et al. 1993; Croft et al. 2001).

N100 and P300 evoked potentials

The N100 wave has provided a useful index of attentional allocation, often measured with simple paradigms requiring the detection of target stimuli among trains of standard stimuli: paradigms most commonly used to assess the P300 to the target or oddball stimuli. Attenuation of the N100 has been found in various schizophrenic subgroups, more so than attenuation of later P200 and P300 components (Boutros et al. 1997). These reductions have been found in obligate carriers (Frangou et al. 1997) although not in children at genetic risk (Freedman et al. 1988), while patients with SDP have shown results intermediate between schizophrenic patients and controls (Trestman et al. 1996). Waldo et al. (1988) have reported the coexistence of P50 suppression failure and N100 diminution in schizophrenic patients, whereas in those relatives with P50 suppression impairment the N100 amplitudes were larger than normal, interpreted as a compensatory mechanism.

Amplitude reduction of the P300 is often found in schizophrenia (McCarley et al. 1993), in patients with schizotypal personality disorder (Blackwood et al. 1986; Trestman et al. 1996) as well as in borderline personality disorder (Blackwood et al. 1986). While P300 reduction has been assumed to accompany negative or deficit symptoms, there is as yet no clear symptom relation in schizophrenia (Gruzelier 1999a) or schizotypal personality disorder (Siever 1991), although in the New York High-Risk Project a negative social–interpersonal dimension was associated with P300 and verbal working memory deficits (Squires-Wheeler et al. 1997). A cognitive measure of allusive thinking has also been found to correlate with P300 amplitude reduction in students (Kutcher et al. 1989).

Lateral asymmetry in the P300 may more readily yield syndrome relations in the schizophrenia spectrum (Strik et al. 1994; Gruzelier et al. 1999b). In the latter study activated–withdrawn syndrome relations were associated with P300 asymmetry and they were also found to hold for the earlier N100 and P200 components, suggestive of a generalized thalamocortical activation imbalance rather than a circumscribed memory deficit often theoretically associated with the P300 deficit.

Eye movements

Of theoretical relevance to disorders of visual perception and attention, eye movement recording has disclosed a range of abnormalities in schizophrenia and family members. One takes the form of deviant smooth pursuit eye tracking through intrusive and anticipatory saccadic eye movements (Grove et al. 1991; Clementz et al. 1994; Ross et al. 1996, 1998), another a failure to inhibit reflexive saccades following instruction (Clementz et al. 1994; Katsanis et al. 1997; McDowell & Clementz 1997). In support of a genetic vulnerability factor disinhibition along with a failure to suppress anticipatory saccades in smooth pursuit has been found to characterize those parents with a history of chronic schizophrenia in comparison to their spouses without a family history (Ross et al. 1998).

Tracking abnormalities have been found in patients with SPD and not in other personality disorders, and have been associated with schizotypy in college students (Siever et al. 1984, 1989, 1990a). Evidence of a functional basis to the deficit follows demonstration in recent-onset schizophrenia of improvement by attentional manipulations, suggesting an association with diminished voluntary attention in keeping with frontal involvement in smooth pursuit (White & Yee 1997).

Syndromal considerations have linked poor tracking with negative symptoms through association with the Chapman scales of physical anhedonia (Simons & Katkin 1985) and social anhedonia (Clementz et al. 1992), and in clinical samples with deficit-like rather than psychotic-like symptoms (Siever 1991; Siever et al. 1993). Perceptual aberration has been implicated along with physical anhedonia as a correlate of poor eye tracking in students (Simons & Katkin 1985; O'Driscoll et al. 1998), while O'Driscoll et al. (1998) found perceptual aberrations to accompany both antisaccade and smooth pursuit deficits.

Information processing and cognitive function

Visual processing

Clinical evidence, such as Klosterkotter et al.'s (1992) report that visual symptoms far outnumbered auditory symptoms in predicting the development of first-rank symptoms in first-episode schizophrenia when combined with experimental results on visual processing, is stimulating new research on the schizophrenia spectrum. Visual processing involves complementary and reciprocally related dorsal magnocellular (fast/transient cell) and the ventral parvocellular (slow/sustained cell) systems (Breitmeyer & Ganz 1976). The magnocellular transient-processing channel (retinal gangion, lateral geniculate nucleus, striate, prestriate, superior temporal sulcus, posterior parietal cortex) exhibits selectivity for low spatial frequencies by virtue of its high temporal resolution and primarily responds to the movement of stimuli and their appearance/disappearance. The magnocellular system is specialized for the precise timing of visual events, playing a major part in motion perception, spatial location and eye movement control including smooth pursuit eye movements. This system is not specific to vision but is also involved in the very rapid temporal coding required for the coherence of visual, auditory and olfactory perception, for cross-modal integration and for motor control. The parvocellular pathway (retinal ganglion, striate, prestriate, inferior temporal cortex) is a sustained-processing channel favouring high spatial frequencies having a low spatial resolution and is involved in pattern analysis. It is concerned with object recognition, colour perception and high-resolution form perception.

Magnocellular function deficits in motion sensitivity have been found in both schizophrenic patients with positive or mixed positive/negative symptoms and in dyslexic subjects, who have often been characterized by positive symptom schizotypy (Richardson et al. 1994). Motion sensitivity together with visual direction sense was also found to be impaired in students with positive features of schizotypy but not in those with negative features (Richardson & Gruzelier 1994). A comparison of magnocellular tasks of motion perception and location with parvocellular tasks of spatial frequency and pattern finding deficits implicated the magno and not the parvo system (O'Donnell et al. 1996). In the same study, more severe than the perceptual impairment in motion detection was a recognition deficit involving working memory which was attributed to prefrontal involvement.

Both magno and parvo systems are dynamically involved in backward masking. This is the phenomenon where the presentation of a stimulus following a target at short interstimulus intervals has the effect of hampering or masking target detection, the interference seemingly working backwards in time. The transient system first locates the target and responds to its offset, having meanwhile given over identifying the target to the sustained system. More than one abnormality has been disclosed in schizophrenia (Braff et al. 1991; Green et al. 1994; Slaghuis & Bakker 1995). In keeping with a parvocellular abnormality, some patients have abnormal threshold durations for identifying the target stimulus without the mask (critical stimulus duration) which suggests longer iconic persistence, also demonstrated with two-pulse temporal resolution measures. This deficit appears to be associated with negative rather than positive symptoms (Gruzelier 1999b).

Magnocellular deficits have been more commonly invoked as an explanation for the masking deficits. The nature of such an aberrant transient system deficit is unclear, but its disruptive consequences suggest overactivity of some kind: easily triggered transients, abnormally potent transients, prolonged transient channel activity or additive transient susceptibility, i.e. susceptibility to multiple transient bursts in a short period of time (Merritt & Balogh 1989). Masking deficits have coexisted with both positive and negative symptoms in schizophrenic patients and in association with the unreality dimension of schizotypy (Saccuzzo et al. 1981; Merritt & Balogh 1989; Schuck & Lee 1989), yet there is a clear preference in the reports towards an association with positive symptoms and positive features of schizotypy.

Green et al. (1997) went on to delineate early sensory–perceptual components from the later attentional disengagement components in backward masking, comparing siblings with schizophrenia and unaffected siblings. Masking deficits relating to both magnocellular and parvocellular systems were disclosed, with the earlier sensory–perceptual components providing the vulnerability marker in the unaffected siblings.

Frontal and executive functions

An implication from more than one investigation of early stages of information processing where higher cognitive functions were also examined was that predisposition to schizophrenia resided with lower level processes while higher cognitive deficits were necessary for the manifestation of psychosis (Harris et al. 1996; Green et al. 1997). This attractive hypothesis has not been confirmed. Cognitive deficits have been well documented in schizotypy, although severity of deficit does appear frequently to be greater in schizophrenia than in schizotypy, at least when the conclusion is based on group comparisons.

Deficits include executive functions involving the frontal lobe such as set changing and perseveration measured with the WCST, which have characterized many schizophrenic patients, patients with SPD and schizotypes in the normal population (Lyons et al. 1991; Raine et al. 1992; Battaglia et al. 1994; Trestman et al. 1995; Voglmaier et al. 1997). In studies of patients and their relatives, a range of higher level cognitive deficiencies have been reported including set alternation frequency, verbal fluency, abstraction, verbal memory and Trail Making (Franke et al. 1993; Keefe et al. 1994).

Addressing the question of specificity, Tien et al. (1992) found by assessing the type of error made on the WCST that perseveration was associated with schizotypal traits as distinct from paranoid and schizoid traits. Similarly, Keefe et al. (1994) found relatives of patients with schizophrenia to have more perseverative errors than other personality disorders, to sort fewer categories and to take more time to complete Trail Making B, although they were no different in verbal fluency or in general intelligence. These results were similar to those found in schizotypal patients by Trestman et al. (1995). A failure in maintaining response set on the WCST has been found to characterize high-scoring students on the perceptual aberration scale (Park et al. 1995).

Continuous performance test

Executive functions include the control and maintenance of attention. A widely used behavioural measure of sustained attention is the CPT. This involves the random brief rapid visual presentation of letters or digits with the instruction to press a key to target stimuli. The task may be made more difficult by degrading stimuli that place a load on perceptual processing or by increasing the load on working memory. Deficits have been demonstrated in schizophrenia, including patients in remission, in children with a schizophrenic parent and other first-degree relatives and in SPD patients (Cornblatt & Keilp 1994; Roitman et al. 1997). The deficits tend not to increase within the session, implying that the disability is not one of sustaining attention per se.

In support of perceptual involvement, an association between CPT deficit and schizotypy in the form of perceptual aberration (PAS) as well as the negative Schizotypal Personality Questionnaire (SPQ) (Raine 1991) interpersonal factor was shown in a Taiwanese study (Chen et al. 1997). Furthermore, when combined with poor CPT performance the similar schizotypy features of perceptual distortion and social anhedonia have characterized subjects performing poorly on frontal lobe tests including the WCST, Trail Making and verbal fluency (Obiols et al. 1999). This is in keeping with frontal lobe involvement in components of the task involving working memory and the control of attention.

Thought disorder and disinhibition

Another type of attentional deficit is distractability which is thought to underpin cognitive disorganization including thought disorder. These features form a major component of positive schizophrenic symptomatology and have been considered one fundamental aspect of schizotypy exemplified by Meehl's (1962) concept of cognitive slippage. At the same time this is one of the least well-defined aspects of schizotypy. The syndrome constellation may include distractability, odd speech, disorganization, cognitive activation and disinhibition, together with odd behaviour and non-conformity.

A diversity of measures has been applied to schizotypy. Using a Thought Disorder Index (TDI) derived from the Rorschach test which reflects a loosening of associations, abnormalities have been found in both clinical SPD and schizophrenia, as well as in siblings of schizophrenic patients and non-clinical samples with high perceptual aberration scores (Edell 1987; Hain et al. 1995; Coleman et al. 1996). Communication deviance has been examined in the parents of schizophrenic patients where it was found to be associated with both schizotypy and distractability (Docherty et al. 1998). Another approach has been to explore mentalizing or the ability to maintain representations of mental states of oneself and others. Using a false-belief picture sequencing task, normal subjects were categorized according to mentalizing ability and examined for differences in SPQ factors (Langdon & Coltheart 1999). In different experiments, the interpersonal factor and the cognitive–perceptual/disorganized factors were implicated. The pattern of deficits supported an impairment in inferring and representing mental states as distinct from executive planning or a failure of disengagement.

A number of cognitive disinhibitory deficits have been examined and, on the whole, they have been associated with positive symptoms. One such phenomenon is latent inhibition. By virtue of repeated pre-exposure to a stimulus without reinforcement consequences, the learning of subsequent associations with the stimulus is retarded. This has been studied as an animal model for schizophrenia because the dopamine agonist amphetamine disrupts latent inhibition and is reversed by typical neuroleptics. However, evidence of a disruption of latent inhibition in schizophrenia is controversial with both affirmative (Baruch et al. 1988a; Gray et al. 1995) and negative reports (Lubow et al.

1987; Swerdlow et al. 1995). Consideration of the conflicting evidence has led to the attribution of latent inhibition disruption to a highly circumscribed aspect of the early schizophrenic process, one without, as yet, any clearly demarcated symptom or process correlates. Latent inhibition has also been associated with the predominantly positive symptom Claridge Schizotypal Personality (STA) scale (Baruch et al. 1988b; Lipp & Vaitl 1992) and with Eysenck's Psychoticism measure (Baruch et al. 1988b).

Cognitive disinhibition manifested by reduced negative priming has also been associated with positive symptoms in schizophrenia (Beech et al. 1989; Williams 1995), in schizotypy in the normal population (Peters et al. 1994; Moritz & Mass 1997) as well as in the relatives of schizophrenic and neurotic patients (Claridge & Beech 1996). Disinhibition has also been implicated in an analysis of the content of verbal fluency tests (Duchene et al. 1998), which disclosed that high-scoring subjects on the magical ideation scale produced more low-frequency words, interpreted as a disinhibition of semantic networks that may underpin thought disorder and creativity.

Memory

Consistent with the view that explicit declarative memory is one of the cardinal neuropsychological deficits in schizophrenia (Gruzelier et al. 1988; Saykin et al. 1994), declarative memory has been found deficient in relatives (Keefe et al. 1994) and in siblings with a schizotypal personality (Cannon et al. 1994). In contrast to this, implicit memory may not be affected (Ferraro & Okerlund 1995). Furthermore, reduced performance on the California Verbal Learning Test has been demonstrated in SPD patients compared with other personality disorders. This deficit has been found accompanied by WCST deficits but not by a range of other deficits interpreted as a profile in support of a left temporofrontal deficit (Voglmaier et al. 1997).

Working memory which involves frontal functions has been found deficient in schizophrenia (Park & Holzman 1992; Keefe et al. 1997) and in first-degree relatives (Park et al. 1995). In relation to schizotypy with a battery of cognitive tasks verbal working memory was found in SPD patients to be mid-way between that of normal subjects and schizophrenic patients, as was general intellectual performance together with recognition memory, abstract reasoning, cognitive inhibition and measures of attention (Cadenhead et al. 1999). Visuospatial working memory impairment has also been identified in SPD patients and the extent found to be greater than in other personality disorders (Roitman et al. 2000). Working memory was identified as the source of the visuospatial deficit rather than perceptual abilities per se (Farmer et al. 2000).

At the same time, perceptual symptoms have been associated with working memory deficits. Working memory deficits have been shown to be related to both positive unreality (PAS, magical ideation or MIS) and social anhedonia features of schizotypy, as well as correlating with WCST performance in support of frontal involvement (Gooding et al. 1999). In normal schizotypes identified by PAS, working memory deficits were disclosed on a delayed spatial response task (Park *et al.* 1995). The working memory deficit was accompanied by set maintenance deficits on the WCST, whereas in a subsequent report the same subjects failed to show verbal working memory deficits (Lenzenweger & Gold 2000). Conflicts as to the verbal or non-verbal nature of the working memory deficit may arise from differences between studies in the composition of various dimensions of schizotypy.

Lateralization

Left hemisphere dysfunction has been a widely researched hypothesis in schizophrenia and while there is a good deal of support for left temporolimbic deficits, functional deficits in the right hemisphere have also been disclosed, and there is some structural evidence of a loss of normal asymmetry in the planum temporale (Gruzelier 1999a). As in schizophrenia, reports in schizotypy on the nature and direction of functional asymmetries have diverged. Claridge and co-workers, with predominantly positive schizotypy scales (STA), have reported evidence with a range of techniques for an imbalance in excitation–inhibition: the right hemisphere excitatory and the left inhibitory. A deficiency in left hemisphere-mediated smooth pursuit has characterized schizotypy measured with the MMPI (Kelly & Bakan 1999). Males with MIS have disclosed olfactory detection deficits implicating the left temporal lobe (Mohr *et al.* 2001), while in females MIS has been associated with excess left hemisphere inhibition indexed by right hemi-space neglect with a modified Corsi block task (Nalcaci *et al.* 2000). In contrast, Raine and Manders (1988) reported neuropsychological evidence for the opposite state of imbalance, as has Jutai (1989), while Goodarzi *et al.* (2000) found a global perceptual processing deficit implicating the right hemisphere in association with unusual experiences and the STA scale.

Consideration of syndrome relations may unravel some of the complexity in the laterality of functional deficits in the schizophrenia spectrum (Gruzelier 1999a). Characterizing schizophrenic patients on the basis of cognitive or electrophysiological asymmetry delineated a positive activated syndrome which was accompanied by left > right functional preference, and a negative withdrawn syndrome accompanied by right > left functional preference activity (Gruzelier *et al.* 1988, 1999a, c; Gruzelier 1999a). Hallucinations and delusions of first-rank were independent of these two syndromes, and constituted a third syndrome which showed inconsistent associations with functional asymmetry.

A similar three-factor solution of activated, withdrawn and unreality factors was demonstrated in schizotypy in the normal population measured with the Raine SPQ accompanied by Thayer activation scales (Gruzelier 1996). Furthermore, tests of verbal and non-verbal recognition memory in schizotypy disclosed the same activated–withdrawn syndrome asymmetry relations as in schizophrenia, with unreality showing inconsistent relations with asymmetry (Gruzelier *et al.* 1995; Gruzelier &

Doig 1996). Congruent relations with a test of lateral visual direction sense, a putative magnocellular measure, were also disclosed with the Oxford–Liverpool Inventory psychosis-proneness scales (OLIFE; Gruzelier & Richardson 1994; Mason *et al.* 1997), as were relations with electrodermal asymmetries in relation both to self-reported social anhedonia in unmedicated schizophrenic patients (Gruzelier & Davis 1995) and to positive schizotypal features in the normal population (Mason *et al.* 1997). Prospective evidence arose serendipitously from a student whose outlying face > word asymmetry predicted a withdrawn/unreality syndrome profile in subsequent first and second schizophrenic episodes (Gruzelier *et al.* 1995).

There is a range of evidence in support of an association between inconsistent functional lateralization and the unreality dimension. High-scoring subjects on MIS were equipotential for either visual field in a lexical decision task on which low-scoring subjects showed a right visual field advantage (Leonhard & Brugger 1998). Inconsistent handedness (as distinct from strong left-handedness) has been associated with unreality and unusual experiences (Richardson 1994; Gruzelier & Doig 1996; Shaw *et al.* 2001). In fact, the incidence and impact of non-righthandedness assessed by handedness questionnaires has been one of the more replicable neurocognitive findings in schizotypy (Chapman & Chapman 1985; Kelly & Coursey 1992; Kim *et al.* 1992; Richardson 1994; Gruzelier & Doig 1996; Shaw *et al.* 2001). This supports the role of developmental influences, as does the ontology of functional asymmetry.

Animal and human evidence shows that functional asymmetries are subject to the influence of genes, hormones and early experiences, and remain vulnerable to stressors throughout the life span (Gruzelier 1999a). Of importance to the nature of the activated and withdrawn syndrome asymmetry findings, it has been shown that after birth and prior to the development of both language and visuoconstructive skills in children, spontaneous asymmetries in gesture and emotion have been documented, described as influencing the approach–withdrawal balance in social encounters (Trevarthen 1996). Also relevant to schizotypy and Meehl's concept of schizotaxia may be the developmental processes that determine variations in neuronal connectivity such as synaptogenesis influenced by pubertal timing. Replicable associations with early and late pubertal timing when compared with normal maturation have been shown with the unreality dimension of schizotypy (Gruzelier & Kaiser 1996; Kaiser & Gruzelier 1999a), while some implications for brain connectivity were supported through measurement of evoked potential latencies and EEG connectivity through coherence in response to photic driving (Kaiser & Gruzelier 1996, 1999b).

Neurochemistry

The dopamine (DA) hypothesis that the schizophrenic process is secondary to an excess of dopamine has long been the cornerstone of research into the pathophysiology of schizophrenia. Although supported, at least in part, by the efficacy of neuroleptic medication with its dopamine blockade mechanism, the DA hypothesis has failed to provide a satisfactory explanation for the pathogenesis of schizophrenia. However, evidence from a variety of postmortem, metabolite and imaging studies suggests dopaminergic abnormalities in schizophrenia (Davis et al. 1991). There are reports of increased cerebrospinal fluid (CSF) homovanillic acid (HVA) in paranoid schizophrenia, with reductions in chronic deficit symptom schizophrenics (Davidson & Davis 1988). Among medication-free schizophrenic patients, plasma HVA concentrations correlate with clinical severity. Clinical improvement associated with medication has been reported as associated with higher baseline and lower post-treatment plasma HVA levels (Pickar et al. 1984; Davis et al. 1985, 1991). The current interpretation of the DA hypothesis posits differences in dopaminergic function among brain regions, with an excess of dopamine in subcortical areas and cortical hypodopaminergia. Deafferentation of limbic DA systems associated with higher cortical impairment may result in disinhibition of limbic DA systems with increased receptor responsiveness and release of dopamine (Davis et al. 1991). The more recent convincing evidence of hyperdopaminergic presynaptic activity in relation to negative symptoms in the prefrontal lobes and positive symptoms in the mesolimbic system are described in detail in Chapter 20.

Schizotypal personality disorder provides a unique opportunity to study the function of the dopaminergic system in relation to schizophrenia-associated psychopathology given the relative absence of confounding variables. Initial studies in this population suggested increases in plasma HVA in clinically selected SPD patients compared with other personality disorder patients or controls. These increases were associated with a number of psychotic-like symptoms; when data analysis included these symptoms as a covariate, the difference between the groups was no longer apparent (Siever et al. 1993). Similar results have been found using CSF HVA. In SPD patients who are relatives of schizophrenics, psychotic-like symptoms were also associated with increases in plasma HVA; however, the net plasma HVA concentrations were lower in the SPD group than in the relatives with no personality disorder or other personality disorders (Amin et al. 1997). This SPD group seems to display primarily deficit-like symptoms and plasma HVA levels were inversely correlated with these symptoms, which may account for the lower mean plasma HVA values (Amin et al. 1997). Some studies also suggest reduced plasma HVA associated with poor performance on cognitive testing in SPD (Siever et al. 1993). Overall, these studies suggest increases in plasma HVA associated with positive symptoms and decreases with negative symptoms and cognitive impairment in SPD.

Studies by our group of plasma response to physiological stressors (a 2-deoxyglucose infusion) (Goodman et al. 2000) and single photon emission computerized tomography (SPECT)/D-amphetamine studies carried out in collaboration with Laruelle et al. at Columbia University of subcortical dopamine release following amphetamine infusions both sug-

gest that SPD patients have subcortical dopamine that is decreased compared to schizophrenic patients and more like that of normal controls (O'Flynn et al. 2001). These findings suggest that decreased frontal dopaminergic activity is associated with deficit symptoms and cognitive impairment, while increased subcortical dopaminergic activity correlates with psychotic symptoms, and that SPD patients may be less likely to experience psychotic symptoms than schizophrenic patients if they are administered dopaminergic agents (Abi-Dhargam et al. 1998; Siever et al. 2002).

In a series of studies involving the administration of a dopaminergic challenge in the form of amphetamine in a placebo-controlled paradigm, when administered 30 mg amphetamines, SPD patients showed a significant improvement in performance on the WCST; those patients with the lowest scores on placebo showed the most improvement on amphetamine (Siegel et al. 1996). Further study also showed improved performance on tests of visuospatial working memory and attentional capacity (the Dot test and CPT respectively) in SPD patients compared with those with other personality disorders (Kirrane et al. 2000). It is of note that there were no changes in positive symptoms in SPD patients in these studies, in contrast to studies of schizophrenic patients where worsening is reported in almost half of those tested. Also relevant is the improvement in negative symptoms in SPD patients. Taken together, these findings raise the intriguing possibility that SPD patients may have a better-buffered subcortical dopaminergic system, which protects them against subcortical overactivity associated with psychosis.

Imaging studies (see also Chapter 22)

Structural imaging

One of the first and most consistent observations of altered brain function in schizophrenia was an increase in the size of the ventricular : brain ratio (VBR). Both an increased VBR and evidence of cortical atrophy on computerized axial tomography (CAT) scans have been associated with the deficit-like symptoms of schizophrenia, impairment of cognitive function, decreased dopaminergic activity and poor outcome in schizophrenic patients (Shelton & Weinberger 1986).

A growing body of work has begun to identify both neuroanatomic similarities and differences between SPD and schizophrenia and similarities and differences in the regions that are activated during cognitive task performance in the two disorders. An increased VBR has been demonstrated in SPD as in schizophrenia (Cazzulo et al. 1991; Siever et al. 1995; Buchsbaum et al. 1997a; Silverman et al. 1998). Our group has reported that an increased VBR involving the lateral ventricle and the frontal horn correlated with increased perseverative errors on the WCST, and frontal horn VBR correlated with an increased omission error rate in the degraded stimulus CPT (Siever et al. 1993; Buchsbaum et al. 1997a).

Frontal lobe volume is decreased in schizophrenics but does not appear to be reduced in schizotypals compared with controls (Buchsbaum *et al.* 2002). Recent magnetic resonance imaging (MRI) studies by our group and others have confirmed that SPD patients, like schizophrenic patients, have decreased grey matter volume in the left superior temporal gyrus and other parts of the temporal lobe (Dickey *et al.* 1999; Downhill *et al.* 2000). Preliminary studies suggest that while tests of executive function such as the WCST, as well as the deficit-like symptoms of SPD, correlate inversely with frontal lobe volume, the volume of the temporal lobe gyrus is inversely associated with performance on verbal learning tasks with the disorganized symptoms of SPD (McCarley *et al.* 1996).

MRI studies have also shown a decrease in the size of the splenium of the corpus callosum (which connects the inferior temporal and part of the superior temporal regions) (Downhill *et al.* 2000) and the presence of cavum septum pellucidi (Kwon *et al.* 1998); these abnormalities were intermediate between schizophrenics and controls which suggests that alteration in mid-line structures during the course of neurodevelopment may play a part in the pathogenesis of schizophrenia spectrum disorders (Kwon *et al.* 1998).

Another area of interest in schizophrenia is the thalamus. The thalamus is both the major relay station of sensory perceptual information to the cortex and an important reciprocal participant in cortical activation. MRI studies have generally shown a reduction in thalamic size in schizophrenia (Andreasen *et al.* 1998). This appears to be independent of neuroleptic medication (Buchsbaum *et al.* 1996). The medial dorsal nucleus of the thalamus, associated closely with prefrontal cortex, is reduced in schizophrenic but not SPD patients, while pulvinar, more closely linked to temporal cortex, is reduced in both cohorts (Byne *et al.* 2001). In the striatum, the putamen is significantly smaller in SPD subjects than in controls, consistent with reduced dopaminergic activity, while in schizophrenic patients the putamen is larger than in controls (Shihabuddin *et al.* 2001).

Taken together, structural imaging studies suggest that: there are reductions in grey matter in the temporal lobes and pulvinar of the thalamus in both schizophrenic and SPD patients; there is diminished interhemispheric connectivity in both disorders, possibly more severe in schizophrenia; in SPD, the putamen may be reduced in size compared with both schizophrenics and controls; and schizophrenic patients have reduced prefrontal volume and associated medial dorsal nucleus (MDN) of thalamus while these structures may be normal in schizophrenic patients.

Functional imaging

Studies have been carried out to test the possibility that SPD patients have the ability to utilize brain regions not normally recruited for specific cognitive functions in order to compensate for deficits of dysfunction in the primary region usually associated with that cognitive function.

A SPECT study comparing regional cerebral blood flow (rCBF) in SPD subjects and normal controls during performance of the WCST found that the frontal region of greatest activation in control subjects was the precentral gyrus, whereas in SPD patients activation was greatest in the middle frontal gyrus (Buchsbaum *et al.* 1997b). In normal subjects, task performance was correlated with left prefrontal cortex (PFC) activation but this was not the case for SPD subjects. This population showed a positive correlation between good WCST performance and cerebral blood flow (CBF) in the right inferior frontal gyrus and poor performance correlated with CBF in the right middle frontal gyrus, which is part of the dorsolateral prefrontal cortex. This suggests that SPD patients recruit different frontal regions for WCST performance than do controls; this may represent a compensatory mechanism.

A positron emission tomography (PET) study carried out in our laboratory, which examined activation of thalamic nuclei during a serial word list learning task, found decreased relative metabolism in the MDN bilaterally in schizophrenic patients but not in SPD patients or normal controls (Hazlett *et al.* 1999). During performance of the same task, SPD patients showed an increase in glucose metabolic rate (GMR) in the ventral putamen compared with controls, consistent with decreased dopaminergic activity, while schizophrenic patients showed decreased GMR compared with controls in that region (Shihabuddin *et al.* 2001). These findings raise the possibility that cognitive impairment in schizophrenia and SPD may be associated in part with anomalous prefrontal cortical activity, activity which is diminished overall in schizophrenia, but may reflect islands of preserved or compensatory function in SPD. They also suggest that there is reduced subcortical dopaminergic activity in SPD compared with schizophrenic patients during cognitive task performance.

Treatment studies

Although most schizotypal subjects have never been treated, studies of the treatment of SPD have been influenced by the biological and phenomenological similarities between SPD and schizophrenia. Several studies suggest that treatment with neuroleptic medication can reduce some of the symptoms of SPD, particularly the psychotic-like symptoms and social anxiety associated with the disorder. Low-dose thioxanthene significantly reduced the symptoms of ideas of reference, illusions and social isolation when compared with placebo in patients with SPD and borderline personality disorder (Goldberg *et al.* 1986). Patients with more severe symptoms were especially responsive to thioxanthene. A 2-week treatment with low-dose haloperidol resulted in significant decreases in ideas of reference, odd communication and social isolation in 17 patients with schizotypal personality disorder (Hymowitz *et al.* 1986). Benefits have also been shown with risperidone (Szigethy & Schulz 1997). A recent placebo-controlled study by our group of low-dose risperidone in SPD showed improved Positive and Negative Syndrome Scale (PANSS) general, positive and negative symptom scores (Koenigsberg *et al.* 2002). One of the difficulties in treating SPD patients with conventional neuroleptic medications is that the side-effects may overwhelm the treatment benefits. Thus, while low-dose dopamine blockade may have a mild symptom-reducing effect in some patients, particularly those with more severe symptom profiles, non-compliance may reduce the overall effectiveness of neuroleptics in SPD.

It would be desirable to find pharmacological interventions that would enhance the functioning of SPD patients by reducing their deficit-like symptoms and enhancing cognitive performance. One potential intervention may involve the activation of dopamine function. As reflected by their poor performance on cognitive tests such as the WCST requiring frontal activation, some SPD patients may have the reduced cognitive functions found in schizophrenia, yet they do not manifest psychotic symptoms. Treatment of these patients with dopamine-enhancing agents may enhance cognitive function without inducing psychosis. In one study at our centre, SPD patients showed an improvement in WCST performance following administration of 30 mg amphetamine in placebo-controlled fashion, with the worst performers on placebo showing the most improvement (Siegel et al. 1996). In another overlapping series of patients, the same amphetamine dose resulted in reduction in errors on the working memory test in schizotypal patients, whereas no such difference was observed in other personality-disordered patients (Kirrane et al. 2000). Amphetamine compared with placebo also resulted in improvement on a verbal learning test and in performance on the CPT in SPD patients but not in other personality-disordered controls. Amphetamine acts largely through D_1 receptors in the frontal cortex. D_1 receptors are known to modulate the performance of visuospatial working memory in primates (Williams & Goldman-Rakic 1995). Amphetamine may also serve to enhance cortical dopaminergic transmission and may be important for performance on the CPT. Dopaminergic modulation may also enhance verbal learning through subcortical frontal and temporal connections. Results from our studies suggest that dopaminergic enhancement may indeed be of benefit in reducing cognitive impairment in SPD without inducing psychosis. Dopaminergic agents warrant further investigation in the treatment of SPD.

Outcome

As with schizophrenia, the outcome of SPD is extremely variable. Owing to the severity of deficit-like symptoms, many SPD patients are presumed to have poor social outcomes but these presumptions are biased by the same flaw as those in schizophrenia, i.e. only those patients who remain in treatment remain in the study. This is a particularly confounding variable in SPD where only a small proportion of patients come to treatment.

SPD patients have been shown to have an outcome that is more similar to that of chronic schizophrenia than to that of borderline personality disorder (McGlashan 1986). One study that compared the outcome of personality-disordered patients found that at follow-up SPD patients had the poorest ratings on global

functioning, social activity and social adjustment (Mehlum et al. 1991). Other findings have indicated that patients who meet criteria for both schizotypal and borderline personality disorders are more similar to patients with borderline personality than to 'pure' schizotypal patients. While the capacity of these 'mixed' patients for more intimate relationships seemed poorer than that of pure borderline patients, their social and social functioning was less isolative than that of patients with pure SPD. Thus, comorbid borderline symptoms may confer some protection for SPD patients by reducing the impact of severe social isolation.

A further confounder in assessing SPD outcome is that it is unclear what percentage is suffering from prodromal schizophrenia. Estimates from a follow-up study of young adults diagnosed as SPD suggest that about 25% went on to develop schizophrenia (Schulz & Soloff 1987). In the Chestnut Lodge study, 17% of the SPD sample was later diagnosed as schizophrenic (Fenton & McGlashan 1989). However, other samples have shown a much lower prevalence. Paranoid ideation, magical thinking and social isolation have been reported as predictors of the later onset of schizophrenia in SPD patients (Fenton & McGlashan 1989).

Caution needs to be exercised in predicting the outcome of SPD. Diagnostic criteria for the condition have been evolving and study results need to be interpreted in the light of the diagnostic criteria at the time the study was carried out. It is also possible that the diagnosis of SPD may actually encompass different subtypes with potentially different outcomes, e.g. those patients who have a family history of schizophrenia and those who do not. Finally, many of this population remain undiagnosed and those who come to clinical attention may be a self-selecting population. Further studies are needed to clarify these issues before any conclusions can be drawn on the outcome of SPD.

Integration of pathophysiology

SPD patients share many phenomenological, genetic, cognitive and biological traits with schizophrenia. By definition, SPD patients do not develop the persistent psychosis associated with schizophrenia. This fact, together with the lack of institutionalization and exposure to psychoactive medication in this population, makes them an ideal group to study for clues as to the pathophysiology of schizophrenia.

While sharing many of the cognitive deficits, the asocial behaviour and social detachment observed in schizophrenia, SPD patients exhibit only psychotic-like symptoms without overt hallucinations and delusions, even after pharmacological challenge. SPD patients appear to be biologically buffered against the emergence of psychosis. It is possible that the two groups share a common neurodevelopmentally based disorder of cortical organization and function, manifest as impairment in verbal and working memory and attention as well as in social deficit symptoms, but may be less likely to show the subcortical overactivity associated with psychosis that is seen in schizophrenia.

One possible pathophysiological model of the schizophrenia

spectrum disorders is based on preclinical studies demonstrating that lesions or abnormalities in one region of the brain may result in abnormal function in other regions, a particularly appealing model when placed in a neurodevelopmental context. Evidence shows, for example, that neonatal lesions in the temporal or hippocampal regions may result in frontal cortical dysfunction (Lipska *et al.* 1993), while prefrontal cortical deficits in dopaminergic activity may result in striatal overactivity in the dopaminergic system (Pycock *et al.* 1980). In this way, genetically based or neurodevelopmental insults in lateral regions of the brain may propagate through prefrontal cortex to affect subcortical regions. Schizophrenic patients may be more susceptible to the downstream effects of these insults, either because of differing genetic susceptibilities or degree of insult. SPD patients show reductions in volume and metabolic activity in temporal cortex, which are quantitatively similar to those seen in schizophrenic patients. These reductions are associated with schizotypal symptomatology and cognitive deficits. SPD patients also show significant reductions in frontal volume compared with controls and impairment on tasks sensitive to frontal cortical dysfunction milder than but similar to the impairment found in schizophrenic patients (Trestman *et al.* 1995). Both SPECT and PET functional imaging studies suggest that SPD patients, like schizophrenic patients, do not activate the dorsolateral prefrontal cortex during WCST as much as controls do. However, they do activate other prefrontal regions, which schizophrenics and controls do not, thereby suggesting the ability to recruit alternative brain regions as a compensatory mechanism in SPD. The cognitive dysfunction on the frontal-related tasks may be associated with reduced indices of dopaminergic activity (Siever *et al.* 1993). Reduced dopaminergic activity in the frontal cortex has been hypothesized to result in increased striatal dopaminergic activity on the basis of a 'disinhibition' by the frontal cortical deficits (Kolachana *et al.* 1996). It is hypothesized that schizophrenic patients are much more susceptible to this 'deafferentation' than are schizotypal patients and are more likely to show subcortical dopaminergic overactivity, particularly on provocation (Csernansky *et al.* 1991). Data to date suggest that SPD patients do not develop psychotic symptoms following amphetamine administration, in contrast to schizophrenic patients (Lieberman *et al.* 1987). Additionally, also in contrast to schizophrenic patients, SPD patients demonstrate diminished rather than increased striatal metabolic activity and reductions in striatal volumes compared with both normal controls and schizophrenic patients (the latter are increased compared with controls). These data are compatible with the hypothesis that schizophrenic patients may be more likely to upregulate their dopamine systems in response to dopaminergic deficits or receptor blockade.

Neurochemical imaging studies combine with these data to suggest the hypothesis that SPD patients have a lesser likelihood than schizophrenic patients of increased phasic dopamine release in the striatum and that this reduced potential for dopaminergic activation may be an important factor that protects SPD patients from developing psychosis.

Conclusions

SPD characterized in patients, as well as schizotypal tendencies characterized in high-scoring normal individuals by schizotypy questionnaires, may be phenomenologically, genetically, biologically and cognitively related to schizophrenia as part of a schizophrenia spectrum. SPD patients have a milder although similar symptom profile yet fail to develop persistent psychosis, even with provocation.

How then does vulnerability give way to the process of schizophrenia? Some hypotheses may be dismissed based on our review of the various neurocognitive studies. First, all existing putative experimental psychophysiological and neurophysiological correlates of schizophrenia are shared with schizotypy. Accordingly, schizotypy may not be distinguished from psychosis by preservation of one particular class of correlates, such as the lower level processes of sensory gating. Secondly, while group comparisons sometimes show that deficits in schizophrenia may be more severe than in schizotypy, the overlap in distribution of scores indicates that severity of impairment on any one vulnerability indicator does not appear capable of providing a diagnostically reliable tool.

What then is the nature of the compensatory process or processes that provide a buffer against schizophrenia? One promising approach lies in the assessment of multiple neurophysiological, psychophysiological and neurobiological correlates. This strategy has already provided a number of suggestive findings that require further investigation. For example, indices of subcortical dopamine raise the possibility that schizotypal individuals may be better 'buffered' in this system than schizophrenic patients. Do schizotypal individuals have compensatory pockets of ability of a superior kind which accompany disabilities in other domains? Another concerns evidence showing that while vulnerability is typically manifested at lower sensory levels of processing, the nature of any coexisting higher level processing deficit may be of greater magnitude. The question then arises as to whether a further loss of top-down influences may be the precursor of the schizophrenic process? A third concerns the lack of evidence of unitary disabilities that can unify the diversity of symptoms and signs. Although such a possibility should not be dismissed entirely for deficits in lower and higher levels of processing have been found to be correlated, and, if found to be independent of general intelligence, would be in keeping with at least one such general process.

Our review of findings has also disclosed that greater homogeneity of results follows subclassification of subjects on factorial, syndromal or dimensional bases. The threefold classification of the deficit-like symptoms of social and emotional withdrawal, cognitive disorganization/disinhibition and unreality or psychotic-like symptoms has been heuristic, yet at the same time these descriptors are blanket terms. Elucidation of neurocognitive correlates will follow further cognitive neuropsychological analysis and fractionation, such as the differentiation of magical ideation from perceptual aberration both covered by umbrella concepts of psychotic-like or unreality experiences.

The problems of heterogeneity and the allied issue of diagnostic specificity are among the most pressing in research on the schizophrenia spectrum. Their study promotes the teasing apart of multiple domains of pathophysiological dysfunction. The study of schizotypal individuals offers the methodological advantage of providing an opportunity to obtain a more homogeneous behavioural sample ascertained through questionnaire assessment of a large number of normal individuals or clinical assessment of community volunteers. In addition, this advantage may be combined with the relative freedom in schizotypal individuals from the confounds of hospitalization, medication, chronic psychosis and other consequences of a long-term psychiatric diagnosis. By combining this strategy with the study of SPD patients, who also suffer fewer of the confounds encountered with schizophrenic patients, valuable insights may be provided into the pathophysiology of schizophrenia.

References

Abi-Dhargam, A., Gil, R., Krystal, J. et al. (1998) Increased striatal dopamine transmission in schizophrenia: confirmation in a second cohort. American Journal of Psychiatry 155, 761–767.

American Psychiatric Association (1980) Diagnostic and Statistical Manual of Mental Disorders, 3rd edn. American Psychiatric Association, Washington DC.

American Psychiatric Association (1994) Diagnostic and Statistical Manual of Mental Disorders, 4th edn. American Psychiatric Association, Washington DC.

Amin, F., Siever, L.J., Silverman, J.M. et al. (1997) Plasma HVA in Schizotypal Personality Disorder Plasma Homovanillic Studies in Schizophrenia, Implications for Presynaptic Dopamine Dysfunction (eds A.J. Fruedhoff & F. Amin), pp. 133–149. Progress in Psychiatry Series, American Psychiatric Press, Washington, DC.

Andreasen, N.C., Paradiso, S. & O'Leary, D.S. (1998) 'Cognitive dysmetria' as an integrative theory of schizophrenia: a dysfunction in cortical-subcortical-cerebullar circuitry? Schizophrenia Bulletin 24, 203–218.

Baron, M., Gruen, R., Rainer, J.D. et al. (1982) Schizoaffective illness, schizophrenia, and affective disorders: morbidity risk and genetic transmission. Acta Psychiatrica Scandinavica 65, 253–262.

Barthell, C. & Holmes, D. (1968) High school yearbooks: a non-reactive measure of social isolation in graduates who later became schizophrenic. Journal of Abnormal Psychology 78, 313–316.

Baruch, I., Hemsley, D.R. & Gray, A. (1988a) Differential performance of acute and chronic schizophrenics in a latent inhibition task. Journal of Nervous and Mental Disease 176, 598–606.

Baruch, I., Hemsley, D.R. & Gray, A. (1988b) Latent inhibition and 'psychotic proneness' in normal subjects. Personality and Individual Differences 1988, 777–783.

Battaglia, M., Abbruzzese, M., Ferri, S. et al. (1994) An assessment of the Wisconsin Card Sorting Test as an indicator of liability to schizophrenia. Schizophrenia Research 14, 39–45.

Battaglia, M., Bernardeschi, L. Franchini, L. et al. (1995) A family study of schizotypal disorder. Schizophrenia Bulletin 21, 33–46.

Battaglia, M., Cavallini, M.C., Macciardi, F. & Bellodi, L. (1997) The structure of DSM-IIIR schizotypal personality disorder diagnosed by direct interview. Schizophrenia Bulletin 23, 83–92.

Beech, A., Powell, T., McWilliam, J. & Claridge, G. (1989) Evidence of reduced 'cognitive inhibition' in schizophrenia. British Journal of Clinical Psychology 28, 109–116.

Bentall, R.P., Claridge, G.S. & Slade, P.D. (1989) The multidimensional nature of schizotypal traits: a factor analytic study with normal subjects. British Journal of Clinical Psychology 28, 363–375.

Bernstein, D.P., Useda, D. & Siever, L.J. (1996) Paranoid personality disorder. In: DSM-IV Sourcebook, Vol. 2 (eds T.A. Widiger, A.J. Frances, H.A. Pincus, R. Ross, M.B. First & W.W. Davis), pp. 665–674. American Psychiatric Association, Washington, DC.

Blackwood, D.H.R., St Clair, D.M. & Kutcher, S.P. (1986) P300 event-related potential abnormalities in borderline personality disorder. Biological Psychiatry 21, 557–560.

Bleuler, E. (1950) Dementia Praecox or the Group of Schizophrenias. International Universities Press, New York.

Bolino, F., Manna, V. DiCicco, L. et al. (1992) Startle reflex habituation in functional psychoses: a controlled study. Neuroscience Letters 145, 126–128.

Bolino, F., Di Michele, V., DiCicco, L. et al. (1994) Sensorimotor gating and habituation evoked by electro-cutaneous stimulation in schizophrenia. Biological Psychiatry 36, 670–679.

Boutros, N.N., Nasrallah, H., Leighty, R. et al. (1997) Auditory evoked potentials: clinical versus research applications. Psychiatry Research 24, 183–195.

Bower, E.M., Schellhammer, T.A. & Daily, J.A. (1960) School characteristics of male adolescents who later become schizophrenic. American Journal of Orthopsychiatry 30, 712–729.

Braff, D.L., Saccucco, D.P., Geyer & M.A. (1991) Information processing dysfunctions in schizophrenia: studies of visual backward masking, sensorimotor gating, and habituation. In: Handbook of Schizophrenia, Vol. 5 Neuropsychology, Psychophysiology and Information Processing (eds S.R. Steinhauser, J.H. Gruzelier & J. Zubin), pp. 303–334. Elsevier, Amsterdam.

Braff, D.L., Grillon, C. & Geyer, M.A. (1992) Gating and habituation of the startle reflex in schizophrenic patients. Archives of General Psychiatry 49, 206–215.

Breitmeyer, B. & Ganz, L. (1976) Implications of sustained and transient channels for theories of visual pattern masking. Psychological Review 83, 1–36.

Buchsbaum, M.S., Someya, T. & Tang, C.Y. (1996) PET and MRI of the thalamus of never-medicated patients with schizophrenia. American Journal of Psychiatry 153, 191–199.

Buchsbaum, M.S., Yang, S., Hazlett, E. et al. (1997a) Ventricular volume and asymmetry in schizotypal personality disorder and schizophrenia assessed with magnetic resonance imaging. Schizophrenia Research 27, 45–53.

Buchsbaum, M.S., Trestman, R.J., Hazlett, E. et al. (1997b) Regional cerebral blood flow during the Wisconsin Card Sort test in schizotypal personality disorder. Schizophrenia Research 27, 21–28.

Buchsbaum, M.S., Nenadic, I., Hazlett, E. et al. (2002) Differential metabolic rates in prefrontal and temporal Brodman areas in schizophrenia and schizotypal personality disorder. Schizophrenia Research 54, 141–150.

Byne, W., Buchsbaum, M.S., Kemether, E. et al. (2001) MRI assessment of medial and dorsal pulvinar nuclei of the thalamus in schizophrenia and schizotypal personality disorder. Archives of General Psychiatry 58, 133–140.

Cadenhead, K.S., Geyer, M.A. & Braff, D.L. (1993) Impaired startle prepulse inhibition and habituation in patients with schizotypal personality disorder. American Journal of Psychiatry 150, 1862–1867.

Cadenhead, K.S., Perry, W. & Braff, D.L. (1996) The relationship of information-processing deficits and clinical symptoms in schizotypal personality disorder. *Biological Psychiatry* **40**, 853–858.

Cadenhead, K.S., Perry, W., Shafer, K. & Braff, D.L. (1999) Cognitive functions in schizotypal personality disorder. *Schizophrenia Research* **37**, 123–132.

Cadenhead, K.S., Light, G.A., Geyer, M.A. & Braff, D.L. (2000) Sensory gating deficits assessed by the P50 event-related potential in subjects with schizotypal personality disorder. *American Journal of Psychiatry* **157**, 55–59.

Cannon, T.D., Mednick, S.A. & Parnas, J. (1990) Antecedents of predominantly negative- and predominantly positive-symptom schizophrenia in a high risk population. *Archives of General Psychiatry* **47**, 622–632.

Cannon, T.D., Zorrilla, L.E., Shtasel, D. *et al.* (1994) Neuropsychological functioning in siblings discordant for schizophrenia and healthy volunteers. *Archives of General Psychiatry* **51**, 651–661.

Cazzulo, V.A., Giobbio, G.M. *et al.* (1991) Cerebral structural abnormalities in schizophreniform disorder and in schizophrenia spectrum disorders. In: *Advances in Neuropsychiatry and Psychopharmacology* (eds C.A. Tamminga & S.C. Schulz).

Chapman, L.J. & Chapman, J.P. (1985) Psychosis proneness. In: *Controversies in Schizophrenia: Changes and Constancies* (ed. M. Alpert), pp. 157–174. Guilford Press, New York.

Chapman, L.J., Chapman, J.P. & Raulin, M.L. (1976) Scales for physical and social anhedonia. *Journal of Abnormal Psychology* **85**, 374–382.

Chapman, L.J., Chapman, J.P. & Raulin, M.L. (1978) Body-image aberration in schizophrenia. *Journal of Abnormal Psychology* **87**, 399–407.

Chen, W.J., Hsiao, C.K. & Lin, C.C. (1997) Schizotypy in community samples: the three-factor structure and correlation with sustained attention. *Journal of Abnormal Psychology* **106**, 649–654.

Claridge, G. & Beech, A. (1996) Schizotypy and lateralised negative priming in schizophrenics' and neurotics' relatives. *Personality and Individual Differences* **20**, 193–199.

Claridge, G. & Broks, P. (1984) Schizotypy and hemisphere function I. Theoretical considerations and the measurement of schizotypy. *Personality and Individual Differences* **5**, 633–648.

Clementz, B.A., Grove, W.M., Iacono, W.G. & Sweeney, J. (1992) Smooth pursuit eye movement dysfunction and liability for schizophrenia: implications for genetic modelling. *Journal of Abnormal Psychology* **101**, 117–129.

Clementz, B.A., McDowell, J.E. & Zisook, S. (1994) Saccadic system functioning among schizophrenia patients and their first-degree biological relatives. *Journal of Abnormal Psychology* **103**, 277–287.

Clementz, B.A., Geyer, M.A. & Braff, D.L. (1998) Poor P50 suppression among schizophrenia patients and their first-degree biological relatives. *American Journal of Psychiatry* **155**, 1691–1694.

Cohen, L.J., Hollander, E., DeCaria, C.M. *et al.* (1996) Specificity of neuropsychological impairment in obsessive–compulsive disorder: a comparison with social phobic and normal control subjects. *Journal of Neuropsychiatry and Clinical Neurosciences* **8**, 82–85.

Coleman, M.J., Levy, D.L., Lenzenweger, M.F. & Holzman, P.S. (1996) Thought disorder, perceptual aberrations, and schizotypy. *Journal of Abnormal Psychology* **105**, 469–473.

Cornblatt, B.A. & Kellp, J.G. (1994) Impaired attention, genetics and the pathophysiology of schizophrenia. *Schizophrenia Bulletin* **20**, 31–46.

Croft, R.J., Lee, A., Bertolot, J. & Gruzelier, J.H. (2001) Associations of P50 suppression and habituation with perceptual and cognitive features of 'unreality' in schizotypy. *Biological Psychiatry* **50**, 441–446.

Crow, T.J., Done, D.J. & Sacker, A. (1995) Birth cohort study of the antecedents of psychosis: ontogeny as witness to phylogenetic origins. In: *Search for the Causes of Schizophrenia*, Vol. 3 (eds H. Haefner & W.F. Gattaz), pp. 3–20. Springer, Berlin.

Csernansky, J., Murphy, G. & Faustman, W. (1991) Limbic/mesolimbic connections and the pathogenesis of schizophrenia. *Biological Psychiatry* **30**, 383–400.

Davidson, M. & Davis, K.L. (1988) A comparison of plasma homovanillic concentrations in schizophrenics and normal controls. *Archives of General Psychiatry* **45**, 561–563.

Davis, K.L., Davidson, M., Mohs, R.C. *et al.* (1985) Plasma homovanillic acid concentration and the severity of schizophrenic illness. *Science* **227**, 1601–1602.

Davis, K.L., Kahn, R.S., Ko. G. & Davidson, M. (1991) Dopamine and schizophrenia: a reconceptualisation. *American Journal of Psychiatry* **148**, 1474–1486.

Dawson, M.E., Hazlett, A.E., Filion, D.L. *et al.* (1993) Attention and schizophrenia: impaired modulation of the startle reflex. *Journal of Abnormal Psychology* **102**, 633–641.

Dickey, C.C., McCarley, R.W., Volgmaier, M., *et al.* (1999) Schizotypal personality disorder and MRI abnormalities of temporal lobe grey matter. *Biological Psychiatry* **45**, 1393–1402.

Docherty, N.M., Rhinewine, J.P., Labhart, R.P. & Gordinier, S.W. (1998) Communication disturbances and family psychiatric history in parents of schizophrenic patients. *Journal of Nervous and Mental Disease* **186**, 761–768.

Downhill, J.E., Buchsbaum, M.S., Wei, T.S. *et al.* (2000) Temporal lobe volume determined by magnetic resonance imaging in schizotypal personality disorder and schizophrenia. *Schizophrenia Research* **42**, 193–208.

Duchene, A., Graves, R.E. & Brugger, P. (1998) Schizotypal thinking and associative processing: a response commonality analysis of verbal fluency. *Journal of Psychiatry and Neuroscience* **23**, 56–60.

Eckblad, M. & Chapman, L.J. (1983) Magical ideation as an indicator of schizotypy. *Journal of Consulting and Clinical Psychology* **51**, 215–225.

Edell, W.S. (1987) Role of structure in disordered thinking in borderline and schizophrenic disorders. *Journal of Personality Assessment* **51**, 23–41.

El-Guebaly, N., Offord, D.R., Sullivan, K.T. & Lynch, G.W. (1978) Psychosocial adjustment of the offspring of psychiatric inpatients: the effect of alcoholic, depressive, and schizophrenic parentage. *Canadian Psychiatric Association Journal* **23**, 281–289.

Farmer, C.M., O'Donnell, B.F., Niznikiewicz, M.A. *et al.* (2000) Visual perception and working memory in schizotypal personality disorder. *American Journal of Psychiatry* **157**, 781–788.

Fenton, T.S. & McGlashan, T.H. (1989) Risk of schizophrenia in character disordered patients. *American Journal of Psychiatry* **146**, 1280–1284.

Ferraro, R.R. & Okerlund, M. (1995) Implicit memory of nonclinical schizotypal individuals. *Perceptual and Motor Skills* **80**, 371–376.

Fish, B. (1986) Antecedents of an acute schizophrenic break. *Journal of the American Academy of Child Psychiatry* **25**, 595–600.

Flach, K.A., Adler, L.E., Gerhardt, G.A. *et al.* (1996) Sensory gating in a computer model of the CA3 neural network of the hippocampus. *Biological Psychiatry* **40**, 1230–1245.

Foerster, A., Lewis, S., Owen, M. & Murray, R. (1991a) Premorbid adjustment and personality in psychosis: effects of sex and diagnosis. *British Journal of Psychiatry* **158**, 171–176.

Foerster, A., Lewis, S., Owen, M. & Murray, R. (1991b) Low birth weight and a family history of schizophrenia predict poor premorbid functioning in psychosis. *Schizophrenia Research* **5**, 13–20.

Frangos, E., Athenassanas, G., Tsitouorides, S., Katsanou, N. &

Alexandrakou, P. (1985) Prevalence of DSM-III schizophrenia among first-degree relatives of schizophrenic probands. *Acta Psychiatrica Scandinavica* **72**, 382–386.

Frangou, S., Sharma, T., Alarcon, G. *et al.* (1997) The Maudsley Family Study. II. Endogenous event-related potentials in familial schizophrenia. *Schizophrenia Research* **23**, 45–53.

Franke, P., Maier, W., Hardt, J. & Hain, C. (1993) Cognitive functioning and anhedonia in subjects at risk for schizophrenia. *Schizophrenia Research* **10**, 77–84.

Freedman, R., Coon, H., Myles-Worsley, M. *et al.* (1997) Linkages of a neurophysiological deficit in schizophrenia to chromosome 15 locus. *Proceedings of the National Academy of Sciences, USA* **94**, 587–592.

Freedman, L.R., Rock, D., Roberts, S.A., Cornblatt, B.A. & Erlenmeyer-Limling, L. (1998) The New York High-Risk Project: attention, anhedonia and social outcome. *Schizophrenia Research* **30**, 1–9.

Gershon, E.S., DeLisi, L.E., Hamovit, J. *et al.* (1988) A controlled family study of chronic psychoses. *Archives of General Psychiatry* **45**, 328–336.

Glish, M.A., Erlenmeyer-Kimling, L. & Watt, N.F. (1982) Parental assessment of the social and emotional adaptation of children at high risk for schizophrenia. In: *Advances in Child Clinical Psychology* (eds B. Lahey & A. Kazdin). Wiley, New York.

Goldberg, S.C., Schulz, C., Schulz, M. *et al.* (1986) Borderline and schizotypal personality disorders treated with low dose thioxene vs. placebo. *Archives of General Psychiatry* **43**, 680–686.

Goodarzi, M.A., Wykes, T. & Hemsley, D.R. (2000) Cerebral lateralization of global–local processing in people with schizotypy. *Schizophrenia Research* **45**, 115–121.

Gooding, D.C., Kwapil, T.R. & Tallent, K.A. (1999) Wisconsin Card Sorting Test deficits in schizotypic individuals. *Schizophrenia Research* **40**, 201–209.

Goodman, M., Mitropoulou, V., New, A.S., Koeningsberg, H. & Siever, L.J. (2000) Frontal cortex dysfunction and dopaminergic activity in schizophrenia spectrum. *Biological Psychiatry* **47**, 34S.

Gray, N.S., Pilowsky, L.S., Gray, J.A. & Kerwin, R.W. (1995) Latent inhibition in drug naïve schizophrenics: relationship to duration of illness and dopamine D$_2$ binding using SPET. *Schizophrenia Research* **17**, 95–107.

Green, M.F., Nuechterlein, K.H. & Mintz, J. (1994) Backward masking in schizophrenia and mania. II. Specifying the visual channels. *Archives of General Psychiatry* **51**, 945–951.

Green, M.F., Nuechterlein, K.H. & Breitmeyer, B. (1997) Backward masking performance in unaffected siblings of schizophrenic patients: evidence for a vulnerability indicator. *Archives of General Psychiatry* **54**, 465–472.

Griffith, J.M., O'Neill, J.E., Petty, F. *et al.* (1998) Nicotinic receptor desensitization and sensory gating deficits in schizophrenia. *Biological Psychiatry* **44**, 98–106.

Grillon, C., Ameli, R., Charney, D.S., Krystal, J. & Braff, D. (1992) Startle gating deficits occur across prepulse intensities in schizophrenic patients. *Biological Psychiatry* **32**, 939–943.

Grove, W.M., Lebow, B.S., Clementz, B.A. *et al.* (1991) Familial prevalence and coaggregation of schizotypy indicators: a multitrait family study. *Journal of Abnormal Psychology* **100**, 115–121.

Gruzelier, J.H. (1996) The factorial structure of schizotypy. I. Affinities and contrasts with syndromes of schizophrenia. *Schizophrenia Bulletin* **22**, 611–620.

Gruzelier, J. (1999a) Functional neuro-psychophysiological asymmetry in schizophrenia: a review and reorientation. *Schizophrenia Bulletin* **25**, 91–120. (Special issue on Lateralization.)

Gruzelier, J. (1999b) A review of the implications of early sensory processing and subcortical involvement for cognitive dysfunction in schizophrenia. In: *Review of Psychiatry* (ed. J. Oldham), pp. 29–76. American Psychiatric Association, Washington, DC.

Gruzelier, J.H. (2002) A Janusian perspective on the nature, development and structure of schizophrenia and schizotypy. *Schizophrenia Research* **54**, 95–103.

Gruzelier, J. & Davis, S. (1995) Social and physical anhedonia in relation to cerebral laterality and electrodermal habituation in unmedicated psychotic patients. *Psychiatry Research* **56**, 163–172.

Gruzelier, J. & Doig, A. (1996) The factorial structure of schizotypy. II. Patterns of cognitive asymmetry, arousal, handedness and gender. *Schizophrenia Bulletin* **22**, 621–634.

Gruzelier, J.H. & Kaiser, J. (1996) Syndromes of schizotypy and timing of puberty. *Schizophrenia Research* **21**, 183–194.

Gruzelier, J. & Raine, A. (1994) Schizophrenia, schizotypal personality, syndromes, cerebral lateralisation and electrodermal activity. *International Journal of Psychophysiology* **16**, 1–16.

Gruzelier, J. & Richardson, A. (1994) Patterns of cognitive asymmetry and syndromes of psychosis-proneness. *International Journal of Psychophysiology* **18**, 217–226. (Special issue on Developmental Psychopathology.)

Gruzelier, J.H., Seymour, K., Wilson, L., Jolley, T. & Hirsch, S. (1988) Impairments on neuropsychological tests of temporo-hippocampal and fronto-hippocampal functions and word fluency in remitting schizophrenia and affective disorders. *Archives of General Psychiatry* **45**, 623–629.

Gruzelier, J., Burgess, A., Stygall, J., Irving, G. & Raine, A. (1995) Patterns of cerebral asymmetry and syndromes of schizotypal personality. *Psychiatry Research* **56**, 71–79.

Gruzelier, J., Richardson, A. & Wilson, L. (1999a) Cognitive asymmetry patterns in schizophrenia: retest reliability and syndrome-related modifiability with recovery. *International Journal of Psychophysiology* **34**, 323–332. (Special issue on Laterality and Psychopathology.)

Gruzelier, J., Kaiser, J., Richardson, A. *et al.* (1999b) Opposite patterns of P300 asymmetry in schizophrenia are syndrome related. *International Journal of Psychophysiology* **34**, 276–282. (Special issue on Laterality and Psychopathology.)

Gruzelier, J., Wilson, L., Liddiard, D., Peters, E. & Pusavat, L. (1999c) Cognitive asymmetry patterns in schizophrenia: active and withdrawn syndromes and sex differences as moderators. *Schizophrenia Bulletin* **25**, 349–362.

Gruzelier, J.H., Jamieson, G.A., Croft, R.J., Kaiser, J. & Burgess, A.F. (2002) Personality Syndrome Questionnaire: reliability, validity and experimental evidence. *International Journal of Psychophysiology*, in press.

Gunderson, J.G., Siever, L.J. & Spaulding, E. (1983) The search for the schizotype: crossing the border again. *Archives of General Psychiatry* **40**, 15–22.

Hain, C., Maier, W., Hoechst-Janneck, S. & Franke, P. (1995) Subclinical thought disorder in first-degree relatives of schizophrenic patients: results from a matched-pairs study with the Thought Disorder Index. *Acta Psychiatria Scandinavica* **92**, 305–309.

Harris, J.G., Adler, L.E., Young, D.A. *et al.* (1996) Neuropsychological dysfunction in parents of schizophrenics. *Schizophrenia Research* **20**, 253–260.

Hazlett, E., Buchsbaum, M.S., Byne, E. *et al.* (1999) Three-dimensional analysis with MRI and PET of the size, shape and function of the thalamus in the schizophrenia spectrum. *American Journal of Psychiatry* **156**, 1190–1199.

Hewitt, J.K. & Claridge, G.S. (1989) The factor structure of schizotypy in a normal population. *Personality and Individual Differences* **10**, 323–329.

Hogg, B., Jackson, H.J., Rudd, R.P. & Edwards, J. (1990) Diagnosing personality disorders in recent-onset schizophrenia. *Journal of Nervous and Mental Disease* **178**, 194–199.

Huber, G. (1997) The heterogeneous course of schizophrenia. *Schizophrenia Research* **28**, 177–185.

Hymowitz, P., Francis, A., Jacobsberg, L.B., Sickles, M. & Hoyt, R. (1986) Neuroleptic treatment of schizotypal personality disorders. *Comprehensive Psychiatry* **27**, 267–271.

Ingraham, L.J. & Kety, S. (2000) Adoption studies of schizophrenia. *American Journal of Medical Genetics* **97**, 18–22.

Jorgensen, A. & Parnas, J. (1990) The Copenhagen high risk study: premorbid and clinical dimensions of maternal schizophrenia. *Journal of Nervous and Mental Disease* **178** (6), 370–376.

Jutai, J.W. (1989) Spatial attention in hypothetically psychosis-prone college students. *Psychiatry Research* **27**, 207–215.

Kaiser, J. & Gruzelier, J.H. (1996) Timing of puberty and EEG coherence during photic stimulation. *International Journal of Psychophysiology* **21**, 135–149.

Kaiser, J. & Gruzelier, J.H. (1999a) Timing of puberty and syndromes of schizotypy: a replication. *International Journal of Psychophysiology* **34**, 237–248. (Special issue on Laterality and Psychopathology.)

Kaiser, J. & Gruzelier, J. (1999b) Effects of pubertal timing on EEG coherence and P3 latency. *International Journal of Psychophysiology* **34**, 225–236. (Special issue on Laterality and Psychopathology.)

Kalus, O., Bernstein, D.P. & Siever, L.J. (1996) Schizoid personality disorder. In: *DSM-IV Sourcebook*, Vol. 2 (eds T.A. Widiger, A.J. Frances, H.A. Pincus, R. Ross, M.B. First & W.W. Davis), pp. 675–684. American Psychiatric Association, Washington, DC.

Karper, L.P., Freeman, G.K., Grillon, C. *et al.* (1996) Preliminary evidence of an association between sensorimotor gating and distractibility in psychosis. *Journal of Neuropsychiatry and Clinical Neurosciences* **8**, 60–66.

Katsanis, J., Kortenkamp, S., Iacono, W.G. & Grove, W.M. (1997) Antisaccade performance in patients with schizophrenia and affective disorder. *Journal of Abnormal Psychology* **106**, 468–472.

Kavoussi, R.J. & Siever, L.J. (1992) Overlap between borderline and schizotypal personality disorders. *Comprehensive Psychiatry* **33**, 7–12.

Keefe, R., Lees-Roitman, S. & Dupre, R. (1997) Performance of patients with schizophrenia on a pen and paper visuospatial working memory task with short delay. *Schizophrenia Research* **26**, 9–14.

Keefe, S.R., Silverman, J.M., Roitman, S.E. *et al.* (1994) Performance of nonpsychotic relatives of schizophrenic patients on cognitive tests. *Psychiatry Research* **53**, 1–12.

Kelly, M.P. & Bakan, P. (1999) Eye tracking in normals: spem asymmetries and association with schizotypy. *International Journal of Neuroscience* **98**, 27–81.

Kelly, M.P. & Coursey, R.D. (1992) Lateral preference and neuropsychological correlates of schizotypy. *Psychiatry Research* **41**, 115–135.

Kendler, K.S. (1985) Diagnostic approaches to schizotypal personality disorder: a historical perspective. *Schizophrenia Bulletin* **11**, 538–553.

Kendler, K.S. (1988) Familial aggregation of schizophrenia and schizophrenia spectrum disorders: evaluation of conflicting results. *Archives of General Psychiatry* **45**, 377–383.

Kendler, K.S. & Hewitt, J.K. (1992) The structure of self-report schizotypy in twins. *Journal of Personality Disorders* **6**, 1–17.

Kendler, K.S., Gruenberg, A.M. & Strauss, J.S. (1981) An independent analysis of the Copenhagen sample of the Danish adoption study of schizophrenia. II. The relationship between schizotypal personality disorder and schizophrenia. *Archives of General Psychiatry* **38**, 982–987.

Kendler, K.S., Ochs, A.L., Gorman, A.M. *et al.* (1991) The structure of schizotypy: a multitrait twin study. *Psychiatry Research* **36**, 19–36.

Kendler, K.S., McGuire, M., Gruenberg, A.M. *et al.* (1993a) The Roscommon Family Study. III. Schizophrenia-related personality disorders in relatives. *Archives of General Psychiatry* **50**, 781–788.

Kendler, K.S., McGuire, M., Gruenberg, A.M. *et al.* (1993b) The Roscommon Family Study. I. Methods, diagnosis of probands and risk of schizophrenia in relatives. *Archives of General Psychiatry* **50**, 527–540.

Kendler, K.S., Gruenberg, A.M. & Kinney, D.K. (1994) Independent diagnosis of adoptees and relatives as defined by DSM-III in the provincial and national samples of the Danish adoption study of schizophrenia. *Archives of General Psychiatry* **51**, 456–468.

Kety, S.S., Rosenthal, D., Wender, P.H. *et al.* (1975) Mental illness in the biological and adoptive families of adopted individuals who have become schizophrenic: preliminary report based o psychiatric interviews. In: *Genetic Research in Psychiatry* (eds R.R. Fieve, D. Rosenthal & H. Brill), pp. 147–165. Johns Hopkins University Press, Baltimore.

Kim, D., Raine, A., Triphon, N. & Green, M.F. (1992) Mixed handedness and features of schizotypal personality in a nonclinical sample. *Journal of Nervous and Mental Disease* **180**, 133–135.

Kirrane, M., Mitropoulou, V., Nunn, M. *et al.* (2000) Effects of amphetamine on visuospatial working memory in schizophrenia spectrum personality disorder. *Neuropsychopharmacology* **22**, 14–18.

Klosterkotter, J., Breuer, H., Gross, G. *et al.* (1992) New approaches to early recognition of idiopathic psychoses. In: *Schizophrenia and Affective Psychoses: Nosology in Contemporary Psychiatry* (eds F.P. Ferro, A.E. Haynal & N. Sartorius), pp. 111–120. J. Libbey, Rome.

Koenigsberg, H.W., Reynolds, D. Goodman, M. *et al.* (2002) Risperidone in the treatment of schizotypeal personality disorder. *Journal of Clinical Psychiatry* (in press).

Kolachana, B., Saunders, R., Bachevalier, J. & Weinberger, D. (1996) Abnormal prefrontal cortical regulation of striatal dopamine release after neonatal medial temporal-limbic lesions in rhesus monkeys. *Abstracts for the Society for Neuroscience* **22**, 1974.

Kraepelin, E. (1919/1971) *Manic-Depressive Insanity and Paranoia*. Translated by R.M. Barclay. E. & S. Livingstone, Edinburgh.

Kretschmer, E. (1921) *Physique and Character*. Translated 1936. Kegan Paul, London.

Kutcher, S.P., Blackwood, D.H.R., Gaskell, D.F., Muir, W.J. & St. Clair, D.M. (1989) Auditory P300 does not differentiate borderline personality disorder from schizotypal personality disorder. *Biological Psychiatry* **26**, 766–774.

Kwon, J.S., Shenton, M.E., Hirayasu, Y. *et al.* (1998) MRI study of cavum septum pellucidi in schizophrenia, affective disorder and schizotypal personality disorder. *American Journal of Psychiatry* **155**, 509–515.

Langdon, R. & Coltheart, M. (1999) Mentalising, schizotypy, and schizophrenia. *Cognition* **71**, 43–71.

Lenzenweger, M.E. & Gold, J.M. (2000) Auditory working memory and verbal recall memory in schizotypy. *Schizophrenia Research* **42**, 101–110.

Leonhard, D. & Brugger, P. (1998) Creative, paranormal and delusional thought: a consequence of right hemisphere semantic activation? *Neuropsychiatry, Neuropsychology and Behavioral Neurology* **11**, 177–183.

Lieberman, J.A., Kane, J.M. & Alvir, R. (1987) Provocative tests with psychostimulant drugs in schizophrenia. *Psychopharmacology* **91** (4), 415–433.

Lipp, O.V. & Vaitl, D. (1992) Latent inhibition in human Pavlovian conditioning: effect of additional stimulation after preexposure and relation to schizotypal traits. *Personality and Individual Differences* **13**, 1003–1012.

Lipska, B.K., Jaskiw, G.E. & Weinberger, D.R. (1993) Postpubertal emergence of hyperresponsiveness to stress and to amphetamine after neonatal excitotoxic hippocampal damage: a potential animal model of schizophrenia. *Neuropsychopharmacology* **9**, 67–75.

Lipska, B.K., Swerdlow, N.R., Geyer, M.A. *et al.* (1995) Neonatal excitotoxic hippocampal damage in rats causes post-pubertal changes in prepulse inhibition of startle and its disruption by apomorphine. *Psychopharmacology* **122**, 35–43.

Lubow, R.E., Weiner, I., Schlossberg, A. & Baruch, I. (1987) Latent inhibition and schizophrenia. *Bulletin of the Psychonomic Society* **25**, 464–467.

Lyons, M., Merla, M.E., Young, L. & Kremen, W. (1991) Impaired neuropsychological functioning in symptomatic volunteers with schizotypy: preliminary findings. *Biological Psychiatry* **30**, 424–426.

McCarley, R.W., Shenton, M.E., O'Donnell, B.F. *et al.* (1993) Auditory P300 abnormalities and left posterior superior temporal gyrus volume reduction in schizophrenia. *Archives of General Psychiatry* **50**, 190–197.

McCarley, R.W., Shenton, M.E., O'Donnell, B., Dickey, C.C. & Holinger, R. (1996) Schizophrenia spectrum disorders: electrophysiological and structural MRI features. 20th Annual Collegium Internationale Neuro-Psychopharmalogicum Congress, Melbourne, Australia.

McDowell, J. & Clementz, B. (1997) The effect of fixation condition manipulations on antisaccade performance in schizophrenia: studies of diagnostic specificity. *Experimental Brain Research* **115**, 333–344.

McGlashan, T.H. (1986) Schizotypal personality disorder, Chestnut Lodge follow-up study. VI. Long-term follow-up perspective. *Archives of General Psychiatry* **43**, 329–334.

Maier, W., Lichterman, D., Minges, J. *et al.* (1993) Continuity and discontinuity of affective disorders and schizophrenia: results of a controlled family study. *Archives of General Psychiatry* **50**, 871–883.

Maier, W., Lichterman, D., Minges, J. *et al.* (1994) Personality disorders among the relatives of schizophrenic patients. *Schizophrenia Bulletin* **20**, 481–493.

Mason, O., Claridge, G. & Clark, K. (1997) Electrodermal relationships with personality measures of psychosis-proneness in psychotic and normal subjects. *International Journal of Psychophysiology* **27**, 137–146.

Meehl, P.E. (1962) Schizotaxia, schizotypy, schizophrenia. *American Psychologist* **17**, 827–839.

Mehlum, L., Friis, S., Irion, T. *et al.* (1991) Personality disorders 2–5 years after treatment: a prospective follow-up study. *Acta Psychiatrica Scandinavica* **84**, 72–77.

Merritt, R.D. & Balogh, D.W. (1989) Backward masking spatial frequency effects among hypothetically schizotypal individuals. *Schizophrenia Bulletin* **15**, 573–583.

Michael, C.M., Morris, D.P. & Soroker, E. (1957) Follow-up studies of shy, withdrawn children. II. Relative incidence of schizophrenia. *American Journal of Orthopsychiatry* **27**, 331–337.

Mohr, C., Rohrenbach, C.M., Laska, M. & Brugger, P. (2001) Unilateral olfactory perception and magical ideation. *Schizophrenia Research* **47**, 255–264.

Moritz, S. & Mass, R. (1997) Reduced cognitive inhibition in schizotypy. *British Journal of Clinical Psychology* **36**, 365–376.

Muntaner, C., Garcia-Sevilla, L., Alberto, A. & Torrubia, R. (1988) Personality dimensions, schizotypal and borderline personality traits and psychosis proneness. *Personality and Individual Differences* **9**, 257–268.

Nalcaci, E., Kalaycioglu, C., Cicek, M. & Budanur, O.E. (2000) Magical ideation and right-sided hemispatial inattention on a spatial working memory task: influences of sex and handedness. *Perceptual and Motor Skills* **91**, 883–892.

Obiols, J.E., Serrano, F., Caparros, B., Subira, S. & Barrantes, N. (1999) Neurological soft signs in adolescents with poor performance on the continuous performance test: markers of liability for schizophrenia spectrum disorders? *Psychiatry Research* **86**, 217–228.

O'Donnell, D.F., Swearer, J.M., Smith, L.T. *et al.* (1996) Selective deficits in visual perception and recognition in schizophrenia. *American Journal of Psychiatry* **153**, 687–692.

O'Driscoll, G.A., Lenzenweger, M.F. & Holzman, P.S. (1998) Antisaccades and smooth pursuit eye tracking and schizotypy. *Archives of General Psychiatry* **55**, 837–843.

O'Flynn, K., Koenigsberg, H.W., Abi Dhargam, A. *et al.* (2001) Striatal dopaminergic activity in schizotypal personality disorder. *Abstract of the 56th Annual Meeting of the Society of Biological Psychiatry* **49**, Abstract 424.

Olin, S.S. & Mednick, S.A. (1996) Risk factors of psychosis: Identifying vulnerable populations premorbidly. *Schizophrenia Bulletin* **22**, 223–240.

Olin, S.S., Raine, A., Cannon, T.D. *et al.* (1997) Childhood behavior precursors of schizotypal personality disorder. *Schizophrenia Bulletin* **23**, 93–103.

O'Neal, P. & Robins, L.N. (1958) Childhood patterns predictive of adult schizophrenia: a 30-year follow-up study. *American Journal of Psychiatry* **115**, 385–391.

Park, S. & Holzman, P.S. (1992) Schizophrenics show spatial working memory deficits. *Archives of General Psychiatry* **49**, 975–982.

Park, S., Holzman, P.S. & Lenzenweger, M.F. (1995) Individual differences in spatial working memory in relation to schizotypy. *Journal of Abnormal Psychology* **104**, 355–363.

Parnas, J. & Jorgensen, A. (1989) Pre-morbid psychopathology in schizophrenia spectrum. *British Journal of Psychiatry* **155**, 623–627.

Parnas, J., Schulsinger, F., Schulsinger, H., Mednick, S.A. & Teasdale, T.W. (1982) Behavioral precursors of schizophrenia spectrum. *Archives of General Psychiatry* **39**, 658–664.

Peralta, V., Cuesta, M.J. & de Leon, J. (1991) Premorbid personality and positive and negative symptoms in schizophrenia. *Acta Psychiatrica Scandanavica* **84**, 336–339.

Peters, E.R., Pickering, A.D. & Hemsley, D.R. (1994) 'Cognitive inhibition' and positive symptomatology in schizotypy. *British Journal of Clinical Psychology* **33**, 33–48.

Pickar, D., Labarac, R., Linnoila, M. *et al.* (1984) Neuroleptic-induced decrease in plasma homovanillic acid and antipsychotic activity in schizophrenic patients. *Science* **225**, 954–956.

Pycock, C.J., Kerwin, R.W. & Carter, C.J. (1980) Effects of lesions of cortical dopamine terminals on subcortical dopamine receptors in rats. *Nature* **286**, 74–77.

Raine, A. (1991) The SPQ: a scale for the assessment of schizotypal personality based on DSM-IIIR criteria. *Schizophrenia Bulletin* **17**, 555–564.

Raine, A. & Allbutt, J. (1989) Factors of schizoid personality. *British Journal of Clinical Psychology* **28**, 31–40.

Raine, A. & Lencz, T. (1995) Conceptual; and theoretical issues in schizotypal personality disorder research. In: *Schizotypal Personality* (eds A. Raine, T. Lencz & S. Mednick), pp. 3–15. Cambridge University Press, Cambridge.

Raine, A. & Manders, D. (1988) Schizoid personality, inter-hemispheric transfer, and left hemisphere over-activation. *British Journal of Clinical Psychology* 27, 333–347.

Raine, A., Sheard, C., Reynolds, G.P. & Lencz, T. (1992) Pre-frontal structural and functional deficits associated with individual differences in schizotypal personality. *Schizophrenia Research* 7, 237–247.

Raine, A., Lencz, T. & Mednick, S.A., eds. (1995) *Schizotypal Personality*. Cambridge University Press, UK.

Raine, A., Benishay, D., Lencz, T. & Scarpa, A. (1997) Abnormal orienting in schizotypal personality disorder. *Schizophrenia Bulletin* 23, 75–82.

Richardson, A.J. (1994) Dyslexia, handedness and syndromes of psychosis-proneness. *International Journal of Psychophysiology* 18, 251–263.

Richardson, A. & Gruzelier, J. (1994) Visual processing, lateralisation and syndromes of schizotypy. *International Journal of Psychophysiology* 18, 227–240. (Special issue on Developmental Psychopathology.)

Ricks, D.F. & Berry, J.C. (1970) Family and symptom patterns that precede schizophrenia. In: *Life History Research in Psychopathology*, Vol. 1. (eds M. Roff & D.F. Ricks), pp. 3–18. University of Minnesota Press, Minneapolis.

Robins, L.N. (1966) *Deviant Children Grown Up*. Williams & Wilkins, Baltimore.

Roff, J.D., Knight, R. & Wertheim, E. (1976) Disturbed preschizophrenics: childhood symptoms in relation to adult outcome. *Journal of Nervous and Mental Disease* 162, 274–281.

Roitman, S.E., Cornblatt, B.A., Bergman, A. et al. (1997) Attentional functioning in schizotypal personality disorder. *American Journal of Psychiatry* 154, 655–660.

Roitman, S.E., Mitropoulou, V., Keefe, R.S. et al. (2000) Visuospatial working memory in schizotypal personality disorder patients. *Schizophrenia Research* 41, 447–455.

Ross, R.G., Hommer, D., Radant, A., Roath, M. & Freedman, R. (1996) Early expression of smooth-pursuit eye movement abnormalities in children of schizophrenic parents. *Journal of the American Academy of Child and Adolescent Psychiatry* 35, 941–949.

Ross, R.G., Olincy, A., Harris, J.G. et al. (1998) Anticipatory saccades during smooth pursuit eye movements and familial transmission of schizophrenia. *Biological Psychiatry* 44, 690–697.

Saykin, A.J., Shtasel, D.L., Gur, R.E. et al. (1994) Neuropsychological deficits in neuroleptic naïve patients with first episode schizophrenia. *Archives of General Psychiatry* 51, 124–131.

Schuck, J.R. & Lee, R.G. (1989) Backward masking, information processing, and schizophrenia. *Schizophrenia Bulletin* 15, 491–500.

Schulz, P.M. & Soloff, P.H. (1987) Still borderline after all these years. 140th Annual Meeting of the American Psychiatric Association, Chicago, IL.

Schulz, P.M., Schulz, S.C., Goldberg, S.C. et al. (1986) Diagnoses of the relatives of schizotypal outpatients. *Journal of Nervous and Mental Disorders* 174, 457–463.

Schwarzkopf, S.B., Lamberti, J.S. & Smith, D.A. (1993) Concurrent assessment of acoustic startle and auditory P50 evoked potential measures of sensory inhibition. *Biological Psychiatry* 33, 815–828.

Shaw, J., Claridge, G. & Clark, K. (2001) Schizotypy and the shift from dextrality: a study of handedness in a large non-clinical sample. *Schizophrenia Research* 50, 181–189.

Shelton, R.C. & Weinberger, D.R. (1986) X-ray computerized tomography studies in schizophrenia: a review & synthesis. In: *The Neurology of Schizophrenia* (eds H.A. Nasrallah & D.R. Weinberger), pp. 207–250. Elsevier, New York.

Shihabuddin, L., Buchsbaum, M.S., Hazlett, E. et al. (2001) Striatal size and relative glucose metabolic rate in schizotypal personality disorder and schizophrenia. *Archives of General Psychiatry* 58 (9), 877–884.

Siegel, B.V., Trestman, R.L., O'Flaithbheartaigh, S. et al. (1996) D-amphetamine challenge effects on Wisconsin Card Sort test: performance in schizotypal personality disorder. *Schizophrenia Research* 20, 29–32.

Siegel, C., Waldo, M., Mizner, G., Adler, L.E. & Freedman, R. (1984) Deficits in sensory gating in schizophrenic patients and their relatives: evidence obtained with auditory evoked responses. *Archives of General Psychiatry* 41, 607–612.

Siever, L.J. (1991) The biology of the boundaries of schizophrenia. In: *Advances in Neuropsychiatry and Psychopharmacology*, Vol. 1, *Schizophrenia Research* (eds C.A. Tamminga & S.C. Schulz), pp. 181–191. Raven Press, New York.

Siever, L.J., Coursey, R.D., Alterman, I.S., Buchsbaum, M.S. & Murphy, D.L. (1984) Impaired smooth-pursuit eye movement: vulnerability marker for schizotypal personality disorder in a normal volunteer population. *American Journal of Psychiatry* 141, 1560–1566.

Siever, L.J., Coursey, R.D., Alterman, I.S. et al. (1989) Clinical, psychophysiologic, and neurologic characteristics of volunteers with impaired smooth pursuit eye movements. *Biological Psychiatry* 26, 35–51.

Siever, L.J., Keefe, R., Bernstein, D.P. et al. (1990a) Eye tracking impairment in clinically identified schizotypal personality disorder patients. *American Journal of Psychiatry* 147, 740–745.

Siever, L.J., Silverman, J.M., Horvath, T.B. et al. (1990b) Increased morbid risk for schizophrenia-related disorders in relatives of schizotypal personality disordered patients. *Archives of General Psychiatry* 47, 634–640.

Siever, L.J., Kalus, O.F. & Keeffe, R.S.E. (1993) The boundaries of schizophrenia. *Psychiatry Clinics of North America* 16 (2), 217–244.

Siever, L.J., Rotter, M., Losonczy, M. et al. (1995) Lateral ventricular enlargement in schizotypal personality disorder. *Psychiatry Research* 57, 109–118.

Siever, L.J., Bernstein, D.P. & Silverman, J.M. (1996) Schizotypal personality disorder. In: *DSM-IV Sourcebook*, Vol. 2 (eds T.A. Widiger, A.J. Frances, H.A. Pincus et al.), pp. 685–701. American Psychiatric Association, Washington.

Siever, L.J., Koenigsberg, H.W., Harvey, P. et al. (2002) Cognitive and brain function in schizotypal personality disorder. *Schizophrenia Research* 54, 157–167.

Silverman, J.M., Smith, C.J., Guo, S.L. et al. (1998) Lateral ventricular enlargement in schizophrenic probands and their siblings with schizophrenia-related disorders. *Biological Psychiatry* 43, 97–106.

Simons, R.F. & Katkin, W. (1985) Smooth pursuit eye movements in subjects reporting physical anhedonia and perceptual aberrations. *Psychiatry Research* 14, 275–289.

Slaghuis, W.L. & Bakker, V.J. (1995) Forward and backward visual masking of contour by light in positive- and negative-symptom schizophrenia. *Journal of Abnormal Psychology* 104, 41–54.

Squires-Wheeler, E., Skodol, A.E., Friedman, D. & Erlenmeyer-Kimling, L. (1988) The specificity of DSM-III Schizotypal personality traits. *Psychological Medicine* 18, 757–765.

Squires-Wheeler, E., Skodol, A.E., Bassett, A. & Erlenmeyer-Kimling, L. (1989) DSM-IIIR schizotypal personality traits in offspring of schizophrenic disorder, affective disorder, and normal control parents. *Journal of Psychiatric Research* 23, 229–239.

Squires-Wheeler, E., Skodol, A.E. & Erlenmeyer-Kimling, L. (1992) The assessment of schizotypal features over two points in time. *Schizophrenia Research* 6, 75–85.

Squires-Wheeler, E., Friedman, D., Amminger, G.P. *et al.* (1997) Negative and positive dimensions of schizotypal personality disorder. *Journal of Personality Disorders* 11, 285–300.

Strik, W.K., Dierks, T., Franzek, E. Stober, G., & Maurer, K. (1994) P300 asymmetries in schizophrenia revisited with reference independent methods. *Psychiatry Research: Neuroimaging* 55, 153–166.

Swerdlow, N.R. & Geyer, M.A. (1998) Using an animal model of deficient sensorimotor gating to study the pathophysiology and new treatments of schizophrenia. *Schizophrenia Bulletin* 24, 285–301.

Swerdlow, N.R., Filion, D., Geyer, M.A. *et al.* (1995) 'Normal' personality correlates of sensorimotor, cognitive, and visuospatial gating. *Biological Psychiatry* 37, 286–299.

Szigethy, E.M. & Schulz, S.C. (1997) Risperidone in comorbid borderline personality disorder and dysthymia. *Journal of Clinical Psychopharmacology* 17, 326–327.

Tien, A.Y., Costa, P.T. & Eaton, W.W. (1992) Couariance of personality, neurocognition, and schizophrenia spectrum traits in the community. *Schizophrenia Research* 7, 149–158.

Torgersen, S., Onstad, S., Skre, I., Edvardsen, J. & Kringlen, E. (1993) 'True' schizotypal personality disorder: a study of co-twins and relatives of schizophrenic probands. *American Journal of Psychiatry* 150, 1661–1667.

Trestman, R.L., Keefe, R.S.E., Mitropoulou, V. *et al.* (1995) Cognitive function and biological correlates of cognitive performance in schizotypal personality disorder. *Psychiatry Research* 59, 127–136.

Trestman, R.L., Horvath, T., Kalus, O. *et al.* (1996) Event-related potentials in schizotypal personality disorder. *Journal of Neuropsychiatry and Clinical Neuroscience* 8, 33–40.

Trevarthen, C. (1996) Lateral asymmetries in infancy: implications for the development of the hemispheres. *Neuroscience and Biobehavioural Reviews* 20, 571–586.

Venables, P.H., Wilkins, S., Mitchell, D.A., Raine, A. & Bailes, K. (1990) A scale for the measurement of schzotypy. *Personality and Individual Differences* 11, 481–495.

Voglmaier, M.M., Seidman, L.J., Salisbury, D. & McCarley, R.W. (1997) Neuropsychological dysfunction in schizotypal personality disorder: a profile analysis. *Biological Psychiatry* 41, 530–540.

Waldo, M.C., Adler, L.E. & Freedman, R. (1988) Defects in auditory sensory gating and their apparent compensation in relatives of schizophrenics. *Schizophrenia Research* 1, 19–24.

Waldo, M.C., Carey, G., Myles-Worsley, M. *et al.* (1991) Codistribution of a sensory gating deficit and schizophrenia in multi-affected families. *Psychiatry Research* 39, 257–268.

Waldo, M.C., Cawthra, E., Adler, L.E. *et al.* (1994) Auditory sensory gating, hippocampal volume, and catecholamine metabolism in schizophrenics and their siblings. *Schizophrenia Research* 12, 93–106.

Warnken, R.G. & Seiss, T.F. (1965) The use of the cumulative record in the prediction of behavior. *Personnel and Guidance Journal* 31, 231–237.

Watt, N.F. (1978) Patterns of childhood social development in adult schizophrenics. *Archives of General Psychiatry* 35, 160–165.

Webb, C.T. & Levinson, D.F. (1993) Schizotypal and paranoid personality disorder in the relatives of patients with schizophrenia and affective disorders: a review. *Schizophrenia Research* 11, 81–92.

Weintraub, S. & Neal, J.M. (1984) Social behavior of children at risk for schizophrenia. In: *Children at Risk for Schizophrenia: a Longitudinal Perspective* (eds N.F. Watt, E.J. Anthony, L.C. Wynne & J.E. Rolf), pp. 279–285. Cambridge University Press, New York.

White, P.M. & Yee, C.M. (1997) Effects of attentional and stressor manipulations on the P50 gating response. *Psychophysiology* 34, 703–711.

Williams, G.V. & Goldman-Rakic, P.S. (1995) Modulation of memory fields by dopamine D_1 receptors in prefrontal cortex. *Nature* 376, 572–575.

Williams, L.M. (1995) Further evidence for a multidimensional personality disposition to schizophrenia in terms of cognitive inhibition. *British Journal of Clinical Psychology* 34, 193–213.

Course and outcome of schizophrenia

H. Häfner and W. an der Heiden

Introduction, 101
    Time trends, 101
Methodological aspects of course and outcome
    research, 102
    Measures for describing course and outcome, 112
Diagnosis, clinical subtypes, empirical symptom
    dimensions and their course, 113
    Positive and negative symptoms, 114
    Course of negative symptoms and cognitive
        impairment, 115
    Course of cognitive impairment and brain
        anomalies, 116
    Course of empirical symptom dimensions and
        clusters, 117
    Early course of schizophrenia (prodromal stage
        and first psychotic episode), 118

Stages in the development of schizophrenia, 120
    Early and later course of depressive symptoms,
        121
    Suicide in the course of schizophrenia, 123
Short- and medium-term social course of
    schizophrenia, 123
Short- and medium-term symptom-related course of
    schizophrenia, 125
    Prognostic indicators, 126
Comorbidity with alcohol and drug abuse, 127
Long-term course of schizophrenia, 127
    Geographical variation of course and outcome in
        schizophrenia, 129
Quality of life, 130
Conclusions, 130
References, 131

Introduction

Studies on the natural history of schizophrenia aim at shedding light on the variance in the natural course and outcome, on the spectrum of consequences of the disorder as well as on the factors influencing these dimensions. Kraepelin (1893), preoccupied with the course of dementia praecox throughout his professional life, was believed to have found the basis for this 'disease entity' in the combination of symptomatology and course. Eventually, his belief was shaken when he came to realize the great variety of courses (Kraepelin 1920).

All recent longitudinal studies have, of necessity, examined the treated rather than the natural course of schizophrenia. The only exceptions have been the studies following up placebo controls; unfortunately, all these are limited to highly selected patient groups with a maximum follow-up of 2 years because they have been carried out to assess the efficacy of therapeutic interventions.

Time trends

A selection of first-admission cohorts of patients with schizophrenia from different countries shows that since the turn of the nineteenth century the length of hospital stay has decreased progressively (Fig. 8.1). Decreasing lengths of stay after first admission for schizophrenia have been reported by several authors, for example Ødegård (1964), who compared data from the national Norwegian case register for cohorts of patients discharged in the periods 1936–42, 1945–52 and 1955–59.

Influenced as they are by disease-independent factors, time trends in the frequency and length of hospital stay hardly pro-

vide reliable indicators of the course of the illness, an der Heiden *et al.* (1995), in the Mannheim follow-up study covering 15.6 years, demonstrated a widening gap between mean symptom scores, which remained stable, and a continued decrease in days per year spent in inpatient treatment. Simultaneously, outpatient treatment contacts increased, reflecting the change that has taken place in the system of care, while the illness course has remained the same.

More or less comparable outcome indicators are provided by rates of recovery or good outcome. Shepherd *et al.* (1989) reviewed selected twentieth century outcome studies of schizophrenia and found a substantial increase in recovery rates since the 1950s. In contrast, Warner (1985), in his more comprehensive but still selective review, came to the conclusion that the recovery rate had scarcely improved since the early years of the twentieth century.

A meta-analysis (Hegarty *et al.* 1994) of 320 longitudinal studies of a century that fulfilled minimum methodological standards found a recovery rate of 35% for the period 1895–1955 and a clearly higher rate of 49% for 1956–85, possibly indicating the success of neuroleptics. However, in the following period of novel antipsychotics, 1986–92, the rate fell back to 36%.

These data are not reliable enough to allow conclusions on possible time trends of the course of schizophrenia. One reason is that the diagnostic criteria have clearly changed over these periods (Loranger 1990; Stoll *et al.* 1993). Furthermore, Hegarty *et al.* (1994) pointed out that not a single study they reviewed was based on a truly representative cohort.

M. Bleuler (1968) noted that the proportion of good outcomes had remained stable, but the number of 'catastrophic' and chronic cases had decreased since the beginning of the

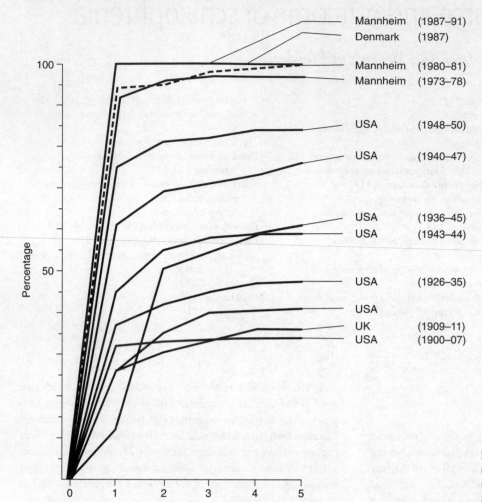

Fig 8.1 Percentage of first admissions for schizophrenia discharged within 5 years (based on Brown 1960, supplemented by data for Mannheim and Denmark). (After Häfner & an der Heiden 1982.)

twentieth century. This sounds plausible considering the fact that psychotic symptoms and episodes can be cured or alleviated by antipsychotic drugs. A gradual disappearance of extremely severe forms of schizophrenia, e.g. life-threatening catatonia, with the improvement in early recognition and the availability of efficacious antipsychotic medication and intensive care has been reported from Germany by Häfner and Kasper (1982). However, the remedies currently available reduce neither predisposition to the illness nor the deficit syndrome in the long term. Since the mid twentieth century the system of care provided for people with schizophrenia, time spent in hospital in particular and, as a result, the social biographies of persons affected have undergone marked changes, as outpatient treatment and complementary care have become more and more widespread.

Methodological aspects of course and outcome research

Systematic studies into the medium- and long-term course of schizophrenia require considerable effort. This explains why

only few studies meet the time-consuming methodological requirements.

A review of 44 long-term follow-up studies, over 10 years or more (an der Heiden 1996), shows considerable variance in the proportion of good outcome in schizophrenia (Fig. 8.2). Factors explaining part of the variance are differences in the outcome measures, in the diagnostic criteria and in the study populations.

Methodological requirements for longitudinal studies into schizophrenia have been proposed by several authors (Robins 1979; Ram *et al.* 1992; Jablensky 1995; Gaebel & Frommann 2000; Häfner 2000). To ensure the validity and comparability of the results, the following are the main requirements to observe.

1 The *inclusion criteria* – diagnosis is the most important – determining what will be studied.

2 To define *diagnosis* only cross-sectional criteria should be adopted. Course-related criteria, such as Criterion C1 – persistance of symptoms for at least 6 months – for an American Psychiatric Association DSM-IIIR (1987) or DSM-IV (American Psychiatric Association 1994) diagnosis of schizophrenia, leads

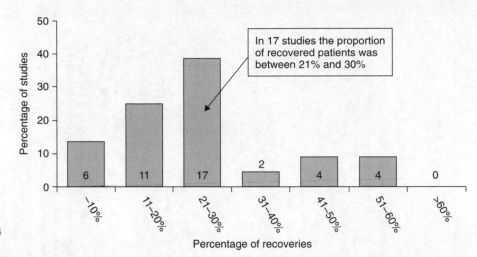

Fig 8.2 Proportion of recovered patients in 44 long-term studies.

to the exclusion of acute cases with predominantly good outcomes.

3 Only if the cohort at entry into a longitudinal study is *representative* of all cases diagnosed with schizophrenia in a given population or of a precisely defined subgroup of these cases, e.g. late-onset schizophrenia, will the study results be valid for all cases of the disorder or for the subgroup in question.

Because of an annual incidence rate of as low as 1–2 cases per 10 000 population it is impractical to try to reach first episodes of schizophrenia in large enough numbers by door-to-door surveys. For this reason, index cases are usually recruited from treatment services. It remains a controversial question whether a treated incidence calculated from inpatient data is a valid estimate of the true incidence. According to the few comparative studies addressing this question, the risk for persons with schizophrenia of coming in contact with inpatient services ranges from 50% to 100% (Link & Dohrenwend 1980; Engelhardt *et al.* 1982; von Korff *et al.* 1985; Goldacre *et al.* 1994; Geddes & Kendell 1995; Thornicroft & Johnson 1996). As the proportion of cases in inpatient care decreases with the increasing proportion of patients cared for in outpatient services, case recruitment should be extended to outpatient services as well. In countries with a hospital-centred system of mental health care, a practical alternative to a field study is to recruit first admissions for schizophrenia from all the mental hospitals serving a defined population or from case registers.

However, the representativeness of samples is bound to be limited if probands are recruited from hospitals not seeing the entire spectrum of schizophrenic illness. Some of the famous US long-term follow-up studies (Table 8.1) recruited their samples from among long-stay inpatients (Breier *et al.* 1991) 'who had not improved sufficiently with chlorpromazine' (Harding *et al.* 1987a) or from among wealthy long-stay inpatients of a private mental hospital (McGlashan 1984a).

Of great importance for the external validity of study results is the question of whether the samples assessed at follow-up are representative of the initial samples. This requirement is difficult to fulfil, particularly in studies covering long periods of time (Riecher-Rössler & Rössler 1998; Häfner & an der Heiden 2000).

In pure outcome studies an initial assessment is compared with a follow-up. Follow-up studies try either to identify trends from at least three cross-sectional assessments or to analyse changes between at least two cross-sections by using a retrospective approach (Robins 1979; Ram *et al.* 1992; Häfner & an der Heiden 2000). A criterion of the quality of follow-up studies that has been paid only little attention, as the great variation in the follow-up periods in Table 8.1 shows (an der Heiden 1996), is that follow-up periods should be identical in length for all the individuals included in a study. If changes are expected to occur in the illness course, and this is a basic hypothesis of all follow-up studies, designs not paying attention to this rule are bound to produce distorted results.

For this same reason, entering subjects at different stages of illness progression should be avoided (Jablensky 1995). In short-term follow-up studies looking into the early stages of illness, rapid changes and much variability can be expected so great care should be taken to avoid variation in the early follow-up periods. Only recently have the requirements of commencing studies at identical stages of illness and of using identical follow-up periods become fulfilled in a few longitudinal studies, e.g. WHO Determinants of Outcome of Severe Mental Disorders Study: 2 and 5 years (Jablensky *et al.* 1992), WHO Disability Study: 13–15 years (Schubart *et al.* 1986; an der Heiden *et al.* 1995; Mason *et al.* 1996; Sartorius *et al.* 1996; Wiersma *et al.* 1998; Häfner *et al.* 1999b).

In studies on the natural course of schizophrenia, the follow-up period ideally begins with the onset of the disorder. As it is not yet possible to predict the onset of schizophrenia with certainty, the first hospital admission is usually chosen as the starting point. Usually triggered by psychotic episodes, first and subsequent admissions take place at illness stages with maximum symptom presentation (Häfner *et al.* 1995). When an initial assessment conducted on hospital admission is compared with a

Table 8.1 Studies on long-term course of schizophrenia (after an der Heiden 1996).

Source	Study/subjects	Design	Diagnosis	N: beginning/end	Follow-up	Course/outcome dimensions; main instruments	Course	Outcome
Bleuler (1972)	Burghölzli study; hospital patients; 31.5% with first admissions	'Real-time' prospective study	Schizophrenia according to Bleuler criteria	216/208 (205)	>20 years	Psychopathological status; social and occupational development; assessment of 'end state' (during the last 5 years)	Eight course types: 4 simple courses – acute or chronic with severe end states, 13%; acute or chronic with mild end states, 25%; 3 undulating courses – severe end states, 9%; mild end states, 27%; recovery, 22%; atypical courses – 4%	(In 152 patients) severe end states, 24%; moderate end states, 24%; mild end states, 33%; recovery, 20%
Bottlender et al. (1999)	Inpatients with first admission to a psychiatric hospital	'Catch-up' prospective study; single follow-up assessment	Diagnosis according to ICD-9: 295, 297, 298.39	245/145	15 years after first hospital admission	AMDP: paranoid-hallucinatory syndrome, depressive syndrome, negative syndrome, 'deficit'-syndrome GAS	–	Average GAS-score, 55.8; negative symptoms, 52.4%; 'deficit' syndrome, 26.2%
Breier et al. (1991)	NIMH Longitudinal Study of Chronic Schizophrenia; 'chronically ill' hospital population	'Catch-up' prospective study; single follow-up assessment	Chronic/subchronic schizophrenia or schizoaffective disorder according to RDC	74/58	On average 13 years after illness onset, resp. 2–12 years after index treatment	Symptomatology; functioning; treatment history BPRS, SANS; LOFS, GAS, WCS	No reduction in symptomatology, instead of this increase during the first 10 years	GAS-score: poor 35%; moderate 62%; good 3% BPRS-total score: poor 38%; moderate 53%; good 10% SANS total score: poor 48%; moderate 36%; good 15% Global outcome: poor 42%; moderate 38%; good 21%
Carpenter & Strauss (1991)	Washington IPSS cohort; hospital population (no evidence of continuous psychosis for longer than 3 years)	'Real-time' prospective study; 3 follow-up assessments: 2, 5 and 11 years	At least one psychotic symptom; schizophrenia, manic-depressive illness, personality disorder according to DSM-II	131/53 (40 with DSM-II schizophrenia)	11 years after index treatment	Duration of inpatient treatment; social relationships; occupational functioning; severity of symptoms DIS; LOFS	No indication for either significant amelioration or deterioration in the period between 5- and 11-year follow-up; many patients tend to reach a plateau of psychopathology early in the course of the illness	Outcome domains of functioning are only moderately correlated
Changhui et al. (1995)	WHO ISoS Study; epidemiologically defined population irrespective of duration of illness	'Catch-up' prospective study; single follow-up assessment	Schizophrenia according to ICD-9	91/56 (55)	12 years after index assessment	Global functioning; social disability; psychological impairments; positive/negative symptoms DAS, GAF, LCS,PIRS, PSE-9, SANS	Simple course, 51.8%; episodic course, 7.1%; neither episodic nor simple, 7.1%; no psychotic episode during follow-up period, 33.9%	GAF-score: good outcome, 32.1%; fair outcome, 16.1%; poor outcome, 41.1%; very poor outcome, 10.7% SANS total score ≥3: 80% PIRS total score ≥2: 74.5% PSE total score ≥11: 60% DAS total score ≥2: 75%
Ciompi & Müller (1976)	Lausanne study; former hospital patients aged <65 at first admission and ≥65 at follow-up	'Catch-up' prospective study; single follow-up assessment	Definition of schizophrenia according to Kraepelin and E. & M. Bleuler	1642/289	36.9 years (median) after index admission	Course and 'end state' criteria according to Bleuler (1972); social adjustment; global psychological status	Simple-progredient courses, 43%; undulating courses, 50%; uncertain, 7%	(Continuous status during the last 5 years) poor end states, 18%; fair end states, 24%; mild end states, 22%; recovered, 27%; uncertain, 9%

Author (year)	Sample/cohort	Diagnosis	N	Follow-up	Assessment		Results
Dube et al. (1984)	Agra IPSS cohort; WHO ISoS study; patients with first contact and illness onset within 1 year before index assessment	Clinical diagnosis of schizophrenia (72.1%), manic-depressive psychosis (20%), psychoneurosis (7.9%)	140/79 (46 = 74.2% with schizophrenia)	13–14 years	Global functioning; symptomatology PSE-9, PPHS	–	(In 46 schizophrenic patients) 'normal', 59%; 'neurotic', 2%; residual states, 20%; schizophrenia, 13%; manic-depressive psychosis, 7%
Eaton et al. (1992a, b)	3 case register cohorts (Victoria, Australia/Denmark/Salford, UK); patients, who received a diagnosis of schizophrenia in a hospital setting during a period of observation of some 23 years	Schizophrenia according to ICD-8, DSM-I	1850	At least 16 years (Salford: 14 years) after discharge for first hospitalization for schizophrenia	Hospital readmissions	–	The probability for readmission decreases significantly with the passage of time; risk for readmission is highest in the first month after discharge; as a tendency duration of community tenure during hospital stays seems to lengthen over time
Ganev et al. (1998); Ganev (2000)	WHO disability study/WHO ISoS study; schizophrenics in inpatient and outpatient treatment from a defined catchment area; illness onset no longer than 2 years before index treatment; age between 15 and 44 years at index admission	Clinical diagnosis of schizophrenia; Schneiderian first rank symptoms; ICD-9 295, 297, 298.3, 298.4, 298.8, 298.9	60/55	16 years after index treatment	Psychopathology, social disability; psychological impairments PSE-9, PHSD, PIRS, DAS, LCS, GAF	–	Course of psychotic illness during 2 years before long-term follow-up: continuously psychotic, 45.5%; episodic course, 12.7%; no symptoms, 38.2%; negative symptoms, 63%; 64.8% with continuous; 13% with intermittent neuroleptic treatment; 74.5% without inpatient treatment GAF score 31–50: 50.9%
Gmür (1991)	2 cohorts of chronically ill patients: (i) night-clinic patients (average duration of illness 18 years); (ii) hospital patients (average duration of illness 15 years)	Diagnosis of schizophrenia according to Bleuler; PSE-CATEGO diagnosis schizophrenia (based on case history records)	46 night clinic +46 hospital patients/ 39 + 44	12 years after index admission (15–18 years after first manifestation)	Psychopathology; social adjustment (among others: work situation; social contacts; sexuality) FBF2	Decline in number and duration of acute episodes, as well as in number and duration of hospital stays; decreasing ability to work; increasing prominence of residual symptoms during quiescent intervals; no differences between the two cohorts	Conspicuous psychopathology: cohort (i), 66.5%; cohort (ii), 64.4%. Work situation: disability pension, 71.8% vs. 62%; employed, 33.3% vs. 35.5%. Relationships: married, 7.7% vs. 20%; living alone, 45.4% vs. 44.4%; no friends or acquaintances, 43.6% vs. 35.6%

Table 8.1 (cont.)

Source	Study/subjects	Design	Diagnosis	N: beginning /end	Follow-up	Course/outcome dimensions; main instruments	Course	Outcome
Harding et al. (1987a); see also Harding et al. (1987b); Harding (1988); Childers & Harding (1990)	Vermont Longitudinal Study; long-stay patients, 'who had not improved sufficiently with chlorpromazine'	'Real-time' prospective study; 2 follow-up assessments: 5–10 years and 20–25 years after discharge from index admission	Chronically ill patients; 79.2% with DSM-I diagnosis schizophrenia	269/168	On average 32 years after index assessment (range: 22–62 years)	Among others: utilization of treatment/social services; residence; work; finances; social support system; competence; community involvement; psychopathology; medication VCQ-I; VCQ-C; GAS; LOFS	–	One-half to two-thirds of the patients achieved considerable improvement/recovery Living conditions: independent housing, 50.3%; boarding home, 39.8%; hospital, 3.1%; nursing homes, 4.3%; other setting, 2.5% Employment status: employed (half of them classified as working in unskilled jobs) 26%; unemployed, 33% GAS score ≥62 (generally functioning 'pretty well'), 68% Overall functioning (LOFS), slight or no impairment, 55%
van der Heiden et al. (1995, 1996)	WHO Disability Study/WHO ISoS Study; hospital patients from a defined catchment area; illness onset no longer than 1 year before index admission; age at index admission: 15–44 years	'Real-time' prospective study; 9 follow-up assessments: 6, 12, 18, 24 months, 3 years, 5, 14, 14.9, 15.6 years	Clinical diagnosis of schizophrenia; Schneiderian first-rank symptoms	70/56 (14-year follow-up)/ 51 (15.6 years)	14 years +18 months after index admission	Among others: living conditions; social contacts; need for inpatient/outpatient care; work situation; negative symptoms; social disability; psychological impairments PSE-9; DAS-M; PIRS; BPRS; SANS; IRAOS-C	Significant decrease in need for inpatient treatment with the passage of time; no change in the number of patients with significant psychopathology (PSE-DAH) and psychological impairments (PIRS); significant increase in the number of patients with social disability (DAS-M)	(9-month interval after 14-year follow-up) significant positive and/or negative symptoms, 60.7%; clinically inconspicuous with neuroleptic treatment, 12.5%; recovered, 26.8%
Helgason (1990)	Epidemiologically based cohort with first inpatient/ outpatient contacts	'Real-time' prospective study; 2 follow-up assessments: 6–7 years, 21 years	ICD-8/9; Schneiderian first-rank symptoms	107/82	21 years	Mental state; ability to work; social interaction	–	Mental state: no/minor symptoms of psychopathology/ no treatment, 30%; obvious symptoms, inpatient treatment <2 months/year, 50%; severe symptoms, inpatient treatment >2 months/year, 21% Social interaction: normal/few but close friends, 55%;

Study	Sample	Design	Criteria	n	Follow-up	Assessment	Outcome
							tendency towards or social isolation, 45% Employment: employed full-time/<6 months/year, 33%; <6 months/year/unemployed, 67%
Huber *et al.* (1979)	Bonn study (67% first admissions)	'Catch-up' prospective study; single follow-up assessment	Criteria of schizophrenia according to K. Schneider and M. & E. Bleuler	758/502	On average 22.4 years (range: 9–59 years) after index admission	Course types considering both the kind of course and psychopathological outcome ('end states') according to M. Bleuler (1972)	Complete remisssion, 22.1%; non-characteristic residual syndromes, 43.2%; characteristic residual syndromes, 34.7%
							12 course types: monophasic course type, 10%; polyphasic course type, 12.1%; chronic pure psychoses, 4.2%, one manifestation to pure residues, 6.2%; phasic-'schubförmig' to pure residues, 10%; 'schubförmig' with second positive bend to pure residues, 5.8%; 'schubförmig/simple to structural deformities, 6.2%; simple to pure residues, 5.4%; 'schubförmig' to pure residues, 12.9%; 'schubförmig' to mixed residues, 9.6%,simple to mixed residues, 7.2%; 'schubförmig'/simple to typically schizophrenic defect psychoses, 10.5%
Leon (1989)	Former IPSS cohort; WHO ISoS study; age of patients at inclusion between 15 and 44 years	'Real-time' prospective study; 3 follow-up assessments: 2, 5 and 10 years	Clinical diagnosis of schizophrenia; diagnosis of schizophrenia according to PSE-9 (ICD-7/8)	101/84 (74)	10 years after index assessment	Psychopathology; social disability; psychological impairments; inpatient treatment DAS, PIRS, PSE-9; SEA, SAF, SPHS, Global outcome assessment: 1 complete recovery (no psychotic symptoms); 2 partial recovery (no psychotic symptoms, but symptoms of neurosis/adaptive problems); 3 covert (inactive) psychosis presence of psychotic characteristics, in a covert way); 4 residual state (usually negative symptoms); 5 overt psychosis (clear presence of psychotic symptoms); 6 deterioration (severe disability of mental functions)	Global course description, based on the analysis of all available clinical information: (1) single episode, 8%; (2) episodic, occasional, 13%; (3) episodic, recurrent, 20%; (4) mixed, with recovery, 8%; (5) recurrent, progressive, 4%; (6) mixed, without recovery, 12%; (7) continuous, fluctuating, 9%; (8) continuous, stationary, 13%; (9) continuous, severe, 13% (1) complete recovery, 43.4%; (2) partial recovery, 7.9%; (3) covert psychosis, 15.8%; (4) residual state, 7.9%; (5) overt psychosis, 14.5%; (6) deterioration, 10.5%

Table 8.1 (cont.)

Source	Study/subjects	Design	Diagnosis	N: beginning /end	Follow-up	Course/outcome dimensions; main instruments	Course	Outcome
Marengo et al. (1991)	Chicago follow-up study; hospital population, 39% with first hospital admission	'Real-time' prospective study; 3 follow-up assessments in 2–3 year intervals	Diagnosis of schizophrenia according to RDC	?/74	On average 8 years after index-admission/10 years after first hospital admission	Course and 'end state' criteria according to M. Bleuler (1972); psychopathology; inpatient data; drug treatment; social adaptation SADS; PSE-9 (modified); Katz and Lyerly Adjustment Scales		(1) Acute onset – undulating course – recovered/mild outcome, 10.8%; (2) acute onset – undulating course – moderately severe outcome, 9.5%; (3) acute onset – simple course – recovered/mild outcome, 6.8%; (4) acute onset – simple course – moderately severe outcome, 13.5%; (5) chronic onset – undulating course – recovered/mild outcome, 6.8%; (6) chronic onset – undulating course – moderately severe outcome, 12.2%; (7) chronic onset – simple course – recovered/mild outcome, 4.1%; (8) chronic onset – simple course – moderately severe outcome, 36.5%
Marneros et al. (1991)	Köln Study; patients from a hospital psychiatric clinic during 1950–79; illness duration not considered	'Catch-up' prospective study; single follow-up assessment	Schizophrenia; schizoaffective disorders, affective disorders; diagnosis according to DSM-III (modified)	(Only schizophrenics) 189/148	23 years (range: 10–50 years) after first manifestation	6 course types, considering pre-episodic alterations and persisting alterations during course/at long-term follow-up; outcome considering psychopathology, social disability, psychological impairments; outcome criteria according to Huber et al. (1979) PSE-9, DAS, PIRS, GAS	(Only schizophrenics) type 1: no enduring pre-episodic alterations/no persisting alterations, 7%; type 2: enduring pre-episodic alterations/no persisting alterations, 0%; type 3: no enduring pre-episodic alterations/persisting alterations during course, 15%; type 4: enduring pre-episodic alterations/persisting alterations during course, 8%; type 5: enduring pre-episodic alterations/persisting alterations since onset, 43%; type 6: enduring pre-episodic alterations/persisting alterations since onset, 28%	(Only schizophrenics) psychopathological outcome (criteria according to Huber): complete remission, 7%; uncharacteristic residues, 51%; characteristic schizophrenic residues, 42%
Mason et al. (1995)	Former WHO Determinants of Outcome Study (incidence) cohort; WHO ISoS study; patients with a first contact with a psychiatric service; age: 15–54 years	'Real-time' prospective study; 2 follow-up assessments: 2 and 13 years	ICD-9 diagnosis schizophrenia	67/58	13 after index assessment	Psychopathology, social disability, living conditions, employment, treatment, assessment of illness course over 2 years before long-term follow-up PSE-9, SANS, LCS, BRS, DAS, GAF	Type of course over last 2 years: episodic, 10%; continuous, 34%; neither episodic nor continuous, 3%; never psychotic, 52%	Severity of psychotic symptoms in the last month (Bleuler's scale): recovered, 56%; mild, 12%; moderate, 26%; severe, 5% Social disability (GAF); nil/mild (score 61–90), 49%; moderate/severe (score 1–60), 51%

Author (year)	Sample / cohort	Type of study	N	Diagnosis	Follow-up	Measures	Results		Outcome
Maurer (1995)	Epidemiologically based cohort with first hospital admission from the Danish case register	Case register analysis	1169 (thereof 475 with ICD 295)	Schizophrenia, paranoid syndrome, acute paranoid reaction, borderline psychosis according to ICD-8	10–11 years after index admission	Treatment episodes (readmission rate, number of inpatient episodes, duration of hospital stays)	(Only ICD 295) 58.1% (men, 58.0%; women, 58.1%) have at least 1 readmission; number of episodes on average 3.1 (men), 2.9 (women) Cumulative total duration of treatment episodes: 533 (men); 445 days (women)	–	Treatment with neuroleptics over the last 2 years: never, 24%; sometimes, 7%; most of the time, 64% Complete recovery (no symptoms/no disability/no treatment), 17%
McGlashan (1984a, b; 1986)	Chestnut Lodge Follow-up Study; chronically ill long-stay patients from a private clinic; discharge between 1950 and 1974 (minimum length of stay 90 days) plus inpatient sample with admission between 1945 and 1970	'Catch-up' prospective study; single follow-up assessment	616/446 (403 interviewed; thereof 163 with diagnosis of schizophrenia)	Schizophrenia, schizophreniform psychosis, schizoaffective psychosis, uni-/bipolar affective disorder, schizotypal, 'borderline' personality according to DSM-III; diagnosis of schizophrenia according to Feighner or RDC or 'New Haven' criteria, u. a.	On average 15 years (range 2–32 years) after discharge (?)	38 course and outcome characteristics from the domains of employment, treatment, family, social relationships, psychopathology, global level of functioning, plus 33 'psychodynamic' outcome criteria (5-point scales: 0 [poor] –4 [good]) Strauss–Carpenter scale	–		(Only 163 schizophrenics) living conditions at time of follow-up: hospital/sheltered environment, 37%; family of origin, 12%; alone, 28%; with friends, 5%; own family, 18% Clinical global functioning: continuously incapacitated, 41%; marginal, 23%; moderate, 23%; good, 8%; recovered, 6%
Ogawa et al. (1987)	Patients discharged from a neuropsychiatric department in the period from 1958–64 (79% first admissions)	'Real-time' prospective study; 2 (?) follow-up assessments: 5 years (?), 21–27 years	140/105 (98)	ICD-9 diagnosis schizophrenia	On average 23.6 years after index treatment (range: 21–27 years), resp. 26.4 years after illness onset (range: 21–47 years)	Social adjustment, psychopathology; ESAS; global assessment of outcome (psychopathology): recovered = no positive symptoms; improved = mild positive and/or negative symptoms; unimproved = remarkable positive and/or negative symptoms; course assessment: 'end state' criteria according to Bleuler (1972) for the last 5 years	–		'End states' (only 71 patients): recovery, 32%; mild chronic, 25%; moderately severe chronic, 25%; severe chronic, 17% Social adjustment: self-supportive, 47%; semi-self-supportive, 8%; socially adjusted to family/community, 11%; maladjusted, 3%; hospitalized, 31% Psychopathology: recovered, 31%; improved, 46%; unimproved, 23%; under psychiatric care, 66%; neuroleptic drugs, 64%

Table 8.1 (cont.)

Source	Study/subjects	Design	Diagnosis	N: beginning /end	Follow-up	Course/outcome dimensions; main instruments	Course	Outcome
Thara et al. (1994)	Madras longitudinal study; first-onset patients	'Real-time' prospective study; 3 follow-up assessments: 2, 5 and 10 years	Schizophrenia according to ICD-9	90/76	10 years after index assessment	Psychopathology; treatment; course types as defined in the IPSS IFS; PSE-9; PPHS	Complete recovery without relapse, 14.5%; no relapses, but with residual symptoms, 2.6%; one or more relapses, complete remissions, 48.7%; one or more relapses, incomplete remissions, 27.6%; continuously psychotic, 6.6%	Status at follow-up: psychotic 22% (7% continuously since inclusion into the study)
Tsoi & Wong (1991)	First admissions to a psychiatric hospital in Singapore; age range: 15–39 years	'Real-time' prospective study; 3 follow-up assessments: 5, 10 and 15 years	Schizophrenia according to ICD-9	330/224	15 years after index treatment	Psychiatric treatment; employment	Treatment and employment; status at 3 points in time: (1) 5 years; (2) 10 years; (3) 15 years after index treatment: in treatment: (1) 45%; (2), 40%; (3) 45%; employed: (1) 55%; (2) 54%; (3) 48%; inpatient treatment: (1) 15%; (2) 17%; (3) 17%; no readmissions in 15, 34%; 1–5 readmission, 45%; 6–10 readmissions, 12%; more than 10 readmission, 11%	–

AMDP, Befundbogen (Arbeitsgemeinschaft für Methodik und Diagnostik in der Psychiatrie 1995); BPRS, Brief Psychiatric Rating Scale (Overall & Gorham 1962); BRS, Broad Rating Schedule (WHO 1992); DAS, Disability Assessment Schedule (WHO 1988); DAS-M, Disability Assessment Schedule – Mannheim Version (Jung et al. 1989); DIS, Diagnostic Interview Schedule (Robins et al. 1981); FBF2, Frankfurt Symptoms Questionnaire (Süllwold 1977); GAF, Global Assessment of Functioning Scale (American Psychiatric Association 1987); GAS, Global Assessment Scale (Endicott et al. 1976); IFS, Interim Follow-up Schedule (Sartorius et al. 1986); IPSS, International Pilot Study of Schizophrenia; IRAOS, Instrument for the Retrospective Assessment of the Onset of Schizophrenia (Häfner et al. 1992); ISoS, International Study on Schizophrenia; Katz and Lyerly Adjustment Scales (Katz & Lyerly 1963); LCS, Life Chart Schedule (WHO 1992); LOFS, Level of Functioning Scale (Hawk et al. 1975); PHSD, Past History and Sociodemographic Description Schedule (WHO 1977); PPHS, Psychiatric and Personal History Schedule (WHO 1978b); PSE-9, Present State Examination (Wing et al. 1974); PIRS, Psychological Impairment Rating Schedule (Biehl et al. 1989); PSE-DAH, Present State Examination – Delusional and Hallucinatory Syndromes; RDC, Research Diagnostic Criteria (Spitzer et al. 1978); SADS, Schedule for Affective Disorders and Schizophrenia (Endicott & Spitzer 1978); SAF, Self-Assessment Form (WHO 1979); SANS, Scale for the Assessment of Negative Symptoms (Andreasen 1989); SEA, Subjective Experience Account (WHO 1979); SPHS, Social and Personal History Schedule (WHO 1979); Strauss–Carpenter Scale (Strauss & Carpenter 1972); VCQ-L, Vermont Community Questionnaire (Harding & Brooks 1984); VCQ-C, Vermont Community Questionnaire – cross-sectional interview (Harding & Brooks 1984); WCS, Wisconsin Card Sorting Test (Berg 1948).

Table 8.2 The 14 most frequent symptoms in a cohort of 811 patients with schizophrenia, examined in the WHO International Pilot Study of Schizophrenia (WHO 1979) (from Jablensky 2000).

Symptom	Frequency (%) in the psychotic index episode	Frequency (%) at 2-year follow-up
Ideas of reference	55.1	18.0
Suspiciousness	60.0	25.2
Delusions of reference	50.3	14.2
Delusions of persecution	48.1	12.7
Presence of auditory hallucinations	43.8	11.6
Presence of verbal hallucinations	37.9	10.7
Voices speak to patient	36.3	9.4
Delusional mood	47.5	10.5
Thought alienation	33.5	7.4
Restricted speech	17.5	12.9
Flatness of affect	51.0	27.1
Apathy	30.4	18.8
Lack of insight	82.7	42.5
Inadequate description	67.2	25.2

later follow-up, the result will show an artefact of improvement or recovery, because in the further course of the disorder only about 20% of the patients are bound to be in psychotic episodes (Biehl et al. 1986; Häfner & an der Heiden 1986; Wiersma et al. 1996). Table 8.2 illustrates the 14 symptoms most frequently presented by 811 patients with schizophrenia in the International Pilot Study of Schizophrenia (IPSS; WHO 1979). The almost proportional decrease over 2 years is accounted for by an artefact of illness stage. To prevent this mistake from happening, later follow-up assessments should be compared with assessments conducted after remission of the psychotic episode, e.g. 6 months after first admission (Biehl et al. 1986; Craig et al. 1999; Häfner & an der Heiden 2000).

Ram et al. (1992) have described follow-up studies based on utilization data of services as statistical reports on admissions and discharges. These can be conducted with considerably less effort than epidemiological longitudinal studies based on direct standardized assessments of patients. Drawbacks are the problems of lacking or limited generalizability. For this reason their aims are mostly limited to (i) describing treatment careers as a basis for comparisons over space and time; and (ii) under certain preconditions, to reconstructing the illness course in clinical populations, mostly to find out whether and to what extent patients' needs for treatment and care are met. Especially when based on case-register data from defined catchment areas, analyses of this sort provide valuable information for services planning, but are of secondary importance in research on the natural course of schizophrenia.

A follow-up study in which patients are clinically assessed

directly at follow-up is termed a catch-up prospective study. In these studies case identification takes place at the beginning of the follow-up period (Robins 1979; Ram et al. 1992; Häfner & an der Heiden 2000). The study sample is retrospectively recruited from admission or discharge records and assessed at the beginning of the study, mostly on the basis of case records, then reassessed at follow-up in a clinical interview. This design is also vulnerable to bias, because the representativeness of samples is difficult to ensure. As good cases tend to drop out, chronic cases are usually overrepresented at follow-up (Jablensky 1995). The direct assessment at follow-up makes it possible to reconstruct the illness course retrospectively using suitable instruments.

A retrospective approach with case identification at follow-up (follow-back design) proceeds from an existing study population, e.g. hospital admissions or discharges, and traces illness onset and history from the patients' memory and/or clinical records. This design misses good courses no longer in treatment contact and also leads to a high degree of variability in the lengths of illness courses included. For this reason this design is only rarely used. An example is the investigation of 77 patients with schizophrenia, treated in the course of 1 year, from the Oxford case register in which the lengths of illness varied from 2 to 22 years (Kolakowska et al. 1985).

In prospective studies – Robins (1979) calls them 'real-time' studies – the assessment and the study started at the beginning of the illness. Ideally, both the initial examination and the follow-up assessments are conducted on the same cohort by the same investigators using the same instruments.

All longitudinal studies – including prospective ones – as far as they map the timespan between two assessments, have retrospective components. Ciompi and Müller (1976) conducted a follow-up at 36.9 years (median) after index admission. In the Bonn Study (Huber et al. 1979) the follow-up assessments took place after an average of 22.4 years, in the Northwick Park Study (Johnstone et al. 1992) 3–13 years and in the Chestnut Lodge Study (McGlashan 1984a) an average of 15 years after initial assessment. The Vermont Longitudinal Study comprised two follow-up assessments (Harding et al. 1987a), 5–10 years and 20–25 years after discharge from index treatment.

Studies with a still greater number of follow-up assessments are rare: e.g. in the Washington IPSS study (Carpenter & Strauss 1991) patients were reassessed 2, 5 and 11 years after index treatment, in the ABC (Age, Beginning, Course) Study*6 months, 1, 2, 3 and 5 years after first admission (Häfner et al. 1999b), and the Mannheim WHO cohort was examined at a total of 10 cross-sections over a period of 15.5 years (an der Heiden et al. 1995, 1996).

The ABC Study, to which we will refer in some contexts, was carried out with a population-based sample of 232 patients aged 12–59 years with first illness episodes of broadly defined schizophrenia (ICD-9 diagnoses 295, 297, 298.3, 298.4; WHO 1978a). This sample comprised 84% of all the patients admitted for the first time with a diagnosis of schizophrenia to 10 hospitals serving a semi-rural, semi-urban German population of 1.5 million (Mannheim, Heidelberg and surrounding countryside).

In a retrospective part of the study, data on family background, pre- and perinatal complications, premorbid development, substance and alcohol use, onset and accumulation of symptoms and impairments were collected using the Interview for the Retrospective Assessment of the Onset of Schizophrenia (IRAOS; Häfner *et al.* 1992, 1999a) including a time matrix until first admission. As controls non-schizophrenic individuals drawn from the population register and matched to the probands for age, sex and place of residence were included. Data were collected from three sources: patients, key persons and case records (e.g. from general practitioners) and compared for reliability testing (Maurer & Häfner 1995; for more details see Häfner *et al.* 1993).

At the first cross-section on first admission, patients were assessed using the Present State Examination (PSE: Wing *et al.* 1974), the Scale for the Assessment of Negative Symptoms (SANS: Andreasen 1983), the Psychological Impairments Rating Schedule (PIRS: Biehl *et al.* 1989) and the Psychiatric Disability Assessment Schedule (DAS-M: WHO 1988; Jung *et al.* 1989). The prospective part, conducted in a population-based subsample of 115 patients with first illness episodes, consisted of follow-up assessments at 6 months, 1, 2, 3 and 5 years after first admission using the instruments mentioned above and, additionally, the Follow-up History and Sociodemographic Description Schedule (FU-HSD) (WHO 1980; for more details see Häfner *et al.* 1995, 1998, 1999c). Currently, a controlled 12-year follow-up of the total ABC sample and a study of their children and the non-schizophrenic parents of these children are underway.

Measures for describing course and outcome

The constructs for describing the course and outcome of schizophrenia depend on the issues studied. When the aim is to evaluate treatment measures, standardized illness-course-related indicators of the effectiveness and side-effects of therapies are frequently chosen. In studies on the 'natural' course of schizophrenia, standards are more or less lacking that would allow direct comparisons of the results. One of the reasons is that none of the designs can really do without using retrospective data on varying periods of time (see above).

Most of the instruments used for assessing the course of schizophrenia are cross-sectional in nature. They are aimed at producing data on the current state, usually focusing on periods of 2–4 weeks preceding the interview. For measuring symptoms over several years: (i) information on reliability is scattered (Andreasen *et al.* 1981; Helzer *et al.* 1981; Robins *et al.* 1982; McGuffin *et al.* 1986; Zimmerman *et al.* 1988; Maurer & Häfner 1995); and (ii) information on validity is almost non-existent (an der Heiden & Krumm 1991).

Kraepelin was one of the first who tried to bring some order into the great variety of illness courses in schizophrenia. He proposed only a few categories. The efforts undertaken in his wake on the basis of such – questionably operational – categories as stable, progressing and remittent, or psychosis vs. disability,

have produced typologies of course types whose number ranges from a mere four (Watt *et al.* 1983) to as many as 79 (Huber *et al.* 1979; see also Jansson & Alström 1967; Bleuler 1972; Ciompi & Müller 1976; Leon 1989; Marengo *et al.* 1991; Marneros *et al.* 1991; Thara *et al.* 1994; Changhui *et al.* 1995). Ciompi (1980) added to the two course types – simple and undulatory were used by Kraepelin – two further stages at the beginning and the end: onset (acute, chronic), course type (simple, undulatory) and end state (recovery or mild, moderate or severe). He applied this system to classify 289 patients from the Lausanne study. Attempts to compare the different typologies of the course of schizophrenia (Bleuler 1972; Ciompi & Müller 1976; Harding 1988; Marengo *et al.* 1991) have largely failed to show agreement (Fig. 8.3).

The course of schizophrenia has also been studied on the basis of the need for inpatient treatment (e.g. Daum *et al.* 1977; Engelhardt *et al.* 1982; Gmür 1991; Tsoi & Wong 1991; Eaton *et al.* 1992a,b; Maurer 1995; an der Heiden *et al.* 1995).

Many longitudinal studies focus on outcome. For studies of this type there are approved and reliable instruments available but this approach does not produce comparable results automatically. In Harding *et al.*'s (1987a,b) follow-up study of 269 inpatients with schizophrenia (at follow-up 168) over a period of 32 years, 68% had a good global outcome (Global Assessment Score, GAS ≥61; Endicott *et al.* 1976). In comparison, Breier *et al.*'s (1991) study of 74 (at follow-up 58) chronic patients with schizophrenia over 13 years on average, using the same instrument and measure (GAS score ≥61), yielded a good outcome in only 3%.

The most important clinical indicators of the course of schizophrenia are symptoms, socio-occupational and cognitive functioning, social impairment and disability, demographic and socioeconomic status, illness behaviour and quality of life. Strauss and Carpenter (1972, 1974) distinguish four domains of outcome in schizophrenic illness, which are only loosely connected with one another ('open-linked systems'): social relations, occupational status, treatment and symptomatology. Whether these domains really are more or less independent remains to be clarified. Several studies (Stephens *et al.* 1980; Breier *et al.* 1991; an der Heiden *et al.* 1996) report pronounced associations between symptom measures, negative symptoms in particular, and domains of functioning, while others have failed to show any correlation between changes on different symptom-related or functional dimensions over the illness course (Loebel *et al.* 1992; Tohen *et al.* 1992; Gupta *et al.* 1997). The various domains show great differences in stability, e.g. positive symptoms, which have mainly an episodic course, vs. negative symptoms, occupational and marital status, so that cross-sectional analyses are bound to yield low correlations.

The categories of 'florid' (Kraepelin) or 'acute' (positive–productive) and 'chronic' (primarily negative–unproductive) symptoms have a special role in the description of the course of schizophrenia. They are presumed to be produced by different psychopathological processes (Crow 1980a,b; Andreasen &

	Onset	Course type	End state	Lausanne study	Burghölzli study	Vermont study	Chicago study	ISoS study*
1	Acute	Undulating	Recovery/mild	25.4	30–40 / 25–35	7	10.8	29.4
2	Chronic	Simple	Moderate/severe	24.1	10–20	4	36.5	14.4
3	Acute	Undulating	Moderate/severe	11.9	5	4	9.5	4.9
4	Chronic	Simple	Recovery/mild	10.1	5–10	12	4.1	10.4
5	Chronic	Undulating	Recovery/mild	9.6	–	38	6.8	22.6
6	Acute	Simple	Moderate/severe	8.3	5–15	3	13.5	9.1
7	Chronic	Undulating	Moderate/severe	5.3	–	27	12.2	4
8	Acute	Simple	Recovery/mild	5.3	5	5	6.8	5.3

Fig 8.3 Course types in schizophrenia. On the right, each of the five columns represents a study. The numbers indicate the percentage of patients with the course type depicted on the left, e.g. 7% of the patients in the Vermont Study demonstrated an acute onset, an undulating course and a recovered mild end state (type 1), in contrast to the ISoS Study in which 29.4% of the patients belonged to this course type (based on Harding 1988; data from Chicago and ISoS studies have been added by the authors). *Incidence cohorts only. Lausanne study, Ciompi and Müller (1976); Burghölzli study, Bleuler (1972); Vermont study, Harding *et al.* (1987); Chicago study, Marengo *et al.* (1991); ISoS study, Harrison *et al.* (2001).

Olsen *1982*). Besides these symptoms more or less characteristic anomalies are observed ('impairments'). While the diagnosis is mainly based on symptoms, the psychological impairments (e.g. of attention, cognition, affect, speech) are less specific, because they are also encountered in other disorders, e.g. in major depressive disorder, where they show less severe presentations, and may to some extent result from external factors, e.g. investigator's attitude. Like symptoms and premorbid personality, the behavioural anomalies are classified as disease-inherent factors, i.e. factors characteristic of the disorder and its course (Schubart *et al.* 1986).

To a greater extent than in the origin of 'impairment', external factors – especially patients' social and occupational status – have a role in the emergence of disabilities. Disability is defined as disordered or deficient functioning in the social roles and domains (work, family, social group, etc.) regarded as normal in that society, by the family or social group or by the person affected (DAS; WHO 1988; Jablensky 1978).

For purposes of clinical and rehabilitative practice, additional measures for assessing the course and outcome of schizophrenia are needed, especially because there are methods of therapy and training available that help to reduce symptoms, cognitive and social impairment and to improve the patients' level of social functioning. As a result, there is a growing demand for tools that, in addition to measuring global outcome, allow a differential assessment of indicators of course and outcome and effects of treatment.

Diagnosis, clinical subtypes, empirical symptom dimensions and their course

Without an identifiable aetiology, and a distinct underlying pathophysiology still rather obscure, the disease concept of schizophrenia is currently based on tradition, clinical experience and the operational definitions of the diagnosis derived from this experience (see Chapters 1, 2, 3 and 12). The symptom patterns conventionally diagnosed as schizophrenia and regarded as reliable produce a rather heterogeneous spectrum of illness courses. The few stable patterns of symptoms or functional deficits from the schizophrenia spectrum nourish hopes that they could soon be linked to brain dysfunctions. Perhaps in this way and with increasing clarification of the role of genes it might become possible to break what is currently known as schizophrenia down into definable subentities of dysfunctioning (Jablensky 2000). However, for the time being there is no alternative to an operationally defined disease concept of schizophrenia in studies into the course and outcome of schizophrenia (see Chapter 12).

The international classification systems divide the diagnosis of schizophrenia into subtypes. The subtypes given in the ICD classification (WHO 1993) follow the clinical tradition, whereas those included in DSM-IV (American Psychiatric Association 1994) to some extent take account of symptom dimensions generated by factor analysis. The subtypes are distinguished mainly by their type of early illness course and outcome.

Of the clinically defined subtypes, 'simple type' and 'hebephrenia' mostly have a poor social prognosis, and 'acute catatonia' and 'paranoid psychosis' the most favourable prognosis. Fenton and McGlashan (1991a,b) used three DSM-III-based subtypes in their follow-back study of 187 patients over an average of 19 years: hebephrenia had an insidious onset and a poor prognosis – in accordance with the definition; undifferentiated schizophrenia occupied an intermediate position; and the paranoid subtype tended to a remittent course and minimum disability. In the IPSS (WHO 1979) the ICD-9 subtypes were subjected to empirical testing on the basis of discriminant function analysis. The result was a considerable degree of overlap, particularly between the simple and hebephrenic type on the one hand and paranoid schizophrenia on the other hand (see Chapter 3).

The most simple distinction between subtypes is based on acute vs. insidious onset (Jablensky et al. 1992). A detailed subtyping is yielded by Leonhard's (1966, 1999) classification of 32 symptomatological course units. However, the data available do not provide enough evidence for regarding these subtypes as discrete entities. In clinical practice some of the clinical subtypes can be helpful, despite the occurrence of continuous transitions between the categories, because they provide therapeutic and prognostic information. Jablensky (2000), however, doubts their prognostic power because of the 'scarcity of well-designed longitudinal studies'.

Positive and negative symptoms

An early attempt to divide the symptoms of schizophrenia into dichotomous categories was undertaken by Emil Kraepelin (1893). In the 1970s the terms 'negative' and 'positive' came into use (Jablensky 2000). These stem from Reynolds (1858), the underlying concepts from Jackson's (1887) hierarchical model, according to which deficit symptoms are classified as primary or lower level nervous dysfunctions and secondary symptoms as reflecting responses from a higher level of the central nervous system (for a detailed description of the history of positive and negative symptoms see Chapter 3). This dichotomous distinction of schizophrenic symptoms is clinically useful. It gives the complex psychopathology a simple order and is reflected in different course types, outcomes and therapy responses.

New interest in the positive and negative symptom dimensions was awakened by the speculative model of causality proposed by T. Crow (1980a,b; see also Chapter 3). Crow described a type I (positive) schizophrenia as characterized by hallucinations, delusions and formal thought disorder. He presumed that the underlying cause was a dopaminergic dysfunction and that for this reason type I as a pure type involved no deficits and responded well to antidopaminergic neuroleptic therapy. Type II (negative) schizophrenia was described by Crow as a clinical poverty syndrome (Wing & Brown 1970) involving social withdrawal, avolition, affective blunting and poverty of content and production of thought and speech. He interpreted it as caused by embryonal or perinatal brain lesions. The persistence of these symptoms and their poor therapy response seemed to point to a stable neurodevelopmental deficit.

According to Crow, type I and II were expressions of co-existing, but independent pathophysiological processes, but he did not specify how they were related to one another. Actually, neither cross-sectionally nor over the course of the disorder have these two types turned out to be mutually exclusive (Lindenmayer et al. 1984; Pogue-Geile & Harrow 1985; Biehl et al. 1986; Gross et al. 1986; Deister et al. 1990; Addington & Addington 1991; Häfner & Maurer 1991; Maurer & Häfner 1991; Peralta et al. 1992; Rey et al. 1994; Marneros et al. 1995; Eaton et al. 1995).

A further effort to classify the symptoms of schizophrenia by the positive–negative dichotomy was made by Andreasen and Olsen (1982) by means of factor analysis. They studied a heterogeneous clinical sample comprising first-admitted patients in psychotic episodes and patients with long histories of illness. As expected, replications of their results in homogeneous samples have failed both cross-sectionally and longitudinally over the course of the disorder (Maurer & Häfner 1991; Tandon & Greden 1991). Andreasen and Olsen (1982) posited one single symptom dimension. At the one extreme end of this dimension the authors identified patients with severe purely negative symptoms and at the other extreme patients with purely positive symptoms and they claimed that these extremes were negatively correlated with each other. The negative type was associated with poor premorbid adjustment, low level of social functioning, cognitive impairment and local brain anomalies, and the positive type with less impairment, absence of neuropsychological changes in the brain and a good outcome. In between, the authors believed, there was a mixed group presenting symptoms from both categories. When the results of a follow-up study of 10 first episodes of schizophrenia over 4 years became available, the model was finally abandoned (Andreasen 1990).

A transphenomenal approach to applying the positive–negative dichotomy is the severity–liability model (Gottesman et al. 1987). On a continuum of genetic liability, patients with negative symptoms occupy significantly more unfavourable rankings than patients with purely positive symptoms (Kendler et al. 1983, 1984, 1985; McGuffin et al. 1987; Tsuang et al. 1991; Lenzenweger & Dworkin 1996). Most studies trying to cluster schizophrenic symptoms or to analyse their dimensionality have produced more than two clusters or factors (Liddle &

Barnes 1990; Lenzenweger *et al.* 1991; Löffler & Häfner 1999; see below).

Negative symptoms are a frequent and fairly persistent characteristic of schizophrenia. Mostly emerging at the prodromal stage long before the first psychotic episode (Häfner *et al.* 1995, 1999b), they cannot be just a residuum of a psychotic episode. Carpenter *et al.* (1988) distinguish between primary and secondary negative symptoms. The primary or deficit syndromes, the authors believe, are a persisting environmentally determined characteristic which precedes psychosis onset and frequently persists between the episodes. These syndromes neither respond to traditional antipsychotic treatment nor do they vary with depressive symptoms, anxiety or dosage of medication. Carpenter *et al.* (1988) classify in this primary group anhedonia, flattening and narrowing of affect, poverty of speech, avolition and reduced social activity. For diagnosing the deficit syndrome they developed the Schedule for the Deficit Syndrome (SDS: Kirkpatrick *et al.* 1989). In patients with the deficit syndrome the authors found poor premorbid adjustment, an increased frequency of neurological soft signs and low depression scores (Buchanan *et al.* 1990; Kirkpatrick *et al.* 1996a,b; see also Chapter 3). Jablensky (2000) contends that these authors have failed to validate the existence of the core deficit syndrome. In his opinion it is more plausible to presume a continuum of negative symptomatology with two extremes: a severe deficit syndrome at the one end and a mild negative syndrome, encountered in borderline cases and in character variants, at the other end.

Primary negative symptoms by definition are traits, stable over time and largely independent of environmental factors (Carpenter *et al.* 1988). In contrast, the course and amount of secondary negative symptoms, such as psychomotor poverty/slowness, anergia, social withdrawal and lack of perseverence, are presumed to fluctuate with psychotic episodes, depression, side-effects of medication, substance abuse and physical morbidity (Whiteford & Peabody 1989; Carpenter *et al.* 1991). An attempt to prove the validity of this model in an epidemiological sample of first episodes of schizophrenia over 3 years failed (Maurer & Häfner 1991). All the five SANS sections (Andreasen 1983) – affective flattening, alogia/paralogia, abulia/apathy, anhedonia/asociality and attentional impairment – showed high proportions of both fluctuating and persistent courses (Fig. 8.4). Nevertheless, the picture that emerged from the mean score for each measure of the SANS and the six cross-sectional assessments was one of limited stability. Anhedonia turned out to be the most stable syndrome, showing a persistent course across the six cross-sections in 30%. The course of the secondary or 'non-deficit syndrome' could not be shown to depend on extrinsic factors, as originally expected. In contrast, the subgroup of 'primary' negative symptoms showed significant correlations with these factors (Häfner & Maurer 1997). The authors interpreted this result according to Jablensky's (2000) model: patients with a deficit syndrome are more severely ill than patients presenting 'milder' non-deficit negative symptoms. For this reason they are also more sensitive to adversity.

Course of negative symptoms and cognitive impairment

In the last few years a growing body of evidence has emerged indicating that negative symptoms might have a pathophysiological basis distinct from that of positive symptoms. In this context especially their association with cognitive impairment and brain dysfunctions has been explored (Addington & Addington 1991; Arndt *et al.* 1995; Maziade *et al.* 1996; Tamminga *et al.* 1998).

It can be regarded as an established fact that schizophrenia is frequently associated with neurocognitive dysfunctions. In persons with schizophrenia, compared with healthy controls, typically impairment in attention, working and episodic memory and executive functions occur (Saykin *et al.* 1994; Goldberg *et al.* 1998; Gold *et al.* 1999; Weickert *et al.* 2000). A small proportion of patients, however, independently of their illness stage, exhibit a broad range of severe impairment – of vigilance, neuromotor skills, abstract and conceptual thinking, etc. – in the sense of overall cognitive impairment (see Chapter 10). The amount of cognitive and functional impairment shows a high degree of interindividual variance, ranging from absence of any impairment to presence of severe cognitive deficits.

Patients with schizophrenia usually show 0.5–2 SD below the values for the general population (Lubin *et al.* 1962; Schwartzman & Douglas 1962; Hoff *et al.* 1999). While in most studies an association between positive symptoms and cognitive functioning has failed to emerge (Goldberg *et al.* 1993; Weickert & Goldberg 2000), weak to medium-sized positive correlations have been found between negative symptoms and cognitive deficits. However, these associations explain less than half of the variance in cognitive functioning (Bilder *et al.* 1985, 1995; Shtasel *et al.* 1992; Goldberg & Gold 1995; Paulsen *et al.* 1995; Censitis *et al.* 1997; Norman *et al.* 1997; Sobizack *et al.* 1999; Weickert & Goldberg 2000).

Saykin *et al.* (1994) demonstrated that the profiles of cognitive impairment in 37 new untreated cases of schizophrenia hardly differed from those of a group of unmedicated formerly treated patients with long histories of illness. A similar result has been reported by Albus *et al.* (1996). Sobizack *et al.* (1999) compared 66 first-episode patients and 49 chronic cases of schizophrenia with 40 healthy controls with regard to memory functions, speech and cognitive flexibility/abstraction by administering a comprehensive neuropsychological test battery. They too found no differences in cognitive performance between the first-episode and the previously treated group, but both patient groups differed highly significantly from healthy controls. According to an overview given by Rund (1998) of 15 studies with follow-up periods of at least 1 year, deficits in verbal skills (word meaning, word association, verbal fluency), memory (long- and short-term, spatial and visual) and attentional span are fairly stable over time. Characteristic profiles of cognitive impairment at early stages of schizophrenia indicate fairly reliably – as long as we lack the means of treating them effectively – that cognitive and functional deficits are going to persist

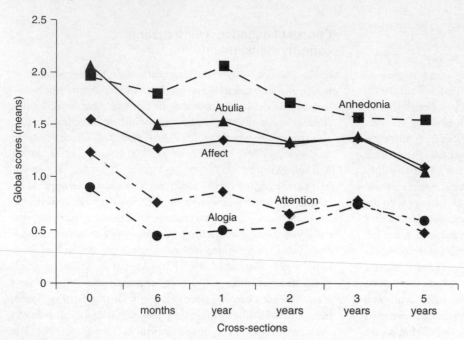

Fig 8.4 Course of negative symptoms – 5 SANS measures – over 5 years after first admission in a representative sample of 115 first illness episodes of schizophrenia. (From Häfner & Maurer 1997.)

in the course of the disorder even in patients receiving antipsychotic therapy (Goldberg *et al.* 1993). Hence, a stable pattern of course of the typical neuropsychological deficits is to be found in most patients and persists until old age. After the first psychotic episode a small group of patients shows, instead of essential improvement, gradual progression in these deficits. Harvey *et al.* (1998, 1999) recently reported that a certain proportion of patients with long illness courses experience mostly slow but serious decline in cognitive and functional abilities in old age, i.e. beyond age 65 years. This form of 'schizophrenia dementia' seems to be free of the pathology encountered in Alzheimer's disease (Harvey *et al.* 1999). The causes of these late neurodegenerative processes are still obscure. In view of the high degree of variance in the age of onset of old-age dementia and the fact that severe forms of schizophrenia frequently persisting almost over lifetime may involve risk factors for dementia – life style, such as lack of mental and physical exercise, long-term institutional care, etc. – a schizophrenia-related late neurodegenerative process cannot yet be regarded as sufficiently established. Further follow-up studies of representative cohorts are needed up until old age as well as studies into the neuropathology of these progressive course types. What Davidson and McGlashan (1997) conclude in their summary of the results from research into the topic continues to hold good, at least for the time being, for the majority of patients with schizophrenia: 'Cognitive deficits, which are associated with negative symptoms . . . constitute a relatively stable dimension over time, showing neither marked deterioration nor improvement, once established early in the course of disorder'.

The stability of the cognitive and neuropsychological impairments over time indicates something about their nature. Unlike abnormalities with a transient occurrence in illness

episodes, deficits consistently diverging from normal levels of functioning can be interpreted as indicating structural changes – in consistency with the assumption of a 'static' encephalopathy – and probably also as stable vulnerability factors (Nuechterlein & Dawson 1984; Rund *et al.* 1997). They correspond to the neurodevelopmental model of schizophrenia (Murray 1994).

Course of cognitive impairment and brain anomalies

Except at the early stages of illness, negative symptoms and neuropsychological deficits do not generally seem to progress. Does this also hold good for the morphological brain anomalies involved? Like cognitive deficits, they are already measurable in the first illness episode (Weinberger 1995). In the majority of studies, their amount shows no correlation with the duration of illness (Lewis 1990; Nair *et al.* 1997; Lawrie & Abukmeil 1998; Johnstone 1999).

There are exceptions, however. In a prospective 5-year follow-up study of 50 first-admission patients with a DSM-IIIR diagnosis of schizophrenia, DeLisi *et al.* (1998), comparing these patients with 20 age-, sex- and IQ-matched controls by means of magnetic resonance imaging (MRI) and automated image analysis, found a fourfold reduction in volume and grey matter in the period studied, but no regional or white matter reduction in subjects with schizophrenia. The widespread cognitive deficits, already present at first admission, remained stable in the course of the disorder and showed no correlation with changes in ventricle size or in grey matter. Verbal memory deficit was the only item showing an increase parallel to brain atrophy. The progression in these brain changes was limited to male patients who showed pronounced neurocognitive changes and did not remit in the 5 years studied. Woods (1998) reported slight increases in morphological brain changes subsequent to the first illness episode in comparison with healthy controls.

From these results it can be concluded that in the majority of cases the destructive phase of schizophrenia, marked by the accumulation of negative symptoms and the decline in cognitive functioning, is mainly confined to the prodromal stage and the first psychotic episode (Häfner *et al.* 1999c). Only in a small proportion of patients with unfavourable illness courses does 'a subtle active brain process seem to be continuing through the first few years of . . . illness causing greater than the normal adult cortical deterioration' (DeLisi *et al.* 1997). But even these progressive brain processes appear not to lead to severe cognitive changes, at least over a period of 5 years under modern conditions of treatment and care. At 0.5–2 SD below the values for control subjects, they seem to remain stable in most patients over the medium-term course studied (Albus *et al.* 1996; DeLisi *et al.* 1997; Hoff *et al.* 1999; Sobizack *et al.* 1999). Over more extended illness courses, however, given the progression in grey matter atrophy, a causal relationship with increasing neuropsychological deficits seems conceivable in a small subgroup of patients. To confirm or refute this assumption, multilevel studies of the type described above over long courses of illness or studies of subsamples at enhanced risk are necessary.

Course of empirical symptom dimensions and clusters (see also Dimensional models in Chapter 3)

Following the early attempts to reduce the diversity of schizophrenic symptoms to a few latent variables by means of explorative analysis of covariance (Lorr *et al.* 1963; WHO 1973) and the analysis of covariance of symptom ratings and neuropsychological variables conducted by Bilder *et al.* (1985), the factor-analytical studies by Liddle (1987a,b) and Liddle and Barnes (1990) have attracted widespread attention. In their three-factor model, which the authors extracted from data on two patient samples with chronic schizophrenia, negative symptoms (affective non-response, apathy, anhedonia) loaded on a single factor (psychomotor poverty). Delusions, hallucinations and psychotic thought disorders loaded on a more restricted psychotic factor (reality distortion). A third factor including speech and thought disorders (inappropriate affect, positive formal thought disorder, bizarre behaviour) the authors called a disorganization syndrome. The negative factor correlated with impairment of conceptual thinking, object naming and long-term memory, and the disorganization factor with impaired concentration, short-term memory and word learning. These two factors were correlated with impaired work and social performance as well as with dysfunctions supposed to be located in two different regions of the frontal lobe (Liddle 1994). The third factor 'reality distortion', was associated with fewer deficits. Bilder *et al.* (1985), also analysing a sample of chronic patients (with 'defect states'), obtained three quite similar clusters of symptoms and neuropsychological deficits (see Chapter 3).

The three-factor model proposed by Liddle has been replicated in several samples on the basis of SANS, the Scale for the Assessment of Positive Symptoms (SAPS: Andreasen 1984) and the Positive and Negative Syndrome Scale (PANSS: Kay *et al.* 1987) data and in some studies in which a depression or a social-dysfunctioning factor has been added, expanded into a four-factor model (Peralta *et al.* 1994; Toomey *et al.* 1997). In most studies the three original factors and – as far as corresponding data have been available – social dysfunctioning (reduced social relationships, instability of work and school performance) as a fourth factor have explained a considerable part of the variance (Kay & Sevy 1990; Keefe *et al.* 1992; Maurer *et al.* 1993; Minas *et al.* 1994; for a review see Peralta *et al.* 1992).

The number of factors required for explaining an optimum degree of the variance depends on the type and number of symptoms fed into the model, on the patient sample studied and the assessment technique adopted (Jablensky 2000). Samples of chronic patients, for example, deliver fewer positive and depressive symptoms than patients in psychotic episodes (Häfner *et al.* 1999c). Instruments providing data on most of the affective symptoms produce a depression factor particularly in first-admission samples (Kay & Sevy 1990; Arora *et al.* 1997; Salokanges 1997; White *et al.* 1997) or an overall neuroticism factor (Rey *et al.* 1994). Davidson and McGlashan (1997), reviewing studies into the domains of functioning, also identified a fourth fairly independent depression dimension. When premorbid data were included (Lenzenweger & Dworkin 1996) 'premorbid social impairment' emerged as a further factor.

The stability of the empirical clusters or symptom dimensions in the course of schizophrenia has not been much studied yet. Arndt *et al.* (1995) showed the validity of the three-factor model over 2 years and Salokangas (1997) over 5 years, both in samples of first-episode patients. The three factors varied independently of each other. In both studies the negative and the delusion factor remained stable until follow-up.

Löffler and Häfner (1999), analysing data collected retrospectively from first admission back to psychosis onset (IRAOS; Häfner *et al.* 1992, 1999a) in 232 first illness episodes of schizophrenia (the population-based ABC sample) and prospectively at six cross-sections over 5 years (PSE: Wing *et al.* 1974; SANS: Andreasen 1983) in a subsample of 115 first-episode cases, compared four models: the severity – liability model (Gottesman *et al.* 1987), Andreasen and Olsen's (1982) bipolar symptom model, Crow's (1980a,b) two-factor model and Liddle and Barnes' (1990) three-factor model – by means of confirmatory factor analysis. Only Liddle and Barnes' three-factor model produced results that were in satisfactory agreement with the data. As expected, all symptoms showed significant positive loadings on the three factors, but the associations with demographic and clinical variables had not much power in discriminating between the three dimensions. The only exceptions were disorganization, associated with a higher degree of familial loading, and the negative factor, which showed significant correlations with pre- and perinatal complications, although the coefficients were low throughout the measurements.

Figure 8.5 illustrates the stability of and the transitions occur-

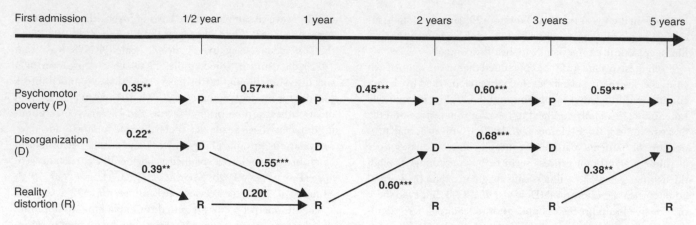

Fig 8.5 Correlations within and between syndrome ratings at 6 points in time over 5 years. The factors were tested by explorative orthogonal factor analysis at each of the five follow-ups – ABC subsample of 115 first illness episodes. Pearson correlations: t $P < 0.1$; * $P < 0.05$; ** $P < 0.01$; *** $P < 0.001$. (From Löffler & Häfner 1999.)

ring between the three factors tested by explorative orthogonal factor analysis at each of the five follow-up assessments. As expected, the factor 'negative symptoms' remained stable and independent of the other factors over the total 5-year period showing highly significant coefficients. The factors 'disorganization' and 'positive symptoms' showed low correlations at the follow-ups. Four of the 10 possible correlations attained significance. Contrary to the two other factors, which showed no prognostic power with respect to social outcome, the presence of negative symptoms at the second follow-up, 6 months after first admission, was a highly significant predictor of the patients' social status up until 3-year follow-up.

The dimensions 'positive symptoms' and 'disorganization' seem not to be separable as two independent and stable factors in the medium-term course. Negative symptoms, stable over time and associated with overall functional impairment and the consequences of the disorder, constitute the only factor that might reflect an independent brain dysfunction persisting at stable values after the first illness episode.

Studying the same sample and the same period of illness, but applying a different methodological approach, Häfner and Maurer (1991) obtained slightly different results: the sum scores for positive and negative symptoms, classified according to the clinical tradition (PSE) and measured on a yearly basis before first admission and in the year preceding first admission on a monthly basis, showed significant positive correlations attaining medium-sized to small coefficients. Similar results have also been reported by Cechnicki and Walczewski (1999) from a controlled prospective investigation with follow-ups at 1, 3 and 7 years and by Biehl *et al.* (1986), who studied a sample of first-admission patients with schizophrenia (PSE-8: 295) prospectively at seven cross-sections over 5 years. Lenzenweger *et al.* (1991) and Löffler and Häfner (1999) have suggested how these seemingly discrepant results might be explained: the two modes of operationalizing positive and negative symptoms differ not only in the underlying methodological procedures. The two-dimensional models differ in how the symptoms pertaining to

the disorganization factor in Liddle's and the other three factor models are classified in the positive and the negative symptom clusters or with the corresponding dimensions. Inadequate affect and bizarre behaviour are usually classified in the positive, positive formal thought disorders in the negative cluster.

Lenzenweger *et al.* (1991) were able to demonstrate that the significant correlations shown by the positive and negative dimensions in Crow's two-factor model are accounted for by this fact. Hence, Fenton and McGlashan (1991b) conclude that the correlations sometimes found between positive and negative symptoms can be explained by their covariation with disorganization symptoms. These findings once more underscore that both the clinical symptom clusters and the latent symptom dimensions are merely heuristic representations of specific patterns of dysfunctioning and impairment and their underlying brain dysfunctions. In contrast, positive symptoms and the disorganization syndrome have been found to show hardly any association with cognitive deficits in the course of the disorder.

Early course of schizophrenia (prodromal stage and first psychotic episode)

In current clinical practice, the first treatment contact is preceded by increasing psychotic symptomatology of a mean duration of about 1 year or more and a prodromal stage of several years. The duration of pretreatment illness is determined by the onset of the disorder, patients' help-seeking behaviour and the availability of care. Prodromal symptoms and behaviours may include mood symptoms (e.g. depression, anxiety, dysphoria and irritability), cognitive symptoms (e.g. distractibility and difficulty concentrating), social withdrawal, obsessive behaviours and attenuated positive symptoms (e.g. illusions, ideas of reference and magical thinking) to name but a few (Yung & McGorry 1996; Davidson & McGlashan 1997; Maurer & Häfner 1997). The duration of untreated psychosis (DUP) or duration of untreated illness (DUI) is seen, although not consistently, as a predictor of an unfavourable illness course (see Table 8.1; Crow *et al.* 1986; Loebel *et al.* 1992; McGorry *et al.* 1996; Wyatt & Henter 1998). The proponents of this hypothesis presume that untreated psychosis may constitute 'an active morbid process' 'toxic' to the brain. If this disease process is not treated with antipsychotics, it might become chronic (Loebel *et al.* 1992; Craig *et al.* 1999; Ho *et al.* 2000).

McGlashan and Johannessen (1996) presume that the plasticity of the brain can be preserved and the condition prevented from deteriorating if the persons affected receive both medication and simultaneous social stimulation at a 'sensitive' stage of the illness. As neuroleptic medications affect only symptom expression and not the underlying biological predisposition, their effects will be limited to the period of their administration. Hence, a positive correlation between a reduced DUP and medium- to long-term outcome might depend on maintenance medication after the end of the period of untreated psychosis (Linszen *et al.* 1998).

In one of the earliest studies Loebel *et al.* (1992), examining 70 patients with a Research Diagnostic Criteria (RDC) diagnosis of schizophrenia or schizoaffective disorder, demonstrated a negative correlation between DUP, time until remission and quality of remission. Bottlender *et al.* (2000) studied, in a sample of 998 first admissions for schizophrenia, how DUP influences various outcome parameters, positive and negative symptoms at discharge from index admission, global level of functioning and length of inpatient treatment. The expected association was observable with all these outcome measures: the longer the DUP, the more pronounced the amount of persisting symptoms and the longer the inpatient treatment.

The expected association was also demonstrated in a study conducted by Haas *et al.* (1998). In 103 patients – of whom 77 had a DSM-IIIR diagnosis of schizophrenia – a significant association was found between DUP (<1 year vs. ≥1 year) and poverty syndrome or reality distortion at discharge from index treatment. Linszen *et al.*'s (1998) study of 63 patients, who had received a combination of inpatient and outpatient treatment, showed that a delay in treatment by more than a year was associated with a poor prognosis (delayed remission of symptoms). Szymanski *et al.* (1996), studying 36 first-episode patients, most of whom had a DSM-IIIR diagnosis of schizophrenia or schizophreniform disorder, demonstrated that an increased DUP was associated with less reduced positive symptoms after 6 months of treatment. McEvoy *et al.* (1991) found in 106 patients – of whom only 32 had not been previously treated with neuroleptics – significant correlations between time to therapy response and length of active illness before hospitalizatton.

The results on the association between DUP and medium-term outcome are less clear-cut. McGorry *et al.* (1996), in their investigation of 200 patients (of whom more than half were patients with schizophrenia or schizophreniform disorder), demonstrated a positive association between DUP on the one hand and positive and negative symptoms, global functioning and quality of life on the other hand 12 months after index assessment. In contrast, three studies found no such association: Craig *et al.* (2000) could not demonstrate any association between illness course and clinical outcome 24 months after first assessment, nor could Ho *et al.* (2000) and Robinson *et al.* (1999a,b). Overall, the studies tend to show that patients with short DUPs respond better to treatment in the first schizophrenic episode, but evidence for a lasting effect on the medium- or long-term illness course has so far refused to emerge.

The findings of significant associations between DUP and short-term effects of therapy are also liable to alternative explanations, because they might have been influenced by third factors. An indication that such influences could be at work is provided by the correlation reported between DUP and negative symptoms (Waddington *et al.* 1995; Scully *et al.* 1997; Binder *et al.* 1998; Haas *et al.* 1998; Larsen *et al.* 1998; Bottlender *et al.* 2000; de Haan *et al.* 2000). An insidious illness onset and an early occurrence of negative symptoms are – regardless of treatment – predictors of a poor course (Ciompi & Müller 1976; Müller *et al.* 1986; Sartorius *et al.* 1986) and an acute onset is a predictor of a favourable illness course, as shown by numerous studies conducted before neuroleptic medications became available (Sartorius *et al.* 1977). Whether it is the duration of the active disease process before the beginning of an efficacious treatment or an unfavourable form of the disorder indicated by an insidious onset that actually determines the poor illness course (Crow *et al.* 1986), could only be shown in controlled intervention trials in early illness. However, such studies are not yet possible for lack of means of sufficiently early case identification. Norman and Malla (2001) thus conclude that it is not yet possible to pass final judgement on the causal relationship between belated treatment onset as a determinant of DUP or DUI and outcome. Hope exists that early detection and early intervention will enable us to reduce at least the pronounced social consequences of the disorder, mostly emerging at this early stage of illness (Häfner *et al.* 1996, 1999b; McGorry *et al.* 1996; McGlashan 1998).

The pretreatment illness course of several years' duration has implications for the interpretation of results from studies that have used first admission as the definition of illness onset. This is the case, for example, with the reports of a significant excess of first admissions for schizophrenia from the lowest social class and their interpretation along the lines of the social causation hypothesis (Faris & Dunham 1939; Kohn 1969; Eaton 1999).

To study the onset of schizophrenia, the transformation from health or from premorbid signs into the prodromal stage in prospective population studies is not practical because of the low incidence rate, the rather poor predictive power of developmental antecedents (Malmberg *et al.* 1998; Jones 1999) and the fact that in about 75% of cases schizophrenia onset occurs with non-specific signs or negative symptoms (Häfner *et al.* 1993). There are two studies that have attempted to investigate this question and with considerable success.

A Swedish conscript study (Malmberg *et al.* 1998) among 50 087 young men aged 18–20 years showed that deficits in socializing are a crucial indicator: the four items 'having fewer than two friends', 'preference for socializing in small groups', 'feeling more sensitive than others' and 'not having a steady girlfriend' were associated with a high relative risk (odds ratio 30.7)* for developing schizophrenia in a period of risk of 13 years. In the total sample, a positive response to all four items predicted psychosis only in 3%, because of the high prevalence of these features in the general population. Davidson et al. (1999) and Rabinowitz et al. (2000) conducted a similar study of 16- to 17-year-old Israeli male conscripts born during a 7-year period in Israel. Using the National Hospitalization Psychiatric Case Register, the authors identifed 692 individuals who had been hospitalized for schizophrenia for the first time in a 9-year period following the initial testing. The results on these persons, who were compared with the entire conscript population and matched controls, pointed in the same direction as the results of the Swedish study. With effect sizes[†] ranging from 0.40 to 0.58, the young males later diagnosed with schizophrenia faired significantly worse in cognitive and behavioural functioning. As in the Swedish study, it was poor social functioning with an effect size difference of 1.25 that turned out to be the main indicator of risk.

First attempts at systematically assessing prodromal signs were made in the context of a targeted antipsychotic therapy of relapses of schizophrenia (Carpenter & Heinrichs 1983; Birchwood et al. 1989; Cutting & Done 1989: Hirsch & Jolley 1989; Gaebel et al. 1993). However, the results were inconsistent, mainly as a result of: (i) differences in the type of prodromal signs included and in the definitions of a psychotic relapse; and (ii) insufficient monitoring of their development over time. Nevertheless, various items from the early scales for psychotic relapses have been incorporated into subsequent instruments for the assessment of onset and early course (Häfner et al. 1992; Maurer & Häfner 1995; Yung et al. 1998; Miller et al. 1999).

The difficulty in generating biological indicators of the onset and early stages of the disorder lies in the fact that current knowledge of the neurobiological disease process is still limited. Most of the biological findings associated with the risk of psychosis are trait factors that appear to be indicators of lifetime risk that may not be causally involved in onset (Cornblatt & Keilp 1994; Cornblatt et al. 1998; Isohanni et al. 1999).

For these reasons psychosis onset is currently depictable only at the level of self-experienced symptoms and observable behaviour. None the less, the monitoring of the neuropsychological and neurophysiological indicators of the disorder from the earliest possible timepoint on is a highly promising approach to modelling the early course of schizophrenia (McGorry et al. 1996; Klosterkötter et al. 1997; Bilder 1998; Cornblatt et al. 1998; Salokangas et al. 1999).

The most frequent initial symptoms mainly belong to two dimensions: a depressive and a negative syndrome. Among these, indicators of cognitive impairment, such as trouble with thinking and concentration and loss of energy, point to early consequences of the disorder (Häfner et al. 1999b,c).

Arranging the earliest symptoms in a time matrix, Häfner et al. (1999c) found, on the basis of IRAOS data collected in the ABC cohort of 232 first episodes of schizophrenia (Häfner et al. 1992), that depressed mood, suicide attempt, loss of self-confidence and feelings of guilt tended to occur 3–5 years before first admission with odds ratios ranging from 3 to 5 compared with controls. In the second time window, 2–4 years before first admission, all the negative symptoms appeared, and it was only in the last year before first admission that positive symptoms emerged. After the first psychotic symptom had appeared, all three symptom categories accumulated rapidly. The climax of the first episode was followed by an almost parallel decrease on all symptom dimensions.

The data were derived from a German population-based sample of 232 first illness episodes of broadly defined schizophrenia (84% of first admissions; Häfner et al. 1993). The prodromal stage, from onset to first psychotic symptom, had a mean duration of 5 years (median: 2.33 years), and the psychotic prestage, from the first positive symptom to the maximum of positive symptoms, of 1.1 years (median: 0.8 years). First admission took place some 2 months later, mostly precipitated by the full-blown psychosis. All the milestones of the early illness course show a significant age difference, widely reported and crucial for the further course of illness, of 3–4 years between the sexes (Hambrecht et al. 1992; Häfner et al. 1995).

The distribution of the durations of early illness course is markedly skewed to the left: 33% of the broadly defined schizophrenias took less than 1 year to develop. Only 18% had an acute type of onset of 4 weeks or less and 68% a chronic type of onset of 1 year or more. Only 6.5% started with positive symptoms, 20.5% presented both positive and negative symptoms within the same month, and 73% had negative or non-specific symptoms, thus experiencing a prodromal stage.

Stages in the development of schizophrenia

Conrad (1958), studying 107 young German soldiers, distinguished four stages of developing schizophrenia.
1 *Trema*, characterized by depression, anxiety, tension, irritability and mysterious experiences.
2 The transition from trema to *apopheny*, which corresponds to the transition from the non-specific prodromal phase to incipient psychosis, is characterized by phenomena occurring without a visible cause.
3 In the third phase, which he called *anastrophae*, these new

---

* The odds ratio (OR) is a measure of the relative risk, i.e. the risk of having a certain characteristic in the index group divided by the risk of having this characteristic in the reference group. If a is the number of people falling ill with schizophrenia in the index group scoring high on the four items defining socializing; and b is the number of people not falling ill with schizophrenia in this group; and if c is the number of people falling ill with schizophrenia in the reference group scoring low on the four items; and d is the number of people not falling ill with schizophrenia in this group, then OR = a : b / c : d.

[†] The effect size (ES) is a measure of the magnitude of an effect; it can be measured as the standardized difference between the means of the index group and the reference group.

experiences are attributed to external causes: delusions and hallucinations. Reality control and insight into illness will be lost.

4 With full-blown psychosis, the stage of *apocalypse* has begun, which refers to the complete loss of structure in perception, experience and thought.

After this psychotic stage the episode may remit in mental consolidation, with patients showing various degrees of functional impairment and residual symptoms. A rare outcome is a further increase in the severity of the psychosis and a transition of the apocalyptic into an often final stage called *catastrophae*, e.g. febrile catatonia, but modern treatment is capable of preventing this stage and its lethal course.

Following Conrad, Docherty *et al.* (1978) proposed four stages of progressive decompensation, which they believed to explain how both first episodes and relapses evolve:

1 overextension;
2 restricted consciousness;
3 disinhibition; and
4 psychotic disorganization.

Hambrecht and Häfner (1993) tested Conrad's phase model on IRAOS data from the ABC Schizophrenia Study. In 73% of the cases trema preceded apopheny, i.e. a prodromal stage and incipient psychosis. Significant transitions from apopheny to the other phases could not be shown to occur.

Both Conrad and Docherty *et al.* proceeded from the assumption that all cases of incipient schizophrenia run through these presumed regular sequences of stages, but this has not been shown to be the case. Nevertheless, quite a number of studies are being conducted with the aim of improving our means of early recognition and prediction of psychosis onset as a basis for early intervention.

Selections of patients with mental disorder in need of treatment and suspected to suffer from schizophrenia (Klosterkötter *et al.* 2001) improve the chances for correct predictions, but reduce the generalizability of the results and their applicability in population-based risk assessments. Applying the concept of self-perceived 'basic disturbances' (Huber 1983) and assessing a sample of 160 such persons using the Bonn Scale for the Assessment of Basic Symptoms (BSABS: Gross *et al.* 1987) – almost 50% of the probands developed a full-blown psychosis during the follow-up period with a mean length of 9.6 years – Klosterkötter *et al.* (2001) demonstrated a high sensitivity (=0.98) but a rather low specificity (=0.59), especially with self-experienced cognitive changes and attenuated positive symptoms.

Enriching the psychosis risk in this way may be sensible in individual intervention studies, provided that precise and reproducible information is given on the high-risk persons studied. However, the 'state approach' (Yung *et al.* 1998) used in many past studies reflects another crucial issue: if the aim is to predict an imminent psychosis onset, as an indication for early intervention, and not only the lifetime risk, a distinction must be drawn between persistent trait markers and truly prodromal signs. This might be possible by mapping symptom accumulation and func-

tional decline (Maurer & Häfner 1995; Cornblatt *et al.* 1998; Yung *et al.* 1998). Applying a series of indicators of an imminent psychosis onset, including a rapid decline in global functioning (a 15-point decrease in the GAF score in 6 weeks), Yung *et al.* (1998) were able to predict psychosis onset in young high-risk individuals (aged 18–30 years) over a period of 1 year in 40% of their cohort.

Early and later course of depressive symptoms

One of the main symptoms of schizophrenia, besides positive, negative and disorganization, is the depressive syndrome. Its frequency naturally depends on the inclusion of the schizoaffective–depressive syndrome. Knights and Hirsch (1981) studied depressive symptoms in the first psychotic episode in a population-based sample with schizophrenia-like disorder. Of all these first admissions, almost all patients had been discharged at 3-month follow-up. On admission depressive and affective symptoms had been as prevalent as psychotic symptoms, whereas at follow-up only depressive and affective symptoms persisted with little reduction, while psychotic symptoms had clearly remitted. The authors concluded that depression is revealed in schizophrenia because, although evident on admission, the symptoms were masked by psychotic symptoms which responded more than the neurotic symptoms. Of the IPSS (WHO 1973) cohort with an ICD-8 diagnosis of schizophrenia (295) who had experienced psychotic symptoms or relapses, 17% experienced clear-cut depressive episodes in a period of 2 years and 15% in a period of 5 years (Sheldrick *et al.* 1977; Leff *et al.* 1992). In a Munich study (Dobmeier *et al.* 2000) conducted among 76 patients with an ICD-10 diagnosis of schizophrenia, assessed at first admission, discharge and 15-year follow-up, depressive symptoms measured by the Calgary Depression Scale (Addington *et al.* 1992) were most frequent in acute psychotic episodes. With remitting psychosis the depression scores fell from about 70% to below 20% and more or less remained at that level without any substantial change in the symptom profile at 15-year follow-up.

In the population-controlled ABC study (Häfner *et al.* 1999c) the maximum of patients with depressive mood, also over 70%, was found in the first psychotic episode, which was in agreement with the findings of Knights and Hirsch (1981) and Dobmeier *et al.* (2000). In the following 5 years a fairly stable proportion of about 20% of the patients were in depressive episodes (according to ICD-10). From their comparable first-episode studies, Biehl *et al.* (1986) and Koreen *et al.* (1993) reported that about 75% of patients presented depressive symptoms in the first psychotic episode and showed a clear tendency to their remission (Hamilton and/or syndrome criteria). At 5-year follow-up, 26% of the patients with psychotic symptoms were rated as concurrently depressed; of the ~8% of patients without psychotic symptoms only 4% (Koreen *et al.* 1993).

Depressive symptoms frequently appear long before the first positive symptoms (McGorry *et al.* 1996; Davidson & McGlashan 1997; Häfner *et al.* 1999b,c). They are the most frequent initial symptoms in schizophrenia, appearing, on average, 5 years before the climax of the first episode. In the ABC cohort, the lifetime prevalence for depressive mood of 2 or more weeks' duration until first admission was 70.2% vs. 19.3% for age- and sex-matched controls from the general population, for feelings of guilt 33.3% vs. 10.5% for controls and for a poor self-confidence 59.4% vs. 12.3% for controls (the symptoms had to persist for at least 2 weeks). The odds ratios for these single symptoms, presumed not to overlap negative symptoms, ranged from 2 to 5. The frequency of attempted suicide at this early illness stage showed an excess of some 40% (Häfner *et al.* 1999b,c; see above).

From these patterns of symptom presentation over time Häfner *et al.* (1999b,c) conclude that the depressive syndrome is, for the most part, a pattern of response of the brain to fairly mild degrees of dysfunction. It seems to be produced by the same neurobiological processes that at a later stage bring forth the characteristic schizophrenic symptoms.

Fenton and McGlashan (1992), looking at a longer period of illness, also found affective and negative symptoms that they did not classify as belonging to the core symptoms of the two main dimensions; e.g. feelings of insufficiency, hopelessness, social withdrawal and rigidity of affect. It is not clear whether these symptoms can be interpreted as expressions of the disorder or as reactions to it. In the course of schizophrenia, reactive depressive symptoms can indeed occur, especially in patients with full insight into their illness (Selten *et al.* 2000) and with unfavourable life situations. Subdepressive symptoms can also result from stressful experiences of acute or chronic life events in the medium-term course of schizophrenia, while no change occurs in the core symptoms of paranoid schizophrenia (Danielyan & Danielyan 1999).

The constructs of a postpsychotic depression (McGlashan & Carpenter 1976), pharmacogenic depression (Helmchen & Hippius 1967) or postremissive depression (Heinrich 1967) have only secondary roles in explaining the occurrence of depressive symptoms in the course of schizophrenia. This was made clear by an early study conducted by Knights and Hirsch (1981) into the course of depressive symptoms before and after the treatment of psychotic episodes. Two plausible explanations have been proposed by Koreen *et al.* (1993): 'Depressive symptoms in schizophrenia may represent a core part of the acute illness or may occur as a subjective reaction to the experience of psychotic decompensation'.

The prognostic value of depression occurring at the initial illness stage is limited to a few clinical variables. Initial depression predicts a greater severity of symptoms in the first episode (CATEGO total score and depression score) (Häfner *et al.* 1999c), but has no effect on depression or on positive symptoms in the further course – which, in the main, tend to show plateaus. In contrast, early-course depression is a significant predictor of reduced negative symptoms, affective flattening in particular, in the medium-term course (Häfner *et al.* 1999c). This is also reflected in the more favourable course of schizoaffective disorder of the depressive type (Johnson 1988).

Depressive symptoms also seem to have an important role as a prodromal stage of relapses. In studies looking at signs that might predict exacerbations during the course of the illness, between 30% and 75% of the patients as well as family informants experienced depressive or dysphoric symptoms as part of the process of schizophrenic decompensation (Herz & Melville 1980; Heinrichs *et al.* 1985; Birchwood *et al.* 1989; Hirsch & Jolley 1989; Kumar *et al.* 1989; Tarrier *et al.* 1991).

Less frequent in schizophrenia than depressive symptoms are manic and hypomanic symptoms. Studies on the course of schizophrenia are consistent in reporting frequencies ranging from 3% to 10% of cases, depending on the definition of these symptoms. They are in part associated with bipolar symptoms (mostly bipolar II) and are primarily episodic or remittent in type. Like bipolar mania, they are associated with the risk of severe social consequences because of ideas of grandeur, disinhibition and reduced impulse control (Marneros *et al.* 1986), but as regards a chronic course with negative symptoms and social impairment, they seem to have a better prognosis than 'pure' schizophrenia.

The catatonic syndrome, one of Kraepelin's subtypes, which was rather frequent before the advent of neuroleptics and still is in some developing countries, has become rare in western Europe and the USA (Häfner & Kasper 1982; Jablensky *et al.* 1993). For this reason, studies looking into this syndrome are rare (Mahendra 1981). Only recently have catatonic features started to attract renewed interest both as aetiologically unspecific symptoms and, first and foremost, as subtypes of Leonhard's nosology (Pfuhlmann & Stöber 2001) comprising motility psychosis, periodic catatonia and systematic catatonia (Stöber & Ungvari 2001). These diagnoses have been found to be both reliable and stable over a 5-year course of illness at one university hospital (Würzburg/Germany) (Franzek & Beckmann 1992). Stöber *et al.* (2000) have even described a susceptibility locus on chromosome 15q15 for periodic catatonia but this finding requires replication.

The only systematic long-term study looking into the stability of the catatonic syndrome within the spectrum of schizophrenic disorders and into the clinical variables involved has been conducted in Croatia. Mimica (1996) and Mimica *et al.* (2001) studied a representative case-register sample of 402 patients with a diagnosis of schizophrenia over a period of 18 years. Of these patients 14.7% received a clinical diagnosis of schizophrenia of the catatonic type (ICD-9: 295.2) at least once in this period. This diagnosis, associated with a significantly lower age at onset and a higher familial loading than the other subtypes of schizophrenia, turned out to be extremely unstable with frequent transitions into other diagnoses. Aggressive behaviour and, hence, hospital admissions were overrepresented in young patients with the catatonic subtype.

Given the scarcity of systematic long-term studies, it is impossible to give a conclusive appraisal of the validity of one or several catatonic subtypes of schizophrenia. The low stability of the syndrome demonstrated in the only large-scale epidemiological long-term study suggests that catatonic symptoms are best interpreted as nosologically unspecific signs.

Suicide in the course of schizophrenid (see also Chapter 12)

It has long been known that schizophrenia is associated with an enhanced risk for both natural and unnatural death (Drake *et al.* 1985; Roy 1986). According to follow-up studies the proportion of patients who have died from suicide – depending on the length of the period studied – ranges from about 5% to about 10% on average. Sartorius *et al.* (1987) found at 5-year follow-up in the WHO Determinants of Outcome Study that nearly 4% of the patients with a diagnosis of schizophrenia had committed suicide. Wilkinson (1982) reported a rate of 8% for suicide from a retrospective case-register-based analysis covering 10–15 years. Of the patients of the Chestnut Lodge Study, 6.4% committed suicide over a mean period of 19 years (Fenton *et al.* 1997). Krausz *et al.* (1995) reported a proportion of 13.5%. Recent long-term studies of first episodes of schizophrenia covering 14–16 years of illness have found proportions ranging from 3–4% (Mason *et al.* 1995; Ganev 2000) to 10% (an der Heiden *et al.* 1996; Wiersma *et al.* 1998). Factors contributing to these differences are missed cases and varying basic risk rates of suicide in the general populations.

On the basis of a meta-analysis of 18 publications, Brown (1997) calculated a crude mortality rate (CMR) of 189 deaths per 10 000 population a year, an aggregate standard mortality rate (SMR) of 151 and a 10-year survival rate of 81%. According to his estimates, 28% of the excess mortality is accounted for by suicide and 12% by accidents. The remaining 60% are attributable to the same causes as in the general population. For suicide alone, Brown reported an SMR of 838. The SMR for unnatural causes of death was significantly higher for men than women and showed a tendency to decrease with age (see also Krausz *et al.* 1995). Similar results have recently been reported by Osby *et al.* (2000) from a linkage study based on the inpatient register and the national cause-of-death register of Stockholm County, Sweden. SMRs, calculated by 5-year age classes and 5-year calendar time periods, were at their highest for suicide as a single cause of death. In this study, though, the rates for women at 19.7 were slightly higher than those for men at 15.7. Baxter and Appleby (1999), combining data from the Salford Psychiatric Case Registers and the NHS Central Registers, also found an excess rate of 11.4 for men and of 13.7 for women.

In their attempt to find out indicators for predicting the risk of suicide, Fenton *et al.* (1997), studying patients from the Chestnut Lodge Study (McGlashan 1984a,b), demonstrated a significant association between a low score for negative symptoms at index admission and death from suicide. Conversely, being classified as belonging to the paranoid schizophrenia subtype was associated with an excess risk of 12% for suicide. Similar results were also reported by Kaplan and Harrow (1996) from their comparison of 70 patients with schizophrenia with 97 depressed patients. While psychotic symptoms, such as delusions and hallucinations, were correlated with a later attempt of suicide, deficit symptoms (psychomotor retardation, concreteness) had

prognostic relevance only in depressed patients. The risk for suicide seems to be highest for patients with the best chances for a good outcome (Fenton 2000). Life events appear to enhance the risk for suicide (Heila *et al.* 1999a), whereas appropriate antipsychotic medication reduces it (Heila *et al.* 1999b).

The excess risk for suicide in schizophrenia seems to decrease exponentially with age (Brown 1997), which can mainly be explained by the high rate of suicide among young patients. The study by Harkavy-Friedman *et al.* (1999) is an exception. The authors found that the risk for suicide was associated neither with demographic factors nor with disease variables, such as length of illness, depression or substance abuse. In contrast, Bartels *et al.* (1992) demonstrated an association between alcohol abuse, depression and an increased risk for suicide: 80% of the variance in suicidal behaviour could be explained by depressive symptoms. Two other reviews (Caldwell & Gottesman 1990; Miles 1997) also came to the conclusion that depressive symptoms are a powerful risk factor for suicide.

Short- and medium-term social course of schizophrenia

Indicators of the social course of schizophrenia are social competence and functioning on the one hand, and social impairment, disability and social disadvantage (e.g. socioeconomic status) on the other. The latter factors are to some extent codetermined by the sociocultural environment. In studies into the social course of schizophrenia, comparisons with controls from the general population are necessary, and the results are expressed as comparing patients with schizophrenia to age- and sex-matched controls.

At first admission, persons with schizophrenia already show a considerable degree of social impairment (Häfner *et al.* 1999b) when compared with age- and sex-matched controls from the population of origin (Table 8.3). As expected, impairment is most pronounced in cases diagnosed by restricted criteria (DSM-IIIR and DSM-IV). Patients with schizophrenia do not show significantly inferior social development, as based on the proportion of probands fulfilling the six major social roles characteristic of the main age of risk for schizophrenia (Häfner *et al.* 1999b; Table 8.3).

Both the ABC study (Häfner *et al.* 1999b) and Salokangas's (1978) first admission study found that in patients diagnosed by broad criteria, the mild retardation or abnormality in neuromotor, cognitive and social development exhibited in childhood and youth (Jones & Done 1997) do not lead to serious social disadvantage before illness onset.

Most of the social impairment in people with schizophrenia occurs between illness onset and the end of the early illness stage (McGorry *et al.* 1996; Häfner *et al.* 1999b; see above for explanation of methodology). The impairments in social functioning and social role performance measured by the DAS (WHO 1988) emerge after the illness onset but between 2 and 4 years before the first admission (Häfner *et al.* 1999b). Most severely affected

Table 8.3 Social role performance at the emergence of the first sign of mental disorder and at first admission for schizophrenia (percentage) in an ABC subsample ($n = 57$) compared with 57 population controls matched for age and sex (after Häfner *et al.* 1999b).

	Subjects (%) fulfilling social role at age by first sign of mental disorder (24.0 years)			Subjects (%) fulfilling social role at age by first admission (30.0 years)		
	Patients ($n = 57$)	Controls ($n = 57$)	*P*	Patients ($n = 57$)	Controls ($n = 57$)	*P*
School education	65	61	NS	93	95	NS
Occupational training	37	44	NS	63	65	NS
Employment	33	42	NS	44	58	t
Own income	37	42	NS	49	74	**
Own accommodation	46	51	NS	63	75	NS
Marriage or stable partnership	47	58	NS	25	68	***

NS, not significant; t: $P < 0.1$; ** $P < 0.01$; *** $P < 0.001$.

are marriage and partnerships. In the ABC sample, 52% of the women and 28% of the men were married or lived in a stable partnership at illness onset, but by the first admission the corresponding figures were 33% for women, compared with 78% for healthy controls, and 17% for men, compared with 60% for controls. These results coincide with findings from the retrospective studies of the early course of schizophrenia conducted by McGorry *et al.* (1996), Yung *et al.* (1998) and McGlashan (1998). Jablensky and Cole (1997) have speculated that marriage might be a factor protecting against the onset of schizophrenia; because of the larger proportion of married women than men, this might account for older age of illness onset for women, but this assumption has found no support in other studies (Jennen-Steinmetz *et al.* 1997). In the main, causality appears to run the other way around (Häfner *et al.* 1999b).

In most cases of schizophrenia, social disability becomes manifest with accumulating negative symptoms and increasing cognitive impairment in the most active phase of the disorder long before the first psychiatric contact (Bilder 1998). According to the few prospective epidemiological studies on the course of schizophrenia extending over up to 5 years after first admission (Biehl *et al.* 1986; Salokangas *et al.* 1987; Shepherd *et al.* 1989; Leary *et al.* 1991; Jablensky *et al.* 1992; Leff *et al.* 1992; Vázquez-Barquero *et al.* 1995; Monking *et al.* 1996; Häfner *et al.* 1999b), the scores and profiles of social disability remain more or less stable after remission of the first episode, i.e. between 6 months and 1.5 years after first admission, as do negative symptoms and cognitive impairment. The studies are also consistent in showing significantly poorer social outcomes for men than women, whereas the symptom-related outcomes show no difference (Häfner *et al.* 1999b).

In almost all studies, a poor premorbid social functioning, the most powerful predictor of social course and outcome in schizophrenia, is contaminated with the prodromal illness stage

(Drues *et al.* 1978; Childers & Harding 1990; Haas & Sweeney 1992; Bailer *et al.* 1996; Maziade *et al.* 1996; Rakfeldt & McGlashan 1996; Asarnow 1999). When the illness starts to interfere with the social biography, it leads to social consequences that depend on the individual's level of social development at illness onset, which is the baseline that the social course is measured against. An early illness onset hits at a low level of social development and presumably cognitive development as well. The disorder impairs further social development and leads to stagnation at this low level. In contrast, a late illness onset at a high level of social development results in social decline (Fig. 8.6). Women, at onset on average 4 years older than men, have attained a higher level of social development than men before falling ill with schizophrenia under the precondition that the educational and occupational chances are the same for both sexes in the population.

In addition, population studies have consistently shown that adolescent and young adult males with schizophrenia show a significantly higher frequency of socially adverse behaviour (e.g. alcohol and drug abuse, self-neglect, aggressive behaviour, lack of interest in a job, reduced leisure activity, poor personal hygiene, etc.) than their female counterparts. Women show a significantly greater social adaptiveness at the early illness stage (Häfner *et al.* 1999b). This difference in illness behaviour reflects a characteristic, age-dependent sex difference in social behaviour. It leads to a reduced compliance with treatment, poor coping behaviour and poor social adjustment in male patients in the course of the disorder. Applying a regression model, Häfner *et al.* (1999b,c) demonstrated that the ability to earn a living 5 years after first admission was significantly predicted by the level of social development at the onset of the psychosis and by illness behaviour in the first episode rather than by age, gender, symptomatology or type of illness onset. Age and gender for their part are significant determinants of sex-specific social behaviour and of the level of social development

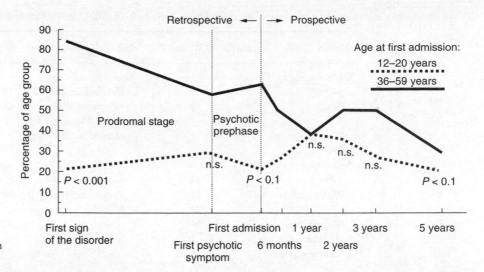

Fig 8.6 The social course of schizophrenia: the ability to earn one's living in two age-of-onset groups (ABC subsample of 115 first illness episodes). The *P*-values test the significance of the difference between the early- and the late-onset group at each point in time.

that patients have attained at illness onset, and it is through these variables that the influence of age and gender on the course and outcome comes about.

Consequently, the significantly poorer social course of schizophrenia in men results from their socially adverse illness behaviour and their lower level of social development at the onset of their illness. Except for the delayed onset in women, probably because of the protective effect of oestrogens, the disorder is similar in core symptoms and course in men and women. As the protective effect of oestrogens in women disappears after menopause and socially adverse male behaviour becomes less frequent with age, women show poorer illness courses in later age while men have milder symptoms and a significantly more favourable course of illness (Opjordsmoen 1998; Häfner *et al.* 1999b,c, 2001).

Further prognostic indicators of the social course are negative symptoms and cognitive impairment. These directly influence social functioning and, hence, the outcome of psychosocial strategies of rehabilitation as well as community outcome (Green 1996). Such patient-related outcome criteria are not the only factors determining community outcome. It also depends on the patients' acceptance in the community, for example on the prevalence of stigma and discrimination, on the availability of good quality care, on the patients' acceptance by their families and, finally, on certain behaviours and personality factors on the patients' part, such as a high communicability versus aggressive behaviour. Most of these factors, again, are associated with gender and more favourable in women than men (Leff 1997; Dörner 1998).

Table 8.4 illustrates the most important variables of social outcome at 5-year follow-up for men and women in an epidemiological sample of 115 first episodes of schizophrenia (cf. Häfner 1999; for sample and design see p. 112). The table makes plain that schizophrenia still is a disorder that entails social loss, even if studied on the basis of a broad definition of

diagnosis including cases of a favourable prognosis and despite the availability of modern methods of treatment.

A radical change for the better in the environment, e.g. by discharge from long-term inpatient treatment into good community care, may even bring about a slight but significant reduction in negative symptoms in the medium-term course (Leff 1997). In fact, it cannot be ruled out that these might be symptoms of institutionalism, described by Wing (1962) as secondary disabilities, which can be brought to remission by resettling the patients in normal stimulating environments. These observations underline the importance of the type of care provided and of the patients' living conditions for course and outcome in schizophrenia.

Short- and medium-term symptom-related course of schizophrenia

Frequency of readmissions or number of days spent in inpatient treatment are no longer regarded as reliable indicators of the course of schizophrenia. According to first-episode studies, the proportion of patients who improve and have no relapses over a 5-year period varies from 21% (Bland & Orn 1978) to 25% (Biehl *et al.* 1986; Maurer & Biehl 1988; Vázquez-Barquero *et al.* 1995) to 30% (Scottish Schizophrenia Research Group 1992). In the WHO cohort (Leff *et al.* 1992) 22% of the patients diagnosed as suffering from schizophrenia according to ICD-9 (295) at entry into the study had experienced no psychotic relapses. A meta-analysis (Hegarty *et al.* 1994) estimates the overall mean proportion of less restrictively defined favourable outcomes at 40% after an average of 6 years of illness.

The proportion of less precisely defined unfavourable outcomes with non-remitting or frequently recurring psychotic symptoms shows more marked variation, ranging from 22% in the WHO cohort to 60% in an der Heiden *et al.*'s study (1996).

Table 8.4 Social outcome in men and women 5 years after first admission for schizophrenia – ABC first-episode subsample ($n = 115$).

Domain	Men (%)	Women (%)	Domain	Men (%)	Women (%)
Marital status[t]			Occupational status[t]		
Married	9	28	Regularly employed	31	42
Single	78	45	Unemployed	43	27
			In rehabilitation/ Occupational therapy	20	9
Living situation: Patient lives[t]					
Alone	15	24	Financial situation*		
With a partner	17	45	Patient earns his or her living	35	58[†]
With parents	53	24			
In sheltered accommodation	11	4			

t: $P < 0.1$; * $P < 0.05$.
[†] Including housewives capable of fulfilling their tasks.

Other investigators have reported proportions varying between these extremes (Salokangas 1978; Carpenter & Kirkpatrick 1988; McGlashan 1988; Schmid et al. 1991; Davidson & McGlashan 1997; Mueser & Tarrier 1998).

Prognostic indicators

Prognostic indicators are studied for two reasons. First, to obtain good prognostic tools for the clinical practice. Such indicators are predominantly characteristics that reflect the disease process because, as a rule, it is possible to predict the further course of a disease from its early stages. The second reason is to generate aetiologically relevant predictors. These predictors must be independent of the disease process. Some of them, e.g. age and gender, are also predictors of the illness onset.

Some prognostic factors are predictive only of certain course and outcome domains. This is the case for example with negative and positive symptoms, which, for the most part, predict only these same dimensions (Strauss & Carpenter 1977; Möller et al. 1982; Pietzcker & Gaebel 1983; Löffler & Häfner 1999). Their predictive power usually decreases with increasing length of illness.

Acute and transient psychoses, which according to Wig and Parhee (1989) show rapid remissions in developing countries (Varma et al. 1996; Craig et al. 1997), have a particularly favourable short- and medium-term prognosis regarding symptomatology, cognitive impairment and social course. That this is also the case in industrialized countries has been shown by Marneros et al. (1991) in a controlled prospective study, the only difference being that these acute syndromes have a considerably lower incidence in the industrialized world. Psychotic symptoms are relevant for the social prognosis only in special cases, e.g. when psychotic episodes are extremely frequent or the

persisting psychotic symptoms particularly severe (Carpenter & Kirkpatrick 1988; McGlashan 1988).

The traditional subtypes, as already mentiond, are only of limited prognostic value (Hargreaves et al. 1977; Strauss & Carpenter 1977; Brockington et al. 1978). In a prospective follow-up study conducted after remission of acute symptoms (6 months after first admission), Ohta et al. (1990) identified three clusters of patients as empirical subtypes on the basis of PANSS data using cluster analysis: 31% with negative symptoms, 32% with persisting delusions and hallucinations and 37% in full remission. As expected, the two symptom-related clusters allowed a fairly reliable prognosis of an elevated relapse rate, higher symptom scores and impaired attention 2 years later.

Poor premorbid functioning (prior to first contact), insidious onset, young age at onset, male gender and not being married have consistently been related to a poor medium-term prognosis of overall outcome (Harrison et al. 1996; Malmberg et al. 1998; Wiersma et al. 2000). Hence, irrespective of their association with the disease process, these factors can be regarded as powerful indicators of the clinical outcome.

With the aim of providing data on all key predictors of 5-year outcome, Möller et al. (1986) studied a sample of hospitalized patients with a diagnosis of schizophrenia according to ICD-9 (295). Of the 17 predictors that the authors tested prospectively only five explained 10–20% of the variance in the general level of functioning (GAS score <50): the duration of occupational disintegration (5 years before admission), impaired working ability (1 year before admission), personality change (1 year before admission), poor psychopathological state at discharge and paranoid tendencies.

A number of predictors have been impossible to replicate. Furthermore, the well-known predictors have rarely explained more than 30% of the total outcome variance (Strauss &

Carpenter 1977; Möller et al. 1986). Therefore, attempts have been made to enhance the accuracy of predictions by pooling various predictors. However, such complex predictor patterns are difficult to use in practice and so they have been incorporated into prognostic scales. Möller and von Zerssen (1995) and Möller et al. (1982, 1984, 1986, 1988) compared six prognostic scales on five dimensions on the basis of product–moment correlations with outcome criteria in their own and in a replication sample at 5-year follow-up. The highest degree of the variance was explained by the Stephens scale and the Strauss–Carpenter scale (Möller et al. 1982, 1984).

Jablensky (2000) has given an overview of the clinically practical, sufficiently validated prognostic indicators, which we have supplemented and adapted to the results of recent predictor studies.

1 Sociodemographic characteristics (gender, age or level of social and cognitive development at psychosis onset.

2 Premorbid personality (schizothymic, schizoid or paranoid).

3 Level of social and occupational functioning prior to illness onset.

4 Past psychotic episodes and successful treatments (rapid remission vs. persisting symptoms).

5 Type of illness onset (acute vs. chronic) and duration of untreated illness.

6 Severe negative symptoms, cognitive and social impairment at the initial illness stage and in the first episode.

7 Illness behaviour (socially adverse behaviour, poor compliance).

8 Cortical atrophy at first admission (Vita et al. 1991; Gattaz et al. 1995).

9 Alcohol and drug abuse, pre- and comorbidly.

Comorbidity with alcohol and drug abuse

The prevalence of alcohol and drug abuse in patients with schizophrenia at the first treatment contact is two- to threefold higher than among controls from the same populations (Mueser et al. 1990, 1992a,b; Addington & Addington 1998; Bühler et al. 2002). Because of an overrepresentation of men among comorbid patients, alcohol and drug abuse has a compounding effect on the sex difference in the social course of schizophrenia. In the short- and medium-term course comorbidity aggravates psychotic symptoms – delusions, hallucinations and thought disorder – increases psychotic relapses but decreases negative symptoms, affective flattening and indifference in particular (Addington & Addington 1998; Bühler et al. 2002). As persons affected appear to suffer less from positive symptoms than from a lack of emotional intensity and pleasure, substance abuse is to some extent also practised as a dysfunctional way of coping with the illness.

Substance abuse leads to reduced compliance with care measures (rehabilitation) and antipsychotic drug treatment (Bühler et al. 2002). In the long term there is an increased risk for social consequences, such as divorce, unemployment and crime

(Mueser et al. 1990, 1992a,b; Addington & Addington 1998; Angermeyer et al. 1998; Brennan et al. 2000).

Long-term course of schizophrenia

The first publications on the long-term course of schizophrenia on the basis of Kraepelin's and Bleuler's diagnostic concept appeared in the 1930s. Mayer-Gross (1932) reports on a 16–17 year follow-up study of 294 patients originally diagnosed with schizophrenia at the psychiatric university hospital in Heidelberg. At follow-up, about 30% were found to be 'practically cured, living at home, socially adjusted', 5% were 'living at home, employed, but poorly socially adjusted', 3.5% were 'living at home, but manifestly ill', 19% were 'in institutions' and, of those, 42.5% of the patients were no longer alive; a majority had died in institutions. Examples of other early studies on the long-term course are those conducted by Langfeldt (1937), Rennie (1939), Hutter (1940), Rupp and Fletcher (1940) and Silverman (1941). All confirm the heterogeneity of illness courses but, because of differences in the diagnostic definitions and study design, valid conclusions cannot be drawn on the proportion with a good outcome or the factors influencing the course of illness (for greater detail see an der Heiden 1996).

In his review published in 1970 Stephens included 31 studies with follow-up periods of at least 5 years. In most cases the clinical diagnosis of schizophrenia was not further specified. Numerous studies have followed. Three large-scale follow-up studies were conducted in German-speaking countries in the 1970s.

Ciompi and Müller (1976) were able to trace from 1642 first admissions in one hospital 289 patients surviving on average 37 years and diagnosed as schizophrenic by Kraepelin's and Bleuler's criteria: 27% of these patients were found to be in full remission and 22% showed only mild impairment, so that in about half the course of the illness and outcome was considered favourable.

Huber et al. (1979) conducted a follow-up investigation of 502 patients from a total of 758 cases with first-rank symptoms admitted to the university psychiatric hospital in Bonn in the period 1945–59. Of these patients 67% were first admissions. At follow-up, an average of 22.4 years later, 22% had remitted, 43% showed, on the basis of the authors' definition, 'uncharacteristic' symptoms and 35% showed 'characteristic' residual syndromes.

Bleuler (1972) re-examined, after an average of 22 years, 208 patients with schizophrenia (66 first admissions) who had been admitted into his Zurich hospital in 1942–43. Bleuler had himself been responsible for these patients' treatment and had stayed in contact with them for over 22 years. His outcome categories are not clear-cut. He considered that about one-half to three-quarters of the patients showed more or less stable conditions after 10 years or more of illness as judged by their overall state of health, their need for treatment in hospital and their social status. One-quarter to one-third Bleuler judged to be fully recovered and between 10% and 20% he classed as having the most severe chronic psychotic symptoms.

All these results are based on interviews conducted by the investigators themselves. The samples were not controlled or representative and had marked variation in their lengths of illness; neither the inclusion diagnoses, the outcome variables nor the assessment instruments were standardized.

The most famous US long-term studies are the Chestnut Lodge Follow-up Study (McGlashan 1984a,b), the Vermont Longitudinal Study (Harding *et al.* 1987a) and the Washington International Pilot Study (Carpenter & Strauss 1991). In the Chestnut Lodge Follow-up Study, 446 patients were included of whom 163 had a diagnosis of schizophrenia. The patients had all been admitted to a very expensive private hospital which emphasized psychodynamic treatment. The patients were reassessed on average 15 years (range 2–32 years) after discharge. They were rated on global functioning at follow-up as showing continued severe impairment (41%), severe impairment (23%), moderate impairment (23%), mild impairment (8%) and no impairment (6%). On average, the patients had spent 25% of the observation period in a 'supervised setting' and had been in work for about 20% of this time. They had 'experienced symptomatic expressions of illness for about 75% of the time'. Broadly, neither significant improvement nor substantial deterioration occurred during the observation period but, as the sample were chronically hospitalized in an expensive psychoanalytically orientated setting, they cannot be regarded as representative.

In the Vermont Longitudinal Study, Harding *et al.* included 168 chronic long-term admissions of whom 72.9% were originally diagnosed as schizophrenic by DSM-I, an unreliable criterion by today's standards. The average follow-up period was 32 years (range 22–62 years). At the end of the observation period about one-half to two-thirds of the patients were rated as 'considerably improved' or 'recovered'. In a later analysis, Harding *et al.* (1987b) and Childers and Harding (1990) rediagnosed schizophrenia for 82 patients by DSM-III; 68% showed no positive or negative (GAS ≥ 61) symptoms at follow-up. The methodological bases of these studies are less rigorous than in the European studies.

In their Washington-based study, Carpenter and Strauss (1991) conducted follow-ups at 2, 5 and 11 years after index assessment in 53 patients from the original sample of 131 patients in the WHO IPSS, of whom 40 had received a DSM-II diagnosis of schizophrenia. These authors, too, found no indication of either improvement or deterioration from 5 to 11-year follow-up. In several cases symptomatology settled on a plateau in the first years following index admission.

In his review of these three and seven other long-term studies from the USA, McGlashan (1988) concludes – as did Bleuler (1972), Huber *et al.* (1979) and Ciompi and Müller (1976) – that, on average, schizophrenia is not a progressive illness. Rather, it frequently reaches a plateau in symptoms after 5–10 years. Over the illness course, even after several years of illness, there is a high degree of interindividual heterogeneity. Part of this heterogeneity is accounted for by differences in the samples studied and the definitions used (psychopathology, sociodemographic characteristics, dimensions of chronicity, etc.). Differences in the systems of care and forms of treatment may also have influenced the results, but these questions are still matters for investigation. There seems to be consensus on the observation that even after several years of illness decisive change may occur in the illness presentation (Harding 1988; Kendell 1988; McGlashan 1988).

In his review, an der Heiden (1996) analysed 59 long-term studies of schizophrenia that covered follow-up periods of 10 years or more on average and were published in the years 1932–96. The overarching finding is the heterogeneity of course and outcome. Given the differences in the study designs, patient samples, timespans covered, course and outcome criteria and lengths of follow-up periods, it is impossible to draw any generally valid conclusions from these results. This was already shown by Fig. 8.2, illustrating the variance in the proportion of recovered patients.

As far as comparisons are feasible, there is only rough agreement between the earlier US and European studies on the long-term course of schizophrenia. Comparing the results of their two studies (Bleuler 1972; Huber *et al.* 1979) Bleuler *et al.* (1976) came to the conclusion that 'statistically over decades of illness, from about the fifth year on, no deterioration, but, rather, improvement in the patients' state occurs'. No improvement was found by Breier *et al.* (1991) in the National Institute of Mental Health Longitudinal Study of Chronic Schizophrenia in the 58 patients of the original 74 patients who were followed up after an average of 13 years. At follow-up there was an increase in symptoms over the first 10 years with an extremely low proportion (3%) of recovery (GAS ≥ 61). On the basis of these results the authors drew a trajectory of the course of schizophrenia, which showed an early stage of deterioration, an intermediate stage of relative stability and an end stage of gradual improvement. Neither the low proportion of good outcomes nor the trajectory of the illness course has been confirmed in recent, methodologically more solid, long-term studies.

Since 1990 prospective long-term studies of schizophrenia have started appearing, some fairly sophisticated in their methodologies. The first was the International Study of Schizophrenia (ISoS; Sartorius *et al.* 1996), co-ordinated by the WHO. Fifteen- and 25-year follow-ups have been conducted on the cohorts of the former IPSS (WHO 1973), the WHO Collaborative Study on the Assessment and Reduction of Social Disability (Jablensky *et al.* 1980) and the Determinants of Outcome of Severe Mental Disorders Study (DOSMED: Sartorius *et al.* 1986). A total of 19 research centres in 16 countries participated in these studies. The results from these studies confirm the heterogeneity of course and outcome (Hopper *et al.* 2000), but demonstrate no early tendency to deterioration after first admission, which is in line with the results of the studies into the medium-term course of schizophrenia.

Ganev (2000) is the only investigator who, reassessing the Sofia sample of the WHO Disability Study (*n* = 55 at follow-up), has reported a favourable long-term outcome of psychotic symptoms: 55% of the patients improved over the first 10 years before follow-up and only 20% deteriorated. Mason *et al.* (1996) from Nottingham (13-year follow-up) and Wiersma *et al.* (1998) from Groningen found no indication of a late recovery. The Groningen study rather showed that chronicity (continued positive or persisting negative symptoms) increased slightly on average and also the length of episodes grew with each episode.

Possibly the most thorough prospective long-term study of population-based first admissions of schizophrenia (ICD-9: 295) has been conducted in the Mannheim cohort (an der Heiden *et al.* 1995), with 10 cross-sections over a period of 15.5 years. The symptom-related course did not show improvement. Social disability deteriorated slightly, but significantly in the final stage (an der Heiden *et al.* 1995; an der Heiden & Häfner 2000). Of the cohort 25% was free of symptoms and, as a result, needed no treatment in the last 9 months before the 15.5-year follow-up; 60% were rated as chronic because of the presence of substantial positive and/or negative symptoms in that same period; 15% were on neuroleptic medication and free of symptoms. Only the patients rated as chronic showed a slight trend towards an increase in positive and negative symptoms over the period studied. The main indicators of social outcome at 15.5-year follow-up in the Mannheim cohort, compared with matched controls, is shown in Table 8.5.

Geographical variation of course and outcome in schizophrenia

The prospective WHO studies (WHO 1973, 1979; Jablensky *et al.* 1992; Leff *et al.* 1992), conducted with culture-independent methods and identical study designs, are consistent in showing that the course of schizophrenia is more favourable at the centres in developing than industrialized countries. This difference proved stable irrespective of the follow-up period. This difference emerged with all the main characteristics of the illness course, e.g. proportion of full recovery vs. that of persisting or episodic symptoms, proportion of time spent with psychotic symptoms vs. time spent without symptoms and social impairment.

Attempts have not succeeded in explaining differences in course and outcome by a more favourable family environment in developing countries and a higher degree of Expressed Emotion (EE) in the industrialized world. Leff *et al.* (1992) and Craig *et al.* (1997) analysed data for 1056 probands of the DOSMED study, for whom sufficient information at 2-year follow-up was available, by applying the recursive partitioning technique for identifying groups of patients with similar outcomes. The authors found that of the centres in industrialized countries, Prague and Nottingham showed fairly favourable profiles of outcome resembling those reported from the centres in developing countries. The second most powerful predictor was type of onset or the proportion of cases with highly acute initial illness.

The first predictor analysis of the long-term course (over 15 and 25 years) on data for the 1633 patients of the ISoS study (Harrison *et al.* 2001) confirmed the relative stability of the differences over any period of illness studied. The most powerful predictor turned out to be type of illness course in the first 2 years after entry into the study. A shorter overall duration of psychotic episodes in this early period of illness predicted lower symptom and disability scores at the long-term follow-up and, as a result, a more favourable overall course of the illness. In the stepwise regression analysis applied in this study, the individual centres

Table 8.5 Sociodemographic outcome indicators of the long-term course of schizophrenia: comparison of 48 (30 male, 18 female) patients with schizophrenia (PSE CATEGO 295) 15.5 years after first admission and 48 controls matched for age, sex and place of residence from the same population of origin (after Weber 1997).

Domain	Patients with schizophrenia (n = 48)		Controls (n = 48)
Marital status/ partnership	52.1	Never married	14.6
	29.2	Married	66.7
	35.4	Lives with a spouse/partner	81.3
	20.8	Lives in a home	–
Employment/financial independence	29.2	No occupational training	10.4
	23.1	Employed	83.5
	62.5	Unemployed	8.4
	73.0	Unable to earn a living	10.5

PSE, Present State Examination (Wing *et al.* 1974).

no longer contributed to the rates of recovery. The only conclusion that can be drawn from this result is that early individual illness course constitutes one of the main factors that determine the course of schizophrenia at later illness stages. Consequently, the transcultural differences in the course of schizophrenia are largely accounted for by differences in the type and severity of cases included in the samples of first-onset patients and only to a lesser extent by differences in environmental factors, which affect the course of schizophrenia only in fully developed illness in the long term.

Quality of life

Besides the classical indicators, constructs such as quality of life (QOL) or life satisfaction have attained special importance in the assessment of the social and clinical outcome of schizophrenia and the evaluation of treatment measures (WHO 1998; Becker *et al.* 1999).

Because quality of life depends not only on the disorder but also on the individual, economic and sociocultural conditions that the patients live in, its assessment requires comparisons with controls from the general population, with people with other illnesses and, more rarely, with the goals and expectations of the patients themselves (Michaelos 1980) or their baseline in the social context (Campbell *et al.* 1976).

Evaluating community-based psychiatric services in the US state of New York, Baker and Intagliata (1982) found out that the persons interviewed, compared with a representative general population sample, were less satisfied particularly with their financial situation and their health. Bigelow *et al.* (1982), studying the effectiveness of the treatment and care provided by community psychiatric services, compared quality of life between psychiatric patients and healthy controls. The authors came to the conclusion that mental health programmes do improve quality of life, but their success varies with the domain as well as type and severity of the problems in question. Lehman (1983) and Lehman *et al.* (1986) compared psychiatric patients in residential care with patients living in the community – of whom one-quarter to one-half had been diagnosed with schizophrenia. Irrespective of the setting, these patients were dissatisfied with their financial situation, and also with the domains of work and security. Nevertheless, psychiatric patients living in the community were generally more satisfied than patients in residential care. Satisfaction depended on the patients' objective situation, and here availability of amenities and comforts in the individual setting played a decisive part.

Subjective quality of life also determines to a high degree how patients rate their experience of their symptoms. Comparable studies have been conducted by von Zerssen and Hecht (1987), who studied the associations between mental health, happiness and life satisfaction; by Huber *et al.* (1988), who compared quality of life between persons with psychiatric illness and healthy individuals; and by Malm *et al.* (1981), Oliver and Mohamad (1992), Mechanic *et al.* (1994) and Priebe *et al.* (1995).

Weber's (1997) investigation of patients from the Mannheim WHO Disability Study cohort at 15.5 years after first admission underlines the importance of individual aspirations and their achievement or non-achievement for the QOL construct. She assessed not only the patients' global life satisfaction, but also the importance of their aspirations in different domains of life and their achievements and their expectations. The age- and gender-matched controls from the general population were clearly more satisfied than the patients with schizophrenia, both overall and in the various life domains studied. The controls had better starting conditions than the patients for attaining their aspirations, they were more confident that the conditions would continue to be favourable in the future and that they would be able to influence the achievement of their goals. Aspirations were equally important to patients and controls.

In summary, there is evidence that the quality of life of people with schizophrenia is impaired, on both subjective and objective criteria, including their work and financial situation (Bengtsson-Tops & Hansson 1999). Their quality of life is reduced by the time of first contact with professional services (Browne *et al.* 2000), but the later outcome depends on their symptoms, the duration of untreated psychosis, and their adjustment preadmission. However, Ho *et al.*'s study (2000) failed to confirm most of these findings.

Becker *et al.* (1998) studied how the size of social network influences quality of life and found that a medium number of social contacts was associated with the highest degree of quality of life.

Assessing 58 patients with schizophrenia in outpatient treatment Rudnick and Kravetz (2001) found that social support seeking may influence outcome favourably, but does not correlate with quality of life. The role of medication was assessed in a survey of 565 patients with schizophrenia in Germany (Angermeyer & Matschinger 2000). The authors came to the conclusion that side-effects of medications such as extrapyramidal motor symptoms affect the patients' quality of life. These results coincide with Sullivan *et al.*'s findings (1992) that the quality of life varies with depressive symptoms, family interaction and side-effects of medications. In contrast, Larsen and Gerlach (1996) found no correlation with the side-effects of neuroleptic depot medication in their sample of 53 chronic cases of schizophrenia, but such results may be accounted for by the type and dosage of medication and the amount of undesirable side-effects.

Conclusions

The last few years of research into the course and outcome of schizophrenia have led us to bid farewell to the traditional long-term studies and their heterogeneous results. Progress in research methods, including precisely defined inclusion criteria (diagnosis without selective course criteria), epidemiological first-episode samples, standardized assessment procedures and prospective, in part controlled, study designs, has yielded increasingly consistent data on the trajectory of the course of schizophrenia. The average course of schizophrenia shows neither progressive deterioration of the type of the Kraepelinean dementia praecox nor pronounced improvement in symptoms and impairments at later stages of the illness. After remission of the first episode, neurocognitive impairments and negative symptoms exhibit a surprising degree of intraindividual stability.

In contrast with the traditional view, schizophrenia now has a life-long perspective. It first appears as subtle deviations in the childhood developmental milestones with mild cognitive, social and emotional anomalies as antecedents of the disorder. The most active part of the disease process occurs in the period from illness onset until the climax of the first psychotic episode, marked by the accumulation of symptoms and of cognitive and social impairment. Even today, treatment usually begins only after most of the social consequences have become reality.

The course of schizophrenia is highly heterogeneous: there are cases that show prodromal stages of several years' duration with increasingly severe negative symptoms, functional impairment and subsequent persisting disability. There are other cases which begin with an acute psychotic episode without any negative symptoms, followed by a sustained remission. There is a small extreme group which shows gradual progression over time. Some of these patients seem to prematurely develop dementia of old age. At present the division of this dimensional spectrum into various diagnoses is of relevance in clinical practice, but not in nosology.

The advance in course and outcome research was made by controlled prospective first-admission studies with data on symptomatology, neuropsychological functioning and morphological changes visible on magnetic resonance tomography (MRT). MRT findings have shown that atrophy appears to progress over time in some patients who have had particularly pronounced cognitive deficits in the first episode. The underlying association with changes in symptoms and neuropsychological functioning and the causal mechanism of these processes, although perhaps not yet sufficiently clarified, are described in many of the chapters which follow.

References

Addington, J. & Addington, D. (1991) Positive and negative symptoms of schizophrenia. Their course and relationship over time. *Schizophrenia Research* 5, 51–59.

Addington, J. & Addington, D. (1998) Effect of substance misuse in early psychosis. *British Journal of Psychiatry* 172 (Suppl. 33), 134–136.

Addington, D., Addington, J., Maticka-Tyndale, E. & Joyce, J. (1992) Reliability and validity of a depression rating scale for schizophrenics. *Schizophrenia Research* 6, 201–208.

Albus, M., Hubmann, W., Ehrenberg, C. *et al.* (1996) Neuropsychological impairment in first-episode and chronic schizophrenic patients. *European Archives of Psychiatry and Clinical Neuroscience* 246, 249–255.

American Psychiatric Association (1987) *DSM-IIIR: Diagnostic and Statistical Manual of Mental Disorders.* American Psychiatric Association, Washington, DC.

American Psychiatric Association (1994) *DSM-IV: Diagnostic and Statistical Manual of Mental Disorders, 4th edition.* American Psychiatric Association, Washington, DC.

Andreasen, N.C. (1983) *The Scale for the Assessment of Negative Symptoms (SANS).* University of Iowa, Iowa City, IA.

Andreasen, N.C. (1984) *The Scale for the Assessment of Positive Symptoms (SAPS).* University of Iowa, Iowa City, IA.

Andreasen, N.C. (1989) Scale for the Assessment of Negative Symptoms (SANS). *British Journal of Psychiatry* 155 (Suppl. 7), 53–58.

Andreasen, N.C. (1990) Positive and negative symptoms: historical and conceptual aspects. In: *Schizophrenia: positive and negative symptoms and syndromes* (ed. N.C. Andreasen), pp. 1–42. Karger, Basel.

Andreasen, N.C. & Olsen, S.A. (1982) Negative vs. positive schizophrenia. *Archives of General Psychiatry* 39, 789–794.

Andreasen, N.C., Grove, W.M., Shapiro, R.W. *et al.* (1981) Reliability of lifetime diagnosis. *Archives of General Psychiatry* 38, 400–405.

Angermeyer, M.C. & Matschinger, H. (2000) Neuroleptika und Lebensqualität: Ergebnisse einer Patientenbefragung. *Psychiatrische Praxis* 27, 64–68.

Angermeyer, M.C., Cooper, B. & Link, B.G. (1998) Mental disorder and violence: results of epidemiological studies in the era of deinstitutionalization. *Social Psychiatry and Psychiatric Epidemiology* 33, 1–6.

Arbeitsgemeinschaft für Methodik und Diagnostik in der Psychiatrie (1995) *Das AMDP-System: Manual zur Dokumentation psychiatrischer Befunde, 5. Auflage.* Springer, Berlin, Heidelberg, New York.

Arndt, S., Andreasen, N.C., Flaum, M., Miller, D. & Nopoulos, P. (1995) A longitudinal study of symptom dimensions in schizophrenia: prediction and patterns of change. *Archives of General Psychiatry* 52, 352–360.

Arora, A., Avasthi, A. & Kulhara, P. (1997) Subsyndromes of chronic schizophrenia: a phenomenological study. *Acta Psychiatrica Scandinavica* 96, 225–229.

Asarnow, R.F. (1999) Neurocognitive impairments in schizophrenia: a piece of the epigenetic puzzle. *European Child and Adolescent Psychiatry* 8 (Suppl. 1), 5–8.

Bailer, J., Brauer, W. & Rey, E.R. (1996) Premorbid adjustment as predictor of outcome in schizophrenia: results of a prospective study. *Acta Psychiatrica Scandinavica* 93, 368–377.

Baker, F. & Intagliata, J. (1982) Quality of life in the evaluation of community support systems. *Evaluation and Program Planning* 5, 69–79.

Bartels, S.J., Drake, R.E. & McHugo, G.J. (1992) Alcohol abuse, depression, and suicidal behavior in schizophrenia. *American Journal of Psychiatry* 149, 394–395.

Baxter, D. & Appleby, L. (1999) Case register study of suicide risk in mental disorders. *British Journal of Psychiatry* 175, 322–326.

Becker, T., Leese, M., Clarkson, P. *et al.* (1998) Links between social network and quality of life: an epidemiologically representative study of psychotic patients in south London. *Social Psychiatry and Psychiatric Epidemiology* 33, 229–304.

Becker, T., Knapp, M., Knudsen, H.C. *et al.* (1999) The EPSILON study of schizophrenia in five European countries: design and methodology for standardising outcome measures and comparing patterns of care and service costs. *British Journal of Psychiatry* 175, 514–521.

Bengtsson-Tops, A. & Hansson, L. (1999) Subjective quality of life in schizophrenic patients living in the community: relationship to clinical and social characteristics. *European Psychiatry* 14, 256–263.

Berg, E.A. (1948) A simple objective treatment for measuring flexibility in thinking. *Journal of General Psychology* 39, 15–22.

Biehl, H., Maurer, K., Schubart, C., Krumm, B. & Jung, E. (1986) Prediction of outcome and utilization of medical services in a prospective study of first onset schizophrenics. *European Archives of Psychiatry and Neurological Sciences* **236**, 139–147.

Biehl, H., Maurer, K., Jablensky, A., Cooper, J.E. & Tomov, T. (1989) The WHO Psychological Impairments Rating Schedule (WHO/PIRS). I. Introducing a new instrument for rating observed behaviour and the rationale of the psychological impairment concept. *British Journal of Psychiatry* **155** (Suppl. 7), 68–70.

Bigelow, L.B., Brodsky, G., Stewart, L. & Olson, M. (1982) The concept and measurement of quality of life as a dependent variable in the evaluation of mental health services. In: *Innovative approaches to mental health evaluation* (eds G.J. Stahler & W.R. Tash), pp. 345–366. Academic Press, New York.

Bilder, R.M. (1998) The neuropsychology of schizophrenia: what, when, where, how? In: *Schizophrene Störungen: State of the Art II* (eds V.W. Fleischhacker, H. Hinterhuber & U. Meise), pp. 155–171. Verlag Integrative Psychiatrie, Innsbruck.

Bilder, R.M., Mukherjee, S., Rieder, R.O. & Pandurangi, A.K. (1985) Symptomatic and neuropsychological components of defect status. *Schizophrenia Bulletin* **11**, 409–419.

Bilder, R.M., Reiter, G., Bates, J.A., Willson, D.F. & Lieberman, J.A. (1995) Neuropsychological profiles of first-episode schizophrenia. *Schizophrenia Research* **15**, 109.

Binder, J., Albus, M., Hubmann, W. *et al.* (1998) Neuropsychological impairment and psychopathology in first-episode schizophrenic patients related to the early course of illness. *European Archives of Psychiatry and Clinical Neuroscience* **248**, 70–77.

Birchwood, M.J., Smith, J., Macmillan, F. *et al.* (1989) Predicting relapse in schizophrenia: the development and implementation of an early signs monitoring system using patients and families as observers, a preliminary investigation. *Psychological Medicine* **19**, 649–656.

Bland, R.C. & Orn, H. (1978) 14-year outcome in early schizophrenia. *Acta Psychiatrica Scandinavica* **58**, 327–338.

Bleuler, M. (1968) A 23-year longitudinal study of 208 schizophrenics and impressions in regard to the nature of schizophenia. In: *The Transmission of Schizophrenia* (eds D. Rosenthal & S.S. Kety), pp. 3–12. Pergamon Press, Oxford.

Bleuler, M. (1972) *Die schizophrenen Geistesstörungen im Lichte langjähriger Kranken- und Familiengeschichten.* Thieme, Stuttgart.

Bleuler, M., Huber, G., Gross, G. & Schüttler, R. (1976) Der langfristige Verlauf schizophrener Psychosen. *Nervenarzt* **47**, 477–481.

Bottlender, R., Wegner, U., Wittmann, J., Strauß, A. & Möller, H.-J. (1999) Deficit syndromes in schizophrenic patients 15 years after their first hospitalization: preliminary results of a follow-up study. *European Archives of Psychiatry and Clinical Neuroscience* **249** (Suppl. 4), 27–36.

Bottlender, R., Strauss, A. & Möller, H.-J. (2000) Impact of duration of symptoms prior to first hospitalization on acute outcome in 998 schizophrenic patients. *Schizophrenia Research* **44**, 145–150.

Breier, A., Schreiber, J.L., Dyer, J. & Pickar, D. (1991) National Institute of Mental Health longitudinal study of chronic schizophrenia: prognosis and predictors of outcome. *Archives of General Psychiatry* **48**, 239–246.

Brennan, P.A., Mednick, S.A. & Hodgins, S. (2000) Major mental disorders and criminal violence in à Danish birth cohort. *Archives of General Psychiatry* **57**, 494–500.

Brockington, I.F., Kendell, R.E. & Leff, J.P. (1978) Definitions of schizophrenia: concordance and prediction of outcome. *Psychological Medicine* **8**, 387–398.

Brown, G.W. (1960) Length of hospital stay and schizophrenia: a review of statistical studies. *Acta Psychiatrica et Neurologica Scandinavica* **35**, 414–430.

Brown, S. (1997) Excess mortality of schizophrenia: a meta-analysis. *British Journal of Psychiatry* **171**, 502–508.

Browne, S., Clarke, M., Gervin, M. *et al.* (2000) Determinants of quality of life at first presentation with schizophrenia. *British Journal of Psychiatry* **176**, 173–176.

Buchanan, R.W., Kirkpatrick, B., Heinrichs, D.W. & Carpenter, W.T. (1990) Clinical correlates of the deficit syndrome of schizophrenia. *American Journal of Psychiatry* **147**, 290–294.

Bühler, B., Hambrecht, M., Löffler, W., an der Heiden, W. & Häfner, H. (2002) Precipitation and determination of the onset and course of schizophrenia by substance abuse: a retrospective and prospective study of 232 population-based first illness episodes. *Schizophrenia Research* **54**, 243–251.

Caldwell, C.B. & Gottesman, I.I. (1990) Schizophrenics kill themselves too: a review of risk factors for suicide. *Schizophrenia Bulletin* **16**, 571–589.

Campbell, A., Converse, R.E. & Rodgers, W.L. (1976) *The Quality of American Life: Perception, Evaluations, and Satisfactions.* Russell Sage Foundation, New York.

Carpenter, W.T. & Heinrichs, D.W. (1983) Early intervention, time-limited, targeted pharmacotherapy of schizophrenia. *Schizophrenia Bulletin* **9**, 533–542.

Carpenter, W.T. & Kirkpatrick, B. (1988) The heterogeneity of the long-term course of schizophrenia. *Schizophrenia Bulletin* **14**, 645–652.

Carpenter, W.T. & Strauss, J.S. (1991) The prediction of outcome in schizophrenia. IV. Eleven-year follow-up of the Washington IPSS cohort. *Journal of Nervous and Mental Disease* **179**, 517–525.

Carpenter, W.T., Heinrichs, D.W. & Wagman, A.M.I. (1988) Deficit and nondeficit forms of schizophrenia: the concept. *American Journal of Psychiatry* **145**, 578–583.

Carpenter, W.T., Buchanan, R.W., Kirkpatrick, B., Thaker, G. & Tamminga, C. (1991) Negative symptoms: a critique of current approaches. In: *Negative Versus Positive Schizophrenia* (eds A. Marneros, N.C. Andreasen & M.T. Tsuang), pp. 126–133. Springer, Berlin, Heidelberg, New York.

Cechnicki, A. & Walczewski, K. (1999) *Dynamic of positive and negative syndrome in schizophrenia: prospective study.* In: *Psychiatry on new thresholds. Abstracts of the XI World Congress of Psychiatry, Hamburg, August 6–11, 1999* (eds J. López-Ibor, N. Sartorius, W. Gaebel & C. Haasen).

Censitis, D.M., Ragland, J.D., Gur, R.C. & Gur, R.E. (1997) Neuropsychological evidence supporting a neurodevelopmental model of schizophrenia: a longitudinal study. *Schizophrenia Research* **24**, 289–298.

Changhui, C., Weixi, Z. & Shuren, L. (1995) Clinical features and outcome of schizophrenia at 12-years follow-up: a report from Chinese partner of the WHO Coordinated Study on the Long-term Course and Outcome of Schizophrenia. Paper presented at the 3rd Meeting of Investigators of ISoS, Bologna, Italy, September 25–27, 1995.

Childers, S.E. & Harding, C.M. (1990) Gender, premorbid social functioning, and long-term outcome in DSM-III schizophrenia. *Schizophrenia Bulletin* **16**, 309–318.

Ciompi, L. (1980) Catamnestic long-term study on the course of life and aging of schizophrenics. *Schizophrenia Bulletin* **6**, 606–618.

Ciompi, L. & Müller, C. (1976) *Lebensweg und Alter der Schizophrenen.* Springer, Berlin.

Conrad, K. (1958) *Die beginnende Schizophrenie.* Thieme, Stuttgart.

Cornblatt, B.A. & Keilp, J.G. (1994) Impaired attention, genetics, and the pathophysiology of schizophrenia. *Schizophrenia Bulletin* **20**, 31–46.

Cornblatt, B., Obuchowski, M., Schnur, D.B. & O'Brian, J. (1998) Hillside study of risk and early detection in schizophrenia. *British Journal of Psychiatry* **172** (Suppl. 3), 26–32.

Craig, T.J., Siegel, C., Hopper, K., Lin, S. & Sartorius, N. (1997) Outcome in schizophrenia and related disorders compared between developing and developed countries: a recursive partitioning re-analysis of the WHO DOSMeD data. *British Journal of Psychiatry* **170**, 229–233.

Craig, T.J., Fennig, S., Tanenberg, K.M. & Bromet, E.J. (1999) Six-month clinical status as a predictor of 24-month clinical outcome in first-admission patients with schizophrenia. *Annals of Clinical Psychiatry* **11**, 197–203.

Craig, T.J., Bromet, E.J., Fennig, S. *et al.* (2000) Is there an association between duration of untreated psychosis and 24-month clinical outcome in a first-admission series? *American Journal of Psychiatry* **157**, 60–66.

Crow, T.J. (1980a) Molecular pathology of schizophrenia: more than one disease process. *British Medical Journal* **260**, 66–68.

Crow, T.J. (1980b) Positive and negative schizophrenic symptoms and the role of dopamine. *British Journal of Psychiatry* **137**, 383–386.

Crow, T.J., MacMillan, J.F., Johnson, A.L. & Johnstone, E.C. (1986) The Northwick Park Study of first episodes of schizophrenia. II. A randomized controlled trial of prophylactic neuroleptic treatment. *British Journal of Psychiatry* **148**, 120–127.

Cutting, J. & Dunne, F. (1989) Subjective experience of schizophrenia. *Schizophrenia Bulletin* **15**, 217–231.

Danielyan, A. & Danielyan, K. (1999) *Paranoid schizophrenia and chronic stressful experience.* In: *Psychiatry on new thresholds. Abstracts of the XI World Congress of Psychiatry, Hamburg, August 6–11, 1999* (eds J. López-Ibor, N. Sartorius, W. Gaebel & C. Haasen).

Daum, C.M., Brooks, G.W. & Albee, G.W. (1977) Twenty year follow-up of 253 schizophrenic patients originally selected for chronic disability: pilot study. *Psychiatric Journal of the University of Ottawa* **2**, 129–132.

Davidson, L. & McGlashan, T.H. (1997) The varied outcomes of schizophrenia. *Canadian Journal of Psychiatry* **42**, 34–43.

Davidson, M., Reichenberg, A., Rabinowitz, J. *et al.* (1999) Behavioral and intellectual markers for schizophrenia in apparently healthy male adolescents. *American Journal of Psychiatry* **156**, 1328–1335.

Deister, A., Marneros, A., Rohde, A., Staab, B. & Jünemann, H. (1990) Long-term outcome of affective, schizoaffective and schizophrenic disorders: a comparison. In: *Affective and schizoaffective disorders* (eds A. Marneros & M.T. Tsuang), pp. 157–167. Springer, Berlin, Heidelberg, New York.

DeLisi, L.E., Sakuma, M., Tew, W. *et al.* (1997) Schizophrenia as a chronic active brain process: a study of progressive brain structural change subsequent to the onset of schizophrenia. *Psychiatry Research* **74**, 129–140.

DeLisi, L.E., Sakuma, M., Ge, S. & Kushner, M. (1998) Association of brain structural change with the heterogeneous course of schizophrenia from early childhood through 5 years subsequent to a first hospitalization. *Psychiatry Research* **84**, 75–88.

Dobmeier, P., Bottlender, R., Wittmann, J. *et al.* (2000) Depressive Symptome bei schizophrenen Erkrankungen: Ergebnisse der Münchner 15-Jahres-Katamnese. In: *Methodik von Verlaufs- und Therapiestudien in Psychiatrie und Psychotherapie* (eds W. Maier, R.R. Engel & H.-U. Möller), pp. 179–188. Hogrefe, Göttingen.

Docherty, J.P., van Kammen, D.P., Siris, S.G. & Marder, S.R. (1978) Stages of onset of schizophrenic psychosis. *American Journal of Psychiatry* **135**, 420–426.

Dörner, K. (1998) *Ende der Veranstaltung: Anfänge der Chronisch-Kranken-Psychiatrie.* Verlag Jakob von Hoddis, Gütersloh.

Drake, R.E., Gates, C., Whitaker, A. & Cotton, P.G. (1985) Suicide among schizophrenics: a review. *Comprehensive Psychiatry* **26**, 90–100.

Drues, J., Hargreaves, W.A., Glick, I.D. & Klein, D.F. (1978) Premorbid asocial adjustment and outcome in schizophrenia. *Journal of Nervous and Mental Disease* **166**, 881–884.

Dube, K.C., Kumar, N. & Dube, S. (1984) Long term course and outcome of the Agra cases in the International Pilot Study of Schizophrenia. *Acta Psychiatrica Scandinavica* **70**, 170–179.

Eaton, W.W. (1999) Evidence for universality and uniformity of schizophrenia around the world: assessment and implications. In: *Search for the Causes of Schizophrenia.* Vol. IV. *Balance of the Century* (eds W.F. Gattaz & H. Häfner), pp. 21–33. Steinkopff Verlag, Darmstadt.

Eaton, W.W., Bilker, W., Haro, J.M. *et al.* (1992a) Long-term course of hospitalization for schizophrenia. II. Change with passage of time. *Schizophrenia Bulletin* **18**, 229–241.

Eaton, W.W., Mortensen, P.B., Herrman, H. *et al.* (1992b) Long-term course of hospitalization for schizophrenia. I. Risk for rehospitalization. *Schizophrenia Bulletin* **18**, 217–227.

Eaton, W.W., Thara, R., Federman, B., Melton, B. & Liang, K.Y. (1995) Structure and course of positive and negative symptoms in schizophrenia. *Archives of General Psychiatry* **52**, 127–134.

Endicott, J. & Spitzer, R.L. (1978) A diagnostic interview: the schedule for affective disorders and schizophrenia. *Archives of General Psychiatry* **35**, 837–844.

Endicott, J., Spitzer, R.L., Fleiss, J.L. & Cohen, J. (1976) The Global Assessment Scale: a procedure for measurement overall severity of psychiatric disturbance. *Archives of General Psychiatry* **33**, 766–771.

Engelhardt, D.M., Rosen, B., Feldman, J., Engelhardt, J.A.Z. & Cohen, P. (1982) A 15-year follow-up of 646 schizophrenic outpatients. *Schizophrenia Bulletin* **8**, 493–503.

Faris, R.E.L. & Dunham, H.W. (1939) *Mental Disorders in Urban Areas: An Ecological Study of Schizophrenia and Other Psychosis.* University of Chicago Press, Chicago.

Fenton, W.S. (2000) Depression, suicide, and suicide prevention in schizophrenia. *Suicide and Life Threatening Behaviour* **30**, 34–49.

Fenton, W.S. & McGlashan, T.H. (1991a) Natural history of schizophrenia subtypes. I. Longitudinal study of paranoid, hebephrenic, and undifferentiated schizophrenia. *Archives of General Psychiatry* **48**, 969–977.

Fenton, W.S. & McGlashan, T.H. (1991b) Natural history of schizophrenia subtypes. II. Positive and negative symptoms and long-term course. *Archives of General Psychiatry* **48**, 978–986.

Fenton, W.S. & McGlashan, T.H. (1992) Testing systems for assessment of negative symptoms in schizophrenia. *Archives of General Psychiatry* **49**, 179–184.

Fenton, W.S., McGlashan, T., Victor, B.J. & Blyler, C.R. (1997) Symptoms, subtype, and suicidality in patients with schizophrenia spectrum disorders. *American Journal of Psychiatry* **154**, 199–204.

Franzek, E. & Beckmann, H. (1992) Reliability and validity of the Leonhard classification tested in a 5-year follow-up study of 50 chronic schizophrenics. In: *Schizophrenia and Affective Psychoses: Nosology in Contemporary Psychiatry* (eds F.P. Ferrero, A.E. Haynal & N. Sartorius), pp. 67–72. John Libbey CIC, New York.

Gaebel, W. & Frommann, N. (2000) Long-term course in schizophrenia: concepts, methods and research strategies. *Acta Psychiatrica Scandinavica* **102** (Suppl. 407), 49–53.

Gaebel, W., Frick, U., Kopke, W. *et al.* (1993) Early neuroleptic intervention in schizophrenia: are prodromal symptoms valid predictors of relapse? *British Journal of Psychiatry* **163** (Suppl. 23), 8–12.

Ganev, K. (2000) Long-term trends of symptoms and disability in schizophrenia and related disorders. *Social Psychiatry and Psychiatric Epidemiology* **35**, 389–395.

Ganev, K., Onchev, G. & Ivanov, P. (1998) A 16-year follow-up study of schizophrenia and related disorders in Sofia, Bulgaria. *Acta Psychiatrica Scandinavica* 98, 200–207.

Gattaz, W.F., Brunner, J., Schmitt, A. & Maras, A. (1995) Increased breakdown of membrane phospholipids in schizophrenia: implications for the hypofrontality hypothesis. In: *Search for the Causes of Schizophrenia*, Vol. III. (eds H. Häfner & W.F. Gattaz), pp. 215–226. Springer, Berlin, Heidelberg, New York.

Geddes, J.R. & Kendell, R.E. (1995) Schizophrenic subjects with no history of admission to hospital. *Psychological Medicine* 25, 859–868.

Gmür, M. (1991) The 12-year clinical course of schizophrenia. *Social Psychiatry and Psychiatric Epidemiology* 26, 202–211.

Gold, A., Arndt, S., Nopoulos, P., O'Leary, D.S. & Andreasen, N.C. (1999) Longitudinal study of cognitive function in first-episode and recent-onset schizophrenia. *American Journal of Psychiatry* 156, 1342–1348.

Goldacre, M., Shiwach, R. & Yeates, D. (1994) Estimating incidence and prevalence of treated psychiatric disorders from routine statistics: the example of schizophrenia in Oxfordshire. *Journal of Epidemiology and Community Health* 48, 318–322.

Goldberg, T.E. & Gold, J.M. (1995) Neurocognitive deficits in schizophrenia. In: *Schizophrenia* (eds S.R. Hirsch & D.R. Weinberger), pp. 146–162. Blackwell Science, London.

Goldberg, T.E., Gold, J.M., Greenberg, R. *et al.* (1993) Contrasts between patients with affective disorders and patients with schizophrenia on a neuropsychological test battery. *American Journal of Psychiatry* 150, 1355–1362.

Goldberg, T.E., Patterson, K., Taqqu, Y. & Wilder, K. (1998) Capacity limitations in short-term memory in schizophrenia. *Psychological Medicine* 28, 665–673.

Gottesman, I.I., McGuffin, P. & Farmer, A.E. (1987) Clinical genetics as clue to the 'real' genetics of schizophrenia (a decade of modest gains while playing for a time). *Schizophrenia Bulletin* 13, 23–47.

Green, M.F. (1996) What are the functional consequences of neurocognitive deficits in schizophrenia. *American Journal of Psychiatry* 153, 321–330.

Gross, G., Huber, G. & Schüttler, R. (1986) Long-term course of Schneiderian schizophrenia. In: *Schizoaffective psychoses* (eds A. Marneros & M.T. Tsuang), pp. 164–178. Springer, Berlin, Heidelberg, New York.

Gross, G., Huber, G., Klosterkötter, J. & Linz, M. (1987) *Bonner Skala für die Beurteilung von Basissymptomen (BSABS: Bonn Scale for the Assessment of Basic Symptoms)*. Springer, Berlin, Heidelberg, New York.

Gupta, S., Andreasen, N.C., Arndt, S. *et al.* (1997) The Iowa Longitudinal Study of Recent Onset Psychosis: one-year follow-up of first episode patients. *Schizophrenia Research* 23, 1–13.

de Haan, L., van der Gaag, M. & Wolthaus, J. (2000) Duration of untreated psychosis and the long-term course of schizophrenia. *European Psychiatry* 15, 264–267.

Haas, G.L. & Sweeney, J.A. (1992) Premorbid and onset features of first-episode schizophrenia. *Schizophrenia Bulletin* 18, 373–386.

Haas, G.L., Garratt, L.S. & Sweeney, J.A. (1998) Delay to first antipsychotic medication in schizophrenia: impact on symptomatology and clinical course of illness. *Journal of Psychiatric Research* 32, 151–159.

Häfner, H. (2000) Methodische Probleme der Forschung am Verlauf der Schizophrenie. In: *Methodik von Verlaufs- und Therapiestudien in der Psychiatrie und Psychotherapie* (eds W. Maier, R.R. Engel & H.-U. Möller), pp. 5–18. Hogrefe, Göttingen.

Häfner, H. & an der Heiden, W. (1982) Evaluation gemeindenaher Versorgung psychisch Kranker. *Archiv für Psychiatrie und Nervenkrankheiten* 232, 71–95.

Häfner, H. & an der Heiden, W. (1986) The contribution of European case registers to research on schizophrenia. *Schizophrenia Bulletin* 12, 26–51.

Häfner, H. & an der Heiden, W. (2000) Methodische Probleme der Verlaufsforschung an der Schizophrenie. *Fortschritte der Neurologie, Psychiatrie* 68, 193–205.

Häfner, H. & Kasper, S. (1982) Akute lebensbedrohliche Katatonie: Epidemiologische und klinische Befunde. *Nervenarzt* 53, 385–394.

Häfner, H. & Maurer, K. (1991) Are there two types of schizophrenia? True onset and sequence of positive and negative syndromes prior to first admission. In: *Negative Versus Positive Schizophrenia* (eds A. Marneros, N.C. Andreasen & M.T. Tsuang), pp. 134–159. Springer, Berlin, Heidelberg, New York.

Häfner, H. & Maurer, K. (1997) Klinische Epidemiologie der schizophrenen Negativsymptomatik: viele Fragen, wenig Antworten. In: *Impulse für die klinische Psychologie* (eds B. Rockstroh, T. Elbert & H. Watzl), pp. 43–69. Hogrefe, Göttingen.

Häfner, H., Riecher-Rössler, A., Hambrecht, M. *et al.* (1992) IRAOS: an instrument for the assessment of onset and early course of schizophrenia. *Schizophrenia Research* 6, 209–223.

Häfner, H., Maurer, K., Löffler, W. & Riecher-Rössler, A. (1993) The influence of age and sex on the onset and early course of schizophrenia. *British Journal of Psychiatry* 162, 80–86.

Häfner, H., Maurer, K., Löffler, W. *et al.* (1995) Onset and early course of schizophrenia. In: *Search for the Causes of Schizophrenia*. Vol. III. (eds H. Häfner & W.F. Gattaz), pp. 43–66. Springer, Berlin, Heidelberg, New York.

Häfner, H., Maurer, K., Löffler, W. & Nowotny, B. (1996) Der Fruhverlauf der Schizophrenie. *Zeitschrift für Medizinische Psychologie* 5, 22–31.

Häfner, H., an der Heiden, W., Behrens, S. *et al.* (1998) Causes and consequences of the gender difference in age at onset of schizophrenia. *Schizophrenia Bulletin* 24, 99–113.

Häfner, H., Löffler, W., Maurer, K., Riecher-Rössler, A. & Stein, A. (1999a) *IRAOS: Interview für die retrospektive Erfassung des Krankheitsbeginns und -verlaufs bei Schizophrenie und anderen Psychosen.* Huber, Bern, Göttingen, Toronto.

Häfner, H., Maurer, K., Löffler, W. *et al.* (1999b) Onset and prodromal phase as determinants of the course. In: *Search for the Causes of Schizophrenia*. Vol. IV. *Balance of the Century* (eds W.F. Gattaz & H. Häfner), pp. 35–58. Steinkopff, Darmstadt.

Häfner, H., Löffler, W., Maurer, K., Hambrecht, M. & an der Heiden, W. (1999c) Depression, negative symptoms, social stagnation and social decline in the early course of schizophrenia. *Acta Psychiatrica Scandinavica* 100, 105–118.

Häfner, H., Löffler, W., Riecher-Rössler, A. & Häfner-Ranabauer, W. (2001) Schizophrenie und Wahn im höheren und hohen Lebensalter. *Nervenarzt* 72, 347–357.

Hambrecht, M. & Häfner, H. (1993) 'Trema, Apophänie, Apokalypse' – Ist Conrads Phasenmodell empirisch begründbar? *Fortschritte der Neurologie, Psychiatrie* 61, 418–423.

Hambrecht, M., Maurer, K., Häfner, H. & Sartorius, N. (1992) Transnational stability of gender differences in schizophrenia? An analysis based on the WHO Study on Determinants of Outcome of Severe Mental Disorders. *European Archives of Psychiatry and Clinical Neuroscience* 242, 6–12.

Harding, C.M. (1988) Course types in schizophrenia: an analysis of European and American studies. *Schizophrenia Bulletin* 14, 633–643.

Harding, C.M. & Brooks, G.W. (1984) Life assessment of a cohort of chronic schizophrenics discharged twenty years ago. In: *The Handbook of Longitudinal Research*. Vol. II. (eds S.A. Mednick, M. Harway & K. Finello), pp. 375–393. Praeger, New York.

Harding, C.M., Brooks, G.W., Ashikaga, T., Strauss, J.S. & Breier, A.

(1987a) The Vermont longitudinal study of persons with severe mental illness. I. Methodology, study sample, and overal status 32 years later. *American Journal of Psychiatry* **144**, 718–726.

Harding, C.M., Brooks, G.W., Ashikaga, T., Strauss, J.S. & Breier, A. (1987b) The Vermont longitudinal study of persons with severe mental illness. II. Long-term outcome of subjects who retrospectively met DSM-III criteria for schizophrenia. *American Journal of Psychiatry* **144**, 727–735.

Hargreaves, W.A., Glick, I.D., Drues, J., Showstack, J.A. & Feigenbaum, E. (1977) Short vs. long hospitalization: a prospective controlled study. VI. Two-year follow-up results for schizophrenics. *Archives of General Psychiatry* **34**, 305–311.

Harkavy-Friedman, J.M., Restifo, K., Malaspina, D. *et al.* (1999) Suicidal behavior in schizophrenia: characteristics of individuals who had and had not attempted suicide. *American Journal of Psychiatry* **156**, 1276–1278.

Harrison, G., Croudace, T., Mason, P., Glazebrook, C. & Medley, I. (1996) Predicting the long-term outcome of schizophrenia. *Psychological Medicine* **26**, 697–705.

Harrison, G., Hopper, K., Craig, T. *et al.* (2001) Recovery from psychotic illness: a 15 and 25 year international follow-up study. *British Journal of Psychiatry* **178**, 506–517.

Harvey, P.D., Howanitz, E., Parrella, M., White, L. & Davidson, M. (1998) Symptoms, cognitive functioning, and adaptive skills in geriatric patients with lifelong schizophrenia: a comparison across treatment sites. *American Journal of Psychiatry* **155**, 1080–1086.

Harvey, P.D., Parrella, M., White, L. *et al.* (1999) Convergence of cognitive and adaptive decline in late-life schizophrenia. *Schizophrenia Research* **35**, 77–84.

Hawk, A.B., Carpenter, W.T. & Strauss, J.S. (1975) Diagnostic criteria and 5-year outcome in schizophrenia: a report from the International Pilot Study of Schizophrenia. *Archives of General Psychiatry* **32**, 343–347.

Hegarty, J.D., Baldessarini, R.J., Tohen, M., Waternaux, C. & Oepen, G. (1994) One hundred years of schizophrenia: a meta-analysis of the outcome literature. *American Journal of Psychiatry* **151**, 1409–1416.

an der Heiden, W. (1996) Der Langzeitverlauf der schizophrenen Psychosen: eine Literaturübersicht. *Zeitschrift für Medizinische Psychologie* **5**, 8–21.

an der Heiden, W. & Häfner, H. (2000) The epidemiology of onset and course of schizophrenia. *European Archives of Psychiatry and Clinical Neuroscience* **250**, 292–303.

an der Heiden, W. & Krumm, B. (1991) The course of schizophrenia: some remarks on a yet unsolved problem of data collection. *European Archives of Psychiatry and Clinical Neuroscience* **240**, 303–306.

an der Heiden, W., Krumm, B., Müller, S. *et al.* (1995) Mannheimer Langzeitstudie der Schizophrenie: Erste Ergebnisse zum Verlauf der Erkrankung über 14 Jahre nach stationärer Erstbehandlung. *Nervenarzt* **66**, 820–827.

an der Heiden, W., Krumm, B., Müller, S. *et al.* (1996) Eine prospektive Studie zum Langzeitverlauf schizophrener Psychosen: Ergebnisse der 14-Jahres-Katamnese. *Zeitschrift für Medizinische Psychologie* **5**, 66–75.

Heila, H., Heikkinen, M.E., Isometsa, E.T. *et al.* (1999a) Life events and completed suicide in schizophrenia: a comparison of suicide victims with and without schizophrenia. *Schizophrenia Bulletin* **25**, 519–531.

Heila, H., Isometsa, E.T., Henriksson, M.M. *et al.* (1999b) Suicide victims with schizophrenia in different treatment phases and adequacy of antipsychotic medication. *Journal of Clinical Psychiatry* **60**, 200–208.

Heinrich, K. (1967) Zur Bedeutung des postremissiven Erschöpfungs-Syndroms für die Rehabilitation Schizophrener. *Nervenarzt* **38**, 487–491.

Heinrichs, D.W., Cohen. B.P. & Carpenter, W. T. (1985) Early insight

and the management of schizophrenic decompensation. *Journal of Nervous and Mental Disease* **173**, 133–138.

Helgason, L. (1990) Twenty years' follow-up of first psychiatric presentation for schizophrenia: what would have been prevented? *Acta Psychiatrica Scandinavica* **81**, 231–235.

Helmchen, H. & Hippius, H. (1967) Depressive Syndrome im Verlauf neuroleptischer Therapie. *Nervenarzt* **38**, 455–458.

Helzer, J.E., Robins, L.N., Croughan, J.L. & Welner, A. (1981) Renard Diagnostic Interview: its reliability and procedural validity with physicians and lay interviewers. *Archives of General Psychiatry* **38**, 393–398.

Herz, M.I. & Melville, C. (1980) Relapse in schizophrenia. *Amercian Journal of Psychiatry* **137**, 801–805.

Hirsch, S.R. & Jolley, A.G. (1989) The dysphoric syndrome in schizophrenia and its implications for relapse. *British Journal of Psychiatry* **155** (Suppl. 5), 46–50.

Ho, B.C., Andreasen, N.C., Flaum, M., Nopoulos, P. & Miller, D. (2000) Untreated initial psychosis: its relation to quality of life and symptom remission in first-episode schizophrenia. *American Journal of Psychiatry* **157**, 808–815.

Hoff, A.L., Sakuma, M., Wieneke, M. *et al.* (1999) Longitudinal neuropsychological follow-up study of patients with first-episode schizophrenia. *American Journal of Psychiatry* **156**, 1336–1341.

Hopper, K., Harrison, G., Janca, A. & Sartorius, N. (2000) *Prospects for recovery from schizophrenia – an international investigation: Report from the WHO-Collaborative Project, the International Study of Schizophrenia.* Psychosocial Press, Westport.

Huber, D., Henrich, G. & Herschbach, P. (1988) Measuring the quality of life: a comparison between physically and mentally chronically ill patients and healthy persons. *Pharmacopsychiatria* **21**, 453–455.

Huber, G. (1983) Das Konzept substratnaher Basissymptome und seine Bedeutung für Theorie und Praxis schizophrener Erkrankungen. *Nervenarzt* **54**, 23–32.

Huber, G., Gross, G. & Schüttler, R. (1979) *Schizophrenie: Eine verlaufs- und sozialpsychiatrische Langzeitstudie.* Springer, Berlin.

Hutter, S. (1940) Beitrag zur Prognose der Schizophrenie. *Archiv für Psychiatrie und Nervenkrankheiten* **112**, 562–612.

Isohanni, M., Isohanni, I., Järvelin, M.R. *et al.* (1999) *Childhood and adolescent predictors of schizophrenia.* In: *Psychiatry on new thresholds. Abstracts of the XI World Congress of Psychiatry, Hamburg, August 6–11, 1999* (eds J. López-Ibor, N. Sartorius, W. Gaebel & C. Haasen).

Jablensky, A. (1978) Review of proposed study design. Paper presented at a meeting of investigators at WHO, Genf, February 2, 1978.

Jablensky, A. (1995) Schizophrenia: the epidemiological horizon. In: *Schizophrenia* (eds S.R. Hirsch & D.R. Weinberger), pp. 206–252. Blackwell Science, Oxford.

Jablensky, A. (2000) Symptome schizophrener Störungen. In: *Psychiatrie der Gegenwart.* Vol. 5, 4th edn (eds H. Helmchen, F. Henn, H. Lauter & N. Sartorius), pp. 3–51. Springer, Berlin.

Jablensky, A. & Cole, S.W. (1997) Is the earlier age at onset of schizophrenia in males a confounded finding? Results from a cross-cultural investigation. *British Journal of Psychiatry* **170**, 234–240.

Jablensky, A., Schwarz, R. & Tomov, T. (1980) WHO collaborative study on impairments and disabilities associated with schizophrenic disorders: a preliminary communication: objectives and methods. *Acta Psychiatrica Scandinavica* (Suppl. 285), 152–163.

Jablensky, A., Sartorius, N., Ernberg, G. *et al.* (1992) Schizophrenia: manifestations, incidence and course in different cultures. A World Health Organization Ten-Country Study. *Psychological Medicine* (Suppl. 20).

Jablensky, A., Hugler, H., von Cranach, M. & Kalinov, K. (1993) Kraepelin revisited: a reassessment and statistical analysis of dementia praecox and manic-depressive insanity in 1908. *Psychological Medicine* **23**, 843–858.

Jackson, J.H. (1887) Remarks on the evolution and dissolution of the nervous system. *Journal of Mental Science* **33**, 25–48.

Jansson, B. & Alström, J. (1967) The relation between prognosis, symptoms and background factors in suspected schizophrenic insufficiencies in young people. *Acta Psychiatrica Scandinavica* **43** (Suppl. 198), 1–96.

Jennen-Steinmetz, C., Löffler, W. & Häfner, H. (1997) Demography and age at onset of schizophrenia. *British Journal of Psychiatry* **170**, 485.

Johnson, D.A.W. (1988) The significance of depression in the prediction of relapse in chronic schizophrenia. *British Journal of Psychiatry* **152**, 320–323.

Johnstone, E.C. (1999) Brain imaging and function: the balance of the century. In: *Search for the Causes of Schizophrenia. Vol. IV. Balance of the Century* (eds W.F. Gattaz & H. Häfner), pp. 293–305. Steinkopff Verlag, Darmstadt.

Johnstone, E.C., Frith, C.D., Crow, T.J. *et al.* (1992) The Northwick Park 'Functional' Psychosis Study: diagnosis and outcome. *Psychological Medicine* **22**, 331–346.

Jones, P.B. (1999) Longitudinal approaches to the search of the causes of schizophrenia: past, present and future. In: *Search for the Causes of Schizophrenia Vol IV. Balance of the Century* (eds W.F. Gattaz & H. Häfner), pp. 91–119. Steinkopff Verlag, Darmstadt.

Jones, P.B. & Done, D.J. (1997) From birth to onset: a developmental perspective of schizophrenia in two national birth cohorts. In: *Neurodevelopmental and Adult Psychopathology* (eds M.S. Keshavan & R.M. Murray), pp. 119–136. Cambridge University Press, Cambridge.

Jung, E., Krumm, B., Biehl, H., Maurer, K. & Bauer-Schubart, C. (1989) *DAS – Mannheimer Skala zur Einschätzung sozialer Behinderung.* Beltz, Weinheim.

Kaplan, K.J. & Harrow, M. (1996) Positive and negative symptoms as risk factors for later suicidal activity in schizophrenics. *Suicide and Life Threatening Behaviour* **26**, 105–121.

Katz, M.M. & Lyerly, S.B. (1963) Methods for measuring adjustment and social behavior in the community. I. Rationale, description, discriminative validity, and scale development. *Psychological Reports* **13**, 503–535.

Kay, S.R. & Sevy, S. (1990) Pyramidical model of schizophrenia. *Schizophrenia Bulletin* **16**, 537–545.

Kay, S.R., Fiszbein, A. & Opler, L.A. (1987) The Positive and Negative Syndrome Scale (PANSS) for schizophrenia. *Schizophrenia Bulletin* **13**, 261–276.

Keefe, R.S.E., Harvey, P.D., Lenzenweger, M.F. *et al.* (1992) Empirical assessment of the factorial structure of clinical symptoms in schizophrenia: negative symptoms. *Psychiatry Research* **44**, 153–165.

Kendell, R.E. (1988) Long-term followup studies: a commentary. *Schizophrenia Bulletin* **14**, 663–667.

Kendler, K.S., Gruenberg, A.M. & Tsuang, M.T. (1983) *The specificity of DSM-III schizotypal symptoms.* Proceedings of the 135th Annual Meeting of the American Psychiatric Association, APA, Washington, 1983.

Kendler, K.S., Masterson, C.C., Ungaro, R. & Davis, K.L. (1984) A family history study of schizophrenia-related personality disorders. *American Journal of Psychiatry* **141**, 424–427.

Kendler, K.S., Masterson, C.C. & Davis, K.L. (1985) Psychiatric illness in first-degree relatives of patients with paranoid psychosis, schizophrenia and medical illness. *British Journal of Psychiatry* **147**, 524–531.

Kirkpatrick, B., Buchanan, R.W., McKenney, P.D., Alphs, L.D. & Carpenter, W.T. (1989) The Schedule for the Deficit Syndrome: an instrument for research in schizophrenia. *Psychiatry Research* **30**, 119–123.

Kirkpatrick, B., Amador, X.F., Flaum, M. *et al.* (1996a) The deficit syndrome in the DSM-IV Field Trial. I. Alcohol and other drug abuse. *Schizophrenia Research* **20**, 69–77.

Kirkpatrick, B., Amador, X.F., Yale, S.A. *et al.* (1996b) The deficit syndrome in the DSM-IV Field Trial. II. Depressive episodes and persecutory beliefs. *Schizophrenia Research* **20**, 79–90.

Klosterkötter, J., Schultze-Lutter, F., Gross, G., Huber, G. & Steinmeyer, E.M. (1997) Early self-experienced neuropsychological deficits and subsequent schizophrenic diseases: an 8-year average follow-up prospective study. *Acta Psychiatrica Scandinavica* **95**, 396–404.

Klosterkötter, J., Hellmich, M., Steinmeyer, E.M. & Schultze-Lutter, F. (2001) Diagnosing schizophrenia in the initial prodromal phase. *Archives of General Psychiatry* **58**, 158–164.

Knights, A. & Hirsch, S.R. (1981) 'Revealed' depression and drug treatment for schizophrenia. *Archives of General Psychiatry* **38**, 806–811.

Kohn, M. (1969) *Class and Conformity: a Study of Values.* Dorsey Press, Homewood, IL.

Kolakowska, T., Williams, A.O., Ardern, M. *et al.* (1985) Schizophrenia with good and poor outcome. I. Early clinical features, response to neuroleptics and signs of organic dysfunction. *British Journal of Psychiatry* **146**, 229–239.

Koreen, A.R., Siris, S.G., Chakos, M. *et al.* (1993) Depression in first-episode schizophrenia. *American Journal of Psychiatry* **150** 1643–1648.

Kraepelin, E. (1893) *Psychiatrie: Ein Lehrbuch für Studierende und Ärzte, 4 edn.* Barth, Leipzig.

Kraepelin, E. (1920) Die Erscheinungsformen des Irreseins. *Zeitschrift für die gesamte Neurologie und Psychiatrie* **62**, 1–29.

Krausz, M., Müller-Thomsen, T. & Haasen, C. (1995) Suicide among schizophrenic adolescents in the long-term course of illness. *Psychopathology* **28**, 95–103.

Kumar, S., Thara, R. & Rajkumar, S. (1989) Coping with symptoms of relapse in schizophrenia. *European Archives of Psychiatry and Neurological Science* **239**, 213–215.

Langfeldt, G. (1937) The prognosis in schizophrenia and the factors influencing the course of the disease. *Acta Psychiatrica et Neurologica Scandinavica* (Suppl. XIII).

Larsen, E.B. & Gerlach, J. (1996) Subjective experience of treatment, side-effects, mental state and quality of life in chronic schizophrenic out-patients treated with depot neuroleptics. *Acta Psychiatrica Scandinavica* **93**, 381–388.

Larsen, T.K., Johannessen, J.O. & Opjordsmoen, S. (1998) First-episode schizophrenia with long duration of untreated psychosis: pathways to care. *British Journal of Psychiatry* **172**, 45–52.

Lawrie, S.M. & Abukmeil, S.S. (1998) Brain abnormality in schizophrenia: a systematic and quantitative review of volumetric magnetic resonance imaging studies. *British Journal of Psychiatry* **172**, 110–120.

Leary, J., Johnstone, E.C. & Owens, D.G. (1991) Disabilities and circumstances of schizophrenic patients: a follow-up study. II. Social outcome. *British Journal of Psychiatry* **159** (Suppl. 13), 13–20.

Leff, J.P. (1997) *Care in the Community: Illusion or Reality?* John Wiley & Sons, Chichester.

Leff, J.P., Sartorius, N., Jablensky, A., Korten, A. & Ernberg, G. (1992) The International Pilot Study of Schizophrenia: five-year follow-up findings. *Psychological Medicine* **22**, 131–145.

Lehman, A.F. (1983) The well-being of chronic mental patients: assessing their quality of life. *Archives of General Psychiatry* **40**, 369–373.

Lehman, A.F., Possidente, S. & Hawker, F. (1986) The quality of life of chronic patients in a state hospital and in community residences. *Hospital and Community Psychiatry* **37**, 901–907.

Lenzenweger, M.F. & Dworkin, R.H. (1996) The dimensions of schizophrenia phenomenology: not one or two, at least three, perhaps four. *British Journal of Psychiatry* **168**, 432–440.

Lenzenweger, M.F., Dworkin, R.H. & Wethington, E. (1991) Examining the underlying structure of schizophrenic phenomenology: evidence for a three-process model. *Schizophrenia Bulletin* **17**, 515–524.

Leon, C.A. (1989) Clinical course and outcome of schizophrenia in Cali, Colombia: a 10-year follow-up study. *Journal of Nervous and Mental Disease* **177**, 593–606.

Leonhard, K. (1966) *Aufteilung der Endogenen Psychosen*. Akademie Verlag, Berlin.

Leonhard, K. (1999) *Classification of Endogenous Psychoses and their Differentiated* Etiology. *2nd edn.* Springer, *Berlin, Heidelberg, New York.*

Lewis, S.W. (1990) Computerised tomography in schizophrenia 15 years on. *British Journal of Psychiatry* **157** (Suppl. 9), 16–24.

Liddle, P.F. (1987a) Schizophrenic syndromes, cognitive performance and neurological dysfunction. *Psychological Medicine* **17**, 49–57.

Liddle, P.F. (1987b) The symptoms of chronic schizophrenia: a re-examination of the positive–negative dichotomy. *British Journal of Psychiatry* **151**, 145–151.

Liddle, P.F. (1994) Volition and schizophrenia in psychological medicine. In: *The Neuropsychology of Schizophrenia* (eds A.S. David & J.C. Cutting), pp. 39–49. Lawrence Erlbaum, Hove.

Liddle, P.F. & Barnes, T.R.E. (1990) Syndromes of chronic schizophrenia. *British Journal of Psychiatry* **157**, 558–561.

Lindenmayer, J.P., Kay, S.R. & Opler, L.A. (1984) Positive and negative subtypes in acute schizophrenia. *Comprehensive Psychiatry* **25**, 455–464.

Link, B.G. & Dohrenwend, B.P. (1980) Formulation of hypotheses about the ratio of untreated to treated cases in the true prevalence studies of functional psychiatric disorders in adults in the United States. In: *Mental Illness in the United States: Epidemiological Estimates* (eds B.P. Dohrenwend, B.S. Dohrenwend, G.M. Schwartz *et al.*), pp. 133–149. New York, Praeger.

Linszen, D., Lenior, M., de Haan, L., Dingemans, P. & Gersons, B. (1998) Early intervention, untreated psychosis and the course of early schizophrenia. *British Journal of Psychiatry* **172** (Suppl. 33), 84–89.

Loebel, A.D., Lieberman, J.A., Alvir, J.M.J. *et al.* (1992) Duration of psychosis and outcome in first-episode schizophrenia. *American Journal of Psychiatry* **149**, 1183–1188.

Loranger, A.W. (1990) The impact of DSM-III on diagnostic practice in a university hospital: a comparison of DSM-II and DSM-III in 10 914 patients. *Archives of General Psychiatry* **47**, 672–675.

Lorr, M., Klett, C.J. & McNair, D.M. (1963) *Syndromes of Psychosis*. Pergamon Press, New York.

Löffler, W. & Häfner, H. (1999) Dimensionen der schizophrenen Symptomatik: Vergleichende Modellprüfung an einem Erstepisodensample. *Nervenarzt* **70**, 416–429.

Lubin, A., Gieseking, G.F. & Williams, H.L. (1962) Direct measurement of cognitive deficit in schizophrenia. *Journal of Consulting and Clinical Psychology* **26**, 139–143.

Mahendra, B. (1981) Where have all the catatonics gone? *Psychological Medicine* **11**, 669–671.

Malm, U., May, P.R.A. & Dencker, S.J. (1981) Evaluation of the quality of life of the schizophrenic outpatient: a checklist. *Schizophrenia Bulletin* **7**, 477–487.

Malmberg, A., Lewis, G., David, A. & Allebeck, P. (1998) Premorbid adjustment and personality in people with schizophrenia. *British Journal of Psychiatry* **172**, 308–313.

Marengo, J.T., Harrow, M., Sands, J. & Galloway, C. (1991) European versus US data on the course on schizophrenia. *American Journal of Psychiatry* **148**, 606–611.

Marneros, A., Rohe, A., Deister, A. & Risse, A. (1986) Schizoaffective disorders: the prognostic value of the affective component. In: *Schizoaffective Psychoses* (eds A. Marneros & M.T. Tsuang), pp. 155–163. Springer, Berlin.

Marneros, A., Deister, A. & Rohde, A. (1991) *Affektive, schizoaffektive und schizophrene Psychosen: Eine vergleichende Langzeitstudie.* Springer, Berlin.

Marneros, A., Rohde, A. & Deister, A. (1995) Psychotic continuum under longitudinal considerations. In: *Psychotic Continuum* (eds A. Marneros, N.C. Andreasen & M.T. Tsuang), pp. 17–30. Springer, Berlin.

Mason, P., Harrison, G., Glazebrook, C., Medley, I., Dalkin, T. & Croudace, T. (1995) Characteristics of outcome in schizophrenia at 13 years. *British Journal of Psychiatry* **167**, 596–603.

Mason, P., Harrison, G., Glazebrook, C., Medley, I. & Croudace, T. (1996) The course of schizophrenia over 13 years: a report from the International Study on Schizophrenia (ISoS) coordinated by the World Health Organization. *British Journal of Psychiatry* **169**, 580–586.

Maurer, K. (1995) *Der geschlechtsspezifische Verlauf der Schizophrenie über 10 Jahre.* Dr Kovac, Hamburg.

Maurer, K. & Biehl, H. (1988) Klinikaufenthalte und produktive Rückfälle bei ersterkrankten Schizophrenen: Determinanten des Zeitverlaufs zwischen stationären Aufnahmen bzw. schizophrenen Reziduven über fünf Jahre. *Nervenheilkunde* **7**, 279–290.

Maurer, K. & Häfner, H. (1991) Dependence, independence or interdependence of positive and negative symptoms. In: *Negative Versus Positive Schizophrenia* (eds A. Marneros, N.C. Andreasen & M.T. Tsuang), pp. 160–182. Springer, Berlin.

Maurer, K. & Häfner, H. (1995) Methodological aspects of onset assessment in schizophrenia. *Schizophrenia Research* **15**, 265–276.

Maurer, K. & Häfner, H. (1997) Die retrospektive Erfassung der Negativsymptomatik im Frühverlauf der Schizophrenie. In: *Negativsymptomatik bei Schizophrenie* (ed. H. Gerbaldo), pp. 13–29. Steinkopff Verlag, Darmstadt.

Maurer, K., Häfner, H. & Löffler, W. (1993) The influence of age and gender on schizophrenic syndromes over three years: results from the Mannheim ABC Schizophrenia Study. Poster presented at the WPA Symposium Changing the course and outcome of mental disorders, Groningen, September 1–3, 1993.

Mayer-Gross, W. (1932) Die Klinik [der Schizophrenie]. In: *Handbuch der Geisteskrankheiten. Band IX, Spezieller Teil V: Die Schizophrenie* (ed. O. Bumke), p. 293–578. Springer, Berlin.

Maziade, M., Bouchard, S., Gingras, N. *et al.* (1996) Long-term st ability of diagnosis and symptom dimensions in a systematic sample of patients with onset of schizophrenia in childhood and early adolescence. II. Postitive–negative distinction and childhood predictors of adult outcome. *British Journal of Psychiatry* **169**, 371–378.

McEvoy, J.P., Schooler, N.R. & Wilson, W.H. (1991) Predictors of therapeutic response to haloperidol in acute schizophrenia. *Psychopharmacology Bulletin* **27**, 97–101.

McGlashan, T.H. (1984a) The Chestnut Lodge follow-up study. I. Follow-up methodology and study sample. *Archives of General Psychiatry* **41**, 573–585.

McGlashan, T.H. (1984b) The Chestnut Lodge follow-up study. II. Long-term outcome of schizophrenia and the affective disorders. *Archives of General Psychiatry* **41**, 586–601.

McGlashan, T.H. (1986) The prediction of outcome in chronic schizophrenia. IV. The Chestnut Lodge follow-up study. *Archives of General Psychiatry* **43**, 167–176.

McGlashan, T.H. (1988) A selective review of recent North American long-term followup studies of schizophrenia. *Schizophrenia Bulletin* **14**, 515–542.

McGlashan, T.H. (1998) Early detection and intervention of schizophrenia: rationale and research. *British Journal of Psychiatry* **172** (Suppl. 33), 3–6.

McGlashan, T.H. & Carpenter, W.T. (1976) Postpsychotic depression in schizophrenia. *Archives of General Psychiatry* **33**, 231–239.

McGlashan, T.H. & Johannessen, J.O. (1996) Early detection and intervention with schizophrenia: rationale. *Schizophrenia Bulletin* **22**, 201–222.

McGorry, P.D., Edwards, J., Mihalopoulos, C., Harrigan, S.M. & Jackson, H.J. (1996) EPPIC: An evolving system of early detection and optimal management. *Schizophrenia Bulletin* **22**, 305–326.

McGuffin, P., Katz, R. & Aldrich, J. (1986) Past and Present State Examination: the assessment of 'lifetime ever psychopathology. *Psychological Medicine* **16**, 461–465.

McGuffin, P., Farmer, A.E. & Gottesman, I.I. (1987) Is there really a split in schizophrenia? The genetic evidence. *British Journal of Psychiatry* **150**, 581–592.

Mechanic, D., McAlpine, D., Rosenfield, S. & Davis, D. (1994) Effects of illness attribution and depression on the quality of life among persons with serious mental illness. *Social Science and Medicine* **39**, 155–164.

Michaelos, A.L. (1980) Satisfaction and happiness. *Social Indicators Research* **8**, 385–422.

Miles, C.P. (1977) Conditions predisposing to suicide: a review. *Journal of Nervous and Mental Disease* **164**, 231–246.

Miller, T.J., McGlashan, T.H., Woods, S.W. *et al.* (1999) Symptom assessment in schizophrenic prodromal states. *Psychiatric Quarterly* **70**, 273–287.

Mimica, N. (1996) Schizophrenia and its catatonic subtype instability during long-term follow-up. *Schizophrenia Research* **18**, 118.

Mimica, N., Folnegovic-Smalc, V. & Folnegovic, Z. (2001) Catatonic schizophrenia in Croatia. *European Archives of Psychiatry and Neurological Sciences* **251** (Suppl. 1), 17–20.

Minas, I.H., Klimidis, S., Stuart, G.W., Copolov, D.L. & Singh, B.S. (1994) Positive and negative symptoms in the psychoses: principal component analysis of items from the Scale of the Assessment of Positive Symptoms and the Scale for the Assessment of Negative Symptoms. *Comprehensive Psychiatry* **35**, 135–144.

Monking, H.S., Staroste, A. & Buiker, B.M. (1996) Über die soziale Situation schizophrener Patienten im Verlauf einer 8-Jahres-Katamnese und die Bedeutung von Angehörigen für die psychosoziale Integration. [The social status of schizophrenic patients during the course of 8 years catamnesis and significance of relatives for psychosocial integration]. *Psychiatrische Praxis* **23**, 282–284.

Möller, H.-J. & von Zerssen, D. (1995) Course and outcome of schizophrenia. In: *Schizophrenia* (eds S.R. Hirsch & D.R. Weinberger), pp. 106–127. Blackwell Science, Oxford.

Möller, H.-J., von Zerssen, D., Werner-Eilert, K. & Wüschner-Stockheim, M. (1982) Outcome in schizophrenia and similar paranoid psychosis. *Schizophrenia Bulletin* **8**, 99–108.

Möller, H.-J., Scharl, W. & von Zerssen, D. (1984) Strauss-Carpenter-Skala: Überprüfung ihres prognostischen Wertes für das 5-Jahres-'Outcome' schizophrener Patienten. *European Archives of Psychiatry and Neurological Sciences* **234**, 112–117.

Möller, H.-J., Schmid-Bode, W. & von Zerssen, D. (1986) Prediction of long-term outcome in schizophrenia by prognostic scales. *Schizophrenia Bulletin* **12**, 225–235.

Möller, H.-J., Schmid-Bode, W., Cording-Tommel, C. *et al.* (1988) Psychopathological and social outcome in schizophrenia versus affective/schizoaffective psychoses and prediction of poor outcome in schizophrenia: results from a 5–8 year follow-up. *Acta Psychiatrica Scandinavica* **77**, 379–389.

Mueser, K.T. & Tarrier, N. (1998) *Handbook of Social Functioning in Schizophrenia*. Allyn Bacon, Boston.

Mueser, K.T., Yarnold, P.R., Levinson, D.F. *et al.* (1990) Prevalence of substance abuse in schizophrenia: demographic and clinical correlates. *Schizophrenia Bulletin* **16**, 31–56.

Mueser, K.T., Bellack, A.S. & Blanchard, J.J. (1992a) Comorbidity of schizophrenia and substance abuse: implications for treatment. *Journal of Consulting and Clinical Psychology* **60**, 845–856.

Mueser, K.T., Yarnold, P.R. & Bellack, A.S. (1992b) Diagnostic and demographic correlates of substance abuse in schizophrenia and major affective disorder. *Acta Psychiatrica Scandinavica* **85**, 48–55.

Murray, R.M. (1994) Neurodevelopmental schizophrenia: the rediscovery of dementia praecox. *British Journal of Psychiatry* (Suppl. 5), 6–12.

Müller, P., Guenther, U. & Lohmeyer, J. (1986) Behandlung und Verlauf schizophrener Psychosen über ein Jahrzehnt. *Nervenarzt* **57**, 332–341.

Nair, T.R., Christensen, J.D., Kingsbury, S.J. *et al.* (1997) Progression of cerebroventricular enlargement and the subtyping of schizophrenia. *Psychiatry Research* **74**, 141–150.

Norman, R.M. & Malla, A.K. (2001) Duration of untreated psychosis: a critical examination of the concept and its importance. *Psychological Medicine* **31**, 381–400.

Norman, R.M., Malla, A.K., Morrison-Stewart, S.L. *et al.* (1997) Neuropsychological correlates of syndromes in schizophrenia. *British Journal of Psychiatry* **170**, 134–139.

Nuechterlein, K.H. & Dawson, M.E. (1984) A heuristic vulnerability/stress model of schizophrenic episodes. *Schizophrenia Bulletin* **10**, 300–312.

Ogawa, K., Miya, M., Watarai, A. *et al.* (1987) A long-term follow-up study of schizophrenia in Japan: with special reference to the course of social adjustment. *British Journal of Psychiatry* **151**, 758–765.

Ohta, Y., Nagata, K., Yoshitake, K. *et al.* (1990) Changes in negative symptoms of schizophrenic patients two years later. *Japanese Journal of Psychiatry and Neurology* **44**, 521–529.

Oliver, J.P. & Mohamad, H. (1992) The quality of life of the chronically mentally ill: a comparison of public, private and voluntary residential provisions. *British Journal of Social Work* **22**, 391–404.

Opjordsmoen, S. (1998) Delusional disorders. I. Comparative long-term outcome. *Acta Psychiatrica Scandinavica* **80**, 603–612.

Osby, U., Correia, N., Brandt, L., Ekbom, A. & Sparen, P. (2000) Mortality and causes of death in schizophrenia in Stockholm county, Sweden. *Schizophrenia Research* **45**, 21–28.

Overall, J.E. & Gorham, D.R. (1962) The Brief Psychiatric Rating Scale. *Psychological Reports* **10**, 799–812.

Ødegård, Ø. (1964) Patterns of discharge from Norwegian psychiatric hospitals before and after the introduction of psychotropic drugs. *American Journal of Psychiatry* **120**, 772–778.

Paulsen, J.S., Heaton, R.K., Sadek, J.R. *et al.* (1995) The nature of learning and memory impairments in schizophrenia. *Journal of the International Neuropsychological Society* **1**, 88–99.

Peralta, V., de Leon, J. & Cuesta, M.J. (1992) Are there more than two syndromes in schizophrenia? A critique of the positive–negative dichotomy. *British Journal of Psychiatry* **161**, 335–343.

Peralta, V., Cuesta, M.J. & de Leon, J. (1994) An empirical analysis of latent structures underlying schizophrenic symptoms. *Biological Psychiatry* **36**, 726–736.

Pfuhlmann, B. & Stöber, G. (2001) The different conceptions of catatonia: historical overview and critical discussion. *European Archives of Psychiatry and Clinical Neuroscience* **251** (Suppl. 1). 1–4.

Pietzcker, A. & Gaebel, W. (1983) Prediction of 'natural' course, relapse and prophylactic response in schizophrenic patients. *Pharmacopsychiatria* **16**, 206–211.

Pogue-Geile, M.F. & Harrow, M. (1985) Negative symptoms in schizophrenia: their longitudinal course and prognostic significance. *Schizophrenia Bulletin* 11, 427–439.

Priebe, S., Gruyters, T., Heinze, M., Hoffmann, C. & Jäkel, A. (1995) Subjektive Evaluationskriterien in der psychiatrischen Versorgung: Erhebungsmethoden für Forschung und Praxis. *Psychiatrische Praxis* 22, 140–144.

Rabinowitz, J., Reichenberg, A., Weiser, M. *et al.* (2000) Cognitive and behavioural functioning in men with schizophrenia both before and shortly after first admission to hospital: cross-sectional analysis. *British Journal of Psychiatry* 177, 26–32.

Rakfeldt, J. & McGlashan, T.H. (1996) Onset, course, and outcome of schizophrenia. *Current Opinion in Psychiatry* 9, 73–76.

Ram, R., Bromet, E.J., Eaton, W.W., Pato, C. & Schwartz, J.E. (1992) The natural course of schizophrenia: a review of first admission studies. *Schizophrenia Bulletin* 18, 185–217.

Rennie, T.A.C. (1939) Follow-up study of five hundred patients with schizophrenia admitted to the hospital from 1913 to 1923. *Archives of Neurology and Psychiatry* 42, 877–891.

Rey, E.R., Bailer, J., Bräuer, W. *et al.* (1994) Stability trends and longitudinal correlations of negative and positive syndromes within a three-year follow-up of initially hospitalized schizophrenics. *Acta Psychiatrica Scandinavica* 90, 405–412.

Reynolds, J.R. (1858) On the pathology of convulsions, with special reference to those of children. *Liverpool Medical and Chirurgical Journal* 2, 1–14.

Riecher-Rössler, A. & Rössler, W. (1998) The course of schizophrenic psychoses: what do we really know? A selective review from an epidemiological perspective. *European Archives of Psychiatry and Clinical Neuroscience* 248, 189–202.

Robins, L.N. (1979) Longitudinal methods in the study of normal and pathological development. In: *Psychiatrie der Gegenwart. Forschung und Praxis, Grundlagen und Methoden der Psychiatrie, Bd.I* (eds K.P. Kisker, J.-E. Meyer, C. Müller & E. Strömgren), pp. 627–684. Springer, Berlin.

Robins, L.N., Helzer, J.E., Croughan, J.L., Williams, J.B.W. & Spitzer, R.L. (1981) *NIMH Diagnostic Interview Schedule: Version III.* National Institute of Mental Health, Washington.

Robins, L.N., Helzer, J.E., Ratcliff, K.S. & Seyfried, W. (1982) Validity of the Diagnostic Interview Schedule, Version II: DSM-III diagnosis. *Psychological Medicine* 12, 855–870.

Robinson, D.G., Woerner, M.G., Alvir, J.M. *et al.* (1999a) Predictors of relapse following response from a first episode of schizophrenia or schizoaffective disorder. *Archives of General Psychiatry* 56, 241–247.

Robinson, D.G., Woerner, M.G., Alvir, J.M. *et al.* (1999b) Predictors of treatment response from a first episode of schizophrenia or schizoaffective disorder. *American Journal of Psychiatry* 156, 544–549.

Roy, A. (1986) Suicide in schizophrenia. In: *Suicide* (ed. A. Roy), pp. 97–112. Williams & Wilkins, Baltimore, MD.

Rudnick, A. & Kravetz, S. (2001) The relation of social support-seeking to quality of life in schizophrenia. *Journal of Nervous and Mental Disease* 189, 258–262.

Rund, B.R. (1998) A review of longitudinal studies of cognitive functions in schizophrenia patients. *Schizophrenia Bulletin* 24, 425–435.

Rund, B.R., Landro, N.I. & Orbeck, A.L. (1997) Stability in cognitive dysfunctions in schizophrenic patients. *Psychiatry Research* 69, 131–141.

Rupp, C. & Fletcher, E.K. (1940) A five to ten year follow-up study of 641 schizophrenic cases. *American Journal of Psychiatry* 86, 877–888.

Salokangas, R.K.R. (1978) *Psychosocial prognosis in schizophrenia.* Annales Universitatis Turkuensis, Turun Yliopisto, Turku.

Salokangas, R.K.R. (1997) Structure of schizophrenic symptomatology and its changes over time: prospective factor-analytical study. *Acta Psychiatrica Scandinavica* 95, 32–39.

Salokangas, R.K.R. Stengard, E., Rääköläinen, V. & Kaljonen, I.A.H. (1987) *New schizophrenic patients and their families [English summary].* In: *Reports of Psychiatria Fennica* 78, pp. 119–216. Foundation for Psychiatric Research in Finland.

Salokangas, R.K.R., Honkonen, T. & Stengard, E. (1999) *Discharged schizophrenic patients in the community: implications for service development* [Abstract]. *WPA Section Symposium From Epidemiology to Clinical Practice, Turku/Finland, August 1–4, 1999.*

Sartorius, N., Jablensky, A. & Shapiro, R.W. (1977) Two-year follow-up of the patients included in the WHO International Pilot Study of Schizophrenia. *Psychological Medicine* 7, 529–541.

Sartorius, N., Jablensky, A., Korten, A. *et al.* (1986) Early manifestation and first-contact incidence of schizophrenia in different cultures: a preliminary report on the initial evaluation phase of the WHO Collaborative Study on determinants of outcome of severe mental disorders. *Psychological Medicine* 16, 909–928.

Sartorius, N., Jablensky, A., Ernberg, G. *et al.* (1987) Course of schizophrenia in different countries: some results of a WHO international comparative 5-year follow-up study. In: *Search for the Causes of Schizophrenia* Vol. I, (eds H. Häfner, W.F. Gattaz & W. Janzarik), Springer, Berlin, Heidelberg, New York, pp. 107–113.

Sartorius, N., Gulbinat, W.H. Harrison, G., Laska, E. & Siegel, C. (1996) Long-term follow-up of schizophrenia in 16 countries: a description of the International Study of Schizophrenia conducted by the World Health Organization. *Social Psychiatry and Psychiatric Epidemiology* 31, 249–258.

Saykin, A.J., Shtasel, D.L., Gur, R.E. *et al.* (1994) Neuropsychological deficits in neuroleptic naive patients with first-episode schizophrenia. *Archives of General Psychiatry* 51, 124–131.

Schmid, G.B., Stassen, H.H., Gross, G., Huber, G. & Angst, J. (1991) Long-term prognosis of schizophrenia. *Psychopathology* 24, 130–140.

Schubart, C., Schwarz, R., Krumm, B. & Biehl, H. (1986) *Schizophrenie und Soziale Anpassung.* Springer, Berlin.

Schwartzmann, A.E. & Douglas, V.I. (1962) Intellectual loss in schizophrenia, part II. *Canadian Journal of Psychology* 16, 161–168.

Scottish Schizophrenia Research Group (1992) The Scottish first episode schizophrenia study. VIII. Five-year follow-up: clinical and psychosocial findings. The Scottish Schizophrenia Research Group. *British Journal of Psychiatry* 161, 496–500.

Scully, P.J., Coakley, G., Kinsella, A. & Waddington, J.L. (1997) Psychopathology, executive (frontal) and general cognitive impairment in relation to duration of initially untreated versus subsequently treated psychosis in chronic schizophrenia. *Psychological Medicine* 27, 1303–1310.

Selten, J.-P., Wiersma, D. & van den Bosch, J. (2000) Clinical predictors of discrepancy between self-ratings and examiner ratings for negative symptoms. *Comprehensive Psychiatry* 41, 191–196.

Sheldrick, C., Jablensky, A., Sartorius, N. & Shepherd, M. (1977) Schizophrenia succeeded by affective illness; catamnestic study and statistical enquiry. *Psychological Medicine* 7, 619–624.

Shepherd, M., Watt, D., Falloon, I.R.H. & Smeeton, N. (1989) The natural history of schizophrenia: a five-year follow-up study of outcome and prediction in a representative sample of schizophrenics. *Psychological Medicine* (Suppl. 15).

Shtasel, D.L., Gur, R.E., Gallacher, F. *et al.* (1992) Phenomenology and functioning in first-episode schizophrenia. *Schizophrenia Bulletin* 18, 449–462.

Silverman, D. (1941) Prognosis in schizophrenia; a study of 271 cases. *Psychiatric Quarterly* 15, 477–493.

Sobizack, N., Albus, M., Hubmann, W. *et al.* (1999)

Neuropsychologische Defizite bei ersterkrankten schizophrenen Patienten. *Nervenarzt* **70**, 408–415.

Spitzer, R.L., Endicott, J. & Robins, E. (1978) Research Diagnostic Criteria – rationale and reliability. *Archives of General Psychiatry* **35**, 773–782.

Stephens, J.H. (1970) Long-term course and prognosis in schizophrenia. *Seminars in Psychiatry* **2**, 464–485.

Stephens, J.H., Ota, K.Y. & Carpenter, W.T. (1980) Diagnostic criteria for schizophrenia: prognostic implications and diagnostic overlap. *Psychiatry Research* **2**, 1–12.

Stoll, A.L., Tohen, M., Baldessarini, R.J. *et al.* (1993) Shifts in diagnostic frequencies of schizophrenia and major affective disorders at six North American psychiatric hospitals, 1972–88. *American Journal of Psychiatry* **150**, 1668–1673.

Stöber, G. & Ungvari, G.S. (2001) Catatonia: a new focus of research. *European Archives of Psychiatry and Clinical Neuroscience* **251** (Suppl. 1).

Stöber, G., Saar, K., Rüschendorf, F. *et al.* (2000) Splitting schizophrenia: periodic catatonia-susceptibility locus on chromosome 15q15. *American Journal of Human Genetics* **67**, 1201–1207.

Strauss, J.S. & Carpenter, W.T. (1972) The prediction of outcome in schizophrenia. I. Characteristics of outcome. *Archives of General Psychiatry* **27**, 739–746.

Strauss, J.S. & Carpenter, W.T. (1974) Characteristic symptoms and outcome in schizophrenia. *Archives of General Psychiatry* **30**, 429–434.

Strauss, J.S. & Carpenter, W.T. (1977) The prediction of outcome in schizophrenia. III. Five-year outcome and its predictors. *Archives of General Psychiatry* **34**, 159–163.

Sullivan, G., Wells, K.B. & Leake, B. (1992) Clinical factors associated with better quality of life in a seriously mentally ill population. *Hospital and Community Psychiatry* **43**, 794–798.

Süllwold, L. (1977) *Symptome Schizophrener Erkrankungen*. Springer, Berlin.

Szymanski, S.R. Cannon, T.D., Gallacher, F., Erwin, R.J. & Gur, R.E. (1996) Course of treatment response in first-episode and chronic schizophrenia. *American Journal of Psychiatry* **153**, 519–525.

Tamminga, C.A., Buchanan, R.W. & Gold, J.M. (1998) The role of negative symptoms and cognitive dysfunction in schizophrenia outcome. *International Clinical Psychopharmacology* **13** (Suppl. 3), 21–26.

Tandon, R. & Greden, J.F. (1991) Negative symptoms of schizophrenia: the need for conceptual clarity. *Biological Psychiatry* **30**, 321–325.

Tarrier, N., Barraclough, C. & Bamrah, J.S. (1997) Prodromal signs of relapse in schizophrenia. *Social Psychiatry and Psychiatric Epidemiology* **26**, 157–161.

Thara, R., Henrietta, M., Joseph, A., Rajkumar, S. & Eaton, W.W. (1994) Ten-year course of schizophrenia: the Madras longitudinal study. *Acta Psychiatrica Scandinavica* **90**, 329–336.

Thornicroft, G. & Johnson, S. (1996) True versus treated prevalence of psychosis: the Prism Case Identification Study. *European Psychiatry* **11** (Suppl. 4), 185.

Tohen, M., Stoll, A.L., Strakowski, S.M. *et al.* (1992) The McLean First-Episode Psychosis Project: six-month recovery and recurrence outcome. *Schizophrenia Bulletin* **18**, 273–282.

Toomey, R., Kremen, W.S., Simpson, J.C. *et al.* (1997) Revisiting the factor structure for positive and negative symptoms: evidence from a large heterogeneous group of psychiatric patients. *American Journal of Psychiatry* **154**, 371–377.

Tsoi, W.F. & Wong, K.E. (1991) A 15-year follow-up study of Chinese schizophrenic patients. *Acta Psychiatrica Scandinavica* **84**, 217–220.

Tsuang, M.T., Gilbertson, M.W. & Faraone, S.V. (1991) Genetic transmission of negative and positive symptomes in the biological relatives of schizophrenics. In: *Negative Versus Positive Schizophrenia* (eds A.

Marneros, N.C. Andreasen & M.T. Tsuang), pp. 265–291. Springer, Berlin, Heidelberg, New York.

Varma, V.K., Malhotra, S. & Yao, E.S. (1996) Course and outcome of acute non-organic psychotic states. *Indian Psychiatric Quarterly* **67**, 195–207.

Vazquez-Barquero, J.L., Cuesta-Nunez, M.J., de la Varga, M. *et al.* (1995) The Cantabria first episode schizophrenia study: a summary of general findings. *Acta Psychiatrica Scandinavica* **91**, 156–162.

Vita, A., Dieci, M., Giobbio, G.M. *et al.* (1991) CT scan abnormalities and outcome of chronic schizophrenia. *American Journal of Psychiatry* **148**, 1577–1579.

von Korff, M., Nestadt, G., Romanoski, A. *et al.* (1985) Prevalence of treated and untreated DSM-III schizophrenia: results of a two-stage community survey. *Journal of Nervous and Mental Disease* **173**, 577–581.

von Zerssen, D. & Hecht, H. (1987) Gesundheit, Glück, Zufriedenheit im Lichte einer katamnestischen Erhebung an psychiatrischen Patienten und gesunden Probanden. *Psychotherapie und Medizinische Psychologie* **37**, 83–96.

Waddington, J.L., Youssef, H.A. & Kinsella, A. (1995) Sequential cross-sectional and 10 year prospective study of severe negative symptoms in relation to duration of initially untreated psychosis in chronic schizophrenia. *Psychological Medicine* **25**, 849–857.

Warner, R. (1985) *Recovery from Schizophrenia: Psychiatry and Political Economy.* Routledge & Kegan Paul, London, Boston, Henley.

Watt, D.C., Katz, K. & Shepherd, M. (1983) The natural history of schizophrenia: a 5-year prospective follow-up of a representative sample of schizophrenics by means of a standardized clinical and social assessment. *Psychological Medicine* **13**, 663–670.

Weber, I. (1997) *Die Lebenszufriedenheit einer Kohorte Schizophrener 15, 5 Jahre nach stationärer Erstaufnahme.* Doctoral dissertation, Fakultät für Klinische Medizin Mannheim der Ruprecht-Karls-Universität Heidelberg.

Weickert, T.W. & Goldberg, T.E. (2000) Neuropsychologie der Schizophrenie. In: *Psychiatrie der Gegenwart. Vol 5, 4th edn* (eds H. Helmchen, F. Henn, H. Lauter & N. Sartorius), pp. 163–180. Springer, Berlin, Heidelberg, New York.

Weickert, T.W. Goldberg, T.E. Gold, J.M., Bigelow, L.B., Egan, M.F. & Weinberger, D.R. (2000) Cognitive impairments in patients with schizophrenia displaying preserved and compromised intellect. *Archives of General Psychiatry* **57**, 907–913.

Weinberger, D.R. (1995) Schizophrenia as a neurodevelopmental disorder. In: *Schizophrenia* (eds S.R. Hirsch & D.R. Weinberger) pp. 293–323. Blackwell, Oxford.

White, L., Harvey, P.D., Opler, L. & Lindenmayer, J.P. (1997) Empirical assessment of the factorial structure of clinical symptoms in schizophrenia: a multisite, multimodel evaluation of the factorial structure of the Positive and Negative Syndrome Scale. The PANSS Study Group. *Psychopathology* **30**, 263–274.

Whiteford, H.A. & Peabody, C.A. (1989) The differential diagnosis of negative symptoms in chronic schizophrenia. *Australian and New Zealand Journal of Psychiatry* **23**, 491–496.

WHO (1973) *The International Pilot Study of Schizophrenia. Vol. 1.* WHO, Geneva.

WHO (1977) *Past History and Sociodemographic Description Schedule (PHSD), 3rd draft.* WHO, Geneva.

WHO (1978a) *Mental Disorders: Glossary and Guide to Their Classification in Accordance with the Ninth Revision of the International Classification of Diseases.* WHO, Geneva.

WHO (1978b) *Psychiatric and Personal History Schedule.* WHO 5365 MNH (10/78), Geneva.

WHO (1979) *Schizophrenia: An International Follow-Up Study.* Wiley, New York.

WHO (1980) *Follow-up History and Sociodemographic Description Schedule (FU-HSD)*. WHO, Geneva.

WHO (1988) *Psychiatric Disability Assessment Schedule (WHO/DAS)*. WHO, Geneva.

WHO (1992) *Life Chart Schedule*. WHO, Geneva.

WHO (1993) *The ICD-10 Classification of Mental and Behavioural disorders: Diagnostic Criteria for Research*. WHO, Geneva.

WHO (1998) The World Health Organization Quality of Life Assessment (WHOQOL): development and general psychometric properties. *Social Science and Medicine* **46**, 1569–1585.

Wiersma, D., Giel, R., de Jong, A., Nienhuis, F.J. & Slooff, C.J. (1996) Assessment of the need for care 15 years after onset of a Dutch cohort of patients with schizophrenia, and an international comparison. *Social Psychiatry and Psychicatric Epidemiology* **31**, 114–121.

Wiersma, D., Nienhuis, F.J., Slooff, C.J. & Giel, R. (1998) Natural course of schizophrenic disorders: a 15-year followup of a Dutch incidence cohort. *Schizophrenia Bulletin* **24**, 75–85.

Wiersma, D., Wanderling, J., Dragomirecka, E. *et al.* (2000) Social disability in schizophrenia: its development and prediction over 15 years in incidence cohorts in six European centres. *Psychological Medicine* **30**, 1155–1167.

Wig, N.N. & Parhee, R. (1989) Acute and transient psychoses: a view from the developing countries. In: *International Classification in Psychiatry: Unity and Diversity* (eds J.E. Mezzich & M. Cranach), pp. 115–121. Cambridge University Press, Cambridge.

Wilkinson, D.G. (1982) The suicide rate in schizophrenia. *British Journal of Psychiatry* **140**, 138–141.

Wing, J.K. (1962) Institutionalism in mental hospitals. *British Journal of Social and Clinical Psychology* **1**, 38–51.

Wing, J.K. & Brown, G.W. (1970) *Institutionalism and Schizophrenia: A Comparative Study of Three Mental Hospitals 1960–1968*. Cambridge University Press, London.

Wing, J.K., Cooper, J.E. & Sartorius, N. (1974) *Measurement and Classification of Psychiatric Symptoms*. Cambridge University Press, London.

Woods, B.T. (1998) Is schizophrenia a progressive neurodevelopmental disorder? Toward a unitary pathogenetic mechanism. *American Journal of Psychiatry* **155**, 1661–1670.

Wyatt, R.J. & Henter, I.D. (1998) The effects of early and sustained intervention on the long-term morbidity of schizophrenia. *Journal of Psychiatric Research* **32**, 169–177.

Yung, A.R. & McGorry, P.D. (1996) The prodromal phase of first-episode psychosis: past and current conceptualizations. *Schizophrenia Bulletin* **22**, 353–370.

Yung, A.R. Phillips, L.J., McGorry, P.D. *et al.* (1998) Prediction of psychosis: a step towards indicated prevention of schizophrenia. *British Journal of Psychiatry* **172** (Suppl. 33), 14–20.

Zimmerman, M., Coryell, W., Pfohl, B. & Stangl, D. (1988) The reliability of the Family History Method for psychiatric diagnosis. *Archives of General Psychiatry* **45**, 320–322.

9 Depression and schizophrenia

S.G. Siris and C. Bench

Incidence and prevalence of 'depression' in schizophrenia, 143
Differential diagnosis of depression in schizophrenia, 143
  Organic factors, 143
  Neuroleptic-induced dysphoria, 143
  Akinesia and akathisia, 150
  Negative symptoms, 150
  Disappointment reactions, 151
  Prodrome of psychotic relapse, 151
  Schizoaffective disorder, 151
  Independent diathesis for depression, 151
Clinical validation of depression in schizophrenia, 152
  Prognosis, 152

Suicide, 152
Life events, 152
Biological validation of depression in schizophrenia, 152
  Brain structure and function, 153
  Endocrine and biochemical measures, 154
  Genetic studies, 154
Treatment implications, 155
  Antipsychotic medications, 155
  Antidepressant medications, 156
  Lithium, 160
  Psychosocial interventions, 160
Conclusions, 160
References, 160

Kraeplin's astute separation, over 100 years ago, of what we now know as mood disorders from what we now know as schizophrenia forms the conceptual basis of much of modern psychiatric nosology. Nevertheless, the fact remains, and has been noted for many years, that a substantial proportion of patients with schizophrenia, no matter how defined, suffer from 'depression-like' symptomatology during the longitudinal course of their disorder.

Early on, Bleuler noted that symptoms of depression often occur during the course of schizophrenia (Bleuler 1950). Later, in the middle years of the twentieth century, the concept of depression in schizophrenia became largely steeped in psychoanalytically influenced writings. Mayer-Gross discussed depression in schizophrenia as being a denial of the future or a reaction of despair to the psychotic experience (McGlashan & Carpenter 1976a). Others found themes of loss to be central to the dynamics of depressed schizophrenic patients (Semrad 1966; Roth 1970; Miller & Sonnenberg 1973). Semrad (1966) also considered that these patients' depressions represented important progress out of a more pathological narcissistic regressed state which more immediately followed the florid psychosis, although he also considered this state to be influenced by pain and/or the despair of an 'empty ego.' Both he and Eissler (1951) were of the opinion that the occurrence of depression in schizophrenia represented a moment of psychotherapeutic opportunity, with the possibility of insight and mastery which would attend the less primitive defensive state which was then manifest. In this regard, depression was interpreted as having positive prognostic significance.

Later, however, more data-based research was conducted documenting the course, frequency and intensity of depression in schizophrenia (Bowers & Astrachan 1967; McGlashan & Carpenter 1976b; Siris 1991; Siris *et al.* 2001). As the definitions of both depression and schizophrenia became progressively operationalized over time, and as the medication treatment of the subjects involved in studies became more highly controlled, investigations began to indicate that the outcomes are often less favourable in those schizophrenic patients who manifest depression during the longitudinal course of their disorders. Such depressions were noted to be associated with higher risks of relapse or rehospitalization (Mandel *et al.* 1982; Roy *et al.* 1983; Johnson 1988; Birchwood *et al.* 1993), as well as with an increased rate of suicide (Roy *et al.* 1983; Drake & Cotton 1986; Caldwell & Gottesman 1990; Siris 2001a).

Through the years, various descriptors have been applied to states of depression occurring in the course of schizophrenia, and nosological agreement has been difficult to come by. Although the designation is controversial and may even be misleading, a full depressive syndrome presenting in the longitudinal course of schizophrenia has often come to be called 'postpsychotic depression'. Indeed, despite the problems with its name, 'postpsychotic depression' has been listed as a diagnosis in ICD-10, and is also included in the appendix of DSM-IV. Previously, although 'postpsychotic depression' *per se* had not been discussed in either ICD or DSM manuals, 'depression superimposed on residual schizophrenia' was included as a diagnostic category in the Research Diagnostic Criteria (RDC) (Spitzer *et al.* 1978).

However named, depressive-like symptomatology has clearly played a part in the devastating long-term character of schizophrenia. The subjective state involved leads to great personal suffering, both for afflicted patients and for their families. No doubt the mood state, loss of energy, impairment in concentration and diminution of self-confidence also contribute materially to the tremendous loss of social and vocational capacity which these individuals experience, and which become such an important component of the morbidity with which they suffer.

Incidence and prevalence of 'depression' in schizophrenia

Over three dozen studies have been published and reviewed concerning the occurrence of depression-like symptomatology over the longitudinal course of schizophrenia (Siris 1991, 2000; Andreasen *et al.* 1995; Lindenmayer *et al.* 1995; Müller & Wetzel 1998; Norman *et al.* 1998). These studies vary substantially in a number of characteristics, including the definition employed for schizophrenia, the definition of depression, the observational interval and the treatment situation of the patients. One thing that is remarkable is that no matter what the definitions or conditions, all studies found at least some meaningful rate of depression in the course of schizophrenia.

The rate of depression described in all these studies varied substantially. The lowest rates were 6% (in a cross-sectional assessment carried out with the Hamilton Depression Rating Scale (HAM-D) of chronically hospitalized 'Kraepelinian' schizophrenic patients; Tapp *et al.* 1994) and 7% (in a cross-sectional assessment study of chronically hospitalized DSM-III schizophrenic patients, which nevertheless emphasized postpsychotic depression's distinct nature from 'negative symptoms'; Hirsch *et al.* 1989). The highest rates were 65% (in a study which followed 'Feighner criteria' schizophrenic patients for whom an effort had been made to exclude neuroleptic-induced akinesia, with ratings at least every 3 months, for 3 years after they had been free of acute psychotic symptoms; Johnson 1988) and 75% (in a study which followed 'first break' schizophrenic patients with repeated prospective assessments for as long as 5 years and counted them as being depressed if they met either of two definitions for depression; Koreen *et al.* 1993). The apparent large difference between these figures is ascribable, at least in part, to the fact that the first two studies represented a determination of point prevalence while the latter two studies involved a cumulative prevalence over 3 and 5 years, respectively.

The modal rate for the occurrence of depression in schizophrenia for all these various investigations was approximately 25%, a rate which has consistently seemed to be a benchmark in such reports over the course of time (Winokur 1972; McGlashan & Carpenter 1976a; Johnson 1981a; Mandel *et al.* 1982; Siris 1991, 2000). Table 9.1 describes the studies that have reported incidence or prevalence figures for episodes of depression in the course of schizophrenia as defined by recent common criteria such as DSM-III, DSM-IIIR, DSM-IV, RDC, ICD, Present State Examination (PSE), International Pilot Study of Schizophrenia (IPSS), New Haven Index, Feighner, CATEGO or Schneiderian First Rank. The very diversity of diagnostic criteria for schizophrenia and depression, and the variety of patient settings and means of observation, support the broad generalizability of the concept that some form or forms of phenotypic 'depression' occur in the longitudinal course of a substantial proportion of patients with schizophrenia.

These studies of rates of occurrence of depression in schizophrenia in study populations are complemented by the findings of a recent wide survey of practising psychiatrists (Siris *et al.*

2001). That study described a 33% rate of depression in first admission schizophrenic patients, a 38% rate in acute relapse schizophrenic patients and a 29% rate in chronic stable schizophrenia.

Additionally of interest is that women have often been described as being more likely than men to manifest depression (McGlashan & Bardenstein 1990; Emsley *et al.* 1999), depressed mood (Goldstein & Link 1988) or dysphoria (Goldstein *et al.* 1990) in the course of schizophrenia. Other reports, however, have not found a difference between the sexes when such issues are examined (Haas *et al.* 1990; Shtasel *et al.* 1992; Häfner *et al.* 1994; Addington *et al.* 1996a).

Differential diagnosis of depression in schizophrenia

Organic factors

There are many potential aetiologies for depression, or a phenocopy of depression, in schizophrenia (Bartels & Drake 1989). The first potential origin which needs to be considered is the set of organic causes for a depressive syndrome (Bartels & Drake 1988; Siris 2000). Organic aetiologies of a depressive syndrome can arise from medical conditions, such as anaemias, carcinomas, endocrinopathies, metabolic abnormalities, infectious diseases, autoimmune, cardiovascular or neurological disorders. Commonly prescribed medications such as sedative hypnotics, β-blockers, various other antihypertensive medications, antineoplastic agents, barbiturates, non-steroidal anti-inflammatory agents, sulphonamides and indometacin, or from the discontinuation of certain other prescribed medications, such as corticosteroids or psychostimulants, can also predispose to a depression syndrome. Substances of abuse can also have a role in the creation of depressed states, either through their acute use, chronic use or discontinuation. Alcohol can contribute to a depression-like state through either acute or chronic use. Chronic cannabis use can lead to an anergic state which shares many features with depression; the withdrawal state from cocaine involves well-described depressive phenomenology. Withdrawal from two commonly used legal substances, caffeine or nicotine (both often used to excess by schizophrenic patients), can also lead to dysphoric states which can be confused with depression (Griffiths & Mumford 1995; Dalack *et al.* 1998).

Neuroleptic-induced dysphoria

One relevant and frequently asked question concerns whether or not neuroleptic medications themselves can contribute to a 'depressed' state in schizophrenic patients (Awad 1993), and impairments in quality of life related to neuroleptic-induced dysphoria have, indeed, been reported (Browne *et al.* 1998). This is a plausible question on a theoretical level because neuroleptic medications blockade dopamine receptors, and dopamine receptors are known to be involved in brain pathways

Table 9.1 Studies reporting incidence or prevalence of secondary depression in cases of schizophrenia diagnosed by popular criteria. (Modified and supplemented after Siris 1991.)

Study (n)	Definition of psychosis	Definition of 'postpsychotic' interval	Definition of depression	Percentage depressed	Comment
McGlashan & Carpenter (1976b) n = 30	IPSS: more than 90% chance of schizophrenia	Cross-sectional assessment at discharge and at 1-year follow-up	'Depression' as per PSE	43% at discharge 50% cummulative as per 1-year follow-up	Depression dimension of PSE had a bimodal distribution
Weissman et al. (1977) n = 50	Outpatients with New Haven Schizophrenia Index diagnosis of schizophrenia	Point prevalence	Raskin Scale score of 7 or more	28%	No differences in demography of depressed group
Van Putten & May (1978) n = 94	Newly admitted patients with Feighner criteria for schizophrenia	Length of acute hospital stay	Increase in BPRS depression scale rating	38%	57% for patients with akinesia 22% for patients without akinesia
Knights et al. (1979) n = 37	CATEGO criteria: 87% = unequivocal schizophrenia	6 months or until relapse while on depot neuroleptic	PSE-based depression rating scale	54%	43% had onset or increase in depression ratings during interval
Roy (1980) n = 100	DSM-III chronic paranoid schizophrenia	Chart review for mean of 6 years	DSM-III for major depressive disorder, secondary type	30%	Depressed mood as assessed by PSE: 9% depressed at follow-up
Johnson (1981a) Cohort A: n = 41	Schizophrenia diagnosis based on Schneiderian first-rank symptoms	Cohort A: 2 months prospective prevalence study	Cohort A: HAM-D and/or BDI = 15 or more	Cohort A: 24%	The risk of an episode of depression was three times the risk of an episode of psychosis for patients maintained on depot neuroleptic
Cohort B: n = 100	Outpatients free of acute symptoms for at least 3 months	Cohort B: Cross-sectional prevalence	Cohort B: Nurses' rating and self-rating	Cohort B: 26%	

Study	Sample/diagnosis	Assessment	Criteria/instrument	Result	Comments
Cohort C: n = 30	Patients maintained on depot neuroleptic	Cohort C: 2-year follow-up	Cohort C: HAM-D and/or BDI = 15 or more	Cohort C: 50% excluding episodes associated with psychotic relapse	34% appeared depressed to staff 40% manifested subjective sadness
Siris et al. (1981) n = 50	Acutely admitted inpatients diagnosed by RDC	Duration of hospitalization after resolution of flagrant psychotic symptoms	RDC for major or minor depression by chart review of symptoms	6% major depression 22% minor depression	More early parental loss among patients with depression
Roy (1981) n = 100	DSM-III for schizophrenia	Chart review: 4–10 years	Treated for depression by antidepressants or ECT	39%	17% developed new episodes of depression
Möller & von Zerssen (1982) n = 81	Inpatients with schizophrenia (77%) or paranoid psychosis (23%) by ICD criteria	Point prevalence at hospital discharge	3 consecutive Actual Mood Scores at or above 21	23%	
Guze et al. (1983) and Martin et al. (1985) n = 44	Feighner criteria for schizophrenia	Retrospective survey at 6–12 year follow-up point	Feighner criteria for depression	57%	Criteria were not exactly those of Feighner, but were extremely close to those
Summers et al. (1983) Cohort A: n = 161	RDC for schizophrenia Cohort A: chronic	Cohort A: at admission to aftercare	Cohort A: SCL-90 scales	Cohort A: as a group, schizophrenics more depressed than normals	Acute and chronic patients found to have comparable depression symptoms after hospitalization
Cohort B: n = 72	Cohort B: acute	Cohort B: past month assessment (average 2.13 year post discharge)	Cohort B: two composite depression scales from KAS	Cohort B: 37% poor 68% poor or equivocal	
Watt & Shepherd (1983) (as reported in Roy 1986) n = 121	Chronic schizophrenia (PSE criteria)	PSE at admission and 1 month, 1 year, and 5 years after discharge	PSE assessment of depression syndrome	40% at 1 month and 1 year ('severe' in 1/4 of these) 19% at 5 years	Prospective epidemiological study

Table 9.1 (cont.)

Study (n)	Definition of psychosis	Definition of 'postpsychotic' interval	Definition of depression	Percentage depressed	Comment
Munro et al. (1984) n = 100	Outpatients with DSM-III for schizophrenia	Clinic cross-sectional prevalence	Carroll Rating Scale	41%	10% severe depression 18% moderate depression 13% mild depression
Leff et al. (1988) n = 31	Newly admitted patients with PSE/CATEGO definition of schizophrenia	Until discharged or until 6 months	Depressed mood as assessed by PSE	45%	Patients were not on neuroleptics. Correlation between improvement in depressive symptoms and in psychosis suggested depression was an 'integral part' of these cases
Johnson (1988) n = 80	Feighner criteria for schizophrenia. Presence of Schneiderian first-rank symptoms	Period began when patients were free of all acute symptoms. Period A: 0–12 months. Period B: 12–36 months (ratings at least every 3 months)	Altered mood state lasting at least 7 days with HAM-D and BDI each more than 15. Meet DSM-III for depression	13–30% for period A. 65% for period B	Akinesia excluded by physical examination for parkinsonism. Risk of psychotic relapse was significantly higher for patients depressed in 2nd or 3rd year, than for patients depressed 1st year or not depressed
Kulhara et al. (1989) n = 95	Outpatients with ICD-9 diagnosis of schizophrenia	Cross-sectional assessment	Finding of depressed mood on PSE instrument	32%	Only 12 patients had no depressive symptoms as assessed by the BPRS and/or PSE
Hirsch et al. (1989)	DSM-III for schizophrenia. Also: Cohort A: thought by nurses to be 'depressed'	Cohort A & B: cross-sectional assessment	Cohort A: HAM-D & BDI	Cohort A: 7%	Depressive symptoms are less common in chronic schizophrenic inpatients than would be predicted if they were a manifestation of negative symptoms or neuroleptic-induced parkinsonism. Depressed patients had more auditory hallucinations in Cohort B
Cohort A: n = 46					

Study	Sample	Design	Depression measure	Prevalence	Comments
Cohort B: n = 196 (also Barnes et al. 1989) Cohort C: n = 44	Cohort B: long-stay inpatients Cohort C: outpatients with no florid symptoms in previous 6 months	Cohort C: repeated bimonthly assessments for 1 year while randomly assigned to depot neuroleptic or placebo	Cohort B: item 23 ('depression') of PSE Cohort C: depression item = 2 or more on Manchester Scale	Cohort B: 13% Cohort C: 73% of psychotic relapses were preceded prodromal symptoms which included depression	
Bandelow et al. (1990) n = 364	ICD-9 and RDC for schizophrenia	Point prevalence 3 months after discharge and stabilization on neuroleptic medication for an acute psychotic episode	BPRS anxious depression scale equal to or greater than 10	19.5%	Two other scales for depression rated between 26.6% and 42.8% of patients as depressed, depending on cut-off scores. 35.7% of patients were rated as depressed when a milder BPRS cut-off was employed
Addington & Addington (1990) n = 50	Schizophrenia by DSM-III criteria	Point prevalence among consecutive admissions	'Depressive episode' by DSM-III criteria, based on PSE interview	24%	Statistically significant, but weak, correlations between depression rating scales and presence of major depressive episode
Brier et al. (1991) n = 58	RDC diagnosis of schizophrenia (n = 42) or schizoaffective disorder (mostly schizophrenic) (n = 16, of whom 12 were depressed type)	Average follow-up period = 6 ± 3 years	Episode of major depression as diagnosed by RDC	24%	38% of the sample had made at least one suicide attempt
Lindenmayer et al. (1991) n = 240	Inpatients (mostly chronic) with a diagnosis of schizophrenia by DSM-III criteria	Point-prevalence study	'Severe' PANSS depression component ≥ 19; 'mild to moderate' 11–18	5% severe depression 52% mild to moderate	Patients rated high in depression tended also to exhibit greater amounts of positive symptoms
Birchwood et al. (1993) n = 49	CATEGO class 's' for schizophrenia	Randomly selected from urban outpatient 'depot' treatment clinic	Score of at least 15 on the BDI	29%	Patients with lesser sense of control concerning their illness were more likely to manifest depression
Koreen et al. (1993) n = 70	'First break', RDC for schizophrenia (77%) or schizo-affective disorder (23%)	Repeated prospective assessment at weekly intervals during acute treatment, and monthly intervals thereafter up to 5 years	Syndromal criteria for depression and/or Extracted Hamilton Rating Scale for Depression based on a SADS interview	75% (met one or the other criteria at some point) 22% (met both criteria concurrently at some point)	26% of ratings for patients who were psychotic noted concurrent depression vs. 4% concurrent depression for patients noted to be non-psychotic at that rating point

Table 9.1 (cont.)

Study (n)	Definition of psychosis	Definition of 'postpsychotic' interval	Definition of depression	Percentage depressed	Comment
Tapp et al. (1994) $n = 91$	DSM-IIIR and RDC by SADS for schizophrenia	Not stated	HAM-D rating (not further specified)	37% (for 'non-Kraepelinian') 6% (for 'Kraepelinian')	More depression in non-Kraepelinian than in Kraepelinian group
Harrow et al. (1994) $n = 54$	RDC diagnosis of schizophrenia	Prevalence during 1 year preceding follow-up interview Follow-up interview was an average of 4.5 years after hospital discharge for index psychotic episode	Presence of a full depressive syndrome by RDC	37%	Patients receiving neuroleptics were more likely to have depression ($P < 0.01$) or experience anhedonia ($P < 0.001$). Depression finding remains when psychosis was controlled for
Mauri et al. (1995) $n = 43$	Chronic schizophrenic inpatients (DSM-IIIR criteria) during an acute exacerbation phase	Prevalence at baseline and after 6 weeks of neuroleptic treatment	BPRS depression subscale HAM-D	16.3% for moderate symptoms of depression 23.2% for mild symptoms of depression	All patients were medication-free for at least 3 weeks. All patients then treated with haloperidol with no other psychotropic or anticholinergic drug allowed
Markou (1996) $n = 94$	Schizophrenia (DSM-IIIR criteria) 50 inpatients and 44 outpatients of a chronic hospital	Point-prevalence assessment	'Significant depression' was a HAM-D score > 17; 'mild to moderate depression' was a HAM-D between 10 and 17	Inpatients: 10% – significant 42% – mild to moderate Outpatients: 4.5% – significant 48% – mild to moderate	A significant correlation was found between the negative subscale of the PANSS and the measure of depression ($r = 0.301, P = 0.003$)
Wassink et al. (1997, 1999) $n = 62$	Recent onset schizophrenia (DSM-III, R or DSM-IV criteria)	Point-prevalence at presentation	DSM-IV criteria for major depressive episode	35%	Patients with depression had more severe initial symptoms, but were not different on premorbid, demographic, or outcome variables

Study	Sample	Assessment	Definition of depression	Prevalence	Comments
Müller & Wetzel (1998) $n=132$	Acute schizophrenia diagnosed by DSM-IIIR criteria	Point-prevalence assessment	Score of 14 or more on the BRMES	42%	Data analysis suggest three factors: retardation, depressive core symptoms, and accessory depressive symptoms
Sands & Harrow (1999) $n=70$	RDC for schizophrenia	Follow-up assessment 7.5 years after hospital discharge. Assessment covers the previous year	Full depressive syndrome or subsyndromal by RDC (subsyndromal is depressed mood and two or three other depressive symptoms or four or more depressive symptoms without depressed mood)	36% (full depressive syndrome) 14% (subsyndromal depression)	Only 35% of a cohort of 46 patients among whom the evaluation had been performed were free of the depression syndrome or subsyndrome for the years preceding a 4.5-year evaluation and the 7.5-year evaluation
Zisook et al. (1999) $n=60$	Outpatients with schizophrenia (DSM-IIIR or DSM-IV criteria) between the ages of 45 and 79	Point-prevalence study	Score of 17 or more on the HAM-D	20% of the women 7% of the men	Note that, in this sample, 15 patients (25%) were taking adjunctive antidepressant medication. 63% of the men and 60% of the women had HDRS scores from 7 to 16
Baynes et al. (2000) $n=120$	Stable outpatients with chronic schizophrenia by DSM-IIIR criteria	Point prevalence	A score of 17 or more on the BDI	13.3% (24.2% had a BDI score 10–16)	If patients already on antidepressants or lithium were excluded, depression rate rose to 14.8%

BDI = Beck Depression Inventory; BPRS = Brief Psychiatric Rating Scale; BRMES = Bech-Rafaelsen Melancholia Scale; DSM = Diagnostic and Statistic Manual; HAM-D = Hamilton Depression Rating Scale; ICD = International Classification of Diseases; IPSS = International Pilot Study of Schizophrenia; KAS = Katz Adjustment Scale; n = number of subjects in the study; PANSS = Positive and Negative Symptom Scale; PSE = Present State Examination; RDC = Research Diagnostic Criteria; SADS = Schedule for Affective Disorders and Schizophrenia; SCL = Symptom Check List.

which mediate 'reward' (Wise 1982; Harrow *et al.* 1994). The reasoning is that, if a neuroleptic interfered with the experience of reward or pleasure, the resultant experience of relative anhedonia could become a phenocopy of a depressed state. Interestingly, a large prospective study found that patients who were maintained on neuroleptic medication manifest more depression than those who were randomized to receive neuroleptic medication only on an 'early intervention' or 'crisis intervention' basis, and patients in that study were found to have lower depression ratings after being taken off neuroleptic medication (Bandelow *et al.* 1992). Another well-designed study specifically comparing anhedonia in schizophrenic patients on vs. off neuroleptics found significantly more anhedonia as well as more depression in those patients who were being treated with neuroleptics (Harrow *et al.* 1994). Notably, several much earlier reports had also implicated neuroleptics as an aetiological agent for depression among schizophrenic patients (DeAlarcon & Carney 1969; Floru *et al.* 1975; Galdi *et al.* 1981; Johnson 1981b; Galdi 1983).

The majority of evidence, however, has tended to refute the notion that appropriately administered neuroleptic medication causes a full depressive state to emerge in schizophrenic patients (Knights & Hirsch 1981; Moller & Von Zerssen 1986; Siris 1991, 2000). This negative evidence comes from three perspectives. First, evaluating psychotic schizophrenic patients throughout the course of treatment for their acute episodes has revealed that the greatest levels of depressive symptomatology exist at the height of the psychosis, and tend to resolve, although often at a slower rate than the psychosis, when the psychosis is treated with a neuroleptic agent (Knights & Hirsch 1981; Möller & von Zerssen 1982; Strian *et al.* 1982; Szymanski *et al.* 1983; Leff *et al.* 1988; Hirsch *et al.* 1989; Green *et al.* 1990; Nakaya *et al.* 1997). These observations oppose the notion that depression is caused by neuroleptics by demonstrating that depressive symptomatology was present before the neuroleptic was administered, and that levels of depression actually decrease as the patient comes under treatment with these compounds. Secondly, a number of studies have found that, when patients being treated with neuroleptics were compared with patients not being treated with neuroleptics, the patients treated with neuroleptics were not observed to be more depressed (Hirsch *et al.* 1973, 1989; Wistedt & Palmstierna 1983; Hogarty & Munetz 1984). Thirdly, when schizophrenic patients with and without depression were compared with each other, in most studies the depressed group was not found to be receiving higher doses of neuroleptic drugs or to have higher neuroleptic blood levels (Roy *et al.* 1983; Roy 1984; Berrios & Bulbena 1987; Siris *et al.* 1988a; Barnes *et al.* 1989; Bandelow *et al.* 1990, 1992; Tugg *et al.* 1997; Peralta & Cuesta 1999; Zisook *et al.* 1999). On the other hand, at least one study did find a positive relationship between haloperidol plasma levels and depressive symptoms in the context of a positive association between extrapyramidal and depressive symptoms (Krakowski *et al.* 1997), and another study found a trend level association

between degree of depression and neuroleptic dose (Perenyi *et al.* 1998). Thus, this 'preponderance of the evidence' refutation of the hypothesis that neuroleptic drugs can cause depression is not entirely conclusive, especially in the presence of one well-designed prospective positive study (Harrow *et al.* 1994), and we certainly cannot rule out the possibility that neuroleptics might not be an important contributing factor to depression in certain individual cases.

Akinesia and akathisia

Antipsychotic drugs may clearly be a factor in generating depression-like states when depressive-like features occur in association with the extrapyramidal neuroleptic side-effects of akinesia and akathisia. Neuroleptic-induced akinesia, a syndrome of reduced spontaneity as well as reduced generalized motor activity, at times can produce a rather exact phenocopy of depression, even when muscle stiffness or cogwheeling is not present (Rifkin *et al.* 1975, 1978; Van Putten & May 1978; Martin *et al.* 1985; Bermanzohn & Siris 1992). This phenocopy includes blue mood as well as reduced energy, pessimism and anhedonia, and is principally differentiated from depression by its responsiveness to antiparkinsonian medication, which is usually not thought to be a treatment for other forms of 'depression'. Akinesia may be particularly problematic in terms of its diagnosis when it occurs in an insidious or subtle form, or when it occurs in the absence of large muscle extrapyramidal signs such as shuffling gait or reduced arm swing. Unfortunately, most of the studies of depression in the course of schizophrenia have made little effort to evaluate the potential presence of neuroleptic-induced akinesia or to rule it out as a confounding factor.

Neuroleptic-induced akathisia is another extrapyramidal side-effect which can easily be confused with depression. It is easy to diagnose in its blatant form, because of prominent motor restlessness, but equally easy to misdiagnose in its subtle form where the patient may be more dysphoric than outwardly restless (Van Putten 1975; Siris 1985; Halstead *et al.* 1994). Patients with less blatant akathisia may still be prone, however, to subtle behavioural excesses such as overtalkativeness or wandering into other people's territory. Dysphoria is often associated with akathisia, and dysphoric akathisia can be easily mistaken for agitated depression. Indeed, the dysphoria of akathisia may be intense, and both suicidal ideation and suicidal behaviour have been associated with this state (Shear *et al.* 1983; Drake & Ehrlich 1985).

Negative symptoms

The negative symptom syndrome of schizophrenia can also present in a way which resembles depression in a number of crucial respects (Crow 1980; Andreasen & Olsen 1982; Carpenter *et al.* 1985; Siris *et al.* 1988b; Kulhara *et al.* 1989; Bermanzohn & Siris 1992; Siris 2000), although clear distinctions may also be evident (Barnes *et al.* 1989; Lindenmayer *et al.* 1991;

Norman & Malla 1991; Kuck *et al.* 1992; Kibel *et al.* 1993). Clinical features such as anhedonia, anergia, social withdrawal and poor motivation may be common between these two states (Bermanzohn & Siris 1992; Sax *et al.* 1996). However, Barnes *et al.* (1989) and Baynes *et al.* (2000) found very little overlap between the diagnosis of the negative symptoms of schizophrenia and diagnosis of depression in chronic inpatients, and some investigators (Norman & Malla 1991, 1994; Sax *et al.* 1996; Nakaya *et al.* 1997; Zisook *et al.* 1999), but not others (Dollfus *et al.* 1993), have found correlations between depression and positive symptoms, perhaps particularly suspiciousness (Kirkpatrick *et al.* 1996; Baynes *et al.* 2000), in schizophrenia.

With careful attention, depression and negative symptoms in schizophrenia need not ordinarily be confused. The symptom which is most likely to set these two conditions apart is blue mood, a clinical feature which is generally present in depression. The negative symptom syndrome, on the other hand, is usually marked by blunted affect.

As one prominent hypothesis concerning the pathogenesis of negative symptoms involves it representing a hypodopaminergic state (Davis *et al.* 1991), it is conceivable that neuroleptic medications, at more than the required dosage, may exacerbate this condition, thereby contributing to the reputation of neuroleptic agents as being 'depressogenic'.

Disappointment reactions

Schizophrenic patients often have a considerable amount to feel disappointed about in the ways in which their lives are progressing (or not progressing), and they may certainly manifest this psychological reaction. An acute disappointment reaction may occur in reaction to any event which goes awry in an individual's life. Operationally, this is most easily distinguished from other forms of depression by the presence of an immediate stressful event and the fact that the reaction is transient – seldom lasting more than a week or two. The chronic variety of disappointment reaction, known as the demoralization syndrome (Frank 1973; Klein 1974), can be more difficult to distinguish from depression. In this situation, patients may become chronically discouraged and dispirited on the basis of repeated failures or losses and/or the impression that important life goals have become impossible to achieve. 'Insight' (Peralta & Cuesta 1994; Kemp & Lambert 1995; Smith *et al.* 2000) or self-awareness of symptoms or psychological deficits may have an important role (Liddle *et al.* 1993; Lysaker *et al.* 1995) and a sense of incompetence may also be prominently involved (deFigueiredo 1993). Of interest, in this regard, is the observation that schizophrenic patients who feel less of a sense of control concerning their illness have been noted to be more prone to experience depression (Birchwood *et al.* 1993; Hoffmann *et al.* 2000). From a clinical perspective, demoralization reactions may be particularly worth diagnosing, because they may represent a condition particularly amenable to psychosocial treatments and supports.

Prodrome of psychotic relapse

Depression has been described as a common symptom which may be manifest by schizophrenic patients during the process of decompensation into a new psychotic episode (Docherty *et al.* 1978; Herz & Melville 1980; Herz 1985; Johnson 1988; Subotnik & Nuechterlein 1988; Hirsch & Jolley 1989; Green *et al.* 1990; Malla & Norman 1994; Tollefson *et al.* 1999). In these cases, the dysphoric state is often accompanied by social withdrawal, anxiety and/or other stigmata such as hypervigilance suggestive of early manifestations of psychosis, but the differential diagnosis may be difficult. Because of this possibility, the lowering of neuroleptic dosage is not necessarily advisable for schizophrenic patients with newly emergent depressive-like symptomatology. Rather, increased monitoring and non-specific support may be the indicated intervention. Initiation of antidepressant medications for patients already in the process of undergoing a psychotic decompensation may have contributed to the early impression, not subsequently validated, that antidepressant medications may be psychotogenic in schizophrenic patients even if neuroleptic medication treatment is maintained (Siris *et al.* 1978).

Schizoaffective disorder

Another condition involving the syndrome of depression and the phenotypic psychosis of schizophrenia, which belongs in the differential diagnosis of secondary depression in schizophrenia, occurs in schizoaffective disorder. In this instance, the full depressive syndrome coincides with the florid psychotic syndrome in ways which have been variously defined over the years and according to different diagnostic schemes (Levitt & Tsuang 1988; Coryell *et al.* 1990; Taylor 1992). Because the definition of the requisite level of psychotic symptomatology coexisting with depression has differed according to the diagnostic system employed, the technical boundary between schizoaffective disorder and secondary depression in residually psychotic schizophrenic patients has also varied. Conceptually though, the pertinent issue is that a full depression syndrome coincides with the appropriate manifestations of psychosis during at least a part of an episode of schizoaffective depression (Siris & Lavin 1995; Siris 1996). Schizoaffective disorder additionally enters into the differential diagnosis of postpsychotic depression in schizophrenia in that episodes of secondary depression can also occur in the course of schizoaffective disorder.

Independent diathesis for depression

Separate from schizoaffective disorder, although perhaps related to it, is the concept that some patients with the diathesis for schizophrenia may also, independently, have the biological diathesis for depression. On purely statistical grounds, the chance occurrence of depression in schizophrenia would be expected to happen at the same rate as in the general population, an interaction which could account for occasional cases. But the construct has also been put forward, based on the stress–vulnerability model of schizophrenia (Zubin & Spring 1977; Nuechterlein & Dawson 1984), that interaction between the two diatheses could account for more cases presenting with both depression and schizophrenia than would be expected by chance alone (Siris 2000, 2001b). This possibility results from the observation that the vulnerability to psychosis appears to occur on a continuum in the population, with a tiny fraction having extreme vulnerability and the vast majority having very low vulnerability. In between, there is a limited, but meaningful, portion of the population with a more moderate, but real, level of psychotic vulnerability. Whereas, in the absence of some other major stressor, only those individuals with extreme vulnerability would become psychotic, in the presence of a major stressor the more moderately vulnerable could also be recruited into the phenotypically psychotic group. The occurrence of major depression, in essence, could represent one such major stressor on both a biological and psychosocial level. As a result, more than the expected by chance number of phenotypically schizophrenic patients would be predicted to manifest depressive syndromes as well. Such a hypothesis would be consistent with the common finding of depressive symptoms occurring during the prodrome of psychotic episodes. It also would be consistent with the findings that dysphoria is more associated with positive than with negative symptoms in schizophrenia (Norman & Malla 1994; Sax et al. 1996) and that adjunctive antidepressant maintenance treatment, designed to prevent the recurrence of depression in schizophrenic individuals with histories of postpsychotic depression, apparently may be protective in reducing the rate of psychotic exacerbations (Siris et al. 1994).

Clinical validation of depression in schizophrenia

Prognosis

The literature concerning the prognostic implications of depressive symptomatology in schizophrenia is complicated by a timing issue: do the depressive symptoms coincide with the psychosis or occur apart from it (Siris 1991, 2000). Although depressive symptoms coinciding with the psychosis carry favourable prognostic implications (McGlashan & Carpenter 1976a; Emsley et al. 1999), such symptoms presenting in intervals during which the patient is not psychotic have been found to predict oppositely (Bartels & Drake 1988; Becker 1988). Specifically, those patients who manifest secondary depressions in schizophrenia have been noted to be more likely to experience psychotic relapse, even when 'prodromal' depressive symptomatology has been accounted for (Falloon et al. 1978; Mandel et al. 1982), and 'major depression' in schizophrenia has also been independently associated with early hospital readmission (Olfson et al. 1999). Consistent with this unfavourable impli-

cation is the observation that postpsychotic depression in schizophrenia is also associated with other negative predictors of outcome, such as poor premorbid adjustment and insidious onset of the first or index psychotic episodes (Moller & von Zerssen 1986).

Suicide

The most blatantly disastrous outcome in schizophrenia is suicide, an event which tragically is not rare and which has been estimated to be the way in which between 2% and 13% of schizophrenic lives end (Tsuang 1978; Black et al. 1985; Drake et al. 1985; Nyman & Jonsson 1986; Roy 1986; Black & Fisher 1992; Krausz et al. 1995; Meltzer & Okayli 1995; Fenton et al. 1997; Stephens et al. 1997, 1999; Inskip et al. 1998; Wiersma et al. 1998; Siris 2001a). This figure has often been interpreted as being approximately 10% (Miles 1977; Caldwell & Gottesman 1990). The rates of suicide attempts in schizophrenia are even higher, with estimates ranging from 18% to 55% (Roy 1986; Breier et al. 1991; Asnis et al. 1993; Cohen et al. 1994; Gupta et al. 1998). A greater number of schizophrenic suicides (Roy 1982, 1986; Drake et al. 1985; Drake & Cotton 1986; Dassori et al. 1990; Heilä et al. 1997; Saarinen et al. 1999; Stephens et al. 1999) and suicide attempters (Roy 1986; Prasad & Kumar 1988; Addington & Addington 1992; Bartels et al. 1992; Cohen et al. 1994; Jones et al. 1994) have been found to have past or recent histories of depressive symptomatology, especially psychological aspects such as hopelessness (Drake et al. 1984; Drake & Cotton 1986; Caldwell & Gottesman 1990; Addington & Addington 1992; Meltzer & Okayli 1995; Saarinen et al. 1999) and loss (Caldwell & Gottesman 1990; Heilä et al. 1999; Saarinen et al. 1999). Suicidal ideation has also been found to be associated with depression in schizophrenia (Barnes et al. 1989; Bartels et al. 1992).

Life events

More undesirable events, more exit events, and more life events altogether have been observed in those schizophrenic patients who manifest secondary depressions (Roy 1981). Additionally, schizophrenic patients with secondary depressions have been found to have had histories of more early parental loss (Roy 1980, 1981; Roy et al. 1983).

Biological validation of depression in schizophrenia

A relatively small number of studies have investigated biological correlates of depression within schizophrenia, either at the symptom or diagnosis level. Even fewer have set out a priori to identify patients on the basis of their comorbidity with depression; rather the vast majority have investigated post hoc the relationship of the measures made with depression subscale scores.

Brain structure and function

Structural imaging

Computerized tomography (CT) and magnetic resonance imaging (MRI) in schizophrenia have produced convincing evidence of increased ventricular volume and decreased cortical volume, with greatest reductions in temporal lobe volume. That regional changes are related to characteristic clinical features of the disorder is an attractive hypothesis. To date, the most consistent relationship found has been between ventricular enlargement and negative symptoms. Far fewer studies have shown significant correlations between regional cerebral *volume* and negative symptoms. A single study (Kohler *et al.* 1998b) examined a priori the effect of depressive symptoms in 64 patients with schizophrenia categorized according to their HAM-D scores into HAM-Hi (>18) or HAM-Lo (<18) groups. The more depressed schizophrenic patients had significantly higher temporal lobe volume, although the effect size was small. Gur *et al.* (2000) found that women but not men with schizophrenia had reduced orbitofrontal cortex volume and that lower volume in this region was associated with higher depression ratings on the HAM-D. On the basis of the studies performed to date, it is fair to conclude that there are no consistently demonstrated structural anatomic correlates of depression in schizophrenia. Data-leads methods of image analysis similar to those used in functional imaging will offer greater opportunities for the identification of clinical correlates of structural changes (Wright *et al.* 1999). Chapter 22 contains a wider discussion of the application of brain imaging to schizophrenia research.

Functional neuroimaging

Functional neuroimaging can be broadly divided into two techniques:
1 'brain mapping', which measures regional cerebral blood flow (rCBF) or metabolism as an index of local neural activity; and
2 neurochemical imaging, in which the specific uptake and binding of radiolabelled tracer compounds is measured.

Brain mapping studies

In primary depression, there is reasonable consistency in the finding of functional abnormalities in key regions of prefrontal and limbic cortex and connected subcortical structures (Drevets 1998). In schizophrenia, it has been demonstrated that functional abnormalities may relate to specific symptoms such as hallucinations (McGuire *et al.* 1993) or syndromes (Liddle *et al.* 1992). Furthermore, observed patterns of functional abnormality may be specific to symptoms across diagnoses (Dolan *et al.* 1993). However, as with structural imaging, very few functional imaging studies in schizophrenia have specifically looked for correlates of depression. No activation studies have addressed this issue. Kohler *et al.* (1998b) used fluo-

rodeoxyglucose positron emission tomography (FDG-PET) to examine 29 schizophrenic patients categorized according to HAM-D scores into HAM-Hi (>18) or HAM-Lo (<18) groups. These data showed no main effect attributable to depression, but the HAM-Hi group had a relatively lower left–right anterior cingulate metabolic ratio. This result is consistent with the left lateralized decrease in dorsal cingulate function seen in some studies of primary depression (Bench *et al.* 1992). Further studies are required before conclusions can be drawn as to whether depression in schizophrenia has well-defined neural correlates and how the pattern of function compares with that seen in primary depression and with other syndromes of schizophrenia.

Neurochemical imaging

Neurochemical imaging relies on the availability of suitable radioligands to measure physiological processes, biochemical pathways and receptor systems of interest. Hypothesis-led attempts to relate neurochemical imaging to depressive symptoms in schizophrenia have been very limited.

Dopamine synthesis

Striatal uptake of the PET tracer [^{18}F]fluorodopa reflects the synthesis rate of dopamine in the terminals of nigrostriatal fibres. Studies using this method generally agree that acute schizophrenia is associated with increased fluorodopa uptake. In 10 neuroleptic-naive patients, Hietala *et al.* (1999) found that positive symptoms correlated positively with basal ganglia fluorodopa uptake, whereas there was a highly *negative* correlation between core depressive symptoms (guilt and depression subscales of the Positive and Negative Symptom Scale, PANSS) and left striatal fluorodopa uptake. This correlation remained high even after exclusion of three schizoaffective patients.

Dopamine receptors

Two recent meta-analyses of studies of dopamine D_2-receptors suggest that a small increase in striatal D_2 density is found in some patients with schizophrenia (Laruelle 1998; Zakzanis & Hansen 1998). In primary depression, increased D_2 density has also been described (D'haenen & Bossuyt 1994) with a positive association with psychomotor retardation (Ebert *et al.* 1996; Shah *et al.* 1997). The relationship between D_2 binding and depression in schizophrenia is less clear. Two studies in drug-free patients both suggest that decreased dopaminergic function may mediate negative symptoms, with no data presented for depressive symptoms (Martinot *et al.* 1994; Knable *et al.* 1997). In patients treated with olanzapine or risperidone, de Haan *et al.* (2000) found that negative symptom ratings (from the PANSS) and Montgomery–Åsberg depression rating scale scores both correlated with D_2-receptor occupancy. These authors suggested that the relationship between higher D_2-receptor occupancy, psychopathology and subjective experience may have important implications for dosing strategies and compliance with antipsychotic medication.

Dopamine release

Dopamine receptor imaging techniques may be adapted to provide a measure of stimulant-induced dopamine release. Studies by two independent groups have demonstrated that medication-free patients with acute schizophrenia have exaggerated amphetamine-induced dopamine release (Breier *et al.* 1997; Abi-Dargham *et al.* 1998; Laruelle *et al.* 1999). Furthermore, these changes correlate with an increase in positive symptoms and a smaller decrease in negative symptoms. As yet no analysis of the change in depressive symptoms has been reported, but this requires further investigation.

Serotonergic system

The hypothesis of a serotonin dysfunction in schizophrenia has been examined in several PET studies. Of the four published studies to examine cortical 5-HT_{2A}-receptors (Trichard *et al.* 1998; Lewis *et al.* 1999; Ngan *et al.* 2000; Verhoeff *et al.* 2000) only Ngan *et al.* found the decrease in prefrontal cortical receptor density predicted by previous postmortem studies. The study by Lewis *et al.* explicitly rated depressive symptoms but no relationship was found with 5-HT_{2A} binding. Laruelle *et al.* (2000) found that the density of brainstem serotonin transporters was unaltered in 24 patients with schizophrenia and not related to symptomatology; depression was not explicitly examined.

Neuropsychology

A single study has been found which examines a priori the effect of depression in schizophrenia on neuropsychological performance. Kohler *et al.* (1998a) examined 128 patients with schizophrenia, categorized according to HAM-D scores into HAM-Hi (>18) or HAM-Lo (<18) groups, on a battery of neuropsychological tests. HAM-Hi patients had a higher score for delusions but the groups were otherwise well matched. The neuropsychological battery revealed that women in the HAM-Hi group were impaired on the vigilance component of the Continuous Performance Task (CPT). While it is tempting to suggest that this deficit is linked to the anatomical changes in the prefrontal cortex in women with schizophrenia previously described, it is impossible to draw any firm conclusions from this single study.

Endocrine and biochemical measures

Inconsistent results have been reported in the several studies which have examined the results of the dexamethasone suppression test (DST) in schizophrenic patients with secondary depressions (Siris *et al.* 1984; Siris 1991). One confounding variable in these investigations may have been the failure to control for the effects of antiparkinsonian or other anticholinergic medications on dexamethasone suppression. Recently, Ismail *et al.* (1998) found very low rates of non-suppression in a group of 64 schizophrenic patients, 36% of whom fulfilled criteria for major depression. Only one study has been reported concerning the thyrotropin-releasing hormone (TRH) test in postpsychotic depressed schizophrenic patients (Siris *et al.* 1991b). Although that study showed rates of blunted response comparable with that of patients with primary depression, it contained no control group of non-depressed schizophrenic patients. The finding of higher levels of platelet monoamine oxidase (MAO) activity in patients with schizophrenia-related depression (Schildkraut *et al.* 1980) has not been replicated.

Genetic studies

Family studies

Several family studies have examined the relationships between schizophrenia and affective disorder. Kendler *et al.* (1993) reported a familial association between schizophrenia and psychotic affective illness, but not with affective illness in general, and Maier *et al.* (1993) found a familial relationship between schizophrenia and unipolar depressive disorder. Kendler *et al.* (1996) also found a relationship with psychotic affective illness in the parents of offspring with schizophrenia. However, most family studies of schizophrenia do not look specifically for an association between comorbid depression in schizophrenia, either at the symptoms or diagnosis level, with depression in other family members. Kendler and Hays (1983) found that schizophrenic patients who have first-degree relatives with unipolar depression have a significantly higher likelihood of developing a depression syndrome following the resolution of a psychotic episode. On the other hand, two relatively small studies ($n = 44$ and $n = 70$) failed to find significant differences in rates of primary affectively disordered relatives between schizophrenic patients with and without depression (Guze *et al.* 1983; Berrios & Bulbena 1987). One unique study found a relationship between neuroleptic-induced depressive symptomatology and those schizophrenic patients who had depressed relatives (Galdi *et al.* 1981).

Sibling pair studies

DeLisi *et al.* (1987) found a significant intrapair association for the occurrence of RDC major depression in 53 sibling pairs with RDC schizophrenia or schizoaffective disorder, and Kendler *et al.* (1997) found significant associations for the severity of depressive symptoms in 256 sibling pairs with DSM-IIIR schizophrenia. In contrast, Cardno *et al.* (1998) found no familial aggregation of presence/absence of depressive episodes in their sample of 109 sibling pairs with DSM-IV schizophrenia or schizoaffective disorder.

Molecular genetic studies

In linkage studies, large families with several affected members are studied to try to find a genetic marker that cosegregates with the disease. The power of linkage studies may be increased by using phenotypes that include key dimensions of gene expression which may act as quantitative traits (Brzustowicz *et al.* 1997). Asherson *et al.* (1998) have implicated markers on chromosome 4p in the expression of schizophrenia with significant affective symptoms, while Kendler *et al.* (2000) reported that patients from families with evidence for linkage to chromosome 8p displayed fewer depressive symptoms.

In association studies, the frequency of various alleles of a gene that is suspected of involvement in the pathogenesis of the disorder is examined in a series of subjects with schizophrenia as compared with a control group. As in linkage studies, interest has been growing in utilizing phenotypes other than diagnosis, such as neurocognitive measures, brain imaging abnormalities and symptom domains including depression (Malhotra 2001). For example, Serretti *et al.* (1996) developed a phenotype definition based on symptomatological factors within the major psychoses of excitement, depression, delusions and disorganization. This group and others have examined a number of genes for their relationship with symptomatology including depression within major psychoses. Although this is a promising approach, to date only negative studies have been published for the serotonin transporter gene (Serretti *et al.* 1999a) and dopamine D_3 and D_4 receptors (Serretti *et al.* 1999b,c).

Treatment implications

The existence of a syndrome of depression in schizophrenia raises several important implications for treatment. A newly emergent syndrome of depression in a patient with schizophrenia is certainly cause for an increased level of observation, attention and support. Increased frequency of outpatient appointments and contact with families or residential providers is indicated, and interventions which solve problems, increase structure and decrease both biological and psychosocial stresses are useful. If the appearance of depressive symptomatology was a product of a transient disappointment reaction, such interventions may prove to be adequate.

Antipsychotic medications

As noted in the differential diagnosis above, a manifestation of 'depression' in schizophrenia may represent an early stage in the process of decompensation into a new episode of psychosis. In a closely followed patient, a new psychotic episode will soon declare itself with an increase in psychotic symptoms such as hallucinations, delusions, overinterpretation of perceptions or events, derailment of thought processes, or illogical or magical thinking. If such proves to be the case, augmentation or change of antipsychotic medication may be called for. Intercepting and treating new episodes of psychosis quickly may substantially curtail both psychiatric and social morbidity and it is a crucial objective in the longitudinal treatment of individuals with schizophrenia. Whether to increase dosage or to change antipsychotic medication will need to be decided on an individual basis, with consideration given to past treatment response to particular antipsychotic agents at particular dosage, current pattern and severity of side-effects and level of patient acceptability for

these, and plasma levels of medications for those which have available meaningful levels. Assessment of proper medication compliance is always an important issue in such a situation.

When a new state of depression in schizophrenia persists or becomes chronic in a patient who is not manifesting florid psychotic symptomatology, reduction of the dosage of neuroleptic medication should be considered if the patient is being treated with a conventional neuroleptic agent (i.e. a 'typical' antipsychotic agent). Although evidence remains divided with regard to whether standard neuroleptic agents can cause an otherwise characteristic depressed illness in schizophrenic patients, standard neuroleptic drugs certainly may at least have a role in generating syndromes which mimic depression. These include akinesia, akathisia and, perhaps, even the 'negative symptoms' state. Therefore, when treating non-acute episodes of depression in schizophrenia, an effort should be made to decrease the neuroleptic dosage to the lowest level consistent with maintaining remission from flagrant psychotic symptomatology. Indeed, the minimizing of neuroleptic dosage in this manner is generally advocated for the long-term maintenance of patients with schizophrenia as a means of reducing side-effects and optimizing psychosocial functioning (Kane *et al.* 1983; Marder *et al.* 1987).

The obvious alternative to continuing treatment with a standard neuroleptic agent when an enduring pattern of depression has emerged in a patient with schizophrenia is to switch the patient to a so-called 'atypical' antipsychotic agent (Siris 2000). First, atypical antipsychotics have been shown to demonstrate a much more favourable extrapyramidal side-effect profile than standard neuroleptics (Chouinard *et al.* 1993; Marder & Meibach 1994; Peuskens 1995; Borison *et al.* 1996; Tandon *et al.* 1997). Because akinesia and akathisia figure quite prominently in the manifestation of depression-like symptomatology in schizophrenia, this atypical antipsychotic benefit alone could account for much of the more favoured 'depression' findings which have been observed following the use of these agents (Siris 2000). Secondly, in light of atypical antipsychotic agents relying much less on dopaminergic blockade for their therapeutic effect (Meltzer *et al.* 1989; Deutch *et al.* 1991; Seeger *et al.* 1995; Jones 1997; Tandon *et al.* 1997), they would be much less likely to be responsible for a dopamine-blockade-induced anhedonia, which could then either directly or indirectly contribute to depressive symptomatology. Thirdly, atypical antipsychotics have been widely reported to be superior in the treatment of negative symptoms of schizophrenia (Kane *et al.* 1988; Chouinard *et al.* 1993; Marder & Meibach 1994; Buchanan 1995; Möller *et al.* 1995; Beasley *et al.* 1996; Borison *et al.* 1996; Tandon *et al.* 1997; Tollefson & Sanger 1997; Tollefson *et al.* 1997). Again, this could generate a more favourable depression profile in patients either directly, in the case where negative symptoms present a phenocopy of depression, or indirectly, where patients are discouraged by their negative symptoms and manifest depression secondarily.

The above factors (and possibly other factors as well) are likely to be contributors to the observation that atypical antipsychotic agents may be associated with superior outcomes in schizophrenia, as suggested by quality of life measures (Franz *et al.* 1997; Tollefson & Andersen 1999; Voruganti *et al.* 2000). If this is the case, it is logical that both acute and chronic disappointment reactions would be reduced when atypical antipsychotic medications are employed. Beyond this, there is the possibility that atypical antipsychotics may have some direct antidepressant activity on their own. This has been suggested by the results of a number of controlled studies (Azorin 1995; Meltzer & Okayli 1995; Beasley *et al.* 1996; Tandon *et al.* 1997; Tollefson *et al.* 1997, 1998a,b; Keck *et al.* 1998; Walker *et al.* 1998; Daniel *et al.* 1999) but, in light of all the above-mentioned confounding issues, it still remains to be definitively determined (Siris 2000).

Antidepressant medications

After the possibilities of impending psychotic relapse and transient disappointment reaction have been accounted for, and an effort has been made to rule out neuroleptic-induced akinesia or akathisia through appropriate adjustments of medication, the efficacy of treatment with antidepressant medication must be considered. Studies addressing this question have had mixed results, but are generally regarded as being favourable (Plasky 1991; Siris 1991, 2000; Levinson *et al.* 1999). Table 9.2 reviews the double-blind, placebo-controlled studies which have been reported concerning the addition of an adjunctive antidepressant medication in cases of secondary depression in schizophrenia.

Most of the negative reports in Table 9.2 have design issues which make their interpretation difficult. These include brief duration of treatment (4 weeks), low antidepressant dosage (maprotiline as low as 50 mg/day), antidepressant dosage which may be too high for some patients (nortriptyline 150 mg/day, especially in the presence of a concomitant neuroleptic which could reduce metabolism), antidepressant medication being given to patients on one antipsychotic agent while placebo is given to patients receiving a different antipsychotic, or a small n limiting the power of the comparison. The studies in Table 9.2 which are positive have fewer limitations of design, although even the most favourable-appearing study (Siris *et al.* 1987) demonstrated 'much improved' responses in fewer than half (42%) of the patients treated with adjunctive antidepressant. Additionally, the large majority of studies in Table 9.2 did not make an attempt to rule out the syndrome of akinesia in their design, so their results have to be interpreted in that light. Finally, the study by Kramer *et al.* (1989) differs from most of the others in that it involved patients who were floridly psychotic at the time of the treatment trial (acutely admitted patients with schizoaffective depressions). The fact that these patients did not benefit from the addition of an antidepressant to their neuroleptic regimen may relate to their being flagrantly psychotic at the time of the trial (Siris 1991).

In general, outpatients in the studies in Table 9.2 did better with an adjunct antidepressant than inpatients did (Fisher Exact Test for this question, $P = 0.015$, for those studies in Table 9.2 which specified whether inpatients or outpatients were involved). However, it is unclear why that is the case. It might be a result of outpatients being likely to have less florid psychotic symptoms, or it might be because of other factors such as more constructive and/or less problematic outlets being available in the outpatient setting for the expression of restored energy.

It is more difficult to assess the impact of adjunctive antidepressant medications in double-blind studies that involved more unselected populations of schizophrenic patients, because absence of depression may have left little or no room for improvement in this dimension, but even in this case there have been some reported improvements (Taiminen *et al.* 1997).

MAO inhibitor antidepressants have not been adequately studied in schizophrenic patients with depressions. Of possible relevance, however, is a double-blind adjunctive tranylcypromine study which found this MAO inhibitor to be of benefit for schizophrenic patients with negative symptoms (Bucci 1987). Preliminary results have suggested that selegiline, an MAO-B inhibitor, may have value as an adjunctive treatment for negative symptoms (Perenyi *et al.* 1992; Bodkin *et al.* 1996), but interpretation of these results is complicated by the fact that selegiline has antiparkinsonian properties (Parkinson Study Group 1993) and the effects being observed may therefore represent treatment of akinesia. One double-blind study which did not show a favourable impact of selegiline on negative symptoms (Goff *et al.* 1993) was fundamentally a study of tardive dyskinesia and had the weakness, for these purposes, of not having originally selected the patients for the presence of negative symptoms, but another negative double-blind study, while small and therefore lacking in statistical power ($n = 16$), did not suffer from this limitation (Jungerman *et al.* 1999). The reversible MAO-A inhibitor meclobemide also appeared to be beneficial in one small open study of adjunctive treatment for negative symptoms (Silver *et al.* 1999).

Several double-blind studies have indicated that an adjunctive serotonin reuptake-inhibitor (SSRI) (Silver & Nassar 1992; Spina *et al.* 1994; Goff *et al.* 1995; Silver & Shmugliakov 1998) or possibly a tricyclic (Collins & Dundas 1967; Siris *et al.* 1991a) or similar (Yamagami & Soejima 1989; Decina *et al.* 1994) antidepressant may be of use in ameliorating negative symptoms in some schizophrenic patients (Evins & Goff 1996), although other double-blind studies have not found such an effect (Buchanan *et al.* 1996; Salokangas *et al.* 1996; Taiminen *et al.* 1997; Lee *et al.* 1998; Arango *et al.* 2000). Careful distinctions would have to be made to differentiate improvements in negative symptoms from improvements in depression among such individuals (Goff & Evins 1998), and the use of instruments which are specifically targeted to depression in schizophrenia may be helpful in targeting these changes (Addington *et al.* 1996b; Collins *et al.* 1996). Otherwise, while the use of antidepressant agents in the absence of antipsychotic drugs is certainly not recommended in patients with schizophrenia (Siris *et al.* 1978), there have not been direct studies of the impact of antidepressant agents on chronic symptoms of schizophrenia

Table 9.2 Double-blind studies of antidepressants in 'depressed' schizophrenic patients. (Modified and supplemented after Siris 1991.)

Study (n)	Patients	Antipsychotic	Antidepressant	Duration	Result
Singh et al. (1978) n = 60	Schizophrenia by Feighner criteria Chronic patients with symptoms of depression HAM-D score >18 Inpatients	Previous phenothiazine continued	Trazodone 300 mg/day or placebo	6 weeks	Trazadone favoured by HAM-D and CGI scale changes No significant differences in BPRS
Prusoff et al. (1979) n = 35	Schizophrenia by New Haven Index criteria A score of at least 7 on the Raskin Depression Rating Scale Outpatients	Perphenazine 16–48 mg/day	Amitriptyline 100–200 mg/day or placebo	1, 2, 4 or 6 months	With amitriptyline: some decrease in depression ratings some increase in thought disorder and agitation ratings improvement in social well-being overall impression: mildly positive
Waehrens & Gerlach (1980) n = 17	'Schizophrenia' (no criteria given) Chronic and 'emotionally withdrawn 'Long-term' inpatients (cross-over design)	Continuation of previous neuroleptics	Maprotiline 50–200 mg/day or placebo	8 weeks	No benefit found from addition of maprotiline
Johnson (1981a) n = 50	Schizophrenia by Feighner or Schneiderian symptoms BDI score 15 or more for episode of 'acute' depression All 'chronic' patients (unstated if inpatients or outpatients)	Fluphenazine decanoate or flupenthixol decanoate (doses not specified)	Nortriptyline 150 mg/day or placebo	5 weeks	No statistically significant benefit to depression from adding nortriptyline, though 40% placebo response rate would make such a finding difficult to detect Increased side-effects with nortriptyline
Kurland & Nagaraju (1981) n = 22	Schizophrenia (no criteria given) HAM-D score of 18 or more Patients treated with antiparkinsonian medications were specifically excluded Inpatients	Chlorpromazine 75–300 mg/day or haloperidol 6–15 mg/day	Viloxazine to 300 mg/day maximum in final week only or placebo	4 weeks	No differences between groups Majority of patients in both groups improved
Becker (1983) n = 52	Schizophrenia by RDC RDC for major depressive syndrome (superimposed on schizophrenia) Inpatients	Chlorpromazine 100–1200 mg/day or thiothixene 5–60 mg/day	Imipramine 150–250 mg/day for patients on chlorpromazine, or placebo for patients on thiothixene	4 weeks (after 2 weeks drug free)	Both treatments effective compared with baseline on BPRS and HAM-D but neither treatment statistically superior to the other More sedative and autonomic side-effects with chlorpromazine–imipramine combination

Table 9.2 (cont.)

Study (n)	Patients	Antipsychotic	Antidepressant	Duration	Result
Siris *et al.* (1987a) *n* = 33	Schizophrenia or schizoaffective disorder by RDC (non-psychotic or residually psychotic) RDC for major or minor depression Depression unresponsive to benztropine 2 mg p.o. t.i.d. Outpatients	Fluphenazine decanoate – clinically adjusted stable weekly dose	Imipramine 150–200 mg/day or placebo	6 weeks	Imipramine group superior on global measure (CGI) and depression scales No difference between groups in psychosis or side-effects
Dufresne *et al.* (1988) *n* = 38	Schizophrenia by DSM-III Superimposed atypical affective disorder (equivalent to DSM-III major depression) Inpatients	Thiothixene – clinically adjusted stable dose	Bupropion 150–750 mg/day flexible dose or placebo	4 weeks	Both groups improved, but placebo group improved more Majority of bupropion-treated patients dropped out
Siris *et al.* (1989, 1994) *n* = 24	Schizophrenia or schizoaffective disorder by RDC (non-psychotic or residually psychotic) RDC for major depression History of favourable response to adjunctive imipramine (150–300 mg/day) Outpatients	Fluphenazine decanoate – clinically adjusted stable dose	Six months open continuation treatment with imipramine 100–300 mg/day, then either maintained on imipramine or tapered to placebo double-blind for 1 year	18 months	Significantly more relapses into depression in group tapered to adjunctive placebo than in those maintained on adjunctive imipramine (*P* < 0.001) No exacerbation of psychosis while on adjunctive imipramine Significantly fewer episodes of psychotic exacerbation in group maintained on adjunctive imipramine (*P* < 0.02)
Kramer *et al.* (1989) *n* = 58	Initial DSM-III diagnosis of schizophrenia RDC for schizophrenia disorder (mainly schizophrenic), depressive subtype HAM-D score >17 Treated with benztropine 2–8 mg/day Inpatients, actively psychotic	Haloperidol 0.4 mg/kg/day p.o.	Amitriptyline 3.5 mg/kg/day, Desipramine 3.5 mg/kg/day, or placebo	4 weeks	Neither addition of amitriptyline nor desipramine showed significant therapeutic advantage. Patients treated with antidepressant tended to score worse at the end on BPRS hallucinatory behaviour and thinking disturbance

Table 9.2 (cont.)

Study (n)	Patients	Antipsychotic	Antidepressant	Duration	Result
Müller-Siecheneder *et al.* (1998) n = 19	Inpatient admissions with schizophrenia or schizophreniform disorder by DSM-IIIR, who had scores of at least 15 on the BRMES and a score of at least 3 on the BRMES depression item	Risperidone 2–12 mg/day (mean = 6.9) vs. haloperidol 2.5–15 mg/day (mean = 9.0)	Amitriptyline 50–300 mg/day for the haloperidol group only	6 weeks	Decreases in the BRMES and BPRS scores were greater in the haloperidol/amitriptyline group, but this finding did not achieve statistical significance ($P = 0.11$ and 0.17, respectively). (Small n limits the power of this comparison, which was part of a much larger study involving patients with combined psychotic and depressive syndromes, the results of which were statistically significant)
Kirli & Çaliskan (1998) n = 40	Schizophrenia with postpsychotic depressive disorder according to DSM-IV HAM-D score of 14 or more No mention if inpatient or outpatient	Continuation of previous antipsychotic regimen (mean equivalent haloperidol dose = 6 mg/day)	Sertraline 50 mg/day vs. imipramine 150 mg/day	5 weeks	Significant reduction in HAM-D score in both groups ($P < 0.01$) in both groups after 5 weeks Significant reduction after 2 weeks in sertraline group only ($P < 0.05$). CGI improvement ($P < 0.01$) for sertraline beginning after first week and for imipramine after 2 weeks No placebo control group
Cooper *et al.* (2000) n = 24	Stable outpatients diagnosed with schizophrenia by DSM-IIIR criteria BPRS Depression item >3 and BDI >14	On stable antipsychotic medication (otherwise unstated)	Sertraline 'up to 100 mg daily' vs. placebo	Unstated	BDI score fell 15.8% in the sertraline group vs. 6.0% in the placebo group ($P < 0.05$). On CGI Change Scale 10/12 on sertraline improved vs. 4/12 on placebo ($P < 0.01$)
Vlokh *et al.* (2000) n = 40	Clinic patients with schizophrenia (criteria not stated), who also had 'depressions' (criteria not stated)	Unstated	Sertraline (doses not stated) vs. placebo	Mean course of treatment = 6 weeks	'Positive dynamics' on basis of HAM-D evaluation in 56.7% of sertraline-treated patients vs. 10.5% of placebo patients (no statistics reported)

BDI = Beck Depression Inventory; BMRES = Bech-Rafaelsen Melancholia Scale; BPRS = Brief Psychiatric Rating Scale; CGI = Clinical Global Impression; DSM = Diagnostic and Statistical Manual; HAM-D = Hamilton Depression Rating Scale; n = number of subjects; RDC = Research Diagnostic Criteria.

other than depression or negative symptoms among patients undergoing maintenance treatment with antipsychotic medication. The assessments of schizophrenic patients with depression or negative symptoms who have received antidepressant medication as an adjunct to an antipsychotic compound, however, have not suggested that ill effects have resulted. The reader is referred to Chapter 25 on the maintenance treatment of schizophrenia for additional discussion of negative and other chronic symptoms of schizophrenia and their treatments.

When adding adjunctive antidepressant medication to antipsychotic medication, the prescriber needs to be cognizant of the possibility that each of these drugs can potentially influence the metabolism of the other. The combination of neuroleptics plus tricyclic antidepressants has been described as raising blood levels in the past (Vandel *et al.* 1979; Nelson & Jatlow 1980; Siris *et al.* 1988c,d), and combinations involving more recently introduced compounds may do the same (Centorrino *et al.* 1996; Ereshefsky 1996). Appropriate cautions include conservatism in terms of rapidity of dosage increase, alertness to side-effects and adverse reactions, awareness of the potential for prolonged medication half-lives, sensitivity to pre-existing conditions which could be problematic (such as heart or liver disease), and monitoring of plasma concentrations where appropriate and available.

Large prospective controlled studies involving the combination of an antidepressant medication with an atypical antipsychotic medication have not as yet been published. It is tempting to extrapolate from the literature regarding standard neuroleptic agents that there might be a useful role for this combination, and clinicians in the field seem to be utilizing such combinations already (Siris *et al.* 2001), but a conclusive assessment is not yet available.

Lithium

Most of the studies involving the use of lithium in schizophrenia have involved the acute treatment of psychotic exacerbations, rather than its use in the maintenance phase of treatment (Christison *et al.* 1991; Plasky 1991), and the most frequently cited predictors of favourable response are excitement, overactivity and euphoria. Little evidence has been gathered concerning the use of lithium when depressive symptoms appear in schizophrenia (Levinson *et al.* 1999). Nevertheless, one small study has identified depressive symptomatology as a positive prognosticator of adjunctive lithium response in schizophrenia (Lerner *et al.* 1988). Previous affective episodes, family history of affective disorder and an overall episodic course may also be favourable indicators (Atre-Vaidya & Taylor 1989). It is therefore reasonable to attempt a trial of adjunctive lithium in patients with postpsychotic depression who have been otherwise non-responsive, especially if there are any other features of bipolar disorder involved in the clinical picture or if there is a family history suggestive of bipolar disorder. Similarly, it is rational to try lithium in addition to an adjunctive antidepressant for schizophrenic patients whose depression does not respond, although, again, specific documentation for this approach does not exist in the literature. Support for the use and safety of lithium, in patients who have both affective and psychotic characteristics, derives from the fact that it may be useful in patients with the closely related symptomatology of schizoaffective disorder (Siris 1996).

Psychosocial interventions

Although psychosocial interventions have not specifically been studied in a controlled fashion in schizophrenic patients with depression, it is clear that appropriate psychosocial approaches can be valuable in the long-term management of schizophrenia (Hogarty *et al.* 1986), and these benefits would logically be expected to be extended to schizophrenic patients with depressions. Such interventions include skill building, psychoeducation, stress reduction, problem-solving and family work aimed at reducing expressed emotion. Appropriate structure and support, along with treatments aimed at building self-esteem and realistic components of hope and confidence, may also be quite useful. Schizophrenic patients with depressions would appear to be particularly likely to benefit from such interventions because of their otherwise compromised status and fragility.

Conclusions

Depressive syndromes occur frequently during the longitudinal course of schizophrenia. These states are associated with considerable morbidity and even the risk of mortality. They carry important prognostic implications, and a number of differential diagnostic alternatives must be considered to undertake their treatment most usefully. Their proper understanding may also have heuristic relevance.

References

Abi-Dargham, A., Gil, R., Krystal, J. *et al.* (1998) Increased striatal dopamine transmission in schizophrenia: confirmation in a second cohort. *American Journal of Psychiatry* 155, 761–767.

Addington, D. & Addington, J. (1990) Depression dexamethasone nonsuppression and negative symptoms in schizophrenia. *Canadian Journal of Psychiatry* 35, 430–433.

Addington, D.E. & Addington, J.M. (1992) Attempted suicide and depression in schizophrenia. *Acta Psychiatrica Scandinavica* 85, 288–291.

Addington, D., Addington, J. & Patten, S. (1996a) Gender and affect in schizophrenia. *Canadian Journal of Psychiatry* 41, 265–268.

Addington, D., Addington, J. & Atkinson, M. (1996b) A psychometric comparison of the Calgary Depression Scale for Schizophrenia and the Hamilton Depression Rating Scale. *Schizophrenia Research* 19, 205–212.

Andreasen, N.C. & Olsen, S. (1982) Negative symptoms in schizophrenia: definition and reliability. *Archives of General Psychiatry* 39, 789–794.

Andreasen, N.C., Arndt, S., Alliger, R., Miller, D. & Flaum, M. (1995) Symptoms of schizophrenia: methods, meanings, and mechanisms. *Archives of General Psychiatry* 52, 341–351.

Arango, C., Kirkpatrick, B. & Buchanan, R.W. (2000) Fluoxetine as an adjunct to conventional antipsychotic treatment of schizophrenia patients with residual symptoms. *Journal of Nervous and Mental Disease* 188, 50–53.

Asherson, P., Mant, R., Williams, N. *et al.* (1998) A study of chromosome 4p markers and dopamine D5 receptor gene in schizophrenia and bipolar disorder. *Molecular Psychiatry* 3, 310–320.

Asnis, G.M., Friedman, T.A., Sanderson, W.C. *et al.* (1993) Suicidal behaviors in adult psychiatric outpatients. I. Description and prevalence. *American Journal of Psychiatry* 150, 108–112.

Atre-Vaidya, N. & Taylor, M.A. (1989) Effectiveness of lithium and schizophrenia: do we really have an answer? *Journal of Clinical Psychiatry* 50, 170–173.

Awad, A.G. (1993) Subjective response to neuroleptics in schizophrenia. *Schizophrenia Bulletin* 19, 609–618.

Azorin, J.M. (1995) Long-term treatment of mood disorders in schizophrenia. *Acta Psychiatrica Scandanavica* 91 (Suppl.), 20–23.

Bandelow, B., Müller, P., Gaebel, W. *et al.* (1990) Depressive syndromes in schizophrenic patients after discharge from hospital. *European Archives of Psychiatry and Clinical Neuroscience* 240, 113–120.

Bandelow, B., Müller, P., Frick, U. *et al.* (1992) Depressive syndromes in schizophrenic patients under neuroleptic therapy. *European Archive of Psychiatry and Clinical Neuroscience* 241, 291–295.

Barnes, T.R.E., Curson, D.A., Liddle, P.F. & Patel, M. (1989) The nature and prevalence of depression in chronic schizophrenic in-patients. *British Journal of Psychiatry* 154, 486–491.

Bartels, S.J. & Drake, R.E. (1988) Depressive symptoms in schizophrenia: comprehensive differential diagnosis. *Comprehensive Psychiatry* 29, 467–483.

Bartels, S.J. & Drake, R.E. (1989) Depression in schizophrenia: current guidelines to treatment. *Psychiatric Quarterly* 60, 337–357.

Bartels, S.J., Drake, R.E. & McHugo, G.J. (1992) Alcohol abuse, depression, and suicidal behavior in schizophrenia. *American Journal of Psychiatry* 149, 394–395.

Baynes, D., Mulholland, C., Cooper, S.J. *et al.* (2000) Depressive symptoms in stable chronic schizophrenia: prevalence and relationship to psychopathology and treatment. *Schizophrenia Research* 45, 47–56.

Beasley, C.M., Tollefson, G., Tran, P. *et al.* (1996) Olanzapine versus placebo and haloperidol: acute phase results of the North American double-blind olanzapine trial. *Neuropsychopharmacology* 14, 111–123.

Becker, R.E. (1983) Implications of the efficacy of thiothixene and a chlorpromazine–imipramine combination for depression in schizophrenia. *American Journal of Psychiatry* 140, 208–211.

Becker, R.E. (1988) Depression in schizophrenia. *Hospital and Community Psychiatry* 39, 1269–1275.

Bench, C.J., Friston, K.J., Brown, R.G. *et al.* (1992) The anatomy of melancholia: focal abnormalities of cerebral blood flow in major depression. *Psychological Medicine* 22, 607–615.

Bermanzohn, P.C. & Siris, S.G. (1992) Akinesia: a syndrome common to parkinsonism, retarded depression, and negative symptoms. *Comprehensive Psychiatry* 33, 221–232.

Berrios, G.E. & Bulbena, A. (1987) Post psychotic depression: the Fulbourn cohort. *Acta Psychiatrica Scandinavica* 76, 89–93.

Birchwood, M., Mason, R., Macmillan, F. & Healy, J. (1993) Depression, demoralization and control over psychotic illness: a comparison of depressed and non-depressed patients with a chronic psychosis. *Psychological Medicine* 23, 387–395.

Black, D.W. & Fisher, R. (1992) Mortality in DSM-IIIR schizophrenia. *Schizophrenia Research* 7, 109–116.

Black, D.W., Winokur, G. & Warrack, G. (1985) Suicide in schizophrenia: the Iowa record linkage study. *Journal of Clinical Psychiatry* 46, 14–17.

Bleuler, E. (1950) *Dementia Praecox or the Group of Schizophrenias*, p. 208. International Universities Press, New York.

Bodkin, A., Cohen, B.M., Salomon, M.S. *et al.* (1996) Treatment of negative symptoms in schizophrenia and schizoaffective disorder by selegiline augmentation of antipsychotic medication: a pilot study examining the role of dopamine. *Journal of Nervous and Mental Disease* 184, 295–301.

Borison, R.L., Arvanitis, L.A. & Miller, B.G. (1996) ICI 204,636, an atypical antipsychotic: efficacy and safety in a multicenter, placebo-controlled trial in patients with schizophrenia. *Journal of Clinical Psychopharmacology* 16, 158–169.

Bowers, M.D. & Astrachan, B.M. (1967) Depression in acute schizophrenic psychosis. *American Journal of Psychiatry* 123, 976–979.

Breier, A., Schreiber, J.L., Dyer, J. & Pickar, D. (1991) National Institute of Mental Health longitudinal study of chronic schizophrenia: prognosis and predictors of outcome. *Archives of General Psychiatry* 48, 239–246.

Breier, A., Su, T.-P., Saunders, R. *et al.* (1997) Schizophrenia is associated with elevated amphetamine-induced synaptic dopamine concentrations: evidence from a novel positron emission tomography method. *Proceedings of the National Academy of Science USA* 94, 2569–2574.

Browne, S., Garavan, J., Gervin, M. *et al.* (1998) Quality of life in schizophrenia: insight and subjective response to neuroleptics. *Journal of Nervous and Mental Disease* 186, 74–78.

Brzustowicz, L.M., Honer, W.G., Chow, E.W. *et al.* (1997) Use of a quantitative trait to map a locus associated with severity of positive symptoms in familial schizophrenia to chromosome 6p. *American Journal of Human Genetics* 61, 1388–1396.

Bucci, L. (1987) The negative symptoms of schizophrenia and monamine oxidase inhibitors. *Psychopharmacology* 91, 104–108.

Buchanan, R.W. (1995) Clozapine: efficacy and safety. *Schizophrenia Bulletin* 21, 579–591.

Buchanan, R.W., Kirkpatrick, B., Bryant, N., Ball, P. & Brier, A. (1996) Fluoxetine augmentation of clozapine treatment in patients with schizophrenia. *American Journal of Psychiatry* 153, 1625–1627.

Caldwell, C.B. & Gottesman, I.I. (1990) Schizophrenics kill themselves too: a review of risk factors for suicide. *Schizophrenia Bulletin* 16, 571–589.

Cardno, A.G., Jones, L.A., Murphy, K.C. *et al.* (1998) Sibling pairs with schizophrenia or schizoaffective disorder: associations of subtypes, symptoms and demographic variables. *Psychological Medicine* 28, 815–823.

Carpenter, W.T. Jr, Heinrichs, D.W. & Alphs, L.D. (1985) Treatment of negative symptoms. *Schizophrenia Bulletin* 11, 440–452.

Centorrino, F., Baldessarini, R.J., Frankenburg, F.R. *et al.* (1996) Serum levels of clozapine and norclozapine in patients treated with selective serotonin reuptake inhibitors. *American Journal of Psychiatry* 153, 820–822.

Chouinard, G., Jones, B., Remington, G. *et al.* (1993) A Canadian multicenter placebo-controlled study of fixed doses of risperidone and haloperidol in the treatment of chronic schizophrenic patients. *Journal of Clinical Psychopharmacology* 13, 25–40.

Christison, G.W., Kirch, D.G. & Wyatt, R.J. (1991) When symptoms persist: choosing among alternative somatic treatments for schizophrenia. *Schizophrenia Bulletin* 17, 217–240.

Cohen, S., Lavelle, J., Rich, C.L. & Bromet, E. (1994) Rates and correlates of suicide attempts in first-admission psychotic patients. *Acta Psychiatrica Scandinavica* 90, 167–171.

Collins, A.A., Remington, G., Coulter, K. & Birkett, K. (1996) Depression in schizophrenia: a comparison of three measures. *Schizophrenia Research* 20, 205–209.

Collins, A.D. & Dundas, J. (1967) A double-blind trial of amitriptyline/perphenazine, perphenazine, and placebo in chronic withdrawn inert schizophrenics. *British Journal of Psychiatry* 113, 1425–1429.

Cooper, S.J., Mulholland, C., Lynch, G., Baynes, D. & King, D.J. (2000) Sertraline in the treatment of depressive symptoms in stable, chronic schizophrenia: a placebo controlled trial [Abstract]. *Schizophrenia Research* 41, 209.

Coryell, W., Keller, M., Lavori, P. & Endicott, J. (1990) Affective syndromes, psychotic features, and prognosis. I. Depression. *Archives of General Psychiatry* 47, 651–657.

Crow, T.J. (1980) Molecular pathology of schizophrenia: more than one disease process? *British Medical Journal* 280, 66–68.

Dalack, G.W., Healy, D.J. & Meador-Woodruff, J.H. (1998) Nicotine dependence in schizophrenia: clinical phenomena and laboratory findings. *American Journal of Psychiatry* 155, 1490–1501.

Daniel, D.G., Zimbroff, D.L., Potkin, S.G. et al. & the Ziprasidone Study Group (1999) Ziprasidone 80 mg/day and 160 mg/day in the acute exacerbation of schizophrenia and schizoaffective disorder: a 6-week placebo-controlled trial. *Neuropsychopharmacology* 20, 491–505.

Dassori, A.M., Mezzich, J.E. & Keshavan, M. (1990) Suicidal indicators in schizophrenia. *Acta Psychiatrica Scandanavica* 81, 409–413.

Davis, K.L., Kahn, R.S., Ko, G. & Davidson, M. (1991) Dopamine in schizophrenia: a review and reconceptualization. *American Journal of Psychiatry* 148, 1474–1486.

DeAlarcon, R. & Carney, M.W.P. (1969) Severe depressive mood changes following slow-release intramuscular fluphenazine injection. *British Medical Journal* 3, 564–567.

Decina, P., Mukherjee, S., Bocola, V. et al. (1994) Adjunctive trazodone in the treatment of negative symptoms of schizophrenia. *Hospital and Community Psychiatry* 45, 1220–1223.

DeLisi, L.E., Goldin, L.R., Maxwell, E., Kazuba, D.M. & Gershon, E.S. (1987) Clinical features of illness in siblings with schizophrenia or schizoaffective disorder. *Archives of General Psychiatry* 44, 891–896.

Deutch, A.Y., Moghaddam, B., Innes, R.B. et al. (1991) Mechanisms of actions of atypical antipsychotic drugs: implications for novel therapeutic strategies for schizophrenia. *Schizophrenia Research* 4, 121–156.

D'haenen, H.A. & Bossuyt, A. (1994) Dopamine D_2 receptors in depression measured with single photon emission tomography. *Biological Psychiatry* 35, 128–132.

Docherty, J.P., van Kammen, D.P., Siris, S.G. & Marder, S.R. (1978) Stages of onset of schizophrenic psychosis. *American Journal of Psychiatry* 135, 420–426.

Dolan, R.J., Bench, C.J., Liddle, P.F. et al. (1993) Dorsolateral prefrontal cortex dysfunction in the major psychoses; symptom or disease specificity? *Journal of Neurology, Neurosurgery and Psychiatry* 56, 1290–1294.

Dollfus, S., Petit, M. & Menard, J.F. (1993) Relationship between depressive and positive symptoms in schizophrenia. *Journal of Affective Disorders* 28, 61–69.

Drake, R.E. & Cotton, P.G. (1986) Depression, hopelessness and suicide in chronic schizophrenia. *British Journal of Psychiatry* 148, 554–559.

Drake, R.E. & Ehrlich, J. (1985) Suicide attempts associated with akathisia. *American Journal of Psychiatry* 142, 499–501.

Drake, R.E., Gates, C., Cotton, P.G. & Whitaker, A. (1984) Suicide among schizophrenics: who is at risk? *Journal of Nervous and Mental Disease* 172, 613–617.

Drake, R.E., Gates, C., Whitaker, A. & Cotton, P.G. (1985) Suicide among schizophrenics: a review. *Comprehensive Psychiatry* 26, 90–100.

Drevets, W.C. (1998) Functional neuroimaging studies of depression: the anatomy of melancholic. *Annual Reviews of Medicine* 49, 341–361.

Dufresne, R.L., Kass, D.J. & Becker, R.E. (1988) Bupropion and thiothixene versus placebo and thiothixene in the treatment of depression in schizophrenia. *Drug Development Research* 12, 259–266.

Ebert, D., Feistel, H., Loew, T. & Pirner, A. (1996) Dopamine and depression: striatal dopamine D_2 receptor SPECT before and after antidepressant therapy. *Psychopharmacology* 126, 91–94.

Eissler, K.R. (1951) Remarks on the psycho-analysis of schizophrenia. *International Journal of Psychoanalysis* 32, 139–156.

Emsley, R.A., Oosthuizen, P.P., Joubert, A.F., Roberts, M.C. & Stein, D.J. (1999) Depressive and anxiety symptoms in patients with schizophrenia and schizophreniform disorder. *Journal of Clinical Psychiatry* 60, 747–751.

Ereshefsky, L. (1996) Pharmacokinetics and drug interactions: update for new antipsychotics. *Journal of Clinical Psychiatry* 57 (Suppl. 11), 12–25.

Evins, A.E. & Goff, D.C. (1996) Adjunctive antidepressant drug therapies in the treatment of negative symptoms of schizophrenia. *CNS Drugs* 6, 130–147.

Falloon, I., Watt, D.C. & Shepherd, M. (1978) A comparative controlled trial of pimozide and fluphenazine decanoate in the continuation therapy of schizophrenia. *Psychological Medicine* 8, 59–70.

Fenton, W.S., McGlashan, T.H., Victor, B.J. & Blyler, C.R. (1997) Symptoms, subtype, and suicidality in patients with schizophrenia spectrum disorders. *American Journal of Psychiatry* 154, 199–204.

deFigueiredo, J.M. (1993) Depression and demoralization: phenomenologic differences and research perspectives. *Comprehensive Psychiatry* 34, 308–311.

Floru, L., Heinrich, K. & Wittek, F. (1975) The problem of postpsychotic schizophrenic depressions and their pharmacological induction. *International Pharmacopsychiatry* 10, 230–239.

Frank, J.D. (1973) *Persuasion and Healing*. Johns Hopkins University Press, Baltimore.

Franz, M., Lis, S., Pluddemann, K. & Gallhofer, B. (1997) Conventional versus atypical neuroleptics: subjective quality of life in schizophrenic patients. *British Journal of Psychiatry* 170, 422–425.

Galdi, J. (1983) The causality of depression in schizophrenia. *British Journal of Psychiatry* 142, 621–625.

Galdi, J., Rieder, R.O., Silber, D. & Bonato, R.R. (1981) Genetic factors in the response to neuroleptics in schizophrenia: a pharmacogenetic study. *Psychological Medicine* 11, 713–728.

Goff, D.C. & Evins, A.E. (1998) Negative symptoms in schizophrenia: neurobiological models and treatment response. *Harvard Review of Psychiatry* 6, 59–77.

Goff, D.C., Renshaw, P.F., Sarid-Segal, O. et al. (1993) A placebo-controlled trial of selegiline (L-depreyl) in the treatment of tardive dyskinesia. *Biological Psychiatry* 33, 700–706.

Goff, D.C., Midha, K.K., Sarid-Segal, O., Hubbard, J.W. & Amico, E. (1995) A placebo-controlled trial of fluoxetine added to neuroleptic in patients with schizophrenia. *Psychopharmacology* 117, 417–423.

Goldstein, J.M. & Link, B.G. (1988) Gender and the expression of schizophrenia. *Journal of Psychiatric Research* 22, 141–155.

Goldstein, J.M., Santangelo, S.L., Simpson, J.C. & Tsuang, M.T. (1990) The role of gender in identifying subtypes of schizophrenia: a latent class analytic approach. *Schizophrenia Bulletin* 16, 263–275.

Green, M.F., Nuechterlein, K.H., Ventura, J. & Mintz, J. (1990) The temporal relationship between depressive and psychotic symptoms in recent-onset schizophrenia. *American Journal of Psychiatry* 147, 179–182.

Griffiths, R.R. & Mumford, G.K. (1995) Caffeine: a drug of abuse? In: *Psychopharmacology: the Fourth Generation of Progress* (eds F.E. Bloom & D.J. Kupfer), pp. 1699–1713. Raven Press, New York.

Gupta, S., Black, D.W., Arndt, S., Hubbard, W.C. & Andreasen, N.C. (1998) Factors associated with suicide attempts among patients with schizophrenia. *Psychiatric Services* 49, 1353–1355.

Gur, R.E., Cowell, P.E., Latshaw, A. *et al.* (2000) Reduced dorsal and orbital prefrontal gray matter volumes in schizophrenia. *Archives of General Psychiatry* 57, 76–768.

Guze, S.B., Cloninger, C.R., Martin, R.L. & Clayton, P.J. (1983) A follow-up and family study of schizophrenia. *Archives of General Psychiatry* 40, 1273–1276.

de Haan, L., Lavalaye, J., Linszen, D., Dingemans, P.M.A.J. & Booij, J. (2000) Subjective experience and striatal dopamine D$_2$ receptor occupancy in patients with schizophrenia stabilized with olanzapine or risperidone. *American Journal of Psychiatry* 157, 1019–1020.

Haas, G.L., Glick, I.D., Clarkin, J.F., Spencer, J.H. & Lewis, A.B. (1990) Gender and schizophrenia outcome: a clinical trial of an inpatient family intervention. *Schizophrenia Bulletin* 16, 277–292.

Häfner, H., Maurer, K., Löffler, W. *et al.* (1994) The epidemiology of early schizophrenia: influence of age and gender on onset and early course. *British Journal of Psychiatry* 164 (Suppl. 23), 29–38.

Halstead, S.M., Barnes, T.R.E. & Speller, J.C. (1994) Akathisia: pre-valence and associated dysphoria in an in-patient population with chronic schizophrenia. *British Journal of Psychiatry* 164, 177–183.

Harrow, M., Yonan, C.A., Sands, J.F. & Marengo, J. (1994) Depression in schizophrenia: are neuroleptics, akinesia, or anhedonia involved? *Schizophrenia Bulletin* 20, 327–338.

Heilä, H., Isometsä, E.T., Henriksson, M.M. *et al.* (1997) A nationwide psychological autopsy study on age- and sex-specific clinical characteristics of 92 suicide victims with schizophrenia. *American Journal of Psychiatry* 154, 1235–1242.

Heilä, H., Heikkinen, M.E., Isometsä, E.T. *et al.* (1999) Life events and completed suicide in schizophrenia: a comparison of suicide victims with and without schizophrenia. *Schizophrenia Bulletin* 25, 519–531.

Herz, M. (1985) Prodromal symptoms and prevention of relapse in schizophrenia. *Journal of Clinical Psychiatry* 46 (11), 22–25.

Herz, M. & Melville, C. (1980) Relapse in schizophrenia. *American Journal of Psychiatry* 137, 801–805.

Hietala, J., Syvälahti, E., Vilkman, H. *et al.* (1999) Depressive symptoms and presynaptic dopamine function in neuroleptic-naive schizophrenia. *Schizophrenia Research* 35, 41–50.

Hirsch, S.R. & Jolley, A.G. (1989) The dysphoric syndrome in schizophrenia and its implications for relapse. *British Journal of Psychiatry* 155 (Suppl. 5), 46–50.

Hirsch, S.R., Gaind, R., Rohde, P.D., Stevens, B.C. & Wing, J.T. (1973) Outpatient maintenance of chronic schizophrenic patients with long-acting fluphenazine: double-blind placebo trial. *British Medical Journal* 1, 633–637.

Hirsch, S.R., Jolley, A.G., Barnes, T.R.E. *et al.* (1989) Dysphoric and depressive symptoms in chronic schizophrenia. *Schizophrenia Research* 2, 259–264.

Hoffmann, H., Kupper, Z. & Kunz, B. (2000) Hopelessness and its impact on rehabilitation outcome in schizophrenia: an exploratory study. *Schizophrenia Research* 43, 147–158.

Hogarty, G.E. & Munetz, M.R. (1984) Pharmacogenic depression among outpatient schizophrenic patients: a failure to substantiate. *Journal of Clinical Psychopharmacology* 4, 17–24.

Hogarty, G.E., Anderson, C.M., Reiss, D.J. *et al.* (1986) Family psychoeducational, social skills training, and maintenance chemotherapy in the aftercare treatment of schizophrenia. I. One-year effects of a controlled study on relapse and expressed emotion. *Archives of General Psychiatry* 43, 633–642.

Inskip, H.M., Harris, E.C. & Barraclough, B. (1998) Lifetime risk of suicide for affective disorder, alcoholism and schizophrenia. *British Journal of Psychiatry* 172, 35–37.

Ismail, K., Murray, R.M., Wheeler, M.J. & O'Keane, V. (1998) The dexamethasone suppression test in schizophrenia. *Psychological Medicine* 28, 311–317.

Johnson, D.A.W. (1981a) Studies of depressive symptoms in schizophrenia. *British Journal of Psychiatry* 139, 89–101.

Johnson, D.A.W. (1981b) Depressions in schizophrenia: some observations on prevalence, etiology, and treatment. *Acta Psychiatrica Scandinavica* 63 (Suppl. 291), 137–144.

Johnson, D.A.W. (1988) The significance of depression in the prediction of relapse in chronic schizophrenia. *British Journal of Psychiatry* 152, 320–323.

Jones, H. (1997) Risperidone: a review of its pharmacology and use in the treatment of schizophrenia. *Journal of Serotonin Research* 4, 17–28.

Jones, J.S., Stein, D.J., Stanley, B. *et al.* (1994) Negative and depressive symptoms in suicidal schizophrenics. *Acta Psychiatrica Scandinavica* 89, 81–87.

Jungerman, T., Rabinowitz, D. & Klein, E. (1999) Depreyl augmentation for treating negative symptoms of schizophrenia: a double-blind, controlled study. *Journal of Clinical Psychopharmacology* 19, 522–525.

Kane, J.M., Rifkin, A., Woerner, M. *et al.* (1983) Low dose neuroleptic treatment of outpatient schizophrenics. I. Preliminary results for relapse rates. *Archives of General Psychiatry* 40, 893–896.

Kane, J., Honigfeld, G., Singer, J. & Meltzer, H. (1988) Clozapine for the treatment-resistant schizophrenic: a double-blind comparison with chlorpromazine. *Archives of General Psychiatry* 45, 789–796.

Keck, P., Buffenstein, A., Ferguson, J. *et al.* (1998) Ziprasidone 40 and 120 mg/day in the acute exacerbation of schizophrenia and schizoaffective disorder: a 4-week placebo-controlled trial. *Psychopharmacology (Berl)* 140, 173–184.

Kemp, R.A. & Lambert, T.J.R. (1995) Insight in schizophrenia and its relationship to psychopathology. *Schizophrenia Research* 18, 21–28.

Kendler, K.S. & Hays, P. (1983) Schizophrenia subdivided by the family history of affective disorder: a comparison of symptomatology and cause of illness. *Archives of General Psychiatry* 40, 951–955.

Kendler, K.S., McGuire, M., Gruenberg, A.M. *et al.* (1993) The Roscommon family study. I. methods, diagnosis of probands, and risk of schizophrenia in relatives. *Archives of General Psychiatry* 50, 527–540.

Kendler, K.S., Karkowski-Shuman, L. & Walsh, D. (1996) The risk for psychiatric illness in siblings of schizophrenics: the impact of psychotic and non-psychotic affective illness and alcoholism in parents. *Acta Psychiatrica Scandinavica* 94, 49–55.

Kendler, K.S., Karkowski-Shuman, L., O'Neill, A. *et al.* (1997) Resemblance of psychotic symptoms and syndromes in affected sibling pairs from the Irish study of high-density schizophrenia families: evidence for possible etiologic heterogeneity. *American Journal of Psychiatry* 154, 191–198.

Kendler, K.S., Myers, J.M., O'Neill, F.A. *et al.* (2000) Clinical features of schizophrenia and linkage to chromosomes 5q, 6p, 8p, and 10p in the Irish study of high-density schizophrenia families. *American Journal of Psychiatry* 157, 402–408.

Kibel, D.A., Laffont, I. & Liddle, P.F. (1993) The composition of the negative syndrome of chronic schizophrenia. *British Journal of Psychiatry* 162, 744–750.

Kirkpatrick, B., Amador, X.F., Yale, S.A. *et al.* (1996) The deficit syndrome in the DSM-IV field trial. II. Depressive episodes and persecutory beliefs. *Schizophrenia Research* 20, 79–90.

Kirli, S. & Çaliskan, M. (1998) A comparative study of sertraline versus imipramine in postpsychotic depressive disorder of schizophrenia. *Schizophrenia Research* 33, 103–111.

Klein, D.F. (1974) Endomorphic depression: a conceptual and terminological revision. *Archives of General Psychiatry* **31**, 447–454.

Knable, M.B., Egan, M.F., Heinz, A. *et al.* (1997) Altered dopaminergic function and negative symptoms in drug-free patients with schizophrenia: [^{123}I]-iodobenzamine SPECT study. *British Journal of Psychiatry* **171**, 574–577.

Knights, A. & Hirsch, S.R. (1981) 'Revealed' depression and drug treatment for schizophrenia. *Archives of General Psychiatry* **38**, 806–811.

Knights, A., Okasha, M.S., Salih, M.A. & Hirsch, S.R. (1979) Depressive and extrapyramidal symptoms and clinical effects: a trial of fluphenazine versus flupenthixol in maintenance of schizophrenic out-patients. *British Journal of Psychiatry* **135**, 515–523.

Kohler, C., Gur, R.C., Swanson, C.L., Petty, R. & Gur, R.E. (1998a) Depression in schizophrenia. I. Association with neuroopsychological deficits. *Biological Psychiatry* **43**, 165–172.

Kohler, C., Swanson, C.L., Gur, R.C., Mozley, L.H. & Gur, R.E. (1998b) Depression in schizophrenia. II. MRI and PET findings. *Biological Psychiatry* **43**, 173–180.

Koreen, A.R., Siris, S.G., Chakos, M. *et al.* (1993) Depression in first-episode schizophrenia. *American Journal of Psychiatry* **150**, 1643–1648.

Krakowski, M., Czobor, P. & Volavka, J. (1997) Effect of neuroleptic treatment on depressive symptoms in acute schizophrenic episodes. *Psychiatric Research* **71**, 19–26.

Kramer, M.S., Vogel, W.H., DiJohnson, C. *et al.* (1989) Antidepressants in 'depressed' schizophrenic inpatients: a controlled trial. *Archives of General Psychiatry* **46**, 922–928.

Krausz, M., Müller-Thomsen, T. & Hassen, C. (1995) Suicide among schizophrenic adolescents in the long-term course of illness. *Psychopathology* **28**, 95–103.

Kuck, J., Zisook, S., Moranville, J.T., Heaton, R.K. & Braff, D.L. (1992) Negative symptomatology in schizophrenic outpatients. *Journal of Nervous and Mental Disease* **180**, 510–515.

Kulhara, P., Avasthi, A., Chadda, R. *et al.* (1989) Negative and depressive symptoms in schizophrenia. *British Journal of Psychiatry* **154**, 207–211.

Kurland, A.A. & Nagaraju, A. (1981) Viloxazine and the depressed schizophrenic: methodological issues. *Journal of Clinical Pharmacology* **21**, 37–41.

Laruelle, M. (1998) Imaging dopamine neurotransmission in schizophrenia: a review and meta-analysis. *Quarterly Journal of Nuclear Medicine* **42**, 211–221.

Laruelle, M., Abi-Dargham, A., Gil, R., Kegeles, L. & Innis, R. (1999) Increased dopamine transmission in schizophrenia: relationship to illness phases. *Biological Psychiatry* **46**, 56–72.

Laruelle, M., Abi-Dargham, A., van Dyck, C. *et al.* (2000) Dopamine and serotonin transporters in patients with schizophrenia: an imaging study with [^{123}]-CIT. *Biological Psychiatry* **47**, 371–379.

Lee, M.S., Kim, Y.K., Lee, S.K. & Suh, K.Y. (1998) A double-blind study of adjunctive sertraline in haloperidol-stabilized patients with chronic schizophrenia. *Journal of Clinical Psychopharmacology* **18**, 399–403.

Leff, J., Tress, K. & Edwards, B. (1988) The clinical course of depressive symptoms in schizophrenia. *Schizophrenia Research* **1**, 25–30.

Lerner, Y., Mintzer, Y. & Schestatzky, M. (1988) Lithium combined with haloperidol in schizophrenic patients. *British Journal of Psychiatry* **153**, 359–362.

Levinson, D.F., Umapathy, C. & Musthaq, M. (1999) Treatment of schizoaffective disorder and schizophrenia with mood symptoms. *American Journal of Psychiatry* **156**, 1138–1148.

Levitt, J.J. & Tsuang, M.T. (1988) The heterogeneity of schizoaffective disorder: implications for treatment. *American Journal of Psychiatry* **145**, 926–936.

Lewis, R., Kapur, S., Jones, C. *et al.* (1999) Serotonin 5-HT$_2$ receptors in schizophrenia: a PET study unsing [^{18}F]setoperone in neuroleptic-naive patients and normal subjects. *American Journal of Psychiatry* **156**, 72–78.

Liddle, P.F., Friston, K.J., Frith, C.D. *et al.* (1992) Patterns of cerebral blood flow in schizophrenia. *British Journal of Psychiatry* **160**, 179–186.

Liddle, P.F., Barnes, T.R.E., Curson, D.A. & Patel, M. (1993) Depression and the experience of psychological deficits in schizophrenia. *Acta Psychiatrica Scandanavica* **88**, 243–247.

Lindenmayer, J.-P., Grochowski, S. & Kay, S.R. (1991) Schizophrenic patients with depression: psychopathological profiles and relationship with negative symptoms. *Comprehensive Psychiatry* **32**, 528–533.

Lindenmayer, J.P., Grochowski, S. & Hyman, R.B. (1995) Five factor model of schizophrenia: replication across samples. *Schizophrenia Research* **14**, 229–234.

Lysaker, P.H., Bell, M.D., Bioty, S.M. & Zito, W.S. (1995) The frequency of associations between positive and negative symptoms and dysphoria in schizophrenia. *Comprehensive Psychiatry* **36**, 113–117.

McGlashan, T.H. & Bardenstein, K.K. (1990) Gender differences is affective, schizoaffective, and schizophrenic disorders. *Schizophrenia Bulletin* **16**, 319–329.

McGlashan, T.H. & Carpenter, W.T. Jr (1976a) Postpsychotic depression in schizophrenia. *Archives of General Psychiatry* **33**, 231–239.

McGlashan, T.H. & Carpenter, W.T. Jr (1976b) An investigation of the post psychotic depressive syndrome. *American Journal of Psychiatry* **133**, 14–19.

McGuire, P.K., Shah, G.M.S. & Murray, R.M. (1993) Increased blood flow in Broca's area during auditory hallucinations in schizophrenia. *Lancet* **342**, 703–706.

Maier, W., Lichtermann, D., Minges, J. *et al.* (1993) Continuity and discontinuity of affective disorders and schizophrenia: results of a controlled family study. *Archives of General Psychiatry* **50**, 871–883.

Malhotra, A. (2001) The genetics of schizophrenia. *Current Opinion in Psychiatry* **14**, 3–7.

Malla, A.K. & Norman, R.M.G. (1994) Prodromal symptoms in schizophrenia. *British Journal of Psychiatry* **164**, 287–293.

Mandel, M.R., Severe, J.B., Schooler, N.R., Gelenberg, A.J. & Mieske, M. (1982) Development and prediction of post-psychotic depression in neuroleptic-treated schizophrenics. *Archives of General Psychiatry* **39**, 197–203.

Marder, S.R. & Meibach, R.C. (1994) Risperidone in the treatment of schizophrenia. *American Journal of Psychiatry* **151**, 825–835.

Marder, S.R., Van Putten, T., Mintz, J. *et al.* (1987) Low- and conventional-dose maintenance therapy with fluphenazine decanoate: two year outcome. *Archives of General Psychiatry* **44**, 518–521.

Markou, P. (1996) Depression in schizophrenia: a descriptive study. *Australian and New Zealand Journal of Psychiatry* **30**, 354–357.

Martin, R.L., Cloninger, R.C., Guze, S.B. & Clayton, P.J. (1985) Frequency and differential diagnosis of depressive syndromes in schizophrenia. *Journal of Clinical Psychiatry* **46** (11), 9–13.

Martinot, J.L., Paillère-Martinot, M.L., Loc'h, C. *et al.* (1994) Central D$_2$ receptors and negative symptoms of schizophrenia. *British Journal of Psychiatry* **164**, 27–34.

Mauri, M.C., Bravin, S., Fabiano, L. *et al.* (1995) Depressive symptoms and schizophrenia: a psychopharmacological approach. *L'Encephale* **21**, 555–558.

Meltzer, H.Y. & Okayli, G. (1995) Reduction of suicidality during clozapine treatment of neuroleptic-resistant schizophrenia: impact on risk-benefit assessment. *American Journal of Psychiatry* **152**, 183–190.

Meltzer, H.Y., Matsubara, S. & Lee, J.C. (1989) Classification of typical and atypical antipsychotic drugs on the basis of dopamine D_1, D_2 and serotonin$_2$ pKi values. *Journal of Pharmacology and Experimental Therapeutics* **25**, 238–246.

Miles, C. (1977) Conditions predisposing to suicide: a review. *Journal of Nervous and Mental Disease* **164**, 221–246.

Miller, J.B. & Sonnenberg, S.M. (1973) Depression following psychotic episodes: a response to the challenge of change? *Journal of the American Academy of Psychoanalysis* **1**, 253–270.

Möller, H.J. & von Zerssen, D. (1982) Depressive states occurring during the neuroleptic treatment of schizophrenia. *Schizophrenia Bulletin* **8**, 109–117.

Möller, H.J. & von Zerssen, D. (1986) Depression in schizophrenia. In: *Handbook of Studies on Schizophrenia, Part 1* (eds G.D. Burrows, T.R. Norman & G. Rubinstein), pp. 183–191. Elsevier, Amsterdam.

Möller, H.J., Muller, H., Borison, R., Schooler, N.R. & Chouinard, G. (1995) A path analytical approach to differentiate between direct and indirect drug effects on negative symptoms in schizophrenic patients: a re-evaluation of the North American risperidone study. *European Archives of Clinical Neuroscience* **245**, 45–49.

Müller, M.J. & Wetzel, H. (1998) Dimensionality of depression in acute schizophrenia: a methodological study using the Bech–Rafaelsen Melancholia Scale (BRMES). *Journal of Psychiatric Research* **32**, 369–378.

Müller-Siecheneder, F., Müller, M.J., Hillert, A. *et al.* (1998) Risperidone versus haloperidol and amitriptyline in the treatment of patients with a combined psychotic and depressive syndrome. *Journal of Clinical Psychopharmacology* **18**, 111–120.

Munro, J.G., Hardiker, T.M. & Leonard, D.P. (1984) The dexamethasone suppression test in residual schizophrenia with depression. *American Journal of Psychiatry* **141**, 250–252.

Nakaya, M., Ohmori, K., Komahashi, T. & Suwa, H. (1997) Depressive symptoms in acute schizophrenic inpatients. *Schizophrenia Research* **25**, 131–139.

Nelson, J.C. & Jatlow, P.I. (1980) Neuroleptic effect on desipramine steady-state plasma concentrations. *American Journal of Psychiatry* **137**, 1232–1234.

Ngan, E.T.C., Yatham, L.N., Ruth, T.J. & Liddle, P.F. (2000) Decreased serotonin 2A receptor densities in neuroleptic-naive patients with schizophenia: a PET study using [^{18}F]setoperone. *American Journal of Psychiatry* **157**, 1016–1018.

Norman, R.M.G. & Malla, A.K. (1991) Dysphoric mood and symptomatology in schizophrenia. *Psychological Medicine* **21**, 897–903.

Norman, R.M.G. & Malla, A.K. (1994) Correlations over time between dysphoric mood and symptomatology in schizophrenia. *Comprehensive Psychiatry* **35**, 34–38.

Norman, R.M.G., Malla, A.K., Cortese, L. & Diaz, F. (1998) Aspects of dysphoria and symptoms of schizophrenia. *Psychological Medicine* **28**, 1433–1441.

Nuechterlein, K.H. & Dawson, M.D. (1984) A heuristic vulnerability/stress model of schizophrenic episodes. *Schizophrenia Bulletin* **10**, 300–312.

Nyman, A.K. & Jonsson, H. (1986) Patterns of self-destructive behaviour in schizophrenia. *Acta Psychiatrica Scandinavica* **73**, 252–262.

Olfson, M., Mechanic, D., Boyer, C.A. *et al.* (1999) Assessing clinical predictions of early rehospitalization in schizophrenia. *Journal of Nervous and Mental Disease* **187**, 721–729.

Parkinson Study Group (1993) Effects of tocopherol and deprenyl on the progression of disability in early Parkinson's disease. *New England Journal of Medicine* **328**, 176–183.

Peralta, V. & Cuesta, M.J. (1994) Lack of insight: its status within schizophrenic psychopathology. *Biological Psychiatry* **36**, 559–561.

Peralta, V. & Cuesta, M.J. (1999) Negative, parkinsonian, depressive and catatonic symptoms in schizophrenia: a conflict of paradigms revisited. *Schizophrenia Research* **40**, 245–253.

Perenyi, A., Goswami, U., Frecska, E. & Arato, M. (1992) L-deprenyl in treating negative symptoms of schizophrenia. *Psychiatry Research* **42**, 189–191.

Perenyi, A., Norman, T., Hopwood, M. & Burrows, G. (1998) Negative symptoms, depression and parkinsonian symptoms in chronic, hospitalised schizophrenic patients. *Journal of Affective Disorders* **48**, 163–169.

Peuskens, J. (1995) Risperidone in the treatment of patients with chronic schizophrenia: a multinational, multi-center, double-blind, parallel group study versus haloperidol. *British Journal of Psychiatry* **166**, 712–726.

Plasky, P. (1991) Antidepressant usage in schizophrenia. *Schizophrenia Bulletin* **17**, 649–657.

Prasad, A.J. & Kumar, N. (1988) Suicidal behavior in hospitalized schizophrenics. *Suicide and Life-Threatening Behavior* **18**, 265–269.

Prusoff, B.A., Williams, D.H., Weissman, M.M. & Astrachan, B.M. (1979) Treatment of secondary depression in schizophrenia. *Archives of General Psychiatry* **36**, 569–575.

Rifkin, A., Quitkin, F. & Klein, D.F. (1975) Akinesia: a poorly recognized drug-induced extrapyramidal behavioral disorder. *Archives of General Psychiatry* **32**, 672–674.

Rifkin, A., Quitkin, F., Kane, J., Struve, F. & Klein, D.F. (1978) Are prophylactic antiparkinsonian drugs necessary? A controlled study of procyclidine withdrawal. *Archives of General Psychiatry* **35**, 483–489.

Roth, S. (1970) The seemingly ubiquitous depression following acute schizophrenic episodes, a neglected area of clinical discussion. *American Journal of Psychiatry* **127**, 51–58.

Roy, A. (1980) Depression in chronic paranoid schizophrenia. *British Journal of Psychiatry* **137**, 138–139.

Roy, A. (1981) Depression in the course of chronic undifferentiated schizophrenia. *Archives of General Psychiatry* **38**, 296–297.

Roy, A. (1982) Suicide in chronic schizophrenia. *British Journal of Psychiatry* **141**, 171–177.

Roy, A. (1984) Do neuroleptics cause depression? *Biological Psychiatry* **19**, 777–781.

Roy, A. (1986) Depression, attempted suicide, and suicide in patients with chronic schizophrenia. *Psychiatric Clinics of North America* **9**, 193–206.

Roy, A., Thompson, R. & Kennedy, S. (1983) Depression in chronic schizophrenia. *British Journal of Psychiatry* **142**, 465–470.

Saarinen, P.I., Lehtonen, J. & Lönnqvist, J. (1999) Suicide risk in schizophrenia: an analysis of 17 consecutive suicides. *Schizophrenia Bulletin* **25**, 533–542.

Salokangas, R.K.R., Saarijärvi, S., Taiminen, T. *et al.* (1996) Citalopram as an adjuvant in chronic schizophrenia: a double-blind placebo-controlled study. *Acta Psychiatrica Scandinavica* **94**, 175–180.

Sands, J.R. & Harrow, M. (1999) Depression during the longitudinal course of schizophrenia. *Schizophrenia Bulletin* **25**, 157–171.

Sax, K.W., Strakowski, S.M., Keck, P.E. *et al.* (1996) Relationships amond negative, positive, and depressive symptoms in schizophrenia and psychotic depression. *British Journal of Psychiatry* **168**, 68–71.

Schildkraut, J.J., Orsulak, P.J., Schatzberg, A.F. & Herzog, J.M. (1980)

Platelet monoamine oxidase activity in subgroups of schizophrenic disorders. *Schizophrenia Bulletin* 6, 220–225.

Seeger, T.F., Seymour, P.A., Schmidt, A.W. *et al.* (1995) Ziprasidone (CP-88,059): a new antipsychotic with combined dopamine and serotonin receptor antagonist activity. *Journal of Pharmacology and Experimental Therapeutics* 275, 101–113.

Semrad, E.V. (1966) Long-term therapy of schizophrenia: formulation of the clinical approach. In: *Psychoneuroses and Schizophrenia* (ed. G. Usdin), pp. 155–173. J.B. Lippincott, Philadelphia.

Serretti, A., Macciardi, F.M. & Smeraldi, E. (1996) Identification of symptomatologic patterns common to major psychoses: proposal for a phenotype definition. *American Journal of Medical Genetics* 67, 393–400.

Serretti, A., Catalano, M. & Smeraldi, E. (1999a) Serotonin transporter gene is not associated with symptomatology of schizophrenia. *Schizophrenia Research* 35, 33–39.

Serretti, A., Lattuada, E., Cusin, C. *et al.* (1999b) Dopamine D$_3$ receptor gene not associated with symptomatology of major psychoses. *American Journal of Medical Genetics* 88, 476–480.

Serretti, A., Cusin, C., Lattuada, E. *et al.* (1999c) No interaction between serotonin transporter gene and dopamine receptor D$_4$ gene in symptomatology of major psychoses. *American Journal of Medical Genetics* 88, 481–485.

Shah, P.J., Ogilvie, A.D., Goodwin, G.M. & Ebmeier, K.P. (1997) Clinical and psychometric correlates of dopamine D$_2$ binding in depression. *Psychological Medicine* 27, 1247–1256.

Shear, K., Frances, A. & Weiden, P. (1983) Suicide associated with akathisia and depot fluphenazine treatment. *Journal of Clinical Psychopharmacology* 3, 235–236.

Shtasel, D.L., Gur, R.E., Gallacher, F., Heimberg, C. & Gur, R.C. (1992) Gender differences in the clinical expression of schizophrenia. *Schizophrenia Research* 7, 225–231.

Silver, H. & Nassar, A. (1992) Fluvoxamine improves negative symptoms in treated chronic schizophrenia: an add-on double-blind, placebo-controlled study. *Biological Psychiatry* 31, 698–704.

Silver, H. & Shmugliakov, N. (1998) Augmentation with fluvoxamine but not maprotiline improves negative symptoms in treated schizophrenia: evidence for a specific serotonergic effect from a double-blind study. *Journal of Clinical Psychopharmacology* 18, 208–211.

Silver, H., Aharon, N., Hausfater, N. & Jhahah, N. (1999) The effect of augmentation with moclobemide on symptoms of schizophrenia. *International Clinical Psychopharmacology* 14, 193–195.

Singh, A.N., Saxena, B. & Nelson, H.L. (1978) A controlled clinical study of trazodone in chronic schizophrenic patients with pronounced depressive symptomatology. *Current Therapeutics Research* 23, 485–501.

Siris, S.G. (1985) Akathisia and 'acting-out. *Journal of Clinical Psychiatry* 46, 395–397.

Siris, S.G. (1991) Diagnosis of secondary depression in schizophrenia: implications for DSM-IV. *Schizophrenia Bulletin* 17, 75–98.

Siris, S.G. (1996) The treatment of schizoaffective disorder. In: *Current Psychiatric Therapy II* (ed. D.L. Dunner), pp. 196–201. W.B. Saunders, Philadelphia.

Siris, S.G. (2000) Depression in schizophrenia: perspective in the era of 'atypical' antipsychotic agents. *American Journal of Psychiatry* 157, 1379–1389.

Siris, S.G. (2001a) Suicide and schizophrenia. *Journal of Psychopharmacology* 15, 129–137.

Siris, S.G. (2001b) Depression in the course of schizophrenia. In: *Schizophrenia and Comorbid Conditions: Diagnosis and Treatment* (eds. M.Y. Hwang & P.C. Bermanzohn), pp. 31–56. American Psychiatric Press, Washington, DC.

Siris, S.G. & Lavin, M.R. (1995) Schizoaffective disorder, schizophreniform disorder, and acute psychotic disorder. In: *Comprehensive Textbook of Psychiatry* Vol. 1, 6th edn (eds H.I. Kaplan & B.J. Sadock), pp. 1019–1031, Williams & Wilkins, Baltimore.

Siris, S.G., van Kammen, D.P. & Docherty, J.P. (1978) The use of antidepressant medication in schizophrenia: a review of the literature. *Archives of General Psychiatry* 35, 1368–1377.

Siris, S.G., Harmon, G.K. & Endicott, J. (1981) Postpsychotic depressive symptoms in hospitalized schizophrenic patients. *Archives of General Psychiatry* 38, 1122–1123.

Siris, S.G., Rifkin, A., Reardon, G.T. *et al.* (1984) The dexamethasone suppression test in patients with post-psychotic depressions. *Biological Psychiatry* 19, 1351–1356.

Siris, S.G., Morgan, V., Fagerstrom, R., Rifkin, A. & Cooper, T.B. (1987) Adjunctive imipramine in the treatment of post-psychotic depression: a controlled trial. *Archives of General Psychiatry* 44, 533–539.

Siris, S.G., Strahan, A., Mandeli, J., Cooper, T.B. & Casey, E. (1988a) Fluphenazine decanoate dose and severity of depression in patients with post-psychotic depression. *Schizophrenia Research* 1, 31–35.

Siris, S.G., Adan, F., Cohen, M. *et al.* (1988b) Post-psychotic depression and negative symptoms: an investigation of syndromal overlap. *American Journal of Psychiatry* 145, 1532–1537.

Siris, S.G., Adan, F., Lee, A. *et al.* (1988c) Patterns of plasma imipramine/desipramine concentrations in patients receiving concomitant fluphenazine decanoate. *Journal of Clinical Psychiatry* 49, 64–65.

Siris, S.G., Sellew, A.P., Frechen, K. *et al.* (1988d) Antidepressants in the treatment of post-psychotic depression in schizophrenia: drug interactions and other considerations. *Journal of Clinical Chemistry* 34, 837–840.

Siris, S.G., Cutler, J., Owen, K. *et al.* (1989) Adjunctive imipramine maintenance in schizophrenic patients with remitted post-psychotic depressions. *American Journal of Psychiatry* 146, 1495–1497.

Siris, S.G., Bermanzohn, P.C., Gonzalez, A. *et al.* (1991a) The use of antidepressants for negative symptoms in a subset of schizophrenic patients. *Psychopharmacology Bulletin* 27, 331–335.

Siris, S.G., Frechen, K., Strahan, A. *et al.* (1991b) Thyroid-releasing hormone test in schizophrenic patients with post-psychotic depression. *Progress in Neuro-Psychopharmacology and Biological Psychiatry* 15, 369–378.

Siris, S.G., Bermanzohn, P.C., Mason, S.E. & Shuwall, M.A. (1994) Maintenance imipramine for secondary depression in schizophrenia: a controlled trial. *Archives of General Psychiatry* 51, 109–115.

Siris, S.G., Addington, D., Azorin, J.-M. *et al.* (2001) Depression in schizophrenia: recognition and management in the USA. *Schizophrenia Research* 47, 185–197.

Smith, T.E., Hull, J.W., Israel, L.M. & Willson, D.F. (2000) Insight, symptoms, and neurocognition in schizophrenia and schizoaffective disorder. *Schizophrenia Bulletin* 26, 193–200.

Spina, E., DeDomenico, P., Ruello, C. *et al.* (1994) Adjunctive fluoxetine in the treatment of negative symptoms in chronic schizophrenic patients. *International Clinical Psychopharmacology* 9, 281–285.

Spitzer, R.L., Endicott, J. & Robins, E. (1978) Research Diagnostic Criteria: rationale and reliability. *Archives of General Psychiatry* 35, 773–782.

Stephens, J.H., Richard, P. & McHugh, P.R. (1997) Long-term follow-up of patients hospitalized for schizophrenia, 1913–40. *Journal of Nervous and Mental Disease* 185, 715–721.

Stephens, J.H., Richard, P. & McHugh, P.R. (1999) Suicide in patients hospitalized for schizophrenia, 1913–40. *Journal of Nervous and Mental Disease* 187, 10–14.

Strian, F., Heger, R. & Klicpera, C. (1982) The time structure of depressive mood in schizophrenic patients. *Acta Psychiatrica Scandinavica* 65, 66–73.

Subotnik, K.L. & Nuechterlein, K.H. (1988) Prodromal signs and symptoms of schizophrenic relapse. *Journal of Abnormal Psychology* 97, 405–412.

Summers, F., Harrow, M. & Westermeyer, J. (1983) Neurotic symptoms in the postacute phase of schizophrenia. *Journal of Nervous and Mental Disease* 171, 216–221.

Szymanski, H.V., Simon, J.C. & Gutterman, N. (1983) Recovery from schizophrenic psychosis. *American Journal of Psychiatry* 140, 335–338.

Taiminen, T., Syvälahti, E., Saarijärvi, S. *et al.* (1997) Citalopram as an adjuvant in schizophrenia: further evidence for a sertonergic dimension in schizophrenia. *International Clinical Psychopharmacology* 12, 31–35.

Tandon, R., Harrigan, E. & Zorn, S.H. (1997) Ziprasidone: a novel antipsychotic with unique pharmacology and therapeutic potential. *Journal of Serotonin Research* 4, 159–177.

Tapp, A., Tandon, R., Douglass, A. *et al.* (1994) Depression in severe chronic schizophrenia. *Biological Psychiatry* 35, 667.

Taylor, M.A. (1992) Are schizophrenia and affective disorder related? A selective literature review. *American Journal of Psychiatry* 149, 22–32.

Tollefson, G.D. & Andersen, S.W. (1999) Should we consider mood disturbance in schizophrenia as an important determinant of quality of life? *Journal of Clinical Psychiatry* 60 (Suppl. 5), 23–29.

Tollefson, G.D. & Sanger, T.M. (1997) Negative symptoms: a path analytic approach to a double-blind, placebo- and haloperidol-controlled clinical trial with olanzapine. *American Journal of Psychiatry* 154, 466–474.

Tollefson, G.D., Beasley, C.M. Jr, Tran, P.V. *et al.* (1997) Olanzapine versus haloperidol in the treatment of schizophrenia and schizoaffective and schizophreniform disorders: results of an international collaborative trial. *American Journal of Psychiatry* 154, 457–465.

Tollefson, G.D., Sanger, T.M., Beasley, C.M. & Tran, P.V. (1998a) A double-blind, controlled comparison of the novel antipsychotic olanzapine versus haloperidol or placebo on anxious and depressive symptoms accompanying schizophrenia. *Biological Psychiatry* 43, 803–810.

Tollefson, G.D., Sanger, T.M., Lu, Y. & Thieme, M.E. (1998b) Depressive signs and symptoms in schizophrenia: a prospective blinded trial of olanzapine and haloperidol. *Archives of General Psychiatry* 55, 250–258.

Tollefson, G.D., Andersen, S.W. & Tran, P.V. (1999) The course of depressive symptoms in predicting relapse in schizophrenia: a double-blind, randomized comparison of olanzapine and risperidone. *Biological Psychiatry* 46, 365–373.

Trichard, C., Paillère-Martinot, M.-L., Attar-Levy, D. *et al.* (1998) No sertonin 5-HT$_{2A}$ receptor density abnormality in the cortex of schizophrenic patients studied with PET. *Schizophrenia Research* 31, 13–17.

Tsuang, M.T. (1978) Suicide in schizophrenics, manics, depressives, and surgical controls. *Archives of General Psychiatry* 35, 153–155.

Tugg, L.A., Desai, D., Predergast, P. *et al.* (1997) Relationship between negative symptoms in chronic schizophrenia and neuroleptic dose, plasma levels and side effects. *Schizophrenia Research* 25, 71–78.

Vandel, B., Vandel, S., Allers, G., Bechtel, P. & Volmat, R. (1979) Interaction between amitriptyline and phenothiazine in man: effect on plasma concentration of amitriptyline and its metabolite nortriptyline and the correlation with clinical response. *Psychopharmcology* 65, 187–190.

Van Putten, T. (1975) The many faces of akathisia. *Comprehensive Psychiatry* 16, 43–47.

Van Putten, T. & May, P.R.A. (1978) 'Akinetic depression' in schizophrenia. *Archives of General Psychiatry* 35, 1101–1107.

Verhoeff, N.P.L.G., Meyer, J.H., Kecojevic, A. *et al.* (2000) A voxel-by-voxel analysis of [^{18}F]septoperone PET data shows no substantial serotonin 5-HT$_{2A}$ receptor changes in schizophrenia. *Psychiatry Research Neuroimaging* 99, 123–135.

Vlokh, I., Mikhnyak, S. & Kachura, O. (2000) Zoloft in management of depression in schizophrenia [Abstract]. *Schizophrenia Research* 41, 209.

Voruganti, L., Cortese, L., Oyewumi, L. *et al.* (2000) Comparative evaluation of conventional and novel antipsychotic drugs with reference to their subjective tolerability, side-effect profile and impact on quality of life. *Schizophrenia Research* 43, 135–145.

Waehrens, J. & Gerlach, J. (1980) Antidepressant drugs in anergic schizophrenia: a double-blind cross-over study with maprotiline and placebo. *Acta Psychiatrica Scandinavica* 61, 438–444.

Walker, A.M., Lanza, L.L., Arellano, F. & Rothman, K.J. (1998) Mortality in current and former users of clozapine. *Epidemiology* 8, 671–679.

Wassink, T.H., Rose, S., Flaum, M. & Andreasen, N.C. (1997) The prevalence and predictive validity of early depressive symptoms in the course of schizophrenia. *Schizophrenia Research* 24, 25.

Wassink, T.H., Flaum, M., Nopoulos, P. & Andreasen, N.C. (1999) Prevalence of depressive symptoms early in the course of schizophrenia. *American Journal of Psychiatry* 156, 315–316.

Weissman, M.M., Pottenger, M., Kleber, H. *et al.* (1977) Symptom patterns in primary and secondary depression: a comparison of primary depressives with depressed opiate addicts, alcoholics, and schizophrenics. *Archives of General Psychiatry* 34, 854–862.

Wiersma, D., Nienhuis, F.J., Sloof, C.J. & Giel, R. (1998) Natural course of schizophrenic disorders: a 15-year followup of a Dutch incidence cohort. *Schizophrenia Bulletin* 24, 75–85.

Winokur, G. (1972) Family history studies. VIII. Secondary depression is alive and well. *Diseases of the Nervous System* 33, 94–99.

Wise, R.A. (1982) Neuroleptics and operant behavior: the anhedonia hypothesis. *Behavioral and Brain Sciences* 5, 39–87.

Wistedt, B. & Palmstierna, T. (1983) Depressive symptoms in chronic schizophrenic patients after withdrawal of long-acting neuroleptics. *Journal of Clinical Psychiatry* 44, 369–371.

Wright, I.C., Ellison, Z.R., Sharma, T. *et al.* (1999) Mapping of grey matter changes in schizophrenia. *Schizophrenia Research* 35, 1–14.

Yamagami, S. & Soejima, K. (1989) Effect of maprotiline combined with conventional neuroleptics against negative symptoms of chronic schizophrenia. *Drugs under Experimental and Clinical Research* 15, 171–176.

Zakzanis, K.K. & Hansen, K.T. (1998) Dopamine D$_2$ densities and the schizophrenic brain. *Schizophrenia Research* 32, 201–206.

Zisook, S., McAdams, L.A., Kuck, J. *et al.* (1999) Depressive symptoms in schizophrenia. *American Journal of Psychiatry* 156, 1736–1743.

Zubin, J. & Spring, B. (1977) Vulnerability: a new view of schizophrenia. *Journal of Abnormal Psychology* 86, 103–126.

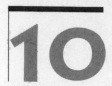

10 Neurocognitive deficits in schizophrenia

T.E. Goldberg, A. David and J.M. Gold

Course of cognitive impairment, 168
Core neurocognitive deficits, 169
  Attention, 169
  Episodic memory, 170
  Executive function and working memory, 170
Differential deficits and neuropsychiatry
  comparative studies, 171
Concurrent and predictive validity of
  neuropsychological impairment, 172

Treatment effects on cognition in schizophrenia:
  atypical neuroleptic medications, 173
Novel approaches, 175
  Neuropsychological investigations of psychotic
   symptoms, 175
  Cognition as an intermediate phenotype, 179
Conclusions, 179
References, 180

Abnormalities in attentional, associative and volitional cognitive processes have been considered central features of schizophrenia since the original clinical descriptions of Kraepelin (1919/1971) and Bleuler (1950). The application of formal psychological assessment techniques in hundreds of studies in dozens of independent laboratories over the past 70 years has more than amply documented that such abnormalities are common occurrences in patients with the disorder. For example, nearly 60 years ago, Rappaport *et al.* (1945/46) published *Diagnostic Psychological Testing*, an influential work reporting findings from the application of a broad test battery to a wide variety of psychiatric patients. In describing deteriorated chronic schizophrenic patients, they noted that such patients had their greatest impairments in 'judgement, attention, concentration, planning ability and anticipation'. They further commented on the memory difficulties, inadequate concept formation and general intellectual inefficiency of patients with schizophrenia. Although interpreted within a psychodynamic framework and prior to the narrowing of the diagnostic conceptualization of schizophrenia and introduction of modern pharmacotherapy, the empirical observations made in the early 1940s are remarkably consistent with current findings. Indeed, we would suggest that the vast body of data on cognitive functioning in schizophrenia has been remarkably uniform over many years. What has changed is the significance attributed to these results.

In the last 15 years, the routine use of clinical neuropsychological assessment and experimental neuropsychological paradigms has offered a new look to accounts of schizophrenia. Indeed, recent studies have thrown light on several of the more problematic facets of the disorder. In particular, they have made important contributions to understanding the course of cognitive impairment, the specificity of profiles of cognitive impairment to schizophrenia and the prognostic importance of deficits. More recently still, the putative importance of cognitive impairment in understanding cardinal symptoms of schizophrenia and in understanding the genetics of schizophrenia is coming to be appreciated. In this chapter we attempt to address some of the classical issues inherent in neurocognitive approaches to schizophrenia and present newer componential accounts of impairments in attention, working memory and episodic memory. Additionally, there have been several novel applications of neurocognition in schizophrenia, including relating impairments to symptoms and using impairments as intermediate phenotypes in genetic studies, which are reviewed.

Course of cognitive impairment

Subtle attenuations in premorbid developmental milestones and cognitive and academic functions have been demonstrated in schizophrenia that date to the 'prodromal' period or before (David *et al.* 1997; Jones & Cannon 1998; Davidson *et al.* 1999). After clinical onset the course of schizophrenia has sometimes been considered similar to that of progressive dementia in that there is relentless social and presumably cognitive decline. However, there are a great many neuropsychological studies that do not support this view (Heaton & Drexler 1987) and a broad literature can be drawn upon to support a different account which emphasizes features in the course consistent with the notion of 'static encephalopathy'. Within the first few years of their clinical illness, patients typically perform poorly on a wide range of tests which include those assessing memory, executive functions and attentional abilities (Goldberg & Weinberger 1988; Saykin *et al.* 1994; Censits *et al.* 1997; Gold *et al.* 1999). In this period, variability in repeated assessment might also occur, as patients' scores may even improve slightly (Sweeney *et al.* 1991). Longitudinal studies of armed forces personnel, prior to the onset of illness and during its active phase, are consistent with results that suggest relatively abrupt declines in functioning. Thus, on armed forces ability tests, patients performed similarly to their controls in the premorbid period and then displayed significant decrements of near 0.5 standard deviation (SD) after the onset of illness (Lubin *et al.* 1962; Schwartzman & Douglas 1962).

Crucially, deterioration does not appear to occur during the early chronic phase of the illness. It thus appears to be self-arresting. For instance, over intervals of 8 years, the performance of patients did not decline on tests such as the Wechsler Adult Intelligence Scale and Halstead–Reitan measures when assessed longitudinally (Smith 1964; Klonoff *et al.* 1970; Rund 1998). In several large cross-sectional studies using tests known to be sensitive to progressive dementias, using IQ or using variants of the Halstead–Reitan Battery, no differences were found between patients with longer durations of illness and those with shorter durations above and beyond ageing (Goldstein & Zubin 1990; Heaton *et al.* 1994; Hyde *et al.* 1994; Mockler *et al.* 1997). On the other hand, Harvey *et al.* (1998a,b) have strongly argued that some although not all patients suffer a very gradual but demonstrable decline in cognitive abilities throughout adulthood on such screening instruments as the Mini Mental Status Examination, and in late life more striking declines in cognitive and functional status. However, the role of chronic institutionalization is not completely understood.

Several correlation studies have not supported cognitive deteriorations with increasing chronicity. In perhaps the best of these, Gold *et al.* (1999) in a large and well-characterized sample found that associations between duration of illness and cognitive level were weak and non-significant (but see Cuesta *et al.* 1998).

Results which support the notion that schizophrenia is a static encephalopathy are also consistent with the observation of Kraepelin (1919/1971): 'As a rule, if no essential improvement intervenes in at most two or three years after the appearance of the more striking morbid phenomena, a state of weak mindedness will be developed, which usually changes only slowly and insignificantly'. Shakow (1946) also noted that, despite individual variations in course, 'the most frequent type is that which resembles temporally the process of oblivescence, a considerable drop at first with the tapering off through a slowed period to a stable level'.

Core neurocognitive deficits

Despite the difficult methodological issues involved in establishing differential deficits, the clinical interpretation of test data can often point to multiple studies that converge on a set of frequent, severe and selective deficits. In our view, patients with schizophrenia typically demonstrate abnormalities in attention/executive function and memory which stand out against a background of diffuse impairment. Although this view cannot, at present, be proven, the apparent impairments in these cognitive functions are of interest in relation to other neurobiological findings in the illness, such as structural abnormalities of the temporal lobe, dysfunctional activation of the prefrontal cortex and abnormalities in catecholamine function.

Attention

Even the casual observer may often be struck by deficits in the capacity of patients to cull information from their environment. Simply put, patients do not seem to focus attention, to anticipate and to sustain concentration. Moreover, they sometimes appear to be preoccupied with internal stimuli at the expense of salient environmental events, or are easily distracted by external stimuli. While such observations, both historical and clinical, have been broadly supported by numerous studies of sustained and selective attention, the precise nature of the impairments has been more difficult to articulate. One of the early experimental studies of attention, devised by Shakow (1979), found that patients with schizophrenia demonstrate slowed reaction time and, moreover, could not improve their performance even when intervals between warning and stimulus were both predictable and long. Thus, patients appeared to be unable to sustain attention, compromising their readiness to respond across longer time intervals. In another set of attentional paradigms, schizophrenic patients had deficits maintaining vigilance during a continuous performance test involving specific combinations of stimuli (Mirsky 1988). Patients typically failed to respond to target stimuli and also responded inappropriately to lures, thereby making both omission and commission errors. However, the meaning of these studies is unclear. Shakow's results might have been caused by failures in context or working memory, resulting in loss of the warning cue's readying function, while Continuous Performance Test (CPT) errors may be caused in part by deficiencies in encoding information or biasing perceptual modules to targets, such that patients were unable to make decisions based on an adequate representation of the stimulus (Elevåg *et al.* 2000e).

It is clear that attention is not a unitary construct, but it is unclear whether there is a particular dimension that is maximally impaired in schizophrenia. Posner and Dehaene (1994) developed an elegant model of the components of spatial attention. An initial examination of this model in schizophrenia was potentially promising: Posner *et al.* (1988) reported that schizophrenic patients displayed an asymmetrical slowing in response to stimuli that appeared in the right visual field after so-called invalid cues for a response. However, attempts to replicate this study have not met with success (e.g. Gold *et al.* 1992). Another aspect of attention involves selective attention. In the Stroop test, an exemplar of this class of tests, a prepotent response must be inhibited and a less salient conflicting response made (e.g. stating the colour of the word 'green' when it is printed in red ink). Several studies have found that patients display an increased cost in the incongruent condition or an increased advantage in the congruent condition (Perlstein *et al.* 1998; Elevåg *et al.* 2000a).

It is also important to consider the extent to which attention is modularized; that is, attentional impairments may or may not disrupt many other cognitive functions. One might assume that poor attention would prevent many types of information from being processed fully. However, correlational studies have generally suggested that attentional dysfunction explains only a small portion of the variance in other cognitive functions (Kenny & Meltzer 1991). Perhaps this should not come as a complete surprise, as patients with well-documented attentional deficit disorders often display many areas of intact cognitive function (Barkley *et al.* 1990). It remains to be seen whether this is because of the properties of the distributed neural system underlying attention (Mesulum 1985) or whether it simply reflects some dissociation between the ecology of the testing situation and the rest of an individual's environment.

Episodic memory

Episodic memory involves binding items and spatiotemporal context to form an episode that can be more or less permanently stored. It is critical in the acquisiton of new information. Its function in schizophrenia was one of the first cognitive abilities to be studied (Hull 1917). The results of numerous studies since then, however, have been difficult to characterize from a cognitive science perspective. Patients with schizophrenia generally remember stories, verbal paired associates and visual designs more poorly than do normal subjects and differences between normal controls and patients may be large (Saykin et al. 1991; Gold et al. 1994). Rate of learning may be abnormal. Thus, Paulsen et al. (1995) found that a large sample of patients exhibited reduced learning slopes when a list of words was repeated over multiple trials. In tests of recognition memory in which retrieval strategies are minimized, patients are generally impaired, but perhaps less so than in free recall (Calev 1984; Gold et al. 1992; Paulsen et al. 1995). Deficits have been attributed not only to consolidation impairments, but to inefficient encoding (Traupmann 1980), poor use of retrieval strategies in effortful recall (Goldberg et al. 1989), rapid forgetting (Sengel & Lovalla 1983; McKenna et al. 1990) and differences between impaired conscious recall and a gross sense of familiarity with the material (Danion et al. 1999).

More recently, Elvevåg et al. (2000b; Elvevåg & Goldberg, unpublished data) have re-examined the possibility that a specific stage of mnemonic processing is disrupted in schizophrenia. They used deep and shallow levels of processing to examine encoding, an 'AB$_R$' paradigm (in which verbal paired associates were first learned and then followed by trials in which pairs were 'shuffled', creating interference and the necessity to 'unlearn') to examine the effects of interference of prior learning, and false memory to examine semantic context effects. They found that these cognitive manipulations exerted the same effect in patients as they did in normal controls, although patients performed more poorly overall. These results suggest that patients do not have qualitative abnormalities in mnemonic processing; rather, consistently poorer performance may be one of degree.

A conservative summary statement is probably in order: schizophrenic patients demonstrate clear deficits in episodic memory measures, i.e. they have difficulty retrieving episodes of experience within distinct spatiotemporal contexts. This is probably a function of multiple factors.

Executive function and working memory

Clinicians have frequently observed that schizophrenic patients have difficulty generating and implementing plans. Patients also appear to have difficulty solving problems whose solutions are not readily apparent, or when they must rely upon novel recom-

binations of existing knowledge. From the neuropsychological standpoint, such deficits are often considered to be 'executive' in nature, in the sense that they involve use of information rather than fundamental processing of the information. Formal tests of analogues of these abilities have usually revealed deficits in patients. For instance, Fey (1951) demonstrated that schizophrenic patients have performance deficits on the Wisconsin Card Sorting Test (WCST) of abstraction, set shifting and response to feedback. More recent studies (Goldberg et al. 1987) have also shown that chronic schizophrenic patients performed poorly on the WCST and had difficulty learning the task even when instructions were provided, suggesting that their capacity to maintain information 'on-line' was reduced.

Studies of verbal tasks also reveal deficits in working memory. Gold et al. (1994) found that schizophrenic patients performed more poorly than patients with temporal lobe epilepsy on tests demanding working memory from the Wechsler Adult Intelligence Scale–Revised. There are multiple reports of poor performance by patients with schizophrenia on variants of the Brown–Peterson task. This task involves remembering a short list of words over a brief delay (e.g. 12 s) during which interpolated distractor activities draw off 'processing resources' and/or prevent covert rehearsal of the to-be-remembered material. Goldberg et al. (1998) showed that patients were inordinately sensitive to interference, large set sizes and notably delay.

In a study involving simultaneous storage and processing of information, Gold et al. (1997) used a working memory task that required ordering short sequences of randomly presented numbers and letters (the so-called letter–number span). Patients fared poorly. Moreover, the degree of impairment was highly correlated with a test of problem solving and rule learning: the WCST. The relationship suggests that both tests, very different in their surface characteristics, may call upon a specialized computational workspace in which material must not only be maintained, but manipulated or transformed.

Several studies of schizophrenia have indicated that patients have impairments on even very basic tests of working memory. Park et al. (1995) showed that on oculomotor delayed response, a probe of prefrontal cortical function adapted from non-human primates, patients scored poorly. The finding was confirmed by Fleming et al. (1997) using a test of memory for patterns and locations. Simple short-term working memory for verbal memory indexed by digit span and involving only veridical reproduction of the items and their sequence has been repeatedly found to be impaired in schizophrenia. Indeed, a meta-analysis indicated that the effect size of the difference between normal controls and patients was large and highly significant (Aleman et al. 1999).

Much recent work has focused on a task requiring both intradimensional and extradimensional (ID/ED) set shifting which reflects, at least in part, a componential version of the WCST. In intradimensional shifts, subjects are required to change their response set to an alternative design within a category (e.g. a new exemplar of a line design) while an irrelevant dimension (e.g. shape), which had been introduced earlier, continues to be ignored. At a later stage, an extradimensional shift is demanded as new exemplars are again introduced but subjects are now required to respond to the previously irrelevant dimension (e.g. shapes rather than lines). Subjects make decisions that were based on feedback after each trial. Chronic schizophrenic patients displayed markedly impaired attentional set shifting on the ID/ED task. Pantelis *et al.* (1999) reported that patients with schizophrenia demonstrated a significantly higher rate of attrition at the intradimensional shift stage compared with frontal lobe patients and they were similarly impaired in comparison to frontal lobe patients on the extradimensional shift stage (Pantelis *et al.* 1999). Chronic patients were also impaired on spatial memory span and spatial working memory tasks. The Tower of London test, which involves planning and memory, was impaired in patients with schizophrenia as they made fewer perfect solutions and required more moves and time to complete the task. Thus, patients with schizophrenia showed an overall deficit in executive function, often greater than that observed in patients with frontal lobe lesions (Pantelis *et al.* 1997).

Several studies have indicated that working memory impairment is present in schizophrenia, even in relatively intellectually intact individuals. For instance, Pantelis *et al.* (1999) found that while patients with high IQ performed better than patients with low IQ, performance was still remarkably abnormal. Their performances at the intradimensional shifting stage were below that of normals and markedly below that of normals in extradimensional shifting. Elliott *et al.* (1995) were able to confirm these results, even in patients with preserved intellectual function (IQs greater than 100). Weickert *et al.* (2000) used a different methodology to come to similar conclusions. They found that patients with developmentally compromised intellectual function, normal premorbid intellectual function that declined significantly (the modal subgroup in this study) and with preserved intellectual function (i.e. both current and putative premorbid IQ were normal) displayed deficits compared with a normal control group on WCST's measure of perseveration. Thus, impaired executive function appears to be a core deficit in that it is present irrespective of IQ pattern.

Differential deficits and neuropsychiatry comparative studies

One of the goals of neuropsychological and cognitive research in schizophrenia is to identify abnormalities in particular cognitive processes that are linked to specific brain regions or systems. The neuropsychologically based search for such a 'fundamental' deficit or deficits faces a basic methodological challenge. As noted by Chapman and Chapman (1973), patients with schizophrenia tend to perform more poorly than normal controls on a wide variety of tasks. They demonstrate a 'generalized' deficit whose origin remains undetermined. Such a deficit might conceivably reflect the experience of institutionalization, failures in co-operation or diffuse brain dysfunction. Of greater theoretical

interest, however, is the existence of 'differential' deficits, i.e. deficits more severe than might be anticipated on the basis of the generalized deficit. Such differential deficits could provide evidence of regionally specific neurocognitive impairment with implications for understanding schizophrenic pathology and pathophysiology. Current clinical assessment test batteries are not capable of rigorously supporting inferences of differential deficit. To demonstrate differential deficit adequately, tasks should be matched on the basis of difficulty level and reliability, so that ceiling effects or measurement error do not skew the results. Very few matched tasks have been developed (Calev 1984) and these tasks have generally not been incorporated into standard clinical assessment batteries or experimental procedures. Certainly, findings that patients perform worse on an easier task than a harder task (e.g. semantic fluency is more impaired than letter fluency; Gourovitch *et al.* 1996) strengthen the interpretation of results.

Another aspect of task matching that is frequently overlooked involves the dispersion of test scores. Some tests are constructed such that it is difficult to score more than 2 SD below the normal control mean, while on many other tests it is possible to score several standard deviations below normal (Randolph *et al.* 1993). Therefore, one could conclude incorrectly that an individual's performance on the latter group is worse than on the former group of tests. It should be recognized that when a difference is found between groups, that difference is valid in terms of its existence. On the other hand, claims that one impaired performance is necessarily more deficient than another impaired performance, or that a normal performance is 'truly' normal, are not valid if tasks are not matched. In summary, the interpretation of neuropsychological findings remains largely a matter of clinical judgement, a process which has clear limitations for supporting more specific inferences about areas of maximal dysfunction in a population with widespread cognitive difficulties.

There are no easy solutions to these problems of measurement. One statistical approach involves comparing the residuals from a regression line that is derived from two variables of interest (Chapman & Chapman 1989). In patients with verified neurological disorders, an approach that has been fruitful in identifying differential deficit patterns involves a search for double dissociations (Teuber 1955; Shallice 1988). In this method, two patient groups are compared on two tests. If one group outperforms the other on the first test, but is itself outperformed on the second, then one infers that the groups have a differential profile of performance. This latter approach, underutilized in previous schizophrenia research, has recently been used by Gold *et al.* (1994) in a study of temporal lobe epilepsy and schizophrenia and by Goldberg *et al.* (1990a) in a study of Huntington's disease and schizophrenia. In the former, patients with schizophrenia had worse attentional but better semantic functioning than did patients with left temporal lobe epilepsy. In the latter, patients with schizophrenia had worse attentional but better visual spatial functioning in comparison with patients with Huntington's disease. While the double dissociation approach is not immune to psychometric artefacts (i.e. one test being 'harder' than the other), it appears to have a distinct advantage over studies comparing patients and normal controls.

Nevertheless, strong claims have been made that schizophrenic cognitive impairment reflects generalized impairment. The argument has been made on psychometric grounds through the use of carefully selected tests (Blanchard and Neale 1994) and by way of the use of large normative databases for the Halstead–Reitan Battery (Braff *et al.* 1991). However, careful clinical analysis of results may suggest otherwise. Using tests with well-established brain–behaviour relationships, Kolb and Whishaw (1983) proposed that schizophrenia reflected executive-memory (i.e. frontomedial temporal lobe) dysfunction. In a series of detailed case studies, Shallice *et al.* (1991) observed consistent evidence for executive dysfunction. Weickert *et al.* (2000) showed that the modal patient in a series of 117 consecutively admitted patients exhibited rather circumscribed executive, attentional and memory impairments, although a significant minority of patients exhibited a diffuse pattern of cognitive impairment. Moreover, these results are not subject to criticisms about difficulty level and dispersion, given that they derive from subgroups obtained from a single 'population'. Importantly, deficits in working memory and cognitive control over attentional processes were present even when IQ was preserved.

The identification of a characteristic neurocognitive profile of schizophrenia relative to other disorders provides useful information concerning the fundamental validity of the accumulated neurocognitive findings. Differences in overall global impairment (i.e. level) may have important implications for everyday functioning. Differences in profile of impairment (i.e. shape) may help to sharpen the discussion of anatomical implications of deficits and identify useful measures for intermediate phenotypes in genetic linkage or association studies. Furthermore, these comparative differential deficits derived from comparative studies could provide targets for rehabilitative and pharmacological treatment efforts.

In particular, the comparison of schizophrenic patients and patients with mood disorders offers some insight into the clinical importance of neuropsychological functioning, given the fact that the outcome of schizophrenia is worse in terms of social and vocational functioning than that observed in mood disorders. If the disability of schizophrenic patients reflects neuropsychological impairment, then one would expect formal testing to distinguish the diagnostic groups. The results of a study by Goldberg *et al.* (1993a) support this view. A schizophrenic group performed significantly below affective groups (unipolar and bipolar) on tests of attention and psychomotor speed, verbal and visual memory, and problem solving and abstraction. Values of IQ were also low in the schizophrenic group and appeared to have deteriorated from a normal premorbid level. Moreover, when the analysis was restricted to patients with IQ scores of 90 or more, the patients with schizophrenia still performed more poorly than did the mood disorder group on the

WCST and visual memory tests, suggesting that inadequacy of global cognitive competence was not the sole source of the intergroup difference.

While affective psychoses have come under increasing scrutiny in terms of their cognitive relations to schizophrenia, in a recent review of the literature that directly compared patients with bipolar disorder to schizophrenia, Goldberg (1999) concluded that the results provide support for the view that patients with bipolar disorders suffer less severe cognitive impairments than do patients with schizophrenia. While several studies have found the groups to be equivalent in impairment, no study has found bipolar patients to be consistently worse than patients with schizophrenia (with the possible exception of backward masking); indeed, the majority of studies have found that schizophrenic patients have worse cognitive function. With respect to profile, patients with schizophrenia appear to have more severe and more frequent working memory impairments. However, it is important to note that patients with affective psychosis have cognitive impairment.

Concurrent and predictive validity of neuropsychological impairment

Neurocognitive deficits may be a rate-limiting factor in the rehabilitation of patients with schizophrenia. For instance, in a study of patients receiving clozapine, Goldberg *et al.* (1993b) observed that while patients' symptoms improved markedly over the 15-month study period, the patients still required supervised living arrangements and could not work in high-level competitive situations. Because their neuropsychological profile remained impaired and unchanged, neurocognitive deficits might have accounted for some of the continuing disabilities. Strong concurrent relations between the global level of functioning and specific neurocognitive test scores have been found (Goldberg *et al.* 1990b, 1995). In a monozygotic (MZ) twin study in which patients were concordant for schizophrenia (thus controlling for genome, educational and family environment, experience of illness and medication), cognitive measures, which included memory for stories from the Wechsler memory scale, verbal fluency, WCST and IQ, of intratwin pair differences were strongly and significantly associated with differences in social and vocational functioning as measured by the global assessment scale (GAS). In addition, in MZ twins concordant for schizophrenia, a group in whom symptomatology was similar, as was the experience of having a chronic illness, differences in a set of cognitive measures (trails, IQ, WCST and memory quotient) accounted for over 95% of the variance in intrapair differences in GAS scores.

In several important meta-analyses, Green (1996) has convincingly shown that executive and attentional impairments account for about 20% of functional outcome, while both short- and long-term memory account for about 30% and 40%, respectively, of the variance in a variety of functional outcome domains. In this type of analysis, the combined sample sizes were large and the relationships between neurocognition and functional outcome were highly significant. Global indicators of cognitive impairment showed even stronger relationships with outcome.

In contrast, psychotic symptoms (hallucinations and delusions) are not strong predictors and correlates of functional outcome (Green *et al.* 2000). Negative symptoms have higher correlations with functional outcome than positive symptoms, but across studies the relationships are neither stronger nor more consistent than those for neurocognitive deficits (Dickerson *et al.* 1996; Velligan *et al.* 1997; Harvey *et al.* 1998a). The relative contributions of symptoms and neurocognition to functional outcome have only rarely been directly compared with appropriate statistical analyses, including multiple regression. In those studies that have made comparisons, the neurocognitive contributions to outcome were stronger than those from positive symptoms. While negative symptoms covaried to at least a modest extent with neurocognition (Dickerson *et al.* 1996; Velligan *et al.* 1997), their relationship to function appear to be mediated through statistical overlap; i.e. they did not make independent contributions to explain outcome variance.

It is likely that some cognitive domains have direct causal relationships on daily functions, while others may be related to functional outcome through mediators, such as social cognition or the appropriate timely application of knowledge and reasoning to problem solving.

Treatment effects on cognition in schizophrenia: atypical neuroleptic medications

The vast majority of studies published over the last 4 decades examining aspects of neurocognitive performance in patients with schizophrenia have been conducted with samples of patients studied while they were receiving antipsychotic medications. This had led to a persistent concern articulated in the literature that it was not possible to determine, in principle, if the impairments observed were fully attributable to the illness, the impact of antipsychotic medication (and related side-effects) or some combination of the two (Spohn *et al.* 1985; Spohn & Strauss 1989). This concern, coupled with evidence that treatment with conventional antipsychotic agents led to the development of tardive dyskinesia in a significant number of patients, was the context for a series of independent extensive narrative literature reviews written in the 1980s and early 1990s examining the cognitive effects of conventional antipsychotics (Heaton & Crowley 1981; Medalia *et al.* 1988; Spohn & Strauss 1989; Cassens *et al.* 1990; King 1990; Bilder *et al.* 1992). The reviews of this large literature, spanning from the late 1950s through the 1980s, came to remarkably similar conclusions: there was little convincing evidence that treatment with conventional antipsychotics had significant cognitive benefits or costs. Costs observed in motor performance were often attributed to ex-

trapyramidal symptoms, and possible memory 'costs' were often thought to be brought about by the impact of anticholinergic medications used as adjunctive treatments. Benefits were most frequently, but not always, reported on tasks requiring sustained attention or resisting the impact of distracting stimuli. However, new meta-analyses (T.E. Goldberg, unpublished; Keefe & Harvey 2001) suggest modest improvements with typical or atypical neuroleptic medications in higher level cognitive domains. These reviews, combined with studies documenting substantial impairment in neuroleptic naïve first-episode samples (Saykin *et al.* 1994), as well as an attenuated pattern of impairment among untreated non-psychotic first-degree relatives (Cannon *et al.* 1994; Faraone *et al.* 1995; Egan *et al.* 2001), all support the basic notion that the cognitive impairments observed in samples of medicated patients could be reliably attributed to the illness and did not represent medication-related artefacts.

Moreover, while the results from studies examining the cognitive effects of conventional agents appear to be highly reproducible, there are a number of reasons to regard conclusions drawn from this literature with skepticism. As noted by reviewers, the methodological quality of the vast majority of studies in the area was quite poor, limiting confidence in the validity of conclusions that can be drawn. Sample sizes were typically small, doses were frequently higher (or uncontrolled) than contemporary clinical practice, and many studies failed to control for the expected gains brought about by repeated testing (e.g. many studies failed to use either control groups or alternative forms for testing materials). In addition, although the relationship between symptom severity and cognitive performance is typically quite modest, it is clearly unidirectional, with better performance associated with reduced symptom severity in the vast majority of studies (Strauss 1993). Thus, the clinical symptomatic benefits of antipsychotic treatment should again lead to an expectation of enhanced performance, albeit indirect, relative to unmedicated performance levels. Beyond the methodological limitations of the literature, there is an increasing appreciation for the role of dopamine in mediating aspects of cognition, including working memory and the processing of error and reward signals (Müller *et al.* 1998; Schultz 1998). Indeed, it would be surprising if nearly complete blockade of D_2 receptors, as achieved by conventional antipsychotic agents at high doses, did not have cognitive consequences. Recent work in non-human primates demonstrating a substantial deficit in working memory performance following treatment with D_2 blocking agents, an effect that was partially alleviated by treatment with a D_1 agonist, illustrates both the prominent role of dopamine in cortical function and the complexity of receptor interactions in the intact brain (Castner *et al.* 2000).

These lingering qualms about the cognitive effects of conventional antipsychotics have been magnified by the introduction of a number of new generation or 'atypical' antipsychotics. The receptor affinities of these compounds differ from one another substantially (Bymaster *et al.* 1996). However, they share the ability to achieve an antipsychotic effect largely in the absence of extrapyramidal side-effects resulting from striatal D_2 blockade. Although there is ongoing debate about the possible mechanism(s) of action of the newer agents, it is clear that chronic blockade of upwards of 80% of D_2 receptors is not required for antipsychotic efficacy, as had been thought to be the case for conventional antipsychotics (Kapur & Seeman 2000; Kapur et al. 2000a,b). Along with reduced side-effect burden, there are claims that the second-generation agents may offer cognitive advantages relative to conventional agents, and may in fact even be cognitive 'enhancers'. Given this linkage between cognitive impairment and functional outcomes, the demonstration of a clear cognitive benefit resulting from treatment with new generation compounds would represent a dramatic step forward in schizophrenia therapeutics.

The available literature examining the cognitive effects of new generation antipsychotics has many of the methodological problems of the older literature: small (and likely unrepresentative) samples, uncontrolled practice effects in test–retest designs and few examples of random assignment double-blind within subject designs. Given the extensive industry sponsorship of studies examining cognitive effects of new generation compounds, there is an additional concern about possible reporting biases. Despite these limitations, the available literature, as recently reviewed by Keefe et al. (1999) and Meltzer and McGurk (1999), supports a number of broad conclusions. Most importantly, there is fairly consistent evidence that patients treated with new generation compounds demonstrate better cognitive performance than comparator groups (often the baseline performance of the same patients) receiving conventional agents. Such improvements have been noted following treatment with all of the new agents currently on the market including clozapine, olanzapine, risperidone and quetiapine. With one major exception discussed below, these advantages have been documented relative to conventional agents. Without head-to-head trials of new generation compounds, it is premature to draw conclusions about possible differential cognitive efficacy of the new agents, or possible differential effects of individual drugs on specific cognitive functions. Given the limitations of the literature at this point, it is only possible to address broad general issues. Most importantly, it appears that the cognitive benefits of new generation compounds are generally modest, with patients continuing to demonstrate marked impairments in most key domains of cognitive functioning relative to normal control subjects. Unfortunately, only one study has investigated if this subtle cognitive advantage impacts functional outcome. Buchanan et al. (1994) reported that the magnitude of change in memory performance following clozapine treatment was correlated with changes in clinical ratings of quality of life (although memory functioning did not improve significantly). This promising result has yet to be replicated or extended to specific functional outcomes of interest including degree of residential independence or vocational performance.

There is one likely exception to the generalization that new generation agents offer a modest advantage for cognitive performance relative to conventional antipsychotics. Freedman et al. have reported in a series of studies that patients with schizophrenia, and a significant number of their first-degree relatives, demonstrate an electrophysiological abnormality which has been named P50 (Freedman et al. 1997; Adler et al. 1998). This abnormality is elicited when pairs of auditory stimuli are presented; normal subjects demonstrate a reduced eletrophysiological response to the second stimuli, whereas patients fail to modulate/inhibit this response. Unlike conventional antipsychotics, both clozapine and risperidone appear to partially, if not largely, normalize this impairment (Nagamoto et al. 1996; Yee et al. 1998; Light et al. 2000). Thus, it may not be possible to document this genetically transmitted abnormality in patients treated with at least some of the new generation compounds, potentially limiting the further development of this promising and important line of research.

The most provocative study of new generation agents was recently published by Purdon et al. (2000) in a double-blind study comparing the cognitive effects of olanzapine, risperidone and haloperidol. They reported statistically significant advantages of olanzapine relative to both risperidone and haloperidol on a broad array of cognitive measures. Cognitive benefits of olanzapine were observed following 6 weeks of treatment, with further gains noted on later retest occasions. What is particularly noteworthy about this study is that the magnitude of change with olanzapine treatment on multiple tests was quite large: effect sizes >0. 6 were observed on measures of motor performance, verbal learning, perseverative behaviour, non-verbal fluency, visual perception and visual construction. There was much less evidence of a benefit of risperidone relative to haloperidol, in contrast to other published studies (Green et al. 1997; Kern et al. 1998, 1999). There are a number of potential methodological problems with the Purdon et al. study, chief among them the very high attrition rate over the course of the trial complicating the interpretation of results, particularly from the last two testing occasions, resulting in a very small sample. Whatever the limitations, this study raises the possibility that olanzapine may have a substantial cognitive advantage relative to both a conventional agent, haloperidol, and another new generation agent, risperidone. It clearly remains to be determined if the results of this important 'outlier' study can be independently replicated.

However, the issue remains of how to understand the implications of the cognitive advantage of new generation agents. Based on the available literature, it appears that several agents offer at least modest benefits, possibly in somewhat different cognitive domains, perhaps supporting a claim that these agents enhance cognitive function. A number of mechanisms have been speculatively proposed to explain the findings, including the role of 5-HT_{2A}-receptors, acetylcholine and D_1 (Keefe et al. 1999; Meltzer & McGurk 1999). Thus, different specific mechanisms would need to be invoked for the different compounds, given their differing affinities for these receptor systems. Although these mechanisms may prove to be important, it is striking that the most obvious possibility has rarely been discussed: each of the new generation agents achieves antipsychotic effects without inducing D_2-mediated extrapyramidal symptoms. Thus, the common 'cognitive denominator' of these agents may be reduced – or more transient – D_2 blockade relative to conventional agents (Kapur & Seeman 2000). If this speculative formulation were correct, it would suggest that the new generation drugs are advantageous because they do not exact a cognitive cost, whether it be directly on cortical information processing or more indirectly on subcortical motor speed and initiation. This formulation would suggest that the frequently observed advantage of new generation agents relative to conventional antipsychotics on measures of psychomotor speed and response production could be an indirect benefit: it may result from the removal of an adverse effect of high levels of chronic D_2 blockade on frontal–striatal systems. In addition, benefits observed on retesting could represent normal practice effects, with enhanced performance following multiple exposures to a number of testing instruments and procedures. Although a crucial form of learning, the biological implications of a restoration of practice effects vs. the direct enhancement of impaired neural systems may be different. The restoration of practice effects could result from the removal of an iatrogenic impediment; actual enhancement suggests a direct pharmacological benefit.

Pharmacology provides a specific window on the underlying neurobiology of the illness. Indeed, the failure of conventional agents to improve cognitive performance, despite being largely effective in the treatment of positive symptoms, was a critical piece of evidence that the symptomatic and cognitive features of the illness were partially independent. Thus, an accurate understanding of the cognitive effects of new generation agents is critical in guiding future drug development. If the cognitive benefits of new generation agents result from an actual enhancement of cortical function, then these agents might rightfully be considered as 'antischizophrenia' drugs rather than as antipsychotics. Alternatively, if the apparent advantage results from a lack of 'cost', then the mechanisms implicated in the clinical efficacy of the new agents are unlikely to prove to be important in the development of future cognitive enhancement treatment strategies.

Novel approaches

Neuropsychological investigations of psychotic symptoms

Is there a relationship between cognitive deficits and symptoms or syndromes within the schizophrenic group of disorders? Liddle (1987a) examined the relationships between symptoms rated on a symptomatic assessment scale (Krawiecka) in 40 patients with chronic schizophrenia, and demonstrated that symptoms segregated into three syndromes:
1 psychomotor poverty (reduced speech, lack of spontaneous movement and blunting of affect);
2 disorganization (inappropriate affect, poverty of content of speech, and disturbances in the form of thought); and

3 reality distortion (delusions and hallucinations).
Examination of the correlations between syndrome severity and performance on a range of well-standardized clinical neuropsychological tests revealed that each of the syndromes was associated with a specific pattern of neuropsychological impairment (Liddle 1987b). Whereas the psychomotor poverty syndrome was associated with poor performance in tests of conceptual thinking, object naming and long-term memory, the two syndromes linked with the presence of positive symptoms were associated with a different pattern of cognitive dysfunction. The disorganization syndrome was associated with poor performance in tests of concentration, immediate recall and word learning, and the reality distortion syndrome was associated with poor figure ground perception. A similar approach using factor analysis was undertaken by Basso et al. (1998) with 62 schizophrenia patients on whom a wide variety of clinical, demographic and neuropsychological measures were available. Negative symptoms were associated with a range of abnormalities such as impaired global IQ, executive function, motor skill, vigilance, attention and memory indices, while disorganization correlated with a subset of these (IQ, attention and motor tasks). Psychotic symptoms did not correlate with the standard tests.

Other research has focused on specific symptoms to understand their neuropsychological basis. This endeavour requires a shift away from the search for 'deficits' and requires a wider conception of cognitive processes, including excesses as well as deficits, dysfunctions and abnormal interactions (see Halligan & David, 2001) in order to generate mechanistic accounts of symptoms.

Hallucinations

There have been no convincing studies to suggest that auditory verbal hallucinations (AVHs) correlate with deficits on standard neuropsychological tests, unlike, for example, negative symptoms (for review see above and David & Cutting 1994).

Hemisphere dysfunction in auditory hallucinations has been examined utilizing the technique of dichotic listening. This entails competition between the right and left hemispheres in the identification of auditory stimuli presented simultaneously, one to each ear. When the stimuli are words or consonant–vowel syllables, input to the left hemisphere predominates, especially in right-handers. This right ear–left hemisphere advantage appears to be attenuated in patients who are hallucination-prone (Green et al. 1994; Bruder et al. 1995) and correlates with symptom severity (Levitan et al. 1999). This pattern could be interpreted as a left hemisphere abnormality with or without overactivity of the right hemisphere. Recent functional magnetic resonance imaging work has shown that the right hemisphere shows more activity relative to the left in response to external speech (Woodruff et al. 1997), while activity during hallucinations in the single cases studied has a right temporal cortex emphasis (Woodruff et al. 1995; Lennox et al. 1999).

Language and hallucinations

Schizophrenic auditory hallucinations, the characteristic 'voices' talking to or about the subject, have a precise content which is often highly personalized to the voice-hearer (Nayani & David 1996). It has been suggested that consistency of semantic content of AVHs leads the voice-hearer to personify the experience (Hoffman *et al*. 1994). Often, a complex relationship develops between the patient and 'the voices' – usually that of the powerless and the powerful, respectively (Chadwick & Birchwood 1994). This is in contradistinction to the idea that hallucinations are the random productions of a disordered neocortex, but rather that they are intimately linked with language perception and expression systems (David 1994a).

Inner speech

The observation that the universal experience of inner speech resembles some AVHs continues to stimulate neurocognitive research. A single case study of a woman with continuous hallucinations showed that inner speech or, more specifically, short-term maintenance of phonological representations, can coexist with AVHs (David & Lucas 1993). This implies that AVHs are not synonymous with inner speech in any simple sense. A battery of short-term memory tests requiring an intact phonological store was used in a group comparison of schizophrenic patients who had recently reported hallucinations vs. patients who had not (Haddock *et al*. 1995). The authors tested the general hypothesis that any abnormality could affect monitoring of inner speech leading to an increased vulnerability to AVHs. The results showed that all patients performed less well than controls but there was no significant interaction with the presence or absence of hallucinations. Similarly, verbal transformation effect (the sensation that when a word like 'life' is repeated over and over, it turns into 'fly') has been used in this context and most recent findings suggest that hallucinators are no more prone to the effect than controls. However, Haddock *et al*. (1995) demonstrated that this effect is vulnerable to motivational factors (i.e. suggestion). In contrast, a separate case study suggested that thought insertion (a pathological experience akin to hearing voices) does appear to be incompatible with effective short-term or working memory (David 1994b).

Evans *et al*. (2000) carried out an in-depth study of seven patients with no history of AVH and 12 with a strong history of AVH using auditory imagery paradigms which tapped into the functioning of the 'inner ear', the 'inner voice' and the 'inner ear–inner voice' partnership. These included parsing meaningful letter strings, pitch judgements, verbal transformations and a range of tasks requiring phonological judgements. The results showed a wide range of abilities and deficits in both groups but no clear pattern and hence do not support an abnormality in inner speech and phonological processing in patients vulnerable to AVHs. However, problems in attribution of inner speech, for example, or theories of hallucinations based on lower level

perceptual or physiological processes are not ruled out (see below).

Reality or source monitoring

The problem of deciding whether one imagined hearing a voice or heard someone else speaking, and, if the latter, deciding who it was, falls under the rubric of source (or reality) monitoring (Johnson *et al*. 1988). Hallucinations and delusions of control can therefore be conceived of as failures of source monitoring – either because of a general failure and hence source confusion or a systematic failure or bias so that imagined voices (planned utterances) tend to be remembered as 'heard'. The first empirical test of this was by Bentall *et al*. (1991) and the results somewhat equivocal, with hallucinators being no more prone to monitoring errors than other groups. Morrison and Haddock (1997) introduced an innovation to this paradigm by examining source monitoring for words with emotional content. They found that such words tended to disrupt source monitoring but only in terms of *immediate* ratings of subjective ownership. Seal *et al*. (1997) manipulated several task parameters including emotional content and found trends toward more self-to-other misattributions in hallucinators ($n = 6$) vs. non-hallucinators ($n = 11$). Other research using similar methodology has shown that patients with schizophrenia may well be prone to making source monitoring errors but the relationship to hallucinations has not emerged (Vinogradov *et al*. 1997). Indeed, a confounding effect of low IQ (Vinogradov *et al*. 1997) and poor verbal memory (Seal *et al*. 1997) has been problematic. In perhaps the most complete study to date, Keefe *et al*. (1999) used a systematic multinomial model to dissect memory level and source and found that patients not only had difficulty remembering both internal and external sources, but showed a bias in reporting that stimuli came from external sources. Unfortunately, only weak relations with various positive symptoms were discerned.

Frith's model (1987, 1992) proposes that source monitoring is achieved by a corollary discharge-like mechanism whereby ownership of a speech act is signalled at the intention stage. The hypothesized failure of this mechanism in AVHs was tested by Cahill *et al*. (1996) using distorted auditory feedback. The aim was to produce a dissonance between external and 'internal' monitoring. Reliance solely on the external route would lead to the attribution of an alien source to the heard speech. By lowering or raising the pitch of the patient's speech, the authors did indeed induce hallucination-like experiences. However, this tendency correlated more strongly with the presence of delusions than hallucinations. Johns and McGuire (1999) repeated the experiment using 10 schizophrenia patients with hallucinations (and delusions) and eight with delusions alone, plus normal volunteers. The results showed that, while uncertainty as to the source of the speech was a feature of both schizophrenia groups, external attribution was more common in the hallucinators, a tendency more evident when derogatory material was heard. Goldberg *et al*. (1997) used delayed auditory feedback on the assumption that the dysfluency this usually causes is a result of the mismatch between planned and perceived speech output. The authors argued that if the speech production is not anticipated (because of a disconnection between intentions and the monitored output) then this adverse effect on speech should be *less* in those with hallucinations compared with those without. The results showed the opposite: speech output was even more affected in the hallucinators and patients with delusions of control. However, the role of attention in this paradigm has been questioned, although it is unclear why this effect would specifically impact hallucinations.

Indirect psychological evidence for a failure in self-monitoring comes from examining speech repairs, especially when these occur rapidly, often within a word, before external acoustic feedback can have come into play. Leudar *et al.* (1994) found that internal error detection occurred much less commonly in schizophrenic patients compared with normal controls. However, there was no difference between patients with and without AVHs.

In summary, inner speech itself appears not to be differentially impaired in hallucinators while there is some inconsistent support for reality monitoring errors. Data on auditory feedback are contradictory.

Delusions

Delusions represent a core feature of psychosis, and are especially evident in schizophrenia. There have been several cognitive models proposed to explain delusion formation. One explanation is that they result from the natural interpretations of abnormal experiences (Maher 1974). However, delusions can occur in the absence of abnormal perceptions and vice versa, and different delusional beliefs can be present in various subjects with abnormal perceptions (Chapman & Chapman 1988). Other theories of delusion formation have therefore emphasized abnormalities in attentional bias, such as increased attention to threatening stimuli in patients with persecutory delusions. Evidence for this includes the significantly longer time that patients with persecutory delusions require to name the print colours of threatening compared with depressive and neutral words in an emotional Stroop test (Kaney & Bentall 1989), and demonstrations of preferential recall of threat-related propositions in a story recall task (Kaney *et al.* 1992). It has also been proposed that patients with persecutory delusions have abnormal attributional processes, making external attributions for negative events and internal attributions for positive events (Kaney & Bentall 1989) and that this acts as a 'self-serving bias' (Kaney & Bentall 1990).

Reasoning

More recent studies have examined the nature of reasoning biases in patients with delusions about non-persecutory themes. Leafhead *et al.* (1996) employed the emotional Stroop paradigm to investigate the attentional bias in a patient with the Cotard delusion, the belief that one is dead. The patient was found to

have increased attention to death-related words. Rossell *et al.* (1998) administered a sentence verification task to patients with delusions. When asked to judge whether statements were real (true), e.g. 'fish swim in rivers', unlikely, e.g. 'passengers have sex on trains' or nonsense (untrue), e.g. 'the bible is a car catalogue', the deluded subjects, whose overall performance matched that of controls, made significantly more incorrect responses to sentences that had an emotional content congruent with their delusional beliefs, especially in the intermediate unlikely category. These findings suggest that reasoning abnormalities in deluded patients become particularly evident with tasks related to the theme of the delusional belief, and also indicate the presence of disturbed higher order semantic processes in these patients. However, it is unclear if delusions cause misinterpretations or misinterpretations cause delusions, or if delusional subjects are relatively preoccupied with certain emotional themes.

Early work suggested that delusions were the consequence of faulty syllogistic reasoning (von Domarus 1944):

I am a man
Napoleon is a man
I am Napoleon.

A recent investigation of logical reasoning ability, including conditional and syllogistic (Evans *et al.* 1993) reasoning tasks, has demonstrated that such reasoning is not impaired in relatively high-functioning deluded patients – at least no more than in non-deluded patients (Kemp *et al.* 1997). Relatively difficult problems were given, such as:

No religious people are criminals
Some priests are criminals
then
Some religious people are not priests (true/false)
or
Some priests are not religious people (true/false).

All subjects tended to be swayed by their common-sense understanding rather than working through the problems logically. In keeping with this, J. Slater, B. Elvevåg and T.E. Goldberg (submitted) found that formal reasoning in patients and normal controls was highly correlated with general intelligence for relationally complex sentences, but not classic working memory measures.

Further studies have emphasized abnormalities in hypothesis testing in deluded patients, with patients with persecutory delusions requiring less information before reaching a conclusion than non-deluded controls – based on judgements of probability of occurrence (Huq *et al.* 1988; Garety *et al.* 1991). Tasks have involved being presented with a bead of one of two colours and judging from which of two jars the bead was most likely to have come, given the known proportion of each coloured bead in the two jars. Deluded patients tended to reach a judgement after a single bead had been presented while controls tended to wait for more beads before deciding the jar of origin. More naturalistic versions of the task have also been devised and the results are similar (Dudley *et al.* 1997). These and similar tasks have shown that patients are more inclined to stick to their hypotheses even in the presence of negative feedback (Young & Bentall 1995). However, recent extensions of this work have failed to confirm the link between performance on such tests and delusions *per se* (Mortimer *et al.* 1996) as opposed to major mental illness.

It is unclear whether these perceptual and reasoning biases lead to predisposition and formation of persecutory delusions or maintain delusions once formed, or are correlates of other cognitive characteristics of delusional patients that are not the causes of the delusions. Indeed, the difficulty in distinguishing between the effects of beliefs on current perception and reasoning and the effects of the latter on belief formation has been highlighted in the investigation of delusional misidentification, in which it has been argued that abnormal beliefs distort current perceptual experiences in a top-down fashion (Fleminger 1994). Delusions may be conceived of as a content-specific reasoning problem. Nevertheless, the extent of reasoning deficits may be slight compared with the fixity and 'irrationality' of abnormal beliefs.

Other approaches to delusions

David and Howard (1994) employed a type of reality monitoring methodology to study cognitively intact patients with delusional memories. The phenomenal characteristics of each person's delusional memory were contrasted with a real memorable event and a fantasy. It was found that delusional memories were more vivid and tangible than even real events (although delusions tended to be 'rehearsed' more mentally) and this vividness could lead to reality confusion. However, a detailed case study approach revealed coincident reasoning aberrations as well, for example, on the cognitive estimates task.

Other psychophysiological methods have been employed to aid the understanding of delusions. Monitoring directed attention in subjects in real time – an 'on-line' measurement of attention – has the advantage over off-line measures in that it allows the presence of 'abnormal' information processing strategies. The measurement of visual scan paths is one method that has potential as a monitor of real-time visual information processing. The visual scan path is, literally, a map which traces the direction and extent of gaze when an individual comprehends a complex scene (Noton & Stark 1971): i.e. a psychophysiological 'marker' of sensory input and directional attention on viewing a stimulus.

A small number of studies have investigated visual scan paths in schizophrenic subjects (Phillips & David 1994). A relationship between symptomatology and viewing strategy has been demonstrated, with the presence of positive symptoms associated with increased scanning and negative symptoms with increased staring (Gaebel *et al.* 1987; Streit *et al.* 1997). While these studies have demonstrated abnormalities in viewing strategies in schizophrenic patients *per se*, others have aimed to investigate specific abnormalities in the visual scan paths (i.e. specific attentional deficits) in deluded schizophrenic patients compared with non-deluded schizophrenics (Phillips & David 1994, 1997, 1998). These studies have demonstrated that deluded schizophrenic patients employ abnormal strategies when viewing salient visual stimuli, e.g. human faces – viewing non-

feature areas to a significantly greater extent than both well-matched non-deluded schizophrenics and normal controls. Such strategies 'normalize' with recovery. One interpretation of these findings is that deluded schizophrenic patients rely on less salient visual information when appraising complex stimuli compared with controls.

Conclusions

The negative symptoms of schizophrenia seem by their very nature to be eminently reducible to cognitive deficits, although there is a danger of circularity (e.g. reduced verbal fluency correlating with poverty of speech). However, linking cognitive abnormalities with positive symptoms has proven to be a challenge. It appears that standard neuropsychological tests lack the specificity and sensitivity to shed light on the cognitive basis of such phenomena as hallucinations and delusions. More successes have been claimed when individual symptoms or symptom complexes have been the focus of investigation coupled with the use of experimental tasks with a sound theoretical basis. Contrasting individual cases with clear-cut phenomenology and relatively few intellectual impairments is a strategy worth employing. Within-subject design with and without the symptoms of interest is another potentially powerful approach. Finally, the remit of neuropsychology needs to expand into social psychology and take account of concepts such as attribution and bias.

Thought disorder

Recent attempts to understand the cognitive underpinnings of thought disorder (i.e. disorganized speech characterized by derailments, tangential responses and poverty of content) in schizophrenia have focused on abnormalities in the semantic memory system. Such formulations generally propose that 'spreading activation' through a network of features or representations based on meaning is abnormal. The construct itself (spreading activation) is usually measured by a cognitive paradigm involving priming, in which one word primes the recognition of a second word because they are related in some way. However, it has been unclear if these abnormalities are caused by failures in controlled processing or automatic processing and even whether the abnormalities reflect too much or too little priming. Moreover, the exact relation of these semantic processing measures to clinical ratings of thought disorder is equivocal. Many of these issues have been covered in detail in recent reviews (Spitzer 1998; Goldberg & Weinberger 2000).

Novel work by Goldberg *et al.* may be helpful in homing on the signal in this rather noisy area of research. Using changes in medication status in patients (unmedicated vs. medicated) to produce changes in thought disorder, they found that not only did the degree of priming change with medication status independent of changes in reaction time, but also that changes in priming significantly and selectively covaried with clinical ratings of disorganized speech (Goldberg & Weinberger 2000).

Thus, improvements in thought disorder were correlated with increases in priming effects. Several negative findings were also important: neither attention nor working memory improved and neither did verbal comprehension nor naming. These results indicate that thought disorder:

1 is not secondary to general cognitive impairments; but
2 may be caused by a specific abnormality in the semantic system, involving not the integrity of representations but access to connectivity among representations.

In a further refinement of this notion, Elvevåg et al. (unpublished data) found that representation (of numbers) in a task requiring numerosity judgements was intact in patients, while priming between 'adjacent' whole numbers was reduced in patients compared with normal controls. However, this work is preliminary and awaits replication.

Cognition as an intermediate phenotype

Genetic linkage studies using diagnosis as a phenotype have generally been disappointing (Egan & Weinberger 1997). One possible reason for this is that individuals do not inherit schizophrenia *per se* but a variety of information processing deficits out of which schizophrenia emerges. In a study of MZ twins discordant for schizophrenia, Goldberg et al. (1995) found subtle attenuations of performance in the otherwise well cotwins when compared with normal twins on neurocognitive measures indexing working memory, speed of information processing and episodic memory. More recently, Cannon et al. (2000), using population-based samples of discordant MZ and dizygotic (DZ) twins, compellingly demonstrated that compromises in frontal-lobe-type cognitive impairments are heritable in schizophrenia. Indeed, the unaffected twins of MZ and DZ pairs, in whom the other member was schizophrenic, differed in step-wise fashion from normal twins on such tasks as impairment in spatial working memory, divided attention, choice reaction time and intrusion errors.

Investigators in the Clinical Brain Disorders Branch of the National Instiue of Mental Health have reported a series of studies of cognitive assessments in a large sample of siblings. Their sample consisted of 147 patients with schizophrenia, 193 of their siblings and 47 controls. The IQ of index cases was 94, for their siblings was 107 and for controls was 108. The percentage of siblings carrying a schizophrenic spectrum diagnosis was relatively low – under 5%. Egan et al. (2000) assessed relative risk of the CPT test of attention and encoding, given that prior work from other groups had suggested that this type of test might be sensitive to certain cognitive impairments in relatives of patients. In a version of the test which included flanking distracters, they found that 50% of patients, 24% of siblings and 18% of controls performed 1 SD below the control mean using d' as a dependent measure. Compared with controls, a subgroup of 97 siblings of patients who performed the CPT abnormally also had significantly reduced CPT performance. Examination of a continuous working memory test, the so-called N-back, which demands rapid and precise encoding of stimuli

and their temporal order, resistance to interference and maintenance, revealed that relative risk for impairment in siblings was high and that the sibling group as a whole was significantly impaired compared with normal controls, suggesting that such deficits were familial and probably related to genetic risk for schizophrenia (T.E. Goldberg, M.F. Egan and D.R. Weinberger, submitted). Moreover, the impairments were not redundant with diagnosis, because the sibling sample was purified in that individuals with psychosis or spectrum diagnoses were excluded.

Impairments in several other domains of cognition have also been observed in many studies of patients with schizophrenia. These include working memory/executive function, verbal memory, language, oculomotor scanning/psychomotor speed and general intelligence. To assess the suitability of cognitive function for use as phenotypes in genetic studies, relative risk (RR) was estimated in the aforementioned cohort of siblings (Egan et al., 2001). They hypothesized that RR of cognitive dysfunction would be moderate and that different subgroups of families would demonstrate different patterns of impairment. Relative risk was estimated using cut-off scores of 1 and 2 SD below the control mean. Patients performed significantly worse than controls on all tests except Wide Range Achievement Test (WRAT). The entire sibling group demonstrated impaired performance on WCST, verbal fluency and Trails B. Siblings of patients with impaired performance also showed deficits in the verbal list learning and memory for stories. Again using 1 SD as the cut-off for affected status, the RR to siblings was elevated on the Trails B (RR = 3.8). Increased RRs were also seen for list learning, WCST, letter fluency and memory for stories scores (RRs were approximately 2.0, $P < 0.05$). Using 2 SD as the cut-off, RRs were generally higher. Correlations between tests of different cognitive functions were generally weak, suggesting that they measure relatively independent processes; multiple regression analysis also demonstrated that impairment on one test did not predict impairment on another test in the sibling group. In general, siblings had 1–2 impaired scores, schizophrenic cases had 4 and normal controls had 0 or 1 for the following measures: verbal list learning, trailmaking, card sorting and IQ decline. Ultimately, it is hoped that using cognitive phenotypes may reduce clinical and genetic heterogeneity and improve the power of genetic studies of schizophrenia.

Conclusions

This chapter has attempted to demonstrate that cognitive paradigms can be utilized to constrain thinking about schizophrenia (for instance, course), make important observations about what is 'wrong' with patients (in the sense of core impairments) and be used in novel ways to provide novel mechanistic accounts of symptoms or reductionistic accounts of the aetiology of the disorder. The modal pattern of the developmental trajectory of cognitive impairment reflects deterioration from some higher level of functioning and then stabilization, as consistent with a static encephalopathy. Working memory and episodic memory dysfunctions are prominent. Working memory impairments in particular may be found independent of IQ. These impairments are heritable and may provide an intermediate phenotype for association or linkage studies not redundant with diagnosis. Because these deficits may account for some of the social and vocational morbidity associated with schizophrenia, they should probably be considered as targets for various remediation modalities, including novel cognitive-enhancing 'antischizophrenia' medications.

References

Adler, L.E., Olincy, A., Waldo, M. *et al.* (1998) Schizophrenia, sensory gating, and nicotinic receptors. *Schizophrenia Bulletin* **24**, 189–202.

Aleman, A., Hijman, R., de Haan, E.H. & Kahn, R.S. (1999) Memory impairment in schizophrenia: a meta-analysis. *American Journal of Psychiatry* **156**, 1358–1366.

Barkley, R.A., DuPaul, G.J. & McMurray, M.B. (1990) Comprehensive evaluation of attention deficit disorder with and without hyperactivity as defined by research criteria. *Journal of Consulting and Clinical Psychology* **58**, 775–789.

Basso, M.R., Nasrallah, H.A., Olson, S.C. & Bornstein, R.A. (1998) Neuropsychological correlates of negative, disorganized and psychotic symptoms in schizophrenia. *Schizophrenia Research* **31**, 99–111.

Bentall, R., Baker, G. & Havers, S. (1991) Reality monitoring and psychotic hallucinations. *British Journal of Clinical Psychology* **30**, 213–222.

Bilder, R.M., Turkel, E., Lipschutz-Broch, L. & Lieberman, J.A. (1992) Antipsychotic medication effects on neuropsychological functions. *Psychopharmacology Bulletin* **28**, 353–366.

Blanchard, J.J. & Neale, J.M. (1994) The neuropsychological signature of schizophrenia: generalized or differential deficit? *American Journal of Psychiatry* **151**, 40–48.

Bleuler, E. (1950) *Dementia Praecox or the Group of Schizophrenia*. International Universities Press, New York.

Braff, D.L., Heaton, R., Kuck, J. *et al.* (1991) The generalized pattern of neuropsychological deficits in outpatients with chronic schizophrenia with heterogeneous Wisconsin Card Sorting Test results. *Archives of General Psychiatry* **48**, 891–898.

Bruder, G., Rabinowicz, E., Towey, J. *et al.* (1995) Smaller right ear (left hemisphere) advantage for dichotic fused words in patients with schizophrenia. *American Journal of Psychiatry* **152**, 932–935.

Buchanan, R.W., Holstein, C. & Breier, A. (1994) The comparative efficacy and long-term effect of clozapine treatment on neuropsychological test performance. *Biological Psychiatry* **36**, 717–725.

Bymaster, F.P., Calligaro, D.O., Falcone, J.F. *et al.* (1996) Radioreceptor binding profile of the atypical antipsychotic olanzapine. *Neuropsychopharmacology* **14**, 87–96.

Cahill, C., Silbersweig, D. & Frith, C. (1996) Psychotic experiences induced in deluded patients using distorted auditory feedback. *Cognitive Neuropsychiatry* **1**, 201–211.

Calev, A. (1984) Recall and recognition in mildly disturbed schizophrenics: the use of matched tasks. *Psychological Medicine* **14**, 425–429.

Cannon, T.D., Zorrilla, L.E., Shtasel, D. *et al.* (1994) Neuropsychological functioning in siblings discordant for schizophrenia and healthy volunteers. *Archives of General Psychiatry* **51**, 651–661.

Cannon, T.D., Huttunen, M.O., Lonnqvist, J. *et al.* (2000) The inheritance of neuropsychological dysfunction in twins discordant for schizophrenia. *American Journal of Human Genetics* **67**, 369–382.

Cassens, G., Inglis, A.K., Applebaum, P.S. & Gutheil, T.G. (1990) Neuroleptics. effects on neuropsychological function in chronic schizophrenic patients. *Schizophrenia Bulletin* **16**, 477–499.

Castner, S.A., Williams, G.V. & Goldman-Rakic, P.S. (2000) Reversal of antipsychotic-induced working memory deficits by short-term dopamine D$_1$ receptor stimulation. *Science* **287**, 2020–2022.

Censits, D.M., Ragland, J.D., Gur, R.C. & Gur, R.E. (1997) Neuropsychological evidence supporting a neurodevelopmental model of schizophrenia. *Schizophrenia Research* **24**, 289–298.

Chadwick, P. & Birchwood, M. (1994) The omnipotence of voices: a cognitive approach to auditory hallucinations. *British Journal of Psychiatry* **164**, 190–201.

Chapman, L.J. & Chapman, J.P. (1973) Problems in the measurement of cognitive deficit. *Psychological Bulletin* **79**, 380–385.

Chapman, L.J. & Chapman, J.P. (1988) The genesis of delusions. In: *Delusional Beliefs* (eds T.F. Oltmanns & B.A. Maher), pp. 167–211. Wiley, New York.

Chapman, L.J. & Chapman, J.P. (1989) Strategies for resolving the heterogeneity of schizophrenics and their relatives using cognitive measures. *Journal of Abnormal Psychology* **98**, 571–366.

Cuesta, M.J., Peralta, V. & Zarzuela, A. (1998) Illness duration and neuropsychological impairments in schizophrenia. *Schizophrenia Research* **33**, 141–150.

Danion, J.M., Rizzo, L. & Bruant, A. (1999) Functional mechanisms underlying impaired recognition memory and conscious awareness in patients with schizophrenia. *Archives of General Psychiatry* **56**, 639–644.

David, A.S. (1994a) The neuropsychology of auditory–verbal hallucinations. In: *The Neuropsychology of Schizophrenia* (eds A. David & J. Cutting), pp. 269–312. Lawrence Erlbaum, Hove.

David, A.S. (1994b) Thought echo reflects the activity of the phonological loop. *British Journal of Clinical Psychology* **33**, 81–83.

David, A.S. & Cutting, J.C. (eds) (1994) *The Neuropsychology of Schizophrenia*. Lawrence Erlbaum Associates, Hillsdale, NJ.

David, A.S. & Halligan, P.W. (2000) Cognitive neuropsychiatry: potential for progress. *Journal of Neuropsychiatry and Clinical Neurosciences* **12**, 506–510.

David, A.S. & Howard, R. (1994) An experimental phenomenological approach to delusional memory in schizophrenia and late paraphrenia. *Psychological Medicine* **24**, 515–524.

David, A.S. & Lucas, P. (1993) Auditory–verbal hallucinations and the phonological loop: a cognitive neuropsychological study. *British Journal of Clinical Psychology* **32**, 431–441.

David, A.S., Malmberg, A., Brandt, L., Allebeck, P. & Lewis, G. (1997) IQ and risk for schizophrenia: a population-based cohort study. *Psychological Medicine* **27**, 1311–1323.

Davidson, M., Reichenberg, A., Rabinowitz, J. *et al.* (1999) Behavioral and intellectual markers for schizophrenia in apparently healthy male adolescents. *American Journal of Psychiatry* **156**, 1328–1335.

Dickerson, F., Boronow, J.J., Ringel, N. & Parente, F. (1996) Neurocognitive deficits and social functioning in outpatients with schizophrenia. *Schizophrenia Research* **21**, 75–83.

von Domarus, E. (1944) The specific laws of logic in schizophrenia. In: *Language and Thought in Schizophrenia*, pp. 104–114. University of California Press, Berkeley, CA.

Dudley, R.E.J., John, C.H., Young, A.W. & Over, D.E. (1997) Normal and abnormal reasoning in people with delusions. *British Journal of Clinical Psychology* **36**, 243–258.

Egan, M.F. & Weinberger, D.R. (1997) Neurobiology of schizophrenia. *Current Opinions in Neurobiology* 7, 701–707.

Egan, M.F., Goldberg, T.E., Gscheidle, T. *et al.* (2000) Relative risk of attention deficits in siblings of patients with schizophrenia. *American Journal of Psychiatry* 157, 1309–1316.

Egan, M.F., Goldberg, T.E., Gscheidle, T. *et al.* (2001) Relative risk for cognitive impairments in siblings of patients with schizophrenia. *Biological Psychiatry* 50, 98–107.

Elliott, R., McKenna, P.J., Robbins, T.W. & Sahakian, B.J. (1995) Neuropsychological evidence for frontostrial dysfunction in schizophrenia. *Psychological Medicine* 25, 619–630.

Elvevåg, B., Duncan, J. & McKenna, P.J. (2000a) The use of cognitive context in schizophrenia: an investigation. *Psychological Medicine* 30, 885–897.

Elvevåg, B., Egan, M.F. & Goldberg, T.E. (2000b) Paired-associate learning and memory interference in schizophrenia. *Neuropsychologia* 38, 1565–1575.

Elvevåg, B., Weinberger, D.R., Egan, M.F. & Goldberg, T.E. (2000c) Memory for temporal oderd in schizophrenia. *Schizophrenia Research* 46, 187–193.

Elvevåg, B., Weinberger, D.R. & Goldberg, T.E. (2000d) Short-term memory for serial order in schizophrenia: a detailed examination of error types. *Neuropsychology* 15, 128–135.

Elvevåg, B., Weinberger, D.R., Suter, J.C. & Goldberg, T.E. (2000e) Continuous performance test and schizophrenia: a test of stimulus-response compatibility, working memory, response readiness, or none of the above? *American Journal of Psychiatry* 157, 772–780.

Evans, C., McGuire, P. & David, A.S. (2000) Is auditory imagery defective in patients with auditory hallucinations? *Psychological Medicine* 30, 137–148.

Evans, J.StB.T., Newstead, S.E. & Byrne, R.M.J. (1993) *Human Reasoning*. Erlbaum, Hove.

Faraone, S.V., Seidman, L.J., Kremen, W.S. *et al.* (1995) Neuropsychological functioning among the non-psychotic relatives of schizophrenic patients: a diagnostic efficacy analysis. *Journal of Abnormal Psychology* 104, 286–304.

Fey, E.T. (1951) The performance of young schizophrenics and young normals on the Wisconsin Card Sorting Test. *Journal of Consulting Psychology* 15, 311–319.

Fleming, K., Goldberg, T.E., Binks, S. *et al.* (1997) Visuospatial working memory in patients with schizophrenia. *Biological Psychiatry* 41, 43–49.

Fleminger, S. (1994) Top-down processing and delusional misidentification. In: *The Neuropsychology of Schizophrenia* (eds A.S. David & J.C. Cutting), pp. 161–167. Lawrence Erlbaum, Hove.

Freedman, R., Coon, H., Myles-Worsley, M. *et al.* (1997) Linkage of a neurophysiological deficit in schizophrenia to a chromosome 15 locus. *Proceedings of the National Academy of Sciences, USA* 94, 587–592.

Frith, C.D. (1987) The positive and negative symptoms of schizophrenia reflect impairments in the perception and initiation of action. *Psychological Medicine* 17, 631–648.

Frith, C. (1992) *Cognitive Neuropsychology of Schizophrenia*. Erlbaum, Hove.

Gaebel, W., Ulrich, G. & Frick, K. (1987) Visuomotor performance of schizophrenic patients and normal controls in a picture viewing task. *Biological Psychiatry* 22, 1227–1237.

Garety, P.A., Hemsley, D.R. & Wessely, S. (1991) Reasoning in deluded schizophrenic and paranoid patients: biases in performance on a probabilistic inference task. *Journal of Nervous and Mental Disease* 179, 194–201.

Gold, J.M., Randolph, C., Coppola, R. *et al.* (1992) Visual orienting in schizophrenia. *Schizophrenia Research* 7, 203–209.

Gold, J.M., Hermann, B.P., Wyler, A. *et al.* (1994) Schizophrenia and temporal lobe epilepsy: a neuropsychological study. *Archives of General Psychiatry* 51, 265–272.

Gold, J.M., Carpenter, C., Randolph, C., Goldberg, T.E. & Weinberger, D.R. (1997) Auditory working memory and Wisconsin Card Sorting Test performance in schizophrenia. *Archives of General Psychiatry* 54, 159–165.

Gold, S., Arndt, S., Nopoulos, P., O'Leary, D.S. & Andreasen, N.C. (1999) Longitudinal study of cognitive function in first-episode and recent-onset schizophrenia. *American Journal of Psychiatry* 156, 1342–1348.

Goldberg, T.E. (1999) Some fairly obvious distinctions between schizophrenia and bipolar disorder. *Schizophrenia Research* 39 (2), 161–162.

Goldberg, T.E. & Weinberger, D.R. (1988) Probing prefrontal function in schizophrenia with neuropsychological paradigms. *Schizophrenia Bulletin* 14, 179–183.

Goldberg, T.E. & Weinberger, D.R. (2000) Thought disorder in schizohrenia: a reappraisal of older formulations and an overview of some recent studies. *Cognitive Neuropsychiatry* 5, 1–19.

Goldberg, T.E., Weinberger, D.R., Berman, K.F., Pliskin, N. & Podd, M. (1987) Possible evidence for dementia of the prefrontal type in schizophrenia? *Archives of General Psychiatry* 44, 1008–1014.

Goldberg, T.E., Weinberger, D.R., Pliskin, N.H., Berman, K.F. & Podd, M. (1989) Recall memory deficits in schizophrenia: a possible manifestation of frontal lobe dysfunction. *Schizophrenia Research* 2, 251–225.

Goldberg, T.E., Berman, K.F., Mohr, E. & Weinberger, D.R. (1990a) Regional cerebral blood flow and cognitive function in Huntington's disease and schizophrenia. *Archives of Neurology* 47, 418–422.

Goldberg, T.E., Ragland, D.R., Gold, J.M. *et al.* (1990b) Neuropsychological assessment of monozygotic twins discordant for schizophrenia. *Archives of General Psychiatry* 47, 1066–1072.

Goldberg, T.E., Gold, J.M., Greenberg, R. *et al.* (1993a) Contrasts between patients with affective disorder and patients with schizophrenia on a neuropsychological screening battery. *American Journal of Psychiatry* 150, 1355–1362.

Goldberg, T.E., Greenberg, R. & Griffin, S. (1993b) The impact of clozapine on cognition and psychiatric symptoms in patients with schizophrenia. *British Journal of Psychiatry* 162, 43–48.

Goldberg, T.E., Torrey, E.F., Gold, J.M. *et al.* (1995) Genetic risk of neuropsychological impairment in schizophrenia: a study of monozygotic twins discordant and concordant for the disorder. *Schizophrenia Research* 17, 77–84.

Goldberg, T.E., Gold, J.M., Coppola, R. & Weinberger, D.R. (1997) Unnatural practices, unspeakable actions: a study of delayed auditory feedback in schizophrenia. *American Journal of Psychiatry* 154, 858–860.

Goldberg, T.E., Patterson, K., Taqqu, Y., Wilder, K. & Weinberger, D.R. (1998) Capacity limitations in schizophrenia: tests of competing hypotheses. *Psychological Medicine* 28, 665–673.

Goldstein, G. & Zubin, J. (1990) Neuropsychological differences between young and old schizophrenics with and without associated neurological dysfunction. *Schizophrenia Research* 3, 117–120.

Gourovitch, M.L., Weinberger, D.R. & Goldberg, T.E. (1996) Verbal fluency deficits in patients with schizophrenia: semantic fluency is differentially impaired as compared with phonologic fluency. *Neuropsychology* 6, 573–577.

Green, M.F. (1996) What are the functional consequences of neurocognitive deficits in schizophrenia? *American Journal of Psychiatry* 153, 321–330.

Green, M.F., Hugdahl, K. & Mitchell, S. (1994) Dichotic listening during auditory hallucinations in patients with schizophrenia. *American Journal of Psychiatry* 151, 357–362.

Green, M.F., Marshall, B.D.J., Wirshing, W.C. *et al.* (1997) Does risperidone improve verbal working memory in treatment-resistant schizophrenia? *American Journal of Psychiatry* 154, 799–804.

Green, M.F., Kern, R.S., Braff, D.L. & Mintz, J. (2000) Neurocognitive deficits and functional outcome in schizophrenia: are we measuring the 'right stuff'? *Schizophrenia Bulletin* 26, 119–136.

Haddock, G., Slade, P.D. & Bentall, R.P. (1995) Auditory hallucinations and the verbal transformation effect: the role of suggestions. *Personality and Individual Differences* 19, 301–306.

Halligan, P.W. & David, A. S. (2001) Cognitive neuropsychiatry: towards a scientific psychoathology. *Nature Reviews. Neuroscience* 2, 209–215.

Harvey, P.D., Howanitz, E., Parrella, M. *et al.* (1998a) Symptoms, cognitive functioning, and adaptive skills in geriatric patients with lifelong schizophrenia: a comparison across treatment sites. *American Journal of Psychiatry* 155, 1080–1086.

Harvey, P.D., Parrella, M., White, L. *et al.* (1998b) Convergence of cognitive and adaptive decline in late-life schizophrenia. *Schizophrenia Research.* 35, 77–84.

Heaton, R.K. & Crowley, T.J. (1981) Effect of psychiatric disorders and their somatic treatments on neuropsychological test results. In: *Handbook of Clinical Neuropsychology* (eds S. Filskov & T.J. Boll), pp. 481–525. John Wiley, New York.

Heaton, R.K. & Drexler, M. (1987) Clinical neuropsychological findings in schizophrenia and aging. In: *Schizophrenia and Aging: Schizophrenia, Paranoia and Schizophreniform* (eds N.E. Miller & G.D. Cohen), pp. 145–161. Guilford Press, New York.

Heaton, R., Paulsen, J.S., McAdams, L.A. *et al.* (1994) Neuropsychological deficits in schizophrenics: relationship to age, chronicity and dementia. *Archives of General Psychiatry* 51, 469–476.

Hoffman, R.E., Oates, E., Hafner, J., Hustig, H.H. & McGlashan, T.H. (1994) Semantic organization of hallucinated 'voices' in schizophrenia. *American Journal of Psychiatry* 151, 1229–1230.

Hull, C.L. (1917) The formation and retention of associations among the insane. *American Journal of Psychology* 28, 419–435.

Huq, S.F., Garety, P.A. & Hemsley, D.R. (1988) Probabilistic judgments in deluded and non-deluded subjects. *Quarterly Journal of Experimental Psychology* 40A (4), 801–812.

Hyde, T.M., Nawroz, S., Goldberg, T.E. *et al.* (1994) Is there cognitive decline in schizophrenia: a cross-sectional study. *British Journal of Psychiatry* 164, 494–500.

Johns, L.C. & McGuire, P.K. (1999) Verbal self-monitoring and auditory hallucinations in schizophrenia. *Lancet* 353, 469–470.

Johnson, M.K., Foley, M.A. & Leach, K. (1988) The consequence for memory of imagining in another person's voice. *Memory and Cognition* 16, 337–342.

Jones, P. & Cannon, M. (1998) The new epidemiology of schizophrenia. *Psychiatric Clinics in North America* 21, 1–25.

Kaney, S. & Bentall, R.P. (1989) Persecutory delusions and attributional style. *British Journal of Medical Psychology* 62, 191–198.

Kaney, S. & Bentall, R.P. (1990) Persecutory delusions and the self-serving bias: evidence from a contingency judgment task. *Journal of Nervous and Mental Disease* 180, 773–780.

Kaney, S., Wolfenden, M., Dewey, M.E. & Bentall, R.P. (1992) Persecutory delusions and the recall of threatening and non-threatening propositions. *British Journal of Clinical Psychology* 31, 85–87.

Kapur, S. & Seeman, P. (2000) Antipsychotic agents differ in how fast they come off the dopamine D_2 receptors: implications for atypical antipsychotic action. *Journal of Psychiatry and Neuroscience* 25, 161–166.

Kapur, S., Zipursky, R., Jones, C. *et al.* (2000a) Relationship between dopamine D_2 occupancy, clinical response, and side effects: a double-blind PET study of first-episode schizophrenia. *American Journal of Psychiatry* 157, 514–520.

Kapur, S., Zipursky, R., Jones, C. *et al.* (2000b) A positron emission tomography study of quetiapine in schizophrenia: a preliminary finding of an antipsychotic effect with only transiently high dopamine D_2 receptor occupancy. *Archives of General Psychiatry* 57, 553–559.

Keefe, R.S.E. & Harvey, P.D. (2001) Studies of cognitive change in patients with schizophrenia following novel and antipsychotic treatment. *American Journal of Psychiatry* 158, 176–284.

Keefe, R.S.E., Silva, S.G., Perkins, D.O. & Lieberman, J.A. (1999) The effects of atypical antipsychotic drugs on neurocognitive impairment in schizophrenia: a review and meta-analysis. *Schizophrenia Bulletin* 25, 201–222.

Kemp, R., Chua, S., McKenna, P. & David, A.S. (1997) Reasoning and delusions. *British Journal of Psychiatry* 170, 398–405.

Kenny, J.T. & Meltzer, H.Y. (1991) Attention and higher cortical functions in schizophrenia. *Journal of Neuropsychiatry* 3, 269–275.

Kern, R.S., Green, M.F., Marshall, B.D. *et al.* (1998) Risperidone vs. haloperidol on reaction time, manual dexterity, and motor learning in treatment-resistant schizophrenia patients. *Biological Psychiatry* 44, 726–732.

Kern, R.S., Green, M.F., Marshall, B.D. *et al.* (1999) Risperidone vs. haloperidol on secondary memory: can newer antipsychotics medications aid learning? *Schizophrenia Bulletin* 25, 223–232.

King, D.J. (1990) The effect of neuroleptics on cognitive and psychomotor function. *British Journal of Psychiatry* 157, 799–811.

Klonoff, H., Hutton, G.H. & Fibiger, C.H. (1970) Neuropsychological patterns in chronic schizophrenia. *Journal of Nervous and Mental Disease* 150, 291–300.

Kolb, B. & Whishaw, I.Q. (1983) Performance of schizophrenic patients on tests sensitive to left or right frontal temporal, and parietal function in neurologic patients. *Journal of Nervous and Mental Disease* 171, 435–443.

Kraepelin, E. (1919/1971) *Dementia Praecox and Paraphrenia* (ed. G.M. Robertson), Translated by R.M. Barclay & R.E. Krieger. Huntington, New York.

Leafhead, K.M., Young, A.W. & Szulecka, T.K. (1996) Delusions demand attention. *Cognitive Neuropsychiatry* 1, 5–16.

Lennox, B.R., Bert, S., Park, B.G., Jones, P.B. & Morris, P.G. (1999) Spatial and temporal mapping of neural activity associated with auditory hallucinations. *Lancet* 353, 644.

Leudar, I., Thomas, P. & Johnston, M. (1994) Self-monitoring in speech production: effects of verbal hallucinations and negative symptoms. *Psychological Medicine* 24, 749–761.

Levitan, C., Ward, P.B. & Catts, S.V. (1999) Superior temporal gyral volumes and laterality correlates of auditory hallucinations in schizophrenia. *Biological Psychiatry* 46, 955–962.

Liddle, P.F. (1987a) The symptoms of chronic schizophrenia: a re-examination of the positive–negative dichotomy. *British Journal of Psychiatry* 151, 145–151.

Liddle, P.F. (1987b) Schizophrenic syndromes, cognitive performance and neurological dysfunction. *Psychological Medicine* 17, 49–57.

Light, G.A., Geyer, M.A., Clementz, B.A. *et al.* (2000) Normal P50 suppression in schizophrenia patients treated with atypical antipsychotic medications. *American Journal of Psychiatry* 157, 767–771.

Lubin, A., Gieseking, G.F. & Williams, H.L. (1962) Direct measurement of cognitive deficit in schizophrenia. *Journal of Consulting, Psychology* 26, 139–143.

Maher, B.A. (1974) Delusional thinking and perceptual disorder. *Journal of Individual Psychology* 30, 85–95.

McKenna, P.J., Tarnlvn, D., Lund, C.E. *et al.* (1990) Amnesic syndrome in schizophrenia. *Psychological Medicine* 20, 967–972.

Medalia, A., Gold, J. & Merriam, A. (1988) The effects of neuroleptics on neuropsychological test results in schizophrenia. *Archives of Clinical Neurology* 3, 249–271.

Meltzer, H.Y. & McGurk, S.R. (1999) The effects of clozapine, risperidone, and olanzapine on cognitive function in schizophrenia. *Schizophrenia Bulletin* 25 (2), 233–256.

Mesulum, M.M. (1985) *Principles of Behavioral Neurology*. F.A. Davis Company, Philadelphia, PA.

Mirsky, A.F. (1988) Research on schizophrenia in the NIMH Laboratory of Psychology and Psychopathology, 1954–87. *Schizophrenia Bulletin* 14, 151–156.

Mockler, D., Riordan, J. & Sharma, T. (1997) Memory and intellectual deficits do not decline with age in schizophrenia. *Schizophrenia Research* 26, 1–7.

Morrison, A.P. & Haddock, G. (1997) Cognitive factors in source monitoring and auditory hallucinations. *Psychological Medicine* 27, 669–679.

Mortimer, A.M. *et al.* (1996) Delusions in schizophrenia: a phenomenological and psychological exploration. *Cognitive Neuropsychiatry* 1, 289–304.

Müller, U., von Cramon, D.Y. & Pollmann, S. (1998) D_1- versus D_2-receptor modulation of visuospatial working memory in humans. *Journal of Neuroscience* 18, 2720–2728.

Nagamoto, H.T., Adler, L.E., Hea, R.A. *et al.* (1996) Gating of auditory P50 in schizophrenics: unique effects of clozapine. *Biological Psychiatry* 40, 181–188.

Nayani, T.H. & David, A.S. (1996) The auditory hallucination: a phenomenological survey. *Psychological Medicine* 26, 177–189.

Norton, D. & Stark, L. (1971) Eye movements and visual perception. *Scientific American* 224, 35–43.

Pantelis, C., Barnes, T.R., Nelson, H.E. *et al.* (1997) Frontal–striatal cognitive deficits in patients with chronic schizophrenia. *Brain* 120, 1823–1843.

Pantelis, C., Barber, F.Z., Barnes, T.R. *et al.* (1999) Comparison of set-shifting ability in patients with chronic schizophrenia and frontal lobe damage. *Schizophrenia Research* 37, 251–270.

Park, S., Holzman, P.S. & Goldman-Rakic, P.S. (1995) Spatial working memory deficits in the relatives of schizophrenic patients. *Archives of General Psychiatry* 52, 821–828.

Paulsen, J.S., Heaton, R.K., Sadek, J.R. *et al.* (1995) The nature of learning and memory impairments in schizophrenia. *Journal of International Neuropsychology Society* 1, 88–99.

Perlstein, W.M., Carter, C.S., Barch, D.M. & Baird, J.W. (1998) The Stroop task and attention deficits in schizophrenia. a critical evaluation of card and single-trial Stroop methodologies. *Neuropsychology* 12, 414–425.

Phillips, M.L. & David, A.S. (1994) Understanding the symptoms of schizophrenia using visual scan paths. *British Journal of Psychiatry* 165, 673–675.

Phillips, M.L. & David, A.S. (1997) Visual scan paths are abnormal in deluded schizophrenics. *Neuropsychologia* 35, 99–105.

Phillips, M.L. & David, A.S. (1998) Abnormal visual scan paths: a psychophysiological marker of delusions in schizophrenia. *Schizophrenia Research* 29, 235–245.

Posner, M.I. & Dehaene, S. (1994) Attentional networks. *Trends in Neuroscience* 17, 75–79.

Posner, M.I., Early, T.S., Reiman, E., Pardo, P.J. & Dhawan, I.M. (1988) Asymmetries in hemispheric control of attention in schizophrenia. *Archives of General Psychiatry* 45, 814–821.

Purdon, S.E., Jones, B.D.W., Stip, E. *et al.* (2000) Neuropsychological change in early phase schizophrenia during 12 months of treatment with olanzapine, risperidone, or haloperidol. *Archives of General Psychiatry* 57, 249–258.

Randolph, C., Goldberg, T.E. & Weinberger, D.R. (1993) The neuropsychology of schizophrenia. In: *Clinical Neuropsychology*, 3rd edn (eds K.M. Heilman & E. Valenstein), pp. 499–522. Oxford, New York.

Rappaport, D., Gill, M. & Schafer, R. (1945/46) *Diagnostic Psychological Testing*. Year Book, Chicago.

Rossell, S.L., Shapleske, J. & David, A.S. (1998) Sentence verification and delusions: a content-specific deficit. *Psychological Medicine* 28, 1189–1198.

Rund, B.R. (1998) A review of longitudinal studies of cognitive functions in schizophrenia patients. *Schizophrenia Bulletin* 24, 425–435.

Saykin, J.A., Gur, R.C., Gur, R.E. *et al.* (1991) Neuropsychological function in schizophrenia: selective impairment in memory and learning. *Archives of General Psychiatry* 48, 618–624.

Saykin, A.J., Shtasel, D.L., Gur, R.E. *et al.* (1994) Neuropsychological deficits in neuroleptic naïve patients with first-episode schizophrenia. *Archives of General Psychiatry* 51, 124–131.

Schultz, W. (1998) Predictive reward signal of dopamine neurons. *Journal of Neurophysiology* 80, 1–27.

Schwartzman, A.E. & Douglas, V.I. (1962) Intellectual loss in schizophrenia. II. *Canadian Journal of Psychology* 16, 161–168.

Seal, M.L., Crowe, S.F. & Cheung, P. (1997) Deficits in source monitoring in subjects with auditory hallucinations may be due to differences in verbal intelligence and verbal memory. *Cognitive Neuropsychiatry* 2, 273–290.

Sengel, R.A. & Lovalla, W.R. (1983) Effects of cueing on immediate and recent memory in schizophrenics. *Journal of Nervous and Mental Disease* 171, 426–430.

Shakow, D. (1946) The nature of deterioration in schizophrenic conditions. *Nervous and Mental Disease Monographs*, 70.

Shakow, D. (1979) *Adaptation in Schizophrenia: the Theory of Segmental Set*. John Wiley, New York.

Shallice, T. (1988) *From Neuropsychology to Mental Structure*. Cambridge University Press, Cambridge.

Shallice, T., Burgess, P.W. & Frith, C.D. (1991) Can the neuropsychological case-study approach be applied to schizophrenia? *Psychological Medicine* 21, 661–673.

Smith, A. (1964) Mental deterioration in chronic schizophrenia. *Journal of Nervous and Mental Disease* 39, 479–487.

Spitzer, M. (1997) A cognitive neuroscience view of schizophrenic thought disorder. *Schizophrenia Bulletin* 23, 29–50.

Spohn, H.E. & Strauss, M.E. (1989) Relation of neuroleptic and anticholinergic medication to cognitive function in schizophrenia. *Journal of Abnormal Psychology* 98, 367–380.

Spohn, H.E., Coyne, L., Lacoursiere, R. *et al.* (1985) Relation of neuroleptic dose and tardive dyskinesia to attention, information-processing, and psychophysiology in medicated schizophrenics. *Archives of General Psychiatry* 42, 849–859.

Strauss, M.E. (1993) Relations of symptoms to cognitive deficits in schizophrenia. *Schizophrenia Bulletin* 19, 215–231.

Streit, M., Woelwer, W. & Gaebel, W. (1997) Facial-affect recognition and visual scanning behaviour in the course of schizophrenia. *Schizophrenia Research* 24, 311–317.

Sweeney, J.A., Haas, G.L., Keilp, J.G. & Long, M. (1991) Evaluation of the stability of neuropsychological functioning after acute episode of schizophrenia: 1-year follow-up, study. *Psychiatry Research* **38**, 63–76.

Teuber, H.L. (1955) Physiological psychology. *Annual Review of Psychology* **9**, 267–298.

Traupmann, K.L. (1980) Encoding processes and memory for categorically related word by schizophrenic patients. *Journal of Abnormal Psychology* **89**, 704–716.

Velligan, D.I., Mahurin, R.K., Diamond, P.L. *et al.* (1997) The functional significance of symptomatology and cognitive function in schizophrenia. *Schizophrenia Research* **25**, 21–31.

Vinogradov, S., Willis-Shore, J., Poole, J.H. *et al.* (1997) Clinical and neurocognitive aspects of source monitoring errors in schizophrenia. *American Journal of Psychiatry* **154**, 1530–1537.

Weickert, T.W., Goldberg, T.E., Gold, J.M. *et al.* (2000) Cognitive impairments in patients with schizophrenia displaying preserved and compromised intellect. *Archives of General Psychiatry* **57**, 907–913.

Woodruff, P., Brammer, M., Mellers, J. *et al.* (1995) Auditory hallucinations and perception of external speech. *Lancet* **346**, 1035.

Woodruff, P.W.R., Wright, I.C., Bullmore, E.T. *et al.* (1997) Auditory hallucinations and the temporal cortical response to speech in schizophrenia: a functional magnetic resonance imaging study. *American Journal of Psychiatry* **154**, 1676–1682.

Yee, C.M., Nuechterlein, K.H., Morris, S.E. & White, P.M. (1998) P50 suppression in recent-onset schizophrenia: clinical correlates and risperidone effects. *Journal of Abnormal Psychology* **107**, 691–698.

Young, H.F. & Bentall, R.P. (1995) Hypothesis testing in patients with persecutory delusions: comparison with depressed and normal subjects. *British Journal of Clinical Psychology* **34**, 353–369.

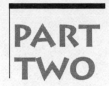

PART TWO

Biological Aspects

11 The secondary schizophrenias

T.M. Hyde and S.W. Lewis

Terminology and classification, 187
How common are secondary
    schizophrenias?, 188
Inferring cause and effect, 189
The co-occurrence of schizophrenia-like symptoms
    and organic brain disease, 190
Epilepsy, 191
Cerebral trauma, 191
Cerebrovascular disease, 192
Demyelinating diseases, 192
Metabolic and autoimmune disorders, 193

Encephalitis and other infections of the central
    nervous system, 193
Sex chromosome abnormalities, 194
Associations with Mendelian disorders, 194
Tumours and other space-occupying lesions, 196
Phenomenology of primary vs. secondary
    schizophrenia, 197
Excluding secondary schizophrenia in practice:
    physical investigations, 198
Conclusions, 198
References, 199

Schizophrenia is a behavioural disorder that is a diagnosis of exclusion. There are no established laboratory tests, neuroimaging studies, electrophysiological paradigms or neuropsychological testing batteries that can explicitly confirm this disorder to the exclusion of phenocopies. This was explicitly recognized by Kraepelin and Bleuler, and particularly by Schneider, as a caveat in the delineation of his first-rank symptoms.

The existence of a disparate range of brain disorders that can, uncommonly, give rise to schizophrenia-like symptomatology presents psychiatry with a problem and an opportunity. On the one hand, it poses nosological dilemmas about the limits of the definition of schizophrenia; on the other, it provides insights into the biological mechanisms underlying the generation of schizophrenic symptoms.

This chapter first outlines the nosological challenges and how recent classification systems have dealt with these, distinguishing secondary schizophrenia-like psychoses arising from defined neuropathological processes and those secondary to cerebral complications of systemic illness. Secondly, it attempts to estimate the prevalence of such secondary schizophrenias in relation to schizophrenia in general. Thirdly, it examines the evidence for symptomatic differences between secondary and primary schizophrenia and discusses their clinical diagnosis. Finally, the chapter reviews broadly which specific brain diseases seem to present a particularly increased risk of schizophrenic symptoms.

Terminology and classification

In the past, schizophrenia has belonged to a class of disorders conventionally known as 'functional psychoses' and this was the terminology that held sway in ICD-9 (World Health Organization 1978). Although the ICD-9 had several disadvantages, most particularly the absence of clearly defined reliable operational diagnostic criteria, one potential advantage was the adherence to a descriptive pattern of phenomenological definition. Thus, the term 'organic', as opposed to 'functional', was not intended to imply an organic aetiology, but specifically to describe a set of symptoms of cognitive impairment such as disorientation, reduced level of consciousness and impairments of memory. This allowed schizophrenia secondary to coarse brain disease to be classed under the rubric of schizophrenia, with appropriate subdiagnosis according to the pathology of the causative agent or disease. In DSM-III and DSM-IIIR, the term 'organic' was redefined in an important way, so as to imply an organic aetiology, rather than to describe particular symptoms in the mental state. Thus, separate categories of 'organic mental disorders' were introduced. Cases of psychosis without cognitive impairment, but in the presence of 'evidence from the history, physical examination or laboratory tests of a specific organic factor judged to be aetiologically related', were now called 'organic delusional syndrome' or 'organic hallucinosis', depending on the predominant symptoms. Nevertheless, in DSM-III it was acknowledged that symptoms in these 'organic' mental disorders could be 'essentially identical with schizophrenia'. This convention put the diagnostician in the problematic position of having to rename a syndrome whenever a likely organic cause became apparent (Lewis *et al.* 1987).

In so far as all behavioural disorders have a biological component, the differentiation between *schizophrenia-like* symptoms arising from a definite cause and those with an obscure aetiology is an inherently dissatisfying process. As we better define the biological basis of psychosis in schizophrenia, the aetiology of these pathological processes will become apparent. As it now stands, in a sense, schizophrenia is a term reserved for those 'idiopathic' cases of chronic psychosis.

Potential problems with the term 'organic' are exemplified by treatment of the term in the ICD-10 (World Health Organization 1992), particularly in the section on 'Other organic mental disorders' (F06). It is worthwhile examining this in a little detail so as to advance the argument that the term organic should be abandoned as a descriptor for schizophrenias caused by coarse brain disease. The ICD-10 use of the term organic introduces a paradox that is referred to in the text thus: 'use of the term organic does not imply that conditions elsewhere in this classification are non-organic'. Moreover, the criteria put forward in ICD-10 by which to identify disorders such as organic schizophrenia-like disorder are not strictly logical. One of the two requirements to justify a diagnosis is 'a temporal relationship (weeks or a few months) between the development of the underlying disease and the onset of the syndrome'. In reality, this time-scale limits inclusion to what are essentially precipitating factors rather than true causes which, as will be discussed later in the chapter, seem often to take several years before generating schizophrenia-like symptoms. A further limitation of the notion of splitting off 'organic' schizophrenias from schizophrenia in general is that our knowledge base as to the epidemiology of the first group, and of the relationship in general between the two groups, is very limited. The greatest difficulty in confidently diagnosing a case of organic schizophrenia-like disorder is in the attribution of the symptoms to a particular organic cause. This is seldom simple, particularly because there may be little time congruence between onset of the physical disorder and onset of the schizophrenic symptoms. It is this difficulty in attribution that seems to have led to the comparatively poor interrater reliability reported in recent field trials of ICD-10 for these organic categories, as compared with their 'functional' counterparts (Sartorius *et al.* 1993).

Spitzer *et al.* (1992) argued cogently for retiring the term 'organic mental disorders'. In this review we shall follow their lead. They asserted that the term 'organic' has insoluble problems attached to it and for this reason another term should be chosen. They considered the term 'symptomatic', but noted that this can be ambiguous and proposed that the term 'secondary' should be used instead. Secondary disorders should be distinguished from substance-induced disorders and are recognized if they are caused by medical disorders that are classified outside the mental disorder section of the ICD. Schizophrenic symptoms can thus be categorized in any individual case to being primary, or secondary 'to a non-psychiatric medical disorder', or substance-induced.

The DSM-IV (American Psychiatric Association 1994) has adopted this approach, which harks back to the phenomenological basis of classification in ICD-9. Sensibly, the introduction to the organizational plan in DSM-IV states that 'the term organic mental disorder is no longer used in DSM-IV because it incorrectly implies that the other mental disorders in the manual do not have a biologic basis.' Thus, schizophrenic symptoms secondary to a non-psychiatric medical disorder are now headed under the section 293.8 'psychotic disorder due to a general medical condition'.

Secondary schizophrenias can be thought of as falling into two categories:
1 Where the psychotic symptoms arise from the cerebral involvement of a systemic illness known to affect the brain. This is the category headed 293.8 in DSM-IV.
2 Where schizophrenic symptoms arise in the context of a demonstrable, often clinically unsuspected, neuropathologically defined disorder that is not part of an ongoing systemic disease process.

This latter area has become considerably more important since the advent of high-resolution neuroimaging techniques in the past 20 years. In the DSM-IV, this category is subsumed into the general class of psychotic disorders due to a general medical condition. This is paradoxical because many of these disorders are restricted to the central nervous system, such as neoplasms and cerebrovascular disease.

In reviewing the literature regarding the association between psychosis and coarse brain disease, another problem frequently arises. Over the decades, the term psychosis has been applied to a wide variety of signs and symptoms. Defined criteria for primary schizophrenia have only been commonly agreed upon in the past 30 years. Even within this period, the criteria have been significantly modified. The details of case reports must be scrutinized carefully. For example, a problem arises in differentiating disorders with prominent psychotic features from delirium. Most reserve the term delirium for an agitated confusional state, with prominent sensory illusions and misperceptions. In fact, there is significant overlap between the clinical signs and symptoms of delirium, primary schizophrenia and the secondary schizophrenias. A relatively abrupt onset and short time course helps differentiate delirium from the other two entities when reported in the literature. Frequently, however, many so-called secondary schizophrenias are actually delirious states, such as the encephalopathy associated with sepsis in the elderly.

How common are secondary schizophrenias?

Given the disputes over definition and diagnosis, it is not surprising that there is little known about the detailed epidemiology of secondary schizophrenia. One difficulty in estimating prevalence is the problem of definition: how confident can one be that the well-defined brain disease is truly responsible for the presenting schizophrenic symptoms? A second difficulty is that the closer one looks, the more likely it is that structural pathology will be revealed. The widespread availability of high-resolution brain imaging techniques has shown that unsuspected cerebral lesions occur in a small but significant number of patients with schizophrenic symptoms. Most structural brain imaging research in psychosis has concentrated rather on minor quantitative changes involving widened fluid spaces and reduced volume of particular structures in the medial temporal lobe. These minor quantitative changes would not usually be reported as abnormal by most clinical radiologists. However, there are a handful of reports in the literature of gross focal brain lesions in schizophrenia.

Three larger imaging studies using X-ray-based computerized tomography (CT) enable an estimate to be made of the prevalence of such unequivocal focal lesions in schizophrenia. Owens *et al.* (1980) in their series of 136 schizophrenic patients found 'unsuspected intracranial pathology' as a focal finding on CT in 12 cases (9%), after excluding lesions resulting from leucotomy. This was a relatively elderly sample: five of these 12 cases were

Table 11.1 Laterality, locus and nature of focal lesions found on computerized tomography in 13 of 228 schizophrenic patients. (From Lewis 1990.)

Site	Number	Nature of lesion
Right-sided		
Frontal	1	Low attenuation
Parietal	3	Calcified mass (1)
		Porencephalic cyst (1)
		Low attenuation (1)
Temporal	1	Old abscess cavity
Left-sided		
Frontoparietal	1	Low attenuation
Temporal	3	Arachnoid cyst (2)
		Calcification (1)
Occipitotemporal	1	Arachnoid cyst
Midline	1	Septal cyst
Bilateral	2	Occipital low attenuation (1)
		Parasagittal calcification (1)

aged over 65. Lewis (1990) examined a series of 228 Maudsley Hospital patients who met Research Diagnostic Criteria (RDC) for schizophrenia and who had been consecutively scanned for clinical reasons. Patients with a history of epilepsy or intracranial surgery, or who were aged over 65 at the time of scan, were excluded. The original scan reports were examined and the films of those not unequivocally normal were reappraised by a neuroradiologist blind to the original report. In 41 patients the scan showed a definite intracranial abnormality. This was in the nature of enlarged fluid spaces in 28 cases, but in 13 patients (6%) there was a discrete focal lesion. These lesions varied widely in location and probable pathology (Table 11.1), although left temporal and right parietal regions were most commonly implicated.

The third study (S. Lewis & M. Reveley, unpublished data) was an attempt to examine a geographically defined sample of schizophrenic patients, ascertained as part of a large multidisciplinary survey (Brugha *et al.* 1988). All Camberwell residents who, on a particular census day, were aged between 18 and 65 and were in regular contact with any psychiatric day service were approached. Of 120 eligible people, 83 consented to CT and psychiatric interview. Fifty of these met RDC for schizophrenia or schizoaffective disorder. In four of these 50 patients (8%) were found clinically unsuspected focal lesions: low density in the right caudate head; a left occipital–temporal porencephalic cyst; low-density regions in the right parietal lobe; and agenesis of the corpus callosum (see below). None of 50 matched healthy volunteers showed focal pathology on CT.

Given the differences in the nature of the patient samples, these three studies are in rough agreement about the prevalence of unexpected focal abnormalities on CT: between 6% and 9%. One magnetic resonance imaging (MRI) study has also examined the issue of the prevalence of focal abnormalities in schizophrenia. Given the higher resolution of MRI technology, one might predict a higher lesion detection rate than with CT. O'Callaghan *et al.* (1992) scanned 47 patients under the age of 65 meeting DSM-III criteria for schizophrenia, with 25 matched controls. Four patients (9%) were revealed to have unsuspected lesions of a neurodevelopmental type: one partial agenesis of the corpus callosum; two cases of marked asymmetric dilatation of the left lateral ventricle (one with an associated porencephalic cyst); and one cerebellar hypoplasia.

The only epidemiologically sound and well-executed study to report prevalence figures for secondary schizophrenias of the type produced by systemic physical illness is the study by Johnstone *et al.* (1987). The study examined a sample of 328 consecutive patients presenting with a first episode of schizophrenia between the age of 15 and 70 years. Patients were screened clinically, without routine diagnostic neuroimaging, for the presence of organic illnesses that the authors judged were 'of definite or possible aetiological significance'. Thirteen patients fell into the category of substance-induced schizophrenia, including one patient who was judged to have developed schizophrenia-like symptoms secondary to treatment with steroids. Nine patients (3%) were regarded as falling into the category of schizophrenia secondary to non-psychiatric medical disorders. These comprised three cases of tertiary syphilis, two cases of neurosarcoidosis, one case of multisystem autoimmune disease including systemic lupus erythematosus, one case of carcinoma of the bronchus with a secondary right parietal and frontal brain infarction, one of cerebral cysticercosis and one of chronic thyrotoxicosis. In these cases, neurological signs were the exception rather than the rule and a history of epilepsy was noted in only one case. Over half of the cases had migrated from developing countries and had presumably been at increased risk of untreated infections and other disorders. No case had a family history of schizophrenia. Two additional aspects of their data that were not specifically commented on by the authors were the relatively late age at onset of these nine cases (range 29–59 years) and, curiously, that all nine cases were female.

Inferring cause and effect

The establishment of a cause–effect relationship between a particular organic disease or lesion and schizophrenic symptoms in clinical practice can be very difficult. Table 11.2 gives general criteria by which observations are used in disease models to support the existence of a causal relationship. As can be seen, in the case of secondary schizophrenias several of these criteria are difficult to fulfil. Neurodevelopmental formulations of aetiology in schizophrenia generally are relatively recent, but mean that the temporality criterion can be difficult to demonstrate if the cause arises many years before the schizophrenic symptoms. None the less, there are clear instances in the literature of cause being attributed where it is by no means clear that the lesion predated the schizophrenia. For example, several old

Table 11.2 General criteria to support causal relationships used in disease models.

Criterion	Observation	Comments regarding schizophrenia
Temporality	Cause precedes effect	Cause may be several years earlier
		Problems with cross-sectional surveys of schizophrenic patients: temporality must be inferred
Consistency	Repeatedly observed	Many observations are anecdotal, single-case reports
Strength	Large relative risk	Relative risk difficult to establish because associations are often rare; best established for epilepsy
Dose–response	Larger exposure to cause associated with larger effect	May not hold for schizophrenia where specific subtle lesion may be important
Reversibility	Reduced exposure to cause associated with reduced effect	Not shown
Specificity	One cause leads to one effect	Several different causes with no clear common pathology; each cause can have different neuropsychiatric effects
Analogy	Similar exposure gives known effects	Closest analogy probably epilepsy; variety of causes, latent period, pleiomorphic behavioural syndrome
Biological plausibility	Makes sense	Neurodevelopmental model facilitates understanding of mechanisms; but what about non-neurodevelopmental causes?

postmortem studies disclosed brain tumours in schizophrenic patients without evidence that the tumour predated the psychiatric symptoms (Davison & Bagley 1969). In addition to the problems noted in Table 11.2, there are other difficulties in many cases. In some instances both the physical disease and the schizophrenic symptoms may result from another underlying cause. Epilepsy might be the best example of this, where both the symptoms of epilepsy – itself a syndrome – and schizophrenia may arise from some underlying brain disease, rather than epilepsy causing schizophrenia directly. Drug treatments of the physical disorder can also predispose to psychotic symptomatology; e.g. steroids and amphetamines (in the case of narcolepsy). A further possible confounding factor is that some aspect of preschizophrenic personality might predispose to health-endangering behaviours, e.g. head injury. Despite all these caveats, a number of different physical disorders have, down the years, been linked to the emergence of secondary schizophrenia.

The co-occurrence of schizophrenia-like symptoms and organic brain disease

In 1969 Kenneth Davison and Christopher Bagley published an extensive review of the world literature, backed with some 800 references, of the co-occurrence of schizophrenia-like symptoms and organic disease. This review remains a landmark in the field. It took as its starting point the operational criteria for schizophrenia of the 1957 WHO Committee, which were adapted slightly by Davison and Bagley so that their case material included cases which today would broadly be headed under the

rubric of schizophrenia and paranoid psychosis. Criteria also included the absence of impaired consciousness and the absence of prominent affective symptoms. The authors concluded that the occurrence of schizophrenia-like symptoms exceeded chance expectation in many organic central nervous system disorders and that, where a discrete lesion was present, those in the temporal lobe and diencephalon seemed to be particularly significant.

Davison and Bagley reviewed the evidence for the association between schizophrenia and a large range of individual central nervous system disorders. Epilepsy was statistically associated with schizophrenia-like psychosis, particularly where a temporal lobe lesion existed. Head injury was also a risk factor for psychosis, again with a possible association with temporal lobe lesions. Severe closed head injury with diffuse cerebral damage was related to early development of psychotic symptoms. Encephalitic disorders, cerebral syphilis, Wilson's disease, Huntington's disease, Friedreich's ataxia, vitamin B_{12} deficiency, subarachnoid haemorrhage and cerebral tumour also seemed to be associated with an increased risk of schizophrenia-like symptoms. They found much less evidence to implicate other central nervous system disorders such as multiple sclerosis, motor neurone disease and Parkinson's disease.

Not surprisingly, 20 years later, a few of Davison and Bagley's conclusions might be amended. For example, their association between narcolepsy and psychosis most likely reflects a side-effect of amphetamines used in treatment, rather than the disease itself. The correlation between cerebral tumour and schizophrenia-like symptoms is weak. Many such instances could be better explained as chance association, unless the tumours were of the type whose natural history was very long-standing, such as hamartomas of the temporal lobe. Conversely, new evidence for these and other disorders being associated is now available, and is reviewed below.

Epilepsy

Estimates of the incidence of schizophrenic symptoms in temporal lobe epilepsy vary widely (reviewed in Hyde & Weinberger 1997), and are obviously sensitive to artefacts of ascertainment. Roberts *et al.* (1990) reported that 25 out of his consecutive autopsy series of 249 cases (10%) had a lifetime history of psychotic symptoms. Trimble (1988) estimated that patients with epilepsy were at three- to ninefold increased risk of schizophrenia-like psychoses.

The definitive case series of 69 patients by Slater and Beard (1963) noted that classical Schneiderian 'positive' symptoms were predominant, often without negative symptoms. Additionally, psychoses frequently arose in the context of a normal premorbid personality, without a family history of schizophrenia. An association between medial temporal lobe, particularly dominant temporal lobe, epilepsy and Schneiderian symptoms does seem to exist. Flor-Henry's initial report (1969) about laterality actually contained 19 cases of left and 12 cases of right temporal lobe involvement (most cases had bilateral involvement), a similar proportion to Slater and Beard's original series (36 left, 32 right). The 10 independent series to examine the laterality issue do show a trend towards left-sided predominance, as reviewed by Trimble (1990). None the less, the observation that about one-sixth of patients with schizophrenic psychoses of epilepsy had only right temporal lobe involvement detracts from the hypothesis that left temporal involvement is necessary: involvement of either side may be sufficient.

In temporal lobe epilepsy with psychosis, neurodevelopmental lesions in the temporal lobe such as hamartomas, rather than the early acquired lesion of mesial temporal sclerosis, are over-represented. Taylor (1975) compared a series of 47 temporal lobectomy patients with hamartomas and focal dysplasias in the resected temporal lobe with 41 patients with mesial temporal sclerosis. Of the former group 23% had histories of psychosis, compared with 5% in the latter group: psychosis was particularly common in left-handed females. Roberts *et al.* (1990) noted that in 16 of 249 cases schizophrenic symptoms were present preoperatively; in a further nine they emerged postoperatively. Schizophrenic symptoms were more commonly found in those epilepsies associated with lesions originating *in utero* or perinatally, which were physiologically active at a relatively early age, as inferred from a comparatively early age at first seizure. The medial temporal lobe was most often involved. An unusual neurodevelopmental tumour, the ganglioglioma (also known as the dysembryoplastic neuroepithelioma, or DNET), was specially associated with heightened risk of psychosis, especially after surgical resection (Andermann *et al.* 1999). The reason for this association is unclear.

Two competing hypotheses attempt to explain the association between epilepsy and schizophrenic symptoms. Either both sets of symptoms arise from a common underlying cerebral pathology, usually in the temporal lobe, or, less plausibly, the schizophrenic symptoms arise out of a process of progressive facilitation of subthreshold electrical activity ('kindling'). The relationship between the timing of seizures and the emergence of schizophrenic symptoms can vary. Classically, the schizophrenic symptoms emerge as interictal phenomena, although occasionally schizophreniform symptoms are part of a postictal psychosis or even an ictal phenomenon during partial complex seizures (Mace 1993). The scalp EEG usually shows no change during interictal schizophrenic psychosis, which argues against the notion of kindling being an important mechanism. Stevens (1992) has advanced a third, neurodevelopmental explanation of the link between epilepsy and schizophrenia, proposing that abnormal neuronal regeneration and connectivity develops in adolescence in some individuals with epilepsy that predisposes to schizophrenic symptoms. Many cases of partial complex seizures develop in late childhood and early adolescence (Mendez *et al.* 1993). Importantly, most cases of schizophrenia develop slightly later, in late adolescence and early adulthood. The overlap in the timing of the appearance of seizures and psychosis is congruent with the notion of neurodevelopmental pathology. More refined electrophysiological studies, perhaps using magnetoencephalography, may be the most promising avenue to explore the anatomical and physiological links between schizophrenic symptoms and epilepsy (Mace 1993).

Cerebral trauma

Head injury is a ubiquitous experience, but in its more severe forms causes lasting pathological change. The most comprehensive psychiatric study of brain-injured patients is the national Finnish cohort of war veterans described by Achté *et al.* (1969, 1991). Of these, 762 (7.6%) were described as having psychotic disorders, although systematic evaluation was lacking. Delusional disorder appeared to be the most common form of psychosis (Achté *et al.* 1991). In his earlier report, Achté *et al.* (1969) found that temporal lobe injury was the site most frequently associated with the subsequent development of psychosis. Gualtieri and Cox (1991) estimated that traumatic brain injury increases risk of psychosis by two- to fivefold. Many years often elapse between the head injury and the emergence of psychotic symptoms. Buckley *et al.* (1993) ascertained three cases of schizophrenia and two cases of schizoaffective disorder in whom the psychosis followed a severe head injury (loss of consciousness greater than 4 h). MRI showed no abnormality in the two schizoaffective patients. Left temporal gliosis and/or atrophy was consistently found in the three schizophrenic patients. Psychosis followed injury at intervals of 1, 7 and 19 years in these patients. Risk factors for psychosis following traumatic brain injury include pre-existing neurological disorders, head injury earlier than adolescence and male gender (Fujii & Ahmed 2001).

Once again, especially with a history of closed head injury in childhood, it is unclear if the head injury is causative or an unrelated comorbidity. Any time a significant head injury occurs prior to the time period of greatest liability towards the development of primary schizophrenia, its role in the production of chronic psychosis is questionable. However, in the initial Achté et al. (1969) study, paranoid and schizophrenic psychoses occurred in 4.1% of the patients, a much higher percentage than would have been expected by chance alone.

Cases where psychosis arises in patients with patterns of acquired brain injury, through trauma or vascular damage, can lead to hypotheses about the possible nature of functional brain abnormalities crucial to schizophrenia. A small number of case reports suggest that, given a specific pattern of brain injury in adult life, schizophrenia can result. Burke et al. (1999) described a schizophrenic illness arising in a case 8 years after a left frontal infarct at age 16. Pang and Lewis (1996) described a case of combined injury to left temporal and ablation of left dorsolateral frontal cortex in a 23-year-old man which appeared to 'convert' pre-existing bipolar disorder to chronic schizophrenia. G.E. Jaskiw and J.F. Kenny (submitted) reported schizophrenia arising in a 34-year-old man 1 year after combined injury to left anterior temporal lobe and frontal cortex. It is known that combined lesions of mesial temporal and prefrontal cortex in the rat lead to increased dopaminergic transmission in the ventral striatum of the rat (Lipska et al. 1994) and this may be the mechanism at work in these cases.

Cerebrovascular disease

There is a time-honoured saying in clinical neurology that neuroanatomy is learned 'one stroke at a time'. In the unusual circumstances where psychosis develops after a stroke, traditional clinical–pathological correlations coupled with modern neuroimaging techniques may elucidate the neuroanatomy of psychosis. Miller et al. (1991) assessed 24 consecutively ascertained patients with 'late-life psychosis', defined as DSM-IIIR schizophrenia, schizophreniform or delusional disorder, or unspecified psychosis of at least 4 weeks' duration, beginning over the age of 45. MRI scans were obtained to rule out structural lesions, and compared with a series of 72 healthy controls. A known history of neurological disease was an exclusion criterion in all subjects. Unsuspected cortical or subcortical white matter infarcts were seen in 25% of the patients, compared with 6% of controls. The largest regional difference between patients and controls was in the temporal lobe. Another two patients showed radiological changes suggesting dementia: one a cerebellar tumour and one post-traumatic brain injury. Delusions and hallucinations occur in early Alzheimer's disease in about 50% of cases (Chen et al. 1991). Moreover, ischaemic cerebrovascular disease occurs in the same age range as Alzheimer's disease and can be a comorbid condition. More often than not,

Alzheimer's disease probably underlies the psychotic symptoms. Autopsy is usually the only way to definitively differentiate these processes, unless the psychotic symptoms occur in close relation to the timing of the stroke. Again, this is a fertile area for research into the pathogenesis of psychotic symptoms (Zubenko et al. 1991).

A number of case reports suggest that schizophreniform symptoms can appear as a result of cerebral infarction, even in patients where comorbid Alzheimer's disease is unlikely. Miller et al. (1989) described five cases of subfrontal white matter infarction leading to psychosis. Ischaemic subfrontal damage also appears to lead to psychosis in young adults. Hall and Young (1992) described an acute schizophreniform psychosis with blunted affect, thought disorder and auditory hallucinations in a 23-year-old man, attributed to a ruptured cerebral aneurysm in the left frontal lobe. Case reports such as this need to be viewed critically, however, as schizophrenia arises with great frequency in this age range. Bouckoms et al. (1986) described a delusional disorder appearing shortly after subarachnoid haemorrhage in a 66-year-old woman, associated with significant impairment of frontal lobe function on neuropsychological testing. Price and Mesulam (1985) presented five cases of right hemispheric infarction with primary psychiatric manifestations. However, only one was a convincing association between infarction and psychosis. In the others, the infarction could not be clearly identified by CT scan, the time between infarction and the appearance of psychosis was extremely delayed, or the psychiatric symptoms were atypical for a psychotic disorder. Levine and Finklestein (1982) described eight cases of hallucinations often accompanied by delusional thoughts, following either intracerebral haemorrhage, infarction or cerebral contusion. Applying more rigorous criteria, four of these cases occurred between the ages of 35 and 65 years of age, making it unlikely that comorbid primary schizophrenia or Alzheimer's disease was confounding their analysis. In all cases, the lesions were localized to the right temporoparietooccipital region.

Demyelinating diseases

Multiple sclerosis (MS) has been associated with a variety of psychiatric sequelae, most commonly affective syndromes. Stevens (1988) noted superficial epidemiological similarities between MS and schizophrenia, proposing that both disorders might have a similar immunological cause. However, MS and schizophrenia have markedly different clinical profiles, and the neuropathological substrate of MS has nothing in common with that of schizophrenia. Moreover, Davison and Bagley (1969) proffered that there was little evidence for increased risk of schizophrenic symptoms in MS. However, recent reports suggest that schizophrenia can arise secondary to MS, but only in rare cases. Temporal lobe demyelination may be the mediating link (Ron & Logsdail 1989). Feinstein et al. (1992) compared MRI findings in 10 psychotic and 10 non-psychotic MS patients: the psychotic patients tended to show more lesions around the temporal horns bilaterally, a similar finding to Reischies *et al.* (1988) and Honer *et al.* (1987). Feinstein *et al.* noted that the symptoms of schizophrenia began relatively late (mean age 36) in their sample, although were typical of schizophrenia thereafter, and postulated that long-standing strategically placed lesions were crucial in the development of psychosis. However, both MS and schizophrenia often begin in the third decade of life, and coincidence should not be confused with causality.

Schizophrenic symptoms have also been noted in rarer demyelinating syndromes (Neumann *et al.* 1988). Schilder's disease is a progressive usually fatal demyelinating disease of children and adolescents which is sporadic and probably related to MS. Occasional reports with schizophrenic symptoms exist (Davison & Bagley 1969; Ramani 1981). A review of reported cases (Ramani 1981) confirmed primary frontal lobe involvement in those cases presenting with psychoses.

Metachromatic leucodystrophy (MLD) is a rare autosomal recessive demyelinating disorder with a particularly strong association with psychosis. Deficiency of arylsulphatase-A is the basic biochemical defect, which leads to progressive demyelination. The inheritance shows incomplete penetrance and the extent of arylsulphatase-A deficiency seems to dictate age at onset. Hyde *et al.* (1992) reviewed the published case reports on MLD, 129 definite cases, and noted that when the onset occurred in adolescence or early adulthood (10–30 years) hallucinations or delusions occurred in over 50% of cases and a clinical diagnosis of primary schizophrenia was made in 35%. Complex auditory hallucinations typical of schizophrenia were commonly reported and other motor as well as negative symptoms also occurred. Hyde *et al.* (1992) argued that the high frequency of schizophrenic symptoms seen in MLD reflected its neuropathological origins in the periventricular frontal white matter. Progressive extension posteriorly heralds the appearance of more formal neurological signs. These observations led to the authors' hypothesis that dysfunctional subcortical pathways linking frontal cortex with normal functioning temporolimbic cortex are crucial to the production of schizophrenic symptoms.

Arylsulphatase-A abnormalities in the absence of clinical MLD have occasionally been reported in schizophrenic samples (Manowitz *et al.* 1981). Adrenoleucodystrophy (ALD) is a separate group of disorders, the main subtype of which involves an X-linked deficit in the breakdown of very-long-chain fatty acids. Three cases have been described with schizophrenic symptoms (Kitchin *et al.* 1987).

Metabolic and autoimmune disorders

Metabolic disorders rarely induce psychotic symptoms; more commonly, such disorders are associated with depression or delirium. For example, thyroid-related psychoses are most usually affectively based (Davis 1989). Hyperparathyroidism, usually an adenoma leading to hypercalcaemia, often causes psychiatric symptoms, although again convincing schizophrenic symptoms seem to be rare (Johnson 1975; Alarcon & Franceschini 1984; Ebel *et al.* 1992). Organic mental states with delirium or depressive symptoms are more commonly seen (Gatewood *et al.* 1975). Vitamin B_{12} deficiency can present with mental changes, although psychosis is unusual. Zucker *et al.* (1981) reviewed the literature and found only 15 cases of 'B_{12} psychosis' responding to B_{12} replacement: most of these were depressive disorders. B_{12} deficiency may more often be an effect, rather than a cause, of schizophrenic symptoms.

It has been recognized only relatively recently that cerebral systemic lupus erythematosus (SLE) can give schizophrenia-like symptoms (MacNeil *et al.* 1976). Attributing causation in individual cases can be difficult: SLE is common, with variable course and symptoms and its first-line treatment, steroids, can produce psychotic symptoms. Additionally, cerebral involvement more often produces seizures and delirium rather than pure psychotic symptoms. Childhood Sydenham's chorea, an immunologically mediated complication of rheumatic fever with probable basal ganglia involvement, may predispose to later schizophrenia (Wilcox & Nasrallah 1986). Paraneoplastic encephalopathies are uncommon poorly understood complications of non-central nervous system tumours, possibly mediated by tumour-directed antibodies. They can, rarely, cause schizophrenic symptoms, seemingly mediated by limbic inflammation (Van Sweden & Van Peteghem 1986).

Encephalitis and other infections of the central nervous system

Wilson (1976) reported three cases of viral encephalitis presenting as psychosis. Limbic encephalitis is most often associated with psychotic symptoms. Many viruses are known to cause limbic encephalitis (Glaser & Pincus 1969; Damasio & Hoesen 1985). In a review of 22 cases, Torrey (1986) noted reports of a variety of neuropathic viruses causing encephalitis leading to psychotic symptoms: Epstein–Barr, cytomegalovirus, rubella, herpes simplex and measles. Nunn *et al.* (1986) reported four cases of adulttype arising in children after viral encephalitic illnesses of varying pathology: rubella, measles, varicella and herpes simplex. Psychosis in Epstein–Barr virus infection is unusual (Leavell *et al.* 1986) and most commonly depressive in form (Rubin 1978; White & Lewis 1987).

Subacute sclerosing panencephalitis (SSPE) is a rare presentation of measles infection of the central nervous system, secondary to an aberrant form of the virus. It presents as a progressive neurological disorder (Koehler & Jakumeit 1976), with a clinical onset usually in early adult life or before, although often years after the initial measles infection. Two case histories are typical: symptoms of schizophrenia (Duncalf *et al.* 1989) or delusional disorder (dysmorphophobia: Salib 1988) presenting in young adults, with the emergence of rapidly progressive neurological signs several months later and death within a year. A report of schizophreniform psychosis more directly following measles infection (Stoler *et al.* 1987) was criticized for failing conclusively to demonstrate brain involvement with the virus (McCune 1987). Sporadic reports of schizophrenia in other infective and inflammatory conditions exist. *Borrelia* encephalitis (neuro-Lyme disease) is a recently described cause of schizophrenic symptoms which apparently responds to antibiotic therapy (Barnett *et al.* 1991). Neurocysticercosis results from invasion of the central nervous system with *Taenia solium* larvae, producing cysts, nodules, fibrosis and hydrocephaly. Schizophrenia-like complications are apparently not uncommon, although this contention deserves more research (Tavares *et al.* 1993). Childhood encephalitis has emerged as a clear-cut but rare risk factor for adult schizophrenia, conferring a fivefold relative risk in epidemiological cohort studies.

Psychotic symptoms can arise in the context of HIV infection, usually AIDS (McDaniel *et al.* 1997). Harris *et al.* (1991) reviewed the literature, as well as the histories of a cohort of 124 HIV-infected patients followed up for 6 years, for new-onset psychosis, after excluding cases where psychotic symptoms arose out of substance abuse or delirium. Psychotic symptoms usually took the form of acute-onset delusions, hallucinations and bizarre behaviour, most often in the context of a mood disturbance, particularly mania or hypomania. Typical schizophrenic symptoms in clear consciousness were rarely described. In a follow-up report, Sewell *et al.* (1994) examined the characteristics of psychosis in HIV-infected individuals. In addition to hallucinations and delusions, the majority of patients had substantial mood symptoms. The psychotic patients also had high rates of previous substance abuse. The pathogenesis of psychosis in the setting of HIV infection has yet to be established.

Sex chromosome abnormalities

Minimal evidence links sex chromosome abnormalities with schizophrenia-like disorders. The first report linked an XXXY genotype to schizophrenia (Money & Hirsch 1963). Most of the reports are single case studies. For example, Turner's syndrome (45 XO) has been associated with schizophrenia in about 10 cases. However, studies with large sample sizes (Nielsen & Stradiot 1987) have not disclosed an increased incidence of schizophrenia in Turner's syndrome: two cases in 968 female schizophrenic patients (Kaplan & Cotton 1968); or one case in 3558 (Akesson & O'Landers 1969), with a likely incidence rate for Turner's being 0.01% of live female births. The coincidence is so low that Bamrah and MacKay (1989) speculated that Turner's syndrome was actually protective against schizophrenia. The issue is complicated by the heterogeneity of Turner's: only half of cases are 45 XO, the rest being mosaics or having a structurally abnormal X chromosome (Fishbain 1990).

There is little evidence associating more unusual sex chromosome abnormalities with schizophrenia-like syndromes. Other sex chromosome abnormalities reported with schizophrenia include an XX male (Muller & Endres 1987) and an XO/XY mosaic with basal ganglia calcification (Deckert *et al.* 1992).

Schizophrenia has been described in Noonan's syndrome (Turner's phenotype with normal karyotype: Krishna *et al.* 1977) and in 47 XYY males (Faber & Abrams 1975; Dorus *et al.* 1977). Of 20 psychotic males with Klinefelter's syndrome (47 XXY) described by Sorensen and Nielsen (1977), five fulfil criteria for schizophrenia. The authors surprisingly concluded that this was insufficient evidence for genuine association. XXXY associations have also been reported. More recently, DeLisi *et al.* (1994) found that the XXX and XXY karyotypes are more common in the schizophrenic population. In his review of the area, Propping (1983) considered that the Klinefelter karyotype and the XXX karyotype were the two sex chromosomal abnormalities that had the strongest association with schizophrenia. From the data available, Propping estimated that for both XXY and XXX the risk of schizophrenia was increased threefold. DeLisi *et al.* (1991) concurred with this conclusion, citing it as evidence for possible linkage of schizophrenia to the X chromosome.

Associations with Mendelian disorders

Propping's (1983) review discussed possible associations between a variety of Mendelian disorders and schizophrenia. Table 11.3 summarizes Propping's conclusions, dividing such disorders into probable and possible associations with increased risk of schizophrenia. Linkage and association studies have been undertaken at many laboratories and clinical centres around the world to identify candidate genes or chromosomal regions conferring an increased risk for schizophrenia or some of its biological components, such as abnormal frontal lobe function on neuropsychological testing batteries (Risch 1990; Egan *et al.* 2000).

The association of Huntington's disease with an increased risk of schizophrenia is well established. Huntington's disease, an autosomal dominant disorder with complete penetrance, localized to chromosome 4, is the first major neurological disorder with a well-characterized genetic defect (Gusella *et al.* 1983). Schizophrenic symptoms were reported in 5–11% of Huntington's patients in those six series each comprising at least 50 cases reviewed in Hyde *et al.* (1992). The reviews by Davison (1983) and Naarding *et al.* (2001) quote similar prevalence figures. Weinberger (1987) noted the age-related risk of psychosis in Huntington's disease, suggesting that psychosis most often appears in the third decade of life, like primary schizophrenia itself. However, developmental changes in the central nervous system immediately before or around this time of life may predispose towards the appearance of psychotic symptoms from a variety of causes, not just genetic abnormalities.

Acute intermittent porphyria is an autosomal dominant disorder of porphyrin metabolism resulting from a deficiency of the enzyme porphobilinogen deaminase. Acute intermittent porphyria may present with episodic psychiatric symptoms. Additionally, psychotropic medications may precipitate or exacerbate an acute attack. Psychiatric symptoms include

Table 11.3 Inherited disorders with an increased risk of schizophrenia. (Adapted from Propping 1983.)

Highly probable
Acute intermittent porphyria
Familial basal ganglia calcification
Huntington's disease
Metachromatic leucodystrophy
Porphyria variegata
Velocardiofacial syndrome

Possible
Congenital adrenal hyperplasia
Erythropoietic porphyria
Fabry's disease
Familial ataxia/spinocerebellar degeneration
Gaucher's disease, adult type
G6PD deficiency
Haemochromatosis
Homocystinuria
Hyperasparaginaemia
Ichthyosis vulgaris
Kartaneger's syndrome
Kufs disease
Laurence–Moon–Biedl syndrome
Niemann–Pick type C disease
Oculocutaneous albinism
Phenylketonuria
Sex chromosome anuoploides
Wilson's disease

G6PD, glucose-6-phosphate dehydrogenase.

psychosis, depression, anxiety and/or delirium. Tishler *et al.* (1985) screened 3867 psychiatric inpatients for acute intermittent porphyria and found a prevalence of 0.21%, higher than the general population. Most of the patients had symptoms of agitated psychosis, apathy or depression, with neuropsychological impairment. In rare cases, acute intermittent porphyria may cause a transient schizophrenia-like state; however, most of the attacks are of relatively short duration. Unlike schizophrenia, with treatment, many individuals with porphyria are relatively normal between acute attacks. The link between the acute intermittent porphyria and psychosis has fuelled recent searches for linkage of schizophrenia to chromosome 11, home of both the D_2 receptor and porphobilinogen deaminase gene. Nevertheless, at least in one study, no linkage has been established (Moises *et al.* 1991). This is not surprising given the rarity of acute intermittent porphyria even in the general psychiatric population.

It is likely that the alleged association between Wilson's disease (hepatolenticular degeneration) and schizophrenic symptoms has been overemphasized. Wilson's disease is an autosomal recessive disease of copper transport linked to chromosome 13 (Frydman *et al.* 1985). Although Wilson's original series included two patients with schizophrenic symptoms, the 520 case reports up to 1959 included only eight convincing cases (Davison

& Bagley 1969). Dening (1985) and Dening and Berrios (1989) reviewed psychiatric symptomatology in a series of 195 cases. Hallucinations occurred in only two cases, delusions in three. Personality and mood disorders are much more common.

Homocystinuria is an autosomal recessive disorder characterized by an abnormality in methionine metabolism. It is often caused by a defect in the gene for methylenetetrahydrofolate reductase, an essential enzyme in folate metabolism. The gene is located on chromosome 1p36.3 (Gaughan *et al.* 2000). Homocystinuria is often associated with mental retardation, seizures and an increased risk of stroke. While some have associated homocystinuria with schizophrenia, literature reviews do not substantiate this assertion, except in unusual cases (Bracken & Coll 1985; Abbott *et al.* 1987; Regland *et al.* 1997). Interestingly, the increase in schizophrenia in cohorts exposed to famine in early gestation in the Dutch 'hunger winter' of 1944–45 has been attributed to folate deficiency. In these cases, it is believed that folate deficiency produced subtle abnormalities of cerebral development, which did not become manifest until early adulthood (Susser *et al.* 1996).

Niemann–Pick type C disease is an autosomal recessive disorder starting in adolescence or early adulthood. Vertical gaze abnormalities, ataxia and extrapyramidal signs predominate. Cataplexy and seizures often appear as the disease evolves. Psychosis may be the initial manifestation of the disease in some cases, leading to the misdiagnosis of primary schizophrenia (Turpin *et al.* 1991). The diagnosis is made by bone marrow biopsy, which reveals sea-blue histiocytes.

Oculocutaneous albinism is an unusual genetic disorder. Cosegregation of schizophrenia and oculocutaneous albinism has been described repeatedly (Baron 1976; Clarke & Buckley 1989); interestingly, neurodevelopmental abnormalities, particularly of projections to the visual association cortex, occur in albinism (Clarke & Buckley 1989). A common biochemical defect may underlie the pigmentary and psychiatric manifestations of this disorder. How the genetic defect in this form of albinism translates into neurodevelopmental abnormalities remains to be explained.

A variety of genetic disorders have been linked to schizophrenia in selected pedigrees. Although these may be chance associations, it is possible that the specific genetic defect may have protean manifestations. In most cases, the psychotic symptoms begin during the traditional window of vulnerability to schizophrenia, in the late second and third decades of life. Two families in which the autosomal dominant connective tissue disorder Marfan's syndrome cosegregated with schizophrenia have been described (Sirota *et al.* 1990), plus one additional case (Romano & Linares 1987). Two autosomal recessive syndromes causing progressive sensorineural deafness and blindness have been described in large pedigrees cosegregating with schizophrenia: Usher's syndrome (Sharp *et al.* 1993). A family with multiple instances of the X-linked Alport's syndrome and psychosis has been described (Shields *et al.* 1990). Recent interest has also focused on the risk of psychoses in families affected by Wolfram syndrome, an autosomal recessive disorder characterized by juvenile-onset diabetes mellitus and progressive bilateral optic nerve atrophy (Swift *et al.* 1990). Tuberous sclerosis is an unusual autosomal dominant disorder characterized by the development of slow-growing hamartomatous tumours in many organs, including the brain. This disorder has been linked to genetic defects on chromosomes 9 and 16 (Jones *et al.* 1997). Schizophrenia-like symptoms have been reported and seem to be linked with tumours affecting the medial temporal lobe (Heckert *et al.* 1972). Bilateral calcification in the temporal lobe was probably the mediating link in a patient with psychotic symptoms in the context of a long-standing autosomal illness, lipoid proteinosis (Emsley & Paster 1985). Better understanding of the precise genetic defect in each of these disorders, and the impact of the defect upon the development and integrity of the central nervous system, might offer intriguing clues into the neurobiology of schizophrenia.

Two unusual genetically based neurodevelopmental disorders have attracted attention as being associated with a schizophrenia-like phenotype. Each involves a disturbance of neuronal migration and is potentially informative about the pathogenesis of schizophrenia. Kallman's syndrome is characterized by anosmia with hypogonadism. The anosmia is a result of a neurodevelopmental failure in the olfactory tracts. The hypogonadism is a result of low hypothalamic secretion of gonadotrophic-releasing hormone. The X-linked subtype is caused by a mutation at Xp22.3; autosomal subtype also exists. Parallels between Kallmann's syndrome and schizophrenia have been drawn in the literature (Cowen & Green 1993), because patients with schizophrenia have relative anosmia and reduced fertility. However, O'Neill *et al.* (1999) found no mutations of the relevant gene (*KAL-X*) in nine schizophrenic patients with Kallmann-type symptoms. The authors concluded that such a mutation rarely, if ever, causes schizophrenia. The first recorded case of DSM-IV schizophrenia arising in a young man with a history of Kallmann's syndrome has recently been described (N. Nuttall, S. Sandhu, J. Stirling, D. Craufurd & S.W. Lewis, submitted). The parallels between the phenotype of Kallman's syndrome and schizophrenia are weak. Schizophrenic subjects do not have obvious pathology in the olfactory tracts or hypogonadism. Their reduced reproductive rate may be more aptly ascribed to their deficits in social function, rather than gonadal dysfunction. It is not surprising that O'Neill *et al.* found no mutations in the relevant gene. The description of a single individual with Kallmann's syndrome and schizophrenia is most likely serendipitous.

Velocardiofacial syndrome (VCFS) is a genetic disorder characterized by craniofacial structural abnormalities, cardiac defects and learning disabilities. In addition, children and adolescents with VCFS have smaller cerebellar, pontine, temporal lobe and hippocampal volumes than normal controls (Eliez *et al.* 2001a,b). VCFS is usually associated with deletion mutations of chromosome 22q11, the same region which includes the gene for catechol-*O*-methyl transferase (COMT), an enzyme involved in the metabolism of dopamine. VCFS is associated with high rates of schizophrenia. Fluorescence *in situ* hybridiza-

tion is the best technique to identify the deletion mutations and confirm the diagnosis of VCFS (Larson & Butler 1995). The largest series examined to date was 50 cases in the UK ascertained mainly through clinical genetic services (Murphy *et al.* 1999). Of these, 15 had a history of a psychotic disorder, and 12 of these met DSM-IV criteria for schizophrenia (24%). In samples of subjects with schizophrenia and clinical features suggestive of VCFS, raised rates of 22q11 deletions have been found (Bassett *et al.* 1998). Interestingly, although the genetic defect and the dysmorphic changes are present from birth, psychotic symptoms do not develop until early adulthood. This illustrates the principle that psychosis only appears in an age-specific window of vulnerability, suggesting an interaction between genetic defects and the natural biology of human brain maturation. Clearly, the discovery of the exact genetic defect leading to psychosis in VCFS is paramount in understanding this syndrome. The role of COMT in the induction of psychosis in VCFS remains speculative at this time.

Tumours and other space-occupying lesions

Routine non-invasive imaging in the clinical assessment of schizophrenia, as well as prospective research, has led to increasing numbers of case reports of more or less unusual cerebral lesions in schizophrenia (Lewis 1989). In most cases these are clinically unsuspected, in that there was no history of neurological symptoms nor neurological signs on examination. Such lesions have been described in many parts of the brain and are of different pathologies. Some lesions are likely to be coincidental. Lesions falling into this category include the small cerebral infarcts and white matter abnormalities on MRI that are seen predominantly in older patients, and which are also seen in normal controls. If numerous, these are often linked to a history of cerebrovascular disease. A retrospective study of 731 psychiatric patients referred for MRI found that patients with psychotic symptoms had the lowest frequency of MRI-identified pathology (Wahlund *et al.* 1992).

Very rarely, unsuspected slow-growing cerebral tumours can present with schizophrenic symptoms. In the series reported by Malamud (1967), these symptoms were most common in tumours affecting the temporal lobe and cingulate gyrus. Frontal tumours have less frequently been implicated (Andy *et al.* 1981). A more extensive review was published by Lisanby *et al.* (1998). They noted that psychosis associated with brain tumour is more common above 50 years of age, although they fail to mention that brain tumours themselves are more common above this age. In their review, like Malamud, tumours located in the temporal lobe are more commonly associated with psychotic symptoms. Given the preponderance of evidence implicating the temporal lobe in the pathophysiology of primary schizophrenia, this localization is not surprising.

When reviewing case reports, there often is difficulty ascribing psychotic symptoms directly to the effects of the tumour itself on adjacent brain structures. For example, a suprasellar germinoma presented with a complex constellation of psychiatric symptoms, including psychosis (Mordecai *et al.* 2000). While the tumour involved the frontal lobes, basal ganglia and brainstem, areas implicated in the pathophysiology of psychosis, it had other profound effects. There were marked disturbances in the neuroendocrine axis. Additionally, there may have been a component of reactive depression. In summary, while tumours may be associated with schizophrenia-like presentations, this is a rare phenomenon, and the presentation may be secondary to remote effects from the tumour. A more intriguing case involved a 26-year-old woman with a 7-year history of auditory hallucinations and paranoia. After resection of meningioma located in the antrum of the right lateral ventricle with extension into the corpus callosum and periventricular white matter, the patient's psychosis completely remitted (Lisanby *et al.* 1998). The complete remission off medication suggests that the tumour was definitively the aetiology of her psychosis.

Occult brain lesions found in association with schizophrenia are often those that can be classified as neurodevelopmental anomalies of one type or another. These include aqueduct stenosis (Reveley & Reveley 1983), arachnoid cysts (Lanczik *et al.* 1989), porencephalic cysts (O'Callaghan *et al.* 1992) and cerebrovascular malformations including congenital arteriovenous malformations in the temporal lobe (Vaillant 1965) and the midline great vein of Galen (Remington & Jeffries 1984). Despite cases of familial basal ganglia calcification being reported in association with schizophrenia (Propping 1983), two large studies have found no association in general between basal ganglia calcification and schizophrenia in large samples of psychiatric patients (Casanova *et al.* 1990; Philpot & Lewis 1990).

Probably the most intriguing subclass of neurodevelopmental lesions reported in association with schizophrenia is midline anomalies associated with the septum pellucidum and adjacent corpus callosum. The first case description of complete agenesis of the corpus callosum (Lewis *et al.* 1987) has been followed by further cases of callosal agenesis, usually involving partial agenesis of the anterior part of the corpus callosum (Velek *et al.* 1988; Swayze *et al.* 1990; O'Callaghan *et al.* 1992). In so far as the corpus callosum is concerned, abnormalities in the projections of the frontal lobes, which have been implicated in the pathophysiology of schizophrenia by neuroimaging, neuropsychological and neuropathological studies, may produce a phenotypic copy of schizophrenia.

In addition to abnormalities of the corpus callosum, other midline malformations have been associated with schizophrenia. An initial CT report of six cases of developmental cavum septum pellucidum (Lewis & Mezey 1985) has been complemented by a combined MRI and postmortem study reporting a surprisingly high prevalence of varying degrees of this anomaly in schizophrenic patients compared with controls (DeGreef *et al.* 1992). Congenital absence of the septum pellucidum has also been described in schizophrenia (George *et al.* 1989). Midline pathology common in schizophrenic subjects includes non-specific abnormalities of the septum pellucidum, cavum

vergae, cavum septum pellucidum and agenesis of the corpus callosum (Scott *et al.* 1993). These abnormalities are more common in women than men. More work is needed in this area. It is unclear whether such neurodevelopmental lesions are in some way directly conferring an increased risk of schizophrenia or whether they are merely signals of a more general neurodevelopmental brain abnormality, whose critical site of action is actually elsewhere. In any event, these lesions usually develop *in utero*, and are relatively 'silent' for several decades before the onset of schizophrenia-like symptoms. This lag reinforces the notion that there is a crucial interface between a static pathological lesion and normal maturational brain processes in the production of psychosis.

Phenomenology of primary vs. secondary schizophrenia

Both brain imaging and clinical studies point to a prevalence rate of 5–8% for psychoses of likely identifiable organic aetiology amongst series of relatively unselected patients. If this is the case, is it possible to distinguish the minority of organic cases on clinical grounds alone?

The short answer is no, in that there is a large overlap in presenting symptoms between functional and organic psychoses. Nevertheless, several studies have compared symptom profiles in the two groups and some general differences do emerge. In their review of the literature, Davison and Bagley (1969) compared rates of individual psychotic symptoms in 150 reported cases of various organic schizophrenia-like psychoses with a series of 475 patients with functional schizophrenia reported by other authors. Of 14 clinical features compared, seven occurred significantly less frequently in the organic group: flat or incongruous affect; passivity feelings; thought disorder; auditory hallucinations; tactile hallucinations; schizoid premorbid personality; and family history of schizophrenia.

Catatonic symptoms were reported more frequently in organic cases. Of the organic group 64% showed Schneiderian first-rank symptoms, although this feature was not recorded in the control group. These results are intriguing, although they represent a retrospective survey of a varied collection of different case reports.

Cutting (1987) compared the Present State Examination (PSE)-rated symptomatology of 74 cases of organic psychosis with 74 cases of RDC acute schizophrenia, all prospectively interviewed. Like Davison and Bagley, he found auditory hallucinations to be less common in the organic group. Delusions were also less frequently found, although simple persecutory delusions were actually more common in the organic group. Contrary to the findings of Davison and Bagley, Schneiderian symptoms were rare in the organic group (3%). Thought disorder and visual hallucinations were more common. Cutting also noted a difference in the content of the phenomenology. Whereas delusions of the first rank were unusual in organic cases, in nearly one-half of the deluded organic patients, two delusional themes were patent: either belief of imminent misadventure to others, or bizarre occurrences in the immediate vicinity. Few non-organic schizophrenic patients showed these features. Cutting offers possible explanations for these organic themes as being delusional elaborations of deficits of perception, or memory. In the area of perceptual disturbance, the mistaken identity of other people was another theme found more commonly in the organic group.

In the study of Johnstone *et al.* (1988), PSE-rated symptomatology was compared between 23 cases of so-called organic psychosis and 92 non-organic psychoses matched for age, sex and ethnicity conforming to DSM-III criteria for schizophrenia, mania and psychotic depression. The authors found considerable overlap in symptoms. Comparing the organic and schizophrenic (n = 43) groups, nuclear (first rank) schizophrenic symptoms tended to be less frequent in the organic group (50% vs. 74%, $P < 0.06$). Visual hallucinations were more common in the organic group only if consciousness was clouded.

In the series of RDC schizophrenia patients under 65 referred to above, Lewis (1987) compared clinical features of those 41 patients with unequivocally abnormal CT scans to features in the 166 with a normal CT scan. Those with abnormal CT had significantly less evidence of a family history of schizophrenia in first-degree relatives, were more likely to have demonstrated formal thought disorder and more often had EEG abnormalities. Clinical presentation also seemed more atypical in the abnormal scan group, in that these patients were significantly more likely to have received alternative prior hospital diagnoses and a longer interval had intervened before a diagnosis of schizophrenia was made.

Feinstein and Ron (1990) examined the symptomatology in a series of 53 schizophrenic patients ascertained retrospectively, in whom psychotic symptoms arose secondary to overt brain disease. Symptom patterns were compared with normative data derived from the international pilot study of schizophrenia. The only individual symptom difference was an excess of visual hallucinations in the secondary schizophrenia group. Feinstein and Ron (1990) noted a relatively old age at onset (mean of 34 years) and a family history of schizophrenia in first-degree relatives was present in three of 53 cases. A wide variety of organic disease was represented. Overall, 50% of cases had epilepsy, reflecting a referral bias compared with the more representative series of Johnstone *et al.* (1987).

Individual cases included frontal meningioma, cerebral lymphoma, tuberous sclerosis, multiple sclerosis, Huntington's disease, encephalitis, cerebral abscess and hyperparathyroidism. Three cases of schizophrenic symptoms arising after neurosurgical operation were also included. The authors noted the wide variability in brain regions involved with, in particular, no consistent lateralized temporal pathology.

Velocardiofacial syndrome appears to be the organic disorder which confers one of the highest risk for the development of schizophrenia. In their series of VCFS cases, Murphy *et al.* (1999) compared the clinical characteristics of those with schizophrenia to a large series of schizophrenic cases without

Table 11.4 Secondary schizophrenias: suggested screening procedures.

Physical investigations

First line
Neurological history and examination
Full blood count and differential
Erythrocyte sedimentation rate
Electrolytes
Syphilis serology
Thyroid function tests
Liver function panel
Electroencephalography
Urinary drug screen

Second line
Autoantibody titres
Magnetic resonance imaging of the brain
Serum calcium
HIV antibody titres
Arylsulphatase-A levels
Copper and ceruloplasmin levels
Karyotype
Cerebrospinal fluid analyses

VCFS. The VCFS schizophrenic patients had a later age at onset and less negative symptoms than those with primary schizophrenia.

Excluding secondary schizophrenia in practice: physical investigations

Table 11.4 outlines first- and second-line physical investigations which should be considered in new cases of psychosis, including schizophrenia. Of the first-line investigations, some may dispute the need always for syphilis serology and EEG. However, tertiary syphilis still occasionally presents as a psychosis in clinical practice. The EEG is performed to exclude the generalized slowing indicative of diffuse brain disease, or the focal paroxysmal spike-and-wave discharges of an epileptic focus.

The second-line investigations are dependent on other abnormal findings (autoantibodies if raised erythroctye sedimentation rate, chromosome studies if developmental delays or unusual body morphology). In particular, CT or MRI scan is probably only warranted in clinical practice if there are neurological symptoms in the history (e.g. epilepsy), or neurological signs on examination, or with an abnormal EEG.

Conclusions

Clinically unsuspected, usually neurodevelopmental, brain lesions of aetiological relevance occur in 5–10% of schizophrenic illness. Males seem to predominate. There is no indication that the discovery of such a lesion influences treatment in any specific way. The more classical variants of secondary schizophrenias are those psychotic disorders arising in the context of systemic physical disease. The best evidence available is that these account for about 3% of newly presenting schizophrenias. Clinically, it is important to detect this subtype, because recognition and treatment of the primary disorder are needed. The existence of secondary schizophrenias offers several potential avenues to illuminate the cause of primary schizophrenia. The observation of neurodevelopmental lesions was one of the building blocks of the neurodevelopmental model of schizophrenia. Association with Mendelian disorders is currently of interest in the search for candidate chromosomes or chromosomal regions predisposing to primary schizophrenia.

Those disorders which remain unexplained are adult-onset physical disorders which produce secondary schizophrenic symptoms, although the notion of a developmental window may prove important in understanding the onset of these disorders.

References

Abbott, M.H., Folstein, S.E., Abbey, H. & Pyeritz, R.E. (1987) Psychiatric manifestations of homocystinuria due to cystathionine beta-synthase deficiency: prevalence, natural history, and relationship to neurologicl impairmnet and vitamin B$_6$-reponsiveness. *American Journal of Medical Genetics* **26**, 959–969.

Achté, K.A., Hillbom, E. & Aalberg, V. (1969) Psychosis following war brain injuries. *Acta Psychiatrica Scandinavica* **45**, 1–18.

Achté, K., Jarho, L., Kyykka, T. & Vesterinen, E. (1991) Paranoid disorders following war brain damage. *Psychopathology* **24**, 309–315.

Akesson, H.O. & O'Landers, S. (1969) Frequency of negative sex chromatin among women in mental hospitals. *Human Heredity* **19**, 43–47.

Alarcon, R.D. & Franceschini, J.A. (1984) Hyperparathyroidism and paranoid psychosis case report and review of the literature. *British Journal of Psychiatry* **145**, 477–486.

American Psychiatric Association (1994) *Diagnostic and Statistical Manual of Mental Disorders*, 4th edn. American Psychiatric Association, Washington, DC.

Andermann, L.F., Savard, G., Meencke, H.J. *et al.* (1999) Psychosis after resection of ganglioglioma or DNET: evidence for an association. *Epilepsia* **40**, 83–87.

Andy, O.J., Webster, J.S. & Carranza, J. (1981) Frontal lobe lesions and behavior. *Southern Medical Journal* **74**, 968–972.

Bamrah, J.S. & MacKay, M.E. (1989) Chronic psychosis in Turner's syndrome. *British Journal of Psychiatry* **155**, 857–859.

Barnett, W., Sigmund, D., Roelcke, U. & Mundt, C. (1991) Endogenous-like paranoid–hallucinatory syndrome due to borrelia encephalitis. *Nervenarzt* **45**, 445–447.

Baron, M. (1976) Albinism and schizophreniform psychosis: a pedigree study. *American Journal of Psychiatry* **133**, 1070–1073.

Bassett, A.S., Hodgkinson, K., Chow, E.W. *et al.* (1998) 22q11 Deletion syndrome in adults with schizophrenia. *American Journal of Human Genetics* **81**, 328–337.

Bouckoms, A., Martuza, R. & Henderson, M. (1986) Capgras syndrome with subarachnoid hemorrhage. *Journal of Nervous and Mental Disease* **174**, 484–488.

Bracken, P. & Coll, P. (1985) Homocystinuria and schziophrenia: literature review and case report. *Journal of Nervous and Mental Disease* **173**, 51–55.

Brugha, T.S., Wing, J.K., Brewin, L.R. *et al.* (1988) The problems of people in long-term psychiatric care: an introduction to the Camberwell High Contact Survey. *Psychological Medicine* **18**, 457–468.

Buckley, P., Stack, J.P., Madigan, C. *et al.* (1993) Magnetic resonance imaging of schizophrenia-like psychoses associated with cerebral trauma: clinicopathological correlates. *American Journal of Psychiatry* **150**, 146–148.

Burke, J.G., Dersun, S.M. & Reveley, M.A. (1999) Refractory symptomatic schizophrenia resulting from frontal lobe lesion: response to clozapine. *Journal of Psychiatry and Neuroscience* **24**, 456–461.

Casanova, M.F., Prasad, C.N., Waldman, I. *et al.* (1990) No difference in basal ganglia mineralization between schizophrenic and non-schizophrenic patients: a quantitative CT study. *Biological Psychiatry* **27**, 138–142.

Chen, J., Stern, Y., Sano, M. & Mayeux, R. (1991) Cumulative risks of developing extrapyramidal signs, psychosis, or myoclonus in the course of Alzheimer's disease. *Archives of Neurology* **48**, 1141–1143.

Clarke, D.J. & Buckley, M. (1989) Familial association of albinism and schizophrenia. *British Journal of Psychiatry* **155**, 551–553.

Cowen, M.A. & Green, M. (1993) The Kallmann's syndrome variant (KSV) model of the schizophrenias. *Schizophrenia Research* **9**, 1–10.

Cutting, J. (1987) The phenomenology of acute organic psychosis: comparison with acute schizophrenia. *British Journal of Psychiatry* **151**, 324–332.

Damasio, A.R. & Van Hoesen, G.W. (1985) The limbic system and the localisation of herpes simplex encephalitis. *Journal of Neurology, Neurosurgery and Psychiatry* **48**, 297–301.

Davis, A.T. (1989) Psychotic states associated with disorders of thyroid function. *International Journal of Psychiatry in Medicine* **19**, 47–56.

Davison, K. (1983) Schizophrenia-like psychoses associated with organic cerebral disorders: a review. *Psychiatric Developments* **1**, 1–34.

Davison, K. & Bagley, C.R. (1969) Schizophrenia-like psychoses associated with organic disorders of the central nervous system. In: *Current Problems in Neuropsychiatry: Schizophrenia, Epilepsy, the Temporal Lobe* (ed. R. Herrington). Special Publication No. 4, British Journal of Psychiatry, London.

Deckert, J., Strik, W.K. & Fritze, J. (1992) Organic schizophrenic syndrome associated with symmetrical basal ganglia sclerosis and XO/XY-mosaic. *Biological Psychiatry* **31**, 401–403.

DeGreef, G., Bogerts, B., Falkai, P. *et al.* (1992) Increased prevalence of the cavum septum pellucidum in magnetic resonance scans and postmortem brains of schizophrenic patients. *Psychiatry Research* **45**, 1–13.

DeLisi, L.E., Crow, T.J., Davies, K.E. *et al.* (1991) No genetic linkage detected for schizophrenia to Xq27–q28. *British Journal of Psychiatry* **158**, 630–634.

DeLisi, L.E., Friedrich, U., Wahlstrom, J. *et al.* (1994) Schizophrenia and sex chromosome anomalies. *Schizophrenia Bulletin* **20**, 495–505.

Dening, T.R. (1985) Psychiatric aspects of Wilson's disease. *British Journal of Psychiatry* **147**, 677–682.

Dening, T.R. & Berrios, G.E. (1989) Wilson's disease: psychiatric symptoms in 195 cases. *Archives of General Psychiatry* **46**, 1126–1134.

Dorus, E., Dorus, W. & Telfer, M.A. (1977) Paranoid schizophrenia in a 47,XYY male. *American Journal of Psychiatry* **134**, 687–689.

Duncalf, C.M., Kent, J.N., Harbord, M. & Hicks, E.P. (1989) Subacute sclerosing panencephalitis presenting as schizophreniform psychosis. *British Journal of Psychiatry* **155**, 557–559.

Ebel, H., Schlegel, U. & Klosterkotter, J. (1992) Chronic schizophreniform psychoses in primary hyperparathyroidism. *Nervenarzt* **63**, 180–183.

Egan, M.F., Goldberg, T.E., Gscheidle, T. *et al.* (2000) Relative risk of attention deficits in siblings of patients with schizophrenia. *American Journal of Psychiatry* **157**, 1309–1316.

Eliez, S., Schmitt, J.E., White, C.D., Wellis, V.G. & Reiss, A.L. (2001a) A quantitative MRI study of posterior fossa development in velocardiofacial syndrome. *Biological Psychiatry* **49**, 540–546.

Eliez, S., Blasey, C.M., Schmitt, J.E. *et al.* (2001b) Velocardiofacial syndrome: are structural changes in the temporal and mesial temporal regions related to schizophrenia? *American Journal of Psychiatry* **158**, 447–453.

Emsley, R.A. & Paster, L. (1985) Lipoid proteinosis presenting with neuropsychiatric manifestations. *Journal of Neurology, Neurosurgery and Psychiatry* **48**, 1290–1292.

Faber, R. & Abrams, R. (1975) Schizophrenia in a 47,XYY male. *British Journal of Psychiatry* **127**, 401–403.

Feinstein, A. & Ron, M.A. (1990) Psychosis associated with demonstrable brain disease. *Psychological Medicine* **20**, 793–803.

Feinstein, A., du Boulay, G. & Ron, M.A. (1992) Psychotic illness in multiple sclerosis: a clinical and magnetic resonance imaging study. *British Journal of Psychiatry* **161**, 680–685.

Fishbain, D.A. (1990) Chronic psychoses in Turner's syndrome. *British Journal of Psychiatry* **156**, 745–746.

Flor-Henry, P. (1969) Psychosis and temporal lobe epilepsy. *Epilepsia* **10**, 363–395.

Frydman, M., Bonne-Tamir, B., Farber, L.A. *et al.* (1985) Assignment of the gene for Wilson disease to chromosome 13: linkage to the esterase D locus. *Proceedings of the National Academy of Sciences of the USA* **82**, 1819–1821.

Fujii, D.E. & Ahmed, I. (2001) Risk factors in psychosis secondary to traumatic brain injury. *Journal of Neuropsychiatry and Clinical Neurosciences* **13**, 61–69.

Gatewood, J.W., Organ, C.H. & Mead, B.T. (1975) Mental changes associated with hyperparathyroidsm. *American Journal of Psychiatry* **132**, 129–132.

Gaughan, D.J., Barbaux, S., Kluijtmans, L.A. & Whitehead, A.S. (2000) The human and mouse methylenetetrahydrofolate reductase (MTHFR) genes: genomic organization, mRNA structure and linkage to the *CLCN6* gene. *Gene* **257**, 279–289.

George, M.S., Scott, T., Kellner, C.H. & Malcolm, R. (1989) Abnormalities of the septum pellucidum in schizophrenia. *Journal of Neuropsychiatry and Clinical Neurosciences* **1**, 385–390.

Glaser, G.H. & Pincus, J.H. (1969) Limbic encephalitis. *Journal of Nervous and Mental Disease* **149**, 59–67.

Gualtieri, T. & Cox, D.R. (1991) The delayed neurobehavioural sequelae of traumatic brain injury. *Brain Injury* **5**, 219–232.

Gusella, J.F., Wexler, N.S., Conneally, P.M. *et al.* (1983) A polymorphic DNA marker genetically linked to Huntington's disease. *Nature* **306**, 234–238.

Hall, D.P. & Young, S.A. (1992) Frontal lobe cerebral aneurysm rupture presenting as psychosis. *Journal of Neurology, Neurosurgery and Psychiatry* **55**, 1207–1208.

Harris, M.J., Jeste, D.V., Gleghorn, A. & Sewell, D.D. (1991) New-onset psychosis in HIV-infected patients. *Journal of Clinical Psychiatry* **52**, 369–376.

Heckert, E.E., Wald, A. & Romero, O. (1972) Tuberous sclerosis and schizophrenia. *Diseases of the Nervous System* **33**, 439–445.

Honer, W.G., Hurwitz, T., Li, D.K.B., Palmer, M. & Paty, D.W. (1987) Temporal lobe involvement in multiple sclerosis patients with psychiatric disorders. *Archives of Neurology* **44**, 187–190.

Hyde, T.M. & Weinberger, D.R. (1997) Seizures and schizophrenia. *Schizophrenia Bulletin* **23**, 611–622.

Hyde, T.M., Ziegler, J.C. & Weinberger, D.R. (1992) Psychiatric disturbances in metachromatic leukodystrophy: insights into the neurobiology of psychosis. *Archives of Neurology* **49**, 401–406.

Johnson, J. (1975) Schizophrenia and Cushing's syndrome cured by adrenalectomy. *Psychological Medicine* **5**, 165–168.

Johnstone, E.C., Owens, D.G., Frith, C.D. & Crow, T.J. (1987) The relative stability of positive and negative features in chronic schizophrenia. *British Journal of Psychiatry* **150**, 60–64.

Johnstone, E.C., Cooling, N.J., Frith, C.D., Crow, T.J. & Owens, D.G. (1988) Phenomenology of organic and functional psychoses and the overlap between them. *British Journal of Psychiatry* **153**, 770–776.

Jones, A.C., Daniells, C.E., Snell, R.G. *et al.* (1997) Molecular genetic and phenotypic analysis reveals differences between TSC1 and TSC2 associated familial and sporadic tuberous sclerosis. *Human Molecular Genetics* **6**, 2155–2161.

Kaplan, A.R. & Cotton, J.E. (1968) Chromosomal abnormalities in female schizophrenics. *Journal of Nervous and Mental Diseases* **147**, 402–417.

Kitchin, W., Cohen-Cole, S.A. & Mickel, S.F. (1987) Adrenoleukodystrophy: frequency of presentation as a psychiatric disorder. *Society of Biological Psychiatry* **22**, 1375–1387.

Koehler, K. & Jakumeit, U. (1976) Subacute sclerosing panencephalitis presenting as Leonhard's speech-prompt catatonia. *British Journal of Psychiatry* **129**, 29–31.

Krishna, N.R., Abrams, R., Taylor, M.A. & Behar, D. (1977) Schizophrenia in a 46,XY male with the Noonan syndrome. *British Journal of Psychiatry* **130**, 570–572.

Lanczik, M., Fritze, J., Classen, W., Ihl, R. & Maurer, K. (1989) Schizophrenia-like psychosis associated with an arachnoid cyst visualized by mapping of EEG and P300. *Psychiatry Research* **29**, 421–423.

Larson, R.S. & Butler, M.G. (1995) Use of fluorescence *in situ* hybridization (FISH) in the diagnosis fo DiGeorge sequence and related diseases. *Diagnostic and Molecular Pathology* **4**, 274–278.

Leavell, R., Ray, C.G., Ferry, P.C. & Minnich, L.L. (1986) Unusual acute neurologic presentations with Epstein–Barr virus infection. *Archives of Neurology* **43**, 186–188.

Levine, D.N. & Finklestein, S. (1982) Delayed psychosis after right temporoparietal stroke or trauma: relation to epilepsy. *Neurology* **32**, 267–273.

Lewis, S.W. (1987) *Schizophrenia with and without intracranial abnormalities on CT scan.* M. Phil thesis, University of London.

Lewis, S.W. (1989) Congenital risk factors for schizophrenia. *Psychological Medicine* **19**, 5–13.

Lewis, S.W. (1990) Computed tomography in schizophrenia fifteen years on. *British Journal of Psychiatry* **157** (Suppl. 9), 16–24.

Lewis, S.W. & Mezey, G.C. (1985) Clinical correlates of septum pellucidum cavities: an unusual association with psychosis. *Psychological Medicine* **15**, 43–54.

Lewis, S.W., Reveley, A.M., Reveley, M.A., Chitkara, B. & Murray, R.M. (1987) The familial–sporadic distinction in schizophrenia research. *British Journal of Psychiatry* **151**, 306–313.

Lipska, B.K., Jaskiw, G.E. & Weinberger, D.R. (1994) The effects of combined prefrontal cortical and hippocampal damage on dopamine-related behaviors in rats. *Pharmacological Biochemistry and Behavior* **48**, 1053–1057.

Lisanby, S.H., Kohler, C., Swanson, C.L. & Gur, R.E. (1998) Psychosis secondary to brain tumor. *Seminars in Clinical Neuropsychiatry* **3**, 12–22.

McCune, N. (1987) Schizophreniform episode following measles infection. *British Journal of Psychiatry* **151**, 558–559.

McDaniel, J.S., Purcell, D.W. & Farber, E.W. (1997) Severe mental illness and HIV-related medical and neuropsychiatric sequelae. *Clinical Psychology Review* **17**, 311–325.

Mace, C.J. (1993) Epilepsy and schizophrenia. *British Journal of Psychiatry* **163**, 439–445.

MacNeil, A., Grennan, D.M., Ward, D. & Dick, W.C. (1976) Psychiatric problems in systemic lupus erythematosus. *British Journal of Psychiatry* **128**, 442–445.

Malamud, N. (1967) Psychiatric disorder with intracranial tumours of limbic system. *Archives of Neurology* **18**, 113–123.

Manowitz, P., Goldstein, L. & Nora, R. (1981) An arylsulfatase-A variant in schizophrenic patients: preliminary report. *Biological Psychiatry* **16**, 1107–1113.

Mendez, M.F., Grau, R., Doss, R.C. & Taylor, J.L. (1993) Schizophrenia in epilepsy: seizure and psychosis variables. *Neurology* **43**, 1073–1077.

Miller, B.L., Lesser, I.M., Boone, K. *et al.* (1989). Brain white-matter lesions and psychosis. *British Journal of Psychiatry* **155**, 73–78.

Miller, B.L., Lesser, I.M., Boone, B.K. *et al.* (1991) Brain lesions and cognitive function in late-life psychosis. *British Journal of Psychiatry* **158**, 76–82.

Moises, H.W., Gelernter, J., Giuffra, L.A. *et al.* (1991) No linkage between D_2 dopamine receptor gene region and schizophrenia. *Archives of General Psychiatry* **48**, 643–647.

Money, J. & Hirsch, S.R. (1963) Chromosome anomalies, mental deficiency and schizophrenia. *Archives of General Psychiatry* **7**, 242–251.

Mordecai, D., Shaw, R.J., Fisher, P.G. *et al.* (2000) Case study: suprasellar germinoma presenting with psychotic and obsessive–compulsive symptoms. *Journal of the American Academy of Child and Adolescent Psychiatry* **39**, 116–119.

Muller, N. & Endres, M. (1987) An XX male with schizophrenia: a case of personality development and illness similar to that in XXY males. *Journal of Clinical Psychiatry* **48**, 379–380.

Murphy, K.C., Jones, L.A. & Owen, M.J. (1999) High rates of schizophrenia in adults with velocardiofacial syndrome. *Archives of General Psychiatry* **56**, 940–945.

Naarding, P., Kremer, H.P.H. & Zitman, F.G. (2001) Huntington's disease: a review of the literature on prevalence and treatment of neuropsychiatric phenomena. *European Psychiatry* **16**, 439–445.

Neumann, P.E., Mehler, M.F., Horoupian, D.S. & Merriam, A.E. (1988) Atypical psychosis with disseminated subpial demyelination. *Archives of Neurology* **45**, 634–636.

Nielsen, J. & Stradiot, M. (1987) Transcultural study of Turner's syndrome. *Clinical Genetics* **32**, 260–270.

Nunn, K.P., Lask, B. & Cohen, M. (1986) Viruses, neurodevelopmental disorder and childhood psychoses. *Journal of Child Psychology and Psychiatry* **27**, 55–64.

O'Callaghan, E., Buckley, P., Redmond, O. *et al.* (1992) Abnormalities of cerebral structure on MRI: interpretation in relation to the neurodevelopmental hypothesis. *Journal of the Royal Society of Medicine* **85**, 227–231.

O'Neill, M., Brewer, W., Thornley, C. *et al.* (1999) Kallmann syndrome gene (*KAL-X*) is not mutated in schizophrenia. *American Journal of Medical Genetics* **88**, 34–37.

Owens, D.G.C., Johnstone, E.C., Bydder, G.M. *et al.* (1980) Unsuspected organic disease in chronic schizophrenia demonstrated by computed tomography. *Journal of Neurology, Neurosurgery and Psychiatry* **43**, 1065–1069.

Pang, A. & Lewis, S.W. (1996) Bipolar affective disorder minus left prefrontal cortex equals schizophrenia. *British Journal of Psychiatry* **168**, 647–650.

Philpot, M. & Lewis, S.W. (1990) Psychopathology of basal ganglia calcification. *Behavioural Neurology* **2**, 227–234.

Price, B.H. & Mesulam, M.M. (1985) Psychiatric manifestations of right hemispheric infarctions. *Journal of Nervous and Mental Disease* **173**, 610–614.

Propping, P. (1983) Genetic disorders presenting as schizophrenia: Karl Bonhoffers early view of the psychoses in the light of medical genetics. *Human Genetics* **65**, 1–10.

Ramani, S.V. (1981) Psychosis associated with frontal lobe lesions in Schilder's cerebral sclerosis: a case report with CT scan evidence. *Journal of Clinical Psychiatry* **42**, 250–252.

Regland, B., Germgard, T., Gottfries, C.G., Grenfeldt, B. & Koch-Schmidt, A.C. (1997) Homozygous thermolabile methylenetretrahydrofolate reductase in schizophrenia-like psychosis. *Journal of Neural Transmission* **104**, 931–941.

Reischies, F.M., Baum, K., Brau, H. *et al.* (1988) Cerebral magnetic resonance imaging findings in multiple sclerosis: relation to disturbance of affect, drive and cognition. *Archives of Neurology* **45**, 1114–1116.

Remington, G. & Jeffries, J.J. (1984) The role of cerebral arteriovenous malformations in psychiatric disturbances: case report. *Journal of Clinical Psychiatry* **45**, 226–229.

Reveley, A.M. & Reveley, M.A. (1983) Aqueduct stenosis and schizophrenia. *Journal of Neurology, Neurosurgery and Psychiatry* **46**, 18–22.

Risch, N. (1990) Genetic linkage and complex diseases, with special reference to psychiatric disorders. *Genetics Epidemiology* **7**, 17–45.

Roberts, C.W., Dane, D.J., Bauton, C. & Crow, T.J. (1990) A 'mock-up' of schizophrenia: temporal lobe epilepsy and schizophrenia-like psychosis. *Biological Psychiatry* **1990**, 127–143.

Romano, J. & Linares, R.L. (1987) Marfan syndrome and schizophrenia: a case report. *Archives of General Psychiatry* **44**, 190–192.

Ron, M.A. & Logsdail, S.J. (1989) Psychiatric morbidity in multiple sclerosis: a clinical and MRI study. *Psychological Medicine* **19**, 887–895.

Rubin, R.L. (1978) Adolescent infectious mononucleosis with psychosis. *Journal of Clinical Psychiatry* **39**, 773–775.

Salib, E.A. (1988) SSPE presenting as a schizophrenia-like state with bizarre dysmorphophic features. *British Journal of Psychiatry* **152**, 709–710.

Sartorius, N., Kaelber, C.T., Cooper, J.E. *et al.* (1993) Progress toward achieving a common language in psychiatry: results from the field trials accompanying the clinical guidelines of mental and behaviourial disorders in ICD-10. *Archives of General Psychiatry* **50**, 115–124.

Scott, T.F., Price, T.R., George, M.S., Brillman, J. & Rothfus, W. (1993) Midline cerebral malformations and schizophrenia. *Journal of Neuropsychiatry and Clinical Neuroscience* **5**, 287–293.

Sewell, D.D., Jeste, D.V., Atkinson, J.H. *et al.* (1994) HIV-associated psychosis: a study of 20 cases. San Diego HIV Neurobehavioral Research Center Groups. *American Journal of Psychiatry* **151**, 237–242.

Sharp, C.W., Muir, W.J., Blackwood, D.H. *et al.* (1993) Schizophrenia: a neuropsychiatric phenotype of the Usher syndrome type 3 allele. *Schizophrenia Research* **9**, 125.

Shields, G.W., Pataki, C. & DeLisi, E. (1990) A family with Alport syndrome and psychosis. *Schizophrenia Research* **3**, 235–239.

Sirota, P., Frydman, M. & Sirota, L. (1990) Schizophrenia and Marfan syndrome. *British Journal of Psychiatry* **157**, 433–436.

Slater, E. & Beard, A.W. (1963) The schizophrenia-like psychoses of epilepsy. *British Journal of Psychiatry* **109**, 95–112.

Sorensen, K. & Nielsen, J. (1977) Twenty psychotic males with Klinefelter's syndrome. *Acta Psychiatrica Scandinavica* **56**, 249–255.

Spitzer, R.H., First, M.B., Williams, J.B.W. *et al.* (1992) Now is the time to retire the term 'organic mental disorders'. *American Journal of Psychiatry* **149**, 240–244.

Stevens, J.R. (1988) Schizophrenia and multiple sclerosis. *Schizophrenia Bulletin* 14, 231–241.

Stevens, J.R. (1992) Abnormal reinnervation as a basis for schizophrenia: a hypothesis. *Archives of General Psychiatry* 49, 235–243.

Stoler, M., Meshulam, B., Zoldan, J. & Sirota, P. (1987) Schizophreniform episode following measles infection. *British Journal of Psychiatry* 150, 861–862.

Susser, E., Neugebauer, R., Hoek, H.W. *et al.* (1996) Schizophrenia after prenatal famine. *Archives of General Psychiatry* 53, 25–31.

Swayze, V.W., Andreasen, N.C., Ehrhardt, J.C. *et al.* (1990) Developmental abnormalities of the corpus callosum in schizophrenia. *Archives of Neurology* 47, 805–808.

Swift, R.G., Sadler, D.B. & Swift, M. (1990) Psychiatric findings in Wolfram syndrome homozygotes. *Lancet* 336, 667–669.

Tavares, A.R., Pinto, D.C., Lemow, A. & Nascimento, E. (1993) Lesion localization in schizophrenia-like disorder associated with neurocysticerosis. *Schizophrenia Research* 9, 111.

Taylor, D. (1975) Factors influencing the occurrence of schizophrenia-like psychoses in temporal lobe epilepsy. *Psychological Medicine* 1, 247–253.

Tishler, P.V., Woodward, B., O'Connor, J. *et al.* (1985) High prevalence of intermittent acute porphyria in a psychiatric patient population. *American Journal of Psychiatry* 142, 1430–1436.

Torrey, E.F. (1986) Functional psychosis and viral encephalitis. *Integrated Psychiatry* 4, 224–236.

Trimble, M.R. (1988) *Biological Psychiatry*. John Wiley, Chichester.

Trimble, M.R. (1990) First-rank symptoms of Schneider: a new perspective? *British Journal of Psychiatry* 156, 195–200.

Turpin, J.C., Masson, M. & Baumann, N. (1991) Clinical aspects of Niemann–Pick type C disease in the adult. *Developmental Neuroscience* 13, 304–306.

Vaillant, G. (1965) Schizophrenia in a woman with temporal lobe arteriovenous malformations. *British Journal of Psychiatry* 111, 307–308.

Van Sweden, B. & Van Peteghem, P. (1986) Psychopathology in paraneoplastic encephalopathy: an electroclinical observation. *Journal of Clinical Psychiatry* 47, 267–268.

Velek, M., White, L.E. Jr, Williams, J.P., Stafford, R.L. & Marco, L.A. (1988) Psychosis in a case of corpus callosum agenesis. *Alabama Medicine* 58, 27–29.

Wahlund, L.-O., Agartz, I., Sääf, J., Wetterberg, L. & Marions, O. (1992) MRI in psychiatry: 731 cases. *Psychiatry Research* 45, 139–140.

Weinberger, D.R. (1987) Implications of normal brain development for pathogenesis of schizophrenia. *Archives of General Psychiatry* 44, 660–669.

White, P.D. & Lewis, S.W. (1987) Delusional depression following infectious mononucleosis. *British Medical Journal* 295, 297–298.

Wilcox, J.A. & Nasrallah, H.A. (1986) Sydenham's chorea and psychosis. *Neuropsychobiology* 15, 13–14.

Wilson, L.G. (1976) Viral encephalopathy mimicking functional psychosis. *American Journal of Psychiatry* 133, 165–170.

World Health Organization (1978) *The ICD-9 Classification of Mental and Behaviourial Disorders*. WHO, Geneva.

World Health Organization (1992) *The ICD-10 Classification of Mental and Behaviourial Disorders*. WHO, Geneva.

Zubenko, G.S., Moossy, J., Martinez, A.J. *et al.* (1991) Neuropathologic and neurochemical correlates of psychosis in primary dementia. *Archives of Neurology* 48, 619–624.

Zucker, D.K., Livingston, R.L., Nakra, R. & Clayton, P.J. (1981) B_{12} deficiency and psychiatric disorders: case report and literature review. *Biological Psychiatry* 16, 197–205.

The epidemiological horizon

A. Jablensky

Sources of variation in the epidemiology of
  schizophrenia related to the method of
  investigation, 203
  Case finding, 204
  Diagnosis, 205
  Investigators, 206
  Instruments, 206
  Measures of morbidity, 207
Descriptive epidemiology of schizophrenia, 207
  Prevalence, 207
  Incidence, 209
  Morbid risk (disease expectancy), 211
  Populations and groups with high and low rates of
    schizophrenia, 211
  Secular trends in the incidence and prevalence of
    schizophrenia, 212
Comorbid association with other diseases, 213
  Comorbidity with substance use, 213
Mortality, 214
Fertility, 215

Analytical epidemiology of schizophrenia: risk
  factors and antecedents, 215
  Age and sex, 215
  Genetic risk, 216
  Children at high genetic risk, 217
  Obstetric complications, 218
  Maternal influenza and other pre- and postnatal
    infections, 219
  Other prenatal exposures, 219
  The early rearing environment, 219
  Premorbid traits and social impairment, 220
  Premorbid intelligence (IQ), 220
  Neurocognitive and neurophysiological markers,
    220
  Social class, 221
  Urban birth, 221
  Season of birth, 221
  Marital status, 222
  Migrant status and ethnic minorities, 222
Prospects for epidemiology in the search for the
  causes of schizophrenia, 223
References, 223

Establishing the epidemiological 'signature' of a disease – its frequency in specified populations, geographical spread and spatial distribution, temporal variation, and associations with comorbid conditions and risk factors – is an essential step towards unravelling its causes and a prerequisite for its ultimate prevention and control. In a number of instances, the epidemiological mapping of a syndrome has revealed patterns suggestive of possible causation and narrowed down the search area for subsequent clinical and laboratory research. The classic examples of successful application of the epidemiological method include pellagra, rubella encephalopathy, the fetal alcohol syndrome and kuru. Attempts to apply this approach to the study of schizophrenia have not met with comparable success although epidemiological investigations into the schizophrenic disorders have been conducted for over a century. A principal source of difficulty is the nature of the disease concept of schizophrenia itself. The attributes defining schizophrenia are primarily inferential and depend critically on self-reported subjective experience; the underlying structural and functional pathology remains hypothetical and there is no objective diagnostic test or easily measurable biological marker that could provide a secure anchor point for epidemiological field research. As pointed out by Jaspers (1963), the disease concept of schizophrenia is 'an idea in Kant's sense', i.e. a guiding methodological principle helping to organize knowledge which should not be mistaken for a tangible piece of empirical reality.

Notwithstanding occasional proposals to scuttle the very concept of schizophrenia because of its elusive nature, there is an increasing acceptance of the notion that schizophrenia is, in a genetic sense, one of the *complex* diseases – characterized by a non-Mendelian pattern of transmission, polygenic or oligogenic basis, incomplete penetrance, possible non-allelic heterogeneity, and a significant non-genetic contribution to its phenotypic expression. Advancing the understanding of the neurobiology of such a complex disorder with ill-defined phenotype boundaries requires an epidemiological horizon for the planning and interpretation of genetic, neuropathological and neurophysiological research. No less important is the demand for an epidemiological resource that would aid clinicians in making evidence-based diagnostic and treatment decisions. In reviewing the existing vast and often inconsistent epidemiological information about schizophrenia, it is therefore essential to identify findings that are replicable and likely to be valid, despite the variation in concepts and research methods that still confound the field. The present chapter surveys a broad range of topics which add up to a composite epidemiological picture of a complex disease. Special attention is given to findings reported in the last few years and to the epidemiological implications of recent clinical and biological research.

Sources of variation in the epidemiology of schizophrenia related to the method of investigation

The measurement of the prevalence, incidence and morbid risk of schizophrenia depends critically on: (i) the capacity to identify in a given population all affected individuals (or the great majority of them); and (ii) the availability of a diagnostic system which will select 'true' cases corresponding to established clinical concepts. The first prerequisite refers to the sensitivity of the case finding and the second to the specificity of disease category allocation needed to minimize false-positive diagnoses.

Case finding

The majority of case finding designs fall into three groups:
1 case detection in clinical populations;
2 population surveys: door-to-door or representative samples; and
3 birth cohort studies.

Cases in treatment contact

At any given time, psychiatric hospital or outpatient populations contain substantial percentages of persons with the diagnosis of schizophrenia. This provides a relatively easy access to cases for epidemiological investigation. However, the probability of being in treatment depends on nosocomial factors such as availability and accessibility of services, their location and the rate of their utilization by population groups. Hospital samples rarely are representative of all the persons with a given disorder. The age and sex distribution, marital state, socioeconomic status, ethnicity and severity of illness in hospital samples often differ from those characterizing the larger pool of people in the community exhibiting the disorder of interest. The extent of the selection bias affecting clinical populations may vary widely from one setting to another (e.g. in a developing country compared with an industrialized country) and between different points in time.

Under the rare circumstances of stable social conditions, adequate service provision, and lack of major changes in legislation, admission policies and treatment philosophy, the presumption that the great majority of people with schizophrenic disorders eventually get admitted to hospital (Ødegaard 1952) may be justified. At present, such conditions hardly obtain anywhere. As a general trend, mental health care is moving away from the hospital into the community. It has been shown that an increasing number of patients with schizophrenia are being managed on an outpatient basis without admission to hospital. Over 50% of first-episode patients with schizophrenia in Nottingham, UK, are not admitted within 3 months of their first contact with a primary care facility (Harrison et al. 1991). Therefore, epidemiological case finding for schizophrenia that is restricted to hospital admissions is liable to be methodologically flawed.

The deficiencies of case finding through hospitals can be overcome by extending the case detection network to community mental health services, general practitioners, private providers and charity organizations. An example of such extension of case finding into the community is provided by a recent Australian national prevalence survey of psychoses (Jablensky et al. 2000) in which the great majority (82%) of cases were identified through non-hospital services and agencies. Another approach to case finding is by using psychiatric case registers, where such facilities exist. Registers collate data from multiple sources, including outpatient and rehabilitation services. The cumulative nature of the data and the capacity for record linkage to other databases make registers highly effective tools for many types of epidemiological research. However, the advantages of the case registers do not offset the problem that an unknown number of persons with schizophrenia never contact the psychiatric services. The proportion of people with schizophrenia who never consult has been estimated at about 17% in the USA (Link & Dohrenwend 1980). There is no evidence that persons with schizophrenia who are not in contact with the mental health services are treated by other agencies such as general practitioners or private psychiatrists. In both Denmark (Munk-Jørgensen & Mortensen 1992) and the UK (Bamrah et al. 1991), the number of patients with schizophrenia managed solely by general practitioners was found to be negligible, although it may have increased during the last decade.

Short of a door-to-door community survey, no standard method of estimating the 'hidden' schizophrenic morbidity is available. The presence of such latent morbidity needs to be taken into account in the planning of epidemiological surveys of schizophrenia. Its size is likely to be increasing as a result of diverse reasons including the spread of alternative treatments, the existence of cult or religious groups providing niches to people with unconventional beliefs and the marginalization of the destitute and homeless in the big cities.

Door-to-door and sample surveys

The field survey method has produced some of the most robust epidemiological data on schizophrenia. An early version of the survey method was used by Brugger (1931) in his investigations of the prevalence of psychoses in Thuringia and Bavaria. The method was applied with great success by Scandinavian investigators in the 1930s to 1960s (Strömgren 1938; Sjögren 1948; Bremer 1951; Essen-Möller et al. 1956; Hagnell 1966; Bøjholm & Strömgren 1989). In the majority of these studies, a single investigator, or a small group of researchers, interviewed and diagnosed nearly every member of a well-defined community, usually of a small size. Several of the Scandinavian studies were prospective and the original population was re-examined after intervals of 10 or more years. While the completeness of case finding and thoroughness of assessment are probably unsurpassed, the representativeness of results obtained from selected small communities is problematic.

A viable substitute for the complete census of a population is the sample survey in which a probability sample is drawn and interviewed to establish point or lifetime prevalence. Examples include the National Institute of Mental Health (NIMH) Epidemiological Catchment Area (ECA) study in which some 20 000 persons at five sites in the USA were interviewed (Robins & Regier 1991); the National Comorbidity Survey (Kessler et al.

1994) based on a national probability sample of 5877 US residents; and the Australian National Mental Health Survey (Andrews *et al.* 2001), in which a national probability sample of 10 641 adults was interviewed. A remarkable feature of these major surveys is that all three used a common method of case detection and diagnosis, based on versions of the same generic diagnostic instrument (administered by lay interviewers). However, because all three were designed as general mental morbidity surveys, the numbers of identified cases of schizophrenia were too small for epidemiological and clinical analysis. In the instance of the Australian survey, a separate in-depth study of 'low-prevalence' disorders, including schizophrenia and other psychoses, was conducted on a stratified sample of 980 cases drawn from a census of 3800 individuals found to be screen-positive for psychosis (Jablensky *et al.* 2000).

Birth cohorts

The birth cohort study can be a particularly effective method for determining incidence and morbid risk because its results produce a 'natural' morbidity and mortality life table. The method was first applied to the major psychoses by Klemperer (1933), who took from the birth registers a random sample of 1000 individuals born in Germany in 1881–90 and attempted to trace them as adults in their fourth decade of life. Because of the high cohort attrition levels that typically affect mobile populations, he succeeded in tracing only 44% and in interviewing a total of 271 probands or key informants. However, there are examples of remarkable success when the method is applied to 'captive' populations such as island inhabitants. Fremming (1947) in Denmark, Helgason (1964) and Helgason and Magnusson (1989) in Iceland were able to trace 92–99% of the members of birth cohorts and to estimate the lifetime morbid risk for schizophrenia. More recent examples of successful use of the method include the search for developmental precursors of adult schizophrenia using prospectively collected data from the UK 1946 birth cohort of the National Survey of Health and Development (NSHD; $n = 5362$; Jones *et al.* 1994; Cannon *et al.* 1996); the UK 1958 birth cohort of the National Child Development Study (NCDS; $n = 15 398$; Done *et al.* 1994); and the North Finland 1966 birth cohort ($n = 11 017$; Isohanni *et al.* 1998; Jones *et al.* 1998). Samples from two birth cohorts in the USA, the National Collaborative Perinatal Project 1959–66 ($n = 9236$; Cannon *et al.* 2000) and the Child Health and Development Study 1960–67 ($n = 19 044$; Susser *et al.* 2000), have recently been drawn for follow-up studies focusing on prenatal, perinatal and early childhood influences on the development of schizophrenia. Birth cohort samples of this kind are eminently suited for the testing of hypotheses about risk factors, especially if the original data collection included biological samples such as frozen blood or placenta specimens. However, their main limitation stems from: (i) the long 'latency' period before follow-up studies can generate schizophrenia incidence data; and (ii) the relatively small yield of cases of schizophrenia (81 cases by age 43 in the NSHD; 45 cases by age 23 in the NCDS; 76 cases by age 28 in the

Finnish cohort study). The latter factor restricts the range of data analyses because of limited statistical power.

Variants of the cohort design include follow-up studies of individuals who had undergone some kind of assessment at a specified age. Examples are a Swedish study including 50 087 men given a psychological examination as army conscripts at age 18–20 during 1969–70 and followed up through the national psychiatric case register until 1983 (Malmberg *et al.* 1998), and a similar Israeli study based on a preconscription cognitive and behavioural assessment during 1985–91 of 9724 male adolescents aged 16–17 and a follow-up through the psychiatric case register (Davidson *et al.* 1999). Follow-up studies of cohorts defined by a particular maternal exposure at a given time, e.g. the offspring of pregnant women exposed to acute undernutrition during the 1945 Dutch 'hunger winter' (Susser & Lin 1992), the stress of the 5-day *blitzkrieg* against Holland in 1940 (van Os & Selten 1998), radiation from the Nagasaki A-bomb in 1945 (Imamura *et al.* 1999), or prenatal rubella (Brown *et al.* 2001) provide further examples of rich research opportunities using cohort data.

Diagnosis

Diagnostic concepts have a critical role in the epidemiology of schizophrenia because: (i) a proportion of the variation in results of individual studies is caused by variation in diagnostic concepts and practices; (ii) the diagnostic classification of cases may not be comparable across studies; and (iii) in any particular study the diagnosis of schizophrenia may include or exclude conditions of uncertain nosological status such as acute schizophreniform episodes, schizoaffective disorders or other 'spectrum' disorders. In addition, the question of how and by whom the diagnosis was made is an important qualifier of the reported results.

Diagnosis-related bias is usually difficult to detect in past epidemiological research. Until the late 1960s, diagnostic rules were seldom explicitly stated and the description of assessment methods often lacked sufficient detail. As demonstrated by the US–UK diagnostic study (Cooper *et al.* 1972), concepts of schizophrenia in two different psychiatric cultures diverged to an extent that practically invalidated the comparisons. The World Health Organization (WHO) International Pilot Study of Schizophrenia (IPSS; World Health Organization 1973, 1979) examined the diagnostic variation across nine countries by applying a computerized reference classification, CATEGO (Wing *et al.* 1974), in addition to the clinical diagnoses made locally by psychiatrists. It transpired, reassuringly, that psychiatrists in the majority of settings were using similar diagnostic concepts of schizophrenia, broadly corresponding to the Kraepelin–Bleuler tradition. In most settings the core diagnostic concept of schizophrenia does not seem to have undergone major changes over time. In a reanalysis of Kraepelin's original cases from 1908, Jablensky *et al.* (1993) demonstrated that clinical data on dementia praecox and manic-depressive psychosis collected early this century could be coded and analysed in terms of CATEGO syndromes and that the agreement between the 1908 diagnosis of dementia praecox and the CATEGO classification of the same cases was 88.6%.

Since 1980, the comparability of epidemiological data on schizophrenia over time has been affected by the adoption of operational diagnostic criteria such as the Research Diagnostic Criteria (RDC), DSM-III, DSM-IIIR and DSM-IV. The introduction of such criteria has helped to resolve some old, and to create some new, diagnostic problems with epidemiological implications. Brockington et al. (1978) applied 10 different definitions of schizophrenia to the same clinical material and obtained an 11-fold difference in the frequency of the disorder, depending on the criteria chosen. Similarly, Stephens et al. (1982), using nine diagnostic systems, established that only 7% of the cases were diagnosed as schizophrenic by all systems. The DSM-III requirement of 6 months' prior duration of symptoms and an upper age limit at 45 for a first diagnosis of schizophrenia excluded from the incidence estimates as many as two-thirds of the cases which met the ICD-9 glossary definition of the disorder. ICD-10, which requires only 4 weeks' symptom duration, agrees well with DSM-IIIR and DSM-IV on the classification of 'core' cases of schizophrenia but the classifications may produce discrepant results in atypical or milder cases (Jablensky et al. 1999). Such differences may be relatively unimportant for clinical practice but are likely to result in serious bias in epidemiological and genetic studies. The inclusion of the 6 months' symptom duration criterion in the DSM classification aims to increase the homogeneity of patient samples and to minimize the false-positive diagnoses. However, this is not an unequivocal advantage for epidemiology. The application of restrictive diagnostic criteria at the case finding stage of surveys is likely to exclude potential 'true' cases that fall short of meeting the full set of criteria on initial examination. As a rule, initial overinclusion of false-positives is less damaging than exclusion of false-negatives in two-stage surveys because, once properly assessed at the second stage, false-positives can be eliminated from data analysis. In contrast, erroneously rejected cases are unlikely ever to be retrieved. Until the aetiology of schizophrenia is elucidated, or a validating pathognomonic lesion is established, the decision as to what constitutes 'true' schizophrenia will remain arbitrary. With regard to epidemiological studies, less restrictive criteria are preferable to strict exclusion rules because they allow for a broader spectrum of outcomes at the endpoint of observation. This greater variation at endpoint should help to identify outcome-based subgroups and to relate their characteristics to the initial symptoms and to various risk factors.

Investigators

Epidemiological studies of schizophrenia vary with regard to how and by whom potential cases are identified and diagnosed. Many of the earlier European studies had been carried out by a single investigator (usually a psychiatrist) or by a small group of researchers. This had the advantage of diagnostic consistency, although systematic bias could not be excluded. Clinician-led studies are less common in current research, where multicentre collaborative designs, large samples and cost considerations limit the use of such strategies. Lay interviewers or professionals other than psychiatrists are increasingly involved in case finding and interviewing, and the clinicians' role is often restricted to a diagnostic review of cases. The effects of interviewer-related variation (e.g. professional vs. lay interviewers) have only been studied in a limited way (Robins 1989). However, there is an increasing concern that lay interviewers using structured diagnostic interviews in community surveys are liable to commit response errors, especially regarding the rating of symptom severity (Regier et al. 1998).

Instruments

Instruments used in epidemiological research into the psychotic disorders differ with regard to purpose and scope, sources of data, output format and user. At a basic conceptual level, the most widely used current diagnostic instruments fall into three categories.

The first category comprises tools designed for screening for psychosis as part of two-phase surveys. At present, there is no generally agreed validated set of screening criteria that could serve as a 'gold standard' in case finding for schizophrenia. Based on a reanalysis of ECA data, Eaton et al. (1991) have suggested that a combination of DSM-III criterion A and 16 items from the Diagnostic Interview Schedule (DIS; Robins et al. 1988) might be capable of identifying two-thirds of the psychotic cases in a community survey, and that the addition of a single question about past psychiatric hospitalization could increase the 'hit' rate to nearly 90%. However, such a screening device is yet to be tested. A psychosis screening questionnaire (PSQ) developed for use by lay interviewers (Bebbington & Nayani 1995) has been shown to perform with a satisfactory positive predictive value of 91.2% and negative predictive value of 98.4%.

The second category of assessment tools includes fully structured interviews, such as the NIMH DIS (Robins et al. 1981) and the related WHO–Alcohol, Drug Abuse, and Mental Health Administration (ADAMHA) Composite International Diagnostic Interview (CIDI; Robins et al. 1988). Both have been designed to match specifically the diagnostic criteria of DSM-IIIR and ICD-10. These instruments were designed for use by non-psychiatric interviewers and clinical judgement is not required in their administration and scoring.

The third category includes semistructured interview schedules such as the Present State Examination (PSE; Wing et al. 1974) and the Schedules for Clinical Assessment in Neuropsychiatry (SCAN; Wing et al. 1990, 1998), which cover a very broad range of psychopathology and require clinical judgement for their administration and scoring. The data elicited by the SCAN can be processed by computer diagnostic algorithms providing ICD-10, DSM-IIIR and DSM-IV diagnoses.

Each type of instrument has both advantages and disadvantages. The main advantage of the DIS/CIDI is that it can be used by lay interviewers who have received brief (2 week) training. It has been shown as capable of achieving high interrater reliability and of generating standard diagnoses in a single-stage survey design. However, the range of psychopathology covered by DIS/CIDI and other similar instruments is restricted to the diagnostic system with which such instruments are interlocked. A major disadvantage is that their clinical validity, in terms of sensitivity and specificity in diagnosing schizophrenia, is questionable. The PSE-SCAN type of interview, on the other hand, allows a great amount of descriptive information to be collected and processed in alternative ways. Both the reliability and validity of the PSE are to a large extent a function of the training and skills of the interviewer. The main disadvantages of the PSE-SCAN system are that the interview is time-demanding, and that making a proper diagnosis often requires collateral information that may only be obtainable in a clinical setting. However, it should be noted that an abbreviated survey version of SCAN, which partly overcomes these limitations, is already available (Brugha *et al.* 1999).

Measures of morbidity

Depending on the type of cases included in the numerator and the time period covered, different aspects of morbidity are captured by indices of prevalence, incidence and morbid risk (disease expectancy). However, problems often arise in relation to the denominator (i.e. the population base from which the cases are recruited). Using as a denominator the total population size (all age groups) is appropriate when 'burden of disease' or service needs are being estimated. The total population is not an appropriate base when the objective is to measure incidence because the probabilities of disease onsets are not evenly distributed over the life span. The denominator therefore should reflect the pooled risks of developing schizophrenia within a given population and exclude age groups for which the risk equals or approximates zero. Three methods can be used to achieve this, depending on the design of the study. First, age correction can be applied, setting the lower limit for schizophrenia risk at 15 years. The upper limit is often set at age 54, but there is no reason why it could not be higher. Secondly, when determining cumulative incidence (morbid risk) in cohort studies, both the numerator and the denominator need to be adjusted by weighting each affected person in the numerator for average life expectancy at the age of ascertainment (or at the age at death for patients who had died prior to survey), as well as by adjusting the denominator for persons who had died as unaffected prior to the survey. Weinberg's abridged method of estimating person-years of exposure (*Bezugsziffer*, BZ) to the risk of disease (Weinberg 1925; Reid 1960) is still widely used. Thirdly, to enable comparisons of rates, the denominator may need to be recalculated to a standard population by direct or indirect standardization.

Although relatively simple statistical methods are available for standardization and adjustment, they have been inconsistently applied in schizophrenia research. Lack of proper standardization of morbidity measures introduces uncontrolled variation and may compromise the validity of comparisons across different studies. In the last decade, the epidemiological analysis of schizophrenia has been showing a trend towards increased use of statistical procedures that are currently standard in the epidemiology of other non-communicable diseases, such as relative risk, incidence ratios, multivariate regression, proportional hazards models, survival analysis, etc. This signals a gradual transition from descriptive to analytical or risk factor epidemiology of the disorder.

Descriptive epidemiology of schizophrenia

The descriptive epidemiology of schizophrenia still contains gaps but the contours of the overall picture have been laid down and enable some tentative conclusions.

Prevalence

The prevalence of a disorder is defined as the number of cases (per 1000 persons at risk) present in a population at a given time or over a defined period. Point prevalence refers to cases which are active (i.e. symptomatic) on a given date, or within a brief interval, with a census date as midpoint. Because cases in remission will usually be missed in a point prevalence survey, the assessment of the present mental state in census or birth cohort studies needs to be supplemented with information about past episodes of the disorder. This results in a lifetime prevalence index, or proportion of survivors affected (PSA). In disorders tending towards a continuous course, such as schizophrenia, point and lifetime prevalence estimates are closely similar or identical. The index of period prevalence, i.e. the number of cases per 1000 population that are active during a specified period (e.g. 6 months or 1 year) is less useful because it confounds point prevalence with incidence.

An overview of selected prevalence studies of schizophrenia spanning a period of some 60 years is given in Table 12.1. The studies differ in their methodology but have in common a high intensity of case finding (many of them were census investigations). Several studies included repeat surveys in which the original population was re-examined at some later time (the resulting follow-up prevalence figures are indicated in the table by an arrow).

The majority of the studies have produced prevalence figures in the range 1.4–4.6 per 1000 population at risk. Considering the many possible sources of variation, this range is fairly narrow. However, similar prevalence figures may mask important differences in incidence rates between populations with different mortality experiences, age structures and migration rates. Crude prevalence figures are difficult to interpret in the absence of such background demographic data. Therefore, it is unwarranted to assume that the modal prevalence rate emerging from the studies listed in Table 12.1, i.e. 1.4–4.6 per 1000, is the unqualified, 'true' rate of schizophrenia in those populations.

Table 12.1 Selected prevalence studies of schizophrenia.

Study	Country	Population	Method	Prevalence per 1000 population at risk
Surveys in developed countries				
Brugger (1931)	Germany	Area in Thuringia ($n = 37\,561$); age 10+	Census	2.4 (point)
Strömgren (1938); Bøjholm & Strömgren (1989)	Denmark	Island population ($n = 50\,000$)	Repeat census	3.9 → 3.3 (point)
Lemkau *et al.* (1943)	USA	Household sample	Census	2.9 (point)
Essen-Möller *et al.* (1956); Hagnell (1966)	Sweden	Community in southern Sweden	Repeat census	6.7 → 4.5 (point)
Crocetti *et al.* (1971)	Croatia	Sample of 9201 households	Census	5.9 (point)
Rotstein (1977)	Russia	Population sample ($n = 35\,590$)	Census	3.8 (lifetime)
Robins & Regier (1991)	USA	Aggregated data across five ECA sites	Sample survey	7.0 (point) 15.0 (lifetime)
Kendler & Walsh (1995)	Ireland	Roscommon County ($n = 32\,775$)	Register-based family study	Lifetime: 5.4 (males) 4.3 (females)
Jeffreys *et al.* (1997)	UK	London health district ($n = 112\,127$)	Census; interviews of a sample ($n = 172$)	5.1 (point)
Jablensky *et al.* (2000)	Australia	Four urban areas ($n = 1\,084\,978$)	Census; interviews of a sample ($n = 980$)	3.1–5.9 (point)* 3.9–6.9 (1 year)[†]
Surveys in developing countries				
Rin & Lin (1962); Lin *et al.* (1989)	Taiwan	Population sample	Repeat census	2.1 → 1.4 (point)
Bash & Bash-Liechti (1969)	Iran	Rural area ($n = 11\,585$)	Census	2.1 (point)
Dube & Kumar (1972)	India	Four areas in Agra ($n = 29\,468$)	Census	2.6 (point)
ICMR (1988)	India	Rural area ($n = 46\,380$)	Census	2.2 (point)
Padmavathi *et al.* (1987)	India	Urban ($n = 101\,229$)	Census	2.5 (point)
Salan (1992)	Indonesia	Slum area in West Jakarta ($n = 100\,107$)	Two-stage survey: (a) key informants (b) interview	1.4 (point)
Lee *et al.* (1990)	Korea	Urban and rural	Census	Lifetime: 3.0 (urban) 4.0 (rural)
Chen *et al.* (1993)	Hong Kong	Community sample ($n = 7229$)	DIS interviews	Lifetime: 1.2 (males) 1.3 (females)
Waldo (1999)	Kosrae (Micronesia)	Island population ($n = 5500$)	Key informants and clinic records; some interviews	6.8 (point), age 15+
Kebede & Alem (1999)	Ethiopia	District ($n = 227\,135$) south of Addis Ababa; mixed urban and rural	Two-stage survey: (a) door-to-door and key informants (b) SCAN interviews	7.1 (point), age 15–49

* All psychoses.
[†] Schizophrenia and other non-affective psychoses.

Incidence

The incidence rate of schizophrenia (annual number of new cases in a defined population per 1000 individuals at risk) is of greater interest than prevalence because its variation is far more sensitive to the effects of causal and risk factors. The estimation of incidence depends critically on the capacity to pinpoint disease onset or inception. There is no agreed definition of inception of schizophrenia and the idea of onset as some kind of a point event raises fundamental difficulties. Because the timing of the 'true' onset of the still hypothetical neural dysfunction that underlies schizophrenia is unknown, investigators have to operate with proxy events. The social onset (appearance of conspicuous behavioural abnormalities leading to consultation, admission or other action) rarely coincides with the onset of the earliest symptoms enabling a diagnosis of the disorder; the diagnostic symptoms are in many cases preceded by a prodromal subclinical phase of varying duration. Precursors of schizophrenia including developmental delays, cognitive abnormalities and behavioural oddities may appear very early in life but, at present, such developmental precursors cannot serve as reference points for dating onset (such precursors can only be identified *post hoc*). Thus, any point on the continuum spanning the prodromal phase, the appearance of psychotic symptoms and the social onset could be arbitrarily designated as the beginning of a schizophrenic illness. This continuum may extend over 2–6 years (Häfner *et al.* 1993) and inconsistencies in the ascertainment of the onset in individual cases may result in unreliable incidence estimates within or across studies. It is clearly important for epidemiology to design and agree on a procedure that ensures consistency in defining onset, e.g. as the point in time when the disorder becomes diagnosable according to specified criteria. A convention addressing this problem has not yet been adopted in incidence studies of schizophrenia. In many studies, the first hospital admission is still being used as an index of onset. This is difficult to sustain in view of the wide variation across individuals, settings and time as regards the time lag between first appearance of symptoms and first admission. A better approximation to the time of onset is provided by the first contact, i.e. the point at which some 'helping agency' is contacted by an individual with incipient psychotic illness. The majority of first contacts are ambulatory and often precede admission to hospital by many months. In a number of instances hospitalization may not take place at all. A version of this method was used in the WHO 10-country study (Jablensky *et al.* 1992) in which case finding targeted prospectively over 2 years first contacts with a variety of services, including many non-medical ones.

Table 12.2 presents the essential features of 11 incidence studies of schizophrenia. Leaving aside the rates based on the RDC or DSM-III definition of schizophrenia, the first admission and first contact rates range from 0.17 to 0.54 per 1000 population per year, i.e. show a threefold difference. There is a very close concordance among the Scandinavian rates (0.20–0.27

per 1000), which is probably because of the nearly complete enumeration of the cases, uniform diagnostic practices and accurate denominator data. Some of the lowest rates in Table 12.2 originate from studies involving non-European populations, e.g. Hindu and Moslem Indians in Mauritius (0.14 and 0.09 per 1000), as well as indigenous people in Taiwan (0.17 per 1000). Because the Mauritius data are on first hospital admissions, the low rates may have resulted from a nosocomial threshold. This does not apply to the Taiwan data, which were collected in a community survey. Two recent studies employing a polydiagnostic (International Classification of Diseases (ICD), RDC and DSM-III) classification illustrate the impact of the restrictive diagnostic criteria which, compared with ICD-9, leads to a threefold drop in the incidence rate for the same population.

To date, the only study that has generated directly comparable incidence data for different populations by using identical case finding and diagnostic procedures prospectively and simultaneously in 12 catchment areas is the WHO 10-country investigation (Sartorius *et al.* 1986; Jablensky *et al.* 1992). Incidence estimates in the WHO study were based on first-in-lifetime contacts with 'helping agencies' in the area (including traditional healers in the developing countries) which were screened and monitored over a 2-year period. Potential cases and key informants were interviewed using standardized instruments, and the onset of psychotic symptoms diagnostic of schizophrenia was ascertained for the majority of the patients (1022 out of the total 1379). For 86% of the 1022 patients the first appearance of diagnostic symptoms of schizophrenia was within a year of the first contact and therefore the first-contact rate could serve as a reasonable approximation to the onset rate. The rates for eight catchment areas are shown in Table 12.3.

The differences between the rates for broadly (ICD-9) defined schizophrenia were significant ($P < 0.001$, two-tailed test) while those for the narrow, or 'nuclear', schizophrenia syndrome were not significant. No consistent differences were found between cases meeting the broad clinical criteria and the cases classified by the computer algorithm CATEGO as 'nuclear' schizophrenia (class S +) with regard to the course and outcome of the disorder or the type of onset (acute or insidious). Therefore, the similar incidence rates across the study areas do not imply that schizophrenia is homogeneous with regard to its prognosis in those populations, nor is there a reason to assume that the cases meeting the narrow S + criteria are in any sense phenotypically 'purer' expressions of schizophrenia, in contrast to cases meeting the broader clinical criteria but not S + 0. The salient aspect of the WHO findings is not the lack of statistically significant differences in the rates of CATEGO S + schizophrenia, but rather the narrow range of variation (0.16–0.42 per 1000) in the incidence of schizophrenia when standard case definitions, case finding procedures and assessment methods are used across very different populations. In recent years, replications of the design and methods of the WHO have been carried out with very similar results by investigators in India, the Caribbean and the UK (Table 12.3).

Table 12.2 Selected incidence studies of schizophrenia.

Study	Country	Population	Method	Annual rate per 1000
Surveys in industrialized countries				
Ødegaard (1946a)	Norway	Total population	First admissions 1926–35 ($n = 14231$)	0.24
Helgason (1964)	Iceland	Total population	First admissions 1966–67 ($n = 2388$)	0.27
Häfner & Reimann (1970)	Germany	City of Mannheim ($n = 330000$)	Case register	0.54
Lieberman (1974)	Russia	Moscow district ($n = 248000$)	Follow-back of prevalent cases	0.20 (male) 0.19 (female)
Castle *et al.* (1991)	UK	London (Camberwell)	Case register	0.25 (ICD) 0.17 (RDC) 0.08 (DSM-III)
Nicole *et al.* (1992)	Canada	Area in Quebec ($n = 338300$)	First admissions	0.31 (ICD) 0.09 (DSM-III)
McNaught *et al.* (1997)	UK	London health district ($n = 112127$)	2 censuses, 5 years apart	0.21 (DSM-IIIR)
Brewin *et al.* (1997)	UK	Nottingham	2 cohorts of first contacts (1978–80 and 1992–94)	$0.25 \rightarrow 0.29$ (all psychoses) $0.14 \rightarrow 0.09$ (ICD-10 schizophrenia)
Surveys in developing countries				
Raman & Murphy (1972)	Mauritius	Total population ($n = 257000$)	First admissions	0.24 (Africans) 0.14 (Indian Hindus) 0.09 (Indian Moslems)
Lin *et al.* (1989)	Taiwan	3 communities ($n = 39024$)	Household survey	0.17
Rajkumar *et al.* (1993)	India	Area in Madras ($n = 43097$)	Door-to-door survey and key informants	0.41
Hickling & Rodgers-Johnson (1995)	Jamaica	Total population ($n = 2.46$ million)	First contacts	0.24 ('broad') 0.21 ('restrictive')
Mahy *et al.* (1999)	Barbados	Total population ($n = 262000$)	First contacts	0.32 ('broad') 0.28 ('restrictive')

First-episode psychosis

The increased interest in the early detection and treatment of first episodes of psychosis has been bolstered by the hypothesis that the course and outcome of the early stages of a schizophrenic illness may have a pathoplastic effect on its subsequent course. More specifically, it has been proposed that excitotoxic neurotransmitter release and neuroendocrine stress responses during an early episode of manifest psychosis may induce irreversible changes in the connectivity between neural networks (Lieberman 1999). As an extension of this hypothesis, it has been suggested that a behavioural or pharmacological interven-tion prior to the onset of psychotic symptoms might delay or, in some cases, prevent the onset of schizophrenia (McGorry *et al.* 1996). Some evidence has been presented that a longer period between the first onset of psychotic symptoms and the initiation of treatment (duration of untreated psychosis, or DUP) correlates with increased time to remission and poor response to treatment (Loebel *et al.* 1992), but several other studies have failed to replicate this effect. None of the hypotheses referred to above have been properly tested, yet some studies focusing on the earliest manifestations of psychosis have highlighted novel phenomena, such as a preonset deterioration in cognitive performance which then remains static (Goldberg *et al.* 1993), early

Table 12.3 Annual incidence rates per 1000 population at risk, age 15–54, for a 'broad' and a 'narrow' case definition of schizophrenia (WHO 10-country study).

Country	Area	'Broad' definition (ICD-9)			'Restrictive' definition (CATEGO S+)		
		Male	Female	Both sexes	Male	Female	Both sexes
Denmark	Aarhus	0.18	0.13	0.16	0.09	0.05	0.07
India	Chandigarh (rural area)	0.37	0.48	0.42	0.13	0.09	0.11
	Chandigarh (urban area)	0.34	0.35	0.35	0.08	0.11	0.09
Ireland	Dublin	0.23	0.21	0.22	0.10	0.08	0.09
Japan	Nagasaki	0.23	0.18	0.20	0.11	0.09	0.10
Russia	Moscow	0.25	0.31	0.28	0.03	0.03	0.02
UK	Nottingham	0.28	0.15	0.22	0.17	0.12	0.14
USA	Honolulu	0.18	0.14	0.16	0.10	0.08	0.09

co-occurrence of both 'positive' and 'negative' symptoms (Gupta *et al.* 1997a), significant decline in social functioning (Häfner *et al.* 1999), and a general malleability of dysfunction through appropriate behavioural interventions and low-dose time-limited pharmacological treatment (Szymanski *et al.* 1996). All this suggests that clinical research bridging the gap between epidemiological investigations of risk factors or antecedents of disease and individual pathways to psychotic illness may contribute importantly to the understanding and management of the early course of schizophrenia.

Morbid risk (disease expectancy)

Morbid risk is the probability (expressed as a percentage) that an individual born into a particular population or group will develop the disease if he/she survives through the entire period of risk for that disease (15–54 in the instance of schizophrenia). If age- and sex-specific incidence rates are available, lifetime disease expectancy can be estimated directly by summing up the rates across the age groups within the period of risk. An indirect approximation to disease expectancy can be obtained from census data using the so-called abridged method of Weinberg (1925):

$$P = \frac{A}{B - \left(B_0 + \frac{1}{2}B_m\right)},$$

where P is disease expectancy (%), A the number of prevalent cases, B the total population surveyed, B_0 persons who have not yet entered the risk period and B_m persons within the risk period.

A modification of Weinberg's method, proposed by Strömgren (1935) and by Bøjholm and Strömgren (1989), weights the numerator for the excess mortality observed among schizophrenic patients. Whether estimated directly from age-specific incidence rates, or indirectly from prevalence data, disease expectancy enables a more reliable comparison of the occurrence of schizophrenia in different populations than the prevalence or incidence rates. Notwithstanding different methods of data collection, the figures suggest considerable consistency of the disease expectancy of schizophrenia across populations and over time. Excluding the northern Swedish isolate and a few other 'outliers', the highest risk ratio (highest–lowest morbid risk) is about 5.0; for the WHO 10-country study it is 2.9 (ICD-9 schizophrenia) and 2.0 (CATEGO S+). Most studies have produced morbid risk estimates in the range 0.50–1.60. Therefore, the often quoted 'rule of thumb' that the morbid risk for schizophrenia is about 1% seems to be consistent with the evidence.

Populations and groups with high and low rates of schizophrenia

The question of whether significant differences exist among populations in the 'true' rate of schizophrenia (Torrey 1987) has no simple answer. Depending on the population size or samples being compared, statistically significant differences are bound to occur. Whether such differences are epidemiologically meaningful is open to interpretation. Because many confounding factors and selection bias can inflate or deflate the incidence and morbid risk estimates, comparisons of schizophrenia rates across populations should be interpreted with caution, taking into account the methods applied and the demography of the populations concerned. For example, it would be a mistake to interpret the sevenfold difference in the estimated population incidence of schizophrenia reported from two of the ECA study sites as evidence of large variation in the incidence of schizophrenia in the USA (Tien & Eaton 1992). The high rates reported from the ECA study in the USA (Robins & Regier 1991), coupled with a 13-fold difference in the rates for age group 18–24 across the sites, remain unexplained. Above all, inconsistencies in the administration of the diagnostic instrument by lay interviewers are likely to have affected the diagnostic classification of cases. In the National Comorbidity Survey (NCS), diagnoses of 'non-affective psychosis' by computer algorithm based on CIDI (a derivative of the DIS) were found to agree poorly with clinicians' diagnoses based on telephone reinterviews, and to result in discrepant estimates of the lifetime prevalence of both 'narrowly' and 'broadly' defined non-affective psychotic illness (Kendler *et al.* 1996a). A different problem is highlighted by a recent incidence study based on a 1959–67 birth cohort in Alameda County, CA, USA (Bresnahan *et al.* 2000). The study reported unusually high rates for males aged 15–29 but, because of the wide confidence intervals, the authors could not rule out the possibility that the high male rates may have resulted from chance.

With such methodological caveats, true 'outlier' populations nevertheless do exist. Very high rates (2–3 times the national or regional rate) have been reported for population isolates, such as an area in northern Sweden (Böök *et al.* 1978) and several areas in Finland (Hovatta *et al.* 1999). High rates have also been described in an area in Croatia, characterized by a high level of emigration during the nineteenth and early twentieth century (Crocetti *et al.* 1971). Certain migrant populations, e.g. the African-Caribbeans in the UK (Harrison *et al.* 1997), and the Surinamese in the Netherlands (Selten *et al.* 1997), have been reported to have an unusually high prevalence of schizophrenia, exceeding 5–7 times the average rate in the general population of the host country, as well as the rate in the country of origin.

At the other extreme, a virtual absence of schizophrenia and a moderate or high rate of depression have been observed among the Hutterites in South Dakota, a Protestant sect whose members live in closely knit endogamous communities, largely sheltered from the outside world (Eaton & Weil 1955; Torrey 1995; Nimgaonkar *et al.* 2000). Negative selection for schizoid individuals who fail to adjust to the communal lifestyle and eventually migrate without leaving progeny has been suggested, but not definitively proven, as an explanation. Low rates have also been reported for certain Pacific Island populations (Rin & Lin 1962) but uncertainties about the completeness of case finding makes the interpretation of such reports problematic. Two surveys in Taiwan (see Table 12.2), separated by 15 years during which major social changes took place, found that the prevalence of schizophrenia decreased from 2.1 to 1.4 per 1000. In both surveys, the aboriginal Taiwanese had significantly lower rates than the mainland Chinese who had migrated to the island after World War II.

The general conclusion is that according to the great majority of studies, the prevalence and incidence rates of schizophrenia are similar across populations. However, a small number of populations have been identified that clearly deviate from this central tendency. The magnitude of these deviations is modest compared with the differences observed across populations with regard to other multifactorial diseases such as diabetes, ischaemic heart disease or cancer, where 10- to 30-fold differences in prevalence across populations are not uncommon. Such 'outlier' population groups with high or low incidence of schizophrenia are of considerable interest as potentially informative settings for the search for susceptibility genes, as well as for studies of culture–gene interactions over multiple generations.

Secular trends in the incidence and prevalence of schizophrenia

The rarity of descriptions of schizophrenia in the medical literature before the eighteenth century has led to speculation that the condition had not existed (Torrey 1980), or was rare (Hare 1983), until the industrial revolution. The earliest references to psychotic states clearly matching the clinical picture of schizophrenia can be found in Pinel (1803) and Haslam (1809). Examination of the nineteenth century asylum statistics suggests that 'monomaniac insanity', 'delusional insanity' and 'ordinary dementia' (i.e. the diagnostic groups likely to contain schizophrenic patients in the pre-Kraepelinian era) composed between 5.3% and 18.9% of all institutionalized patients (Jablensky 1986). The records of the Munich University Psychiatric Clinic under the direction of Kraepelin in 1908 indicate that in the course of a year dementia praecox accounted for only 9.1% of the first admissions among men and for 7.3% among women (Jablensky *et al.* 1993). It is likely that during much of the nineteenth century schizophrenia was less conspicuous than it is today, because of the much higher prevalence of organic brain diseases such as general paresis. The hypothesis that schizophrenia is of recent origin is not plausible, considering the genetics of the disorder and its similar rates of occurrence in diverse populations. However, it is possible that the number of people diagnosed and hospitalized as schizophrenic increased rapidly during the early decades of the twentieth century. Whether the increase was real (e.g. resulting from a decreasing mortality, rising incidence, or both) or spurious (increased use of the diagnosis, social pressure to institutionalize the mentally ill) remains unclear.

The question of whether long-term trends in the incidence of schizophrenia can be detected has attracted interest following reports since 1985 indicating a 40% or more reduction in the first admissions with a diagnosis of schizophrenia in Denmark, UK and New Zealand over the last three decades. A decline in the hospitalization rate for schizophrenia was first reported by Weeke and Strömgren (1978), who noted that the national census of hospitalized patients with schizophrenia in Denmark had dropped from 6200 in 1957 to 4500 in 1972. The more recent data can be summed up as follows: (i) a trend of diminishing administrative incidence rates (both first hospital admissions and first contacts with a psychiatric case register) has been demonstrated but the data are inconsistent as regards the age- and sex-specific rate reduction; (ii) this trend has been found in large national databases, e.g. in Denmark, Scotland, England and Wales, but has not been consistently replicated at local or regional level: two case registers have identified a downward trend (Eagles *et al.* 1988; de Alarcon *et al.* 1992), another two have shown increases (Castle *et al.* 1991; Bamrah *et al.* 1991), and one has reported no change (Harrison *et al.* 1991); (iii) studies in which research diagnoses (RDC, DSM-III or CATEGO) were made (Bamrah *et al.* 1991; Castle *et al.* 1991) have shown no decline in rates; (iv) in the areas where reduction of schizophrenia has been reported, there have been during the same period concomitant reductions in the total number of beds and first admissions; (v) in several areas increases have been reported in the mortality of schizophrenic patients (Munk-Jørgensen & Mortensen 1992), in the diagnoses of paranoid and reactive psychoses or borderline states on first admission (Munk-Jørgensen 1986; Der et al. 1990; Harrison et al. 1991) and in the delay between first outpatient contact and first hospital admission (Harrison et al. 1991). Although a trend of diminishing rates of schizophrenia cannot be excluded, the combined effect of several factors could explain the observed changes: variations in the definition of first admission or first contact; changes in diagnostic practices over time; changes in the treatment modalities and settings; increases in the mortality of schizophrenic patients; and changes in the age composition of the populations concerned. An increasing reluctance to make a diagnosis of schizophrenia on first admission has been noted among Danish psychiatrists (Munk-Jørgensen 1986) and the same may be occurring in the diagnostic practice in other countries. The reported size of the compensatory increase of other diagnoses on first admission is sufficient to account for the drop in schizophrenia diagnoses. In addition, the time lag in the diagnosis of schizophrenia, which in many instances amounts to years after the first service contact, may artificially depress the first admission rates for the most recent years of the observation period. The gradual 'disappearance' of schizophrenia therefore is a rather unlikely hypothesis.

Comorbid association with other diseases

The concept of comorbidity refers to the simultaneous presence in an individual of two or more nosologically different disorders which may be either coincident or causally related. In schizophrenia, comorbidity comprises: (i) relatively common medical problems and diseases that tend to occur among schizophrenic patients more frequently as a consequence of dysfunctional behaviour, poor self-care or medical neglect; and (ii) specific disorders that may have a putative pathogenetic relationship with schizophrenia itself.

Physical disease is common among patients with schizophrenia but is rarely diagnosed. Between 46% and 80% of inpatients, and between 20% and 43% of outpatients with schizophrenia, have been found in different surveys to have concurrent medical illnesses. In 46% of the patients a physical illness was thought to aggravate the mental state, and in 7% it was life-threatening (Adler & Griffith 1991). In a study of acute admissions of patients with schizophrenia, 10% were found to be dehydrated, 33% had hypokalaemia and 66% had elevated serum muscle enzymes (Hatta et al. 1999). Schizophrenic patients have a dramatically increased risk of poisoning with psychotropic drugs (50-fold for men and 20-fold for women, according to Mäkikirö et al. 1998). In addition to a generally increased susceptibility to infection, especially pulmonary tuberculosis prior to hospitalization (Baldwin 1979), schizophrenic patients have higher than expected rates of

diabetes, arteriosclerotic disease and myocardial infarction (Saugstad & Ødegaard 1979), middle ear disease (Mason & Winton 1995), irritable bowel syndrome (Gupta et al. 1997b), some rare genetic or idiopathic disorders such as acute intermittent porphyria (Crimlisk 1997) and HIV (5–7% estimated prevalence in patients with schizophrenia in the USA; Sewell 1996). This heavy burden of medical morbidity remains largely under-recognized because schizophrenic patients with comorbid conditions are usually excluded from research studies (Jeste et al. 1996).

'Negative' comorbidity (i.e. a lower than expected rate of occurrence of diseases) has been demonstrated for rheumatoid arthritis (Österberg 1978; Eaton et al. 1992), although a recent record linkage study (Lauerma et al. 1998) failed to replicate this. Several population-based record linkage studies have shown that schizophrenic patients have a significantly lower incidence of cancer, compared with the general population (Dupont et al. 1986; Mortensen 1994; Lawrence et al. 2000a). The lower rates are particularly pronounced for lung cancer in male patients. There is no obvious explanation for this finding but some protective effect of long-term neuroleptic medication has been suggested (Mortensen 1987).

Numerous studies have reported a significantly increased frequency of dysmorphic features and minor physical anomalies, including high-steepled palate, malformed ears, epicanthus, single palmar crease and finger and toe abnormalities, which may result from deviations in fetal development during the first gestational trimester (Murphy & Owen 1996; Ismail et al. 1998). A variety of rare organic brain disorders and anomalies have been described to occur in association with schizophrenia, including basal ganglia calcification (Francis & Freeman 1984; Flint & Goldstein 1992), aqueductus Sylvii stenosis (Reveley & Reveley 1983; Roberts et al. 1983; O'Flaithbheartaigh et al. 1994), cerebral hemiatrophy (Puri et al. 1994; Honer et al. 1996), corpus callosum agenesis (Lewis et al. 1988), schizencephaly (Alexander et al. 1997), septal cysts (Lewis & Mezey 1985), acute intermittent porphyria (Propping 1983), coeliac disease (Dohan 1966), and Marfan syndrome (Sirota et al. 1990). Most of these associations have been observed in single case studies; epidemiological evidence of a higher than chance co-occurrence with schizophrenia has so far only been provided for epilepsy (Bruton et al. 1994; Bredkaer et al. 1998) and metachromatic leukodystrophy (Hyde et al. 1992).

Comorbidity with substance use

Substance abuse is by far the most common comorbid problem among schizophrenic patients (Strakowski et al. 1993; Rosenthal 1998) and involves alcohol, stimulants, anxiolytics, hallucinogens, antiparkinsonian drugs, as well as caffeine and tobacco. In the WHO 10-country study (Jablensky et al. 1992), a history of alcohol use in the year preceding the first contact was elicited in 57% of the male patients, and in three of the study areas drug abuse (mainly cannabis and cocaine) was reported by 24–41% of the patients. Cannabis abuse exacerbates the symptoms, may precipitate relapse (Linszen *et al.* 1994) and was a significant predictor of poor 2-year outcome in the WHO study. Heavy cannabis use prior to the manifest onset of psychotic symptoms has been consistently reported in over 60% of patients with a first episode of schizophrenia (Allebeck *et al.* 1993; Silver & Abboud 1994). In a recent Australian prevalence study of psychoses (Jablensky *et al.* 2000), 38.7% of the male patients and 17.0% of the female patients with schizophrenia had a comorbid lifetime diagnosis of substance abuse or dependence. The prevalence of cigarette smoking among schizophrenia patients was 73.2% in males and 56.3% in females (compared with 27.3% and 20.3%, respectively, in the general population).

The interactions between the pharmacological effects of drugs of abuse and the neurocognitive deficits that are thought to be intrinsic to schizophrenia remain little understood (Tracy *et al.* 1995). Recent research on the interactions between the nicotinic receptor and the glutamatergic and dopaminergic systems has led to the hypothesis that smoking in schizophrenic patients might be an attempt at self-medication reinforced by the modulatory and short-term normalizing effect of nicotine on neurocognitive deficits such as defective sensory gating (Dalack *et al.* 1998). Endogenous cannabinoids, which downregulate gamma-aminobutyric acid (GABA) release in hippocampal neurones (Wilson & Nicoll 2001), have been found elevated in schizophrenia patients independent of recency of cannabis use, suggesting an abnormality in cannabinoid receptors and signalling (Leweke *et al.* 1999). However, the question of whether excessive cannabis use can precipitate or advance the onset of a schizophrenic illness in vulnerable individuals, or is a self-medication phenomenon analogous to nicotine abuse and secondary to a developing psychosis, has not been unequivocally answered. Studies using small samples suggest that, among acutely psychotic patients, cannabis users are more likely to have a higher familial risk of schizophrenia than non-users (McGuire *et al.* 1995). In a recent study using an epidemiological design, the prevalence of cannabis use in a relatively large sample of first-episode patients (*n* = 232) was 13%, twice that found among matched normal controls. Approximately equal proportions among the early psychosis patients had been using cannabis for several years prior to the onset of symptoms, had started using it concurrently with the development of psychosis and had initiated cannabis use following the onset of schizophrenia (Hambrecht & Häfner 2000). Thus, analysis of the temporal sequence of cannabis use and psychosis onset appears unlikely to help resolve the causality issue without recourse to biological vulnerability markers, such as polymorphisms in the cannabinoid receptor type 1 (*CNR1*) gene that may characterize a particular 'cannabis-sensitive' subset of schizophrenia patients (Krebs *et al.* 2002).

Mortality

Excess mortality among schizophrenic patients has been docu-

mented by epidemiological studies on large cohorts. National case register data for Norway indicate that while the total mortality of psychiatric patients decreased between 1926–41 and 1950–74, the relative mortality of patients with schizophrenia remained unchanged at a level more than twice that of the general population (Ødegaard 1946a). Results from more recent cohort and record linkage studies in European countries and North America suggest that the excess mortality of people with schizophrenia is not decreasing and may, indeed, be increasing (Lawrence *et al.* 2000b; Ösby *et al.* 2000). Successive Danish national cohorts (Mortensen & Juel 1993) show an alarming trend of increasing mortality in first-admission patients with schizophrenia. The 5-year cumulated standard mortality ratio (SMR) increased from 530 (males) and 227 (females) in 1971–73 to 779 (males) and 452 (females) in 1980–82. Particularly striking was the SMR of 164 for male schizophrenics in the first year after the diagnosis was made. A meta-analysis of 18 studies (Brown 1997) resulted in a crude mortality rate of 189 deaths per 10 000 population per year and a 10-year survival rate of 81%. Current SMRs for patients with schizophrenia are of the order of 260–300, which corresponds to more than 20% reduction in life expectancy compared with the general population (S. Brown *et al.* 2000). SMRs as high as 376 (men) and 314 (women) have been observed among homeless people with schizophrenia (Babidge *et al.* 2001). The significantly higher mortality among males, as compared with females, is almost entirely explained by excess suicides and accidents. Unnatural causes apart, there is a nearly fivefold increase (SMR 468) of 'avoidable' natural deaths, caused by hypertension, cerebrovascular disease and smoking-related disease (S. Brown *et al.* 2000). The phenomenon of 'sudden unexplained death' among schizophrenic patients (Appleby *et al.* 2000) may be related to cardiotoxic effects of antipsychotic drugs, especially in patients receiving more than one antipsychotic concurrently (Waddington *et al.* 1998). The single most common cause of death among schizophrenic patients at present is suicide (aggregated SMR 960 in males and 680 in females) which accounts, on average, for 28% of the excess mortality in schizophrenia (Mortensen & Juel 1993). The actual mortality as a result of suicide is likely to be higher because a proportion of the deaths classified as accidental or of undetermined cause are probably suicides. Thus, the suicide rate in schizophrenic patients is at least equal to, or may be higher than, the suicide rate in major depression. Several risk factors have been suggested as relatively specific to schizophrenic suicide: being young and male, experiencing a chronic disabling illness with multiple relapses and remissions, realistic awareness of the deteriorating course of the condition, comorbid substance use and loss of faith in treatment (Caldwell & Gottesman 1990). Data from Scotland (Geddes & Juszczak 1995) point to a trend of an increasing suicide rate in schizophrenic patients, mostly within the first year after discharge. This trend seems to parallel the significant reductions in the number of psychiatric beds. Whether this new wave of increasing suicide mortality can be attributed to the transition from hospital to community management of schizophrenia remains to be established.

Fertility

The low fertility of men and women diagnosed with schizophrenia has been extensively documented by Essen-Möller (1935), Larson and Nyman (1973) and Ødegaard (1980). The average number of children fathered by schizophrenic men was 0.9 in Sweden, and the average number of live births over the entire reproductive period of women treated for schizophrenia in Norway during 1936–75 was 1.8, compared with 2.2 for the general female population. Similar results have been reported from Germany (Hilger *et al.* 1983) and Australia (McGrath *et al.* 1999). Yet this phenomenon does not seem to be either universal or consistent over time. According to the WHO 10-country study (Jablensky *et al.* 1992), the fertility of women with schizophrenia in India did not differ from that of women in the general population within the same age groups and geographical areas. An increase in the fertility of women with schizophrenia has been observed in recent decades (Nimgaonkar *et al.* 1997) and is likely to be sustained as a result of the deinstitutionalization of the mentally ill. Although men with schizophrenia continue to be reproductively disadvantaged, at least two studies (Lane *et al.* 1995; Waddington & Youssef 1996) have found a higher than average fertility among married schizophrenic men. The results of studies which have examined the fertility of biological relatives of probands with schizophrenia suggest that clinically asymptomatic parents and siblings of patients have higher than average fertility (Fañanás & Bertranpetit 1995; Srinivasan & Padmavati 1997). Such findings are sometimes invoked to explain the maintenance of a stable incidence of schizophrenia in populations despite the reduced fertility of affected probands.

Analytical epidemiology of schizophrenia: risk factors and antecedents

Risk factors influence the probability of occurrence of a disease or its outcome without necessarily being direct causes. Because the strongest proof of causation is the experiment, the identification of risk factors that are modifiable by intervention and may result in a reduced incidence or a better outcome is the ultimate aim of risk factor epidemiology. This is still a remote aim in schizophrenia but current research is beginning to address the issue. The epidemiological classification of initiating pathogenetic and interacting risk factors (Khoury *et al.* 1993) is not readily applicable to schizophrenia, as the role of many putative risk factors is still insufficiently understood. A provisional grouping of such factors into familial, sociodemographic, pre-, peri- and early postnatal, neurodevelopmental and neurocognitive variables may be more appropriate to the present state of knowledge (Table 12.4).

Age and sex

There is abundant evidence that schizophrenia may have its onset at almost any age – in childhood as well as past middle age

– although the vast majority of onsets fall within the interval of 15–54 years of age. Neither childhood-onset schizophrenia (onset before age 12) nor late-onset schizophrenia (onset after age 50) present with any clinical features or risk factors that are qualitatively distinct from those characterizing schizophrenia arising in young adults (Brodaty *et al.* 1999; Nicolson & Rapoport 1999; Palmer *et al.* 2001), with the possible exception of psychotic disorganization symptoms being more likely to characterize early-onset cases and systematized paranoid delusions being predominant in late-onset cases (Häfner *et al.* 2001). With regard to age at onset, schizophrenia appears to be a continuum, where variation is consistent with a model incorporating random developmental effects and environmental experiences unique to the individual (Kendler *et al.* 1996b).

Onsets in men peak steeply in the age group 20–24; thereafter the rate of inception remains more or less constant at a lower level. In women, a less prominent peak in the age group 20–24 is followed by an increase in incidence in age groups older than 35. While the age-specific incidence up to the mid-thirties is significantly higher in men, the male–female ratio becomes inverted with age, reaching 1 : 1.9 for onsets after age 40 and 1 : 4 or even 1 : 6 for onsets after age 60. Scandinavian population-based studies which have followed up cohorts at risk into a very old age (over 85) reported a higher cumulated lifetime risk in women, compared with men (Helgason & Magnusson 1989). In the WHO 10-country study (Jablensky *et al.* 1992), the cumulated risks for males and females up to age 54 were approximately equal.

An earlier age at onset in men than in women has been reported in over 50 studies (Häfner *et al.* 1998) and such observations have stimulated theorizing and empirical studies into a possible protective effect of oestrogen via reduction of the sensitivity of the D_2 receptor in the brain (Häfner *et al.* 1998). Data from the WHO 10-country study (Jablensky & Cole 1997) show that age at onset is influenced by multiple interacting factors including sex, premorbid personality traits, family history of psychosis and marital status. The unconfounding of such interactions resulted in a significant attenuation of the effect of sex on age at onset. Thus, the observed sex difference in age at onset is unlikely to be an invariant biological characteristic of the disease. Within families with two or more affected members with schizophrenia, no significant differences in age at onset have been found between male and female siblings (DeLisi *et al.* 1987; Albus & Maier 1995) and, in some populations, e.g. India, the male–female difference in the frequency of onsets in the younger age groups is attenuated or even inverted (Murthy *et al.* 1998).

There is therefore no unequivocal evidence of consistent sex differences in the symptoms of schizophrenia, including the frequency of positive and negative symptoms. Although sex differences have been described in relation to premorbid adjustment (better premorbid functioning in women), occurrence of brain abnormalities (more frequent in men), course (a higher percentage of remitting illness episodes and shorter hospital stay in women) and outcome (higher survival rate in the community, less

Table 12.4 Risk factors and antecedents of schizophrenia.

Risk factor or antecedent	Estimated effect size (odds ratio or relative risk)	Reference
Familial (family member with schizophrenia)		
Biological parent	7.0–10.0	Mortensen *et al.* (1999)
Two parents	29.0	Kringlen *et al.* 1978)
Monozygotic twin	40.8	Cardno *et al.* (1999)
Dizygotic twin	5.3	Cardno *et al.* (1999)
Non-twin sibling	7.3	Gottesman *et al.* (1987)
Second-degree relative	1.6–2.8	Gottesman *et al.* (1987)
Social and demographic		
Low socioeconomic status	3.0	Eaton (1974)
Single marital status	3.9	van Os *et al.* (2000)
Stressful life events	1.5	
Migrant/minority status (e.g. African-Caribbeans in UK)	>7.0	Harrison *et al.* (1997)
Urban birth	2.1–4.2	Mortensen *et al.* (1999)
		Eaton *et al.* (2000)
Winter birth	1.1	Mortensen *et al.* (1999)
Prenatal, perinatal and early postnatal		
Obstetric complications ('non-optimality' summary score)	4.6	Hultman *et al.* (1997)
Maternal respiratory infection, second trimester	2.1	A.S. Brown *et al.* (2000)
Birth weight < 2000 g	3.0	Byrne *et al.* (2000)
Birth weight < 2500 g	2.9	Wahlbeck *et al.* (2001)
Severe malnutrition during pregnancy	2.6	Susser & Lin (1992)
Gestation < 37 weeks	2.5	Ichiki *et al.* (2000)
Perinatal hypoxic brain damage	4.6–6.9	Zornberg *et al.* (2000)
		Jones *et al.* (1998)
Neurodevelopmental and neurocognitive		
Early CNS infection	4.8	Rantakallio *et al.* (1997)
Epilepsy	11.1	Mäkikyrö *et al.* (1998)
Low IQ (< 74)	8.6	David *et al.* (1997)
Difficulty in maintaining close personal relationships	30.7	Malmberg *et al.* (1998)
Preference for solitary play, age 4–6	2.1	Jones *et al.* (1994)
Speech and educational problems, age < 12	2.8	Jones *et al.* (1994)
Low score on Continuous Performance Test	3.3	Egan *et al.* (2000)

disability in women), such differences are consistent with normal sexual dimorphism in brain development (Noupoulos *et al.* 2000), as well as with learned gender-assigned social roles, and do not invoke the need for a sex-specific aetiological factor.

Genetic risk

The contribution of genetic liability to the aetiology of schizophrenia is one of the few firmly established facts about the disorder. As pointed out by Shields (1977), 'no environmental indicator predicts a raised risk of schizophrenia in small or moderate-sized samples of persons not already known to be genetically related to a schizophrenic'. The genetic epidemiology of schizophrenia is underpinned by heritability estimates from twin, adoptive and family studies which have been consistently at 0.80 or higher (Cardno *et al.* 1999). Because the concordance rate in monozygotic twins (MZ) does not exceed 50%,

it is widely assumed that environmental factors also contribute to its pathogenesis, but no single environmental variable has yet been demonstrated to be either necessary or sufficient for causation. Three models of the joint effects of genotype and environment have been proposed (Kendler & Eaves 1986):

1 the effects of predisposing genes and environmental factors are additive and increase the risk of disease in a linear fashion;

2 genes control the sensitivity of the brain to environmental insults; and

3 genes influence the likelihood of an individual's exposure to environmental pathogens, e.g. by fostering certain personality traits.

Attempts to identify major genetic loci by linkage analysis of multiply affected pedigrees or of affected sib pairs have produced inconsistent results. Few of the positive linkage findings have stood the test of replication (DeLisi & Crow 1999). Similarly, numerous association studies have been beset with problems of type I or II error brought about by population stratification, diagnostic misclassification and questionable biological plausibility of the candidate genes. The majority of investigators today share the view that schizophrenia is one of the genetically complex disorders, characterized by oligo- or polygenic inheritance, likely locus heterogeneity, incomplete penetrance and high population frequency of the disease-causing alleles (Hyman *et al.* 1999). The relationship between genotype and phenotype in schizophrenia is likely to be mediated by complex causal pathways involving gene–gene and gene–environment interactions, 'programmable' neural substrate and stochastic events. Under such circumstances, the gene effects might be too weak to be detectable through the clinical diagnostic phenotype in any but very large samples (Lander & Schork 1994).

In view of such constraints, alternative clinical and epidemiological strategies have been proposed in order to circumvent the need for excessively large pooled samples (such samples may be confounded by latent population differences and by variations in ascertainment methods and diagnostic assessment). One such strategy aims at resolving the locus heterogeneity problem through search and investigation of genetically homogeneous populations in which schizophrenia segregates in multiply affected family groups of common ancestry – as is the case in isolates or rare sporadic lineages. Schizophrenia in such families is more likely to be linked to a small number of predisposing loci, some of which may be of moderate to strong effect, detectable by screening for alleles shared among affected individuals originating from common ancestors. To date, this strategy has produced mixed results, indicating that multiple susceptibility loci operate even in isolated populations (Hovatta *et al.* 1999). However, at least one study has detected linkage to a major susceptibility locus (Brzustowicz *et al.* 2000).

Another strategy proceeds from the assumption that the ICD-10 or DSM-IV clinical diagnoses of schizophrenia and its 'spectrum' satellites, such as schizotypal disorder, schizoaffective disorder and other non-affective psychosis, may not represent relevant phenotypes for genetic research. Because of the multiple pathways that lead from genotype to phenotype, and from structural brain abnormalities to behavioural expression, the observable clinical phenotypes are likely to be heavily confounded with 'downstream' epigenetic events that make it hard for the currently available methods of genetic analysis to detect the primary genetic defect. This has led to an exploration of alternative 'correlated' phenotypes (or 'endophenotypes'), such as neurocognitive abnormalities or temperament and character traits that are known to be associated with schizophrenia and may be expressed in both affected individuals and their asymptomatic biological relatives. Correlated phenotypes have the advantage of higher penetrance and more clearly definable patterns of inheritance. There have been promising attempts to detect genetic linkage using neurobehavioural markers (Freedman *et al.* 2000).

A genetic epidemiological criterion for the gain in power to detect linkage by using correlated phenotypes, regardless of the mode of transmission, is the magnitude of the risk (or prevalence) ratio (λ_s) between the prevalence of the trait or abnormality in the first-degree relatives of affected probands and its prevalence in the general population (Risch 1997). To increase the power to detect linkage, λ_s, for a 'correlated' phenotype should be well in excess of the risk ratio for clinically manifest schizophrenia (usually estimated at 10.0). A number of neurocognitive and personality traits, associated with schizophrenia, appear to meet this criterion (Faraone *et al.* 1995) and therefore should be explored as candidate phenotypes. A prerequisite for the application of this approach is the establishment of population prevalences for such phenotypes in epidemiological samples. A step in this direction has been made recently with regard to a measure of attention dysfunction (Chen *et al.* 1998).

Children at high genetic risk

Studies of children born to parents diagnosed with schizophrenia (mothers, in the majority of studies) have highlighted a range of early developmental abnormalities that could be markers of increased risk of adult schizophrenia. Studies in the USA (Fish 1977; Goldstein 1987; Erlenmeyer-Kimling *et al.* 1997), Denmark (Schulsinger *et al.* 1984), Sweden (McNeil & Kaij 1987) and Israel (Mirsky *et al.* 1995) have examined in prospective case–control designs a total of 230 high-risk (HR) children of schizophrenic parent(s), 248 children of parents with other psychiatric disorders and 392 control children born to parents with no psychiatric disorder. In reviewing the data, Fish *et al.* (1992) proposed a syndrome of 'pandysmaturation' (PDM), defined as a transient retardation of motor and visual development, an abnormal pattern of functional test scores on cross-sectional developmental examinations, and a retardation of skeletal growth. PDM could be a marker of a neurointegrative defect and a precursor of schizotypal traits. PDM may develop *in utero* and in such cases it is associated with low birth weight, but obstetric complications do not lead to PDM in the absence of genetic risk. The schizophrenic parent effect has been identified as the only 'robust and direct predictor of adult psychiatric outcomes' in another HR study in which 18% of the offspring of schizophrenic parent(s) had developed schizophrenic illnesses after 19 years of follow-up, compared with 7% psychosis in the offspring of parent(s) with affective disorders and 2% in the control group (Erlenmeyer-Kimling *et al.* 1991). The PDM syndrome remains as a promising developmental marker of high risk for schizophrenia because it is relatively specific to the biological offspring of parent(s) with schizophrenia. However, it is not known if PDM can be reliably diagnosed in large samples. Furthermore, it is not known how frequently it occurs in non-HR subjects, and whether its causation is primarily genetic or environmental (e.g. resulting from parenting disrupted by psychosis). Further research could clarify these issues and explore the potential use of PDM as an intermediate phenotype for genetic research.

Individuals at high genetic risk who develop schizophrenia as adults are more likely to manifest: (i) neurocognitive deficits; and (ii) difficulties in social interaction during childhood and adolescence, compared with individuals at high risk who do not develop schizophrenia. Thus, in the Israeli High-Risk Study cohort, poor scores on attention tasks obtained in childhood were associated with schizophrenia spectrum disorders at ages 26 and 32 (Mirsky et al. 1995). In a reanalysis of the Copenhagen High-Risk Study (Cannon et al. 1990), in which 207 children of schizophrenic women and 104 controls had been assessed at age 15 and reassessed 10 years later, poor social competence, passivity and social isolation in adolescence predicted predominantly negative symptoms, while overactive behaviour and aggressiveness predicted positive symptoms in the 15 high-risk subjects who developed schizophrenia by age 25 (Cannon et al. 1990). In addition to genetic risk, a possible role of non-genetic factors was suggested in this study by the increased incidence of perinatal complications and enlarged third ventricle in the negative symptom subgroup, and of a history of an unstable early rearing environment in the positive symptom subgroup.

Obstetric complications

Maternal obstetric complications (OC), a focus of research since the 1960s (Lane & Albee 1966; Stabenau & Pollin 1967; Mednick 1970), are widely cited as an established risk factor in schizophrenia (Cannon 1997). Several explanatory models have been proposed:

1 Severe OC, such as perinatal hypoxia and a resulting hippocampal damage, can prepare the ground for adult schizophrenia even if genetic liability is weak or absent.
2 Genetic predisposition sensitizes the developing brain to lesions resulting from randomly occurring less severe OC.
3 Genetic predisposition to schizophrenia leads to abnormal fetal development which in turn causes OC.
4 Maternal constitutional factors, partially influenced by genes, such as small physique or proneness to risk behaviour (drug use, smoking during pregnancy), increase the risk of OC and fetal brain damage.

The testing of these hypotheses presupposes epidemiological and clinical samples, as well as animal models (Bernstein et al. 1999; Mallard et al. 1999). A total of 34 studies and databases have been examined by Geddes and Lawrie (1995) and by Verdoux et al. (1997) using meta-analysis techniques and a comprehensive review has been published by McNeil et al. (2000). Although significant associations have been found between complications of pregnancy and adult schizophrenia, the effects observed are inconsistent and indicate significant interstudy heterogeneity. A large number of published case–control studies, reporting positive findings of an association between OC and schizophrenia, are of small sample size and have used parental interviews as the source of OC data. OC histories based on maternal recall have been shown to have methodological limitations (Cantor-Graae et al. 1998). For these reasons, the standards for this type of research should involve:

1 birth cohorts or large populations samples;

2 prospectively recorded pregnancy and birth data; and
3 use of standardized scales enabling comparisons of data across studies.

While a number of studies in the last decade have met the first two criteria, there is still no generally adopted framework for summarizing, analysing and reporting OC data; this limits the interpretation of findings.

Positive findings that have emerged from population-based studies with prospectively collected OC data include:

1 perinatal brain injury involving hypoxia (Jones et al. 1998; Cannon et al. 2000; Zornberg et al. 2000);
2 low birth weight (Jones et al. 1998; Ichiki et al. 2000; Wahlbeck et al. 2001);
3 gestation < 37 weeks and/or small for gestational age (Jones et al. 1998; Hultman et al. 1999; Ichiki et al. 2000; Wahlbeck et al. 2001);
4 low maternal body mass index (Sacker et al. 1995; Wahlbeck et al. 2001); and
5 combinations of the above, plus specific OC events, such as bleeding and placentation abnormalities (Jones et al. 1988; Hultman et al. 1999).

Although all of the above epidemiological studies report significant associations between one or more OC risk factor and subsequent schizophrenia, no obvious pattern or hierarchy of causal pathways can be inferred from these studies, nor is it possible to conclude whether the effects of individual OCs are additive or interactive. The interpretation of the OC findings is further complicated by the fact that at least two recent population-based studies have failed to identify any significant associations with schizophrenia (Byrne et al. 2000; Kendell et al. 2000). It is difficult to answer conclusively the question about possible interactions between familial risk of schizophrenia and the effects of OCs on the manifestation of the disease in adult life. Studies on monozygotic twins discordant for schizophrenia (Cantor-Graae et al. 1994; Torrey et al. 1994) found a significant intratwin pair effect for minor physical anomalies in the cotwin who subsequently developed schizophrenia but not for OCs, including birth weight. A recent linkage study between the Danish twin resister and the psychiatric case register reported a significantly greater rate of first admissions for schizophrenia in members of dizygotic, but not monozygotic, twin pairs when compared with the general population (Kläning 1999). Because maternal age, physique, parity, as well as a maternal genetic factor, are all known to influence dizygotic twinning but have no effect on monozygotic twinning, assessment of OCs in dizygotes may offer an additional paradigm for studies aiming to disentangle the complex relationships between OCs and genetic liability in schizophrenia.

Overall, the many inconsistencies among the findings of individual studies evoke a critical appraisal of the whole field (Crow 2000) and caution against an unqualified acceptance of OC as a proven risk factor in schizophrenia. To clarify their role should remain an important priority for epidemiological research.

Maternal influenza and other pre- and postnatal infections

In utero exposure to influenza has been implicated as a risk factor since a report that an increased proportion of adult schizophrenia in Helsinki was associated with presumed second trimester *in utero* exposure to the 1957 A2 influenza epidemic (Mednick *et al*. 1988). Over 40 studies have subsequently attempted to replicate the putative link between maternal influenza and schizophrenia, using designs ranging from interviews with mothers of probands with schizophrenia to complex statistical analyses of large databases linking the incidence of schizophrenia in birth cohorts to measures of mortality or morbidity associated with documented influenza epidemics. Putative ascertainment of influenza on the basis of retrospective recall has been shown to result in 70% false-positive self-diagnosis when questionnaire responses were correlated with individual serological findings (Elder *et al*. 1996). Reports from studies utilizing this method are unlikely to be valid. Several studies correlating schizophrenia incidence in population databases with influenza epidemics (Barr *et al*. 1990; Sham *et al*. 1992; Adams *et al*. 1993; Takei *et al*. 1994; Kunugi *et al*. 1995) have produced results supporting the original Finnish findings. However, as argued by Crow (1994), statistical overanalysis may have resulted in false-positive findings. More recently, negative results have been reported from an increasing number of studies based on large epidemiological samples, some from populations previously implicated in the reports on positive findings (Grech *et al*. 1997; Morgan *et al*. 1997; Battle *et al*. 1999; Selten *et al*. 1999a; Mino *et al*. 2000). While all of the population-based studies were 'ecological' in design (in the sense that information on actual individual exposure was not available), the only two studies to date (Crow & Done 1992; Cannon *et al*. 1996) in which data on actually infected pregnant women were accessed by the investigators found no increase in the risk of schizophrenia among the offspring. These negative results are consistent with the failure of studies using polymerase chain reaction to detect influenza virus-specific nucleic acid sequences in brain tissue or cerebrospinal fluid from patients with schizophrenia (Sierra-Honigmann *et al*. 1995; Taller *et al*. 1996). The balance of evidence therefore does not support the hypothesis of a significant contribution of *in utero* exposure to influenza to the aetiology of schizophrenia.

The more general issue of pre- or postnatal exposure to infection as a risk factor has not been laid to rest. A recent analysis of data from a well-documented birth cohort (A.S. Brown *et al*. 2000) suggests that second trimester exposure to respiratory infections (including tuberculosis, influenza, pneumonia and upper respiratory tract infections) may be associated with increased incidence of schizophrenia spectrum disorders in the offspring. In a follow-up study of the children of a cohort of women clinically and serologically documented with prenatal rubella, Brown *et al*. (2001) reported increased risk of schizophrenia spectrum disorders. Postnatal central nervous system

infections in children followed up to age 14 in the North Finland 1966 birth cohort was associated with a significant odds ratio of 4.8 for subsequent schizophrenia (Rantakallio *et al*. 1997). An association between Borna disease virus and both schizophrenia and affective disorders has been suggested by several serological studies but this line of investigation is still in an early stage (Taieb *et al*. 2001). The extent to which such research is capable of discovering true causal contributions to schizophrenia, in the absence of a more advanced pathogenetic understanding of the role of genetic factors, remains debatable (DeLisi 1996).

Other prenatal exposures

A variety of other prenatal exposures have been explored in 'opportunistic' epidemiological studies making use of documented historic cohorts. Fetal vulnerability to acute maternal starvation during the first trimester, with an increased subsequent risk of schizophrenia, has been suggested by a study of the offspring of Dutch women exposed to severe wartime famine in 1944–45. Severe food deprivation (<4200 kJ/day) during the first trimester was associated with an increased relative risk of 2.6 for narrowly defined schizophrenia in female offspring (Susser & Lin 1992) and a relative risk of 2.0 for schizotypal personality disorder (Hoek *et al*. 1996). Another Dutch study has attempted to evaluate the effect of maternal stress on the risk of schizophrenia in the offspring, using the five-day German *blitzkrieg* against the Netherlands in May 1940 as a proxy measure of stress exposure during pregnancy. A small but statistically significant increase in RR (risk ratio 1.28) was found for first trimester exposure (van Os & Selten 1998). Another Dutch stress exposure study (the 1953 flood catastrophe in the south-west of the Netherlands; Selten *et al*. 1999b) failed to find a significant association between maternal stress and non-affective psychoses in the offspring. The lifetime prevalence of schizophrenia among 1867 people prenatally exposed to the 1945 atomic bomb explosion over Nagasaki was examined by Imamura *et al*. (1999) and found to be 0.96%, i.e. not different from the expected rate in non-exposed populations.

The early rearing environment

Support for an effect of the early rearing environment on the risk of developing schizophrenia comes from a recent study of a Finnish sample of 179 adopted-away children of schizophrenic parents (a high-risk group) and a matched control sample of adoptees at no increased genetic risk (Tienari 1991; Wahlberg *et al*. 1997). Psychosis or severe personality disorder was diagnosed in 34 out of 121 HR subjects followed up for 5–7 years after the initial assessment, compared with 24 out of 150 controls. While the rates of adult psychosis or severe personality disorder were significantly higher in the HR group compared with the control group, the difference was entirely attributable to the subset of HR children who grew up in dysfunctional adoptive families – a result consistent with the model of genetic control of the sensitivity to the environment.

Premorbid traits and social impairment

Schizoid (Kretschmer 1936) or schizotypal (Meehl 1962) premorbid traits have been thought to express a predisposition to schizophrenia. Estimates of the frequency of schizotypal personality disorder among siblings of schizophrenic patients are of the order of 17% (Kendler *et al.* 1984; Baron *et al.* 1985) but epidemiological data on its occurrence in the general population are lacking. The association between early schizoid or schizotypal traits and the risk of adult schizophrenia is not restricted to HR populations, such as offspring of schizophrenic parents. Evidence of early developmental peculiarities in children who develop schizophrenia as adults has been provided by prospectively collected data on a national birth cohort in the UK (Jones *et al.* 1994). Preschizophrenic children had an excess (odd ratios 2.1–5.8) of speech and educational problems, social anxiety and preference for solitary play. The Swedish cohort study of 50 087 men conscripted into the army at age 18–20 and followed up over 15 years (Malmberg *et al.* 1998) found that poor social adjustment during childhood and adolescence was significantly more common among the 195 individuals who subsequently developed schizophrenia than among the rest of the cohort. Positive scores on four variables (having fewer than two friends, preference for socializing in small groups, feeling excessively sensitive and not having a steady girlfriend) were strongly associated with schizophrenia in later life but, because a high proportion of the cohort scored positive on at least one item, the predictive value of this set of variables was negligible. Similar results (deficits in social functioning and organizational ability, as well as low test scores on all measures) were reported from the Israeli conscript study (Davidson *et al.* 1999).

On balance, there is converging evidence that a cluster of behavioural traits broadly similar to adult schizoid or schizotypal personality traits and to some of the negative symptoms of schizophrenia can be detected during childhood and adolescence in a proportion of the people who develop schizophrenia in adult life. However, there is no conclusive evidence on the extent to which such traits are genetically or environmentally determined.

Premorbid intelligence (IQ)

The association between mental retardation and schizophrenia was first highlighted by Kraepelin (1919), who estimated that about 7% of the cases of dementia praecox evolved on the basis of intellectual impairment and introduced the term *Pfropfschizophrenie* (engrafted schizophrenia) for a subtype characterized by early onset, negativism and stereotypies. A deficit in intellectual performance antedating by many years the onset of schizophrenia was described by Lane and Albee (1964). More recently, the concept has been revived and partially validated (Doody *et*

al. 1998; Sanderson *et al.* 2001) in a study which identified a comorbid pattern of mild learning disability, neurological symptoms and schizophrenia-like psychosis segregating in multiply affected families with high rates of chromosomal abnormalities. Independently of the notion of a discrete subtype of schizophrenia characterized by intellectual impairment, a strong relationship between low IQ and risk of schizophrenia has been demonstrated in the Swedish (David *et al.* 1997) and the Israeli conscript studies (Davidson *et al.* 1999). After controlling for confounding effects in the Swedish cohort, the risk of schizophrenia increased linearly with the decrement of IQ (compared with an IQ > 126 as the baseline, the odds ratio for schizophrenia increased from 3.5 for IQ 90–95 to 8.6 for IQ < 74). The prevalence of borderline intellectual disability among patients with psychoses has been estimated at 18% (Hassiotis *et al.* 1999).

The relationship between low IQ and risk of schizophrenia is among the most robust findings in the risk factor epidemiology of the disorder and merits further study with a view to its genetic determinants and pathogenetic implications.

Neurocognitive and neurophysiological markers

Cognitive impairment in the domains of attention control, verbal memory, spatial working memory and executive function – all compromising the ability to select task-relevant response strategies and to recruit appropriate neural circuits (Gold & Weinberger 1995) – represent a stable core feature of schizophrenia and are relatively independent of the symptom dimension. Specific deficits in sustained attention (Cornblatt & Keilp 1994; Egan *et al.* 2000), verbal fluency (Chen *et al.* 2000), event-related brain potentials (Freedman *et al.* 1996; Frangou *et al.* 1997; Javitt *et al.* 1997; Michie *et al.* 2000) and saccadic eye movement control (Clementz *et al.* 1994) have been found in clinical and laboratory research to be common in schizophrenic patients and in a proportion of their clinically normal biological relatives, but rare in control subjects drawn from the general population. Their sensitivity and specificity as risk predictors in schizophrenia needs to be investigated in larger population samples. Family and field studies employing the Continuous Performance Test (CPT) suggest that versions of this task involving an increased processing load (engaging working memory) may be a particularly sensitive measure of sustained attention as one of the core deficits characterizing schizophrenia. In a proportion of the clinically asymptomatic first-degree relatives of probands with schizophrenia, CPT performance is within the range of the affected probands. Estimates of relative risk for CPT as a neurocognitive trait vary in different studies between a low $\lambda_s = 2.1$–3.3 (Egan *et al.* 2000) and a high $\lambda_s = 15$–30 (Chen *et al.* 1998). In the latter study, the heritability of CPT performance has been estimated at 0.48–0.62. Should CPT and other neurocognitive variables be further validated by epidemiological studies as biological markers of schizophrenia, the power of risk prediction at the level of the individual may increase substantially.

Social class

Since the 1930s, numerous studies in North America and Europe have consistently found that the economically disadvantaged social groups contribute disproportionately to the first admission rate for schizophrenia. Two explanatory hypotheses, of social causation ('breeder') and of social selection ('drift'), were originally proposed (Mischler & Scotch 1983). According to the social causation theory, the socioeconomic adversity characteristic of lower class living conditions could precipitate psychosis in genetically vulnerable individuals who have a constricted capacity to cope with complex or stressful situations. In the 1960s this theory was considered refuted by a single study which found that the social class distribution of schizophrenic patients' fathers did not deviate from that of the general population, and that the excess of low socioeconomic status among schizophrenic patients was mainly attributable to individuals who had drifted down the occupational and social scale prior to the onset of psychosis (Goldberg & Morrison 1963) – a tendency that has been confirmed in more recent prospective studies focusing on the prodromal period (Häfner et al. 1999). Generally, aetiological research in schizophrenia in the last decades has tended to ignore 'macrosocial' risk factors. However, the possibility remains that social stratification and socioeconomic status are important in the causation of schizophrenia but the effect manifests in ways that do not conform to the earlier theories. An example of this is the finding, reported from the North Finland 1966 birth cohort (Mäkikirö et al. 1997), that the cumulative incidence of early-onset schizophrenia was significantly higher among individuals whose fathers had attained status and achievement, placing them into the highest social class. Upward occupational mobility in fathers was found to be associated with acculturation stress and high levels of psychopathology which might exacerbate latent predisposition to psychosis in the offspring. However, this remains speculative and more refined research tools may be needed to tackle the issue.

Urban birth

The nineteenth century hypothesis that urban environments increase the risk of psychosis (Freeman 1994) has been revived in recent years. The 'urban drift', resulting in a higher density of cases of psychosis in inner city areas, has been extensively documented since the 1930s (Faris & Dunham 1939) and was mainly interpreted in socioeconomic and behavioural terms (availability of cheap accommodation, attraction of an anonymous lifestyle). Recently, the focus has shifted towards presumed exposure to physicochemical and infectious risk factors. In a reanalysis of archival material (the US 1880 census data on 'insanity'), Torrey et al. (1997a) found that urban residence was associated with an odds ratio of 1.66 for psychosis and semiurban residence with an odds ratio of 1.46, when completely rural counties were used as the baseline for comparisons. The authors speculate that the greater likelihood of infectious and toxic insults on the brain (e.g. lead exposure) in urban settings might be part of the explanation.

The crucial distinction between urban birth and urban residence was introduced in the epidemiological literature only in the 1960s (Astrup & Ødegaard 1961). Marcelis et al. (1999) analysed by place of birth all first admissions for schizophrenia and other psychoses in the Netherlands between 1942 and 1978. A graded measure to urban exposure was found, suggesting a linear relationship between urban birth and moderate but statistically significant increases in the incidence of schizophrenia, affective psychoses and other psychoses, with the effect size increasing in successive birth cohorts. In two record linkage studies across the Danish civil registration system, the medical birth register and the national psychiatric case register, Mortensen et al. (1999) and Eaton et al. (2000) calculated an $RR = 2.4$–4.2 for schizophrenia prevalence of those born in the capital Copenhagen as compared with rural births. In terms of population attributable risk, urban birth accounted for 34.6% of all cases of schizophrenia in Denmark – in contrast to history of schizophrenia in a first-degree relative which, with $RR = 9.3$, accounted for only 5.5% of the cases. The presumed urban birth risk factor was not mediated by obstetric complications.

In interpreting these findings, it is important to take into consideration that genetic predisposition to schizophrenia may remain unexpressed in gene carriers; therefore the comparison of risks attributable to familial occurrence of schizophrenia and place of birth is problematic. Moreover, the nature of the suspected 'urban risk factor' remains cryptic and the possibility that it is a proxy for multiple interacting factors, including selective urban–rural and rural–urban migration of individuals varying in their 'load' of schizophrenia predisposing genes, cannot be excluded. As pointed out by Verheij et al. (1998) in a study of urban–rural variations in general health status in the Netherlands, migration processes may cause spurious findings in cross-sectional research into the relation between urbanicity and health. Therefore, the existence of an 'urban risk factor' for schizophrenia remains unproven.

Season of birth

Seasonality of schizophrenic births was first described by Tramer (1929). The current interest in the phenomenon dates back to the 1960s (Barry & Barry 1961). A 5–8% excess of schizophrenic births in winter–spring has been reported by a large number of studies (reviewed by Bradbury & Miller 1985; Torrey et al. 1997b). The effect seems to be present in the northern but not in the southern hemisphere, where studies (reviewed by McGrath & Welham 1999) have failed to demonstrate a consistent seasonal effect. Seasonality fluctuations of births are not specific to schizophrenia and have been described in bipolar affective disorder, autism, attention deficit disorder, alcoholism, stillbirths, diabetes, Alzheimer's disease and Down's syndrome. Many of the studies are methodologically vulnerable with regard to sample size, sampling bias or statistical analysis. Furthermore, the evidence for a seasonal factor associated with the risk for schizophrenia and operating at birth has been weakened, although not invalidated, by the argument that it could be an artefact of the so-called age-incidence and age-prevalence effect (Dalen 1975; Lewis & Griffin 1981): because the risk of onset of schizophrenia rises rapidly from age 15 onwards, 'older' individuals born in the early months of each calender year will have a higher rate of onset of schizophrenia than 'younger' individuals born late in the same year. Nevertheless, a relative excess of winter births among people with schizophrenia still seems to be a valid and robust finding. Kendell and Adams (1991) calculated year-to-year and month-to-month variation in schizophrenic births between 1914 and 1960 for all patients admitted to hospitals in Scotland since 1963 ($n = 13\,661$). A Poisson distribution fitted to the data indicated a significant deviation from the expected chance fluctuations. This deviation, entirely limited to the months February–May, in which the rates of schizophrenic births increased by 7%, needs discussion. Similar findings were reported by Mortensen et al. (1999) on the basis of a large Danish cohort.

Notwithstanding the fact that seasonality of schizophrenia births has been extensively documented and cannot be explained away as a statistical artefact, the understanding of its underlying causes has hardly progressed since the phenomenon was first described. Various explanations have been proposed. According to the procreational habits hypothesis, parents of schizophrenic patients are more likely to have a seasonal pattern of sexual activity and conception, with a peak in the summer months (Hare & Price 1968). Some evidence consistent with this hypothesis (a slight winter–spring excess of births of both patients and their unaffected siblings) has been reported by Suvisaari et al. (2001). Other theories include 'seasonal ovopathy' involving increased risk of chromosomal anomalies because of delayed ovulation (Pallast et al. 1994). A range of noxious influences capable of causing fetal damage have also been proposed, including seasonal viral infections, extremes of temperature, seasonal variation in nutrition or vitamin levels, exposure to insecticides and birth trauma. None have yet been identified and it is unlikely that the problem will be resolved by further studies of the effect itself. Seasonality of births is likely to be a distant echo of the impact of such risk factors that will remain hidden, although their nature may not be entirely novel and surprising. Therefore, a reversal of the strategy may be more productive: instead of focusing on seasonality of births, research should systematically examine risk factors known to disrupt normal fetal brain development for seasonal effects in their operation.

Marital status

Marital status is a strong predictor of psychiatric hospitalization (Jarman et al. 1992). In schizophrenia, it is significantly associated with measures of incidence, age at onset, and course and outcome. Single men and, to a lesser degree, single women tend to be over-represented among first admissions or first contacts (68% and 39%, respectively, in the WHO 10-country study;

Jablensky et al. 1992). Riecher-Rössler et al. (1992) found a 12-fold higher first admission rate for single men when compared with married men, and a 3.3 times higher rate for single women when compared with married women. Being single was associated with 50-fold higher odds of developing schizophrenia in males and 15-fold higher odds in women during the 1-year follow-up of the Epidemiological Catchment Area study (Tien & Eaton 1992). This is not sufficient to prove that being single is an independent antecedent risk factor (or that being married is a protective risk modifier) because both overt schizophrenia and preschizophrenic traits and impairments reduce the chances of getting married. Schizophrenic patients living in a stable marital or other partnership may be a positively selected group with a milder form of the disease (Ødegaard 1946b). Evidence that being married (or living with a partner) can delay the onset of schizophrenia in males, and thus act as a risk modifier, was obtained from the WHO 10-country study after unconfounding the effects of gender, premorbid personality traits, family history of psychosis and marital status on age at onset. (Jablensky & Cole 1997). An interaction between single marital status and a neighbourhood environment characterized by a high degree of social isolation was significantly associated with incidence of schizophrenia in a recent Dutch study (van Os et al. 2000).

Migrant status and ethnic minorities

Since the publication of the first report on an increased morbidity of psychoses among African-Caribbean immigrants to the UK (Hemsi 1967), an increasing number of studies have pointed to exceptionally high incidence rates of schizophrenia (about 6.0 per 10 000) in the African-Caribbean population in the UK (Bhugra et al. 1997; Harrison et al. 1997). This excess morbidity is not restricted to recent immigrants and is, in fact, higher in the British-born second generation of migrants. Similar findings of nearly fourfold excess over the general population rate have been reported for the Dutch Antillean and Surinamese immigrants in Holland (Selten et al. 1997). In spite of much research effort focusing on this phenomenon, its causes remain almost entirely obscure. Little evidence has been presented to support suggestions that these psychotic illnesses might be better explained as acute transient psychoses or drug-induced psychoses. It seems that neither the psychopathology nor the course and outcome of these disorders presents any atypical features that would sufficiently set them apart from ICD-10 or DSM-IIIR schizophrenia (Harrison et al. 1999; Hutchinson et al. 1999), although one report (Hickling et al. 1999) indicated poor diagnostic agreement ($\kappa = 0.45$) between a Jamaican psychiatrist and a group of British psychiatrists assessing the same cases. Incidence studies in the Caribbean (Hickling & Rodgers-Johnson 1995; Bhugra et al. 1999) do not indicate any excess schizophrenia morbidity in the indigenous populations from which migrants are recruited. Explanations in terms of biological risk factors, such as an increased incidence of obstetric complications or maternal influenza, have so far found no support (Hutchinson et al. 1997; Selten et al. 1998). Hypotheses involving psychosocial risk factors, such as lack of a supportive community structure, acculturation stress, demoralization cause by racial discrimination and blocked opportunities for upward social mobility, have been proposed (Bhugra *et al.* 1999) but none has yet been adequately tested. A potentially important finding in need of replication is the significant increase of schizophrenia among the siblings of second-generation African-Caribbean schizophrenic probands, compared with the incidence of schizophrenia in the siblings of white patients (Hutchinson *et al.* 1996). 'Horizontal' increases in the morbid risk usually suggest that environmental factors may be modifying (increasing) the penetrance of the predisposition to disease in gene carriers. Although psychosocial stress is most likely a factor affecting the majority of African-Caribbeans in the UK, there is at present no plausible mechanism linking such stress selectively to schizophrenia. Unexplored gene–environment interactions, involving various infectious, nutritional or toxic environmental factors, remain a possibility.

Prospects for epidemiology in the search for the causes of schizophrenia

After nearly a century of epidemiological research, essential questions about the nature and causes of schizophrenia still remain unanswered. Nevertheless, important insights into this complex disorder have been gained from population-based studies. Two major conclusions stand out. First, the clinical syndrome of schizophrenia is robust and can be identified reliably in diverse populations. This suggests that a common pathophysiology and underlying genetic predisposition are likely to underlie the spectrum of manifestations of schizophrenia. On balance, the evidence suggests that no major differences in incidence and disease risk can be found across populations at the level of large population aggregates. However, the study of 'atypical' populations, such as genetic isolates or minority groups, may be capable of detecting unusual variations in the incidence of schizophrenia that could provide novel clues to the aetiology and pathogenesis of the disorder. Notwithstanding the difficulties currently accompanying the genetic dissection of complex disorders, novel methods of genetic analysis will eventually identify genomic regions and loci predisposing to schizophrenia. The majority are likely to be of small effect, although one cannot rule out the possibility that genes of moderate or even major effects will also be found, especially in relation to the neurophysiological abnormalities associated with schizophrenia. Clarifying the function of such genes will be a complex task. Part of the solution is likely to be found in the domain of epidemiology because establishing their population frequency and associations with a variety of phenotypic expressions, including personality traits, is a prerequisite for understanding their causal role.

The second conclusion is that no single environmental risk factor of major effect on the incidence of schizophrenia has yet been discovered. Further studies using large samples are required to evaluate potential risk factors, antecedents and predictors for which the present evidence is inconclusive. Assuming that the methodological pitfalls of risk factor epidemiology (such as the 'ecological fallacy') can be avoided, and that a number of environmental variables of small to moderate effect will eventually be identified as risk factors, epidemiology will usefully complement genetic research that implicates multiple genes of small to moderate effect. Current epidemiological research is making use of large existing databases such as cumulative case registers or birth cohorts to test hypotheses about risk factors in case–control designs. Methods and models of genetic epidemiology are increasingly being integrated within population-based studies. These trends predict an important role for epidemiology in the coming era of molecular biology of mental disorders. The complementarity between genetics and epidemiology will provide tools for unravelling the gene–environment interactions that are likely to be the key to the aetiology of schizophrenia. The molecular epidemiology of schizophrenia may be the next major chapter in the search for its causes and cures.

References

Adams, W., Kendell, R.E., Hare, E.H. & Munk-Jørgensen, P. (1993) Epidemiological evidence that maternal influenza contributes to the aetiology of schizophrenia. *British Journal of Psychiatry* 163, 522–534.

Adler, L.E. & Griffith, J.M. (1991) Concurrent medical illness in the schizophrenic patient: epidemiology, diagnosis and management. *Schizophrenia Research* 4, 91–107.

de Alarcon, J., Seagroatt, V., Sellar, C. & Goldacre, M. (1992) Evidence for decline in schizophrenia [Abstract]. *Schizophrenia Research* 6, 100–101.

Albus, M. & Maier, W. (1995) Lack of gender differences in age at onset in familial schizophrenia. *Schizophrenia Research* 18, 51–57.

Alexander, R.C., Patkar, A.A., Lapointe, J.S., Flynn, S.W. & Honer, W.G. (1997) Schizencephaly associated with psychosis. *Journal of Neurology, Neurosurgery and Psychiatry* 63, 373–375.

Allebeck, P., Adamsson, C., Engström, A. & Rydberg, U. (1993) Cannabis and schizophrenia: a longitudinal study of cases treated in Stockholm County. *Acta Psychiatrica Scandinavica* 88, 21–24.

Andrews, G., Henderson, S. & Hall, W. (2001) Prevalence, comorbidity, disability and service utilisation: overview of the Australian National Mental Health Survey. *British Journal of Psychiatry* 178, 145–153.

Appleby, L., Thomas, S., Ferrier, N. *et al.* (2000) Sudden unexplained death in psychiatric in-patients. *British Journal of Psychiatry* 176, 405–406.

Astrup, C. & Ødegaard, Ø. (1961) Internal migration and mental illness in Norway. *Psychiatric Quarterly* 34, 116–130.

Babidge, N.C., Buhrich, N. & Butler, T. (2001) Mortality among homeless people with schizophrenia in Sydney, Australia: a 10-year follow-up. *Acta Psychiatrica Scandinavica* 103, 105–110.

Baldwin, J.A. (1979) Schizophrenia and physical disease. *Psychological Medicine* 9, 611–618.

Bamrah, J.S., Freeman, H.L. & Goldberg, D.P. (1991) Epidemiology of schizophrenia in Salford, 1974–84. *British Journal of Psychiatry* 159, 802–810.

Baron, M., Gruen, R., Asnis, L. & Lord, S. (1985) Familial transmission of schizotypal and borderline personality disorders. *American Journal of Psychiatry* **142**, 927–934.

Barr, C.E., Mednick, S.A. & Munk-Jorgensen, P. (1990) Exposure to influenza epidemics during gestation and adult schizophrenia. *Archives of General Psychiatry* **47**, 869–874.

Barry, H. & Barry, H. Jr (1961) Season of birth: an epidemiological study in psychiatry. *Archives of General Psychiatry* **5**, 100–108.

Bash, K.W. & Bash-Liechti, J. (1969) Psychiatrische Epidemiologie in Iran. In: *Perspektiven der heutigen Psychiatrie* (ed. H.E. Ehrhard), pp. 313–320. Gerhards, Frankfurt.

Battle, Y.L., Martin, B.C., Dorfman, J.H. & Miller, L.S. (1999) Seasonality and infectious disease in schizophrenia: the birth hypothesis revisited. *Journal of Psychiatric Research* **33**, 501–509.

Bebbington, P. & Nayani, T. (1995) The Psychosis Screening Questionnaire. *International Journal of Methods in Psychiatric Research* **5**, 11–19.

Bernstein, H.G., Grecksch, G., Becker, A., Hollt, V. & Bogerts, B. (1999) Cellular changes in rat brain areas associated with neonatal hippocampal damage. *Neuroreport* **10**, 2307–2311.

Bhugra, D., Hilwig, M., Hossein, B. *et al.* (1997) Incidence and outcome of schizophrenia in Whites, African-Caribbeans and Asians in London. *Psychological Medicine* **27**, 791–798.

Bhugra, D., Mallett, R. & Leff, J. (1999) Schizophrenia and African-Caribbeans: a conceptual model of aetiology. *International Review of Psychiatry* **11**, 145–152.

Bøjholm, S. & Strömgren, E. (1989) Prevalence of schizophrenia on the island of Bornholm in 1935 and in 1983. *Acta Psychiatrica Scandinavica* **79** (Suppl. 348), 157–166.

Böök, J.A., Wetterberg, L. & Modrzewska, K. (1978) Schizophrenia in a North Swedish geographical isolate, 1900–77: epidemiology, genetics and biochemistry. *Clinical Genetics* **14**, 373–394.

Bradbury, T.N. & Miller, G.A. (1985) Season of birth in schizophrenia: a review of the evidence, methodology and etiology. *Psychological Bulletin* **98**, 569–594.

Bredkær, S., Mortensen, P.B. & Parnas, J. (1998) Epilepsy and non-organic non-affective psychosis: national epidemiologic study. *British Journal of Psychiatry* **172**, 235–238.

Bremer, J. (1951) A social-psychiatric investigation of a small community in Northern Norway. *Acta Psychiatrica et Neurologica Scandinavica Supplement* **62**.

Bresnahan, M.A., Brown, A.S., Schaefer, C.A. *et al.* (2000) Incidence and cumulative risk of treated schizophrenia in the Prenatal Determinants of Schizophrenia study. *Schizophrenia Bulletin* **26**, 297–308.

Brewin, J., Cantwell, R., Dalkin, T. *et al.* (1997) Incidence of schizophrenia in Nottingham. *British Journal of Psychiatry* **171**, 140–144.

Brockington, I.F., Kendell, R.E. & Leff, J.P. (1978) Definitions of schizophrenia: concordance and prediction of outcome. *Psychological Medicine* **8**, 387–398.

Brodaty, H., Sachdev, P., Rose, N., Rylands, K. & Prenter, L. (1999) Schizophrenia with onset after age 50 years. I. Phenomenology and risk factors. *British Journal of Psychiatry* **175**, 410–415.

Brown, A.S., Schaefer, C.A., Wyatt, R.J. *et al.* (2000) Maternal exposure to respiratory infections and adult schizophrenia spectrum disorders: a prospective birth cohort study. *Schizophrenia Bulletin* **26**, 287–295.

Brown, A.S., Cohen, P., Harkavy-Friedman, J. *et al.* (2001) Prenatal rubella, premorbid abnormalities, and adult schizophrenia. *Biological Psychiatry* **49**, 473–486.

Brown, S. (1997) Excess mortality of schizophrenia. *British Journal of Psychiatry* **171**, 502–508.

Brown, S., Inskip, H. & Barraclough, B. (2000) Causes of the excess mortality of schizophrenia. *British Journal of Psychiatry* **177**, 212–217.

Brugger, C. (1931) Versuch einer Geisteskrankenzählung in Thüringen. *Zeitschrift für die gesamte Neurologie und Psychiatrie* **133**, 252–390.

Brugha, T.S., Nienhuis, F., Bagchi, D., Smith, J. & Meltzer, H. (1999) The survey form of SCAN: the feasibility of using experienced lay survey interviewers to administer a semi-structured systematic clinical assessment of psychotic and non-psychotic disorders. *Psychological Medicine* **29**, 703–711.

Bruton, C.J., Stevens, J.R. & Frith, C.D. (1994) Epilepsy, psychosis and schizophrenia. *Neurology* **44**, 34–42.

Brzustowicz, L.M., Hodgkinson, K.A., Chow, E.W., Honer, W.G. & Bassett, A.S. (2000) Location of a major susceptibility locus for familial schizophrenia on chromosome 1q21–q22. *Science* **288**, 678–682.

Byrne, M., Browne, R., Mulryan, N. *et al.* (2000) Labour and delivery complications and schizophrenia. *British Journal of Psychiatry* **176**, 531–536.

Cannon, M., Cotter, D., Coffey, V.P. *et al.* (1996) Prenatal exposure to the 1957 influenza epidemic and adult schizophrenia: a follow-up study. *British Journal of Psychiatry* **168**, 368–371.

Caldwell, C.B. & Gottesman, I.I. (1990) Schizophrenics kill themselves too: a review of risk factors for suicide. *Schizophrenia Bulletin* **16**, 571–589.

Cannon, T.D. (1997) On the nature and mechanisms of obstetric influences in schizophrenia: a review and synthesis of epidemiologic studies. *International Review of Psychiatry* **9**, 387–397.

Cannon, T.D., Mednick, S.A. & Parnas, J. (1990) Antecedents of predominantly negative- and predominantly positive-symptom schizophrenia in a high-risk population. *Archives of General Psychiatry* **47**, 622–632.

Cannon, T.D., Rosso, I.M., Hollister, J.M. *et al.* (2000) A prospective cohort study of genetic and perinatal influences in the etiology of schizophrenia. *Schizophrenia Bulletin* **26**, 351–366.

Cantor-Graae, E., McNeil, T.F., Fuller Torrey, E. *et al.* (1994) Link between pregnancy complications and minor physical anomalies in monozygotic twins discordant for schizophrenia. *American Journal of Psychiatry* **151**, 1188–1193.

Cantor-Graae, E., Cardenal, S., Ismail, B. & McNeil, T.F. (1998) Recall of obstetric events by mothers of schizophrenic patients. *Psychological Medicine* **28**, 1239–1243.

Cardno, A.G., Marshall, E.J., Coid, B. *et al.* (1999) Heritability estimates for psychotic disorders: the Maudsley twin psychosis series. *Archives of General Psychiatry* **56**, 162–168.

Castle, D., Der Wessely, S.G. & Murray, R.M. (1991) The incidence of operationally defined schizophrenia in Camberwell, 1965–84. *British Journal of Psychiatry* **159**, 790–794.

Chen, C.N., Wong, J., Lee, N. *et al.* (1993) The Shatin community mental health survey in Hong Kong. II. Major findings. *Archives of General Psychiatry* **50**, 125–133.

Chen, W.J., Liu, S.K., Chang, C.J. *et al.* (1998) Sustained attention deficit and schizotypal personality features in non-psychotic relatives of schizophrenic patients. *American Journal of Psychiatry* **155**, 1214–1220.

Chen, Y.L.R., Chen, Y.H.E. & Lieh, M.F. (2000) Semantic verbal fluency deficit as a familial trait marker in schizophrenia. *Psychiatry Research* **95**, 133–148.

Clementz, B.A., McDowell, J.E. & Zisook, S. (1994) Saccadic system functioning among schizophrenia patients and their first-degree biological relatives. *Journal of Abnormal Psychology* **103**, 277–287.

Cooper, J.E., Kendell, R.E., Gurland, B.J. *et al.* (1972) *Psychiatric Diagnosis in New York and London.* Oxford University Press, London.

Cornblatt, B.A. & Keilp, J.G. (1994) Impaired attention, genetics, and the pathophysiology of schizophrenia. *Schizophrenia Bulletin* **20**, 31–46.

Crimlisk, H.L. (1997) The little imitator: porphyria – a neuropsychiatric disorder. *Journal of Neurology, Neurosurgery and Psychiatry* **62**, 319–328.

Crocetti, G.J., Lemkau, P.V., Kulcar, Z. & Kesic, B. (1971) Selected aspect of the epidemiology of psychoses in Croatia, Yugoslavia. II. The cluster sample and the results of the pilot survey. *American Journal of Epidemiology* **94**, 126–134.

Crow, T.J. (1994) Prenatal exposure to influenza as a cause of schizophrenia. *British Journal of Psychiatry* **164**, 588–592.

Crow, T.J. (2000) Do obstetric complications really cause psychosis? Why it matters: invited commentary. *British Journal of Psychiatry* **176**, 527–529.

Crow, T.J. & Done, D.J. (1992) Prenatal exposure to influenza does not cause schizophrenia. *British Journal of Psychiatry* **161**, 390–393.

Dalack, G.W., Healy, D.J. & Meador-Woodruff, J.H. (1998) Nicotine dependence in schizophrenia: clinical phenomena and laboratory findings. *American Journal of Psychiatry* **155**, 1490–1501.

Dalen, P. (1975) *Season of Birth: A Study of Schizophrenia and Other Mental Disorders*. North Holland, Amsterdam.

David, A.S., Malmberg, A., Brandt, L., Allebeck, P. & Lewis, G, (1997) IQ and risk for schizophrenia: a population-based cohort study. *Psychological Medicine* **27**, 1311–1323.

Davidson, M., Reichenberg, A., Rabinowitz, J. *et al.* (1999) Behavioral and intellectual markers for schizophrenia in apparently healthy male adolescents. *American Journal of Psychiatry* **156**, 1328–1335.

DeLisi, L.E. (1996) Is there a viral or immune dysfunction etiology to schizophrenia? Re-evaluation a decade later. *Schizophrenia Research* **22**, 1–4.

DeLisi, L.E. & Crow, T.J. (1999) Chromosome Workshops 1998: current state of psychiatric linkage. *American Journal of Medical Genetics* **88**, 215–218.

DeLisi, L.E., Goldin, L.R., Maxwell, M.E., Kazuba, D.M. & Gershon, E.S. (1987) Clinical features of illness in siblings with schizophrenia or schizoaffective disorder. *Archives of General Psychiatry* **44**, 891–896.

Der, G., Gupta, S. & Murray, R.M. (1990) Is schizophrenia disappearing? *Lancet* **335**, 513–516.

Dohan, F.C. (1966) Cereals and schizophrenia: data and hypothesis. *Acta Psychiatrica Scandinavica* **42**, 125–152.

Done, D.J., Crow, T.J., Johnstone, E.C. & Sacker, A. (1994) Childhood antecedents of schizophrenia and affective illness: social adjustment at ages 7 and 11. *British Medical Journal* **309**, 699–703.

Doody, G.A., Johnstone, E.C., Sanderson, T.L., Cunningham Owens, D.G. & Muir, W.J. (1998) 'Pfropfschizophrenie' revisited: schizophrenia in people with mild learning disability. *British Journal of Psychiatry* **173**, 145–153.

Dube, K.C. & Kumar, N. (1972) An epidemiological study of schizophrenia. *Journal of Biosocial Science* **4**, 187–195.

Dupont, A., Jensen, O.M., Stromgren, E. & Jablensky, A. (1986) Incidence of cancer in patients diagnosed as schizophrenic in Denmark. In: *Psychiatric Case Registers in Public Health* (eds S.H. ten Horn, R. Giel & W. Gulbinat), pp. 229–239. Elsevier, Amsterdam.

Eagles, J.M., Hunter, D. & McCance, C. (1988) Decline in the diagnosis of schizophrenia among first contacts with psychiatric services in north-east Scotland, 1969–84. *British Journal of Psychiatry* **152**, 793–798.

Eaton, W.W. (1974) Residence, social class, and schizophrenia. *Journal of Health and Social Behavior* **15**, 289–299.

Eaton, J.W. & Weil, R.Y. (1955) *Culture and Mental Disorders*. Free Press, Glencoe, IL.

Eaton, W.W., Romanoski, A., Anthony, J.C. & Nestadt, G. (1991) Screening for psychosis in the general population with a self-report interview. *Journal of Nervous and Mental Disease* **179**, 689–693.

Eaton, W.W., Hayward, C. & Ram, R. (1992) Schizophrenia and rheumatoid arthritis: a review. *Schizophrenia Research* **6**, 181–192.

Eaton, W.W., Mortensen, P.B. & Frydenberg, M. (2000) Obstetric factors, urbanization and psychosis. *Schizophrenia Research* **43**, 117–123.

Egan, M.F., Goldberg, T.E., Gscheidle, T. *et al.* (2000) Relative risk of attention deficits in siblings of patients with schizophrenia. *American Journal of Psychiatry* **157**, 1309–1316.

Elder, A.G., O'Donnell, B., McCruden, E.A.B., Symington, I.S. & Carman, W.F. (1996) Incidence and recall of influenza in a cohort of Glasgow healthcare workers during the 1993–94 epidemic: results of serum testing and questionnaire. *British Medical Journal* **313**, 1241–1242.

Erlenmeyer-Kimling, L., Rock, D., Squires-Wheeler, E., Roberts, S. & Yang, J. (1991) Early life precursors of psychiatric outcomes in adulthood of subjects at risk for schizophrenia or affective disorders. *Psychiatry Research* **39**, 239–256.

Erlenmeyer-Kimling, L., Adamo, U.H., Rock, D. *et al.* (1997) The New York High-Risk project: prevalence and comorbidity of Axis I disorders in offspring of schizophrenic patients at 25-year follow-up. *Archives of General Psychiatry* **54**, 1096–1102.

Essen-Möller, E. (1935) Untersuchungen über die Fruchtbarkeit gewisser Gruppen von Geisteskranken. *Acta Psychiatrica et Neurologica Scandinavica Supplement* 8.

Essen-Möller, E., Larsson, H., Uddenberg, C.E. & White, G. (1956) Individual traits and morbidity in a Swedish rural population. *Acta Psychiatrica et Neurologica Scandinavica Supplement* 100.

Fañanás, L. & Bertranpetit, J. (1995) Reproductive rates in families of schizophrenic patients in a case–control study. *Acta Psychiatrica Scandinavica* **91**, 202–204.

Faraone, S.V., Kremen, W.S., Lyons, M.J. *et al.* (1995) Diagnostic accuracy and linkage analysis: how useful are schizophrenia spectrum phenotypes? *American Journal of Psychiatry* **152**, 1286–1290.

Faris, R.E.L. & Dunham, H.W. (1939) *Mental Disorders in Urban Areas*. University of Chicago Press, Chicago.

Fish, B. (1977) Neurobiologic antecedents of schizophrenia in children: evidence for an inherited, congenital neurointegrative defect. *Archives of General Psychiatry* **34**, 1297–1313.

Fish, B., Marcus, J., Hans, S.L., Auerbach, J.G. & Perdue, S. (1992) Infants at risk for schizophrenia: sequelae of a genetic neurointegrative defect. *Archives of General Psychiatry* **49**, 221–235.

Flint, J. & Goldstein, L.H. (1992) Familial calcifraction fo the basal ganglia: a case report and reivew of the literature. *Psychological Medicine* **22**, 581–595.

Francis, A. & Freeman, H. (1984) Psychiatric abnormality and brain calcification over four generations. *Journal of Nervous and Mental Disease* **172**, 166–170.

Frangou, S., Sharma, T., Alarcon, G. *et al.* (1997) The Maudsley Family Study. II. Endogenous event-related potentials in familial schizophrenia. *Schizophrenia Research* **23**, 45–53.

Freedman, R., Adler, L.E., Myles-Worsley, M. *et al.* (1996) Inhibitory gating of an evoked response to repeated auditory stimuli in schizophrenic and normal subjects. *Archives of General Psychiatry* **53**, 1114–1121.

Freedman, R., Adams, C.E., Adler, L.E. *et al.* (2000) Inhibitory neurophysiological deficit as a phenotype for genetic investigation of schizophrenia. *American Journal of Medical Genetics* **97**, 58–64.

Freeman, H. (1994) Schizophrenia and city residence. *British Journal of Psychiatry* **164** (Suppl. 23), 39–50.

Fremming, K.H. (1947) Sygdomsrisikoen for sindslidelser og andre sjaelige abnormtilstande i den Danske gennemshitbefolkning. *Paa grundlag af en katamnestisk underøgelsse af 5500 personer født I, 1883–87*. Munksgaard, Copenhagen.

Geddes, J.R. & Juszczak, E. (1995) Period trends in rate of suicide in first 28 days after discharge from psychiatric hospital in Scotland, 1968–92. *British Medical Journal* **311**, 357–360.

Geddes, J.R. & Lawrie, S.M. (1995) Obstetric complications and schizophrenia: a meta-analysis. *British Journal of Psychiatry* **167**, 786–793.

Gold, J.M. & Weinberger, D.R. (1995) Cognitive deficits and the neurobiology of schizophrenia. *Current Opinion in Neurobiology* **5**, 225–230.

Goldberg, E.M. & Morrison, S.L. (1963) Schizophrenia and social class. *British Journal of Psychiatry* **109**, 785–802.

Goldberg, T.E., Hyde, T.M., Kleinman, J.E. & Weinberger, D.R. (1993) Course of schizophrenia: neuropsychological evidence for a static encephalopathy. *Schizophrenia Bulletin* **19**, 797–804.

Goldstein, M. (1987) The UCLA high-risk project. *Schizophrenia Bulletin* **13**, 505–514.

Gottesman, I.I., McGuffin, P. & Farmer, A.E. (1987) Clinical genetics as clues to the 'real' genetics of schizophrenia. *Schizophrenia Bulletin* **13**, 23–47.

Grech, A., Takei, N. & Murray, R.M. (1997) Maternal exposure to influenza and paranoid schizophrenia. *Schizophrenia Research* **26**, 121–125.

Gupta, S., Andreasen, N.C., Arndt, S. *et al.* (1997a) The Iowa Longitudinal Study of Recent Onset Psychosis: one-year follow-up of first episode patients. *Schizophrenia Research* **23**, 1–13.

Gupta, S., Masand, P.S., Kaplan, D., Bhandary, A. & Hendricks, S. (1997b) The relationship between schizophrenia and irritable bowel syndrome (IBS). *Schizophrenia Research* **23**, 265–268.

Häfner, H. & Reimann, H. (1970) Spatial distribution of mental disorders in Mannheim, 1965. In: *Psychiatric Epidemiology* (eds. E.H. Hare & J.K. Wing), pp. 341–354. Oxford University Press, London.

Häfner, H., Maurer, K., Löffler, W. & Riecher-Rössler, A. (1993) The influence of age and sex on the onset and early course of schizophrenia. *British Journal of Psychiatry* **162**, 80–86.

Häfner, H., Hambrecht, M., Löffler, P., Munk-Jørgensen, P. & Riecher-Rössler, A. (1998) Is schizophrenia a disorder of all ages? A comparison of first episodes and early course across the life-cycle. *Psychological Medicine* **28**, 351–365.

Häfner, H., Löffler, W., Maurer, K., Hambrecht, M. & van der Heiden, W. (1999) Depression, negative symptoms, social stagnation and social decline in the early course of schizophrenia. *Acta Psychiatrica Scandinavica* **100**, 105–118.

Häfner, H., Löffler, W., Riecher-Rössler, A. & Häfner-Ranabauer, W. (2001) Schizophrenie und Wahn im höheren und hohen Lebensalter. *Nervenarzt* **72**, 347–357.

Hagnell, O. (1966) *A Prospective Study of the Incidence of Mental Disorder*. Svenska Bokforlaget, Lund.

Hambrecht, M. & Häfner, H. (2000) Cannabis, vulnerability, and the onset of schizophrenia: an epidemiological perspective. *Australian and New Zealand Journal of Psychiatry* **34**, 468–475.

Hare, E. (1983) Was insanity on the increase? *British Journal of Psychiatry* **142**, 439–445.

Hare, E.H. & Price, J.S. (1968) Mental disorder and season of birth: comparison of psychoses with neuroses. *British Journal of Psychiatry* **115**, 533–540.

Harrison, G., Cooper, J.E. & Gancarczyk, R. (1991) Changes in the administrative incidence of schizophrenia. *British Journal of Psychiatry* **159**, 811–816.

Harrison, G., Glazebrook, C., Brewin, J. *et al.* (1997) Increased incidence of psychotic disorders in migrants from the Caribbean to the United Kingdom. *Psychological Medicine* **27**, 799–806.

Harrison, G., Amin, S., Singh, S., Croudace, T. & Jones, P. (1999) Outcome of psychosis in people of African-Caribbean family origin. *British Journal of Psychiatry* **175**, 43–49.

Haslam, J. (1809) *Observations on Madness and Melancholy*, 2nd edn. Callow, London.

Hassiotis, A., Ukoumunne, O., Tyrer, P. *et al.* (1999) Prevalence and characteristics of inpatients with severe mental illness and borderline intellectual functioning. *British Journal of Psychiatry* **175**, 135–140.

Hatta, K., Takahashi, T., Nakamura, H. *et al.* (1999) Laboratory findings in acute schizophrenia. *General Hospital Psychiatry* **21**, 220–227.

Helgason, T. (1964) Epidemiology of mental disorders in Iceland. *Acta Psychiatrica Scandinavica Supplement* **173**.

Helgason, T. & Magnusson, H. (1989) The first 80 years of life: a psychiatric epidemiological study. *Acta Psychiatrica Scandinavica* **79** (Suppl. 348), 85–94.

Hemsi, L.K. (1967) Psychiatric morbidity of West Indian immigrants. *Social Psychiatry* **2**, 95–100.

Hickling, F.W. & Rodgers-Johnson, P. (1995) The incidence of first contact schizophrenia in Jamaica. *British Journal of Psychiatry* **167**, 193–196.

Hickling, F.W., McKenzie, K., Mullen, R. & Murray, R. (1999) A Jamaican psychiatrist evaluates diagnoses at a London psychiatric hospital. *British Journal of Psychiatry* **175**, 283–285.

Hilger, T., Propping, P. & Haverkamp, F. (1983) Is there an increase of reproductive rates in schizophrenics? *Archiv für Psychiatrie und Nervenkrankheiten* **233**, 177–186.

Hoek, H.W., Susser, E., Buck, K.A. *et al.* (1996) Schizoid personality disorder after prenatal exposure to famine. *American Journal of Psychiatry* **153**, 1637–1639.

Honer, W.G., Kopala, L.C., Locke, J.J. & Lapointe, J.S. (1996) Left cerebral hemiatrophy and schizophrenia-like psychosis in an adolescent. *Schizophrenia Research* **20**, 231–234.

Hovatta, I., Varilo, T., Suvisaari, J. *et al.* (1999) A genomewide screen for schizophrenia genes in an isolated Finnish subpopulation, suggesting multiple susceptibility loci. *American Journal of Human Genetics* **65**, 1114–1124.

Hultman, C.M., Öhman, A., Cnattingius, S., Wieselgren, I.M. & Lindström, L.H. (1997) Prenatal and neonatal risk factors for schizophrenia. *British Journal of Psychiatry* **170**, 128–133.

Hultman, C.M., Sparén, P., Takei, N., Murray, R.M. & Cnattingius, S. (1999) Prenatal and perinatal risk factors for schizophrenia, affective psychosis, and reactive psychosis of early onset: case–control study. *British Medical Journal* **318**, 421–426.

Hutchinson, G., Takei, N., Fany, T.A. *et al.* (1996) Morbid risk of schizophrenia in first-degree relatives of White and African-Caribbean patients with psychosis. *British Journal of Psychiatry* **169**, 776–780.

Hutchinson, G., Takei, N., Bhugra, D. *et al.* (1997) Increased rate of psychosis among African-Caribbeans in Britain is not due to an excess of pregnancy and birth complications. *British Journal of Psychiatry* **171**, 145–147.

Hutchinson, G., Takei, N., Sham, P., Harvey, I. & Murray, R.M. (1999) Factor analysis of symptoms in schizophrenia: differences between White and Caribbean patients in Camberwell. *Psychological Medicine* **29**, 607–612.

Hyde, T.M., Ziegler, J.C. & Weinberger, D.R. (1992) Psychiatric disturbances in metachromatic leukodystrophy. *Archives of Neurology* **49**, 401–406.

Hyman, S. (1999) Introduction to the complex genetics of mental disorders. *Biological Psychiatry* **45**, 518–521.

Ichiki, M., Kunugi, H., Takei, N. *et al.* (2000) Intra-uterine physical growth in schizophrenia: evidence confirming excess of premature birth. *Psychological Medicine* **30**, 597–604.

Indian Council of Medical Research (ICMR) (1988) *Multi-Centered Collaborative Study of Factors Associated with Course and Outcome of Schizophrenia.* ICMR, New Delhi.

Imamura, Y., Nakane, Y., Ohta, Y. & Kondo, H. (1999) Lifetime prevalence of schizophrenia among individuals prenatally exposed to atomic bomb radiation in Nagasaki City. *Acta Psychiatrica Scandinavica* **100**, 344–349.

Ismail, B., Cantor-Graae, E. & McNeil, T.F. (1998) Minor physical abnormalities in schizophrenic patients and their siblings. *American Journal of Psychiatry* **155**, 1695–1702.

Isohanni, I., Jarvelin, M.R., Nieminen, P. *et al.* (1998) School performance as a predictor of pychiatric hospitalizaiton in adult life. A 28-year follow-up in the Northern Finland 1966 Birth Cohort. *Psychological Medicine* **28**, 967–974.

Jablensky, A. (1986) Epidemiology of schizophrenia: a European perspective. *Schizophrenia Bulletin* **12**, 52–73.

Jablensky, A. & Cole, S.W. (1997) Is the earlier age at onset of schizophrenia in males a confounded finding? Results from a cross-cultural investigation. *British Journal of Psychiatry* **170**, 234–240.

Jablensky, A., Sartorius, N., Ernberg, G. *et al.* (1992) Schizophrenia: manifestations, incidence and course in different cultures: a World Health Organization 10-Country Study. *Psychological Medicine.* Monograph (Suppl. 20). Cambridge University Press, Cambridge.

Jablensky, A., Hugler, H., von Cranach, M. & Kalinov, K. (1993) Kraepelin revisited: a reassessment and statistical analysis of dementia praecox and manic-depressive insanity in 1908. *Psychological Medicine* **23**, 843–858.

Jablensky, A., McGrath, J., Herrman, H. *et al.* (1999) *People Living with Psychotic Illness: an Australian Study 1997–98.* National Survey of Mental Health and Wellbeing Report 4. Commonwealth of Australia, Canberra.

Jablensky, A., McGrath, J., Herrman, H. *et al.* (2000) Psychotic disorders in urban areas: an overview of the Study of Low Prevalence Disorders. *Australian and New Zealand Journal of Psychiatry* **34**, 221–236.

Jarman, B., Hirsch, S., White, P. & Driscoll, R. (1992) Predicting psychiatric admission rates. *British Medical Journal* **304**, 1146–1151.

Jaspers, K. (1963) *General Psychopathology.* Manchester University Press, Manchester.

Javitt, D.C., Strous, R.D., Cowan, N., Grochowski, S. & Ritter, W. (1997) Impaired precision, but normal retention, of auditory sensory ('echoic') memory information in schizophrenia. *Journal of Abnormal Psychology* **106**, 315–324.

Jeffreys, S.E., Harvey, C.A., McNaught, A.S. *et al.* (1997) The Hampstead Schizophrenia Survey 1991. I. Prevalence and service use comparisons in an inner London health authority, 1986–91. *British Journal of Psychiatry* **170**, 301–306.

Jeste, D.V., Gladsjo, J.A., Lindamer, L.A. & Lacro, J.P. (1996) Medical comorbidity in schizophrenia. *Schizophrenia Bulletin* **22**, 413–430.

Jones, P., Rodgers, B., Murray, R. & Marmot, M. (1994) Child developmental risk factors for adult schizophrenia in the British 1946 birth cohort. *Lancet* **344**, 1398–1402.

Jones, P.B., Rantakallio, P., Hartikainen, A.L., Isohanni, M. & Sipila, P. (1998) Schizophrenia as a long-term outcome of pregnancy, delivery, and perinatal complications: a 28-year follow-up of the 1966 North Finland general population birth cohort. *American Journal of Psychiatry* **155**, 355–364.

Kebede, D. & Alem, A. (1999) Major mental disorders in Adis Ababa, Ethiopia. I. Schizophrenia, schizoaffective and cognitive disorders. *Acta Psychiatrica Scandinavica* **100**, 11–17.

Kendell, R.E. & Adams, W. (1991) Unexplained fluctuations in the risk for schizophrenia by month and year of birth. *British Journal of Psychiatry* **158**, 758–763.

Kendell, R.E., McInneny, K., Juszczak, E. & Bain. M. (2000) Obstetric complications and schizophrenia. *British Journal of Psychiatry* **176**, 516–522.

Kendler, K.S. & Eaves, L.J. (1986) Models for the joint effect of genotype and environment on liability to psychiatric illness. *American Journal of Psychiatry* **143**, 279–289.

Kendler, K.S. & Walsh, D. (1995) Gender and schizophrenia: results of an epidemiologically based family study. *British Journal of Psychiatry* **167**, 184–192.

Kendler, K.S., Masterson, C.C., Ungaro, R. & Davis, K.L. (1984) A family history study of schizophrenia-related personality disorders. *American Journal of Psychiatry* **141**, 424–427.

Kendler, K.S., Gallagher, T.J., Abelson, J.M. & Kessler, R.C. (1996a) Lifetime prevalence, demographic risk factors, and diagnostic validity of non-affective psychosis as assessed in a US community sample: the National Comorbidity Survey. *Archives of General Psychiatry* **53**, 1022–1031.

Kendler, K.S., Karkowski-Shuman, L. & Walsh, D. (1996b) Age at onset in schizophrenia and risk of illness in relatives. *British Journal of Psychiatry* **169**, 213–218.

Kessler, R.C., McGonagle, K.A., Zhao, S. *et al.* (1994) Lifetime and 12-month prevalence of DSM-IIIR psychiatric disorders in the United States. *Archives of General Psychiatry* **51**, 8–19.

Khoury, M.J., Beaty, T.H. & Cohen, B.H. (1993) *Fundamentals of Genetic Epidemiology*, pp. 59–61. Oxford University Press, New York.

Kläning, U. (1999) Greater occurrence of schizophrenia in dizygotic but not monozygotic twins. *British Journal of Psychiatry* **175**, 407–409.

Klemperer, J. (1933) Zur Belastungsstatistik der Durchschnittsbevölkerung: Psychosehäufigkeit unter 1000 stichprobemässig ausgelesenen Probanden. *Zeitschrift für die gesamte Neurologie und Psychiatrie* **146**, 277–316.

Kraepelin, E. (1919) *Dementia Praecox and Paraphrenia.* Livingstone, Edinburgh.

Krebs, M.O., Leroy, S., Duaux, E. *et al.* (2002) Vulnerability to cannabis, schizophrenia and the (ATT) N polymorphism of the cannabinoid receptor type 1 gene [Abstract]. *Schizophrenia Research* **53** (Suppl.), 72.

Kretschmer, E. (1936) *Physique and Character*, 2nd edn. Trubner, New York.

Kringlen, E. (1978) Adult offspring of two psychotic parents, with special reference to schizophrenia. In: *The Nature of Schizophrenia* (eds L.C. Wynne, R.L. Cromwell & S. Matthysse), pp. 9–24. Wiley, New York.

Kunugi, H., Nanko, S., Takei, N. *et al.* (1995) Schizophrenia following *in utero* exposure to the 1957 influenza epidemics in Japan. *American Journal of Psychiatry* **152**, 450–452.

Lander, E.S. & Schork, N.J. (1994) Genetic dissection of complex traits. *Science* **265**, 2037–2048.

Lane, A., Byrne, M., Mulvany, F. *et al.* (1995) Reproductive behaviour in schizophrenia relative to other mental disorders: evidence for increased fertility in men despite decreased marital rate. *Acta Psychiatrica Scandinavica* **91**, 222–228.

Lane, E. & Albee, G.W. (1964) Early childhood intellectual differences between schizophrenic adults and their siblings. *Journal of Abnormal and Social Psychology* 68, 193–195.

Larson, C.A. & Nyman, G.E. (1973) Differential fertility in schizophrenia. *Acta Psychiatrica Scandinavica* 9, 272–280.

Lauerma, H., Lehtinen, V., Joukamaa, M. *et al.* (1998) Schizophrenia among patients treated for rheumatoid arthritis and appendicitis. *Schizophrenia Research* 29, 255–261.

Lawrence, D., Holman, C.D.J., Jablensky, A., Threfall, T.J. & Fuller, S.A. (2000a) Excess cancer mortality in Western Australian psychiatric patients due to higher case fatality rates. *Acta Psychiatrica Scandinavica* 101, 382–388.

Lawrence, D., Jablensky, A.V., Holman, C.D.J. & Pinder, T.J. (2000b) Mortality in Western Australian psychiatric patients. *Social Psychiatry and Psychiatric Epidemiology* 35, 341–347.

Lee, C.K., Kwak, Y.S., Yamamoto, J. *et al.* (1990) Psychiatric epidemiology in Korea. *Journal of Nervous and Mental Disorders* 178, 242–252.

Lemkau, P., Tietze, C. & Cooper, M. (1943) A survey of statistical studies on the prevalence and incidence of mental disorder in sample populations. *Public Health Reports* 58, 1909–1927.

Leweke, F.M., Giuffrida, A., Wurster, U., Emrich, H.M. & Piomelli, D. (1999) Elevated endogenous cannabinoids in schizophrenia. *Neuroreport* 10, 1665–1669.

Lewis, M.S. & Griffin, T. (1981) An explanation for the season of birth effect in schizophrenia and certain other diseases. *Psychological Bulletin* 89, 589–596.

Lewis, S.W. & Mezey, G.C. (1985) Clinical correlates of septum pellucidum cavities: an unusual association with psychosis. *Psychological Medicine* 15, 43–54.

Lewis, S.W., Reveley, A.M., David, A.S. & Ron, M.A. (1988) Agenesis of the corpus callosum and schizophrenia. *Psychological Medicine* 18, 341–347.

Lieberman, Y.I. (1974) The problem of incidence of schizophrenia: material from a clinical and epidemiological study [in Russian]. *Zhurnal Nevropatologii I Psikhiatrii* 74, 1224–1232.

Lieberman, J.A. (1999) Is schizophrenia a neurodegenerative disorder? A clinical and neurobiological perspective. *Biological Psychiatry* 46, 729–739.

Lin, T.Y., Chu, H.M., Rin, H. *et al.* (1989) Effects of social change on mental disorders in Taiwan: observations based on a 15-year follow-up survey of general populations in three communities. *Acta Psychiatrica Scandinavica* 79 (Suppl. 348), 11–34.

Link, B. & Dohrenwend, B.P. (1980) Formulation of hypotheses about the ratio of untreated to treated cases in the true prevalence studies of functional psychiatric disorders in adults in the United States. In: *Mental Illness in the United States: Epidemiologic Estimates* (eds B.P. Dohrenwend, B.S. Dohrenwend, M.S. Gould *et al.*), pp. 133–148. Praeger, New York.

Linszen, D.H., Dingemans, P.M. & Lenior, M.E. (1994) Cannabis abuse and the course of recent-onset schizophrenic disorders. *Archives of General Psychiatry* 51, 273–279.

Loebel, A.D., Lieberman, J.A., Alvir, J.M.J. *et al.* (1992) Duration of psychosis and outcome in first-episode schizophrenia. *American Journal of Psychiatry* 149, 1183–1188.

McGorry, P.D., Edwards, J., Mihalopoulos, C., Harrigan, S.M. & Jackson, H.J. (1996) EPPIC: an evolving system of early detection and optimal management. *Schizophrenia Bulletin* 22, 305–326.

McGrath, J.J. & Welham, J.L. (1999) Season of birth and schizophrenia: a systematic review and meta-analysis of data from the Southern Hemisphere. *Schizophrenia Research* 35, 237–242.

McGrath, J.J., Hearle, J., Jenner, L. *et al.* (1999) The fertility and fecundity of patients with psychoses. *Acta Psychiatrica Scandinavica* 99, 441–446.

McGuire, P.K., Jones, P., Harvey, I. *et al.* (1995) Morbid risk of schizophrenia for relatives of patients with cannabis-associated psychosis. *Schizophrenia Research* 15, 277–281.

McNaught, A., Jeffreys, S.E., Harvey, C.A. *et al.* (1997) The Hampstead Schizophrenia Survey 1991. II. Incidence and migration in inner London. *British Journal of Psychiatry* 170, 307–311.

McNeil, T.F. & Kaij, L. (1987) Swedish high-risk study: sample characteristics at age 6. *Schizophrenia Bulletin* 13, 373–381.

McNeil, T.F., Cantor-Graae, E. & Ismail, B. (2000) Obstetric complications and congenital malformations in schizophrenia. *Schizophrenia Research* 31, 166–178.

Mahy, E., Mallett, R., Leff, J. & Bhugra, D. (1999) First contact rate incidence of schizophrenia on Barbados. *British Journal of Psychiatry* 175, 28–33.

Mäkikirö, T., Isohanni, M., Moring, J. *et al.* (1997) Is a child's risk of early onset schizophrenia increased in the highest social class? *Schizophrenia Research* 23, 245–252.

Mäkikirö, T., Karvonen, J.T., Hakko, H. *et al.* (1998) Comorbidity of hospital-treated psychiatric and physical disorders with special reference to schizophrenia: a 28 year follow-up of the 1966 Northern Finland general population birth cohort. *Public Health* 112, 221–228.

Mallard, E.C., Rehn, A., Rees, S., Tolcos, M. & Copolov, D. (1999) Ventriculomegaly and reduced hippocampal volume following intrauterine growth-restriction: implications for the aetiology of schizophrenia. *Schizophrenia Research* 40, 11–21.

Malmberg, A., Lewsi, G., David, A. & Allebeck, P. (1998) Premorbid adjustment and personality in people with schizophrenia. *British Journal of Psychiatry* 172, 308–313.

Marcelis, M., Takei, N. & van Os, J. (1999) Urbanization and risk for schizophrenia: does the effect operate before or around the illness onset? *Psychological Medicine* 29, 1197–1203.

Mason, P.R. & Winton, F.E. (1995) Ear disease and schizophrenia: a case–control study. *Acta Psychiatrica Scandinavica* 91, 217–221.

Mednick, S.A. (1970) Breakdown in individuals at high risk for schizophrenia: possible predispositional perinatal factors. *Mental Hygiene* 54, 50–63.

Mednick, S.A., Machon, R.A., Huttunen, M.O. & Bonett, D. (1988) Adult schizophrenia following prenatal exposure to an influenza epidemic. *Archives of General Psychiatry* 45, 189–192.

Meehl, P.E. (1962) Schizotaxia, schizotypy, schizophrenia. *American Psychologist* 17, 827–838.

Michie, P.T., Budd, T.W., Todd, J. *et al.* (2000) Duration and frequency mismatch negativity in schizophrenia. *Clinical Neurophysiology* 111, 1054–1065.

Mino, Y., Oshima, I., Tsuda, T. & Okagami, K. (2000) No relationship between schizophrenic birth and influenza epidemics in Japan. *Journal of Psychiatric Research* 34, 133–138.

Mirsky, A.F., Ingraham, L.J. & Kugelmass, S. (1995) Neuropsychological assessment of attention and its pathology in the Israeli cohort. *Schizophrenia Bulletin* 21, 193–204.

Mischler, E.G. & Scotch, N.A. (1983) Sociocultural factors in the epidemiology of schizophrenia: a review. *Psychiatry* 26, 315–351.

Morgan, V., Castle, D., Page, A. *et al.* (1997) Influenza epidemics and incidence of schizophrenia, affective disorders and mental retardation in Western Australia: no evidence of a major effect. *Schizophrenia Research* 26, 25–39.

Mortensen, P.B. (1987) Neuroleptic treatment and other factors modifying cancer risk in schizophrenic patients. *Acta Psychiatrica Scandinavica* 75, 585–590.

Mortensen, P.B. (1994) The occurrence of cancer in first admitted schizophrenic patients. *Schizophrenia Research* 12, 185–194.

Mortensen, P.B. & Juel, K. (1993) Mortality and causes of death in first admitted schizophrenic patients. *British Journal of Psychiatry* 163, 183–189.

Mortensen, P.B., Pedersen, C.B., Westergaard, T. *et al.* (1999) Effects of family history and place and season of birth on the risk of schizophrenia. *New England Journal of Medicine* 340, 603–608.

Munk-Jørgensen, P. (1986) Decreasing first-admission rates of schizophrenia among males in Denmark from 1970 to 1984. *Acta Psychiatrica Scandinavica* 73, 645–650.

Munk-Jørgensen, P. & Mortensen, P.B. (1992) Incidence and other aspects of the epidemiology of schizophrenia in Denmark, 1971–87. *British Journal of Psychiatry* 161, 489–495.

Murphy, K.C. & Owen, M.J. (1996) Minor physical anomalies and their relationship to the aetiology of schizophrenia. *British Journal of Psychiatry* 168, 139–142.

Murthy, G.V.S., Janakiramaiah, N., Gangadhar, B.N. & Subbarrishna, D.K. (1998) Sex difference in age at onset of schizophrenia: discrepant findings from India. *Acta Psychiatrica Scandinavica* 97, 321–325.

Nicole, L., Lesage, A. & Lalonde, P. (1992) Lower incidence and increased male : female ratio in schizophrenia. *British Journal of Psychiatry* 161, 556–557.

Nicolson, R. & Rapoport, J.L. (1999) Childhood-onset schizophrenia: rare but worth studying. *Biological Psychiatry* 46, 1418–1428.

Nimgaonkar, V.L., Ward, S.E., Agarde, H., Weston, N. & Ganguli, R. (1997) Fertility in schizophrenia: results from a contemporary US cohort. *Acta Psychiatrica Scandinavica* 95, 364–369.

Nimgaonkar, V.L., Fujiwara, T.M., Dutta, M. *et al.* (2000) Low prevalence of psychoses among the Hutterites, an isolated religious community. *American Journal of Psychiatry* 157, 1065–1070.

Noupoulos, P., Flaum, M., O'Leary, D. & Andreasen, N.C. (2000) Sexual dimorphism in the human brain: evaluation of tissue volume, tissue composition and surface anatomy using magnetic resonance imaging. *Psychiatry Research* 98, 1–13.

O'Flaithbheartaigh, S., Williams, P.A. & Jones, G.H. (1994) Schizophrenic psychosis and associated aqueduct stenosis. *British Journal of Psychiatry* 164, 684–686.

Ødegaard, Ø. (1946a) A statistical investigation of the incidence of mental disorder in Norway. *Psychiatric Quarterly* 20, 381–401.

Ødegaard, Ø. (1946b) Marriage and mental disease: a study in social psychopathology. *Journal of Mental Science* 92, 35–59.

Ødegaard, Ø. (1952) The incidence of mental diseases as measured by census investigations versus admission statistics. *Psychiatric Quarterly* 26, 212–218.

Ødegaard, Ø. (1980) Fertility of psychiatric first admissions in Norway, 1936–75. *Acta Pychiatrica Scandinavica* 62, 212–220.

van Os, J. & Selten, J.P. (1998) Prenatal exposure to maternal stress and subsequent schizophrenia. The May 1940 invasion of the Netherlands. *British Journal of Psychiatry* 172, 324–326.

van Os, J., Driessen, G., Gunther, N. & Delespaul, P. (2000) Neighbourhood variation in incidence of schizophrenia: evidence for person–environment interaction. *British Journal of Psychiatry* 176, 243–248.

Ösby, U., Correia, N., Brandt, L., Ekbom, A. & Sparén, P. (2000) Mortality and causes of death in schizophrenia in Stockholm County, Sweden. *Schizophrenia Research* 45, 21–28.

Österberg, E. (1978) Schizophrenia and rheumatic disease. *Acta Psychiatrica Scandinavica* 58, 339–359.

Padmavathi, R., Rajkumar, S., Kumar, N., Manoharan, A. & Kamath, S. (1987) Prevalence of schizophrenia in an urban community in Madras. *Indian Journal of Psychiatry* 31, 233–239.

Pallast, E.G.M., Jongbloet, P.H., Straatman, P.H. & Zielhuis, G.A. (1994) Excess seasonality of births among patients with schizophrenia and seasonal ovopathy. *Schizophrenia Bulletin* 20, 269–275.

Palmer, B.W., McClure, F.S. & Jeste, D.V. (2001) Schizophrenia in late life: findings challenge traditional concepts. *Harvard Review of Psychiatry* 9, 51–58.

Pinel, P. (1803) *Nosographie philosophique: ou la methode de l'analyse apliquée a la médecine*, 2nd edn, Vol. 3. Brosson, Paris.

Propping, P. (1983) Genetic disorders presenting as 'schizophrenia': Karl Bonhoeffer's early view of the psychosis in the light of medical genetics. *Human Genetics* 65, 1–10.

Puri, B.K., Hall, A.D. & Lewis, S.W. (1994) Cerebral hemiatrophy and schizophrenia. *British Journal of Psychiatry* 165, 403–405.

Rajkumar, S., Padmavathi, R., Thara, R. & Sarada Menon, M. (1993) Incidence of schizophrenia in an urban community in Madras. *Indian Journal of Psychiatry* 35, 18–21.

Raman, A.C. & Murphy, H.M.M. (1972) Failure of traditional prognostic indicators in Afro-Asian psychotics: results from a long-term follow-up study. *Journal of Nervous and Mental Disease* 154, 238–247.

Rantakallio, P., Jones, P., Moring, J. & von Wendt, L. (1997) Association between central nervous system infections during childhood and adult onset schizophrenia and other psychoses: a 28-year follow-up. *International Journal of Epidemiology* 26, 837–843.

Regier, D.A., Kaelber, C.T., Rae, D.S. *et al.* (1998) Limitations of diagnostic criteria and assessment instruments for mental disorders: implications for research and policy. *Archives of General Psychiatry* 55, 109–115.

Reid, D.D. (1960) *Epidemiological Methods in the Study of Mental Disorders*. Public Health Papers No. 2. World Health Organization, Geneva.

Reveley, A.M. & Reveley, M.A. (1983) Aqueduct stenosis and schizophrenia. *Journal of Neurology, Neurosurgery and Psychiatry* 46, 18–22.

Riecher-Rössler, A., Fatkenheuer, B., Löffler, W., Maurer, K. & Häfner, H. (1992) Is age of onset in schizophrenia influenced by marital status? *Social Psychiatry and Psychiatric Epidemiology* 27, 122–128.

Rin, H. & Lin, T.Y. (1962) Mental illness among Formosan aborigines as compared with the Chinese in Taiwan. *Journal of Mental Science* 198, 134–146.

Risch, N. (1997) Evolving methods in genetic epidemiology. II. Genetic linkage from an epidemiological perspective. *Epidemiologic Reviews* 19, 24–32.

Roberts, J.K.A., Trimble, M.R. & Robertson, M. (1983) Schizophrenic psychosis associated with aqueduct stenosis in adults. *Journal of Neurology, Neurosurgery and Psychiatry* 46, 892–898.

Robins, L.N. (1989) Diagnostic grammar and assessment: translating criteria into questions. *Psychological Medicine* 19, 57–68.

Robins, L.N., Helzer, J.E., Croughan, J. *et al.*(1981) National Institute of Mental Health Diagnostic Interview Schedule. Its History, characteristics, and validity. *Archives of General Psychiatry* 38, 381–389.

Robins, L.N. & Regier, D.A., eds (1991) *Psychiatric Disorders in America: the Epidemiologic Catchment Area Study*, pp. 1–10. Free Press, New York.

Robins, L.N., Wing, J.K., Wittchen, H.U. *et al.* (1988) The Composite International Diagnostic Interview: an epidemiologic instrument suitable for use in conjunction with different diagnostic systems and in different cultures. *Archives of General Psychiatry* 45, 1069–1077.

Rosenthal, R.N. (1998) Is schizophrenia addiction prone? *Current Opinion in Psychiatry* 11, 45–48.

Rotstein, V.G. (1977) Material from a psychiatric survey of sample groups from the adult population in several areas of the USSR [in Russian]. *Zhurnal Nevropatologii i Psikhiatrii* 77, 569–574.

Sacker, A., Done, J., Crow, T.J. & Golding, J. (1995) Antecedents of schizophrenia and affective illness: obstetric complications. *British Journal of Psychiatry* 166, 734–741.

Salan, R. (1992) Epidemiology of schizophrenia in Indonesia (the Tambora I study). *ASEAN Journal of Psychiatry* 2, 52–57.

Sanderson, T.L., Doody, G.A., Best, J., Owens, D.G.C. & Johnstone, E.C. (2001) Correlations between clinical and historical variables, and cerebral structural variables in people with mild intellectual disability and schizophrenia. *Journal of Intellectual Disability Research* 45, 89–98.

Sartorius, N., Jablensky, A., Korten, A. *et al.* (1986) Early manifestations and first-contact incidence of schizophrenia in different cultures: a preliminary report on the initial evaluation phase of the WHO Collaborative Study on Determinants of Outcome of Severe Mental Disorders. *Psychological Medicine* 16, 909–928.

Saugstad, L.F. & Ødegaard, Ø. (1979) Mortality in psychiatric hospitals in Norway, 1950–74. *Acta Psychiatrica Scandinavica* 59, 431–447.

Schulsinger, F., Parnas, J., Petersen, E.T. *et al.* (1984) Cerebral ventricular size in the offspring of schizophrenic mothers. *Archives of General Psychiatry* 41, 602–606.

Selten, J.P., Slaets, J. & Kahn, R.S. (1997) Schizophrenia in Surinamese and Dutch Antillean immigrants to the Netherlands: evidence of an increased incidence. *Psychological Medicine* 27, 807–811.

Selten, J.P., Slaets, J. & Kahn, R. (1998) Prenatal exposure to influenza and schizophrenia in Surinamese and Dutch Antillean immigrants to the Netherlands. *Schizophrenia Research* 30, 101–103.

Selten, J.P., Brown, A.S., Moons, K.G.M. *et al.* (1999a) Prenatal exposure to the 1957 influenza pandemic and non-affective psychosis in the Netherlands. *Schizophrenia Research* 38, 85–91.

Selten, J.P., van der Graaf, Y., van Duursen, R., Gispen-de Wied, C. & Kahn, R.S. (1999b) Psychotic illness after prenatal exposure to the 1953 Dutch flood disaster. *Schizophrenia Research* 35, 243–245.

Sewell, D.D. (1996) Schizophrenia and HIV. *Schizophrenia Bulletin* 22, 465–473.

Sham, P.C., O'Callaghan, E., Takei, N. *et al.* (1992) Schizophrenia following prenatal exposure to influenza epidemics between 1939 and 1960. *British Journal of Psychiatry* 160, 461–466.

Shields, J. (1977) High risk for schizophrenia: genetic considerations. *Psychological Medicine* 7, 7–10.

Sierra-Honigmann, A.M., Carbone, K.M. & Yolken, R.H. (1995) Polymerase chain reaction (PCR) search for viral nucleic acid sequences in schizophrenia. *British Journal of Psychiatry* 166, 55–60.

Silver, H. & Abboud, E. (1994) Drug abuse in schizophrenia: comparison of patients who began drug abuse before their first admission with those who began abusing drugs after their first admission. *Schizophrenia Research* 13, 57–63.

Sirota, P., Frydman, M. & Sirota, L. (1990) Schizophrenia and Marfan syndrome. *British Journal of Psychiatry* 157, 433–436.

Sjögren, T. (1948) Genetic-statistical and psychiatric investigations of a West Swedish population. *Acta Psychiatrica et Neurologica Scandinavica Supplement* 52.

Srinivasan, T.N. & Padmavati, R. (1997) Fertility and schizophrenia: evidence for increased fertility in the relatives of schizophrenic patients. *Acta Psychiatrica Scandinavica* 96, 260–264.

Stabenau, J.R. & Pollin, W. (1967) Early characteristics of monozygotic twins discordant for schizophrenia. *Archives of General Psychiatry* 17, 723–734.

Stephens, J.H., Astrup, C., Carpenter, W.T., Shaffer, J.W. & Goldberg, J. (1982) A comparison of nine systems to diagnose schizophrenia. *Psychiatry Research* 6, 127–143.

Strakowski, S.M., Tohen, M., Stoll, A.L. *et al.* (1993) Comorbidity in psychosis at first hospitalization. *American Journal of Psychiatry* 150, 752–757.

Strömgren, E. (1935) Zum Ersatz des Weinbergschen 'abgekurzten Verfahren': Zugleich ein Beitrag zur Frage der Erblichkeit des Erkrankungsalters bei der Schizophrenie. *Zeitschrift für die gesamte Neurologie und Psychiatrie* 153, 784–797.

Strömgren, E. (1938) Beiträge zur psychiatrischen Erblehre, auf Grund von Untersuchungen an einer Inselbevölkerung. *Acta Psychiatrica et Neurologica Scandinavica Supplement* 19.

Susser, E.S. & Lin, S.P. (1992) Schizophrenia after prenatal exposure to the Dutch hunger winter of 1944–45. *Archives of General Psychiatry* 49, 983–988.

Susser, E.S., Schaefer, C.A., Brown, A.S., Begg, M.D. & Wyatt, R.J. (2000) The design of the prenatal determinants of schizophrenia study. *Schizophrenia Bulletin* 26, 257–273.

Suvisaari, J.M., Haukka, J.K. & Lönnqvist, J.K. (2001) Season of birth among patients with schizophrenia and their siblings: evidence for the procreational habits hypothesis. *American Journal of Psychiatry* 158, 754–757.

Szymanski, S.R., Cannon, T.D., Gallacher, F., Erwin, R.J. & Gur, R.E. (1996) Course of treatment response in first-episode and chronic schizophrenia. *American Journal of Psychiatry* 153, 519–525.

Taieb, O., Baleyte, J.M., Mazet, P. & Fillet, A.M. (2001) Borna disease virus and psychiatry. *European Psychiatry* 16, 3–10.

Takei, N., Sham, P., O'Callaghan, E. *et al.* (1994) Prenatal exposure to influenza and the development of schizophrenia: is the effect confined to females? *American Journal of Psychiatry* 151, 117–119.

Taller, A., Asher, D.M., Pomeroy, K.L. *et al.* (1996) Search for viral nucleic acid sequences in brain tissues of patients with schizophrenia using nested polymerase chain reaction. *Archives of General Psychiatry* 53, 32–40.

Tien, A.Y. & Eaton, W.W. (1992) Psychopathologic precursors and sociodemographic risk factors for the schizophrenia syndrome. *Archives of General Psychiatry* 49, 37–46.

Tienari, P. (1991) Interaction between genetic vulnerability and family environment: the Finnish adoptive family study of schizophrenia. *Acta Psychiatrica Scandinavica* 84, 460–465.

Torrey, E.F. (1980) *Schizophrenia and Civilization*. Jason Aronson, New York.

Torrey, E.F. (1987) Prevalence studies of schizophrenia. *British Journal of Psychiatry* 150, 598–608.

Torrey, E.F. (1995) Prevalence of psychosis among the Hutterites: a reanalysis of the 1950–53 study. *Schizophrenia Research* 16, 167–170.

Torrey, E.F., Taylor, E.H., Bracha, H.S. *et al.* (1994) Prenatal origin of schizophrenia in a subgroup of discordant monozygotic twins. *Schizophrenia Bulletin* 20, 423–432.

Torrey, E.F., Bowler, A.E. & Clark, K. (1997a) Urban birth and residence as risk factors for psychoses: an analysis of 1880 data. *Schizophrenia Research* 25, 169–176.

Torrey, E.F., Miller, J., Rawlings, R. & Yolken, R.H. (1997b) Seasonality of births in schizophrenia and bipolar disorder: a review of the literature. *Schizophrenia Research* 28, 1–38.

Tracy, J.I., Josiassen, R.C. & Bellack, A.S. (1995) Neuropsychology of dual diagnosis: understanding the combined effects of schizophrenia and substance use disorders. *Clinical Psychology Review* 15, 67–97.

Tramer, M. (1929) Über die biologische Bedeutung des Geburtsmonats, insbesondere für die Psychosenerkrankung. *Schweizer Archiv für Neurologie, Neurochirurgie und Psychiatrie* 24, 17–24.

Verdoux, H., Geddes, J.R., Takei, N. *et al.* (1997) Obstetric complications and age at onset in schizophrenia: an international collaborative meta-analysis of individual patient data. *American Journal of Psychiatry* **154**, 1220–1227.

Verheij, R.A., van de Mheen, H.D., de Bakker, D.H., Groenewegen, P.P. & Mackenbach, J.P. (1998) Urban–rural variations in health in the Netherlands: does selective migration play a part? *Journal of Epidemiology and Community Health* **52**, 487–493.

Waddington, J.L. & Youssef, H.A. (1996) Familial-genetic and reproductive epidemiology of schizophrenia in rural Ireland: age at onset, familial morbid risk and parental fertility. *Acta Psychiatrica Scandinavica* **93**, 62–68.

Waddington, J.L., Youssef, H.A. & Kinsella, A. (1998) Mortality in schizophrenia. *British Journal of Psychiatry* **173**, 325–329.

Wahlbeck, K., Forsén, T., Osmond, C., Barker, D.J. & Eriksson, J.G. (2001) Association of schizophrenia with low maternal body mass index, small size at birth, and thinness during childhood. *Archives of General Psychiatry* **58**, 48–52.

Wahlberg, K.E., Wynne, L.C., Oja, H. *et al.* (1997) Gene–environment interaction in vulnerability to schizophrenia: findings from the Finnish Adoptive Family Study of Schizophrenia. *American Journal of Psychiatry* **154**, 355–362.

Waldo, M.C. (1999) Schizophrenia in Kosrae, Micronesia: prevalence, gender ratios, and clinical symptomatology. *Schizophrenia Research* **35**, 175–181.

Weeke, A. & Strömgren, E. (1978) Fifteen years later: a comparison of patients in Danish psychiatric institutions in 1957, 1962, 1967 and 1972. *Acta Psychiatrica Scandinavica* **57**, 129–144.

Weinberg, W. (1925) Methoden und Technik der Statistik mit besonderer Berücksichtigung der Sozialbiologie. *Handbuch der Sozialen Hygiene und Gesundheitsfürsorge*. Band I. Springer, Berlin.

World Health Organization (1973) *Report of the International Pilot Study of Schizophrenia*, Vol. I. World Health Organization, Geneva.

World Health Organization (1979) *Schizophrenia. An International Follow-Up Study*. Wiley, Chichester.

Wilson, R.I. & Nicoll, R.A. (2001) Endogenous cannabinoids mediate retrograde signalling at hippocampal synapses. *Nature* **410**, 588–592.

Wing, J.K., Cooper, J.E. & Sartorius, N. (1974) *The Measurement and Classification of Psychiatric Symptoms*. Cambridge University Press, Cambridge.

Wing, J.K., Babor, T., Brugha, T. *et al.* (1990) SCAN: Schedules for Clinical Assessment in Neuropsychiatry. *Archives of General Psychiatry* **47**, 589–593.

Wing, J.K., Sartorius, N. & Üstün, T.B. (1998) *Diagnosis and Clinical Measutrement in Psychiatry: A Reference Manual for SCAN*. Cambridge University Press, Cambridge.

Zornberg, G.L., Buka, S.L. & Tsuang, M.T. (2000) Hypoxic-ischemia fetal/neonatal complications and risk of schizophrenia and other non-affective psychoses: a 19-year longitudinal study. *American Journal of Psychiatry* **157**, 196–202.

13 Risk factors for schizophrenia: from conception to birth

J.J. McGrath and R. M. Murray

What is a risk factor? 232
Proxy markers of disturbed early development, 232
   Minor physical abnormalities, 232
   Dermatoglyphic features, 233
The search for candidate exposures, 236
   Season of birth, 236
   Place of birth, 236
Pregnancy and birth complications, 236
   Determining exposure status, 236
   Specific pregnancy and birth complications, 239

Demographic and clinical correlates of
   pregnancy and birth complications in
   schizophrenia, 240
   Putative mechanism of action, 240
Prenatal infection, 241
Prenatal nutrition, 241
Prenatal stress, 244
Conclusions, 244
Acknowledgements, 245
References, 245

The neurodevelopmental hypothesis of schizophrenia can be traced back to the end of the nineteenth century (Lewis 1989), but re-emerged in the mid-1980s (Weinberger 1987; Murray *et al.* 1988; Lyon *et al.* 1989). In short, the rediscovered hypothesis regards schizophrenia as a distal consequence of disturbed brain development during the pre- or perinatal period, but does not specify the nature of the early brain disruption, nor define the pathogenesis of the disorder. The neurodevelopmental hypothesis has heuristic appeal in that it directs attention to early life exposures, decades before the onset of the clinical syndrome. However, it has become clear that the model proposed in the 1980s was oversimplistic, and therefore contemporary revisions of the hypothesis regard neurodevelopmental deviance as one component of a more complex aetiology. Thus, the 'developmental risk factor' model talks in terms of an interaction between early and late risk factors, and of a cascade of increasing deviance finally culminating in psychosis (McDonald *et al.* 1999; Murray & Fearon 1999).

The sturdiest of the known risk factors for schizophrenia is the presence of an affected relative. The evidence for a genetic contribution to schizophrenia is addressed in Chapter 14, but it is worth noting here that this may operate in part through one or more of the genes involved in the control of early brain development (Jones & Murray 1991). In this chapter we concentrate on non-genetic risk factors that operate prior to or around birth. The first section examines minor physical anomalies and quantitative measures of dysmorphogenesis as risk indicators (i.e. proxy markers) of developmental disturbance. Subsequently, we examine the broad clues provided by epidemiology that allow us to generate candidate exposures, and detail the evidence for several of these candidates (e.g. pregnancy and birth complications, prenatal infection, prenatal nutrition).

What is a risk factor?

In recent times there has been an effort to clarify terminology surrounding risk factors (Susser 1991; Kraemer *et al.* 1997). Variables that correlate with an outcome, but do not precede the outcome, are sequelae and should not be labelled risk factors. Variables that precede an outcome, but are not causally related to that outcome, are defined as risk indicators or proxy markers. The term 'risk modifying factor' should be reserved for factors that appear to operate within the causal chain (contribute to the outcome). In neurodevelopmental models of schizophrenia, we are looking for distal or 'upstream' risk modifying variables. These factors may operate directly or indirectly. Risk modifying factors can be fixed (e.g. gender) or variable (alcohol intake), endogenous (e.g. genetic factors) or exogenous (e.g. obstetric complications), protective or adverse.

Proxy markers of disturbed early development

Minor physical abnormalities

In the late nineteenth century, Thomas Clouston noted that palatal abnormalities (steep narrow-roofed palates) were more common in those patients he regarded as having 'adolescent insanity' – a type of psychosis that he considered had a strong familial tendency (Clouston 1891). Since then, a sizeable body of research has examined minor physical anomalies (MPAs) in schizophrenia and other psychiatric disorders. MPAs are subtle variations in soft-tissue, cartilaginous and bony structures that are the result of an uncertain mix of genetic and environmental factors that operate prenatally. They include variations in the shape and proportions of the head, face, mouth, fingers, hands and toes. Variations of dermatoglyphics (e.g. finger and palm prints) can also be included under this broad heading.

Minor physical anomalies are of interest because they may serve as persistent markers or 'fossilized' evidence of deviant development in fetal life and, in particular, as markers of early events that could have impacted on brain development. They may arise from teratogenic or genetic factors. The latter may result from a general vulnerability to developmental disruption, or to more specific genes underlying infrequent phenotypic variants. The nature of the MPAs may provide clues to the timing of the disruption (e.g. the major features of the palate are essentially complete by 16–17 weeks).

Table 13.1 lists the key findings of studies that have compared the prevalence of MPAs in schizophrenic patients vs. well controls. Overall, the majority of studies indicate an excess of MPAs in schizophrenia (Gualtieri et al. 1982; Lohr & Flynn 1993; Cantor-Graae et al. 1994; Green et al. 1994; Lane et al. 1997; Lohr et al. 1997; Griffiths et al. 1998; Ismail et al. 2000; McGrath et al. 2002) but two studies failed to find an association (McNeil et al. 1992; Alexander et al. 1994). However, high rates of MPAs are by no means specific to schizophrenia or psychosis, being found in a range of other neurodevelopmental disorders such as mental retardation (Alexander et al. 1994), cerebral palsy (Illingworth 1979; Coorssen et al. 1992) and schizotypal personality disorder (Weinstein et al. 1999).

The Waldrop scale (Waldrop et al. 1968), while widely used to assess MPAs from a broad qualitative perspective, is acknowledged to be unsatisfactory by most authors in the field. As a result of problems with the reliance on qualitative measures, two groups have used quantitative craniofacial measures in order to examine dysmorphogenesis. Lane et al. (1997) included quantitative anthropomorphic measures in their study of 174 patients with schizophrenia and 80 control subjects. They reported an overall elongation of the mid- and lower face, widening of the skull base and a concentration of qualitative MPAs in the eyes, ears and mouth in the patient group. McGrath et al. (2002) replicated these findings in a group of 303 subjects with psychotic disorders and 313 well controls. The odds of having a psychotic disorder were increased in those with wider skull bases, smaller lower facial heights, protruding ears, and shorter and wider palates. The ratio of skull width : length was significantly larger in those with psychotic disorders compared to the well controls.

Waddington et al. (1999) have drawn attention to the close links between brain growth and development of the face. The relationship between wider skulls and shorter middle/lower faces noted in the two studies examining craniofacial measures in schizophrenia has also been noted by research on variation in, and evolution of, the human skull (Weidenreich 1941; Enlow & Bhatt 1984; Enlow 1990; Cheverud et al. 1992; Lieberman et al. 2000). Exposures that can impact on these structures include prenatal viral exposures, obstetric complications, general nutritional deficiencies and low vitamin D (Engstrom et al. 1982; Sperber 1989).

Uncommon genetic disorders that may be associated with MPAs have also received increasing attention in recent times. Velocardiofacial syndrome (VCFS) is caused by a microdeletion in the long arm of chromosome 22 and is associated with an increased frequency of schizophrenia and bipolar mood disorder (Gothelf et al. 1999). Waddington et al. (1999) have

suggested that genes involved in craniofacial development warrant close inspect in schizophrenia research. Also, informative craniofacial quantitative measures (e.g. skull base width, facial heights) may serve as useful correlated phenotypes in genetic studies of psychosis (Pulver 2000).

Some investigators have tried to characterize those patients with schizophrenia with high total MPA scores. Studies have shown that patients with high MPA scores tend to have more orofacial tardive dyskinesia (Waddington et al. 1995), have impaired performance on neurognitive tasks (O'Callaghan et al. 1991a; McGrath et al. 1995) and are more likely to be male (O'Callaghan et al. 1991a; Griffiths et al. 1998). This clinical profile has features in common with early descriptions of dementia praecox (Murray 1994).

The relationship between MPAs and the family history of schizophrenia and/or other psychiatric conditions is still not clear, with one group reporting higher MPAs in those with a positive family history (O'Callaghan et al. 1991a), while others have reported either no association (McGrath et al. 1995) or an excess of MPAs in those without a family history (Griffiths et al. 1998). Two studies have compared MPAs in patients with schizophrenia vs. their unaffected siblings. Both studies found that patients had higher total MPA scores compared to the sibling group (Green et al. 1994; Ismail et al. 1998). The study by Ismail et al. also found that siblings had higher total MPA scores compared to well controls, and that while MPA scores were positively correlated within families, there was little correlation in the specific nature of MPAs between patients and their unaffected siblings. These findings suggest (but do not prove) that those with higher total MPA scores have a general developmental instability related to genetic factors but, in the absence of other non-genetic factors, this vulnerability is not sufficient to lead to schizophrenia.

The results concerning age of onset have also been inconsistent, with some groups reporting an association between higher total MPA scores and earlier age of onset (Green et al. 1989; McGrath et al. 2002), while others find no such association (O'Callaghan et al. 1991a; Lohr & Flynn 1993; McGrath et al. 1995; Akabaliev & Sivkov 1998).

Dermatoglyphic features

Many dermatoglyphic features also provide clues to early developmental disturbances because most of these features have stabilized by the second trimester. Quantitative features include measures related to ridge counts (e.g. total ridge count, differences between right- and left-hand total ridge counts, ridge counts between tri-radii at the base of the first and second fingers) and angles related to the shape of the palm and the hand. Qualitative features include the assessment of finger pad patterns (e.g. loops, whorls), palmar creases and ridge dissociations.

Several investigators have found significant group differences when comparing schizophrenia patients vs. well controls on various measures derived from finger and hand prints (Markow &

Table 13.1 Minor physical anomalies and schizophrenia.

Reference	Samples	Method	Comment
Gualtieri *et al.* (1982)	n = 64 Sz n = 127 other psychiatric disorders n = 171 controls	Subset of Waldrop scale	Highest scores found in the Sz group. Significantly higher scores in Sz compared to controls. High scores also in hyperkinetic and autistic children
Guy *et al.* (1983)	n = 40 Sz	Waldrop scale	The patient group had higher rates of MPAs than unpublished norms
Green *et al.* (1989)	n = 67 Sz n = 88 controls	Waldrop scale	Sz had significantly more abnormalities. Patients had high incidence of mouth abnormalities. Younger age of onset for the high MPA group
O'Callaghan *et al.* (1991)	n = 41 Sz	Waldrop scale	Higher levels of MPAs were associated with positive family history, male sex, poor score on test of mental flexibility, and presence of PBCs. No association with age of onset
McNeil *et al.* (1992)	n = 84 offspring of women with non-organic psychosis n = 100 offspring of controls	Congenital malformations Ekelund system	No significant difference between the groups. Suggests that the higher rates of MPAs in Sz are due more to PBCs than genes
Alexander *et al.* (1994)	n = 41 Sz n = 8 BAD n = 19 mentally retarded n = 14 controls	Waldrop scale	An increased prevalence of minor physical anomalies was found in the mentally retarded adults relative to the other groups. There was a non-significant trend for the total mean Waldrop score of the schizophrenic group to be higher than the mean score of the normal group
Lohr and Flynn (1993)	n = 118 Sz n = 33 mood disorders n = 31 controls	Waldrop scale	Sz (but not mood disorders) had more anomalies than controls. Patients with tardive dyskinesia had more MPAs than those without tardive dyskinesia. In Sz, MPAs were unrelated to severity of psychopathology, age of onset, positive/negative symptoms or socio-economic status
Cantor-Graae *et al.* (1994)	n = 22 discordant MZ pairs n = 10 concordant MZ pairs n = 6 control MZ pairs	Waldrop scale plus additional items	Trend for higher total MPA scores in affected vs. non-affected discordant Sz MZ twin. In the overall group, those with pregnancy and birth complications had more MPAs
Green *et al.* (1994)	n = 63 Sz n = 33 sibs n = 26 BAD n = 9 sibs n = 40 controls	Modified Waldrop scale	Sz had higher MPAs than controls and BAD. Those with Sz pts had higher MPA scores than their sibs; sibs did not differ from controls
McGrath *et al.* (1995)	n = 79 Sz n = 31 SA n = 24 mania n = 13 major dep n = 8 organic psychosis n-2 other organic psychosis n = 63 controls	Modified Waldrop scale	MPAs not associated with any particular psychotic disorder. For white subjects, the Sz group had more MPAs than controls. For males there was a weak association between MPAs and family history of major psychiatric disorder. Those with more MPAs had more admissions and longer admissions. MPAs were not associated with gender, age at onset, negative symptoms, premorbid functioning/intelligence, PBCs and selected CT scan variables

Table 13.1 (cont.)

Reference	Samples	Method	Comment
Lane et al. (1997)	n = 174 Sz n = 80 controls	Modified Waldrop and craniofacial and bodily quantitative measures	Patients had significantly higher MPA scores and displayed multiple anomalies of the craniofacial region with an overall narrowing and elongation of the mid-face and lower face. Twelve craniofacial anomalies independently distinguished patients from controls and these variables correctly classified 95% of patients and 80% of control subjects
Lohr et al. (1997)	n = 15 Sz onset after 45 + year n = 8 Sz onset before 45 years n = 11 Alzheimer's n = 11 depression n = 15 controls		Early and late-onset Sz and unipolar depression had more MPAs than normal comparisons Alzheimer's were no different from well controls
Akabaliev and Sivkov (1998)	n = 42 Sz n = 36 controls	Waldrop scale	Sz had more anomalies of head (mouth, ears and eyes) than controls. Higher MPA scores were associated with later birth order. No association with age at onset or season of birth
Ismail et al. (1998)	n = 60 Sz n = 21 non-psychotic sibs n = 75 controls	Waldrop scale and other MPA items	Higher MPA scores found in Sz and their sibs when compared to controls in all body areas, with Sz having higher scores than sibs. Higher MPA scores shared by patients and their sibs but little similarity in specific anomalies within families. MPAs frequently found in, but not limited to, head region
Griffiths et al. (1998)	n = 32 Sz (familial) n = 63 1st degree rel (familial) n = 28 Sz (sporadic) n = 44 1st degree rel (sporadic) n = 47 controls	Weighted Waldrop scale	Compared prevalence of MPAs in familial and sporadic Sz and their 1st degree relatives The Sz group had increased MPAs. More MPAs in sporadic group patients (those without a positive family history of Sz). The group difference was significant for males; trend for females Patients with Sz and a positive family history and the sibling group did not differ from well controls
McGrath et al. (2002)	n = 310 psychosis n = 313 controls	Modified Waldrop scale and craniofacial quantitative measures	Psychosis group had higher MPA total score. The odds of having a psychotic disorder were increased in those with wider skull bases, smaller lower facial heights, protruding ears, and shorter and wider palates. The ratio of skull width/skull length was significantly larger in those with psychotic disorders compared to the well controls. Earlier age of onset was associated with more MPAs and with smaller skull width/length ratios

Sz = schizophrenia, MPA = minor physical anomaly, PBCs = pregnancy and birth complications, BAD = bipolar affective disorder, MZ = monozygotic, sibs = sibling, SA = schizoaffective psychosis, CT = computerized tomography.

Gottesman 1989; Fananas et al. 1990; Bracha et al. 1991; Mellor 1992; Cannon et al. 1994). Fananas et al. have been the main contributors to the recent literature on this subject (Fananas et al. 1990, 1996a,b; Van Os et al. 1997, 2000; Gutierrez et al. 1998; Rosa et al. 2000a). In their twin studies, qualitative dermatoglyphic features (ridge dissociation and palmar creases) were significantly more likely to be found in the affected cotwin in monozygotic twins discordant for psychosis (Rosa et al. 2000b).

In summary, the excess of MPAs and dermatoglyphic abnor-malities in schizophrenia provides tantalizing but tangential evidence about the earliest phases of the pathogenesis of schizo-phrenia. The role of genes and/or teratogens in the production of the MPAs and dermatoglyphic abnormalities may shed light on their parallel role in the orderly development of the brain. How-ever, despite the theoretical association between MPAs and brain development, attempts to link MPAs to adult brain struc-ture and function have been disappointing, with no associations found between MPAs and selected measures derived from computerized tomography (McGrath et al. 1995), magnetic resonance spectroscopy (Buckley *et al.* 1994) or hippocampal or ventricle size (McNeil *et al.* 2000). However, Fananas and colleagues (Van Os *et al.* 2000; Rosa *et al.* 2001) have reported a relationship between abnormalities in dermatoglyphics (a-b-ridge count) and ventricular volume as measured on magnetic resonance imaging (MRI) scans.

The search for candidate exposures

Season of birth

One of the most consistently replicated epidemiological features of schizophrenia is the slight excess of births in the late winter and spring in the northern hemisphere; many studies also show a small decrement in births in the late summer–autumn (Bradbury & Miller 1985; Torrey *et al.* 1997). In one of the most impressive studies, which was based on a comprehensive Danish record-linkage study, Mortensen *et al.* (1999) found that the small seasonal excess of schizophrenia births (relative risk = 1.11) was associated with a sizeable (10.5%) population attributable fraction (PAF) for the disorder. The reason for this high PAF is, of course, that birth in late winter–spring is such a common exposure.

While data on the season of birth effect in the northern hemisphere population are quite robust, the same cannot be said for the southern hemisphere. A meta-analysis performed on data from southern hemisphere studies (in Australia, South Africa and the Reunion Islands) did not support a season of birth effect (McGrath & Welham 1999). There have also been some suggestions of a decrease in the magnitude of the season of birth effect over time in the northern hemisphere (Eagles *et al.* 1995; Suvisaari *et al.* 2000).

Explanations proposed for the seasonal effect range from unusual parental procreational habits to a variety of more specific candidate risk-modifying variables. Candidate exposures that have been proposed as underlying the season of birth effect include perinatal viral exposures (Torrey *et al.* 1997) and various nutritional deficiencies.

Place of birth

Several groups have suggested that being born and/or raised in urban regions is associated with an increased risk of developing schizophrenia compared to rural regions (Lewis *et al.* 1992; O'Callaghan *et al.* 1992a; Takei *et al.* 1992). The quality of evidence for place of birth as a risk factor is now more robust following the publication of two major population-based studies: one from Holland (Marcelis *et al.* 1998a) and one from Denmark (Mortensen *et al.* 1999). The relative risk of developing schizophrenia when born in the city vs. being born in the country is about 2.4. However, as urban-birth is relatively frequent, the two studies reported the PAF for this variable to be substantial (about 30%). Place of birth could be a proxy marker for a risk-modifying variable operating at or before birth. However,

because most people who are born in a city are also brought up there, it is difficult to disentangle pre- and perinatal effects from those operating later in childhood. Indeed, there is some recent evidence that the more years spent in an urban area during childhood, the greater the risk of developing schizophrenia (Pedersen & Mortensen 2001).

Pregnancy and birth complications

There is considerable evidence that pregnancy and birth complications (PBCs) are detrimental to the health of the developing fetus and, in particular, its neurodevelopment (Low *et al.* 1985; Taylor *et al.* 1985; Paneth & Pinto-Martin 1991). It seems obvious therefore to examine the possible role of PBCs in increasing the risk of later schizophrenia.

A substantial body of research is now available that examines the association between PBCs and schizophrenia. Key details from some of these studies are summarized in Table 13.2. The studies have employed a range of designs (e.g. case–control studies, cohort studies), measures of the exposure (based on maternal recall, records, midwife notes, different scoring systems) and measures of the outcome (diagnosis confirmed on interview, register-based diagnosis). Meta-analyses of these data are now available (Geddes & Lawrie 1995; Verdoux *et al.* 1997; Geddes *et al.* 1999). Overall, there is robust evidence that PBCs have a significant but modest effect in increasing the risk of later schizophrenia (odds ratio of about 2).

Determining exposure status

Many studies have relied upon maternal recall to evaluate PBCs (Pollack *et al.* 1966), and the Lewis–Murray scale (Owen *et al.* 1988) has been widely used for this purpose (McCreadie *et al.* 1992; Marcelis *et al.* 1998b). However, studies that have compared maternal recall and birth records have found discrepancies between the two methods (O'Callaghan *et al.* 1990; Cantor-Graae *et al.* 1998; Buka *et al.* 2000) and there is general agreement that birth records provide a more reliable source of data. The majority of the studies in Table 13.2 have been able to access birth records (which themselves can vary in detail and reliability).

Methods to score PBCs have also been refined in recent years with the development of more detailed operationalized systems (McNeil & Sjostrom 1995) and of scoring systems related to pathological processes such as hypoxia/ischaemia (Zornberg *et al.* 2000). The hope has been that an 'ideal' scoring system may allow the identification of particular types of PBCs related to the risk of schizophrenia. However, it is likely that our ability to fractionate PBCs into pathophysiological domains (e.g. infection, inflammation, hypoxia/ischaemia, undernutrition) does not adequately reflect the complex interconnected nature of events that disturb maternal–fetal homeostasis. Also, traditional items included as PBCs are clearly only a small subset of all teratogens. It seems likely that many exposures that impact on

Table 13.2 The association between pregnancy and birth complications and schizophrenia.

Reference	Samples	Source of PBC information Research design	Conclusions
Pollack et al. (1966)	n = 33 Sz n = 33 well sibs	Maternal recall Case–control study	Non-significant trend for more PBCs in the Sz group
Lane and Albee (1966)	n = 52 Sz n = 115 well sibs	Birth records Case–control study	The Sz group had significantly lower birth weight and had higher rates of prematurity
Woerner et al. (1971)	n = 34 Sz n = 42 well sibs	Birth records Case–control study	Non-significant trend for lower birth weight in the Sz group
Woerner et al. (1973)	n = 46 Sz n = 37 well sibs n = 17 affected sibs	Maternal recall and birth records Case–control study	The Sz group had more PBCs than well sibs
McNeil and Kaij (1978)	n = 54 process Sz n = 46 Sz-like psychoses n = 100 controls	Birth records Case–control study	Process Sz group had more PBCs
Jacobsen and Kinney (1980)	n = 63 Sz n = 63 controls	Birth records Case–control study	The Sz group had significantly more PBCs
Parnas et al. (1982)	n = 12 Sz n = 25 schizotypal n = 55 controls	Birth records Case–control study	The Sz group had more PBCs, the schizotypal group had least PBCs. All subjects had mothers with Sz
Lewis and Murray (1987)	n = 955 psychiatric patients	Maternal recall Case–control study	The patients with Sz had more PBCs than other psychiatric patients
Schwarzkopf et al. (1989)	n = 15 Sz n = 6 schizoaffective n = 10 BAD	Maternal recall Case–control study	The Sz and schizoaffective groups had significanly more perinatal complications than the bipolar group
Eagles et al. (1990)	n = 27 Sz n = 27 well sibs	Birth records Case–control study	The Sz group had significantly more PBCs than the well sibls
Done et al. (1991)	n = 57 Sz n = 32 affective disorder n = 16980 full cohort	Birth records Birth cohort	The Sz group did not have an excess of PBCs, however, the affective psychoses group had decreased length of gestation and increased rates of Vitamin K administration at birth
Foerster et al. (1991)	n = 45 Sz n = 28 affective disorders	Maternal recall Case–control study	The Sz group had significantly more PBCs than the affective group
O'Callaghan et al. (1992)	n = 65 Sz n = 65 controls	Birth records Case–control study	The Sz group, especially males, had an excess of PBCs. Those with PBCs had an earlier age of onset
McCreadie et al. (1992)	n = 54 Sz n = 114 sibs (4 with Sz)	Maternal recall Case–control study	No difference found in levels of PBCs between the groups
Heun and Maier (1993)	n = 47 Sz and schizoaffective n = 70 sibs	Maternal recall Case–control study	Patients had more often suffered perinatal complications (42%) than their sibs (29%)
Stober et al. (1993)	n = 80 Sz n = 80	Maternal recall Case–control study	Patients had more PBCs compared to well controls as assessed by two different PBC scales
Verdoux and Bourgeois (1993)	n = 23 Sz n = 23 BAD n = 23 controls	Maternal recall Case–control study	The Sz group had significantly more PBCs than the BAD and the well sibs

Table 13.2 (cont.)

Reference	Samples	Source of PBC information Research design	Conclusions
Gunther-Genta et al. (1994)	$n = 23$ Sz $n = 40$ well sibs	Birth records Case–control study	The patients with Sz had more frequent umbilical cord complications and atypical presentations, as well as higher scores on a scale measuring PBCs linked to possible neonatal asphyxia
Rifkin et al. (1994)	$n = 110$ Sz $n = 100$ controls	Maternal recall Case–control study	The patients with Sz were more likely to have been of lower birth weight. In schizophrenic men, lower birth weight was correlated with poorer premorbid social and cognitive ability, and with impairment in adult cognitive function
Kunugi et al. (1996)	$n = 59$ Sz $n = 31$ healthy sibs $n = 108$ well controls	Birth records Case–control study	Female patients with Sz had experienced significantly more perinatal complications than their sibs and controls
Hollister et al. (1996)	$n = 1867$ Sz males only	Birth records Case–control study nested within hospital-based cohort	Incidence of Sz significantly higher in the Rh-incompatible group compared with Rh-compatible group
Hultman et al. (1997)	$n = 107$ psychotic disorders (82 with Sz) $n = 214$ controls	Birth records Case–control study	Higher total PBC score was associated with Sz A disproportionate birth weight for body length and small head circumference were the strongest independent risk factors for Sz
Jones et al. (1998)	$n = 76$ Sz $n = 11017$ total cohort	Birth records Birth cohort	Combination of low birth weight (<2.5 kg) and short gestation (<37 weeks) was more common among the Sz
Marcelis et al. (1998)	$n = 151$ psychosis $n = 100$ controls	Maternal recall Case–control study	Familial morbid risk of Sz and related psychosis was not associated with PBCs, where there was a positive association with PBCs and familial morbid risk of affective psychosis
Alvir et al. (1999)	$n = 59$ Sz	Birth records Case–control study	A history of PBCs predicted poor response to treatment in the first episode of Sz
Hultman et al. (1999)	$n = 167$ Sz $n = 198$ affective psychosis $n = 292$ reactive psychosis $n = 3285$ controls	Birth records Population-based Case–control study	Sz was associated with multiparity and maternal bleeding during the pregnancy. For males, small for gestational age was associated with Sz. Affective psychosis was associated with uterine atony. Reactive psychosis was associated with later birth order
Nicolson et al. (1999)	$n = 36$ Sz $n = 35$ sib controls	Interview and birth records Case–control study	No significant differences between case and controls in rates of OCs. Patients with OCs did not have early age of onset of Sz
Gunduz et al. (1999)	$n = 61$ Sz $n = 26$ schizoaffective $n = 28$ affective psychosis $n = 21$ controls	Birth records and interview Case–control study	No significant group differences identified

Table 13.2 (cont.)

Reference	Samples	Source of PBC information Research design	Conclusions
Preti *et al.* (2000)	$n = 44$ Sz $n = 44$ controls	Birth records Case–control study	Sz spectrum patients were more likely than controls to have experienced PBCs
Ichiki *et al.* (2000)	$n = 312$ Sz $n = 517$ controls	Birth records Case–control study	Sz have more preterm birth (< 36 weeks), low birth weight, and smaller head circumference than controls
Byrne *et al.* (2000)	$n = 413$ Sz $n = 413$ controls	Birth records Case–control study	No group difference found. Males with early onset Sz had more PBCs compared to their well, matched controls
Eaton *et al.* (2000)	$n = 132$ Sz $n = 1266$ controls	Birth records Case–control study nested within birth cohort	PBCs were associated with Sz, but the relationship of urban birth to Sz was unaffected by adjustment for obstetric complications
Kendell *et al.* (2000)	$n = 296$ Sz probands $n = 296$ controls	Birth records Case–control study nested within birth cohort	No significant association was observed between OCs and Sz probands in 1971–74 birth cohort
Kendell *et al.* (2000)	$n = 156$ Sz probands $n = 156$ controls	Birth records Case–control study nested within birth cohort	Emergency Caesarean section and labour lasting over 12 h were significantly more common in the Sz probands in 1975–78 birth cohort
Schaefer *et al.* (2000)	$n = 63$ Sz $n = 6570$ controls	Birth records Birth cohort	High maternal prepregnant BMI (>30.0), compared to average BMI, was significantly associated with Sz
Brown *et al.* (2000)	$n = 71$ Sz $n = 7725$ controls	Birth records Birth cohort	Second trimester exposure to respiratory infection associated with a significant risk of Sz spectrum disorder
Zornberg *et al.* (2000)	$n = 693$ Sz and non-affective psychoses	Maternal recall and birth records Cohort	There was an elevated, graded and independent risk of Sz and non-affective psychoses association with antecedent hypoxic-ischaemia-related fetal/neonatal complications
Wahlbeck *et al.* (2001)	$n = 114$ Sz or schizoaffective disorder $n = 7086$ total cohort	Birth records Cohort study	Mothers of cases had lower BMI. Cases had lower birth weight, were shorter and had lower placental weight
Rosso *et al.* (2000)	$n = 80$ Sz $n = 56$ sib controls $n = 26273$ total cohort	Maternal recall and birth records Birth records Case–control study nested within birth cohort	Hypoxia-associated PBCs significantly increased the odds of early onset but not later-onset Sz, after prenatal infection and fetal growth retardation were controlled

Sz = schizophrenia, sibs = siblings, PBCs = pregnancy and birth complications, BAD = bipolar affective disorder, BMI = body mass index.

the very early development of the brain are 'silent' and, as such, are not open to measurement with available technology (Niswander & Kiely 1991).

Specific pregnancy and birth complications

Mindful of these caveats, the majority of studies, using various sources of data and various scoring methods, have supported an association between the presence of PBCs and an increased risk of schizophrenia. The specific PBCs implicated have included low birth weight (Lane & Albee 1966; Woerner *et al.* 1971; Rifkin *et al.* 1994), prematurity and 'small for dates' status (McNeil & Kaij 1978; Jones *et al.* 1998; Ichiki *et al.* 2000), pre-eclampsia (McNeil & Kaij 1978; Dalman *et al.* 1999), prolonged labour (McNeil & Kaij 1978; Kendell *et al.* 2000), asphyxia and hypoxia-related PBCs (McNeil & Kaij 1978;

Rosso *et al.* 2000; Zornberg *et al.* 2000), antepartum haemorrhage (Hultman *et al.* 1997, 1999), rhesus incompatibility (Hollister *et al.* 1996), both high (Jones *et al.* 1998; Schaefer *et al.* 2000) and low (Wahlbeck *et al.* 2001) body mass index (BMI), multiparity (Hultman *et al.* 1999) and fetal distress (O'Callaghan *et al.* 1991a). In an individual-patient meta-analysis including 700 schizophrenia subjects and 835 controls, Geddes *et al.* (1999) reported that there were significant associations between schizophrenia and premature rupture of the membranes, gestational age less than 37 weeks and the use of resuscitation or incubator. There was a trend level association between low birth weight (less than 2500 g) and schizophrenia.

However, not all studies have been positive (Done *et al.* 1991; McCreadie *et al.* 1992; Gunduz *et al.* 1999; Byrne *et al.* 2000; Kendell *et al.* 2000). What are we to make of these apparent contradictions? First, there is wide consensus about the lack of specificity and predictive power of PBCs. Most fetuses exposed to the broad range of PBCs do not develop schizophrenia and most patients with schizophrenia have not had overt PBCs. Goodman (1988) concluded that PBCs (as currently detected) increase the risk of schizophrenia from about 0.6 to only about 1.5% and the individual-patient meta-analysis found very low attributable fractions for the handful of individual PBCs that were significantly associated with schizophrenia (Geddes *et al.* 1999).

Demographic and clinical correlates of pregnancy and birth complications in schizophrenia

It seems that only some PBCs have a risk-increasing effect, and even these are only indirect indicators of likely hazards to the developing brain. In addition, any increased risk may be for a subtype of schizophrenia rather than the whole spectrum of conditions. Thus, a number of studies suggest that PBCs are particularly associated with schizophrenia of severe rather than mild type (McNeil & Kaij 1978), male sex (O'Callaghan *et al.* 1991a) and early onset (Verdoux *et al.* 1997). Rifkin *et al.* (1994) found that low birth weight in male (but not female) schizophrenics was associated with cognitive and social impairment in childhood, and cognitive defects and negative symptoms in adult life. These findings are reminiscent of the evidence that PBCs predict increasing risk of cognitive impairment in the general population (Stewart *et al.* 1999; Seidman *et al.* 2000).

There is no doubt that in the general population of infants and children, exposure to obstetric hazards is associated with an increased risk of brain injury and of resultant neurological and neuropsychological deficits. Furthermore, the anatomical sequelae of the brain injury persist into adolescence. Thus, Stewart *et al.* (1999) noted that over half of the MRI scans of a cohort of adolescents (mean age 15 years) who had been born before 32 weeks were rated as abnormal by neuroradiologists, compared with only 5% of controls. Increased ventricular volume, corpus callosal abnormalities and white matter lesions were particularly common in the preterm adolescents. Subsequent volumetric analysis on the same subjects revealed decrements in whole brain volume, grey matter and hippocampi as well as strikingly increased ventricular volume, findings reminiscent of, but more severe than, those found in schizophrenia (Nosarti *et al.* 2001).

Many studies have therefore attempted to relate obstetric complications to brain structure in patients with schizophrenia. Several groups have reported an association between the presence of PBCs and either enlarged ventricles or wider sulci and fissures (Roberts 1980; Reveley *et al.* 1984; Schulsinger *et al.* 1984; Silverton *et al.* 1985; DeLisi *et al.* 1986; Turner *et al.* 1986; Lewis & Murray 1987; Owen *et al.* 1988; Cannon *et al.* 1989; Pearlson *et al.* 1989; Smith *et al.* 1998; Stefanis *et al.* 1999). These studies included different designs and a range of brain measures, and included high-risk offspring of schizophrenics and twins. On the other hand, many studies have found no association between PBCs and increased ventricular volume in schizophrenia (DeLisi *et al.* 1988; Nimgaonkar *et al.* 1988; Johnstone *et al.* 1989; Kaiya *et al.* 1989; Reddy *et al.* 1990; Nasrallah *et al.* 1991; Harvey *et al.* 1993).

Some studies found that PBCs were more common among individuals with schizophrenia without a family history of the illness (McNeil & Kaij 1978; Lewis & Murray 1987). Against this are reports that PBCs are only of aetiological importance in those individuals who already carry some genetic predisposition to schizophrenia (Schulsinger *et al.* 1987; Cannon 1997). One study reported that the individuals with schizophrenia who had an obvious genetic predisposition were more prone to develop increased ventricular and decreased hippocampal volume in response to obstetric complications (Cannon *et al.* 1989).

Stefanis *et al.* (1999) selected patients with schizophrenia without any family history of the disorder but who had been exposed to PBCs. Those with a history of PBCs had decreased hippocampal volume, especially on the left. McNeil *et al.* (2000) have shown that in monozygotic twins discordant for schizophrenia, the differences in brain structure are largely explained by exposure to delivery complications in the affected twins.

Putative mechanism of action

The direction of causality between PBCs and risk of schizophrenia remains open to question. A century ago, Freud noted that the links between cerebral palsy and birth complications may be the result of pre-existing abnormalities of brain development causing the birth complications (Freud 1897). A pre-existing neural defect can be the cause of PBCs (Nelson & Ellenberg 1986) and, in theory, it is possible that the postulated neurodevelopmental abnormality underlying schizophrenia is directly or indirectly the cause of the increase rates of PBCs. Nevertheless, McNeil and Cantor-Graae (1999) provide arguments against this being the case in schizophrenia.

A common denominator of many PBCs is their ability to produce fetal hypoxia. As with all lesions of the developing brain, the long-term sequelae of hypoxia depend not only on the extent of the damage (the 'dose') but also on the timing of the event. For example, prior to the last few weeks of gestation, the cerebral vasculature is fragile and more sensitive to perturbations of oxygenation. Haemorrhages and secondary ischaemic damage at this stage may result in periventricular leucomalacia, a potential antecedent of ventricular enlargement (Leichty *et al.* 1983). Hypoxia later in gestation can result in more damage to the cortex, especially the hippocampus and subiculum, as well as the more familiar patterns of 'watershed' infarcts seen in adults (Lewis & Owen 1989). In brief, PBCs may impact on the complex temporal and spatial cascade of brain development via a multitude of mechanisms including cell proliferation, cell migration, cell differentiation, synaptic connectivity and apoptosis (see Chapter 17).

There is good evidence that PBCs are associated with an increased risk of schizophrenia, and robust evidence that they are associated with a broad range of adverse neurocognitive outcomes. The links between PBCs and schizophrenia raise the question of whether there may be candidate genes that mediate the brain's vulnerability to hypoxic–ischaemic damage (Cannon 1997). They also indicate the potential value of seeking practical ways to reduce the incidence of PBCs for women with schizophrenia and consequently high-risk fetuses (Barkla & McGrath 2000; McGrath 2000).

Prenatal infection

One possible cause of the late winter–spring excess of schizophrenic births is maternal exposure to winter-borne viruses. Many groups have now examined prenatal exposure to influenza as a candidate risk factor for schizophrenia. A number of studies have suggested that fetuses exposed to the 1957 A2 influenza pandemic during the second trimester have an increased risk of schizophrenia (Mednick *et al.* 1988, 1990a, 1993; O'Callaghan *et al.* 1991b; Fahy *et al.* 1992; Kunugi *et al.* 1992, 1995; McGrath *et al.* 1994; Izumoto *et al.* 1999). Furthermore, the link with influenza exposure has also been found when the relationship between influenza epidemics and schizophrenic births was assessed over several decades (Watson *et al.* 1984). Several of the studies have found an effect for female but not for male schizophrenics (Table 13.3).

While the body of evidence linking influenza epidemics and increased risk of schizophrenia seems impressive, there are also many studies that have not identified an association (Crow *et al.* 1991; Torrey *et al.* 1992; Erlenmeyer-Kimling *et al.* 1994; Selten & Slaets 1994; Susser *et al.* 1994; Takei *et al.* 1995; Cannon *et al.* 1996; Grech *et al.* 1997; Morgan *et al.* 1997; Battle *et al.* 1999; Westergaard *et al.* 1999; Mino *et al.* 2000). How can we reconcile this literature? While animal experiments have improved the biological plausibility of prenatal influenza as a factor impacting on brain development (Fatemi *et al.* 1999, 2000), the lack of consistency across the studies has seriously weakened the case that prenatal exposure to the influenza virus,

per se, is causally related to schizophrenia (McGrath & Castle 1995). When assessing this literature it is important to recall that most of the studies are ecological (i.e. it is known that the population were exposed to influenza during a certain period, but not specifically that the mothers of people who later developed schizophrenia contracted it). It should also be noted that some of the studies lack adequate power to detect true but small effects.

Schizophrenia births have been found to be increased in association with epidemics of other prenatal infectious agents: diphtheria, measles, varicella and polio (Watson *et al.* 1984; Torrey *et al.* 1988). Prenatal exposure to poliovirus has been associated with increased schizophrenia births in a population-based Finnish study (Suvisaari *et al.* 1999). In a rare study with individual data on maternal antibody levels, an association between rubella and schizophrenia has been found (Brown *et al.* 2000).

In summary, in spite of the inconsistencies in the data, infective agents remain attractive candidate exposures from a public health perspective, because of the potential to avert cases by vaccination.

Prenatal nutrition

There has been considerable interest in recent years in the impact of prenatal nutrition and various adult-onset disorders such as diabetes, cardiovascular disease and hypertension – the so-called 'Barker hypothesis' (Barker 1992). Even in the absence of overt nutritional deficits, supplementing nutrition before and after birth warrants consideration. For example, supplementing folate to women periconceptually is associated with a reduction in the incidence of neural tube defects in their offspring (Scott *et al.* 1994). Recent evidence from a randomized controlled trial of nutritional supplements for preterm infants found not only that cognitive outcomes (measured at age 7 years) were superior in the group allocated the enriched infant formulae, but this group also had less cerebral palsy (Lucas *et al.* 1998). This study suggested that suboptimal nutrition during a critical period of brain growth could impair functional compensation in those sustaining an earlier brain insult.

Because the role of diet in crucial phases of development can have important neurological consequences for the offspring (Stein & Susser 1985), by inference prenatal nutritional deprivation is a biologically plausible risk factor for schizophrenia (Brown *et al.* 1996). While studies of the incidence of schizophrenia in developing nations (where more fetuses are exposed to poor nutrition) do not appear to show higher rates, there remains the possibility that deficits in specific micronutrients may have a role.

Susser *et al.* (1996) identified an increased risk of schizophrenia in the offspring of women who were pregnant during a famine in Holland during World War II. A range of adverse health outcomes have been associated with exposure to this prenatal famine (e.g. neural tube defect and intellectual handicap).

Table 13.3 The association between prenatal exposure to influenza epidemics and schizophrenia.

Reference	Location	Epidemics	Base sample size*	Comment
Watson et al. (1984)	Minnesota, USA	1916–58	3246	Association with diphtheria, pneumonia and influenza
Torrey et al. (1988)	10 states USA	1920–55	2519	Associations found with measles, polio, varicella-zoster, but only trend-level associations with influenza
Mednick et al. (1988, 1990b)	Helsinki, Finland	1957	1781 (subset)	Second-trimester exposure associated with increased risk of being admitted to a psychiatric hosptial with a diagnosis of schizophrenia
Kendell and Kemp (1989)	Edinburgh, Scotland	1957 1919–20	2371 13540	Edinburgh data showed an association with 6th-month exposure for the 1957 epidemic which was not found for Scotland as a whole. No association found with 1919–20 epidemic
Torrey et al. (1992)	10 states USA	1957	43814	No associations found
O'Callaghan et al. (1991a)	England and Wales	1957	1670 (subset)	Associations between exposure during the 5th month, especially for females
Crow et al. (1991)	UK	1957	30724 cohort study	No associations found using record linkage with a large birth cohort
Kunugi et al. (1992)	Japan	1957	836 (subset)	Associations with exposure during second trimester
Fahy et al. (1992)	Afro-Caribbeans in England	1957	1722	Associations between exposure during second trimester found in Afro-Caribbean patients
McGrath et al. (1994)	Queensland, Australia	1954 1957 1959	7858	Associations between exposure during second trimester after the 1954 (mainly males) and the 1957 (mainly females) epidemics. No associations found after the 1959 epdemic
Sham et al. (1992)	England and Wales	1939–60	14830	Associations between exposure during 3rd and 7th months
Barr et al. (1990)	Denmark	1911–50	7239	Association found for exposure during 6th month of gestation
Morris et al. (1993)	Ireland	1921–71	2846	Association found for exposure in late third trimester
Adam et al. (1993)	Denmark Scotland England	1911–65 1932–60 1921–60	18723 16960 22021	1957 data demonstrate second trimester associations for all three countries. General association between epidemics and schizophrenia only found

Table 13.3 (cont.)

Reference	Location	Epidemics	Base sample size*	Comment
				in the English data (lag of 2 and 3 months)
Takei *et al.* (1994)	England and Wales	1938–65	3 827	Association with second-trimester exposure
Erlenmeyer-Kimling *et al.* (1994)	Croatia	1957	1 816	No association found between influenza and schizophrenia births
Selten and Slaets (1994)	The Netherlands	1957	4 634	No association between influenza and schizophrenia found
Susser *et al.* (1994)	The Netherlands	1957 i	991	No association between influenza and schizophrenia found
Kunugi *et al.* (1995)	Japan	1957	1 284	Increased risk of schizophrenia in females exposed to the epidemic during the 5th month of gestation. No association found for male births and influenza epidemics
Takei *et al.* (1995)	The Netherlands	1947–69	10 630	No association between influenza and schizophrenia found. Trend level association between influenza and higher schizophrenia 3 months later
Cannon *et al.* (1996)	Ireland	1957	525 cohort study	No association found, however this study lacked power to detect true small effect
Takei *et al.* (1996)	Denmark	1915–70	9 462	Exposure to influenza epidemics in the 6th month of gestation associated with increased risk of schizophrenia. Population attributable fraction was estimated to be 1.4%
Grech *et al.* (1997)	England and Wales	1923–65	17 247	No association between prenatal exposure to influenza epidemics and proportion of patients with paranoid schizophrenia compared to other schizophrenia
Morgan *et al.* (1997)	Western Australia	1950–60	804 (subset)	No association between influenza and schizophrenia, but a link between influenza and mental retardation was found
Battle *et al.* (1999)	Georgia, USA	1948–65	11 736	No association found between influenza and schizophrenia, nor measles and schizophrenia

Table 13.3 (cont.)

Reference	Location	Epidemics	Base sample size*	Comment
Izumoto et al. (1999)	Japan Kochi	1957	941	Increased risk of schizophrenia in females exposed to the epidemics during the 5th month of gestation. No association found for male births and influenza epidemics
Westergaard et al. (1999)	Denmark	1950–88	2 669 from cohort 1.7 million	No association between influenza and schizophrenia found
Mino et al. (2000)	Japan (whole country, Kanto, Shikoku/ Kyusu areas)	1957/58 1962 1965	2 715	No association between influenza and schizophrenia found for any of the analyses

* Total sample of patients with schizophrenia (exposed and non-exposed) for case–control studies; total number of births for cohort studies.

Low maternal late-pregnancy BMI, and low weight at birth and during infancy have been associated with schizophrenia (Wahlbeck et al. 2001).

Low prenatal vitamin D has also been proposed as a candidate risk-modifying factor for schizophrenia (McGrath 1999). This hypothesis could explain the excess of winter–spring births (vitamin D levels fluctuate across the seasons, falling to their lowest levels in later winter–early spring), and the increased rate of schizophrenia births in urban vs. rural setting (those in the city have less ultraviolet radiation, and thus have lower vitamin D levels). However, no direct evidence is yet available to test this hypothesis.

In summary, while the evidence implicating prenatal nutrition as a risk factor in schizophrenia is still scant, it is an attractive candidate for universal intervention. Better maternal nutrition is safe, relatively cheap and could improve a range of health outcomes in the offspring, making this a cost-effective public health intervention (Rose 1992).

Prenatal stress

Huttunen and Niskanen (1978) reported an increased risk of schizophrenia in the offspring of women whose husbands had been killed in the Finnish–Russian war. Extreme prenatal maternal stress is a biologically plausible risk factor, and recently a study from Denmark reported an association between prenatal maternal life events (e.g. severe emotional stress such as bereavement was associated with cranial–neural-crest malformations; Hansen et al. 2000). However, the relative lack of data limits the conclusions that can be drawn regarding prenatal stress as a risk factor for schizophrenia.

Conclusions

Susser (1991) has pointed out that an association between a variable and a disease can be weighed up with respect to its strength and specificity, consistency (replicability and survivability), predictive performance and coherence (theoretical or general biological coherence). With respect to schizophrenia, the neurodevelopmental model has considerable coherence, with evidence from a range of sources including clinical studies of minor physical anomalies and epidemiological studies of pre- and perinatal exposures. Numerous variables have been proposed as candidate teratogens but none of these rate well on specificity or predictive performance.

As we reflect on our ability to identify individual pre- and perinatal risk factors for schizophrenia, it is sobering to examine the situation with another neurodevelopmental disorder, cerebral palsy. The Collaborative Perinatal Project examined a broad range of candidate risk factors in over 54 000 pregnancies (Nelson & Ellenberg 1986). When all the predictors were combined they appeared to explain only 37% of the cases of cerebral palsy, and the overwhelming majority of children in the group at highest risk did not in fact turn out to have cerebral palsy. The state of knowledge concerning the prenatal risk factors for cerebral palsy reminds us that the problem lies not so much in the neurodevelopmental model as in our current ignorance of the factors that can impact on the orderly development of the brain and, as a consequence, our ability to measure them. Clearly, our current methods of assessing neurodevelopment are crude in the extreme.

In order to progress in this field, we need to first go beyond investigating proxies for causal risk factors (e.g. season of birth). Then, instead of the small and underpowered studies we are used to in schizophrenia research, we need to initiate well-designed studies on the large scale now commonplace in cancer or heart disease epidemiology. Epidemiological research can serve to 'sharpen the focus', allowing candidate risk factors to be identified, but history has shown that risk-factor epidemiology can sometimes enter cycles of uninformative replications (called 'circular epidemiology') (Kuller 1999). For example, 'season of birth' has been studied as a risk factor for 80 years, with little real progress in identifying the underlying risk-modifying exposure.

Therefore, some research groups are now looking to developments in obstetric and neonatal medicine to elucidate the acute neurochemical and pathological consequences of various putative insults. Others are testing novel candidate exposures in animal models. For example, the impact of candidate exposures on neuronal development can be examined *in vitro* and in whole animal studies (with analyses ranging from gene expression profiling to behaviours such as prepulse inhibition). For example, animal models in schizophrenia research have included early lesioning of selected brain areas (Lipska *et al.* 1993), prenatal exposure to specific viruses such as influenza (Fatemi *et al.* 1999) and Borna virus (Hornig *et al.* 1999) and prenatal hypoxic/ischaemic insults (Mallard *et al.* 1999). The potential to extend this type of research with the use of genetic 'knock-out' mice (looking for gene–environment interactions) and gene expression profiling (cross-referencing altered gene expression in animal experiments with gene expression studies in schizophrenia vs. well controls) offer powerful new tools to the neuroscience community. In addition, dialogue between those involved in risk factor epidemiology and developmental neurobiology can illuminate new clues about the potential timing of exposures (e.g. vulnerable periods of brain development) and broad classes of exposures (e.g. exposures that may impact on neural apoptosis, migration).

One particular question that deserves attention is whether the teratogens that impair neurodevelopment result in lesions that directly cause psychotic symptoms several decades later. This view, sometimes characterized as the 'doomed from the womb' model, suggests that the nature of the lesion is such that it inevitably produces schizophrenia. The alternative to this deterministic model is one that postulates an early lesion that induces more general neurodevelopmental impairment. This, in turn, leads to childhood deficits in cognition and behaviour that interact iteratively with a broader range of variables (biological, psychological and social) that are also known to directly or indirectly influence brain functioning. Depending on the 'fit' between the child and the environment, the child may go on to develop schizophrenia. In other words, factors that impact between conception and birth may be neither necessary nor sufficient 'causes' of schizophrenia, but in some cases be key initiating events in a complex multidetermined cascade of risk factors. The authors tend towards the later model but, whichever proves to be the case, we look forward to a time when we will be able to use the knowledge we have gained to introduce rational attempts at the primary prevention of schizophrenia.

Acknowledgements

The authors are grateful to Sukanta Saha and Joy Welham for their assistance with this chapter, and to the Stanley Foundation for financial support.

References

Adams, W., Kendell, R.E., Hare, E.H. & Munk-Jorgensen, P. (1993) Epidemiological evidence that maternal influenza contributes to the aetiology of schizophrenia: an analysis of Scottish, English and Danish data. *British Journal of Psychiatry* 163, 522–534.

Akabaliev, V. & Sivkov, S. (1998) Minor physical anomalies in schizophrenia. *Folia Medical (Plovdiv)* 40, 39–45.

Alexander, R.C., Mukherjee, S., Richter, J. & Kaufmann, C.A. (1994) Minor physical anomalies in schizophrenia. *Journal of Nervous and Mental Disease* 182, 639–644.

Alvir, J.M., Woerner, M.G., Gunduz, H., Degreef, G. & Lieberman, J.A. (1999) Obstetric complications predict treatment response in first-episode schizophrenia. *Psychological Medicine* 29, 621–627.

Barker, D.J.P. (1992). *Fetal and Infant Origins of Adult Disease*, 1st edn. British Medical Journal, London.

Barkla, J.M. & McGrath, J.J. (2000) Antenatal needs of women with schizophrenia. In: *Women and Schizophrenia* (eds D. Castle, J. McGrath & J. Kulkarni), pp. 67–78. Cambridge University Press, Cambridge.

Barr, C.E., Mednick, S.A. & Munk-Jorgensen, P. (1990) Exposure to influenza epidemics during gestation and adult schizophrenia: a 40-year study. *Archives of General Psychiatry* 47, 869–874.

Battle, Y.L., Martin, B.C., Dorfman, J.H. & Miller, L.S. (1999) Seasonality and infectious disease in schizophrenia: the birth hypothesis revisited. *Journal of Psychiatrics Research* 33, 501–509.

Bracha, H.S., Torrey, E.F., Bigelow, L.B., Lohr, J.B. & Linington, B.B. (1991) Subtle signs of prenatal maldevelopment of the hand ectoderm in schizophrenia: a preliminary monozygotic twin study. *Biological Psychiatry* 30, 719–725.

Bradbury, T.N. & Miller, G.A. (1985) Season of birth in schizophrenia: a review of evidence, methodology, and etiology. *Psychological Bulletin* 98, 569–594.

Brown, A.S., Susser, E.S., Butler, P.D. *et al.* (1996) Neurobiological plausibility of prenatal nutritional deprivation as a risk factor for schizophrenia. *Journal of Nervous and Mental Disease* 184, 71–85.

Brown, A.S., Cohen, P., Greenwald, S. & Susser, E. (2000) Non-affective psychosis after prenatal exposure to rubella. *American Journal of Psychiatry* 157, 438–443.

Buckley, P.F., Moore, C., Long, H. *et al.* (1994) 1H-magnetic resonance spectroscopy of the left temporal and frontal lobes in schizophrenia: clinical, neurodevelopmental, and cognitive correlates. *Biological Psychiatry* 36, 792–800.

Buka, S.L., Goldstein, J.M., Seidman, L.J. & Tsuang, M.T. (2000) Maternal recall of pregnancy history: accuracy and bias in schizophrenia research. *Schizophrenia Bulletin* 26, 335–350.

Byrne, M., Browne, R., Mulryan, N. *et al.* (2000) Labour and delivery complications and schizophrenia: case–control study using contemporaneous labour ward records. *British Journal of Psychiatry* 176, 531–536.

Cannon, T.D. (1997) On the nature and mechanisms of obstetric influences in schizophrenia; a review and synthesis of epidemiologic studies. *International Review of Psychiatry* 9, 387–397.

Cannon, T.D., Mednick, S.A. & Parnas, J. (1989) Genetic and perinatal determinants of structural brain deficits in schizophrenia. *Archives of General Psychiatry* 46, 883–889.

Cannon, M., Byrne, M., Cotter, D. *et al.*. (1994) Further evidence for anomalies in the hand-prints of patients with schizophrenia: a study of secondary creases. *Schizophrenia Research* 13, 179–184.

Cannon, M., Cotter, D., Coffey, V.P. *et al.* (1996) Prenatal exposure to the 1957 influenza epidemic and adult schizophrenia: a follow-up study. *British Journal of Psychiatry* 168, 368–371.

Cantor-Graae, E., McNeil, T.F., Torrey, E.F. *et al.* (1994) Link between pregnancy complications and minor physical anomalies in monozygotic twins discordant for schizophrenia. *American Journal of Psychiatry* 151, 1188–1193.

Cantor-Graae, E., Cardenal, S., Ismail, B. & McNeil, T.F. (1998) Recall of obstetric events by mothers of schizophrenic patients. *Psychological Medicine* 28, 1239–1243.

Cheverud, J.M., Kohn, L.A., Konigsberg, L.W. & Leigh, S.R. (1992) Effects of fronto-occipital artificial cranial vault modification on the cranial base and face. *American Journal of Physical Anthropology* 88, 323–345.

Clouston, T.S. (1891) *The Neuroses of Development: the Morison Lectures for 1890*. Oliver & Boyd, Edinburgh.

Coorssen, E.A., Msall, M.E. & Duffy, L.C. (1992) Multiple minor malformations as a marker for prenatal etiology of cerebral palsy. *Developmental Medicine and Child Neurology* 33, 730–736.

Crow, T.J., Done, D.J. & Johnstone, E.C. (1991) Schizophrenia and influenza. *Lancet* 338, 116–117.

Dalman, C., Allebeck, P., Cullberg, J., Grunewald, C. & Koster, M. (1999) Obstetric complications and the risk of schizophrenia: a longitudinal study of a national birth cohort. *Archives of General Psychiatry* 56, 234–240.

DeLisi, L.E., Goldin, L.R., Hamovit, J.R. *et al.* (1986) A family study of the association of increased ventricular size with schizophrenia. *Archives of General Psychiatry* 43, 148–153.

DeLisi, L.E., Dauphinais, I. & Gershon, E.S. (1988) Perinatal complications and reduced size of brain limbic structures in familial schizophrenia. *Schizophrenia Bulletin* 14, 185–191.

Done, D.J., Johnstone, E.C., Frith, C.D. *et al.* (1991) Complications of pregnancy and delivery in relation to psychosis in adult life: data from the British perinatal mortality survey sample. *British Medical Journal* 302, 1576–1580.

Eagles, J.M., Gibson, I., Bremner, M.H. *et al.* (1990) Obstetric complications in DSM-III schizophrenics and their siblings. *Lancet* 335, 1139–1141.

Eagles, J.M., Hunter, D. & Geddes, J.R. (1995) Gender-specific changes since 1900 in the season-of-birth effect in schizophrenia [see comments]. *British Journal of Psychiatry* 167, 469–472.

Eaton, W.W., Mortensen, P.B. & Frydenberg, M. (2000) Obstetric factors, urbanization and psychosis. *Schizophr Research* 43, 117–123.

Engstrom, C., Magnusson, B.C. & Linde, A. (1982) Changes in craniofacial suture metabolism in rats fed a low calcium and vitamin D-deficient diet. *Journal of Anatomy* 134, 443–458.

Enlow, D.H. (1990) *Facial Growth*, 3rd edn. W.B. Saunders, Philadelphia.

Enlow, D.H. & Bhatt, M.K. (1984) Facial morphology variations associated with headform variations. *Journal of Charles Tweed Foundation* 12, 21–23.

Erlenmeyer-Kimling, L., Folnegovic, Z., Hrabak-Zerjavic, V. *et al.* (1994) Schizophrenia and prenatal exposure to the 1957, A2 influenza epidemic in Croatia. *American Journal of Psychiatry* 151, 1496–1498.

Fahy, T.A., Jones, P.B., Sham, P.C. & Murray, R.M. (1992) Schizophrenia in afro-Carribeans in the UK following prenatal exposure to the 1957, A2 influenza epdiemic. *Schizophrenia Research* 6, 98–99.

Fananas, L., Moral, P. & Bertranpetit, J. (1990) Quantitative dermatogyphics in schizophrenia: study of family history subgroups. *Human Biology* 62, 421–427.

Fananas, L., Gutierrez, B., Bosch, S., Carandell, F. & Obiols, J.E. (1996a) Presence of dermatoglyphic ridge dissociation in a schizotypy-affected subject in a pair of discordant MZ twins. *Schizophrenia Research* 21, 125–127.

Fananas, L., Van Os, J., Hoyos, C. *et al.* (1996b) Dermatoglyphic a-b ridge count as a possible marker for developmental disturbance in schizophrenia: replication in two samples. *Schizophrenia Research* 20, 307–314.

Fatemi, S.H., Emamian, E.S., Kist, D. *et al.* (1999) Defective corticogenesis and reduction in Reelin immunoreactivity in cortex and hippocampus of prenatally infected neonatal mice. *Molecular Psychiatry* 4, 145–154.

Fatemi, S.H., Cuadra, A.E., El Fakahany, E.E., Sidwell, R.W. & Thuras, P. (2000) Prenatal viral infection causes alterations in nNOS expression in developing mouse brains. *Neuroreport* 11, 1493–1496.

Foerster, A., Lewis, S., Owen, M. & Murray, R. (1991) Low birth weight and a family history of schizophrenia predict poor premorbid functioning in psychosis. *Schizophrenia Research* 5, 13–20.

Freud, S. (1897) *Infantile Cerebral Paralysis*. Translated by L.A. Russin, [*Die infantile cerebrallähmung*]. University of Miami Press, Coral Cables.

Geddes, J.R. & Lawrie, S.M. (1995) Obstetric complications and schizophrenia: a meta-analysis. *British Journal of Psychiatry* 167, 786–793.

Geddes, J.R., Verdoux, H., Takei, N. *et al.* (1999) Schizophrenia and complications of pregnancy and labour: an individual patient data meta-analysis. *Schizophrenia Bulletin* 1999, 25, 413–423.

Goodman, R. (1988) Are complications of pregnancy and birth causes of schizophrenia? *Developmental Medicine and Child Neurology* 30, 391–395.

Gothelf, D., Frisch, A., Munitz, H. *et al.* (1999) Clinical characteristics of schizophrenia associated with velocardiofacial syndrome. *Schizophrenia Research* 35, 105–112.

Grech, A., Takei, N. & Murray, R.M. (1997) Maternal exposure to influenza and paranoid schizophrenia. *Schizophrenia Research* 26, 121–125.

Green, M.F., Satz, P., Gaier, D.J., Ganzell, S. & Kharabi, F. (1989) Minor physical anomalies in schizophrenia. *Schizophrenia Bulletin* 15, 91–99.

Green, M.F., Satz, P. & Christenson, C. (1994) Minor physical anomalies in schizophrenia patients, bipolar patients, and their siblings. *Schizophrenia Bulletin* 20, 433–440.

Griffiths, T.D., Sigmundsson, T., Takei, N. *et al.* (1998) Minor physical anomalies in familial and sporadic schizophrenia: the Maudsley family study. *Journal of Neurology, Neurosurgery and Psychiatry* 64, 56–60.

Gualtieri, C.T., Adams, A., Shen, C.D. & Loiselle, D. (1982) Minor physical anomalies in alcoholic and schizophrenic adults and hyperactive and autistic children. *American Journal of Psychiatry* 139, 640–643.

Gunduz, H., Woerner, M.G., Alvir, J.M., Degreef, G. & Lieberman, J.A. (1999) Obstetric complications in schizophrenia, schizoaffective disorder and normal comparison subjects. *Schizophrenia Research* 40, 237–243.

Gunther-Genta, F., Bovet, P. & Hohlfeld, P. (1994) Obstetric complications and schizophrenia: a case–control study. *British Journal of Psychiatry* 164, 165–170.

Gutierrez, B., van Os, J., Valles, V. *et al.* (1998) Congenital dermatoglyphic malformations in severe bipolar disorder. *Psychiatry Research* 78, 133–140.

Guy, J.D., Majorski, L.V., Wallace, C.J. & Guy, M.P. (1983) The incidence of minor physical anomalies in adult male schizophrenics. *Schizophrenia Bulletin* 9, 571–582.

Hansen, D., Lou, H.C. & Olsen, J. (2000) Serious life events and congenital malformations: a national study with complete follow-up. *Lancet* 356, 875–880.

Harvey, I., de Boulay, G., Wicks, D. *et al.* (1993) Reduction of cortical volume in schizophrenia on magnetic resonance imaging. *Psychological Medicine* 23, 591–604.

Heun, R. & Maier, W. (1993) The role of obstetric complications in schizophrenia. *Journal of Nervous and Mental Disease* 181, 220–226.

Hollister, J.M., Laing, P. & Mednick, S.A. (1996) Rhesus incompatibility as a risk factor for schizophrenia in male adults. *Archives of General Psychiatry* 53, 19–24.

Hornig, M., Weissenbock, H., Horscroft, N. & Lipkin, W.I. (1999) An infection-based model of neurodevelopmental damage. *Proceedings of the National Academy of Sciences of the USA* 96, 12102–12107.

Hultman, C.M., Ohman, A., Cnattingius, S., Wieselgren, I.M. & Lindstrom, L.H. (1997) Prenatal and neonatal risk factors for schizophrenia. *British Journal of Psychiatry* 170, 128–133.

Hultman, C., Sparen, P., Takei, N., Murray, R.M. & Cnattingius, S. (1999) Prenatal and perinatal risk factors for schizophrenia, affective psychosis, and reactive psychosis for early onset: case–control study. *British Medical Journal* 318, 421–426.

Huttunen, M.O. & Niskanen, P. (1978) Prenatal loss of father and psychiatry disorders. *Archives of General Psychiatry* 35, 429–431.

Ichiki, M., Kunugi, H., Takei, N. *et al.* (2000) Intra-uterine physical growth in schizophrenia: evidence confirming excess of premature birth. *Psychological Medicine* 30, 597–604.

Illingworth, R.S. (1979) Why blame the obsetrician? *British Medical Journal* 1, 797–801.

Ismail, B., Cantor-Graae, E. & McNeil, T.F. (1998) Minor physical anomalies in schizophrenic patients and their siblings. *American Journal of Psychiatry* 155, 1695–1702.

Ismail, B., Cantor-Graae, E. & McNeil, T.F. (2000) Minor physical anomalies in schizophrenia: cognitive, neurological and other clinical correlates. *Journal of Psychiatrics Research* 34, 45–56.

Izumoto, Y., Inoue, S. & Yasuda, N. (1999) Schizophrenia and the influenza epidemics of 1957 in Japan. *Biological Psychiatry* 46, 119–124.

Jacobsen, B. & Kinney, D.K. (1980) Perinatal complications in adopted and non-adopted schizophrenics and their controls: preliminary results. *Acta Psychiatrica Scandinavica* 285 (Suppl.), 337–351.

Johnstone, E.C., Owens, D.G.C., Bydder, G.M. *et al.* (1989) The spectrum of structural brain changes in schizophrenia: age of onset as a predictor of cognitvie and clinical impairments and their correlates. *Psychological Medicine* 19, 91–103.

Jones, P. & Murray, R.M. (1991) The genetics of schizophrenia is the genetics of neurodevelopment. *British Journal of Psychiatry* 158, 615–623.

Jones, P.B., Rantakallio, P., Hartikainen, A.L., Isohanni, M. & Sipila, P. (1998) Schizophrenia as a long-term outcome of pregnancy, delivery, and perinatal complications: a 28-year follow-up of the 1966 north Finland general population birth cohort. *American Journal of Psychiatry* 155, 355–364.

Kaiya, H., Uematsu, M., Ofuji, M. *et al.* (1989) Computerised tomogra-phy in schizophrenia: familial versus non-familial forms of illness. *British Journal of Psychiatry* 155, 444–450.

Kendell, R.E. & Kemp, I.W. (1989) Maternal influenza in the etiology of schizophrenia. *Archives of General Psychiatry* 46, 878–882.

Kendell, R.E., McInneny, K., Juszczak, E. & Bain, M. (2000) Obstetric complications and schizophrenia: two case–control studies based on structured obstetric records. *British Journal of Psychiatry* 176, 516–522.

Kraemer, H.C., Kazdin, A.E., Offord, D.R. *et al.* (1997) Coming to terms with the terms of risk. *Archives of General Psychiatry* 54, 337–343.

Kuller, L.H. (1999) Circular epidemiology [see comments]. *American Journal of Epidemiology* 150, 897–903.

Kunugi, H., Nanko, S. & Takei, N. (1992) Influenza and schizophrenia in Japan. *British Journal of Psychiatry* 161, 274–275.

Kunugi, H., Nanko, S., Takei, N. *et al.* (1995) Schizophrenia following *in utero* exposure to the 1957 influenza epidemics in Japan. *American Journal of Psychiatry* 152, 450–452.

Kunugi, H., Nanko, S., Takei, N. *et al.* (1996) Perinatal complications and schizophrenia: data from the *Maternal and Child Health Handbook* in Japan. *Journal of Nervous and Mental Disease* 184, 542–546.

Lane, A., Kinsella, A., Murphy, P. *et al.* (1997) The anthropometric assessment of dysmorphic features in schizophrenia as an index of its developmental origins. *Psychological Medicine* 27, 1155–1164.

Lane, E.A. & Albee, G.W. (1966) Comparative birth weight of schizophrenics and their siblings. *Journal of Psychology* 64, 227–231.

Leichty, E.A., Gilmore, R.L., Bryson, C.Q. & Bull, J. (1983) Outcome of high-risk neonates with ventriculomegaly. *Developmental Medicine and Child Neurology* 25, 162–168.

Lewis, G., David, A. & Andreasson, S.A.P. (1992) Schizophrenia and city life. *Lancet* 340, 137–140.

Lewis, S.W. (1989) Congenital risk factors for schizophrenia. *Psychological Medicine* 19, 5–13.

Lewis, S.W. & Murray, R.M. (1987) Obstetric complications, neurodevelopmental deviance, and risk of schizophrenia. *Journal of Psychiatric Research* 21, 413–421.

Lewis, S.W., Owen, M.J. & Murray, R.M. (1989) Obstetric complications and schizophrenia: methodology and mechanisms. In: *Schizophrenia: Scientific Progress* (eds S.C. Schulz & C.A. Tamminga), pp. 56–68. Oxford University Press, Oxford.

Lieberman, D.E., Pearson, O.M. & Mowbray, K.M. (2000) Basicranial influence on overall cranial shape. *Journal of Human Evolution* 38, 291–315.

Lipska, B.K., Jaskiw, G.E. & Weinberger, D.R. (1993) Postpubertal emergence of hyperresponsiveness to stress and to amphetamine after neonatal excitotoxic hippocampal damage: a potential animal model of schizophrenia. *Neuropsychopharmacology* 9, 67–75.

Lohr, J.B. & Flynn, K. (1993) Minor physical anomalies in schizophrenia and mood disorders. *Schizophrenia Bulletin* 19, 551–556.

Lohr, J.B., Alder, M., Flynn, K., Harris, M.J. & McAdams, L.A. (1997) Minor physical anomalies in older patients with late-onset schizophrenia, early-onset schizophrenia, depression, and Alzheimer's disease. *American Journal of Geriatrics Psychiatry* 5, 318–323.

Low, J.A., Galbraith, R.S., Muir, D.W. *et al.* (1985) The contribution of fetal–newborn complications to motor and cognitive deficits. *Developmental Medicine and Child Neurology* 27, 578–587.

Lucas, A., Morley, R. & Cole, T.J. (1998) Randomised trail of early diet in preterm babies and later intelligence quotient. *British Medical Journal* 317, 1481–1487.

Lyon, M., Barr, C.E., Cannon, T.D., Mednick, S.A. & Shore, D. (1989) Fetal neurodevelopment and schizophrenia. *Schizophrenia Bulletin* 15, 149–161.

McCreadie, R.G., Hall, D.J., Berry, I.J. *et al.* (1992) The Nithdale schizophrenia surveys. X. Obstetric complications, family history and abnormal movements. *British Journal of Psychiatry* **161**, 799–805.

McDonald, C., Fearon, P. & Murray, R.M. (1999) Neurodevelopmental hypothesis of schizophrenia 12 years on: data and doubts. In: *Childhood Onset of Adult Psychopathology* (ed. J. Rapopart), pp. 193–220. American Psychiatric Press, Washington.

McGrath, J. (1999) Hypothesis: is low prenatal vitamin D a risk-modifying factor for schizophrenia? *Schizophrenia Research* **40**, 173–177.

McGrath, J. (2000) Universal interventions for the primary prevention of schizophrenia. *Australian and New Zealand Journal of Psychiatry* **34**, 58–64.

McGrath, J. & Castle, D. (1995) Does influenza cause schizophrenia? A five year review. *Australian and New Zealand Journal of Psychiatry* **29**, 23–31.

McGrath, J.J. & Welham, J.L. (1999) Season of birth and schizophrenia: a systematic review and meta-analysis of data from the southern hemisphere. *Schizophrenia Research* **35**, 237–242.

McGrath, J., El-Saadi, O., Grim, V. *et al.* (2002) Minor physical anomalies and quantitative measures of the head and face in psychosis. *Archives of General Psychiatry* **59**, 458–464.

McGrath, J.J., Pemberton, M.R., Welham, J.L. & Murray, R.M. (1994) Schizophrenia and the influenza epidemics of 1954, 1957 and 1959: a southern hemisphere study. *Schizophrenia Research* **14**, 1–8.

McGrath, J.J., Van Os, J., Hoyos, C. *et al.* (1995) Minor physical anomalies in psychoses: associations with clinical and putative aetiological variables. *Schizophrenia Research* **18**, 9–20.

McNeil, T.F. & Cantor-Graae, E. (1999) Does pre-existing abnormality cause labor–delivery complications in fetuses who will develop schizophrenia? *Schizophrenia Bulletin* **25**, 425–435.

McNeil, T.F. & Kaij, L. (1978) Obstetric factors in the development of schizophrenia: complications in the births of preschizophrenics and in reproductions by schizophrenic parents. In: *The Nature of Schizophrenia: New Approaches to Research and Treatment*, 1st edn. (eds L.C. Wynne, R.L. Cromwell & S. Matthysse), pp. 401–429. John Wiley, New York.

McNeil, T.F. & Sjostrom, K. (1995) *The McNeil–Sjostrom Scale for Obstetric Complications*. Department of Psychiatry, Lund University, Malmo.

McNeil, T.F., Blennow, G. & Lundberg, L. (1992) Congenital malformations and structural developmental anomalies in groups at high risk for psychosis. *American Journal of Psychiatry* **149**, 57–61.

McNeil, T.F., Cantor-Graae, E. & Weinberger, D.R. (2000) Relationship of obstetric complications and differences in size of brain structures in monozygotic twin pairs discordant for schizophrenia. *American Journal of Psychiatry* **157**, 203–212.

Mallard, E.C., Rehn, A., Rees, S., Tolcos, M. & Copolov, D. (1999) Ventriculomegaly and reduced hippocampal volume following intrauterine growth-restriction: implications for the aetiology of schizophrenia. *Schizophrenia Research* **40**, 11–21.

Marcelis, M., Navarro-Mateu, F., Murray, R., Selten, J.-P. & Van Os, J. (1998a) Urbanization and psychosis: a study of 1942–78 birth cohorts in the Netherlands. *Psychological Medicine* **28**, 871–879.

Marcelis, M., Van Os, J., Sham, P. *et al.* (1998b) Obstetric complications and familial morbid risk of psychiatric disorders. *American Journal of Medical Genetics* **81**, 29–36.

Markow, T.A. & Gottesman, I.I. (1989) Fluctuating dermatoglyphic asymmetry in psychotic twins. *Psychiatry Research* **29**, 37–43.

Mednick, S.A., Machón, R.A., Huttunen, M.O. & Bonett, D. (1988) Adult schizophrenia following prenatal exposure to an influenza epidemic. *Archives of General Psychiatry* **45**, 189–192.

Mednick, S.A., Machon, R.A., Huttunen, M.O. & Barr, C.E. (1990a) Influenza and schizophrenia: Helsinki vs. Edinburgh. *Archives of General Psychiatry* **47**, 875–878.

Mednick, S.A., Machon, R.A. & Huttunen, M.O. (1990b) An update on the Helsinki Influenza Project. *Archives of General Psychiatry* **47**, 292.

Mednick, S.A., Huttunen, M.O. & Machón, R.A. (1994) Prenatal influenza infections and adult schizophrenia. *Schizophrenia Bulletin* **20**, 263–267.

Mellor, C.S. (1992) Dermatoglyphic evidence of fluctuating asymmetry in schizophrenia [see comments]. *British Journal of Psychiatry* **160**, 467–472.

Mino, Y., Oshima, I., Tsuda, T. & Okagami, K. (2000) No relationship between schizophrenic birth and influenza epidemics in Japan. *Journal of Psychiatric Research* **34**, 133–138.

Morgan, V., Castle, D., Page, A. *et al.* (1997) Influenza epidemics and incidence of schizophrenia, affective disorders and mental retardation in Western Australia: no evidence of a major effect. *Schizophrenia Research* **26**, 25–39.

Morris, M., Cotter, D., Takei, N. *et al.* (1993) An association between schizophrenic births and influenza deaths in Ireland in the years 1921–71. *Schizophrenia Research* **9**, 137.

Mortensen, P.B., Pedersen, C.B., Westergaard, T. *et al.* (1999) Effects of family history and place and season of birth on the risk of schizophrenia. *New England Journal of Medicine* **340**, 603–608.

Murray, R.M. (1994) Neurodevelopmental schizophrenia: the rediscovery of dementia praecox. *British Journal of Psychiatry Supplement* **6**, 12.

Murray, R.M. & Fearon, P. (1999) The developmental 'risk factor' model of schizophrenia. *Journal of Psychiatric Research* **33**, 497–499.

Murray, R.M., Lewis, S.W., Owen, M.J. & Foerster, A. (1988) The neurodevelopmental origins of dementia praecox. In: *Schizophrenia: The Major Issues* (eds P. Bebbington & P. McGuffin), pp. 90–106. Heinemann, London.

Nasrallah, H.A., Schwarzkopf, S.B., Olson, S.C. & Coffman, J.A. (1991) Perinatal brain injury and cerebellar vermal lobules I–X in schizophrenia. *Biological Psychiatry* **29**, 567–574.

Nelson, K.B. & Ellenberg, J.H. (1986) Antecendents of cerebral palsy: multivariate analysis of risk. *New England Journal of Medicine* **315**, 81–86.

Nicolson, R., Malaspina, D., Giedd, J.N. *et al.* (1999) Obstetrical complications and childhood-onset schizophrenia. *American Journal of Psychiatry* **156**, 1650–1652.

Nimgaonkar, V.L., Wessely, S. & Murray, R.M. (1988) Prevalence of familiality, obstetric complications, and structural brain damage in schizophrenic patients. *British Journal of Psychiatry* **153**, 191–197.

Niswander, K. & Kiely, R.M. (1991) Intrapartum asphyxia and cerebral palsy. In: *Reproductive and Perinatal Epidemiology*, 1st edn. (ed. M. Kiely), pp. 357–368. CRC Press, Boca Ranton.

Nosarti, C.A.I., Asady, M.H., Rifkin, L., Stewart, A. & Murray, R.M. (2001) Brain abnormalities as measured by magnetic resonance imaging (MRI) in very preterm adolescents: a model for schizophrenia? *Schizophrenia Research* **49**, 162.

O'Callaghan, E., Larkin, C. & Waddington, J.L. (1990) Obstetric complications in schizophrenia and the validity of maternal recall. *Psychological Medicine* **20**, 89–94.

O'Callaghan, E., Larkin, C., Kinsella, A. & Waddington, J.L. (1991a) Familial, obstetric, and other clinical correlates of minor physical anomalies in schizophrenia. *American Journal of Psychiatry* **148**, 479–483.

O'Callaghan, E., Sham, P., Takei, N., Glover, G. & Murray, R.M. (1991b) Schizophrenia after prenatal exposure to 1957, A2 influenza epidemic. *Lancet* 337, 1248–1250.

O'Callaghan, E., Colgan, K., Cotter, D. *et al.* (1992a) Evidence for confinement of winter birth excess in schizophrenia to those born in cities. *Schizophrenia Research* 6, 102.

O'Callaghan, E., Gibson, T., Colohan, H.A. *et al.* (1992b) Risk of schizophrenia in adults born after obstetric complications and their associatin with early onset of illness: a controlled study. *British Medical Journal* 305, 1256–1259.

Owen, M.J., Lewis, S.W. & Murray, R.M. (1988) Obstetric complications and schizophrenia: a computed tomographic study. *Psychological Medicine* 18, 331–339.

Paneth, N. & Pinto-Martin, J. (1991) The epidemiology of germinal matrix/intraventricular hemorrhage. In: *Reproductive and Perinatal Epidemiology* (ed. M. Kiely), pp. 371–399. CRC Press, Boca Ranton.

Parnas, J., Schulsinger, F., Teasdale, T.W. *et al.* (1982) Perinatal complications and clinical outcome within the schizophrenia spectrum. *British Journal of Psychiatry* 140, 416–420.

Pearlson, G.D., Kim, W.S., Kubos, K.L. *et al.* (1989) Ventricle–brain ratio; computed tomographic density, and brain area in 50 schizophrenics. *Archives of General Psychiatry* 46, 690–697.

Pedersen, C.B. & Mortensen, P.B. (2001) Evidence of a dose–response relationship between urbanicity during upbringing and schizophrenia risk. *Archives of General Psychiatry* 58, 1039–1046.

Pollack, M., Woerner, M.G., Goodman, W. & Greenberg, I.M. (1966) Childhood developmental patterns of hospitalized adult schizophrenic and non-schizophrenic patients and their siblings. *American Journal of Orthopsychiatry* 36, 510.

Preti, A., Cardascia, L., Zen, T. *et al.* (2000) Risk for obstetric complications and schizophrenia. *Psychiatry Research* 96, 127–139.

Pulver, A.E. (2000) Search for schizophrenia susceptibility genes. *Biological Psychiatry* 47, 221–230.

Reddy, R., Mukherjee, S., Schnur, D.B., Chin, J. & Degreef, G. (1990) History of obstetric complications, family history, and CT scan findings in schizophrenic patients. *Schizophrenia Research* 3, 311–314.

Reveley, A.M., Reveley, M.A. & Murray, R.M. (1984) Cerebral ventricular enlargement in non-genetic schizophrenia: a controlled twin study. *British Journal of Psychiatry* 144, 89–93.

Rifkin, L., Lewis, S.W., Jones, P.B., Toone, B.K. & Murray, R.M. (1994) Low birth weight and schizophrenia. *Schizophrenia Research* 11, 94.

Roberts, J. (1980) *The use of the CT scanner in psychiatry.* MPhil thesis, University of London.

Rosa, A., Fananas, L., Marcelis, M. & Van Os, J. (2000a) a-b Ridge count and schizophrenia. *Schizophrenia Research* 46, 285–286.

Rosa, A., Fananas, L., Bracha, H.S., Torrey, E.F. & Van Os, J. (2000b) Congenital dermatoglyphic malformations and psychosis: a twin study. *American Journal of Psychiatry* 157, 1511–1513.

Rosa, A., Marcelis, M., Suckling, J. *et al.* (2001) Replication of an association between cerebral and dermatoglyphic abnormalities pointing to a possible early prenatal origin of psychosis. *Schizophrenia Research* 49, 164.

Rose, G. (1992) *The Strategy of Preventive Medicine.* Oxford University Press, Oxford.

Rosso, I.M., Cannon, T.D., Huttunen, T. *et al.* (2000) Obstetric risk factors for early-onset schizophrenia in a Finnish birth cohort. *American Journal of Psychiatry* 157, 801–807.

Schaefer, C.A., Brown, A.S., Wyatt, R.J. *et al.* (2000) Maternal prepregnant body mass and risk of schizophrenia in adult offspring. *Schizophrenia Bulletin* 26, 275–286.

Schulsinger, F., Parnas, J., Petersen, E.T. *et al.* (1984) Cerebral ventricular size in the offspring of schizophrenic mothers: a preliminary study. *Archives of General Psychiatry* 41, 602–606.

Schulsinger, F., Parnas, J., Mednick, S., Teasdale, T.W. & Schulsinger, H. (1987) Heredity–environment interaction and schizophrenia. *Journal of Psychiatric Research* 21, 431–436.

Schwarzkopf, S.B., Nasrallah, H.A., Olson, S.C., Coffman, J.A. & McLaughlin, J.A. (1989) Perinatal complications and genetic loading in schizophrenia: preliminary findings. *Psychiatry Research* 27, 233–239.

Scott, J.M., Weir, D.G., Molloy, A. *et al.* (1994) *Folic Acid Metabolism and Mechanisms of Neural Tube Defects.* John Wiley, West Sussex.

Seidman, L.J., Buka, S.L., Goldstein, J.M. *et al.* (2000) The relationship of prenatal and perinatal complications to cognitive functioning at age 7 in the New England cohorts of the National Collaborative Perinatal Project. *Schizophrenia Bulletin* 26, 309–321.

Selten, J.P. & Slaets, J.P. (1994) Evidence against maternal influenza as a risk factor for schizophrenia. *British Journal of Psychiatry* 164, 674–676.

Sham, P.C., O'Callaghan, E., Takei, N. *et al.* (1992) Schizophrenia following prenatal exposure to influenza epidemics between 1939 and 1960 [see comments]. *British Journal of Psychiatry* 160, 461–466.

Silverton, L., Finello, K.M., Mednick, S.A. & Schulsinger, F. (1985) Low birth weight and ventricular enlargement in a high-risk sample. *Journal of Abnormal Psychology* 94, 405–409.

Smith, G.N., Kopala, L.C., Lapointe, J.S. *et al.* (1998) Obstetric complications, treatment response and brain morphology in adult-onset and early-onset males with schizophrenia. *Psychological Medicine* 28, 645–653.

Sperber, G.H. (1989) *Craniofacial Embryology,* 4th edn. Wright, London.

Stefanis, N., Frangou, S., Yakeley, J. *et al.* (1999) Hippocampal volume reduction in schizophrenia: effects of genetic risk and pregnancy and birth complications. *Biological Psychiatry* 46, 697–702.

Stein, Z. & Susser, M. (1985) Effects of early nutrition on neurological and mental competence in human beings. *Psychological Medicine* 15, 717–726.

Stewart, A.L., Rifkin, L., Amess, P.N. *et al.* (1999) Brain structure and neurocognitive and behavioural function in adolescents who were born very preterm. *Lancet* 353, 1653–1657.

Stober, G., Franzek, E. & Beckmann, H. (1993) Pregnancy and labor complications – their significance in the development of schizophrenic psychoses. *Fortschritte der Neurologie-Psychiatrie* 61, 329–337.

Susser, E., Lin, S.P., Brown, A.S., Lumey, L.H. & Erlenmeyer-Kimling, L. (1994) No relation between risk of schizophrenia and prenatal exposure to influenza in Holland. *American Journal of Psychiatry* 151, 922–924.

Susser, E., Neugebauer, R., Hoek, H. *et al.* (1996) Schizophrenia after prenatal famine: further evidence. *Archives of General Psychiatry* 53, 25–31.

Susser, M. (1991) What is a cause and how do we know one? A grammar for pragmatic epidemiology. *American Journal of Epidemiology* 133, 635–648.

Suvisaari, J., Haukka, J., Tanskanen, A., Hovi, T. & Lonnqvist, J. (1999) Association between prenatal exposure to poliovirus infection and adult schizophrenia. *American Journal of Psychiatry* 156, 1100–1102.

Suvisaari, J.M., Haukka, J.K., Tanskanen, A.J. & Lonnqvist, J.K. (2000) Decreasing seasonal variation of births in schizophrenia. *Psychological Medicine* 30, 315–324.

Takei, N., O'Callaghan, E., Sham, P., Glover, G. & Murray, R.M. (1992)

Winter birth excess in schizophrenia: its relationship to place of birth. *Schizophrenia Research* **6**, 102.

Takei, N., Sham, P., O'Callaghan, E., Glover, G. & Murray, R.M. (1994) Prenatal influenza and schizophrenia: is the effect confined to females? *American Journal of Psychiatry* **151**, 117–119.

Takei, N., Van Os, J. & Murray, R.M. (1995) Maternal exposure to influenza and risk of schizophrenia: a 22 year study from the Netherlands. *Journal of Psychiatric Research* **29**, 435–445.

Takei, N., Mortensen, P.B., Klaening, U. *et al.* (1996) Relationship between *in utero* exposure to influenza epidemics and risk of schizophrenia in Denmark. *Biological Psychiatry* **40**, 817–824.

Taylor, D.J., Howie, P.W., Davidson, J., Davidson, D. & Drillien, C.M. (1985) Do pregnancy complications contribute to neurodevelopmental disability? *Lancet* **i**, 713–716.

Torrey, E.F., Rawlings, R. & Waldman, I.N. (1988) Schizophrenic births and viral diseases in two states. *Schizophrenia Research* **1**, 73–77.

Torrey, E.F., Bowler, A.E. & Rawlings, R. (1992) Schizophrenia and the 1957 influenza epidemic. *Schizophrenia Research* **6**, 100.

Torrey, E.F., Miller, J., Rawlings, R. & Yolken, R.H. (1997) Seasonality of births in schizophrenia and bipolar disorder: a review of the literature. *Schizophrenia Research* **28**, 1–38.

Turner, S.W., Toone, B.K. & Brett-Jones, J.R. (1986) Computerised tomographic scan changes in early schizophrenia: preliminary findings. *Psychological Medicine* **16**, 219–225.

Van Os, J., Fananas, L., Cannon, M., Macdonald, A. & Murray, R. (1997) Dermatoglyphic abnormalities in psychosis: a twin study. *Biological Psychiatry* **41**, 624–626.

Van Os, J., Woodruff, P.W., Fananas, L. *et al.* (2000) Association between cerebral structural abnormalities and dermatoglyphic ridge counts in schizophrenia. *Comprehensive Psychiatry* **41**, 380–384.

Verdoux, H. & Bourgeois, M. (1993) A comparative study of obstetric history in schizophrenics, bipolar patients and normal subjects. *Schizophrenia Research* **9**, 67–69.

Verdoux, H., Geddes, J.R., Takei, N. *et al.* (1997) Obstetric complications and age at onset in schizophrenia: an international collaborative meta-analysis of individual patient data [see comments]. *American Journal of Psychiatry* **154**, 1220–1227.

Waddington, J.L., O'Callaghan, E., Buckley, P. *et al.* (1995) Tardive dyskinesia in schizophrenia: relationship to minor physical anomalies, frontal lobe dysfunction and cerebral structure on magnetic resonance imaging. *British Journal of Psychiatry* **167**, 41–44.

Waddington, J.L., Lane, A., Scully, P. *et al.* (1999) Early cerebro-craniofacial dysmorphogenesis in schizophrenia: a lifetime trajectory model from neurodevelopmental basis to 'neuroprogressive' process. *Journal of Psychiatric Research* **33**, 477–489.

Wahlbeck, K., Forsen, T., Osmond, C., Barker, D.J. & Eriksson, J.G. (2001) Association of schizophrenia with low maternal body mass index, small size at birth, and thinness during childhood. *Archives of General Psychiatry* **58**, 48–52.

Waldrop, M.F., Pedersen, F.A. & Bell, R.Q. (1968) Minor physical anomalies and behavior in preschool children. *Child Development* **39**, 391–400.

Watson, C.G., Kucala, T., Tilleskjor, C. & Jacobs, L. (1984a) Schizophrenic birth seasonality in relation to the incidence of infectious diseases and temperature extremes. *Archives of General Psychiatry* **41**, 85–90.

Watson, C.G., Kucala, T., Tilleskjor, C. & Jacobs, L. (1984b) Schizophrenic birth seasonality in relation to the incidence of infectious diseases and temperature extremes. *Archives of General Psychiatry* **41**, 85–90.

Weidenreich, F. (1941) The brain and its role in the phylogenetic transformation of the human skull. *Transactions of the American Philosophical Society,* **31**(5), 321–442.

Weinberger, D.R. (1987) Implications of normal brain development for the pathogenesis of schizophrenia. *Archives of General Psychiatry* **44**, 660–669.

Weinstein, D.D., Diforio, D., Schiffman, J., Walker, E. & Bonsall, R. (1999) Minor physical anomalies, dermatoglyphic asymmetries, and cortisol levels in adolescents with schizotypal personality disorder. *American Journal of Psychiatry* **156**, 617–623.

Westergaard, T., Mortensen, P.B., Pedersen, C.B., Wohlfahrt, J. & Melbye, M. (1999) Exposure to prenatal and childhood infections and the risk of schizophrenia: suggestions from a study of sibship characteristics and influenza prevalence. *Archives of General Psychiatry* **56**, 993–998.

Woerner, M.G., Pollack, M. & Klein, D.F. (1971) Birth weight and length in schizophrenics, personality disorders, and their siblings. *British Journal of Psychiatry* **118**, 461–464.

Woerner, M.G., Pollack, M. & Klein, D.F. (1973) Pregnancy and birth complications in psychiatric patients: a comparison of schizophrenic and personality disorder patients with their siblings. *Acta Psychiatrica Scandinavica* **49**, 712–721.

Zornberg, G.L., Buka, S.L. & Tsuang, M.T. (2000) Hypoxic–ischemia-related fetal/neonatal complications and risk of schizophrenia and other non-affective psychoses: a 19-year longitudinal study. *American Journal of Psychiatry* **157**, 196–202.

14 Genetics and schizophrenia

B. Riley, P.J. Asherson and P. McGuffin

Early family studies, 251
More recent family studies, 252
Twin studies, 252
  Criticisms of twin studies, 254
Adoption studies, 255
What is the mode of transmission?, 256
  Single gene models, 256
  Multifactorial threshold model, 256
  Mixed models, 257
  Models involving gene or allele interaction
    effects, 257
Aetiological heterogeneity, 257
Linkage and association studies, 258
  DNA markers, 260
  Problems in linkage analysis, 261
Linkage studies in schizophrenia, 262
  Chromosome 5, 262

Chromosome 22q, 263
Chromosome 8p, 263
Chromosome 6p, 264
Chromosome 10p, 264
Chromosome 6q, 264
Chromosome 13q, 264
Chromosome 15q13–q14, 265
Chromosome 18, 265
Chromosome 1q, 265
X chromosome, 265
Other chromosomal regions, 266
Association studies, 266
  Association studies in schizophrenia, 267
Molecular neurobiology, 268
Genetic counselling, 268
Conclusions, 269
References, 269

It has long been recognized that schizophrenia runs in families, and there is compelling evidence from family twin and adoption studies that inherited genetic factors are important (McGue & Gottesman 1991). Such evidence and the enormous rate of progress in molecular methods have together led to a great deal of activity over the last 10–15 years, with probably more researchers engaged in genetic studies than at any time in the history of the disorder. However, before discussing molecular genetics – a comparative recent arrival on the scene – it is necessary to review the 'classical' genetic methods of study.

Early family studies

The first systematic family study was published by Rudin in 1916, who found that dementia praecox was more common among the siblings of probands than in the general population. Following this, a large study of over a thousand schizophrenic probands was published by Kallman in 1938, which showed that both siblings and offspring had increased rates of the disorder.

These early workers recognized the need for systematically ascertaining index cases or probands for family studies in order to ensure that the cases were representative of schizophrenia as a whole. In most studies this was done by taking consecutive admissions referred to a clinic. They also recognized that in order to make accurate estimates of the lifetime expectancy or morbid risk to various classes of relatives, they had to take account of the age of those being studied and make appropriate corrections. This is important when considering the status of unaffected relatives, some of whom will be too young to have entered the age of risk, while others who are within the age of

risk may develop the disorder in the future. Only those who are beyond the age of risk can be unequivocally classified as unaffected. Lifetime expectancy for a particular class of relatives can therefore be calculated by dividing the number of affecteds by an age-corrected total. The method most often used is Weinberg's shorter method, the denominator being known as the *Bezugsziffer* (BZ), but more complicated approaches include so-called life table methods (Slater & Cowie 1971).

The results of all Western European studies from before the current era of operational diagnostic criteria, looking at the frequency of the disorder among various classes of relatives, has been summarized by Gottesman and Shields (Table 14.1). In order to interpret these data, comparisons must be made with the morbid risk in the general population, which is generally thought to be in the region of 1%. Shields calculated a lifetime risk of 0.86% using the Camberwell Register of all known hospital contacts within a borough of London, while Essen-Moller, who personally studied a small rural population in southern Sweden, found a lifetime risk of 1.39% (Gottesman & Shields 1982).

These studies clearly show that the risk of developing schizophrenia is increased among the relatives of schizophrenic probands, but there are some apparent anomalies. The first is that while the risk to siblings and offspring of a schizophrenic is in the order of 10%, the risk to the parent of a schizophrenic is only about 6%. This finding is likely to be explained by reduced fecundity which follows the development of schizophrenia, because illness among parents of index cases occurs mainly in those who developed the disease after they had children. It has been calculated that if this were taken into account, the risk among parents would be about 11% (Essen-Moller 1955). This decrease in reproduction may also account for the finding in

Table 14.1 Lifetime expectancy (morbid risk) of schizophrenia in the relatives of schizophrenics.

Type of relative	Number at risk (BZ)	Lifetime expectancy (%)	Correlation in liability (r)*
First-degree			
Parent	8020.0	5.6	0.30
Siblings	9920.7	10.1	0.48
Siblings with one schizophrenic parent	623.5	16.7	0.57
Children	1577.6	12.9	0.50
Children with both parents schizophrenic	134.0	46.3	0.85
Second-degree			
Half siblings	499.5	4.2	0.24
Uncle/aunts	2421.0	2.4	0.14
Nephews/nieces	3965.5	3.0	0.18
Grandchildren	739.5	3.7	0.22
Third-degree			
Cousins	1600.5	2.4	0.14

*Correlation in liability assuming general population morbid risk of 1%.

some studies that mothers of schizophrenic probands are more likely to be affected than fathers, because women tend to have a later age of onset and tend to have children at an earlier age than men. The alternative suggestions that affected women are either more 'schizophrenogenic' or pass on a greater genetic liability than affected men are both unlikely, because if we take as our starting point affected parents, the risk among the offspring is no greater for affected women than affected men (Gottesman & Shields 1982).

More recent family studies

Investigators studying the familiality of schizophrenia more recently have used standardized methods of assessment and explicit operationalized diagnostic criteria. They have also been rigorous in their methodology, using appropriate control samples and assessing relatives blind to proband diagnosis. The use of carefully collected control samples has proved to be important because there have been reports of lifetime risks for schizophrenia among first-degree relatives much lower than those found in earlier studies. Kendler *et al.* (1985) reported a lifetime risk of only 3.7% among first-degree relatives using DSM-III criteria of schizophrenia. However, this must be compared with a lifetime risk among controls of 0.2%. When other non-affective psychosis and schizoaffective disorder were considered, the lifetime risk in first-degree relatives of schizophrenics increased to 8.6%. Gershon *et al.* (1988) have reviewed the results of family studies using modern diagnostic criteria and found a wide range of lifetime risks reported in the first-degree relatives of schizophrenics probands, from 3.1% to 16.9%. However, as in the study of Kendler *et al.*, where control samples had been coll-

ected, there were substantially higher lifetime risks among the relatives of schizophrenics.

The reason for these highly variable results appears to be that different investigators have chosen to use different diagnostic criteria. This problem comes about because, while there are numerous explicit diagnostic criteria which can all be reliably assessed, it is not at all clear which of these (if any) is the most valid. As can be seen in the study of Kendler *et al.*, when using DSM-III criteria, the breadth of the criteria used to assign an individual as affected has a large impact upon the final result. It has been suggested that in order to overcome this problem researchers should collect data in such a way that they can apply many different operational criteria to the same dataset (McGuffin & Owen 1991). This 'polydiagnostic' approach would enable researchers in different centres and countries to make direct comparisons of their results. For this reason this approach has been adopted by many groups in Europe and the USA who are carrying out linkage and association studies of schizophrenia (Leboyer & McGuffin 1991).

These studies clearly demonstrate that schizophrenia tends to cluster within families, but do not provide any evidence about the relative contributions of genetic vs. environmental components. To answer the question of whether 'nature', 'nurture' or both bring about familial aggregation we have to turn to other 'classical' genetic approaches: twin and adoption studies.

Twin studies

The main strategy in twin studies is to compare the concordance for the disease between members of monozygotic (MZ) twin pairs and members of dizygotic (DZ) twin pairs. As MZ twins

Table 14.2 Studies in monozygotic and dizygotic twins.

Study	Monozygotic (MZ)			Dizygotic (DZ)		
	No.	Proband-wise concordance (%)	r	No.	Proband-wise concordance (%)	r
Tienari (1971)	17	35	0.78	20	13	0.50
Kringlen (1976)	55	45	0.85	90	15	0.56
Fischer (1971)	21	56	0.90	141	27	0.70
Pollin *et al.* (1969)	95	43	0.83	125	9	0.41
Gottesman & Shields (1972)	22			33		
Weighted		58	0.91		12	0.48
Average		46	0.85		14	0.52

are genetically identical, whereas DZ twins share on average 50% of their genes, greater MZ than DZ concordance will reflect genetic influence, provided that both MZ and DZ twins share their environment to approximately the same extent.

Data from five 'classical' twin studies, which ascertained probands systematically from twin registries, are shown in Table 14.2. The results, while based on small samples, are consistent between studies, showing MZ concordance rates about three times as high as DZ concordance rates. These studies used national registries (Fischer 1971; Tienari 1971; Kringlen 1976), a consecutive hospital registry of twins (Gottesman & Shields 1972) and a registry of US military veterans (Pollin *et al.* 1969). Systematic ascertainment is essential in twin studies in order to avoid the substantial biases that can occur from selective ascertainment. These biases arise from the preferential selection of the most prominent twin pairs, which are likely to be monozygotic and concordant for the disorder. The results are expressed as proband-wise concordance rates, which are calculated by dividing the number of affected cotwins by the total number of cotwins. On statistical grounds, this method of calculating concordance rates is preferable to the pair-wise method, which calculates the proportion of affected pairs, because individuals within a twin pair may be ascertained independently as two separate probands. The proband-wise method has the effect of providing an unbiased assessment of morbid risk for each cotwin, which can then be compared with the morbid risk to other relatives and the general population.

Like early family studies, the diagnosis of individuals in these studies was not based upon modern operationalized diagnostic criteria, and they were therefore open to the criticism of diagnostic unreliability. This problem prompted a reassessment of the case material from the Maudsley Hospital twin series, which had originally been studied by Gottesman and Shields (1972) applying operational criteria (McGuffin *et al.* 1984; Farmer *et al.* 1987). By using a polydiagnostic approach these workers were able to compare the effect of different diagnostic criteria in producing the highest estimates of genetic parameters such as the MZ/DZ ratio and heritability (or proportion of variances

accounted for by genes). Their results showed that Schneider's first-rank symptoms were excessively restrictive and gave no evidence of genetic determination, while the St Louis criteria (Feighner *et al.* 1972) and Research Diagnostic Criteria (Spitzer *et al.* 1978) defined highly 'genetic' forms of the disease. Using DSM-III criteria, the best estimate of heritability was in the order of 80%.

The first study to use modern criteria from the outset was carried out in Norway (Onstad *et al.* 1991). The concordance rates found in this study are very close to those found when Farmer applied DSM criteria (Table 14.3). An attempt was also made to define the most genetically determined definition of schizophrenia by both of these research groups. They considered the effect of varying the definition of affected status on the MZ/DZ ratio by broadening the diagnosis to include other psychotic and affective disorders. Both groups found that including schizoaffective disorder, atypical psychosis and schizotypy gave the greatest difference between MZ and DZ concordance rates, whereas further broadening of the definition to include affective disorders and personality disorders greatly increased the DZ concordance rate resulting in a lowering of the MZ/DZ ratio. These results are pertinent to the question of how to define the phenotype for genetic analysis, in which the ability to define precisely what is being inherited greatly increases the chances of detecting genes. The MZ/DZ ratio is a rather crude way of determining what is inherited, but in keeping with earlier observations of Gottesman and Shields (1972) the results suggest that the 'most genetic' definition is not restricted to tightly defined schizophrenia alone, but on the other hand is not excessively broad.

More recently, there have been five further twin studies where the cases have been defined using operational criteria (Table 14.4). One of these was an updating and extension of the Maudsley series. Cardno *et al.* (1999a) found proband-wise concordances of 20/47 (43%) in MZ twins compared with 0/50 (0%) in DZ twins using DSM-IIIR criteria. For ICD-10 defined schizophrenia, the rates were 21/50 (42%) in MZ twins and 1/58 (2%) in DZ twins. Applying genetic model fitting they estimated that the broad heritability, or proportion of variation in

Table 14.3 Proband-wise concordance for operationally defined schizophrenia.

Reference	Criteria	Monozygotic (MZ)		Dizygotic (DZ)	
		No.	Concordance (%)	No.	Concordance (%)
Farmer *et al.* (1987)	DSM-III	21	48	21	10
Onstad *et al.* (1991)	DSM-IIIR	31	48	28	4

Table 14.4 Twin studies 1996–99 (modified from Cardno & Gottesman 2000).

Authors	Country	Ascertainment	Diagnostic criteria	MZ concordance (%)	DZ concordance (%)	Heritability (%)
Kläning (1996)	Denmark	Population register	ICD-10	7/16 (44)	2/19 (11)	83
Cannon *et al.* (1998)	Finland	Population register	ICD-8/ DSM-IIIR	40/87 (46)	18/195 (9)	
Franzek & Beckmann (1998)	Germany	Hospital admissions	DSM-IIIR	20/31 (65)	7/25 (28)	
Cardno *et al.* (1999a)	UK	Hospital register	DSM-IIIR ICD-10	20/47 (43) 21/50 (42)	0/50 (0) 1/58 (2)	84 83
Tsujita *et al.* (1992)	Japan	Hospital admissions	DSM-IIIR	11/22 (50)	1/7 (14)	
Combined			DSM-IIIR ICD-10	57/114 (50) 28/66 (42.4)	4/97 (4.1) 3/77 (3.9)	88 83

liability, to schizophrenia was about 84% for the DSM-IIIR and 83% for the ICD-10 definition of schizophrenia. Interestingly, the model fitting analyses also suggested the presence of non-additive genetic effects, something that we return to later in the chapter when we consider modes of transmission.

Subsequently, Cardno and Gottesman (2000) combined their own data with those from the four other studies giving a pooled MZ proband-wise concordance of 50% and a DZ concordance of 4.1% for DSM-IIIR schizophrenia. Using ICD-10 criteria, the pooled concordances were 42.4% for MZ and 3.9% for DZ twins. Again model fitting gave very high heritability estimates of 88% for DSM-IIIR criteria and 83% for ICD-10. For both sets of criteria, the remainder of the variance was explained by non-shared environment. That is, shared environmental effects appeared to play no part in causing twin similarity with respect to liability to schizophrenia.

Criticisms of twin studies

Twin studies have been criticized for making the assumption that the environments are equal between members of MZ and DZ twins: MZ twins are more likely to dress alike, have similar interests and be treated in the same way than DZ twins. The argument is that the 'microenvironment' of MZ and DZ twins

differs, and this could account for the increased concordance rates among MZ pairs. There is no direct evidence for this hypothesis, while on the other hand there is some evidence against it from data on MZ twins reared apart (MZA). Gottesman and Shields (1982) reviewed all systematic twin studies of schizophrenia and found 12 MZA pairs. Seven (58%) were concordant for the disorder, a rate similar to MZ twins reared together, suggesting that a shared environment contributed little to the development of the disorder.

An alternative hypothesis is that there are other non-genetic factors which occur more commonly between MZ twins. It has been suggested that birth trauma, where the risk is higher in MZ than DZ twins, may predispose to schizophrenia. However, this is unlikely to account for greater MZ than DZ concordance because there is little evidence that twins in general have a higher risk for schizophrenia than other members of the population (Gottesman & Shields 1982). Only one study gave evidence for an increased rate of schizophrenia in twins, and this was found only in DZ pairs, counter to the prediction of the hypothesis above (Kläning 1996).

However, there has been a continued interest in the relationship between the development of schizophrenia, subtle neurological signs and birth trauma. Twins discordant for schizophrenia have been examined for brain abnormalities using computerized tomography (CT) (Reveley *et al.* 1982) and magnetic resonance imaging (MRI) (Suddath *et al.* 1990). These studies show that individuals with schizophrenia have larger cerebral ventricles than their unaffected cotwins. Other studies have examined series of unrelated schizophrenics and show that ventricular enlargement is found in at least a proportion of acute-onset first episode cases (Turner *et al.* 1986). These observations have led some to propose that where there is evidence of such brain changes, schizophrenia is likely to be the result of intrauterine infection, birth complications or other trauma affecting neurodevelopment. Because it is no longer feasible to reject the view that inherited genetic factors are of major importance in the aetiology of schizophrenia, it has been proposed that there are in effect two separate mechanisms: one predominantly genetic and the other predominantly non-genetic (Murray *et al.* 1985). If this were the case, we would expect that at least a proportion of those MZ twins discordant for schizophrenia would have the 'non-genetic' form of schizophrenia. However, the evidence from the study of twins does not support this view. Early evidence was provided by Luxenberger (1928), who showed that the relatives of discordant MZ pairs had an equally high risk for schizophrenia as the relatives of concordant twin pairs. Further evidence was provided by Fischer (1971), and this work has been subsequently expanded and updated by Gottesman and Bertelsen (1989). The results are shown in Table 14.4 and show that in discordant MZ pairs there is an equally high risk among the offspring of the affected as among the offspring of the unaffected cotwin. By contrast, discordant DZ twins show a marked difference in the risks of schizophrenia among the offspring.

Although a smaller but similar study by Kringlen and Cramer (1989) produced less clear-cut results, the data of Gottesman and Bertelsen strongly argue for two important principles. First, non-genetic forms of the disorder (phenocopies), if they exist, are relatively uncommon. Secondly, genotypes which give susceptibility to schizophrenia may not be expressed. As we shall see later, this is important for linkage analysis where genetic parameters must be estimated.

Adoption studies

Adoption studies are also important in distinguishing inherited from non-inherited factors. These studies use various strategies, giving compelling evidence that schizophrenia has an important genetic component.

The first major adoption study was carried out by Heston (1966). He was able to study the adopted-away offspring of 47 schizophrenic mothers and compare them to an age- and sex-matched group of adopted-away offspring of psychiatrically well mothers. The schizophrenic mothers all gave birth within Oregon State mental hospitals at a time when it was the state law that their offspring must be fostered or adopted within 72 h of birth. At the time of the study, the offspring had all entered the age of risk for schizophrenia and Heston, along with two other

psychiatrists, made diagnoses blind to the parental diagnosis. Among the offspring of the 47 schizophrenic mothers, five (10.6%; 16% after age correction) were themselves schizophrenic compared with none of the offspring of the psychiatrically well mothers.

Rosenthal *et al.* (1971), using a similar approach, were able to obtain subjects from Danish adoption registrars. This had the advantage over Heston's study that most of the affected parents gave up their children for adoption before their first admissions and about one-third of the affected parents were fathers. This provided safeguards against illness in adoptees being either a result of early contact with an overtly schizophrenic parent, or intrauterine maternal environment. These researchers thought that a variety of conditions, especially 'borderline schizophrenia' and schizoid or paranoid traits, might be biologically similar to more narrowly defined schizophrenia and they used the term 'schizophrenia spectrum disorder' (SSD) to describe this group of disorders. Their initial report found that three of the offspring of schizophrenic parents developed schizophrenia, compared with none of 47 matched controls. When they later extended the study and considered SSD, they found that 13 (18.8%) of 69 adoptees of schizophrenic parents had SSD compared with eight (10.1%) of 79 matched controls.

These researchers were also able to employ a 'cross-fostering' study design (Wender *et al.* 1974). Here, they considered the rate of SSD among the adopted offspring of affected parents, and were able to obtain a sample of 28 individuals whose biological parents were normal but who were adopted by parents one of whom later developed schizophrenia. In this comparison group 10.7% of the offspring were diagnosed as having SSD, a figure very close to that found among the 79 matched controls.

An alternative approach is the 'adoptees family study' design (Kety *et al.* 1976), where the probands are individuals who were adopted in early life and subsequently developed schizophrenia. A comparison is then made between the rate of schizophrenia among the biological and adoptive relatives. It was found that 20.3% of 118 biological parents of adopted-away schizophrenics had SSD, compared with only 5.8% of 224 adoptive parents of schizophrenics and parents of control adoptees.

More recently, the results of Kety's study have been re-examined using more explicit and stricter criteria (Kendler & Gruenberg 1984). This reanalysis served to emphasize the genetic relationship by increasing the separation between the different groups studied. Kendler took DSM-III schizophrenia and DSM-III schizotypal personality disorder as the definition of an affected case and found that 13.3% of 105 biological relatives of adopted-away schizophrenics were affected, compared with only 1.3% of the 224 adoptive parents.

The most recent adoption study was carried out in Finland by Tienari (1991). The author has promised further analyses, combining attempts to incorporate more detailed family environmental measures with genetic analyses, but the results reported so far are in line with previous adoptee studies in showing a lifetime prevalence of 9.4% in the adopted-away offspring of schizophrenic parents and a lifetime prevalence in control adoptees of 1.2%. In addition, this study attempts to measure environmental influences in detail. Interestingly, the preliminary results regarding family environment show a significant association between the genetic predisposition to schizophrenia and psychological abnormalities in adopting parents, a result that, it could be argued, indicates the importance of psychological environmental factors in the aetiology of schizophrenia. This will need to be reconciled, if it is confirmed in more definitive analyses, with the twin model fitting results suggesting no effect of shared environment on twin concordance.

What is the mode of transmission?

It is clear from the preceding discussion that family, twin and adoption studies demonstrate the existence of inherited genetic factors in the aetiology of schizophrenia. However, analyses of families segregating schizophrenia and studies of the risks to various classes of relatives are unable to demonstrate a simple Mendelian mode of transmission. In other words, the pattern of inheritance is complex or irregular and it is not clear whether familial clustering in schizophrenia is brought about by one gene, a few genes or many genes. Attempts to define the mode of transmission are important for two main reasons. First, the knowledge of how many genes are involved and the size of their effect determines the approach taken to their eventual isolation. Secondly, in order to perform linkage analysis, the genetic parameters of penetrance and gene frequency must be defined.

Single gene models

In the simplest models, single genes are considered to be the sole source of genetic influence resulting in resemblance among relatives. These are termed single major locus (SML) models. If this were the situation in schizophrenia, how could we account for the irregular pattern of transmission observed? One possible explanation is variable expressivity. An example of this is tuberous sclerosis in which an affected individual may show occult skin lesions only visible with a Woods lamp, whereas in others a severe condition with multiple skin tumours and systemic involvement can occur. Likewise, it has been suggested that schizophrenia might be a single gene dominant disorder with highly variable expression, ranging from a 'core' syndrome through milder schizoid traits to a range of minor psychological characteristics among relatives (Heston 1970). Another possible explanation for irregular transmission of a single gene disorder is reduced *penetrance*. Penetrance is the degree to which phenotype is determined by genotype. In classical Mendelian disorders, penetrance is close to or equal to 100%. Reduced penetrance implies that less than 100% of people carrying a disease-causing genotype will develop the disease. Indeed, evidence from the study of discordant MZ twin pairs strongly suggests that this is the case, because the risk in offspring of the unaffected cotwin is as high as that in the offspring of the affected twin (see Table 14.4; Gottesman & Bertelsen 1989).

Slater (1958) proposed a gene with intermediate penetrance for schizophrenia with 100% penetrance in homozygotes and 16% penetrance in heterozygotes. This 'intermediate' model, although a poor fit statistically (McGuffin & Owen 1991), in fact turns out to be close to that suggested by the use of more sophisticated computer model fitting (Elston & Campbell 1970).

However, it has been pointed out by James (1971) that attempts to fit a single gene model to data in pairs of relatives may give misleading results because of mathematical underidentification (i.e. there is not enough information to specify all of the parameters that specify the model). This problem can be partly overcome by constraining parameter values to within biologically meaningful limits (i.e. between 0 and 1 for penetrances and gene frequencies). However, on doing this and testing a general SML model on published Western European data, O'Rourke *et al.* (1982) showed that single gene inheritance provided a mathematically unsatisfactory explanation and McGue *et al.* (1985) showed that an SML model could be rejected statistically.

Multifactorial threshold model

Under a polygenic or multifactorial liability/threshold (MFT) model, genetic factors are assumed to be brought about by the additive effect of many genes at different loci. In other words, several or many genes, each of small effect, combine additively with the effects of non-inherited factors to influence liability to schizophrenia. Liability to develop the disorder is considered to be a continuously distributed variable in the population and individuals who develop the disorder are considered to have liability above a threshold value along that continuum (Falconer 1965; Gottesman & Shields 1967).

The MFT model of inheritance can account for the observed risks to different classes of relatives, which appears to decline exponentially as you pass from monozygous twins, to first-, to second- and then to third-degree relatives. This is explained by a reduction in the genetic risk because of a shift of the liability curve with successive generations, as the number of shared genes reduces from 1 to 1/2 to 1/4 to 1/8 and so on. There are several other observations which best fit an MFT model. For example, the risk for schizophrenia in an individual increases with the number of affected relatives and schizophrenia persists in the population despite selective disadvantage (e.g. reduced fecundity) conferred by the condition. Finally, if severity of the condition is related to the degree of liability for the disorder, this would explain the observation that concordance in twins or first-degree relatives increases with severity of the disorder in the proband.

However, it is important to note that although McGue *et al.* (1985) were unable to reject the MFT model statistically, the observed data do not fit this model well. Such comparisons of model and observed data are made with the goodness-of-fit test, which asks how similar observed and predicted patterns of risk are, and assesses the probability that the model is generating the observed data. A *P*-value of 0.05 in such a test indicates that the observed data would only be generated by the model 5% of the time, and is taken as significant evidence that the model is incorrect. McGue *et al.* found that the observed risks in relatives would only occur 6–7% of the time if the MFT model was the true generating model, very close to the limit of what is conventionally regarded as acceptable. This, together with the more recent twin analysis by Cardno *et al.* (1999a), suggests that the mode of transmission of schizophrenia is more complicated than a purely additive combination of gene effects as dictated by the classic MFT model.

Mixed models

What is now referred to as a 'mixed model' (Morton & MacLean 1974) was first proposed as an explanation for the transmission of schizophrenia by Meehl (1973). He suggested that the expression of a single major gene is modified by interaction or coaction with a number of other genes, each having only a small effect on their own. There have been several studies of the mixed model in schizophrenia (Carter & Chung 1980; Risch & Baron 1984; Vogler *et al.* 1990) where iterative procedures have been used to define the model of 'best fit'. These tests provide some evidence in favour of MFT over SML models, but they have been inconclusive and, while they do not support SML models, they lack power to differentiate mixed vs. MFT models. Perhaps the best evidence against a mixed model comes from recent linkage studies involving large numbers of families (see below), which have failed to find any genes of large effect across the disorder as a whole. It is possible that mixed models (and the major genes they hypothesize) may account for a small minority of families.

Models involving gene or allele interaction effects

The classic polygenic (or multifactorial) model of complex diseases (Falconer 1965) assumes that many genes of small effect simply add together to contribute a liability to disorder. An alternative explanation is that some of the genetic effects are non-additive. The two types of non-additive effects that can occur are allele–allele interaction within a single gene (*dominance*) and interactions between different genes (*epistasis*). In a dominant system, one allele of a gene exerts a stronger effect on the resulting phenotype than the other allele does, and the phenotype of the heterozygote is shifted away from the mean of the two homozygotes. In an epistatic system, different genes, each with their own contribution to liability, have a multiplicative interaction and the total liability from n genes is greater than the sum of the n individual liabilities. Earlier we noted that the twin analyses of Cardno *et al.* (1999a) found non-additive effects in schizophrenia. In fact Cardno *et al.* found evidence suggestive of dominance effects. However, in practice in twin analyses it is difficult to distinguish between epistasis and dominance.

One of the implications of postulating epistasis is that just a few genes, an oligogenic model, could explain all of the differences between the risk of disorder in relatives of schizophrenics and that in the population at large. Risch (1990) defined the

quantity λ_R, the ratio of risks in relatives of type R to the population risk. $(\lambda_R - 1)$ decreases by a factor of 2 with each degree of kinship for monogenic or additive polygenic traits, and by a factor of more than 2 for polygenic traits with epistasis. The fall-off in concordance rates for a trait in first-, second- and third-degree relatives allows estimation of the number of different genetic loci involved and their interaction type. Data from US schizophrenics and their relatives are most consistent with several epistatically interacting loci (Risch 1990). Basic modelling with minimal assumptions shows that as the number of loci increases, the risk-bearing alleles at those loci become very common in the population, of the order of 14–20% (Riley *et al.* 1997).

Such loci show smaller effects when examined singly than additively interacting ones, because the proportion of total risk associated with a single locus in an epistatic system is less than that for a single locus in an additive system with the same n genes. Such loci must also be biologically related – functionally, temporally or spatially. Epistatic interaction is only possible if the *genotype* (the two *alleles*, or variable forms, of a gene) or *phenotype* (the observable effect of the genotype) from one gene exerts an effect on the genotype or phenotype from another. Modelling such synergistic interaction for hypothesis testing or data analysis is much more complex than modelling additive interaction, because the risk for particular genotypes (the penetrance) at different loci must be defined, and this requires specifying the loci and genotypes, and their contribution a priori. At our current stage in studies of most complex genetic traits, where the individual genes contributing to risk are unknown, this is clearly not possible.

Aetiological heterogeneity

So far it has proven impossible to demonstrate clearly which genetic model is most applicable to schizophrenia (McGue & Gottesman 1991). Furthermore, most studies aimed at defining the mode of inheritance consider schizophrenia as a unitary disorder, whereas in reality there may well be genetic heterogeneity as has now been demonstrated in a number of other common genetic disorders. One of the best examples of this is Alzheimer's disease, in which genes on chromosome 21 (amyloid precursor protein) (Goate *et al.* 1991) and chromosome 14 (Van Broeckhoven *et al.* 1992) have been detected that may be the main determinants of genetically different forms of the disease in individuals from multiply affected families. Interestingly, the illness differs in these 'familial Alzheimer's disease' (FAD) cases from that more commonly found by having an earlier age of onset and more rapidly progressive course. Other common disorders, such as non-insulin-dependent diabetes (NIDDM), coronary artery disease and breast cancer, also display this type of heterogeneity with a small proportion of multiply affected families characterized by early age of onset resulting from a highly penetrant single gene defect.

In schizophrenia there are a number of pedigrees that are highly loaded with affected individuals and have a 'dominant-like' appearance (McGuffin & Owen 1991). It is entirely possible that in these rare families single genes are the sole or main source of resemblance between relatives. The observation that affected individuals from multiply affected families on average show an earlier age of onset than seen in those with schizophrenia among the general population lends some support for the existence of major genes in such families. However, this finding is equally compatible with polygenic inheritance (Walsh *et al.* 1993) or with genetic mechanisms such as *anticipation*.

Much has been written about anticipation and dynamic mutations in schizophrenia. The term anticipation, meaning earlier onset and more severe course in successive generations, now known to be brought about by unstable expanding trinucleotide repeat sequences, was first put forward in the context of 'inherited insanity' (Mott 1910). Some studies have shown evidence for earlier onset and more severe course measured by age of first, and total frequency of, hospitalization in the schizophrenic offspring of schizophrenics (Asherson *et al.* 1994; Bassett & Honer 1994; Chotai *et al.* 1995; Yaw *et al.* 1996; Gorwood *et al.* 1997; Imamura *et al.* 1998; Heiden *et al.* 1999) but these results need to be treated cautiously because of a variety of potential biases originally pointed out by Penrose (Asherson *et al.* 1994).

There may be more than one mutation at a single genetic locus (*allelic heterogeneity*) and different pedigrees may segregate completely different disease genes (*locus heterogeneity*). Furthermore, as single genes are unlikely to account for all cases of schizophrenia, aetiological heterogeneity might exist with different forms resulting from mixed genetic and environmental effects. As we shall see below, the combined results of both modelling and molecular genetic studies seem to be most consistent with aetiological heterogeneity resulting from different subsets (in a patient or family) of a larger pool of predisposing genes (in a population) combined with varying environmental effects.

Linkage and association studies

The two main strategies employed to locate disease genes with DNA markers are positional cloning (linkage analysis) and association studies. In order to understand these methods it is essential to understand the concepts of *crossover* and *recombination* (Fig. 14.1). During meiosis (cell division resulting in the production of eggs or sperm) there is physical exchange of material, or crossover, between the chromosome pairs. Recombination, the occurrence of new chromosomes with alleles at some loci from one of the parental chromosomes and alleles at some loci from the other parental chromosome, is observed genetically and is the result of this crossover. If two genetic loci are on different chromosomes the probability that they are inherited together will be 0.5. This phenomenon of *independent assortment*, as Mendel described it, is also true for two loci far apart on the same chromosome when there is an even chance that they will be separated by crossovers at meiosis. On the other hand, linkage is observed between two loci when they are in such close proximity on the same chromosome that

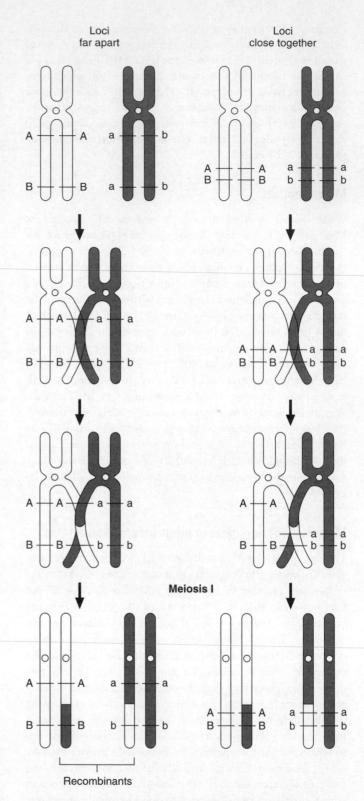

Fig 14.1 Recombination between homologous chromosomes in meiosis. The left diagram illustrates two loci which are far apart on the same chromosome. These loci have an even chance that they will be separated by crossovers at meiosis. On the right, the two loci are close together so they are less likely to recombine.

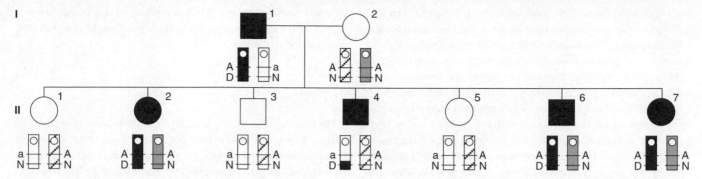

Fig 14.2 Linkage between a disease gene and marker locus close together on the same chromosome. Allele D is a dominantly inherited disease gene, whereas N is the normal allele at the disease locus. A and a are alternative alleles at a marker locus. Individuals indicated by a solid symbol are affected by disease. Among three of the four affected offspring, the disease gene (D) is inherited with the marker allele A. The three unaffected offspring inherit the normal allele (N) along with the marker allele a. These individuals demonstrate linkage between the two loci. However, individual II-4 is a recombinant because D has been inherited along with a; crossover has occurred between the disease locus and marker locus in the paternal meiosis.

their alleles are separated by crossing over less than half the time. In other words there is a departure from the law of independent assortment (see Fig. 14.2).

In linkage analysis, the approximate distance between two linked loci can be estimated by observing the number of individuals within a sibship where recombination has occurred and calculating the recombination fraction θ; i.e. the number of recombinants divided by the total number within the sibship. Thus, $\theta = 1/2$ indicates that there is independent assortment, but where $\theta < 1/2$ the loci are linked. Genetic distance is usually expressed in centimorgans (cM), where 1 cM is equivalent to a 1% chance of recombination between two loci. The most common method of estimating the degree of support for linkage is to calculate log of the odds (LOD) scores, abbreviated as Z, as below.

In practice, the LOD score is plotted for a range of possible values of θ between zero and 0.5. Where the maximum LOD score is obtained provides the maximum likelihood (or best fit) estimate of θ. By convention, for simple Mendelian traits, a LOD score of 3 or more, corresponding to odds favouring linkage of 1000:1 or greater, is taken as acceptable evidence that linkage is present. Linkage analysis also allows for *heterogeneity*, more than one gene producing the same phenotype, provided that within families the gene causing disease is the same one. Here, the likelihood ratio is maximized over two parameters, the recombination fraction, θ, and the proportion of families linked, α, and results from these analyses are referred to as HLODs.

Non-parametric methods, based on testing for deviations from expected allele-sharing distributions, avoid many of the problems (discussed below) of linkage analysis. One alternative approach for detecting linkage is the study of affected sibling pairs (Penrose 1935; Green & Woodrow 1977). This approach is much simpler and is based upon the assumption that two siblings both affected with the same disorder will share one or more susceptibility loci. This method compares the distribution of marker alleles inherited by the affected siblings with that expected under random segregation. Statistical tests then assess whether alleles are shared *identical by state* (IBS) beyond chance expectation. Unlike the LOD score approach, it is not model-dependent and therefore does not require the specification of genetic parameters. A drawback is that large samples are required, especially in the face of genetic heterogeneity, and the method cannot estimate the distance between the disease gene and the marker.

However, because marker alleles are *not* the gene of interest, it is more compelling to see that affected relatives share alleles inherited from the same source *identical by descent* (IBD). Not only siblings, but all classes of relatives have predefined probabilities of sharing zero, one or two marker alleles at a random locus. The most common non-parametric method currently used is the non-parametric linkage (NPL) score, a multipoint IBD approach (Kruglyak *et al.* 1996) that considers all loci simultaneously to examine for excess sharing in affected relative pairs IBD. When the data are fully informative, and often they are not, the method specifies exactly which of the distinct founder alleles each individual has inherited at every point in the linear map of marker loci.

Numerous authors have suggested that linkage tests for complex traits be interpreted relative to the probability of observing results by chance in a complete screen of the genome (Morton 1955; Lander & Kruglyak 1995). Lander and Kruglyak suggest that nominal *P*-values of 0.000049 (for parametric analysis) or 0.000022 (for non-parametric analysis) will be observed by chance in 5% of genome screens, giving an approximate cut-off for 'significance' in linkage studies. This is equivalent to a LOD of 3.3 or an NPL of 3.6, very similar to Morton's original proposal for Mendelian traits. Nominal *P*-values of 0.0017 and 0.00074 will be observed by chance once per genome scan, and they suggest these as cut-offs for 'suggestive' linkage, equivalent to a LOD of 1.9 or an NPL of 2.2. Few linkage studies of schizophrenia have ever produced 'significant' results under these criteria (for an exception see Chromosome 1, below). Even the original report on chromosome 6p from the Irish sample (see Chromosome 6, below), which did achieve this level of significance, would require correction for the numerous models tested.

In contrast, association studies compare the frequencies of marker alleles in a group of affected individuals and a sample of controls without the disease or drawn from the general population. A statistically significant difference suggests either very tight linkage resulting in *linkage disequilibrium* between a marker allele and the disease mutation, or that a marker allele itself confers susceptibility to disease. Linkage disequilibrium refers to the phenomena of two loci being so close together on a chromosome (1 cM apart or less) that they are not separated by recombination over many generations. Alleles at the two loci will therefore appear to be associated, even in individuals from different families. A recent example of this is the population association between a marker near to the insulin gene and IDDM. This finding has led to identification of mutations within the insulin gene, which have a definite role in the aetiology of diabetes.

Linkage studies are more difficult to carry out because they involve the study of multiply affected pedigrees, which are more difficult to collect than the unrelated individuals required for association studies. However, linkage is a powerful technique for locating genes of major effect and a single DNA marker may give information over a large genetic distance. In contrast, association studies are able to identify genes of small effect (Edwards 1965; Nothen *et al.* 1993) if the mutation rates of both the DNA marker and the disease gene are sufficiently low.

DNA markers

Investigators working before DNA markers became readily accessible were restricted to the use of 'classical' genetic markers, such as red blood cell antigens (ABO, MNS and Rhesus) and the human leucocyte antigens (HLA) (McGuffin *et al.* 1992). However, these are limited in number and informativity and unlikely to lead to the eventual location of disease genes. The revolution in molecular genetics, which has resulted in the localization of a host of disease genes, has followed the discovery of techniques for measuring variation within genomic DNA. Variation is common in genomes and methods have been developed to exploit these differences. At loci where variation occurs there will be two or more different sequences or *alleles*, which are inherited in a simple Mendelian fashion and behave as codominant markers. Loci at which two or more of the alleles have frequencies of at least 1% are described as polymorphisms. It is important that marker loci show a high degree of polymorphism because this increases the chance of there being a different allele on each of the parental chromosomes (i.e. the parents are heterozygous at the marker locus). Where the parent is homozygous at a marker locus, the cosegregation of that locus and a putative disease locus cannot be examined, so the meioses are not informative for linkage.

The detection of one class of DNA markers depends on the use of restriction endonucleases (REs), which are enzymes isolated from bacteria that cut DNA according to a specific base sequence; for example, one of these enzymes recognizes and cuts only at the sequence:

GAATTC

CTTAAG.

The specific sequences where REs cut are known as restriction sites. Where variation in base sequence creates or deletes one of these restriction sites, DNA fragments of different lengths are produced known as *restriction fragment length polymorphisms* (RFLPs). The standard method used to detect RFLPs is known as Southern blotting, named after its author E.M. Southern. In this technique, genomic DNA is incubated with the RE. The resulting fragments are then separated according to size on an agarose gel. The DNA is then transferred from the gel to a nylon membrane to produce a long-lasting copy of the DNA fragment pattern. A piece of DNA complementary to the region of the polymorphism is then labelled with the isotope ^{32}P and used as a probe. The probe binds or hybridizes to the fragments on the nylon membrane, to produce a pattern of bands on an autoradiograph.

More recently, it has been found that between restriction sites and within non-coding regions of genomic DNA there are multiple repeats of nucleotide sequences. The number of repeats of the core sequence can be highly variable and are inherited in a Mendelian fashion. Some of these sequences are located only at one locus on a pair of homologous chromosomes – the so-called *variable number of tandem repeats* (VNTR). Most of these VNTR markers are located in the subtelomeric region of the chromosome, so limiting their usefulness in mapping studies.

A subset of VNTR markers consisting of 1–4 base pair (bp) repeat units is one of the most useful tools to genetic mappers, as they are widely distributed throughout the human genome. These units are known as *microsatellites* or *simple sequence repeat* (SSR) polymorphisms. These tandem repeats of di-, tri- or tetranucleotides often show length polymorphism. Generally, the longer the run of perfect repeat units the more polymorphic the marker, and sequences with 12 or fewer repeats are usually not polymorphic. On average, one microsatellite greater than 19 bp in length is found every 6000 base pairs (6 kb).

The most common of these repeat units is the AC repeat, one of which occurs approximately every 30 kb (Weber & May 1989). All SSRs can be analysed relatively simply by amplifying a small segment of DNA that contains the repeat unit and a little sequence on either side. This is only possible using the polymerase chain reaction (PCR), an innovation which has revolutionized molecular biology (Mullis & Faloona 1987). In this technique, the starting material is total genomic DNA which can be extracted easily from whole blood. Two primers are made, which are small stretches of about 20 DNA bases, complementary to sequences flanking the region to be amplified. The total DNA is heated and then cooled, which first separates the usually doubly stranded DNA into single strands and then allows the primers to bind onto their complementary flanking sites. By adding a mixture of precursors for the four DNA bases (2'-deoxyribonucleoside 5'-triphosphates) and a heat-resistant polymerase (usually Taq polymerase), a new strand of DNA is synthesized between the two primers. The process is then repeated many times over, each step doubling the number of double-stranded target molecules, so that a rapid amplification of the target region is achieved. The amplified fragments can then be separated on a gel by electrophoresis so that different length fragments can be identified. The benefits of this method are that very small amounts of DNA are needed initially and it results in the amplification of specified regions. In addition, the method is relatively easy, rapid and can be automated.

It has been calculated that the number of polymorphic AC repeat sequences in the human genome will be around 12 000. Assuming a total genetic length of 3300 cM, these markers would yield genetic maps with average resolution of approximately 0.3–0.5 cM (White & Lalouel 1988).

More recently, the importance of another kind of DNA variation, the single nucleotide polymorphism (SNP), has been recognized. The publication of draft versions of the human genome (Lander *et al.* 2001; Venter *et al.* 2001) has provided an enormous amount of data about the base-by-base variability of the human genome. Some now think that the key step will not be the sequencing of the first human genome, but rather the sequencing of numerous genomes and the identification of the several million base pairs that differ between us (McGuffin *et al.* 2001). As of early 2001, there were 1.65 million non-redundant SNPs deposited in dbSNP, the public SNP database, of which approximately 80% are true polymorphisms (as opposed to errors in the draft genome sequence) and about 50% have frequencies of the rarer allele large enough (20% or greater) to make them useful for fine mapping of genetic loci (Marth *et al.* 2001). Again assuming a map of total length 3300 cM, these numbers would yield a map with average resolution of 0.004 cM (or about 4 kb pairs based on the average figure of ~ 1 megabase per cM).

Problems in linkage analysis

The current emphasis on linkage analysis in schizophrenia research assumes that genes of major effect exist in at least some families. However, we cannot be certain of this and even if major genes contribute to liability in schizophrenia in some multiply affected families, it seems likely that the most common mode of transmission is either polygenic or oligogenic. In addition, to carry out linkage analysis, penetrance values and frequency of the disease gene must be specified. Failure to specify them accurately reduces the power to detect linkage leading to false-negative findings (Clerget-Darpoux *et al.* 1986; Ott 1991). There are also the uncertainties concerning aetiological heterogeneity. Interpretation of positive LOD scores under these circumstances is very difficult (Ott 1991) and, as we shall see, even seemingly very high LOD scores found in a schizophrenia linkage study have turned out to be false-positive results. On the other hand, it is equally difficult to interpret negative results, which can only exclude regions of the genome assuming specific

genetic models. Additionally, it has been shown recently that even with large numbers of families, chance variation in the location estimate (essentially the chromosomal position) of a LOD score is significant, making both positioning of results from individual studies and interpretation of replication studies difficult and unreliable (Roberts *et al.* 1999).

There are substantial problems with the linkage analysis of complex traits, whether undertaken by parametric or non-parametric means. Classical genetic illnesses are assumed to have a single faulty gene, located at a single place on a chromosome. Because these illnesses are rare, the rare risk allele must segregate from parents with a family history into affected offspring, or arise as an even rarer *de novo* mutation. By following the segregation of marker alleles from the affected lineage into offspring, chromosome regions in which affected offspring inherit one marker allele and unaffected offspring the other can be identified. Likelihood-based tests can be maximized over one or more parameters, so the focus is often the relative likelihood of one parameter value compared with another, expressed as a likelihood ratio. In LOD score analyses, the likelihood ratio is maximized over θ, the rate of recombination, which increases with the physical distance between loci. More than one gene can produce the same phenotype, and LOD score analyses which allow for aetiological heterogeneity are maximized over both θ and the proportion of families linked to a given locus, α.

Recombination in the search for disease genes is an *apparent* event between real genetic marker alleles and the conceptual alleles 'affected' and 'unaffected'. In real terms, what is being examined is whether affected members of a family share one of the two possible alleles they can inherit and unaffected members the other. Differences between affected individuals or similarities between an affected and an unaffected individual appear in the calculation as recombinations, increasing θ artificially. This can be partly overcome by treating all unaffected relatives as unknown, the *affected only* analysis, but this leaves several problems just in considering the affected members of a family.

First, in a disease with multiple common inputs, no two individuals (even in the same family) need to share input from any individual gene (because there are many genes) or from one particular lineage (because the risk alleles at all these genes are relatively common). Secondly, this will increase apparent recombination, even in affected-only analyses, inflating the apparent distance between marker and disease and making accurate positioning of a putative gene impossible. Thirdly, it will unavoidably decrease the magnitude of the statistic: because the LOD score is the log of a ratio, as the value of θ increases toward 0.5, the value of the ratio decreases towards 1, and that of the statistic decreases towards 0.

The inescapable conclusion is that while parametric linkage analysis is extremely powerful for monogenic traits, much of its power is lost in complex traits. Multipoint parametric linkage analysis, a powerful tool for defining regions of the genome which *do not* contain the single gene responsible for a monogenic trait, has been shown to be statistically invalid for polygenic traits (Risch & Giuffra 1992).

The non-parametric IBD method is also not ideal, however, because the high population frequency of risk alleles and the apparently large number of predisposing genes means that risk alleles may be inherited from different parents or in different genes. Additionally, two different groups have shown that when data are not fully informative, the NPL test is overly conservative (Davis & Weeks 1997; Kong & Cox 1997).

These problems may at first sight seem to preclude the successful application of linkage analysis to schizophrenia. However, we have also seen that this disorder can occur in large pedigrees with multiple affected members, and these may be segregating single disease genes with more regular modes of transmission. These loaded families are atypical, and the resulting Mendelian appearance can be misleading (Sturt & McGuffin 1985), but no bias with respect to detection of linkage should be introduced (Ott 1991).

Broadly, there are two approaches to searching for major genes conferring liability to schizophrenia. The first is to try to focus on a specific region or locus which appears promising. Several clues, such as cytogenetic abnormalities or other genetic disorders co-occurring with schizophrenia, as well as targeting genes which are a priori good candidates (i.e. search for proteins which might plausibly be involved in aetiology), have been followed up by investigators and these will be described later. However, the issue of whether or not major genes for schizophrenia exist within these families may only be resolved following a second approach, which is to perform a systematic screening of the entire genome in a large sample of multiply affected families. Because the genome spans a genetic distance of approximately 3000 cM and each DNA marker should be informative for 10 cM either side of itself, most genome screens use a total of 300 markers evenly spaced throughout the genome. Although an enormous undertaking, this is a common study design. Studies using 3000 markers, for a resolution of 1 cM, have also been undertaken. The development of maps of highly informative SSR markers throughout the genome and the use of automated PCR technology now makes this entirely possible (Dib et al. 1996).

The possibility of genome-wide searches for linkage disequilibrium has been proposed in the past (McGuffin et al. 1992) but this has usually been dismissed as unfeasible. Recent advances encourage greater optimism; testing every gene in the genome for association may ultimately be more practical than a linkage approach (Risch & Merikangas 1996). For example, a locus with genotype relative risk (GRR) of 1.5 would require 950–2200 trios (parents and one affected child) or 500–900 sib pairs for detection, compared with a sample size of 18 000–68 000 families required to detect linkage. However, not every gene in the genome is yet known or characterized, so this approach is not yet practicable. High-density high-throughput mapping may be available soon using methods that detect single nucleotide polymorphisms on microarrays. Other methods using DNA pooling are already being employed in attempts to screen whole chromosomes for linkage disequilibrium with complex traits (Fisher et al. 1999; Hill et al. 1999). The most im-

portant realization is that, even for allelic association studies, the necessary sample sizes are far larger than has previously been thought.

Linkage studies in schizophrenia

Early linkage studies, before DNA markers became available, used classical markers. Studies with HLA showed promise when a maximum LOD score of 2.57 was obtained at a recombination fraction of 0.15 between a broadly defined phenotype 'schizotaxia' (similar to Kety's schizophrenia spectrum disease) and HLA (Turner 1979). The analysis assumed an autosomal dominant mode of transmission. However, these findings were not replicated by a further four linkage studies and a 'model free' sib-pair analysis which showed substantial evidence against linkage. Studies with other classical markers have not provided evidence of linkage. Such early attempts must now, with hindsight, be viewed as optimistic. Indeed, taken together the linkage results using classical markers could at best scan about 6% of the genome (McGuffin & Sturt 1986; Owen & McGuffin 1991).

The major change that occurred in the 1980s and 1990s was the discovery of a new generations of DNA markers and the construction of more detailed and complete linkage maps. There have subsequently been many studies using DNA markers. Indeed, linkage analysis has, over the past decade and a half, been one of the most intensive areas of research in schizophrenia. Despite the high volume of activity, discerning a signal or signals among the noise has proven very difficult (Riley & McGuffin 2000). Here we review the findings in the main regions of interest which have been implicated in more than one study.

Chromosome 5

The segregation of a chromosomal abnormality such as a translocation or deletion with the disorder may provide clues to the localization of disease genes. This is because the altered segment of chromosome may contain a disrupted gene (the disruption of which is pathogenic) or because the disease gene is nearby and in linkage with the chromosomal lesion. In 1988, Bassett et al. reported a Canadian family of oriental origin in which a young man who was schizophrenic and his schizophrenic uncle both had a partial trisomy of the long (q) arm of chromosome 5 resulting from an unbalanced translocation. In one of the first linkage studies of schizophrenia ever undertaken, data from seven families of UK and Icelandic origin gave a LOD of 6.49 using a very broad definition at marker p105–599Ha on chromosome 5q11–q13 (Sherrington et al. 1988). Numerous replication studies failed to support this finding and a combined reanalysis of published data effectively ruled out straightforward linkage heterogeneity (Aschauer et al. 1990; Crowe et al. 1991; Campion et al. 1992a). Follow-up and reanalysis of the original 'linked' pedigrees, using more informative markers, have confirmed that the original results were falsely positive (Kalsi et al. 1999).

Errors can be easily introduced by mistyping individuals, transferring incorrect genotype data onto computer files and lack of strict blindness between investigators carrying out marker analysis and those making clinical diagnosis. There are many other problems which beset the study of complex disorders such as unknown mode of inheritance, late age of onset and variable expressivity and uncertainties in diagnosis. To overcome these problems, multiple tests using a range of parameters are often employed. In the study of Sherrington *et al.* this process may have acted to falsely inflate the LOD score, although it has been suggested that this alone could not have generated LOD scores of the size observed (McGuffin *et al.* 1990; J. Ott, personal communication).

Two groups have subsequently found suggestive evidence of linkage on chromosome 5q22–q31 in a region that appears distinct from either of those in the earlier study. Data from the western Irish sample gave an HLOD of 3.04 in this region (Straub *et al.* 1997b). Results were positive (although of variable magnitude) across the entire set of 14 markers spanning 45 cM of this region. Markers in the same region gave positive results first in a sample of 14 families from Germany, with a LOD of 1.8, and then in a sample of 44 families from Germany and Israel (including four from the first sample), with a marker 2 cM away, also with a LOD of 1.8. This value dropped to 1.27 when the four families common to both samples were removed. Sib pair analyses of the 44 family sample gave evidence for excess allele sharing across a region of 8 cM from D5S666 to D5S658 which includes the markers IL9 and D5S393. Excess allele sharing peaked at 61.5% ($P < 0.005$) for marker D5S399 (Schwab *et al.* 1997). The second multicentre collaborative study did not find additional support for this region (Levinson *et al.* 2000).

Chromosome 22q

Several reports from independent samples initially suggested that loci at chromosome 22q12–q13.1 might be linked to susceptibility to schizophrenia, with the result that this small chromosome has been one of the most intensively studied for putative schizophrenia susceptibility genes. Early results in a genome screen of families from the USA gave a LOD of 1.54 for 22q13, which increased to 2.82 after maximizing the LOD score over several parameters (Pulver *et al.* 1994b). The strongest results came from allele sharing analysis and gave a *P*-value of 0.009 (Lasseter *et al.* 1995). In an independent sample of US families, first round genome screen data produced a LOD of 1.45 and further analyses of these families with a dense map of markers across the region yielded a LOD of 2.09 (Coon *et al.* 1994).

A collaboration involving four centres, and containing 256 pedigrees from Europe and the USA, examined three loci on 22q12–q13 and found negative LODs across this set, both in the total and the individual samples (Pulver *et al.* 1994a). A large collaborative study using non-parametric analysis on the combined samples of 11 different groups found 252 alleles shared vs. 188 not shared ($\chi^2 = 9.31$, $P = 0.001$) at one locus in the 292 complete sib pairs available (Gill *et al.* 1996). However, using

the relationship between excess proportion of alleles shared IBD and the parameters of a single locus model (Suarez *et al.* 1978), the authors conclude that it is likely to be responsible for no more than 2% of the total variance in liability for schizophrenia. Further reports, split evenly between positive and negative results for the region, have continued to appear, both direct replication attempts and data from other genome screens (Kalsi *et al.* 1995a; Vallada *et al.* 1995; Riley *et al.* 1996a; Straub *et al.* 1997a; Hallmayer *et al.* 1998; Levinson *et al.* 1998; Shaw *et al.* 1998).

Velocardiofacial syndrome (VCFS, including DiGeorge's syndrome) is associated with haploinsufficiency of genes at chromosome 22q11 because of submicroscopic deletions (Kelly *et al.* 1993), and it was noted that early linkage results for schizophrenia were near this region (Pulver *et al.* 1994b). Ten per cent of VCFS patients present with a psychotic phenotype (Shprintzen *et al.* 1992). This region also contains the gene for catechol-O-methyl transferase (*COMT*) located at 22q11, which has been suggested (Dunham *et al.* 1992) to be involved in the psychiatric symptoms observed in VCFS, and which is known to be functionally as well as genetically polymorphic (Weinshilboum & Raymond 1977). In studies of VCFS patients, rates of schizophrenia or schizoaffective disorder from 25% to 29% have been found (Pulver *et al.* 1994c; Murphy & Owen 1997). Numerous studies of polymorphisms in this gene have been performed with mixed results. Although most studies of the *COMT* gene have tested for association with the low activity allele, a recent report suggests that the high activity allele, through its increased capacity for the catabolism of dopamine and specifically via this increased catabolism in the prefrontal cortex, may slightly increase the risk of schizophrenia (Egan *et al.* 2001).

Chromosome 8p

Data from one of the two studies which first suggested linkage to chromosome 22q also showed very significant excess allele sharing and small positive LOD scores on chromosome 8p22–p21 (Pulver *et al.* 1995). Across a region of 10 cM containing six markers, affected sib-pair analysis gave *P*-values of between 0.00004 and 0.0097. Parametric analysis yielded LOD scores between 2.2 and 2.35, depending on the model in affected pedigree members only. The Schizophrenia Linkage Collaborative Group study found an HLOD of 2.22 in the independent samples only, and 3.06 when the original families were included (Levinson *et al.* 1996). Allele sharing was higher in the original families alone at 70.4% shared (multipoint maximum likelihood score (MLS) = 2.90, $P = 0.0002$) than in the replication samples (54.1%, MLS = 1.58, $P = 0.005$) or the combined data (55.3%, MLS = 2.73, $P = 0.0003$). This analysis method is similar to the NPL test, but is an earlier version (Kruglyak & Lander 1995). Preliminary data from a denser map of markers in the original sample showed an HLOD of 5.12 with 58% of families linked and an NPL of 3.73, $P = 0.00014$, close to the end of the original region of interest in this sample (Dombroski *et al.* 1997). Data from an independent sample gave a LOD of 3.49, but this decreased to 2.13 in a multipoint analysis (Brzustowicz *et al.* 1999).

Chromosome 6p

Analyses of a 265 family cohort from western Ireland found a maximum HLOD score of 3.51 with 15% of families linked (Straub *et al.* 1995). To date, six independent reports of analyses of this region of 6p have been published. Three of these (Gurling *et al.* 1995; Mowry *et al.* 1995; Riley *et al.* 1996b) found strongly negative LOD scores in the region which become very weakly positive only at large values of Θ, and three (Antonarakis *et al.* 1995; Moises *et al.* 1995; Schwab *et al.* 1995) supported the original finding. The Schizophrenia Linkage Collaborative Group study, which contained data from most of the samples above, examined the region 6p24–p22 and found some support for a susceptibility locus in this region. Across the set of markers tested, allele sharing (again using the multipoint maximum likelihood method) of 55.9% and an MLS of 2.19, $P = 0.001$, was found at in the replication sample only, and MLS = 2.68, $P = 0.0004$ in the replication sample plus the Irish families (Levinson *et al.* 1996). It is also of interest to note that eye tracking dysfunction, a widely used secondary phenotype for schizophrenia, has been mapped to chromosome 6p although at a fairly large distance (approximately 30 cM) from the peak in the Irish data (Arolt *et al.* 1996).

McGuffin and Sturt (1986) reviewed linkage and association results from the 'premolecular' era of classical genetic markers. The most consistent result was an association with the histocompatibilty allele *HLA-A9*, found in seven out of nine studies, but this finding was complicated in a number of ways. Positive results were found only for paranoid subtypes of schizophrenia and there was no overall support from linkage studies (McGuffin *et al.* 1983). Recent studies, while not ruling out a role for HLA, have tended to focus on other components of the HLA complex and on potential mediating mechanisms such as susceptibility to viral infections *in utero* (Wright *et al.* 1998). The findings are nevertheless of some interest in view of the results on chromosome 6p.

Chromosome 10p

Another independent genome screen of 43 US families of European descent gave suggestive evidence on chromosome 10p15–q21 (Faraone *et al.* 1998). Across a set of nine markers, NPL scores were consistently above 2.0 (P-values < 0.03), with a peak of 3.36 ($P = 0.0004$). Data from the western Irish (Straub *et al.* 1998) and German and Israeli (Schwab *et al.* 1998) samples supported linkage of schizophrenia to this same region. These results were unusual and particularly exciting because of the close agreement in location shown by different samples using different diagnostic and analytical approaches. A second multicentre collaborative study found rather modest support for linkage to this region with significant evidence for heterogeneity between samples (Levinson *et al.* 2000).

Chromosome 6q

A sample of 53 US families of mixed ethnicity containing a total of 81 affected sib pairs provided evidence for a susceptibility locus on chromosome 6q21–q22.3 (Cao *et al.* 1997). This study is unique in that a second independent sample of families held by the same researchers was used to replicate the finding internally. In the first sample, excess allele sharing among affected siblings at one locus was 69% IBD sharing ($P = 0.00024$). In the replication data set, 69 families containing 109 affected sib pairs gave maximum IBD allele sharing between 62% ($P = 0.0009$) and 64% ($P = 0.0004$) across a set of three markers. A total of seven markers spanning approximately 3.5 cM gave sharing between 55% and 65%, and P-values < 0.04. A follow-up study by the same group found positive but less significant maxima using a third independent sample, with 62% IBD sharing ($P = 0.022$) (Martinez *et al.* 1999). Combining the data from both replication samples, the interval between two of the markers used previously gave a LOD of 3.82 and IBD sharing of 63.8% ($P = 0.000014$). Data from the African American pedigrees in the National Institute of Mental Health/Millenium schizophrenia genome screen also provided support for these findings (Kaufmann *et al.* 1998). The second multicentre collaborative study found support for linkage to this region with empirical P-values of < 0.002 with the original sample included and 0.004 without it, again with significant evidence for heterogeneity between samples (Levinson *et al.* 2000). A recent study found further evidence for linkage in this region in a very large Swedish pedigree (Lindholm *et al.* 2001).

Chromosome 13q

Data from a mixed sample of 11 UK and two Japanese families initially suggested the possibility of a schizophrenia susceptibility locus on chromosome 13q14.1–q32 (Lin *et al.* 1995), already an area of interest because of the presence of the 5-HT$_{2A}$ receptor gene (Williams *et al.* 1997). Preliminary data from two other groups gave some initial support (Antonarakis *et al.* 1996; Kalsi *et al.* 1996). A further study by the original group using an independent sample of 34 Taiwanese and 10 UK families yielded negative LOD sores over most of the region, except for a single marker which gave a LOD of 1.06 (Lin *et al.* 1997). However, when data from both samples were combined and families of European and Asian origin were analysed separately, the European pedigrees gave an HLOD of 1.41 at one locus with 100% of families suggesting involvement and 1.54 at a second 30% of families linked. A multipoint model free (MFLOD) analysis (Curtis & Sham 1995) of the European sample yielded a LOD of 2.58 around two markers located at 13q32. Positive scores were found around these two markers, but they were separated by a region where the values of both statistics dropped almost to zero. Other studies have been mixed, with two supporting this region (Blouin *et al.* 1998; Shaw *et al.* 1998), two giving weak positive results (Straub *et al.* 1997a; Riley *et al.* 1998) and two giving negative data (Jensen *et al.* 1998; Barden *et al.* 1999). Recently, three point analyses using pairs of adjacent markers in a sample of 21 narrowly defined Canadian pedigrees gave an HLOD of 4.42 with 65% of families linked at marker D13S793 (Brzustowicz *et al.* 1999). The second multicentre collaborative study did not find additional support for this region (Levinson *et al.* 2000).

Chromosome 15q13–q14

The first evidence for a possible chromosome 15 schizophrenia susceptibility locus was the report of linkage of the p50 sensory gating deficit (an evoked potential abnormality which is common in schizophrenics and relatively rare in controls, and which segregates as a single gene trait in families) to chromosome 15q13–q14 (Freedman *et al.* 1997). In nine US families, a marker within the α7 nicotinic cholinergic receptor subunit gene (*CHRNA7*) gave a LOD of 5.3 when tested against the sensory gating phenotype, and 1.33 when tested against schizophrenia. This gene is an attractive candidate because of the high incidence of smoking in schizophrenics (De Leon *et al.* 1995), because both nicotine (Adler *et al.* 1993) and clozapine (Nagamoto *et al.* 1996) ameliorate the sensory gating deficit, and because the secondary phenotype common in schizophrenics is strongly linked to this region.

Data from South African Bantu families in a dense map of markers at 1 cM intervals around this gene showed some evidence in support of this finding, with positive NPL results across the entire map (Riley *et al.* 2000). Analyses by the original group in an independent sample showed 58% IBD allele sharing (*P* < 0.0024) at D15S1360 (Leonard *et al.* 1998). Two studies have failed to find any evidence for involvement of this locus in five families from eastern Canada (Neves-Pereira *et al.* 1998) and 54 families from the Maryland sample (Curtis *et al.* 1999).

Chromosome 18

Initial interest in chromosome 18 began with several reports of the co-occurrence of psychiatric disorders and chromosomal anomalies (Bassett 1992; Calzolari *et al.* 1996; Mors *et al.* 1997), and was strengthened by the initial report of linkage between this chromosome and bipolar disorder (BP) (Berrettini *et al.* 1997). Data from chromosome 18 in schizophrenic families comes partly from the inclusion of data from all chromosomes in whole genome screens, and partly from replication attempts, because of the possible overlap between BP and schizophrenia. Two initial replication attempts following the putative BP linkage gave no evidence of linkage between schizophrenia and chromosome 18 (DeLisi *et al.* 1995; Fang *et al.* 1995). In contrast, data from the families in the German/Israeli sample gave a LOD of 3.1 when both schizophrenics and affective disorder cases were included in the analysis, and using the schizophrenics alone (Wildenauer *et al.* 1997). Transmission disequilibrium studies of the 124 base pair (bp) allele in a polymorphism in the α subunit gene of the olfactory G-protein (GOLF) showed 41 transmitted and 13 non-transmitted (*P* = 0.0007) considering

schizophrenia and schizoaffective disorder, and 45 transmitted and 13 non-transmitted (*P* = 0.00012) when the affective disorder cases were included.

Chromosome 1q

Interest in chromosome 1 in schizophrenia began with reports of a balanced 1:11 translocation segregating with serious mental illness in a large pedigree from Scotland (St Clair *et al.* 1990), although this region was not studied in the same intensive manner as the region around the chromosome 11 breakpoint, which contains the dopamine D_2 receptor gene (*DRD2*). Numerous studies of the chromosome 11 region were undertaken and gave no evidence for linkage in other family samples (Gill *et al.* 1993; Su *et al.* 1993; Zhe Wu *et al.* 1993; Kalsi *et al.* 1995c; Mulcrone *et al.* 1995). The chromosome 1 breakpoint lies at 1q42.1, and two groups had reported preliminary suggestive linkage findings in this region. A three-stage genome screen of a population isolate from Finland gave a LOD of 3.82 in this region in the dense-mapping third stage of the genome screen (Hovatta *et al.* 1999). Another sample also gave some preliminary evidence for this region, with an NPLZ of 1.39, *P* = 0.084, at D1S304 (1q44) (Blouin *et al.* 1998). Recently, two genes directly disrupted by the translocation were cloned (Millar *et al.* 2000a,b) although their function remains to be described in detail. It seems likely that the effect of the translocation, and the disruption of surrounding genes, is specific to this large pedigree and not a common susceptibility factor in schizophrenia, but the characterization of the disrupted genes may identify sequences or gene families relevant to more common psychoses, and the linkage evidence may suggest other variants in these genes which predispose to schizophrenia. In one of the most significant reported findings ever seen in linkage studies of schizophrenia, a third group found a LOD score of 5.79 in a different region at chromosome 1q22 (Brzustowicz *et al.* 2000).

X chromosome

The X chromosome was initially hypothesized as a potential source of genetic liability because of the well-documented differences between the sexes for various aspects of schizophrenia, including higher concordance in same sex twin pairs, age of onset (which is generally lower in males) and the greater risk if a female, rather than a male, relative is affected (reviewed by Crow 1988). A pseudoautosomal locus for a schizophrenia susceptibility gene that would account for these differences was suggested (Crow *et al.* 1989). An early study using sib-pair analysis reported evidence of excess sharing at DXYS14 (Collinge *et al.* 1991), which was supported in one non-parametric replication (D'Amato *et al.* 1992), but was not supported by a number of other studies using both parametric and non-parametric analyses (Asherson *et al.* 1992; Wang *et al.* 1993; Barr *et al.* 1994; Crow *et al.* 1994; Kalsi *et al.* 1995b; Maier *et al.* 1995).

A large collaborative study examining markers within band

Xp11 near the *MAO* loci found a LOD of 1.97 under a dominant model for DXS7 in a set of 92 sib pairs selected for maternal inheritance. In a second analysis, 34 families not selected for inheritance pattern gave a LOD of 2.16 at *MAOB* under a dominant model (Dann *et al.* 1997). Results from a number of recent genome screens have suggested a possible X chromosome locus, but these results are of weaker magnitude than the most positive loci in these studies (Paterson *et al.* 1999).

Other chromosomal regions

Other reports have implicated numerous other chromosomes: chromosome 2, based on a balanced 2:18 translocation (Maziade *et al.* 1993) and supported by some linkage evidence (Aschauer *et al.* 1993; Coon *et al.* 1998; Levinson *et al.* 1998; Shaw *et al.* 1998), although this was spread over an enormous region of approximately 100 cM of chromosome 2, from 2p22–q21; chromosome 4 (Kaufmann *et al.* 1998; Hovatta *et al.* 1999); chromosome 5p (Silverman *et al.* 1996; Garver *et al.* 1998); chromosome 7 (Blouin *et al.* 1998); chromosome 9, in two different locations, one centromeric (Moises *et al.* 1995; Levinson *et al.* 1998; Hovatta *et al.* 1999), and one at the telomere of the p-arm (Riley *et al.* 1997; Kaufmann *et al.* 1998).

Overall, the collected data from linkage studies of schizophrenia are not in good agreement about the involvement of any region. This is likely to be a result of the small GRR associated with any individual gene contributing to susceptibility to schizophrenia. The numbers of families required to detect linkage vs. association depend strongly on both the GRR and the population frequency of the risk allele, which is likely to be relatively high for schizophrenia susceptibility loci (Risch & Merikangas 1996). If GRR for a particular genotype is 4 and the allele frequency in the population is between 10% and 50%, then the number of families required is roughly 200–300, a large but just about practical sample size. However, if the GRR is 2 (and the frequency is in the same range) then the number of families increases to 2500–5400. If the GRR drops to 1.5, the number of families increases to 18 000–68 000, which is clearly not practical. GRR can be converted into the relative risk measure most widely used currently: λ_s (Scott *et al.* 1997). If GRR is < 2, λ_s is < 1.3. The data for schizophrenia are most compatible with several genes all having λ_s less than 2 (Risch 1990), and the sample sizes currently held appear to be inadequate to generate unequivocal results.

Results are also often of lesser magnitude when new data are added to the sample, as in the collaborative replication study of chromosomes 3, 6 and 8 (Levinson *et al.* 1996). The simplest interpretation of these differences is random variation in the inputs to the disease found in any given sample. Simulation studies suggest that in a polygenic disease, initial positive findings may be difficult to replicate, and require much larger samples than the original, because detection of linkage with any one of several susceptibility loci is always more probable than replication of just one specific locus (Suarez *et al.* 1995).

It has become clear over the last 10 years that mutations in the coding sequence of genes are not the only way to produce illness. Much of what we currently know about complex trait genetics comes from the study of insulin-dependent diabetes mellitus (IDDM). In genome-wide studies, affected sib pairs share alleles IBD significantly more often than expected by chance at numerous loci. After the HLA region on chromosome 6 (responsible for the autoimmune destruction of the pancreatic β cells), the locus with the greatest degree of excess sharing was the insulin gene on chromosome 11 (Davies *et al.* 1994). This locus had long shown association with IDDM (Bell *et al.* 1984) but had been excluded from linkage using parametric analysis (Hitman *et al.* 1985; Ferns *et al.* 1986; Elbein *et al.* 1988; Donald *et al.* 1989). Further, the effect at the insulin gene is now known to be a quantitative one. A VNTR polymorphism lies between the promoter and the start of the first exon (Bell *et al.* 1982), and IDDM susceptibility at this locus is determined by this VNTR (Bennett *et al.* 1995). Transcription of the insulin gene (and thus insulin expression) is regulated by alleles of this VNTR (Kennedy *et al.* 1995), and *all* alleles of this variable DNA region are within the range of normal variation.

Association studies

While linkage analysis enables the detection of genes of major effect, it will not detect genes of small effect contributing in an additive or interactive way with other genes or with genes plus environment. However, genes of minor effect have been successfully isolated in a number of other complex genetic disorders, such as the transforming growth factor α (TGF-α) gene in cleft lip and palate (Holder *et al.* 1992), the glucokinase and glycogen synthase genes in NIDDM (Chiu *et al.* 1993) and IDDM (Bell *et al.* 1984) and the myelin basic protein gene in multiple sclerosis (Tienari *et al.* 1992), using association methods.

Association studies in schizophrenia using DNA markers have unfortunately thrown up a number of contradictory results. This has been in part because of the problems of diagnosis and the question of comparability of patient populations from different centres. However, the major confounding factor in these studies is the selection of controls which can result in so-called stratification effects. The problem is that there may be a section of the population in which a particular marker and a certain disorder are common without there being any causal relationship. For example, HLA BW16 is more common in Ashkenazi Jews, so that an excess of Jewish patients in an affected sample could lead to the false conclusion that an association exists between the disorder and that antigen. A recent solution to this problem is to compare the frequencies of the parental alleles not inherited by an affected individual with the alleles that are inherited, thus providing a perfectly matched internal control in the *transmission disequilibrium test* (TDT) (Falk & Rubinstein 1987). The samples for this approach are, however, less easy to collect than those for traditional association studies.

Another problem is the statistical handling of results. Because the prior probability of obtaining a true association is extremely remote, the conventional level of statistical significance ($P < 0.05$) is probably not sufficiently stringent. In addition, account must be made of the use of multiple markers in these studies. A conservative correction is to multiply the obtained P-value by the number of markers tested.

The task of carrying out a systematic search for association throughout the entire genome would involve the use of a very large series of markers, each showing linkage disequilibrium with its neighbours. While this is at present an impossibly large amount of work, it is likely to become increasingly feasible as automated technology is developed. For the moment, the best strategy is probably to focus upon markers that are close to or within candidate genes.

An alternative to the use of DNA markers resulting from variations in non-coding sequences in the vicinity of candidate genes is the study of sequence *variations that affect protein structure or expression* (VAPSEs) (Sobell *et al.* 1992) and to look for these gene mutations directly among schizophrenic probands. This has the advantage that a VAPSE disease association is not affected by recombination and directly identifies the pathogenic mutation. On the other hand, if the VAPSE is not the pathogenic mutation itself, it may well be very close to a mutation within the same gene that is pathogenic or in linkage disequilibrium with a mutation in a nearby gene. The problem here is that we understand little about the pathophysiology of schizophrenia and plausible candidate genes are few and far between.

Association studies in schizophrenia

Early association studies in schizophrenia used classical markers such as the ABO and other blood groups and the HLA system. The results of these studies are inconsistent but when considered overall no clear evidence for association has been found (McGuffin & Sturt 1986). The main reasons for this, multiple testing and stratification, are discussed above.

An interesting finding was of association between a subtype of schizophrenia (paranoid schizophrenia) and HLA A9 in seven out of nine studies. Combining the data and applying a correction for multiple testing gave a P-value of 0.0003 (McGuffin & Sturt 1986). However, several conflicting findings have been found. Two groups found A9 to be decreased in paranoid schizophrenia compared with controls (Miyanaga *et al.* 1984; Rudduck 1984), while others using samples from the same countries found A9 to be increased (Eberhard *et al.* 1975; Asaka *et al.* 1981). A9 consists of two subspecificities: AW23 and AW24. Two studies suggested an association with AW23 (Crowe *et al.* 1979; Asaka *et al.* 1981), while others found a stronger relationship with AW24 (Ivanyi *et al.* 1983). More recently, a study found no association between paranoid schizophrenia and either AW23 or AW24 (Alexander *et al.* 1990). Another recent study of 33 pedigrees collected in France failed to find evidence of linkage between HLA and the schizophrenic phenotype (Campion *et al.* 1992b). In addition, they performed an association study using pooled data from six independent studies and were unable to show a significant excess of HLA A9 in the affected group, but they did not subdivide their sample into paranoid vs. hebephrenic subforms.

Disturbances in dopamine neurotransmission and dopamine receptors have long been postulated to underlie schizophrenia and genes coding for dopamine receptors have been targeted as candidates. Until recently, two types of dopamine receptor had been identified, known as D_1 and D_2, which differ from each other functionally, with D_1 suppressing adenylate cyclase and D_2 stimulating adenylate cyclase. However, recent work in this field has identified a further three dopamine receptor genes known as D_3, D_4 and D_5 (Sunahara *et al.* 1990; Van Tol *et al.* 1991; Sokoloff *et al.* 1992). D_3 and D_4 have a similar structure to D_2 and bind D_2-selective ligands, while D_5 is similar in structure to D_1. It was thought that the therapeutic effects of antipsychotic drugs are related to their high affinity for D_2 receptors, and this view has been revised to include D_3 and D_4.

The D_3 receptor may be of particular interest because its expression is restricted to limbic regions implicated in schizophrenia. Furthermore, expression of D_3 in brain is, unlike D_1 and D_2, increased by both typical and atypical neuroleptics (Buckland *et al.* 1993; see below). The gene for this receptor has been localized to the long arm of chromosome 3 (Le Coniat *et al.* 1991) and contains a polymorphic site in its coding region which gives rise to a glycine to serine substitution and results in a restriction site for the enzyme BalI (Lannfelt *et al.* 1992). Study of this polymorphism is an example of the VAPSE approach in a candidate gene.

Initially, two independent groups from Wales and France carried out studies of this polymorphism in the dopamine D_3-receptor gene in samples of patients with DSM-IIIR schizophrenia and normal controls (Crocq *et al.* 1992). In both studies, more patients than controls were homozygotes of either type ($P = 0.005$, $P = 0.008$). Pooling of the data gave a highly significant result ($P = 0.0001$) with a relative risk of schizophrenia in homozygotes of 2.61 (95% confidence intervals 1.60–4.26). There have subsequently been many attempts to replicate this finding with variable and, to an extent, controversial results. There is little doubt that some of the 'negative' studies (in common with many allegedly negative association results) have simply not had enough power to detect the originally reported effect. Williams *et al.* (1998) have performed a meta-analysis of over 30 case–control studies and observed an odds ratio of 1.21 for the association between schizophrenia and homozygosity at the BalI D_3 polymorphism, which, although a smaller effect than that originally reported, was highly significant. There was no evidence of publishing bias (preferential publishing of positive results). The same authors also undertook a family-based association analysis using TDT, which guards against spurious positive results arising from recently mixed populations, a phenomenon called population stratification (McGuffin *et al.* 1994b). The TDT also showed a significant excess of homozygotes among schizophrenics.

Another potentially interesting candidate gene is the serotonin receptor 5-HT$_{2A}$ gene. The 5-HT$_{2A}$ receptor is one of the sites of action of 'atypical' neuroleptics and a multicentre

European study (Williams *et al.* 1996) found a significant excess of the 2 allele of a polymorphism 5-HT$_{2A}$ T102C in the first exon or coding region of the gene among schizophrenics compared with controls. Again, other groups reported both replications and failure to replicate. Williams *et al.* (1997) performed a meta-analysis combining the findings on nearly 200 patients and a similar number of controls. The odds ratio once more turned out to be small but the result was of a highly significant association and no suggestion of distortion by publication bias.

Numerous other candidate genes, based either on biochemistry or location near linkage signals, have been investigated for allele or genotype association with schizophrenia. Many of these have had an initial report of association with no positive replications. For example, porphobilinogen deaminase (*PBGD*) was of interest briefly because of its location on chromosome 11. Several polymorphisms were identified within this gene, and an initial report (Sanders *et al.* 1993) suggested strong association between schizophrenia and one of these markers. In seeking to replicate this finding, Owen *et al.* (1992) found no evidence for allelic association between the PBGD gene and schizophrenia.

Phospholipase A2 (*PLA2*) is a key enzyme in the metabolism of phospholipids. PLA2 is enriched in neuronal membranes and has an essential role in the functioning of membrane structures in the brain. A disordered phospholipid metabolism has been postulated in schizophrenia (Gattaz *et al.* 1990), and there is evidence for increased PLA2 activity in schizophrenic cases (Noponen *et al.* 1993; Gattaz *et al.* 1995). Two reports show association between marker alleles in this gene and schizophrenia (Hudson *et al.* 1996; Peet *et al.* 1998), while three do not (Price *et al.* 1997; Strauss *et al.* 1999; Frieboes *et al.* 2001).

Markers in the *NOTCH4* gene, located on chromosome 6p in the major histocompatibility (MHC) region, gave a *P*-value of 0.000036 for a single marker and 0.0000078 for a two-marker haplotype in a recent report (Wei & Hemmings 2000). This level of significance suggests an odds ratio of 2.7 conferred by the associated alleles, which would correspond to a large population-attributable risk, and a major locus for schizophrenia susceptibility (Sklar *et al.* 2001). Replication studies of this locus in three independent family samples and a case–control sample of diverse ethnic origin (Sklar *et al.* 2001), a Scottish population-based case–control sample (McGinnis *et al.* 2001) and a Japanese case–control sample (Ujike *et al.* 2001) failed to show any evidence for the association.

Earlier we discussed the controversy surrounding the idea that anticipation occurs in schizophrenia and mentioned that in several other diseases involving the nervous system that are more simply transmitted via single genes the phenomenon of anticipation is now known to have a molecular basis. This is the result of unstable or dynamic mutations involving trinucleotide repeat sequences that can increase in length over generations. Examples include Huntington's disease, mytonic dystrophy and fragile X mental retardation. Could such mechanisms also occur in more complex polygenic or oligogenic systems such as those involved in schizophrenia? *Repeat expansion detection* (RED) analysis allows a search for trinucleotide expansion occurring

anywhere in the genome and, applied to schizophrenia, has provided evidence of larger repeats *somewhere* in the genomes of schizophrenics than controls (Schalling *et al.* 1993). Where that *somewhere* might be is still unknown but one candidate is a gene that codes for a calcium gated ion channel called *hKCa3* (Bowen *et al.* 1998). There is some evidence that long trinucleotide repeats in *hKCa3* are particularly associated with negative symptoms of schizophrenia (Cardno *et al.* 1999b).

Molecular neurobiology

Molecular techniques have also resulted in major advances to our understanding of neurobiology, much of which may be of relevance in schizophrenia. For example, the cloning of five separate dopamine receptor genes along with genes coding for enzymes and other proteins involved in dopaminergic transmission has opened up new approaches to examining hypotheses involving the dopamine system.

The expression of these genes can be studied in animals exposed to antipsychotic drugs in order to examine the mechanisms involved in their therapeutic action. Buckland *et al.* (1993) have studied the effect in rat brain of chronic treatment (32 days) with the 'atypical' antipsychotics sulpiride and clozapine. They demonstrated that dopamine D$_3$ receptor messenger ribonucleic acid (mRNA) levels increased by fourfold, whereas no effect was observed on the mRNA levels encoding D$_1$ or D$_2$ receptors, or tyrosine hydroxylase. They postulate that D$_3$ receptor mRNA may be associated with the therapeutic action of antipsychotic drugs. These results contrast with other studies which have shown increases in both D$_2$ and D$_3$ mRNA with 'typical' neuroleptics such as chlorpromazine and haloperidol.

A different approach is to look for variations within these genes that may be associated with drug responsiveness. Of recent interest has been the drug clozapine, which is widely reported to reduce symptoms of schizophrenia that are unresponsive to other antipsychotic medication (McKenna & Bailey 1993). However, some patients remain unresponsive to clozapine and it has been suggested that response to this drug may be related to variation of the D$_4$ receptor. This view arises from the observations that clozapine has a particularly high affinity for D$_4$ receptors and that the D$_4$ receptor shows a high degree of variation (Van Tol *et al.* 1992). Clozapine and other 'atypical' antipsychotics also tend to show a high affinity for 5-HT$_{2A}$ receptors and it is of interest that treatment response may be predicted by genetic profiling, i.e. genotyping patients over a number of polymorphisms in genes encoding serotonergic and dopaminergic receptors (Arranz *et al.* 2000).

Genetic counselling

At present, it is not possible to determine the specific risk that a particular individual will develop schizophrenia. Because of the complex mode of inheritance and variable expressivity of the disorder, the only reasonable information to provide to relatives regarding recurrence risks of the disorder in other family members is based upon the empirical data from family studies. Probably the most useful figures are those provided by Gottesman (1991) based upon a compilation of results from many Western European studies (see Table 14.1). Despite this there is a definite role for counselling based upon an informed and responsible approach (McGuffin *et al*. 1994a).

There is now considerable experience in genetic counselling and the principal approaches are the same regardless of the disorder in question. Most counsellors take a non-directive educational approach (Harper *et al*. 1988). The aim is to impart accurate information and help the counsellee to fully understand the risks and potential burdens so that they can make an informed decision. It is important to emphasize that it is the counsellee who must make the ultimate decisions.

Most of those who seek counselling are concerned about the potential risks to their children or, if they are an unaffected relative, about their own chances of developing the disorder. At present the only information that is useful to impart comes from empirical sources (i.e. family, twin and adoption studies). For example, a couple planning a family, one of whom has a parent with schizophrenia, would be informed that the average risk to each of their children is about 3% or three times that in the general population. In some rare cases the counsellee may come from a family which has multiple affected members and gives the appearance of Mendelian transmission. However, in our current state of knowledge it would be wrong to assume that this is the case because these loaded families would also be expected to exist as a result of multifactorial/polygenic inheritance. In these families the risks to relatives appear to increase in relation to the number of affected family members and decrease in relation to the number of well family members (Gottesman 1991).

Empirical data also tell us that schizophrenia is in most, if not all, cases, a complex disease with both inherited and non-inherited causative factors. In schizophrenia the nature of these non-inherited factors remains controversial (McGuffin *et al*. 1995) and some, such as exposure of the fetus to viral infections, are not easily avoided. On the other hand, it would be useful to advise relatives of patients with schizophrenia to avoid the 'experimental' use of drugs such as LSD, PCP, cocaine and amphetamine, because they may be especially vulnerable to drug-precipitated psychoses as a result of high genetic loading.

In the future, advances in our understanding of the molecular basis of schizophrenia may allow the use of prenatal and presymptomatic testing. The complexity of this disorder suggests that in most cases it will not be possible to attain high levels of predictive certainty, but there may be rare families that show true single gene inheritance and here accurate testing is a realistic possibility. The issues are best exemplified by work with relatives and patients from families with Huntington's disease. Until recently, risk calculations in this disorder relied upon DNA marker testing involving the genotyping of individuals in several generations, although the identification of the disease causing mutation (Huntington's Disease Collaborative Research Group 1993) makes a specific test in individuals possible. Predictive testing is usually carried out in specialist centres with expert counselling. Counsellees are given advice prior to testing to allow them to make an informed decision about the usefulness of such testing. In one series (Tyler *et al*. 1992), out of 238 initial requests for testing, only 40 results were eventually given out as a result of such pretest counselling. We would suggest that if presymptomatic or prenatal testing were possible in schizophrenia, similar principles should be adopted. This would involve skilled counselling, with adequate consideration given to the severity of the disorder, the age of onset, variable expressivity and other aspects of the phenotype. This would allow counsellees to be fully informed before making any final decisions.

Conclusions

Family, twin and adoption studies provide compelling evidence that schizophrenia has an important genetic component and quantitative analyses suggest that most of the variance in liability to the disorder (perhaps 80% or more) is accounted for by genetic factors. However, the pattern of transmission in families is complex and, although some multigeneration pedigrees with a Mendelian-like appearance exist, they are very much the exception rather than the rule. It seems likely that schizophrenia at a molecular level will turn out to be heterogeneous, even though so far attempts to relate clinical heterogeneity to aetiological heterogeneity have failed. This may partly account for the disappointingly inconclusive results of attempts to resolve the mode (or modes) of transmission statistically. However, it now seems that genes of major effect are rare in schizophrenia and that most cases are polygenic (or oligogenic) in origin. Such susceptibility loci are more difficult to detect and localize using molecular genetic approaches and this almost certainly accounts for the current complexity of linkage and association study results. Nevertheless, the detection and identification of susceptibility loci is now becoming increasingly feasible and it seems probable that schizophrenia, like many other common familial disorders, will have a molecular basis that will begin to be understood within the foreseeable future.

References

Adler, L.E., Hoffer, L.D., Wiser, A. & Freedman, R. (1993) Normalization of auditory physiology by cigarette smoking in schizophrenic patients. *American Journal of Psychiatry* 150, 1856–1861.

Alexander, R.C., Coggiano, M., Daniel, D.G. & Wyatt, R.J. (1990) HLA antigens in schizophrenia. *Psychiatry Research* 31, 221–233.

Antonarakis, S.E., Blouin, J.-L., Pulver, A.E. *et al*. (1995) Schizophrenia susceptibility and chromosome 6p24–22. *Nature Genetics* 11, 235–236.

Antonarakis, S.E., Blouin, J.L., Curran, M. *et al*. (1996) Linkage and sib-pair analysis reveal a potential schizophrenia susceptibility gene on chromosome 13q32. *American Journal of Human Genetics* 59, A210.

Arolt, V., Lencer, R., Nolte, A. *et al.* (1996) Eye tracking dysfunction is a putative phenotypic susceptibility marker of schizophrenia and maps to a locus on chromosome 6p in families with multiple occurrence of the disease. *American Journal of Medical Genetics and Neuropsychiatric Genetics* 67, 564–579.

Arranz, M.J., Munro, J., Birkett, J. *et al.* (2000) Pharmacogenetic prediction of clozapine response. *Lancet* 355, 1615–1616.

Asaka, A., Okazaki, Y., Namura, I. *et al.* (1981) Study of HLA antigens among Japanese schizophrenics. *British Journal of Psychiatry* 138, 498–500.

Aschauer, H.N., Aschauer-Treiber, G., Isenberg, K.E. *et al.* (1990) No evidence for linkage between choromosome 5 markers and schizophrenia. *Human Heredity* 40, 109–115.

Aschauer, H.N., Fischer, G., Isenberg, K.E. *et al.* (1993) No proof of linkage between schizophrenia-related disorders including schizophrenia and chromosome 2q21 region. *European Archives of Psychiatry and Clinical Neuroscience* 243, 193–198.

Asherson, P., Parfitt, E., Sargeant, M. *et al.* (1992) No evidence for a pseudoautosomal locus for schizophrenia linkage analysis of multiply affected families. *British Journal of Psychiatry* 161, 63–68.

Asherson, P., Walsh, C., Williams, J. *et al.* (1994) Imprinting and anticipation: are they relevant to genetic studies of schizophrenia? *British Journal of Psychiatry* 164, 619–624.

Barden, N., Morissette, J., Blaveri, K. *et al.* (1999) Chromosome 13 workshop report. *American Journal of Medical Genetics and Neuropsychiatric Genetics* 88, 260–262.

Barr, C.L., Kennedy, J.L., Pakstis, A.J. *et al.* (1994) Linkage study of a susceptibility locus for schizophrenia in the pseudoautosomal region. *Schizophrenia Bulletin* 20, 277–286.

Bassett, A.S. (1992) Chromosomal aberrations and schizophrenia: autosomes. *British Journal of Psychiatry* 161, 323–334.

Bassett, A.S. & Honer, W.G. (1994) Evidence for anticipation in schizophrenia. *American Journal of Human Genetics* 54, 864–870.

Bell, G.I., Selby, M. & Rutter, W.J. (1982) The highly polymorphic region near the human insulin gene is composed of simple tandemly repeating sequences. *Nature* 395, 31–35.

Bell, G.I., Horita, S. & Karam, J.H. (1984) A polymorphic locus near the human insulin gene is associated with insulin-dependent diabetes mellitus. *Diabetes* 33, 176–183.

Bennett, S.T., Lucassen, A.M., Gough, S.C.L. *et al.* (1995) Susceptibility to human type I diabetes at IDDM2 is determined by tandem repeat variation at the insulin gene minisatellite locus. *Nature Genetics* 9, 284–292.

Berrettini, W.H., Ferraro, T.N., Goldin, L.R. *et al.* (1997) A linkage study of bipolar illness. *Archives of General Psychiatry* 54, 27–35.

Blouin, J.L., Dombroski, B.A., Nath, S.K. *et al.* (1998) Schizophrenia susceptibility loci on chromosomes 13q32 and 8p21. *Nature Genetics* 20, 70–73.

Bowen, T., Guy, C.A., Craddock, N. *et al.* (1998) Further support for an association between a polymorphic CAG repeat in the *hKCa3* gene and schizophrenia. *Molecular Psychiatry* 3, 266–269.

Brzustowicz, L.M., Honer, W.G., Chow, E.W.C. *et al.* (1999) Linkage of familial schizophrenia to chromosome 13q32. *American Journal of Human Genetics* 65, 1096–1103.

Brzustowicz, L.M., Hodgkinson, K.A., Chow, E.W.C., Honer, W.G. & Bassett, A.S. (2000) Location of a major susceptibility locus for familial schizophrenia on chromosome 1q21–q22. *Science* 288, 678–682.

Buckland, P.R., O'Donovan, M.C. & McGuffin, P. (1993) Clozapine and sulpiride up-regulate dopamine D_3 receptor mRNA levels. *Neuropharmacology* 32, 901–907.

Calzolari, E., Aiello, V., Palazzi, P. *et al.* (1996) Psychiatric disorder in a familial 15; 18 translocation and sublocalization of myelin basic protein to 18q22.3. *American Journal of Medical Genetics and Neuropsychiatric Genetics* 67, 154–161.

Campion, D., D'Amato, T., Laklou, H. *et al.* (1992a) Failure to replicate linkage between chromosome 5q11–q13 markers and schizophrenia in 28 families. *Psychiatry Research* 44, 171–179.

Campion, D., Leboyer, M., Hillaire, D. *et al.* (1992b) Relationship of HLA to schizophrenia not supported in multiplex families. *Psychiatry Research* 41, 99–105.

Cannon, T.D., Kaprio, J., Lonnqvist, J., Huttunen, M. & Koskenvuo, M. (1998) The genetic epidemiology of schizophrenia in a Finnish twin cohort: a population-based modeling study. *Archives of General Psychiatry* 55, 67–74.

Cao, Q., Martinez, M., Zhang, J. *et al.* (1997) Suggestive evidence for a schizophrenia susceptibility locus on chromosome 6q and a confirmation in an independent series of pedigrees. *Genomics* 43, 1–8.

Cardno, A.G. & Gottesman, I.I. (2000) Twin studies of schizophrenia: from bow-and-arrow concordances to Star Wars Mx and functional genomics. *American Journal of Medical Genetics* 97, 12–17.

Cardno, A.G., Marshall, E.J., Cold, B. *et al.* (1999a) Heritability estimates for psychotic disorders: the Maudsley Twin psychosis series. *Archives of General Psychiatry* 56, 162–168.

Cardno, A.G., Bowen, T., Guy, C.A. *et al.* (1999b) CAG repeat length in the *hKCa3* gene and symptom dimensions in schizophrenia. *Biological Psychiatry* 45, 1592–1596.

Carter, C.L. & Chung, C.S. (1980) Segregation analysis of schizophrenia under a mixed genetic model. *Human Heredity* 30, 350–356.

Chiu, K.C., Tanizawa, Y. & Permutt, M.A. (1993) Glucokinase gene variants in the common form of NIDDM. *Diabetes* 42, 579–582.

Chotai, J., Engstrom, C., Ekholm, B. *et al.* (1995) Anticipation in Swedish families with schizophrenia. *Psychiatric Genetics* 5, 181–186.

Clerget-Darpoux, F., Goldin, L.R. & Gershon, E.S. (1986) Clinical methods in psychiatric genetics. III. Environmental stratification may simulate a genetic effect in adoption studies. *Acta Psychiatrica Scandinavica* 74, 305–311.

Collinge, J., DeLisi, L.E., Boccio, A. *et al.* (1991) Evidence for a pseudoautosomal locus for schizophrenia using the method of affected sibling pairs. *British Journal of Psychiatry* 158, 624–629.

Coon, H., Holik, J., Hoff, M. *et al.* (1994) Analysis of chromosome 22 markers in nine schizophrenia pedigrees. *American Journal of Medical Genetics* 54, 72–79.

Coon, H., Myles-Worsley, M., Tiobech, J. *et al.* (1998) Evidence for a chromosome 2p13–14 schizophrenia susceptibility locus in families from Palau, Micronesia. *Molecular Psychiatry* 3, 521–527.

Crocq, M.-A., Mant, R., Asherson, P. *et al.* (1992) Association between schizophrenia and homozygosity at the dopamine D_3 receptor gene. *Journal of Medical Genetics* 29, 858–860.

Crow, T.J. (1988) Sex chromosomes and psychosis: the case for a pseudoautosomal locus. *British Journal of Psychiatry* 153, 675–683.

Crow, T.J., DeLisi, L.E. & Johnstone, E.C. (1989) Concordance by sex in sibling pairs with schizophrenia is paternally inherited: evidence for a pseudoautosomal locus. *British Journal of Psychiatry* 155, 92–97.

Crow, T.J., DeLisi, L.E., Lofthouse, R. *et al.* (1994) An examination of linkage of schizophrenia and schizoaffective disorder to the pseudoautosomal region (Xp22.3). *British Journal of Psychiatry* 164, 159–164.

Crowe, R.R., Black, D.W., Wesner, R. *et al.* (1991) Lack of linkage to chromosome 5q11–q13 markers in six schizophrenia pedigrees. *Archives of General Psychiatry* 48, 357–361.

Crowe, R.R., Thompson, J.S., Flink, R. & Weinberger, B. (1979) HLA antigens and schizophrenia. *Archives of General Psychiatry* 36, 231–233.

Curtis, D. & Sham, P.C. (1995) Model-free linkage analysis using likelihoods. *American Journal of Human Genetics* 57, 703–716.

Curtis, L., Blouin, J.L., Radhakrishna, U. *et al.* (1999) No evidence for linkage between schizophrenia and markers at chromosome 15q13–14. *American Journal of Medical Genetics and Neuropsychiatric Genetics* 88, 109–112.

D'Amato, T., Campion, D., Gorwood, P. *et al.* (1992) Evidence for a pseudoautosomal locus for schizophrenia. II. Replication of a nonrandom segregation of alleles at the *DXYS14* locus. *British Journal of Psychiatry* 161, 59–62.

Dann, J., DeLisi, L.E., Devoto, M. *et al.* (1997) A linkage study of schizophrenia to markers within Xp11 near the *MAOB* gene. *Psychiatry Research* 70, 131–143.

Davies, J.L., Kawaguchi, Y., Bennett, S.T. *et al.* (1994) A genome-wide search for human type 1 diabetes susceptibility genes. *Nature* 371, 130–136.

Davis, S. & Weeks, D.E. (1997) Comparison of nonparametric statistics for detection of linkage in nuclear families: single marker evaluation. *American Journal of Human Genetics* 61, 1431–1444.

De Leon, J., Dadvand, M., Canuso, C. *et al.* (1995) Schizophrenia and smoking: an epidemiological survey in a state hospital. *American Journal of Psychiatry* 152, 453–455.

DeLisi, L.E., Lofthouse, R., Lehner, T. *et al.* (1995) Failure to find a chromosome 18 pericentric linkage in families with schizophrenia. *American Journal of Medical Genetics and Neuropsychiatric Genetics* 60, 532–534.

Dib, C., Faure, S., Fizames, C. *et al.* (1996) A comprehensive genetic map of the human genome based on 5264 microsatellites. *Nature* 380, 152–154.

Dombroski, B.A., Ton, C.C., Nath, S.K. *et al.* (1997) A susceptibility locus for schizophrenia on chromosome 8p. *American Journal of Medical Genetics and Neuropsychiatric Genetics* 74, 668.

Donald, J.A., Barendse, W. & Cooper, D.W. (1989) Linkage studies of HLA and insulin gene restriction fragment length polymorphisms in families with IDDM. *Genetic Epidemiology* 6, 77–81.

Dunham, I., Collins, J., Wadey, R. & Scambler, P. (1992) Possible role for COMT in psychosis associated with velocardiofacial syndrome. *Lancet* 340, 1361–1362.

Eberhard, G., Franzen, G. & Low, B. (1975) Schizophrenia susceptibility and HL-A antigen. *Neuropsychobiology* 1, 211–217.

Edwards, T.H. (1965) The meaning of the associations between blood groups and disease. *Annals of Human Genetics* 29, 77–83.

Egan, M.F., Goldberg, T.E., Kolachana, B.S. *et al.* (2001) Effect of *COMT* Val108/158 Met genotype on frontal lobe function and risk for schizophrenia. *Proceedings of the National Academy of Sciences of the USA* 98, 6917–6922.

Elbein, S.C., Corsetti, L., Goldgar, D., Skolnick, M. & Permutt, M.A. (1988) Insulin gene in familial NIDDM: lack of linkage in Utah mormon pedigrees. *Diabetes* 37, 569–576.

Elston, R.C. & Campbell, M.A. (1970) Schizophrenia: evidence for the major gene hypothesis. *Behavior Genetics* 1, 3–10.

Essen-Moller, E. (1955) The calculation of morbid risk in parents of index cases, as applied to a family sample of schizophrenics. *Acta Genetica et Statistica Medica* 5, 334–342.

Falconer, D.S. (1965) The inheritance of liability to certain diseases, estimated from the incidence among relatives. *Annals of Human Genetics* 29, 51–76.

Falk, C.T. & Rubinstein, P. (1987) Haplotype relative risks: an easy reliable way to construct a proper control sample for risk calculations. *Annals of Human Genetics* 51, 227–233.

Fang, N., Coon, H., Hoff, M. *et al.* (1995) Search for a schizophrenia susceptibility gene on chromosome 18. *Psychiatric Genetics* 5, 31–35.

Faraone, S.V., Matise, T., Svrakic, D. *et al.* (1998) Genome scan of European-American schizophrenia pedigrees: results of the NIMH Genetics Initiative and Millennium Consortium. *American Journal of Medical Genetics and Neuropsychiatric Genetics* 81, 290–295.

Farmer, A.E., McGuffin, P. & Gottesman, I.I. (1987) Twin concordance for DSM-III schizophrenia: scrutinizing the validity of the definition. *Archives of General Psychiatry* 44, 634–640.

Feighner, J.P., Robins, E., Guze, S.B. *et al.* (1972) Diagnostic criteria for use in psychiatric research. *Archives of General Psychiatry* 26, 57–63.

Ferns, G.A.A., Hitman, G.A. & Trembath, R. (1986) DNA polymorphic haplotypes on the short arm of chromosome 11 and the inheritance of type I diabetes mellitus. *Journal of Medical Genetics* 23, 210–216.

Fischer, M. (1971) Psychoses in the offspring of schizophrenic monozygotic twins and their normal co-twins. *British Journal of Psychiatry* 118, 43–52.

Fisher, P.J., Turic, D., Williams, N.M. *et al.* (1999) DNA pooling identifies QTLs on chromosome 4 for general cognitive ability in children. *Human Molecular Genetics* 8, 915–922.

Franzek, E. & Beckmann, H. (1998) Different genetic background of schizophrenia spectrum psychoses: a twin study. *American Journal of Psychiatry* 155, 76–83.

Freedman, R., Coon, H., Myles-Worsley, M. *et al.* (1997) Linkage of a neurophysiological deficit in schizophrenia to a chromosome 15 locus. *Proceedings of the National Academy of Sciences of the USA* 94, 587–592.

Frieboes, R.M., Moises, H.W., Gattaz, W.F. *et al.* (2001) Lack of association between schizophrenia and the phospholipase-A (2) genes cPLA2 and sPLA2. *American Journal of Medical Genetics* 105, 246–249.

Garver, D.L., Barnes, R., Holcombe, J. *et al.* (1998) Genome-wide scan and schizophrenia in African Americans. *American Journal of Medical Genetics and Neuropsychiatric Genetics* 81, 454–455.

Gattaz, W.F., Nevalainen, T.J. & Kinnunen, P.K.J. (1990) Possible involvement of phospholipase A2 in the pathogenesis of schizophrenia. *Fortschritte der Neurologie und Psychiatrie* 58, 148–153.

Gattaz, W.F., Schmitt, A. & Maras, A. (1995) Increased platelet phospholipase A2 activity in schizophrenia. *Schizophrenia Research* 16, 1–6.

Gershon, E.S., DeLisi, L.E., Hamovit, J. *et al.* (1988) A controlled family study of chronic psychoses: schizophrenia and schizoaffective disorder. *Archives of General Psychiatry* 45, 328–336.

Gill, M., McGuffin, P., Parfitt, E. *et al.* (1993) A linkage study of schizophrenia with DNA markers from the long arm of chromosome 11. *Psychological Medicine* 23, 27–44.

Gill, M., Vallada, H., Collier, D. *et al.* (1996) A combined analysis of D22S278 marker alleles in affected sib-pairs: support for a susceptibility locus for schizophrenia at chromosome 22q12. *American Journal of Medical Genetics and Neuropsychiatric Genetics* 67, 40–45.

Goate, A., Chartier-Harlin, M.C., Mullan, M. *et al.* (1991) Segregation of a missense mutation in the amyloid precursor protein gene with familial Alzheimer's disease [see comments]. *Nature* 349, 704–706.

Gorwood, P., Leboyer, M., Falissard, B. *et al.* (1997) Further epidemiological evidence for anticipation in schizophrenia. *Biomedicine and Pharmacotherapy* 51, 376–380.

Gottesman, I.I. (1991) *Schizophrenia Genesis.* W.H. Freeman, New York.

Gottesman, I.I. & Bertelsen, A. (1989) Confirming unexpressed genotypes for schizophrenia: risks in the offspring of Fischer's Danish identical and fraternal discordant twins. *Archives of General Psychiatry* 46, 867–872.

Gottesman, I.I. & Shields, J. (1967) A polygenic theory of schizophrenia. *Proceedings of the National Academy of Sciences of the USA* 58, 199–205.

Gottesman, I.I. & Shields, J. (1972) *Schizophrenia and Genetics: a Twin Study Vantage Point*. Academic Press, London.

Gottesman, I.I. & Shields, J. (1982) *Schizophrenia: the Epigenetic Puzzle*. Cambridge University Press, Cambridge.

Green, J.R. & Woodrow, J.C. (1977) Sibling method for detecting HLA-linked genes in the disease. *Tissue Antigens* 31, 31–35.

Gurling, H., Kalsi, G., Chen, A.H.S. *et al.* (1995) Schizophrenia susceptibility and chromosome 6p24–22. *Nature Genetics* 11, 234–235.

Hallmayer, J., Schwab, S., Albus, M. *et al.* (1998) A potential schizophrenia susceptibility locus for schizophrenia on 22q12–q13: re-evaluation in 72 families. *American Journal of Medical Genetics and Neuropsychiatric Genetics* 81, 529.

Harper, P.S., Quarrell, O.W. & Youngman, S. (1988) Huntington's disease: prediction and prevention. *Philosophical Transactions of the Royal Society of London B: Biological Science* 319, 285–298.

Heiden, A., Willinger, U., Scharfetter, J. *et al.* (1999) Anticipation in schizophrenia. *Schizophrenia Research* 35, 25–32.

Heston, L.L. (1966) Psychiatric disorders in foster home reared children of schizophrenic mothers. *British Journal of Psychiatry* 112, 819–825.

Heston, L.L. (1970) The genetics of schizophrenic and schizoid disease. *Science* 167, 249–256.

Hill, L., Craig, I.W., Asherson, P. *et al.* (1999) DNA pooling and dense marker maps: a systematic search for genes for cognitive ability. *Neuroreport* 10, 843–848.

Hitman, G.A., Tarn, A.C. & Winter, R.M. (1985) Type 1 (insulin-dependent) diabetes and a highly variable locus close to the insulin gene on chromosome 11. *Diabetologia* 28, 218–222.

Holder, S.E., Vintiner, G.M., Farren, B., Malcolm, S. & Winter, R.M. (1992) Confirmation of an association between RFLPs at the transforming growth factor-alpha locus and non-syndromic cleft lip and palate. *Journal of Medical Genetics* 29, 390–392.

Hovatta, I., Varilo, T., Suvisaari, J. *et al.* (1999) A genome-wide screen for schizophrenia genes in an isolated Finnish subpopulation suggesting multiple susceptibility loci. *American Journal of Human Genetics* 65, 1114–1124.

Hudson, C.J., Kennedy, J.L., Gotowiec, A. *et al.* (1996) Genetic variant near cytosolic phospholipase A2 associated with schizophrenia. *Schizophrenia Research* 21, 111–116.

Huntington's Disease Collaborative Research Group (1993) A novel gene containing a trinucleotide repeat that is expanded and unstable on Huntington's disease chromosomes. *Cell* 72, 971–983.

Imamura, A., Honda, S., Nakane, Y. & Okazaki, Y. (1998) Anticipation in Japanese families with schizophrenia. *Journal of Human Genetics* 43, 217–223.

Ivanyi, P., Droes, J., Schreuder, G.M., D'Amaro, J. & van Rood, J.J. (1983) A search for association of HLA antigens with paranoid schizophrenia: A9 appears as a possible marker. *Tissue Antigens* 22, 186–193.

James, J.W. (1971) Frequency in relatives for an all-or-none trait. *Annals of Human Genetics* 35, 47–49.

Jensen, J., Coon, H., Hoff, M. *et al.* (1998) Search for a schizophrenia susceptibility gene on chromosome 13. *Psychiatric Genetics* 8, 239–243.

Kalsi, G., Brynjolfsson, J., Butler, R. *et al.* (1995a) Linkage analysis of chromosome 22q12–13 in a United Kingdom/Icelandic sample of 23 multiplex schizophrenia families. *American Journal of Medical Genetics and Neuropsychiatric Genetics* 60, 298–301.

Kalsi, G., Curtis, D., Brynjolfsson, J. *et al.* (1995b) Investigation by linkage analysis of the XY pseudoautosomal region in the genetic susceptibility to schizophrenia. *British Journal of Psychiatry* 167, 390–393.

Kalsi, G., Mankoo, B.S., Curtis, D. *et al.* (1995c) Exclusion of linkage of schizophrenia to the gene for the dopamine D2 receptor (*DRD2*) and

chromosome 11q translocation sites. *Psychological Medicine* 25, 531–537.

Kalsi, G., Chen, C.H., Smyth, C. *et al.* (1996) Genetic linkage analysis in an Icelandic/British sample fails to exclude the putative chromosome 13q14.1–q32 schizophrenia susceptibility locus. *American Journal of Human Genetics* 59, A388.

Kalsi, G., Mankoo, B., Curtis, D. *et al.* (1999) New DNA markers with increased informativeness show diminished support for a chromosome 5q11–13 schizophrenia susceptibility locus and exclude linkage in two new cohorts of British and Icelandic families. *Annals of Human Genetics* 63, 235–247.

Kaufmann, C.A., Suarez, B., Malaspina, D. *et al.* (1998) NIMH genetics initiative millennium schizophrenia consortium: linkage analysis of African-American pedigrees. *American Journal of Medical Genetics and Neuropsychiatric Genetics* 81, 282–289.

Kelly, D., Goldberg, R., Wilson, D. *et al.* (1993) Confirmation that the velocardiofacial syndrome is associated with haplo-insufficiency of genes at chromosome 22q11. *American Journal of Medical Genetics* 45, 308–312.

Kendler, K.S. & Gruenberg, A.M. (1984) An independent analysis of the Danish Adoption Study of schizophrenia. VI. The relationship between psychiatric disorders as defined by DSM-III in the relatives and adoptees. *Archives of General Psychiatry* 41, 555–564.

Kendler, K.S., Masterson, C.C. & Davis, K.L. (1985) Psychiatric illness in first-degree relatives of patients with paranoid psychosis, schizophrenia and medical illness. *British Journal of Psychiatry* 147, 524–531.

Kennedy, G.C., German, M.S. & Rutter, W.J. (1995) The minisatellite in the diabetes susceptibility locus IDDM2 regulates insulin transcription. *Nature Genetics* 9, 293–298.

Kety, S.S., Rosenthal, D., Wender, P.H., Schulsinger, F. & Jacobsen, B. (1976) Mental illness in the biological and adoptive families of adopted individuals who have become schizophrenic. *Behavior Genetics* 6, 219–225.

Kläning, U. (1996) *Schizophrenia in twins: incidence and risk factors*. PhD thesis, University of Aarhus, Denmark.

Kong, A. & Cox, N.J. (1997) Allele-sharing models: LOD score and accurate linkage tests. *American Journal of Human Genetics* 61, 1179–1188.

Kringlen, E. (1976) Twins: still our best method. *Schizophrenia Bulletin* 2, 429–433.

Kringlen, E. & Cramer, G. (1989) Offspring of monozygotic twins discordant for schizophrenia. *Archives of General Psychiatry* 46, 873–877.

Kruglyak, L. & Lander, E.S. (1995) Complete multipoint sib-pair analysis of qualitative and quantitative traits. *American Journal of Human Genetics* 57, 439–454.

Kruglyak, L., Daly, M.J., Reeve-Daly, M.P. & Lander, E.S. (1996) Parametric and non-parametric linkage analysis: a unified multipoint approach. *American Journal of Human Genetics* 58, 1347–1363.

Lander, E. & Kruglyak, L. (1995) Genetic dissection of complex traits: guidelines for interpreting and reporting linkage results. *Nature Genetics* 11, 241–247.

Lander, E.S., Linton, L.M., Birren, B. *et al.* and the International Human Genome Sequencing Consortium (2001) Initial sequencing and analysis of the human genome. *Nature* 409, 860–921.

Lannfelt, L., Sokoloff, P. & Martres, M.P. (1992) Amino-acid substitution in the dopamine D3 receptor as a ueful polymorphism for investigating psychiatric disorders. *Psychiatric Genetics* 2, 249–256.

Lasseter, V.K., Pulver, A.E., Wolyniec, P. *et al.* (1995) Follow-up report of potential linkage for schizophrenia on chromosome 22q. Part III. *American Journal of Medical Genetics* 60, 172–173.

Leboyer, M. & McGuffin, P. (1991) Collaborative strategies in the molecular genetics of the major psychoses. *British Journal of Psychiatry* **158**, 605–610.

Le Coniat, M., Sokoloff, P., Hillion, J. *et al.* (1991) Chromosomal localization of the human D$_3$ dopamine receptor gene. *Human Genetics* **87**, 618–620.

Leonard, S., Gault, J., Moore, T. *et al.* (1998) Further investigation of a chromosome 15 locus in schizophrenia: analysis of affected sibpairs from the NIMH genetics initiative. *American Journal of Medical Genetics and Neuropsychiatric Genetics* **81**, 308–312.

Levinson, D.F., Wildenauer, D.B., Schwab, S.G. *et al.* (1996) Additional support for schizophrenia linkage on chromosomes 6 and 8: a multicenter study. *American Journal of Medical Genetics and Neuropsychiatric Genetics* **67**, 580–594.

Levinson, D.F., Mahtani, M.M., Nancarrow, D.J. *et al.* (1998) Genome scan of schizophrenia. *American Journal of Psychiatry* **155**, 741–750.

Levinson, D.F., Holmans, P., Straub, R.E. *et al.* (2000) Multicenter linkage study of schizophrenia candidate regions on chromosomes 5q, 6q, 10p, and 13q: schizophrenia linkage collaborative group III. *American Journal of Human Genetics* **67**, 652–663.

Lin, M.W., Curtis, D., Williams, N. *et al.* (1995) Suggestive evidence for linkage of schizophrenia to markers on chromosome 13q14.1–q32. *Psychiatric Genetics* **5**, 117–126.

Lin, M.W., Sham, P., Hwu, H.G. *et al.* (1997) Suggestive evidence for linkage of schizophrenia to markers on chromosome 13 in Caucasian but not Oriental populations. *Human Genetics* **99**, 417–420.

Lindholm, E., Ekholm, B., Shaw, S. *et al.* (2001) A schizophrenia-susceptibility locus at 6q25, in one of the world's largest reported pedigrees. *American Journal of Human Genetics* **69**, 96–105.

Luxenberger, H. (1928) Vorlaufizer Bericht uber psychiatrische Serien Untersuchungen an Zwillinger. *Zeitschift Fur Gesante Neurologie und Psychiatrie* **116**, 297–326.

McGinnis, R.E., Fox, H., Yates, P. *et al.* (2001) Failure to confirm NOTCH4 association with schizophrenia in a large population-based sample from Scotland. *Nature Genetics* **28**, 128–129.

McGue, M. & Gottesman, I. (1991) The genetic epidemiology of schizophrenia and the design of linkage studies. *European Archives of Psychiatry and Clinical Neuroscience* **240**, 174–181.

McGue, M., Gottesman, I. & Rao, D.C. (1985) Resolving genetic models for the transmission of schizophrenia. *Genetic Epidemiology* **2**, 99–110.

McGuffin, P. & Owen, M. (1991) The molecular genetics of schizophrenia: an overview and forward view. *European Archives of Psychiatry and Clinical Neuroscience* **240**, 169–173.

McGuffin, P. & Sturt, E. (1986) Genetic markers in schizophrenia. *Human Heredity* **36**, 461–465.

McGuffin, P., Festenstein, H. & Murray, R. (1983) A family study of HLA antigens and other genetic markers in schizophrenia. *Psychological Medicine* **13**, 31–43.

McGuffin, P., Farmer, A.E. & Gottesman, I.I. (1984) Twin concordance for operationally defined schizophrenia: confirmation of familiality and heritability. *Archives of General Psychiatry* **41**, 541–545.

McGuffin, P., Sargeant, M., Hetti, G. *et al.* (1990) Exclusion of a schizophrenia susceptibility gene from the chromosome 5q11–q13 region: new data and a reanalysis of previous reports. *American Journal of Human Genetics* **47**, 524–535.

McGuffin, P., Owen, M. & Gill, M. (1992) Molecular genetics of schizophrenia. In: *Genetic Research in Psychiatry* (eds I. Mendlewicz & H. Hippius), pp. 25–48. Springer-Verlag, Berlin.

McGuffin, P., Asherson, P., Owen, M. & Farmer, A. (1994a) The strength of the genetic effect: is there room for an environmental influence in the aetiology of schizophrenia? *British Journal of Psychiatry* **164**, 593–599.

McGuffin, P., Owen, M.J., O'Donovan, M.C., Thapar, A. & Gottesman, I.I. (1994b) *Seminars in Psychiatric Genetics*. Gaskell, London.

McGuffin, P., Owen, M.J. & Farmer, A.E. (1995) Genetic basis of schizophrenia. *Lancet* **346**, 678–682.

McGuffin, P., Riley, B. & Plomin, R. (2001) Genomics and behavior: toward behavioral genomics. *Science* **291**, 1232–1249.

McKenna, P.J. & Bailey, P.E. (1993) The strange story of clozapine. *British Journal of Psychiatry* **162**, 32–37.

Maier, W., Schmidt, F., Schwab, S.G. *et al.* (1995) Lack of linkage between schizophrenia and markers at the telomeric end of the pseudoautosomal region of the sex chromosomes. *Biological Psychiatry* **37**, 344–347.

Marth, G., Yeh, R., Minton, M. *et al.* (2001) Single-nucleotide polymorphisms in the public domain: how useful are they? *Nature Genetics* **27**, 371–372.

Martinez, M., Goldin, L.R., Cao, Q. *et al.* (1999) Follow-up study on a susceptibility locus for schizophrenia on chromosome 6q. *American Journal of Medical Genetics and Neuropsychiatric Genetics* **88**, 337–343.

Maziade, M., Debraekeleer, M., Genest, P. *et al.* (1993) A balanced 2:18 translocation and familial schizophrenia: falling short of an association. *Archives of General Psychiatry* **50**, 73–75.

Meehl, P.E. (1973) *Psychodiagnosis: Selected Papers*. University of Minnesota Press, Minneapolis.

Millar, J.K., Christie, S., Semple, C.A.M. & Porteous, D.J. (2000a) Chromosomal location and genomic structure of the human translin-associated factor X gene (*TRAX*; *TSNAX*) revealed by intergenic splicing to *DISC1*, a gene disrupted by a translocation segregating with schizophrenia. *Genomics* **67**, 69–77.

Millar, J.K., Wilson-Annan, J.C., Anderson, S. *et al.* (2000b) Disruption of two novel genes by a translocation co-segregating with schizophrenia. *Human Molecular Genetics* **9**, 1415–1423.

Miyanaga, K., Machiyama, Y. & Juji, T. (1984) Schizophrenic disorders and HLA-DR antigens. *Biological Psychiatry* **19**, 121–129.

Moises, H.W., Yang, L., Kristbjarnarson, H. *et al.* (1995) An international two-stage genome-wide search for schizophrenia susceptibility genes. *Nature Genetics* **11**, 321–324.

Mors, O., Ewald, H., Blackwood, D. & Muir, W. (1997) Cytogenetic abnormalities on chromosome 18 associated with bipolar affective disorder or schizophrenia. *British Journal of Psychiatry* **170**, 278–280.

Morton, N.E. (1955) Sequential tests for the detection of linkage. *American Journal of Human Genetics* **7**, 277–318.

Morton, N.E. & MacLean, C.J. (1974) Analysis of family resemblance. III. Complex segregation of quantitative traits. *American Journal of Human Genetics* **26**, 489–503.

Mott, F.W. (1910) Hereditary aspects of nervous and mental diseases. *British Medical Journal* **2**, 1013.

Mowry, B.J., Nancarrow, D.J., Lennon, D.P. *et al.* (1995) Schizophrenia susceptibility and chromosome 6p24–22. *Nature Genetics* **11**, 233–234.

Mulcrone, J., Whatley, S.A., Marchbanks, R. *et al.* (1995) Genetic linkage analysis of schizophrenia using chromosome 11q13–24 markers in Israeli pedigrees. *American Journal of Medical Genetics and Neuropsychiatric Genetics* **60**, 103–108.

Mullis, K.B. & Faloona, F.A. (1987) Specific synthesis of DNA *in vitro* via a polymerase-catalyzed chain reaction. *Methods in Enzymology* **155**, 335–350.

Murphy, K.C. & Owen, M.J. (1997) The behavioral phenotype in velo-cardiofacial syndrome. *American Journal of Medical Genetics and Neuropsychiatric Genetics* **74**, 660.

Murray, R.M., Lewis, S.W. & Reveley, A.M. (1985) Towards an aetiological classification of schizophrenia. *Lancet* **1**, 1023–1026.

Nagamoto, H.T., Adler, L.E., Hea, R.A. *et al.* (1996) Gating of auditory

P50 in schizophrenics: unique effects of clozapine. *Biological Psychiatry* 40, 181–188.

Neves-Pereira, M., Bassett, A.S., Honer, W.G. *et al.* (1998) No evidence for linkage of the *CHRNA7* gene region in Canadian schizophrenia families. *American Journal of Medical Genetics and Neuropsychiatric Genetics* 81, 361–363.

Noponen, M., Sanfilipo, M., Samanich, K. *et al.* (1993) Elevated PLA2 activity in schizophrenics and other psychiatric patients. *Biological Psychiatry* 34, 641–649.

Nothen, M.M., Propping, P. & Fimmers, R. (1993) Association versus linkage studies in psychosis genetics. *Journal of Medical Genetics* 30, 634–637.

Onstad, S., Skre, I., Torgersen, S. & Kringlen, E. (1991) Twin concordance for DSM-IIIR schizophrenia. *Acta Psychiatrica Scandinavica* 83, 395–401.

O'Rourke, D.H., Gottesman, I.I., Suarez, B.K., Rice, J. & Reich, T. (1982) Refutation of the general single-locus model for the etiology of schizophrenia. *American Journal of Human Genetics* 34, 630–649.

Ott, J. (1991) *Analysis of Human Genetic Linkage.* Johns Hopkins University Press, Baltimore.

Owen, M.J. & McGuffin, P. (1991) DNA and classical genetic markers in schizophrenia. *European Archives of Psychiatry and Clinical Neuroscience* 240, 197–203.

Owen, M.J., Mant, R., Parfitt, E. *et al.* (1992) No association between RFLPs at the porpholbilinogen deaminase gene and schizophrenia. *Human Genetics* 90, 131–132.

Paterson, A.D., DeLisi, L., Faraone, S.V. *et al.* (1999) Sixth World Congress of Psychiatric Genetics X chromosome workshop. *American Journal of Medical Genetics and Neuropsychiatric Genetics* 88, 279–286.

Peet, M., Ramchand, C.N., Lee, J. *et al.* (1998) Association of the Ban I dimorphic site at the human cytosolic phospholipase A2 gene with schizophrenia. *Psychiatric Genetics* 8, 191–192.

Penrose, L.S. (1935) The detection of autosomal linkage in data which conists of pairs of brothers and sisters of unspecified parentage. *Annals of Eugenics* 6, 133–138.

Pollin, W., Allen, M.G., Hoffer, A., Stabenau, J.R. & Hrubec, Z. (1969) Psychopathology in 15 909 pairs of veteran twins: evidence for a genetic factor in the pathogenesis of schizophrenia and its relative absence in psychoneurosis. *American Journal of Psychiatry* 126, 597–610.

Price, S.A., Fox, H., St Clair, D. & Shaw, D.J. (1997) Lack of association between schizophrenia and a polymorphism close to the cytosolic phospholipase A2 gene. *Psychiatric Genetics* 7, 111–114.

Pulver, A.E., Karayiorgou, M., Lasseter, V.K. *et al.* (1994a) Follow-up of a report of a potential linkage for schizophrenia on chromosome 22q12–q13.1: Part II. *American Journal of Medical Genetics* 54, 44–50.

Pulver, A.E., Karayiorgou, M., Wolyniec, P.S. *et al.* (1994b) Sequential strategy to identify a susceptibility gene for schizophrenia: report of potential linkage on chromosome 22q12–q13.1: Part 1. *American Journal of Medical Genetics* 54, 36–43.

Pulver, A.E., Nestadt, G., Goldberg, R. *et al.* (1994c) Psychotic illness in patients diagnosed with velocardiofacial syndrome and their relatives. *Journal of Nervous and Mental Disease* 182, 476–478.

Pulver, A.E., Lasseter, V.K., Kasch, L. *et al.* (1995) Schizophrenia: a genome scan targets chromosomes 3p and 8p as potential sites of susceptibility genes. *American Journal of Medical Genetics and Neuropsychiatric Genetics* 60, 252–260.

Reveley, A.M., Reveley, M.A., Clifford, C.A. & Murray, R.M. (1982) Cerebral ventricular size in twins discordant for schizophrenia. *Lancet* 1, 540–541.

Riley, B.P. & McGuffin, P. (2000) Linkage and associated studies of schizophrenia. *American Journal of Medical Genetics Seminars in Medical Genetics* 97, 23–44.

Riley, B., Mogudi-Carter, M., Jenkins, T. & Williamson, R. (1996a) No evidence for linkage of chromosome 22 markers to schizophrenia in southern African Bantu-speaking families. *American Journal of Medical Genetics and Neuropsychiatric Genetics* 67, 515–522.

Riley, B.P., Rajagopalan, S., Mogudi-Carter, M., Jenkins, T. & Williamson, R. (1996b) No evidence for linkage of chromosome 6p markers to schizophrenia in Southern African Bantu-speaking families. *Psychiatric Genetics* 6, 41–49.

Riley, B.P., Tahir, E., Rajagopalan, S. *et al.* (1997) A linkage study of the N-methyl-D-aspartate receptor subunit gene loci and schizophrenia in southern African Bantu-speaking families. *Psychiatric Genetics* 7, 57–74.

Riley, B.P., Lin, M.W., Mogudi-Carter, M. *et al.* (1998) Failure to exclude a possible schizophrenia susceptibility locus on chromosome 13q14.1–q32 in Southern African Bantu-speaking families. *Psychiatric Genetics* 8, 155–162.

Riley, B.P., Makoff, A., Mogudi-Carter, M. *et al.* (2000) Haplotype transmission disequilibrium and evidence for linkage of the *CHRNA7* gene region to schizophrenia in southern African Bantu families. *American Journal of Medical Genetics and Neuropsychiatric Genetics* 96, 196–201.

Risch, N. (1990) Linkage strategies for genetically complex traits. I. Multilocus models. *American Journal of Human Genetics* 46, 222–228.

Risch, N. & Baron, M. (1984) Segregation analysis of schizophrenia and related disorders. *American Journal of Human Genetics* 36, 1039–1059.

Risch, N. & Giuffra, L. (1992) Model misspecification and multipoint linkage analysis. *Human Heredity* 42, 77–92.

Risch, N. & Merikangas, K. (1996) The future of genetic studies of complex human diseases. *Science* 273, 1516–1517.

Roberts, S.B., MacLean, C.J., Neale, M.C., Eaves, L.J. & Kendler, K.S. (1999) Replication of linkage studies of complex traits: an examination of variation in location estimates. *American Journal of Human Genetics* 65, 876–884.

Rosenthal, D., Wender, P.H., Kety, S.S., Welner, J. & Schulsinger, F. (1971) The adopted-away offspring of schizophrenics. *American Journal of Psychiatry* 128, 307–311.

Rudduck, C. (1984) *Genetic markers and schizophrenia.* Thesis, University of Lund.

Sanders, A.R., Rincon-Limas, D.E., Chakraborty, R. *et al.* (1993) Association between genetic variation at the porpholbilinogen deaminase gene and schizophrenia. *Schizophrenia Research* 8, 211–221.

Schalling, M., Hudson, T.J., Buetow, K.H. & Housman, D.E. (1993) Direct detection of novel expanded trinucleotide repeats in the human genome. *Nature Genetics* 4, 135–139.

Schwab, S.G., Albus, M., Hallmayer, J. *et al.* (1995) Evaluation of a susceptibility gene for schizophrenia on chromosome 6p by multipoint affected sib-pair linkage analysis. *Nature Genetics* 11, 325–327.

Schwab, S.G., Eckstein, G.N., Hallmayer, J. *et al.* (1997) Evidence suggestive of a locus on chromosome 5q31 contributing to susceptibility for schizophrenia in German and Israeli families by multipoint affected sib-pair linkage analysis. *Molecular Psychiatry* 2, 156–160.

Schwab, S.G., Hallmayer, J., Albus, M. *et al.* (1998) Further evidence for a susceptibility locus on chromosome 10p14–p11 in 72 families with schizophrenia by non-parametric linkage analysis. *American Journal of Medical Genetics and Neuropsychiatric Genetics* 81, 302–307.

Scott, W.K., Pericak-Vance, M.A., Haines, J.L. *et al.* (1997) Genetic analysis of complex diseases. *Science* 275, 1327–1330.

Shaw, S.H., Kelly, M., Smith, A.B. *et al.* (1998) A genome-wide search for schizophrenia susceptibility genes. *American Journal of Medical Genetics and Neuropsychiatric Genetics* **81**, 364–376.

Sherrington, R., Brynjolfsson, J., Petursson, H. *et al.* (1988) Localization of a susceptibility locus for schizophrenia on chromosome 5. *Nature* **336**, 164–167.

Shprintzen, R.J., Goldberg, R., Golding-Kushner, K.J. & Marion, R.W. (1992) Late-onset psychosis in the velocardiofacial syndrome. *American Journal of Medical Genetics* **42**, 141–142.

Silverman, J.M., Greenberg, D.A., Altstiel, L.D. *et al.* (1996) Evidence of a locus for schizophrenia and related disorders on the short arm of chromosome 5 in a large pedigree. *American Journal of Medical Genetics and Neuropsychiatric Genetics* **67**, 162–171.

Sklar, P., Schwab, S.G., Williams, N.M. *et al.* (2001) Association analysis of *NOTCH4* loci in schizophrenia using family and population-based controls. *Nature Genetics* **28**, 126–128.

Slater, E. (1958) The monogenic theory of schizophrenia. *Acta Genetica* **8**, 50–56.

Slater, E. & Cowie, V. (1971) *The Genetics of Mental Disorder*. Oxford University Press, Oxford.

Sobell, J.L., Heston, L.L. & Sommer, S.S. (1992) Delineation of genetic predisposition to multifactorial disease: a general approach on the threshold of feasibility. *Genomics* **12**, 1–6.

Sokoloff, P., Giros, B., Martres, M.P. *et al.* (1992) Localization and function of the D_3 dopamine receptor. *Arzneimittel Forschung* **42**, 224–230.

Spitzer, R.L., Endicott, J. & Robins, E. (1978) Research diagnostic criteria: rationale and reliability. *Archives of General Psychiatry* **35**, 773–782.

St Clair, D., Blackwood, D., Muir, W. *et al.* (1990) Association within a family of a balanced autosomal translocation with major mental illness. *Lancet* **336**, 13–16.

Straub, R.E., MacLean, C.J., O'Neill, F.A. *et al.* (1995) A potential vulnerability locus for schizophrenia on chromosome 6p24–22: evidence for genetic heterogeneity. *Nature Genetics* **11**, 287–293.

Straub, R.E., MacLean, C.J., O'Neill, F.A., Walsh, D. & Kendler, K.S. (1997a) Genome scan for schizophrenia genes: a detailed progress report in an Irish cohort. *American Journal of Medical Genetics and Neuropsychiatric Genetics* **74**, 558.

Straub, R.E., MacLean, C.J., O'Neill, F.A., Walsh, D. & Kendler, K.S. (1997b) Support for a possible schizophrenia vulnerability locus in region 5q22–31 in Irish families. *Molecular Psychiatry* **2**, 148–155.

Straub, R.E., MacLean, C.J., Martin, R.B. *et al.* (1998) A schizophrenia locus may be located in region 10p15–p11. *American Journal of Medical Genetics and Neuropsychiatric Genetics* **81**, 296–301.

Strauss, J., Zhang, X.R., Barron, Y., Ganguli, R. & Nimgaonkar, V.L. (1999) Lack of association between schizophrenia and a pancreatic phospholipase A-2 gene (*PLA2G1B*) polymorphism. *Psychiatric Genetics* **9**, 153–155.

Sturt, E. & McGuffin, P. (1985) Can linkage and marker association resolve the genetic aetiology of psychiatric disorders? Review and argument. *Psychological Medicine* **15**, 455–462.

Su, Y., Burke, J., O'Neill, F.A. *et al.* (1993) Exclusion of linkage between schizophrenia and the D_2 dopamine receptor gene region of chromosome 11q in 112 Irish multiplex families. *Archives of General Psychiatry* **50**, 205–211.

Suarez, B.K., Rice, J. & Reich, T. (1978) The generalized sib-pair IBD distribution: its use in the detection of linkage. *Annals of Human Genetics* **42**, 87–94.

Suarez, B., Hampe, C.L. & van Eerdewegh, P. (1995) Problems of replicating linkage claims in psychiatry. In: *New Genetic Approaches to Mental Disorders* (eds E.S. Gershon & C.R. Cloninger), pp. 23–46. American Psychiatric Press, Washington, DC.

Suddath, R.L., Christison, G.W., Torrey, E.F., Casanova, M.F. & Weinberger, D.R. (1990) Anatomical abnormalities in the brains of monozygotic twins discordant for schizophrenia. *New England Journal of Medicine* **322**, 789–794.

Sunahara, R.K., Niznik, H.B., Weiners, D.M. *et al.* (1990) Human dopamine D_1 receptor encoded by an intronless gene on chromosome 5. *Nature* **347**, 80–83.

Tienari, P. (1971) Schizophrenia and monozygotic twins. *Psychiatria Fennica* **2**, 97–104.

Tienari, P. (1991) Interaction between genetic vulnerability and family environment: the Finnish adoptive family study of schizophrenia. *Acta Psychiatrica Scandinavica* **84**, 460–465.

Tienari, P.J., Wikstrom, J., Sajantila, A., Palo, J. & Peltonen, L. (1992) Genetic susceptibility to multiple sclerosis linked to myelin basic protein gene. *Lancet* **340**, 987–991.

Tsujita, T., Okazaki, Y., Fujimaru, K. *et al.* (1992) Twin concordance rates of DSM-IIIR schizophrenia in a new Japanese sample. *Abstracts of the Seventh International Congress on Twin Studies, Tokyo. Japan* **152**.

Turner, S.W., Toone, B.K. & Brett-Jones, J.R. (1986) Computerized tomographic scan changes in early schizophrenia: preliminary findings. *Psychological Medicine* **16**, 219–225.

Turner, W.J. (1979) Genetic markers for schizotaxia. *Biological Psychiatry* **14**, 177–206.

Tyler, A., Morris, M., Lazarou, L. *et al.* (1992) Presymptomatic testing for Huntington's disease in Wales 1987–90. *British Journal of Psychiatry* **161**, 481–488.

Ujike, H., Takehisa, Y., Takaki, M. *et al.* (2001) *NOTCH4* gene polymorphism and susceptibility to schizophrenia and schizoaffective disorder. *Neuroscience Letters* **301**, 41–44.

Vallada, H.P., Gill, M., Sham, P. *et al.* (1995) Linkage studies on chromosome 22 in familial schizophrenia. *American Journal of Medical Genetics and Neuropsychiatric Genetics* **60**, 139–146.

Van Broeckhoven, C., Backhovens, H., Cruts, M. *et al.* (1992) Mapping of a gene predisposing to early-onset Alzheimer's disease to chromosome 14q24.3. *Nature Genetics* **2**, 335–339.

Van Tol, H.H., Bunzow, J.R., Guan, H.C. *et al.* (1991) Cloning of the gene for a human dopamine D_4 receptor with high affinity for the antipsychotic clozapine. *Nature* **350**, 610–614.

Van Tol, H.H., Wu, C.M., Guan, H.C. *et al.* (1992) Multiple dopamine D_4 receptor variants in the human population. *Nature* **358**, 149–152.

Venter, J.C., Adams, M.D., Myers, E.W. *et al.* (2001) The sequence of the human genome. *Science* **291**, 1304–1351.

Vogler, G.P., Gottesman, I.I., McGue, M.K. & Rao, D.C. (1990) Mixed-model segregation analysis of schizophrenia in the Lindelius Swedish pedigrees. *Behavior Genetics* **20**, 461–472.

Walsh, C., Asherson, P. & Sham, P. (1993) Familial schizophrenia shows no gender difference in age of onset. *Schizophrenia Research* **9**, 127.

Wang, Z.W., Black, D., Andreasen, N. & Crowe, R.R. (1993) Pseudoautosomal locus for schizophrenia excluded in 12 pedigrees. *Archives of General Psychiatry* **50**, 199–204.

Weber, J.L. & May, P.E. (1989) Abundant class of human DNA polymorphisms which can be typed using the polymerase chain reaction. *American Journal of Human Genetics* **44**, 388–396.

Wei, J. & Hemmings, G.P. (2000) The *NOTCH4* locus is associated with susceptibility to schizophrenia. *Nature Genetics* **25**, 376–377.

Weinshilboum, R.M. & Raymond, F.A. (1977) Inheritance of low erythrocyte catechol-O-methyltransferase in man. *American Journal of Medical Genetics* **29**, 125–135.

Wender, P.H., Rosenthal, D., Kety, S.S., Schulsinger, F. & Welner, J.

(1974) Crossfostering: a research strategy for clarifying the role of genetic and experiential factors in the etiology of schizophrenia. *Archives of General Psychiatry* 30, 121–128.

White, R. & Lalouel, J.M. (1988) Chromosome mapping with DNA markers. *Scientific American* 258, 40–48.

Wildenauer, D., Hallmayer, J., Schwab, S. *et al.* (1997) 18p-Support for a locus conferring susceptibility to functional psychoses as evidenced by linkage and linkage disequilibrium studies in families with schizophrenia. *American Journal of Medical Genetics and Neuropsychiatric Genetics* 74, 676–677.

Williams, J., Spurlock, G., McGuffin, P. *et al.* (1996) Association between schizophrenia and T102C polymorphism of the 5-hydroxytryptamine type 2a-receptor gene. European Multicentre Association Study of Schizophrenia (EMASS) Group. *Lancet* 347, 1294–1296.

Williams, J., McGuffin, P., Nothen, M. & Owen, M.J. (1997) Meta-analysis of association between the 5-HT (2a) receptor T102C polymorphism and schizophrenia. *Lancet* 349, 1221.

Williams, J., Spurlock, G., Holmans, P. *et al.* (1998) A meta-analysis and transmission disequilibrium study of association between the dopamine D_3 receptor gene and schizophrenia. *Molecular Psychiatry* 3, 141–149.

Wright, P., Dawson, E., Donaldson, P.T. *et al.* (1998) A transmission/disequilibrium study of the DRB1*04 gene locus on chromosome 6p21.3 with schizophrenia. *Schizophrenia Research* 32, 75–80.

Yaw, J., Myles-Worsley, M., Hoff, M. *et al.* (1996) Anticipation in multiplex schizophrenia pedigrees. *Psychiatric Genetics* 6, 7–11.

Zhe Wu, W., Black, D., Andreasen, N.C. & Crowe, R.R. (1993) A linkage study of chromosome 11q in schizophrenia. *Archives of General Psychiatry* 50, 212–216.

15 Intermediate phenotypes in genetic studies of schizophrenia

M.F. Egan, M. Leboyer and D.R. Weinberger

Methodological issues, 278
  Assumptions, 278
  Characteristics of intermediate phenotypes, 278
  Determining genetic variance for intermediate phenotypes, 279
  Design of genetic studies using intermediate phenotypes, 280
Eye tracking dysfunction, 281
  Studies of eye tracking dysfunction in patients with schizophrenia, 281
  Family studies of eye tracking dysfunction, 283

Genetic models of eye tracking dysfunction, 284
  Summary, 284
Clinical phenotypes, 285
Neurochemical phenotypes, 286
Electrophysiological markers, 286
Neuroimaging phenotypes, 287
Cognitive phenotypes, 289
Other phenotypes, 291
Conclusions, 291
References, 292

Recent advances in molecular genetics have produced break-throughs in the genetics of complex traits such as diabetes, coronary heart disease and Alzheimer's disease. By contrast, molecular genetic studies of schizophrenia have not yet had similar successes. This may in part be a result of obstacles that complicate efforts to identify genes for any complex disorder such as unknown mode of inheritance, genetic heterogeneity, phenocopies, incomplete penetrance and variable expressivity (Pauls 1993; Lander & Schork 1994). These issues are described in more detail elsewhere in this volume (see Chapter 14). A second obstacle is the uncertainty of the heritable phenotype. Tsuang *et al.* (1993) have pointed out that ambiguities in identifying the phenotype may be the 'rate-limiting step' in psychiatric genetic studies. Indeed, although reliable diagnostic criteria and structured psychiatric interviews have been used in psychiatric genetics, little is known about how to choose the diagnostic system that best describes the most heritable form of the illness or most heritable aspects of psychopathology. Within apparently affected subjects various types of phenotypic misclassification reduce the power of linkage studies because of phenocopies or genetic heterogeneity. For example, family studies of schizophrenic probands have revealed that familial/genetic aspects of schizophrenia were more apparent when broadening the affected status to include subsyndromal variants such as schizophrenia-like personality disorders (schizotypal, paranoid and schizoid personality disorders). However, broadening the definition of affected status might increase the risk of false-positive misclassification, which can dramatically confound linkage studies. Furthermore, using multiple diagnostic classifications in a linkage study inflates the number of comparisons (e.g. Straub *et al.* 1995), raising the possibility of type I errors.

To minimize imprecision introduced by categorical diagnoses, new strategies have been described aiming at identifying more elemental neurobiological traits related to genetic risk for schizophrenia, so-called endophenotypes or, more aptly, inter-mediate phenotypes (Egan & Weinberger 1997; Leboyer *et al.* 1998). Intermediate phenotypes may be any neurobiological measure related to the underlying molecular genetics of the illness, including biochemical, endocrinological, neurophysiological, neuroanatomical or neuropsychological markers. A true intermediate phenotype, by virtue of being closer to the direct effects of susceptibility alleles, should have a simpler genetic architecture, with individual loci contributing a greater percentage of total phenotypic variance than one could hope to find with the more complex clinical phenotypes. This simpler genetic architecture thus increases the power of both linkage and association studies. For example, endophenotypes might be underlined by a Mendelian inheritance pattern which would considerably diminish the sample size required to detect the responsible genetic mutation (Freedman *et al.* 1999). Furthermore, because biological measures are more tractable for molecular research, a set of compelling candidate genes can be more readily generated, relative to clinical phenotypes, for association studies. Thus, using intermediate phenotypes is a promising strategy to enhance the power of both linkage and association studies of schizophrenia.

There are several examples from somatic diseases where biological measures helped in defining the genetic basis of the illness in molecular terms. For instance, understanding the mode of inheritance of idiopathic haemochromatosis was unclear until serum iron concentration was selected as a biological indicator of intrinsic liability to the disease. Including serum iron in the analysis uncovered a linkage with the HLA-A locus (Lalouel *et al.* 1985). To identify a genetic susceptibility factor in juvenile myoclonic epilepsy, investigators chose a subclinical trait (i.e. a characteristic EEG abnormality) as an endophenotype in affected and non-affected family members and found linkage to chromosome 6 (Greenberg *et al.* 1988). Focusing on families with the highest serum glucose levels as a specific phenotype led to the discovery of a genetic deficit underlying type 2 diabetes (Mahtani *et al.* 1996).

One way to conceptualize this approach is to view schizophrenia as emerging from the interaction of a variety of elementary neurobiological abnormalities, each underlined by specific defects in a unique set of candidate genes, and interacting with non-genetic factors (Fig. 15.1). If this is the case, then it becomes clear how measuring intermediate phenotypes can improve the power to find genes. Studies of family members of patients with schizophrenia have often found that even relatives with no psychiatric disease may have one of a number of subtle neurobiological alterations typically seen in patients. This suggests, but does not prove, that intermediate phenotypes may exist. To date, such studies have provided a variety of potential intermediate phenotypes, but only two have been related to specific genes. Freedman *et al.* (1997) found linkage between a deficit in the inhibition of the P50 waveform of the auditory evoked response to repeated auditory stimuli and markers near the α7 nicotinic acid receptor gene. More recently, Egan *et al.* (2001b) found evidence for an association between the high activity valine at codon 108 (158 for the membrane-bound protein) allele of the gene for *COMT* and several measures of prefrontal function. The *COMT* valine allele, in contrast to the methionine allele, was also weakly associated with schizophrenia. These initial successes demonstrate the plausibility of this approach.

In this chapter, we review the existing literature on intermediate phenotypes associated with schizophrenia. First, we review methodological issues in genetic studies using intermediate phenotypes. Next we describe studies of family members that have employed a variety of methodologies including clinical, cognitive, electrophysiology, biochemical, structural or functional brain imaging.

Methodological issues

Assumptions

Using biological measures in genetic studies assumes that genes increase susceptibility to schizophrenia by virtue of their effects on these measures (Fig. 15.1). Just as increased serum cholesterol is a risk factor for coronary artery disease, one assumes that the putative intermediate phenotype fits in the causal chain between gene, protein, physiology and manifest illness. This assumption could be wrong, in that many schizophrenia genes may not exert any impact except in conjunction with one another to produce a single final common pathophysiology (Fig. 15.2). This approach also assumes that the genetic architecture of a given measure is simpler or more approachable than schizophrenia itself, which could also be wrong. For example, IQ is lower in patients with schizophrenia but it is very possible that the genetic architecture of IQ is more complex than that of schizophrenia.

Characteristics of intermediate phenotypes

Quantitative measures vary in their suitability for use in genetic studies. Two useful characteristics of intermediate phenotypes are high test–retest reliability and stability over time. Variance as a result of measurement error and other state-dependent processes are forms of environmental variance that reduce the genetic component of total phenotypic variance. This in turn reduces one's power to detect genes. In other words, poor reliability or stability adds 'noise'. Related to this, measures should be relatively unaffected by neuroleptics and other medications, as

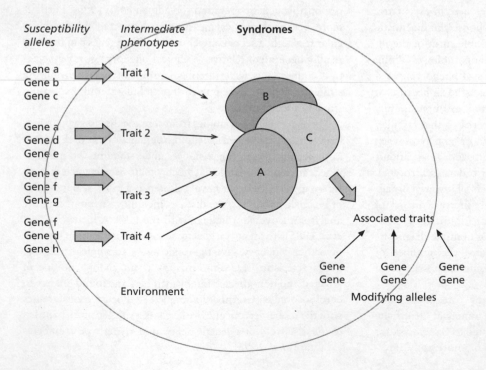

Fig 15.1 Intermediate phenotypes are biological measures more closely related to the effects of genes that increase risk for illness in complex genetic disorders such as schizophrenia. These measures can increase the power for finding disease genes because of their simpler genetic architecture and because often their underlying molecular biology is more certain, providing a stronger basis for selecting candidate genes.

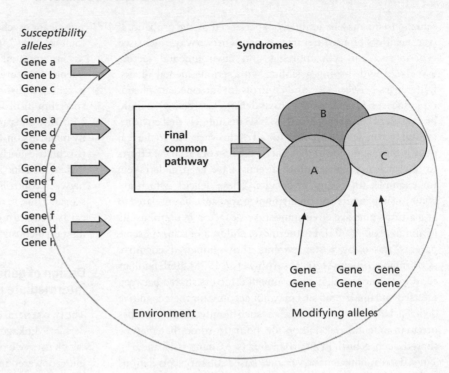

Fig 15.2 An alternative model of a complex genetic disorder. In this model, susceptibility genes act in concert to produce a final common pathway and a clinical phenotype. By themselves, genes or groups of genes do not produce specific detectable effects on biological measures. In this case, the intermediate phenotype approach is not useful.

this increases environmental and reduces genetic components of variance. Unfortunately, these data are lacking for many candidate phenotypes discussed below. Given the high rates of tobacco, caffeine and alcohol use in patients, if these substances markedly impact on a phenotypic measure, the increased environmental variance may dilute genetic effects. While patients using these substances could be excluded, this will increase ascertainment difficulties.

Biological traits that have an approachable neurobiology, e.g. through animal models, neuroimaging, etc., have an added advantage because they offer more obvious molecular targets for association studies. For example, sensory gating has been examined in an animal model and a prime candidate gene has been shown to be related to this phenotype (Freedman *et al.* 1997). In contrast, phenotypes such as paranoia or hallucinations are not amendable to molecular studies using animal models. Phenotypes that appear to be related to a critical aspect of the neurobiology and morbidity may have certain advantages over those whose role in the illness is vague. For example, cognitive deficits, such as impaired working memory, appear to predict outcome (Goldberg *et al.* 1995; Green 1996) and may have a key role in pathophysiology (Weinberger 1987). In contrast, it is unclear if correcting eye tracking deficits would have any detectable impact on illness or outcome. Alternatively, eye tracking deficits may be a surrogate measure for a broader deficit in prefrontal function. Finally, to be useful, intermediate phenotypes *per se* must offer some additional genetic information beyond psychiatric diagnosis. A biological test with 100% sensitivity and specificity for schizophrenia may not offer any additional genetic information beyond what one could already obtain with diagnosis.

Determining genetic variance for intermediate phenotypes

Many biological aspects of schizophrenia may be related to environmental factors, such as chronic illness or neuroleptic treatment, rather than to schizophrenia genes. Thus, a critical issue in selecting an intermediate phenotype for genetic studies is to demonstrate a significant genetic component related to risk for schizophrenia. The traditional genetic epidemiological approach is to study a variety of relatives (i.e. first, second and third degree), spouses and adoptees to infer the genetic and environmental components of total phenotypic variance (Plomin *et al.* 1990; Falconer & Mackay 1996). These studies have essentially not been performed to any significant degree for most putative intermediate phenotypes. The overwhelming majority of studies have looked exclusively at siblings and/or parents. Correlations between first-degree relatives set an upper limit on heritability (Falconer & Mackay 1996). Such studies of first-degree relatives are unable to exclude shared environment as a cause for family correlations. However, there are reasons, at least for some phenotypes, to think that shared environment has only a small role and that much of the variance in familial correlations is brought about by genetic factors that increase risk for schizophrenia.

Data from family studies suggest that familial aggregation of schizophrenia is largely accounted for by genetic and not environmental factors (Rao *et al.* 1981; McGue & Gottesman 1989). In other words, there are no environmental factors shared between siblings that increase risk for schizophrenia (Plomin *et al.* 1990; Cannon *et al.* 1998a). This implies that all environmental variance related to increased risk for schizophrenia may be uniquely experienced by the proband. If true, healthy siblings differ from controls in two ways: increased genetic risk for schizophrenia and environmental factors associated with having a sibling with serious mental illness. Differences between sibs and controls for intermediate phenotypic measures, such as cognitive deficits (see below), should be a result of one of these factors. It seems unlikely that environmental factors would account for all of this variance, so the real issue is the magnitude of the genetic portion of variance. Efforts to test such hypotheses more directly have been undertaken; for example, for cognitive deficits. These deficits, which are common in patients and their siblings, appear to be unrelated to at least one putative environmental risk factor, *in utero* insults (Cannon *et al.* 2000a). Furthermore, children of schizophrenic parents raised by foster parents show impaired cognitive performance on some tests (Asarnow *et al.* 1978). Both findings support the notion that environmental factors shared between affected and unaffected sibs may not account for their cognitive deficits. However, in contrast to such family studies, studies of environmental risk factors do point to some that may be shared, such as birth in an urban area (see Chapters 12 and 31). Thus, determining genetic variance based solely on correlations between first-degree relatives, which is the most commonly used method, involves assumptions that may be somewhat inaccurate.

Most studies of intermediate phenotypes begin by looking for a difference between first-degree relatives and controls. Some family cohorts have included relatives who do not have schizophrenia spectrum disorders. One advantage to studying these subjects is that affected sib pairs may share a variety of illness-related environmental factors impacting on neurobiological measures. Thus, studies of only affected sib pairs could be misleading and underestimate environmental components of phenotypic variance. A second advantage to studying 'healthy' relatives is that they are far easier to ascertain than affected sib pairs. The strength of genetic effect can be estimated using the intraclass correlation coefficient (ICC) or relative risk measures. The former is the classic method used with quantitative traits. Relative risk (percentage sibs 'affected'/percentage controls 'affected'), on the other hand, reduces quantitative to qualitative measures, thus 'throwing away' information; however, using relative risk to look specifically for degree of *impairment* (e.g. 1 SD below the control mean) may provide additional evidence that *impairment* itself is heritable (Egan *et al.* 2000, 2001a). For most biological traits, such as cognitive performance, prior studies have already clearly demonstrated a genetic component. Deriving an ICC value from families with schizophrenia does not directly address the question of the heritability of impaired function.

A recurring theme in the sections below relates to the difficulties with replication. Several factors may be involved. First, initial reports of putative intermediate phenotypes typically include small numbers of subjects that are not systematically ascertained. Secondly, control groups are sometimes poorly described. More recent studies have screened out controls with

significant psychopathology or recruit controls with higher IQs than relatives, often from the hospital staff (referred to herein as 'supernormal' controls). In contrast, family cohorts are frequently mixtures of parents and siblings with a variety of psychiatric disorders, including depression and schizophrenia spectrum disorders. While it is critical to describe the normal control group carefully, failure to match control subjects to family members on variables such as age, gender, education, IQ or psychiatric morbidity may introduce bias by reducing neurobiological deficits in the control group, increasing differences between controls and sibs and artificially elevating relative risk scores. Thus, in comparing studies below, specific methodological aspects are highlighted when appropriate in an effort to shed light on inconsistent findings.

Design of genetic studies using intermediate phenotypes

The two general approaches to finding genes for complex disorders are linkage and association (see Chapter 14). Linkage, which uses two or more members from the same family, may be underpowered relative to association studies for complex traits (Risch & Merikangas 1996), although for phenotypes with a simple mode of inheritance this may not be the case. For example, abnormal sensory gating, assessed using the P50 wave, appears to have a simple Mendelian inheritance pattern in families studied thus far. Most of the intermediate phenotypes described below, however, do not have a clear genetic architecture and seem likely to be at least oligogenic or polygenic. Therefore, using linkage with densely affected family members may not be optimal for some phenotypes. A second concern with linkage is that using either elderly or very young subjects in multigenerational families can introduce additional variance from ageing and developmental processes. Using age as a covariate may not adequately adjust measures because they may have a non-linear relationship to age. Thus, it may be difficult, for example, to attribute enlarged ventricles in elderly subjects to the effects of schizophrenia genes, in contrast to ageing, medical illness, etc. A second linkage design, using affected sib pairs, can also be difficult given the high rates of drug and alcohol abuse that confound most phenotypic measures described below. Excluding such subjects makes recruiting adequate numbers extremely difficult. An alternate strategy is to use quantitative genetic methods with unaffected and affected sibs. One example of this type of study uses extreme discordant sib pairs, which may provide much of the power in genetic analyses of unselected sib pairs (Risch & Zhang 1995).

Some of the limitations of linkage can be avoided using association methods, which include case–control and family-based designs and both qualitative (e.g. diagnoses) or quantitative traits. Briefly, with case–control designs, gene frequencies are compared between probands and controls, but poor matching for ethnicity (or population stratification) can produce spurious results. Using additional genetic markers to test for such stratification (Pritchard & Rosenberg 1999; Pritchard *et al.* 2000) may circumvent this problem. Family-based designs use genotypes of family members as controls, including parents (for qualitative phenotypes; Spielman *et al.* 1993) or siblings (for qualitative or quantitative measures; Allison *et al.* 1999). Given that age is likely to affect many intermediate phenotypes, using sibs may provide an advantage over multigenerational designs. Such sib pairs could also be used for sib linkage analyses, such as the extreme discordant method. However, recruitment is more difficult with family-based designs, but allows one to assess familiality of putative intermediate phenotypes if not previously known. Finally, future studies are likely to involve a combination of linkage and association, whereby case–control samples are compared for all genetic variation. This approach takes advantage of linkage disequilibrium to look for haplotypes shared by affected subjects more often than controls.

Eye tracking dysfunction

Abnormalities in eye tracking are one of the first and most extensively studied candidate intermediate phenotypes in schizophrenia. Observed early in the twentieth century, eye tracking dysfunction (ETD) was rediscovered by Holzman (Holzman *et al.* 1973) who also noted impairment in unaffected relatives (Holzman *et al.* 1974). The initial excitement that ETD may identify a simple Mendelian trait related to risk for schizophrenia (Holzman *et al.* 1988) gradually gave way as additional studies produced conflicting findings. A review of this extensive literature highlights many of the issues that confront and confound studies of intermediate phenotypes. For example, which measures should be used? Is ETD affected by neuroleptics? To what degree is ETD genetic and how is it related to risk for schizophrenia? Unfortunately, despite many years of intensive effort, it remains uncertain how useful ETD may be for finding susceptibility genes for schizophrenia.

Studies of eye tracking dysfunction in patients with schizophrenia

Over 100 studies have been published on ETD in patients with schizophrenia, addressing issues ranging from frequency, specificity, effects of medications, familiality and underlying neurobiology. An important consideration in evaluating and comparing these studies is the methods used to record eye movements, the task employed, outcome measures and the nature of the control and patient groups. Electro-oculography and, more recently, high-resolution infrared oculography have been the primary methods used to assess and quantify ETD. Qualitative ratings of how closely the eye tracks the target have been advanced as a dependable method of assessing overall performance, but such measures do little to clarify the precise mechanism underlying global impairment. Consequently, most recent studies include a variety of quantitative parameters. The two most frequently studied aspects of eye tracking are the smooth pursuit and saccade systems (Table 15.1; for review see Levy *et al.* 1993). Gain,

Table 15.1 Eye tracking measures.

Gain: speed of eye relative to speed of target

Root mean square (RMS) error: measure of how closely the eye is foveated on the target throughout the task
Example: Gain (eye speed) may closely match target speed but consistently lag behind target. In this case gain would be normal while RMS error would be reduced

Saccades: rapid movement of eye toward a target
Example: during eye tracking, the eye may jump ahead of target (anticipatory saccade) or, if gain is reduced and the eye falls behind the target, a 'catch-up' saccade can bring the eye back to the target
Saccades may have varying amplitudes. 'Small' saccades are generally those that travel less than 4° of the visual field

Antisaccade task: subjects have to move eyes rapidly to a specified location on the *opposite* side of the visual field from a remembered target. This task is very difficult, particularly for patients. One must inhibit the initial temptation to look towards the remembered target

or speed of the eye, is a measure of the smooth pursuit system and is slowed in patients. Saccades are very rapid movements used to move the eye quickly toward a target, such as when one hears a voice and rapidly turns the eye to the estimated position of the speaker. Patients with schizophrenia, during smooth pursuit, follow the target slowly and often show compensatory saccades to catch-up to the target ('catch-up saccades') (Levy *et al.* 1994). Subjects may also move ahead of the target ('anticipatory saccades'). Thus, the most commonly reported pattern in patients is reduced gain, with a compensatory increase in catch-up saccades to correct the increasing error in eye position (Levy *et al.* 1994). Some studies have reported normal gain and a primary deficit in intrusive saccades (Levin *et al.* 1982). Another frequently used outcome measure is root mean square (RMS) error, which captures how closely the eye remains foveated on the target and is thus reduced by slow gain and saccades that move the fovea off target. RMS error is typically reduced in patients but does not distinguish which system is responsible for the impairment. Estimates of the frequency of ETD (typically using qualitative ratings, gain and/or RMS error) in patients with schizophrenia range from 20% to 80%. Reasons for this large range are unclear but may be related to differences in methodology, the measures used and/or ascertainment issues (see below).

Other abnormalities in eye movement during visual tasks have also been found. For example, simple fixation, or the ability to stay focused on a fixed target, may be impaired in patients (Amador *et al.* 1995). Patients also simply spend less time engaged in pursuit tasks (Friedman *et al.* 1995). Increased small-amplitude saccades, increased phase lag and increased intrusive saccades have been reported as well (Levy *et al.* 1994). In an 'antisaccade' task, subjects must produce a 'volitional' saccade in the direction opposite to the target (McDowell & Clementz 1996). Patients and relatives have difficulty in this (Clementz 1998). Yet another type of eye tracking abnormality, again for 'volitional' saccades, is the memory-guided saccade generated during an oculomotor delayed response task (Park *et al.* 1995; McDowell & Clementz 1996). These additional abnormalities, while promising intermediate phenotypes, appear to involve more than simple eye movements. For example, the delayed response tasks are likely to involve the spatial working memory system. Performance of these other tasks may also be impaired in relatives, and thus serve as potential intermediate phenotypes. The focus of this review is primarily on the more widely studied eye tracking measures derived from sinusoidal tracking tasks.

A number of studies have examined whether ETD is secondary to non-specific factors related to psychiatric illness. One of the most important confounds is treatment with neuroleptic medications. The effects of neuroleptics on ETD have been investigated using a variety of study designs. First, investigators have looked at patients treated chronically with neuroleptics who have been withdrawn for brief periods (several weeks). Most find that eye tracking is no different or may be slightly better when on medications compared with performance when off medications (Holzman *et al.* 1974; Spohn *et al.* 1988; Litman *et al.* 1989). One exception is the atypical neuroleptic clozapine which appears to reduce gain and increase saccade number, perhaps because of its antihistaminic properties (Litman *et al.* 1994). Other atypical antipsychotic drugs do not appear to impair eye tracking although data on this issue are limited (Hutton *et al.* 2001). A second study design is to examine patients early in their illness. ETD, and reduced gain in particular, is seen both in drug-naïve patients as well as treated and untreated first break patients, compared with controls. Thirdly, several studies have found that first episode and/or drug-naïve patients are no different on ETD parameters, including gain, when directly compared with chronic patients withdrawn from medications (Sweeney *et al.* 1994b, 1998, 1999). Fourthly, patients followed over time show that eye tracking abnormalities appear trait-like, remaining stable over extended periods even during marked changes in clinical status (Campion *et al.* 1992; Gooding *et al.* 1994; Sweeney *et al.* 1994b; Yee *et al.* 1998). On the other hand, some studies have suggested that neuroleptics could produce a mildly deleterious effect on eye tracking. For example, chronically treated patients have worse gain compared with first episode patients and chronically ill patients off neuroleptics (Campion *et al.* 1992; Hutton *et al.* 2001). This could be as a result of either some illness-related deterioration or a deleterious effect of long-term neuroleptic treatment. Alternatively, this could be interpreted as a cohort effect. Furthermore, normal controls given haloperidol show increased saccades and worse qualitative performance, although it is unclear whether gain is affected (Malaspina *et al.* 1994). ETD is seen in patients with Parkinsonism and is ameliorated with dopamine agonists (Kuechenmeister *et al.* 1977), suggesting that the reduced dopamine neurotransmission from neuroleptics could produce some ETD. Overall, while these data are consistent with a possible slight deleterious effect of neuroleptics on eye tracking, it seems unlikely that ETD seen in patients with schizophrenia is solely brought about by neuroleptic treatment.

In contrast to neuroleptics, other medications may be more liable to impair some eye tracking measures. Following up on reports of ETD in bipolar patients, several studies have found evidence that lithium can interfere with eye tracking (Levy *et al.* 1985; Holzman *et al.* 1991), although other studies have not (Iacono *et al.* 1992; Gooding *et al.* 1993). Impaired pursuit can also be a result of inattention, fatigue and sedating drugs, such as benzodiazepines (Yee *et al.* 1987). Furthermore, ETD may not be specific to schizophrenia, and has been reported in patients with mood disorders in some (Sweeney *et al.* 1994a, 1999), but not all studies (Levy *et al.* 1985; Iacono *et al.* 1992; for review see Levy *et al.* 1994). Some aspects of ETD can be improved with tasks that increase attention, but the basic deficit in smooth pursuit persists (Sweeney *et al.* 1994a). These studies suggest that to reduce non-genetic sources of variance for eye tracking, subjects should be studied off non-neuroleptic medications when possible and when in a euthymic and rested state. Finally, another potentially important confound is nicotine use. Nicotine withdrawal worsens eye tracking while nicotine administration improves it. The role of smoking in familial eye tracking studies has not been systematically addressed.

One attractive feature of classical eye tracking measures, such as gain and saccades, is that the neurobiology of these systems is increasingly well understood. Visual information from the occipital lobe is processed for motion and target speed in the medial temporal visual area in primates and its likely analogue in humans, the posterior inferior temporal sulcus. From there, visual motion information is relayed to several additional areas, including the middle superior temporal area, and then on to both the frontal eye fields and the posterior parietal cortex. Specific lesions in these areas in primates and humans produce different patterns of abnormalities in smooth pursuit and saccades; those of the frontal lobes most closely mirror the ETD seen in schizophrenia (MacAvoy & Bruce 1995; Lekwuwa & Barnes 1996). Experiments in patients to tease out which mechanisms are responsible have been mixed. Some data suggest that the primary deficit may be underactivation of the frontal eye fields (Sweeney *et al.* 1998, 1999; O'Driscoll *et al.* 1999). Others have found impaired perception of target velocity, referable to the temporal lobe (Chen *et al.* 1999a,b). The saccade system seems intact in some ways. For example, saccade accuracy to catch-up with a rapidly moving target appears normal. On the other hand, patients sometimes show more intrusive saccades, suggesting impaired inhibition. Thus, the exact nature of ETD in patients remains unclear and the idea that several processes are abnormal remains a very real possibility. These include impaired gain, increased intrusive saccades, reduced fixation and overall reduced attentional capacity to stay engaged in the task. This may not be so surprising given the number of temporal and prefrontal abnormalities seen in patients using other functional measures of the neural networks involving these brain regions.

Family studies of eye tracking dysfunction

The history of ETD studies in family members begins in the early 1970s. An initial series of compelling studies by Holzman *et al.* suggested that ETD was common in family members, was unique to schizophrenia and could be accounted for by a single dominant gene. Subsequent studies with improved methods and larger sample sizes began to steadily erode the strength of these findings. Differences in methods and ascertainment may account for some of these discrepancies and are highlighted below. By far the largest number of family studies have looked at smooth pursuit and measures derived from it, including qualitative measures, RMS error and, more recently, gain. Regarding ascertainment, many studies have used 'supernormal' control groups. To the extent that intermediate phenotypes are related to psychopathology, this ascertainment strategy may overestimate the frequency of abnormalities in family members and spuriously increase relative risk estimates. A second confound is age. A number of studies have shown that ETD, similar to other intermediate phenotypic measures, increases in normal subjects with increasing age. Some studies have compared parents of probands with younger controls, which also may artificially increase rates of ETD.

Data from the first 15 years of family studies indicated that ETD was very common in schizophrenia and their relatives. In Holzman's initial family study, 53–86% of probands, who were acutely psychotic inpatients ($n = 40$) or chronically institutionalized inpatients ($n = 29$), had ETD. The group of relatives included 35 psychiatrically healthy first-degree family members (aged 17–60) who were compared with a younger psychiatrically screened control group. Qualitative measures ('normal' vs. 'deviant') were used; 15 out of 34 relatives (42.8%) were classified as 'deviant' compared with only six out of 72 normal controls (8.3%) (Holzman *et al.* 1974, 1988). This yields a relative risk of 5 or more, less than that for schizophrenia but still substantial and consistent with a strong genetic trait. Kuechenmeister *et al.* (1977) were the first to attempt to replicate this finding in a small group of parents, again using qualitative scores, who were compared with age- and gender-matched controls (10 per group). While the mean scores were different between groups, the percentage of 'deviant' parents was not given. A third study found that 39% of 44 first-degree relatives had ETD, using a qualitative scoring method, compared with an age-matched 'supernormal' control group (Siegel *et al.* 1984). Two subsequent small studies reported ETD in teenage offspring (Mather 1985) but not parents (Whicker *et al.* 1985) of subjects with schizophrenia. In another study of parents, Holzman found only 34% (13/38) had ETD compared with 10% (2/21) of parents of bipolar probands using cut-off criteria established from a large control group of unstated age (Holzman *et al.* 1984). Holzman also examined offspring of patients with schizophrenia: 27% had ETD (Holzman *et al.* 1988). Remarkably, the pedigrees used for this study showed that at least two male probands had eight and nine offspring, respectively, highly unusual for schizophrenia, suggesting they were very atypical. Thus, over the first 15 years

of research on ETD, rates in relatives ranged from 27% to 43%, while the only reported rate in a control group was 8% in a 'supernormal' group of only 72 subjects.

Efforts to analyse the nature of ETD using quantitative measures in somewhat larger cohorts of patients and family members followed. Clementz *et al.* (1990) investigated ETD in a group of 24 patients recently admitted to the Payne Whitney Clinic, 58 first-degree relatives (mean age = 44.1), the majority of whom were parents, and a 'supernormal' control group (mean age = 38.9) screened for psychiatric disorders. 'Unaffected' relatives had impaired pursuit gain compared with the control group, and relatives with schizophrenia spectrum disorders (11/58) had even more impaired gain. Anticipatory saccades followed a similar pattern. Next, Grove *et al.* (1991) measured RMS error, gain and anticipatory saccades in 46 relatives (parents and siblings mixed) compared with 18 'supernormal' controls, with mean ages not given. They found no difference between these two groups in RMS error but gain was worse in relatives with a moderate effect size. Remarkably, the low sib intraclass correlations suggested that the heritability of gain was essentially zero! In an important epidemiological study, Iacono *et al.* (1992) studied ETD in 482 subjects, including 157 probands with psychiatric disorders. Only 51 patients with schizophrenia and 52 of their relatives were included. Over 40% of the relatives had a variety of psychiatric disorders compared with none in the younger 'supernormal' control group. RMS error, the primary outcome measure, was worse in patients with schizophrenia and their relatives. Furthermore, the distribution was skewed and appeared to fit a two-component model best. Using 2 SD as the cut-off, only 20% of probands and relatives had ETD compared with no more than 7% in non-schizophrenic patient groups and controls. This suggests a relative risk of roughly 3. Clementz, in an effort to replicate this finding, reanalysed data from two prior studies (Clementz *et al.* 1990; Grove *et al.* 1991) and also found a bimodal distribution. Furthermore, Clementz *et al.* found a relatively low prevalence of ETD in patients (20–37%) and relatives (19–22%). Finally, Blackwood *et al.* (1991), in the largest study to date, examined ETD in 151 non-schizophrenic subjects from 20 families (each with at least two index cases) compared with a 'supernormal' control group ($n = 135$). Relatives of patients with schizophrenia showed a bimodal distribution of ETD (using log of signal/noise ratio). Of the 107 relatives with no psychiatric history, 15 fell 2 SD below the control mean, compared with roughly 20% of probands and 5% of controls. This also suggests a relative risk of roughly 3, albeit in a markedly different family cohort. Thus, three relatively large studies, with different ascertainment methods, are consistent in suggesting that ETD is present in a fairly small percentage of patients and relatives. These are considerably smaller frequencies than suggested in earlier studies by Holzman *et al.* However, similar to earlier studies, they often employ younger 'supernormal' control groups, and thus may overestimate the magnitude of risk to family members.

Several more recent studies have failed to shed further light on the prevalence, relative risk or heritability of ETD (Amador *et al.* 1995; Thaker *et al.* 1996; Kinney *et al.* 1998; Ross *et al.* 1998). In a relatively large cohort, Keefe *et al.* (1997) studied 83 non-psychotic first-degree relatives (mostly siblings) from 38 families, compared with 45 'supernormal' controls. Data were analysed only for between 46 and 64 relatives and 25–35 controls, and it is unclear how well these subgroups were matched for age. No group differences were found in gain or large amplitude saccades, although qualitative ratings were markedly worse in relatives. These studies continue to suggest that family members have subtle ETD, but the magnitude of the effect is generally weak and the use of 'supernormal' controls raises questions even about this.

Twin studies have been used to assess the heritability of ETD but results are difficult to interpret. Holzman examined two separate but small samples of monozygotic (MZ) and dizygotic (DZ) twins. In the first study of 11 MZ twins (four at least 'partially' concordant for schizophrenia) and 15 DZ twins (one pair 'partially' concordant), five of seven MZ pairs and seven of 13 DZ pairs were concordant for ETD. Although these ratios are not significantly different, the results were described as supporting a genetic hypothesis (Holzman *et al.* 1977); however, they equally support a non-genetic hypothesis. In their second twin study, which included subjects with schizophrenia and other psychotic disorders, seven of 10 MZ twins pairs were concordant for 'good' and three of three were concordant for 'bad' eye tracking. In the DZ group, 10 pairs were concordant (five for 'good', three for 'bad' tracking) (Holzman *et al.* 1980). These rates are again not significantly different but were again interpreted as indicating that ETD is partly genetic. In a third study of 12 discordant MZ twins compared with 12 control twin pairs, Litman *et al.* (1997) found no differences in scores from the unaffected cotwins of discordant pairs compared with controls. This suggests that the penetrance for ETD is no different from that for the clinical phenotype but the data are not suitable for estimating genetic portion of total phenotypic variance in the population. Overall, the twin data, even when combined, are not sufficient to permit an estimation of how this putative trait is related to genetic risk for schizophrenia.

Genetic models of eye tracking dysfunction

Despite the uncertainties, family data have been used to develop genetic models relating ETD to risk for schizophrenia. It is worth noting that studies of normal twins indicate that eye tracking *per se* is likely to have a genetic component (Iacono & Lykken 1979a,b), although this does not indicate that poor tracking is related to genetic risk for schizophrenia. Holzman *et al.* first suggested that a single dominant gene (frequency 0.09) with no phenocopies could account for their data and may produce ETD in schizophrenia. This seems overly optimistic, if for no other reason than the many reports that ETD phenocopies can be produced by a variety of drugs, ageing and psychi-

atric states. They further suggested that such a gene produced a latent trait with variable phenotypic expression, accounting for observations of normal eye tracking in some patients who had family members with poor eye tracking. Iacono *et al.* (1992) noted that their finding of a bimodal distribution was also consistent with a single gene. Similarly, Clementz *et al.* (1992) combined data from two studies (Clementz *et al.* 1990; Grove *et al.* 1991) and found evidence consistent with a single dominant gene for both RMS error and gain, but not for anticipatory saccades or signal/noise ratios. Interestingly, they reported that sib correlations were significantly higher than parent–offspring correlations for gain and RMS error, a pattern indicating a dominance component of genetic variance, which is not shared by parent–offspring pairs. On the other hand, Grove *et al.* (1992) reported the opposite. They combined three samples (from Iacono, Clementz and Grove) and applied segregation analysis using RMS error and Elston's SAGE program. In this sample, they found parent–offspring correlations of 0.29 and sib correlations of 0.32, which were not different and are not consistent with a dominance genetic component. Their data fit best a mixed model which includes a major gene effect and polygenic component and rejects a simple polygenic model, but not oligogenic models (Grove *et al.* 1992). Despite the heuristic value of such modelling, the results are critically dependent on the accuracy of correlations between various types of relatives, which are based on very small sample sizes relative to those needed to estimate family correlations with confidence. Secondly, correlations between parents and offspring can be confounded by age much more than sib–sib correlations, adding further noise to genetic modelling. Overall, it remains unclear exactly what the genetic architecture of ETD is and how many genes contribute to both ETD and risk for schizophrenia.

Summary

The vast literature on ETD demonstrates the vicissitudes associated with searching for intermediate phenotypes associated with schizophrenia. While it appears unlikely that ETD is caused solely by neuroleptics or other non-specific factors related to chronic mental illness, the critical issue of whether relatives have increased rates of ETD remains uncertain. Most family studies do show increased rates, but frequency estimates have steadily eroded over time and the persistent use of 'supernormal' control groups leaves some room for doubt. It seems very possible that ETD is present in some family members, but the effect size may be small and the relative risk is likely to be 3 or less. Whether gain, RMS error, qualitative ratings or some other measure best captures the genetic component of variance is unclear. Genetic modelling, while initially suggesting a single major dominant gene, has been based on relatively small sample sizes and is plagued by other methodological problems, such as confounds caused by age. Thus, it seems increasingly doubtful that a single gene will explain more than a small portion of variance in ETD. One published linkage study, which attempted to use eye tracking to improve power, has demonstrated enthusiasm for this approach but has not been replicated and has not led to the discovery of a specific gene (Arolt *et al.* 1996). On the other hand, the physiology of eye tracking is increasingly well understood and functional variants in obvious candidate genes can now be examined to assess their effects on this phenotype.

Clinical phenotypes (see also Chapter 7)

Odd personalities among the biological relatives of schizophrenic subjects have been observed both by Kraepelin (1919) and Bleuler (1911). These observations have had a key role in the definition of the DSM-III (American Psychiatric Association 1968) criteria for schizotypal personality. In addition to the diagnostic criteria, self-report scales have been developed to quantitatively assess schizotypy and the different aspects of proneness to psychosis. Definitions of schizotypy and the different instruments used vary. In particular, the hypothesis of anhedonia being a quantitative family marker has received thorough exploration since the work of Meehl (1962), who used the term 'schizotype' to refer to individuals who possess underlying vulnerability for schizophrenia. Meehl recommended assessing schizotypic signs through objective measures rather than clinical judgement. Chapman and Chapman (1984) found that individuals who were identified by high scores on their Social Anhedonia Scale (SAS), Physical Anhedonia Scale (PAS), Perceptual Aberration Scale (PABS) or Magical Ideation Scale (MIS) differed from controls on a variety of schizotypal features and identify subjects showing deficits in sustained attention similar to those in schizophrenics (Lenzenweger *et al.* 1991). Ten years later, the Chapman scales that showed the best predictive validity were the MIS and the SAS, whereas the PAS and the Impulsive Nonconformity Scale were not effective predictors of psychosis proneness (Chapman *et al.* 1994). Heritability studies have also been conducted using sibling intraclass correlation analysis. A greater heritability has been found for the PAS and for the PABS rather than for the SAS and the MIS (Clementz *et al.* 1991; Berenbaum & McGrew 1993; Lyons *et al.* 1995).

Using a family design, five studies have tested the Chapman self-rating scales to assess anhedonia among relatives of schizophrenic probands compared with relatives of controls. Katsanis *et al.* (1990) examined 44 relatives of schizophrenic probands and 160 normal subjects. The relatives of schizophrenic patients had higher scores on physical and social anhedonia but lower on perceptual aberration. Grove *et al.* (1991) showed that relatives of schizophrenic patients ($n = 61$) scored higher on physical anhedonia than normal controls ($n = 18$). Clementz *et al.* (1991) found that relatives of schizophrenic patients ($n = 146$) scored higher on physical anhedonia and lower on perceptual aberration than 178 normal controls. Franke *et al.* (1993) found that compared with 32 controls, healthy siblings of schizophrenic patients had higher levels of social anhedonia but similar levels of perceptual aberration. Kendler *et al.* (1996) showed that only relatives of schizophrenic patients scored higher on social anhedonia than relatives of three other proband groups (other non-affective psychoses, psychotic affective illness and non-psychotic affective illness). Altogether, fairly consistent results have shown that anhedonia scales (physical and/or social), but not PABS or MIS constitute useful indicators of liability among relatives of schizophrenic probands. It should also be noted that several authors have found significant correlations between scores on both physical and social anhedonia (Clementz *et al.* 1991; Grove *et al.* 1991; Kendler *et al.* 1991), while MIS and PABS are highly correlated and form a 'positive schizotypy 'dimension. It is thus likely that the more negative schizotypal traits such as social anhedonia are better indices of the familial liability to schizophrenia than are more psychotic-like traits such as magical thinking or illusions.

Meaningful dimensions of symptoms in schizophrenia have recently focused on the characterization of positive symptoms (e.g. disorganized thinking, hallucinations and delusions) and negative symptoms (e.g. anhedonia, limited speech and social withdrawal). The Scale for the Assessment of Negative Symptoms (SANS) and the Scale for the Assessment of Positive Symptoms (SAPS) are commonly used to rate these symptoms (Andeasen *et al.* 1982). Negative symptoms are more stable over time than positive symptoms (Addington & Addington 1991) and seem to be the main source of familial aggregation in schizophrenia. A twin study by Dworkin and Lenzenweger (1984) found an increased concordance rate for schizophrenic twins with two or more negative symptoms, but not for positive symptoms. They also found that negative symptoms, but not positive symptoms, were correlated between pairs concordant for schizophrenia. Sautter *et al.* (1987) found that a family history of schizophrenia correlated with negative symptoms. Kay *et al.* (1986) also reported that negative symptoms were positively correlated with a family history of major psychiatric disorders, but negatively with a family history of affective disorders. Tsuang *et al.* (1993) showed that negative symptom ratings are higher for the relatives of schizophrenics, whereas positive symptoms were similar for the relatives of schizophrenic patients and depressive controls. These findings suggest that negative symptoms could reflect familial liability to schizophrenia, whereas positive symptoms reflect a clinical endophenotype common both to affective disorders and to schizophrenia. Indeed, several studies have demonstrated a familial relationship between schizophrenia and affective disorders, in particular with psychotic affective disorders (Taylor *et al.* 1993). Thus, one might hypothesize that the shared phenotype might be represented by positive symptoms. Bruztowicz *et al.* (1997) provided the first evidence of the interest of using a quantitative dimensional approach in linkage study. Positive linkage with chromosome 6p markers was obtained only when using as phenotype scores on positive symptoms both among schizophrenic patients and their non-affected relatives. Negative linkage results were obtained with negative scores or with a classical nosographical approach.

Neurochemical phenotypes

(see also Chapter 16)

Investigation of neurochemical abnormalities among unaffected relatives of schizophrenic patients is a convenient method to explore biochemical predisposition to schizophrenia in natural conditions, without any pharmacological challenge and in the absence of confounding factors such as chronicity of illness or effects of medication. Dopamine (DA) abnormalities have been explored in non-psychotic relatives as negative and positive symptoms are hypothesized to be caused by decreased and increased brain DA functions.

Amin et al. (1999) showed that healthy first-degree relatives of schizophrenic patients (n = 55) had decreased plasma homovanillic acid (HVA), the major DA metabolite, compared with 20 normal subjects. This finding is supported by similar results in a subgroup of relatives (Waldo et al. 1992). Such decreased plasma HVA in relation to negative symptoms is hypothesized to be a result of mesocortical DA activity, but it is unclear whether and to what degree plasma HVA is a measure of central DA function. In schizophrenic patients, proteins involved in DA uptake and metabolism have been extensively studied; i.e. platelet monamine oxidase-B (MAO-B), D_2 lymphocyte binding sites, positron emission tomography (PET) studies of DA receptors and measures of prolactin (PRL) or growth hormone (GH) have been used for assessment of static and dynamic DA function, but so far there have been very few studies of these parameters in unaffected relatives of schizophrenic patients. Increased densities of postsynaptic DA function [^{3}H]spiperone binding sites on lymphocytes have been reported in one-third of the well relatives of schizophrenic probands (Bondy & Ackenheil 1987). Sautter et al. (1987) have investigated the familiality of the GH response to apomorphine in patients with schizophrenia. They found that the GH response differentiated the relative risk of schizophrenia in families; probands with high GH response had the lowest familial risk. Regarding serotonergic parameters, two studies have reported higher cerebrospinal fluid 5-hydroxyindoleacetic acid (5-HIAA) concentrations in schizophrenic patients with a strong positive family history of schizophrenia (Sedvall & Wode-Helgodt 1980). To our knowledge, studies of neuroendocrine measures of 5-hydroxytryptamine (5-HT) function and platelet markers of 5-HT function have not yet been undertaken in individuals at risk for schizophrenia.

Electrophysiological markers

Cognitive event-related potentials (ERPs) have been widely used as potential indicators of risk for schizophrenia (for review see Friedman & Squires-Wheeler 1994). ERPs are usually measured in terms of amplitude, latency and topography of a component. ERPs elicited by infrequent auditory targets, for example during an oddball paradigm, are characterized successively by an early component, N100, which reflects the sensory analysis of the physical parameters of the stimulus (Näätänen & Picton 1987), then N200, which reflects selective attention processes conducting to stimulus categorization, which is followed by P300 classically related to the postperceptual updating of short-term working memory traces of expected environmental stimuli (Donchin & Isreal 1980). The ERP technique is a safe non-invasive approach to the study of psychophysiological correlates of human mental processes. However, several methodological issues have to be taken into account to infer an underlying physiological deficit, such as whether to use single or several electrode sites and the need to control for age, as amplitude and latency differ as a function of increasing age (Pfefferbaum et al. 1984).

The most robust ERP abnormality in patients with schizophrenia is that of reduced P300 amplitude and increased latency using an oddball paradigm (for review see Friedman & Squires-Wheeler 1994). This finding has been reported in both medicated and unmedicated schizophrenic patients using an auditory modality, whereas the visual modality varies and may serve as a state marker (Duncan et al. 1987; Pfefferbaum et al. 1989; St Claire et al. 1989). Altogether, the abnormal auditory P300 waveform in schizophrenics appears to be independent of medication effect, clinical state (Blackwood et al. 1987), duration of symptoms and clinical subtype of the illness (St Clair et al. 1989). However, reduced P300 is not specific to schizophrenia as it has been reported in a variety of different disorders such as dementia (Pfefferbaum et al. 1984), alcoholism (Porjesz et al. 1980) and bipolar disorder (Muir et al. 1991; Souza et al. 1995). Discrepant results have been obtained concerning the observation of a reduction in the P300 amplitude over the left, compared with the right, temporal scalp in schizophrenic subjects. This finding was originally reported by Morstyn et al. (1983), but has not always been replicated (Pfefferbaum et al. 1989).

High-risk studies provided evidence that P300 abnormalities can be considered as vulnerability indicators. Schreiber et al. (1991) have reported a prolonged P300 latency in the offspring of schizophrenic patients, but no difference for P300 amplitude. Kidogami et al. (1991) observed a reduction in P300 amplitude in the schizophrenic sample and their relatives compared with controls. Blackwood et al. (1991) found P300 amplitude reduction and latency prolongation in the schizophrenia sample and half of their non-schizophrenic relatives showed prolonged P300 latency. However, in those two studies, P300 latency values were not age-adjusted and a single electrode was used. Furthermore, no difference between offspring of schizophrenics and controls was reported by Friedman et al. (1986). Latency prolongation or amplitude reduction has not been observed in schizotypal individuals (Condray & Steinhauser 1992) who are supposed to share genetic variance with schizophrenia. Squires-Wheeler et al. (1993) did not find a link between reduced P300 amplitude in adolescents at risk for schizophrenia and those who become schizophrenic in young adulthood. Thus, on the basis of the existing literature, which is based on small sample size, there is mixed evidence regarding whether P300 abnormalities can be considered as marker traits.

Other abnormalities of the components of the ERPs have been observed in schizophrenia. The negative component peaking at about 100 ms following auditory stimuli (N100) is also reduced in schizophrenia in the auditory but not the visual component (Roth *et al.* 1980). Frontal N100 and parietal P300 component reductions have also been observed in high-risk children compared with controls (Schreiber *et al.* 1992). Schizophrenic patients and their relatives showed similar amplitude reduction and latency prolongation of the N100, N200 and P300 waves compared with controls (Frangou *et al.* 1997). However, N100 reduction is not specific to schizophrenia as it is also observed in patients with major depressive disorder. N100 reduction might be the result of an overlapping component, the processing negativity, which is elicited during selective attention paradigms and appears to be reduced in schizophrenia patients (Michie *et al.* 1990; Shelley *et al.* 1999). A reduction in processing negativity is consistent with deficits in selective attention, which have been proposed to account for some schizophrenic symptomatology.

One of the most promising ERP phenotypes comes from studies of the P50 waveform. This paradigm examines P50 amplitude to two consecutive simple auditory stimuli (usually a clicking noise) (Freedman *et al.* 1983; Siegel *et al.* 1984). The clicks are separated by several hundred milliseconds. The normal response is for subjects to have a reduced P50 response to the second click, suggesting that this repeated stimulus is actively suppressed, perhaps because it is less relevant, and is referred to as sensory gating. Patients with schizophrenia and roughly 50% of their first-degree relatives seem to have impaired sensory gating in this paradigm, as demonstrated by a failure to suppress the P50 wave amplitude to the second click relative to the first. There is some controversy regarding whether the schizophrenia-related deficit represents a 'gating' phenomenon. Some studies have reported that the amplitude from the second click is the same in patients and controls, while the amplitude and/or latency of the first click is altered in patients, perhaps accounting for the decreased ratio (Jin & Potkin 1996; Jin *et al.* 1997). Failure of sensory gating in this paradigm has also been reported in acutely manic patients. It appears to be state-dependent in affective disorders but a stable trait abnormality in families with a schizophrenic proband (Baker *et al.* 1987). The neurobiology of sensory gating has been examined in rodent models and is critically dependent on cholinergic input to the hippocampus (Luntz-Leybman *et al.* 1992). This input is mediated in part by the α7 nicotinic receptor. Remarkably, the P50 phenotype has been used in linkage studies and has shown linkage to a marker very close to the gene for the α7 nicotinic receptor with the 15q32 region (Freedman *et al.* 1997). This constitutes one of the most impressive and successful uses of intermediate phenotypes to dissect the genetics of schizophrenia. However, it remains uncertain exactly what aspect of this gene is responsible for impaired gating and how it contributes to the clinical syndrome of schizophrenia (for discussion see Adler *et al.* 1998).

Neuroimaging phenotypes
(see also Chapter 22)

Neuroimaging techniques have been relatively underutilized in the search for intermediate phenotypes associated with schizophrenia. Nevertheless, they hold significant promise, as such measures appear, at least prima facie, to be closer to the biological effects of genes. Neuroimaging parameters are likely to be less subject to confounds related to understanding directions, motivation and other vicissitudes of testing that might affect, for example, eye tracking and neuropsychological tests. A recent demonstration of the surprising power of neuroimaging measures comes from a study of the effects of *COMT* genotype on prefrontal function (Egan *et al.* 2001b). In this study, the effects of the val108/158met polymorphism, which has a profound effect on enzyme activity and prefrontal dopamine catabolism, could be detected using functional magnetic resonance imaging (fMRI) measures of prefrontal efficiency during a working memory task with as few as 15 subjects. In contrast, several hundred subjects were needed to detect this effect using scores from the working memory task. This suggests that the fMRI-derived measures of frontal lobe function are much closer to the direct effects of *COMT*, compared with test scores. Efforts to uncover other neuroimaging phenotypes have generated promising leads. However, many of these studies have suffered some of the same methodological confounds seen with other techniques, such as small sample sizes and the use of 'supernormal' control groups. By far the most intensive efforts have been directed towards structural measures derived from computerized tomography (CT) and magnetic resonance imaging (MRI) scans. fMRI and magnetic resonance spectroscopy (MRS) have also been used in a handful of studies, while methods involving radioactive ligands, such as PET and single photon emission computerized tomography (SPECT), have not.

Structural measures derived from CT and MR images seem prime candidates to serve as intermediate phenotypes, given their hypothesized role in the pathophysiology of schizophrenia (see Chapter 22). However, the results from different studies are not consistent and no clear phenotype has emerged. In the first CT study of family members, Weinberger *et al.* (1981) found increased lateral ventricular size in 12 siblings compared with a well-matched control group. Ill siblings had larger ventricles compared with well siblings, who in turn had larger ventricles than controls, suggesting a relationship to genetic risk for schizophrenia. On the other hand, there was no correlation between ill and well siblings, indicating a lack of genetic effect. A second study by DeLisi *et al.* (1986) found just the opposite. Ten non-psychotic siblings were compared with 20 controls. Both groups included subjects with a variety of non-psychotic psychiatric disorders. No differences were seen on several volumetric measures between sibs and controls. However, there was clearly an effect of family membership on ventricular size in schizophrenic families (DeLisi *et al.* 1986). In a third study, DeLisi *et al.* looked at 11 sib pairs concordant for schizophrenia and found significant correlations for some measures, e.g. left posterior hippocampal volume, but not others, e.g. total left hippocampal volume (DeLisi *et al.* 1988). The small sample size makes these results and their anatomical specificities seem somewhat unreliable.

In a fourth and more ambitious CT study, Cannon *et al.* (1989) looked at 34 offspring who had either one or two parents with schizophrenia. Most of these offspring also had a schizophrenia spectrum diagnosis themselves. The authors found that increasing lateral ventricular size and reduced cortical volume were associated with increasing genetic risk (i.e. having a father with spectrum disorder) for schizophrenia. While consistent with a genetic effect, this could also be because of shared environmental effects of having two ill parents or simply as a result of confounds of the illness itself, because the offspring had high rates of schizophrenia spectrum disorder (Cannon *et al.* 1989, 1993). Looking at the factor structure of these CT measurements, Cannon *et al.* (1989) found two factors: one for cortical volumetric deficits and a second for lateral and third ventricular enlargement. Prospectively ascertained labour and delivery complications were correlated with the ventricular factor but not the cortical factor, suggesting two independent processes. Cannon *et al.* (1993) expanded their sample in a remarkable second study of 97 offspring, and found similar results. Genetic risk for schizophrenia again predicted cortical and ventricular volumetric abnormalities, and the latter interacted with labour and delivery complications. This was seen in the total group as well as a group including only the new subjects, and even when patients with schizophrenia were excluded. These provocative findings were, nevertheless, somewhat clouded by possible methodological issues, such as the inclusion of subjects with organic brain syndromes and head injury, and the inherent imprecision of CT. Finally, a recent CT study by Silverman *et al.* (1998) reported essentially no differences between siblings ($n = 69$) and controls ($n = 22$), although a very strong correlation was found between family members, confirming that there is a family component for ventricular size *per se*. In this study, lateral ventricular enlargement was seen in probands compared with siblings but not controls, suggesting an atypical proband group. Overall, the CT literature provides support for the notion that structural abnormalities commonly seen in patients, such as ventricular enlargement, may also be present in family members; however, the findings are highly inconsistent, making it difficult to draw firm conclusions.

Despite improved resolution of MRI, studies using this technique have also been inconclusive. Initial series of reports were encouraging but were difficult to interpret because of small sample sizes. For example, Dauphinais *et al.* (1990) examined 12 sib pairs concordant for schizophrenia. While several volumetric abnormalities were found, only reduced volume of the cerebral hemisphere was familial. Waldo *et al.* (1994) used MRI to measure hippocampal and amygdala volume in 20 healthy sibs and 43 controls. A strong effect of family on hippocampal volume was observed in schizophrenic families, suggesting a genetic component for this trait, but no differences were observed between sibs and controls. Seidman *et al.* (1997) found

reduced subcortical grey matter and lateral ventricular enlargement in a cohort of six healthy siblings, while Keshavan *et al.* (1997) found reduced left amygdala volume, enlarged third ventricular volume and smaller total brain volume in a group of 11 offspring (mean age 15.1 years) of schizophrenic mothers.

Several larger and better designed MRI studies followed. In an important partial replication of their original CT studies, Cannon *et al.* (1998b) reported reduced cortical grey volume in sibs compared with a well-matched control group. The sibling group included 60 non-psychotic subjects largely past the age of risk. Sibs did not differ from controls on ventricular volume, a measure that combined lateral and third ventricular volumes. In a second large MRI study (Sharma *et al.* 1998), 57 unaffected relatives (parents and siblings) from 16 families with at least two affected subjects were compared with a younger supernormal control group. Relatives had enlarged left but not right lateral ventricles. No difference in cortical grey or white matter volume was observed between patients, relatives and controls. In contrast, Lawrie *et al.* (1999) found reduced thalamic as well as amygdala–hippocampal volume in 100 subjects at 'high risk' (two relatives with schizophrenia) compared with a 'supernormal' control group. A weak trend ($P = 0.09$) was found for reduced left prefrontal volume but there was no difference in lateral ventricular volume. Many of these young at-risk subjects are likely to later develop schizophrenia, suggesting that these findings could be antecedents to the illness itself. In a follow-up study with an expanded sample size, similar findings were reported (Lawrie *et al.* 2001). Reduced amygdala–hippocampal volume was also recently reported in a small sample of healthy adult siblings ($n = 20$) compared with a well-matched control group (O'Driscoll *et al.* 2001) and in a cohort ($n = 28$) of healthy parents, sibs and adult children (Seidman *et al.* 1999). Finally, Staal *et al.* (1998, 2000) found only third ventricular enlargement and reduced thalamic volume in 16 healthy siblings compared with a carefully matched control group. Remarkably, no differences were seen between sibs and controls for volumes of a number of other structures, including the lateral ventricles, the hippocampi, and prefrontal grey or white matter (Staal *et al.* 2000). Thus, at least three fairly large studies of subjects with increased genetic risk for schizophrenia have reported three different abnormalities:

1 reduced cortical grey matter volume;
2 enlarged lateral ventricles; and
3 reduced amygdala–hippocampal and thalamic volume.

The third finding has also been seen in two smaller subsequent studies. Of the three large studies, two used 'supernormal' controls, which should accentuate differences between relatives and controls. While the reasons for the lack of replication are uncertain, these results indicate that structural measures are not robust discriminators of family members from controls.

Structural imaging studies of twins provide another avenue to explore genetic aspects of volumetric alterations but fail to clarify whether these measures are good intermediate phenotypes. Reveley *et al.* (1982) in a CT study of 11 MZ and eight DZ healthy twin pairs showed that lateral ventricular size is highly heritable. In a small sample of seven MZ pairs of twins discordant for schizophrenia, they also found high heritability (70% and above) which was less than the heritability estimated for normal twins (87–98%). Affected MZ twins generally had larger ventricles relative to their unaffected cotwin, who in turn tended to have increased ventricular size relative to normal twin pairs, suggesting that part of the ventricular enlargement in schizophrenia is genetic. Suddath et al. (1990), using MRI, looked at 15 discordant MZ twin pairs and found that affected twins had larger lateral and third ventricles and smaller rostral hippocampi. Similar findings emerged when the data set was expanded to 22 MZ discordant pairs (McNeil 2000). Unfortunately, the authors did not look at differences between the unaffected twin and controls or correlations between pairs, leaving it unclear whether these abnormalities were familial. Baare et al. (2001) replicated these findings to some degree in a study of 15 MZ and 14 DZ discordant twin pairs. They also reported reduced hippocampal, intracranial and frontal lobe volumes in the MZ twin pairs. The correlation coefficients suggested that the discordant MZ twins were much more similar for most structural measures compared with the discordant DZ twins, although confidence intervals were very large, making conclusions difficult. Nevertheless, this careful comparison provides additional support for the notion that prefrontal, intracranial and whole brain volume reductions could be useful intermediate phenotypes. Overall, both CT and MRI structural studies indicate that some volumetric abnormalities, such as ventricular enlargement or reduced cortical or mesial temporal volume, may be present in family members, but the inconsistencies suggest that the effect size may be small and that further study is needed.

Volumetric data from structural scans have been used to derive measures of asymmetry and to test these as potential intermediate phenotypes. For example, Frangou (1997) looked at volume and asymmetry of the planum temporale in 32 patients, 55 of their non-psychotic first-degree relatives and 39 controls. They found no difference between the control group and relatives or patients. DeLisi (1997) looked at sylvian fissure asymmetry in 14 pairs of schizophrenia siblings and found a meagre yet significant effect of family for one of three measures, consistent with a possible genetic component. Asymmetry based on volumetric measures does not seem to be a robust intermediate phenotype.

Only a handful of studies have looked at neuroimaging parameters other than volumetric measures. Klemm et al. (2001) used phosphorus-31 magnetic resonance spectroscopic imaging (MRSI) to study 14 first-degree relatives (sibs and offspring) compared with 14 age-matched controls. Relatives had increased phosphodiesters, interpreted by the authors as suggesting increased breakdown of phospholipids in the prefrontal cortex. Keshavan et al. (1997) found a trend for reduced cingulate N-acetylaspartate (NAA) measures in a small group ($n = 10$) of young offspring of schizophrenic mothers. Callicott et al. (1998a), in by far the largest cohort of siblings studied with MRSI to date, looked at 60 healthy siblings compared with 66 controls. Siblings had significant reduced hippocampal NAA

measures, with relative risk estimates ranging from 3.8 to 9, depending on the criteria to define abnormal NAA (e.g. 1 or 2 SD below the control mean.). Block et al. (2000) found no differences in NAA levels in a cohort of 35 non-psychotic family members but only looked in the prefrontal cortex. Of note, Callicott et al. also found no reductions in sib prefrontal cortex. Two groups have reported abnormalities in prefrontal physiology in family members. First, Blackwood et al. (1999) noted reduced prefrontal blood flow in a cohort of 36 first-degree relatives using SPECT. Similarly, abnormalities in prefrontal blood flow ('inefficiency') were seen by Callicott et al. (1998b) using fMRI. As noted above, this phenotype was useful in demonstrating the effect of COMT val158met genotype on prefrontal function.

In summary, neuroimaging methods have been used to elucidate several potential intermediate phenotypes. Data from structural measures, particularly MRI studies, have provided some evidence of abnormalities including ventricular enlargement, reduced cortical volume and reduced mesial temporal volume, which vary from study to study. This troubling lack of consistency could either be a result of subtle methodological differences between studies, such as ascertainment issues, or may indicate that these are not robust phenotypes. Several other measurements, including neurochemical measurements from MRSI and physiological measures from fMRI, seem very promising but replications in large samples with well-matched control groups are needed.

Cognitive phenotypes

Neuropsychological deficits are a prominent dimension of schizophrenia and may account for a substantial portion of the functional impairments in daily living (see Chapter 10). An impressive number of studies of first-degree relatives also indicate that cognitive impairments may be familial and that the pattern of such deficits is similar to, albeit less severe than, that seen in patients themselves (Cannon et al. 1994; Kremen et al. 1994). Furthermore, the shared variance between tests of different cognitive domains is small, suggesting that there may be several cognitive phenotypes suitable for use as intermediate phenotypes (Egan et al. 2001a). Studies of neuropsychological deficits share some of the same problems described above for studies of other intermediate phenotypes, such as the use of 'supernormal' controls and inconsistent results. However, overall matching with controls is generally better than that seen in other studies: subjects with Axis I disorders are excluded but siblings with Axis II disorders are included, whereas controls with these disorders are not. Such studies of 'healthy' sibs and their matched 'supernormal' controls therefore are less likely to overestimate differences between sibs and controls. Furthermore, while inconsistencies exist, the majority of studies are positive, suggesting that the differences are real.

The earliest family studies focused on 'at-risk' children of schizophrenic mothers. These children exhibited a variety of behavioural abnormalities including impaired attention (Fish

1977; Parnas *et al.* 1982). Studies using more rigorous neuropsychological testing, such as the continuous performance tests (CPT), soon followed (Nuechterlein & Dawson 1984; Cornblatt & Keilp 1994). 'At-risk' children do poorly on these tests, particularly on harder versions (Grunebaum *et al.* 1974; Asarnow *et al.* 1977; Rutschmann *et al.* 1977, 1986). The type of CPT used may be important, because more difficult CPT tasks are likely to involve cognitive demands beyond pure attention. Some versions (e.g. the identical pairs (IP) version) have significant working memory loads, which may therefore confound impaired attention with impaired working memory. Adult siblings largely past the age of risk for schizophrenia have also shown impairment on CPT performance, again primarily with more difficult versions (Nuechterlein & Dawson 1984; Mirsky *et al.* 1992; Franke *et al.* 1993; Cornblatt & Keilp 1994). Studies using simpler versions of the CPT have been mixed. One recent large study using well-matched controls found no overall differences between sibs ($n = 193$) and controls ($n = 47$) (Egan 2000), although sibs of probands with impaired attention were worse as a group compared with controls. Two studies have reported a trend for impaired attention in sibs (Keefe *et al.* 1997; Laurent *et al.* 2000), while five have reported marked impairments (Maier *et al.* 1992; Cannon *et al.* 1994; Finkelstein *et al.* 1997; Chen *et al.* 1998; Saoud *et al.* 2000). The reasons for discrepancies between studies are unclear. Some studies used 'supernormal' control groups (Finkelstein *et al.* 1997; Keefe *et al.* 1997) and have included sib groups with relatively high rates of schizophrenia spectrum disorders, such as personality disorders (Cannon *et al.* 1994; Finkelstein *et al.* 1997; Keefe *et al.* 1997). Some studies include both parents and siblings, leading to possible bias as a result of age effects (Chen *et al.* 1998).

Several studies have tried to quantify the magnitude of the familial effect on impaired attention. Grove *et al.* (1991) estimated heritability of CPT performance in 61 first-degree relatives using the ICC and found $h^2 = 0.79$, suggesting a substantial genetic component. A second study of a Taiwanese cohort (parents and siblings, $n = 148$) using the 1–9 version with degraded stimuli (Chen *et al.* 1998) found very high rates of impairment in relatives compared with controls. Relative risk of 'impaired attention' was 18–130, depending on the cut-off criteria, which is dramatically higher than the relative risk for schizophrenia itself. In contrast, a second large study of 193 siblings in a US cohort (Egan *et al.* 2000) found only slightly increased relative risk in a subgroup of siblings. The marked differences in these relative risk values could be a result of confounds such as ethnicity, recruitment biases, education and type of relatives (parent or sib) studied. Overall, it remains possible that subtle deficits in attention are present in siblings, or at least in a subgroup, that these deficits are not simply antecedents of illness and that CPT measures could serve as a useful intermediate phenotype, but the effect seems weak.

Soon after impaired attention was noted, a variety of additional cognitive deficits were reported in family members. In general, these include cognitive tasks referable to prefrontal and mesial temporal structures. Prefrontal deficits were seen using several tests, most notably the Wisconsin Card Sort Test (WCST) but also tests of verbal fluency and the 'N back' working memory task. Secondly, tests of declarative memory, such as the Wechsler Memory Scale, revised version (WMS-R) or the California Verbal List Test (CVLT), have also tended to be abnormal in first-degree family members. Thirdly, scores on the Trail Making tests, including A and B versions, are reduced, implicating oculomotor scanning/psychomotor speed. Poor Trails B performance, while a crude measure sensitive to many neurological insults, is also seen with prefrontal deficits. Other abnormalities have also been reported, although less consistently (Kremen *et al.* 1994).

Studies employing fairly comprehensive neuropsychological batteries, while somewhat inconsistent, suggest the effect size in the moderate range for several tests with abnormalities seen even in psychiatrically healthy relatives. First, Pogue-Geile *et al.* (1991), in 40 non-schizophrenic sibs, and then Franke *et al.* (1992, 1993), in 33 healthy sibs, both found impaired performance on the WCST, Trails B and verbal fluency compared with well-matched control groups. On the other hand, Scarone *et al.* (1993) found no differences in WCST in 35 well siblings compared with matched but supernormal controls. Yurgelun-Todd and Kinnney (1993) found lower scores on the WCST but not Trails B in a group of 15 healthy sibs. Shedlack *et al.* (1997) found essentially no differences between 14 well siblings from multiplex families and well-matched 'supernormal' controls on verbal memory. In contrast, Cannon *et al.* (1994) found impaired performance on a large battery of tests including attention, working memory/executive function and verbal memory in 16 non-schizophrenic siblings, but six of 16 had definite or likely schizotypal personality disorder compared with 'supernormal' controls. Larger studies have more consistently found differences. Keefe *et al.* (1994), in a cohort of 54 non-psychotic first-degree relatives, found impaired performance on Trails B and verbal fluency (both letter and category), but not on the WCST, compared with 'supernormal' controls. Faraone *et al.* (1995) found impairments in abstraction, verbal memory and attention in a group of 35 non-psychotic first-degree relatives similar to the results of Toomey *et al.* (1998), who found impaired working memory (WCST) and verbal memory in an overlapping sample of 54 first-degree healthy relatives. Both studies apparently used the same well-matched control group, screened using the Minnesota Multiphasic Personality Inventory (MMPI). Egan *et al.* (2001a), in a study of 193 siblings compared with a closely matched control group, found deficits on WCST, Trails B and CVLT, whether or not subjects with schizophrenia spectrum disorders were included in these groups. Thus, as studies have included larger groups of siblings, more consistent differences have emerged and implicate the same brain regions and cognitive functions that are typically seen in patients with schizophrenia, including prefrontal cortex/working memory and ventral temporal lobe/declarative memory.

Two major studies have examined cognitive deficits in twins. In the first study of discordant twins, Goldberg *et al.* (1993, 1994, 1995), using a wide neuropsychological battery, found that unaffected MZ twins have subtle cognitive deficits for the WMS-R, with trends for impairment on WCST perseverative errors (PE) and Trails A ($P < 0.05$) (Goldberg *et al.* 1995). A second study of 18 MZ and 34 DZ discordant twin pairs examined the relationship between cognitive deficits and genetic risk for schizophrenia using canonical discriminant analysis (Cannon *et al.* 2000b). Four tests contributed unique genetic variance to increased risk for schizophrenia. These tests were spatial working memory (visual span test of the WMS-R), divided attention (using a Brown–Peterson dual-task paradigm), intrusions during recall of a word list (CVLT) and choice reaction time (using a Posner paradigm related to the CPT). It is unclear whether the same group differences were seen with these MZ twins compared with the Goldberg sample. In Cannon's analysis, verbal memory was more impaired in affected MZ subjects, relative to cotwins, suggesting an effect of unique environmental variance related to illness. While these data leave open the question of which tests are most informative for genetic studies, the conclusions are similar to those of other relatives in one important respect. Several domains of cognition are impaired, including working memory/executive function and some aspects of verbal recall and attention, which are related to genetic risk for schizophrenia.

Finding deficits on several neuropsychological tests does not necessarily mean that these measure independent traits. An alternative possibility is that impairments are found on different tests because of one underlying abnormality. Attempts to address this question, using several statistical approaches, suggest that this is not the case. For example, correlations between measures are generally low in these groups (Yurgelun-Todd & Kinney 1993; Keefe *et al.* 1994). On the other hand, Toomey *et al.* (1998) found fairly high correlations between attention and verbal memory and between attention and abstraction in a cohort of 54 first-degree relatives, but no significant correlation between WCST and memory measures (on the WMS-R). Egan *et al.* (2001a), using multiple regression, found only modest shared variance (less than 15% in siblings) between measures of working memory, verbal memory and psychomotor speed. Using factor analysis, Mirsky *et al.* (1991) and Kremen *et al.* (1992) found that WCST and Trails B load on different factors, similar to Egan *et al.* (2001a). Finally, Cannon *et al.* (2000b), in a critical analysis of MZ and DZ twins, found evidence for four distinct independent cognitive deficits using canonical discriminant analysis. In non-patient populations, factor analysis has consistently shown that most of the variance on tests of different cognitive domains load significantly on the first factor, often referred to as 'g'. In contrast, analyses of patient and sib groups, which include subjects with a variety of impairments, tend to find somewhat less loading on the first factor and more evidence of additional orthogonal factors where both patients and siblings have lower scores than controls. Overall, these results suggest that several independent domains of cognitive dysfunction are related to genetic risk for schizophrenia and that correlation and factor analytic studies could show different results because of different patterns of impairments.

Is it plausible to use neuropsychological phenotypes to find schizophrenia genes? Support for this approach comes from a recent finding by Egan *et al.* (2001b) using working memory and the WCST as the phenotype. One attractive aspect of using working memory is that the neurobiology is increasingly well understood (Williams & Goldman-Rakic 1995; Goldman-Rakic *et al.* 1996). Specifically, D_1-mediated dopamine neurotransmission at glutamatergic neurones in the prefrontal cortex is critical. While there is essentially no known genetic variance affecting D_1-receptor function or other factors modulating dopamine prefrontal tone, an important exception is COMT. This enzyme is critical for inactivating released dopamine (Karoum *et al.* 1994) and knock-outs show increased prefrontal dopamine (Gogos *et al.* 1998), a regional specificity that is likely to be caused by the paucity of the dopamine transporter in prefrontal cortex (Sesack *et al.* 1998). Also, remarkably, several studies in animals and humans suggest that reduced COMT activity improves working memory (Kneavel *et al.* 2000). The val/met polymorphism produces a dramatic effect on COMT enzyme activity (Weinshilboum & Dunnette 1981). Thus, the *val* allele would be expected to be related to relatively reduced working memory. In a cohort of 175 patients, 200 siblings and 45 controls, Egan *et al.* (2001b) found that the COMT genotype was associated with working memory; subjects with the *val* allele had worse scores. Furthermore, the *val* allele was associated with schizophrenia using the transmission disequilibrium test (TDT). Thus, this intermediate phenotype pointed to gene and mechanism of action, making the weak association much more plausible.

Other phenotypes

A variety of other abnormalities found in patients with schizophrenia have also been examined in relatives. These include measures such as handedness, neurological signs (Egan *et al.* 2001c), minor physical anomalies (Ismail *et al.* 1998), finger ridge counts (Davis & Bracha 1996) and others. In general, these studies are relatively small, very few or inconclusive.

Conclusions

Do intermediate phenotypes exist and can they be used to find genes that increase risk for schizophrenia.? The substantial body of research reviewed above suggest that the answer to both is a qualified yes. Many phenotypic measures have been examined in relatives of patients with schizophrenia and many differences have been reported when compared with controls. Unfortunately, replication has often been difficult. Studies of eye tracking dysfunction, the archetypical intermediate phenotype, demonstrate many of the vicissitudes that can lead to inconsistent and misleading results. One reason for the inconsistencies seems to be ascertainment. Because both age and psychopathology may be related to intermediate phenotypic measures, relatives and controls should be matched closely on age and psychiatric status. Other variables may also be relevant, such as gender, IQ, smoking or others. Eye tracking dysfunction remains a viable candidate phenotype and has been used successfully in one linkage study, but it appears that the genetic architecture is more complex than initially imagined and the likely contribution of eye tracking dysfunction genes to risk for schizophrenia is far from clear.

Data on clinical phenotypes suggest that negative symptoms may be an important focus for future research, although the lack of neurobiological models for negative symptoms could reduce their utility and it is unclear if the genetics of negative symptoms are any more tractable than that of schizophrenia itself. The use of neurochemical and neuroimaging phenotypes is in its infancy, but both seem to be promising areas for future research. Studies using electrophysiological markers, such as those related to P300 waveform, have been plagued by inconsistencies. One bright spot has been the use of the P50 waveform and the sensory gating paradigm. Neuropsychological abnormalities, which are more reliably found in relatives, in contrast to many other phenotypic measures, also hold promise for the future. Sensory gating and working memory measures have been used to demonstrate the effects of two genes, the $\alpha7$ nicotinic receptor and *COMT*, on biology and risk for schizophrenia. While replication is needed, these findings provide some validation for the utility of this approach. Clearly, further work is needed to describe more elementary phenotypes that are related to mechanisms relevant for neural function and that have simpler genetic architecture. For example, deficits in memory could be caused by abnormal encoding, early or late phases of long-term potentiation (LTP), or to other factors related to dendrite formation and stabilization in response to learning (see e.g. Milner *et al.* 1998). Deficits in prefrontal function may be related to processes, such as neuronal migration, or presynaptic dopamine input. Unfortunately, at present, there are no methods to study such elemental phenotypes in human subjects.

Several problems confront future studies using intermediate phenotypes. First, it is unclear whether any of these phenotypes will provide substantially simpler genetic architecture. Most are themselves complex. Secondly, given the unknown genetic architecture, it is difficult to predict how many subjects are required to detect quantitative trait loci that account for only a few per cent of total phenotypic variance. Thirdly, intermediate phenotypes are also plagued with problems of phenocopies. Neurobiological abnormalities may occur because of medications, drug abuse or other problems associated with chronic mental illness. Finally, the relationship between various measures is also uncertain, and some are bound to overlap, wholly or in part.

Beyond the methodological problems, inconsistencies and weak findings in family studies of intermediate phenotypes may indicate something about the neurobiology of genetic risk for schizophrenia. The effects of susceptibility genes on psychiatrically healthy relatives, who must have some of these genes, seems slight. This could be because of a variety of factors, such as the need for specific environmental triggers or other genetic loci

acting in a multiplicative or epistatic fashion. A second factor could be heterogeneity. If there are different neurobiological pathways to develop schizophrenia, only some families will demonstrate some abnormalities. This could dilute the findings in relatives if all types are lumped together. Overall, it remains uncertain how useful intermediate phenotypes will be to find genes. It is very possible that the bulk of schizophrenia susceptibility genes may be found using traditional methods without these measures. On the other hand, given the difficulties encountered using psychiatric nosology and the dramatic advances in molecular neuroscience, which offer increasingly attractive candidate genes for phenotypes such as verbal and working memory, intermediate phenotypes remain attractive targets for genetic studies of schizophrenia.

References

Addington, J. & Addington, D. (1991) Positive and negative symptoms of schizophrenia. Their course and relationship over time. *Schizophrenia Research* 5, 51–59.

Adler, L.E., Olincy, A., Waldo, M. *et al.* (1998) Schizophrenia, sensory gating, and nicotinic receptors. *Schizophrenia Bulletin* 24, 189–202.

Allison, D.B., Heo, M., Kaplan, N. & Martin, E.R. (1999) Sibling-based tests of linkage and association for quantitative traits. *American Journal of Human Genetics* 64, 1754–1763.

Amador, X.F., Malaspina, D., Sackeim, H.A. *et al.* (1995) Visual fixation and smooth pursuit eye movement abnormalities in patients with schizophrenia and their relatives. *Journal of Neuropsychiatry and Clinical Neuroscience* 7, 197–206.

American Psychiatric Association. (1994) *Diagnostic and Statistical Manual of Mental Disorders*, 4th edn (DSM-IV). American Psychiatric Association, Washington, DC.

Amin, E., Silverman, J.M., Siever, L.J. *et al.* (1999) Genetic antecedents of dopamine dysfunction in schizophrenia. *Biological Psychiatry* 45, 1143–1150.

Andreasen, N.C. & Olsen, S. (1982) Negative v positive schizophrenia. Definition and validation. *Archives of General Psychiatry* 39, 789–794.

Arolt, V., Lencer, R., Nolte, A. *et al.* (1996) Eye tracking dysfunction is a putative phenotypic susceptibility marker of schizophrenia and maps to a locus on chromosome 6p in families with multiple occurrence of the disease. *American Journal of Medical Genetics* 67, 564–579.

Asarnow, R.F., Steffy, R.A., MacCrimmon, D.J. & Cleghorn, J.M. (1977) An attentional assessment of foster children at risk for schizophrenia. *Journal of Abnormal Psychology* 86, 267–275.

Asarnow, R.F., Steffy, R.A., MacCrimmon, D.J. *et al.* (1978) The McMaster Waterloo project. In: *An Attentional and Clinical Assessment of Foster Children at Risk for Schizophrenia. The Nature of Schizophrenia: New Approaches to Research and Treatment.* (eds L.C. Wynne, R.L. Cromwell & S. Matthysse), pp. 339–358. Wiley, New York.

Baare, W.F., van Oel, C.J., Hulshoff Pol, H.E. *et al.* (2001) Volumes of brain structures in twins discordant for schizophrenia. *Archives of General Psychiatry* 58, 33–40.

Baker, N., Adler, L.E., Franks, R.D. *et al.* (1987) Neurophysiological assessment of sensory gating in psychiatric inpatients: comparison between schizophrenia and other diagnoses. *Biological Psychiatry* 22, 603–617.

Berenbaum, H. & McGrew, J. (1993) Familial resemblance of schizotypic traits. *Psychological Medicine* 23, 327–333.

Blackwood, D.H., Whalley, L.J., Christie, J.E. *et al.* (1987) Changes in auditory P3 event-related potential in schizophrenia and depression. *British Journal of Psychiatry* 150, 154–160.

Blackwood, D.H., St Clair, D.M., Muir, W.J. & Duffy, J.C. (1991) Auditory P300 and eye tracking dysfunction in schizophrenic pedigrees. *Archives of General Psychiatry* 48, 899–909.

Blackwood, D.H., Glabus, M.F., Dunan, J. *et al.* (1999) Altered cerebral perfusion measured by SPECT in relatives of patients with schizophrenia: correlations with memory and P300. *British Journal of Psychiatry* 175, 357–366.

Bleuler, E. (1911) Dementia praecox oder Die Gruppe der Schizophrenien. In: *Handbuch der Psychiatrie, hrsg. Von G. Aschaffenburg,* Deiticke.

Block, W., Bayer, T.A., Tepest, R. *et al.* (2000) Decreased frontal lobe ratio of N-acetyl aspartate to choline in familial schizophrenia: a proton magnetic resonance spectroscopy study. *Neuroscience Letters* 289, 147–151.

Bondy, B. & Ackenheil, M. (1987) ^{3}H-Spiperone binding sites in lymphocytes as possible vulnerability marker in schizophrenia. *Journal of Psychiatric Research* 21, 521–529.

Brzustowicz, L.M., Honer, W.G., Chow, E.W. *et al.* (1997) Use of a quantitative trait to map a locus associated with severity of positive symptoms in familial schizophrenia to chromosome 6p. *American Journal of Human Genetics* 61, 1388–1396.

Callicott, J.H., Egan, M.F., Bertolino, A. *et al.* (1998a) Hippocampal N-acetyl aspartate in unaffected siblings of patients with schizophrenia: a possible intermediate neurobiological phenotype. *Biological Psychiatry* 44, 941–950.

Callicott, J., Egan, M., Mattay V. *et al.* (1998b) Altered prefrontal cortical function in unaffected siblings of patients with schizophrenia. *Neuroimage* 7, S895.

Campion, D., Thibaut, F., Denise, P. *et al.* (1992) SPEM impairment in drug-naive schizophrenic patients: evidence for a trait marker. *Biological Psychiatry* 32, 891–902.

Cannon, T.D., Mednick, S.A. & Parnas, J. (1989) Genetic and perinatal determinants of structural brain deficits in schizophrenia. *Archives of General Psychiatry* 46, 883–889.

Cannon, T.D., Mednick, S.A., Parnas, J. *et al.* (1993) Developmental brain abnormalities in the offspring of schizophrenic mothers. I. Contributions of genetic and perinatal factors. *Archives of General Psychiatry* 50, 551–564.

Cannon, T.D., Zorrilla, L.E., Shtasel, D. *et al.* (1994) Neuropsychological functioning in siblings discordant for schizophrenia and healthy volunteers. *Archives of General Psychiatry* 51, 651–661.

Cannon, T.D., Kaprio, J., Lonnqvist, J., Huttunen, M. & Koskenvuo, M. (1998a) The genetic epidemiology of schizophrenia in a Finnish twin cohort: a population-based modeling study. *Archives of General Psychiatry* 55, 67–74.

Cannon, T.D., van Erp, T.G., Huttunen, M. *et al.* (1998b) Regional gray matter, white matter, and cerebrospinal fluid distributions in schizophrenic patients, their siblings, and controls. *Archives of General Psychiatry* 55, 1084–1091.

Cannon, T.D., Bearden, C.E., Hollister, J.M. *et al.* (2000a) Childhood cognitive functioning in schizophrenia patients and their unaffected siblings: a prospective cohort study. *Schizophrenia Bulletin* 26, 379–393.

Cannon, T.D., Huttunen, M.O., Lonnqvist, J. *et al.* (2000b) The inheritance of neuropsychological dysfunction in twins discordant for schizophrenia. *American Journal of Human Genetics* 67, 369–382.

Chapman, L.J. & Chapman, J.P. (1984) Psychosis proneness. In: *Con-troversies in Schizophrenia: Changes and Constancies* (ed. M. Alpert), pp. 157–174. Guilford, New York.

Chapman, L.J., Chapman, J.P., Kwapil, T.R., Eckblad, M. & Zinser, M.C. (1994) Putatively psychosis-prone subjects 10 years later. *Journal of Abnormal Psychology* 103, 171–183.

Chen, W.J., Liu, S.K., Chang, C.J. *et al.* (1998) Sustained attention deficit and schizotypal personality features in non-psychotic relatives of schizophrenic patients. *American Journal of Psychiatry* 155, 1214–1220.

Chen, Y., Levy, D.L., Nakayama, K. *et al.* (1999a) Dependence of impaired eye tracking on deficient velocity discrimination in schizophrenia. *Archives of General Psychiatry* 56, 155–161.

Chen, Y., Palafox, G.P., Nakayama, K. *et al.* (1999b) Motion perception in schizophrenia. *Archives of General Psychiatry* 56, 149–154.

Clementz, B.A. (1998) Psychophysiological measures of (dis) inhibition as liability indicators for schizophrenia. *Psychophysiology* 35, 648–668.

Clementz, B.A., Sweeney, J.A., Hirt, M. & Haas, G. (1990) Pursuit gain and saccadic intrusions in first-degree relatives of probands with schizophrenia. *Journal of Abnormal Psychology* 99, 327–335.

Clementz, B.A., Grove, W.M., Katsanis, J. & Iacono, W.G. (1991) Psychometric detection of schizotypy: perceptual aberration and physical anhedonia in relatives of schizophrenics. *Journal of Abnormal Psychology* 100, 607–612.

Condray, R. & Steinhauer, S.R. (1992) Schizotypal personality disorder in individuals with and without schizophrenic relatives: similarities and contrasts in neurocognitive and clinical functioning. *Schizophrenia Research* 7, 33–41.

Cornblatt, B.A. & Keilp, J.G. (1994) Impaired attention, genetics, and the pathophysiology of schizophrenia. *Schizophrenia Bulletin* 20, 31–46. [Published erratum appears in *Schizophrenia Bulletin* 1994; 20, 248.]

Dauphinais, I.D., DeLisi, L.E., Crow, T.J. *et al.* (1990) Reduction in temporal lobe size in siblings with schizophrenia: a magnetic resonance imaging study. *Psychiatry Research* 35, 137–147.

Davis, J.O. & Bracha, H.S. (1996) Prenatal growth markers in schizophrenia: a monozygotic co-twin control study. *American Journal of Psychiatry* 153, 1166–1172.

DeLisi, L.E., Goldin, L.R., Hamovit, J.R. *et al.* (1986) A family study of the association of increased ventricular size with schizophrenia. *Archives of General Psychiatry* 43, 148–153.

DeLisi, L.E., Dauphinais, I.D. & Gershon, E.S. (1988) Perinatal complications and reduced size of brain limbic structures in familial schizophrenia. *Schizophrenia Bulletin* 14, 185–191.

DeLisi, L.E., Sakuma, M., Kushner, M. *et al.* (1997) Anomalous cerebral asymmetry and language processing in schizophrenia. *Schizophr Bull* 23, 255–271.

Donchin, E. & Isreal, J.B. (1980) Event-related potentials and psychological theory. *Progress in Brain Research* 54, 697–715.

Duncan, C.C., Perlstein, W.M. & Morihisa, J.M. (1987) The P300 metric in schizophrenia: effects of probability and modality. *Electroencephalogr and Clinical Neurophysiology* 40, 670–674.

Dworkin, R.H. & Lenzenweger, M.F. (1984) Symptoms and the genetics of schizophrenia: implications for diagnosis. *American Journal of Psychiatry* 141, 1541–1546.

Egan, M.F. & Weinberger, D.R. (1997) Neurobiology of schizophrenia. *Current Opinions in Neurobiology* 7, 701–707.

Egan, M.F., Goldberg, T.E., Gscheidle, T. *et al.* (2000) Relative risk of attention deficits in siblings of patients with schizophrenia. *American Journal of Psychiatry* 157, 1309–1316.

Egan, M.F., Goldberg, T.E., Gscheidle, T. *et al.* (2001a) Relative risk for cognitive impairments in siblings of patients with schizophrenia. *Biological Psychiatry* 50, 98–107.

Egan, M.F., Goldberg, T.E., Kolachana, B.S. *et al.* (2001b) Effect of COMT Val108/158Met genotype on frontal lobe function and risk for schizophrenia. *Proceedings of the National Academy of Sciences of the USA* 98, 6917–6922.

Egan, M.F., Hyde, T.M., Bonomo, J.B. *et al.* (2001c) Relative risk of neurological signs in siblings of patients with schizophrenia. *American Journal of Psychiatry* 158, 1827–1834.

Falconer, D.S. & Mackay, T.F.C. eds. (1996) *Introduction to Quantitative Genetics*, Vol. 4, Longman, Essex.

Faraone, S.V., Seidman, L.J., Kremen, W.S. *et al.* (1995) Neuropsychological functioning among the nonpsychotic relatives of schizophrenic patients: a diagnostic efficiency analysis. *Journal of Abnormal Psychology* 104, 286–304.

Finkelstein, J.R., Cannon, T.D., Gur, R.E., Gur, R.C. & Moberg, P. (1997) Attentional dysfunctions in neuroleptic-naive and neuroleptic-withdrawn schizophrenic patients and their siblings. *Journal of Abnormal Psychology* 106, 203–212.

Fish, B. (1977) Neurobiologic antecedents of schizophrenia in children: evidence for an inherited, congenital neurointegrative defect. *Archives of General Psychiatry* 34, 1297–1313.

Frangou, S., Sharma, T., Sigmudsson, T. *et al.* (1997) The Maudsley Family Study. 4. Normal planum temporale asymmetry in familial schizophrenia. A volumetric MRI study. *British Journal of Psychiatry* 170, 328–333.

Franke, P., Maier, W., Hain, C. & Klingler, T. (1992) Wisconsin Card Sorting Test: an indicator of vulnerability to schizophrenia? *Schizophrenia Research* 6, 243–249.

Franke, P., Maier, W., Hardt, J. & Hain, C. (1993) Cognitive functioning and anhedonia in subjects at risk for schizophrenia. *Schizophrenia Research* 10, 77–84.

Freedman, R., Adler, L.E., Waldo, M.C., Pachtman, E. & Franks, R.D. (1983) Neurophysiological evidence for a defect in inhibitory pathways in schizophrenia: comparison of medicated and drug-free patients. *Biological Psychiatry* 18, 537–551.

Freedman, R., Coon, H., Myles-Worsley, M. *et al.* (1997) Linkage of a neurophysiological deficit in schizophrenia to a chromosome 15 locus. *Proceedings of the National Academy of Sciences of the USA* 94, 587–592.

Freedman, R., Adler, L.E. & Leonard, S. (1999) Alternative phenotypes for the complex genetics of schizophrenia. *Biological Psychiatry* 45, 551–558.

Friedman, D. & Squires-Wheeler, E. (1994) Event-related potentials (ERPs) as indicators of risk for schizophrenia. *Schizophrenia Bulletin* 20, 63–74.

Friedman, D., Cornblatt, B., Vaughan, H. Jr & Erlenmeyer-Kimling, L. (1986) Event-related potentials in children at risk for schizophrenia during two versions of the continuous performance test. *Psychiatry Research* 18, 161–177.

Friedman, L., Jesberger, J.A., Siever, L.J. *et al.* (1995) Smooth pursuit performance in patients with affective disorders or schizophrenia and normal controls: analysis with specific oculomotor measures, RMS error and qualitative ratings. *Psychological Medicine* 25, 387–403.

Gogos, J.A., Morgan, M., Luine, V. *et al.* (1998) Catechol-O-methyltransferase-deficient mice exhibit sexually dimorphic changes in catecholamine levels and behavior. *Proceedings of the National Academy of Sciences of the USA* 95, 9991–9996.

Goldberg, T.E., Torrey, E.F., Gold, J.M. *et al.* (1993) Learning and memory in monozygotic twins discordant for schizophrenia. *Psychological Medicine* 23, 71–85.

Goldberg, T.E., Torrey, E.F., Berman, K.F. & Weinberger, D.R. (1994)

Relations between neuropsychological performance and brain morphological and physiological measures in monozygotic twins discordant for schizophrenia. *Psychiatry Research* 55, 51–61.

Goldberg, T.E., Torrey, E.F., Gold, J.M. *et al.* (1995) Genetic risk of neuropsychological impairment in schizophrenia: a study of monozygotic twins discordant and concordant for the disorder. *Schizophrenia Research* 17, 77–84.

Goldman-Rakic, P.S., Bergson, C., Mrzljak, L. & Williams G.V. (1996) Dopamine receptors and cognitive function in nonhuman primates. In Neve, K.A. & Neve, R.L. (eds), *The Dopamine Receptors*. New Jersey.: Human Press/Totowa, pp 499–522.

Gooding, D.C., Iacono, W.G., Katsanis, J., Beiser, M. & Grove, W.M. (1993) The association between lithium carbonate and smooth pursuit eye tracking among first-episode patients with psychotic affective disorders. *Psychophysiology* 30, 3–9.

Gooding, D.C., Iacono, W.G. & Beiser, M. (1994) Temporal stability of smooth-pursuit eye tracking in first-episode psychosis. *Psychophysiology* 31, 62–67.

Green, M.F. (1996) What are the functional consequences of neurocognitive deficits in schizophrenia? *American Journal of Psychiatry* 15, 321–330.

Greenberg, D.A., Delgado-Escueta, A.V., Widelitz, H. *et al.* (1988) Juvenile myoclonic epilepsy (JME) may be linked to the BF and HLA loci on human chromosome 6. *American Journal of Medical Cenetics* 31, 185–192.

Grove, W.M., Lebow, B.S., Clementz, B.A. *et al.* (1991) Familial prevalence and coaggregation of schizotypy indicators: a multitrait family study. *Journal of Abnormal Psychology* 100, 115–121.

Grove, W.M., Clementz, B.A., Iacono, W.G. & Katsanis, J. (1992) Smooth pursuit ocular motor dysfunction in schizophrenia: evidence for a major gene. *American Journal of Psychiatry* 149, 1362–1368.

Grunebaum, H., Weiss, J.L., Gallant, D. & Cohler, B.J. (1974) Attention in young children of psychotic mothers. *American Journal of Psychiatry* 131, 887–891.

Holzman, P.S., Proctor, L.R. & Hughes, D.W. (1973) Eye-tracking patterns in schizophrenia. *Science* 181, 179–181.

Holzman, P.S., Proctor, L.R., Levy, D.L. *et al.* (1974) Eye-tracking dysfunctions in schizophrenic patients and their relatives. *Archives of General Psychiatry* 31, 143–151.

Holzman, P.S., Kringlen, E., Levy, D.L. *et al.* (1977) Abnormal-pursuit eye movements in schizophrenia: evidence for a genetic indicator. *Archives of General Psychiatry* 34, 802–805.

Holzman, P.S., Kringlen, E., Levy, D.L. & Haberman, S.J. (1980) Deviant eye tracking in twins discordant for psychosis: a replication. *Archives of General Psychiatry* 37, 627–631.

Holzman, P.S., Solomon, C.M., Levin, S. & Waternaux, C.S. (1984) Pursuit eye movement dysfunctions in schizophrenia: family evidence for specificity. *Archives of General Psychiatry* 41, 136–139.

Holzman, P.S., Kringlen, E., Matthysse, S. *et al.* (1988) A single dominant gene can account for eye tracking dysfunctions and schizophrenia in offspring of discordant twins [see comments]. *Archives of General Psychiatry* 45, 641–647.

Holzman, P.S., O'Brian, C. & Waternaux, C. (1991) Effects of lithium treatment on eye movements. *Biological Psychiatry* 29, 1001–1015.

Hutton, S.B., Crawford, T.J., Gibbins, H. *et al.* (2001) Short- and long-term effects of antipsychotic medication on smooth pursuit eye tracking in schizophrenia. *Psychopharmacology* 157, 284–291.

Iacono, W.G. & Lykken, D.T. (1979a) Electro-oculographic recording and scoring of smooth pursuit and saccadic eye tracking: a parametric study using monozygotic twins. *Psychophysiology* 16, 94–107.

Iacono, W.G. & Lykken, D.T. (1979b) Eye tracking and psychopathology: new procedures applied to a sample of normal monozygotic twins. *Archives of General Psychiatry* 36, 1361–1369.

Iacono, W.G., Moreau, M., Beiser, M., Fleming, J.A. & Lin, T.Y. (1992) Smooth-pursuit eye tracking in first-episode psychotic patients and their relatives. *Journal of Abnormal Psychology* **101**, 104–116.

Ismail, B., Cantor-Graae, E. & McNeil, T.F. (1998) Minor physical anomalies in schizophrenic patients and their siblings. *American Journal of Psychiatry* **155**, 1695–1702.

Jin, Y. & Potkin, S.G. (1996) P50 changes with visual interference in normal subjects: a sensory distraction model for schizophrenia. *Clinical Electroencephalography* **27**, 151–154.

Jin, Y., Potkin, S.G., Patterson, J.V. *et al.* (1997) Effects of P50 temporal variability on sensory gating in schizophrenia. *Psychiatry Research* **70**, 71–81.

Karoum, F., Chrapusta, S.J. & Egan, M.F. (1994) 3-Methoxytyramine is the major metabolite of released dopamine in the rat frontal cortex: reassessment of the effects of antipsychotics on the dynamics of dopamine release and metabolism in the frontal cortex, nucleus accumbens, and striatum by a simple two pool model. *Journal of Neurochemistry* **63**, 972–979.

Katsanis, J., Iacono, W.G. & Beiser, M. (1990) Anhedonia and perceptual aberration in first episode psychotic patients and their relatives. *Journal of Abnormal Psychology* **99**, 202–206.

Kay, S.R., Fiszbein, A., Lindenmayer, J.P. & Opler, I.A. (1986) Positive and negative syndromes in schizophrenia as a function of chronicity. *Acta Psychiatrica Scandinavica* **74**, 507–518.

Keefe, R.S., Silverman, J.M., Roitman, S.E. *et al.* (1994) Performance of non-psychotic relatives of schizophrenic patients on cognitive tests. *Psychiatry Research* **53**, 1–12.

Keefe, R.S., Silverman, J.M., Mohs, R.C. *et al.* (1997) Eye tracking, attention, and schizotypal symptoms in nonpsychotic relatives of patients with schizophrenia [see comments]. *Archives of General Psychiatry* **54**, 169–176.

Kendler, K.S., Ochs, A.L., Gorman, A.M. *et al.* (1991) The structure of schizotypy: a pilot multitrait twin study. *Psychiatry Research* **36**, 19–36.

Kendler, K.S., Thacker, L. & Walsh, D. (1996) Self-report measures of schizotypy as indices of familial vulnerability to schizophrenia. *Schizophrenia Bulletin* **22**, 511–520.

Keshavan, M.S., Montrose, D.M., Pierri, J.N. *et al.* (1997) Magnetic resonance imaging and spectroscopy in offspring at risk for schizophrenia: preliminary studies. *Progress in Neuropsychopharmacology and Biological Psychiatry* **21**, 1285–1295.

Kidogami, Y., Yoneda, H., Asaba, H. & Sakai, T. (1991) P300 in first degree relatives of schizophrenics. *Schizophrenia Research* **6**, 9–13.

Kinney, D.K., Levy, D.L., Yurgelun-Todd, D.A., Tramer, S.J. & Holzman, P.S. (1998) Inverse relationship of perinatal complications and eye tracking dysfunction in relatives of patients with schizophrenia: evidence for a two-factor model. *American Journal of Psychiatry* **155**, 976–978.

Klemm, S., Rzanny, R., Riehemann, S. *et al.* (2001) Cerebral phosphate metabolism in first-degree relatives of patients with schizophrenia. *American Journal of Psychiatry* **158**, 958–960.

Kneavel, M., Gogos, J., Karayiorgou, K. & Luine, V. (2000) *Interaction of COMT Gene Deletion and Environment on Cognition*, abstract 571.20. Society for Neuroscience, 30th Annual Meeting.

Kraepelin, E. (1919) *Dementia Praecox and Paraphrenia*. Livingstone, Edinburgh.

Kremen, W.S., Tsuang, M.T., Faraone, S.V. & Lyons, M.J. (1992) Using vulnerability indicators to compare conceptual models of genetic heterogeneity in schizophrenia. *Journal of Nervous and Mental Disease* **180**, 141–152.

Kremen, W.S., Seidman, L.J., Pepple, J.R. *et al.* (1994) Neuropsychological risk indicators for schizophrenia: a review of family studies. *Schizophrenia Bulletin* **20**, 103–119.

Kuechenmeister, C.A., Linton, P.H., Mueller, T.V. & White, H.B. (1977) Eye tracking in relation to age, sex, and illness. *Archives of General Psychiatry* **34**, 578–579.

Lalouel, J.M., Le Mignon, L. Simon, M. *et al.* (1985) Genetic analysis of idiopathic hemochromatosis using both qualitative (disease status) and quantitative (serum iron) information. *American Journal of Human Genetics* **37**, 700–718.

Lander, E.S. & Schork, N.J. (1994) Genetics dissection of complex traits. *Science* **265**, 2037–2048.

Laurent, A., Biloa-Tang, M., Bougerol, T. *et al.* (2000) Executive/attentional performance and measures of schizotypy in patients with schizophrenia and in their non-psychotic first-degree relatives. *Schizophrenia Research* **46**, 269–283.

Lawrie, S.M., Whalley, H., Kestelman, J.N. *et al.* (1999) Magnetic resonance imaging of brain in people at high risk of developing schizophrenia. *Lancet* **353**, 30–33.

Lawrie, S.M., Whalley, H.C., Abukmeil, S.S. *et al.* (2001) Brain structure, genetic liability, and psychotic symptoms in subjects at high risk of developing schizophrenia. *Biological Psychiatry* **49**, 811–823.

Leboyer, M., Bellivier, F., Nosten-Bertrand, M. *et al.* (1998) Psychiatric genetics: search for phenotypes. *Trends in Neuroscience* **21**, 102–105.

Lekwuwa, G.U. & Barnes, G.R. (1996) Cerebral control of eye movements. I. The relationship between cerebral lesion sites and smooth pursuit deficits. *Brain* **119**, 473–490.

Lenzenweger, M.E. Cornblatt, B.A. & Putnick, M. (1991) Schizotypy and sustained attention. *Journal of Abnormal Psychology* **100**, 84–89.

Levin, S., Jones, A., Stark, L., Merrin, E.L. & Holzman, P.S. (1982) Identification of abnormal patterns in eye movements of schizophrenic patients. *Archives of General Psychiatry* **39**, 1125–1130.

Levy, D.L., Dorus, E., Shaughnessy, R. *et al.* (1985) Pharmacologic evidence for specificity of pursuit dysfunction to schizophrenia: lithium carbonate associated with abnormal pursuit. *Archives of General Psychiatry* **42**, 335–341.

Levy, D.L., Holzman, P.S., Matthysse, S. & Mendell, N.R. (1993) Eye tracking dysfunction and schizophrenia: a critical perspective [see comments]. *Schizophrenia Bulletin* **19**, 461–536. [Published erratum appears in *Schizophrenia Bulletin* 1993; **19**, 685.]

Levy, D.L., Holzman, P.S., Matthysse, S. & Mendell, N.R. (1994) Eye tracking and schizophrenia: a selective review. *Schizophrenia Bulletin* **20**, 47–62.

Litman, R.E., Hommer, D.W., Clem, T. *et al.* (1989) Smooth pursuit eye movements in schizophrenia: effects of neuroleptic treatment and caffeine. *Psychopharmacological Bulletin* **25**, 473–478.

Litman, R.E., Hommer, D.W., Radant, A., Clem, T. & Pickar, D. (1994) Quantitative effects of typical and atypical neuroleptics on smooth pursuit eye tracking in schizophrenia. *Schizophrenia Research* **12**, 107–120.

Litman, R.E., Torrey, E.F., Hommer, D.W. *et al.* (1997) A quantitative analysis of smooth pursuit eye tracking in monozygotic twins discordant for schizophrenia. *Archives of General Psychiatry* **54**, 417–426.

Luntz-Leybman, V., Bickford, P.C. & Freedman, R. (1992) Cholinergic gating of response to auditory stimuli in rat hippocampus. *Brain Research* **587**, 130–136.

Lyons, M.J., Toomey, R., Faraone, S.V. *et al.* (1995) Correlates of psychosis proneness in relatives of schizophrenic patients. *Journal of Abnormal Psychology* **104**, 390–394.

MacAvoy, M.G. & Bruce, C.J. (1995) Comparison of the smooth eye tracking disorder of schizophrenics with that of non-human primates with specific brain lesions. *International Journal of Neuroscience* **80**, 117–151.

McDowell, J.E. & Clementz, B.A. (1996) Ocular-motor delayed-response task performance among schizophrenia patients. *Neuropsychobiology* **34**, 67–71.

McGue, M. & Gottesman, I.I. (1989) Genetic linkage in schizophrenia: perspectives from genetic epidemiology. *Schizophrenia Bulletin* **15**, 453–464.

McNeil, T.E., Cantor-Graae, E. & Weinberger, D.R. (2000) Relationship of obstetric complications and differences in size of brain structures in monozygotic twin pairs discordant for schizophrenia. *American Journal of Psychiatry* **157**, 203–212.

Mahtani, M.M., Widen, E., Lehto, M. *et al.* (1996) Mapping of a gene for type 2 diabetes associated with an insulin secretion defect by a genome scan in Finnish Families. *Nature Genetics* **14**, 90–94.

Maier, W., Franke, P., Hain, C., Kopp, B. & Rist, F. (1992) Neuropsychological indicators of the vulnerability to schizophrenia. *Progress in Neuropsychopharmacology and Biological Psychiatry* **16**, 703–715.

Malaspina, D., Colemann, E.A., Quitkin, M. *et al.* (1994) Effects of pharmacologic catecholamine manipulation on smooth pursuit eye movements in normals. *Schizophrenia Research* **13**, 151–159.

Mather, J.A. (1985) Eye movements of teenage children of schizophrenics: a possible inherited marker of susceptibility to the disease. *Journal of Psychiatric Research* **19**, 523–532.

Meehl, P.E. (1962) Schizotaxia, schizotypy, schizophrenia. *American Psychologist* **17**, 827–839.

Michie, P.T., Fox, A.M., Ward, P.B., Catts, S.V. & McConaghy, N. (1990) Event-related potential indices of selective attention and cortical laterlization in schizophrenia. *Psychophysiology* **27**, 209–227.

Milner, B., Squire, L.R. & Kandel, E.R. (1998) Cognitive neuroscience and the study of memory. *Neuron* **20**, 445–468.

Mirsky, A.F., Anthony, B.J., Duncan, C.C., Ahearn, M.B. & Kellam, S.G. (1991) Analysis of the elements of attention: a neuropsychological approach. *Neuropsychology Review* **2**, 109–145.

Mirsky, A.F., Lochhead, S.J., Jones, B.P. *et al.* (1992) On familial factors in the attentional deficit in schizophrenia: a review and report of two new subject samples. *Journal of Psychiatric Research* **26**, 383–403.

Morstyn, R., Duffy, E.H. & McCarley, R.W. (1983) Altered topography of EEG spectral content in schizophrenia. *Electroencephalography and Clinical Neurophysiology* **56**, 263–271.

Muir, W.J., St Clair, D.M. & Blackwood, D.H. (1991) Long-latency auditory event-related potentials in schizophrenia and in bipolar and unipolar affective disorder. *Psychological Medicine* **21**, 867–879.

Naatanen, R. & Picton, T. (1987) The N1 wave of the human electric and magnetic response to sound: a review and an analysis of the component structure. *Psychophysiology* **24**, 375–425.

Nuechterlein, K.H. & Dawson, M.E. (1984) Information processing and attentional functioning in the developmental course of schizophrenic disorders. *Schizophrenia Bulletin* **10**, 160–203.

O'Driscoll, G.A., Benkelfat, C., Florencio, P.S. *et al.* (1999) Neural correlates of eye tracking deficits in first-degree relatives of schizophrenic patients: a positron emission tomography study. *Archives of General Psychiatry* **56**, 1127–1134.

O'Driscoll, G.A., Florencio, P.S., Gagnon, D. *et al.* (2001) Amygdala–hippocampal volume and verbal memory in first-degree relatives of schizophrenic patients. *Psychiatry Research* **107**, 75–85.

Park, S., Holzman, P.S. & Goldman-Rakic, P.S. (1995) Spatial working memory deficits in the relatives of schizophrenic patients. *Archives of General Psychiatry* **52**, 821–828.

Pauls, D. (1993) Behvioural disorders: lessons in linkage. *Nature Genetics* **3**, 4–5.

Parnas, J., Schulsinger, F., Schulsinger, H., Mednick, S.A. & Teasdale, T.W. (1982) Behavioral precursors of schizophrenia spectrum: a prospective study. *Archives of General Psychiatry* **39**, 658–664.

Pfefferbaum, A., Wenegrat, B.G., Ford, J.M., Roth, W.T. & Kopell, B.S. (1984) Clinical application of the P3 component of event-related potentials. II. Dementia. depression and schizophrenia. *Electroencephalography and Clinical Neurophysiology* **59**, 104–124.

Pfefferbaum, A., Ford, J.M., White, P.M. & Roth, W.T. (1989) P3 in schizophrenia is affected by stimulus modality, response requirements, medication status, and negative symptoms. *Archives of General Psychiatry* **46**, 1035–1144.

Plomin, R., DeFries, J.C. & McClearn, G.E. (1990) *Behavioral Genetics*, 2nd edn. W.H. Freeman, New York.

Pogue-Geile, M.F., Garrett, A.H., Brunke, J.J. & Hall, J.K. (1991) Neuropsychological impairments are increased in siblings of schizophrenic patients [Abstract]. *Schizophrenia Research* **4**, 390.

Porjesz, B., Begleiter, H. & Samuelly, I. (1980) Cognitive deficits in chronic alcoholics and elderly subjects assessed by evoked brain potentials. *Acta Psychiatrica Scandinavica* **286** (Suppl.), 15–29.

Pritchard, J.K. & Rosenberg, N.A. (1999) Use of unlinked genetic markers to detect population stratification in association studies. *American Journal of Human Genetics* **65**, 220–228.

Pritchard, J.K., Stephens, M. & Donnelly, P. (2000) Inference of population structure using multilocus genotype data. *Genetics* **155**, 945–959.

Rao, D.C., Morton, N.E., Gottesman, I.I. & Lew, R. (1981) Path analysis of qualitative data on pairs of relatives: application to schizophrenia. *Human Heredity* **31**, 325–333.

Reveley, A.M., Reveley, M.A., Clifford, C.A. & Murray, R.M. (1982) Cerebral ventricular size in twins discordant for schizophrenia. *Lancet* **1**, 540–541.

Risch, N. & Merikangas, K. (1996) The future of genetic studies of complex human diseases [see comments]. *Science* **273**, 1516–1517.

Risch, N. & Zhang, H. (1995) Extreme discordant sib pairs for mapping quantitative trait loci in humans. *Science* **268**, 1584–1589.

Ross, R.G., Olincy, A., Harris, J.G. *et al.* (1998) Anticipatory saccades during smooth pursuit eye movements and familial transmission of schizophrenia. *Biological Psychiatry* **44**, 690–697.

Roth, W.T., Pfefferbaum, A., Horvath, T.B., Berger, P.A. & Kopell, B.S. (1980) P3 reduction in auditory evoked potentials of schizophrenics. *Electroencephalography Clinical Neurophysiology* **49**, 497–505.

Rutschmann, J., Cornblatt, B. & Erlenmeyer-Kimling, L. (1977) Sustained attention in children at risk for schizophrenia: report on a continuous performance test. *Archives of General Psychiatry* **34**, 571–575.

Rutschmann, J., Cornblatt, B. & Erlenmeyer-Kimling, L. (1986) Sustained attention in children at risk for schizophrenia: findings with two visual continuous performance tests in a new sample. *Journal of Abnormal Child Psychology* **14**, 365–385.

Saoud, M., d'Amato, T., Gutknecht, C. *et al.* (2000) Neuropsychological deficit in siblings discordant for schizophrenia. *Schizophrenia Bulletin* **26**, 893–902.

Sautter, E., Garver, D.L., Zemlan, E.P. & Hirschowitz, J. (1987) Growth hormone response to apomorphine and family patterns of illness. *Biological Psychiatry* **22**, 717–724.

Sautter, E.J., McDermott, D.E. & Garver, D.L. (1987) Familial and social determinants of outcome. Presented as new research at the annual meeting of the American Psychiatric Association. May 12, 1987, Chicago, IL.

Scarone, S., Abbruzzese, M. & Gambini, O. (1993) The Wisconsin Card Sorting Test discriminates schizophrenic patients and their siblings. *Schizophrenia Research* **10**, 103–107.

Schreiber, H., Stolz-Born, G., Rothmeier, J. *et al.* (1991) Endogenous event-related brain potentials and psychometric performance in children at risk for schizophrenia. *Biological Psychiatry* **30**, 177–189.

Schreiber, H., Stolz-Born, G., Kornhuber, H.H. & Born, J. (1992) Event-related potential correlates of impaired selective attention in children at high risk for schizophrenia. *Biological Psychiatry* **32**, 634–651.

Sedvall, G.C. & Wode-Helgodt, B. (1980) Aberrant monoamine

metabolite levels in CSF and family history of schizophrenia. Their relationships in schizophrenic patients. *Archives of General Psychiatry* 37, 1113–1116.

Seidman, L.J., Faraone, S.V., Goldstein, J.M. *et al.* (1997) Reduced subcortical brain volumes in nonpsychotic siblings of schizophrenic patients: a pilot magnetic resonance imaging study. *American Journal of Medical Genetics* 74, 507–514.

Seidman, L.J., Faraone, S.V., Goldstein, J.M. *et al.* (1999) Thalamic and amygdala–hippocampal volume reductions in first-degree relatives of patients with schizophrenia: an MRI-based morphometric analysis. *Biological Psychiatry* 46, 941–954.

Sesack, S.R., Hawrylak, V.A., Matus, C., Guido, M.A. & Levey, A.I. (1998) Dopamine axon varicosities in the prelimbic division of the rat prefrontal cortex exhibit sparse immunoreactivity for the dopamine transporter. *Journal of Neuroscience* 18, 2697–2708.

Sharma, T., Lancaster, E., Lee, D. *et al.* (1998) Brain changes in schizophrenia: volumetric MRI study of families multiply affected with schizophrenia – the Maudsley Family Study 5. *British Journal of Psychiatry* 173, 132–138.

Shedlack, K., Lee, G., Sakuma, M. *et al.* (1997) Language processing and memory in ill and well siblings from multiplex families affected with schizophrenia. *Schizophrenia Research* 25, 43–52.

Shelley, A.M., Silipo, G. & Javitt, D.C. (1999) Diminished responsiveness of ERPs in schizophrenic subjects to changes in auditory stimulation parameters: implications for theories of cortical dysfunction. *Schizophrenia Research* 37, 65–79.

Siegel, C., Waldo, M., Mizner, G., Adler, L.E. & Freedman, R. (1984) Deficits in sensory gating in schizophrenic patients and their relatives: evidence obtained with auditory evoked responses. *Archives of General Psychiatry* 41, 607–612.

Silverman, J.M., Smith, C.J., Guo, S.L. *et al.* (1998) Lateral ventricular enlargement in schizophrenic probands and their siblings with schizophrenia-related disorders. *Biological Psychiatry* 43, 97–106.

Souza, V.B., Muir, W.J., Walker, M.T. *et al.* (1995) Auditory P300 event-related potentials and neuropsychological performance in schizophrenia and bipolar affective disorder. *Biological Psychiatry* 37, 300–310.

Spielman, R.S., McGinnis, R.E. & Ewens, W.J. (1993) Transmission test for linkage disequilibrium: the insulin gene region and insulin-dependent diabetes mellitus (IDDM). *American Journal of Human Genetics* 52, 506–516.

Spohn, H.E., Coyne, L. & Spray, J. (1988) The effect of neuroleptics and tardive dyskinesia on smooth-pursuit eye movement in chronic schizophrenics. *Archives of General Psychiatry* 45, 833–840.

Squires-Wheeler, E., Friedman, D., Skodol, A.E. & Erlenmeyer-Kimling, L. (1993) A longitudinal study relating P3 amplitude to schizophrenia spectrum disorders and to global personality functioning. *Biological Psychiatry* 33, 774–785.

Staal, W.G., Hulshoff Pol, H.E., Schnack, H., van der Schot, A.C. & Kahn, R.S. (1998) Partial volume decrease of the thalamus in relatives of patients with schizophrenia. *American Journal of Psychiatry* 155, 1784–1786.

Staal, W.G., Hulshoff Pol, H.E., Schnack, H.G. *et al.* (2000) Structural brain abnormalities in patients with schizophrenia and their healthy siblings. *American Journal of Psychiatry* 157, 416–421.

St Clair, D., Blackwood, D. & Muir, W. (1989) P300 abnormality in schizophrenic subtypes. *Journal of Psychiatric Research* 23, 49–55.

Straub, R.E., MacLean, C.J., O'Neill, F.A. *et al.* (1995) A potential vulnerability locus for schizophrenia on chromosome 6p24-22: evidence for genetic heterogeneity [see comments]. *Nature Genetics* 11, 287–293.

Suddath, R.L., Christison, G.W., Torrey, E.F., Casanova, M.F. & Weinberger, D.R. (1990) Anatomical abnormalities in the brains of monozygotic twins discordant for schizophrenia. *New England Journal of Medicine* 322, 789–794.

Sweeney, J.A., Clementz, B.A., Haas, G.L. *et al.* (1994a) Eye tracking dysfunction in schizophrenia: characterization of component eye movement abnormalities, diagnostic specificity, and the role of attention. *Journal of Abnormal Psychology* 103, 222–230.

Sweeney, J.A., Haas, G.L., Li, S. & Weiden, P.J. (1994b) Selective effects of antipsychotic medications on eye-tracking performance in schizophrenia. *Psychiatry Research* 54, 185–198.

Sweeney, J.A., Luna, B., Haas, G.L. *et al.* (1999) Pursuit tracking impairments in schizophrenia and mood disorders: step-ramp studies with unmedicated patients. *Biological Psychiatry* 46, 671–680.

Sweeney, J.A., Luna, B., Srinivasagam, N.M. *et al.* (1998) Eye tracking abnormalities in schizophrenia: evidence for dysfunction in the frontal eye fields. *Biological Psychiatry* 44, 698–708.

Taylor, M., Berenbaum, S., Jampala, V. & Cloninger, R. (1993) Are schizophrenia and affective disorder related? Preliminary data from a family study? *American Journal of Psychiatry* 150, 278–285.

Thaker, G.K., Cassady, S., Adami, H., Moran, M. & Ross, D.E. (1996) Eye movements in spectrum personality disorders: comparison of community subjects and relatives of schizophrenic patients. *American Journal of Psychiatry* 153, 362–368.

Toomey, R., Faraone, S.V., Seidman, L.J. *et al.* (1998) Association of neuropsychological vulnerability markers in relatives of schizophrenic patients. *Schizophrenia Research* 31, 89–98.

Tsuang, M. (1993) Genotypes, phenotypes and the brain: a search for commections in schizophrenia. *British Journal of Psychiatry* 163, 299–307.

Waldo, M., Gerhardt, G., Baker, N. *et al.* (1992) Auditory sensory gating and catecholamine metabolism in schizophrenic and normal subjects. *Psychiatry Research* 44, 21–32.

Waldo, M.C., Cawthra, E., Adler, L.E. *et al.* (1994) Auditory sensory gating, hippocampal volume, and catecholamine metabolism in schizophrenics and their siblings. *Schizophrenia Research* 12, 93–106.

Weinberger, D.R. (1987) Implications of normal brain development for the pathogenesis of schizophrenia. *Archives of General Psychiatry* 44, 660–669.

Weinberger, D.R., DeLisi, L.E., Neophytides, A.N. & Wyatt, R.J. (1981) Familial aspects of CT scan abnormalities in chronic schizophrenic patients. *Psychiatry Research* 4, 65–71.

Weinshilboum, R. & Dunnette, J. (1981) Thermal stability and the biochemical genetics of erythrocyte catechol-O-methyl-transferase and plasma dopamine-beta-hydroxylase. *Clinical Genetics* 19, 426–437.

Whicker, L., Abel, L. & Dell'Osso, L. (1985) Smooth pursuit eye movements in the parents of schizophrenics. *Neuro-Ophthalmology* 5, 1–8.

Williams, G.V. and Goldman-Rakic P.S. (1995) Modulation of memory fields by dopamine D1 receptors in prefrontal cortex. [see comments]. *Nature* 376, 572–5.

Yee, C.M., Nuechterlein, K.H. & Dawson, M.E. (1998) A longitudinal analysis of eye tracking dysfunction and attention in recent-onset schizophrenia. *Psychophysiology* 35, 443–451.

Yee, R.D., Baloh, R.W., Marder, S.R. *et al.* (1987) Eye movements in schizophrenia. *Investigative Ophthalmology and Visual Science* 28, 366–374.

Yurgelun-Todd, D.A. & Kinney, D.K. (1993) Patterns of neuropsychological deficits that discriminate schizophrenic individuals from siblings and control subjects. *Journal of Neuropsychiatry and Clinical Neuroscience* 5, 294–300.

16 Electrophysiology of schizophrenia

D.F. Salisbury, S. Krljes and R.W. McCarley

The electroencephalogram, 298
  Event-related potentials, 298
The place of electrophysiology in the neuroimaging
  spectrum, 298
Event-related potentials in schizophrenia, 299
  Overview, 299
  History of event-related potential research in
    schizophrenia, 299

Current event-related potential research in
  schizophrenia, 300
Magnetoencephalography – a complement to
  electroencephalography, 306
Conclusions, 307
Acknowledgements, 307
References, 307

The electroencephalogram (EEG) was the first physiological technique used to examine brain activity in schizophrenia and has evolved into a powerful method for studying brain information processing activity. In today's world of multimodal imaging, the EEG is still unsurpassed in providing real-time, millisecond resolution of normal and pathological brain processing, literally at the speed of thought. This chapter discusses the application of this technique to schizophrenia research. The first section begins with an introduction to some basic concepts of electrophysiology.

The electroencephalogram

Cognitive events are subserved by neurones in the brain and this electrical activity may be recorded from the electrodes placed on the surface of the scalp. In general, the EEG derives from summated dendritic inhibitory and excitatory postsynaptic activity in neurones, primarily pyramidal cells in the cortex of the brain. It is important to emphasize that the EEG does not typically reflect neuronal discharges, because they are usually too brief and too asynchronous. (As an aside, we note that blood oxygenation level-dependent (BOLD) functional magnetic resonance imaging (fMRI) 'activation' similarly mainly reflects postsynaptic potential (PSP) activity, which is metabolically most demanding and necessitates the increased blood flow, but not action potential activity, which is metabolically much less demanding.)

The EEG primarily reflects the activity generated in the large dendritic trees of pyramidal cells, with an especially strong representation of activity in dendrites orientated in parallel, perpendicular to the plane of the scalp surface. One of the main limitations of the EEG technique is a difficulty in assessing the source of the recorded activity. For example, generators in different brain locations can produce the same EEG scalp recorded signal. To combat this problem various source localization techniques are employed.

Event-related potentials

The EEG reflects the activity of many groups of neurones, representing brain operations related to a variety of ongoing events, such as breathing, seeing, hearing and thinking, as well as different processing modes of large groups of nerve cells. One of the important advances in EEG-based research was the development of a technique to isolate brain activity related to specific events from the background EEG. Using various averaging techniques, it is possible to visualize small potentials related to one of the many different brain operations reflected in the EEG. Typically, these events are related to the specific processing of certain stimuli in the stimulus field, i.e. the events in the environment impinging upon the individual. Signal averaging isolates the brain activity related to specific events by recording small portions (epochs) of the EEG each time a specific stimulus is presented. The stimulus is presented many times, thus a large number of EEG epochs are recorded. For each epoch, there are two types of activity:

1 the activity specifically related to the stimulus; and
2 the activity related to the other ongoing processes in the brain.
The former activity is said to be time-locked, with all the activity in sensory system relay and processing areas occurring at roughly the same time after each stimulus is presented. Hence, at any specific point in time after the presentation of the stimulus, time-locked event-related activity will be temporally stable from one trial to the next. The latter activity will be, by definition, random with respect to the stimulus. By averaging together all the epochs, the time-locked event-related activity will remain stable, because it occurs at roughly the same time from trial to trial, while the rest of the EEG activity is averaged out. The time-locked brain activity that remains is referred to as the event-related potential (ERP) waveform, and each of the various positive or negative events that comprise it are referred to as event-related potentials. The reader desiring more information regarding EEG and ERP theory and techniques is referred to Regan (1989).

The place of electrophysiology in the neuroimaging spectrum

In recent years many new means of measuring brain structure and function have been developed. Some image the structure of the brain: X-ray-based techniques (e.g. computerized axial tomography or CAT scans) and nuclear magnetic field-based techniques (e.g. magnetic resonance imaging or MRI). These structural techniques have high spatial resolution and provide detailed information about the static structure of the brain. However, they provide little information about brain activity, as they provide only a snapshot of brain tissue rather than a series of measures of brain physiology.

A second class of brain imaging techniques measure brain functional activity. These functional techniques assay brain activity based on blood oxygenation level, an indirect measure of brain activity (BOLD fMRI), or on positron emission tomography (PET), which uses radioactive-labelled substances to measure metabolism ($[^{18}]$fluorodeoxyglucose or $[^{18}F]$2DG), blood flow ($[^{15}O]$water) or receptor occupancy (labelled ligands) as well as single photon emission tomography (SPECT). It is an important point that fMRI haemodynamic signals and $[^{15}O]H_2O$ PET, as well as $[^{18}F]$2DGPET metabolic measures, all primarily derive from PSP activity and not neuronal discharge, because PSP activity is metabolically most demanding on the neurone and also evokes most of the blood flow changes (Logothetis *et al.* 2001). Thus, 'activation', as is commonly used in neuroimaging, mainly reflects PSPs (often from input to the region) and not neuronal discharge. These techniques provide relatively good spatial resolution (although not as good as structural MRI) but their temporal resolution (in the second range) is at best several thousand-fold less than electrophysiological measures, which provide resolution within a few milliseconds. The interested reader is referred to Raichle (1998) and Rauch and Renshaw (1995) for further information regarding different imaging modalities, as well as to other chapters in this volume.

In contrast with its superior temporal resolution, the EEG's spatial resolution is limited, because the source of the voltage fluctuations at the scalp cannot be precisely identified as coming from particular brain regions. It seems intuitively obvious that 'multimodal' imaging (combining EEG and other modalities with higher spatial resolution) has advantages, particularly when coupled with knowledge of plausible locations of brain activity based on depth EEG recordings in patients being prepared for surgery, and from experimental animal data on the origin of certain potentials.

Event-related potentials in schizophrenia

Overview

This section discusses some key issues in the history of ERP research in schizophrenia, and then focuses on three auditory ERPs of particular relevance to current schizophrenia research (gamma-band oscillations, mismatch negativity and P300). We conclude this section with a brief overview of other ERPs that have been studied in schizophrenia patients, and implications of ERP findings to the overall knowledge on schizophrenia. While we focus on ERP measures in schizophrenia in this chapter, we

note that other EEG measures have been studied extensively. For example, measures of resting level EEG and techniques for analysing the data, such as measuring the relative amounts of activity in each constituent frequency band, called quantitative electroencephalography (Q-EEG), have led to interesting findings regarding brain–behaviour relationships in schizophrenia. The interested reader is referred to John *et al.* (1994).

The vast majority of ERP studies in schizophrenia have been conducted on chronically ill patients who have had persistent symptoms for many years. Thus, many studies may be confounded by the fact that chronicity itself may lead to secondary effects on brain physiology because of the possible effects of long-term medication, poor diet, understimulating environment and comorbidity (e.g. use of illicit drugs, poor general health). Such factors could affect the brain independently of any disease process and it is difficult to identify which effects arise from chronicity factors as opposed to those directly related to a schizophrenic disease process.

A physiological abnormality in chronically ill patients that is also present at the onset of the disease cannot be caused by the secondary effects associated with chronicity. Whatever abnormal brain process gives rise to schizophrenia at the time of first overt psychosis should give clues as to the primary brain pathology of schizophrenia, highlighting the importance of research on first episode and unmedicated patients.

History of event-related potential research in schizophrenia

The technique for signal averaging the EEG to reveal ERPs was developed in the late 1950s, and the brain potentials related to the stimulus parameters, the so-called sensory potentials, were recorded in schizophrenia patients as early as 1959 (Shagass 1968). Much of the ERP work in schizophrenia throughout the 1960s and 1970s focused on the evoked potentials – those brain potentials elicited by repetitive stimuli in some sensory modality. The major interest was in N100, a negative-going brain potential arising approximately 100 ms after the onset of a stimulus. N100 amplitude (size) and latency (timing) are tied to stimulus intensity in several different modalities; thus N100 is referred to as a sensory potential. N100 was shown to be of smaller amplitude and greater variability in schizophrenia patients in the auditory modality (Saletu *et al.* 1971), visual modality (Shagass 1977) and the somatosensory modality (Shagass *et al.* 1974). However, results were far from uniform. Some groups reported larger ERP amplitudes in patients (Shagass 1968) while others reported no differences between patients and controls (Domino *et al.* 1979). Studies were motivated in large part by the theory that patients with schizophrenia were unable to filter irrelevant stimuli from the environment and were swamped or overloaded with stimuli seeking access to higher order cognitive processing resources (McGhie & Chapman 1961; Venables 1964). The size of the ERPs was thus thought to reflect either abnormally large signals (either pathological at the sensory channel or abnormally 'augmented') which forced their processing rather than filtration, or abnormally small signals which reflected the active 'reducing' of input by schizophrenics as a defensive adjustment to an abnormal filter (see e.g. Schooler *et al.* 1976). By the late 1970s, it was apparent from controlled methodology and from technological improvements that the signals were, in general, reduced in schizophrenia. Shagass *et al.* also argued, somewhat presciently, that the lateralized pattern of abnormalities in N100 in all modalities indicated a left hemisphere abnormality in schizophrenia.

As the intellectual attractiveness of theories of augmenting and reducing decreased, and the notion that changes in N100 amplitude reflected the operations of selective attention was replaced by the idea that changes in N100 were likely caused by other coincident preattentive signals (e.g. mismatch negativity), interest in these potentials waned in the 1980s, although there has been a recent renaissance of research into basic sensory processing ERPs in schizophrenia, as discussed below. Analysis of sensory evoked potentials was largely replaced by a focus on P300, which was robustly reduced in patients and clearly linked to the operations of selective attention and processing of infrequent stimuli (the reader is referred to reviews of ERP research by Buchsbaum 1977; Roth 1977; Shagass 1979).

Sutton *et al.* (1965), using a prediction paradigm wherein subjects tried to guess which of two stimuli was going to be presented, described a brain potential that was related to the cognitive activity of the subject, rather than directly to the characteristics of the stimulus. This revolutionary finding revealed a brain potential, an objective physiological event, related to the internal operations of the subject. This ERP, eventually termed the P3 or P300 (for the third positive potential or the positive potential at 300 ms after the stimulus, respectively), was found to be intimately tied to the selective attention paid to rare external events by the subjects in tasks where they had to use information about the stimulus. Roth and Cannon (1972), the first to examine P300 in schizophrenia, reported that P300 was reduced relative to controls. Levit *et al.* (1973) also showed a reduction of P300 in schizophrenia. This finding has subsequently been termed the most robust physiological finding of any abnormality in schizophrenia. However, reduction of P300 is not pathognomonic to schizophrenia as it is also reduced in other psychiatric diseases, such as bipolar disorder and Alzheimer's dementia. More specific alterations of the total scalp field, or regionally specific topographic differences, by contrast, may be specifically associated with different psychiatric diseases, as discussed below in the section entitled 'P300'.

Although P300 amplitude varies with the amount of attention paid to a task, there is only moderate improvement in P300 amplitude when there is symptom resolution in schizophrenia (Ford *et al.* 1994; Turetsky *et al.* 1998): the reduction of P300 in schizophrenia is largely trait-like, rather than state-like. Even with improvement in symptoms, the P300 of patients rarely reaches normal levels. Hence, P300 amplitude might reflect abnormalities of an enduring aspect of the disease pathology. By contrast, P300 latency, which is occasionally reported as prolonged in schizophrenia (Blackwood *et al.* 1991), is intimately

tied to attention and task performance and may be more state-like in nature (Salisbury *et al.* 1994a).

Current event-related potential research in schizophrenia

Because space limitations preclude discussion of all ERPs currently being investigated in schizophrenia, this section focuses on the three ERPs currently being researched by the authors and also under examination in other laboratories. We briefly discuss other potentials at the end of the section. Each of the three ERPs can be related to an increasingly more complex stage of information processing in the brain. We chose the auditory modality because it is one of the most affected in schizophrenia, as evinced in the primacy of auditory hallucinations and speech/language pathology. It is our hypothesis that schizophrenia involves abnormalities in auditory processing from the most simple to the most complex level, and that the anatomical substrates in the neocortical temporal lobe, most carefully investigated in the superior temporal gyrus, themselves evince reduction in grey matter neuropil volume.

The first ERP we consider is the steady-state gamma-band response. Gamma-band refers to a brain oscillation at and near the frequency of 40 hertz (hz) or 40 times per second, while 'steady state' refers to its being elicited by a stimulus of the same frequency. The second ERP discussed is mismatch negativity (MMN), an ERP related to the automatic sensory memory detection of a stimulus that deviates from a repetitive pattern, regardless of whether the subject is actively trying to detect the deviant stimulus or not. The last potential considered reflects the active, deliberate and conscious detection and processing of a deviant or 'oddball' stimulus by the subject. This ERP is called the P3 or P300, and is one of the most widely studied physiological events in schizophrenia, as well as one of the most robustly abnormal measures of brain activity in that disorder. ERPs provided the first objective physiological measure of brain activity related to mental cognitive events, joined later by PET and regional cerebral blood blow (rCBF) studies, and only recently by fMRI. As previously noted, the temporal resolution of ERPs, in the order of milliseconds, far surpasses the temporal resolution of fMRI (in the order of many seconds). In addition, ERPs are more sensitive to neural activation than is fMRI. The spatial resolution of fMRI surpasses that of ERPs, but combination of MRI and ERPs informed by intracortical recordings provides the greatest accuracy in modelling localized brain activity *in vivo*. This approach is particularly fruitful in brain disorders where abnormalities are thought to be localized to specific areas from which arise certain ERPs. As a case in point, schizophrenia is likely to involve abnormalities in temporal lobe areas that generate P300, and structural abnormalities in these areas are strongly related to abnormalities of the brain activity thought to arise there (see below).

Gamma activity

At the cellular level, gamma-band activity is an endogenous

brain oscillation thought to reflect the synchronizing of activity in several columns of cortical neurones, or between cortex and thalamus, with this synchronization facilitating communication. At the cognitive level, work in humans suggests that gamma activity reflects the convergence of multiple processing streams in cortex, giving rise to a unified percept. A simple example is a 'firetruck', where a particular combination of form perception, motion perception and auditory perception are melded to form this percept. Gamma activity at its simplest, however, involves basic neural circuitry composed of projection neurones, usually using excitatory amino acid (EAA) neurotransmission, linked with inhibitory γ-aminobutyric acid (GABA) interneurones. Studies of gamma activity in schizophrenia aim to determine if there is a basic circuit abnormality present, such as a deficiency in recurrent inhibition, postulated by a number of workers (see review in McCarley *et al.* 1996).

Kwon *et al.* (1999) began the study of gamma in schizophrenia using an exogenous input of 40 Hz auditory clicks, leading to a steady-state gamma response. The magnitude of the brain response was measured by power, the amount of EEG energy at a specific frequency, with the degree of capability of gamma driving being reflected in the power at and near 40 Hz.

As shown in Fig. 16.1, schizophrenia patients had – compared with healthy controls – a markedly reduced power at 40 Hz input, although showing normal driving at slower frequencies which indicated that this was not a general reduction in power, but one specific to the gamma band.

Moreover, the phase–response curve, a description of the relationship between the timing of each stimulus and the EEG response, suggested that it was an intrinsic oscillator that was being driven. This was because the time duration between the stimulus and the EEG response, as the 40 Hz stimulation continued, was reduced to a duration too short to be explained by simple conduction to the auditory cortex. This phase–response curve is very common when an external signal drives a 'tuned oscillator', much as auditory stimuli can set in motion a tuning fork, which oscillates (resonates) at a particular frequency. The abnormal amplitude and phase–response in schizophrenic patients raised the possibility that there was an intrinsic deficit in brain circuitry supporting 40 Hz oscillations. Were this to be

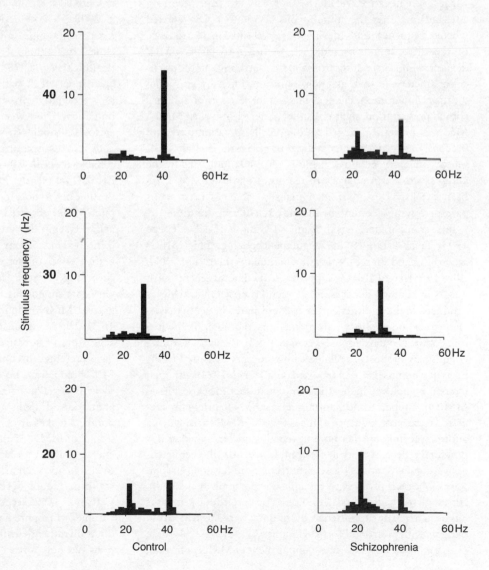

Fig 16.1 Mean power spectra for the EEG recorded to trains of clicks at three different stimulus rates: 40 Hz stimulation (upper); 30 Hz stimulation (middle); and 20 Hz stimulation (lower). The schizophrenic patients (*n* = 15; right column) show decreased power at 40 Hz stimulation compared with control subjects (*n* = 15; left column), but there was no difference between groups at lower frequencies of stimulation. (Adapted from Kwon *et al.* 1999.)

confirmed, it would be an important addition to our knowledge about schizophrenia.

However, it remains to be determined if this deficiency in externally driven gamma implies a deficiency in gamma-band synchronization which occurs endogenously in the course of perception as when, for example, a certain pattern of spots embedded in a field of spots is suddenly perceived to be a Dalmatian dog. Thus, the next phase of gamma research in schizophrenia will be evaluating this kind of gamma, also known as evoked gamma. At present, few studies have been conducted. Baldeweg et al. (1998) presented evidence of increased gamma-band activity during somatic hallucinations in a case report. Kissler et al. (2000) reported reduced gamma activity and reversed hemispheric asymmetry in chronically ill patients during a mental arithmetic task. Clearly, more work needs to be carried out regarding endogenous gamma oscillations in schizophrenia.

Mismatch negativity

MMN is a negative, relatively short-latency (e.g. occurring 150–250 ms after the stimulus onset) auditory ERP elicited when infrequent sounds (deviants) are presented in the sequence of repetitive sounds (standards). In order to elicit MMN, deviant sounds may differ from the standards in a simple physical characteristic such as pitch, duration, intensity or spatial location. In addition, changes in abstract features of auditory stimuli presentation, such as distinct patterns, also elicit MMN. MMN is primarily evoked automatically, preattentively and preconsciously and is thus thought to reflect the operations of sensory memory, a kind of memory of past stimuli used by the auditory cortex in analysis of temporal patterns. MMN has been extensively studied in humans to changes in stimulus parameters, most commonly to tone pitch or tone duration.

Intracranial recordings in animals (Kraus et al. 1994; Csepe 1995; Javitt et al. 1996), magnetoencephalographic (MEG) recordings and source localization in humans (Hari et al. 1984; Alho 1995) have led to the supposition of bilateral generators of MMN in auditory cortices. It has been proposed that MMN is produced in the auditory cortex by a mismatch between the deviant tone and auditory sensory memory representing the features of the standard tone (Naatanen 1992). Recently, a frontal component supposedly related to involuntary attention to the deviant stimulus has been reported (Giard et al. 1994), although it remains unclear whether this component should be considered MMN or a separate mechanism such as the N2b originally suggested to be a consequence of the activity of MMN arising from auditory cortex. Furthermore, it remains unclear whether this potential reflects activity in prefrontal cortex or whether it arises in secondary auditory association cortex in the anterior temporal lobe that projects to the anterior portions of the scalp. Although still controversial, the notion of a prefrontal generator has been partially supported by the findings of reduced MMN in patients with prefrontal cortical lesions (Alho et al. 1994; Alain et al. 1998), as well as selective impairment of MMN at frontal,

but not mastoid, sites in patients with schizophrenia (Baldeweg et al. 2002).

MMN has been suggested to reflect the activity of N-methyl-D-aspartate (NMDA) channel-mediated influx of current flow in supragranular cortical layers. Studies carried out in monkeys showed that deviants elicited MMN-like activity in the supragranular (surface) layers of primary auditory cortex, and further that this activity was obliterated by application of NMDA-specific antagonists (Javitt et al. 1996). Umbricht et al. (2000) showed reduced MMN in normal subjects following the administration of ketamine, an NMDA receptor antagonist.

Not surprisingly, given the long-standing interest in early sensory gating abnormalities and the more recent interest in NMDA abnormalities in schizophrenia, MMN has been investigated in schizophrenia to determine whether such an index of early stimulus processing was disrupted. Most studies of MMN have shown reductions in chronically ill schizophrenia patients, generally in the order of 40–50% in the study of pitch deviants (Fig. 16.2). Some studies have reported correlations between the severity of negative symptoms and reduced MMN amplitude at a frontal recording site (Catts et al. 1995; Javitt et al. 2000a). The reduction of MMN in chronically ill schizophrenia patients appears to be trait-like and not ameliorated by either typical (haloperidol) or atypical (clozapine) medication (Umbricht et al. 1998). MMN characteristics have only recently been reported in first episode patients. Javitt et al. (2000a) reported marginally significant ($P = 0.06$) MMN reductions in outpatients who were within 3 years of their first psychotic episode, although these patients were not necessarily recorded at their first hospitalization.

Salisbury et al. (2002) recently reported that pitch MMN was normal very early in the course of schizophrenia, i.e. at the time of first hospitalization (Fig. 16.2) Thus, the reduction in pitch MMN observed in chronically ill patients is not apparent at the first episode (often empirically defined as the first hospitalization). Thus, it may be related to a progressive neurodegenerative effect of the disease, or possibly to some secondary chronicity variable. Umbricht et al. (2002) presented preliminary data supporting the finding of Salisbury et al. (2002) of a normal MMN amplitude in first-episode schizophrenia (Fig. 16.3). The recent-onset group also showed a reduced MMN, suggesting progressive changes in pathology. Salisbury et al. have presented preliminary longitudinal data to suggest that MMN reductions become apparent within the first 2 years of schizophrenia onset in patients who displayed a normal MMN at first episode (Salisbury et al. 2001). While their small subject numbers makes any conclusion tentative, it does raise the possibility of MMN as an index of neurodegeneration in the early course of the disorder (Fig. 16.2), although effects secondary to chronicity, such as the onset of an antipsychotic mediation regimen, cannot be ruled out. It is interesting to note that Catts et al. (1995) reported an MMN reduction in unmedicated chronic schizophrenia patients, which suggests that disease duration rather than medication may be related to MMN reductions. We note further that there is evidence that tone duration

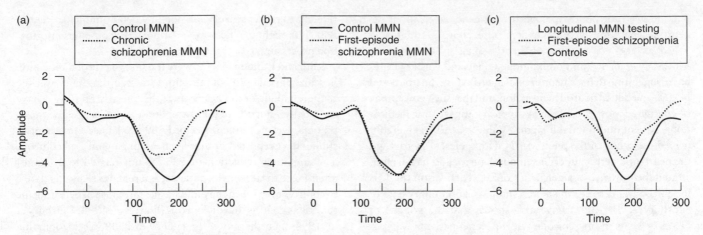

Fig 16.2 (a) Reduced MMN amplitude to pitch deviants in chronic schizophrenia patients. (b) Normal MMN amplitude to pitch deviants in first episode schizophrenia patients. (c) Longitudinal testing of first episode schizophrenia patients 1.5 years later indicates reduction in MMN amplitude to pitch deviants not present at first hospitalization.

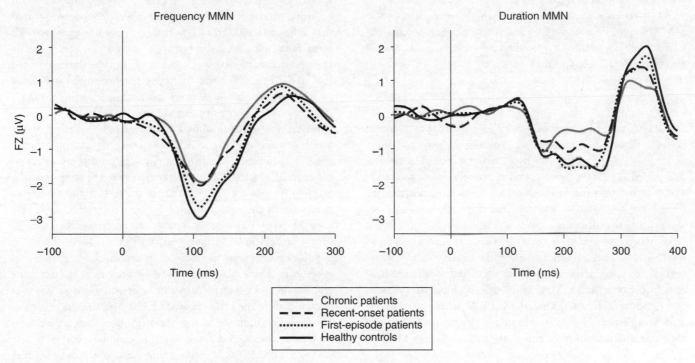

Fig 16.3 Frequency and duration MMN difference waves for chronic patients, recent-onset patients and healthy controls. (Adapted from Umbricht *et al.* 2002.)

MMN may be more sensitive to schizophrenic pathology than pitch MMN.

Reports of normal MMN amplitudes in first episode schizophrenia with an apparent progression of MMN reduction longitudinally suggest that MMN abnormalities develop as a consequence of disease onset. The direct genetic contribution to this reduction remains unclear, given reports of MMN reduction in a small sample of first-degree relatives of schizophrenic patients (Jessen *et al.* 2001). The data from first episode patients indicate a minimal early developmental component, because the MMN in these patients is apparently of normal amplitude at first hospitalization.

Because MMN may reflect, in part, NMDA-mediated activity and this receptor has an important role in cortical excitation and brain development, it is tempting to speculate about an NMDA-related abnormality active during the early course of the illness. If the preliminary data of Salisbury *et al.* (2001) (Fig. 16.2) are supported by subsequent work indicating that MMN undergoes a process of active reduction during the first few years after symptom onset and this is not simply drug-related, then there is the possibility that the MMN, especially the pitch MMN, might serve as an index of disease progression in the superior temporal gyrus. Further, the presence of an active phase of neurodegeneration around the time of first hospitalization would underline the need for pharmacological treatment, especially if the neurodegeneration were dependent on excitatory amino-acid neurotoxicity, as a number of theories suggest (see review in McCarley *et al.* 1996). For example, Olney and Farber (1995) have suggested that schizophrenia may involve postpubertal NMDA-mediated neurodegeneration, and that such effects may be countered most effectively by atypical antipsychotic medications. Recent multimodal imaging (Wible *et al.* 2001) has confirmed the origin of the pitch MMN within Heschl's gyrus and the nearby posterior superior temporal gyrus, and has demonstrated the presence of a deficiency of fMRI activation (BOLD) in schizophrenia to the mismatch stimulus. Preliminary data of Salisbury *et al.* (2001) have also shown that the volume of Heschl's gyrus in first episode schizophrenia patients was significantly correlated with MMN amplitude ($r = -0.68$, $P < 0.05$), even though neither measure was abnormal in the group as a whole. Those patients with the largest Heschl's gyrus volumes had the largest (most negative) MMN amplitudes (Fig. 16.4). It remains to be determined whether the reduction in MMN amplitude over the first few years after first hospitalization for schizophrenia is related to progressive reductions of grey matter in Heschl's gyrus.

P300

The P300 is an ERP that occurs to a stimulus that a subject actively detects and processes. Typically, a low-probability event among another frequently occurring standard stimulus is designated the target. Subjects must actively detect the target stimulus. It differs from the typical MMN paradigm in that the stimuli are presented at a slower rate (typically around 1 per second) and the subject is actively attending the stimuli. P300 is larger when the stimulus is rarer, and thus is typically evoked by 'oddball' stimulus paradigms, much like MMN. Thus, P300 is sensitive to cognitive processes that necessitate selective attention, by contrast with MMN, which reflects automatic orientating responses and is occluded by ERPs reflecting selective attention. Hence, P300 reflects brain activity related to complex cognitive operations on the part of the subject. Where MMN is

thought to reflect sensory memory, by definition preconscious, P300 is thought to reflect an updating of the conscious information processing stream and of expectancy.

Roth and Cannon (1972) were the first to report a reduction in schizophrenia of P300 amplitude in recording sites over the sagittal midline of the head. Since then, nearly all studies have reported a reduction of P300 amplitude in subjects with schizophrenia. Delays in the onset of P300 are less certain, as most studies have reported similar latencies in patients and controls. The amplitude reduction of P300 is not related to a lack of attention to the task in the patients, as it remains reduced relative to controls even when the patients' performance in detecting the tones is as good as that of controls (Ford *et al.* 1994; Salisbury *et al.* 1994a). Furthermore, the latency of P300 in schizophrenia patients does vary with task difficulty, as in controls, but the amplitude remains reduced. Thus, P300 amplitude is robustly reduced in chronically ill schizophrenia patients. This widespread P300 reduction also appears to be trait-like and an enduring feature of the disease. Ford *et al.* (1994) demonstrated that although P300 showed moderate amplitude increases with symptom resolution, it did not approach normal values during these periods of remission. Umbricht *et al.* (1998) have reported that atypical antipsychotic treatment led to a significant increase of P300 amplitudes in patients with schizophrenia, although this response was not normalized.

In addition to the midline P300 reductions described above and broad reductions of P300 over both left and right hemispheres, chronically ill schizophrenic subjects display an asymmetry in P300 with smaller voltage over the left temporal lobe vs. right (Fig. 16.5). This left temporal P300 amplitude abnormality (from the mid-temporal T3 site) correlates negatively with the extent of psychopathology, as reflected in thought disorder and delusions (McCarley *et al.* 1993).

P300 likely reflects the activity of several different bilateral generators. There is clear evidence for activity in inferior parietal lobule and posterior superior temporal gyrus (STG) that corresponds to the scalp recorded P300. There is less evidence, but suggestive none the less, of a contribution from dorsolateral prefrontal cortex and from anterior cingulate cortex to the scalp-recorded P300. It is likely that many of the deep sources that generate P300-like activity do not propagate to the scalp (e.g. hippocampus).

The left temporal P300 amplitude reduction correlates positively with the grey matter volume of left posterior STG, one of the generator sites of P300, and an area also intimately related to language processing and thinking (McCarley *et al.* 1993). The volume of cortical grey matter in left STG volume is, in turn, correlated negatively with measures of thought disorder (Shenton *et al.* 1992) and the severity of auditory hallucinations (Barta *et al.* 1990). Therefore, abnormal left temporal P300 may reflect underlying STG abnormality and index the severity of psychopathology, and serve as a physiological tie between underlying brain pathology and behavioural psychopathology.

Salisbury *et al.* (1998) showed that the overall P300 reduction across the whole surface of the scalp was present in first episode

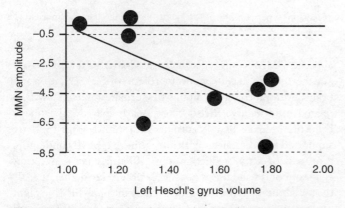

Fig 16.4 MMN amplitude in first episode schizophrenia patients is significantly correlated with the underlying grey matter volume of Heschl's gyrus, which contains primary auditory cortex.

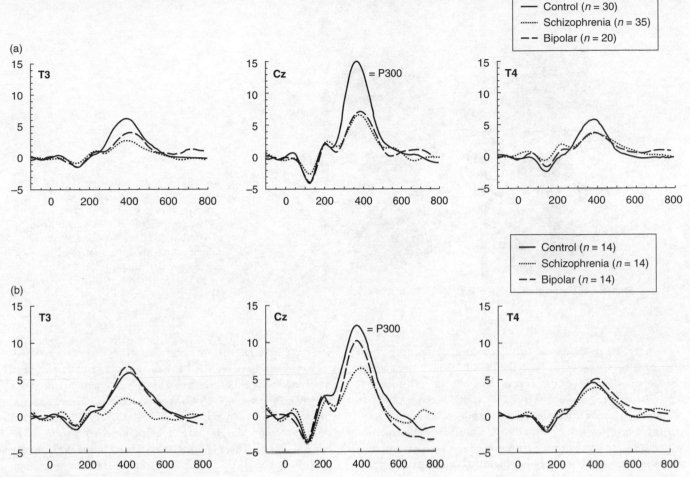

Fig 16.5 (a) P300 is broadly reduced in chronically ill schizophrenia (and psychotic mania) but is asymmetrically reduced on the left only in schizophrenia (T3 site). (b) First episode schizophrenia patients show the same overall and left-sided P300 reductions as do chronically ill patients. Note: T3 site overlies left middle temporal gyrus, T4 overlies right middle temporal gyrus, and Cz overlies sensorimotor cortex at the sagittal and coronal midpoint of the skull (vertex). (Adapted from Salisbury *et al.* 1998; 1999.)

schizophrenia patients, albeit to a lesser degree than in chronically ill patients, as was the same left-hemisphere localized deficit. Both first episode and chronically ill schizophrenia patients show an altered scalp topography of P300, with greater reduction over the left temporal areas (Fig. 16.6). Quantitative volumetric MRI studies have shown that the first episode schizophrenia patients show, in comparison to healthy control and manic first episode patients, a specific reduction in the cortical grey matter volume of posterior superior temporal gyrus, greatest on the left, and of planum temporale, again greatest on the left, as do chronically ill patients compared with controls (Hirayasu *et al.* 1998). Furthermore, as in chronically ill patients, the volumes in posterior STG and planum temporale, which likely contain one of several generators of P3, correlate positively with the left temporal scalp area P3 (McCarley *et al.* 2002). This programme of research has illuminated the specificity of significant left posterior superior temporal lobe involvement in schizophrenia during the early course of the disease, which highlights a possible aetiological role for dysfunction of

these cortical areas in the disease. As in this selective illustration, the examination of first episode patients is crucially important in determining whether some pathological findings in chronically ill patients are present at disease onset and thus intrinsic to the disorder, rather than a secondary consequence of chronicity, such as a long exposure to neuroleptic medication.

Other ERPs in schizophrenia

Other ERPs are the focus of intense research in schizophrenia patients, but space limitations preclude extensive discussion of them here. Several of these potentials have been related to the search for an electrophysiological concomitant of an early sensory gating deficit in schizophrenia. These include, for example, the startle response, where the size of a blink to an acoustic probe is measured. Schizophrenia patients appear to be unable to modify their large startle response when forewarned that a probe is coming, by contrast with controls (Braff *et al.* 1978).

(a)

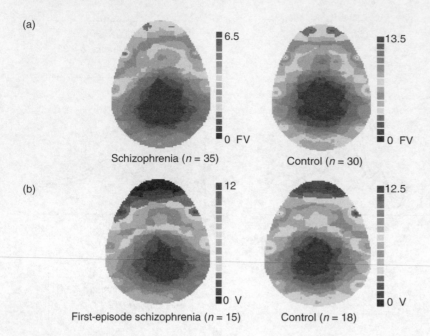

Schizophrenia (*n* = 35)   Control (*n* = 30)

(b)

First-episode schizophrenia (*n* = 15)   Control (*n* = 18)

Fig 16.6 Topographic maps of P300 scalp distribution. (a) Chronically ill schizophrenia patients show more oval P300 maxima, skewed to the right relative to controls. (b) The same left-sided reduction and skewed distribution is present in first episode schizophrenia. (Adapted from Salisbury *et al.* 1998; 1999). P300 voltage topography (peak ± 25 ms).

Another ERP thought to be sensitive to an early sensory gating abnormality in schizophrenia is the P50. In the sensory gating paradigm, an auditory click is presented to a subject, eliciting a positive deflection about 50 ms after stimulus onset, the P50 component. After a brief interval (about 500 ms), a second click elicits a much smaller amplitude P50 in normal adult subjects, who are said to show normal gating: the first stimulus inhibits, or closes, the gate to neurophysiological processing of the second stimulus. Patients with schizophrenia, on the other hand, show less reduction in P50 amplitude to the second click, which is referred to as a failure in gating (Freedman *et al.* 1983). This gating deficit occurs in about half of first-degree relatives of a schizophrenic patient, suggesting that it may index a genetic factor in schizophrenia in the absence of overt psychotic symptoms (Waldo *et al.* 1991). While patients with affective disorder may show a gating deficit, the deficit does not persist after successful treatment, whereas in patients with schizophrenia the deficit occurs in both medicated and unmedicated patients and persists after symptom remission (Freedman *et al.* 1983; Adler & Waldo 1991).

The gating effect is thought to take place in temporal lobe structures, possibly the medial temporal lobe (Adler *et al.* 1985). P50 gating is enhanced by nicotinic cholinergic mechanisms, and it is possible that smoking in patients with schizophrenia is a form of self-medication (McCarley *et al.* 1996). Freedman *et al.* (1994) have shown that blockade of the α7 nicotinic receptor, localized to hippocampal neurones, causes loss of the inhibitory gating response to auditory stimuli in an animal model. The failure of inhibitory mechanisms to gate sensory input to higher order processing may result in 'sensory flooding', which Freedman suggests may underlie many of the symptoms of schizophrenia.

The N100 has recently received renewed interest in schizophrenia. The majority of studies using various experimental paradigms have reported a reduction of N100 amplitude in medicated and medication-free schizophrenic patients (Ogura *et al.* 1991; Boutros *et al.* 1997). The underlying basis of this dysfunction was also investigated. Shelley *et al.* (1999) argued that this abnormality was related to a deficit in current flow in underlying neurones. This hypothesis was tested in monkeys, where applications of phencyclidine (PCP), an NMDA receptor antagonist, blocked the normal increase in N100 amplitude with increasing inter-stimulus interval (ISI) (Javitt *et al.* 2000b). Further studies have been interested in the behaviour of the responses as stimulus parameters change. Adler *et al.* (1990) showed that N100 in schizophrenia patients was less influenced by intensity and ISI than N100 in controls. A recent study measured visual evoked potentials in first episode patients, and reported no evidence of reductions in N100 (Katsanis *et al.* 1996). No other study has examined N100 in first episode patients. One other potential, the N200, is thought to relate to the initial categorization of stimuli in the selective attention stream. Studies have reported reduced amplitudes and increased latencies of N200 in schizophrenia (Salisbury *et al.* 1994b; Laurent *et al.* 1999). Unlike the P300, the deficit of the N200 amplitude is not ameliorated by antypsychotic treatment (Umbricht *et al.* 1998). However, the abnormality of N200 in schizophrenia is still not well understood and further studies are needed to address this issue.

Magnetoencephalography – a complement to electroencephalography

Magnetoencephalography (MEG) is the measure of magnetic fields generated by the brain. A key difference in the physical source of the MEG as contrasted to the EEG is that the MEG is sensitive to cells which lie tangential to the brain surface and consequently have magnetic fields orientated tangentially. Cells with a radial orientation (perpendicular to the brain surface) do not generate signals detectable with MEG. The EEG and MEG are complementary in that the EEG is most sensitive to radially orientated neurones and fields. This distinction arises because magnetic fields are generated at right angles to electrical fields. One major advantage that magnetic fields have over electrical potentials is that, once generated, they are relatively invulnerable to intervening variations in the media they traverse (i.e. the skull, grey and white matter, and cerebrospinal fluid), unlike electrical fields, which are 'smeared' by different electrical conductivities. This has made MEG a favourite for use in source localization, where attention has been especially focused on early potentials.

Perhaps because of the expense and non-mobility of the recording equipment needed for MEG, there has been relatively little work using MEG in schizophrenia to replicate and extend the findings of ERPs. A search of Medline revealed only 23 published studies using MEG measures of brain activity in schizophrenia. Studies have shown interesting results. Reite *et al.* (1999) demonstrated that the M100 component (the magnetic analogue to the N100) showed less interhemispheric asymmetry in schizophrenics and had different source orientations in the left hemisphere. The recent review by Reite *et al.* (1999) should be consulted for more details of the work on MEG in schizophrenia.

To summarize the studies to date, most have focused on M100. Results show a great degree of consistency across laboratories. The M100 shows abnormalities, particularly in the left hemisphere, with an altered dipole location (shifted anteriorly), and reduced asymmetry for right-ear stimuli in schizophrenia patients.

Conclusions

ERPs provide the greatest temporal resolution of all current functional imaging techniques. When coupled with information about likely generator sites from intracortical recordings, lesion studies and fMRI, and with spatially accurate measures of brain structure from high-resolution MRI, ERPs greatly contribute to the elucidation of brain function, essentially detecting physiology at the speed of thought. Further, ERPs allow for the elucidation of information processing long before any overt behaviour on the part of the subject. Both exogenous and endogenous ERPs are abnormal in chronically ill schizophrenia patients. These ERPs have help to direct investigations of specific cortical regions, which has identified pathophysiology specific to schizophrenia compared with affective psychosis. The concurrent investigation of ERPs and MRI in chronically ill and first episode patients has allowed for the detection of those abnormalities that are present at disease onset and those that appear to develop with disease course. For the latter abnormalities, such a demonstration immediately suggests the importance

of developing psychopharmacological interventions, which might counter at least some of the symptoms that develop with the disease course.

Acknowledgements

This work was supported in part by VA MERIT (R.W.M.) and Schizophrenia Center Awards (R.W.M.) from the Department of Veterans Affairs, the National Institute of Mental Health (MH 40977 R.W.M.), and the National Alliance for Research in Schizophrenia and Depression (D.F.S.).

References

Adler, L.E. & Waldo, M.C. (1991) Counterpoint: sensory gating-hippocampal model of schizophrenia,. *Schizophrenia Bulletin* 17, 19–24.

Adler, L.E., Waldo, M.C. & Freeman, R. (1985) Neurophysiological studies of sensory gating in schizophrenia: comparison of auditory and visual responses. *Biological Psychiatry* 20, 1284–1296.

Adler, G., Adler, J., Schenk, M. & Armbruster, B. (1990) Influence of stimulation parameters on auditory stimulus processing in schizophrenia and major depression: an evoked potential study. *Acta Psychiatrica Scandinavica* 81, 453–458.

Alain, C., Woods, D.L. & Knight, R.T. (1998) A distributed cortical network for auditory sensory memory in humans. *Brain Research* 812, 23–37.

Alho, K. (1995) Cerebral generators of mismatch negativity (MMN) and its magnetic counterpart (MMNm) elicited by sound changes. *Ear and Hearing* 16, 38–51.

Alho, K., Woods, D.L., Algazi, A., Knight, R.T. & Naatanen, R. (1994) Lesions of frontal cortex diminish the auditory mismatch negativity. *Electroencephalography and Clinical Neurophysiology* 91, 353–362.

Baldeweg, T., Spence, S., Hirsch, S.R. & Gruzelier, J. (1998) Gamma-band electroencephalographic oscillations in a patient with somatic hallucinations. *Lancet* 352, 620–621.

Baldeweg, T., Klugman, A., Gruzelier, J.H. & Hirsch, S.R. (2002). Impairment in frontal but not temporal components of mismatch negativity in schizophrenia. *International Journal of Psychophysiology* 43, 111–122.

Barta, P.E., Pearlson, G.D., Powers, R.E., Richards, S.S. & Tune, L.E. (1990) Auditory hallucinations and smaller superior temporal gyral volume in schizophrenia. *American Journal of Psychiatry* 147, 1457–1462.

Blackwood, D.H.R., St. Clair, D.M., Muir, W.J. & Duffy, J.C. (1991) Auditory P300 and eye tracking dysfunction in schizophrenic pedigrees. *Archives of General Psychiatry* 48, 899–909.

Boutros, N., Nasrallah, H., Leighty, R. *et al.* (1997) Auditory evoked potentials, clinical vs. research applications. *Psychiatry Research* 69, 183–195.

Braff, D., Stone, C., Callaway, E. *et al.* (1978) Prestimulus effects on human startle reflex in normals and schizophrenics. *Psychophysiology* 15, 339–343.

Buchsbaum, M. (1977) The middle evoked response components and schizophrenia. *Schizophrenia Bulletin* 3, 93–104.

Catts, S.V., Shelley, A.M., Ward, P.B. *et al.* (1995) Brain potential evidence for an auditory sensory memory deficit in schizophrenia. *American Journal of Psychiatry* 152, 213–219.

Csepe, V. (1995) On the origin and development of the mismatch negativity. *Ear Hear* **16**, 91–104.

Domino, E.F., Demetriou, S., Tuttle, T. & Klinge, V. (1979) Comparison of the visually evoked response in drug-free chronic schizophrenic patients and normal controls. *Electroencephalography and Clinical Neurophysiology* **46**, 123–137.

Ford, J.M., White, P.M., Csernansky, J.G. *et al.* (1994) ERPs in schizophrenia: effects of antipsychotic medication. *Biological Psychiatry* **36**, 153–170.

Freedman, R.F., Adler, L., Waldo, M., Oachtman, E. & Franks, R. (1983) Neurophysiological evidence for a defect in inhibitory pathways in schizophrenia: comparison of medicated and drug-free patients. *Biological Psychiatry* **18**, 537–551.

Freedman, R.F., Adler, L.E., Bickford, P. *et al.* (1994) Schizophrenia and nicotinic receptors. *Harvard Review of Psychiatry* **2**, 179–192.

Giard, M.H., Perrin, F., Echallier, J.F. *et al.* (1994) Dissociation of temporal and frontal components in the human auditory N1 wave: a scalp current density and dipole model analysis. *Electroencephalography and Clinical Neurophysiology* **92**, 238–252..

Hari, R., Hamalainen, M., Ilmoniemi, R. *et al.* (1984) Responses of the primary auditory cortex to pitch changes in a sequence of tone pips: neuromagnetic recordings in man. *Neuroscience Letters* **50**, 127–132.

Hirayasu, Y., Shenton, M.E., Salisbury, D.F. *et al.* (1998) Lower left temporal lobe MRI volumes in patients with first-episode schizophrenia compared with psychotic patients with first-episode affective disorder and normal subjects. *American Journal of Psychiatry* **155**, 1384–1391.

Javitt, D.C., Steinschneider, M., Schroeder, C.E. & Arezzo, J.C. (1996) Role of cortical N-methyl D-aspartate receptors in auditory sensory memory and mismatch negativity generation: implications for schizophrenia. *Proceedings of the National Academy of Sciences of the USA* **93**, 11962–11967.

Javitt, D.C., Shelley, A.M. & Ritter, W. (2000a) Associated deficits in mismatch negativity generation and tone matching in schizophrenia. *Clinical Neurophysiology* **111**, 1733–1737.

Javitt, D.C., Jayachandra, M., Lindsley, R.W., Specht, C.M. & Schroeder, C.E. (2000b) Schizophrenia-like deficits in auditory P1 and N1 refractoriness induced by the psychotomimetic agent phencyclidine. *Clinical Neurophysiology* **111**, 833–836.

Jessen, F., Fries, T., Kucharski, C. *et al.* (2001) Amplitude reduction of the mismatch negativity in first-degree relatives of patients with schizophrenia. *Neuroscience Letters* **309**, 185–188.

John, E.R., Prichep, L.S., Alper, K.R. *et al.* (1994) Quantitative electrophysiological characteristics and subtyping of schizophrenia. *Biological Psychiatry* **36**, 801–826.

Katsanis, J., Iacono, W.G. & Beiser, M. (1996) Visual event-related potentials in first-episode psychotic patients and their relatives. *Psychophysiology* **33**, 207–217.

Kissler, J., Muller, M.M., Fehr, T., Rockstroh, B.E. & Bert, T. (2000) MEG gamma band activity in schizophrenia patients and healthy subjects in a mental arithmetic task and at rest. *Clinical Neurophysiology* **111**, 2079–2087.

Kraus, N., McGee, T., Carrell, T. *et al.* (1994) Discrimination of speech-like contrasts in the auditory thalamus and cortex. *Journal of Acoustic Society of America* **96**, 2758–2768.

Kwon, J.S., O'Donnell, B.F., Wallenstein, G.V. *et al.* (1999) Gamma frequency-range abnormalities to auditory stimulation in schizophrenia. *Archives of General Psychiatry* **56**, 1001–1005.

Laurent, A., Garcia-Larréa, L., d'Amato, T. *et al.* (1999) Auditory event-related potentials and clinical scores in unmedicated schizophrenic patients. *Psychiatry Research* **87**, 147–157.

Levit, R.A., Sutton, S. & Zubin, J. (1973) Evoked potential correlated of information processing in psychiatric patients. *Psychological Medicine* **3**, 487–494.

Logothetis, N.K., Pauls, J., Augath, M., Trinath, T. & Oeltermann, A. (2001) Neurophysiological investigation of the basis of the fMRI signal. *Nature* **412**, 150–157.

McCarley, R.W., Shenton, M.E., O'Donnell, B.F. *et al.* (1993) Auditory P300 abnormalities and left posterior superior temporal gyrus volume reduction in schizophrenia. *Archives of General Psychiatry* **50**, 190–197.

McCarley, R.W., Hsiao, J.K., Freedman, R., Pfefferbaum, A. & Donchin, E. (1996) Neuroimaging and the cognitive neuroscience of schizophrenia. *Schizophrenia Bulletin* **22**, 703–725.

McCarley, R.W., Salisbury, D.F., Hirayasu, Y. *et al.* (2002) Association between smaller left posterior superior temporal gyrus MRI volume and smaller left temporal P300 amplitude in first episode schizophrenia. *Archives of General Psychiatry* **59**, 321–331.

McGhie, A. & Chapman, J. (1961) Disorders of attention and perception in early schizophrenia. *British Journal of Medical Psychiatry* **34**, 103–116.

Naatanen, R. (1992) *Attention and Brain Function*. Hillsdale, NJ/ Lawrence Erlbaum, Hove.

Ogura, C., Nageishi, Y., Matsubayashi, M. *et al.* (1991) Abnormalities in event-related potentials, N100, P200, P300 and slow wave in schizophrenia. *Japanese Journal of Psychiatry and Neurology* **45**, 57–65.

Olney, J.W. & Farber, N.B. (1995) Glutamate receptor dysfunction and schizophrenia. *Archives of General Psychiatry* **52**, 998–1007.

Raichle, M. (1998) Behind the scence of functional brain imaging: a historical and physiological perspective. *Proceedings of the National Academy of Sciences of the USA* **95**, 765–772.

Rauch, S. & Renshaw, P. (1995) Clinical neuroimaging in psychiatry. *Harvard Review of Psychiatry* **2**, 297–312.

Regan, D. (1989) Human brain electrophysiology. *Evoked-Potentials and Evoked Magnetic Fields in Science and Medicine*. Elsevier, New York.

Reite, M., Teale, P. & Rojas, D.C. (1999) Magnetoencephalography: applications in psychiatry. *Biological Psychiatry* **45**, 1553–1563.

Roth, W.T. (1977) Late event-related potentials and psychopathology. *Schizophrenia Bulletin* **3**, 105–120.

Roth, W.T. & Cannon, E. (1972) Some features of the auditory evoked response in schizophrenics. *Archives of General Psychiatry* **27**, 466–471.

Saletu, B., Itil, T.M. & Saletu, M. (1971) Auditory evoked response, EEG, and thought process in schizophrenia. *American Journal of Psychiatry* **128**, 336–343.

Salisbury, D.F., O'Donnell, B.F., McCarley, R.W. *et al.* (1994a) Parametric manipulations of auditory stimuli differentially affect P3 amplitude in schizophrenics and controls. *Psychophysiology* **31**, 29–36.

Salisbury, D.F., O'Donnell, B.F., McCarley, R.W., Shenton, M.E. & Benavage, A. (1994b) The N2 event-related potential reflects attention deficit in schizophrenia. *Biological Psychology* **39**, 1–13.

Salisbury, D.F., Shenton, M.E., Sherwood, A.R. *et al.* (1998) First episode schizophrenic psychosis differs from first episode affective psychosis and controls in P300 amplitude over left temporal lobe. *Archives of General Psychiatry* **55**, 173–180.

Salisbury, D.F., Bonner-Jackson, A., Griggs, C.B., Shenton, M.E. & McCarley, R.W. (2001) Mismatch negativity in schizophrenia: does MMN amplitude decline with disease duration? *Biological Psychiatry* **49** (Suppl.), 85S.

Salisbury, D.F., Shenton, M.E., Griggs, C.B., Bonner-Jackson, A. & McCarley, R.W. (2002) Mismatch negativity in chronic schizophrenia and first-episode schizophrenia. *Archives of General Psychiatry* **59**, 686–694.

Schooler, C., Buchsbaum, M.S. & Carpenter, W.T. (1976) Evoked response and kinesthetic measures of augmenting/reducing in schizophrenics: replications and extensions. *Journal of Nervous and Mental Disease* **163**, 221–232.

Shagass, C. (1968) Cerebral evoked responses in schizophrenia. *Conditional Reflex* **3**, 205–216.

Shagass, C. (1977) The early potentials. *Schizophrenia Bulletin* **3**, 80–92.

Shagass, C., Soskis, D.A., Straumanis, J.J. & Overton, D.A. (1974) Symptom patterns related to somatosensory evoked response differences within a schizophrenia population. *Biological Psychiatry* **9**, 25–43.

Shelley, A.M., Silipo, G. & Javitt, D.C. (1999) Diminished responsiveness of ERPs in schizophrenic subjects to changes in auditory stimulation parameters: implications for theories of cortical dysfunction. *Schizophrenia Research* **37**, 65–79.

Shenton, M.E., Kikinis, R., Jolesz, F.A. *et al.* (1992) Abnormalities of the left temporal lobe and thought disorder in schizophrenia: a quantitative magnetic resonance imaging study. *New England Journal of Medicine* **327**, 604–612.

Sutton, S., Braren, M., Zubin, J. & John, E.R. (1965) Evoked potential correlates of stimulus uncertainty. *Science* **150**, 1187–1188.

Turetsky, B., Colbath, E.A. & Gur, R.A. (1998) P300 subcomponent abnormalities in schizophrenia. II. Longitudinal stability and relationship to symptom change. *Biological Psychiatry* **43**, 31–39.

Umbricht, D., Javitt, D., Novak, G. *et al.* (1998) Effects of clozapine on auditory event-related potentials in schizophrenia. *Biological Psychiatry* **44**, 716–725.

Umbricht, D., Schmid, L., Koller, R. *et al.* (2000) Ketamine-induced deficits in auditory and visual context-dependent processing in healthy volunteers. *Archives of General Psychiatry* **57**, 1139–1147.

Umbricht, D.C., Javitt, J., Bates, J., Kane, J.A. & Lieberman (2002) Auditory event-related potentials (ERP): indices of both premorbid and illness-related progressive neuropathology in schizophrenia? *Schizophrenia Research* **53** (3), 18.

Venables, P. (1964) Input dysfunction in schizophrenia. In: *Progress in Experimental Personality Research* (ed. B. Maher), pp. 1–47. Academic Press, New York.

Waldo, M.C., Carey, G., Myles-Worsley, M. *et al.* (1991) Codistribution of a sensory gating deficit and schizophrenia in multi-affected families. *Psychiatry Research* **39**, 257–268.

Wible, C., Kubicki, M., Yoo, S. *et al.* (2001) A functional magnetic resonance imaging study of auditory mismatch in schizophrenia. *American Journal of Psychiatry* **158**, 938–943.

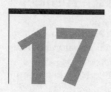

17 Neuropathology of schizophrenia

P.J. Harrison and D.A. Lewis

Neurodegeneration in schizophrenia, 310
  Gliosis, 310
  Alzheimer's disease, 311
The hippocampal formation, 311
  Hippocampal morphometric findings, 312
  Hippocampal synaptic and dendritic
    abnormalities, 312
The prefrontal cortex, 313
  Synaptic abnormalities and the connections of the
    dorsal prefrontal cortex, 314
  Thalamic projections to the prefrontal cortex, 314
  Dorsal prefrontal cortex interneurones and their
    connections, 316
  Prefrontal cortex projections to the thalamus, 317
Neuropathological interpretations, 317

How are the hippocampal and dorsal prefrontal
  cortex changes related? 317
Is there an asymmetry of neuropathology? 317
How are the pathology and the symptoms related?
  317
Do the neuropathological data support a
  neurodevelopmental origin of schizophrenia?
  318
Are the changes specific to schizophrenia? 319
Are the changes brought about by medication?
  319
Will schizophrenia ever be diagnosable down a
  microscope? 319
Conclusions, 320
References, 320

There is no neuropathology of schizophrenia in the sense that there is a neuropathology of Huntington's disease, neurosyphilis or a glioma. However, this stark statement conceals the fact that significant progress has been made in discovering the existence and nature of histological correlates of schizophrenia, both by ruling out certain processes, as well as by providing some intriguing positive results concerning alterations in cortical architecture which may contribute to the anatomical substrate of the disorder.

The recent upturn of fortunes in this field has come about for several reasons. First, accumulating evidence from computerized tomography (CT) and magnetic resonance imaging (MRI) studies of the past 25 years has shown unequivocally that structural brain abnormalities are present in schizophrenia. There must be a histological and, ultimately, a molecular basis for such alterations, and this simple but fundamental point has stimulated neuropathological research. Secondly, lessons have been learned from the earlier generation of studies, which were inadequate by current standards of study design, methodology and statistical analysis. Thirdly, the resurgence of interest has coincided with the rapid progress in neuroscience and molecular biology. These have increased the sophistication of contemporary studies, and have provided a much more powerful range of tools with which to conduct them.

This chapter summarizes the current understanding of the neuropathology of schizophrenia and its interpretation. We have not attempted a comprehensive or historical review, but emphasize those aspects for which there is a convergence and consistency to the findings in order to highlight the key points and major themes; in anatomical terms we have focused on the hippocampal formation, dorsal prefrontal cortex (DPFC) and the thalamus. (For more detailed coverage, including discussion of brain areas not considered here, see Arnold & Trojanowski 1996; Harrison 1999a; Harrison & Roberts 2000. For review of the now largely disregarded early literature, see David 1957.)

Neurodegeneration in schizophrenia

A critical question concerns the neuropathological nature of schizophrenia. In the most basic (and grossly oversimplified) sense, neuropathological processes are either degenerative or developmental. In the former, there are usually cytopathological inclusions (e.g. neurofibrillary tangles, Lewy bodies) and evidence for neuronal and synaptic loss, accompanied by gliosis (reactive astrocytosis). A degenerative process underlies most dementias, as well as the pathology seen after hypoxia, infection and trauma. In the absence of any evidence for abnormalities of this kind, a neurodevelopmental process, in which something goes awry with normal brain maturation, is by default the likely form of pathology to explain a brain disorder. (Weinberger 1987) Because this distinction – despite its limitations – has such important implications for the nature of the disease, we first review the studies which have sought, and failed, to find consistent positive evidence for neurodegeneration in schizophrenia.

Gliosis

In a paper which heralded the start of the current phase of research, Stevens (1982) described reactive astrocytosis in ~70% of her series of cases with schizophrenia. The gliosis was usually located in periventricular and subependymal regions of the diencephalon or in adjacent basal forebrain structures. This finding supported aetiopathogenic scenarios for schizophrenia involving infective, ischaemic, autoimmune or neurodegenerative processes.

In contrast to Stevens' findings, many subsequent investigations of schizophrenia have not found gliosis (Roberts & Harrison 2000). The study of Bruton et al. (1990) was illuminating, finding that gliosis in schizophrenia was only seen in cases exhibiting separate neuropathological abnormalities, such as focal lesions, infarcts and so on, many of which clearly post-dated the onset of psychosis. This suggested strongly that gliosis is not an intrinsic feature of the disease, but is a sign of coincidental or superimposed pathological changes (which occur in a significant minority of cases; Riederer et al. 1995). This view, although now broadly accepted, is subject to qualifications. First, the recognition and definition of gliosis is not as straightforward as sometimes assumed (Stevens et al. 1988, 1992; Da Cunha et al. 1993). Secondly, most studies have focused on the cerebral cortex rather than on the diencephalic regions where the gliosis of Stevens (1982) was concentrated, although the recent study of Falkai et al. (1999) overcomes this limitation. Thirdly, there could be pathological heterogeneity, with a proportion of cases being 'neurodegenerative'; however, the cumulative data suggest that this proportion would have to be small.

The gliosis debate has been stimulated by its implications for the nature of schizophrenia. The gliotic response is said not to occur until the end of the second trimester in utero (Friede 1989). Hence, an absence of gliosis, in the context of other pathological abnormalities, is considered strong evidence for an early neurodevelopmental origin of schizophrenia. However, timing of the developmental onset of the glial response has not been well investigated and so absence of gliosis should not be used to time the pathology of schizophrenia with any certainty. For example, gliotic reactions have been clearly described after amniocentesis needle injury occurring at 16–18 weeks' gestation (Squier et al. 2000). Moreover, gliosis is not always demonstrable or permanent (Kalman et al. 1993). Neither is it thought to accompany programmed cell death (apoptosis) of neurones, which has been hypothesized to be relevant to schizophrenia. Furthermore, it is a moot point whether the subtle kinds of morphometric disturbance to be described, whenever and however they occurred, would be sufficient to trigger detectable gliosis. Thus, the lack of gliosis does not mean, in isolation, that schizophrenia must be a neurodevelopmental disorder of prenatal origin; it is merely one argument in favour of that conclusion (Roberts & Harrison 2000). Certainly, in isolation, an absence of gliosis does not negate models of schizophrenia which include aberrant plasticity and perhaps mild neurotoxic processes in addition to a classically neurodevelopmental process (DeLisi 1997; Lieberman 1999). Addressing this possibility will require study of other glial cell populations, particularly microglia, which provide complementary information about immune and inflammatory processes (Bayer et al. 1999).

Alzheimer's disease

The other area of controversy regarding neurodegenerative processes in schizophrenia concerns the neuropathological explanation for the cognitive deficits of the disorder, and the supposedly greater prevalence of Alzheimer's disease in schizophrenia.

The belief that Alzheimer's disease is more common in schizophrenia originated in the 1930s (Corsellis 1962) and was bolstered by a large, although uncontrolled, study (Prohovnik et al. 1993), and by data implying that antipsychotic drugs might promote Alzheimer-type changes (Wisniewski et al. 1994).

However, a meta-analysis (Baldessarini et al. 1997) and several subsequent studies, which have used sophisticated staining techniques and careful experimental designs, show conclusively that Alzheimer's disease is not more common than expected in schizophrenia (Arnold et al. 1998; Murphy et al. 1998; Purohit et al. 1998; Jellinger & Gabriel 1999). This even applies amongst elderly schizophrenics with moderate to severe dementia and in whom there is no other neurodegenerative disorder apparent (Arnold et al. 1996, 1998; Purohit et al. 1998). Moreover, the evidence does not support the view that antipsychotic drugs predispose to neurofibrillary or amyloid-related pathology (Baldessarini et al. 1997; Harrison 1999b).

The only known neuropathological correlate of dementia in schizophrenia is a small increase in the number of glial fibrillary acidic protein (GFAP)-positive astrocytes, with no change in other immunocytochemical indices of gliosis (Arnold et al. 1996). Apart from this, the severe cognitive impairment observed in chronically hospitalized elderly subjects with schizophrenia remains unexplained. It may just be a more severe manifestation of whatever pathology underlies the disorder itself, or perhaps the brain in schizophrenia is rendered more vulnerable to cognitive impairment in response to a normal age-related amount of neurodegeneration.

The hippocampal formation

In the absence of degenerative changes, attention is now focused on alterations in the neural cytoarchitecture (the morphology and arrangement of neurones), in tandem with studies of synapses and dendrites. The majority of these studies of schizophrenia have been in the hippocampal formation and prefrontal cortex, and the data in these two areas are considered in turn.

The hippocampal formation (hippocampus and parahippocampal gyrus) in the medial temporal lobe has been studied in schizophrenia for three reasons. First, when the current renaissance began 20 years ago, it was the hippocampal formation wherein several of the most striking initial findings were described, and this has continued to be the case (Arnold 1997; Weinberger 1999). The search for histological changes has been encouraged by the demonstration in vivo that hippocampal volume is decreased in first episode (Velakoulis et al. 1999) as well as chronic (Nelson et al. 1998) cases – although the latter has not been consistently shown postmortem. Furthermore, hippocampal proton resonance spectroscopy shows a reduced hippocampal N-acetyl aspartate (NAA) signal, suggestive of a neuronal pathology (Bertolino et al. 1998). Parenthetically, the NAA decrease is also present in first episode schizophrenia, providing some encouragement that complementary morphometric findings to be described below, although made in chronic cases, may also have been present at this time. Secondly, abnormal metabolic activity of the medial temporal lobe is seen in functional imaging studies of schizophrenia, related both to psychotic symptoms (Friston et al. 1992; Tamminga et al. 1992) and attentional/cognitive aspects (Heckers et al. 1998).

Neuropsychological data also implicate hippocampal dysfunction (Saykin *et al.* 1994). Thirdly, the relatively precise circuitry of the hippocampal formation lends itself to studies seeking to investigate neural connectivity, a concept which has become central to pathophysiological theories of schizophrenia (Friston & Frith 1995; Harrison 1999a; Benes 2000); this question is much more difficult to address in most other regions.

Hippocampal morphometric findings

The first influential morphometric abnormality reported in the hippocampus in schizophrenia was that of neuronal disarray. Normally, pyramidal neurones in Ammon's horn are aligned, as in a pallisade, with the apical dendrite orientated towards the stratum radiatum. Kovelman and Scheibel (1984) reported that this orientation was more variable and even reversed in schizophrenia, hence the term neuronal disarray. The disarray was present at the boundaries of CA1 with CA2 and subiculum. They suggested that a developmental migrational disturbance might be responsible. Qualified support for a greater variability of hippocampal neuronal orientation came in subsequent studies from the same group (Altshuler *et al.* 1987; Conrad *et al.* 1991). However, several other groups, using computerized image analysis-assisted measurements of neuronal orientation, have not replicated the observation (Christison *et al.* 1989; Benes *et al.* 1991b; Arnold *et al.* 1995a; Zaidel *et al.* 1997b). It is therefore unlikely that hippocampal neuronal disarray is associated with schizophrenia.

The second oft-cited feature of the hippocampal formation in schizophrenia is that of misplaced and aberrantly clustered neurones in lamina II (pre-α cells) and lamina III of the entorhinal cortex (anterior parahippocampal gyrus), described by Jakob and Beckmann (1986) and replicated by Arnold *et al.* (1991a, 1997). This finding was also interpreted as being developmental in origin and resulting from aberrant neuronal migration; certainly it is difficult to think of another plausible mechanism by which a cell population could show this kind of abnormality. However, other studies, with larger samples, better control groups or methodologies which take into account the significant intrinsic and interindividual heterogeneity of the entorhinal cortex, have not found clear differences (Heinsen *et al.* 1996; Akil & Lewis 1997; Krimer *et al.* 1997; Bernstein *et al.* 1998). Nevertheless, the situation remains controversial. Falkai *et al.* (2000) have recently reported quantitative evidence of abnormally located and smaller sized clusters of neurones in the entorhinal cortex, using a different form of analysis in the same brain series as that of Bernstein *et al.* (1998). It is essential to explain these discrepancies and establish if such abnormalities are or are not seen in the disorder, because their presence would be strong evidence in favour of an early neurodevelopmental origin of schizophrenia (Roberts 1991).

A loss of hippocampal neurones is a third finding sometimes described as a feature of schizophrenia. In fact, only two studies have found reductions in neuronal density (Jeste & Lohr 1989; Jonsson *et al.* 1997) and one reported a lower number of pyramidal neurones (Falkai & Bogerts 1986). In contrast, several have found no change in neuronal density (Falkai &Bogerts 1986; Benes *et al.* 1991b; Arnold *et al.* 1995) and one found a right-sided increase (Zaidel *et al.* 1997a). As well as being contradictory, none of these studies were stereological and so their value is limited by the inherent weaknesses of neuronal counts made in this way. The fact that the single stereological study which has been carried out found no difference in neuronal number or density in any subfield (Heckers *et al.* 1991) supports the view that there is no overall change in neuronal content of the hippocampus in schizophrenia. In this context, single reports of altered neuronal density restricted to a specific neuronal type (Benes *et al.* 1998), subfield or hemisphere (Zaidel *et al.* 1997b) must be replicated before discussion is warranted.

Computerized image analysis made it relatively straightforward to measure the size of neurones, either by tracing around the cell body or by measuring the smallest circle within which it fits, although neither of these approaches produces unbiased estimates of somal size now available with stereological techniques. Three studies, each counting large numbers of neurones, have identified a smaller mean size of hippocampal pyramidal neurones (Benes *et al.* 1991b; Arnold *et al.* 1995; Zaidel *et al.* 1997a). Although different individual subfields reached significance in the latter two studies, the same downward trend was present in all CA fields and in the subiculum. The nonreplications comprise Christison *et al.* (1989) and Benes *et al.* (1998), perhaps because measurements were limited to a restricted subset of neurones. Smaller neuronal size has also been reported in DPFC, as discussed below. A degree of anatomical specificity is apparent, because cell size is unchanged in visual cortex (Rajkowska *et al.* 1998) and in motor cortex (Benes *et al.* 1986; Arnold *et al.* 1995). Finally, Zaidel *et al.* (1997a) found that pyramidal neurones were more elongated (as well as being smaller) in some hippocampal subfields in schizophrenia, which might relate to the abnormalities in dendritic arborization described in the next section.

Hippocampal synaptic and dendritic abnormalities

Changes in neuronal cell body parameters are likely to be a sign and a consequence of alterations in other neuronal compartments and the cytoarchitecture in which they are situated. Neuronal size is related to axonal diameter and other parameters of axodendritic arborization (Gilbert & Kelly 1975; Lund *et al.* 1975; Pierce & Lewin 1994; Hayes & Lewis 1996; Esiri & Pearson 2000), because the vast majority of a neurone's total volume is in its processes (especially axons in the case of projection neurones), and the size of the soma reflects the cellular machinery necessary to support them. Somal size varies normally within as well as between neuronal populations; it also changes (in both directions) in response to altered afferent and efferent connectivity (e.g. shrinkage after retrograde degeneration).

Investigation of synapses in schizophrenia has used various proteins, which are concentrated in presynaptic terminals, to serve as markers (Honer *et al.* 2000; Eastwood & Harrison

2001). First applied to Alzheimer's disease, using the protein synaptophysin, this approach has been validated in various neuropathological and experimental situations (Eastwood *et al.* 1994). Dendrites can also be investigated in an analogous fashion using dendritically located proteins, notably microtubule-associated protein-2 (MAP-2). In addition, the rapid Golgi method can be used, despite limitations, to study dendritic parameters (e.g. spine density, shape analysis) in postmortem material.

Key synaptic and dendritic findings in the hippocampal formation in schizophrenia are as follows (Harrison & Eastwood 2001). Decreased expression of synaptophysin has been found in several studies, with decrements also in other synaptic proteins such as SNAP-25, the synapsins and the complexins (Eastwood & Harrison 1995, 1999; for review see Honer *et al.* 2000). Data in degenerative disorders indicate that these decreases are likely to be a reflection of a lowered density of synapses; however, decreases in synaptic activity, synaptic plasticity (Eastwood & Harrison 1998) or the turnover of these gene products might also contribute to the observations. The affected circuits involve intrinsic hippocampal neurones (in addition to any involvement of neurones projecting into the hippocampal formation), because the level of the encoding messenger RNAs (mRNAs) is also reduced. Some data suggest that excitatory neurones and their synapses may be more affected than inhibitory ones (Harrison & Eastwood 1998), but other data indicate the reverse pattern (Benes *et al.* 1998; Benes 2000) or a similar involvement of both (Eastwood & Harrison 2000). There are complementary data showing hippocampal dendritic alterations in schizophrenia, with decreased immunoreactivity for MAP-2, a dendritic marker (Arnold *et al.* 1991b), as well as reduced density of dendritic spines in subicular neurones (Rosoklija *et al.* 2000). In summary, there is good evidence for synaptic pathology in the hippocampal formation, but the specific characteristics of the alterations remain to be established. These issues are discussed in more detail after description of the main findings in the prefrontal cortex.

The prefrontal cortex

Although studies by Alzheimer identified the dorsal prefrontal cortex (DPFC) as a possible site of pathological alterations in schizophrenia, this brain region did not become a major focus of postmortem studies until the early 1990s. As such, they have lagged behind those of the hippocampal formation, although noteworthy similarities, as well as differences, are becoming apparent between the two areas. The hippocampal findings were described above by taking each type of morphometric alteration in turn; in contrast, the DPFC studies are considered here within the context of how they may contribute to an overall picture of aberrant connectivity. The latter approach represents the prevailing view as to the nature of the anatomical basis of schizophrenia (Lewis 1997; Harrison 1999a).

Investigations of the DPFC in schizophrenia have been motivated by observations that subjects with schizophrenia exhibit both a relative hypometabolism of the DPFC, and impaired performance on cognitive tasks, such as those involving working memory, which are known to depend upon the integrity of DPFC circuitry. The idea that this dysfunction might be attributable to structural abnormalities in the DPFC has been supported by MRI studies which have revealed subtle reductions in grey matter volume of the DPFC in subjects with schizophrenia (McCarley *et al.* 1999). The failure to detect such abnormalities in all studies has been hypothesized to be a consequence of several factors, including volume reductions that approach the level of sensitivity of MRI and the restriction of volumetric changes to certain DPFC regions or gyri (McCarley *et al.* 1999). Consistent with this view, postmortem studies have frequently revealed a 3–12% decreased in cortical thickness in the DPFC in subjects with schizophrenia (Pakkenberg 1993; Daviss & Lewis 1995; Selemon *et al.* 1995; Woo *et al.* 1997a), although these changes were not always statistically significant. In addition, some (Bertolino *et al.* 1996, 2000; Deicken *et al.* 1997), but not all (Stanley *et al.* 1996), *in vivo* proton spectroscopy studies indicate that subjects with schizophrenia have reduced concentrations of DPFC NAA, a putative marker of neuronal and/or axonal integrity. Interestingly, the magnitude of these NAA changes in the DPFC has been correlated with the degree of impaired activation in other brain regions during working memory tasks, raising the possibility that a neuronal abnormality in the DPFC could account for distributed functional disturbances in the working memory network (Bertolino *et al.* 2000).

Other lines of evidence suggest that these changes may reflect disturbances in the synaptic connectivity of the DPFC. Observations by phosphorus-31 spectroscopy that never-medicated schizophrenic subjects have decreased phosphomonoesters and/or increased phosphodiesters in the DPFC have been interpreted as evidence of decreased synthesis and increased breakdown of membrane phospholipids, and consequently of a decreased number of synapses (Keshavan *et al.* 2000). In addition, DPFC levels of synaptophysin, an integral membrane protein of small synaptic vesicles, have been reported to be reduced in subjects with schizophrenia in many (Perrone-Bizzozero *et al.* 1996; Glantz & Lewis 1997; Davidsson *et al.* 1999; Honer *et al.* 1999; Karson *et al.* 1999) but not all studies (Gabriel *et al.* 1997; Eastwood *et al.* 2000). Alterations in other synapse-related proteins have also been described in the DPFC, although these observations are fewer in number and less consistent across studies and prefrontal cortex regions (Thompson *et al.* 1998; Davidsson *et al.* 1999; Karson *et al.* 1999). Finally, reports of increased cell packing density (Daviss & Lewis 1995; Selemon *et al.* 1995, 1998) have been interpreted as evidence that the DPFC neuropil, which is composed of the axon terminals and dendritic spines and shafts that form most cortical synapses, is reduced in schizophrenia (Selemon & Goldman-Rakic 1999).

Thus, various lines of evidence support the hypothesis that schizophrenia is associated with a decrease in the synaptic connectivity of the DPFC, although alternative explanations for these observations need to be considered. For example, some of the data cited above could be explained by a decrease in the number of DPFC neurones. However, the total number of prefrontal cortex neurones was not decreased in subjects with schizophrenia in a study that used an unbiased approach to address this question (Thune *et al*. 1998). In addition, postmortem studies have tended to find either a normal or, as noted above, increased cell packing density in the DPFC (Daviss & Lewis 1995; Selemon *et al*. 1995, 1998; Rajkowska *et al*. 1998). One limitation of these studies is that they may have lacked adequate sensitivity to detect reduced neuronal number or density of small subpopulations of DPFC neurones. Thus, the possibility that schizophrenia is associated with decrements in certain subsets of neurones, such as small neurones in layer 2 (Benes *et al*. 1991a) or the parvalbumin-containing subpopulation of γ-aminobutyric acid (GABA) neurones (Beasley & Reynolds 1997), cannot be excluded. However, the latter abnormality was not observed in another study (Woo *et al*. 1997a), and it should be noted that a reduction in neuronal density when using immunocytochemical markers may reflect an alteration in abundance or antigenicity of the target protein rather than in the number of neurones.

The reduction in DPFC grey matter in schizophrenia could also be caused, at least in part, by smaller neuronal cell bodies. The somal volume of pyramidal cells in deep layer 3 of DPFC area 9 has been reported in two studies to be decreased in subjects with schizophrenia (Rajkowska *et al*. 1998; Pierri *et al*. 2001). As discussed in the section on the hippocampal formation, this reduction may be associated with a decrease in total length of the basilar dendrites of these neurones (Glantz & Lewis 2000; Kalus *et al*. 2000), as well as with the decreased synaptophysin levels mentioned above. In contrast, the size of DPFC GABA neurones does not appear to be reduced in schizophrenia (Benes *et al*. 1986; Woo *et al*. 1997a). In summary, although a reduction in neurone number cannot be completely excluded, the subtle reduction in DPFC grey matter in schizophrenia appears more attributable to a combination of smaller neurones and a decrease in the axon terminals, distal dendrites and dendritic spines (see below) that represent the principal components of cortical synapses.

Synaptic abnormalities and the connections of the dorsal prefrontal cortex

Alterations in DPFC synaptic connectivity in schizophrenia may involve synapses formed by intrinsic axon terminals arising from neurones within the DPFC and/or from extrinsic axon terminals projecting to the DPFC from other cortical regions, the brainstem or the thalamus.

The reduced somal volume of DPFC layer 3 pyramidal cells (Rajkowska *et al*. 1998; Pierri *et al*. 2001), which give rise to a substantial number of intrinsic excitatory synapses (Levitt *et al*. 1993; Pucak *et al*. 1996), suggests that the synapses furnished by the intrinsic axon collaterals of these neurones may be reduced in number in schizophrenia. The results of a recent study using complementary DNA (cDNA) microarray profiling of the ex-

pression of over 7000 genes in DPFC area 9 of subjects with schizophrenia (Mirnics *et al*. 2000) may also be consistent with a disturbance in intrinsic connectivity. For example, among 250 functional gene groups, the most marked changes in expression were found in the group that encode for proteins involved in the regulation of presynaptic neurotransmitter release. Although these findings very likely indicate a general impairment of synaptic transmission within the DPFC in schizophrenia, it remains to be determined whether they represent a 'primary' abnormality intrinsic to the DPFC or a 'secondary' response to deficient inputs from other brain regions. Furthermore, because the specific genes within this group with the most altered levels of expression differed between subjects, it seems unlikely that these findings can be attributed solely to a downregulation of transcription secondary to a diminished number of intrinsic DPFC synapses. Consistent with this interpretation, synaptophysin mRNA levels do not appear to be reduced in the DPFC in schizophrenia (Karson *et al*. 1999; Eastwood *et al*. 2000; Glantz *et al*. 2000), suggesting that the reduced amount of synaptophysin protein in the DPFC may have an extrinsic source. The reduction of synaptophysin mRNA levels in other brain areas in schizophrenia, such as the hippocampal formation, may also be consistent with this view (Eastwood & Harrison 1999). However, whether these transcriptional changes occur in neurones that project to the DPFC, and if so whether they result in reduced levels of synaptophysin protein in the terminal fields of these neurones, has not been assessed.

In terms of subcortical inputs to the DPFC, the dopamine (DA) projections from the mesencephalon may be reduced in number in schizophrenia. The densities of axons immunoreactive for tyrosine hydroxylase, the rate-limiting enzyme in catecholamine synthesis, and the DA membrane transporter, are both decreased in DPFC area 9 of subjects with schizophrenia (Akil *et al*. 1999). In addition, an *in vivo* neuroimaging study reported a reduced density of D_1 receptors in the DPFC of unmedicated subjects with schizophrenia (Okubo *et al*. 1997). Thus, these findings may be in line with other data supporting a hypodopaminergic state in the DPFC in schizophrenia (Weinberger *et al*. 1988; Davis *et al*. 1991). However, the following caveats must be considered:

1 these observations may reflect merely a change in protein markers, and do not necessarily mean that the number of DPFC DA axons is decreased;

2 the reductions in markers of DA axons were confined to the deep cortical layers; and

3 DA axons are estimated to contribute < 1% of cortical synapses (Lewis & Sesack 1997).

Thus, these findings could not alone account for the observed reductions in grey matter volume, or synaptophysin levels, in the DPFC of subjects with schizophrenia.

Thalamic projections to the prefrontal cortex

Various lines of evidence suggest that altered inputs from the thalamus may be one of the major contributors to decreased

Fig 17.1 Schematic diagram summarizing disturbances in the connectivity between the mediodorsal nucleus of the thalamus (MDN) and the dorsal prefrontal cortex (PFC) in schizophrenia. Postmortem studies have reported that subjects with schizophrenia have:

1 decreased number of neurones in the mediodorsal thalamic nucleus;

2 diminished density of parvalbumin-positive varicosities, a putative marker of thalamic axon terminals, selectively in deep layers 3–4, the termination zone of MDN projections to the PFC;

3 preferential reduction in spine density on the basilar dendrites of deep layer 3 pyramidal neurones, a principal synaptic target of the excitatory projections from the MDN;

4 reduced expression of the mRNAs for glutamic acid decarboxylase (GAD_{67}), the synthesizing enzyme for GABA, and the GABA transporter (GAT-1) in a subset of PFC GABA neurones;

5 decreased density of GAT-1-immunoreactive axon cartridges, the distinctive, vertically arrayed axon terminals of GABAergic chandelier neurones, which synapse exclusively on the axon initial segment of pyramidal neurones;

6 decreased dopamine (DA) innervation of layer 6, the principal location of pyramidal neurones that provide corticothalamic feedback projections (see Lewis 2000b for additional details and references). (Adapted from Lewis & Lieberman 2000.)

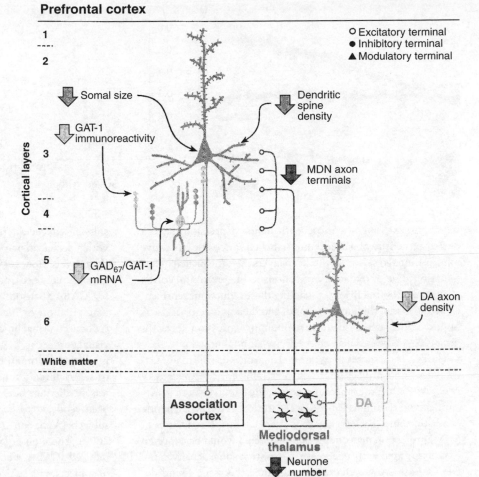

Prefrontal cortex

○ Excitatory terminal
● Inhibitory terminal
▲ Modulatory terminal

Somal size

GAT-1 immunoreactivity

Dendritic spine density

MDN axon terminals

GAD_{67}/GAT-1 mRNA

DA axon density

Association cortex

Mediodorsal thalamus

DA

Neurone number

Cortical layers

White matter

synaptic connectivity within the DPFC (Fig. 17.1). Total thalamic volume is decreased, as determined by a meta-analysis of MRI data (Konick & Friedman 2001), with the reduction also seen in never-medicated subjects (Buchsbaum *et al.* 1996). Thalamic volume correlates with prefrontal white matter volume in schizophrenic subjects (Portas *et al.* 1998), suggesting that a reduction in thalamic volume may be associated with fewer axonal projections to the prefrontal cortex. Consistent with these observations, three postmortem studies, all stereologically based, have found that the mediodorsal thalamic nucleus (MDN), the principal source of thalamic projections to the prefrontal cortex, is reduced by 17–25% in volume and by 27–40% in total neurone number in schizophrenia (Pakkenberg 1990; Popken *et al.* 2000; Young *et al.* 2000; see also Byne *et al.* 2001). The available data also suggest that these abnormalities may be specific for projections to the prefrontal cortex and related cortical regions. For example, reduced cell numbers have also been reported in the anterior thalamic nuclei (which project to the prefrontal cortex and anterior cingulate cortex), whereas the ventral posterior medial nucleus, a sensory relay nucleus, appears unaffected (Popken *et al.* 2000; Young *et al.* 2000). In addition, within the MDN, neurone number is reportedly reduced to a greater extent in the parvocellular and denso-

cellular subdivisions (which project principally to the DPFC) than in the magnocellular subdivision (which projects principally to the orbital and medial prefrontal cortex; Popken *et al.* 2000). Finally, studies in patients who had never received antipsychotics (Pakkenberg 1992) and in monkeys treated for 1 year with haloperidol (Pierri *et al.* 1999a) suggest that these medications do not account for the reduction in MDN neurone number. Despite this weight and convergence of data, a reduction in MDN size and neurone number in schizophrenia must still be considered a provisional finding, partly because there is one large negative study (Cullen *et al.* 2000) and because potentially important confounds, such as comorbid alcoholism (which is associated with prominent MDN pathology), have not been adequately assessed.

Nevertheless, several additional lines of evidence are consistent with a thalamic role in diminished DPFC connectivity in schizophrenia. For example, the density of neurones in the anterior thalamic nuclei that contain parvalbumin (Danos *et al.* 1998), a calcium-binding protein present in thalamic projection neurones (Jones & Hendry 1989), is reported to be reduced in schizophrenia. This observation suggests that it is thalamic neurones, that project to the cortex, and not just thalamic interneurones that are affected. In addition, subjects with

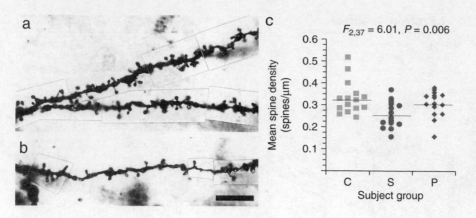

$F_{2,37} = 6.01$, $P = 0.006$

Fig 17.2 Brightfield photomicrographs illustrating Golgi-impregnated basilar dendrites and spines on PFC layer 3 pyramidal neurones from: (a) a normal control subject; and (b) a subject with schizophrenia. Calibration bar = 10 μm. (c) Scatter plot illustrating mean spine densities for 15 pyramidal neurones per subject in the deep portion of layer 3 in PFC area 46. Horizontal lines indicate group means for control (C), schizophrenic (S) and non-schizophrenic psychiatric (P) subjects. (Adapted from Glantz & Lewis 2000.)

schizophrenia, but not those with major depression, have a decreased density of parvalbumin-labelled varicosities (putative axon terminals) selectively in deep layers 3–4, the principal termination zone of thalamic projections to the prefrontal cortex (Cruz *et al.* 2000). However, whether these reductions represent an actual loss of thalamic neurones and their axon terminals, as opposed to a decrease in parvalbumin expression (perhaps because of decreased neuronal activity), is not known.

The dendritic spines of pyramidal neurones are the major target of thalamic projections to the prefrontal cortex (Melchitzky *et al.* 1999). In experimental animals, the elimination of presynaptic axon terminals leads to a resorption of the postsynaptic dendritic spine (Parnavelas *et al.* 1974). Thus, a reduction in MDN projection neurones in schizophrenia would be expected to be associated with a decrease in dendritic spine density in the DPFC. Both studies that have examined this issue found decreased spine density on the basilar dendrites of DPFC layer 3 pyramidal neurones (Garey *et al.* 1998; Glantz & Lewis 2000) (Fig. 17.2). This decrease was most marked for pyramidal neurones whose cell bodies were located in deep layer 3 (Glantz & Lewis 2000), and whose basilar dendrites extend through the laminar zone of termination of projections from the thalamus (Giguere & Goldman-Rakic 1988). These observations are consistent with a reduction in MDN–DPFC connectivity in schizophrenia. However, the presence of more modest reductions in spine density on pyramidal neurones in cortical layers and regions that do not directly receive MDN input suggest that decreased spine density in deep layer 3 may reflect the combined effect of a deficient number of thalamic *and* cortical synapses (Garey *et al.* 1998; Glantz & Lewis 2000). Furthermore, the size of deep layer 3 pyramidal neurones is reported to be reduced in the DPFC of subjects with schizophrenia. Although the possible relationship of these findings to a decrease in MDN inputs is less clear, studies in animals have provided evidence of denervation atrophy of layer 3 pyramidal cells following the loss of other afferent inputs (Wellman *et al.* 1995).

Dorsal prefrontal cortex interneurones and their connections

In the primate visual system, monocular deprivation, which re-

sults in reduced afferent drive from the thalamus, is associated with a decline in markers of activity in cortical GABA neurones (Hendry & Jones 1988), including decreased expression of glutamic acid decarboxylase (GAD_{67}), the synthesizing enzyme for GABA (Benson *et al.* 1994). Although this experimental manipulation of the visual system did not involve a partial reduction in thalamic neurone number, if these findings in the visual cortex can be generalized to a deficient number of MDN projections to the DPFC, then a reduction in GAD_{67} in the DPFC of schizophrenic subjects might be expected. Consistent with this prediction, both GAD_{67} mRNA and protein levels have been reported to be reduced in the DPFC of schizophrenic subjects (Akbarian *et al.* 1995; Guidotti *et al.* 2000; Volk *et al.* 2000). These observations are supported by other evidence of reduced GABA neurotransmission in the cerebral cortex of subjects with schizophrenia, such as a decrease in GABA release and uptake and an increase in the binding of muscimol, but not benzodiazepines, to $GABA_A$ receptors (see Lewis *et al.* 1999 for review). However, rather than a consequence of decreased input from the MDN, the reduction in GAD_{67} levels might also be attributable to other factors, such as a deficiency in reelin expression in schizophrenia (Guidotti *et al.* 2000).

The possibility that these alterations in GABA neurotransmission are a result of a disturbance in cortical circuitry is supported by observations that only a subpopulation of GABA neurones are affected. For example, decreased GAD_{67} mRNA expression in schizophrenia appears to be restricted to approximately 25–30% of DPFC GABA neurones, especially those located in the middle cortical layers (Volk *et al.* 2000). Other studies suggest that the affected subpopulation of GABA neurones includes the chandelier subclass of GABA neurones. The axon terminals of chandelier cells form distinctive vertical arrays (termed cartridges) which synapse exclusively on the axon initial segment of pyramidal neurones (Lewis 1998). Interestingly, expression of the mRNA for the GABA membrane transporter (GAT-1) is also undetectable in approximately 25–30% of DPFC GABA neurones, which have a laminar distribution similar to the neurones with undetectable GAD_{67} mRNA expression (Volk *et al.* 2001). In addition, the density of GAT-1 immunoreactive chandelier neurone axon cartridges is decreased in the DPFC of schizophrenic subjects, with the reduction most evident in the middle cortical layers (Woo *et al.* 1998; Pierri *et al.* 1999b). Together, these findings suggest that chandelier cells contain reduced levels of two proteins critical for GABA neurotransmission, although a morphological alteration in their axon terminals cannot be excluded.

Thus, given the powerful inhibitory control that chandelier neurones exert over pyramidal cell output, decreased excitatory thalamic drive to the DPFC may be partially compensated for by a reduction in chandelier cell-mediated inhibition at the axon initial segment of layer 3 pyramidal cells. This effect could occur via the local axon collaterals of layer 3 pyramidal cells, approximately 50% of which target the dendritic shafts of GABA neurones (Melchitzky *et al.* 2001). However, other potential causes and consequences of the observed alterations in chandelier neurones have not been excluded (see Volk *et al.* 2000 for further discussion).

Prefrontal cortex projections to the thalamus

Together, the data summarized in the preceding two sections converge on the hypothesis that schizophrenia is associated with abnormalities in the projection from the MDN to the DPFC. As in other cortical regions, the connections between the MDN and DPFC are reciprocal, which raises the question of whether abnormalities in thalamocortical projections are paralleled by alterations in corticothalamic projections. Studies which have examined DPFC neurones in layer 6, the principal location of corticothalamic projection neurones, have generally not found evidence of a decrease in neurone size or number (Benes *et al.* 1991a; Selemon *et al.* 1995; Rajkowska *et al.* 1998), although one study (Benes *et al.* 1986) did report decreased neuronal density in layer 6. A reduced density of markers of DA axons was observed selectively in DPFC layer 6 of schizophrenic subjects (Akil *et al.* 1999). Interestingly, the dendritic shafts and spines of pyramidal cells are the principal synaptic targets of DA axon terminals in layer 6, and DA appears to play a critical part in regulating the influence of other inputs on pyramidal cell activity (Goldman-Rakic *et al.* 1989). Thus, a shift in DA neurotransmission in DPFC layer 6 could reflect a change in the modulation of corticothalamic feedback in response to abnormal thalamocortical drive (Akil *et al.* 1999).

Neuropathological interpretations

Having reviewed the major themes in the neuropathology of schizophrenia (summarized in Table 17.1), we end with a brief consideration of some of the diverse, broader interpretational issues raised by these data.

How are the hippocampal and dorsal prefrontal cortex changes related?

Experimental studies in rodents and monkeys show that dysfunction of the DPFC may appear postpubertally following peri-

Table 17.1 Key neurohistopathological findings in schizophrenia.

General
Absence of gliosis
Absence of Alzheimer's disease or other recognized degenerative pathologies

Morphometric findings in hippocampal formation and DPFC
Smaller pyramidal neuronal cell bodies
Increased neuronal packing density (only replicated in DPFC)
Decreased presynaptic protein markers (e.g. SNAP-25, synaptophysin)
Lower density of dendritic spines
Decreased markers of inhibitory neurones and their synaptic terminals (in DPFC)
No overall loss of neurones

Other areas
Mediodorsal thalamic nucleus: decreased volume and neuronal number

For more detailed listings and citations, see text and Harrison (1999a).
DPFC, dorsal prefrontal cortex.

natal lesions of the hippocampus (Weinberger & Lipska 1995; Saunders *et al.* 1998), perhaps because of age-related maturation of hippocampal–frontal pathways. In this respect, the hippocampal pathology of schizophrenia might be considered primary to that in the DPFC, a view supported indirectly in patients by correlations between hippocampal volume and DPFC activity (Weinberger *et al.* 1992). Equally, however, the direction of causality might be reversed, or there may be an independent pathological event which underlies the changes in both regions.

Is there an asymmetry of neuropathology?

A number of postmortem studies, notably of the temporal lobe (Crow *et al.* 1989; Zaidel *et al.* 1997a,b; McDonald *et al.* 2000), and also of the thalamus (Blennow *et al.* 1996), have shown lateralized changes in schizophrenia, as do some of the results from other research modalities (Holinger *et al.* 2000). In this respect there is some neuropathological support for an interaction between cerebral asymmetry and schizophrenia (Crow 1990). However, many other studies find bilateral alterations, or have not been designed to address the question – the latter includes most investigations of the DPFC. Overall, it remains unclear whether the neuropathology of schizophrenia is asymmetrical in some way.

How are the pathology and the symptoms related?

The question of clinicopathological correlations in a broad sense is a basic but neglected issue in the literature. It has several facets.

A neural circuitry-based model of schizophrenia requires an appreciation of the mechanistic relationships between the various abnormalities observed in different components of the circuitry. Specifically, understanding the pathophysiology of schizophrenia (or any other psychiatric disorder) depends ultimately on knowledge of how abnormalities in one brain region or circuitry component produce and/or result from disturbances in others, a task that involves a consideration of cause, consequence and compensation (Lewis 2000a). Does a given abnormality represent a primary pathogenetic event (cause), does it reflect a secondary deleterious event (consequence) or does it reveal a homeostatic response intended to restore normal brain function (compensation)? Distinguishing among these three possibilities for each component of a neural network will be necessary for understanding the pathophysiology of the disease as well as for developing novel therapies designed to correct causes and consequences and/or to augment compensatory responses.

A related issue concerns the correspondence between clinical symptoms and pathological findings. For example, which aspects of the clinical syndrome are most closely related to the pathological findings? To date, the clinical information available and the sample sizes used in postmortem research have been inadequate to allow this issue to be addressed. However, it may be hypothesized that the nature and distribution of pathological changes suggest that they might be particularly related to the cognitive deficits rather than necessarily with the psychotic symptoms (Harrison 1999a). Similarly, based on the current data, it is more parsimonious to postulate a single pathological process which varies in severity between patients with schizophrenia – as is the case with the structural imaging findings – rather than invoking multiple pathologies. Across subjects, there may also be different molecular pathways leading to a common final functional and structural disturbance in brain circuitry (Mirnics et al. 2000). This view does not preclude a different conclusion as new data emerge (e.g. the possibility of a different pathological phenotype in late-onset schizophrenia).

The temporal relationship between neuropathology and the onset of symptoms is unknown, because postmortem studies of first episode patients are impossible in practice. It is only by extrapolation (e.g. from the decreased NAA seen in first episode cases; the lack of correlation of postmortem findings with duration of illness) that the suggestion can be made that the alterations, at least partly, are present at or before the onset of illness and therefore may have a direct causal role. Equally, however, even if some of the neuropathological changes occur later in the illness, this does not negate their importance or imply that they are epiphenomenal. Rather, if this were the case, it might mean that their development was a factor contributing to the course of the illness.

Do the neuropathological data support a neurodevelopmental origin of schizophrenia?

Although the idea that schizophrenia is a late consequence of an early developmental lesion has many merits, it has proven difficult to obtain direct *positive* evidence for a brain abnormality that necessarily supports such a model (i.e. which can confidently be timed to the second trimester, perinatal period,

adolescence, etc.). To date, it remains the lack of evidence *against* there being a progressive or degenerative disease process that, by default, is the strongest pointer towards a neurodevelopmental origin.

The dearth of positive neuropathological support has already been mentioned with regard to the failure to confirm the initial reports of entorhinal dysplasia and hippocampal neurone disarray. Another conceptually attractive finding was the altered distribution of interstitial neurones in the subcortical white matter, because it also strongly suggested an early developmental lesion affecting neuronal migration and/or programmed cell death (Akbarian et al. 1993a,b). However, it is not a feature in the majority of schizophrenic subjects (Akbarian et al. 1996; Anderson et al. 1996; Kirkpatrick et al. 1999; see also Dwork 1997). Instead, the changes which are more robustly demonstrable – smaller neuronal size, loss of synaptic proteins and dendritic spines – affect parameters which are dynamically regulated, and mean that the alterations could arise at any timepoint. For example, synaptic proteins and dendritic spines can be altered by many experimental situations, including neuronal activity, seizures, environmental complexity and hypoxia–ischaemia, as well as by ageing (e.g. Masliah et al. 1993; Saito et al. 1994; Marti et al. 1998; Bravin et al. 1999; Harris 1999). Thus, developmental interpretations of alterations of this kind observed in schizophrenia should be made with due caution.

On the other hand, one should not neglect the corroborative and circumstantial evidence which, complementing the lack of gliosis, supports a developmental basis for the pathological findings in schizophrenia. There are three aspects to consider:
1 The demonstration that the neural pathways implicated in the pathology of schizophrenia show marked developmental changes at relevant time periods. One example is in the hippocampal formation (Benes et al. 1994); another is the circuitry of the primate DPFC. For example, after rising dramatically during the main phase of synaptogenesis in prenatal and early postnatal life, the number of excitatory, but not inhibitory, synapses in the DPFC declines by 50% during adolescence in both monkeys and humans (Huttenlocher 1979; Bourgeois et al. 1994). During this time period, dendritic spine densities decrease (Anderson et al. 1995), but pyramidal neurone size and total dendritic length increase (Lambe et al. 2000). These maturational changes may differ according to the neuronal and synaptic population being considered. For example, there are substantial changes to excitatory, inhibitory and modulatory inputs to pyramidal neurones in deep layer 3 of primate DPFC. The terminals of intrinsic axon collaterals from DPFC layer 3 pyramidal cells may be more extensively pruned than associational cortical projections (Woo et al. 1997b), while serotonergic synapses upon these neurones develop much more rapidly than catecholaminergic ones (Lambe et al. 2000). The apparent laminar specificity of at least some of these changes supports the observations that circuits involving these pyramidal neurones may be preferentially affected in schizophrenia (Lewis 1997). Knowing whether projections from the MDN are particularly vulnerable to this process might provide critical information for

hypotheses regarding the mechanisms underlying disturbances in MDN–DPFC circuitry in schizophrenia.

2 There are studies in schizophrenia of molecules known to be important in one or other aspect of brain maturation (e.g. neuronal migration, synaptogenesis, apoptosis). Reported alterations of reelin, *Wnt* and glycogen synthase kinase 3b expression in schizophrenia exemplify this approach, and there will no doubt be many more as other key developmental genes are investigated (Weickert & Weinberger 1998). The assumption behind these studies is that the altered gene expression seen in schizophrenia is a persistent sign of aberrant neurodevelopment. This interpretation may well be true, but the very fact that a given gene continues to be expressed in the adult brain may also indicate that it has other, non-developmental, functions and therefore a similarly non-developmental implication for schizophrenia. As with morphometric alterations, a convergence and consistency of results will be needed to allow confidence in the developmental explanation.

3 The neuropathological findings in known neurodevelopmental disorders, although far from conclusive in their own right, provide another form of circumstantial support for a developmental interpretation of the schizophrenia data. For example, dendritic arborizations, dendritic proteins and dendritic spine densities are decreased in the cortex in Rett's syndrome and Williams' syndrome (Kaufmann & Moser 2000), dendritic spines are abnormal in fragile X syndrome (Irwin *et al.* 2000) and neuronal size is reduced in Rett's syndrome and autism (Kemper & Bauman 1998). Parenthetically, because these disorders may be considered 'cognitive' rather than 'psychotic', the data are consistent with the suggestion made earlier that the pathological features in schizophrenia might be related to the cognitive aspects of the syndrome.

Are the changes specific to schizophrenia?

The overlap with the morphometric findings reported in several neurodevelopmental disorders raises the issue of diagnostic specificity. Most neuropathological studies of schizophrenia have not included a comparison group comprised of patients with other psychiatric disorders, and so the specificity of many alterations is uncertain.

Of the DPFC findings mentioned, some have been examined for diagnostic specificity, whereas others have not. The reduction in DPFC dendritic spine density on deep layer 3 pyramidal neurones was not found in subjects with major depressive disorders (Glantz & Lewis 2000), and the reduction in density of GAT-1 immunoreactive axon cartridges was not apparent in subjects with non-schizophrenic psychiatric disorders (Pierri *et al.* 1999b). However, other results show a considerable similarity in bipolar disorder and in schizophrenia (Eastwood & Harrison 2000; Guidotti *et al.* 2000), suggesting that there may be overlaps at least in some aspects of pathology between the disorders. At this stage it is impossible to determine whether neuropathology will ultimately support the continuum or the dichotomy view of the functional psychoses. Such clarification

will be aided by the brain series collected by the Stanley Foundation, which comprises matched groups of brains from patients with schizophrenia, bipolar disorder and major depression, as well as controls (Torrey *et al.* 2000).

Are the changes brought about by medication?

Antipsychotic drugs, and other treatments received by patients, are often suspected as contributing to, or even causing, the neuropathological features reported in schizophrenia. Certainly, given that very few subjects in postmortem studies were medication-free at death, and virtually none were medication-naive, it is a difficult possibility to eliminate entirely. However, various experimental and statistical strategies are available, and the data are in fact reassuring: the morphological alterations caused by antipsychotics are largely limited to the basal ganglia, and their characteristics are different from those reported in schizophrenia (Harrison 1999b).

The absence of demonstrable antipsychotic effects on cortical cytoarchitecture is exemplified by findings in the DPFC and MDN. Globally, the increase in DPFC cell packing density seen in subjects with schizophrenia was not found in monkeys treated for 6 months with a variety of antipsychotics (Selemon *et al.* 1999). In addition, treatment of monkeys for 12 months with haloperidol and benzatropine at blood levels known to be therapeutic in humans was not associated with a reduction in the size or total neurone number of the MDN (Pierri *et al.* 1999a). The decreased dendritic spine density also appears to be specific to schizophrenia, in that it was not observed in a psychiatric disorder control group who had received antipsychotics (Glantz & Lewis 2000; Fig. 17.2). The potential influence of antipsychotic drugs on GAT-1-labelled axon cartridges has been examined in several ways (Pierri *et al.* 1999b). Interestingly, the density of labelled cartridges was greater in schizophrenic subjects who were on than off antipsychotic medications at the time of death (although both groups showed reduced levels compared to normal controls). In addition, compared to matched control animals, the density of GAT-1-positive cartridges was elevated in monkeys treated for 1 year with haloperidol. Together, these findings suggest that the pathophysiology of schizophrenia may actually be associated with more marked reductions in GAT-1-immunoreactive cartridge density than those seen in postmortem studies, illustrating that antipsychotic drugs may even attenuate some neuropathological alterations.

There are fewer data on the pathological consequences of other treatments sometimes used in schizophrenia, such as antidepressants and electroconvulsive therapy, but those that exist do not suggest that they are likely to be major confounders (Harrison 1999b).

Will schizophrenia ever be diagnosable down a microscope?

It is quite clear that the existing neuropathological data do not allow this question to be answered. Nevertheless, comparison with Alzheimer's disease is relevant for illustrating the kinds of conditions which would need to be met if it is ever to be answered in the affirmative.

1 In Alzheimer's disease there are reliably identifiable lesions (neurofibrillary tangles, amyloid plaques) that are qualitatively different from normal cytological and histological parameters.

2 These diagnostic lesions have a quantitative relationship to the presence and severity of the clinical syndrome, and their distribution and effect on the cortical circuitry gives a convincing explanation for the features of the syndrome.

3 Key aspects of Alzheimer's disease pathology can now be reproduced in transgenic mice, which develop cognitive impairment; recent data even suggest that the pathology can be reversed, with corresponding improvement in memory performance.

4 The neuropathological picture is clearly different from that of other dementias, and in this sense it is diagnostically specific (although this becomes a circular argument once the disorder is defined by the neuropathology and not the clinical features).

Ultimately, schizophrenia might become, like Alzheimer's disease, a disorder – or disorders – in which neuropathological features are necessary and sufficient for diagnostic purposes. Like Alzheimer's disease, it may also become possible to link the pathology directly to the aetiology, as illustrated by the mice carrying mutations in the causative genes. Alternatively, new approaches, such as gene expression profiling or proteomic strategies, may provide molecular signatures in postmortem tissue that are diagnostic of schizophrenia(s). However, the value of the next generation of postmortem studies of schizophrenia may not rest in the realm of a 'gold standard' for diagnosis, but in the types of pathogenetic or pathophysiological insights that reveal novel targets for pharmacological interventions.

Conclusions

Several histological features have now been observed and replicated in the hippocampal formation and DPFC in schizophrenia (Table 17.1): pyramidal neurones are smaller, dendrites show a lower density of spines and have less extensive arborizations, and presynaptic indices are also decreased. These features together strongly suggest that neural circuits are altered and perhaps 'wired differently' in both of these areas in schizophrenia. In the hippocampal formation, the identity of the affected circuits is unclear, whereas in DPFC there is increasing evidence that it includes thalamocortical afferent connections as well as intrinsic connections between inhibitory interneurones and pyramidal neurones. Changes in the MDN are consistent with the DPFC findings. The spatial distribution of pathological features in schizophrenia beyond these areas remains unclear, although there are many positive findings, not mentioned here, which deserve further study (Arnold & Trojanowski 1996; Harrison 1999a; Benes 2000). The cytoarchitectural findings as a whole, in the absence of any evidence of a degenerative process, support but do not prove a neurodevelopmental origin. Other important

questions remain regarding the specificity, molecular characteristics and interpretation of the pathology. Nevertheless, many of the findings are now reasonably robust and, as such, the main focus of attention is no longer whether there is any neuropathology in schizophrenia, but what its details are and how it relates to the aetiology and clinical features of the syndrome.

References

Akbarian, S., Bunney, W.E. Jr, Potkin, S.G. et al. (1993a) Altered distribution of nicotinamide-adenine dinucleotide phosphate-diaphorase cells in frontal lobe of schizophrenics implies disturbances of cortical development. Archives of General Psychiatry 50, 169–177.

Akbarian, S., Viñuela, A., Kim, J.J. et al. (1993b) Distorted distribution of nicotinamide-adenine dinucleotilde phosphate-diaphorase neurons in temporal lose of schizophrenic implies anomalous cortical development. Archives of General Psychiatry 50, 178–187.

Akbarian, S., Kim, J.J., Potkin, S.G. et al. (1995) Gene expression for glutamic acid decarboxylase is reduced without loss of neurons in prefrontal cortex of schizophrenics. Archives of General Psychiatry 52, 258–266.

Akbarian, S., Kim, J.J., Potikin, S.G. et al. (1996) Maldistribution of interstitial neurons in prefrontal white matter of the brains of schizophrenic patients. Archives of General Psychiatry 53, 425–436.

Akil, M. & Lewis, D.A. (1997) The cytoarchitecture of the entorhinal cortex in schizophrenia. American Journal of Psychiatry 154, 1010–1012.

Akil, M., Pierri, J.N., Whitehead, R.E. et al. (1999) Lamina-specific alteration in the dopamine innervation of the prefrontal cortex in schizophrenic subjects. American Journal of Psychiatry 156, 1580–1589.

Altshuler, L.L., Conrad, A., Kovelman, J.A. & Scheibel, A.B. (1987) Hippocampal pyramidal cell orientation in schizophrenia: a controlled neurohistologic study of the Yakovlev collection. Archives of General Psychiatry 44, 1094–1098.

Anderson, S.A., Classey, J.D., Condé, F., Lund, J.S. & Lewis, D.A. (1995) Synchronous development of pyramidal neuron dendritic spines and parvalbumin-immunoreactive chandelier neuron axon terminals in layer III of monkey prefrontal cortex. Neuroscience 67, 7–22.

Anderson, S.A., Volk, D.W. & Lewis, D.A. (1996) Increased density of microtubule-associated protein 2-immunoreactive neurons in the prefrontal white matter of schizophrenic subjects. Schizophrenia Research 19, 111–119.

Arnold, S.E. (1997) The medial temporal lobe in schizophrenia. Journal of Neuropsychiatry and Clinical Neuroscience 9, 460–470.

Arnold, S.E. & Trojanowski, J.Q. (1996) Recent advances in defining the neuropathology of schizophrenia. Acta Neuropathologica 92, 217–231.

Arnold, S.E., Hyman, B.T., Van Hoesen, G.W. & Damasio, A.R. (1991a) Some cytoarchitectural abnormalities of the entorhinal cortex in schizophrenia. Archives of General Psychiatry 48, 625–632.

Arnold, S.E., Lee, V.M.Y., Gur, R.E. & Trojanowski, J.Q. (1991b) Abnormal expression of two microtubule-associated proteins (MAP2 and MAP5) in specific subfields of the hippocampal formation in schizophrenia. Proceedings of the National Academy of Sciences of the USA 88, 10850–10854.

Arnold, S.E., Franz, B.R., Gur, R.C. et al. (1995) Smaller neuron size in schizophrenia hippocampal subfields that mediate cortical–

hippocampal interactions. *American Journal of Psychiatry* **152**, 738–748.

Arnold, S.E., Franz, B.R., Trojanowski, J.Q., Moberg, P.J. & Gur, R.E. (1996) Glial fibrillary acidic protein-immunoreactive astrocytosis in elderly patients with schizophrenia and dementia. *Acta Neuropathologica* **91**, 269–277.

Arnold, S.E., Ruscheinsky, D.D. & Han, L.Y. (1997) Further evidence of abnormal cytoarchitecure of the entorhinal corex in schizophrenia using spatial point pattern analysises. *Biological Psychiatry* **42**, 639–647.

Arnold, S.E., Trojanowski, J.Q., Gur, R.E. *et al.* (1998) Absence of neurodegeneration and neural injury in the cerebral cortex in a sample of elderly patients with schizophrenia. *Archives of General Psychiatry* **55**, 225–232.

Baldessarini, R.J., Hegarty, J., Bird, E.D. & Benes, F.M. (1997) Meta-analysis of postmortem studies of Alzheimer's disease-like neuropathology in schizophrenia. *American Journal of Psychiatry* **154**, 861–863.

Bayer, T.A., Busiei, R., Havas, L. & Falkai, P. (1999) Evidence for activation of microglia in patients with psychiatric illnesses. *Neuroscience Letters* **271**, 126–128.

Beasley, C.L. & Reynolds, G.P. (1997) Parvalbumin-immunoreactive neurons are reduced in the prefrontal cortex of schizophrenics. *Schizophrenia Research* **24**, 349–355.

Benes, F.M. (2000) Emerging principles of altered neural circuitry in schizophrenia. *Brain Research Reviews* **31**, 251–269.

Benes, F.M., Davidson, J. & Bird, E.D. (1986) Quantitative cytoarchitectural studies of the cerebral cortex of schizophrenics. *Archives of General Psychiatry* **43**, 31–35.

Benes, F.M., McSparren, J., Bird, E.D., SanGiovanni, J.P. & Vincent, S.L. (1991a) Deficits in small interneurons in prefrontal and cingulate cortices of schizophrenic and schizoaffective patients. *Archives of General Psychiatry* **48**, 996–1001.

Benes, F.M., Sorensen, I. & Bird, E.D. (1991b) Reduced neuronal size in posterior hippocampus of schizophrenic patients. *Schizophrenia Bulletin* **17**, 597–608.

Benes, F.M., Turtle, M., Khan, Y. & Farol, P. (1994) Myelination of a key relay zone in the hippocampal formation occurs in the human brain during childhood, adolescence, and adulthood. *Archives of General Psychiatry* **51**, 477–484.

Benes, F.M., Kwok, E.W., Vincent, S.L. & Todtenkopf, M.S. (1998) Reduction of non-pyramidal cells in section CA2 of schizophrenics and manic depressives. *Biological Psychiatry* **44**, 88–97.

Benson, D.L., Huntsman, M.M. & Jones, E.G. (1994) Activity-dependent changes in GAD and preprotachykinin mRNAs in visual cortex of adult monkeys. *Cerebral Cortex* **4**, 40–51.

Bernstein, H.-G., Krell, D., Baumann, B. *et al.* (1998) Morphometric studies of the entorhinal cortex in neuropsychiatric patients and controls: clusters of heterotopically displaced lamina II neurons are not indicative of schizophrenia. *Schizophrenia Research* **33**, 125–132.

Bertolino, A., Nawroz, S., Mattay, V.S. *et al.* (1996) Regionally specific pattern of neurochemical pathology in schizophrenia as assessed by multislice proton magnetic resonance spectroscopic imaging. *American Journal of Psychiatry* **153**, 1554–1563.

Bertolino, A., Callicott, J.H., Elman, I. *et al.* (1998) Regionally specific neural pathology in untreated patients with schizophrenia: a proton magnetic resonance spectroscopic imaging study. *Biological Psychiatry* **43**, 641–648.

Bertolino, A., Esposito, G., Callicott, J.H. *et al.* (2000) Specific relationship between prefrontal neuronal N-acetylaspartate and activation of the working memory cortical network in schizophrenia. *American Journal of Psychiatry* **157**, 26–33.

Blennow, K., Davidsson, P., Gottfries, C.-G., Ekman, R. & Heilig, M. (1996) Synaptic degeneration in thalamus in schizophrenia. *Lancet* **348**, 692–693.

Bourgeois, J.-P., Goldman-Rakic, P.S. & Rakic, P. (1994) Synaptogenesis in the prefrontal cortex of rhesus monkeys. *Cerebral Cortex* **4**, 78–96.

Bravin, M., Morando, L., Vercelli, A., Rossi, F. & Strata, P. (1999) Control of spine formation by electrical activity in the adult rat cerebellum. *Proceedings of the National Academy of Sciences of the USA* **96**, 1704–1709.

Bruton, C.J., Crow, T.J., Frith, C. *et al.* (1990) Schizophrenia and the brain: a prospective cliniconeuropathological study. *Psychological Medicine* **20**, 285–304.

Buchsbaum, M.S., Someya, T., Teng, C.Y. *et al.* (1996) PET and MRI of the thalamus in never-medicated patients with schizophrenia. *American Journal of Psychiatry* **153**, 191–199.

Byne, W., Buchsbaum, M.S., Kemether, E. *et al.* (2001) Magnetic resonance imaging of the thalamic mediodorsal nucles and pulvinar in schizophrenia and schizotypal personality disorder. *Archives of General Psychiatry* **58**, 133–140.

Christison, G.W., Casanova, M.F., Weinberger, D.R., Rawlings, R. & Kleinman, J.E. (1989) A quantitative investigation of hippocampal pyramidal cell size, shape, and variability of orientation in schizophrenia. *Archives of General Psychiatry* **46**, 1027–1032.

Conrad, A.J., Abebe, T., Austin, R., Forsythe, S. & Scheibel, A.B. (1991) Hippocampal pyramidal cell disarray in schizophrenia as a bilateral phenomenon. *Archives of General Psychiatry* **48**, 413–417.

Corsellis, J.A.N. (1962) Mental illness and the ageing brain. *Institute of Psychiatry Maudsley Monographs No. 9.* Oxford University Press, London.

Crow, T.J. (1990) Temporal lobe asymmetries as the key to the etiology of schizophrenia. *Schizophrenia Bulletin* **16**, 433–443.

Crow, T.J., Ball, J., Bloom, S. *et al.* (1989) Schizophrenia as an anomaly of development of cerebral asymmetry. *Archives of General Psychiatry* **46**, 1145–1150.

Cruz, D.A., Melchitzky, D.S., Pierri, J.N. & Lewis, D.A. (2000) Decreased density of putative thalamic axon terminals in the prefrontal cortex in schizophrenia: effect of antipsychotic medication and diagnostic specificity. *Society of Neuroscience Abstracts* **26**, 1564.

Cullen, T.J., Walker, M.A., Roberts, H. *et al.* (2000) The mediodorsal nucleus of the thalamus in schizophrenia: a post-mortem study. *Schizophrenia Research* **41**, 5.

Da Cunha, A., Jefferson, J.J., Tyor, W.R. *et al.* (1993) Gliosis in human brain: relationship to size but not other properties of astrocytes. *Brain Research* **600**, 161–165.

Danos, P., Baumann, B., Bernstein, H.-G. *et al.* (1998) Schizophrenia and anteroventral thalamic nucleus: selective decrease of parvalbumin-immunoreactive thalamocortical projection neurons. *Psychiatry Research: Neuroimaging* **82**, 1–10.

David, G.B. (1957) The pathological anatomy of the schizophrenias. In: *Schizophrenia: Somatic Aspects.* (ed. D. Richter), pp. 93–130. Pergamon, Oxford.

Davidsson, P., Gottfries, J., Bogdanovic, N. *et al.* (1999) The synaptic-vesicle-specific proteins rab3a and synaptophysin are reduced in thalamus and related cortical brain regions in schizophrenic brains. *Schizophrenia Research* **40**, 23–29.

Davis, K.L., Kahn, R.S., Ko, G. & Davidson, M. (1991) Dopamine in schizophrenia: a review and reconceptualization. *American Journal of Psychiatry* **148**, 1474–1486.

Daviss, S.R. & Lewis, D.A. (1995) Local circuit neurons of the prefrontal cortex in schizophrenia: selective increase in the density of calbindin-immunoreactive neurons. *Psychiatry Research* **59**, 81–96.

Deicken, R.F., Zhou, L., Corwin, F., Vinogradov, S. & Weiner, M.W. (1997) Decreased left frontal lobe N-acetylaspartate in schizophrenia. *American Journal of Psychiatry* **154**, 688–690.

DeLisi, L.E. (1997) Is schizophrenia a lifetime disorder or brain plasticity, growth and aging. *Schizophrenia Research* **23**, 119–129.

Dwork, A.J. (1997) Postmortem studies of the hippocampal formation in schizophrenia. *Schizophrenia Bulletin* **23**, 385–402.

Eastwood, S.L. & Harrison, P.J. (1995) Decreased synaptophysin in the medial temporal lobe in schizophrenia demonstrated using immunoautoradiography. *Neuroscience* **69**, 339–343.

Eastwood, S.L. & Harrison, P.J. (1998) Hippocampal and cortical growth-associated protein-43 messenger RNA in schizophrenia. *Neuroscience* **86**, 437–448.

Eastwood, S.L. & Harrison, P.J. (1999) Detection and quantification of hippocampal synaptophysin messenger RNA in schizophrenia using autoclaved, formalin-fixed paraffin wax-embedded sections. *Neuroscience* **93**, 99–106.

Eastwood, S.L. & Harrison, P.J. (2000) Hippocampal synaptic pathology in schizophrenia bipolar disorder and major depression: a study of complexin mRNAs. *Molecular Psychiatry* **5**, 425–432.

Eastwood, S.L. & Harrison, P.J. (2001) Synaptic pathology in the anterior cingulate cortex in schizophrenia and mood disorders: an immunoblotting study of synaptophysin, gap-43 and the complexins and a review. *Brain Research Bulletin* **55**, 569–578.

Eastwood, S.L., Burnet, P.W.J., McDonald, B., Clinton, J. & Harrison, P.J. (1994) Synaptophysin gene expression in human brain: a quantitative *in situ* hybridization and immunocytochemical study. *Neuroscience* **59**, 881–892.

Eastwood, S.L., Cairns, N.J. & Harrison, P.J. (2000) Synaptophysin gene expression in schizophrenia: investigation of synaptic pathology in the cerebral cortex. *British Journal of Psychiatry* **176**, 236–242.

Esiri, M.M. & Pearson, R.C.A. (2000) Perspectives from other diseases and lesions. In: *The Neuropathology of Schizophrenia: Progress and Interpretation* (eds P.J. Harrison & G.W. Roberts), pp. 257–276. Oxford University Press, Oxford.

Falkai, P. & Bogerts, B. (1986) Cell loss in the hippocampus of schizophrenics. *European Archives of Psychiatry and Neurological Science* **236**, 154–161.

Falkai, P., Honer, W.G., David, S. *et al.* (1999) No evidence for astrogliosis in brains of schizophrenic patients: a post-mortem study. *Neuropathology and Applied Neurobiology* **25**, 48–53.

Falkai, P., Schneider-Axmann, T. & Honer, W.G. (2000) Entorhinal cortex pre-alpha cell cluster in schizophrenia: quantitative evidence of a developmental abnormality. *Biological Psychiatry* **47**, 937–943.

Friede, R.J. (1989) *Developmental Neuropathology*. Springer Verlag, Berlin.

Friston, K.J. & Frith, C.D. (1995) Schizophrenia: a disconnection syndrome. *Clinical Neuroscience* **3**, 89–97.

Friston, K.J., Liddle, P.F., Frith, C.D., Hirsch, S.R. & Frackowiak, R.S. (1992) The left medial temporal region and schizophrenia. *Brain* **115**, 367–382.

Gabriel, S.M., Haroutunian, V., Powchik, P. *et al.* (1997) Increased concentrations of presynaptic proteins in the cingulate cortex of subjects with schizophrenia. *Archives of General Psychiatry* **54**, 559–566.

Garey, L.J., Ong, W.Y., Patel, T.S. *et al.* (1998) Reduced dendritic spine density on cerebral cortical pyramidal neurons in schizophrenia. *Journal of Neurology, Neurosurgery and Psychiatry* **65**, 446–453.

Giguere, M. & Goldman-Rakic, P.S. (1988) Mediodorsal nucleus: areal, laminar, and tangential distribution of afferents and efferents in the frontal lobe of rhesus monkeys. *Journal of Comparative Neurology* **277**, 195–213.

Gilbert, C.D. & Kelly, J.P. (1975) The projections of cells in different layers of the cat's visual cortex. *Journal of Comparative Neurology* **63**, 81–106.

Glantz, L.A. & Lewis, D.A. (1997) Reduction of synaptophysin immunoreactivity in the prefrontal cortex of subjects with schizophrenia: regional and diagnostic specificity. *Archives of General Psychiatry* **54**, 943–952.

Glantz, L.A. & Lewis, D.A. (2000) Decreased dendritic spine density on prefrontal cortical pyramidal neurons in schizophrenia. *Archives of General Psychiatry* **57**, 65–73.

Glantz, L.A., Austin, M.C. & Lewis, D.A. (2000) Normal cellular levels of synaptophysin mRNA expression in the prefrontal cortex of subjects with schizophrenia. *Biological Psychiatry* **48**, 389–397.

Goldman-Rakic, P.S., Leranth, C., Williams, S.M., Mons, N. & Geffard, M. (1989) Dopamine synaptic complex with pyramidal neurons in primate cerebral cortex. *Proceedings of the National Academy of Sciences of the USA* **86**, 9015–9019.

Guidotti, A., Auta, J., Davis, J.M. *et al.* (2000) Decrease in reelin and glutamic acid decarboxylase$_{67}$ (GAD$_{67}$) expression in schizophrenia and bipolar disorder. *Archives of General Psychiatry* **57**, 1061–1069.

Harris, K.M. (1999) Structure, development, and plasticity of dendritic spines. *Current Opinion in Neurobiology* **9**, 343–348.

Harrison, P.J. (1999a) The neuropathology of schizophrenia: a critical review of the data and their interpretation. *Brain* **122**, 593–624.

Harrison, P.J. (1999b) The neuropathological effects of antipsychotic drugs. *Schizophrenia Research* **40**, 87–99.

Harrison, P.J. & Eastwood, S.L. (1998) Preferential involvement of excitatory neurons in medial temporal lobe in schizophrenia. *Lancet* **352**, 1669–1673.

Harrison, P.J. & Eastwood, S.L. (2001) Neuropathological studies of synaptic connectivity in the hippocampal formation in schizophrenia. *Hippocampus* **11**, 508–519.

Harrison, P.J. & Roberts, G.W. (2000) *The Neuropathology of Schizophrenia: Progress and Interpretation*. Oxford University Press, Oxford.

Hayes, T.L. & Lewis, D.A. (1996) Magnopyramidal neurons in the anterior motor speech region: dendritic features and interhemispheric comparisons. *Archives of Neurology* **53**, 1277–1283.

Heckers, S., Heinsen, H., Geiger, B. & Beckmann, H. (1991) Hippocampal neuron number in schizophrenia: a stereological study. *Archives of General Psychiatry* **48**, 1002–1008.

Heckers, S., Rauch, S.L., Goff, D.C. *et al.* (1998) Impaired recruitment of the hippocampus during conscious recollection in schizophrenia. *Nature Neuroscience* **1**, 318–323.

Heinsen, H., Gössmann, E., Rüb, U. *et al.* (1996) Variability in the human entorhinal region may confound neuropsychiatric diagnoses. *Acta Anatomica* **157**, 226–237.

Hendry, S.H.C. & Jones, E.G. (1988) Activity-dependent regulation of GABA expression in the visual cortex of adult monkeys. *Neuron* **1**, 701–712.

Holinger, D., Galaburda, A.M. & Harrison, P.J. (2000) Cerebral asymmetry. In: *The Neuropathology of Schizophrenia: Progress and Interpretation* (eds P.J. Harrison & G.W. Roberts), pp. 151–171. Oxford University Press, Oxford.

Honer, W.G., Falkai, P., Chen, C. *et al.* (1999) Synaptic and plasticity-associated proteins in anterior frontal cortex in severe mental illness. *Neuroscience* **91**, 1247–1255.

Honer, W.G., Young, C. & Falkai, P. (2000) Synaptic pathology. In: *The Neuropathology of Schizophrenia: Progress and Interpretation* (eds P.J. Harrison & G.W. Roberts), pp. 105–136. Oxford University Press, Oxford.

Huttenlocher, P.R. (1979) Synaptic density in human frontal cortex: developmental changes and effects of aging. *Brain Research* **163**, 195–205.

Irwin, S.A., Galvez, R. & Greenough, W.T. (2000) Dendritic spine structural anomalies in fragile X mental retardation syndrome. *Cerebral Cortex* **10**, 1038–1044.

Jakob, H. & Beckmann, H. (1986) Prenatal developmental disturbances in the limbic allocortex in schizophrenics. *Journal of Neural Transactions* **65**, 303–326.

Jellinger, K.A. & Gabriel, E. (1999) No increased incidence of Alzheimer's disease in elderly schizophrenics. *Acta Neuropathologica* **97**, 165–169.

Jeste, D.V. & Lohr, J.B. (1989) Hippocampal pathologic findings in schizophrenia: a morphometric study. *Archives of General Psychiatry* **46**, 1019–1024.

Jones, E.G. & Hendry, S.H.C. (1989) Differential calcium binding protein immunoreactivity distinguishes classes of relay neurons in monkey thalamic nuclei. *European Journal of Neuroscience* **1**, 222–246.

Jonsson, S.A.T., Luts, A., Guldberg-Kjaer, N. & Brun, A. (1997) Hippocampal pyramidal cell disarray correlates negatively to cell number: implications for the pathogenesis of schizophrenia. *European Archives of Psychiatry and Neurological Science* **247**, 120–127.

Kalman, M., Csillag, A., Schleicher, A. *et al.* (1993) Long-term effects of anterograde degeneration on astroglial reaction in the rat geniculo-cortico system as revealed by computerized image analysis. *Anatomical Embryology* **187**, 1–7.

Kalus, P., Muller, T.J., Zuschratter, W. & Senitz, D. (2000) The dendritic architecture of prefrontal pyramidal neurons in schizophrenic patients. *Neuroreport* **11**, 3621–3625.

Karson, C.N., Mrak, R.E., Schluterman, K.O. *et al.* (1999) Alterations in synaptic proteins and their encoding mRNAs in prefrontal cortex in schizophrenia: a possible neurochemical basis for 'hypofrontality'. *Molecular Psychiatry* **4**, 39–45.

Kaufmann, W.E. & Moser, H.W. (2000) Dendritic anomalies in disorders associated with mental retardation. *Cerebral Cortex* **10**, 981–991.

Kemper, T.L. & Bauman, M. (1998) Neuropathology of infantile autism. *Journal of Neuropathology and Experimental Neurology* **57**, 645–652.

Keshavan, M.S., Stanley, J.A. & Pettegrew, J.W. (2000) Magnetic resonance spectroscopy in schizophrenia: methodological issues and findings – Part II. *Biological Psychiatry* **48**, 369–380.

Kirkpatrick, B., Conley, R.C., Kakoyannis, A., Reep, R.L. & Roberts, R.C. (1999) Interstitial cells of the white matter in the inferior parietal cortex in schizophrenia: an unbiased cell-counting study. *Synapse* **34**, 95–102.

Konick, L.C. & Friedman, L. (2001) Meta-analysis of thalamic size in schizophrenia. *Biological Psychiatry* **49**, 28–38.

Kovelman, J.A. & Scheibel, A.B. (1984) A neurohistological correlate of schizophrenia. *Biological Psychiatry* **19**, 1601–1621.

Krimer, L.S., Herman, M.M., Saunders, R.C. *et al.* (1997) A qualitative and quantitative analysis of the entorhinal cortex in schizophrenia. *Cerebral Cortex* **7**, 732–739.

Lambe, E.K., Krimer, L.S. & Goldman-Rakic, P.S. (2000) Differential postnatal development of catecholamine and serotonin inputs to identified neurons in prefrontal cortex of rhesus monkey. *Journal of Neuroscience* **20**, 8780–8787.

Levitt, J.B., Lewis, D.A., Yoshioka, T. & Lund, J.S. (1993) Topography of pyramidal neuron intrinsic connections in macaque monkey prefrontal cortex (areas 9 and 46). *Journal of Comparative Neurology* **338**, 360–376.

Lewis, D.A. (1997) Development of the prefrontal cortex during adolescence: insights into vulnerable neural circuits in schizophrenia. *Neuropsychopharmacology* **16**, 385–398.

Lewis, D.A. (1998) Chandelier cells: shedding light on altered cortical circuitry in schizophrenia. *Molecular Psychiatry* **3**, 468–471.

Lewis, D.A. (2000a) Distributed disturbances in brain structure and function in schizophrenia. *American Journal of Psychiatry* **157**, 1–2.

Lewis, D.A. (2000b) Is there a neuropathology of schizophrenia? Recent findings converge on altered thalamic–prefrontal cortical connectivity. *Neuroscientist* **6**, 208–218.

Lewis, D.A. & Lieberman, J.A. (2000) Catching up on schizophrenia: natural history and neurobiology. *Neuron* **28**, 325–334.

Lewis, D.A. & Sesack, S.R. (1997) Dopamine systems in the primate brain. In: *Handbook of Chemical Neuroanatomy* (eds F.E. Bloom, A. Björklund & T. Hökfelt), pp. 261–373. Elsevier Science, Amsterdam.

Lewis, D.A., Pierri, J.N., Volk, D.W., Melchitzky, D.S. & Woo, T.-U. (1999) Altered GABA neurotransmission and prefrontal cortical dysfunction in schizophrenia. *Biological Psychiatry* **46**, 616–626.

Lieberman, J.A. (1999) Is schizophrenia a neurodegenerative disorder? A clinical and neurobiological perspective. *Biological Psychiatry* **46**, 729–739.

Lund, J.S., Lund, R.D., Hendrickson, A.E., Bunt, A.H. & Fuchs, A.F. (1975) The origin of efferent pathways from the primary visual cortex, area 17, of the macaque monkey as shown by retrograde transport of horseradish peroxidase. *Journal of Comparative Neurology* **164**, 287–304.

Marti, E., Ferrer, I., Ballabriga, J. & Blasi, J. (1998) Increase in SNAP-25 immunoreactivity in mossy fibers following transient forebrain ischemia in the gerbil. *Acta Neuropathologica* **95**, 254–260.

Masliah, E., Mallory, M., Hansen, L., DeTeresa, R. & Terry, R.D. (1993) Quantitative synaptic alterations in the human neocortex during normal aging. *Neurology* **43**, 192–197.

McCarley, R.W., Wible, C.G., Frumin, M. *et al.* (1999) MRI anatomy of schizophrenia. *Biological Psychiatry* **45**, 1099–1119.

McDonald, B., Highley, J.R., Walker, M.A. *et al.* (2000) Anamalous asymmetry of fusiform and parahippocampal gyrus gray matter in schizophrenia: a postmortem study. *American Journal of Psychiatry* **157**, 40–47.

Melchitzky, D.S., Sesack, S.R. & Lewis, D.A. (1999) Parvalbumin-immunoreactive axon terminals in monkey and human prefrontal cortex: Laminar, regional and target specificity of Type I and Type II synapses. *Journal of Comparative Neurology* **408**, 11–22.

Melchitzky, D.S., Gonzalez-Burgos, G., Barrionuevo, G. & Lewis, D.A. (2001) Synaptic targets of the intrinsic axon collaterals of supragranular pyramidal neurons in monkey prefrontal cortex. *Journal of Comparative Neurology* **430**, 209–221.

Mirnics, K., Middleton, F.A., Marquez, A., Lewis, D.A. & Levitt, P. (2000) Molecular characterization of schizophrenia viewed by microarray analysis of gene expression in prefrontal cortex. *Neuron* **28**, 53–67.

Murphy, G.M. Jr, Lim, K.O., Wieneke, M. *et al.* (1998) No neuropathologic evidence for an increased frequency of Alzheimer's disease among elderly schizophrenics. *Biological Psychiatry* **43**, 205–209.

Nelson, M.D., Saykin, A.J., Flashman, L.A. & Riordan, H.J. (1998) Hippocampal volume reduction in schizophrenia as assessed by magnetic resoance imaging: a meta-analytic study. *Archives of General Psychiatry* **55**, 433–440.

Okubo, Y., Suhara, T., Suzuki, K. *et al.* (1997) Decreased prefrontal dopamine D_1 receptors in schizophrenia revealed by PET. *Nature* **385**, 634–636.

Pakkenberg, B. (1990) Pronounced reduction of total neuron number in mediodorsal thalamic nucleus and nucleus accumbens in schizophrenics. *Archives of General Psychiatry* **47**, 1023–1028.

Pakkenberg, B. (1992) The volume of the mediodorsal thalamic nucleus in treated and untreated schizophrenics. *Schizophrenia Research* **7**, 95–100.

Pakkenberg, B. (1993) Total nerve cell number in neocortex in chronic schizophrenics and controls estimated using optical disectors. *Biological Psychiatry* **34**, 768–772.

Parnavelas, J.G., Lynch, G., Brecha, N., Cotman, C.W. & Globus, A. (1974) Spine loss and regrowth in hippocampus following deafferentation. *Nature* **248**, 71–73.

Perrone-Bizzozero, N.I., Sower, A.C., Bird, E.D. *et al.* (1996) Levels of the growth-associated protein GAP-43 are selectively increased in association cortices in schizophrenia. *Proceedings of the National Academy of Sciences of the USA* **93**, 14182–14187.

Pierce, J.P. & Lewin, G.R. (1994) An ultrastructural size principle. *Neuroscience* **58**, 441–446.

Pierri, J.N., Melchitzky, D.S. & Lewis, D.A. (1999a) Volume and neuronal number of the primate mediodorsal thalamic nucleus: effects of chronic haloperidol administration. *Society for Neuroscience Abstracts* **25**, 1833.

Pierri, J.N., Chaudry, A.S., Woo, T.-U. & Lewis, D.A. (1999b) Alterations in chandelier neuron axon terminals in the prefrontal cortex of schizophrenic subjects. *American Journal of Psychiatry* **156**, 1709–1719.

Pierri, J.N., Volk, C.L.E., Auh, S., Sampson, A. & Lewis, D.A. (2001) Decreased somal size of deep layer 3 pyramidal neurons in the prefrontal cortex in subjects with schizophrenia. *Archives of General Psychiatry* **58**, 466–473.

Popken, G.J., Bunney, W.E. Jr, Potkin, S.G. & Jones, E.G. (2000) Subnucleus-specific loss of neurons in medial thalamus of schizophrenics. *Proceedings of the National Academy of Sciences of the USA* **97**, 9276–9280.

Portas, C.M., Goldstein, J.M., Shenton, M.E. *et al.* (1998) Volumetric evaluation of the thalamus in schizophrenic male patients using magnetic resonance imaging. *Biological Psychiatry* **43**, 649–659.

Prohovnik, I., Dwork, A.J., Kaufman, M.A. & Wilson, N. (1993) Alzheimer-type neuropathology in elderly schizophrenia patients. *Schizophrenia Bulletin* **19**, 805–816.

Pucak, M.L., Levitt, J.B., Lund, J.S. & Lewis, D.A. (1996) Patterns of intrinsic and associational circuitry in monkey prefrontal cortex. *Journal of Comparative Neurology* **376**, 614–630.

Purohit, D.P., Peri, D.P., Haroutunian, V. *et al.* (1998) Alzheimer disease and related neurodegenerative diseases in elderly patients with schizophrenia: a portmortem neuropathologic study of 100 cases. *Archives of General Psychiatry* **55**, 205–211.

Rajkowska, G., Selemon, L.D. & Goldman-Rakic, P.S. (1998) Neuronal and glial somal size in the prefrontal cortex: a postmortem morphometric study of schizophrenia and Huntington disease. *Archives of General Psychiatry* **55**, 215–224.

Riederer, P., Gsell, W., Calza, L. *et al.* (1995) Consensus on minimal criteria of clinical and neuropathological diagnosis of schizophrenia and affective disorders for post mortem research. Report from the European Dementia and Scizophrenia Network (BIOMED 1). *Journal of Neural Transmission* **102**, 255–264.

Roberts, G.W. (1991) Schizophrenia: a neuropathological perspective. *British Journal of Psychiatry* **158**, 8–17.

Roberts, G.W. & Harrison, P.J. (2000) Gliosis and its implications for the disease process. In: *The Neuropathology of Schizophrenia: Progress and Interpretation* (eds P.J. Harrison & G.W. Roberts), pp. 137–150. Oxford University Press, Oxford.

Rosoklija, G., Toomayan, G., Ellis, S.P. *et al.* (2000) Structural abnormalities of subicular dendrites in subjects with schizophrenia and

mood disorders: preliminary findings. *Archives of General Psychiatry* **57**, 349–356.

Saito, S., Kobayashi, S., Ohashi, Y. *et al.* (1994) Decreased synaptic density in aged brains and its prevention by rearing under enriched environment as revealed by synaptophysin contents. *Journal of Neuroscience Research* **39**, 57–62.

Saunders, R.C., Kolachana, B.S., Bachevalier, J. & Weinberger, D.R. (1998) Neonatal lesions of the medial temporal lobe disrupt prefrontal regulation of striatal dopamine. *Nature* **393**, 169–171.

Saykin, A.J., Shtasel, D.L., Gur, R.E. *et al.* (1994) Neuropsychological deficits in neuroleptic naive patients with first-episode schizophrenia. *Archives of General Psychiatry* **51**, 124–131.

Selemon, L.D. & Goldman-Rakic, P.S. (1999) The reduced neuropil hypothesis: a circuit based model of schizophrenia. *Biological Psychiatry* **45**, 17–25.

Selemon, L.D., Rajkowska, G. & Goldman-Rakic, P.S. (1995) Abnormally high neuronal density in the schizophrenic cortex: a morphometric analysis of prefrontal area 9 and occipital area 17. *Archives of General Psychiatry* **52**, 805–818.

Selemon, L.D., Rajkowska, G. & Goldman-Rakic, P.S. (1998) Elevated neuronal density in prefrontal area 46 in brains from schizophrenic patients: application of a three-dimensional, stereologic counting method. *Journal of Comparative Neurology* **392**, 402–412.

Selemon, L.D., Lidow, M.S. & Goldman-Rakic, P.S. (1999) Increased volume and glial density in primate prefrontal cortex associated with chronic antipsychotic drug exposure. *Biological Psychiatry* **46**, 161–172.

Squier, M., Chamberlain, P., Zaiwalla, Z. *et al.* (2000) Five cases of brain injury following amniocentesis in mid-term pregnancy. *Developmental Medicine and Child Neurology* **42**, 554–560.

Stanley, J.A., Williamson, P.C., Drost, D.J. *et al.* (1996) An *in vivo* proton magnetic resonance spectroscopy study of schizophrenia patients. *Schizophrenia Bulletin* **22**, 597–609.

Stevens, C.D., Altshuler, L.L., Bogerts, B. & Falkai, P. (1988) Quantitative study of gliosis in schizophrenia and Huntington's chorea. *Biological Psychiatry* **24**, 697–700.

Stevens, J.R. (1982) Neuropathology of schizophrenia. *Archives of General Psychiatry* **39**, 1131–1139.

Stevens, J.R., Casanova, M.F., Poltorak, M. & Buchan, G.C. (1992) Comparison of immunocytochemical and Holzer's methods for detection of acute and chronic glioses in human post-mortem material. *Journal of Neuropsychiatry and Clinical Neuroscience* **4**, 168–173.

Tamminga, C.A., Thaker, G.K., Buchanan, R. *et al.* (1992) Limbic system abnormalities identified in schizophrenia using positron emission tomography with fluorodeoxyglucose and neocortical alterations with deficit syndrome. *Archives of General Psychiatry* **49**, 522–530.

Thompson, P.M., Sower, A.C. & Perrone-Bizzozero, N.I. (1998) Altered levels of the synaptosomal associated protein SNAP-25 in schizophrenia. *Biological Psychiatry* **43**, 239–243.

Thune, J.J., Hofsten, D.E., Uylings, H.B.M. & Pakkenberg, B. (1998) Total neuron numbers in the prefrontal cortex in schizophrenia. *Society for Neuroscience Abstracts* **24**, 985.

Torrey, E.F., Webster, M., Knable, M., Johnston, N. & Yoken, R.H. (2000) The Stanley Foundation brain collection and Neuropathology Consortium. *Schizophrenia Research* **44**, 151–155.

Velakoulis, D., Panetelis, C., McGorry, P.D. *et al.* (1999) Hippocampal volume in first-episode psychosis and chronic schizophrenia: a high-resolution magnetic resonance imaging study. *Archives of General Psychiatry* **56**, 133–141.

Volk, D.W., Austin, M.C., Pierri, J.N., Sampson, A.R. & Lewis, D.A. (2000) Decreased GAD$_{67}$ mRNA expression in a subset of prefrontal cortical GABA neurons in subjects with schizophrenia. *Archives of General Psychiatry* **57**, 237–245.

Volk, D.W., Austin, M.C., Pierri, J.N., Sampson, A.R. & Lewis, D.A. (2001) GABA transporter-1 mRNA in the prefrontal cortex in schizophrenia: decreased expression in a subset of neurons. *American Journal of Psychiatry* **158**, 256–265.

Weickert, C. & Weinberger, D.R. (1998) A candidate molecular approach to defining the developmental pathology in schizophrenia. *Schizophrenia Bulletin* **24**, 303–316.

Weinberger, D.R. (1987) Implications of normal brain development for the pathogenesis of schizophrenia. *Archives of General Psychiatry* **44**, 660–669.

Weinberger, D.R. (1999) Cell biology of the hippocampal formation in schizophrenia. *Biological Psychiatry* **45**, 395–402.

Weinberger, D.R. & Lipska, B.K. (1995) Cortical maldevelopment, anti-psychotic drugs, and schizophrenia: a search for common ground. *Schizophrenia Research* **16**, 87–110.

Weinberger, D.R., Berman, K.F. & Illowsky, B.P. (1988) Physiological dysfunction of dorsolateral prefrontal cortex in schizophrenia. III. A new cohort and evidence for a monoaminergic mechanism. *Archives of General Psychiatry* **45**, 609–615.

Weinberger, D.R., Berman, K.F., Suddath, R. & Torrey, E.F. (1992) Evidence of dysfunction of a prefrontal-limbic network in schizophrenia: a magnetic resonance imaging and regional cerebral blood flow study of discordant monozygotic twins. *American Journal of Psychiatry* **149**, 890–897.

Wellman, C.L., Logue, S.F. & Sengelaub, D.R. (1995) Maze learning and morphology of frontal cortex in adult and aged basal forebrain-lesioned rats. *Behavioral Neuroscience* **109**, 837–850.

Wisniewski, H.M., Constantinidis, J., Wegiel, J., Bobinski, M. & Tarnawski, M. (1994) Neurofibrillary pathology in brains of elderly schizophrenics treated with neuroleptics. *Alzheimer Disease and Associated Disorders* **8**, 211–227.

Woo, T.-U., Miller, J.L. & Lewis, D.A. (1997a) Parvalbumin-containing cortical neurons in schizophrenia. *American Journal of Psychiatry* **154**, 1013–1015.

Woo, T.-U., Pucak, M.L., Kye, C.H., Matus, C.V. & Lewis, D.A. (1997b) Peripubertal refinement of the intrinsic and associational circuitry in monkey prefrontal cortex. *Neuroscience* **80**, 1149–1158.

Woo, T.-U., Whitehead, R.E., Melchitzky, D.S. & Lewis, D.A. (1998) A subclass of prefrontal gamma-aminobutyric acid axon terminals are selectively altered in schizophrenia. *Proceedings of the National Academy of Sciences of the USA* **95**, 5341–5346.

Young, K.A., Manaye, K.F., Liang, C.-L., Hicks, P.B. & German, D.C. (2000) Reduced number of mediodorsal and anterior thalamic neurons in schizophrenia. *Biological Psychiatry* **47**, 944–953.

Zaidel, D.W., Esiri, M.M. & Harrison, P.J. (1997a) The hippocampus in schizophrenia: lateralized increase in neuronal density and altered cytoarchitectural asymmetry. *Psychological Medicine* **27**, 703–713.

Zaidel, D.W., Esiri, M.M. & Harrison, P.J. (1997b) Size, shape and orientation of neurons in the left and right hippocampus: investigation of normal asymmetries and alterations in schizophrenia. *American Journal of Psychiatry* **154**, 812–818.

Schizophrenia as a neurodevelopmental disorder

D.R. Weinberger and S. Marenco

Evidence of developmental neuropathology, 327
  Obstetric abnormalities, 327
  Intrauterine infection and abnormal
    nutrition, 329
  Minor physical anomalies, 330
  Premorbid neurological and behavioural
    abnormalities, 331
Evidence of brain tissue abnormalities, 331

Neuroimaging, 331
  Postmortem studies, 336
Evidence against neurodegeneration, 337
Mechanisms of delayed onset, 338
  Candidate maturational processes and clinical
    onset, 341
Conclusions, 341
References, 342

The idea that schizophrenia has its origins in early development dates back at least to the modern classification of the syndrome by Kraepelin and Bleuler, both of whom noted abnormal neurological and behavioural signs in the childhood histories of adult patients. Some of the neuropathological findings reported in the early part of the twentieth century were interpreted as evidence of abnormal brain development (e.g. Southard 1915). Bender (1947), in her landmark study of cases of childhood schizophrenia, argued that the condition was likely to be a developmental encephalopathy. In studies of children of schizophrenic mothers, Fish and Hagin (1972) described a constellation of apparent lags and disruptions in neurological development, which predicted the later emergence of schizophrenia spectrum symptoms; they also proposed abnormal brain development as the cause. Other investigators had emphasized the early childhood social abnormalities of individuals with adult-onset schizophrenia (Watt 1972), also potentially implicating abnormal brain development. In spite of this diverse literature, the general view among psychiatrists and researchers during much of the twentieth century was that schizophrenia occurs principally because of a biological process that happens or is expressed around early adult life, and that clinical remission is related to reversal of this pathological process, while progression of the clinical condition is an expression of continuing progression of the pathology. This view echoed aspects of Kraepelin's codification of schizophrenia as an early dementia ('dementia praecox') and seemed consistent with the clinical fact that many patients with schizophrenia do not have a clearly abnormal premorbid history.

Beginning in the mid-1980s, a broad conceptual shift in thinking about the neurobiology of schizophrenia began to gather momentum, as the possibility of abnormal brain development again became a popular idea and a neurodevelopmental hypothesis of schizophrenia was elaborated and embraced by both the clinical and research communities. A convergence of factors accounted for this conceptual shift: in particular, a growing body of indirect evidence of abnormal brain development in individuals with schizophrenia and the failure of older formulations to capture the meaning and complexity of new data. For example, several longitudinal outcome studies (Bleuler 1941; Tsuang *et al.* 1979; Harding *et al.* 1992) demonstrated that considerable recovery was well within the bounds of schizophrenia, thus undermining the Kraepelinian concept of schizophrenia as a degenerative disease of early adulthood. Even in patients who did not have good outcomes, the pattern of neuropsychological impairment was not a progressively deteriorating one (Aylward *et al.* 1984). The advent of neuroimaging technologies permitted direct *in vivo* brain studies and led to the archival finding of increased cerebral ventricle size – the first unequivocal neurobiological marker of the illness (Johnstone *et al.* 1976; Weinberger *et al.* 1979, 1982a). The fact that this biological abnormality was present from the onset of the illness (Weinberger *et al.* 1982a), that it did not correlate with duration of illness (Weinberger *et al.* 1979) or advance with continuing illness in most longitudinal studies (Illowsky *et al.* 1988) strengthened further the assumption that a neurodegenerative process was not responsible. Evidence that ventricular enlargement was associated with poor premorbid social adjustment during childhood and that ventricular enlargement existed at the time of the first break was interpreted to indicate that the determining biology was present long before the typical clinical onset and was likely to be developmental in origin (Weinberger *et al.* 1980, 1982a). Meanwhile, postmortem histopathology studies were unable to demonstrate evidence of neurodegeneration, and the long-recognized absence of astrogliosis in the schizophrenic brain was now interpreted as further potential evidence that changes in the brain were of developmental origin and thus would not be associated with a gliotic reaction (Weinberger *et al.* 1983; Weinberger 1987).

By the end of the 1980s, a detailed formulation of the neurodevelopmental hypothesis emerged (Weinberger 1986, 1987), which included educated guesses on the distinct roles of cortical and subcortical dopaminergic systems in the brain, and the relationship of limbic and prefrontal cortical pathology to the manifest psychopathology. It was proposed that subtle abnormalities of cortical development, particularly involving limbic and prefrontal cortices and their connectivities, increase risk for the adult emergence of the schizophrenia syndrome.

Dopamine innervation of prefrontal cortex was considered an important factor in prefrontal cortical function related to negative symptoms and cognitive deficits in schizophrenia and to stress-related symptomatic exacerbation. Impaired dopamine function at the prefrontal cortical level also was seen as a factor in upregulating subcortical dopamine activity, perhaps accounting for psychotic symptoms and response to neuroleptic drugs. Moreover, it was proposed that the triggering of the emergence of the syndrome depended on an interaction of the early developmental abnormalities with normal maturation events of early adult life, such as the maturation of intracortical connectivities and of the cortical dopamine system. Neurodevelopmental changes during adulthood were considered as a possible factor in the clinical evolution of the syndrome, as progression of negative symptoms and even some cognitive deficits might represent normal age-related changes in prefrontal cortex, and the tendency for positive symptoms to attenuate with ageing might reflect normal age-related involution of the dopamine system.

The basic concepts elaborated at that time have remained largely relevant to our current state of knowledge, and in fact considerable evidence has accrued to bolster their credibility. Indeed, the heuristic impact of this paradigm shift in thinking about schizophrenia is illustrated by the many new areas of clinical and basic investigation it has spawned, including:

1 epidemiological studies about prenatal, behavioural and developmental factors associated with the illness, which have provided the most compelling evidence in support of the neurodevelopmental hypothesis (see below and Chapters 12 and 13);

2 the elaboration of a spectrum of developmental animal models which have confirmed the neurobiological plausibility of the hypothesis (see Chapter 21);

3 the search for molecular markers of abnormal cortical development in schizophrenic brain tissue (see Chapter 17); and

4 a quest for genes that might increase susceptibility by affecting brain development (see Chapters 14 and 15).

Numerous authors and investigators have made brain development and schizophrenia a centrepiece of their theoretical approach to the disorder (Murray & Lewis 1987; Bogerts 1989; Crow et al. 1989a; Waddington & Youssef 1990; Mednick 1991; Bloom 1993; Cannon et al. 1993; Keshavan & Hogarty 1999).

In the first edition of this book, the chapter on neurodevelopment and schizophrenia reviewed the available evidence supporting the hypothesis and speculated about possible developmental mechanisms of pathogenesis (Weinberger 1995). It focused on four areas:

1 basic aspects of normal brain development, with particular reference to how and when putative abnormalities associated with schizophrenia might occur;

2 neuroimaging and postmortem research data interpreted to represent cerebral maldevelopment;

3 evidence for abnormal environmental factors impacting on early brain development; and

4 mechanisms that might explain how the onset of the illness could be delayed until long after the early pathology occurred.

In this revised edition, we focus on new clinical information that has emerged about brain development and schizophrenia since the early 1990s and consider in detail the implications of these new data on the neurodevelopmental hypothesis. This chapter is not intended as a comprehensive summary of the recent literature, which is also surveyed in other chapters in this volume (specifically, Chapters 12, 13 and 22). In contrast to these chapters, we highlight the problems and inconsistencies in this literature as they relate to the potential neurodevelopmental origins of schizophrenia. As we note, some of the evidence for a neurodevelopmental abnormality has become stronger, e.g. environmental adversity in utero, while other evidence has come under challenge, e.g. from neuroimaging and neuropathology studies.

Evidence of developmental neuropathology

In the past decade, literally hundreds of studies in many countries have been undertaken in the search for evidence of abnormal brain development in patients with schizophrenia. While there is substantial indication that the brains of such patients are not normal and that their developmental histories are not normal, the evidence that abnormal brain development is a risk factor for schizophrenia remains indirect and circumstantial. Thus, numerous in vivo neuroimaging studies have revealed compelling evidence of morphometric changes in the schizophrenic brain (see Chapter 22) and many postmortem studies (see Chapter 17) have found replicable cellular and molecular abnormalities; however, none of the findings can be definitively attributed to a developmental origin. Large epidemiological cohort studies in several countries have confirmed that increased frequency of obstetric complications and abnormal social, motor and cognitive maturation during childhood are associated with emergence of schizophrenia during adulthood (see Chapter 13). However, a direct causative link between these phenomena and abnormal brain development is lacking. We consider now some of the indirect evidence for abnormal early brain development. More detailed discussions of this evidence have appeared in earlier reviews (Marenco & Weinberger 2000; Marenco & Weinberger 2003).

Obstetric abnormalities

The most extensively studied of the early developmental markers are obstetric complications (OCs; see Chapter 13). Beginning in the 1930s (Rosanoff et al. 1934), reports that adult patients with schizophrenia had increased frequency of OCs appeared and, as the neurodevelopmental hypothesis became more popular, the frequency of these reports in the literature has increased dramatically. Many obstetric risk factors have been linked with schizophrenia in one study or another, including pre-eclampsia (Kendell et al. 1996; O'Dwyer 1997), small head circumference (McNeil *et al.* 1993; Kunugi *et al.* 1996), low birth weight (Lane & Albee 1970; Torrey 1977; Jones *et al.* 1998), Rhesus factor incompatibility (Hollister *et al.* 1996), fetal distress (O'Callaghan *et al.* 1992), weight heavy for length (Hultman *et al.* 1997), multiparity, maternal bleeding during pregnancy (Hultman *et al.* 1999), abnormal presentations (Parnas *et al.* 1982; Gunthergenta *et al.* 1994; Verdoux *et al.* 1997) and increased prepregancy body weight (Susser *et al.* 2000). While most of this evidence is based on case–control comparisons, several recent large cohort epidemiological studies are especially noteworthy. Most impressive of these is a study of 500 000 births in Sweden (Dalman *et al.* 1999). It was reported in this study that the relative risk for schizophrenia was increased up to 2.5 times by pre-eclampsia, gestational age below 33 weeks, inertia of labour, vacuum extraction, respiratory illness and low birth weight. Pre-eclampsia, an indicator of fetal malnutrition, emerged after logistical regression as the strongest risk factor, increasing the risk for schizophrenia between 2 and 2.5 times. Extreme prematurity also increased risk for schizophrenia by more than twice. In spite of the impressive statistical results, the absolute number of cases involved was quite small. Out of a total sample of 238 cases of schizophrenia, only 11 had a history of pre-eclampsia, five extreme prematurity and two very low birth weight.

Two large cohort studies were conducted in Finland: one based on a 1960s cohort of 11 000 pregnancies (Jones *et al.* 1998) and another based on 7840 births in Helsinki in 1955 (Rosso *et al.* 2000). Only low birth weight and short gestation conferred increased risk in the first study, while increased scores on an inventory of abnormalities loosely linked to 'hypoxia' (including prematurity, but not birth weight and gestational age) were found to increase risk in the second study, but only after the cases were divided into those with age of onset before age 22. In the group with age of onset after 22, there was no association with OCs. The authors of the first study also noted the curious finding that mothers of patients with schizophrenia reported being depressed during pregnancy more frequently than mothers of probands without the disorder.

Finally, Cannon *et al.* (2000) examined birth records of 9236 births at an inner city hospital in Philadelphia who were followed as part of the US National Collaborative Perinatal Project. They again reported an increased risk associated with their 'hypoxia' scale only in so-called early-onset cases. Several studies, including those of Rosso *et al.* (2000) and Cannon *et al.* (2000), report an apparent dose relationship between number of OCs and risk for schizophrenia (Hultman *et al.* 1997), as if greater intrauterine or perinatal distress accounts for greater brain involvement and ultimate risk for illness. Indeed, earlier clinical correlation studies have tended to find that adult patients with a history of OCs have other evidence associated with poorer outcome, such as a more chronic course (Wilcox & Nasrallah 1987), predominant negative symptoms (Cannon *et al.* 1990), younger age at onset (Smith *et al.* 1998) and more structural abnormalities on magnetic resonance imaging (MRI) scan (McNeil *et al.* 2000).

Notwithstanding the impressive number of positive reports of an association of OCs with risk for schizophrenia, there are important inconsistencies. In particular, there are two recent large case–control studies based on contemporaneous birth records. Byrne *et al.* (2000) found that OCs were more frequent and more severe only in males presenting for psychiatric treatment before the age of 30. Kendell *et al.* (2000) found almost no association between OCs and schizophrenia in an even larger (almost 500 cases) case–control study. These results were in conflict with those obtained 4 years earlier on the same group of subjects (Kendell *et al.* 1996), when fewer schizophrenia cases had passed through the age of risk. Kendell *et al.* (2000) identified a case–control matching algorithm in the earlier positive study that erroneously depressed the frequency of OCs in controls. There are also negative reports among older cohort studies also based on obstetric records (Done *et al.* 1991; Buka *et al.* 1993). Interestingly, a reanalysis of the data in Done *et al.* (1991) by Sacker *et al.* (1995) found that schizophrenia was associated with a higher likelihood of risk behaviour during pregnancy by the mothers, including smoking, drinking, poorer prenatal care, etc. Perhaps such behaviours should qualify as OCs, although they are not included in the scales used in most studies. It should also be noted that later reanalysis after more prolonged follow-up of the cohort originally studied by Buka *et al.* (1993) did show an association of schizophrenia and OCs related to hypoxia (Zornberg *et al.* 2000).

It is likely that the inconsistencies in the literature reflect the relative weakness of the effect size of OCs on risk for schizophrenia. Meta-analyses of this literature have found that, in general, OCs increase risk from 1.3- to twofold (Geddes *et al.* 1999); thus, they account for a relatively small numbers of cases, analogous to estimates of risk attributable to a single genetic locus (Risch 1990). Nevertheless, it is difficult to escape the conclusion that OCs, of various sorts, depending probably on cohort and record-keeping variations, do slightly increase risk for the emergence of schizophrenia in late life. This means that abnormalities of the intrauterine environment can affect fetal development in a manner that has implications for the expression of schizophrenia. However, this broad conclusion may be as far as the association with OCs will ultimately go in clarifying the specific developmental mechanisms related to schizophrenia.

There are a number of problems in interpreting the biological implications of the OC data. In most studies, the assessment of OCs has tended to lump together those occurring at different times during gestation, delivery and the neonatal period. There has been no agreement on what scales to use and whether multiple OCs should be considered as independent measures related to increasing severity of prenatal or perinatal abnormality (McNeil *et al.* 1997). The attribution of specific OCs to specific pathophysiological mechanisms, e.g. prematurity to hypoxia, is suspect. Certainly, OCs are not specific for schizophrenia, and have been associated with increased risk for bipolar disorder (Lewis & Murray 1987; Done *et al.* 1991; Guth *et al.* 1993; Kinney *et al.* 1998; Marcelis *et al.* 1998), although probably less clearly so than with schizophrenia (Verdoux & Bourgeois 1993;

Bain *et al.* 2000), disruptive behaviour in adolescents (Allen *et al.* 1998), antisocial behaviours (Szatmari *et al.* 1986), autism (Bolton *et al.* 1997) and 'minimal brain dysfunction' (Rao 1990) and cerebral palsy (Nelson & Ellenberg 1984; Eschenbach 1997). Why the same pattern of OCs would result in such diverse conditions is unknown. It may well be that many psychiatric disorders have this antecedent and that OCs are generic risk factors for many behavioural complications.

Another confusing aspect of the OC literature that complicates a mechanistic formulation is that the evidence is inconsistent in terms of timing of OCs during pregnancy. It is difficult to understand how causes acting in the second or third trimester or in the perinatal period result in a similar outcome as a disruption in brain development at different times might be expected to result in different outcomes. Indeed, one of the perplexing aspects of the OC literature is the variability from one study to another of which OC confers increased risk. It is also surprising that OCs tend *not* to correlate with other aspects of premorbid abnormal development, such as motor and cognitive function (Cannon 2000). It would be reasonably expected that if OCs relate to schizophrenia in adulthood because of their impact on brain development, they should relate even more strongly to childhood maturational antecedents that are more proximate to the effects of OCs.

It is also unclear why OCs affect some individuals adversely and appear to have no impact in others, probably the majority of people. Several studies have considered the possibility that OCs interact with genetic risk factors. Cannon *et al.* (1993) reported that a relationship with CT abnormalities and OCs was found only in patients with a family history of schizophrenia. However, several other groups have reported the tendency for OCs to segregate with cases lacking a family history (Lewis *et al.* 1989; Cantor-Graae *et al.* 1994). The question of whether the occurrence of OCs *per se* is related to genetic risk for schizophrenia, i.e. whether risk genes for schizophrenia might also be risk genes for causing OCs, has been addressed in several recent studies, with largely negative results (Marcelis *et al.* 1998; Cannon *et al.* 2000). However, it is also clear that schizophrenic mothers, perhaps because of prenatal behavioural risk factors such as smoking and poor prenatal care, have increased frequencies of OCs (Sacker *et al.* 1996; Bennedsen *et al.* 2001).

Finally, a striking omission in almost all of the OC literature is consideration of environmental risk factors such as smoking and drug/alchohol use on pregnancy outcome. It is clear that tobacco and alcohol use affect the frequency of OCs and brain development (Frank *et al.* 2001). The possibility that an association of such behaviours in the mothers of schizophrenic offspring would provide a potential causative mechanism for OCs needs to be considered in future studies. The implications for prevention are also apparent.

In conclusion, while the OC literature does not provide a mechanistic account of how OCs biologically translate into risk for schizophrenia, it does add substantial evidence of a role of a neurodevelopmental abnormality *per se*, and of the plausibility of the neurodevelopmental hypothesis.

Intrauterine infection and abnormal nutrition

While the causes of OCs associated with schizophrenia are unknown, evidence that potential aetiological factors, such as intrauterine infection and abnormal nutrition, may increase risk for schizophrenia provide further support for the neurodevelopmental hypothesis (see also Chapters 12 and 13). Several studies have linked schizophrenia to evidence of adverse maternal nutrition during pregnancy (e.g. Susser *et al.* 1996; Rosso *et al.* 2000; Wahlbeck *et al.* 2001), although the timing of the putative nutritional adversity has been either unspecified or varied. The data related to famine (Susser *et al.* 1996) have not been independently replicated. A more consistent association has been found between some influenza epidemics, especially the one in Europe in 1957, and an excess of births that would later develop schizophrenia (Mednick *et al.* 1988, 1990). This observation has been replicated in several countries, both in the northern (Kendell & Kemp 1989; O'Callaghan *et al.* 1991; Kunugi *et al.* 1995) and the southern hemispheres (McGrath *et al.* 1994). According to these studies, the fetus, judging from its date of birth, should have been in the second trimester of pregnancy when exposed to the virus. However, Crow *et al.* (1992), using the British birth cohort of 1957, found no evidence of such an effect, and other studies have failed to support an association of intrauterine influenza and schizophrenia (Torrey *et al.* 1988; Selten & Slaets 1994; Susser *et al.* 1994; Morgan *et al.* 1997; Westergaard *et al.* 1999). There are only a few studies where an attempt was made to verify whether mothers had actually suffered from a viral infection during their second trimester (Crow *et al.* 1992; Mednick *et al.* 1994; Cannon *et al.* 1996) and the results of these studies are controversial. Moreover, the mechanism by which influenza *in utero* might produce schizophrenia is unclear, as there is little evidence for direct cytotoxicity of the influenza virus in the fetus (Cotter *et al.* 1995) and influenza viral markers have not been found in cerebrospinal fluid or in postmortem brain tissue of patients with schizophrenia (Sierrahonigmann *et al.* 1995; Taller *et al.* 1996). In addition, possible influenza exposure *in utero* has also been linked to affective disorders in the same population of cases exposed to the 1957 epidemic in Finland that generated the initial data for schizophrenia (Machon *et al.* 1997).

In studies that reviewed the effect of influenza epidemics other than the one in 1957, there is even less consistency and preliminary evidence for a causative role of other potential infectious aetiological agents has emerged, including diptheria and pneumonia (Watson *et al.* 1984), measles, polio, varicella and zoonoses (Torrey *et al.* 2000), rubella (Brown *et al.* 2001) and non-specific upper respiratory infections (Brown *et al.* 2000). The data supporting these recent additional associations are discussed in greater detail elsewhere (see Chapter 13; Marenco & Weinberger 2003).

Schizophrenia has been linked in several large unbiased epidemiological studies to urban birth (Marcelis *et al.* 1999; Mortensen *et al.* 1999) and to late winter–early spring season of birth (Mortensen *et al.* 1999; Suvisaari *et al.* 2000, 2001). The evidence for urban birth is particularly intriguing because it is where an individual was born, not raised or lived, that appears to convey the greatest risk. This implicates indirectly obstetric factors, although the specific variables have not been identified. Multiple studies have found evidence of the so-called season of birth effect (Bradbury & Miller 1985; Hafner et al. 1987; Kendell & Kemp 1987; Kendell & Adams 1991; O'Callaghan et al. 1991; Torrey et al. 1993; Mortensen et al. 1999) and the most popular explanation has been increased likelihood of infection during the winter, possibly at a critical period of gestation. However, there are few data directly linking infection rates and season of birth in the same population and fluctuations in epidemic infection rates are unlikely to account for the whole effect (Sham et al. 1992). While O'Callaghan et al. (1991) reported an interaction between the seasonal variation of schizophrenia births and urban births, this was not replicated in a much larger sample (Suvisaari et al. 2000). In general, the seasonality of birth phenomena has been difficult to interpret. There is no consensus in the literature regarding the correlates of seasonal variation in schizophrenia births in terms of other evidence of infection, intrauterine adversity, OCs, later development or manifest symptomatology (for review see Cotter et al. 1996). Moreover, seasonal variation in birth may be present in the population as a whole (Russell et al. 1993) and in other central nervous system conditions such as bipolar disorder, autism, dyslexia and epilepsy (Cotter et al. 1996). There are also unexplained geographical discrepancies in the degree of seasonal variation in birth, with similar data in Japan (Kunugi et al. 1997) and Finland (Suvisaari et al. 2000), but a quite different pattern in Scotland (Eagles et al. 1995).

Several recent studies have explored the possibility that stressful environments experienced by the mother could impact biologically on the developing fetus and increase risk for schizophrenia. For example, Van Os and Selten (1998) have found an association between exposure to aerial bombardment during World War II during the first trimester of pregnancy and subsequent development of schizophrenia. Similarly, Selten et al. (1999) found weak evidence for exposure to a flood in the Netherlands to increase the risk for the development of schizophrenia in offspring. However, these studies did not control for other potential deprivations that may accompany such catastrophes and do not implicate a mechanism for the effect. Nevertheless, it has become popular in psychiatry research almost to the point of faddism to attribute structural changes in brain during development and even later in life to the cellular and molecular sequelae of stress, although the evidence for this possibility is limited.

In summary, over the past decade there has been a dramatic accumulation of data that OCs and intrauterine adversity slightly but significantly increase the risk for adult emergence of schizophrenia. Because these factors are likely to reflect phenomena linked to aspects of brain development, they represent the most substantial evidence that abnormal brain development increases the risk for schizophrenia. However, it is also clear from this extensive literature that there is no specific or consistent developmental factor, nor does there appear to be a specific time or stage in human intrauterine development. This makes it difficult to implicate a specific biological mechanism, or a spe-cific developmental defect, at least across the general population of affected patients. The second trimester may be a particularly vulnerable period of development and the 1957 influenza epidemic might have conferred a particularly clear risk but, at most, this event accounts for a very small minority of patients with the illness. Non-specific insults to the brain (from drug exposure to head trauma to epilepsy) also are sometimes thought to cause schizophrenia-like syndromes in adulthood, which appears to be a particularly vulnerable period of life for the expression of psychotic symptoms regardless of the manner of brain insult (Weinberger 1987; Hyde et al. 1992). Moreover, the same developmental causes that increase risk for schizophrenia may also increase risk for other disorders, including affective psychosis. These results invite reflection upon the notion of specificity of causation and pathogenesis with respect to schizophrenia. It is reasonable to assume that such diverse environmental factors that disrupt the normal programmes of early human brain development have individually varying clinical effects depending on other modifying and protecting factors, including genetic background and environmental aspects of postnatal development.

Minor physical anomalies

The data reviewed thus far suggest that OCs associated with the later development of schizophrenia are quite non-specific. Given this apparent fact, we would expect that the development of other organs might also be affected. Some evidence exists for the occurrence of an excess of physical anomalies outside the brain in patients with schizophrenia (see Chapter 12; Green et al. 1994). These generally range from webbed toes to altered craniofacial morphometry. These putative abnormalities have been interpreted as evidence that brain development also is abnormal.

The physical anomalies that seem to differentiate most clearly patients with schizophrenia from other patient groups are primarily craniofacial. According to Lane et al. (1996), these include palate height, bifid tongue, ear protrusion, supraorbital ridges, eye fissure inclination, epicanthus and widened helix. Interestingly, Kraepelin (1919) cited high palate and low set ears as being over-represented in his patients with schizophrenia. A more recent study (Lane et al. 1997) found that the combination of 12 variables, all related to cranial morphology, allowed a correct classification of 90% of patients with schizophrenia and 80% of a matched sample of controls.

Another interesting putative physical anomaly involves the development of finger and hand print patterns. Altered dermatoglyphic patterns have been reported in patients with schizophrenia, based on quantitative assessment of ridge counts and patterns (Lane et al. 1996; Fearon et al. 2001), including in discordant monozygotic twins (Davis & Bracha 1996). Because such dermatoglyphic patterns are thought to cease development by the third trimester of pregnancy, the variations reported in schizophrenia have been interpreted as further evidence of fetal adversity.

The major limitation of interpreting the physical anomaly data is that their frequency in healthy subjects is sometimes surprisingly high (up to 50% for some craniofacial abnormalities; Lane *et al.* 1997), raising the question of whether they are truly anomalies at all. It should also be noted that subtle effects of medication, including parkinsonism or dyskinesias, which may impact on facial features, have not been ruled out as a possible confounder. Moreover, and perhaps most critical, the interpretation of these studies is based on the assumption that because classical developmental syndromes (e.g. Down's syndrome) are associated with marked qualitative deviations in facial and dermatoglyphic features, quantitative physical deviance, if present in schizophrenia, must also be developmental in origin. This assumption may not be valid for such quantitative measures that vary considerably in the normal population. Thus, minor physical anomalies, if they were valid effects of abnormal organ development, would represent direct evidence of disturbed intrauterine development. We believe that the jury is still out on the interpretation of the minor physical anomaly data.

Premorbid neurological and behavioural abnormalities

If the brains of individuals at risk to manifest schizophrenia have not developed normally, it might be expected that some evidence of subtle abnormalities of nervous system function would be apparent during their childhood before they become clinically ill. In fact, the data from case–control and especially from large epidemiological cohorts are unequivocal that such evidence exists. This evidence includes delayed motor and speech milestones during the first year of life, various deficits in motor and cognitive development throughout childhood and consistent social and educational abnormalities. This evidence is reviewed in detail elsewhere (see Chapters 12 and 13; Marenco & Weinberger 2000). A remarkable aspect to the results, of the large epidemiological studies especially, is their consistency. Virtually every study has found evidence of deficits – subtle but significant – in the premorbid development of individuals who manifest schizophrenia during adulthood. The deficits are especially clear in school performance and other signs of cognitive development, although this may reflect in part that such skills are consistently sampled as outcome measures. Clearly, schizophrenia, as it is currently defined and diagnosed, is a disorder of early adult life, but antecedent abnormalities of cognitive and psychological function are part of the syndrome. Thus, it can be concluded that such antecedents reflect malfunction of certain brain systems from relatively early in life. However, because social and psychological deprivations also can affect cognitive and social development, the specific aetiology of these antecedents of schizophrenia cannot be specified from these studies.

Evidence of brain tissue abnormalities

Neuroimaging

The current incarnation of the neurodevelopmental hypothesis was originally proposed based on some unexpected results from computerized axial tomography (CAT) scan studies of adult patients with schizophrenia. Beginning in 1976 with an *in vivo* study of cerebral ventricular size using the novel method of CAT scanning (Johnstone *et al.* 1976), literally hundreds of reports have appeared of subtle variations in cerebral anatomy associated with schizophrenia, especially enlarged cerebral ventricles. Recent applications of MRI, which allow much more detailed measurements of cortical and subcortical brain structures, have confirmed that volumes of various structures in the brain in schizophrenia are slightly smaller and cerebrospinal fluid spaces are larger than found in comparison control groups (see Chapter 22 for a survey of this literature). Weinberger *et al.* (1979) reported, to their surprise, that ventricular size measured on a CAT scan did not correlate with duration of illness, as would have been expected if the neuropathological process responsible for ventricular enlargement advanced as the illness progressed. They raised the possibility that the underlying process was no longer active, i.e. was non-degenerative. The lack of a correlation between ventricular size and duration of illness has been widely replicated (Raz & Raz 1990), and its interpretation appeared to be supported by the results of several longitudinal studies that followed the same patients for up to 10 years (e.g. Jaskiw *et al.* 1994). Shortly after the initial reports in chronic patients, ventricular enlargement was reported in patients at the onset of psychosis in early adulthood (Weinberger *et al.* 1982a), a finding which also has been frequently confirmed (DeLisi *et al.* 1991; Lieberman *et al.* 1993; Gur *et al.* 1998). Moreover, ventricular enlargement has been shown to correlate with early childhood social adjustment and with OCs (Weinberger *et al.* 1980b; Reveley *et al.* 1984; McNeil *et al.* 2000). Together, these various findings led to the conclusions that ventricular enlargement reflects changes in the brain that predate the adult emergence of the clinical syndrome, appear to be relatively stable during the course of the illness, and may reflect early developmental pathology. These conclusions appeared to support the neurodevelopmental hypothesis, as neurodevelopmental changes in brain anatomy would be expected to be present at the onset of the illness, would correlate with antecedents and, unlike degenerative changes, would remain relatively stable during adulthood.

However, a recent review (Woods 1998) and a new series of longitudinal MRI studies have called into question this assumption, by arguing that changes in extracerebral cerebrospinal fluid could not be developmental in origin (Woods 1998), and by revealing changes in measurements of brain structures (e.g. ventricles, hippocampus) over relatively short periods in patients who have been ill for varying periods of time and at various stages of life (reviewed in Weinberger & McClure 2002). Indeed, these recent MRI studies offer a serious challenge to the neurodevelopmental hypothesis and have generated enthusiasm for resurrecting a neurodegeneration hypothesis of schizophrenia (Miller 1989; Olney & Farber 1995; DeLisi *et al.* 1997; Woods 1998; Lieberman 1999) – harkening back to proposals of Kraepelin and others during the first quarter of the twentieth century that there is destruction of neural tissue associated with psychosis. Several studies also have reported that certain changes frequently observed in chronic patients, such as reduced hippocampal volume, are not characteristic of first episode patients (e.g. DeLisi *et al.* 1995; Laakso *et al.* 2001; Matsumoto *et al.* 2001). While these data from longitudinal studies and from first episode patients do not negate other evidence associating abnormal development with risk for schizophrenia, these MRI data, if valid evidence of neurodegeneration, argue strongly that the neurodevelopmental hypothesis does not capture the complexity of the brain pathology underlying schizophrenia.

The crux of the matter is in the interpretation of MRI measurements. Clearly, quantitative measurements of cerebrospinal fluid spaces and tissue volumes on an MRI scan cannot establish that tissue has degenerated nor, for that matter, that the brain has developed abnormally. This can only be done at the cellular level. MRI measurements during life represent the volume of living structures, which can vary depending not only on changes in neuronal elements, but also on changes in vascularity, perfusion, extracellular constituents, etc. Thus, while brain shrinkage in Alzheimer's disease reflects primarily loss of neuronal elements, this is not true of brain shrinkage that is also seen with MRI in anorexia nervosa, or with steroid administration or with an alcoholic binge, as shrinkage in such instances is largely reversible (Weinberger & McClure 2002). The recent longitudinal MRI data in schizophrenia are notably inconsistent from one study to another and their interpretation as a reflection of neuronal degeneration is implausible in a number of respects (see Table 18.1). For example, while clearly there are some studies that find evidence of changes in MRI volume measurements (DeLisi *et al.* 1992, 1995, 1997, 1998; Nair *et al.* 1997; Rapoport *et al.* 1997; Davis *et al.* 1998; Gur *et al.* 1998; Jacobsen *et al.* 1998; Lieberman *et al.* 2001; Mathalon *et al.* 2001), the results vary considerably from one study to another, even among the positive studies. Some changes, e.g. in temporal lobes, in frontal lobes and in cerebrospinal fluid spaces, have been found in more than one study; however, no two studies have found the same pattern of changes across all measures, and each study appears to have its own unique combination of results. Another important inconsistency in the MRI data concerns the correlations between changes in symptoms and in MRI measurements; these also vary considerably from one study to another. More remarkably, in the majority of studies, patients have actually improved symptomatically while their MRI changes have appeared to progress (Rapoport 1997; DeLisi *et al.* 1998; Gur *et al.* 1998; Jacobsen *et al.* 1998). Clinical improvement is hardly what would be predicted as a result of progressive loss of brain tissue.

Further concerns about the plausibility of MRI volume changes in schizophrenia reflecting neurodegeneration are raised by comparisons with neurological conditions where neurodegeneration is established. The magnitude of the changes reported in the studies purporting to show neurodegeneration in schizophrenia is not trivial. Mathalon *et al.* (2001) claim a 2% per year reduction in frontal grey matter in patients with schizophrenia who have already been ill for an average of 15 years before they were studied. A recent study with very sophisticated image analysis methodology (Thompson *et al.* 2001) reported a 5% per year grey matter loss in many cortical areas. This degree of change is in the range reported in Alzheimer's disease for the hippocampus, a structure that is markedly degenerated in this illness (Laakso *et al.* 2000). Other studies of schizophrenia have reported volume loss in the hippocampus of even greater magnitude, as much as 7% per year (Jacobsen *et al.* 1998). The mesial area of the thalamus was shrinking at the alarming rate of 7% per year in a study of chronic adolescent patients (Rapoport *et al.* 1997). In a study of adolescent patients who had already been ill for several years, the rate of ventricular volume change was 10% per year, translating into a doubling period of only 10 years (Rapoport *et al.* 1997). At this pace, by the time a patient with schizophrenia reached age 60, there would be little brain left. While it has been countered that the progressive MRI changes in schizophrenia may not be linear and may not occur throughout the course of illness (DeLisi 1997; Rapoport *et al.* 1997; Jacobsen *et al.* 1998), the fact that similar MRI changes have been reported in chronic adolescent patients (DeCarli *et al.* 1990; Rapoport *et al.* 1997), in first episode patients in their twenties (Gur *et al.* 1998), in patients in their forties (Mathalon *et al.* 2001) and also in patients in their fifties (Davis *et al.* 1998), makes this *post hoc* explanation seem quite improbable. The magnitude of these MRI changes, if they are the result of neurodegeneration, would be readily observable at the tissue level but, as noted below and elsewhere in this volume (see Chapter 22), tissue evidence of neurodegeneration is generally lacking in schizophrenia.

While it seems implausible that these MRI results represent the effects of neurodegeneration, their true meaning is unclear. We believe that the most likely explanation involves physiological and neuroplasticity changes that have yet to be identified. Potential factors include changes in perfusion associated with functional changes in brain activity, medication effects, drug (including chronic smoking) or alcohol effects, body weight changes, etc. Recent findings that ventricular size can alternatively increase, decrease and then increase again in the same patients scanned repeatedly over just a few months strongly suggest that such changes may reflect physiological variations (DeLisi *et al.* 1998; Garver *et al.* 2000). It is also conceivable that the MRI changes reflect some degree of neuroplastic adaptation to the environment or to the experience of being psychotic or to treatment (e.g. changes in synaptic architecture), but whether such subtle cellular changes would be apparent at the level of a gross anatomical measurement on an MRI scan is uncertain.

Another approach to differentiating MRI changes potentially related to the effects of illness from those related to risk for

Table 18.1 Recent studies showing morphometric changes.

Investigators	Average age at first scan (years)	Average length follow up (years)	Brain region showing progressive change	Maximum percentage change (per year)	Brain region showing no change or opposite change	Correlation with clinical change
DeLisi *et al.* (1992, 1995, 1997, 1998)	26.5	1, 4, 4.7	Left lateral ventricle Left and right cerebral hemispheres Right cerebellum Corpus callosum (isthmus)	(+) 3.0 (−) 1.42 (Right) (−) 2.2 (−) 1.14	Right and left temporal lobes Right and left superior temporal gyrus Right and left hippocampus/amygdala Right and left caudate	No significant correlation between clinical measures and changes in ventricle or cerebral hemisphere volume Overall, symptoms improved in patients
Rapoport *et al.* (1997)	14.8	2	Total cerebrum Lateral ventricles and VBR (left > right) Caudate Globus pallidus Thalamic area	(−) 2.58 (+) 9.7 (−) 4.1 (−) 9.9 (−) 7.1	None	Overall, symptoms improved in patients
Jacobsen *et al.* (1998)	15.2	2	Total cerebrum Right temporal lobe Superior temporal gyrus (total) Superior temporal gyrus (posterior) Right superior temporal gyrus (anterior) Left hippocampus	(−) 2.30 (−) 4.15 (−) 3.7 (−) 4.3 (−) 3.2 (−) 7.15	Left temporal lobe Left superior temporal gyrus (anterior) Left and right amygdala Right hippocampus	No significant correlation between temporal lobe volume decrease and hallucinations, delusions, or negative symptoms Overall, symptoms improved in patients
Nair *et al.* (1997)	31.3	2	Lateral ventricle	(+) 12.48	None	Not reported
Garver *et al.* (2000)	35.8	2.6	None		Lateral ventricle Total brain	Worsening of symptoms correlated with decreased ventricular and increased total brain volume

Table 18.1 *Continued*.

Investigators	Average age at first scan (years)	Average length follow up (years)	Brain region showing progressive change	Maximum percentage change (per year)	Brain region showing no change or opposite change	Correlation with clinical change
Gur *et al.* (1998)	29.2	2.5	Frontal lobe (left > right) Temporal lobe (left > right)	(−) 4.2 (left) (−) 3.4 (left)	Whole brain Cerebral spinal fluid spaces	Improvement in most symptoms correlated with decreased frontal and temporal lobe volumes in previously previously treated patients Overall, symptoms improved in patients
Davis *et al.* (1998)	39.5	5.1	VBR (left > right) in Kraepelinian patients	(+) 3.3	None	No significant correlation between change in VBR and negative symptoms in non-Kraepelinian patients
Lieberman *et al.* (2001)	26	1.5	Cerebral cortex in poor outcome patients Total ventricles in poor outcome patients	(−) 0.42 (females) (−) 5.4 (females)	Caudate nuclei in all patients Hippocampus in all patients Cerebral cortex in all patients Total ventricles in all patients Total ventricles in good outcome patients Cerebral cortex in good outcome patients Hippocampus in poor outcome patients	Total ventricle and cerebral cortex increase correlates with poor outcome Cerebral cortex and hippocampus increase correlates with good outcome
Mathalon *et al.* (2001)	39.4	3.3	Prefrontal sulcii Right prefrontal grey Right frontal sulcii Left frontal grey Posterior superior temporal sulcii Posterior superior temporal grey Left lateral ventricle	(+) 6.63 (left) (−) 2.12 (−) 2.71 (−) 1.72 (+) 9.65 (left) (−) 3.35 (right) (+) 12.96	Left prefrontal grey Left frontal sulcii Right frontal grey Anterior superior temporal sulcii Right anterior superior temporal grey	Overall, symptoms improved in patients

VBR, ventricle-to-brain ratio.

illness is to examine healthy relatives of patients. Presumably, these individuals share risk factors that may operate at the level of brain development, but do not share illness-related epiphenomena. Several studies of family members, especially siblings, have suggested that slightly enlarged ventricles and reduced cortical volumes are found in healthy siblings (see Chapter 15; Weinberger *et al.* 1980b; Seidman *et al.* 1997; Cannon *et al.* 1998). In a recent study of 29 pairs of twins discordant for schizophrenia (15 MZ pairs and 14 DZ pairs) and 29 normal MZ pairs, Baare *et al.* (2001) found evidence of risk and illness-related changes. Slightly smaller intracranial volumes (2%) and larger ventricles were found in the unaffected twin from the discordant MZ pairs but not from the DZ pairs, suggesting that smaller brain growth was related to genetic risk for schizophrenia. Illness was associated with larger changes in brain volume measurements and with reduction in size of other cortical regions (e.g. parahippocampal cortex), suggesting that illness was associated with epigenetic changes affecting brain volume. Because intracranial volume is largely determined early in life, the twin data argue for abnormal brain development being related to genetic risk factors. These data in twins will require replication in larger samples.

While MRI volume measurements are difficult to interpret as evidence for or against pathological brain development, other approaches to analysing MRI scan data may be more informative. For example, several studies have looked at aspects of cortical gyral development. In principle, anomalous gyral patterns would be unequivocal evidence of cortical maldevelopment, as such patterns are almost completely established before birth. However, the results have been inconsistent (Kikinis *et al.* 1994; Kulynych *et al.* 1995a, 1997; Noga *et al.* 1996), and clearly most patients with schizophrenia do not have obvious gyral anomalies (e.g. microgyria, distorted gyri, etc.). Bullmore *et al.* (1998) and Friston and Frith (1995) used statistical methods to analyse the patterns of intercorrelated regional signal intensities on MRI in an effort to test for evidence of dysconnectivity. They reported differences in the intraregional correlation patterns between patients and controls, interpreting their results as evidence of pathological connectivity and presumably abnormal development. The validity of this interpretation of the MRI data is unclear. Several groups have examined the shape of various structures, particularly involving the temporal lobe, arguing that shape may more directly reflect structural development than would volume (Casanova *et al.* 1990; Csernansky *et al.* 1998). While abnormal shape of temporal lobe structures (e.g. hippocampus) was reported in these studies, the validity of the claim that changes in shape are more likely to reflect developmental change than is volume is untested.

Another neuroimaging observation that has been interpreted as reflecting abnormal brain development involves asymmetries of various regional volumes. In some studies, evidence of pathological changes appears to favour the left side of the brain. This has been especially true for the size of the ventricles (Crow *et al.* 1989a,b) and for the volume of the superior temporal gyrus (Shenton *et al.* 1992). Reports of relatively greater reductions in

other regions of left temporal cortex have also appeared (Suddath *et al.* 1990; Shenton *et al.* 2001). Indeed, when asymmetric findings have been reported, they usually involve the left hemisphere. This has prompted some to suggest that this lateralization tendency is consistent with a putative delay in the development of the left hemisphere during the second trimester, leaving it more vulnerable to adverse events that might otherwise affect the brain diffusely (Crow *et al.* 1989a; Roberts 1991). Whether the slight delay in the appearance of surface gyri means that the left hemisphere is developing slower or that it is more vulnerable to injury or vulnerable for a longer period is unknown. Moreover, most of the morphometric studies, even those that report unilateral findings (Crow *et al.* 1989a; Shenton *et al.* 1992), have also observed bilateral changes.

Studies of lateralized cerebral function, such as handedness, dichotic listening asymmetries and lateralized cognitive tasks, have suggested that patients with schizophrenia may be less completely lateralized than normal individuals. Some evidence from positron emission tomography (PET) studies even indicates reversed functional cerebral asymmetries in schizophrenia (Gur & Chin 1999). If these functional asymmetries are related to mechanisms of the development of normal anatomical asymmetries, the findings may have implications for abnormal cerebral development in schizophrenia. In a sense, anatomical asymmetries are closer to the issue of intrauterine development than are other morphometric assessments. They inherently control for individual differences in state variables and other artefacts that can confound measurements of *in vivo* and postmortem specimens, presumably because such variables should not be lateralized. In contrast to asymmetric findings (referred to above), findings of anomalous asymmetries are potentially more understandable as developmental in origin. The research question involved is not whether a pathological process is distributed or affects the brain asymmetrically, but whether the normal programmes that determine healthy asymmetry are disrupted. Because the times of origin of many of the well-characterized normal anatomical asymmetries are known, the time of disruption might be inferred. For instance, normal asymmetries of the Sylvian fissures (Chi *et al.* 1977), of the planum temporale (Wada *et al.* 1975), of the frontal operculum (Chi *et al.* 1977) and of the frontal and occipital lobes (Weinberger *et al.* 1982b) appear during the second trimester of gestation. Therefore, if variations in the appearance of such asymmetries are seen in patients with schizophrenia, this might provide further evidence of adverse development during that period. In general, there have been both positive and negative studies in assessments of various asymmetries, and the reasons for the inconsistencies are uncertain (Luchins *et al.* 1979; Bullmore *et al.* 1995; Kulynych *et al.* 1995b; Kwon *et al.* 1999; Shapleske *et al.* 2001). Even the advent of more sophisticated promising methods of image analysis (Thompson *et al.* 1997) has not resulted in extremely convincing findings. For example, Narr *et al.* (2001a) showed no effect of diagnosis on asymmetries of temporal sulci when comparing 28 patients with schizophrenia and 25 normal controls. On the other hand, they reported that the gyrification complexity of superior frontal cortex appears to be higher in the left hemisphere of patients, while the opposite pattern is true in normal controls. These results need to be replicated and their biological significance remains obscure. In another study on the same group of subjects (Narr *et al.* 2001b), these investigators confirmed with similar methodology that some parts of the ventricles appear to be larger on the left rather than the right hemisphere and that there was some interaction with diagnosis. Moreover, significant interactions of diagnosis and asymmetry were also found for anterior hippocampal size (Narr *et al.* 2001b). Crow has hypothesized that an abnormal frequency of brain asymmetries may be a core feature of schizophrenia and might be genetically determined (reviewed in Crow *et al.* 1996). The possibility that abnormal functional lateralization and anatomical asymmetries might be related to genetic risk for schizophrenia has been looked at with MRI in discordant MZ twins (Bartley *et al.* 1993) and in healthy relatives of patients with schizophrenia (Honer *et al.* 1995; Orr *et al.* 1999; Egan *et al.* 2001b), also with inconsistent results. The hypothesis of Crow further proposes that the development of cerebral asymmetries was a speciation event in human evolution and that psychosis is an inevitable casualty of this biological evolution. This hypothesis lacks consistent support in the literature, disregards evidence that anatomical asymmetries are found in other primates and does not address more generalized deficits in patients with schizophrenia. The arguments related to cerebral asymmetries and risk for schizophrenia are discussed in more detail elsewhere (Elvevåg & Weinberger 1997). Nevertheless, abnormal cerebral asymmetries similar to those reported in schizophrenia have been described in a number of developmental brain conditions, including dyslexia, autism, attention deficit–hyperactivity disorder, Down's syndrome and left-handedness, and may represent a non-specific anatomical sign that programmes of normal cerebral lateralization have been affected during early brain development.

In summary, evidence of cerebral anatomical abnormalities is a consistent finding from neuroimaging of patients with schizophrenia. In the early years of this literature, the correlative data supported the interpretation that the changes might reflect abnormal brain development. However, the data that have emerged from further studies over the past decade have made it impossible to draw strong inferences about the underlying mechanism of pathology. Thus, the MRI database, while offering some evidence in support of the neurodevelopmental hypothesis, especially the intracranial volume data in discordant MZ twins and the cerebral asymmetry results, does not further elucidate the presence or the role of developmental pathology in the pathogenesis of schizophrenia.

Postmortem studies

To the extent that abnormal brain development is inferred from epidemiological studies of developmental risk factors, from observations of physical anomalies and from neuroimaging,

definitive evidence and a mechanistic explication can only emerge from studies of brain tissue. Unfortunately, finding such evidence is not a simple task. It is not clear what specific neuropathological findings would represent an unequivocal indication that abnormal brain development had occurred, and it is not certain whether such changes would be obscured by age, chronic illness or other neuropathological processes encountered during life. Certainly, heterotopias or cytoarchitectural disarray that can only be explained by abnormal neuronal migration or neuronal settling would provide reasonable confirmation. At the molecular level, if the brains of patients with schizophrenia expressed a developmental molecule not normally found in adulthood, or expressed it in a region or structure where it is not normally found, that would be highly suggestive. Such clear findings are currently lacking (see Chapter 17). On the other hand, neuropathological evidence against the neurodevelopmental hypothesis might include pathological gliosis or other cellular and molecular signs of neurodegeneration, both of which are also lacking.

In the first edition of this volume, it was concluded that the most convincing evidence that pathological brain development was associated with schizophrenia came from studies of postmortem brain tissue (Weinberger 1995). This conclusion was based primarily on reports of ectopic cortical neurones and of abnormal cortical cytoarchitecture in prefrontal (Akbarian *et al.* 1993) and entorhinal cortices (Jakob & Beckmann 1986), findings which implicated abnormalities of neuronal migration and settling. While several deficiencies were described in these early reports, it was asserted that, 'if these data can be replicated in methodologically unimpeachable studies, a "smoking gun" will have been identified'. Several carefully conducted studies have attempted such replication and the findings have lost their lustre. In particular, the observations of Jakob and Beckman (1986) of abnormal sulcogyral patterns and cytoarchitectonics of the entorhinal cortex were not confirmed by at least four studies that carefully matched cases and controls for cytoarchitectonic zones along the rostral–caudal axis of the entorhinal cortex (Heinsen *et al.* 1996; Akil & Lewis 1997; Krimer *et al.* 1997; Bernstein *et al.* 1998). These studies further suggested that the original observations of Jakob and Beckman were artefacts of imprecise matching of sections. Likewise, the findings of Akbarian *et al.* (1993), of displaced neurones in deep subcortical white matter suggesting an abnormality in maturation of the cortical subplate, could not be replicated by Anderson *et al.* (1996). In a later report, Akbarian *et al.* (1996) were themselves unable to clearly replicate their own earlier result. In their newer study of 20 schizophrenics and 20 controls, only seven of the 20 schizophrenics demonstrated a 'substantial redistribution' of neurones, and this included five cases from the original report. Thus, only two of the added 15 cases showed the original phenomenon, which was not different from the frequency in controls.

Another approach to exploring brain development and schizo-phrenia is to measure the expression of genes and proteins involved in critical developmental processes such as neuronal migration and synapse formation. Barbeau *et al.* (1995)

found a significant reduction of the polysialylated form of the neural cell adhesion molecule (PSA-NCAM) in the dentate gyrus and the hilus region of the hippocampus, but Vawter *et al.* (1998) found an increase. Hyde *et al.* (1997) found a reduction of limbic system-associated protein (LAMP) in the entorhinal cortex. Impagnatiello *et al.* (1998) found reduced reelin protein in schizophrenia brain. Perrone-Bizzozero *et al.* (1996) found increased expression of GAP-43 protein in prefrontal cortex, but Shannon-Weickert *et al.* (2001) found decreased GAP-43 mRNA content in prefrontal cortex. Studies of gene and protein expression in schizophrenia brains are in their relative early stages and the reasons for the inconsistencies are unclear. More important, however, is that while such trophic and plasticity-related molecules are important in brain development, they also have critical roles in neuronal function throughout life. Thus, attributing differences in the expression of so-called neurodevelopmental molecules to exclusively developmental abnormalities is likely to be incorrect. A similar note of caution applies to interpretations of recent findings of reduced dendritic volume and spine density in schizophrenic cortex (Lewis & Lieberman 2000). Such findings have been taken as evidence in support of the hypothesis of abnormal synaptic pruning during adolescence in schizophrenia (see below). However, spine formation and maintenance is a life-long dynamic process, and spines can literally appear and disappear in a matter of minutes (Toni *et al.* 1999; van Rossum & Hanisch 1999; Segal 2001). Thus, attributing their density in brain tissue from elderly individuals to processes during postnatal or prenatal brain development is problematic.

In conclusion, examination of postmortem tissue in schizophrenia has not to date produced clear evidence of cellular or molecular changes that can be attributed to abnormal brain development. Earlier promising findings of abnormal cortical gyral and cellular architecture have not withstood methodologically rigorous tests. Improved methods of tissue collection and processing and more detailed molecular dissection of cellular phenotype are necessary. On the other hand, as will be discussed in the next section, postmortem tissue studies have not revealed evidence of neuronal degeneration in schizophrenia, which would probably be more readily observed if present than subtle developmental abnormalities. A further note of caution comes from the comparison of neuropathological findings reported in schizophrenia and those that are associated with confirmed perinatal injury and OCs (Marin-Padilla 1997). In general, the latter group of changes are much more severe and easily recognizable than those described in the schizophrenic brain.

Evidence against neurodegeneration

One of the many challenges to a neurodevelopmental formulation of schizophrenia is the apparent deterioration experienced by many patients after the onset of the illness in early adult life. Some patients become dilapidated in many respects during their adult years, and become increasingly resistant to treatment. Such phenomena have been invoked as support for the pos-

sibility that neurodegeneration is an important feature of schizophrenia that either adds to or interacts with putative neurodevelopmental factors (Olney & Farber 1995; Lieberman *et al.* 1996). Indeed, the research data summarized so far as potential evidence for abnormal brain development in schizophrenia might appear relatively inconsequential if objective signs of neurodegeneration were found. However, in postmortem tissue, where such evidence should be most obvious, signs of neurodegeneration have not been observed (see below, and Chapter 17). Thus, the possibility of neurodegeneration in schizophrenia is based largely on two phenomena. First, the apparent progression of clinical aspects of the syndrome in some patients, such as personality deterioration, dilapidation and treatment resistance (Lieberman 1999). While some patients do show such apparent deterioration, overall, the clinical course of most patients with schizophrenia is not chronically deteriorating (Marenco & Weinberger 2000). Moreover, clinical lore is replete with examples of patients who have 'awakening'-like responses to new medications, even from states of extreme clinical deterioration. In longitudinal studies of cognitive function, a relatively direct and objective measure of the integrity of cortical neuronal systems, the weight of the data are against progression, at least during the first 20 or so years of illness (e.g. Heaton *et al.* 2001; reviewed in Rund 1998).

If psychosis is neurotoxic, which has become a popular notion in the literature (Robinson *et al.* 1999a), it might be expected that the longer one goes untreated in a psychotic state, the more obvious would be the signs of such toxicity. Four recent studies examined whether the duration of untreated psychosis had an impact on outcome after treatment, including medication response, cognition, social function, psychopathology and structural measurements on MRI scan (Craig *et al.* 2000; Ho *et al.* 2000; Hoff *et al.* 2000; Verdoux *et al.* 2001). These studies are remarkably consistent in demonstrating no such effect.

The second line of evidence for neurodegeneration is progressive changes of volume measurements in structural MRI studies. The results of these MRI studies do not appear to be plausible indicators of neurodegeneration (see above). Perhaps most clearly against the notion that schizophrenia is associated with degeneration of neural tissue are the results of postmortem studies. The schizophrenic brain typically does not show loss of cortical neurones or gliosis or, for that matter, *any* consistent evidence of degenerating or degenerated neurones (Pakkenberg 1993; Selemon *et al.* 1995; Harrison 1999). It is often stated in the psychiatric literature that these negative findings are consistent with apoptosis (Olney & Farber 1995; Lieberman 1999; Mathalon *et al.* 2001). This assertion is likely to be based on studies of apoptosis in early brain development or in non-central nervous system cancers, some of which are associated with cell death without *inflammation*, and from studies of experimental excitotoxicity that were of only short duration (Fix *et al.* 1993). In pathological brain conditions associated with apoptosis, including ageing, steroid and alchohol toxicity, Alzheimer's disease, Huntington's disease (Zuccato *et al.* 2001) and epilepsy, gliosis is prominent (see Weinberger & McClure 2002 for further discussion). Furthermore, the sine qua non of apoptosis is cell death, and diminished populations of cortical neurones are generally not found in schizophrenic tissue, even in elderly patients who have suffered psychotic symptoms all of their adult lives (Pakkenberg 1993; Selemon *et al.* 1995; Arnold *et al.* 1998; Harrison 1999).

These negative results leave unanswered the question of why some patients appear to deteriorate over time. Many unfortunate human circumstances and behaviours appear to get worse in some individuals during their lifetime (e.g. joblessness and homelessness), without necessarily implicating degeneration of brain tissue. While chronic unemployment may in fact be associated with dynamic changes in synaptic architecture, just as learning new behaviours and habits may involve changes in the connections made between cells, these presumably are *plastic* modifications (i.e. potentially reversible), not toxic degenerations (which usually imply irreversibility). It has become increasingly clear from studies in experimental animals that numerous environmental factors have an impact on neuronal plasticity and can be associated with regression of dendrites and spines. However, these non-degenerative adaptations are potentially reversible – part of how a brain does molecular business with its environment – in contrast to the implications of changes that reflect neurodegeneration.

In summary, while the course of schizophrenia implicates progressive processes in some individuals, the evidence that such processes reflect irreversible degeneration of neuronal elements, analogous to a neurotoxic process, are circumstantial and improbable. In terms of cognitive function and the capacity for clinical recovery, and at the level of cellular and molecular analysis, there is virtually no objective evidence for abnormal neurodegeneration in schizophrenia.

Mechanisms of delayed onset

The possibility that schizophrenia is related to an abnormality of early brain development poses yet another interesting theoretical challenge, for the clinical expression of the illness is delayed typically for about two decades after birth. If a neurological abnormality is present at birth, why is the illness itself not manifested earlier in life and what accounts for its predictable clinical expression in early adulthood? Speculation about the answers to these questions has come primarily from two perspectives:
1 the possibility of an additional pathological process occurring around the time of onset of the clinical illness; and
2 an interaction between a developmental defect and developmental programmes or events that occur in early adult life.

As the foremost proponent of the first perspective, Feinberg (1982) focused on the age of onset of schizophrenia as a clue to neurodevelopmental abnormalities that might explain the illness. He posited that schizophrenia is caused by a defect in adolescent synaptic reorganization, because 'too many, too few, or the wrong synapses are eliminated'. In effect, he argued for a second pathological process, a specific pathology of synaptic elimination not necessarily related to possible maldevelopment *in utero*. His hypothesis does not take into account the neuropathological database (most of which did not exist at the time of his original proposal), and he does not address the biological mechanisms that might be responsible for this putative disorder of synaptic elimination. In light of the extensive database that implicates early developmental abnormalities, this hypothesis requires the occurrence of a second primary pathology. It is also unclear what this pathology would be, in the sense of what would be abnormal about the pruning process. As pruning is presumed to reflect a negative state, i.e. the end result of an absence of sustaining molecular and physiological processes that are required to support a synapse, the pathology would not likely be in the pruning *per se*, but in the mechanisms of synaptic sustenance. Numerous electrophysiological and molecular factors, involving classic neurotransmitters and trophic molecules, participate in the process of synaptic survival and plasticity. Another problem with this hypothesis is that it is unclear how one could directly test it, especially because it accommodates all potential variations (i.e. too much, too little, or the 'wrong' pruning). Nevertheless, the abnormal pruning hypothesis has become very popular over the past decade as an explanation for a variety of clinical phenomena, including cortical thinning on MRI scans (Rapoport *et al.* 1999; Mathalon *et al.* 2001), psychotic psychopathology (McGlashan & Hoffman 2000) and metabolic abnormalities (Keshavan 1999).

Other mechanisms for delayed onset that emphasize a new pathology around the time of clinical onset have been proposed. These include abnormalities of myelination (Benes 1989), of neuronal sprouting (Stevens 1992) and of adverse effects of stress-related neural transmission (Bogerts 1989). Each of these involves a variation on the theme of another abnormality taking place in early adult life. In essence, they are dual pathology hypotheses, either positing that maldevelopment is not sufficient pathology, or is coincidental, or that it is only one of two relatively independent pathologies that characterize the illness.

It is possible that abnormalities of pruning or of other processes related to the formation and maintenance of neuronal connections (e.g. myelination) could be abnormal without implicating a 'second hit' hypothesis. Early maldevelopment may set the stage for secondary synaptic disorganization that has its greatest neurobiological and clinical impact in adolescence. Neuronal circuitry that is anomalous from early in development may have particularly profound implications for eventual connectivity (Schwartz & Goldman-Rakic 1990; Marin-Padilla 1997). It is conceivable therefore that primary developmental defects may lead to the creation of abnormal circuits which compete successfully for survival, while certain normal circuits either do not form or are structurally disadvantaged so that they cannot avoid elimination. This modification of the two-hit hypotheses verges on aspects of the second theoretical perspective on mechanisms of delayed onset.

The second theoretical perspective begins with evidence of abnormal brain development and applies the principle of Occam's razor to accommodate delayed emergence of the syndrome without implicating a second pathology during adolescence. This perspective involves an interaction between cortical maldevelopment *in utero* and normal developmental processes that occur much later (Weinberger 1986, 1987). This view rests on several assumptions: that the clinical implications of a developmental defect vary with the maturational state of the brain; that the neural systems disrupted by the defect in early brain development in schizophrenia are normally late maturing neural systems; and that a defect in the function of these neural systems will not be reliably apparent until their normal time of functional maturation. In other words, it is posited that certain neural systems are primed from early development to have the capacity to malfunction in a manner that accounts for the illness but, until a certain state of postnatal brain development, they either do not malfunction to a clinically significant degree, or their malfunctioning can be compensated for by other systems. The first of these assumptions has been repeatedly validated in developmental neurobiology. Indeed, a fundamental principle of the clinical impact of developmental neuropathology, as exemplified by the landmark work of Kennard (1936), is that in general brain damage is apparent early and tends to become less so over time. The young brain has a greater capacity for functional compensation than does the old brain (Kolb & Whishaw 1989), presumably because immature pathways and connections that are normally transient can be recruited and maintained in order to subserve the functions lost by the damaged circuits (Huttenlocher 1990). It is also a fundamental principle of paediatric neurology that in some cases congenital brain damage can have delayed or varying clinical effects if the neural systems involved are neurologically immature at birth (Adams & Lyons 1982).

In the case of schizophrenia, the 'Kennard principle' appears to be inverted, in that the impact of putative early damage is less apparent early and more apparent late. In this respect, the other two assumptions of this perspective are much more speculative. It is not known whether the principle of clinical effects being delayed until the affected neural systems reach functional maturity applies to those neural systems implicated in schizophrenia. More data are needed about the neural systems that develop abnormally in schizophrenia and about their normal course of functional maturation. However, this has been explored over the past decade in a series of experiments in animal models. Animal models based on a variety of neonatal and prenatal perturbations in cortical connectivity, analogous to what is implicated in schizophrenia, have been created (see Chapter 21; for review see Lipska & Weinberger 2000). These animals, especially those with disconnections involving hippocampal–prefrontal circuits, manifest abnormalities in a number of behaviours and pharmacological responses but not until they reach early adulthood. These results in animals support the biological plausibility of the notion that early developmental changes in cortical circuitry can have a delayed impact on complex behaviours and not become manifest until early adult life.

Data from studies of cortical function in patients with schizophrenia, including neuropsychological testing results (see Chapter 10) and studies of cortical physiology using functional brain imaging techniques (see Chapter 22), indicate that cortical dysfunction is a prominent characteristic of the illness and that prefrontal–temporal functional connectivity is especially affected. Even if cortical maldevelopment is widespread, the functional neural systems that appear to be particularly relevant to the clinical characteristics of schizophrenia are those involved in prefrontal–temporal cortical connectivity (Weinberger *et al.* 1992; Weinberger & Lipska 1995; Friston 1998). If the functional maturation of such connectivity is relatively late, as a number of lines of evidence in human and non-human primates suggest (Bachevalier & Mishkin 1984; Chelune & Baer 1986; Thatcher *et al.* 1987; Buchsbaum *et al.* 1992), then this would fit this delayed-onset model. The molecular events that account for the functional maturation of these systems are complex, and involve stabilization of synapses, growth and modification of dendritic arbors, myelination of intracortical pathways and other processes related to the refinement of cortical connectivity, all of which seem to plateau in early adult life.

Interestingly, while it has been popular in the psychiatric literature to emphasize synaptic pruning as a critical maturational event in adolescent brain development, progressive synaptic events, involved in dendritic and spine elaboration, are probably at least if not even more prominent during adolescence. Synaptic pruning is a relatively circumscribed process in early adulthood in the primate, involving so-called asymmetric synapses, which are presumably excitatory and glutamatergic. GABA-ergic inhibitory connections are not pruned at this time. However, despite evidence for synaptic pruning of certain excitatory inputs in cortical neurones, at least in prefrontal cortex, the overall growth of dendrites and of dendritic spines of pyramidal neurones, which are the postsynaptic targets of excitatory, glutamatergic inputs, actually increase in size and density quite remarkably in early adult life (Lambe *et al.* 2000). This dramatic increase in pyramidal dendritic arborization, combined with continuing myelination of cortical–cortical projections during adolescence, probably accounts for the fact that neuropil actually increases in thickness during this period. It is tempting to conclude from these data that the processes of pruning and of synaptic elaboration, which are clearly occurring in parallel during adolescence, dynamically shape the synaptic landscape into a more mature, efficient and environmentally adapted system. This is consistent with the notion that it is the stabilization of dynamic processes involved in postnatal cortical differentiation that signals the functional maturation of cortex (Rakic *et al.* 1986; Lidow & Rakic 1992). In addition to progressive events at the level of dendritic and spine abundance, cortical inputs from subcortical projection neuronal systems also undergo progressive changes during early adulthood. Recent evidence indicates that in the primate prefrontal cortex, dopamine inputs show a dramatic postnatal developmental elaboration culminating in early adult life (Lambe *et al.* 2000). A similar developmental trajectory is not seen with serotonergic inputs, which appear to reach their adult density level much earlier in development.

In a more psychological vein, prefrontal–temporal connectivity has been viewed as facilitating the use of past experience to guide purposeful behaviour when environmental cues are inadequate or maladaptive (Goldman-Rakic 1987; Weinberger 1993). The stresses of independent adult living might be especially likely to place a premium on this manner of neural function. If the neural systems that permit such highly evolved behaviours are developmentally defective, their malfunction might be occult until either they alone are meant to subserve such functions and other systems can no longer compensate, or until the environmental demands for such behaviour overwhelm their diminished capacity. It is important to note that this view does not predict that illness is inevitable, simply because of the existence of early pathology and of the inevitable maturation of relevant brain systems in early adulthood. Clearly, catalytic events may be critical for many individuals, including environment adversity, stress or substance abuse (Lewis & Gonzalez-Burgos 2000).

These alternative perspectives on mechanisms of delayed onset, although differing on the question of whether neurodevelopmental processes of adolescence are abnormal, share an emphasis on cortical connectivity being abnormal, as do the *in vivo* imaging, neuropsychological and postmortem data (Bunney & Bunney 2000). This raises an additional problem for the explanatory power of neurodevelopmental models of schizophrenia, in that the diagnostic symptoms of the illness, i.e. hallucinations and delusions, have not been classically imputed to cortical dysfunction (Jaskiw & Weinberger 1992). Moreover, it is unclear how this apparent inconsistency could be resolved by the added complexity of the neurodevelopmental frame of reference. Studies of animal models based on developmental cortical injury have helped illustrate at least the biological plausibility of cortical maldevelopment impacting on brain functions thought to be related to psychosis (e.g. dopamine activity). To the extent that hallucinations and delusions respond to antidopaminergic drugs, dysfunction of the dopamine system has been a target outcome measure for the animal studies. In general, this work has demonstrated that such developmental cortical abnormalities impact on the regulation of dopamine activity during adulthood, even in the non-human primate (Bertolino *et al.* 1997; Saunders *et al.* 1998), and that this occurs in a manner analogous to what has been described in patients with schizophrenia.

Further support for the model that developmental pathology can be a primary event underlying secondary emergent psychotic phenomena related to adolescent onset comes from studies of various neurological conditions involving subtle developmental abnormalities of intracortical connections. Psychosis is not uncommon in many such conditions, including developmental epilepsies, mental retardation of various types and cerebral malformations. A hemi-deletion of the long arm of chromosome 22,

the so-called velocardiofacial syndrome (VCFS), has been the subject of much interest in relation to schizophrenia, because a large portion (perhaps as much as 50%) of such cases develop psychiatric disorders, especially psychosis, and because linkage studies of families segregating schizophrenia have identified a potential genetic susceptibility locus in the hemi-deletion region of chromosome 22 (Bassett & Chow 1999). VCFS cases have subtle cerebral malformations and mild mental retardation (Eliez *et al.* 2001). The interesting aspect of this syndrome in terms of the present discussion is that while the changes in the brain are present at birth, and presumably reflect early abnormal brain development, the psychotic symptoms do not emerge until adolescence or early adulthood (Shprintzen *et al.* 1992; Arnold *et al.* 2001). In fact, the same pattern exists for epilepsy and for many other congenital brain disorders associated with psychosis (Weinberger 1987). This suggests, again, that there is an interaction of the developmental changes in the brain with other processes that are critical for the full expression of the behavioural abnormalities and that these processes are expressed or reach a critical stage around early adulthood. The fact that many neurological and developmental syndromes show the same chronological pattern with respect to the onset of psychosis argues that the factors leading to the manifestation of psychosis are generic and not specific to a particular condition. If they are specific to anything, it appears to be to early adult life.

Metachromatic leucodystrophy (MLD), a rare disorder of aryl sulphatase deficiency, is another informative example of this age association and also of the potential importance of functional 'dysconnection' of cortical regions. Hyde *et al.* (1992) have demonstrated that when MLD presents between the ages of 13 and 30, it presents in the majority of cases as a schizophrenia-like illness. Moreover, the clinical presentation is probably more similar to schizophrenia than is seen in any other neurological disease. Patients have disorganized thinking, act bizarrely, have complex delusions and, when hallucinated, invariably have complex Schneiderian-type auditory hallucinations. The condition is often misdiagnosed as schizophrenia, sometimes for years, before neurological symptoms appear. Interestingly, MLD is a pure connectivity disorder in that the neuropathological changes involve white matter. In its early neuropathological stages, when it is most likely to present with psychosis, the changes are especially prominent in subprefrontal white matter. This suggests that a neural dysfunction with a high valence for producing psychotic symptoms is failure of some aspects of prefrontal connectivity, analogous functionally to what has been implicated in schizophrenia.

In the case of MLD, however, this functional 'dysconnection' does not appear to be enough. When MLD presents outside of this critical age range, it almost never presents with psychosis, even though the location of the neuropathology is not age dependent. In other words, the involvement of critical neural systems is not by itself sufficient for the expression of psychosis. An age-related factor that appears to be independent of the illness is also required. Again, because this age association is seen in other diseases and thus transcends specific illness boundaries, it is probably a function of normal postnatal brain maturation.

The MLD example, like the VCFS example, provides another potential insight into how cortical maldevelopment might be a crucial factor in schizophrenia. The distribution of white matter pathology in MLD is not unique to this illness. For example, a similar distribution of changes was produced by prefrontal leucotomies which did not worsen psychosis, and is seen in some other leucoencephalopathies, such as multiple sclerosis (MS). However, MS plaques and leucotomy lesions spare intracortical fibres which are affected in MLD, suggesting that intracortical 'dysconnection' is closer to the source of psychosis. It also suggests, particularly with reference to leucotomy, that 'dysconnection' is more problematic than no connection. The developmental neuropathology described in association with schizophrenia is much more consistent with the possibility of dysconnection than of no connection. Further support for this possibility comes from studies of epilepsy and psychosis in which congenital malformations of the mesial temporal lobe are more likely to be associated with psychosis than are sclerotic lesions (Roberts et al. 1990). The former are also more consistent with the possibility of dysconnection than are the latter. Moreover, temporal lobectomy does not cure psychosis associated with epilepsy, further suggesting that the source of the psychosis is represented as a distributed abnormality.

Candidate maturational processes and clinical onset

Finally, it is of interest to speculate on the critical maturational processes that might interact with the subtle brain developmental abnormalities implicated in schizophrenia. The foregoing discussion militates towards processes involving synaptic plasticity during development and during postnatal life. While schizophrenia may involve genetic variations that impact on the biology of synaptic plasticity (Weinberger 1999), and developmental adversity may disrupt the formation of normal cortical circuitry, the convergence of these risk factors on the processes that hone intracortical connectivity during early adulthood would seem to be the final common pathway for the emergence of the syndrome. We believe that both the genetic risk factors, which may themselves impact on brain development, and environmental adversity during brain development bias the normal molecular processes of postnatal synaptic plasticity towards abnormal connectivity during the early adult years. This biasing effect could operate purely at a cellular and molecular level, i.e. connections that are anomalous do not process signals normally and do not form normal secondary and tertiary connectivities. On the other hand, this biasing effect could also operate at the level of neuronal experience, i.e. anomalous circuits experience (perceive and process) environmental stimuli abnormally, and develop and maintain connections that are normal in terms of their cellular and molecular machinery, but are based on abnormal perception and processing of environmental events. These biasing effects, we surmise, are the proximate causes of the various emergent behavioural and biological phenomena that ultimately result in the diagnosis of schizophrenia (Weinberger et al. 2001).

The recent demonstration of a genetic mechanism of risk for schizophrenia is consistent with and extends much of this speculation. Egan et al. (2001a) recently showed that a functional polymorphism in the gene for COMT slightly increases risk for schizophrenia because the high-risk allele is associated with poorer prefrontal cortical function. This allele appears to lead to more rapid inactivation of prefrontal dopamine and to less efficient prefrontal dopamine signalling and prefrontal cortical function (for detailed discussion see Weinberger et al. 2001). The role of prefrontal function in the expression of the schizophrenic syndrome is presumed to be a biological mechanism through which this genetic effect operates. However, because prefrontal function also impacts adversely on subcortical dopamine regulation, which is implicated in psychosis, the high-risk allele may also act through this process. Consistent with this possibility, Akil et al. (2001) showed that the high-risk COMT allele also is associated with upregulation of tyrosine hydroxylase gene expression in brainstem dopamine neurones in brain tissue of normal subjects. These findings indicate that COMT genotype is one of the inherited factors controlling dopamine neuronal activity and prefrontal cortical function. Thus, an allele of this gene that impacts adversely on both of these processes increases risk for the expression of schizophrenia at the levels of both prefrontal cortical dysfunction and subcortical dopamine dysregulation. The fact that dopaminergic innervation of the prefrontal cortex reaches a peak in early adulthood (Lambe et al. 2000) and that, as shown in the animal models, prefrontal cortical regulation of mesencephalic dopaminergic function also emerges in early adulthood, would suggest that the impact of this genetic factor on these biological mechanisms related to schizophrenia is likely to be clearest on the phenotype of schizophrenia at this time of life. It might also be hypothesized that if the effects of COMT on prefrontal dopamine signalling and subcortical dopamine regulation interact with the cortical elaboration of the dopamine system in early adulthood, then the high-risk COMT allele would predict an earlier age of onset. There is preliminary evidence in support of this prediction (Karayiorgou et al. 1998).

Conclusions

The neurodevelopmental hypothesis of schizophrenia offers a framework for investigation that prompts us to focus on early antecedents and, in particular, on biological events during pregnancy and during early adolescence. It has obvious public health implications in that prevention should start early and include interventions at multiple ages. A vast body of research data supports this contention, but evidence of a 'smoking gun' is lacking and evidence of specificity for schizophrenia is limited.

The extensive data concerning premorbid developmental abnormalities and the remarkable lack of tissue evidence of neuronal loss or of neuronal degeneration allow us to dismiss a purely degenerative hypothesis of schizophrenia. While much evidence points to the last months of gestation as a critical period for vulnerability to potential causes of schizophrenia, there is no clear evidence against a cause operating across infancy and adolescence and possibly through the initial phases of the illness. On the other hand, the evidence in favour of such a postnatal pathological process is meagre. The most parsimonious reduction of the available evidence argues that early developmental abnormalities subtly alter intracortical connectivity which biases postnatal development towards further abnormalities of synaptic maturation and organization in critical cortical circuits and in their subcortical projections, which together increase the risk that schizophrenia will be manifest in early adult life.

While not fully demonstrated, the neurodevelopmental hypothesis remains the most heuristic conceptual framework, with the broadest health policy implications and the most evidence in its favour. Moreover, the neurodevelomental hypothesis provides a theoretical structure that has made it possible to bridge between molecular biology and genetics, systems neuroscience, and clinical psychology. One of the weaknesses of the hypothesis, however, is that it is difficult to disprove. Sparing convincing evidence of a degenerative process or of some other mechanism of pathogenesis that excludes brain development as a factor, the neurodevelopmental hypothesis cannot be easily dismissed. In order to translate the hypothesis into a definitive understanding of schizophrenia pathogenesis, it will be necessary to elaborate the genetic and molecular mechanisms governing brain growth and connectivity and to evaluate the evolution of these processes in individuals who manifest this illness.

References

Adams, R.D. & Lyons, G. (1982) *Neurology of Hereditary Metabolic Diseases of Children*. McGraw-Hill, New York.

Akbarian, S., Vinuela, A., Kim, J.J. *et al*. (1993) Distorted distribution of nicotinamide-adenine dinucleotide phosphate diaphorase neurons in temporal-lobe of schizophrenics implies anomalous cortical development. *Archives of General Psychiatry* 50, 178–187.

Akbarian, S., Kim, J.J., Potkin, S.G. *et al*. (1996) Maldistribution of interstitial neurons in prefrontal white matter of the brains of schizophrenic patients. *Archives of General Psychiatry* 53, 425–436.

Akil, M. & Lewis, D.A. (1997) Cytoarchitecture of the entorhinal cortex in schizophrenia. *American Journal of Psychiatry* 154, 1010–1012.

Akil, M. Rothmond, D.A., Kolachana, B.S. *et al*. (2001) Effect of COMT genotype on tyrosine hydroxylase gene expression in the human mesencephalon. *Society for Neuroscience Abstracts*. http://sfn.scholarone.com/itin2001/

Allen, N.B., Lewinsohn, P.M. & Seeky, J.R. (1998) Prenatal and perinatal influences on risk for psychopathology in childhood and adolescence. *Developmental Psychopathology* 10, 513–529.

Anderson, S.A., Volk, D.W. & Lewis, D.A. (1996) Increased density of microtubule associated protein 2- immunoreactive neurons in the prefrontal white matter of schizophrenic subjects. *Schizophrenia Research* 19, 111–119.

Arnold, P.D., Siegel-Bartelt, J., Cytrynbaum, C., Teshima, I. & Schachar, R. (2001) Velocardiofacial syndrome: implications of microdeletion 22q11 for schizophrenia and mood disorders. *American Journal of Medical Genetics* 105, 354–362.

Arnold, S.E., Trojanowski, J.Q. , Gur, R.E. *et al*. (1998) Absence of neurodegeneration and neural injury in the cerebral cortex in a sample of elderly patients with schizophrenia. *Archives of General Psychiatry* 55, 225–232.

Aylward, E., Walker, E. & Bettes, B. (1984) Intelligence in schizophrenia: meta-analysis of the research. *Schizophrenia Bulletin* 10, 430–459.

Baare, W.F., van Oel, C.J., Hulshoff Pol. H.E. *et al*. (2001) Volumes of brain structures in twins discordant for schizophrenia. *Archives of General Psychiatry* 58, 33–40.

Bachevalier, J. & Mishkin, M. (1984) An early and a late developing system for learning and retention in infant monkeys. *Behavioral Neuroscience* 98, 770–778.

Bain, M., Juszczak, E., McInneny, K. & Kendell, R.E. (2000) Obstetric complications and affective psychoses: two case–control studies based on structured obstetric records. *British Journal of Psychiatry* 176, 523–526.

Barbeau, D., Liang, J.J., Robitaille, Y. Quirion, R. & Srivastava, L.K. (1995) Decreased expression of the embryonic form of the neural cell-adhesion molecule in schizophrenic brains. *Proceedings of the National Academy of Sciences of the USA* 92, 2785–2789.

Bartley, A.J., Jones, D.W., Torrey, E.F. Zigun, J.R. & Weinberger, D.R. (1993) Sylvian fissure asymmetries in monozygotic twins: a test of laterality in schizophrenia. *Biological Psychiatry* 34, 853–863.

Bassett, A.S. & Chow, E.W. (1999) 22q11 Deletion syndrome: a genetic subtype of schizophrenia. *Biological Psychiatry* 46, 882–891.

Bender, L. (1947) Childhood schizophrenia: clinical study of 100 schizophrenic children. *American Journal of Orthopsychiatry* 17, 40–56.

Benes, F.M. (1989) Myelination of cortical–hippocampal relays during late adolescence. *Schizophrenia Bulletin* 15, 585–593.

Bennedsen, B.E., Mortensen, P.B., Olesen, A.V. Henriksen, T.B. & Frydenberg, M. (2001) Obstetric complications in women with schizophrenia. *Schizophrenia Research* 47, 167–175.

Bernstein, H.G., Krell, D., Baumann, B. *et al*. (1998) Morphometric studies of the entorhinal cortex in neuropsychiatric patients and controls: clusters of heterotopically displaced lamina II neurons are not indicative of schizophrenia. *Schizophrenia Research* 33, 125–132.

Bertolino, A., Saunders, R.C., Mattay, V.S. *et al*. (1997) Altered development of prefrontal neurons in rhesus monkeys with neonatal mesial temporo-limbic lesions: a proton magnetic resonance spectroscopic imaging study. *Cerebral Cortex* 7, 740–748.

Bleuler, M. (1941) *Krankheitsverlauf, Persoenlichkeit und Verwandtschaft Schizophrener und Ihre Gegenseitigen Beziehungen*. Georg Thieme, Leipzig.

Bloom, F.E. (1993) Advancing a neurodevelopmental origin for schizophrenia. *Archives of General Psychiatry* 50, 224–227.

Bogerts, B. (1989) The role of limbic and paralimbic pathology in the etiology of schizophrenia. *Psychiatry Research* 29, 255–256.

Bolton, P.F., Murphy, M., Macdonald, H. *et al*. (1997) Obstetric complications in autism: consequences or causes of the condition? *Journal of the American Academy of Child and Adolescent Psychiatry* 36, 272–281.

Bradbury, T.N. & Miller, G.A. (1985) Season of birth in schizophrenia: a review of evidence, methodology, and etiology. *Psychological Bulletin* 98, 569–594.

Brown, A.S., Schaefer, C.A., Wyatt, R.J. *et al*. (2000) Maternal exposure to respiratory infections and adult schizophrenia spectrum disorders: a prospective birth cohort study. *Schizophrenia Bulletin* 26, 287–295.

Brown, A.S., Cohen, P., Harkavy-Friedman, J., *et al.* (2001) Prenatal rubella, premorbid abnormalities, and adult schizophrenia. *Biological Psychiatry* 49, 473–486.

Buchsbaum, M.S., Mansour, C.S. Teng, D.G. *et al.* (1992) Adolescent developmental change in topography of EEG amplitude. *Schizophrenia Research* 7, 101–107.

Buka, S.L., Tsuang, M.T. & Lipsitt, L.P. (1993) Pregnancy/delivery complications and psychiatric diagnosis: a prospective study. *Archives of General Psychiatry* 50, 151–156.

Bullmore, E., Brammer, M., Harvey, I. Murray, R. & Ron, M. (1995) Cerebral hemispheric asym-metry revisited: effects of handedness, gender and schizophrenia measured by radius of gyration in magnetic resonance images. *Psychological Medicine* 25, 349–363.

Bullmore, E.T., Woodruff, P.W.R., Wright, I.C. *et al.* (1998) Does dysplasia cause anatomical dysconnectivity in schizophrenia?. *Schizophrenia Research* 30, 127–135.

Bunney, W.E. & Bunney, B.G. (2000) Evidence for a compromised dorsolateral prefrontal cortical parallel circuit in schizophrenia. *Brain Research Brain Research Review* 31, 138–146.

Byrne, M., Browne, R., Mulryan, N. *et al.* (2000) Labour and delivery complications and schizophrenia: case–control study using contemporaneous labour ward records. *British Journal of Psychiatry* 176, 531–536.

Cannon, M., Cotter, D., Coffey, V.P. *et al.* (1996) Prenatal exposure to the 1957 influenza epidemic and adult schizophrenia: a follow-up study. *British Journal of Psychiatry* 168, 368–371.

Cannon, T.D., Mednick, S.A. & Parnas, J. (1990) Antecedents of predomi-nantly negative-symptom and predominantly positive-symptom schizophrenia in a high-risk population. *Archives of General Psychiatry* 47, 622–632.

Cannon, T.D., Mednick, S.A., Parnas, J. *et al.* (1993) Developmental brain abnormalities in the offspring of schizophrenic mothers. I. Contributions of genetic and perinatal factors. *Archives of General Psychiatry* 50, 551–564.

Cannon, T.D., van Erp, T.G.M., Huttumen, M. *et al.* (1998) Regional gray matter, white matter, and cerebrospinal fluid distributions in schizophrenic patients, their siblings, and controls. *Archives of General Psychiatry* 55, 1084–1091.

Cannon, T.D., Rosso, I.M., Hollister, J.M. *et al.* (2000) A prospective cohort study of genetic and perinatal influences in the etiology of schizophrenia. *Schizophrenia Bulletin* 26, 351–366.

Cantor-Graae, E., McNeil, T.F., Sjostrman, K. Nordstrom, L.G. & Rosenlund, T. (1994) Obstetric complications and their relationship to other etiological risk factors in schizophrenia: case–control study. *Journal of Nervous and Mental Disease* 182, 645–650.

Casanova, M.F., Goldberg, T.E. Suddath, R.L. *et al.* (1990) Quantitative shape analysis of the temporal and prefrontal lobes of schizophrenic patients: a magnetic resonance image study. *Journal of Neuropsychiatry and Clinical Neuroscience* 2, 363–372.

Chelune, G.J. & Baer, R.A. (1986) Developmental norms for the Wisconsin Card Sorting test. *Journal of Clinical and Experimental Neuropsychology* 8, 219–228.

Chi, J.G., Dooling, E.C. & Gilles, F.H. (1977) Left-right asymmetries of the temporal speech areas of the human fetus. *Archives of Neurology* 34, 346–348.

Cotter, D., Takei, N., Farrell, M. *et al.* (1995) Does prenatal exposure to influenza in mice induce pyramidal cell disarray in the dorsal hippocampus. *Schizophrenia Research* 16, 233–241.

Cotter, D., Larkin, C., Waddington, J.L. & O'Callaghan, E. (1996) Season of birth in schizophrenia: clue or cul-de-sac? *The Neurodevelopmental Basis of Schizophrenia* (eds J.L. Waddington & P.F. Buckley), pp. 17–30. R.G. Landes, Georgetown, TX.

Craig, T.J., Bromet, E.J., Fennig, S. *et al.* (2000) Is there an association between duration of untreated psychosis and 24-month clinical outcome in a first-admission series?. *American Journal of Psychiatry* 157, 60–66.

Crow, T.J., Ball, J., Bloom, S. R. *et al.* (1989a) Schizophrenia as an anomaly of development of cerebral asymmetry: a postmortem study and a proposal concerning the genetic basis of the disease. *Archives of General Psychiatry* 46, 1145–1150.

Crow, T.J., Colter, N., Frith, C.D., Johnstone, E.C. & Owens, D.G. (1989b) Developmental arrest of cerebral asymmetries in early onset schizophrenia. *Psychiatry Research* 29, 247–253.

Crow, T.J., Done, D.J. & Johnstone, E.C. (1992) Schizophrenia is not due to maternal influenza in the second (or other) trimester of pregnancy. *Schizophrenia Research* 6, 99–99.

Crow, T.J., Done, D.J. & Sacker, A. (1996) Cerebral lateralization is delayed in children who later develop schizophrenia. *Schizophrenia Research* 22, 181–185.

Csernansky, J.G., Joshi, S., Wang, L. *et al.* (1998) Hippocampal morphometry in schizophrenia by high dimensional brain mapping. *Proceedings of the National Academy of Sciences of the USA* 95, 11406–11411.

Dalman, C., Allebeck, P., Cullberg, J. Grunnewald, C. & Koster, M. (1999) Obstetric complications and the risk of schizophrenia: a longitudinal study of a national birth cohort. *Archives of General Psychiatry* 56, 234–240.

Davis, J.O. & Bracha, H.S. (1996) Prenatal growth markers in schizophrenia: a monozygotic co-twin control study. *American Journal of Psychiatry* 153, 1166–1172.

Davis, K.L., Buchsbaum, M.S., Shihebuddin, L. *et al.* (1998) Ventricular enlargement in poor-outcome schizophrenia. *Biological Psychiatry* 43, 783–793.

DeCarli, C., Kay, J.A., Horowitz, B. & Rapoport, S.I. (1990) Critical analysis of the use of computerized assisted axial tomography to study human brain in aging and dementia of the Alzheimer type. *Neurology* 40, 872–883.

DeLisi, L. (1997) Is schizophrenia a lifetime disorder of brain plasticity, growth, and aging? *Schizophrenia Research* 23, 119–129.

DeLisi, L.E., Stritzke, P.H., Holan, V. *et al.* (1991) Brain morphological-changes in first episode cases of schizophrenia: are they progressive. *Schizophrenia Research* 5, 206–208.

DeLisi, L., Hoff, A.L., Kushner, M., Calev, A. & Stritzke, P. (1992) Left ventricular enlargement associated with diagnostic outcome of schizophreniform disorder. *Biological Psychiatry* 32, 199–201.

DeLisi, L.E., Tew, W., Xie, S.H. *et al.* (1995) A prospective follow-up-study of brain morphology and cognition in first-episode schizophrenic-patients: preliminary findings. *Biological Psychiatry* 38, 349–360.

DeLisi, L.E., Sakuma, M., Tew, W. *et al.* (1997) Schizophrenia as a chronic active brain process: a study of progressive brain structural change subsequent to the onset of schizophrenia. *Psychiatry Research:Neuroimaging* 74, 129–140.

DeLisi, L.E., Sakuma, M., Ge, S. & Kushner, M. (1998) Association of brain structural change with the heterogeneous course of schizophrenia from early childhood through 5 years subsequent to a first hospitalization. *Psychiatry Research: Neuroimaging* 84, 75–88.

Done, D.J., Johnstone, E.C., Frith, C.D. *et al.* (1991) Complications of pregnancy and delivery in relation to psychosis in adult life: data from the British Perinatal-Mortality Survey sample. *British Medical Journal* 302, 1576–1580.

Eagles, J.M., Hunter, D. & Geddes, J.R. (1995) Gender-specific changes since 1900 in the season-of-birth effect in schizophrenia. *British Journal of Psychiatry* 167, 469–472.

Egan, M.F., Goldberg, T.E., Kolachana, B.S. *et al.* (2001a) Effect of

COMT Val108/158 Met genotype on frontal lobe function and risk for schizophrenia. *Proceedings of the National Academy of Sciences of the USA* **98**, 6917–6922.

Egan, M.F., Goldberg, T.E., Gscheidle, T. *et al.* (2001b) Relative risk for cognitive impairments in siblings of patients with schizophrenia. *Biological Psychiatry* **50**, 98–107.

Eliez, S., Antonarakis, S.E. *et al.* (2001) Parental origin of the deletion 22q11.2 and brain development in velocardiofacial syndrome: a preliminary study. *Archives of General Psychiatry* **58**, 64–68.

Elvevåg, B. & Weinberger, D.R. (1997) Commentary: schizophrenia and autism considered as the products of an agnosic right shift gene. *Cognitive Neuropsychiatry* **2**, 221–225.

Eschenbach, D.A. (1997) Amniotic fluid infection and cerebral palsy: focus on the fetus. *Journal of the American Medical Association* **278**, 247–248.

Fearon, P., Lane, A., Airie, M. *et al.* (2001) Is reduced dermatoglyphic a-b ridge count a reliable marker of developmental impairment in schizophrenia?. *Schizophrenia Research* **50**, 151–157.

Feinberg, I. (1982) Schizophrenia: caused by a fault in programmed synaptic elimination during adolescence? *Journal of Psychiatric Research* **17**, 319–334.

Fish, B. & Hagin, R. (1972) Visual-motor disorders in infants at risk for schizophrenia. *Archives of General Psychiatry* **27**, 594–598.

Fix, A., Horn, J.W., Wightman, K.A. *et al.* (1993) Neuronal vacuolization and necrosis induced by the non-competitive N-methyl-D-aspartate (NMDA) antagonist MK(+) 801 (dizocilpine maleate): a light and electron microscopic evaluation of the rat retrosplenial cortex. *Experimental Neurology* **123**, 204–215.

Frank, D.A., Augustyn, M., Knight, W.G., Pell, T. & Zuckerman, B. (2001) Growth, development, and behavior in early childhood following prenatal cocaine exposure: a systematic review. *Journal of the American Medical Association* **285**, 1613–1625.

Friston, K.J. (1998) The disconnection hypothesis. *Schizophrenia Research* **30**, 115–125.

Friston, K.J. & Frith, C.D. (1995) Schizophrenia: a disconnection syndrome? *Clinical Neuroscience* **3**, 89–97.

Garver, D., Nair, T.R., Chrisensen, J.D., Holcomb, J.A. & Kingsbury, S.L. (2000) Brain and ventricular instability during psychotic episodes of the schizophrenias. *Schizophrenia Research* **44**, 11–23.

Geddes, J.R., Verdoux, H., Takei, N. *et al.* (1999) Schizophrenia and complications of pregnancy and labor: an individual patient data meta-analysis. *Schizophrenia Bulletin* **25**, 413–423.

Goldman-Rakic, P.S. (1987) Development of cortical circuitry and cognitive function. *Child and Development* **58**, 601–622.

Green, M.F., Satz, P. & Christenson, C. (1994) Minor physical anomalies in schizophrenia patients, bipolar patients, and their siblings. *Schizophrenia Bulletin* **20**, 433–440.

Gunthergenta, F., Bovet, P. & Hohlfeld, P. (1994) Obstetric complications and schizophrenia: a case–control study. *British Journal of Psychiatry* **164**, 165–170.

Gur, R.E. & Chin, S. (1999) Laterality in functional brain imaging studies of schizophrenia. *Schizophrenia Bulletin* **25**, 141–156.

Gur, R.E., Cowell, P., Turetsky, B.I. *et al.* (1998) A follow-up magnetic resonance imaging study of schizophrenia: relationship of neuroanatomical changes to clinical and neurobehavioral measures. *Archives of General Psychiatry* **55**, 145–152.

Guth, C., Jones, P. & Murray, R. (1993) Familial psychiatric illness and obstetric complications in early-onset affective-disorder: a case–control study. *British Journal of Psychiatry* **163**, 492–498.

Hafner, H., Haas, S., Pfeifer-Kurda M, Eichhorn, S. & Michitsuji, S. (1987) Abnormal seasonality of schizophrenic births: a specific find-ing? *European Archives of Psychiatry Neurological Science* **236**, 333–342.

Harding, C.M., Zubin, J. & Strauss, J.S. (1992) Chronicity in schizophrenia: revisited. *British Journal of Psychiatry* **161**, 27–37.

Harrison, P. (1999) The neuropathology of schizophrenia: a critical review of the data and their interpretation. *Brain* **122**, 593–624.

Heaton, R.K., Gladsjo, J.A., Palmer, B.W. *et al.* (2001) Stability and course of neuropsychological deficits in schizophrenia. *Archives of General Psychiatry* **58**, 24–32.

Heinsen, H., Gossmann, E., Rub, U. *et al.* (1996) Variability in the human entorhinal region may confound neuropsychiatric diagnoses. *Acta Anatomica* **157**, 226–237.

Ho, B.C., Andreasen, N.C., Flaum, M., Nopoulos P. & Miller, D. (2000) Untreated initial psychosis: its relation to quality of life and symptom remission in first-episode schizophrenia. *American Journal of Psychiatry* **157**, 808–815.

Hoff, A.L., Sakuma, M., Razi, K. *et al.* (2000) Lack of association between duration of untreated illness and severity of cognitive and structural brain deficits at the first episode of schizophrenia. *American Journal of Psychiatry* **157**, 1824–1828.

Hollister, J.M., Laing, P. & Mednick, S.A. (1996) Rhesus incompatibility as a risk factor for schizophrenia in male adults. *Archives of General Psychiatry* **53**, 19–24.

Honer, W.G., Bassett, A.S., Squires-Wheeler, E. *et al.* (1995) The temporal lobes, reversed asymmetry and the genetics of schizophrenia. *Neuroreport* **7**, 221–224.

Hultman, C.M., Ohman, A., Cnattingius, S. Wieselgren, I.M. & Lindstrom, L.H. (1997) Prenatal and neonatal risk factors for schizophrenia. *British Journal of Psychiatry* **170**, 128–133.

Hultman, C.M., Sparen, P., Takei, N., Murray, R.M. & Cnattingius, S. (1999) Prenatal and perinatal risk factors for schizophrenia, affective psychosis, and reactive psychosis of early onset: case–control study. *British Medical Journal* **318**, 421–426.

Huttenlocher, P.R. (1990) Morphometric study of human cerebral cortex development. *Neuropsychologia* **28**, 517–527.

Hyde, T.M., Ziegler, J.C. & Weinberger, D.P. (1992) Psychiatric disturbances in metachromatic leukodystrophy: insights into the neurobiology of psychosis [see comments]. *Archives of Neurology* **49**, 401–406.

Hyde, T.M., Bachus, S.E., Levitt, P. *et al.* (1997) Reduction in hippocampal limbic system associated protein (LAMP) mRNA in schizophrenia. *Society for Neuroscience Abstracts*, 2200.

Illowsky, B.P., Juliano, D.M., Bigelow, L.B. & Weinberger, D.R. (1988) Stability of CT scan findings in schizophrenia: results of an 8 year follow-up study. *Journal of Neurology, Neurosurgery and Psychiatry* **51**, 209–213.

Impagnatiello, F., Guidotti, A.R., Pesold, C. *et al.* (1998) A decrease of reelin expression as a putative vulnerability factor in schizophrenia. *Proceedings of the National Academy of Sciences of the USA* **95**, 15718–15723.

Jacobsen, L., Giedd, J.N., Castellanos, F.X. *et al.* (1998) Progressive reduction of temporal lobe structures in childhood-onset schizophrenia. *American Journal of Psychiatry* **155**, 678–685.

Jakob, H. & Beckmann, H. (1986) Prenatal developmental disturbances in the limbic allocortex in schizophrenics. *Journal of Neural Transmission* **65**, 303–326.

Jaskiw, G.E. & Weinberger, D.R. (1992) Ibotenic acid lesions of medial prefrontal cortex augment swim-stress-induced locomotion. *Pharmacological Biochemistry and Behavior* **41**, 607–609.

Jaskiw, G.E., Juliano, D.M., Goldberg, T.E. *et al.* (1994) Cerebral ventricular enlargement in schizophreniform disorder does not progress: a 7 year follow-up study. *Schizophrenia Research* **14**, 23–28.

Johnstone, E.C., Crow, T.J., Frith, C.D., Husband, J. & Kreel L. (1976)

Cerebral ventricular size and cognitive impairment in chronic schizophrenia. *Lancet* **2**, 924–926.

Jones, P.B., Rantakallio, P., Hartikainen, A.L., Isohanni, M. & Sipila, P. (1998) Schizophrenia as a long-term outcome of pregnancy, delivery, and perinatal complications: a 28-year follow-up of the 1966 North Finland general population birth cohort. *American Journal of Psychiatry* **155**, 355–364.

Karayiorgou, M., Gogos, J.A., Galke, B.L. *et al.* (1998) Identification of sequence variants and analysis of the role of the catechol-O-methyltransferase gene in schizophrenia susceptibility. *Biological Psychiatry* **43**, 425–431.

Kendell, R.E. & Adams, W. (1991) Unexplained fluctuations in the risk for schizophrenia by month and year of birth. *British Journal of Psychiatry* **158**, 758–763.

Kendell, R.E. & Kemp, I.W. (1987) Winter-born vs. summer-born schizophrenics. *British Journal of Psychiatry* **151**, 499–505.

Kendell, R.E. & Kemp, I.W. (1989) Maternal influenza in the etiology of schizophrenia. *Archives of General Psychiatry* **46**, 878–882.

Kendell, R.E., Juszczak, E. & Cole, S.K. (1996) Obstetric complications and schizophrenia: a case–control study based on standardised obstetric records. *British Journal of Psychiatry* **168**, 556–561.

Kendell, R.E., McInneny, K., Juszczak, E. & Bain, M. (2000) Obstetric complications and schizophrenia: two case–control studies based on structured obstetric records. *British Journal of Psychiatry* **176**, 516–522.

Kennard, M.A. (1936) Age and other factors in motor recovery from precentral lesions in monkeys. *American Journal of Physiology* **115**, 138–146.

Keshavan, M.S. (1999) Development, disease and degeneration in schizophrenia: a unitary pathophysiological model. *Journal of Psychiatric Research* **33**, 513–521.

Keshavan, M.S. & Hogarty, G.E. (1999) Brain maturational processes and delayed onset in schizophrenia. *Developmental Psychopathology* **11**, 525–543.

Kikinis, R., Shenton, M.E., Gerig, G. *et al.* (1994) Temporal-lobe sulco-gyral pattern anomalies in schizophrenia: an *in vivo* MR 3-dimensional surface rendering study. *Neuroscience Letters* **182**, 7–12.

Kinney, D.K., Yurgelun-Todd, D.A., Tohen, M. & Tramer, S. (1998) Pre- and perinatal complications and risk for bipolar disorder: a retrospective study. *Journal of Affective Disorders* **50**, 117–124.

Kolb, B. & Whishaw, I.Q. (1989) Plasticity in the neocortex: mechanisms underlying recovery from early brain damage. *Progress in Neurobiology* **32**, 235–276.

Kraepelin, E. (1919) *Dementia Praecox and Paraphrenia*. Livingstone, Edinburgh.

Krimer, L.S., Hyde, T.M., Herman, M.M. & Saunders, R.C. (1997) The entorhinal cortex: an examination of cyto- and myeloarchitectonic organization in humans. *Cerebral Cortex* **7**, 722–731.

Kulynych, J.J., Foundas, A.L. & Weinberger, D.R. (1995a) Abnormal cortical gyrification in schizophrenia. *Schizophrenia Research* **15**, 89–89.

Kulynych, J.J., Vladar, K., Fantie, B.D., Jones, D.W. & Weinberger, D.R. (1995b) Normal asymmetry of the planum temporale in patients with schizophrenia: 3-dimensional cortical morphometry with MRI. *British Journal of Psychiatry* **166**, 742–749.

Kulynych, J.J., Luevano, L.F., Jones, D.W. & Weinberger, D.R. (1997) Cortical abnormality in schizophrenia: an *in vivo* application of the gyrification index. *Biological Psychiatry* **41**, 995–999.

Kunugi, H., Nanko, S., Takei, N. *et al.* (1995) Schizophrenia following *in utero* exposure to the 1957 influenza epidemics in Japan. *American Journal of Psychiatry* **152**, 450–452.

Kunugi, H., Takei, N., Murray, R.M., Saito, K. & Nanko, S. (1996) Small head circumference at birth in schizophrenia. *Schizophrenia Research* **20**, 165–170.

Kunugi, H., Nanko, S., Hayashi, N. *et al.* (1997) Season of birth of schizophrenics in a recent Japanese sample. *Psychiatry Clinical Neuroscience* **51**, 213–216.

Kwon, J.S., McCarley, R.W., Hirayasu, Y. *et al.* (1999) Left planum temporale volume reduction in schizophrenia. *Archives of General Psychiatry* **56**, 142–148.

Laakso, M.P., Lehtovirta, M. Partanen, K. Riekkinen, P.J. & Soininen, H. (2000) Hippocampus in Alzheimer's disease: a 3-year follow-up MRI study. *Biological Psychiatry* **47**, 557–561.

Laakso, M.P., Tiihonen, J. Syvalahti, E. *et al.* (2001) A morphometric MRI study of the hippocampus in first-episode, neuroleptic-naive schizophrenia. *Schizophrenia Research* **50**, 3–7.

Lambe, E.K., Krimer, L.S. & Goldman-Rakic, P.S. (2000) Differential postnatal development of catecholamine and serotonin inputs to identified neurons in prefrontal cortex of rhesus monkey. *Journal of Neuroscience* **20**, 8780–8787.

Lane, A., Larkin, C., Waddington, J.L. & O'Callaghan, E. (1996) Dysmorphic features and schizophrenia. In: *The Neurodevelopmental Basis of Schizophrenia* (eds J.L. Waddington & P.F. Buckley), pp. 79–94. R.G. Landes, Georgetown, TX.

Lane, A., Kinsella, A., Murphy, P. *et al.* (1997) The anthropometric assessment of dysmorphic features in schizophrenia as an index of its developmental origins. *Psychological Medicine* **27**, 1155–1164.

Lane, E.A. & Albee, G.W. (1970) The birth weight of children born to schizophrenic women. *Journal of Psychology* **74**, 157–160.

Lewis, D.A. & Gonzalez-Burgos, G. (2000) Intrinsic excitatory connections in the prefrontal cortex and the pathophysiology of schizophrenia. *Brain Research Bulletin* **52**, 309–317.

Lewis, D.A. & Lieberman, J.A. (2000) Catching up on schizophrenia: natural history and neurobiology. *Neuron* **28**, 325–334.

Lewis, S.W. & Murray, R.M. (1987) Obstetric complications, neurodevelopmental deviance, and risk of schizophrenia. *Journal of Psychiatric Research* **21**, 413–421.

Lewis, S.W., Owen, M.J. & Murray, R.M. (1989) Obstetric complications and schizophrenia: methodology and mechanisms. *Schizophrenia: Scientific Progress* (eds S.C. Schultz & C.A. Tamminga), pp. 56–68. Oxford University Press, New York.

Lidow, M.S. & Rakic, P. (1992) Scheduling of monoaminergic neurotransmitter receptor expression in the primate neocortex during postnatal development. *Cerebral Cortex* **2**, 401–416.

Lieberman, J. (1999) Is schizophrenia a neurodegenerative disorder? A clinical and neurobiological perspective. *Biological Psychiatry* **46**, 729–739.

Lieberman, J., Chakos M.A., Wu, H. *et al.* (2001) Longitudinal study of brain morphology in first episode schizophrenia. *Biological Psychiatry* **49**, 487–499.

Lieberman, J.A., Jody, D., Alvir, J.M.J. *et al.* (1993) Brain morphology, dopamine, and eye-tracking abnormalities in first-episode schizophrenia: prevalence and clinical correlates. *Archives of General Psychiatry* **50**, 357–368.

Lieberman, J.A., Koreen, A.R., Chakos, M. *et al.* (1996) Factors influencing treatment response and outcome of first-episode schizophrenia: implications for understanding the pathophysiology of schizophrenia. *Journal of Clinical Psychiatry* **57** (Suppl. 9), 5–9.

Lipska, B.K. & Weinberger, D.R. (2000) To model a psychiatric disorder in animals: schizophrenia as a reality test. *Neuropsychopharmacology* **23**, 223–239.

Luchins, D.J., Weinberger, D.R. & Wyatt, R.J. (1979) Schizophrenia: evidence of a subgroup with reversed cerebral asymmetry. *Archives of General Psychiatry* **36**, 1309–1311.

McGlashan, T.H. & Hoffman, R.E. (2000) Schizophrenia as a disorder of developmentally reduced synaptic connectivity. *Archives of General Psychiatry* 57, 637–648.

McGrath, J.J., Pemberton, M.R., Welham, J.L. & Murray, R.M. (1994) Schizophrenia and the influenza epidemics of 1954, 1957 and 1959: a southern-hemisphere study. *Schizophrenia Research* 14, 1–8.

McNeil, T.F., Cantorgraae, E. & Cardenal, S. (1993) Prenatal cerebral development in individuals at genetic risk for psychosis: head size at birth in offspring of women with schizophrenia. *Schizophrenia Research* 10, 1–5.

McNeil, T.F., Cantor-Graae, E., Nordstrom, L.G. & Rosenlund, T. (1997) Does choice of scale for scoring obstetric complications influence their relationship to other etiological risk factors in schizophrenia? *Journal of Nervous and Mental Disease* 185, 27–31.

McNeil, T.F., Cantor-Graae, E. & Weinberger, D.R. (2000) Relationship of obstetric complications and differences in size of brain structures in monozygotic twin pairs discordant for schizophrenia. *American Journal of Psychiatry* 157, 203–212.

Machon, R.A., Mednick, S.A. & Huttunen, M.O. (1997) Adult major affective disorder after prenatal exposure to an influenza epidemic. *Archives of General Psychiatry* 54, 322–328.

Marcelis, M., van Os, J., Sham, P. *et al.* (1998) Obstetric complications and familial morbid risk of psychiatric disorders. *American Journal of Medical Genetics* 81, 29–36.

Marcelis, M., Takei, N. & van OS, J. (1999) Urbanization and risk for schizophrenia: does the effect operate before or at the time of illness onset?. *Psychological Medicine* 29, 1197–1203.

Marenco, S. & Weinberger, D.R. (2000) The neurodevelopmental hypothesis of schizophrenia: following a trail of evidence from cradle to grave. *Developmental Psychopathology* 12, 501–527.

Marenco, S. & Weinberger, D.R. (2003) Following Ariadne's double stranded thread through early development: will we ever get out of the labirynth? In: *Early Clinical Intervention and Prevention in Schizophrenia* (eds W.S. Stone, S.V. Faraone & M.T. Tsuang). Humana Press, Totowa, NJ, in press.

Marin-Padilla, M. (1997) Developmental neuropathology and impact of perinatal brain damage. II. White matter lesions of the neocortex. *Journal of Neuropathology and Experimental Neurology* 56, 219–235.

Mathalon, D.H., Sullivan, E.V., Lim, K.O. & Pfefferbaum, A. (2001) Progressive brain volume changes and the clinical course of schizophrenia in men: a longitudinal magnetic resonance imaging study. *Archives of General Psychiatry* 58, 148–157.

Matsumoto, H., Simmons, A., Williams, S. *et al.* (2001) Structural magnetic imaging of the hippocampus in early onset schizophrenia. *Biological Psychiatry* 49, 824–831.

Mednick, S.A. (1991) Fetal neural development and adult schizophrenia. *Fetal Neural Development and Adult Schizophrenia* (eds S.A. Mednick, T.D. Cannon, C.E. Barr & M. Lyon) Cambridge University Press, Cambridge.

Mednick, S.A., Machon, R.A. *et al.* (1988) Adult schizophrenia following prenatal exposure to an influenza epidemic. *Archives of General Psychiatry* 45, 189–192.

Mednick, S.A., Machon, R.A. Huttunen, M.O. & Barr, C.E. (1990) Influenza and schizophrenia: Helsinki vs. Edinburgh. *Archives of General Psychiatry* 47, 875–876.

Mednick, S.A., Huttunen, M.O. & Machon, R.A. (1994) Prenatal influenza infections and adult schizophrenia. *Schizophrenia Bulletin* 20, 263–267.

Miller, R. (1989) Schizophrenia as a progressive disorder: relations to EEG, CT, neuropathological and other evidence. *Progress in Neurobiology* 33, 17–44.

Morgan, V., Castle, D., Page, A. *et al.* (1997) Influenza epidemics and incidence of schizophrenia, affective disorders and mental retardation

in Western Australia: no evidence of a major effect. *Schizophrenia Research* 26, 25–39.

Mortensen, P.B., Pedersen, C.B., Westergaard, T. *et al.* (1999) Effects of family history and place and season of birth on the risk of schizophrenia. *New England Journal of Medicine* 340, 603–608.

Murray, R.M. & Lewis (1987) Is schizophrenia a neurodevelopmental disorder? *British Medical Journal* 295, 681–682.

Nair, T.R., Christensen, J.D., Kingsbury, S.J. *et al.* (1997) Progression of cerebroventricular enlargement and the subtyping of schizophrenia. *Psychiatry Research* 74, 141–150.

Narr, K., Thompson, P., Sharma, T. *et al.* (2001a) Three-dimensional mapping of gyral shape and cortical surface asymmetries in schizophrenia: gender effects. *American Journal of Psychiatry* 158, 244–255.

Narr, K.L., Thompson, P.M., Sharma, T. *et al.* (2001b) Three-dimensional mapping of temporo-limbic regions and the lateral ventricles in schizophrenia: gender effects. *Biological Psychiatry* 50, 84–97.

Nelson, K.B. & Ellenberg, J.H. (1984) Obstetric complications as risk factors for cerebral palsy or seizure disorders. *Journal of the American Medical Association* 251, 1843–1848.

Noga, J.T., Bartley, A.J., Jones, D.W., Torrey, E.F. & Weinberger, D.R. (1996) Cortical gyral anatomy and gross brain dimensions in monozygotic twins discordant for schizophrenia. *Schizophrenia Research* 22, 27–40.

O'Callaghan, E., Sham, P., Takei, N., Glover, G.R., Murray, R.M. (1991) Schizophrenia after prenatal exposure to 1957, A2 influenza epidemic. *Lancet* 337, 1248–1250.

O'Callaghan, E., Gibson, T., Colohan, H.A. *et al.* (1992) Risk of schizophrenia in adults born after obstetric complications and their association with early onset of illness: a controlled study. *British Medical Journal* 305, 1256–1259.

O'Dwyer, J.M. (1997) Schizophrenia in people with intellectual disability: the role of pregnancy and birth complications. *Journal of Intellectual Disability Research* 41, 238–251.

Olney, J.W. & Farber, N.B. (1995) Glutamate receptor dysfunction and schizophrenia. *Archives of General Psychiatry* 52, 998–1007.

Orr, K.G., Cannon, M., Giluarry, C.M., Jones, P.B. & Murray, R.M. (1999) Schizophrenic patients and their first-degree relatives show an excess of mixed-handedness. *Schizophrenia Research* 39, 167–176.

Pakkenberg, B. (1993) Total nerve cell number in neocortex in chronic schizophrenics and controls estimated using optical dissectors. *Biological Psychiatry* 34, 768–772.

Parnas, J., Schulsinger, F., Teasdak, T.W. *et al.* (1982) Perinatal complications and clinical outcome within the schizophrenia spectrum. *British Journal of Psychiatry* 140, 416–420.

Perrone-Bizzozero, N.I., Sower, A.C., Bird, E.D. *et al.* (1996) Levels of the growth-associated protein GAP-43 are selectively increased in association cortices in schizophrenia. *Proceedings of the National Academy of Sciences of the USA* 93, 14182–14187.

Rakic, P., Bourgeois, J.P., Eckenhoff, M.F., Zecevic, N. & Goldman-Rakic, P.E. (1986) Concurrent overproduction of synapses in diverse regions of the primate cerebral cortex. *Science* 232, 232–235.

Rao, J.M. (1990) A population-based study of mild mental handicap in children: preliminary analysis of obstetric associations. *Journal of Mental Deficiency Research* 34, 59–65.

Rapoport, J., Giedd, J., Kumra, S. *et al.* (1997) Childhood-onset: progressive ventricular change during adoloescence. *Archives of General Psychiatry* 54, 897–903.

Rapoport, J.L., Giedd, J.N., & Murray, R.M. *et al.* (1999) Progressive cortical change during adolescence in childhood-onset schizophrenia: a longitudinal magnetic resonance imaging study. *Archives of General Psychiatry* 56, 649–654.

Raz, S. & Raz, N. (1990) Structural brain abnormalities in the major psychoses: a quantitative review of the evidence from computerized imaging. *Psychological Bulletin* **108**, 93–108.

Reveley, A.M., Reveley, M.A. & Murrary, R.M. (1984) Cerebral ventricular enlargement in non-genetic schizophrenia: a controlled twin study. *British Journal of Psychiatry* **144**, 89–93.

Risch, N. (1990) Genetic linkage and complex diseases, with special reference to psychiatric disorders. *Genetics Epidemiology* **7**, 3–16; discussion 17–45.

Roberts, G.W. (1991) Schizophrenia: a neuropathological perspective. *British Journal of Psychiatry* **158**, 8–17.

Roberts, G.W., Done, D.J., Bruton, C. & Crow, T.J. (1990) A 'mock up' of schizophrenia: temporal lobe epilepsy and schizophrenia-like psychosis. *Biological Psychiatry* **28**, 127–143.

Robinson, D., Woerner, M.G., Alvir, J.M.J. *et al.* (1999a) Predictors of relapse following response from a first episode of schizophrenia or schizoaffective disorder. *Archives of General Psychiatry* **56**, 241–247.

Robinson, D.G., Woerner, M.G., Alvir, J.M.J. *et al.* (1999b) Predictors of treatment response from a first episode of schizophrenia or schizoaffective disorder. *American Journal of Psychiatry* **156**, 544–549.

Rosanoff, A.J., Handy, L.M., Rosanoff-Plesset, I.R. & Brush, S. (1934) The etiology of so-called schizophrenic psychoses. *American Journal of Psychiatry* **91**, 247–286.

Rosso, I.M., Cannon, T.D., Huttunen, T. *et al.* (2000) Obstetric risk factors for early-onset schizophrenia in a Finnish birth cohort. *American Journal of Psychiatry* **157**, 801–807.

van Rossum, D. & U.K. Hanisch (1999) Cytoskeletal dynamics in dendritic spines: direct modulation by glutamate receptors?. *Trends in Neuroscience* **22**, 290–295.

Rund, B.R. (1998) A review of longitudinal studies of cognitive functions in schizophrenia patients. *Schizophrenia Bulletin* **24**, 425–435.

Russell, D., Douglas, A.S. & Allan, T.M. (1993) Changing seasonality of birth: a possible environmental effect. *Journal of Epidemiology and Community Health* **47**, 362–367.

Sacker, A., Done, D.J. *et al.* (1995) Antecedents of schizophrenia and affective-illness: obstetric complications. *British Journal of Psychiatry* **166**, 734–741.

Sacker, A., Done, D.J., Crow, T.J. & Golding, J. (1996) Obstetric complications in children born to parents with schizophrenia: a meta-analysis of case–control studies. *Psychological Medicine* **26**, 279–287.

Saunders, R.C., Kolachana, B.S., Bachevalier, J. & Weinberger, D.R. (1998) Neonatal lesions of the medial temporal lobe disrupt prefrontal cortical regulation of striatal dopamine. *Nature* **393**, 169–171.

Schwartz, M.L. & Goldman-Rakic, P. (1990) Development and plasticity of the primate cerebral cortex. *Clinical Perinatology* **17**, 83–102.

Segal, M. (2001) Rapid plasticity of dendritic spine: hints to possible functions? *Progress in Neurobiology* **63**, 61–70.

Seidman, L.J., Faraone, S.V., Goldstein, J.M. *et al.* (1997) Reduced subcortical brain volumes in non-psychotic siblings of schizophrenic patients: a pilot magnetic resonance imaging study. *American Journal of Medical Genetics* **74**, 507–514.

Selemon, L.D., Rajkowska, G. & Goldman-Rakic, P.S. (1995) Abnormally high neuronal density in the schizophrenic cortex: a morphometric analysis of prefrontal area-9 and occipital area-17. *Archives of General Psychiatry* **52**, 805–818.

Selten, J. & Slaets, J.P.J. (1994) Evidence against maternal influenza as a risk factor for schizophrenia. *British Journal of Psychiatry* **164**, 674–676.

Selten, J.P., van der Graaf, Y., van Duursen, R., Gispen-delvied, C.C., & Kahn, R.S. (1999) Psychotic illness after prenatal exposure to the 1953 Dutch flood disaster. *Schizophrenia Research* **35**, 243–245.

Sham, P.C., O'Callaghan, E., Takei, N. (1992) Schizophrenia following prenatal exposure to influenza epidemics between 1939 and 1960. *British Journal of Psychiatry* **160**, 461–466.

Shannon-Weickert, C., Webster, M.J., Hyde, T.M. *et al.* (2001) Reduced GAP-43 mRNA in dorsolateral prefrontal cortex of patients with schizophrenia. *Cerebral Cortex* **11**, 136–147.

Shapleske, J., Rossell, S.L., Simmons, A., David, A.S. & Woodruff, P.W. (2001) Are auditory hallucinations the consequence of abnormal cerebral lateralization? A morphometric MRI study of the sylvian fissure and planum temporale. *Biological Psychiatry* **49**, 685–693.

Shenton, M.E., Kikinis, R., Jolesz, F.A. *et al.* (1992) Abnormalities of the left temporal lobe and thought disorder in schizophrenia: a quantitative magnetic resonance imaging study. *New England Journal of Medicine* **327**, 604–612.

Shenton, M.E., Dickey, C.C., Frumin, M. & McCarley, R.W. (2001) A review of MRI findings in schizophrenia. *Schizophrenia Research* **49**, 1–52.

Shprintzen, R.J., Goldberg, R. Golding-Kushner, K.J. & Marion, R.W. (1992) Late-onset psychosis in the velocardiofacial syndrome. *American Journal of Medical Genetics* **42**, 141–142.

Sierrahonigmann, A.M., Carbone, K.M., & Yolken, R.H. (1995) Polymerase chain-reaction (PCR) search for viral nucleic-acid sequences in schizophrenia. *British Journal of Psychiatry* **166**, 55–60.

Smith, G.N., Kopala, L.C., Lapointe, J.S. *et al.* (1998) Obstetric complications, treatment response and brain morphology in adult-onset and early-onset males with schizophrenia. *Psychological Medicine* **28**, 645–653.

Southard, E.E. (1915) On the topographical distribution of cortex lesions and anamolies in dementia praecox, with some account of their functional significance. *American Journal of Insanity* **71**, 603–671.

Stevens, J.R. (1992) Abnormal reinnervation as a basis for schizophrenia: a hypothesis. *Archives of General Psychiatry* **49**, 238–243.

Suddath, R.L., Christison, G.W., Torrey, E.F., Csanova, M.F. & Weinberger, D.R. (1990) Anatomical abnormalities in the brains of monozygotic twins discordant for schizophrenia. *New England Journal of Medicine* **322**, 789–794.

Susser, E., Lin, S.P., Brown, A.S. *et al.* (1994) No relation between risk of schizophrenia and prenatal exposure to influenza in Holland. *American Journal of Psychiatry* **151**, 922–924.

Susser, E., Neugebauer, R., Hoek, H.W. *et al.* (1996) Schizophrenia after prenatal famine: further evidence. *Archives of General Psychiatry* **53**, 25–31.

Susser, E.S., Schaefer, C.A., Brown, A.S., Begg, M.D. & Wyatt, R.J. (2000) The design of the prenatal determinants of schizophrenia study. *Schizophrenia Bulletin* **26**, 257–273.

Suvisaari, J.M., Haukka, J.K., Tanskanen, A.J. & Lonnquist, J.K. (2000) Decreasing seasonal variation of births in schizophrenia. *Psychological Medicine* **30**, 315–324.

Suvisaari, J.M., Haukka, J.K. & Lonnquist, J.K. (2001) Season of birth among patients with schizophrenia and their siblings: evidence for the procreational habits hypothesis. *American Journal of Psychiatry* **158**, 754–757.

Szatmari, P., Reitsma-Street, M. & Offord, D.R. (1986) Pregnancy and birth complications in antisocial adolescents and their siblings. *Canadian Journal of Psychiatry* **31**, 513–516.

Taller, A.M., Asher, D.M., Pomeroy, K.L. *et al.* (1996) Search for viral nucleic acid sequences in brain tissues of patients with schizophrenia using nested polymerase chain reaction. *Archives of General Psychiatry* **53**, 32–40.

Thatcher, R.W., Walker, R.A. & Giudice, S. (1987) Human cerebral hemispheres develop at different rates and ages. *Science* **236**, 1110–1113.

Thompson, P.M., MacDonald, D. Mega, M.S. *et al.* (1997) Detection and mapping of abnormal brain structure with a probabilistic atlas of cortical surfaces. *Journal of computer Assisted Tomography* **21**, 567–581.

Thompson, P.M., Vidal, C. Giedd, J.N. *et al.* (2001) From the cover: mapping adolescent brain change reveals dynamic wave of accelerated gray matter loss in very early-onset schizophrenia. *Proceedings of the National Academy of Sciences of the USA* **98**, 11650–11655.

Toni, N., Buchs, P.A., Nikonenko, I., Bron, C.R. & Muller, D. (1999) LTP promotes formation of multiple spine synapses between a single axon terminal and a dendrite. *Nature* **402**, 421–425.

Torrey, E.F. (1977) Birth weights, perinatal insults, and HLA types: return to 'original din'. *Schizophrenia Bulletin* **3**, 347–351.

Torrey, E.F., Rawlings, R. & Waldman, I.N. (1988) Schizophrenic births and viral diseases in two states. *Schizophrenia Research* **1**, 73–77.

Torrey, E.F., Bowler, A.E., Rawlings, R. & Terrazas, A. (1993) Seasonality of schizophrenia and stillbirths. *Schizophrenia Bulletin* **19**, 557–562.

Torrey, F.E., Rawlings, R. & Yolken, R.H. (2000) The antecedents of psychoses: a case–control study of selected risk factors. *Schizophrenia Research* **46**, 17–23.

Tsuang, M.T., Woolson, R.F. & Fleming, J.A. (1979) Long-term outcome of major psychoses. I. Schizophrenia and affective disorders compared with psychiatrically symptom-free surgical conditions. *Archives of General Psychiatry* **36**, 1295–1301.

Van Os, J. & Selten, J.P. (1998) Prenatal exposure to maternal stress and subsequent schizophrenia: the May 1940 invasion of the Netherlands. *British Journal of Psychiatry* **172**, 324–326.

Vawter, M.P., Cannon-Spoor, H.E., Hemperly, J.J. *et al.* (1998) Abnormal expression of cell recognition molecules in schizophrenia. *Experimental Neurology* **149**, 424–432.

Verdoux, H. & Bourgeois, M. (1993) A comparative study of obstetric history in schizophrenics, bipolar patients and normal subjects. *Schizophrenia Research* **9**, 67–69.

Verdoux, H., Geddes, J.R., Takei, N. *et al.* (1997) Obstetric complications and age at onset in schizophrenia: an international collaborative meta-analysis of individual patient data. *American Journal of Psychiatry* **154**, 1220–1227.

Verdoux, H., Liraud, F., Bergey, C. *et al.* (2001) Is the association between duration of untreated psychosis and outcome confounded? A 2 year follow-up study of first-admitted patients. *Schizophrenia Research* **49**, 231–241.

Wada, J.A., Clarke, R. & Hamm, A. (1975) Cerebral hemispheric asymmetry in humans: cortical speech zones in 100 adults and 100 infant brains. *Archives of Neurology* **32**, 239–246.

Waddington, J.L. & Youssef, H.A. (1990) The lifetime outcome and involuntary movements of schizophrenia never treated with neuroleptic drugs: four rare cases in Ireland. *British Journal of Psychiatry* **156**, 106–108.

Wahlbeck, K., Forsen, T., Osmond, C., Barker, D.J. & Eriksson, J.G. (2001) Association of schizophrenia with low maternal body mass index, small size at birth, and thinness during childhood. *Archives of General Psychiatry* **58**, 48–52.

Watson, C.G., Kucala, T., Tilleskjor, C. & Jacobs, L. (1984) Schizophrenic birth seasonality in relation to the incidence of infectious diseases and temperature extremes. *Archives of General Psychiatry* **41**, 85–90.

Watt, N.F. (1972) Longitudinal changes in the social behavior of children hospitalized for schizophrenia as adults. *Journal of Nervous and Mental Disease* **155**, 42–54.

Weinberger, D.R. (1986) The pathogenesis of schizophrenia: a neurodevelopmental theory. In: *The Neurology of Schizophrenia* (eds H.A.W. Nasrallah & D.R. Weinberger), pp. 397–406. Elsevier, Amsterdam.

Weinberger, D.R. (1987) Implications of normal brain development for the pathogenesis of schizophrenia. *Archives of General Psychiatry* **44**, 660–669.

Weinberger, D.R. (1993) A connectionist approach to the prefrontal cortex. *Journal of Neuropsychiatry and Clinical Neuroscience* **5**, 241–253.

Weinberger, D.R. (1995) Schizophrenia as a neurodevelopmental disorder. In: *Schizophrenia* (ed. S.R. Hirsch), pp. 293–323. Blackwell Science, Oxford.

Weinberger, D.R. (1999) Schizophrenia: new phenes and new genes. *Biological Psychiatry* **46**, 3–7.

Weinberger, D.R. & Lipska, B.K. (1995) Cortical maldevelopment, anti-psychotic drugs, and schizophrenia: a search for common ground. *Schizophrenia Research* **16**, 87–110.

Weinberger, D.R. & McClure, R.K. (2002) Neurotoxicity, neuroplasticity, and MRI morphometry: what's happening in the schizophrenic brain? *Archives of General Psychiatry* **59**, 553–558.

Weinberger, D.R., Torrey, E.F., Neophytides, A.N. & Wyatt, R.J. (1979) Lateral cerebral ventricular enlargement in chronic schizophrenia. *Archives of General Psychiatry* **36**, 735–739.

Weinberger, D.R., Bigelow, L.B.; Kleiman, J.E. *et al.* (1980a) Cerebral ventricular enlargement in chronic schizophrenia: an association with poor response to treatment. *Archives of General Psychiatry* **37**, 11–13.

Weinberger, D.R., Cannon-Spoor, E., Potkin, S.G. & Wyatt, R.J. (1980b) Poor premorbid adjustment and CT scan abnormalities in chronic schizophrenia. *American Journal of Psychiatry* **137**, 1410–1413.

Weinberger, D.R., DeLisi, L.E., Perman, G.P. *et al.* (1982a) Computed tomography in schizophreniform disorder and other acute psychiatric disorders. *Archives of General Psychiatry* **39**, 778–783.

Weinberger, D.R., Luchins, D.J., Morihisa, J. & Wyatt, R.J. (1982b) Asymmetrical volumes of the right and left frontal and occipital regions of the human brain. *Annals of Neurology* **11**, 97–100.

Weinberger, D.R., Wagner, R.L. & Wyatt, R.J. (1983) Neuropathological studies of schizophrenia: a selective review. *Schizophrenia Bulletin* **9**, 193–212.

Weinberger, D.R., Berman, K.F. Suddath, R. & Torrey, E.F. (1992) Evidence of dysfunction of a prefrontal–limbic network in schizophrenia: a magnetic-resonance-imaging and regional cerebral blood-flow study of discordant monozygotic twins. *American Journal of Psychiatry* **149**, 890–897.

Weinberger, D.R., Egan, M.F., Bertolino, A. *et al.* (2001) Prefrontal neurons and the genetics of schizophrenia. *Biological Psychiatry* **50**, 825–844

Westergaard, T., Mortensen, P.B., Pedersen, C.B. Wohlfahrt, J. & Melbye, M. (1999) Exposure to prenatal and childhood infections and the risk of schizophrenia: suggestions from a study of sibship characteristics and influenza prevalence. *Archives of General Psychiatry* **56**, 993–998.

Wilcox, J.A. & Nasrallah, H.A. (1987) Perinatal distress and prognosis of psychotic illness. *Neuropsychobiology* **17**, 173–175.

Woods, B.T. (1998) Is schizophrenia a progressive neurodevelopmental disorder? Toward a unitary pathogenetic mechanism. *American Journal of Psychiatry* **155**, 1661–1670.

Zornberg, G.L., Buka, S.L. & Tsuang, M.T. (2000) Hypoxic-ischemia-related fetal/neonatal complications and risk of schizophrenia and other non-affective psychoses: a 19-year longitudinal study. *American Journal of Psychiatry* **157**, 196–202.

Zuccato, C., Ciammola, A., Rigamouti, D. *et al.* (2001) Loss of Huntington-mediated BDNF gene transcription in Huntington's disease. *Science* **293**, 493–498.

19

The neurochemistry of schizophrenia

B. Moghaddam and J.H. Krystal

Dopamine, 349
Glutamate, 349
  Glutamate receptor genes and binding, 350
  Psychopharmacological studies, 351
Serotonin (5-HT), 352
  5-HT-receptor binding and gene expression, 352
  Psychopharmacological studies, 353
GABA, 354
  Abnormal number or localization of GABA
    neurones, 354

GABA neurone dysfunction, 355
GABA receptors, 356
  Psychopharmacological studies, 356
Acetylcholine, 356
  Cholinergic receptors, 356
  Psychopharmacological studies, 357
Conclusions, 357
References, 357

The discovery in the 1950s that drugs such as reserpine and chlorpromazine could influence the expression of some of the symptoms of schizophrenia led to the development of the concept that 'neurochemical' abnormalities may be associated with this disorder. Contrary to the common belief that the 'dopamine hypothesis' was the first neurochemical hypothesis of schizophrenia to follow the discovery of neuroleptics, the 'serotonin deficiency' and 'norepinephrine-depletion' theories (Brodie 1959) were put forth several years before dopamine was implicated in the mechanisms of action of neuroleptics. These theories originated from observations that, in animals, reserpine reduces brain tissue levels of serotonin (and norepinephrine), leading to the postulation that 'liberation' of active serotonin alleviates the serotonin deficiency suspected to occur during active psychosis. While, given our present state of knowledge, this concept appears far-fetched, the inferential line of reasoning used to justify this theory is still applied today to support the two most influential neurotransmitter theories of schizophrenia: the dopamine (hyperactivity) hypothesis and glutamate (deficiency) hypothesis. Fortunately, however, recent advances made in the fields of molecular and cellular neuroscience and brain imaging methodologies have made it possible to move beyond the indirect approach and discover specific abnormalities in neurotransmitter systems in schizophrenia. The goal of this chapter is to provide the reader with an overview of these recent findings on specific neurotransmitter systems which are contributing to our current understanding of the complex abnormal neurotransmitter dynamics that may lead to expression of schizophrenic symptomotology.

Dopamine

The dopamine hypothesis of schizophrenia remains the most studied neurochemical theory relating to schizophrenia. In its simplest form, this hypothesis proposes that dopamine neurotransmission is hyperactive in schizophrenia (Carlsson 1978). This notion is supported by the fact that antipsychotic drugs block central dopamine receptors, and that their effective therapeutic doses correlate with blockade of dopamine D_2 receptors (Seeman *et al.* 1976). Furthermore, chronic exposure to amphetamines, which are indirect dopamine agonists, produces psychosis (Snyder *et al.* 1974a; see Chapter 20 for a review of dopaminergic involvement in schizophrenia).

Glutamate

The notion that glutamate neurotransmission is involved in the pathophysiology of schizophrenia is hardly academic. After all, the most consistent findings in schizophrenia, across all technical disciplines, have involved abnormalities in the function and organization of association cortices, in particular the prefrontal cortices. Considering that *all* cortical efferents – and the majority of cortical afferents including those from the thalamus and limbic structures – are glutamatergic, it is inevitable that glutamate neurotransmission mediates the abnormal cortical connectivity and functioning suspected to occur in schizophrenia. However, evidence for a glutamatergic involvement in schizophrenia has only begun to surface in the last decade.

The first suggestion of glutamatergic abnormality in schizophrenia was put forth by Kim *et al.* (1980). These authors reported reduced glutamate levels in the cerebral spinal fluid (CSF) of schizophrenics compared to controls, and hence postulated that glutamate neurotransmission may be downregulated in schizophrenia. The CSF findings, however, were not replicated by three other groups (Gattaz *et al.* 1982; Perry 1982; Korpi *et al.* 1987). Even if they were, considering that the majority of glutamate found in the brain is involved in intermediary metabolism and other non-neuronal functions, measures of glutamate levels in the CSF would not be considered an accurate index of glutamate-mediated neurotransmission.

About the same time that the CSF studies were being reported, several laboratories were attempting to characterize the mechanism by which the potent 'schizophrenomimetic' drug phencyclidine (PCP) (Luby *et al.* 1959) binds to brain tissue (Zukin & Zukin 1979). The discovery that PCP reduces glutamate neurotransmission at the *N*-methyl-D-aspartate (NMDA) subtype of the glutamate receptor (Lodge & Anis 1982; Anis *et al.* 1983), and is a potent non-competitive antagonist of the NMDA receptor channel, provided compelling, albeit indirect, support for glutamatergic involvement in schizophrenia and led to the speculation that hypoactive glutamate neurotransmission at the NMDA receptor is involved in schizophrenia (Javitt & Zukin 1991). Subsequently, numerous postmortem studies have reported region-specific changes in different subtypes of glutamate receptors in schizophrenic brains (see below) and the glutamate hypothesis has been modified to incorporate more complex mechanisms (Olney & Farber 1995; Tamminga 1998; Krystal *et al.* 1999b; Goff & Coyle 2001).

Glutamate receptor genes and binding

Until two decades ago, it was thought that glutamate exerted its physiological action solely through receptors that act directly as ion channels. Binding of glutamate to these so-called ionotropic receptors stimulates Ca^{2+} entry into neurones through channels formed either by the receptor itself (as is the case with the NMDA receptor subtype) or by opening voltage-sensitive Ca^{2+} channels which are on the cell membrane. Ionotropic glutamate receptors are classified into three broad subtypes according to their preferential agonists as the NMDA, kainate and α-amino-3-hydroxy-5-methyl-isoxazole propionic acid (AMPA) receptors. The AMPA receptors are composed of at least four subunits derived from a family of four genes termed *gluR1–gluR4*. Kainate receptors are thought to be composed of five identical subunits (homomers) derived from genes termed *gluR5–gluR7* and *KA1–KA2*. The NMDA receptor is composed of four or five subunits derived from fives genes *NR1* and *NR2A–NR2D*. The NR1 subunit, which has several isoforms, is an obligate subunit. Nearly all neurones express AMPA and NMDA receptors and it is estimated that glutamate ionotropic receptors mediate nearly 50% of all synaptic transmission in the mammalian central nervous system.

The classical views of glutamate-mediated neurotransmission were changed in the late 1980s when two research groups independently cloned a novel receptor with high affinity for glutamate which had different functional characteristics than other glutamate receptors (Conn & Pin 1997). In contrast to the rapid excitation and opening of ion channels that was the hallmark of ionotropic glutamate receptor activation, stimulation of these so-called metabotropic receptors indirectly regulated electrical signalling by activation of various second messenger cascades. From a clinical point of view, the discovery of these receptors was important because they activated synaptic transduction mechanisms similar to those of the monoamine neurotransmitters such as dopamine and serotonin, which are the site of action of most known psychotherapeutic drugs. At least eight metabotropic glutamate receptors have been cloned (mGlu1–mGlu8). These receptors share no sequence homology with other known receptors in the nervous system, suggesting that they are members of a new receptor gene family. The eight subtypes of mGlu receptors are currently classified into three groups

(groups I–III). This classification is primarily based on sequence identity: the amino acid sequence homology between mGluR of the same group is about 70%, while between groups the homology is about 40%. The classification is also based on transduction mechanism: stimulation of group I mGlu receptor activates the enzyme phospholipase C which in turn results in breakdown of membrane phospholipid to the second messengers, inositol triphosphate or diacylglycerol. Activation of group II or III receptors results in downregulation of the enzyme adenylate cyclase, resulting in reduced synthesis of the second messenger cyclic adenosine monophosphate (cAMP).

Unlike the monoamine systems, selective glutamate receptor ligands for clinical imaging studies have not been fully developed for routine use in healthy and patient volunteers (Bressan & Pilowsky 2000). Although studies using proton magnetic resonance spectroscopy (MRS) are beginning to provide some valuable functional data on glutamate abnormalities in schizophrenia (Kegeles *et al.* 2000), the primary focus of research on glutamate and schizophrenia remains on postmortem studies.

As would be expected, numerous studies have examined glutamate receptor binding or expression in cortical, striatal and temporal lobe structures in schizophrenic brain (for a recent review see Meador-Woodruff & Healy 2000). The earliest report in the literature using [3H]MK801 (MK801 is a selective non-competitive antagonist of the NMDA receptor) described increased binding in the putamen, but not in the frontal cortex or temporal lobe (Kornhuber *et al.* 1989). Similar increases were reported using [3H]D-aspartate (Aparicio-Legarza *et al.* 1997) but another study failed to replicate the finding in putamen (Noga *et al.* 1997). Studies using [3H]TCP (which, similar to MK801, binds to the PCP site on the NMDA receptor complex) have also resulted in conflicting observations with either no change (Weissman *et al.* 1991) or an increase in binding in orbitofrontal cortex being reported (Simpson *et al.* 1992).

More recent studies have examined the expression of NMDA receptor subunits in schizophrenic brain and have reported several region-specific results. In the prefrontal cortex, Akbarian *et al.* (1996b) found no major changes in any of the NMDA receptor subunits; however, a higher ratio of NR2D to the other NR2 subunits was noted. In the thalamus, a significant reduction in NR1, NR2B and NR2CR subunits has been reported (Ibrahim *et al.* 2000). In a study of prospectively assessed patients, levels of NR1 subunit was shown to be significantly correlated with several measures of cognitive function (global cognitive deterioration, Mini Mental State examination, and National Adult Learning test) in rapid autopsy samples of schizophrenic patients (Humphries *et al.* 1996). Other reports have also demonstrated a downregulation of NR1 in the superior temporal gyrus and hippocampus (Sokolov 1998; Gao *et al.* 2000) and the thalamus (Ibrahim *et al.* 2000) and upregulation of NR2B subunit in the superior temporal cortex (Grimwood *et al.* 1999).

Findings with the AMPA receptor subunits have been more consistent, suggesting a decrease in the expression of several AMPA receptor subunits as well as a decrease in receptor binding in the medial temporal lobe in schizophrenic brains. Decreases in AMPA receptor binding in CA3 and CA4 subfields of hippocampus was first noted by Harrison and coworkers (Kerwin *et al.* 1990; Harrison *et al.* 1991). These findings are consistent with reduced expression of *gluR1* and *gluR2* reported by several laboratories (Harrison *et al.* 1991; Eastwood *et al.* 1995, 1997; Healy *et al.* 1998). In contrast to the temporal lobe regions, one study reported small changes in frontal cortex and striatal regions (Noga *et al.* 2001).

Several other studies have examined kainate receptor binding or messenger RNA (mRNA) levels (Nishikawa *et al.* 1983; Deakin *et al.* 1989; Noga *et al.* 1997; Porter *et al.* 1997; Sokolov 1998; Meador-Woodruff *et al.* 2001). In general, these studies follow the same pattern of change as in AMPA receptor expression, suggesting reduced levels of expression in temporal lobe regions and small increases or no effect in these cortical areas.

Studies examining the expression of the family of metabotropic glutamate receptor have only recently begun and, although there are only a few published studies in this area (Ohnuma *et al.* 1998; Richardson-Burns *et al.* 2000), this is likely to be an active field of research in the future. So far, an increase in mGluR5 in orbitofrontal cortex has been reported (Ohnuma *et al.* 1998).

In addition to glutamate receptors, Coyle and coworkers (Tsai *et al.* 1995) have reported postmortem abnormalities in the expression of the neuropeptide N-acetylaspartyl glutamate (NAAG), which is considered an endogenous ligand for some subtypes of glutamate receptors. This reported increase in the levels of NAAG as well as a decrease in its catabolic enzyme NAALADase in the prefrontal cortex and hippocampus most likely reflects alteration in glutamate neurotransmission in schizophrenia (Coyle 1996).

Despite the above-reported changes in glutamate receptor expression and binding, genetic studies have not yet provided convincing evidence of a functional mutation of glutamate receptor genes in schizophrenia. A linkage study with a genetically isolated African population suggested that an NR1 subunit polymorphism may be associated with predisposition to develop schizophrenia (Riley *et al.* 1997). Other studies, however, have so far reported lack of association with polymorphisms for genes encoding for NR1, NR2B, GluR5, mGluR7 and mGluR8 (Pariseau *et al.* 1994; Bray *et al.* 2000; Nishiguchi *et al.* 2000; Bolonna *et al.* 2001).

Psychopharmacological studies

One of the first 'challenge' studies with schizophrenic subjects involved the use of the drug PCP (Luby *et al.* 1959; Itil *et al.* 1967). PCP (Sernyl) was developed in the 1950s as a general anaesthetic that was devoid of depressant effects on the cardiovascular system. However, intraoperative reactions that included hallucinations and postoperative psychotic states, which in some cases persisted for days, led to its withdrawal from the market in 1965. Luby and several other investigators reported on the effects of subanaesthetic doses of PCP in healthy individuals as well as patients with schizophrenia (Luby *et al.* 1959; Bakker & Amini 1961; Itil *et al.* 1967; Burns & Lerner 1976;

Aniline & Pitts 1982). These reports suggested that PCP produces a behavioural syndrome in non-schizophrenics that closely resembles endogenous symptoms of schizophrenia. These symptoms included: positive symptoms such as paranoia, agitation, auditory hallucination; negative symptoms such as apathy, social withdrawal; and cognitive deficits such as impaired attention. More importantly, in patients with schizophrenia, including chronic stabilized patients, a single dose of PCP produced a profound exacerbation of pre-existing symptoms that lasted for days or months.

The 'schizophrenomimetic' effects of PCP engendered a great deal of interest in understanding its biological actions. In 1979, a high-affinity binding site for PCP was described (Vincent *et al.* 1979; Zukin & Zukin 1979). This 'PCP receptor' was later found to be a binding site in the NMDA receptor ion channel (Javitt *et al.* 1987; Sircar *et al.* 1987; Wong *et al.* 1988), consistent with reports that PCP reduces the excitatory effects of glutamate (Anis *et al.* 1983). Based on these findings, and previous clinical reports indicating that PCP intoxication resembles schizophrenia more closely than the acute paranoid psychosis caused by amphetamines, Javitt and Zukin (1991) proposed that a dysfunction in the NMDA receptor-mediated neurotransmission contributes to pathogenesis of schizophrenia.

NMDA receptor-related hypotheses related to the neurobiology of schizophrenia have been the subject of intense research in the past decade. The interest in this model has been, in part, a result of several recent studies that have established the clinical validity of this model using the PCP analogue, ketamine. At subanaesthetic doses, similar to PCP, ketamine is a relatively selective non-competitive antagonist of the NMDA receptor. However, unlike PCP, ketamine is a widely used anaesthetic with an established record of safety in healthy humans. The original human studies with PCP were descriptive and naturalistic, and hence difficult to interpret in the context of present diagnostic criteria. Using ketamine, a new generation of rigorous clinical pharmacological studies has been performed (Krystal *et al.* 1994; Malhotra *et al.* 1996b; Newcomer *et al.* 1999). These studies used validated measures of assessing signs and symptoms of schizophrenia and therefore provided a thorough documentation of the cognitive and other behavioural effects of ketamine in healthy subjects. The features of the ketamine psychosis can be quite striking. The form and content of thought may be altered, resulting in bizarre, disorganized or concrete ideation, which may be indistinguishable from that seen in some schizophrenic patients. Cognitive functions common for schizophrenic patients in attention, abstract reasoning, the shifting of mental set and memory are observed in healthy subjects administered ketamine. Less common for schizophrenia, ketamine alters perception in most perceptual spheres. During ketamine, time may seem to slow; the shape, colour or vividness of objects may be altered; sounds may be distorted in intensity, content or localization; derealization or depersonalization are also common (Krystal *et al.* 1994).

In addition to studies in healthy volunteers, a very limited number of challenge studies administered ketamine to schizophrenic volunteers who were on antipsychotic medication. In these schizophrenic patients, ketamine produced a brief exacerbation of pre-existing psychotic symptoms (Lahti *et al.* 1995; Malhotra *et al.* 1997). Collectively, the human pharmacological studies, albeit not without ethical concerns, have been invaluable for facilitating translational and hypothesis-driven research on the role of NMDA receptors in normal cognitive functioning and in schizophrenia. This line of research has led to the identification of several novel therapeutic approaches which are in various stages of basic laboratory characterization or clinical trials (Javitt *et al.* 1994; Moghaddam & Adams 1998; Goff *et al.* 1999; Anand *et al.* 2000).

It should be emphasized, however, that while animal and human studies with ketamine and PCP have strongly implicated a role for NMDA receptors in the pathophysiology of schizophrenia, the nature of this NMDA involvement remains unclear. The most simplified hypothesis has been that a reduction in glutamate neurotransmission at the NMDA receptor is responsible for aspects of schizophrenic symptomatology (Javitt & Zukin 1991; Olney & Farber 1995; Tamminga 1998). However, as reviewed above, uniform postmortem or genomic evidence for an NMDA receptor dysfunction has been difficult to identify in schizophrenia. An alternative hypothesis is that secondary effects of systemic NDMA blockade may produce conditions that mimic some aspects of schizophrenic pathophysiology. For example, PCP and ketamine produce a prefrontal cortex-specific activation of glutamate efflux (Moghaddam *et al.* 1997), suggesting that a cortical glutamate hyperactivity (at non-NMDA receptors) may produce some of the schizomimetic effects of these drugs (Moghaddam & Adams 1998; Krystal *et al.* 1999b). Consistent with this mechanism, pharmacological pretreatments that reduce glutamate hyperactivity also ameliorate behavioural effects of PCP or ketamine in animals (Moghaddam & Adams 1998) and humans (Anand *et al.* 2000).

Serotonin (5-HT)

Currently, there is no clear evidence that 5-HT neuronal cytopathology contributes to the pathophysiology of schizophrenia, although alterations in 5-HT neuronal function may be features of the symptoms of schizophrenia and its treatment. 5-HT projections arise from the raphe nuclei and project widely, but not randomly, in the brain (Wilson & Molliver 1991). The single study to report on 5-HT neuronal architecture in brain tissue from schizophrenic patients did not find evidence of abnormal morphology of 5-HT axons within the prefrontal cortex (Akil *et al.* 1999). Other postmortem studies did not find altered levels of cortical or striatal 5-HT metabolites (Crow *et al.* 1979; Joseph *et al.* 1979) or evidence of altered monoamine oxidase (MAO) activity in brain tissue from schizophrenic patients (Meltzer *et al.* 1980; Reveley *et al.* 1981). Many other studies have related clinical characteristics of schizophrenia or its treatment to the CSF levels of 5-HT or its metabolites. This topic, reviewed elsewhere (Widerlov 1988), is beyond the scope of this

review. In the following section, we consider the possibility that schizophrenia may be associated with alterations in the binding properties of 5-HT-receptors, mutations in 5-HT-related genes.

5-HT-receptor binding and gene expression

Studies of postmortem brain tissue from schizophrenic patients reported alterations in several 5-HT receptors. Several studies report upregulation of the density of 5-HT_{1A}-receptor binding in the prefrontal cortex, but not hippocampus, in tissue from schizophrenic patients, although mRNA levels for this receptor were not changed in either region (Hashimoto *et al.* 1991; Burnet *et al.* 1996; Simpson *et al.* 1996; Sumiyoshi *et al.* 1996; Gurevich & Joyce 1997). So far, only one study failed to find changes in the cortical levels of 5-HT_{1A}-receptors in prefrontal cortex tissue from schizophrenic patients (Dean *et al.* 1999b). A single study found no difference in the levels of mRNA for 5-HT_{1A}-receptors in the prefrontal cortical tissue from patients where increased 5-HT_{1A}-receptor binding was measured (Burnet *et al.* 1996). To date, there are no studies suggesting that polymorphisms of the 5-HT_{1A}- or 5-HT_{1B}-receptor genes are related to the diagnosis of schizophrenia or treatment response in this patient group (Erdmann *et al.* 1995; Kawanishi *et al.* 1998; Bruss *et al.* 1999).

Several studies report reductions in the density of 5-HT_{2A}- or 5-HT_{2C}-receptors in cortical and hippocampal tissue from schizophrenic patients (Bennett *et al.* 1979; Mita *et al.* 1986; Arora & Meltzer 1991; Hashimoto *et al.* 1991; Burnet *et al.* 1996; Dean & Hayes 1996; Gurevich & Joyce 1997; Hernandez & Sokolov 2000). Confusion related to these 5-HT_2-receptor subtypes was introduced by the use of non-selective ligands, such as $[^3\text{H}]$lysergic acid diethylamide (LSD), in several of the initial studies (Bennett *et al.* 1979; Whitaker *et al.* 1981; Gurevich & Joyce 1997). As reviewed elsewhere (Abi-Dargham & Krystal 2000), there are mixed findings with postmortem studies of 5-HT_{2A}-preferring ligands, with some studies reporting reductions in cortical receptor density and others not finding diagnosis-related differences. Studies of medicated patients suggest that reported reductions in the density of 5-HT_2-receptors in schizophrenic patients reflect a large and widespread downregulation related to antipsychotic treatment at the time of death and a more modest reduction that shows greater brain regional restriction described in medication-free patients (Gurevich & Joyce 1997). Another factor complicating postmortem studies is that tissue is often collected from medical examiners (coroners). As a result, they may over-represent the population of patients who die from suicide or violent causes. One study noted that patients who died from suicide did not differ from control groups in the density of cortical 5-HT_{2A}-receptors, while those patients who died from natural causes showed reductions in prefrontal 5-HT_{2A}-receptor density (Laruelle *et al.* 1993). Other potential confounds, such as the impact of comorbid substance abuse, cannot be adequately addressed on the basis of the current postmortem literature. Findings from *in vivo* neuroimaging studies have similarly not provided clear evidence of reductions in cortical 5-HT$_2$-receptors. One study reported reductions in 5-HT$_2$ binding (Ngan *et al.* 2000), but no difference was found in four other studies (Trichard *et al.* 1998; Lewis *et al.* 1999b; Okubo *et al.* 2000; Verhoeff *et al.* 2000).

Molecular genetic studies do not yet provide evidence of a functional mutation of 5-HT$_2$-receptor-related genes and schizophrenia. The most intensively studied polymorphism is a T-to-C substitution at nucleotide 102 of the 5-HT$_{2A}$-receptor gene that does not alter the amino acid sequence of this protein. Six studies reported associations between alleles of this gene and the diagnosis of schizophrenia (Erdmann *et al.* 1996b; Inayama *et al.* 1996; Williams *et al.* 1996, 1997; Tay *et al.* 1997; Spurlock *et al.* 1998), while nine others failed to find this relationship (Arranz *et al.* 1996; Malhotra *et al.* 1996a; Nimgaonkar *et al.* 1996; Chen *et al.* 1997; Hawi *et al.* 1997; He *et al.* 1999; Lin *et al.* 1999; Ohara *et al.* 1999; Serretti *et al.* 2000). Because the *T102C* polymorphism was silent, interest shifted to other polymorphisms that were in linkage disequilibrium with this site. An A-to-G substitution in the promoter region of the 5-HT$_{2A}$-receptor gene (*A-1438G*) was also identified, found to have no functional significance and was associated with schizophrenia in one of two studies (Spurlock *et al.* 1998; Ohara *et al.* 1999). Similarly, this polymorphism was not related to the density of 5-HT$_{2A}$-receptors in the frontal cortex of schizophrenic patients (Kouzmenko *et al.* 1999). Two other mutations of the 5-HT$_{2A}$-receptor gene (*Thr25Asn, His452Tyr*) were not associated with schizophrenia in a population that showed an association between the *T102C* allele and schizophrenia (Erdmann *et al.* 1996b).

5-HT$_2$-receptor-related genes also have been implicated in the clinical response to atypical neuroleptic agents. An association was reported between *T102C* or *A-1438G* polymorphisms and clozapine response; however, some of the positive reports are of marginal significance or not replicated internally (Arranz *et al.* 1995, 1998a,b, 2000; Joober *et al.* 1999). Other studies fail to find a link between these polymorphisms and response to typical (Nimgaonkar *et al.* 1996) or atypical antipsychotic drugs (Malhotra *et al.* 1996b; Nimgaonkar *et al.* 1996; Masellis *et al.* 1998; Lin *et al.* 1999). Similarly, a *Cys23Ser* polymorphism of the 5-HT$_{2C}$-receptor gene was not related to clozapine response in schizophrenic patients (Malhotra *et al.* 1996a; Masellis *et al.* 1998).

Several studies have also suggested that the 5-HT transporter (5-HTT) is abnormally expressed in the hippocampus and perhaps other regions in brain tissue from schizophrenic patients. As was recently reviewed (Abi-Dargham & Krystal 2000), several studies report reductions in 5-HTT binding in postmortem tissue in the frontal cortex, although reductions in receptor density were not observed in occipital cortex (Laruelle *et al.* 1993) or hippocampus (Dean *et al.* 1995). A single photon emission computerized tomography (SPECT) study failed to find brainstem alterations in schizophrenic patients using a ligand, [^{123}I]β-CIT, which is not informative in studies of cortical 5-HTT binding (Laruelle *et al.* 2000). New radiotracers are able to provide information about cortical and limbic 5-HTT binding *in*

vivo and the data generated using these tracers should enhance our understanding of this 5-HT binding site. Genetic studies have suggested an association between the long variant of the 5-HTT gene and schizophrenia (Malhotra *et al.* 1998), although negative studies exist (Rao *et al.* 1998; Serretti *et al.* 1999).

To date, no significant postmortem findings have emerged for the 5-HT$_3$- (Abi-Dargham *et al.* 1993) or 5-HT$_4$-receptors (Dean *et al.* 1999a). Also, no significant associations have emerged between markers related to the 5-HT$_3$-, 5-HT$_{5A}$-, 5-HT$_6$-, or 5-HT$_7$-receptor genes and the diagnosis of schizophrenia (Erdmann *et al.* 1996a; Birkett *et al.* 2000; Vogt *et al.* 2000; Niesler *et al.* 2001). Although one 5-HT$_6$-receptor-related marker showed an association with atypical neuroleptic response (Yu *et al.* 1999), no other associations between genes for the 5-HT$_3$ to 5-HT$_7$-receptors have yet emerged (Masellis *et al.* 2001).

Psychopharmacological studies

The study of the behavioural effects of the serotonergic hallucinogens was a fundamental step in the appreciation of the neurochemical basis of psychosis and a potent stimulus for the development of modern psychopharmacology (Gouzoulis-Mayfrank *et al.* 1998; Krystal *et al.* 1999a). Albert Hoffman described his accidental discovery of the psychedelic properties of LSD in these terms:

> Last Friday, April 16, 1943, I was forced to interrupt my work in the laboratory in the middle of the afternoon and proceed home, being affected by a remarkable restlessness, combined with a slight dizziness. At home I lay down and sank into a not unpleasant intoxicated-like condition characterized by an extremely stimulated imagination. In a dreamlike state, with eyes closed (I found the daylight to be unpleasantly glaring), I perceived an uninterrupted stream of fantastic pictures, extraordinary shapes with intense, kaleidoscopic play of colours. After some two hours this condition faded away. (from www.macalester.edu/~psych/whathap/UBNRP/LSD/links.htm)

Subsequent careful study of LSD (Rosenbaum *et al.* 1959; Cohen *et al.* 1962; Freedman 1968), mescaline (Hermle *et al.* 1998), psilocybin (Vollenweider *et al.* 1997; Vollenweider 1998) and N,N-dimethyltryptamine (DMT) (Strassman *et al.* 1994) yielded a consistent picture. These drugs generally produce, in a dose-related fashion, profound sensory distortions and hallucinations, impairments in attention and concentration, mood instability, depersonalization, derealization and formal thought disorder. Drug administration less consistently produces systematized delusions or auditory hallucinations, but these symptoms may emerge in some individuals. Relative to NMDA antagonists, the psychosis associated with the serotonergic hallucinogens is associated with less blunting of affect and cognitive impairment. However, these comparisons are difficult because these effects are dose-dependent and adequate comparison would require a clear reference point and the comparison of multiple doses of each drug.

Clinical studies of these hallucinogenic agents suggest that drugs that block 5-HT$_2$-receptors attenuate their cognitive and perceptual effects. For example, the cognitive and perceptual effects of psilocybin were blocked dose-dependently by ketanserin and risperidone, but not by haloperidol (Vollenweider et al. 1998). Also, the hallucinogenic effects of DMT were potentiated rather than reduced by pretreatment with the 5-HT$_{1A}$ antagonist pindolol (Strassman 1996). These findings are consistent with preclinical studies implicating 5-HT$_2$-receptor stimulation in the cognitive and behavioural effects of serotonergic hallucinogens (Aghajanian & Marek 1999).

The capacity of these 5-HT$_2$ agonists to produce psychosis may have therapeutic implications for schizophrenia. The serotonergic hallucinogens produce psychoses and cognitive impairments that resemble some aspects of schizophrenia, stimulate lasting schizophrenic-like states in a vulnerable subpopulation of individuals exposed to these drugs (Bowers 1987) and may worsen or even reduce symptoms in some schizophrenic patients (Itil et al. 1969). The extent to which the psychotogenic or propsychotic effects of these drugs are attributable to 5-HT$_2$-receptor stimulation suggests a role for 5-HT$_2$-receptor antagonism in the treatment of schizophrenia. Further, elaboration of the circuitry underlying the actions of 5-HT$_2$-receptor stimulation within the cortex suggests that drugs that attenuate glutamate release or attenuate its postsynaptic effects might also have a role in the treatment of schizophrenia (Aghajanian & Marek 2000; Marek et al. 2000). Similarly, interactions between 5-HT$_2$ and dopamine systems may contribute to both symptoms and the treatment of schizophrenia (Abi-Dargham et al. 1997).

Studies employing the 5-HT agonist m-chlorophenylpiperazine (mCPP) supported interest in the contribution of 5-HT systems to the pathophysiology and treatment of this disorder. Although it acts at multiple sites (Hamik & Peroutka 1989; Schoeffter & Hoyer 1989), the behavioural effects of mCPP appear most likely to be mediated by facilitation of 5-HT$_{1B}$- (Meneses et al. 1997; Maurel et al. 1998) or 5-HT$_{2C}$- (Fiorella et al. 1995) receptors (reviewed in Abi-Saab et al. 2002). While behavioural findings across groups were not consistent (Kahn et al. 1992; Owen et al. 1993; Maes & Meltzer 1996; Koreen et al. 1997), three studies found that mCPP increased psychosis and behavioural activation or anxiety in schizophrenic patients (Iqbal et al. 1991; Krystal et al. 1993; Abi-Saab et al. 2002). In contrast, several studies indicate that mCPP does not produce psychosis in healthy subjects (Charney et al. 1987; Kahn & Wetzler 1991; Seibyl et al. 1991; Krystal et al. 1993). The cause of the differential response to mCPP in schizophrenic patients and healthy control subjects is not clear. However, GABA deficits associated with schizophrenia may play a part. For example, pretreatment of healthy subjects with the benzodiazepine inverse agonist iomazenil resulted in a vulnerability to mCPP-induced psychosis (D'Souza et al. 2002). The behavioural and endocrine effects of mCPP in schizophrenic patients were attenuated by treatment with clozapine, but not by haloperidol (Krystal et al. 1990; Breier et al. 1993; Kahn et al. 1993b, 1994; Owen et al. 1993). These effects of mCPP were also attenuated by pretreatment with single doses of ritanserin (Abi-Saab et al. 2002). The adrenocorticotrophic hormone (ACTH) and cortisol response to mCPP in schizophrenic patients also predicted subsequent treatment response in schizophrenic patients (Kahn et al. 1993a; Owen et al. 1993). Unlike a preferential 5-HT$_2$-receptor antagonist in healthy subjects (Seibyl et al. 1991), clozapine treatment completely blocked the prolactin response to mCPP in schizophrenic patients (Kahn et al. 1994).

There is compelling evidence that 5-HT$_2$-receptor antagonism or inverse agonism may contribute to the efficacy of atypical neuroleptic medications. Atypical neuroleptics showed greater affinity for serotonin-2A (5-HT$_{2A}$)-receptors relative to their affinity for D$_2$ receptors (Meltzer et al. 1989). More recently, the clinical profile of the atypical neuroleptic class was attributed to relatively higher levels of occupancy of cortical 5-HT$_{2A}$-receptors relative to their occupancy of striatal D$_2$ receptors at therapeutic doses (Kapur et al. 1999). Recent preclinical data suggest that typical and atypical neuroleptic drugs are inverse agonists at 5-HT$_{2A}$-receptors (Egan et al. 1998), but only atypical neuroleptics cause internalization of these receptors (Willins et al. 1999). In addition, atypical neuroleptics, but not typical neuroleptics, show inverse agonist activity at 5-HT$_{2C}$-receptors (Herrick-Davis et al. 2000) and perhaps the 5-HT$_6$-receptor (Glatt et al. 1995; Frederick & Meador-Woodruff 1999; Zhukovskaya & Neumaier 2000).

GABA

There is now substantial evidence that abnormalities in cortical and limbic GABA neuronal populations are a facet of the neurobiology of schizophrenia. The reader is referred to two excellent recent reviews of this topic for more detail (Lewis 2000; Benes & Berretta 2001).

Abnormal number or localization of GABA neurones

After a series of postmortem studies, it remains unclear whether schizophrenia is associated with a reduction in the number of cortical interneurones, most of which contain GABA as their neurotransmitter. If this deficit exists, it is not likely to be specific to schizophrenia. Reductions in the density of nonpyramidal neurones were reported in layers II–VI of the anterior cingulate cortex and in layer II of the prefrontal cortex (Benes et al. 1991). Reductions in the number of parvalbumin, presumably GABA, neurones in prefrontal cortex were also reported in another laboratory (Beasley & Reynolds 1997). Subsequent studies have not replicated these findings (Akbarian et al. 1995; Arnold et al. 1995; Selemon et al. 1995, 1998; Woo et al. 1997). It is possible that opposing changes in subpopulations of GABA neurones may confound analyses that do not control for these effects. For example, regional reductions in parvalbumin-containing neurones may be accompanied by increases in the density of calretinin-containing neurones (Daviss & Lewis 1995).

Reduction in the density of GABA neurones is found in schizoaffective disorder patients (Benes *et al.* 1991) as well as patients with unipolar and bipolar affective disorder without comorbid schizophrenia (Benes *et al.* 1997; Rajakowska *et al.* 1998). These studies raise the possibility that GABA deficits are a consequence of pathogenic processes related to comorbid mood disorder in schizophrenic patients.

One unresolved issue related to the measurement of GABA neuronal populations is whether there is a disturbance in the migration of GABA neurones within the cortex in early development. There are at least two sources of cortical GABA neurones in development. One population migrates into the cerebral cortex from the lateral ganglionic eminence, a region that becomes the striatum later in development (Anderson *et al.* 1997). A second population, including the Cajal–Retzius cells, is present in layer I. These cells secrete reelin, a substance implicated in the modulation of cellular migration and cortical and hippocampal lamination (Ogawa *et al.* 1995; Del Rio *et al.* 1997). GABAergic abnormalities could arise in schizophrenia as a defect in the secretion of molecules that control the migration of GABA. For example, the reductions in GABA neurones in superficial cortical layers could be consistent with decreases in reelin found in superficial layers of prefrontal cortex in tissue from schizophrenic patients (Impagnatiello *et al.* 1998).

Other interneurone migration abnormalities associated with schizophrenia have less clear aetiologies. For example, two studies suggest that schizophrenia is associated with increased density, 'nests of cells', in the subcortical white matter (Akbarian *et al.* 1993, 1996a). It is conceivable that migration abnormalities contributing to alterations in cell migration contribute to alterations in interneurone density. For example, if the GABA neurones in the deep layers were cells that failed to migrate to positions in more superficial layers, migration deficits could contribute to decreases in GABA neuronal populations that have been reported. However, it is not clear that interneurone migration abnormalities in schizophrenia, if they exist, are specific to this disorder. For example, a growing number of genes have been identified where mutations produce human neural migration disorders (Pilz & Quarrell 1996; Uher & Golden 2000). A neuronal migration disturbance also has been described in the context of velocardiofacial syndrome (22q11 deletion) (Bird & Scambler 2000), a condition associated with schizophrenia. Similarly, environmental insults that may increase risk for schizophrenia may independently produce disturbances in neuronal migration, including prenatal cytomegalovirus infection (Tarantal *et al.* 1998) and prenatal ethanol exposure (Miller 1993; see also Chapter 17).

GABA neurone dysfunction

If GABA neuronal populations were normal in size and in their appropriate locations, abnormalities in the structure or function of GABA neurones might signal abnormalities in the development of the brain and might, in turn, contribute to the dysfunction of neural networks. This section reviews evidence of GABAergic dysfunction in schizophrenia. To our knowledge, published studies have not yet examined whether polymorphisms of genes related to GABA systems are particularly associated with schizophrenia. Therefore, this section focuses on neurobiological studies of postmortem tissue.

Several studies suggest that schizophrenic patients exhibit reductions in the levels of protein or mRNA for glutamate acid decarboxylase (GAD). However, the impact of medication effects on the current findings is not clear. GAD exists in two isoforms, GAD_{65}, primarily localized to axon terminals, and GAD_{67}, which is localized widely within GABA neurones. Most GAD_{67} is active under basal conditions, i.e. present as a holoenzyme saturated with its cofactor pyridoxal phosphate. Only half of GAD_{65} is present in this form (Kaufman *et al.* 1991). Several studies report reductions in GAD_{67} mRNA and protein levels in studies of prefrontal cortex and hippocampal tissue from patients with schizophrenia and bipolar disorder (Akbarian *et al.* 1995; Guidotti *et al.* 2000; Volk *et al.* 2000). In contrast, GAD_{65} protein levels were reported to be reduced in the anterior cingulate in patients with bipolar disorder but not schizophrenia (Todtenkopf & Benes 1998).

Reductions in GAD levels would be expected to reflect a reduction in GAD activity or cortical GABA level. One study failed to find reductions in GAD activity in prefrontal cortex (Bennett *et al.* 1979). However, several studies documented reductions in GABA levels in cortical and subcortical structures (Cross *et al.* 1979; Perry *et al.* 1979). In studies of GAD, neuroleptic effects have received attention as a potential confounding factor. However, mood stabilizing anticonvulsants, commonly prescribed to both schizophrenic and bipolar disorder patients, are of perhaps greater concern as confounding factors. For example, an anticonvulsant that significantly increases synaptic GABA levels by two- to threefold produces up to an 80% drop in cortical GAD_{67} protein levels after a 7-day administration period in animals (Rimvall *et al.* 1993). The effects of long-term anticonvulsant treatment upon GAD mRNA levels are not known. Recent measurements of cortical GABA levels also suggest that benzodiazepine administration reduces cortical GABA level in healthy human subjects (Goddard *et al.* 2002). Thus, additional research is needed to systematically distinguish medication effects from the GAD abnormalities intrinsic to schizophrenia.

Placed in a broader context, GAD_{67} reductions in schizophrenia could reflect an abnormality intrinsic to GABA neuronal terminals, particularly in the chandelier cell subgroup of interneurones. In this regard, several markers associated with GABA terminals are reduced in schizophrenic patients. For example, several studies reported reductions in binding to the GABA transporter (GAT1) in cortical and subcortical structures (Simpson *et al.* 1989; Reynolds *et al.* 1990). Decreases in GAT1 expression show a similar laminar distribution in the prefrontal cortex to reductions in GAD_{67} gene expression (Volk *et al.* 2001). Reductions in cortical GABA content in prefrontal cortex also are associated with reductions in GAT1 mRNA levels (Ohnuma *et al.* 1999). GAT1 labelling was also used to visualize and quantify the axon cartridges from chandelier cells, a sub-population of GABA interneurone that provides an inhibitory input to the initial axon segment of cortical pyramidal neurones. These studies suggest that schizophrenia is associated with a reduction in these axon cartridges in areas 9 and 46 of the prefrontal cortex (Woo *et al.* 1998). The aetiology of these GABAergic abnormalities is not known, but may reflect activity-dependent and activity-independent aspects of neurodevelopment.

GABA receptors

Alterations in the levels of GABA receptor binding, subunit protein levels or subunit mRNA levels might be expected in the cerebral cortex of schizophrenic patients if prominent abnormalities in GABA cellular architecture were associated with this disorder. Benes *et al.* (1992, 1996) described increases in $GABA_A$ receptor binding in superficial layers of the cingulate gyrus and prefrontal cortex, where their earlier studies described reductions in interneurone populations. However, in the hippocampus, regional increases in GABA binding in tissue from schizophrenic patients relative to tissue from comparison subjects were not associated with increases in benzodiazepine binding (Benes *et al.* 1997). Together, these data raise the possibility that reductions in GABA neurone number or function produce an upregulation in $GABA_A$ receptor binding. It is not yet known whether the dissociation of benzodiazepine binding from $GABA_A$ receptor binding reflects abnormal GABA receptor subunit genes, abnormal regulation of GABA receptors, or other regulatory abnormalities. In contrast, $GABA_B$ receptor binding on pyramidal but not interneurones may be reduced in some hippocampal subfields in tissue from schizophrenic patients (Mizukami *et al.* 2000).

Neurochemical brain imaging studies using ligands for the benzodiazepine binding site of the $GABA_A$ receptor may not have provided adequate tests of the hypothesis that GABAergic denervation would produce a highly localized laminar upregulation of $GABA_A$ receptor binding in the frontal or cingulate cortex. None of the published studies to date describe increases in binding in schizophrenic patients (Busatto *et al.* 1997; Abi-Dargham *et al.* 1999; Verhoeff *et al.* 1999). The special resolution of the existing published studies may have been insufficient to resolve highly localized changes in benzodiazepine binding, if they occurred. Also, the reported dissociation between [^{3}H]muscimol and benzodiazepine binding suggests that benzodiazepine ligands may not have been an adequate ligand to quantify $GABA_A$ receptor changes in schizophrenia.

Psychopharmacological studies

Recent reviews highlight the fundamental contributions of GABA neurones within the cortex to cognitive function (Lewis *et al.* 1999a; Benes & Berretta 2001). By implication, these studies suggest that GABAergic abnormalities might contribute to the cognitive functions associated with schizophrenia. To date, there is little direct support for this hypothesis. For example, there are no studies to suggest that benzodiazepines or other anticonvulsants that are commonly added to reduce anxiety, control aggression or achieve mood stabilization produce a specific or generalized enhancement of cognitive function in patients diagnosed with schizophrenia (Wassef *et al.* 1999). Even in epilepsy, where GABA-facilitating agents clearly suppress seizures, impairment rather than enhancement of cognitive function has been an important problem (Trimble 1987).

However, the possibility that GABA deficits might contribute to schizophrenia symptoms is supported by several observations. Benzodiazepines do appear to reduce emotional distress and symptom levels in some patients when added to antipsychotic treatment (Wolkowitz & Pickar 1991). In contrast, the administration of a benzodiazepine partial inverse agonist, iomazenil, may unmask the psychotogenic potential of drugs that are not previously associated with producing psychosis in healthy individuals, such as the serotonin partial agonist mCPP (D'Souza *et al.* 2002).

Acetylcholine

Cholinergic projections to the cortex and basal forebrain have an integral role in the processing of several cognitive constructs that are known to be compromised in schizophrenia (Robbins 1997). Although cholinergic mechanisms have long been implicated in the extrapyramidal side-effects of neuroleptics (Snyder *et al.* 1974b), several indirect lines of evidence have implicated cholineric neurotransmission at both muscarinic and nicotinic receptors in the pathophysiology of schizophrenia (Tandon & Greden 1989; Dalack *et al.* 1998; Sarter & Bruno 1998). These include the extremely high prevalence of smoking in schizophrenia – 90% as compared to the general population rate of 25% – which has implicated the nicotinic cholinergic receptor family in the pathophysiology of schizophrenia (for review see Freedman *et al.* 1994; Dalack *et al.* 1998). In addition, Lewy body dementia, a rare disorder, which is accompanied by high rates (70%) of fluctuating bouts of impaired cognitive functioning and episodic psychosis typified by visual and auditory hallucinations and paranoid delusions, is associated with a primary deficiency in cortical cholinergic processing (Perry & Perry 1995). Although the research efforts involving cholinergic function in schizophrenia have been less prevalent than those involving dopamine, 5-HT and amino acid neurotransmitters, the available data for a cholinergic involvement in schizophrenia are, nevertheless, significant and have engendered a great deal of recent interest.

Cholinergic receptors

The cholinergic nicotinic receptor is a ligand-gated ion channel receptor composed of five subunits which are encoded by separate genes. The two families of neuronal nicotinic receptors are named α and β. There are several types of α (α2–α9) and β

($\beta2$–$\beta4$) subunits. Binding studies have so far demonstrated three types of nicotinic receptors with distinct subunit composition and function. These include:
1 'high affinity nicotine binding sites', which are the most abundant sites in the brain and contain $\alpha4$ and $\beta2$ subunits;
2 'α-bungarotoxin' sites, which are named for their high affinity to bind this snake neurotoxin and are composed exclusively of $\alpha7$ subunits; and
3 'neuronal bungaratoxin sites', which are composed of $\alpha3$ subunits and other, as yet unelucidated, α and β subunits.
Binding studies suggest that schizophrenics may have fewer high affinity nicotine and α-bungarotoxin binding sites in the hippocampus, cortex and striatum (Freedman *et al.* 1995; Breese *et al.* 2000; Durany *et al.* 2000).

The most convincing evidence for a nicotinergic involvement in schizophrenia comes from the seminal studies by Freedman *et al.* (1997) implicating a role for $\alpha7$ nicotinic receptor gene in the auditory sensory gating defect observed in schizophrenia. This defect was shown to be linked to a locus on the long arm of chromosome 15 and the gene for the $\alpha7$ nicotinic receptor subunit, which forms the homomeric α-bungarotoxin-sensitive acetycholine receptors. This finding is consistent with functional data from animal and human studies, suggesting that the $\alpha7$ nicotinic receptor is involved in the auditory evoked potential response, and presents some of the most concrete evidence in the literature implicating a neurotransmitter receptor dysfunction in schizophrenia.

Alteration in muscarinic cholinergic receptor binding in postmortem schizophrenic brains has also been reported. In particular, a recent study (Crook *et al.* 2001) found a decrease in binding of M1 and M4 cholinergic receptors, which are the major receptors mediating postsynaptic excitatory effects of acetylcholine in the prefrontal cortex (Brodmann areas 9 and 46) of schizophrenic brains. A similar decrease was also noted in the putamen (Dean *et al.* 1996).

Psychopharmacological studies

The majority of psychotropical plants with identified hallucinogenic compounds, such as jimson weed, contain high levels of antimuscarinic agents such as atropine and scopolamine (Schultes & Hofmann 1992). Injection of jimson weed has been associated with an intoxicated state which could be misdiagnosed as schizophrenia (Mahler 1976; Shervette *et al.* 1979). Although, unlike amphetamines and ketamine, careful and controlled clinical studies on the behavioural pharmacology of anticholinergic drugs are lacking, the limited available data suggest that anticholinergic drugs such as scopolamine and atropine administered to healthy volunteers, or when used therapeutically, can produce an intoxicated state that is associated with hallucinations and delusions (Ketchum *et al.* 1973; Fisher 1991). Accordingly, activation of cholinergic activity using the acetylcholinesterase inhibitor physostigmine, which is known to ameliorate the hallucinations and delusions associated with Alzheimer's disease, may have therapeutic efficacy for treating the cognitive deficits of schizophrenia (Kirrane *et al.* 2001), although no significant effects have been reported in treating the psychosis associated with schizophrenia (Davis *et al.* 1978; Edelstein *et al.* 1981).

Conclusions

The comprehensive literature summarized in this chapter provides an overview of the complexity of neuronal abnormalities that may be associated with schizophrenia. It is now evident that no single heuristic model involving one or two neurotransmitter systems can explain the pathophysiology of this syndrome. Clearly, the field of schizophrenia research is undergoing a transition of moving from psychopharmacology- and neurochemistry-based models to genetic-based models. However, in view of the consensus that the genetic nature of vulnerability to develop schizophrenia is most likely to involve the complex interaction of several genes and the environment, continued efforts to better understand the neurochemical abnormalities of schizophrenia are necessary to provide leads for candidate genes, and to continue establishing the foundation for novel therapeutic approaches for schizophrenia.

References

Abi-Dargham, A. & Krystal, J. (2000) Serotonin receptors as targets of antipsychotic medications. In: *Neurotransmitter Receptors in Actions of Antipsychotic Medications* (ed. M.S. Lidow), pp. 79–107. CRC Press, Boca Raton, FL.

Abi-Dargham, A., Laruelle, M., Lipska, B. *et al.* (1993) Serotonin 5-HT$_3$ receptors in schizophrenia: a postmortem study of the amygdala. *Brain Research* **616**, 53–57.

Abi-Dargham, A., Laruelle, M., Aghajanian, G.K., Charney, D. & Krystal, J. (1997) The role of serotonin in the pathophysiology and treatment of schizophrenia. *Journal of Neuropsychiatry and Clinical Neurosciences* **9**, 1–17.

Abi-Dargham, A., Laruelle, M., Krystal, J. *et al.* (1999) No evidence of altered *in vivo* benzodiazepine receptor binding in schizophrenia. *Neuropsychopharmacology* **20**, 650–661.

Abi-Dargham, A., Rodenhiser, J., Printz, D. *et al.* (2000) From the cover: increased baseline occupancy of D$_2$ receptors by dopamine in schizophrenia [see comments]. *Proceedings of the National Academy of Sciences of the USA* **97**, 8104–8109.

Abi-Saab, W., Seibyl, J.P., D'Souza, D.C. *et al.* (2002) Ritanserin antagonism of *m*-chlorophenylpiperazine (mCPP) effects in neuroleptic-free schizophrenic patients: support for 5-HT$_2$ receptor modulation of schizophrenia symptoms. *Psychopharmacology* **162**, 55–62.

Aghajanian, G.K. & Marek, G.J. (1999) Serotonin and hallucinogens. *Neuropsychopharmacology* **21**, 16S–23S.

Aghajanian, G.K. & Marek, G.J. (2000) Serotonin model of schizophrenia: emerging role of glutamate mechanisms. *Brain Research – Brain Research Reviews* **31**, 302–312.

Akbarian, S., Vinuela, A., Kim, J.J. *et al.* (1993) Distorted distribution of nicotinamide-adenine dinucleotide phosphate-diaphorase neurons in temporal lobe of schizophrenics implies anomalous cortical development. *Archives of General Psychiatry* **50**, 178–187.

Akbarian, S., Kim, J.J., Potkin, S.G. *et al.* (1995) Gene expression for glutamic acid decarboxylase is reduced without loss of neurons in prefrontal cortex of schizophrenics. *Archives of General Psychiatry* **52**, 258–266.

Akbarian, S., Kim, J.J., Potkin, S.G. *et al.* (1996a) Maldistribution of interstitial neurons in prefrontal white matter of the brains of schizophrenic patients. *Archives of General Psychiatry* **53**, 425–436.

Akbarian, S., Sucher, N.J., Bradley, D. *et al.* (1996b) Selective alterations in gene expression for NMDA receptor subunits in prefrontal cortex of schizophrenics. *Journal of Neuroscience* **16**, 19–30.

Akil, M., Pierri, J.N., Whitehead, R.E. *et al.* (1999) Lamina-specific alterations in the dopamine innervation of the prefrontal cortex in schizophrenic subjects. *American Journal of Psychiatry* **156**, 1580–1589.

Anand, A., Charney, D.S., Oren, D.A. *et al.* (2000) Attenuation of the neuropsychiatric effects of ketamine with lamotrigine: support for hyperglutamatergic effects of N-methyl-D-aspartate receptor antagonists. *Archives of General Psychiatry* **57**, 270–276.

Anderson, S.A., Eisenstat, D.D., Shi, L. & Rubenstein, J.L. (1997) Interneuron migration from basal forebrain to neocortex: dependence on Dlx genes. *Science* **278**, 474–476.

Aniline, O. & Pitts, F.N. Jr (1982) Phencyclidine (PCP): a review and perspectives. *Critical Reviews in Toxicology* **10**, 145–177.

Anis, N.A., Berry, S.C., Burton, N.R. & Lodge, D. (1983) The dissociative anaesthetics, ketamine and phencyclidine, selectively reduce excitation of central mammalian neurones by N-methyl-aspartate. *British Journal of Pharmacology* **79**, 565–575.

Aparicio-Legarza, M.I., Cutts, A.J., Davis, B. & Reynolds, G.P. (1997) Deficits of [³H]D-aspartate binding to glutamate uptake sites in striatal and accumbens tissue in patients with schizophrenia. *Neuroscience Letters* **232**, 13–16.

Arnold, S.E., Franz, B.R., Gur, R.C. *et al.* (1995) Smaller neuron size in schizophrenia in hippocampal subfields that mediate cortical–hippocampal interactions. *American Journal of Psychiatry* **152**, 738–748.

Arora, R.C. & Meltzer, H.Y. (1991) Serotonin₂ (5-HT₂) receptor binding in the frontal cortex of schizophrenic patients. *Journal of Neural Transmission – General Section* **85**, 19–29.

Arranz, M., Collier, D., Sodhi, M. *et al.* (1995) Association between clozapine response and allelic variation in 5-HT$_{2A}$ receptor gene. *Lancet* **346**, 281–282.

Arranz, M.J., Lin, M.W., Powell, J., Kerwin, R. & Collier, D. (1996) 5-HT$_{2A}$ receptor T102C polymorphism and schizophrenia. *Lancet* **347**, 1831–1832.

Arranz, M.J., Munro, J., Owen, M.J. *et al.* (1998a) Evidence for association between polymorphisms in the promoter and coding regions of the 5-HT$_{2A}$ receptor gene and response to clozapine. *Molecular Psychiatry* **3**, 61–66.

Arranz, M.J., Munro, J., Sham, P. *et al.* (1998b) Meta-analysis of studies on genetic variation in 5-HT$_{2A}$ receptors and clozapine response. *Schizophrenia Research* **32**, 93–99.

Arranz, M.J., Munro, J., Birkett, J. *et al.* (2000) Pharmacogenetic prediction of clozapine response. *Lancet* **355**, 1615–1616.

Bakker, C.B. & Amini, F.B. (1961) Observations on the psychotomimetic effects of sernyl. *Comparative Psychiatrics* **2**, 269–280.

Beasley, C.L. & Reynolds, G.P. (1997) Parvalbumin-immunoreactive neurons are reduced in the prefrontal cortex of schizophrenics. *Schizophrenia Research* **24**, 349–355.

Benes, F.M. & Berretta, S. (2001) GABAergic interneurons: implications for understanding schizophrenia and bipolar disorder. *Neuropsychopharmacology* **25**, 1–27.

Benes, F.M., McSparren, J., Bird, E.D., SanGiovanni, J.P. & Vincent, S.L. (1991) Deficits in small interneurons in prefrontal and cingulate cortices of schizophrenic and schizoaffective patients. *Archives of General Psychiatry* **48**, 996–1001.

Benes, F.M., Vincent, S.L., Alsterberg, G., Bird, E.D. & SanGiovanni, J.P. (1992) Increased GABAA receptor binding in superficial layers of cingulate cortex in schizophrenics. *Journal of Neuroscience* **12**, 924–929.

Benes, F.M., Vincent, S.L., Marie, A. & Khan, Y. (1996) Upregulation of GABAA receptor binding on neurons of the prefrontal cortex in schizophrenic subjects. *Neuroscience* **75**, 1021–1031.

Benes, F.M., Wickramasinghe, R., Vincent, S.L., Khan, Y. & Todtenkopf, M. (1997) Uncoupling of GABA (A) and benzodiazepine receptor binding activity in the hippocampal formation of schizophrenic brain. *Brain Research* **755**, 121–129.

Bennett, J.P. Jr, Enna, S.J., Bylund, D.B. *et al.* (1979) Neurotransmitter receptors in frontal cortex of schizophrenics. *Archives of General Psychiatry* **36**, 927–934.

Bird, L.M. & Scambler, P. (2000) Cortical dysgenesis in two patients with chromosome 22q11 deletion. *Clinical Genetics* **58**, 64–68.

Birkett, J.T., Arranz, M.J., Munro, J. *et al.* (2000) Association analysis of the 5-HT$_{5A}$ gene in depression, psychosis and antipsychotic response. *Neuroreport* **11**, 2017–2020.

Bolonna, A.A., Kerwin, R.W., Munro, J., Arranz, M.J. & Makoff, A.J. (2001) Polymorphisms in the genes for mGluR types 7 and 8: association studies with schizophrenia. *Schizophrenia Research* **47**, 99–103.

Bowers, M.B.J. (1987) The role of drugs in the production of schizophreniform psychoses and related disorders. In: *Psychopharmacology: the Third Generation of Progress* (ed. H.Y. Meltzer), pp. 819–823. Raven Press, New York.

Bray, N.J., Williams, N.M., Bowen, T. *et al.* (2000) No evidence for association between a non-synonymous polymorphism in the gene encoding human metabotropic glutamate receptor 7 and schizophrenia. *Psychiatric Genetics* **10**, 83–86.

Breese, C.R., Lee, M.J., Adams, C.E. *et al.* (2000) Abnormal regulation of high affinity nicotinic receptors in subjects with schizophrenia. *Neuropsychopharmacology* **23**, 351–364.

Breier, A., Kirkpatrick, B. & Buchanan, R.W. (1993) Clozapine attenuates *meta*-chlorophenylpiperazine (mCPP)-induced plasma cortisol increases in schizophrenia. *Biological Psychiatry* **34**, 492–494.

Bressan, R.A. & Pilowsky, L.S. (2000) Imaging the glutamatergic system *in vivo*: relevance to schizophrenia. *European Journal of Nuclear Medicine* **27**, 1723–1731.

Brodie, T.M. (1959) Psychopharmacology: an evaluation. In: *Biological Psychiatry* (ed. J.H. Masserman), pp. 264–268. Grune & Stratton, New York.

Bruss, M., Bonisch, H., Buhlen, M. *et al.* (1999) Modified ligand binding to the naturally occurring Cys-124 variant of the human serotonin 5-HT$_{1B}$ receptor. *Pharmacogenetics* **9**, 95–102.

Burnet, P.W., Eastwood, S.L. & Harrison, P.J. (1996) 5-HT$_{1A}$ and 5-HT$_{2A}$ receptor mRNAs and binding site densities are differentially altered in schizophrenia. *Neuropsychopharmacology* **15**, 442–455.

Burns, R. & Lerner, L.S. (1976) Perspectives: acute phencyclidine intoxication. *Clinical Toxicology* **9**, 477–501.

Busatto, G.F., Pilowsky, L.S., Costa, D.C. *et al.* (1997) Correlation between reduced *in vivo* benzodiazepine receptor binding and severity of psychotic symptoms in schizophrenia [see comments]. *American Journal of Psychiatry* **154**, 56–63. [Published erratum appears in *American Journal of Psychiatry* 1997; **154**, 722.]

Carlsson, A. (1978) Antipsychotic drugs, neurotransmitters, and schizophrenia. *American Journal of Psychiatry* **135**, 164–173.

Charney, D.S., Woods, S.W., Goodman, W.K. & Heninger, G.R. (1987) Serotonin function in anxiety. II. Effects of the serotonin agonist MCPP in panic disorder patients and healthy subjects. *Psychopharmacology* **92**, 14–24.

Chen, C.H., Lee, Y.R., Wei, F.C. *et al.* (1997) Lack of allelic association between 102T/C polymorphism of serotonin receptor type 2A gene and schizophrenia in Chinese. *Psychiatric Genetics* **7**, 35–38.

Cohen, B.D., Rosenbaum, G., Luby, E.D. & Gottlieb, J.S. (1962) Comparison of phencyclidine hydrochloride (sernyl) with other drugs: simulation of schizophrenic performance with phencyclidine hydrochloride (sernyl), lysergic acid diethylamide (LSD-25), amobarbital (amytal) sodium. II. Symbolic and sequential thinking. *Archives of General Psychiatry* **6**, 79–85.

Conn, J.P. & Pin, J.-P. (1997) Pharmacology and functions of metabotropic glutamate receptors. *Annual Review of Pharmacology and Toxicology* **37**, 205–237.

Coyle, J. (1996) The glutamatergic dysfunction hypothesis for schizophrenia. *Harvard Review of Psychiatry* **3**, 241–253.

Crook, J.M., Tomaskovic-Crook, E., Copolov, D.L. & Dean, B. (2001) Low muscarinic receptor binding in prefrontal cortex from subjects with schizophrenia: a study of Brodmann's areas 8, 9, 10 and 46 and the effects of neuroleptic drug treatment. *American Journal of Psychiatry* **158**, 918–925.

Cross, A.J., Crow, T.J. & Owen, F. (1979) Gamma-aminobutyric acid in the brain in schizophrenia. *Lancet* **1**, 560–561.

Crow, T.J., Baker, H.F., Cross, A.J. *et al.* (1979) Monoamine mechanisms in chronic schizophrenia: post-mortem neurochemical findings. *British Journal of Psychiatry* **134**, 249–256.

Dalack, G.W., Healy, D.J. & Meador-Woodruff, J.H. (1998) Nicotine dependence in schizophrenia: clinical phenomena and laboratory findings. *American Journal of Psychiatry* **155**, 1490–1501.

Davis, K.L., Berger, P.A., Hollister, L.E. & Defraites, E. (1978) Physostigmine in mania. *Archives of General Psychiatry* **35**, 119–122.

Daviss, S.R. & Lewis, D.A. (1995) Local circuit neurons of the prefrontal cortex in schizophrenia: selective increase in the density of calbindin-immunoreactive neurons. *Psychiatry Research* **59**, 81–96.

Deakin, J., Slater, P., Simpson, M. *et al.* (1989) Frontal cortical and left temporal glutamatergic dysfunction in schizophrenia. *Journal of Neuroscience* **52**, 1781–1786.

Dean, B. & Hayes, W. (1996) Decreased frontal cortical serotonin$_{2A}$ receptors in schizophrenia. *Schizophrenia Research* **21**, 133–139.

Dean, B., Opeskin, K., Pavey, G. *et al.* (1995) [^{3}H]paroxetine binding is altered in the hippocampus but not the frontal cortex or caudate nucleus from subjects with schizophrenia. *Journal of Neurochemistry* **64**, 1197–1202.

Dean, B., Crook, J.M., Opeskin, K. *et al.* (1996) The density of muscarinic M1 receptors is decreased in the caudate–putamen of subjects with schizophrenia [see comments]. *Molecular Psychiatry* **1**, 54–58.

Dean, B., Tomaskovic-Crook, E., Opeskin, K., Keks, N. & Copolov, D. (1999a) No change in the density of the serotonin$_{1A}$ receptor, the serotonin$_4$ receptor or the serotonin transporter in the dorsolateral prefrontal cortex from subjects with schizophrenia. *Neurochemistry International* **34**, 109–115.

Dean, B., Hussain, T., Hayes, W. *et al.* (1999b) Changes in serotonin$_{2A}$ and GABA (A) receptors in schizophrenia: studies on the human dorsolateral prefrontal cortex. *Journal of Neurochemistry* **72**, 1593–1599.

Del Rio, J.A., Heimrich, B., Borrell, V. *et al.* (1997) A role for Cajal–Retzlus cells and reelin in the development of hippocampal connections. *Nature* **385**, 70–74.

D'Souza, D.C., Gil, R., MacDougall, L. *et al.* (2002) GABA–serotonin interactions in healthy subjects: implications for psychosis and dissociation. *Archives of General Psychiatry* in press.

Durany, N., Zochling, R., Boissl, K.W. *et al.* (2000) Human postmortem striatal α4β2 nicotinic acetylcholine receptor density in schizophrenia and Parkinson's syndrome. *Neuroscience Letters* **287**, 109–112.

Eastwood, S.L., McDonald, B., Burnet, P.W. *et al.* (1995) Decreased expression of mRNAs encoding non-NMDA glutamate receptors GluR1 and GluR2 in medial temporal lobe neurons in schizophrenia. *Brain Research – Molecular Brain Research* **29**, 211–223.

Eastwood, S.L., Burnet, P.W. & Harrison, P.J. (1997) GluR2 glutamate receptor subunit flip and flop isoforms are decreased in the hippocampal formation in schizophrenia: a reverse transcriptase-polymerase chain reaction (RT-PCR) study. *Brain Research – Molecular Brain Research* **44**, 92–98.

Edelstein, P., Schultz, J.R., Hirschowitz, J., Kanter, D.R. & Garver, D.L. (1981) Physostigmine and lithium response in the schizophrenias. *American Journal of Psychiatry* **138**, 1078–1081.

Egan, C.T., Herrick-Davis, K. & Teitler, M. (1998) Creation of a constitutively activated state of the 5-hydroxytryptamine$_{2A}$ receptor by site-directed mutagenesis: inverse agonist activity of antipsychotic drugs. *Journal of Pharmacology and Experimental Therapeutics* **286**, 85–90.

Erdmann, J., Shimron-Abarbanell, D., Cichon, S. *et al.* (1995) Systematic screening for mutations in the promoter and the coding region of the 5-HT$_{1A}$ gene. *American Journal of Medical Genetics* **60**, 393–399.

Erdmann, J., Nothen, M.M., Shimron-Abarbanell, D. *et al.* (1996a) The human serotonin 7 (5-HT$_7$) receptor gene: genomic organization and systematic mutation screening in schizophrenia and bipolar affective disorder. *Molecular Psychiatry* **1**, 392–397.

Erdmann, J., Shimron-Abarbanell, D., Rietschel, M. *et al.* (1996b) Systematic screening for mutations in the human serotonin-2A (5-HT$_{2A}$) receptor gene: identification of two naturally occurring receptor variants and association analysis in schizophrenia. *Human Genetics* **97**, 614–619.

Fiorella, D., Rabin, R.A. & Winter, J.C. (1995) The role of the 5-HT$_{2A}$ and 5-HT$_{2C}$ receptors in the stimulus effects of m-chlorophenylpiperazine. *Psychopharmacology* **119**, 222–230.

Fisher, C.M. (1991) Visual hallucinations on eye closure associated with atropine toxicity: a neurological analysis and comparison with other visual hallucinations. *Canadian Journal of Neurological Sciences* **18**, 18–27.

Frederick, J.A. & Meador-Woodruff, J.H. (1999) Effects of clozapine and haloperidol on 5-HT$_6$ receptor mRNA levels in rat brain. *Schizophrenia Research* **38**, 7–12.

Freedman, D.X. (1968) On the use and abuse of LSD. *Archives of General Psychiatry* **18**, 330–347.

Freedman, R., Adler, L.E., Bickford, P. *et al.* (1994) Schizophrenia and nicotinic receptors. *Harvard Review of Psychiatry* **2**, 179–192.

Freedman, R., Hall, M., Adler, L.E. & Leonard, S. (1995) Evidence in postmortem brain tissue for decreased numbers of hippocampal nicotinic receptors in schizophrenia. *Biological Psychiatry* **38**, 22–33.

Freedman, R., Coon, H., Myles-Worsley, M. *et al.* (1997) Linkage of a neurophysiological deficit in schizophrenia to a chromosome 15 locus. *Proceedings of the National Academy of Sciences USA* **94**, 587–592.

Gao, X.M., Sakai, K., Roberts, R.C. *et al.* (2000) Ionotropic glutamate receptors and expression of N-methyl-D-aspartate receptor subunits in subregions of human hippocampus: effects of schizophrenia. *American Journal of Psychiat* **157**, 1141–1149.

Gattaz, W.F., Gattaz, D. & Beckmann, H. (1982) Glutamate in

schizophrenics and healthy controls. *Archiv Fur Psychiatrie und Nervenkrankheiten* **231**, 221–225.

Glatt, C.E., Snowman, A.M., Sibley, D.R. & Snyder, S.H. (1995) Clozapine: selective labeling of sites resembling 5-HT$_6$ serotonin receptors may reflect psychoactive profile. *Molecular Medicine* **1**, 398–406.

Goddard, A.W., Mason, G.F., Rothman, D.L., Behar, K.L. & Krystal, J.H. (2002) Reduced cortical GABA neuronal response to benzodiazepine administration in panic disorder. *Biological Psychiatry* (in press).

Goff, D.C. & Coyle, J.T. (2001) The emerging role of glutamate in the pathophysiology and treatment of schizophrenia. *American Journal of Psychiatry* **158**, 1367–1377.

Goff, D.C., Tsai, G., Levitt, J. *et al.* (1999) A placebo-controlled trial of D-cycloserine added to conventional neuroleptics in patients with schizophrenia [see comments]. *Archives of General Psychiatry* **56**, 21–27.

Gouzoulis-Mayfrank, E., Hermle, L., Thelen, B. & Sass, H. (1998) History, rationale and potential of human experimental hallucinogenic drug research in psychiatry. *Pharmacopsychiatry* **31**, 63–68.

Grimwood, S., Slater, P., Deakin, J.F. & Hutson, P.H. (1999) NR2B-containing NMDA receptors are up-regulated in temporal cortex in schizophrenia. *Neuroreport* **10**, 461–465.

Guidotti, A., Auta, J., Davis, J.M. *et al.* (2000) Decrease in reelin and glutamate acid decarboxylase$_{67}$ (GAD$_{67}$) expression in schizophrenia and bipolar disorder. *Archives of General Psychiatry* **57**, 1061–1069.

Gurevich, E.V. & Joyce, J.N. (1997) Alterations in the cortical serotonergic system in schizophrenia: a postmortem study. *Biological Psychiatry* **42**, 529–545.

Hamik, A. & Peroutka, S.J. (1989) 1-(*m*-chlorophenyl) piperazine (mCPP) interactions with neurotransmitter receptors in the human brain. *Biological Psychiatry* **25**, 569–575.

Harrison, P.J., McLaughlin, D. & Kerwin, R.W. (1991) Decreased hippocampal expression of a glutamate receptor gene in schizophrenia. *Lancet* **337**, 450–452.

Hashimoto, T., Nishino, N., Nakai, H. & Tanaka, C. (1991) Increase in serotonin 5-HT$_{1A}$ receptors in prefrontal and temporal cortices of brains from patients with chronic schizophrenia. *Life Sciences* **48**, 355–363.

Hawi, Z., Myakishev, M.V., Straub, R.E. *et al.* (1997) No association or linkage between the 5-HT$_{2A}$/T102C polymorphism and schizophrenia in Irish families. *American Journal of Medical Genetics* **74**, 370–373.

He, L., Li, T., Melville, C. *et al.* (1999) 102T/C polymorphism of serotonin receptor type 2A gene is not associated with schizophrenia in either Chinese or British populations. *American Journal of Medical Genetics* **88**, 95–98.

Healy, D.J., Haroutunian, V., Powchik, P. *et al.* (1998) AMPA receptor binding and subunit mRNA expression in prefrontal cortex and striatum of elderly schizophrenics. *Neuropsychopharmacology* **19**, 278–286.

Hermle, L., Gouzoulis-Mayfrank, E. & Spitzer, M. (1998) Blood flow and cerebral laterality in the mescaline model of psychosis. *Pharmacopsychiatry* **31**, 85–91.

Hernandez, I. & Sokolov, B.P. (2000) Abnormalities in 5-HT$_{2A}$ receptor mRNA expression in frontal cortex of chronic elderly schizophrenics with varying histories of neuroleptic treatment. *Journal of Neuroscience Research* **59**, 218–225.

Herrick-Davis, K., Grinde, E. & Teitler, M. (2000) Inverse agonist activity of atypical antipsychotic drugs at human 5-hydroxytryptamine$_{2C}$ receptors. *Journal of Pharmacology and Experimental Therapeutics* **295**, 226–232.

Humphries, C., Mortimer, A., Hirsch, S. & de Belleroche, J. (1996)

NMDA receptor mRNA correlation with antemortem cognitive impairment in schizophrenia. *Neuroreport* **7**, 2051–2055.

Ibrahim, H.M., Hogg, A.J. Jr, Healy, D.J. *et al.* (2000) Ionotropic glutamate receptor binding and subunit mRNA expression in thalamic nuclei in schizophrenia. *American Journal of Psychiatry* **157**, 1811–1823.

Impagnatiello, F., Guidotti, A.R., Pesold, C. *et al.* (1998) A decrease of reelin expression as a putative vulnerability factor in schizophrenia. *Proceedings of the National Academy of Sciences of the USA* **95**, 15718–15723.

Inayama, Y., Yoneda, H., Sakai, T. *et al.* (1996) Positive association between a DNA sequence variant in the serotonin 2A receptor gene and schizophrenia. *American Journal of Medical Genetics* **67**, 103–105.

Iqbal, N., Asnis, G.M., Wetzler, S. *et al.* (1991) The MCPP challenge test in schizophrenia: hormonal and behavioral responses. *Biological Psychiatry* **30**, 770–778.

Itil, T.M., Keskiner, A., Kiremitci, N. & Holden, J.M.C. (1967) Effect of phencyclidine in chronic schizophrenics. *Canadian Psychiatric Association Journal* **12**, 209–212.

Itil, T.M., Keskiner, S. & Holden, J.M. (1969) The use of LSD and ditran in the treatment of therapy resistant schizophrenics (symptom provocation approach). *Diseases of the Nervous System* **30** (Suppl.), 93–103.

Javitt, D.C. & Zukin, S.R. (1991) Recent advances in the phencyclidine model of schizophrenia. *American Journal of Psychiatry* **148**, 1301–1308.

Javitt, D.C., Jotkowitz, A., Sircar, R. & Zukin, S.R. (1987) Noncompetitive regulation of phencyclidine/sigma-receptors by the N-methyl-D-aspartate receptor antagonist D-(-)-2-amino-5-phosphonovaleric acid. *Neuroscience Letters* **78**, 193–198.

Javitt, D.C., Zylberman, I., Zukin, S.R., Heresco-Levy, U. & Lindenmayer, J.-P. (1994) Amelioration of negative symptoms in schizophrenia by glycine. *American Journal of Psychiat* **151**, 1234–1236.

Joober, R., Benkelfat, C., Brisebois, K. *et al.* (1999) T102C polymorphism in the 5-HT$_{2A}$ gene and schizophrenia: relation to phenotype and drug response variability. *Journal of Psychiatry and Neuroscience* **24**, 141–146.

Joseph, M.H., Baker, H.F., Crow, T.J., Riley, G.J. & Risby, D. (1979) Brain tryptophan metabolism in schizophrenia: a postmortem study of metabolites of the serotonin and kynurenine pathways in schizophrenic and control subjects. *Psychopharmacology* **62**, 279–285.

Kahn, R.S. & Wetzler, S. (1991) *m*-Chlorophenylpiperazine as a probe of serotonin function. *Biological Psychiatry* **30**, 1139–1166.

Kahn, R.S., Siever, L.J., Gabriel, S. *et al.* (1992) Serotonin function in schizophrenia: effects of *meta*-chlorophenylpiperazine in schizophrenic patients and healthy subjects. *Psychiatry Research* **43**, 1–12.

Kahn, R.S., Siever, L., Davidson, M., Greenwald, C. & Moore, C. (1993a) Haloperidol and clozapine treatment and their effect on *m*-chlorophenylpiperazine-mediated responses in schizophrenia: implications for the mechanism of action of clozapine. *Psychopharmacology* **112**, S90–S94.

Kahn, R.S., Davidson, M., Siever, L. *et al.* (1993b) Serotonin function and treatment response to clozapine in schizophrenic patients. *American Journal of Psychiatry* **150**, 1337–1342.

Kahn, R.S., Davidson, M., Siever, L.J., Sevy, S. & Davis, K.L. (1994) Clozapine treatment and its effect on neuroendocrine responses induced by the serotonin agonist, *m*-chlorophenylpiperazine. *Biological Psychiatry* **35**, 909–912.

Kapur, S., Zipursky, R.B. & Remington, G. (1999) Clinical and theoretical implications of 5-HT$_2$ and D$_2$ receptor occupancy of clozapine, risperidone, and olanzepine in schizophrenia. *American Journal of Psychiatry* **156**, 286–293.

Kaufman, D.L., Houser, C.R. & Tobin, A.J. (1991) Two forms of the gamma-aminobutyric acid synthetic enzyme glutamate decarboxylase have distinct intraneuronal distributions and cofactor interactions. *Journal of Neurochemistry* 56, 720–723.

Kawanishi, Y., Harada, S., Tachikawa, H., Okubo, T. & Shiraishi, H. (1998) Novel mutations in the promoter and coding region of the human 5-HT$_{1A}$ receptor gene and association analysis in schizophrenia. *American Journal of Medical Genetics* 81, 434–439.

Kegeles, L.S., Shungu, D.C., Anjilvel, S. *et al.* (2000) Hippocampal pathology in schizophrenia: magnetic resonance imaging and spectroscopy studies. *Psychiatry Research* 98, 163–175.

Kerwin, R., Patel, S. & Meldrum, B. (1990) Quantitative autoradiographic analysis of glutamate binding sites in the hippocampal formation in normal and schizophrenic brain postmortem. *Neuroscience* 39, 25–32.

Ketchum, J.S., Sidell, F.R., Crowell, E.B. Jr, Aghajanian, G.K. & Hayes, A.H. Jr (1973) Atropine, scopolamine, and ditran: comparative pharmacology and antagonists in man. *Psychopharmacologia* 28, 121–145.

Kim, J., Kornhuber, H., Schmid-Burgk, W. & Holzmuller, B. (1980) Low cerebrospinal fluid glutamate in schizophrenic patients and a new hypothesis on schizophrenia. *Neuroscience Letters* 20, 379–382.

Kirrane, R.M., Mitropoulou, V., Nunn, M., Silverman, J. & Siever, L.J. (2001) Physostigmine and cognition in schizotypal personality disorder. *Schizophr Research* 48, 1–5.

Koreen, A.R., Lieberman, J.A., Alvir, J. & Chakos, M. (1997) The behavioral effect of *m*-chlorophenylpiperazine (mCPP) and methylphenidate in first-episode schizophrenia and normal controls. *Neuropsychopharmacology* 16, 61–68.

Kornhuber, J., Mack-Burkhardt, F., Riederer, P. *et al.* (1989) [^{3}H]MK-801 binding sites in postmortem brain regions of schizophrenic patients. *Journal of Neural Transmission* 77, 231–236.

Korpi, E.R., Kaufmann, C.A., Marnela, K.M. & Weinberger, D.R. (1987) Cerebrospinal fluid amino acid concentrations in chronic schizophrenia. *Psychiatry Research* 20, 337–345.

Kouzmenko, A.P., Scaffidi, A., Pereira, A.M. *et al.* (1999) No correlation between A (-1438) G polymorphism in 5-HT$_{2A}$ receptor gene promoter and the density of frontal cortical 5-HT$_{2A}$ receptors in schizophrenia. *Human Heredity* 49, 103–105.

Krystal, J.H., Seibyl, J.P., Price, L.H. *et al.* (1990) MCPP effects in schizophrenic patients: effects of pharmacotherapy. *Society of Neuroscience Abstracts* 16, 244–246.

Krystal, J.H., Seibyl, J.P., Price, L.H. *et al.* (1993) *m*-Chlorophenylpiperazine effects in neuroleptic-free schizophrenic patients: evidence implicating serotonergic systems in the positive symptoms of schizophrenia. *Archives of General Psychiatry* 50, 624–635.

Krystal, J.H., Karper, L.P., Seibyl, J.P. *et al.* (1994) Subanesthetic effects of the non-competitive NMDA antagonist, ketamine, in humans: psychotomimetic, perceptual, cognitive, and neuroendocrine responses. *Archives of General Psychiatry* 51, 199–214.

Krystal, J.H., Abi-Dargham, A., Laruelle, M. & Moghaddam, B. (1999a) Pharmacologic model psychoses. In: *Neurobiology of Mental Illness* (eds D.S. Charney, E. Nestler & B.S. Bunney), pp. 214–224. Oxford University Press, New York.

Krystal, J.H., D'Souza, D.C., Belge, A. *et al.* (1999b) Therapeutic implications of the hyperglutamatergic effects of NMDA antagonists. *Neuropsychopharmacology* 21, S143–S157.

Lahti, A.C., Holocomb, H.H., Medoff, D.R. & Tammings, C.A. (1995) Ketamine activates psychosis and alters limbic blood flow in schizophrenia. *Neuroreport* 6, 869–872.

Laruelle, M., Abi-Dargham, A., Casanova, M.F. *et al.* (1993) Selective abnormalities of prefrontal serotonergic receptors in schizophrenia: a postmortem study. *Archives of General Psychiatry* 50, 810–818.

Laruelle, M., Abi-Dargham, A., van Dyck, C. *et al.* (2000) Dopamine and serotonin transporters in patients with schizophrenia: an imaging study with [^{123}I]β-CIT. *Biological Psychiatry* 47, 371–379.

Lewis, D.A. (2000) GABAergic local circuit neurons and prefrontal cortical dysfunction in schizophrenia. *Brain Research – Brain Research Reviews* 31, 270–276.

Lewis, D.A., Pierri, J.N., Volk, D.W., Melchitzky, D.S. & Woo, T.U. (1999a) Altered GABA neurotransmission and prefrontal cortical dysfunction in schizophrenia. *Biological Psychiatry* 46, 616–626.

Lewis, R., Kapur, S., Jones, C. *et al.* (1999b) Serotonin 5-HT$_2$ receptors in schizophrenia: a PET study using [^{18}F]setoperone in neuroleptic-naive patients and normal subjects. *American Journal of Psychiatry* 156, 72–78.

Lin, C.H., Tsai, S.J., Yu, Y.W. *et al.* (1999) No evidence for association of serotonin-2A receptor variant (102T/C) with schizophrenia or clozapine response in a Chinese population. *Neuroreport* 10, 57–60.

Lodge, D. & Anis, N.A. (1982) Effects of phencyclidine on excitatory amino acid activation of spinal interneurones in the cat. *European Journal of Pharmacology* 77, 203–204.

Luby, E., Cohen, B., Rosenbaum, G., Gottlieb, J. & Kelley, R. (1959) Study of a new schizophrenomimetic drug: sernyl. *American Medical Association Archives of Neurological Psychiatry* 81, 363–369.

Maes, M. & Meltzer, H.Y. (1996) Effects of *meta*-chlorophenylpiperazine on neuroendocrine and behavioral responses in male schizophrenic patients and normal volunteers. *Psychiatry Research* 64, 147–159.

Mahler, D.A. (1976) Anticholinergic poisoning from Jimson weed. *Journal of the American College of Emergency Physicians* 5, 440–442.

Malhotra, A.K., Goldman, D., Buchanan, R., Breier, A. & Pickar, D. (1996a) 5-HT$_{2A}$ receptor T102C polymorphism and schizophrenia. *Lancet* 347, 1830–1831.

Malhotra, A.K., Pinals, D.A., Weingartner, H. *et al.* (1996b) NMDA receptor function and human coginition: the effects of ketamine in healthy volunteers. *Neuropsychopharmacology* 14, 301–307.

Malhotra, A.K., Pinals, D.A., Adler, C.M. *et al.* (1997) Ketamine-induced exacerbation of psychotic symptoms and cognitive impairment in neuroleptic-free schizophrenics. *Neuropsychopharmacology* 17, 141–150.

Malhotra, A.K., Goldman, D., Mazzanti, C. *et al.* (1998) A functional serotonin transporter (5-HTT) polymorphism is associated with psychosis in neuroleptic-free schizophrenics. *Molecular Psychiatry* 3, 328–332.

Marek, G.J., Wright, R.A., Schoepp, D.D., Monn, J.A. & Aghajanian, G.K. (2000) Physiological antagonism between 5-hydroxytryptamine (2A) and group II metabotropic glutamate receptors in prefrontal cortex. *Journal of Pharmacology and Experimental Therapeutics* 292, 76–87.

Masellis, M., Basile, V., Meltzer, H.Y. *et al.* (1998) Serotonin subtype 2 receptor genes and clinical response to clozapine in schizophrenia patients. *Neuropsychopharmacology* 19, 123–132.

Masellis, M., Basile, V.S., Meltzer, H.Y. *et al.* (2001) Lack of association between the T→C 267 serotonin 5-HT$_6$ receptor gene (HTR6) polymorphism and prediction of response to clozapine in schizophrenia. *Schizophrenia Research* 47, 49–58.

Maurel, S., Schreiber, R. & De Vry, J. (1998) Role of 5-HT$_{1B}$, 5-HT$_{2A}$ and 5-HT$_{2C}$ receptors in the generalization of 5-HT receptor agonists to the ethanol cue in the rat. *Behavioural Pharmacology* 9, 337–343.

Meador-Woodruff, J.H. & Healy, D.J. (2000) Glutamate receptor expression in schizophrenic brain. *Brain Research – Brain Research Reviews* 31, 288–294.

Meador-Woodruff, J.H., Davis, K.L. & Haroutunian, V. (2001) Abnormal kainate receptor expression in prefrontal cortex in schizophrenia. *Neuropsychopharmacology* **24**, 545–552.

Meltzer, H.Y., Jackman, H. & Arora, R.C. (1980) Brain and skeletal muscle monoamine oxidase activity in schizophrenia. *Schizophrenia Bulletin* **6**, 208–212.

Meltzer, H.Y., Matsubara, S. & Lee, J.C. (1989) Classification of typical and atypical antipsychotic drugs on the basis of dopamine D-1, D-2 and serotonin$_2$ pKi values. *Journal of Pharmacology and Experimental Therapeutics* **251**, 238–246.

Meneses, A., Terron, J.A. & Hong, E. (1997) Effects of the 5-HT receptor antagonists GR127935 (5-HT1B/1D) and MDL100907 (5-HT$_{2A}$) in the consolidation of learning. *Behavioural Brain Research* **89**, 217–223.

Miller, M.W. (1993) Migration of cortical neurons is altered by gestational exposure to ethanol. *Alcoholism: Clinical and Experimental Research* **17**, 304–314.

Mita, T., Hanada, S., Nishino, N. *et al.* (1986) Decreased serotonin S2 and increased dopamine D$_2$ receptors in chronic schizophrenics. *Biological Psychiatry* **21**, 1407–1414.

Mizukami, K., Sasaki, M., Ishikawa, M. *et al.* (2000) Immunohistochemical localization of gamma-aminobutyric acid (B) receptor in the hippocampus of subjects with schizophrenia. *Neuroscience Letters* **283**, 101–104.

Moghaddam, B. & Adams, B. (1998) Reversal of phencyclidine effects by a group II metabotropic glutamate receptor agonist in rats. *Science* **281**, 1349–1352.

Moghaddam, B., Adams, B., Verma, A. & Daly, D. (1997) Activation of glutamatergic neurotransmission by ketamine: a novel step in the pathway from NMDA receptor blockade to dopaminergic and cognitive disruptions associated with the prefrontal cortex. *Journal of Neuroscience* **17**, 2921–2927.

Newcomer, J.W., Farber, N.B., Jevtovic-Todorovic, V. *et al.* (1999) Ketamine-induced NMDA receptor hypofunction as a model of memory impairment and psychosis. *Neuropsychopharmacology* **20**, 106–118.

Ngan, E.T., Yatham, L.N., Ruth, T.J. & Liddle, P.F. (2000) Decreased serotonin 2A receptor densities in neuroleptic-naive patients with schizophrenia: a PET study using [^{18}F]setoperone. *American Journal of Psychiatry* **157**, 1016–1018.

Niesler, B., Weiss, B., Fischer, C. *et al.* (2001) Serotonin receptor gene HTR$_{3A}$ variants in schizophrenic and bipolar affective patients. *Pharmacogenetics* **11**, 21–27.

Nimgaonkar, V.L., Zhang, X.R., Brar, J.S., DeLeo, M. & Ganguli, R. (1996) 5-HT$_2$ receptor gene locus: association with schizophrenia or treatment response not detected. *Psychiatric Genetics* **6**, 23–27.

Nishiguchi, N., Shirakawa, O., Ono, H., Hashimoto, T. & Maeda, K. (2000) Novel polymorphism in the gene region encoding the carboxyl-terminal intracellular domain of the NMDA receptor 2B subunit: analysis of association with schizophrenia. *American Journal of Psychiatry* **157**, 1329–1331.

Nishikawa, T., Takashima, M. & Toru, M. (1983) Increased [^{3}H]kainic acid binding in the prefrontal cortex in schizophrenia. *Neuroscience Letters* **40**, 245–250.

Noga, J.T., Hyde, T.M., Herman, M.M. *et al.* (1997) Glutamate receptors in the postmortem striatum of schizophrenic, suicide, and control brains. *Synapse* **27**, 168–176.

Noga, J.T., Hyde, T.M., Bachus, S.E., Herman, M.M. & Kleinman, J.E. (2001) AMPA receptor binding in the dorsolateral prefrontal cortex of schizophrenics and controls. *Schizophrenia Research* **48**, 361–363.

Ogawa, M., Miyata, T., Nakajima, K. *et al.* (1995) The reeler gene-associated antigen on Cajal–Retzius neurons is a crucial molecule for laminar organization of cortical neurons. *Neuron* **14**, 899–912.

Ohara, K., Nagai, M., Tani, K. & Tsukamoto, T. (1999) Schizophrenia and the serotonin-2A receptor promoter polymorphism. *Psychiatry Research* **85**, 221–224.

Ohnuma, T., Augood, S.J., Arai, H., McKenna, P.J. & Emson, P.C. (1998) Expression of the human excitatory amino acid transporter 2 and metabotropic glutamate receptors 3 and 5 in the prefrontal cortex from normal individuals and patients with schizophrenia. *Brain Research – Molecular Brain Research* **56**, 207–217.

Ohnuma, T., Augood, S.J., Arai, H., McKenna, P.J. & Emson, P.C. (1999) Measurement of GABAergic parameters in the prefrontal cortex in schizophrenia: focus on GABA content, GABA (A) receptor α-1 subunit messenger RNA and human GABA transporter-1 (HGAT-1) messenger RNA expression. *Neuroscience* **93**, 441–448.

Okubo, Y., Suhara, T., Suzuki, K. *et al.* (2000) Serotonin 5-HT$_2$ receptors in schizophrenic patients studied by positron emission tomography. *Life Sciences* **66**, 2455–2464.

Olney, J. & Farber, N. (1995) Glutamate receptor dysfunction and schizophrenia. *Archives of General Psychiatry* **52**, 998–1007.

Owen, R.R. Jr, Gutierrez-Esteinou, R., Hsiao, J. *et al.* (1993) Effects of clozapine and fluphenazine treatment on responses to *m*-chlorophenylpiperazine infusions in schizophrenia. *Archives of General Psychiatry* **50**, 636–644.

Pariseau, C., Gregor, P., Myles-Worsley, M. *et al.* (1994) Schizophrenia and glutamate receptor genes. *Psychiatric Genetics* **4**, 161–165.

Perry, E.K. & Perry, R.H. (1995) Acetylcholine and hallucinations: disease-related compared to drug-induced alterations in human consciousness. *Brain and Cognition* **28**, 240–258.

Perry, T.L. (1982) Normal cerebrospinal fluid and brain glutamate levels in schizophrenia do not support the hypothesis of glutamatergic neuronal dysfunction. *Neuroscience Letters* **28**, 81–85.

Perry, T.L., Kish, S.J., Buchanan, J. & Hansen, S. (1979) Gamma-aminobutyric-acid deficiency in brain of schizophrenic patients. *Lancet* **1**, 237–239.

Pilz, D.T. & Quarrell, O.W. (1996) Syndromes with lissencephaly. *Journal of Medical Genetics* **33**, 319–323.

Porter, R.H., Eastwood, S.L. & Harrison, P.J. (1997) Distribution of kainate receptor subunit mRNAs in human hippocampus, neocortex and cerebellum, and bilateral reduction of hippocampal GluR6 and KA2 transcripts in schizophrenia. *Brain Research* **751**, 217–231.

Rajakowaska, G., Selemon, I. & Goldman-Rakic, P. (1998) Neuronal and glial somal size in the prefrontal cortex. A postmortem study of schizophrenia and Huntington disease. *Archives of General Psychiatry* **55**, 215–224.

Rao, D., Jonsson, E.G., Paus, S. *et al.* (1998) Schizophrenia and the serotonin transporter gene. *Psychiatric Genetics* **8**, 207–212.

Reveley, M.A., Glover, V., Sandler, M. & Spokes, E.G. (1981) Brain monoamine oxidase activity in schizophrenics and controls. *Archives of General Psychiatry* **38**, 663–665.

Reynolds, G.P., Czudek, C. & Andrews, H.B. (1990) Deficit and hemispheric asymmetry of GABA uptake sites in the hippocampus in schizophrenia. *Biological Psychiatry* **27**, 1038–1044.

Richardson-Burns, S.M., Haroutunian, V., Davis, K.L., Watson, S.J. & Meador-Woodruff, J.H. (2000) Metabotropic glutamate receptor mRNA expression in the schizophrenic thalamus. *Biological Psychiatry* **47**, 22–28.

Riley, B.P., Tahir, E., Rajagopalan, S. *et al.* (1997) A linkage study of the N-methyl-D-aspartate receptor subunit gene loci and schizophrenia in southern African Bantu-speaking families. *Psychiatric Genetics* **7**, 57–74.

Rimvall, K., Sheikh, S.N. & Martin, D.L. (1993) Effects of increased gamma-aminobutyric acid levels on GAD67 protein and mRNA levels in rat cerebral cortex. *Journal of Neurochemistry* **60**, 714–720.

Robbins, T. (1997) Arousal systems and attentional processes. *Biological Psychiatry* 45, 57–71.

Rosenbaum, G., Cohen, B.D., Luby, E.D., Gottlieb, J.S. & Yelen, D. (1959) Comparison of sernyl with other drugs: simulation of schizophrenic performance with sernyl, LSD-25, and amobarbital (amytal) sodium. I. Attention, motor function, and proprioception. *Archives of General Psychiatry* 1, 651–656.

Sarter, M. & Bruno, J.P. (1998) Cortical acetylcholine, reality distortion, schizophrenia, and Lewy Body Dementia: too much or too little cortical acetylcholine? *Brain and Cognition* 38, 297–316.

Schoeffter, P. & Hoyer, D. (1989) Interaction of arylpiperazines with 5-HT$_{1A}$, 5-HT$_{1B}$, 5-HT$_{1C}$ and 5-HT$_{1D}$ receptors: do discriminatory 5-HT$_{1B}$ receptor ligands exist? *Naunyn-Schmiedeberg's Archives of Pharmacology* 339, 675–683.

Schultes, R.E. & Hofmann, A. (1992) *Plants of the Gods*. Healing Arts Press, Rochester.

Seeman, P., Lee, T., Chau-Wong, M. & Wong, K. (1976) Antispsychotic drug doses and neuroleptic/dopamine receptors. *Nature* 261, 717–719.

Seibyl, J.P., Krystal, J.H., Price, L.H. *et al.* (1991) Effects of ritanserin on the behavioral, neuroendocrine, and cardiovascular responses to *meta*-chlorophenylpiperazine in healthy human subjects. *Psychiatry Research* 38, 227–236.

Selemon, L.D., Rajkowska, G. & Goldman-Rakic, P.S. (1995) Abnormally high neuronal density in the schizophrenic cortex: a morphometric analysis of prefrontal area 9 and occipital area 17. *Archives of General Psychiatry* 52, 805–818; discussion, 819–820.

Selemon, L.D., Rajkowska, G. & Goldman-Rakic, P.S. (1998) Elevated neuronal density in prefrontal area 46 in brains from schizophrenic patients: application of a three-dimensional, stereologic counting method. *Journal of Comparative Neurology* 392, 402–412.

Serretti, A., Catalano, M. & Smeraldi, E. (1999) Serotonin transporter gene is not associated with symptomatology of schizophrenia. *Schizophrenia Research* 35, 33–39.

Serretti, A., Cusin, C., Lorenzi, C. *et al.* (2000) Serotonin-2A receptor gene is not associated with symptomatology of schizophrenia. *American Journal of Medical Genetics* 96, 84–87.

Shervette, R.E. III, Schydlower, M., Lampe, R.M. & Fearnow, R.G. (1979) Jimson 'loco' weed abuse in adolescents. *Pediatrics* 63, 520–523.

Simpson, M.D., Slater, P., Deakin, J.F., Royston, M.C. & Skan, W.J. (1989) Reduced GABA uptake sites in the temporal lobe in schizophrenia. *Neuroscience Letters* 107, 211–215.

Simpson, M.D., Slater, P., Royston, M.C. & Deakin, J.F.W. (1992) Regionally selective deficits in uptake sites for glutamate and gamma-aminobutyric acid in the basal ganglia in schizophrenia. *Psychiatry Research* 42, 273–282.

Simpson, M.D., Lubman, D.I., Slater, P. & Deakin, J.F. (1996) Autoradiography with [^{3}H]8-OH-DPAT reveals increases in 5-HT (1A) receptors in ventral prefrontal cortex in schizophrenia. *Biological Psychiatry* 39, 919–928.

Sircar, R., Rappaport, M., Nichtenhauser, R. & Zukin, S.R. (1987) The novel anticonvulsant MK-801: a potent and specific ligand of the brain phencyclidine/sigma-receptor. *Brain Research* 435, 235–240.

Snyder, S., Banerjee, S. & Yamamura, H. (1974a) Drugs, neurotransmitters and schizophrenia. *Science* 184, 1243–1253.

Snyder, S.H., Greenberg, D. & Yamumura, H.I. (1974b) Antischizophrenic drugs: affinity for muscarinic cholinergic receptor sites in the brain predicts extrapyramidal effects. *Journal of Psychiatrics Research* 11, 91–95.

Sokolov, B.P. (1998) Expression of NMDAR1, GluR1, GluR7, and KA1 glutamate receptor mRNAs is decreased in frontal cortex of 'neuroleptic-free' schizophrenics: evidence on reversible up-regulation by typical neuroleptics. *Journal of Neurochemistry* 71, 2454–2464.

Spurlock, G., Heils, A., Holmans, P. *et al.* (1998) A family based association study of T102C polymorphism in 5-HT$_{2A}$ and schizophrenia plus identification of new polymorphisms in the promoter. *Molecular Psychiatry* 3, 42–49.

Strassman, R.J. (1996) Human psychopharmacology of N,N-dimethyltryptamine. *Behavioural Brain Research* 73, 121–124.

Strassman, R.J., Qualls, C.R., Uhlenhuth, E.H. & Kellner, R. (1994) Dose–response study of N,N-dimethyltryptamine in humans. II. Subjective effects and preliminary results of a new rating scale. *Archives of General Psychiatry* 51, 98–108.

Sumiyoshi, T., Stockmeier, C.A., Overholser, J.C., Dilley, G.E. & Meltzer, H.Y. (1996) Serotonin$_{1A}$ receptors are increased in postmortem prefrontal cortex in schizophrenia. *Brain Research* 708, 209–214.

Tamminga, C.A. (1998) Schizophrenia and glutamatergic transmission. *Critical Reviews in Neurobiology* 12, 21–36.

Tandon, R. & Greden, J.F. (1989) Cholinergic hyperactivity and negative schizophrenic symptoms: a model of cholinergic–dopaminergic interactions in schizophrenia. *Archives of General Psychiatry* 46, 745–753.

Tarantal, A.F., Salamat, M.S., Britt, W.J. *et al.* (1998) Neuropathogenesis induced by rhesus cytomegalovirus in fetal rhesus monkeys (*Macaca mulatta*). *Journal of Infectious Diseases* 177, 446–450.

Tay, A.H., Lim, L.C., Lee, W.L. *et al.* (1997) Association between allele 1 of T102C polymorphism, 5-hydroxytryptamine 2a receptor gene and schizophrenia in Chinese males in Singapore. *Human Heredity* 47, 298–300.

Todtenkopf, M.S. & Benes, F.M. (1998) Distribution of glutamate decarboxylase$_{65}$ immunoreactive puncta on pyramidal and nonpyramidal neurons in hippocampus of schizophrenic brain. *Synapse* 29, 323–332.

Trichard, C., Paillere-Martinot, M.L., Attar-Levy, D. *et al.* (1998) No serotonin 5-HT$_{2A}$ receptor density abnormality in the cortex of schizophrenic patients studied with PET. *Schizophrenia Research* 31, 13–17.

Trimble, M.R. (1987) Anticonvulsant drugs and cognitive function: a review of the literature. *Epilepsia* 28, S37–S45.

Tsai, G., Passani, L.A., Slusher, B.S. *et al.* (1995) Abnormal excitatory neurotransmitter metabolism in schizophrenic brains. *Archives of General Psychiatry* 52, 829–836.

Uher, B.F. & Golden, J.A. (2000) Neuronal migration defects of the cerebral cortex: a destination debacle. *Clinical Genetics* 58, 16–24.

Verhoeff, N.P., Soares, J.C., D'Souza, D.C. *et al.* (1999) [^{123}I]iomazenil SPECT benzodiazepine receptor imaging in schizophrenia. *Psychiatry Research Neuroimaging* 91, 163–173.

Verhoeff, N.P., Meyer, J.H., Kecojevic, A. *et al.* (2000) A voxel-by-voxel analysis of [^{18}F]setoperone PET data shows no substantial serotonin 5-HT (2A) receptor changes in schizophrenia. *Psychiatry Research* 99, 123–135.

Vincent, J.P., Kartalovski, B., Geneste, P., Kamenka, J.M. & Lazdunski, M. (1979) Interaction of phencyclidine ('angel dust') with a specific receptor in rat brain membranes. *Proceedings of the National Academy of Sciences of the USA* 76, 4678–4682.

Vogt, I.R., Shimron-Abarbanell, D., Neidt, H. *et al.* (2000) Investigation of the human serotonin 6 [5-HT$_6$] receptor gene in bipolar affective disorder and schizophrenia. *American Journal of Medical Genetics* 96, 217–221.

Volk, D.W., Austin, M.C., Pierri, J.N., Sampson, A.R. & Lewis, D.A. (2000) Decreased glutamic acid decarboxylase$_{67}$ messenger RNA expression in a subset of prefrontal cortical gamma-aminobutyric acid neurons in subjects with schizophrenia. *Archives of General Psychiatry* 57, 237–245.

Volk, D., Austin, M., Pierri, J., Sampson, A. & Lewis, D. (2001) GABA transporter-1 mRNA in the prefrontal cortex in schizophrenia: decreased expression in a subset of neurons. *American Journal of Psychiatry* **158**, 256–265.

Vollenweider, F.X. (1998) Advances and pathophysiological models of hallucinogenic drug actions in humans: a preamble to schizophrenia research. *Pharmacopsychiatry* **31**, 92–103.

Vollenweider, F.X., Leenders, K.L., Scharfetter, C. *et al.* (1997) Positron emission tomography and fluorodeoxyglucose studies of metabolic hyperfrontality and psychopathology in the psilocybin model of psychosis. *Neuropsychopharmacology* **16**, 357–372.

Vollenweider, F.X., Vollenweider-Scherpenhuyzen, M.F., Babler, A., Vogel, H. & Hell, D. (1998) Psilocybin induces schizophrenia-like psychosis in humans via a serotonin-2 agonist action. *Neuroreport* **9**, 3897–3902.

Wassef, A.A., Dott, S.G., Harris, A. *et al.* (1999) Critical review of GABA-ergic drugs in the treatment of schizophrenia. *Journal of Clinical Psychopharmacology* **19**, 222–232.

Weissman, A.D., Casanova, M.F., Kleinman, J.E., London, E.D. & De Souza, E.B. (1991) Selective loss of cerebral cortical sigma, but not PCP binding sites in schizophrenia. *Biological Psychiatry* **29**, 41–54.

Whitaker, P.M., Crow, T.J. & Ferrier, I.N. (1981) Tritiated LSD binding in frontal cortex in schizophrenia. *Archives of General Psychiatry* **38**, 278–279.

Widerlov, E. (1988) A critical appraisal of CSF monoamine metabolite studies in schizophrenia. *Annals of the New York Academy of Sciences* **537**, 309–323.

Williams, J., Spurlock, G., McGuffin, P. *et al.* (1996) Association between schizophrenia and T102C polymorphism of the 5-hydroxytryptamine type 2a-receptor gene. European Multicentre Association Study of Schizophrenia (EMASS) Group. *Lancet*, **347**, 1294–1296.

Williams, J., McGuffin, P., Nothen, M. & Owen, M.J. (1997) Meta-analysis of association between the 5-HT$_{2A}$ receptor T102C polymorphism and schizophrenia. EMASS Collaborative Group, European Multicentre Association Study of Schizophrenia. *Lancet* **349**, 1221.

Willins, D.L., Berry, S.A., Alsayegh, L. *et al.* (1999) Clozapine and other 5-hydroxytryptamine-2A receptor antagonists alter the subcellular distribution of 5-hydroxytryptamine-2A receptors *in vitro* and *in vivo. Neuroscience* **91**, 599–606.

Wilson, M.A. & Molliver, M.E. (1991) The organization of serotonergic projections to cerebral cortex in primates: regional distribution of axon terminals. *Neuroscience* **44**, 537–553.

Wolkowitz, O.M. & Pickar, D. (1991) Benzodiazepines in the treatment of schizophrenia: a review and reappraisal. *American Journal of Psychiatry* **148**, 714–726.

Wong, E.H., Knight, A.R. & Woodruff, G.N. (1988) [^{3}H]MK-801 labels a site on the N-methyl-D-aspartate receptor channel complex in rat brain membranes. *Journal of Neurochemistry* **50**, 274–281.

Woo, T.U., Miller, J.L. & Lewis, D.A. (1997) Schizophrenia and the parvalbumin-containing class of cortical local circuit neurons. *American Journal of Psychiatry* **154**, 1013–1015.

Woo, T.U., Whitehead, R.E., Melchitzky, D.S. & Lewis, D.A. (1998) A subclass of prefrontal gamma-aminobutyric acid axon terminals are selectively altered in schizophrenia. *Proceedings of the National Academy of Sciences of the USA* **95**, 5341–5346.

Yu, Y.W., Tsai, S.J., Lin, C.H. *et al.* (1999) Serotonin-6 receptor variant (C267T) and clinical response to clozapine. *Neuroreport* **10**, 1231–1233.

Zhukovskaya, N.L. & Neumaier, J.F. (2000) Clozapine downregulates 5-hydroxytryptamine$_6$ (5-HT$_6$) and upregulates 5-HT$_7$ receptors in HeLa cells. *Neuroscience Letters* **288**, 236–240.

Zukin, S.R. & Zukin, R.S. (1979) Specific [^{3}H]phencyclidine binding in rat central nervous system. *Proceedings of the National Academy of Sciences of the USA* **76**, 5372–5376.

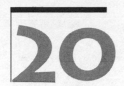

20 Dopamine transmission in the schizophrenic brain

M. Laruelle

Dopaminergic systems in the brain, 366
  Dopaminergic projections, 366
  Dopaminergic receptors, 368
Studies documenting alterations of dopamine
    systems in schizophrenia, 368
  Postmortem studies, 368
  Imaging studies, 370
Discussion, 376
  Cortical regulation of subcortical dopamine
    transmission, 376

Schizophrenia and endogenous sensitization, 378
Beyond the dopaminergic synapse, 379
Dopamine in the history of the schizophrenic
    brain, 379
Conclusions, 380
Acknowledgements, 381
References, 381

The 'classical' dopamine (DA) hypothesis of schizophrenia proposed that hyperactivity of DA transmission is responsible for the positive symptoms (hallucinations, delusions) observed in this disorder (Carlsson & Lindqvist 1963). This hypothesis was supported by the correlation between clinical doses of antipsychotic drugs and their potency to block DA D_2 receptors (Seeman & Lee 1975; Creese *et al.* 1976) and by the psychotogenic effects of DA enhancing drugs (for review see Angrist & van Kammen 1984; Lieberman *et al.* 1987). These critical pharmacological observations suggest, but do not establish, the existence of a dysregulation of DA transmission in schizophrenia.

On the other hand, negative and cognitive symptoms of the illness are generally resistant to treatment by antipsychotic drugs (Keefe *et al.* 1999). Impairment in higher cognitive functions, such as working memory, is one of the most enduring symptoms of schizophrenia and a strong predictor of poor clinical outcome (Green 1996). Functional brain imaging studies suggest that these symptoms might be associated with a dysfunction of the prefrontal cortex (PFC) (for reviews see Weinberger 1987; Knable & Weinberger 1997). Studies in non-human primates demonstrated that a deficit in DA transmission in PFC and lack of stimulation of D_1 receptors (the main DA receptor subtype in the PFC) induce cognitive impairments reminiscent of the ones observed in patients with schizophrenia (Goldman-Rakic & Selemon 1997; Goldman-Rakic 1999; Goldman-Rakic *et al.* 2000). Together, these observations suggest that a deficit in DA transmission at D_1 receptors in the PFC might be implicated in the cognitive impairments and negative symptoms presented by these patients.

Thus, the current view on DA and schizophrenia proposes that schizophrenia might be associated with a dopaminergic imbalance, involving an excess of subcortical DA function and a deficit in cortical DA function: subcortical mesolimbic DA projections might be hyperactive (resulting in hyperstimulation of D_2 receptors and positive symptoms) while mesocortical DA projections to the PFC might be hypoactive (resulting in hypo-

stimulation of D_1 receptors, negative symptoms and cognitive impairment). This view is commonly referred to as the 'revised' dopamine hypothesis of schizophrenia (Weinberger 1987; Davis *et al.* 1991).

Despite decades of effort to generate experimental data supporting these hypotheses, documentation of abnormalities of DA function in schizophrenia has remained elusive. Postmortem studies measuring DA and its metabolites and DA receptors in the brains of schizophrenic patients has yielded inconsistent or inconclusive results (for review see Davis *et al.* 1991). The lack of clear evidence for altered dopaminergic indices in schizophrenia prompted some authors to propose that DA transmission in schizophrenia might be essentially normal and elevated only relative to other systems, such as the glutamatergic or serotonergic system (Carlsson 1988; Meltzer 1989). Under this perspective, the antipsychotic properties of D_2 receptor blockade do not derive from correcting a hyperdopaminergic state, but from re-establishing an appropriate balance between DA and other neuronal systems. Yet, the absence of data supporting the DA hypothesis of schizophrenia might be a result of the difficulty in obtaining a direct measurement of DA transmission in the living human brain. Over the last few years, progress in brain imaging methods has enabled direct measurement of DA transmission at D_2 receptors, and the application of these techniques to the study of schizophrenia has provided new insights into the nature and the role of DA function dysregulation in this illness.

This chapter reviews postmortem and imaging studies that directly evaluated indices of DA transmission in the brain of patients with schizophrenia. We focus on a simple question: what is the current evidence that schizophrenia *per se* is associated with alteration in DA transmission? This chapter focuses special attention on recent brain imaging results aimed at direct measurement of DA transmission. Because these new scanning techniques have been used to study D_2 receptor transmission in subcortical areas (i.e. striatum), the discussion focuses more on

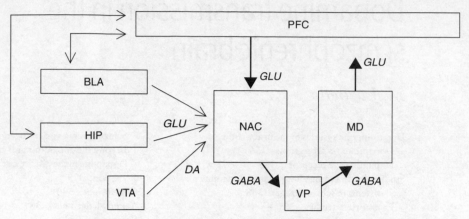

Fig 20.1 Schematic representation of ventral limbic circuits implicated in the positive symptoms of schizophrenia (adapted from Grace *et al.* 1998). The nucleus accumbens (NAC) receives major excitatory inputs from prefrontal cortex (PFC), basolateral amygdala (BLA) and hippocampus (HIP) and DA input from ventral tegmental area (VTA). NAC sends inputs to the ventral pallidum (VP) which projects to the mediodorsal nucleus (MD) of the thalamus. MD provides excitatory inputs back to PFC. The NAC is a crucial node in this circuit where inputs from the PFC are gated by excitatory projections from HIP and BLA and DA projections from VTA. It is proposed that, in schizophrenia, increased DA activity induces perturbation in the information flow within this circuit, in the modulation of this information by hippocampus and amygdala, and in the gating of sensory information by the thalamus. If sustained, the increase in DA activity might lead to neuroplastic changes in this circuit resulting in the emergence of psychotic experience.

subcortical DA systems and their relationships with positive symptoms in schizophrenia. This focus does not imply that the second arm of the imbalance hypothesis (mesocortical DA deficit) is not important. The data supporting this hypothesis are also reviewed. However, direct measurement of DA function in the PFC *in vivo* in humans is not currently feasible and, currently, direct evidence for alteration of DA transmission in the PFC is still limited. Development of new techniques to image DA transmission in the neocortex is under way in several laboratories and will, in the future, provide a more complete picture of alterations of DA systems in schizophrenia.

A review of data on DA parameters in the brain of patients with schizophrenia is preceded by a brief overview of the anatomy and pharmacology of DA systems, to put into context the interpretation and discussion of these results.

Dopaminergic systems in the brain

Dopaminergic projections

Dopaminergic projections are classically divided into nigrostriatal, mesolimbic and mesocortical systems (Lindvall & Björklund 1983). The nigrostriatal system projects from the substantia nigra (SN) to the dorsal striatum, and has been classically involved in cognitive integration, habituation, sensorimotor co-ordination and initiation of movement. The mesolimbic system projects from the ventral tegmental area (VTA) to limbic structures such as ventral striatum (the part of the striatum that is rostral and ventral to the anterior commissure and which includes the nucleus accumbens, shell and core,

and the ventral parts of the caudate and putamen), hippocampus and amygdala. The mesocortical system projects from the VTA to cortical regions, mostly orbitofrontal, medial prefrontal and cingulate cortices, but also to the dorsolateral prefrontal cortex (DLPFC) and temporal and parietal cortex. The mesolimbic and mesocortical systems are involved in regulation of motivation, attention and reward (Mogenson *et al.* 1980).

Corticostriatal–thalamocortical loops are important targets of DA modulation. The general scheme of these loops involves projections from the cortex to striatum to the internal segment of the globus pallidum (GPi) or the SN pars reticulata (SNr) to thalamus and back to the cortex. These loops have been functionally classified into 'limbic' loops (medial prefrontal and orbitofrontal cortex and anterior cingulate cortex–ventral striatum–ventral pallidum–mediodorsal thalamic nuclei–cortex), associative loops (associative areas of the cortex including DLPFC–precommisural putamen and most of the caudate–GPi/SNr–ventral anterior thalamic nuclei–cortex) and motor loops (primary motor cortex, premotor cortex and supplementary motor area–postcommisural putamen and dorsolateral region of the caudate–GPi/SNr–ventral anterior thalamic nuclei–cortex) (Alexander *et al.* 1986; Hoover & Strick 1993; Parent & Hazrati 1995a; Ferry *et al.* 2000; Joel & Weiner 2000). The amygdala and hippocampus also provide significant inputs to the ventral striatum, contributing to information integration into the limbic loop (Everitt *et al.* 1991; Kunishio & Haber 1994; Pennartz *et al.* 1994; Grace 2000). A schematic representation of the limbic loop is provided in Fig. 20.1. Animal studies suggest that the nucleus accumbens is the critical region in which both typical and atypical antipsychotic drugs exert their antipsychotic effects (Chiodo & Bunney 1983; Deutch *et al.* 1991,

1992; Robertson *et al.* 1994), and the connection of this region supports the hypothesis that information processing into the ventral striatum (VST) provides a critical link between limbic and associative cortical areas.

It important to note that these different corticostriatal–thalamocortical loops are not completely segregated parallel loops. While corticostriatal–thalamic loops do generally re-enter the cortical area that provides input to the striatal subregions involved in these loops, thus forming closed circuits and serving segregating processes, they also project back to other areas of the cortex, forming open circuits and serving integrative processes (Joel & Weiner 2000).

Within each loop, the striatum output reaches the GPi/SNr via a direct pathway and via an indirect pathway that traverses the external segment of the globus pallidus (GPe) and the subthalamic nuclei (STN), both pathways providing antagonistic inputs to the GPi/SNr (DeLong *et al.* 1985; Albin *et al.* 1989; Gerfen 1992; Joel & Weiner 2000). The schematic circuitry of these pathways is presented in Fig. 20.2. Corticostriatal projections are glutamatergic, striatopallidal and pallidothalamic projections are GABAergic, and thalamocortical projections are glutamatergic. It follows that activation of striatal neurones of the direct pathway by glutamatergic inputs from the cortex results in decreased activity of the pallidostriatal inhibitory projections to the thalamus, and that the direct pathway is generally considered as stimulatory. Projections from the striatum to the GPe and from the GPe to the STN are GABAergic, and from the STN back to GPe and to GPi/SNr are glutamatergic. Activation of the indirect pathway is generally considered as providing an inhibitory effect of thalamocortical neurones (DeLong *et al.* 1985). The view of the antagonistic nature of the direct/stimulatory pathway vs. the indirect/inhibitory pathway has been criticized as oversimplistic (Parent & Hazrati 1995b). Nevertheless, it is important to keep in mind that activation of medium spiny GABAergic neurones in the striatum by corticostriatal glutamatergic afferents can provide both stimulatory and inhibitory influences on thalamocortical projections (Carlsson *et al.* 1999b).

DA modulates the flow of information within these loops. In primates, DA cells from the VTA projects to the ventral striatum and cortex, the dorsal tier of the SN includes cells that project to all striatal regions and cortex, and the ventral tier of the SN projects widely throughout the dorsal striatum but not to the cortex (for review see Haber & Fudge 1997). The striatum provides GABA projections back to the VTA and SN. Projections from the VST to midbrain DA neurones are not restricted to the VTA and dorsal tier of the SN (where DA neurones projecting to the VST are located), but also terminate in the ventral tier of SN (where DA neurones projecting to the dorsal striatum are located). Based on these observations, Haber proposed that the DA system provides a bridge by which information circulating in the ventral limbic corticostriatal–thalamocortical loops spirals along nigrostriatal loops and feeds into the cognitive and sensory motor loops, translating drives into actions (Haber & Fudge 1997; Haber *et al.* 2000; Joel & Weiner 2000).

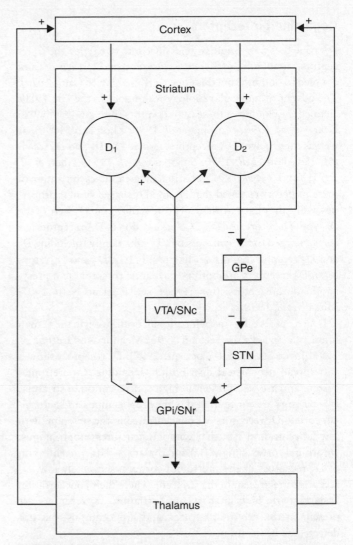

Fig 20.2 Schematic representation of the direct and indirect pathways (adapted from Gerfen 1992; Carlsson *et al.* 1999b) and their modulation by D_1 and D_2 receptors. D_1 receptors are expressed in the dynorphin and substance P expressing striatal GABAergic neurones that provide inhibition to the GABAergic neurones of the internal segment of the globus pallidum (GPi) and the SN pars reticulata (SNr). GPi and SNr provide inhibitory projections to thalamocortical neurones. This direct pathway is stimulatory (even number of GABA neurones). Stimulation of D_1 receptors activates this pathway, and reinforces glutamatergic inputs from the cortex. Thus, glutamate inputs from the cortex and DA input from the VTA and SN pars compacta (SNc) to D_1 receptors act synergistically to activate the direct pathways. D_2 receptors are expressed in enkephalin expressing striatal GABAergic neurones that are the source of the indirect pathway. This pathway sends inhibitory projections to the external segment of the globus pallidus (GPe), which, in turn, sends inhibitory projections to the subthalamic nucleus (STN). STN projections to the GPi/SNr are glutamatergic. This direct pathway is inhibitory (odd number of GABA neurones). Stimulation of D_2 receptors inhibits this pathway, and antagonizes glutamatergic projections from the cortex. Thus, in the indirect pathways, DA oppose the action of glutamatergic cortical afferents via D_2 receptor. This classical scheme is an oversimplification; however, it helps to understand that stimulation of both D_1 and D_2 receptors by DA might be synergistic, despite having opposite intracellular effects and how antipsychotic drugs, by blocking D_2 rather than D_1 receptors, might facilitate the flow of glutamatergic transmission from the cortex.

Dopaminergic receptors

DA receptors were originally classified into two types: the D_1 receptors, stimulating adenylate cyclase; and the D_2 receptors, not coupled to or inhibiting this effector (Kebabian & Calne 1979). The advent of molecular biology techniques in the late 1980s enabled the cloning of these two receptors (Bunzow *et al.* 1988; Dearry *et al.* 1990; Monsma *et al.* 1990; Zhou *et al.* 1990), as well as three newer DA receptors, termed D_3, D_4 and D_5 receptors (Sokoloff *et al.* 1990; Sunahara *et al.* 1991; Tiberi *et al.* 1991; Van Tol *et al.* 1991). Pharmacological characterization of these receptors revealed that D_1 and D_5 shared similar properties, while the pharmacological profiles of D_3 and D_4 were of the D_2 type. Therefore, the D_1–D_2 classification of DA receptors has been enlarged to the concepts of a D_1-like family (including D_1 and D_5 receptors) and a D_2-like family (D_2, D_3 and D_4 receptors). D_2 receptors are both postsynaptic receptors and presynaptic autoreceptors (for review see Palermo-Neto 1997; Missale *et al.* 1998).

DA receptors differ in their regional localization in the human brain (for reviews see Seeman 1992; Meador-Woodruff *et al.* 1996; Joyce & Meador-Woodruff 1997). D_1 receptors show a widespread neocortical distribution, including the prefrontal cortex, and are also present in high concentration in striatum. D_5 receptors are concentrated in the hippocampus and entorhinal cortex. D_2 receptors are concentrated in the striatum, with low concentration in medial temporal structures (hippocampus, entorhinal cortex, amygdala) and thalamus. The concentration of D_2 receptors in the prefrontal cortex is extremely low. D_3 receptors are present in the striatum, where their concentration is particularly high in the ventral striatum. D_4 receptors are present in the prefrontal cortex and hippocampus, but not detected in the striatum.

In the striatum, D_2 receptors are preferentially found in enkephalin-rich GABAergic neurones that participate in the indirect pathways, while D_1 receptors are most abundant in dynorphin/substance P GABAergic neurones that contribute to the direct pathways (Le Moine *et al.* 1990, 1991; Gerfen 1992; Hersch *et al.* 1995). The magnitude of the segregation vs. coexpression of D_1 and D_2 receptors in striatal neurones is still a matter of debate (Surmeier *et al.* 1992, 1996). In the VST, D_3 receptors colocalize preferentially on neurones expressing D_1 receptors (Schwartz *et al.* 1998). The segregation of D_2 and D_1 receptors on different and antagonistic pathways might account for the fact that activation of these receptors is often synergistic at the behavioural level (e.g. stimulation of both D_1 and D_2 receptors stimulate locomotion), while their effects on intracellular signalling (starting with adenylate cyclase activity) are opposite in many regards. For example, stimulation of D_1 and D_2 receptors increases or decreases DARP32 phosphorylation, induces or blocks *c-fos* expression, promotes or inhibits *N*-methyl-D-aspartate (NMDA) receptor function respectively (Nguyen *et al.* 1992; Nishi *et al.* 1997; Konradi 1998; Leveque *et al.* 2000; Dunah & Standaert 2001). Thus, activation of D_2 receptors by DA might provide an inhibitory influence to the indirect pathway and activation of D_1 receptors by DA might provide a stimulatory influence on the direct pathway. Both effects are expected to result in stimulation of thalamocortical neurones (Fig. 20.2).

However, the action of DA on target neurones should not be viewed in terms of simple excitation or inhibition. Unlike classical 'fast' transmitters, DA does not directly gate ion channels, but stimulation of DA G-protein-linked receptor induces a cascade of intracellular signalling that results in modifying the response of the cells to other transmitters. DA is neither 'inhibitory' or 'excitatory', but its action will depend on the state of the neurones at the time of the stimulation (Yang *et al.* 1999). In the striatum, DA modulates the response of GABAergic medium spiny neurones to glutamatergic drive from the cortex. In this structure, it has been proposed that DA is 'reinforcing' (i.e. augmenting) the inhibition of neurones that are inhibited and the excitability of neurones that are excited (Wickens 2000). In this manner, DA acts to gate glutamatergic inputs by increasing their signal/noise ratio. Moreover, DA input might produce long-term changes in the strength of corticostriatal glutamatergic synapses (long-term depression, LTD, and long-term potentiation, LTP) (Arbuthnott *et al.* 2000; Kerr & Wickens 2001), a process which might underlie DA-mediated incentive learning and have a role in the plasticity associated with the emergence of positive symptoms upon prolonged DA hyperactivity.

In the prefrontal cortex, $D_{1/5}$ receptors are localized both on pyramidal cells (dendritic spines and shafts) and on axonal terminals of non-dopaminergic neurones (Smiley *et al.* 1994), while some data suggest that D_4 receptors might be localized on GABA interneurones (Mrzljak *et al.* 1996). DA modulates pyramidal cell excitability, both directly and via GABAergic interneurones (Yang *et al.* 1999). Recent data suggest that DA differently affects GABAergic activity in the PFC via D_1- or D_2-like mechanisms, whereas $D_{1/5}$ and $D_{2/4}$ receptor stimulation enhances or inhibits GABAergic activity respectively. Here again, it has been proposed that DA increases the signal/noise ratio of glutamatergic afferents (Seamans *et al.* 2001).

Studies documenting alterations of dopamine systems in schizophrenia

Postmortem studies

The discovery of the antipsychotic effect of D_2 receptor blockade inspired decades of postmortem research seeking to determine if schizophrenia was associated with alterations of DA transmission parameters. This large body of research has so far failed to provide definitive answers, partly because of the confounding effect of antemortem antipsychotic treatment.

Tissue DA and HVA

Direct measures of tissue content of DA and its metabolites failed to demonstrate consistent and reproducible abnormalities (for review see Cross *et al.* 1981; Reynolds 1989; Davis *et al.* 1991). It should be noted, however, that some studies reported higher DA tissue levels in samples from patients with schizophrenia, compared with controls, in subcortical regions such as caudate (Owen *et al.* 1978), accumbens (Mackay *et al.* 1982) or amygdala (Reynolds 1983), and that no studies reported lower DA content in these regions in patients compared with controls.

D_2 receptors

Increased density of striatal D_2 receptors in patients with schizophrenia measured with [^{3}H]spiperone and other [^{3}H] neuroleptic drugs has been a consistent finding in a large number of postmortem studies (Lee *et al.* 1978; Owen *et al.* 1978; Mackay *et al.* 1982; Cross *et al.* 1983; Seeman *et al.* 1984, 1987; Mita *et al.* 1986; Hess *et al.* 1987; Reynolds *et al.* 1987; Joyce *et al.* 1988). This upregulation was also observed in the SN (Owen *et al.* 1984). However, because chronic neuroleptic administration upregulates D_2 receptor density (Burt *et al.* 1977), it is unclear if these postmortem findings are related to prior neuroleptic exposure or to the disease process *per se*. In light of these very consistent results with [^{3}H]spiperone, it is interesting to note that the striatal binding of [^{3}H]raclopride has been reported to be increased in many studies (Ruiz *et al.* 1992; Sumiyoshi *et al.* 1995; Dean *et al.* 1997; Marzella *et al.* 1997), but normal in several others (Seeman *et al.* 1993; Knable *et al.* 1994; Lahti *et al.* 1996a), even in patients exposed to neuroleptic drugs prior to death. This observation suggests that the increase in [^{3}H]raclopride binding is of lower magnitude than that of [^{3}H]spiperone binding. This discrepancy might simply reflect the observation that, for reasons that are not currently understood, antipsychotic drugs upregulate more [^{3}H]spiperone than [^{3}H]raclopride binding to D_2 receptors (Schoots *et al.* 1995; Tarazi *et al.* 1997).

D_4 receptors

Based on ligand subtraction techniques, several studies reported increased D_4-like receptors in schizophrenia (Seeman *et al.* 1993; Murray *et al.* 1995; Sumiyoshi *et al.* 1995; Marzella *et al.* 1997). These findings, combined with the relative higher affinity of clozapine for D_4 relative to other DA receptors, prompted the hypothesis that D_4 receptors might play a critical part in the pathophysiology of the illness (Seeman *et al.* 1995). Yet, elevation of D_4-like receptors in the striatum of patients with schizophrenia was not confirmed by other studies using the same subtraction technique (Reynolds & Mason 1994; Lahti *et al.* 1996a), nor by one study using the selective D_4 ligand [^{3}H]NGD 94-1 (Lahti *et al.* 1996b). Moreover, the hypothesis that clozapine might act by blocking D_4 receptors (Van Tol *et al.* 1991) was not supported by a clinical trial with the D_4 selective agent L745, 870 (Kramer *et al.* 1997).

D_3 receptors

Gurevich *et al.* (1997) reported a significant increase (almost twofold) in D_3 receptor number in postmortem samples of ventral striata from patients with schizophrenia who were off neuroleptics at the time of death. In contrast, D_3 receptor binding was normal in patients on neuroleptics at the time of death. This finding is particularly interesting because D_3 receptor overexpression does not appear to be a consequence of prior neuroleptic exposure (Joyce & Gurevich 1999). This finding is of potential great significance, given the localization of D_3 receptors in the ventral striatum. In addition, D_3 receptors upregulate in the presence of hyperdopaminergic tone (Fauchey *et al.* 2000), and it is tempting to speculate that the D_3 receptor increase observed in schizophrenia might be secondary to increased dopaminergic tone in the mesolimbic systems. However, D_3 receptor mRNA levels were reported to be normal in the accumbens (Meador-Woodruff *et al.* 1997).

D_1 receptors

Striatal D_1 receptors were generally reported as unaltered in schizophrenia (Pimoule *et al.* 1985; Seeman *et al.* 1987; Joyce *et al.* 1988; Reynolds & Czudek 1988), although one study reported decreased density (Hess *et al.* 1987). In the prefrontal cortex, one study reported no change (Laruelle *et al.* 1990), and one study reported a non-significant increase (Knable *et al.* 1996). D_1 receptor mRNA levels were reported unchanged in both PFC and striatum (Meador-Woodruff *et al.* 1997).

DA transporters

A large number of studies reported unaltered DA transporter (DAT) density in the striatum of patients with schizophrenia. Six out of six postmortem studies of striatal DAT concentration, using a variety of radioligands, reported no alteration in DAT density in striatal tissue of patients with schizophrenia compared with controls: binding of [^{3}H]GBR-12935 (Hirai *et al.* 1988; Czudek & Reynolds 1989; Pearce *et al.* 1990), [^{3}H]mazindol (Joyce *et al.* 1988; Chinaglia *et al.* 1992) and [^{3}H]CFT (Knable *et al.* 1994) was not statistically different in samples from schizophrenic patients compared with controls.

Tyrosine hydroxylase immunolabelling

A recent and interesting postmortem finding regarding DA parameters in patients with schizophrenia is the observation of decreased tyrosine hydroxylase (TH) labelled axons in layers III and VI of the entorhinal cortex (EC) and in layer VI of the PFC, a finding suggesting that schizophrenia might be associated with a deficit in DA transmission in the EC and PFC (Akil *et al.* 1999, 2000). This finding was clearly unrelated to premortem neuroleptic exposure. Benes *et al.* (1997) observed no significant changes in TH positive varicosities in the DLPFC. In the anterior cingulate region (layer II), Benes *et al.* (1997) observed a significant shift in the distribution of TH varicosities from large to small neurones.

In conclusion, postmortem measurements of indices of DA transmission generated two consistent observations in the striatum: (1) the binding of radioligand to D_2-like receptors in the striatum of patients with schizophrenia is increased, but the magnitude of this increase varies with the type of radioligands used, and it is difficult to exclude the contribution of premortem antipsychotic exposure in this set of findings; (2) striatal DAT and D_1 receptor density is unaffected in schizophrenia. Several interesting observations such as the increase in D_3 receptors in the ventral striatum and alteration in TH immunolabelling in several cortical regions do not appear to be consequences of pre-mortem neuroleptic exposure, but these findings have yet to be independently confirmed.

Imaging studies

Imaging studies of DA receptors in schizophrenia

The advent, in the early 1980s, of receptor imaging in living subjects with positron emission tomography (PET) made it possible to evaluate the density of DA receptors and transporters in drug-free and drug-naïve patients with schizophrenia.

Striatal D_2 receptor density in schizophrenia has been extensively studied with PET and single photon emission computerized tomography (SPECT) imaging. Studies comparing parameters of D_2 receptor binding in patients with schizophrenia and healthy controls ($n = 17$ studies) are listed in Table 20.1, and included a total of 245 patients (112 were neuroleptic-naive, and 133 were neuroleptic-free for variable periods of time). These patients were compared with 231 controls, matched for age and sex. Eleven studies used PET and six studies used SPECT. Radiotracers included butyrophenones ([^{11}C]N-methyl-spiperone, [^{11}C]NMSP, $n = 4$; [^{76}Br]bromospiperone, $n = 3$), benzamides ([^{11}C]raclopride, $n = 3$; [^{123}I]IBZM, $n = 5$) or the ergot derivative [^{76}Br]lisuride ($n = 2$).

Only two out of 17 studies detected a significant elevation of D_2 receptor density parameters at a level of $P < 0.05$. However, meta-analysis of the 17 studies reveals a small but significant elevation of D_2 receptors in patients with schizophrenia. If D_2 receptor density did not differ between patients and controls (null hypothesis), one would expect approximately 50% of the studies to report lower D_2 receptor levels in schizophrenics compared with controls. Instead, 13 out of 17 studies reported an increase (although not significant in 11 out of 13 cases), two reported no change, and only two studies reported a decrease in patients compared with controls. This distribution is unlikely ($P < 0.05$, sign test) under the null hypothesis. The average effect size (mean value in schizophrenic group − mean value in control group/SD in control group) of the 17 studies was 0.51 ± 0.76 (SD), and the probability to yield such effect size under the null hypothesis is again < 0.05. The aggregate magnitude of this elevation is thus 51% of the SD of controls. Given an average control SD of 23%, the effect is about 12%. To detect an effect size of 0.51 at 0.05 significance level with a power of 80%, a sample of 64 patients and 64 controls would be needed. Clearly, none of the studies included enough patients to detect this small effect with appropriate power.

No clinical correlates of increased D_2 receptor binding parameters have been reliably identified. Thus, the simplest conclusions from these studies are: that untreated or never-treated patients with schizophrenia show a modest elevation in D_2 receptor density parameters (of about 12%) of undetermined clinical significance; that all studies were underpowered; and that the positive results occasionally reported (Crawley *et al.* 1986; Wong *et al.* 1986) are caused by a sampling effect. These conclusions are reached under the assumptions that all studies measured parameters from the 'same' D_2 receptor population. Clearly, the aggregate D_2 receptor increase reported *in vivo* in drug-free patients is lower than the increase reported in post-mortem studies, supporting the idea that postmortem results were significantly affected by antemortem medications.

Studies performed with butyrophenones ($n = 7$) have an effect size of 0.96 ± 1.05, while studies performed with other ligands (benzamides and lisuride, $n = 10$) have an effect size of 0.20 ± 0.26, a difference that is significant ($P = 0.04$). This observation suggests that the *in vivo* increase in butyrophenone binding might be larger than the increase in benzamide binding. Unfortunately, no studies have been reported in which the same subjects were scanned with both ligands. Such a study is warranted to directly test this proposition. Several hypotheses have been advanced to account for the existence of a differential increase in [^{11}C]NMSP *in vivo* binding in patients with schizophrenia in the face of normal *in vivo* benzamide binding. Because [^{11}C]raclopride and [^{123}I]IBZM bind to D_2 and D_3 receptors while [^{11}C]NMSP bind to D_2, D_3 and D_4 receptors, this difference could reflect a selective elevation of D_4 receptors in schizophrenia (Seeman *et al.* 1993) but this hypothesis has not been substantiated (Lahti *et al.* 1998). Another hypothesis derives from the observation that D_2 receptors, like several G-protein-coupled receptors, exist in monomers, dimers and other oligomeric forms (Ng *et al.* 1994, 1996; Zawarynski *et al.* 1998; Lee *et al.* 2000). Photoaffinity labelling experiments suggested that butyrophenones detect only monomers, while benzamides detect both monomers and dimers. Thus, increased butyrophenone binding and normal benzamide binding might reflect a higher monomer/dimer ratio in schizophrenia. This interesting hypothesis deserves further exploration. A third proposition evolved around the idea that the binding of these ligands would display different vulnerability to competition by endogenous DA (Seeman 1988; Seeman *et al.* 1989). This proposition was based on two assumptions:

1 the concentration of DA in the proximity of D_2 receptors might be higher in patients compared with controls; and
2 [^{11}C]NMSP might be less affected than [^{11}C]raclopride or [^{123}I]IBZM binding by endogenous DA competition.

It follows that D_2 receptor density measured *in vivo* with [^{11}C]raclopride and [^{123}I]IBZM would be 'underestimated' to a greater extent in patients with schizophrenia than in control subjects. This hypothesis played an important part in bringing the endogenous competition concept to the attention of the imaging field (see below).

One PET study with [^{11}C]SCH 23390 reported decreased

Table 20.1 Imaging studies of striatal D_2 receptor parameters in drug-naive and drug-free patients with schizophrenia.

Class radiotracer	Radiotracer	Study	Controls (n)	Patients (n) (DN/DF)*	Method	Outcome	Controls (n) (mean±SD)*	Patients (n) (mean±SD)*	P	Effect size†	Ratio SD
Butyrophenones	[11C]NMSP	(Wong et al. 1986)	11	15 (10/5)	Kinetic	B_{max}	100±50	253±105	<0.05	3.06	2.10
	[76Br]SPI	(Crawley et al. 1986)	8	16 (12/4)	Ratio	S/C	100±14	111±12	<0.05	0.79	0.86
	[76Br]SPI	(Blin et al. 1989)	8	8 (0/8)	Ratio	S/C	100±14	104±14	ns	0.28	1.00
	[76Br]SPI	(Martinot et al. 1990)	12	12 (0/12)	Ratio	S/C	100±11	101±15	ns	0.14	1.41
	[11C]NMSP	(Tune et al. 1993)	17	10 (8/2)	Kinetic	B_{max}	100±80	173±143	0.08	0.91	1.79
	[11C]NMSP	(Nordstrom et al. 1995)	7	7 (7/0)	Kinetic	B_{max}	100±25	133±63	ns	1.33	2.50
	[11C]NMSP	(Okubo et al. 1997)	18	17 (10/7)	Kinetic	k_3	100±21	104±16	ns	0.19	0.74
Benzamides	[11C]Raclopride	(Farde et al. 1990)	20	18 (18/0)	Equilib.	B_{max}	100±29	107±18	ns	0.23	0.63
	[11C]Raclopride	(Hietala et al. 1994)	10	13 (0/13)	Equilib.	B_{max}	100±22	112±43	ns	0.55	1.99
	[123I]IBZM	(Pilowsky et al. 1994)	20	20 (17/3)	Ratio	S/FC	100±8	99±7	ns	-0.07	0.82
	[123I]IBZM	(Laruelle et al. 1996)	15	15 (1/14)	Equilib.	BP	100±26	115±33	ns	0.56	1.25
	[123I]IBZM	(Knable et al. 1997)	16	21 (1/20)	Equilib.	BP	100±29	97±38	ns	-0.12	1.31
	[11C]Raclopride	(Breier et al. 1997)	12	11 (6/5)	Equilib.	BP	100±18	100±30	ns	0.02	1.69
	[123I]IBZM	(Abi-Dargham et al. 2000b)	18	18 (8/10)	Equilib.	BP	100±13	104±14	ns	0.33	1.11
Ergot Alk.	[76Br]Lisuride	(Martinot et al. 1991)	14	19 (10/9)	Ratio	S/C	100±10	104±12	ns	0.45	1.21
	[76Br]Lisuride	(Martinot et al. 1994)	10	10 (2/8)	Ratio	S/C	100±10	100±13	ns	0.00	1.29

DF, drug free; DN, drug naive; Equilib, equilibrium; ns, not significant; B_{max}, maximal density of binding sites; S, striatum; C, cerebellum, k_3, association rate constant; FC, frontal cortex; BP, binding potential.

* Mean normalized to mean of control subjects.

† Effect size calculated as (mean patients – mean controls)/SD controls.

density of D_1 receptors in the PFC of patients with schizophrenia (Okubo *et al.* 1997). No significant differences were found in the other regions examined (anterior cingulate, temporal, occipital and striatum). In addition, low PFC D_1 density was associated with the severity of negative symptoms and poor performance on the Wisconsin Card Sorting Test (WCST). This finding is important because it provides direct evidence for an association between negative symptoms, working memory deficits and selective alteration in prefrontal DA function. However, the camera used in this study had a limited resolution, and the low specific/non-specific ratio of [11C]SCH3390 makes the measurement of D_1 receptor in PFC with this ligand quite vulnerable to noise (Karlsson *et al.* 1997). Several groups are currently attempting to replicate this finding, using better cameras and a superior D_1 receptor radiotracer, [11C]NNC 112 (Abi-Dargham *et al.* 2000a).

Imaging amphetamine-induced DA release in schizophrenia

Neuroreceptor imaging studies with PET and SPECT are classically aimed at measuring neuroreceptor parameters in the living human brain. More recently, several groups demonstrated that, under specific conditions, *in vivo* neuroreceptor binding techniques can also be used to measure acute fluctuations in the concentration of endogenous transmitters in the vicinity of radiolabelled receptors (Dewey *et al.* 1991; Innis *et al.* 1992; Carson *et al.* 1997; Laruelle *et al.* 1997b). Competition between radiotracers and transmitters for binding to neuroreceptors is the principle underlying this approach, although other mechanisms such as agonist-induced receptor internalization might also have a role (for review see Laruelle 2000a). So far, applications of this new paradigm have been mainly developed to study DA transmission at D_2 receptors.

The amphetamine-induced reduction in [123I]IBZM or [11C]raclopride BP has been well validated as an indirect measure of the changes in synaptic DA concentration induced by the challenge (Breier *et al.* 1997; Laruelle *et al.* 1997b; Kegeles *et al.* 1999). Several studies (Table 20.2) reported that amphetamine-induced DA release is increased in patients with schizophrenia compared with matched healthy controls (Laruelle *et al.* 1996, 1999; Breier *et al.* 1997; Abi-Dargham *et al.* 1998). In our sample, the amphetamine-induced reduction in [123I]IBZM BP was $7.5 \pm 7.1\%$ in control subjects ($n = 34$) and $17.1 \pm 13.2\%$ in patients with schizophrenia ($n = 34$, $P = 0.0003$; Fig. 20.3). A similar finding was reported by Breier *et al.* (1997) using [11C]raclopride, PET and a smaller dose of amphetamine (0.2 mg/kg, i.v.). This increased effect of amphetamine on [123I]IBZM BP in patients with schizophrenia was not related to differences in amphetamine plasma disposition, because amphetamine plasma levels were similar in both groups. Provided that the affinity of D_2 receptors for DA is unchanged in this illness (see discussion in Laruelle *et al.* 1999), these data are consistent with increased amphetamine-induced DA release in schizophrenia.

The amphetamine effect on [123I]IBZM BP was similar between chronic/previously treated patients and first episode/neuroleptic-naive patients, and both groups were significantly different from controls. In the previously treated group, no association was found between the duration of the neuroleptic-free period and the amphetamine-induced [123I]IBZM displacement. Together, these data indicated that the exaggerated dopaminergic response to amphetamine exposure was not a prolonged side-effect of previous neuroleptic exposure.

In patients with schizophrenia, the amphetamine challenge induced a significant increase in positive symptoms. The emergence or worsening of positive symptoms was transient, and patients returned to their baseline symptomatology within a few hours of the challenge. We observed a significant correlation between the increase in positive symptoms and the [123I]IBZM displacement ($r = 0.54$, $P = 0.0009$; Fig. 20.4). This result provided direct evidence that exaggerated activation of DA transmission at D_2 receptors mediates the expression of psychotic symptoms following amphetamine challenge. However, DA-mediated stimulation of D_2 receptors explained only about 30% of the variance in the positive symptom changes, indicating that other factors play a part in the exacerbation of these symptoms following amphetamine.

We tested associations between the amphetamine effect on [123I]IBZM BP and several demographic and clinical variables in the patients group, in an attempt to characterize the profile of patients with exaggerated response. Symptom severity *per se* (whether positive or negative symptoms) at baseline was not predictive of the amphetamine effect on D_2 receptor transmission. No association was found between the amphetamine effect and age, gender, race, subject socioeconomic status, familial socioeconomic status, duration of illness or number of previous hospitalizations. However, patients who were experiencing an illness exacerbation (identified by the fact that their admission was motivated by clinical reasons) presented a higher amphetamine-induced [123I]IBZM displacement ($23.7 \pm 13.2\%$, $n = 17$) than patients who were in remission and recruited as outpatients ($10.5 \pm 9.7\%$, $n = 17$, $P = 0.002$). Furthermore, amphetamine-induced [123I]IBZM displacement in remitted patients ($10.5 \pm 9.7\%$, $n = 17$) was not statistically different from controls ($7.5 \pm 7.1\%$, $n = 36$, $P = 0.27$). This observation suggests that dysregulation of DA release in patients with schizophrenia might be present only during episodes of illness exacerbation. Studying the same patients during exacerbation and remission phases is required to confirm this point.

An important question raised by these studies is whether the stress associated with psychiatric hospitalization and/or the scanning procedure might account for the excess DA release measured in patients with schizophrenia, because stress activates DA release (Deutch *et al.* 1990; Kalivas & Duffy 1995). To investigate this potential confounding factor, we recently studied amphetamine-induced DA release in a group of non-psychotic unipolar depressed subjects (Parsey *et al.* 2001). Despite reporting preamphetamine anxiety levels higher than schizophrenic patients, patients with depression showed normal amphetamine-induced displacement of [123I]IBZM.

Table 20.2 Imaging studies of striatal presynaptic DA parameters in drug-naive and drug-free patients with schizophrenia.

Study	Controls (n)	Patients (n) (DN/DF)	Radiotracer (/challenge)	Method	Outcome	Controls (n) (mean ± SD)*	Patients (n) (mean ± SD)*	P	Effect size†	Ratio SD
DOPA decarboxylase activity										
(Reith et al. 1994)	13	5 (4/1)	[^{18}F]DOPA	Kinetic	k_3	100 ± 23	120 ± 15	<0.05	0.91	0.68
(Hietala et al. 1995)	7	7 (7/0)	[^{18}F]DOPA	Graphical	K_i	100 ± 11	117 ± 20	<0.05	1.54	1.82
(Dao-Castellana et al. 1997)	7	6 (2/4)	[^{18}F]DOPA	Graphical	K_i	100 ± 11	103 ± 40	ns	0.30	3.80
(Lindstrom et al. 1999)	10	12 (10/2)	[^{11}C]DOPA	Graphical	K_i	100 ± 17	113 ± 12	<0.05	0.77	0.70
(Hietala et al. 1999)	13	10 (10/0)	[^{18}F]DOPA	Graphical	K_i	100 ± 14	115 ± 28	<0.05	1.09	1.25
Amphetamine-induced DA release										
(Laruelle et al. 1996)	15	15 (2/13)	[^{123}I]IBZM/amphetamine	Equilib.	Delta BP	100 ± 113	271 ± 221	<0.05	1.51	1.95
(Breier et al. 1997)	18	18 (8/10)	[^{11}C]raclopride/amphetamine	Equilib.	Delta BP	100 ± 43	175 ± 82	<0.05	1.73	1.90
(Abi-Dargham et al. 1998)	16	21 (1/20)	[^{123}I]IBZM/amphetamine	Equilib.	Delta BP	100 ± 88	194 ± 145	<0.05	1.07	1.64
Baseline DA concentration										
(Abi-Dargham et al. 2000b)	18	18 (8/10)	[^{123}I]IBZM/αMPT	Equilib.	Delta BP	100 ± 78	211 ± 122	<0.05	1.43	1.57
DAT density										
(Laakso et al. 2000)	9	9 (9/0)	[^{18}F]CFT	Ratio	S/C	100 ± 12	101 ± 13	ns	0.11	1.06
(Laruelle et al. 2000)	22	22 (2/20)	[^{123}I]β-CIT	Equilib.	BP	100 ± 17	93 ± 20	ns	−0.43	1.21

DA, dopamine; DAT, dopamine transporter; DF, drug-free; DN, drug-naive; Equilib., equilibrium; ns, not significant; k_3, rate constant; BP, binding potential; S, striatum; C, cerebellum.

*Mean normalized to mean of control subjects.

†Effect size calculated as (mean patients − mean controls)/SD controls.

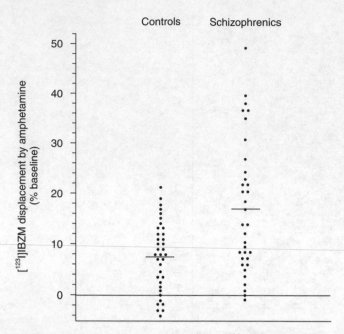

Fig 20.3 Effect of amphetamine (0.3 mg/kg) on [^{123}I]IBZM binding in healthy controls and untreated patients with schizophrenia. The y-axis shows the percentage decrease in [^{123}I]IBZM binding potential induced by amphetamine, which is a measure of the increased occupancy of D$_2$ receptors by DA following the challenge. Increased stimulation of D$_2$ receptors in schizophrenia was associated with transient worsening or emergence of positive symptoms.

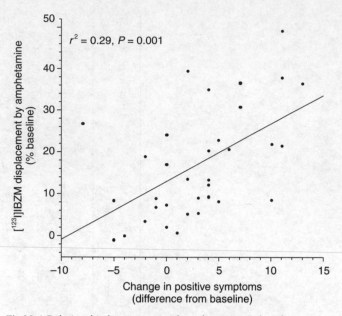

Fig 20.4 Relationship between striatal amphetamine-induced dopamine release (y-axis) and amphetamine-induced changes in positive symptoms measured with the positive subscale of the Positive and Negative Symptom Scale (PANSS) in patients with schizophrenia. Stimulation of D$_2$ receptors was associated with emergence or worsening of positive symptoms and accounted for about 30% of the variance in this behavioural response.

This finding supports the hypothesis that the increased amphetamine effect observed in patients with schizophrenia was not a non-specific consequence of stressful conditions, although it could represent a specific interaction between stress and schizophrenia.

These data are consistent with higher DA output in the striatum of patients with schizophrenia. This phenomenon is probably not a result of increased density of DA terminals. Striatal DA transporters (DATs) are exclusively localized on DA terminals, and the *in vivo* binding of the DAT radioligands [^{123}I]β-CIT (Laruelle *et al.* 2000) or [^{18}F]CFT (Laakso *et al.* 2000) is unaltered in patients with schizophrenia. These *in vivo* observations confirm the postmortem findings of normal DAT density in the striatum of patients with schizophrenia discussed above. In addition, *in vivo* measurement of the vesicular monoamine transporter in the caudate, putamen and ventral striatum with [^{11}C]dihydrotetrabenazine is unaltered in patients with schizophrenia (Taylor *et al.* 2000). We observed no association between amphetamine-induced DA release and DAT density (Laruelle *et al.* 2000). Thus, the increased presynaptic output suggested by the amphetamine studies appears to be associated with a functional dysregulation of DA neurones, rather than an increased number of these neurones.

Imaging baseline DA activity in schizophrenia

A major limitation of the amphetamine studies is that they measured changes in synaptic DA transmission following a non-

physiological challenge (i.e. amphetamine) and did not provide any information about 'baseline' synaptic DA levels (i.e. synaptic DA levels in the absence of pharmacological interventions). Several laboratories reported that, in rodents and non-human primates, acute depletion of synaptic DA is associated with an acute increase in the *in vivo* binding of [^{11}C]raclopride or [^{123}I]IBZM to D$_2$ receptors (Van der Werf *et al.* 1986; Ross & Jackson 1989; Seeman *et al.* 1989; Ross 1991; Young *et al.* 1991; Dewey *et al.* 1992; Ginovart *et al.* 1997). The increased binding was observed *in vivo* but not *in vitro*, indicating that it was not caused by receptor upregulation (Laruelle *et al.* 1997a), but to removal of endogenous DA and unmasking of D$_2$ receptors previously occupied by DA. Using this acute depletion strategy, baseline occupancy of striatal D$_2$ receptors by DA was studied in acute patients with schizophrenia (Abi-Dargham *et al.* 2000b). D$_2$ receptor availability was measured at baseline (i.e. in the absence of any pharmacological intervention) and during acute DA depletion. Acute DA depletion was achieved by administration of high doses of α-MPT for 2 days (Spector *et al.* 1965; Udenfriend *et al.* 1965). Comparing D$_2$ receptor availability at baseline and in the depleted state provided an indirect measure of the proportion of D$_2$ receptors occupied by DA in the baseline state. Removal of endogenous DA by α-MPT increased D$_2$ receptor availability by 9 ± 7% in controls ($n = 18$) and by 19 ± 11% in patients with schizophrenia ($n = 18$, $P = 0.003$). The differential effect of α-MPT between patients and controls was not a result of differences in α-MPT plasma levels. α-MPT effect on D$_2$ receptor availability was not statistically different between drug-naïve ($n = 8$, $17 \pm 6\%$) and previously treated patients ($n = 10$, $20 \pm 15\%$), and both groups were significantly different from controls.

Thus, the results of this study suggest that DA occupies a greater proportion of striatal D_2 receptors in patients with schizophrenia compared with matched control subjects during first episode of illness and subsequent episodes of illness exacerbation. The significance of this result stems from the fact that the paradigm used here reveals D_2 receptor occupancy by DA during the baseline scan, i.e. in the absence of any pharmacological intervention. The result of this study directly supports the classical dopamine hypothesis of schizophrenia, but should be viewed with caution until independently replicated.

The results of the α-MPT study are consistent with results of studies reporting DOPA decarboxylase activity in patients with schizophrenia, using [18F]DOPA (Reith et al. 1994; Hietala et al. 1995, 1999; Dao-Castellana et al. 1997) or [11C]DOPA (Lindstrom et al. 1999). Four out of five studies reported increased accumulation of DOPA in the striatum of patients with schizophrenia (Table 20.2), and the combined analysis of these studies yields an effect size of 0.92 ± 0.45, which is significantly different from zero ($P = 0.01$). While the relationship between DOPA decarboxylase and DA synthesis rate is unclear (DOPA decarboxylase is not the rate-limiting step of DA synthesis), these observations appear consistent with the higher synaptic DA concentration observed in patients with schizophrenia in the α-MPT study.

The term 'baseline' activity used here simply denotes that this study aimed at measuring occupancy of D_2 receptors by DA in the absence of pharmacological challenge. Because patients were studied during an episode of illness exacerbation, the occupancy of D_2 receptors by DA during periods of illness remission remains uncharacterized.

The 'baseline' DA activity studied by the α-MPT paradigm should not be confused with the tonic release described by Grace (1991, 1993) in his model of DA dysregulation associated with schizophrenia. This model rests on the distinction between tonic and phasic DA release. Tonic release refers to the extracellular extrasynaptic DA release, is impulse-independent and regulated by glutamatergic projections from the PFC to DA terminals in striatum. In contrast, the phasic release is the impulse-dependent synaptic DA release. Grace (1991, 1993) speculated that schizophrenia might be associated with low tonic DA activity, resulting from a decreased glutamatergic stimulation. This low DA tonic activity would in turn induce increased phasic DA activity, leading to overstimulation of postsynaptic D_2 receptors and emergence of positive symptoms. The baseline D_2 receptor occupancy by DA measured in the α-MPT study is presumably caused by the temporal and spatial integration of phasic release, as several lines of evidence suggest that the effect measured by these imaging techniques is intra- rather than extrasynaptic (for review and discussion see Laruelle 2000a). Thus, results of the α-MPT are consistent with the Grace (1991, 1993) model.

Importantly, high synaptic DA concentration revealed by the α-MPT paradigm was not associated with global severity of positive symptoms (Abi-Dargham et al. 2000b). Among positive symptoms, only severity of suspiciousness was associated at trend level with high synaptic DA levels, an interesting observation because suspiciousness is probably one of the most 'DA-dependent' dimensions of psychosis (Ellinwood et al. 1973). One of the important functions of subcortical DA is to signal the 'salience' of environmental stimuli (Schultz et al. 1998), and it is relatively easy to comprehend how dysregulation of the DA salience system might lead to suspiciousness, interpretation and paranoia (Ellinwood et al. 1973). None the less, the general lack of correlation between synaptic DA excess and severity of positive symptoms guards against simplistic association between positive symptoms and D_2 receptor stimulation.

This negative result might be a result of the limited resolution of the SPECT camera. Rodent studies suggest that antipsychotic drug action is associated with D_2 receptor antagonism in the mesolimbic (nucleus accumbens) rather than the nigrostriatal (dorsostriatal) DA systems (for review see Deutch 1993). This hypothesis derives mainly from the observation that atypical antipsychotic drugs, such as clozapine, are more potent at affecting DA transmission in the nucleus accumbens compared with the striatum (for review see Abi-Dargham et al. 1997). The limited resolution of the PET or SPECT cameras used in clinical studies so far did not allow distinguishing the respective contributions of the ventral and dorsal striata to the imaging signal. Studies with the newest high-resolution PET cameras recently demonstrated that the signal from ventral and dorsal striata can be reliably identified (Drevets et al. 2001; Mawlawi et al. 2001). Thus, the use of this improved technology will enable comparison of ventral and dorsal striatal DA transmission in schizophrenia. Meanwhile, the specific role of the ventral striatum in the psychotic process remains conjectural.

On the other hand, this negative result might indicate that the severity of positive symptoms rated cross-sectionally at a given point in time depends mostly on factors located downstream from the mesolimbic dopaminergic synapses. The dysfunctional neuronal circuits that underlie the experience of positive symptoms are likely to involve dysregulated information processing in the prefrontal–ventrostriatal–ventropallidal–mediodorsal–thalamoprefrontal loops reviewed above, and their regulation by hippocampal and amygdalar afferents (Grace et al. 1998; O'Donnell & Grace 1998a). Activity in these putative propsychotic neuronal ensembles is under modulatory influence of subcortical DA. A sudden rise in subcortical DA (such as measured following amphetamine) will exacerbate these symptoms, while a sudden decline in DA (such as measured following α-MPT) will blunt their intensity. Thus, psychotic symptomatology includes both DA-dependent and DA-independent components, with the respective contribution of each component varying from patient to patient (and presumably varying with time within the same patient).

Patients included in the α-MPT study completed 6 weeks of antipsychotic medication as inpatients. High synaptic levels of DA at baseline, measured by the α-MPT effect on D_2 receptor

BP, was significantly associated with greater improvement of positive symptoms following 6 weeks of antipsychotic treatment. Thus, the dysregulation of DA transmission revealed by the imaging study was predictive of better response of positive symptoms to antipsychotic treatment. Schizophrenic patients who experienced positive symptoms in the presence of increased DA stimulation of D_2 receptors showed a remarkable and rapid decline in these symptoms following treatment with antipsychotic drugs. Subjects who experienced positive symptoms in the presence of apparently normal stimulation of D_2 receptors by DA showed little improvement of these symptoms following 6 weeks of antipsychotic treatment. The fact that high levels of synaptic DA at baseline predicted better or faster response to atypical antipsychotic drugs (13 out of 14 patients were treated with atypical drugs) also suggests that the D_2 receptor blockade induced by these drugs remains a key component of their initial mode of action.

Contrary to widely accepted views, antipsychotic drugs have only partial efficacy against positive symptoms. A substantial proportion of schizophrenic patients, possibly one-third, remains actively psychotic despite appropriate and prolonged blockade of D_2 receptors (Huckle & Palia 1993; Weiden et al. 1996). The data from the α-MPT study suggest that, in some patients, blockade of D_2 receptors by antipsychotic drugs fails to alter positive symptoms significantly because these symptoms might not be related to excessive stimulation of these receptors by DA.

Discussion

While the studies reviewed above generally confirmed the classical DA hypothesis of schizophrenia, it is important to examine these results in light of the more recent views of schizophrenia as a neurodevelopmental illness, involving dysconnectivity of cortico–subcortical and intracortical networks. In this discussion, we speculate about the possible relationships between the imaging results reviewed above and this contemporary view of schizophrenia. The model proposed here suggests that neurodevelopmental abnormalities of intracortical and corticolimbic connectivity set the stage for the development of intermittent episodes of endogenous sensitization of the mesolimbic DA system that lead to the abnormal gating of information flow in the limbic loops that is underlying the psychotic experience. If sustained, this aberrant gating leads to plastic adaptation and remodelling of these circuits. As a result of these neuroplastic changes, the psychotic symptoms might become independent of sustained DA hyperactivity and resistant to D_2 receptor blockade.

Cortical regulation of subcortical dopamine transmission

While it cannot be definitively ruled out that the DA dysregulation revealed by these studies would stem from a primary abnormality of DA neurones, it seems more likely that these abnormalities are a consequence of cortico–subcortical dysconnectivity. Moreover, given the weight of evidence implicating PFC connectivity as a central deficient node in the schizophrenic brain, it is tempting to speculate that a dysregulation of the firing activity of dopaminergic neurones might stem from a failure of the PFC to regulate this process. In fact, it has long been hypothesized that dysregulation of subcortical DA function in schizophrenia may be secondary to a failure of the PFC to adequately control subcortical dopaminergic function (Weinberger et al. 1986; Grace 1991).

In patients with schizophrenia, low N-acetyl-aspartate (NAA) concentration in the DLPFC, a marker of DLPFC pathology, is associated with increased amphetamine-induced DA release (Bertolino et al. 2000). This result provides direct support to the hypothesis that disinhibition of subcortical DA activity might be secondary to prefrontal pathology in schizophrenia. Yet, the nature of the PFC pathology in schizophrenia and how it might affect subcortical DA function remains to be elucidated.

According to a model introduced by Carlsson et al. (1999b), the PFC modulates activity of midbrain DA neurones via both an activating pathway (the 'accelerator') and an inhibitory pathway ('the brake'), allowing fine tuning of dopaminergic activity by the PFC (Fig. 20.5). The activating pathway is provided by direct and indirect glutamatergic projections onto the dopaminergic cells. These indirect projections are likely to involve the pedunculopontine tegmentum (see discussion and reference in Carr & Sesack 2000). The inhibitory pathway is provided by PFC glutamatergic efferents to midbrain GABAergic interneurones and striatomesencephalic GABA neurones.

The inhibition of dopaminergic cell firing following amphetamine is an important feedback mechanism by which the brain reduces the effect of amphetamine on DA release. The inhibition of dopaminergic cell firing induced by amphetamine is mediated both by stimulation of presynaptic D_2 autoreceptors and by stimulation of this inhibitory pathway (Bunney & Aghajanian 1978; Carlsson et al. 1999b). Following administration of amphetamine (i.e. under conditions in which the inhibitory pathway should be activated), NMDA receptor blockade results in a failure of activation of the inhibitory pathway, resulting in exaggerated amphetamine-induced DA release (Miller & Abercrombie 1996). Kegeles et al. (2000) recently confirmed this mechanism in humans: pretreatment with the NMDA non-competitive antagonist ketamine significantly enhanced amphetamine-induced DA release. The increase in amphetamine-induced DA release induced by ketamine (greater than twofold) was comparable in magnitude to the exaggerated response seen in patients with schizophrenia (Fig. 20.6). These data are consistent with the hypothesis that the alteration of DA release revealed by the amphetamine challenge in schizophrenia results from a disruption of glutamatergic neuronal systems regulating dopaminergic cell activity. Moreover, these data provide a direct link between the DA hypothesis and the NMDA receptor hypofunction hypothesis of schizophrenia (Javitt & Zukin 1991; Olney & Farber 1995; Jentsch & Roth 1999).

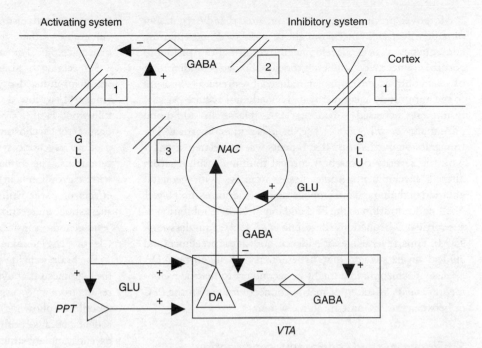

Fig 20.5 Model of modulation of VTA DA cells activity by PFC. Activity of midbrain DA neurones is under dual influence of PFC via activating and inhibitory pathways, allowing fine tuning of dopaminergic activity by the PFC. The activating pathway is provided by glutamatergic projections onto the dopaminergic cells, and the inhibitory pathway is provided by glutamatergic projections to midbrain GABAergic interneurones or striatomesencephalic GABA neurones (see text for description and references). This model predicts that a deficiency in N-methyl-D-aspartate (NMDA) transmission [lesion 1] and/or GABA PFC function [lesion 2] and/or DA PFC function [lesion 3] would result in a failure of the PFC to inhibit subcortical DA activity under conditions of excessive stimulation (such as stress or amphetamine challenge). NAC, nucleus accumbens; PPT, pedunculopontine tegmentum; VTA, ventral tegmental area.

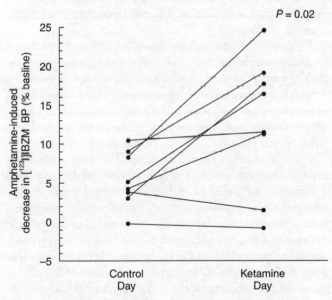

Fig 20.6 Ketamine modulation of striatal amphetamine-induced dopamine release in healthy volunteers, showing a significantly larger release in eight healthy volunteers pretreated with i.v. ketamine compared with control conditions (repeated measures ANOVA, $P = 0.023$). These data indicate that, in humans, amphetamine-induced DA release in the striatum is modulated by glutamatergic circuits involving NMDA transmission.

Alternatively, the failure of PFC control of subcortical DA release might stem from mechanisms other than NMDA hypofunction. For example, glutamatergic projections from the PFC to the VTA are under tonic inhibition by prefrontal GABA (see Karreman & Moghaddam 1996 and references therein). It follows that deficit in GABAergic function in the PFC is also expected to lead to disinhibition of subcortical DA response to amphetamine. Alteration of GABAergic function in the PFC is one of the most consistently noted postmortem abnormalities in schizophrenia. Gene expression for GABA synthetic enzyme glutamic acid decarboxylase-67 ($GABA_{67}$) appears to be reduced in the PFC (Akbarian *et al.* 1995; Volk *et al.* 2000). GABAergic markers in axon terminals of chandelier neurones might be substantially reduced (Woo *et al.* 1998). One study reported decreased density of GABAergic interneurones in PFC in layer II (Benes *et al.* 1991), although this finding has not been replicated (Akbarian *et al.* 1995; Woo *et al.* 1997). Increased binding of the $GABA_A$ receptors was also observed (Hanada *et al.* 1987; Benes *et al.* 1992, 1996), which has been interpreted as a compensatory upregulation induced by GABA deficit.

Since the seminal work of Pycock *et al.* (1980), many laboratories have described the reciprocal and opposite regulations between cortical and subcortical dopaminergic systems: stimulation of cortical DA leads to inhibition of subcortical DA (Kolachana *et al.* 1995; Karreman & Moghaddam 1996), while destruction of cortical DA projections leads to subcortical disinhibition (Deutch *et al.* 1990; Wilkinson 1997). In the cortex, DA has an inhibitory effect on pyramidal neurones that stimulate DA release at the VTA level (Karreman & Moghaddam 1996), an effect mediated in part by DA stimulation of GABAergic interneurones (Deutch 1993). Schizophrenia has been postulated to be associated with a deficit of the prefrontal DA system. Thus, deficits in PFC DA innervation might represent another avenue leading to the disinhibition of subcortical DA revealed by these imaging studies. Figure 20.5 summarizes how these various pathophysiological mechanisms in the PFC might result in disinhibition of subcortical DA neurones.

Moreover, preclinical studies documented that dysregulation of subcortical DA function might be a delayed and enduring consequence of neurodevelopmental abnormalities of limbo-cortical connectivity. Studies in rodents showed that alteration of corticolimbic development induced by prenatal exposure to the antimitotic agent methylazoxymethanol acetate (MAM) results in increased subcortical DA release in adulthood (Watanabe *et al.* 1998). The increase in subcortical DA transmission in MAM-treated rodents was correlated strongly with the severity of cerebral cortical thinning resulting from altered development. Adult rhesus monkeys with neonatal ablation of the amygdala–hippocampal formation exhibit lower NAA concentration in the PFC and impaired PFC inhibition of subcortical DA functions (Bertolino *et al.* 1997; Saunders *et al.* 1998). Thus, several lines of evidence, both at the preclinical and clinical level, suggest that hyperactivity of subcortical DA release in schizophrenia might be secondary to neurodevelopmental events affecting primarily connectivity within the PFC or between the PFC and the limbic system.

Schizophrenia and endogenous sensitization

While the evidence reviewed above is consistent with the model that dysregulation of subcortical DA function in schizophrenia is an enduring consequence of neurodevelopmental abnormalities involving PFC connectivity, these models *per se* do not account for the apparent episodic nature of this dysregulation. In the imaging studies reviewed above, elevated amphetamine-induced DA release was observed only in patients experiencing a first episode of illness or an episode of illness exacerbation, but not in patients studied during a period of illness remission. To confirm this observation by studying the same subjects during and between episodes is warranted. Nevertheless, this observation, combined with the clinical evidence of the fluctuating nature of positive symptomatology, suggests that subcortical hyperdopaminergia is episodic in the schizophrenic brain.

Neurochemical sensitization of mesolimbic DA systems has been proposed by several authors as one mechanism that might underlie the progression of a 'silent' vulnerability into an overt symptomatology, resulting in further 'toxic' effects on the brain (Robinson & Becker 1986; Lieberman *et al.* 1990, 1997; Glenthoj & Hemmingsen 1997; Pierce & Kalivas 1997). Sensitization is a process whereby exposure to a given stimulus such as a drug or a stressor results in an enhanced response to subsequent exposures. This phenomenon has been well characterized in rodents: repeated exposure to psychostimulants such as amphetamine induces an increase in the behavioural (loco-motion) and biochemical (DA release) response to amphetamine, other stimulants, or stressors (for review see Robinson & Becker 1986; Kalivas & Stewart 1991; Kalivas *et al.* 1993; Sorg *et al.* 1994). Under certain conditions, sensitization is a long-lasting adaptation: animals sensitized to stimulants continue to display enhanced response after months of abstinence (Magos 1969; Robinson & Becker 1986). Sensitization is a form of learning behaviour and is essentially a non-homeostatic positive feedback mechanism. Sensitization makes individuals more vulnerable rather than more resistant to a number of pharmacological or environmental stimulations.

Subjects who abused psychostimulants and experienced stimulant-induced psychotic episodes are reported to remain vulnerable to low doses of psychostimulants (Connell 1958; Ellinwood *et al.* 1973; Sato *et al.* 1983). In these subjects, exposure to psychostimulants at doses that do not normally produce psychotic symptoms can trigger recurrence of these symptoms. The similarity between these patients and patients with schizophrenia in terms of vulnerability to the propsychotic effects of psychostimulants has been noted and led to the suggestion that schizophrenia might be associated with an 'endogenous' sensitization process (Lieberman *et al.* 1990; Glenthoj & Hemmingsen 1997).

The brain imaging data reviewed above provide support for the hypothesis that dysfunction of DA systems in schizophrenia results from a process similar to the sensitization phenomenon described following repeated psychostimulant exposure in rodents, because both conditions are associated with increased psychostimulant-induced DA release. In turn, this proposition suggests that neurodevelopmental abnormalities associated with schizophrenia may set the stage for the development of an endogenous sensitization process (Lieberman *et al.* 1997; Laruelle 2000b).

We have reviewed elsewhere (Laruelle 2000b) the preclinical literature suggesting that early brain lesions that affect the development of cortical connectivity might result in enhanced vulnerability to sensitization of mesolimbic DA systems. During late adolescence, alteration in cortical connectivity in schizophrenia might limit the capacity of the brain to modulate stress-related increased activity of mesolimbic DA neurones. This failure of normal homeostatic and buffering mechanisms results in endogenous sensitization of mesolimbic DA neurones, a response not observed in humans under normal circumstances. While increased DA activity is initially associated with environmental stressors, the sensitization process is self-perpetuating and, beyond a given threshold, becomes independent of the environmental factors responsible for its initiation. This positive feedback loop, in which more DA leads to more DA, results ultimately in profound gating alterations in the corticostriatal–thalamocortical loops and expression of positive symptoms.

With treatment, chronic blockade of D_2 receptors and/or neuroleptic-induced depolarization blockade of dopaminergic neurones (Bunney & Grace 1978) might allow a progressive extinction of this sensitized state of the mesolimbic DA system. This proposition is suggested by the failure to detect an increase in amphetamine-induced DA release in currently untreated patients with schizophrenia during periods of illness stabilization. However, the high rate of relapse during prolonged treatment discontinuation suggests that the vulnerability to develop endogenous sensitization remains. Upon environmental, physiological or pharmacological stress, this process might be reactivated, leading to clinical relapse.

Beyond the dopaminergic synapse

The data derived from the brain imaging studies reviewed above are consistent with the hypothesis that subcortical DA transmission mediates the expression of positive symptoms in patients with schizophrenia. However, the data also suggest that a component of the positive symptomatology is independent of increased activity of subcortical DA transmission. First, the increase in DA transmission at striatal D_2 receptors following amphetamine explained only 30% of the variability in the psychotic response to D-amphetamine (Fig. 20.4). Secondly, the severity of positive symptoms was not associated with increased synaptic DA concentration as revealed by the α-MPT challenge (Abi-Dargham et al. 2000b). Thus, a simple relationship between intensity of DA transmission at the D_2 receptors and severity of positive symptoms is an oversimplification. In addition, such a simple relationship is not supported by the delay between D_2 receptor blockade and antipsychotic response, or by resistance of positive symptoms to even sustained dopaminergic blockade in about 25% of patients with schizophrenia (Huckle & Palia 1993).

In this context, it is also important to note a critical difference in the propsychotic effects of DA agonists, on one hand, and NMDA antagonists or 5-HT$_{2A}$ agonists, on the other. In healthy individuals, drugs such as ketamine or lysergic acid diethylamide (LSD) induce a psychotic state immediately upon drug exposure, while sustained administration of DA agonists is typically required for the emergence of psychotic symptoms (for review see Krystal et al. 1999). This time-dependency of DA agonists' psychotogenic effect suggests that some plasticity or neuroadaptation must take place between the hyperstimulation of D_2 receptors and the psychotic experience.

To account for these data, one might speculate that, with time, increased DA activity triggers neuroplastic adaptation 'downstream' from the mesolimbic dopaminergic synapse and that, once established, these neuroplastic changes become independent of increased DA activity. Positive symptom circuits might become 'hard-wired' in prefrontal–ventrostriatal–ventropallidal–mediodorsal–thalamoprefrontal loops described above (Fig. 20.1). The established role of DA in modulating LTP and LTD of glutamatergic synapses (Arbuthnott et al. 2000; Kerr & Wickens 2001) provides a potential cellular mechanism by which sustained excess of DA activity might shape and remodel these circuits. Following this neuroplastic change, excessive DA stimulation maintains the potential to activate these neuronal ensembles (as demonstrated by the relationship between D_2 receptor stimulation and worsening of positive symptoms), but the evidence suggests that, at least in some patients, these symptoms might become independent of continuous DA stimulation (as demonstrated by the observation that some patients exhibit severe positive symptoms in the absence of detectable abnormalities in synaptic DA). Thus, the emergence of treatment-resistant positive symptoms suggests that these symptoms have taken 'a life of their own', i.e. have become independent of DA stimulation. A better understanding of the consequences of sustained dopaminergic activity on the plasticity of prefrontal–striatothalamic loops is needed to further characterize the neurobiological effects of the sustained hyperdopaminergic state.

The ubiquitous role of DA in the creation of these hypothetical psychotic ensembles remains to be established. Whether DA hyperactivity has been present at some point or another in the life of every schizophrenic patient with positive symptoms is quite uncertain. A deficiency in glutamate transmission that would impair appropriate modulation of prefrontal–striatothalamic loops by afferents from the amygdala–hippocampal complex is another mechanism that might induce positive symptoms in the absence of overactivity of DA transmission (Carlsson 1988; Grace et al. 1998; O'Donnell & Grace 1998b). In other terms, endogenous sensitization of dopaminergic systems might represent only one avenue among others leading to chronic and/or recurrent psychotic episodes.

This view is supported by the observation that the acute propsychotic effects of NMDA antagonists in humans (or their putative equivalent manifestation in animals) do not appear to be modulated by increased DA activity or markedly affected by D_2 receptor blockade (for review see Lahti et al. 1995; Moghaddam & Adams 1998; Carlsson et al. 1999a,b; Jentsch & Roth 1999). Clinical and preclinical evidence suggests that NMDA hypofunction, at least acutely, induces psychotic symptoms by mechanisms largely independent of DA. We should note, however, that a DA transmission imbalance (decreased prefrontal activity and increased mesolimbic reactivity) is involved in the effects of prolonged administration of NMDA antagonists such as PCP, effects that more faithfully mimic schizophrenia than the effects of acute NMDA antagonist administration (Jentsch & Roth 1999).

Dopamine in the history of the schizophrenic brain

The general model proposed here predicates that in schizophrenia various clinical and neurobiological periods could be differentiated in relation to subcortical hyperdopaminergia (Fig. 20.7). It might be important to think about DA in schizophrenia within the context of a brain with a history, divided into a predopaminergic, a dopaminergic and a postdopaminergic era. The neurodevelopmental abnormalities associated with schizophrenia do not lead to hyperdopaminergia during childhood, but induce vulnerability to stress-mediated induction of sensitization of mesolimbic DA systems during adolescence. Sustained hyperactivity of DA neurones resulting from this sensitization process leads to neuroplastic changes downstream from the DA synapse. These neuroplastic adaptations underlie the emergence of the psychotic experience. If untreated, activities in these aberrant circuits become 'hard-wired' and independent from increased DA activity. Early treatment will reverse these neuroplastic changes and induce an extinction of the sensitization process. This model clearly supports the rationale for D_2 blockade during periods of illness exacerbation, and for early intervention during prodromal states.

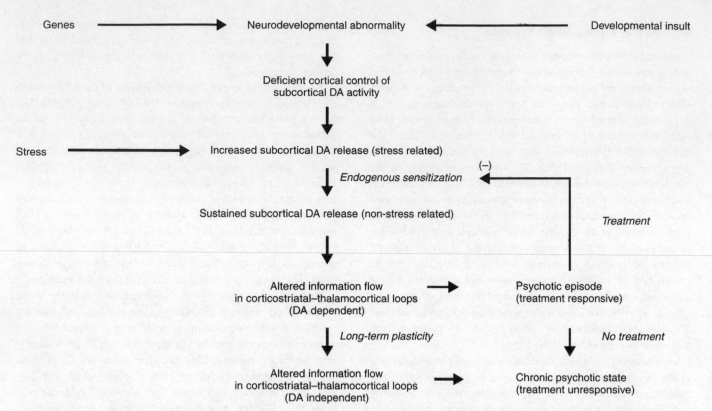

Fig 20.7 Model describing the role of subcortical DA dysregulation in the chain of events leading to clinical expression of positive symptoms in schizophrenia. It is postulated that neurodevelopmental abnormalities, resulting from complex interactions of genetic vulnerability and pre- or perinatal insults, induce, among other consequences, impaired regulation of subcortical DA activity by the prefrontal cortex (see Fig. 20.5). The lack of normal buffering systems results in vulnerability of DA systems to develop a process of endogenous sensitization. Excessive DA activity, initially as a response to stress, initiates a positive feedback loop, in which elevated DA activity becomes self-sustained even in the absence of stressors or other salient stimuli. This excessive DA activity perturbs information flow in corticostriatal–thalamocortical loops (see Fig. 20.1), which results over time in remodelling of these circuits. The hypothetical neuroplastic response to DA hyperactivity mediates alterations of information processing leading to a psychotic episode. D_2 receptor blockade not only recalibrates DA responsivity by interrupting the endogenous DA process, but also reverses the neuroplastic changes that took place downstream from the DA synapse. However, in the absence of treatment, these neuroplastic changes become progressively 'hard-wired', and activity in these re-entrant psychotic ensembles becomes independent of sustained DA activity and unresponsive to D_2 receptor blockade. While this model integrates observations from brain imaging studies of DA synaptic activity in schizophrenia, its speculative nature has to be emphasized. Furthermore, we do not imply that this chain of events is the only avenue leading to emergence of psychotic symptoms in the schizophrenic brain. None the less, it provides a number of testable hypotheses and directions for future research.

This model also calls for new relapse prevention strategies. Currently, pharmacological 'maintenance' during remission phases is based on dopaminergic D_2 receptor blockade. These treatments succeed in preventing the re-emergence of sensitization and in reducing the risk of relapse yet they exert their preventive benefits at the price of inducing a hypodopaminergic state, which is associated with significant adverse effects and lower quality of life. A better understanding of the neurobiological mechanisms that trigger the re-emergence of sensitization might lead to new relapse prevention strategies sparing D_2 receptor function. In other terms, the apparent normality of DA transmission during illness remission might be a more important finding of these imaging studies than the dysregulation during illness exacerbation.

This model also calls for a better understanding of the long-term consequences of exaggerated stimulation of D_2 receptors on cortico–subcortical connectivity. The observation that, in some patients, psychotic symptoms are independent of DA transmission (these symptoms are experienced in the presence of apparently normal levels of synaptic DA and show little or no response to D_2 receptor blockade) is another fundamental observation from these imaging studies. This observation supports the need for the development of new non-dopaminergic therapeutic approaches.

Conclusions

The availability of new imaging methods aiming at measuring presynaptic activity in striatal DA afferents provided data consistent with the view that schizophrenia is associated with hyperactivity of subcortical transmission at D_2 receptors. These results are consistent with the known mode of action of current antipsychotic treatment (D_2 receptor blockade), with the psychotogenic effects of sustained stimulation of DA function by psychostimulants, and with the 'classical' DA hypothesis of schizophrenia derived from these observations. In addition, these results suggest that the DA hyperactivity of subcortical systems is episodic in nature, and accounts for only some aspects of positive symptomatology. These observations have several implications for the development of new treatment strategies.

As a final note, it should be re-emphasized that positive symptoms are only one aspect of the symptomatology presented by these patients. While they might be the most visible expression of the illness, these symptoms are not the most enduring nor the ones associated with most disability, at least in the postneuroleptic era. Cognitive impairments appear to precede and outlive psychotic episodes, and their severity is one of the best predictors of poor outcome (Green 1996). While the brain imaging studies reported here supported the role of subcortical hyperdopaminergic activity in the pathophysiology of positive symptoms, the potential role of prefrontal deficit in DA transmission in the pathophysiology of cognitive impairment remains to be firmly established. The development of new brain imaging techniques enabling the study of prefrontal DA transmission is warranted to explore this other face of the dopaminergic imbalance hypothesis of schizophrenia.

Acknowledgements

Supported by the National Alliance for Research on Schizophrenia and Depression (NARSAD), and the National Institute of Mental Health (K02 MH01603-01).

References

Abi-Dargham, A., Laruelle, M., Aghajanian, G.K., Charney, D. & Krystal, J. (1997) The role of serotonin in the pathophysiology and treatment of schizophrenia. *Journal of Neuropsychology and Clinical Neuroscience* 9, 1–17.

Abi-Dargham, A., Gil, R., Krystal, J. *et al.* (1998) Increased striatal dopamine transmission in schizophrenia: confirmation in a second cohort. *American Journal of Psychiatry* 155, 761–767.

Abi-Dargham, A., Martinez, D., Mawlawi, O. *et al.* (2000a) Measurement of striatal and extrastriatal dopamine D_1 receptor binding potential with [^{11}C]NNC 112 in humans: validation and reproducibility. *Journal of Cerebral Blood Flow Metabolism* 20, 225–243.

Abi-Dargham, A., Rodenhiser, J., Printz, D. *et al.* (2000b) Increased baseline occupancy of D_2 receptors by dopamine in schizophrenia. *Proceedings of the National Academy of Sciences of the USA* 97, 8104–8109.

Akbarian, S., Kim, J.J., Potkin, S.G. *et al.* (1995) Gene expression for glutamic acid decarboxylase is reduced without loss of neurons in prefrontal cortex of schizophrenics. *Archives of General Psychiatry* 52, 258–266.

Akil, M., Pierri, J.N., Whitehead, R.E. *et al.* (1999) Lamina-specific alterations in the dopamine innervation of the prefrontal cortex in schizophrenic subjects. *American Journal of Psychiatry* 156, 1580–1589.

Akil, M., Edgar, C.L., Pierri, J.N., Casali, S. & Lewis, D.A. (2000) Decreased density of tyrosine hydroxylase-immunoreactive axons in the entorhinal cortex of schizophrenic subjects. *Biological Psychiatry* 47, 361–370.

Albin, R.L., Young, A.B. & Penney, J.B. (1989) The functional anatomy of basal ganglia disorders. *Trends in Neuroscience* 12, 366–375.

Alexander, G.E., Delong, M.R. & Stick, P.L. (1986) Parallel organization of functionally segregated circuits linking basal ganglia and cortex. *Annual Review of Neuroscience* 9, 357–381.

Angrist, B. & van Kammen, D.P. (1984) CNS stimulants as a tool in the study of schizophrenia. *Trends in Neuroscience* 7, 388–390.

Arbuthnott, G.W., Ingham, C.A. & Wickens, J.R. (2000) Dopamine and synaptic plasticity in the neostriatum. *Journal of Anatomy* 196, 587–596.

Benes, F.M., McSparren, J., Bird, E.D., Vincent, S.L. & SanGiovani, J.P. (1991) Deficits in small interneurons in schizophrenic cortex. *Archives of General Psychiatry* 48, 996–1001.

Benes, F.M., Vincent, S.L., Alsterberg, G., Bird, E.D. & SanGiovanni, J.P. (1992) Increased GABAa receptor binding in superficial layers of cingulate cortex in schizophrenics. *Journal of Neuroscience* 12, 924–929.

Benes, F.M., Vincent, S.L., Marie, A. & Khan, Y. (1996) Upregulation of GABAA receptor binding on neurons of the prefrontal cortex in schizophrenic subjects. *Neuroscience* 75, 1021–1031.

Benes, F.M., Todtenkopf, M.S. & Taylor, J.B. (1997) Differential distribution of tyrosine hydroxylase fibers on small and large neurons in layer II of anterior cingulate cortex of schizophrenic brain. *Synapse* 25, 80–92.

Bertolino, A., Saunders, R.C., Mattay, V.S. *et al.* (1997) Altered development of prefrontal neurons in rhesus monkeys with neonatal mesial temporolimbic lesions: a proton magnetic resonance spectroscopic imaging study. *Cerebral Cortex* 7, 740–748.

Bertolino, A., Breier, A., Callicott, J.H. *et al.* (2000) The relationship between dorsolateral prefrontal neuronal N-acetylaspartate and evoked release of striatal dopamine in schizophrenia. *Neuropsychopharmacology* 22, 125–132.

Blin, J., Baron, J.C., Cambon, H. *et al.* (1989) Striatal dopamine D_2 receptors in tardive dyskinesia: PET study. *Journal of Neurology, Neurosurgery and Psychiatry* 52, 1248–1252.

Breier, A., Su, T.P., Saunders, R. *et al.* (1997) Schizophrenia is associated with elevated amphetamine-induced synaptic dopamine concentrations: evidence from a novel positron emission tomography method. *Proceedings of the National Academy of Sciences of the USA* 94, 2569–2574.

Bunney, B.S. & Aghajanian, G.K. (1978) D-Amphetamine-induced depression of central dopamine neurons: evidence for mediation by both autoreceptors and a striato-nigral feedback pathway. *Naunyn-Schmiedeberg's Archives of Pharmacology* 304, 255–261.

Bunney, B.S. & Grace, A.A. (1978) Acute and chronic haloperidol treatment: comparison of effects on nigral dopaminergic cell activity. *Life Science* 23, 423–435.

Bunzow, J.R., Van Tol, H.H., Grandy, D.K. *et al.* (1988) Cloning and expression of a rat D_2 dopamine receptor cDNA. *Nature* 336, 783–787.

Burt, D.R., Creese, I. & Snyder, S.S. (1977) Antischizophrenic drugs: chronic treatment elevates dopamine receptors binding in brain. *Science* 196, 326–328.

Carlsson, A. (1988) The current status of the dopamine hypothesis of schizophrenia. *Neuropsychopharmacology* 1, 179–186.

Carlsson, A. & Lindqvist, M. (1963) Effect of chlorpromazine or haloperidol on formation of 3-methoxytyramine and normetanephrine in mouse brain. *Acta Pharmacologica Toxicologica* **20**, 140–144.

Carlsson, A., Hansson, L.O., Waters, N. & Carlsson, M.L. (1999a) A glutamatergic deficiency model of schizophrenia. *British Journal of Psychiatry Supplement* **37**, 2–6.

Carlsson, A., Waters, N. & Carlsson, M.L. (1999b) Neurotransmitter interactions in schizophrenia: therapeutic implications. *Biological Psychiatry* **46**, 1388–1395.

Carr, D.B. & Sesack, S.R. (2000) Projections from the rat prefrontal cortex to the ventral tegmental area: target specificity in the synaptic associations with mesoaccumbens and mesocortical neurons. *Journal of Neuroscience* **20**, 3864–3873.

Carson, R.E., Breier, A., deBartolomeis, A. *et al.* (1997) Quantification of amphetamine-induced changes in [C-11]raclopride binding with continuous infusion. *Journal of Cerebral Blood Flow and Metabolism* **17**, 437–447.

Chinaglia, G., Alvarez, F.J., Probst, A. & Palacios, J.M. (1992) Mesostriatal and mesolimbic dopamine uptake binding sites are reduced in Parkinson's disease and progressive supranuclear palsy: a quantitative autoradiographic study using [^{3}H]mazindol. *Neuroscience* **49**, 317–327.

Chiodo, L. & Bunney, B. (1983) Typical and atypical neuroleptics: differential effects of chronic administration on the activity of A9 and A10 midbrain dopaminergic neurons. *Journal of Neuroscience* **3**, 1607–1619.

Connell, P.H. (1958) *Amphetamine Psychosis*. Chapman and Hill, London.

Crawley, J.C., Owens, D.G., Crow, T.J. *et al.* (1986) Dopamine D_2 receptors in schizophrenia studied *in vivo*. *Lancet* **2**, 224–225.

Creese, I., Burt, D.R. & Snyder, S.H. (1976) Dopamine receptor binding predicts clinical and pharmacological potencies of antischizophrenic drugs. *Science* **19**, 481–483.

Cross, A.J., Crow, T.J. & Owen, F. (1981) ^{3}H-Flupenthixol binding in postmortem brains of schizophrenics: evidence for a selective increase in dopamine D_2 receptors. *Psychopharmacology* **74**, 122–124.

Cross, A.J., Crow, T.J., Ferrier, I.N. *et al.* (1983) Dopamine receptor changes in schizophrenia in relation to the disease process and movement disorder. *Journal of Neural Transmission Supplement* **18**, 265–272.

Czudek, C. & Reynolds, G.P. (1989) [^{3}H]GBR 12935 binding to the dopamine uptake site in postmortem brain tissue in schizophrenia. *Journal of Neural Transmission* **77**, 227–230.

Dao-Castellana, M.H., Paillere-Martinot, M.L., Hantraye, P. *et al.* (1997) Presynaptic dopaminergic function in the striatum of schizophrenic patients. *Schizophrenia Research* **23**, 167–174.

Davis, K.L., Kahn, R.S., Ko, G. & Davidson, M. (1991) Dopamine in schizophrenia: a review and reconceptualization. *American Journal of Psychiatry* **148**, 1474–1486.

Dean, B., Pavey, G. & Opeskin, K. (1997) [H-3]raclopride binding to brain tissue from subjects with schizophrenia: methodological aspects. *Neuropharmacology* **36**, 779–786.

Dearry, A., Gingrich, J.A., Falardeau, P. *et al.* (1990) Molecular cloning and expression of the gene for a human D_1 dopamine receptor. *Nature* **347**, 72–76.

DeLong, M.R., Crutcher, M.D. & Georgopoulos, A.P. (1985) Primate globus pallidus and subthalamic nucleus: functional organization. *Journal of Neurophysiology* **53**, 530–543.

Deutch, A.Y. (1993) Prefrontal cortical dopamine systems and the elaboration of functional corticostriatal circuits: implications for schizophrenia and Parkinson's disease. *Journal of Neural Transmission* **91**, 197–221.

Deutch, A., Clark, W.A. & Roth, R.H. (1990) Prefrontal cortical

dopamine depletion enhances the responsiveness of the mesolimbic dopamine neurons to stress. *Brain Research* **521**, 311–315.

Deutch, A., Moghadam, B., Innis, R. *et al.* (1991) Mechanisms of action of atypical antipsychotic drugs: implication for novel therapeutic strategies for schizophrenia. *Schizophrenia Research* **4**, 121–156.

Deutch, A., Lee, M.C. & Iadarola, M.J. (1992) Regionally specific effects of atypical antipsychotic drugs on striatal fos expression: the nucleus accumbens shell as a locus of antipsychotic action. *Molecular and Cellular Neurosciences* **3**, 332–341.

Dewey, S.L., Logan, J., Wolf, A.P. *et al.* (1991) Amphetamine induced decrease in [^{18}F]-N-methylspiperidol binding in the baboon brain using positron emission tomography (PET). *Synapse* **7**, 324–327.

Dewey, S.L., Smith, G.S., Logan, J. *et al.* (1992) GABAergic inhibition of endogenous dopamine release measured *in vivo* with ^{11}C-raclopride and positron emission tomography. *Journal of Neuroscience* **12**, 3773–3780.

Drevets, W.C., Gautier, C., Price, J.C. *et al.* (2001) Amphetamine-induced dopamine release in human ventral striatum correlates with euphoria. *Biological Psychiatry* **49**, 81–96.

Dunah, A.W. & Standaert, D.G. (2001) Dopamine D_1 receptor-dependent trafficking of striatal nmda glutamate receptors to the postsynaptic membrane. *Journal of Neuroscience* **21**, 5546–5558.

Ellinwood, E.H., Sudilovsky, A. & Nelson, L.M. (1973) Evolving behavior in the clinical and experimental amphetamine model psychosis. *American Journal of Psychiatry* **130**, 1088–1093.

Everitt, B.J., Morris, K.A., O'Brien, A. & Robbins, T.W. (1991) The basolateral amygdala–ventral striatal system and conditioned place preference: further evidence of limbic–striatal interactions underlying reward-related processes. *Neuroscience* **42**, 1–18.

Farde, L., Wiesel, F., Stone-Elander, S. *et al.* (1990) D_2 dopamine receptors in neuroleptic-naive schizophrenic patients: a positron emission tomography study with [^{11}C]raclopride. *Archives of General Psychiatry* **47**, 213–219.

Fauchey, V., Jaber, M., Caron, M.G., Bloch, B. & Le Moine, C. (2000) Differential regulation of the dopamine D_1, D_2 and D_3 receptor gene expression and changes in the phenotype of the striatal neurons in mice lacking the dopamine transporter. *European Journal of Neuroscience* **12**, 19–26.

Ferry, A.T., Ongur, D., An, X. & Price, J.L. (2000) Prefrontal cortical projections to the striatum in macaque monkeys: evidence for an organization related to prefrontal networks. *Journal of Comparative Neurology* **425**, 447–470.

Gerfen, C.R. (1992) The neostriatal mosaic: multiple levels of compartmental organization in the basal ganglia. *Annual Review of Neuroscience* **15**, 285–320.

Ginovart, N., Farde, L., Halldin, C. & Swahn, C.G. (1997) Effect of reserpine-induced depletion of synaptic dopamine on [C-11]raclopride binding to D_2-dopamine receptors in the monkey brain. *Synapse* **25**, 321–325.

Glenthoj, B.Y. & Hemmingsen, R. (1997) Dopaminergic sensitization: implications for the pathogenesis of schizophrenia. *Progress in Neuro-Psychopharmacology and Biological Psychiatry* **21**, 23–46.

Goldman-Rakic, P.S. (1999) The physiological approach: functional architecture of working memory and disordered cognition in schizophrenia. *Biological Psychiatry* **46**, 650–661.

Goldman-Rakic, P.S. & Selemon, L.D. (1997) Functional and anatomical aspects of prefrontal pathology in schizophrenia. *Schizophrenia Bulletin* **23**, 437–458.

Goldman-Rakic, P.S., Muly, E.C. III & Williams, G.V. (2000) D_1 receptors in prefrontal cells and circuits. *Brain Research Review* **31**, 295–301.

Grace, A.A. (1991) Phasic versus tonic dopamine release and the modulation of dopamine system responsivity: a hypothesis for the etiology of schizophrenia. *Neuroscience* **41**, 1–24.

Grace, A.A. (1993) Cortical regulation of subcortical systems and its possible relevance to schizophrenia. *Journal of Neural Transmission* **91**, 111–134.

Grace, A.A. (2000) Gating of information flow within the limbic system and the pathophysiology of schizophrenia. *Brain Research Review* **31**, 330–341.

Grace, A.A., Moore, H. & O'Donnell, P. (1998) The modulation of corticoaccumbens transmission by limbic afferents and dopamine: a model for the pathophysiology of schizophrenia. *Advances in Pharmacology* **42**, 721–724.

Green, M.F. (1996) What are the functional consequences of neurocognitive deficits in schizophrenia? *American Journal of Psychiatry* **153**, 321–330.

Gurevich, E.V., Bordelon, Y., Shapiro, R.M. *et al.* (1997) Mesolimbic dopamine D_3 receptors and use of antipsychotics in patients with schizophrenia: postmortem study. *Archives of General Psychiatry* **54**, 225–232.

Haber, S.N. & Fudge, J.L. (1997) The primate substantia nigra and VTA: integrative circuitry and function. *Critical Reviews in Neurobiology* **11**, 323–342.

Haber, S.N., Fudge, J.L. & McFarland, N.R. (2000) Striatonigrostriatal pathways in primates form an ascending spiral from the shell to the dorsolateral striatum. *Journal of Neuroscience* **20**, 2369–2382.

Hanada, S., Mita, T., Nishino, N. & Tanaka, C. (1987) [^{3}H]muscimol binding sites increased in autopsied brains of chronic schizophrenics. *Life Sciences* **40**, 259–266.

Hersch, S.M., Ciliax, B.J., Gutekunst, C.A. *et al.* (1995) Electron microscopic analysis of D_1 and D_2 dopamine receptor proteins in the dorsal striatum and their synaptic relationships with motor corticostriatal afferents. *Journal of Neuroscience* **15**, 5222–5237.

Hess, E.J., Bracha, H.S., Kleinman, J.E. & Creese, I. (1987) Dopamine receptor subtype imbalance in schizophrenia. *Life Science* **40**, 1487–1497.

Hietala, J., Syvälahti, E., Vuorio, K. *et al.* (1994) Striatal D_2 receptor characteristics in neuroleptic-naive schizophrenic patients studied with positron emission tomography. *Archives of General Psychiatry* **51**, 116–123.

Hietala, J., Syvalahti, E., Vuorio, K. *et al.* (1995) Presynaptic dopamine function in striatum of neuroleptic-naive schizophrenic patients. *Lancet* **346**, 1130–1131.

Hietala, J., Syvalahti, E., Vilkman, H. *et al.* (1999) Depressive symptoms and presynaptic dopamine function in neuroleptic-naive schizophrenia. *Schizophrenia Research* **35**, 41–50.

Hirai, M., Kitamura, N., Hashimoto, T. *et al.* (1988) [^{3}H]GBR-12935 binding sites in human striatal membranes: binding characteristics and changes in parkinsonians and schizophrenics. *Japanese Journal of Pharmacology* **47**, 237–243.

Hoover, J.E. & Strick, P.L. (1993) Multiple output channels in the basal ganglia. *Science* **259**, 819–821.

Huckle, P.L. & Palia, S.S. (1993) Managing resistant schizophrenia. *British Journal of Hospital Medicine* **50**, 467–471.

Innis, R.B., Malison, R.T., Al-Tikriti, M. *et al.* (1992) Amphetamine-stimulated dopamine release competes *in vivo* for [^{123}I]IBZM binding to the D_2 receptor in non-human primates. *Synapse* **10**, 177–184.

Javitt, D.C. & Zukin, S.R. (1991) Recent advances in the phencyclidine model of schizophrenia. *American Journal of Psychiatry* **148**, 1301–1308.

Jentsch, J.D. & Roth, R.H. (1999) The neuropsychopharmacology of phencyclidine: from NMDA receptor hypofunction to the do-

pamine hypothesis of schizophrenia. *Neuropsychopharmacology* **20**, 201–225.

Joel, D. & Weiner, I. (2000) The connections of the dopaminergic system with the striatum in rats and primates: an analysis with respect to the functional and compartmental organization of the striatum. *Neuroscience* **96**, 451–474.

Joyce, J.N. & Gurevich, E.V. (1999) D_3 receptors and the actions of neuroleptics in the ventral striatopallidal system of schizophrenics. *Annals of New York Academy of Sciences* **877**, 595–613.

Joyce, J.N. & Meador Woodruff, J.H. (1997) Linking the family of D_2 receptors to neuronal circuits in human brain: insights into schizophrenia. *Neuropsychopharmacology* **16**, 375–384.

Joyce, J.N., Lexow, N., Bird, E. & Winokur, A. (1988) Organization of dopamine D_1 and D_2 receptors in human striatum: receptor autoradiographic studies in Huntington's disease and schizophrenia. *Synapse* **2**, 546–557.

Kalivas, P.W. & Duffy, P. (1995) Selective activation of dopamine transmission in the shell of the nucleus accumbens by stress. *Brain Research* **675**, 325–328.

Kalivas, P.W. & Stewart, J. (1991) Dopamine transmission in the initiation and expression of drug- and stress-induced sensitization of motor activity. *Brain Research Review* **16**, 223–244.

Kalivas, P.W., Sorg, B.A. & Hooks, M.S. (1993) The pharmacology and neural circuitry of sensitization to psychostimulants. *Behavioral Pharmacology* **4**, 315–334.

Karlsson, P., Farde, L., Halldin, C. & Sedvall, G. (1997) D_1-dopamine receptors in schizophrenia examined by PET. *Schizophrenia Research* **24**, 179.

Karreman, M. & Moghaddam, B. (1996) The prefrontal cortex regulates the basal release of dopamine in the limbic striatum: an effect mediated by ventral tegmental area. *Journal of Neurochemistry* **66**, 589–598.

Kebabian, J.W. & Calne, D.B. (1979) Multiple receptors for dopamine. *Nature* **277**, 93–96.

Keefe, R.S., Silva, S.G., Perkins, D.O. & Lieberman, J.A. (1999) The effects of atypical antipsychotic drugs on neurocognitive impairment in schizophrenia: a review and meta-analysis. *Schizophrenia Bulletin* **25**, 201–222.

Kegeles, L.S., Zea-Ponce, Y., Abi-Dargham, A. *et al.* (1999) Stability of [^{123}I]IBZM SPECT measurement of amphetamine-induced striatal dopamine release in humans. *Synapse* **31**, 302–308.

Kegeles, L.S., Abi-Dargham, A., Zea-Ponce, Y. *et al.* (2000) Modulation of amphetamine-induced striatal dopamine release by ketamine in humans: implications for schizophrenia. *Biological Psychiatry* **48**, 627–640.

Kerr, J.N. & Wickens, J.R. (2001) Dopamine D_1/D_5 receptor activation is required for long-term potentiation in the rat neostriatum *in vitro*. *Journal of Neurophysiology* **85**, 117–124.

Knable, M.B. & Weinberger, D.R. (1997) Dopamine, the prefrontal cortex and schizophrenia. *Journal of Psychopharmacology* **11**, 123–131.

Knable, M.B., Hyde, T.M., Herman, M.M. *et al.* (1994) Quantitative autoradiography of dopamine-D_1 receptors, D_2 receptors, and dopamine uptake sites in postmortem striatal specimens from schizophrenic patients. *Biological Psychiatry* **36**, 827–835.

Knable, M.B., Hyde, T.M., Murray, A.M., Herman, M.M. & Kleinman, J.E. (1996) A postmortem study of frontal cortical dopamine D_1 receptors in schizophrenics, psychiatric controls, and normal controls. *Biological Psychiatry* **40**, 1191–1199.

Knable, M.B., Egan, M.F., Heinz, A. *et al.* (1997) Altered dopaminergic function and negative symptoms in drug-free patients with schizophrenia. [^{123}I]-iodobenzamide SPECT study. *British Journal of Psychiatry* **171**, 574–577.

Kolachana, B.S., Saunders, R. & Weinberger, D. (1995) Augmentation of prefrontal cortical monoaminergic activity inhibits dopamine release in the caudate nucleus: an *in vivo* neurochemical assessment in the rhesus monkey. *Neurosciences* **69**, 859–868.

Konradi, C. (1998) The molecular basis of dopamine and glutamate interactions in the striatum. *Advances in Pharmacology* **42**, 729–733.

Kramer, M.S., Last, B., Getson, A. *et al.* (1997) The effects of a selective D₄ dopamine receptor antagonist (L-745 870) in acutely psychotic inpatients with schizophrenia. *Archives of General Psychiatry* **54**, 567–572.

Krystal, J.H., Abi-Dargham, A., Laruelle, M. & Moghaddam, B. (1999) In: *Neurobiology of Mental Illness* (eds D. Charney, E.J. Nestler & B. Bunney), pp. 214–224. Oxford University Press, New York.

Kunishio, K. & Haber, S.N. (1994) Primate cingulostriatal projection: limbic striatal versus sensorimotor striatal input. *Journal of Comparative Neurology* **350**, 337–356.

Laakso, A., Vilkman, H., Alakare, B. *et al.* (2000) Striatal dopamine transporter binding in neuroleptic-naive patients with schizophrenia studied with positron emission tomography. *American Journal of Psychiatry* **157**, 269–271.

Lahti, A.C., Koffel, B., LaPorte, D. & Tamminga, C.A. (1995) Subanesthetic doses of ketamine stimulate psychosis in schizophrenia. *Neuropsychopharmacology* **13**, 9–19.

Lahti, R.A., Roberts, R.C., Conley, R.R. *et al.* (1996a) D₂-type dopamine receptors in postmortem human brain sections from normal and schizophrenic subjects. *Neuroreport* **7**, 1945–1948.

Lahti, R.A., Roberts, R.C., Conley, R.R. & Tamminga, C.A. (1996b) Dopamine D₂, D₃ and D₄ receptors in human postmortem brain sections: comparison between normals and schizophrenics. *Schizophrenia Research* **18**, 173.

Lahti, R.A., Roberts, R.C., Cochrane, E.V. *et al.* (1998) Direct determination of dopamine D₄ receptors in normal and schizophrenic postmortem brain tissue: a [H-3]NGD-94-1 study. *Molecular Psychiatrics* **3**, 528–533.

Laruelle, M. (2000a) Imaging synaptic neurotransmission with *in vivo* binding competition techniques: a critical review. *Journal of Cerebral Blood Flow and Metabolism* **20**, 423–451.

Laruelle, M. (2000b) The role of endogenous sensitization in the pathophysiology of schizophrenia: implications from recent brain imaging studies. *Brain Research Review* **31**, 371–384.

Laruelle, M., Casanova, M., Weinberger, D. & Kleinman, J. (1990) Postmortem study of the dopaminergic D₁ receptors in the dorsolateral prefrontal cortex of schizophrenics and controls. *Schizophrenia Research* **3**, 30–31.

Laruelle, M., Abi-Dargham, A., van Dyck, C.H. *et al.* (1996) Single photon emission computerized tomography imaging of amphetamine-induced dopamine release in drug-free schizophrenic subjects. *Proceedings of the National Academy of Sciences of the USA* **93**, 9235–9240.

Laruelle, M.D., Souza, C.D., Baldwin, R.M. *et al.* (1997a) Imaging D₂ receptor occupancy by endogenous dopamine in humans. *Neuropsychopharmacology* **17**, 162–174.

Laruelle, M., Iyer, R.N., Al-Tikriti, M.S. *et al.* (1997b) Microdialysis and SPECT measurements of amphetamine-induced dopamine release in non-human primates. *Synapse* **25**, 1–14.

Laruelle, M., Abi-Dargham, A., Gil, R., Kegeles, L. & Innis, R. (1999) Increased dopamine transmission in schizophrenia: relationship to illness phases. *Biological Psychiatry* **46**, 56–72.

Laruelle, M., Abi-Dargham, A., van Dyck, C. *et al.* (2000) Dopamine and serotonin transporters in patients with schizophrenia: an imaging study with [¹²³I]β-CIT. *Biological Psychiatry* **47**, 371–379.

Lee, S.P., O'Dowd, B.F., Ng, G.Y. *et al.* (2000) Inhibition of cell surface expression by mutant receptors demonstrates that D₂ dopamine receptors exist as oligomers in the cell. *Molecular Pharmacology* **58**, 120–128.

Lee, T., Seeman, P., Tourtelotte, W.W., Farley, I.J. & Hornykiewicz, O. (1978) Binding of ³H-neuroleptics and ³H-apomorphine in schizophrenic brains. *Nature* **274**, 897–900.

Le Moine, C., Normand, E., Guitteny, A.F. *et al.* (1990) Dopamine receptor gene expression by enkephalin neurons in rat forebrain. *Proceedings of the National Academy of Sciences of the USA* **87**, 230–234.

Le Moine, C., Normand, E. & Bloch, B. (1991) Phenotypical characterization of the rat striatal neurons expressing the D₁ dopamine receptor gene. *Proceedings of the National Academy of Sciences of the USA* **88**, 4205–4209.

Leveque, J.C., Macias, W., Rajadhyaksha, A. *et al.* (2000) Intracellular modulation of NMDA receptor function by antipsychotic drugs. *Journal of Neuroscience* **20**, 4011–4020.

Lieberman, J.A., Kane, J.M. & Alvir, J. (1987) Provocative tests with psychostimulant drugs in schizophrenia. *Psychopharmacology* **91**, 415–433.

Lieberman, J.A., Kinon, B.L. & Loebel, A.D. (1990) Dopaminergic mechanisms in idiopathic and drug-induced psychoses. *Schizophrenia Bulletin* **16**, 97–110.

Lieberman, J.A., Sheitman, B.B. & Kinon, B.J. (1997) Neurochemical sensitization in the pathophysiology of schizophrenia: deficits and dysfunction in neuronal regulation and plasticity. *Neuropsychopharmacology* **17**, 205–229.

Lindstrom, L.H., Gefvert, O., Hagberg, G. *et al.* (1999) Increased dopamine synthesis rate in medial prefrontal cortex and striatum in schizophrenia indicated by L-(β-11C) DOPA and PET. *Biological Psychiatry* **46**, 681–688.

Lindvall, O. & Björklund, A. (1983) In: *Chemical Neuroanatomy* (ed. P. Emson), pp. 229–255. Raven Press, New York.

Mackay, A.V., Iversen, L.L., Rossor, M. *et al.* (1982) Increased brain dopamine and dopamine receptors in schizophrenia. *Archives of General Psychiatry* **39**, 991–997.

Magos, L. (1969) Persistence of the effect of amphetamine on stereotyped activity in rats. *European Journal of Pharmacology* **6**, 200–201.

Martinot, J.-L., Peron-Magnan, P., Huret, J.-D. *et al.* (1990) Striatal D₂ dopaminergic receptors assessed with positron emission tomography and ⁷⁶Br-bromospiperone in untreated patients. *American Journal of Psychiatry* **147**, 346–350.

Martinot, J.L., Paillère-Martinot, M.L., Loc'h, C. *et al.* (1991) The estimated density of D₂ striatal receptors in schizophrenia: a study with positron emission tomography and ⁷⁶Br-bromolisuride. *British Journal of Psychiatry* **158**, 346–350.

Martinot, J.L., Paillère-Martinot, M.L., Loch, H.C. *et al.* (1994) Central D₂ receptors and negative symptoms of schizophrenia. *British Journal of Pharmacology* **164**, 27–34.

Marzella, P.L., Hill, C., Keks, N., Singh, R. & Copolov, D. (1997) The binding of both [H-3]nemonapride and [H-3]raclopride is increased in schizophrenia. *Biological Psychiatry* **42**, 648–654.

Mawlawi, O., Martinez, D., Slifstein, M. *et al.* (2001) Imaging human mesolimbic dopamine transmission with positron emission tomography. I. Accuracy and precision of D₂ receptor parameter measurements in ventral striatum. *Journal of Cerebral Blood Flow and Metabolism* **21**, 1034–1057.

Meador-Woodruff, J.H., Damask, S.P., Wang, J. *et al.* (1996) Dopamine receptors mRNA expression in human striatum and neocortex. *Neuropsychopharmacology* **15**, 17–29.

Meador-Woodruff, J.H., Haroutunian, V., Powchik, P. *et al.* (1997) Dopamine receptor transcript expression in striatum and prefrontal and occipital cortex: focal abnormalities in orbitofrontal cortex in schizophrenia. *Archives of General Psychiatry* 54, 1089–1095.

Meltzer, H. (1989) Clinical studies on the mechanism of action of clozapine: the dopamine–serotonin hypothesis of schizophrenia. *Psychopharmacology* 99, S18–S27.

Miller, D.W. & Abercrombie, E.D. (1996) Effects of MK-801 on spontaneous and amphetamine-stimulated dopamine release in striatum measured with *in vivo* microdialysis in awake rats. *Brain Research Bulletin* 40, 57–62.

Missale, C., Nash, S.R., Robinson, S.W., Jaber, M. & Caron, M.G. (1998) Dopamine receptors: from structure to function. *Physiological Review* 78, 189–225.

Mita, T., Hanada, S., Nishino, N. *et al.* (1986) Decreased serotonin S_2 and increased dopamine D_2 receptors in chronic schizophrenics. *Biological Psychiatry* 21, 1407–1414.

Mogenson, G.J., Jones, D.L. & Yim, C.Y. (1980) From motivation to action: functional interface between the limbic system and the motor system. *Progress in Neurobiology* 14, 69–97.

Moghaddam, B. & Adams, B.W. (1998) Reversal of phencyclidine effects by a group II metabotropic glutamate receptor agonist in rats. *Science* 281, 1349–1352.

Monsma, F. Jr, Mahan, L.C., McVittie, L.D., Gerfen, C.R. & Sibley, D.R. (1990) Molecular cloning and expression of a D_1 dopamine receptor linked to adenylyl cyclase activation. *Proceedings of the National Academy of Sciences of the USA* 87, 6723–6727.

Mrzljak, L., Bergson, C., Pappy, M. *et al.* (1996) Localization of dopamine D_4 receptors in GABAergic neurons of the primate brain. *Nature* 381, 245–248.

Murray, A.M., Hyde, T.M., Knable, M.B. *et al.* (1995) Distribution of putative D_4 dopamine receptors in postmortem striatum from patients with schizophrenia. *Journal of Neuroscience* 15, 2186–2191.

Ng, G.Y., O'Dowd, B.F., Caron, M. *et al.* (1994) Phosphorylation and palmitoylation of the human D_2L dopamine receptor in Sf9 cells. *Journal of Neurochemistry* 63, 1589–1595.

Ng, G.Y., O'Dowd, B.F., Lee, S.P. *et al.* (1996) Dopamine D_2 receptor dimers and receptor-blocking peptides. *Biochemical and Biophysical Research Communications* 227, 200–204.

Nguyen, T.V., Kosofsky, B.E., Birnbaum, R., Cohen, B.M. & Hyman, S.E. (1992) Differential expression of c-fos and zif268 in rat striatum after haloperidol, clozapine, and amphetamine. *Proceedings of the National Academy of Sciences of the USA* 89, 4270–4274.

Nishi, A., Snyder, G.L. & Greengard, P. (1997) Bidirectional regulation of DARPP-32 phosphorylation by dopamine. *Journal of Neuroscience* 17, 8147–8155.

Nordstrom, A.L., Farde, L., Eriksson, L. & Halldin, C. (1995) No elevated D_2 dopamine receptors in neuroleptic-naive schizophrenic patients revealed by positron emission tomography and [^{11}C] N-methylspiperone [see comments]. *Psychiatry Research* 61, 67–83.

O'Donnell, P. & Grace, A.A. (1998a) Dysfunctions in multiple interrelated systems as the neurobiological bases of schizophrenic symptom clusters. *Schizophrenia Bulletin* 24, 267–283.

O'Donnell, P. & Grace, A.A. (1998b) Phencyclidine interferes with the hippocampal gating of nucleus accumbens neuronal activity *in vivo*. *Neuroscience* 87, 823–830.

Okubo, Y., Suhara, T., Suzuki, K. *et al.* (1997) Decreased prefrontal dopamine D_1 receptors in schizophrenia revealed by PET. *Nature* 385, 634–636.

Olney, J.W. & Farber, N.B. (1995) Glutamate receptor dysfunction and schizophrenia. *Archives of General Psychiatry* 52, 998–1007.

Owen, F., Cross, A.J., Crow, T.J. *et al.* (1978) Increased dopamine-receptor sensitivity in schizophrenia. *Lancet* 2, 223–226.

Owen, R., Owen, F., Poulter, M. & Crow, T.J. (1984) Dopamine D_2 receptors in substantia nigra in schizophrenia. *Brain Research* 299, 152–154.

Palermo-Neto, J. (1997) Dopaminergic systems: dopamine receptors. *Psychiatrics Clinics of North America* 20, 705–721.

Parent, A. & Hazrati, L.N. (1995a) Functional anatomy of the basal ganglia. I. The corticobasal ganglia–thalamocortical loop. *Brain Research Review* 20, 91–127.

Parent, A. & Hazrati, L.N. (1995b) Functional anatomy of the basal ganglia. II. The place of subthalamic nucleus and external pallidum in basal ganglia circuitry. *Brain Research Review* 20, 128–154.

Parsey, R.V., Oquendo, M., Zea-Ponce, Y. *et al.* (2001) Dopamine D_2 receptor availability and amphetamine-induced dopamine release in unipolar depression. *Biological Psychology* 50, 313–322.

Pearce, R.K., Seeman, P., Jellinger, K. & Tourtellotte, W.W. (1990) Dopamine uptake sites and dopamine receptors in Parkinson's disease and schizophrenia. *European Neurology* 30 (Suppl. 1), 9–14.

Pennartz, C.M., Groenewegen, H.J. & Lopes da Silva, F.H. (1994) The nucleus accumbens as a complex of functionally distinct neuronal ensembles: an integration of behavioural, electrophysiological and anatomical data. *Progress in Neurobiology* 42, 719–761.

Pierce, R.C. & Kalivas, P.W. (1997) A circuitry model of the expression of behavioral sensitization to amphetamine-like psychostimulants. *Brain Research Review* 25, 192–216.

Pilowsky, L.S., Costa, D.C., Ell, P.J. *et al.* (1994) D_2 dopamine receptor binding in the basal ganglia of antipsychotic-free schizophrenic patients: an I-123-IBZM single photon emission computerized tomography study. *British Journal of Psychiatry* 164, 16–26.

Pimoule, C., Schoemaker, H., Reynolds, G.P. & Langer, S.Z. (1985) [^{3}H]SCH 23390 labelled D_1 dopamine receptors are unchanged in schizophrenia and Parkinson's disease. *European Journal of Pharmacology* 114, 235–237.

Pycock, C.J., Kerwin, R.W. & Carter, C.J. (1980) Effect of lesion of cortical dopamine terminals on subcortical dopamine receptors in rats. *Nature* 286, 74–77.

Reith, J., Benkelfat, C., Sherwin, A. *et al.* (1994) Elevated dopa decarboxylase activity in living brain of patients with psychosis. *Proceedings of the National Academy of Sciences of the USA* 91, 11651–11654.

Reynolds, G.P. (1983) Increased concentrations and lateral asymmetry of amygdala dopamine in schizophrenia. *Nature* 305, 527–529.

Reynolds, G.P. (1989) Beyond the dopamine hypothesis: the neurochemical pathology of schizophrenia. *British Journal of Psychiatry* 155, 305–316.

Reynolds, G.P. & Czudek, C. (1988) Status of the dopaminergic system in postmortem brain in schizophrenia. *Psychopharmacological Bulletin* 24, 345–347.

Reynolds, G.P. & Mason, S.L. (1994) Are striatal dopamine D_4 receptors increased in schizophrenia? *Journal of Neurochemistry* 63, 1576–1577.

Reynolds, G.P., Czudek, C., Bzowej, N. & Seeman, P. (1987) Dopamine receptor asymmetry in schizophrenia. *Lancet* 1, 979.

Robertson, G.S., Matsumura, H. & Fibiger, H.C. (1994) Induction patterns of Fos-like immunoreactivity in the forebrain as predictors of atypical antipsychotic activity. *Journal of Pharmacology and Experimental Therapy* 271, 1058–1066.

Robinson, T.E. & Becker, J.B. (1986) Enduring changes in brain and behavior produced by chronic amphetamine administration: a review and evaluation of animal models of amphetamine psychosis. *Brain Research Review* 11, 157–198.

Ross, S.B. (1991) Synaptic concentration of dopamine in the mouse striatum in relationship to the kinetic properties of the dopamine receptors and uptake mechanism. *Journal of Neurochemistry* **56**, 22–29.

Ross, S.B. & Jackson, D.M. (1989) Kinetic properties of the *in vivo* accumulation of [^{3}H] (–)-N-propylnorapomorphine in the mouse brain. *Naunyn-Schmiedeberg's Archives of Pharmacology* **340**, 13–20.

Ruiz, J., Gabilondo, A.M., Meana, J.J. & Garcia-Sevilla, J.A. (1992) Increased [^{3}H] raclopride binding sites in postmortem brains from schizophrenic violent suicide victims. *Psychopharmacology* **109**, 410–414.

Sato, M., Chen, C.C., Akiyama, K. & Otsuki, S. (1983) Acute exacerbation of paranoid psychotic state after long-term abstinence in patients with previous methamphetamine psychosis. *Biological Psychiatry* **18**, 429–440.

Saunders, R.C., Kolachana, B.S., Bachevalier, J. & Weinberger, D.R. (1998) Neonatal lesions of the medial temporal lobe disrupt prefrontal cortical regulation of striatal dopamine. *Nature* **393**, 169–171.

Schoots, O., Seeman, P., Guan, H.C., Paterson, A.D. & Vantol, H.H.M. (1995) Long-term haloperidol elevates dopamine D_4 receptors by 2-fold in rats. *European Journal of Pharmacology: Molecular Pharmacology Section* **289**, 67–72.

Schultz, W., Tremblay, L. & Hollerman, J.R. (1998) Reward prediction in primate basal ganglia and frontal cortex. *Neuropharmacology* **37**, 421–429.

Schwartz, J.C., Diaz, J., Bordet, R. *et al.* (1998) Functional implications of multiple dopamine receptor subtypes: the D_1/D_3 receptor coexistence. *Brain Research Review* **26**, 236–242.

Seamans, J.K., Gorelova, N., Durstewitz, D. & Yang, C.R. (2001) Bidirectional dopamine modulation of GABAergic inhibition in prefrontal cortical pyramidal neurons. *Journal of Neuroscience* **21**, 3628–3638.

Seeman, P. (1988) Brain dopamine receptors in schizophrenia: PET problems. *Archives of General Psychiatry* **45**, 598–560.

Seeman, P. (1992) Dopamine receptor sequences. Therapeutic levels of neuroleptics occupy D_2 receptors, clozapine occupies D_4. *Neuropsychopharmacology* **7**, 261–284.

Seeman, P. & Lee, T. (1975) Antipsychotic drugs: direct correlation between clinical potency and presynaptic action on dopamine neurons. *Science* **188**, 1217–1219.

Seeman, P., Ulpian, C., Bergeron, C. *et al.* (1984) Bimodal distribution of dopamine receptor densities in brains of schizophrenics. *Science* **225**, 728–731.

Seeman, P., Bzowej, N.H., Guan, H.C. *et al.* (1987) Human brain D_1 and D_2 dopamine receptors in schizophrenia, Alzheimer's, Parkinson's, and Huntington's diseases. *Neuropsychopharmacology* **1**, 5–15.

Seeman, P., Guan, H.-C. & Niznik, H.B. (1989) Endogenous dopamine lowers the dopamine D_2 receptor density as measured by [^{3}H] raclopride: implications for positron emission tomography of the human brain. *Synapse* **3**, 96–97.

Seeman, P., Guan, H.C. & Van Tol, H.H.M. (1993) Dopamine D_4 receptors elevated in schizophrenia. *Nature* **365**, 411–445.

Seeman, P., Guan, H.C. & Van Tol, H.H. (1995) Schizophrenia: elevation of dopamine D_4-like sites, using [^{3}H]nemonapride and [^{125}I]epidepride. *European Journal of Pharmacology* **286**, R3–R5.

Smiley, J.F., Levey, A.I., Ciliax, B.J. & Goldman-Rakic, P.S. (1994) D_1 dopamine receptor immunoreactivity in human and monkey cerebral cortex: predominant and extrasynaptic localization in dendritic spines. *Proceedings of the National Academy of Sciences of the USA* **91**, 5720–5724.

Sokoloff, P., Giros, B., Martres, M.-P., Bouthenet, M.-L. & Schwartz, J.-C. (1990) Molecular cloning and characterization of a novel dopamine receptor D_3 as a target for neuroleptics. *Nature* **347**, 146–151.

Sorg, B.A., Hooks, M.S. & Kalivas, P.W. (1994) Neuroanatomy and neurochemical mechanisms of time-dependent sensitization. *Toxicology and Industrial Health* **10**, 369–386.

Spector, S., Sjoerdsma, A. & Udenfriend, S. (1965) Blockade of endogenous norepinephrine synthesis by α-methyl-tyrosine, an inhibitor of tyrosine hydroxylase. *Journal of Pharmacology and Experimental Therapy* **147**, 86–95.

Sumiyoshi, T., Stockmeier, C.A., Overholser, J.C., Thompson, P.A. & Meltzer, H.Y. (1995) Dopamine D_4 receptors and effects of guanine nucleotides on [^{3}H]raclopride binding in postmortem caudate nucleus of subjects with schizophrenia or major depression. *Brain Research* **681**, 109–116.

Sunahara, R.K., Guan, H.-C., O'Dowd, B.F. *et al.* (1991) Cloning of the gene for a human dopamine D_5 receptor with higher affinity for dopamine than D_1. *Nature* **350**, 614–619.

Surmeier, D.J., Eberwine, J., Wilson, C.J. *et al.* (1992) Dopamine receptor subtypes colocalize in rat striatonigral neurons. *Proceedings of the National Academy of Sciences of the USA* **89**, 10178–10182.

Surmeier, D.J., Song, W.J. & Yan, Z. (1996) Coordinated expression of dopamine receptors in neostriatal medium spiny neurons. *Journal of Neuroscience* **16**, 6579–6591.

Tarazi, F.I., Florijn, W.J. & Creese, I. (1997) Differential regulation of dopamine receptors after chronic typical and atypical antipsychotic drug treatment. *Neuroscience* **78**, 985–996.

Taylor, S.F., Koeppe, R.A., Tandon, R., Zubieta, J.K. & Frey, K.A. (2000) *In vivo* measurement of the vesicular monoamine transporter in schizophrenia. *Neuropsychopharmacology* **23**, 667–675.

Tiberi, M., Jarvie, K.R., Silvia, C. *et al.* (1991) Cloning, molecular characterization, and chromosomal assignment of a gene encoding a second D_1 dopamine receptor subtype: differential expression pattern in rat brain compared with the D_{1A} receptor. *Proceedings of the National Academy of Sciences of the USA* **88**, 7491–7495.

Tune, L.E., Wong, D.F., Pearlson, G. *et al.* (1993) Dopamine D_2 receptor density estimates in schizophrenia: a positron emission tomography study with ^{11}C-N-methylspiperone. *Psychiatry Research* **49**, 219–237.

Udenfriend, S., Nagatsu, T. & Zaltzman-Nirenberg, P. (1965) Inhibitors of purified beef adrenal tyrosine hydroxylase. *Biochemistry and Pharmacology* **14**, 837–847.

Van der Werf, J.F., Sebens, J.B., Vaalburg, W. & Korf, J. (1986) *In vivo* binding of N-propylnorapomorphine in the rat brain: regional localization, quantification in striatum and lack of correlation with dopamine metabolism. *European Journal of Pharmacology* **87**, 259–270.

Van Tol, H.H.M., Bunzow, J.R., Guan, H-C. *et al.* (1991) Cloning of the gene for a human dopamine D_4 receptor with high affinity for the antipsychotic clozapine. *Nature* **350**, 610–614.

Volk, D.W., Austin, M.C., Pierri, J.N., Sampson, A.R. & Lewis, D.A. (2000) Decreased glutamic acid decarboxylase$_{67}$ messenger RNA expression in a subset of prefrontal cortical γ-aminobutyric acid neurons in subjects with schizophrenia. *Archives of General Psychiatry* **57**, 237–245.

Watanabe, M., Nonaka, R., Hagino, Y. & Kodama, Y. (1998) Effects of prenatal methylazoxymethanol treatment on striatal dopaminergic systems in rat brain. *Neuroscience Research* **30**, 135–144.

Weiden, P., Aquila, R. & Standard, J. (1996) Atypical antipsychotic drugs and long-term outcome of schizophrenia. *Journal of Clinical Psychiatry* **57** (S1), 53–60.

Weinberger, D.R. (1987) Implications of the normal brain development for the pathogenesis of schizophrenia. *Archives of General Psychiatry* **44**, 660–669.

Weinberger, D.R., Berman, K.F. & Zec, R.F. (1986) Physiological dysfunction of dorsolateral prefrontal cortex in schizophrenia. I. Regional cerebral blood flow evidence. *Archives of General Psychiatry* **43**, 114–124.

Wickens, J.R. (2000) In: *Brain Dynamics and the Striatal Complex* (eds R. Miller & J.R. Wickens), pp. 65–76. Academic, Harwood.

Wilkinson, L.S. (1997) The nature of interactions involving prefrontal and striatal dopamine systems. *Journal of Psychopharmacology* **11**, 143–150.

Wong, D.F., Wagner, H.N., Tune, L.E. *et al.* (1986) Positron emission tomography reveals elevated D_2 dopamine receptors in drug-naive schizophrenics. *Science* **234**, 1558–1563.

Woo, T.U., Miller, J.L. & Lewis, D.A. (1997) Schizophrenia and the parvalbumin-containing class of cortical local circuit neurons. *American Journal of Psychiatry* **154**, 1013–1015.

Woo, T.U., Whitehead, R.E., Melchitzky, D.S. & Lewis, D.A. (1998)

A subclass of prefrontal γ-aminobutyric acid axon terminals are selectively altered in schizophrenia. *Proceedings of the National Academy of Sciences of the USA* **95**, 5341–5346.

Yang, C.R., Seamans, J.K. & Gorelova, N. (1999) Developing a neuronal model for the pathophysiology of schizophrenia based on the nature of electrophysiological actions of dopamine in the prefrontal cortex. *Neuropsychopharmacology* **21**, 161–194.

Young, L.T., Wong, D.F., Goldman, S. *et al.* (1991) Effects of endogenous dopamine on kinetics of [3H]methylspiperone and [3H]raclopride binding in the rat brain. *Synapse* **9**, 188–194.

Zawarynski, P., Tallerico, T., Seeman, P. *et al.* (1998) Dopamine D_2 receptor dimers in human and rat brain. *FEBS Letters* **441**, 383–386.

Zhou, Q.Y., Grandy, D.K., Thambi, L. *et al.* (1990) Cloning and expression of human and rat D_1 dopamine receptors. *Nature* **347**, 76–80.

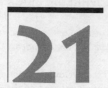

21 Animal models of schizophrenia

B.K. Lipska and D.R. Weinberger

Pharmacological dopamine-based animal
    models, 388
Novel approaches to modelling schizophrenia, 389
Neurodevelopmental models, 390
    Models testing aetiological theories, 390
    Models of disrupted neurogenesis, 391
    Perinatal stress models, 392

Neonatal lesion models, 392
Pharmacological models of glutamatergic
    antagonism, 394
Genetic models, 394
Conclusions, 396
References, 397

Animal models are important in exploring the mechanisms underlying human disease and designing new therapies. However, this approach has not been very popular in psychiatric research as modelling of psychiatric disorders in experimental animals has often been regarded as highly controversial. Schizophrenia is an example of a particularly formidable challenge for animal modelling. It is a complex disorder of unknown origin, characterized by abnormalities of uniquely human behaviours in the realms of perception, thinking and the experience of emotions, and whose onset is virtually restricted to young adulthood. Schizophrenia is an inherently human disease, so it is not possible to reproduce in a rodent, or even in a non-human primate, its most prominent symptoms – hallucinations, delusions and thought disorder. However, recent new evidence about the neurobiology of the condition has generated new avenues of animal research. In this chapter, we present recent achievements in the efforts to model the neurobiology of schizophrenia in animals, consider limitations inherent in any heuristic animal model of this and probably other psychiatric disorders, and discuss the usefulness of a new generation of animal models for testing particular hypotheses about aetiology and pathophysiology of schizophrenia. Parts of this chapter appeared in an earlier version (Lipska & Weinberger 2000).

An animal model may represent a disease on three different levels:

1 it may reproduce inducing factor(s) (e.g. a genetic defect and the subsequent pathological processes underlying the disease);

2 it may mimic phenomenology (e.g. an array of symptoms of schizophrenia); and

3 it may predict responsiveness to already available treatments (e.g. antipsychotic drugs).

Thus, the characteristics of an animal model and its faithfulness vary according to the aspects that it aspires to represent. Models that reconstruct the aetiology and pathophysiological mechanisms of the disease are of the highest order of fidelity; they have so-called 'construct validity'. Models with construct validity usually, although not invariably (see below), possess some degree of face and predictive validity (Kornetsky & Markowitz 1978; McKinney & Moran 1981; Ellenbroek & Cools 1990; Rupniak & Iversen 1993; Costall & Naylor 1995). A good illus-

tration of valid and useful models of complex diseases are the genetic models of diabetes and hypertension: for instance, the db/db mice model of diabetes (Kobayashi *et al.* 2000) and the spontaneously hypertensive rat (SHR) (Patel *et al.* 2000). Unlike these models, which faithfully reproduce relatively clear-cut physiological characteristics (e.g. high blood sugar levels or high blood pressure), models of psychiatric disorders face the unique difficulty of simulating much more complex and less easily defined pathophysiology.

Pharmacological dopamine-based animal models

Traditionally, most animal models of schizophrenia have focused on phenomena linked to dopamine, because the dopaminergic system has been strongly implicated in this disorder, as all effective antipsychotic drugs are antagonists of dopamine receptors, and dopamine agonists induce symptoms that resemble psychosis (Kornetsky & Markowitz 1978; McKinney & Moran 1981; Ellenbroek & Cools 1990; Costall & Naylor 1995; see Table 21.1). For instance, some dopamine-based models involve behavioural paradigms that were inspired by antipsychotic (i.e. antidopaminergic) pharmacology but bear no resemblance to schizophrenia (e.g. antagonism of apomorphine-induced emesis). Others reproduce phenomena isomorphic with selected characteristics of schizophrenia such as motor behaviours (e.g. dopamimetic drugs-induced stereotypies) and information processing deficits (e.g. apomorphine-induced prepulse inhibition of startle (PPI) abnormalities; Costall & Naylor 1995). These dopamine-linked behaviours, although not specific for or uniquely prominent in schizophrenia, can at least be detected and precisely quantified in non-human species and have been useful in screening drugs with a predicted mechanism of action (e.g. dopamine blockade). Thus, models based on perturbing dopamine have no construct validity, limited face validity but relatively good predictive validity. The predictive validity is to be expected given that the models are based on changing dopamine function. However, as 'dopamine-in, dopamine-out' models (i.e. models based on direct pharmacological manipulation of

Table 21.1 Clinical aspects of schizophrenia and relevant behavioural changes in animals.

Schizophrenia: clinical phenomena	Animal models: behavioural changes
1 Psychotic symptoms	Behaviours related to increased dopaminergic transmission: (i) Dopamimetic-induced hyperlocomotion (ii) Reduced haloperidol-induced catalepsy
2 Stereotypic behaviours	Dopamimetic-induced stereotypies
3 Worsening of psychotic symptoms by NMDA antagonists	NMDA antagonist-induced locomotion
4 Vulnerability to stress	Stress-induced hyperlocomotion
5 Information processing deficits	Sensorimotor gating (PPI, P50) deficits
6 Attentional deficits	Deficits in latent inhibition
7 Cognitive deficits	Impaired performance in delayed alternation and spatial memory tests
8 Social withdrawal	Reduced contacts with unfamiliar partners

the dopaminergic system and tests of behavioural outcome related to dopamine function), they precluded exploring other than dopamine-based mechanisms of the disease and discovering novel antipsychotic therapies. Drugs that have emerged as a result of such models all exert antidopaminergic efficacy. Antidopaminergic drugs, however, although ameliorative of some of the symptoms of schizophrenia, do not cure the disease. It has become increasingly clear that models based on direct manipulations of the dopamine system may have exhausted their heuristic potential and that new strategies need to be developed to provide novel targets for the development of more effective therapeutic agents.

Novel approaches to modelling schizophrenia

In the context of our current knowledge about schizophrenia, innovative or heuristic models have several goals:
1 to test the plausibility of theories derived from the emerging research data about the disorder;
2 to probe the explanatory power of new biological findings about the disorder;
3 to uncover mechanisms of schizophrenia-like phenomena; and
4 to suggest potential new treatments.
Thus, a heuristic model, in contrast to a traditional dopamine-based model, needs to evince other schizophrenia-like abnormalities besides the feature that it directly manipulates. For instance, a model based on hippocampal injury would be heuristic if it triggered behavioural and/or molecular changes outside the hippocampus that are associated with schizophrenia, enabled testing of the mechanisms underlying the ensuing changes, and predicted novel therapies based on newly discovered mechanisms.

Recently, as interest in schizophrenia research has shifted

from a principal focus on dopamine to theories of abnormal neurodevelopment, dysfunction of cortical glutamatergic neurones and genetic susceptibility, animal models have followed a similar trend. The novel models considered below are either non-pharmacological or based on pharmacological manipulation of a neurotransmitter other than dopamine. Thus, they have ventured off the beaten path of 'dopamine-in, dopamine-out' models, and offer the potential of elucidating non-dopamine mechanisms of disease and treatment. All animal models of schizophrenia, however, whether new or old, suffer from a generic problem – lack of a straightforward test of fidelity. This is because there is no valid genotype, cellular phenotype or other biological marker that is characteristic of the disorder, and no animal model can fully reproduce the perceptual, cognitive and emotional features of the human illness. In the absence of a pathognomonic marker, a faithful model is expected to reproduce a constellation of behavioural and biological phenomena relevant to schizophrenia. If a model addresses a cluster of relevant changes ranging from anatomical and neurochemical to behavioural and cognitive features, rather than a single or a few non-specific phenomena, then there is a higher probability that the model is heuristic and isomorphic with biological processes related to the human disorder. As new findings about the pathophysiology of schizophrenia emerge, new models increasingly focus on certain cell or tissue phenotypes and a variety of complex behavioural characteristics, in addition to time-honoured effects on dopamine-related function (see Tables 21.1 and 21.2); unfortunately, as shown in the examples below, rarely are multiple phenomena addressed in a single model.

In this chapter, we examine three approaches to creating animal models related to schizophrenia:
1 neurodevelopmental models;
2 glutamatergic hypofunction models; and
3 genetic models.
The first approach is based on experimentally induced disruption of brain development that becomes evident in an adult

Table 21.2 The neonatal ventral hippocampal (VH) lesion model: schizophrenia-like phenomena.

Neonatal VH lesion model	Schizophrenia
Behavioural changes	
Hyperlocomotion to stress	Stress vulnerability
PPI deficits	PPI deficits
LI deficits	LI deficits
Deficits in delayed alternation tests	Working memory deficits
Reduced social contacts	Social withdrawal
Pharmacological responses	
Amphetamine-induced hyperactivity	Enhanced symptomatic response to dopamimetics
Apomorphine-induced stereotypies	Neuroleptic tolerance enhanced
Reduced catalepsy to haloperidol	Symptomatic response to ketamine
MK-801 and PCP-induced hyperactivity	
Molecular changes in the prefrontal cortex	
NAA levels ↓	NAA levels ↓
GAD_{67} mRNA ↓	GAD_{67} mRNA ↓
BDNF mRNA ↓	BDNF mRNA ↓
Changes in synaptic morphology in the prefrontal cortex	
Spine density ↓	Spine density ↓

BDNF, brain-derived neurotrophic factor; GAD_{67}, glutamate decarboxylase-67; LI, latent inhibition; NAA, N-acetylaspartate; PCP, phencyclidine; PPI, prepulse inhibition of startle; ↓ reduced vs. controls.

animal in the form of altered brain neurochemistry and aberrant behaviour (neurodevelopmental models). These models test hypotheses that schizophrenia is caused by a defect in cerebral development (Lillrank *et al.* 1995; Lipska & Weinberger 2000) and, in some instances, test whether the effects of early brain damage could remain inconspicuous until after a considerable delay, as appears to be the case in the human condition (Weinberger 1986, 1987; Murray & Lewis 1987; Bloom 1993). Another popular modelling approach involves pharmacological disruption of brain function and behaviour via N-methyl-D-aspartate (NMDA) antagonists. These models test the hypothesis that dysfunction of glutamate neurotransmission accounts for a variety of schizophrenic phenomena (Javitt & Zukin 1991). Still another effort focuses on the search for susceptibility genes employing modern technologies of genetic engineering (genetic models; Erickson 1996). These models test the clinical evidence that susceptibility genes account for risk for illness and, together with epigenetic/environmental factors, for phenotypic variation. Characteristically, a majority of these new models, despite the diversity of their origins, target components of a common neural circuitry implicated in schizophrenia, i.e. the temporolimbic cortices–nucleus accumbens/striatal complex–thalamus–prefrontal cortex. The involvement of this circuitry

may account for the overlap in 'schizophrenia-like' phenomena at the anatomical, neurochemical or behavioural level that are common to these various models.

Neurodevelopmental models

Models testing aetiological theories

Many epidemiological and clinical correlational studies have been carried out in search of early developmental factors that may predispose to schizophrenia. There have been reports linking schizophrenia to obstetric complications (Woerner *et al.* 1973; DeLisi *et al.* 1988; McNiel 1988; Hultman *et al.* 1997; Dalman *et al.* 1999), *in utero* exposure to alcohol (Lohr & Bracha 1989) and severe malnutrition (Susser & Lin 1992). A number of animal models have been designed to test the plausibility of specific gestational factors having a role in the origin of this disorder. These 'aetiological' models, none of which directly manipulates dopamine, aspire to construct validity and heuristic value because they reproduce putative causes of the disease and theoretically model putative primary pathological mechanisms.

For instance, a gestational malnutrition model (or, more precisely, prenatal protein deprivation that begins prior to and continues throughout pregnancy) results in severe permanent changes in the development of the rat brain (for reviews see Morgane *et al.* 1993; Brown *et al.* 1996). Malnutrition affects neurogenesis, cell migration and differentiation, and leads to deviations in normal brain development, including disrupted formation of neural circuits and neurotransmitter systems (Lewis *et al.* 1979; Cintra *et al.* 1997). Not suprisingly, malnutrition has been shown to have debilitating effects on cognitive function and learning abilities (Tonkiss & Galler 1990). Thus, to some degree these models mimic certain 'face' features of schizophrenia. In contrast to schizophrenia, however, morphological abnormalities are severe and widespread, and the behavioural consequences are varied and inconsistent, perhaps, at least in part, because the impact of malnutrition on brain development is likely to be quite variable and depend on many factors, which have only been explored to a small degree. As a test of the plausibility of the malnutrition theory of schizophrenia this model has limited validity.

Prenatal exposure to influenza virus, another predisposing factor implicated in schizophrenia by several large epidemiological studies (Mednick *et al.* 1988; Kendell & Kemp 1989; O'Callaghan *et al.* 1991; Adams *et al.* 1993), has been shown to induce pyramidal cell disarray in a small subgroup of mice whose mothers were inoculated with the virus (Cotter *et al.* 1995). This developmental defect is somewhat similar to that reported in two studies in the hippocampi of schizophrenic patients (Scheibel & Kovelman 1981; Conrad *et al.* 1991). Another recent report indicates that infection with human influenza of day 9 pregnant mice results in defective corticogenesis as indicated by reduced thickness of the neocortex and hippocampus and by significant reductions of cortical reelin immunoreactivity in the offspring (Fatemi *et al.* 1999). This model thus reproduces a hypothetical causative factor in schizophrenia and has face validity, at least at the level of reduced reelin expression, a neurobiological finding recently explored in brains of patients with schizophrenia (Impagnatiello *et al.* 1998). These are intriguing observations, but more conclusive data on the involvement of reelin in schizophrenia and on the behavioural phenotype of the animal model are required before conclusions about the relevance of this model for schizophrenia can be made.

The plausibility that other, less common, viruses may induce schizophrenia-like changes has also been investigated (Rott *et al.* 1985; Waltrip *et al.* 1995). *In utero* Borna disease virus (BDV), a neurotropic virus with limbic selectivity, damages the hippocampus and prefrontal cortex and results in complex changes in regional dopamine in rats (Solbrig *et al.* 1994, 1996a,b; Hornig *et al.* 1999). While this model may invite further research into the mechanisms involved, notwithstanding convincing evidence of BDV infection in schizophrenia, its relevance to the pathophysiology of schizophrenia seems remote. Another example of a viral model is neonatal infection with lymphocytic choriomeningitis virus (LCMV) which disrupts in adult rats the integrity of γ-aminobutyric acid (GABA)-ergic neurones and excitatory amino acid systems, both implicated in schizophrenia (Pearce *et al.* 1996, 1999). The potential face validity of this model at a cellular level makes it particularly attractive because it addresses two theories about the pathophysiology of schizophrenia: vulnerability of GABAergic interneurones to developmental insult and adolescent vulnerability to excitotoxic injury (Benes *et al.* 1991, 1992; Olney & Farber 1995). Although conceptually appealing, it has yet to address a broader spectrum of aspects of the disorder and its basic construct, LCMV infection, is of dubious relevance to schizophrenia.

The plausibility of obstetric and birth complications is difficult to explore in animals because their causes in schizophrenia are unknown. Nevertheless, studies of models of caesarean birth and of anoxia during birth in rats report changes in limbic dopamine function of adult animals consistent with hyperresponsiveness of the dopamine system to stimulants (Brake *et al.* 1997a,b; El-Khodor & Boksa 1997, 1998). Surprisingly, animals born by caesarean section and not subject to anoxia seem to be even more affected than anoxic rats (El-Khodor & Boksa 1997). If this has bearing on schizophrenia, it would suggest that caesarean section constitutes a greater risk factor than the more dramatic birth trauma of anoxia. In humans, caesarean section is generally assumed to involve less stress to the fetus and has not been noted as one of the obstetric complications linked to schizophrenia. Clearly, more studies are needed to elucidate the mechanisms underlying the caesarean section-related phenomena in animals.

Until a broader array of schizophrenia-related phenomena is assessed in each of these aetiological models, it is premature to draw firm conclusions about whether any reproduces mechanisms underlying the human disorder. Moreover, the validity of these models is tempered by the lack of convincing evidence for the role of any of these various causative factors in schizophrenia, with the possible exception of influenza. However, these models illustrate that certain early developmental insults may permanently disrupt brain function in ways that are similar to some of the phenomena reported in schizophrenia.

Models of disrupted neurogenesis

Several postmortem studies of schizophrenia have reported variations in cortical cytoarchitecture (Arnold *et al.* 1991; Akbarian *et al.* 1993a,b; Kirkpatrick *et al.* 1999), possibly of developmental nature. These reports have inspired models based on disrupted neurogenesis. These models do not attempt to reproduce specific putative causative factors implicated in schizophrenia, but aspire to face validity at the anatomical level by mimicking cellular aberrations that presumably would follow a disruption of early cortical development analogous to what has been described in some of the human postmortem studies. The heuristic framework of these models is that specific prenatal interruptions of cell maturation would result in relevant biological and behavioural changes as the animal matures. Examples include cortical dysgenesis induced by gestational X-ray irradiation (Rakic 1996; Mintz *et al.* 1997; Selemon *et al.* 2000), *in utero* exposure to a mitotic toxin, methylazoxymethanol acetate (MAM), which destroys populations of rapidly dividing neurones (Johnston *et al.* 1988; Talamini *et al.* 1998), and systemic administration of nitric oxide synthase (NOS) inhibitors, which interfere with maturation of neurones and synaptogenesis (Black *et al.* 1999). Animals that have undergone X-ray or MAM manipulations exhibit morphological changes in a broad array of brain structures implicated in schizophrenia, particularly the hippocampus, and frontal and entorhinal cortices. These animals also demonstrate a variety of behavioural alterations such as locomotor hyperactivity, stereotypies, cognitive impairments and disruption of latent inhibition and PPI, and show electrophysiological abnormalities posited to underlie psychomotor disturbances in schizophrenia (Johnston *et al.* 1988; Moore *et al.* 1998; Talamini *et al.* 1998). Male rats exposed to a NOS inhibitor (L-nitroarginine) between 3 and 5 days of life show in adulthood locomotor hypersensitivity to amphetamine and deficits in PPI, but similarly treated females were not found to be affected on these measures (Black *et al.* 1999). These preliminary results are provocative and invite further research.

Models of aberrant neurogenesis, although the data are limited at this time, appear to have potential heuristic value in discovering mechanisms of specific neural circuit disruptions caused by elimination of maturing neurones. There are a number of areas to be pursued including characterizing critical risk periods (specifically, a period corresponding to the second trimester of gestation in humans), critical neuronal populations, molecular adaptations in remaining neurones, etc. These models demonstrate again that perturbation in cortical development can reproduce some of the behavioural characteristics associated with schizophrenia, including those linked to dopamine systems.

Perinatal stress models

This group of models focuses on the long-lasting consequences of stress for brain development and for shaping adult behavioural responses. They have been variably used as models of depression, anxiety and schizophrenia, diseases in which stress has long been thought to have some role. Stress has been postulated as a factor in so-called 'two hit' models of schizophrenia in which two independent insults (e.g. aberrant genetic trait and stressful experience) are thought to be necessary for the occurrence of the disorder. In rodents, early life exposure to experiential stressors such as maternal separation (Liu et al. 1997) and social isolation (Jones et al. 1992; Geyer et al. 1993; Wilkinson et al. 1994) produce numerous hormonal, neurochemical and behavioural changes, including locomotor hyperactivity in a novel environment, maze learning impairments, anxiety, latent inhibition and sensorimotor gating deficits. Of particular interest is that some of these alterations emerge in adult life and can be restored by a wide range of antipsychotics, including various typical and atypical drugs (Varty & Higgins 1995; Bakshi et al. 1998; Ellenbroek et al. 1998). Importantly, the effects of adverse early life events (e.g. maternal separation) on adult reactivity are strongly influenced by genetic as well as non-genomic factors (Zaharia et al. 1996; Anisman et al. 1998; Francis et al. 1999).

These models provide important evidence for an interaction between genetic predisposition and early life experiences and demonstrate that both are involved in shaping the adult stress response system and adult patterns of behaviour. They might thus represent an interesting approach to study the interactions of these variables in schizophrenia.

Neonatal lesion models

Another series of studies have focused on neonatal damage of restricted brain regions in rats (Lipska et al. 1993; Chambers et al. 1996; Flores et al. 1996a; Wan et al. 1996, 1998; Wan & Corbett 1997; Black et al. 1998; Becker et al. 1999; Brake et al. 1999; Grecksch et al. 1999; Schroeder et al. 1999) and in monkeys (Beauregard & Bachevalier 1996; Bertolino et al. 1997; Saunders et al. 1998; Bachevalier et al. 1999). The main objective of many of these studies is to disrupt development of the hippocampus, a brain area consistently implicated in human schizophrenia (Falkai & Bogerts 1986; Jeste & Lohr 1989; Bogerts et al. 1990; Suddath et al. 1990; Eastwood & Harrison 1995, 1998; Eastwood et al. 1995, 1997; Weinberger 1999), and thus disrupt development of the widespread cortical and subcortical circuitry in which the hippocampus participates. The lesions were intended to involve regions of the hippocampus that directly project to the prefrontal cortex, i.e. ventral hippocampus and ventral subiculum (Jay et al. 1989; Carr & Sesack 1996), and that correspond to the anterior hippocampus

in humans, a region that shows anatomical abnormalities in schizophrenia (Suddath et al. 1990).

Neonatal excitotoxic lesions of the rat ventral hippocampus (VH) lead in adolescence or early adulthood to the emergence of abnormalities in a number of dopamine-related behaviours, which bear close resemblance to behaviours seen in animals sensitized to psychostimulants. When tested as juveniles (postnatal day 35), rats with the neonatal VH lesions are less social than controls (Sams-Dodd et al. 1997), but otherwise behave normally in motor tests involving exposure to stress and dopamine agonists. In adolescence and adulthood (postnatal day 56 and older), lesioned animals display markedly changed behaviours thought to be primarily linked to increased mesolimbic/nigrostriatal dopamine transmission (motor hyperresponsiveness to stress and stimulants, enhanced stereotypies). They also show enhanced sensitivity to glutamate antagonists (MK-801 and PCP), deficits in PPI and latent inhibition, impaired social behaviours and working memory problems (Lipska & Weinberger 1993, 1994a,b; Lipska et al. 1995a; Becker et al. 1999; Grecksch et al. 1999; Hori et al. 1999; Al-Amin et al. 2000, 2001), phenomena showing many parallels with schizophrenia. Emergence of the behavioural changes in adolescence appears not to be related to the surge of gonadal hormones during puberty because a similar temporal pattern of abnormalities is observed in animals depleted of gonadal hormones prior to puberty (Lipska & Weinberger 1994b). Notably, removal of prefrontal neurones in adult animals with the earlier hippocampal lesion restores some of the behaviours (i.e. those modulated by but not critically dependent on the prefrontal cortex, such as hyperlocomotion after amphetamine), suggesting that aberrant development of the prefrontal cortex in the context of early damage to the hippocampus may be a critical factor in the expression of the syndrome (Lipska et al. 1998a). In this context, it is important to emphasize that anatomical findings from postmortem studies and neuropsychological and neuroimaging studies of brain function in patients with schizophrenia have implicated prefrontal cortical maldevelopment and a developmental 'dysconnection' of the temporolimbic and prefrontal cortices (for review see Weinberger & Lipska 1995). Although the exact mechanisms of a seemingly similar 'dysconnection' and malfunction of the prefrontal cortex in the VH lesioned rats need to be elucidated, preliminary findings from molecular and electrophysiological studies (such as reduced cortical levels of N-acetylaspartate (NAA), attenuated stress-induced cortical dopamine release, attenuated cortical expression of a membrane glutamate transporter EAAC1 and of a synthetic enzyme for GABA, glutamate decarboxylase-67 (GAD_{67}), reduced brain-derived neurotrophic factor (BDNF) expression, altered cortical expression of transcription factors, c-fos and ΔfosB, as well as altered firing pattern of cortical pyramidal neurones in response to ventral tegmental area (VTA) stimulation) suggest that aberrant cortical dopamine–glutamate–GABA interactions may underlie cortical dysfunction in the neonatally VH lesioned rats (Lipska et al. 1995b; Lee et al. 1998; Ashe et al. 1999; Bertolino et al. 1999; O'Donnell et al. 1999). We have recently reported that excitotoxic prefrontal cortical lesions in adult animals cause downstream striatal NAA losses and reduced GAD_{67} mRNA expression, and suggested that both changes might reflect transsynaptic pathology (Roffman *et al.* 2000). It is possible that similar transsynaptic events occur in response to the neonatal VH lesion but further work is required to determine if and by what mechanisms molecular changes in prefrontal neurones are linked.

It is interesting to note that many of these changes have been reported in stress- and psychostimulant-sensitization models (Feldpausch *et al.* 1998; Gambarana *et al.* 1999; Vanderschuren *et al.* 1999), as well as in patients with schizophrenia (Akbarian *et al.* 1995; Bertolino *et al.* 1998). Subcortical function in the neonatally lesioned rats is also altered in a fashion consistent with at least some reports on behavioural sensitization (Imperato *et al.* 1996; Nestler & Aghajanian 1997; Steiner & Gerfen 1998; Castner *et al.* 2000), i.e. striatal dopamine release is attenuated in response to stress and amphetamine, midbrain expression of the membrane dopamine transporter (DAT) mRNA is reduced, striatal expression of dynorphin (an opioid peptide colocalized with D_1 receptors) and of ΔfosB (a transcription factor sensitive to persistent stimulation) are enhanced (Lipska *et al.* 1998b; Lee *et al.* 1998). However, it should be noted that enhanced rather than attenuated striatal dopamine release has been observed in other paradigms of sensitization to psychostimulants (for review see Spanagel & Weiss 1999) as well as in a subgroup of schizophrenics as evidenced by recent single photon emission computerized tomography (SPECT) studies (Laruelle *et al.* 1996; Breier *et al.* 1997; Abi-Dargham *et al.* 1998). Similarly discrepant are the findings of synaptic morphology – increased synaptic densities, the number of branches and dendritic length are reported in prefrontal cortex in sensitization models (Robinson & Kolb 1997), whereas these dendritic parameters are decreased in schizophrenia (Glantz & Lewis 2000) and in the neonatal hippocampal lesion model (Lipska *et al.* 2001). Nevertheless, an array of behavioural and molecular changes associated with this model suggest that early developmental insult of the ventral hippocampus may facilitate sensitization of the dopamine system, and thereby account for the adult onset of a maladaptive condition characterized by a variety of dopamine-related abnormalities. Similar pathophysiological mechanisms have been hypothesized to underlie schizophrenia (Lieberman *et al.* 1997; Meng *et al.* 1998; Duncan *et al.* 1999). Unlike psychostimulant sensitization models, however, the neonatal lesion model does not target the dopamine system directly and similar sensitization-like phenomena are not seen following an analogous hippocampal lesion in adult animals. It may be of considerable heuristic interest to determine how the developmental lesion initiates the subsequent behavioural and molecular phenomena associated with sensitization.

In terms of the predictive validity of the neonatal VH lesion model, antipsychotic drugs normalize some lesion-induced behaviours (Lipska & Weinberger 1994a; Sams-Dodd *et al.* 1997). Drugs targeting the glutamate system may also prove beneficial; LY293558, an alpha-amino-3-hydroxy-5-methyl-4-isoxazole propionic acid (AMPA) antagonist, is highly efficient in blocking hyperlocomotion in the neonatally lesioned rats at doses that do not affect locomotor activity in controls (Al-Amin *et al.* 2000). Thus, this model may have predictive validity and heuristic potential to identify drugs with new mechanisms of action. The model also appears to mimic a spectrum of neurobiological and behavioural features of schizophrenia, including functional pathology in presumably critical brain regions interconnected with the hippocampal formation and targeted by antipsychotic drugs – the striatum/nucleus accumbens and the prefrontal cortex (see Table 21.2). It is noteworthy that in the non-human primate, early postnatal damage of the hippocampal region also alters development of the dorsal prefrontal cortex and the mechanisms whereby the dorsal prefrontal cortex regulates subcortical dopamine function, phenomena similar to those described in patients with schizophrenia (Bertolino *et al.* 1997, 2000; Saunders *et al.* 1998). Thus, neonatal damage to the hippocampus of the rat appears to reproduce a broad spectrum of schizophrenia-related phenomena, and establishes the neurobiological plausibility of early damage having a delayed impact on neural functions implicated in schizophrenia.

Developmental lesions of other brain structures implicated in schizophrenia and components of a limbic–neocortical circuit (e.g. thalamus, prefrontal cortex) also have been considered as models. For instance, thalamic excitotoxic lesions in PD7 rats result in adult expression of apomorphine- and amphetamine-induced hyperlocomotion (Rajakumar *et al.* 1996). Intracerebroventricular infusions of kainic acid into neonatal (PD7) rats lead in adulthood to a reduction in neural numbers in the dorsal hippocampus, and are associated with changes in the expression of subpopulations of glutamate receptors and immediate early genes (Csernansky *et al.* 1998; Montgomery *et al.* 1999). Neonatal (PD7) excitotoxic damage of the medial prefrontal cortex was reported to produce delayed behavioural effects accompanied by dopamine receptor changes (Flores *et al.* 1996b), although others did not confirm these data (Lipska *et al.* 1998a). The spectrum of behavioural and cellular parameters examined in these models is rather limited at this time.

Another neonatal insult with intriguing implications is selective depletion of serotonin in neonatal rats (by tryptophan hydroxylase inhibitor parachlorophenylalanine (PCPA) that decreases markers of synaptic density in the adult brain, and results in cognitive deficits; Mazer *et al.* 1997). These effects are somewhat similar to those reported in the postmortem schizophrenic brain (Weinberger 1999), but other schizophrenia-relevant aspects need to be tested in this model.

Although developmental lesion models represent a rather crude technique to study the role of particular brain regions, transmitter systems or the connections between them, they have confirmed the plausibility of neurodevelopmental damage having selected deleterious effects after a prolonged period of relative normalcy. In this respect, they appear to have face validity, not only in terms of behavioural, cellular and pharmacological phenomena, but also in terms of the temporal course of the clinical disorder. As models of developmental pathology they certainly lack construct validity, as the schizophrenic brain does not manifest a 'lesion' analogous to any of these models, but they may have heuristic value in discovering molecular consequences of early brain damage and new treatment prospects.

Pharmacological models of glutamatergic antagonism

In addition to the non-pharmacological non-dopaminergic approaches described above, pharmacological blockade of NMDA receptors in adult animals has gained popularity as a model of schizophrenia. Observations that non-competitive NMDA antagonists, such as phencyclidine (PCP) and ketamine, exacerbate some psychotic symptoms in schizophrenic patients and have psychotomimetic effects in normal humans (Krystal *et al.* 1994; Lahti *et al.* 1995) have encouraged speculation that some aspects of schizophrenia may relate to abnormal glutamatergic function. This has been further supported by postmortem studies in schizophrenia showing a variety of changes in the glutamate system, including altered glutamate metabolism and expression of various glutamate receptors (Javitt & Zukin 1991; Akbarian *et al.* 1996; Jentsch & Roth 1999; Weinberger 1999).

In rodents and monkeys, acute subanaesthetic doses of NMDA antagonists produce a constellation of phenomena potentially relevant to schizophrenic symptomatology, including hyperlocomotion, enhanced stereotyped behaviours, cognitive and sensorimotor gating deficits and impaired social interactions. PCP as well as other NMDA antagonists acutely increase extracellular levels of dopamine and glutamate (as well as norepinephrine and acetylcholine) in the prefrontal cortex, and alter firing patterns of dopaminergic and nucleus accumbens neurones (Verma & Moghaddam 1996; O'Donnell & Grace 1998). Repeated administration of PCP can also induce robust behavioural and neurochemical changes even after long-term withdrawal (Jentsch *et al.* 1997, 1998a,b). Of particular interest is differential dysregulation of the firing patterns of mesolimbic and mesocortical dopaminergic neurones by low behaviourally relevant doses of NMDA antagonists. These changes in dopamine cell firing may render them unresponsive or inappropriately responsive to salient environmental stimuli such as stress and reward (Murase *et al.* 1993; Mathe *et al.* 1998). If a similar process underlies psychotic symptoms and cognitive deficits in schizophrenia, the NMDA antagonist model may offer novel treatment strategies targeting glutamate rather than dopamine. Recently, experimental approaches to reverse NMDA antagonist-induced abnormalities have included pharmacological enhancement of NMDA receptor activity, enhancement of metabotropic glutamate receptor (mGluR2) activity, and blockade of AMPA receptors (Moghaddam *et al.* 1997; Moghaddam & Adams 1998), the latter approach shown to be also effective in the neonatal hippocampal lesion model (see above). Thus, a model based on a primary glutamatergic abnormality appears to show important heuristic properties in terms of identifying potential novel therapies. This model may offer insight into molecular adaptations that follow chronic NMDA blockade, and identify new therapeutic targets. Notably, the repeated non-competitive NMDA blockade model, which had also been intensely investigated from the perspective of behavioural sensitization and its role in drug addiction and reward mechanisms (Wolf *et al.* 1993), shares certain behavioural and neurochemical similarities with the neonatal hippocampal lesion model, including cognitive deficits (in particular, in working memory tasks), reduced frontal dopamine transmission (Jentsch *et al.* 1997, 1998a) and reduced GABA activity as indicated by reduced levels of GAD_{67} (Qin *et al.* 1994; Yonezawa *et al.* 1998), and disrupted social behaviours and augmented locomotor responses to stress and amphetamine (Jentsch *et al.* 1998b). The similarities between the models may reflect a common disruption of cortical glutamate–GABA function which may converge towards a common underlying process of behavioural sensitization. Unlike the aetiological or neonatal lesions models, the NMDA antagonist approach does not, however, address the developmental component of schizophrenia.

Genetic models

Schizophrenia is a highly heritable disorder that probably involves multiple genes with small effects across large populations (Kendler *et al.* 1996). Elucidating the roles of the susceptibility genes for this clinically diverse and probably genetically heterogeneous disorder will require considerable effort and is unlikely to be fully resolved soon. Modern technologies, involving targeted gene deletions or gene transfer techniques that have revolutionized experimental medicine, may provide a new generation of animal models for schizophrenia that may help in this daunting task.

Some genetic models for neurological diseases are almost perfect in terms of construct validity because transgenic animals may be, in a sense, 'humanized' by the introduction of human genes involved in the disease or the mutated animal homologues of such genes (Loring *et al.* 1996). However, transgenic models also illustrate that even a highly accurate model in terms of construct validity may fail the test of face validity in terms of a phenotype analogous to the disorder. For instance, the Duchenne's muscular dystrophy mdx mutation mouse model is hardly symptomatic (Erickson 1996), the PDAPP transgenic mouse model of Alzheimer's disease which overexpresses human amyloid precursor protein (Johnson-Wood *et al.* 1997) does not have an isomorphic behavioural phenotype, and the hypoxanthine-guanine phosphoribosyl-transferase (HPRT) knockout mouse has no recognizable phenotype analogous to Lesch–Nyhan disease (Wu & Melton 1993). Behavioural phenotypes of these models are not isomorphic with the disease, because genetic mutation can have remarkably different phenotypes when placed on different genetic backgrounds. However, despite phenotypic dissimilarity, such models are faithful in terms of certain cellular characteristics and can be very useful in illuminating molecular mechanisms leading to pathological changes and in discovering new treatments. This approach is possible only if the disease can be attributed to specific human genes, and thus seems to have limited application in studying schizophrenia or other psychiatric illnesses at the present time.

In an attempt to test the possibility of involvement of various neurotransmitter receptors relevant to schizophrenia (D_1–D_5 subtypes of dopamine receptors, adenosine A2A receptors, α_2-adrenergic receptors and NMDA receptors) and to elucidate their functional roles, investigators have used genetically altered mice in which expression of these receptors was selectively and usually completely suppressed (Sibley 1999). Probably the most intriguing is a recent attempt at targeting the NR1 subunit of the NMDA receptor in a genetic mouse model (Mohn *et al.* 1999), despite lack of direct evidence that an NMDA receptor gene is abnormal in schizophrenia. Mutant mice expressing only 5% of essential NR1 receptors show increased spontaneous hyper-locomotion that attenuates after a single injection of haloperidol and clozapine, and deficits in social and sexual behaviours that respond to acute clozapine treatment. Although some of these behavioural changes suggest increased dopaminergic tone, dopamine release and turnover are not altered in these animals. However, somewhat contrary to the phenotype expected in a schizophrenia model, NR1 mutant mice do not exhibit enhanced responsiveness to the NMDA antagonists MK-801 and PCP. Continued studies of these mice will provide more information about the consequences of dramatic congenital hypo-function of the glutamatergic system and will shed light on interactions of the glutamatergic system with other neurotransmitter systems, but the relevance of this model to schizophrenia is yet unclear. This example underscores a unique problem of modelling the schizophrenic phenotype in animals that even a genetic model cannot escape – lack of pathognomonic neurobiological markers and validation criteria.

Another promising genetic strategy is identification of predisposing candidate genes by selecting rodent lines or strains for particular behavioural traits. Such candidate genes may then be used to identify homologous human genes potentially involved in the aetiology of schizophrenia. For instance, studies in inbred mice strains with deficits in sensory inhibition have indicated that altered expression and function of the α_7 nicotinic cholinergic receptor may be responsible for some auditory sensory gating deficits (Stevens *et al.* 1998). A defect in the so-called 'P50 auditory-evoked response' is found in patients with schizophrenia and in their unaffected relatives (Freedman *et al.* 1987). This evoked potential defect (but not schizophrenia itself because many individuals showing P50 deficits are clinically unaffected) was subsequently linked to a chromosome 15 locus, near the site of the α_7 nicotinic cholinergic receptor gene (Freedman *et al.* 1997). This linkage finding, which echoed data from the earlier mice experiments, suggested that a genetic defect in the α_7 nicotinic cholinergic receptor might be a predisposing factor in schizophrenia. Sequencing of the α_7 nicotinic cholinergic receptor gene in individuals with this phenotype is currently in progress. Another example involves animals bred for high sus-

ceptibility to apomorphine-induced stereotypic behaviours (APO-SUS rats). These animals, in contrast to apomorphine non-responsive (APO-UNSUS) rats, demonstrate various behavioural (e.g. prepulse inhibition and latent inhibition deficits), biochemical (e.g. elevated levels of tyrosine hydroxylase mRNA in the substantia nigra and D_2 receptor binding in the dorsal striatum) and immunological (e.g. reduced sensitivity for rheumatoid arthritis) features implicated in schizophrenia (Ellenbroek *et al.* 1995, 2000). Thus, such behavioural trait-selected animals may be used as models of schizophrenia-prone individuals and provide material for novel gene identification and for candidate gene analyses.

Another model has combined neurodevelopmental and genetic predisposition approaches. Fisher344 rats, a highly stress-responsive inbred strain, show particularly high susceptibility to the behavioural effects of neonatal hippocampal damage. Lewis rats, on the other hand, bred for low stress responsiveness, appear to be resistant to the behavioural consequences of identical lesions (Lipska & Weinberger 1995). This lesion genetic model may be used for identification of candidate genes that mediate behavioural responses to a neonatal hippocampal insult, and that, by extension, might predispose to or modify the expression of schizophrenia.

Because recent data suggest a significant role for neurodevelopmental processes in schizophrenia, another approach to genetic modelling of schizophrenia may focus on manipulating in animals those genes that have a role in neurodevelopment, maintenance of cell–cell connections, and trophic factors (Weickert & Weinberger 1998; see Table 21.3). For instance, in an attempt to alter genes involved in neural migration, neural cell adhesion molecule isoform 180 (*NCAM-180*) gene was deleted in mice. Mice with this selective gene deletion display a marked reduction in the levels of PSA-NCAM (polysialic-acid-rich NCAM), a molecule involved in neuronal regeneration and plasticity, which has also been reported as reduced in the hippocampus of patients with schizophrenia (Barbeau *et al.* 1995). *NCAM-180*-depleted mice are characterized by abnormal migration of neurones within the subventricular zone, altered cytoarchitecture of multiple brain regions, including olfactory bulb, hippocampus and cerebellum, enlarged ventricles and changes in behaviour (PPI deficits) (Tomasiewicz *et al.* 1993; Wood *et al.* 1998). Although some of these changes resemble abnormalities observed in schizophrenia, more thorough phenotypic characterization is needed.

Because the early hippocampal damage models have demonstrated the plausibility of developmental defects in the hippocampus having a delayed impact on other neural circuits and systems (e.g. prefrontal cortex), transgenic models that selectively disrupt development of hippocampal circuitry may turn out to be especially heuristic. In a recent attempt to alter development of the hippocampus, the LIM homeobox *Lhx5* gene was deleted in mice (Zhao *et al.* 1999). The *Lhx5* homozygous mutant embryos showed dramatic defects in hippocampal morphology; however, most of the homozygotes died within a few days after birth. Somewhat less severe changes in hippocampal

Table 21.3 Potential animal models based on genetic manipulation of cellular phenotype.

Molecular changes in schizophrenia	Brain region	Molecular targets for genetic manipulations in animals
Trophic/ECM molecules ↓	Cortex, hippocampus	BDNF, LAMP, PSA-NCAM, reelin[1]
Glutamate function ↓	Cortex, hippocampus	GluR1-4, GluR5-7, NR1-2, KA1-2, GCP II, EAAC1, GLT1, GLAST[2]
GABA function ↓	Cortex, hippocampus	GAD_{67}, GABA(A)[3]
Synaptic markers ↓	Cortex, hippocampus	Synapsin, synaptophysin, SNAP-25, GAT1,3, complexin[4]
Other cellular markers ↓	Cortex, hippocampus	GAP-43, MAPs[5]

BDNF, brain-derived neurotrophic factor; ECM, extracellular matrix; EAAC1, neuronal glutamate transporter; GABA(A), γ-aminobutyric acid A receptors; GAP-43, neuronal growth-associated protein; GAD_{67}, glutamate decarboxylase-67; GAT1,3, GABA transporters; GCP II, glutamate carboxypeptidase II; GLT1, GLAST, glial glutamate transporters; GluR1-4, subunits of AMPA (α-amino-3-hydroxy-5-methyl-4-isoxazolepropionic acid) receptor; GluR5-7 and KA1-2, subunits of kainate receptor; LAMP, limbic system-associated membrane protein, MAP, microtubule-associated protein; NR1-2, subunits of NMDA (N-methyl-D-aspartate) receptor; PSA-NCAM, polysialylated neural cell adhesion molecule; SNAP-25, synaptosomal-associated protein of 25 kDa; ↓ decreased expression or compromised function.

Selected references:

1 Vawter *et al.* (1998); Barbeau *et al.* (1995); Impagnatiello *et al.* (1998); Fatemi *et al.* (1999)
2 Ohnuma *et al.* (1998); Eastwood *et al.* (1995, 1997)
3 Benes *et al.* (1996, 1997); Huntsman *et al.* (1998); Dean *et al.* (1999)
4 Eastwood & Harrison (1995); Glantz & Lewis (1997); Young *et al.* (1998); Harrison & Eastwood (1998); Karson *et al.* (1999)
5 Perrone-Bizzozero *et al.* (1996); Eastwood & Harrison (1998)

development, but still often lethal or too damaging to be considered relevant to schizophrenia, have been reported in mice with null deletions of other homeobox genes (e.g. *Emx2* (Pellegrini *et al.* 1996) and *Lhx2* (Porter *et al.* 1997)) as well as genes involved in neural migration during development (e.g. β subunit of platelet-activating factor acetylhydrolase *Pafah1b1* (or *Lis1*) (Hirotsune *et al.* 1998), cycline-dependent kinase 5 (*Cdk5*) (Ohshima *et al.* 1996), *mdab1* (Sheldon *et al.* 1997) and reeler (Goffinet 1995)). More interesting, because of a more subtle pathology, is a model of heterozygous haploinsufficient reeler mouse (HRM) which expresses 50% of the brain reelin content of a wild-type mouse and exhibits many phenotypic traits reminiscent of neurochemical and neuroanatomical characteristics of schizophrenia (Liu *et al.* 2001). These features include: (i) downregulation of prefrontal cortical GAD_{67} mRNA; (ii) an increase of neuronal packing density and a decrease of cortical thickness; and (iii) a reduction in cortical and hippocampal spine density. Some intriguing behavioural changes, such as increased anxiety, disrupted PPI and cognitive deficits in a radial maze, have also been observed in this model. Another promising strategy might involve conditional reduction (or enhancement) of expression of certain genes restricted to critical periods in development, an approach that has recently been used in a drug addiction model that inducibly overexpresses ΔfosB (Kelz *et al.* 1999). Table 21.3 contains other suggestions for novel models based on transgenic approaches to reproduce specific cellular abnormalities that have been implicated in certain brain regions in schizophrenia; not all of these findings, however, have been independently replicated. Such developmental genetic models may provide new candidate genes for assessment in clinical studies and help to model the cell biology of this complex disorder. Candidate genes selected from their chromosomal position near genetic loci linked to schizophrenia might also be future targets for transgenic models.

Conclusions

The approach to studying the aetiology and pathophysiology of schizophrenia at the level of animal neurobiology has become much more sophisticated. In light of mounting evidence linking schizophrenia to certain neuropathological processes in the brain, heuristic animal models may prove to be important tools in testing new theories about the origin and mechanisms of this disorder. In particular, some of the recent models have confirmed the plausibility of neurodevelopmental insults having prolonged effects on the dopamine system and behaviours relevant to schizophrenia, and supported the notion that disruption of glutamatergic neurotransmission may lead to new approaches to treatment. The neonatal lesion model has suggested that the effects of an early ventral hippocampal insult, rather than being compensated for, precipitate a state remarkably similar to stress- or psychostimulant-induced sensitization, associated with long-lasting maladaptive cellular changes that lead to delayed onset of abnormal behaviours. Mechanisms underlying sensitization to stress, amphetamine, cocaine, opioids or non-competitive NMDA antagonists are not well understood and seem to involve complex changes in multiple neurotransmitter systems, including dopamine, glutamate and GABA. If the effects of sensitization following developmental abnormalities of the cortex are, indeed, involved in the adolescent/adult onset of schizophrenia-like changes in this model, and by extension in schizophrenia, this may underscore the importance of preventive treatment strategies directed at reducing the impact of experiential stressors in predisposed individuals. Findings from the neonatal stress models discussed above might provide clues about the mechanisms of such potential interventions.

Modern technologies that have been successfully applied to animal modelling of genetic neurological diseases may one day also open the door to our understanding of the mechanisms underlying psychiatric disorders. The transgenic murine models, in which mutations homologous to mutations in humans are inserted by transgenesis or by stem cell knockouts, may seem superior to any pharmacological, surgical or experiential models, but they have their own limitations. It is clear that most psychiatric disorders, including schizophrenia, are multifactorial (i.e. multiple genes interact with multiple environmental factors to create a particular phenotype; Egan & Weinberger 1997). Theoretically at least, by choosing the right combination of the mutation and modifier genes as well as appropriate environmental influences on their expression, one might be able to create at the cellular level a high fidelity animal model of such a complex human disease as schizophrenia.

References

Abi-Dargham, A., Gil, R., Krystal, J. *et al.* (1998) Increased striatal dopamine transmission in schizophrenia: confirmation in a second cohort. *American Journal of Psychiatry* 155, 761–767.

Adams, W., Kendell, R.E., Hare, E.H. & Munk-Jorgensen, P. (1993) Epidemiological evidence that maternal influenza contributes to the aetiology of schizophrenia: an analysis of Scottish, English and Danish data. *British Journal of Psychiatry* 163, 169–177.

Akbarian, S., Bunney, W.E. Jr, Potkin, S.G. *et al.* (1993a) Altered distribution of nicotinamide–adenine dinucleotide phosphate-diaphorase cells in frontal lobe of schizophrenics implies disturbances of cortical development. *Archives of General Psychiatry* 50, 169–177.

Akbarian, S., Vinuela, A., Kim, J.J. *et al.* (1993b) Distorted distribution of nicotinamide–adenine dinucleotide phosphate–diaphorase neurons in temporal lobe of schizophrenics implies anomalous cortical development. *Archives of General Psychiatry* 50, 178–187.

Akbarian, S., Kim, J.J., Potkin, S.G. *et al.* (1995) Gene expression for glutamic acid decarboxylase is reduced without loss of neurons in prefrontal cortex of schizophrenics. *Archives of General Psychiatry* 52, 258–266.

Akbarian, S., Sucher, N.J., Bradley, D. *et al.* (1996) Selective alterations in gene expression for NMDA receptor subunits in prefrontal cortex of schizophrenics. *Journal of Neuroscience* 16, 19–30.

Al-Amin, H.A., Weinberger, D.R. & Lipska, B.K. (2000) Exaggerated MK-801-induced motor hyperactivity in rats with the neonatal lesion of the ventral hippocampus. *Behavioral Pharmacology* 11, 269–278.

Al-Amin, H.A., Weickert, C.S., Lillrank, S.M., Weinberger, D.R. & Lipska, B.K. (2001) Delayed onset of enhanced MK-801-induced motor hyperactivity after neonatal lesions of the rat ventral hippocampus. *Biological Psychiatry* 49, 528–539.

Anisman, H., Zaharia, M.D., Meaney, M.J. & Merali, Z. (1998) Do early-life events permanently alter behavioral and hormonal responses to stressors? *International Journal of Developmental Neuroscience* 16, 149–164.

Arnold, S.E., Hyman, B.T., van Hoesen, G.W. & Damasio, A.R. (1991) Some cytoarchitectural abnormalities of the entorhinal cortex in schizophrenia. *Archives of General Psychiatry* 48, 625–632.

Ashe, P., Chlan-Fourney, J., Juorio, A.V., Li, X.-M. & Boulton, A.A. (1999) Brain-derived neurotrophic factor mRNA in rats with neonatal ibotenic acid lesions of the ventral hippocampus. *Society of Neuroscience Abstract* 635.11.

Bachevalier, J., Alvarado, M.C. & Malkova, L. (1999) Memory and socioemotional behavior in monkeys after hippocampal damage incurred in infancy or in adulthood. *Biological Psychiatry* 46, 329–339.

Bakshi, V.P., Swerdlow, N.R., Braff, D.L. & Geyer, M.A. (1998) Reversal of isolation rearing-induced deficits in prepulse inhibition by Seroquel and olanzapine. *Biological Psychiatry* 43, 436–445.

Barbeau, D., Liang, J.J., Robitalille, Y., Quirion, R. & Srivastava, L.K. (1995) Decreased expression of the embryonic form of the neural cell adhesion molecule in schizophrenic brains. *Proceedings of the National Academy of Sciences of the USA* 92, 2785–2789.

Beauregard, M. & Bachevalier, J. (1996) Neonatal insult to the hippocampal region and schizophrenia: a review and a putative animal model. *Canadian Journal of Psychiatry* 41, 446–456.

Becker, A., Grecksch, G., Bernsteinn, H.-G., Hollt, V. & Bogerts, B. (1999) Social behavior in rats lesioned with ibotenic acid in the hippocampus: quantitative and qualitative analysis. *Psychopharmacology* 144, 333–338.

Benes, F.M., McSparren, J., Bird, E.D., San Giovanni, J.P. & Vincent, S.L. (1991) Deficits in small interneurons in prefrontal cortex and anterior cingulate cortices of schizophrenic and schizoaffective patients. *Archives of General Psychiatry* 48, 996–1001.

Benes, F.M., Vincent, S.L., Alsterberg, G., Bird, E.D. & San Giovanni, J.P. (1992) Increased GABA-A receptor binding in superficial laminae in cingulate cortex of schizophrenic brain. *Journal of Neuroscience* 12, 924–929.

Benes, F.M., Vincent, S.L., Marie, A. & Khan, Y. (1996) Up-regulation of GABAA receptor binding on neurons of the prefrontal cortex in schizophrenic subjects. *Neuroscience* 7, 1021–1031.

Benes, F.M., Wickramasinghe, R., Vincent, S.L., Khan, Y. & Todtenkopf, M. (1997) Uncoupling of GABA (A) and benzodiazepine receptor binding activity in the hippocampal formation of schizophrenic brain. *Brain Research* 755, 121–129.

Bertolino, A., Saunders, R.C., Mattay, V.S. *et al.* (1997) Altered development of prefrontal neurons in rhesus monkeys with neonatal mesial temporo-limbic lesions: a proton magnetic resonance spectroscopic imaging study. *Cerebral Cortex* 7, 740–748.

Bertolino, A., Callicott, J.H., Elman, I. *et al.* (1998) Regionally specific neuronal pathology in untreated patients with schizophrenia: a proton magnetic resonance spectroscopic imaging study. *Biological Psychiatry* 43, 641–648.

Bertolino, A., Roffman, J.L., Lipska, B.K. *et al.* (1999) Postpubertal emergence of prefrontal neuronal deficits and altered dopaminergic behaviors in rats with neonatal hippocampal lesions. *Society of Neuroscience Abstract* 520.8.

Bertolino, A., Breier, A., Callicott, J.H. *et al.* (2000) The relationship between dorsolateral prefrontal neuronal N-acetylaspartate and evoked release of striatal dopamine in schizophrenia. *Neuropsychopharmacology* **22**, 125–132.

Black, M.D., Lister, S., Hitchcock, J.M., Giersbergen, P. & Sorensen, S.M. (1998) Neonatal hippocampal lesion model of schizophrenia in rats: sex differences and persistence of effects into maturity. *Drug and Developmental Research* **43**, 206–213.

Black, M.D., Selk, D.E., Hitchcock, J.M., Wetttstein, J.G. & Sorensen, S.M. (1999) On the effect of neonatal nitric oxide synthase inhibition in rats: a potential neurodevelopmental model of schizophrenia. *Neuropharmacology* **38**, 1299–1306.

Bloom, F.E. (1993) Advancing a neurodevelopmental origin of schizophrenia. *Archives of General Psychiatry* **50**, 224–227.

Bogerts, B., Ashtar, M., Degreef, G. *et al.* (1990) Reduced temporal limbic structure volumes on magnetic resonance images in first-episode schizophrenia. *Psychiatrics Research: Neuroimaging* **35**, 1–13.

Brake, W., Noel, M.B., Boksa, P. & Gratton, A. (1997a) Influence of perinatal factors on the nucleus accumbens dopamine response to repeated stress during adulthood: an electrochemical study in rat. *Neuroscience* **77**, 1067–1076.

Brake, W., Boksa, P. & Gratton, A. (1997b) Effects of perinatal anoxia on the locomotor response to repeated amphetamine administration in adult rats. *Psychopharmacology* **133**, 389–395.

Brake, W.G., Sullivan, R.M., Flores, G., Srivastava, L. & Gratton, A. (1999) Neonatal ventral hippocampal lesions attenuate the nucleus accumbens dopamine response to stress: an electrochemical study in the rat. *Brain Research* **831**, 25–32.

Breier, A., Su, T.P., Saunders, R. *et al.* (1997) Schizophrenia is associated with elevated amphetamine-induced synaptic dopamine concentrations: evidence from a novel positron emission tomography method. *Proceedings of the National Academy of Sciences of the USA* **94**, 2569–2574.

Brown, A.S., Susser, E.S., Butler, P.D. *et al.* (1996) Neurobiological plausibility of prenatal nutritional deprivation as a risk factor for schizophrenia. *Journal of Nervous and Mental Disease* **184**, 71–85.

Carr, D.B. & Sesack, S.R. (1996) Hippocampal afferents to the rat prefrontal cortex: Synaptic targets and relation to dopaminergic terminals. *Journal of Comparative Neurology* **369**, 1–15.

Castner, S.A., Al-Tikriti, M.S., Baldwin, R.M. *et al.* (2000) Behavioral changes and [123I]IBZM equilibrium SPECT measurement of amphetamine-induced dopamine release in rhesus monkeys exposed to subchronic amphetamine. *Neuropsychopharmacology* **22**, 4–13.

Chambers, R.A., Moore, J., McEvoy, J.P. & Levin, E.D. (1996) Cognitive effects of neonatal hippocampal lesions in a rat model of schizophrenia. *Neuropsychopharmacology* **15**, 587–594.

Cintra, L., Granados, L., Aguilar, A. *et al.* (1997) Effects of prenatal protein malnutrition on mossy fibers of the hippocampal formation in rats of four age groups. *Hippocampus* **7**, 184–191.

Conrad, A.J., Abebe, T., Ron, A., Forsythe, S. & Scheibel, B. (1991) Hippocampal pyramidal cell disarray in schizophrenia as a bilateral phenomenon. *Archives of General Psychiatry* **48**, 413–417.

Costall, B. & Naylor, R.J. (1995) Animal neuropharmacology and its prediction of clinical response. In: *Schizophrenia* (eds S.R. Hirsch & D.R. Weinberger), pp. 401–424. Blackwell Science, Oxford.

Cotter, D., Takei, N., Farrell, M. *et al.* (1995) Does prenatal exposure to influenza in mice induce pyramidal cell disarray in the dorsal hippocampus? *Schizophrenia Research* **16**, 233–241.

Csernansky, J.G., Csernansky, C.A., Kogelman, L., Montgomery, E.M. & Bardgett, M.E. (1998) Progressive neurodegeneration after intracerebroventricular kainic acid administration in rats: implications for schizophrenia? *Biological Psychiatry* **44**, 1143–1150.

Dalman, C., Allebeck, P., Cullberg, J., Grunewald, C. & Koster, M. (1999) Obstetric complications and the risk of schizophrenia: a longitudinal study of a national birth cohort. *Archives of General Psychiatry* **56**, 234–240.

Dean, B., Hussain, T., Hayes, W. *et al.* (1999) Changes in serotonin2A and GABA (A) receptors in schizophrenia: studies on the human dorsolateral prefrontal cortex. *Journal of Neurochemistry* **72**, 1593–1599.

DeLisi, L.E., Dauphinais, I.D. & Gershon, E.S. (1988) Perinatal complications and reduced size of brain limbic structures in afmilial schizophrenia. *Schizophrenia Bulletin* **14**, 185–191.

Duncan, G.E., Sheitman, B.B. & Lieberman, J.A. (1999) An integrated view of pathophysiological models of schizophrenia. *Brain Research Brain Research Review* **29**, 250–264.

Eastwood, S.L. & Harrison, P.J. (1995) Decreased synaptophysin in the medial temporal lobe in schizophrenia demonstrated using immunoautoradiography. *Neuroscience* **69**, 339–343.

Eastwood, S.L. & Harrison, P.J. (1998) Hippocampal and cortical growth-associated protein-43 messenger RNA in schizophrenia. *Neuroscience* **86**, 437–448.

Eastwood, S.L., McDonald, B., Burnet, P.W. *et al.* (1995) Decreased expression of mRNAs encoding non-NMDA glutamate receptors GluR1 and GluR2 in medial temporal lobe neurons in schizophrenia. *Brain Research Molecular Brain Research* **29**, 211–223.

Eastwood, S.L., Burnet, P.W. & Harrison, P.J. (1997) GluR2 glutamate receptor subunit flip and flop isoforms are decreased in the hippocampal formation in schizophrenia: a reverse transcriptase-polymerase chain reaction (RT-PCR) study. *Brain Research Molecular Brain Research* **44**, 92–98.

Egan, M. & Weinberger, D.R. (1997) Neurobiology of schizophrenia. *Current Opinion in Neurobiology* **7**, 701–707.

El-Khodor, B.F. & Boksa, P. (1997) Long-term reciprocal changes in dopamine levels in prefrontal cortex versus nucleus accumbens in rats born by Cesarean section compared to vaginal birth. *Experimental Neurology* **145**, 118–129.

El-Khodor, B.F. & Boksa, P. (1998) Birth insult increases amphetamine induced responses in the adult rat. *Neuroscience* **87**, 893–904.

Ellenbroek, B.A. & Cools, A.R. (1990) Animal models with construct validity for schizophrenia. *Behavioral Pharmacology* **1**, 469–490.

Ellenbroek, B.A., Geyer, M.A. & Cools, A.R. (1995) The behavior of APO-SUS rats in animal models with construct validity for schizophrenia. *Journal of Neuroscience* **11**, 7604–7611.

Ellenbroek, B.A., van den Kroonenberg, P.T. & Cools, A.R. (1998) The effects of an early stressful life event on sensorimotor gating in adult rats. *Schizophrenia Research* **30**, 251–260.

Ellenbroek, B.A., Sluyter, F. & Cools, A.R. (2000) The role of genetic and early environmental factors in determining apomorphine susceptibility. *Psychopharmacology* **148**, 124–131.

Erickson, R.P. (1996) Mouse models of human genetic disease: which mouse is more like a man? *Bioessays* **18**, 993–998.

Falkai, P. & Bogerts, B. (1986) Cell loss in the hippocampus of schizophrenics. *European Archives of Psychiatry and Neurological Science* **236**, 154–161.

Fatemi, S.H., Emamian, E.S., Kist, D. *et al.* (1999) Defective corticogenesis and reduction in Reelin immunoreactivity in cortex and hippocampus of prenatally infected neonatal mice. *Molecular Psychiatry* **4**, 145–154.

Feldpausch, D.L., Needham, L.M., Stone, M.P. *et al.* (1998) The role of dopamine D_4 receptor in the induction of behavioral sensitization to amphetamine and accompanying biochemical and molecular adaptations. *Journal of Pharmacology and Experimental Therapy* **286**, 497–508.

Flores, G., Barbeau, D., Quirion, R. & Srivastava, L.K. (1996a) Decreased binding of dopamine D3 receptors in limbic subregions after neonatal bilateral lesion of rat hippocampus. *Journal of Neuroscience* **16**, 2020–2026.

Flores, G., Wood, G.K., Liang, J.-J., Quirion, R. & Srivastava, L.K. (1996b) Enhanced amphetamine sensitivity and increased expression of dopamine D$_2$ receptors in postpubertal rats after neonatal excitotoxic lesions of the medial prefrontal cortex. *Journal of Neuroscience* **16**, 7366–7375.

Francis, D., Diorio, J., Liu, D. & Meaney, M.J. (1999) Nongenomic transmission across generations of maternal behavior and stress responses in the rat. *Science* **286**, 1155–1158.

Freedman, R., Adler, L.E., Gerhardt, G.A. *et al.* (1987) Neurobiological studies of sensory gating in schizophrenia. *Schizophrenia Bulletin* **13**, 669–678.

Freedman, R., Coon, H., Myles-Worsley, M. *et al.* (1997) Linkage of a neurophysiological deficit in schizophrenia to a chromosome 15 locus. *Proceedings of the National Academy of Sciences of the USA* **94**, 587–592.

Gambarana, C., Masi, F., Tagliamonte, A. *et al.* (1999) A chronic stress that impairs reactivity in rats also decreases dopaminergic transmission in the nucleus accumbens: a microdialysis study. *Journal of Neurochemistry* **72**, 2039–2046.

Geyer, M.A., Wilkinson, L.S., Humby, T. & Robbins, T.W. (1993) Isolation rearing of rats produces a deficit in prepulse inhibition of acoustic startle similar to that in schizophrenia. *Biological Psychiatry* **34**, 361–372.

Glantz, L.A. & Lewis, D.A. (1997) Reduction of synaptophysin immunoreactivity in the prefrontal cortex of subjects with schizophrenia: regional and diagnostic specificity. *Archives of General Psychiatry* **54**, 943–952.

Glantz, L.A. & Lewis, D.A. (2000) Decreased dendritic spine density on prefrontal cortical pyramidal neurons in schizophrenia. *Archives of General Psychiatry* **57**, 65–73.

Goffinet, A.M. (1995) Developmental neurobiology. A real gene for reeler. *Nature* **374**, 675–676.

Grecksch, G., Bernstein, H.G., Becker, A., Hollt, V. & Bogerts, B. (1999) Disruption of latent inhibition in rats with postnatal hippocampal lesions. *Neuropsychopharmacology* **20**, 525–532.

Harrison, P.J. & Eastwood, S.L. (1998) Preferential involvement of excitatory neurons in medial temporal lobe in schizophrenia. *Lancet* **352**, 1669–1673.

Hirotsune, S., Fleck, M.W., Gambello, M.J. *et al.* (1998) Graded reduction of Pafah1b1 (Lis1) activity results in neuronal migration defects and early embryonic lethality. *Nature Genetics* **19**, 333–339.

Hori, T., Subramaniam, S., Carli, M., Srivastava, L.K. & Quirion, R. (1999) Effects of repeated phencyclidine administration on locomotor activity and forced swimming test in rats with neonatal ventral hippocampal lesions. *Society of Neuroscience Abstract* **635.8**.

Hornig, M., Weissenbock, H., Horscroft, N. & Lipkin, W.I. (1999) An infection-based model of neurodevelopmental damage. *Proceedings of the National Academy of Sciences of the USA* **96**, 12102–12107.

Hultman, C.M., Ohman, A., Cnattingius, S., Wieselgren, I.M. & Lindstrom, L.H. (1997) Prenatal and neonatal risk factors for schizophrenia. *British Journal of Psychiatry* **170**, 128–133.

Huntsman, M.M., Tran, B.V., Potkin, S.G., Bunney, W.E. Jr & Jones, E.G. (1998) Altered ratios of alternatively spliced long and short gamma2 subunit mRNAs of the gamma-amino butyrate type A receptor in prefrontal cortex of schizophrenics. *Proceedings of the National Academy of Sciences of the USA* **95**, 15066–15071.

Impagnatiello, F., Guidotti, A.R., Pesold, C. *et al.* (1998) A decrease of reelin expression as a putative vulnerability factor in schizophrenia. *Proceedings of the National Academy of Sciences of the USA* **95**, 15718–15723.

Imperato, A., Obinu, M.C., Carta, G. *et al.* (1996) Reduction of dopamine release and synthesis by repeated amphetamine treatment: role in behavioral sensitization. *European Journal of Pharmacology* **317**, 231–237.

Javitt, D.C. & Zukin, S.R. (1991) Recent advances in the phencyclidine model of schizophrenia. *American Journal of Psychiatry* **148**, 1301–1308.

Jay, T.M., Glowinski, J. & Thierry, A.-M. (1989) Selectivity of the hippocampal projection to the prelimbic area of the prefrontal cortex in the rat. *Brain Research* **505**, 337–340.

Jentsch, J.D. & Roth, R.H. (1999) The neuropsychopharmacology of phencyclidine: from NMDA receptor hypofunction to the dopamine hypothesis of schizophrenia. *Neuropsychopharmacology* **20**, 201–225.

Jentsch, J.D., Tran, A., Le, D., Joungren, K.D. & Roth, R.H. (1997) Subchronic phencyclidine administration reduces mesoprefrontal dopamine utilization and impairs prefrontal cortical-dependent cognition in the rat. *Neuropsychopharmacology* **17**, 92–99.

Jentsch, J.D., Redmond, D.E., Elsworth, J.D. *et al.* (1998a) Enduring cognitive deficits and cortical dopamine dysfunction in monkeys after long-term administration of phencyclidine. *Science* **277**, 953–955.

Jentsch, J.D., Taylor, J.R. & Roth, R.H. (1998b) Subchronic phencyclidine administration increases mesolimbic dopaminergic system responsivity and augments stress- and psychostimulant-induced hyperlocomotion. *Neuropsychopharmacology* **19**, 105–113.

Jeste, D.V. & Lohr, J.B. (1989) Hippocampal pathologic findings in schizophrenia: a morphometric study. *Archives of General Psychiatry* **46**, 1019–1024.

Johnson-Wood, K., Lee, M., Motter, R. *et al.* (1997) Amyloid precursor protein processing and Aβ42 deposition in a transgenic mouse model of Alzheimer disease. *Proceedings of the National Academy of Sciences of the USA* **94**, 1550–1555.

Johnston, M.V., Barks, J., Greenmyre, T. & Silverstein, F. (1988) Use of toxins to disrupt neurotransmitter circuitry in the developing brain. *Progress in Brain Research* **73**, 425–446.

Jones, G.H., Hernandez, T.D., Kendall, D.A., Marsden, C.A. & Robbins, T.W. (1992) Dopaminergic and serotonergic function following isolation rearing in rats: study of behavioral responses and postmortem and *in vivo* neurochemistry. *Pharmacology, Biochemistry and Behavior* **43**, 17–35.

Karson, C.N., Mrak, R.E., Schluterman, K.O. *et al.* (1999) Alterations in synaptic proteins and their encoding mRNAs in prefrontal cortex in schizophrenia: a possible neurochemical basis for 'hypofrontality'. *Molecular Psychiatry* **4**, 39–45.

Kelz, M.B., Chen, J., Carlezon, W.A. Jr *et al.* (1999) Expression of the transcription factor deltaFosB in the brain controls sensitivity to cocaine. *Nature* **401**, 272–276.

Kendell, R.E. & Kemp, I.W. (1989) Maternal influenza in the etiology of schizophrenia. *Archives of General Psychiatry* **46**, 878–882.

Kendler, K.S., MacLean, C.J., O'Neill, F.A. *et al.* (1996) Evidence for a schizophrenia vulnerability locus on chromosome 8p in the Irish study of high-density schizophrenia families. *American Journal of Psychiatry* **153**, 1534–1540.

Kirkpatrick, B., Conley, R.C., Kakoyannis, A., Reep, R.L. & Roberts, R.C. (1999) Interstitial cells of the white matter in the inferior parietal cortex in schizophrenia: an unbiased cell-counting study. *Synapse* **34**, 95–102.

Kobayashi, K., Forte, T.M., Taniguchi, S. *et al.* (2000) The db/db mouse, a model for diabetic dyslipidemia: molecular characterization and effects of Western diet feeding. *Metabolism* **49**, 22–31.

Kornetsky, C. & Markowitz, R. (1978) Animal models of schizophrenia. In: *Psychopharmacology: a Generation of Progress* (eds M.A. Lipton, A. DiMascio & K.F. Killam), pp. 583–593. Raven Press, New York.

Krystal, J.H., Karper, L.P., Seibyl, J.P. *et al.* (1994) Subanesthetic effects of the noncompetitive NMDA antagonist, ketamine, in humans: psychotomimetic, perceptual, cognitive, and neuroendocrine responses. *Archives of General Psychiatry* 51, 199–214.

Lahti, A.C., Koffel, B., LaPorte, D. & Tamminga, C.A. (1995) Subanesthetic doses of ketamine stimulate psychosis in schizophrenia. *Neuropsychopharmacology* 13, 9–19.

Laruelle, M., Abi-Dargham, A., van Dyck, C.H. *et al.* (1996) Single photon emission computerized tomography imaging of amphetamine-induced dopamine release in drug-free schizophrenic subjects. *Proceedings of the National Academy of Sciences of the USA* 93, 9235–9240.

Lee, C.J., Binder, T., Lipska, B.K. *et al.* (1998) Neonatal ventral hippocampal lesions produce an elevation of Δ-FosB-like protein(s) in the rodent neocortex. *Society of Neuroscience Abstract* 24, 489.

Lewis, P., Patel, A. & Balazs, R. (1979) Effect of undernutrition on cell generation in the adult rat brain. *Brain Research* 168, 186–189.

Lieberman, J.A., Sheitman, B.B. & Kinon, B.J. (1997) Neurochemical sensitization in the pathophysiology of schizophrenia: deficits and dysfunction in neuronal regulation and plasticity. *Neuropsychopharmacology* 17, 205–229.

Lillrank, S.M., Lipska, B.K. & Weinberger, D.R. (1995) Neurodevelopmental animal models of schizophrenia. *Clinical Neuroscience* 3, 98–104.

Lipska, B.K. & Weinberger, D.R. (1993) Delayed effects of neonatal hippocampal damage on haloperidol-induced catalepsy and apomorphine-induced stereotypic behaviors in the rat. *Developmental Brain Research* 75, 13–222.

Lipska, B.K. & Weinberger, D.R. (1994a) Subchronic treatment with haloperidol or clozapine in rats with neonatal excitotoxic hippocampal damage. *Neuropsychopharmacology* 10, 199–205.

Lipska, B.K. & Weinberger, D.R. (1994b) Gonadectomy does not prevent novelty- or drug-induced hyperresponsiveness in rats with neonatal excitototxic hippocampal damage. *Developmental Brain Research* 78, 253–258.

Lipska, B.K. & Weinberger, D.R. (1995) Genetic variation in vulnerability to the behavioral effects of neonatal hippocampal damage in rats. *Proceedings of the National Academy of Sciences of the USA* 92, 8906–8910.

Lipska, B.K. & Weinberger, D.R. (2000) To model a psychiatric disorder in animals: schizophrenia as a reality test. *Neuropsychopharmacology* 23, 223–239.

Lipska, B.K., Jaskiw, G.E. & Weinberger, D.R. (1993) Postpubertal emergence of hyperresponsiveness to stress and to amphetamine after neonatal hippocampal damage: a potential animal model of schizophrenia. *Neuropsychopharmacology* 9, 67–75.

Lipska, B.K., Swerdlow, N.R., Geyer, M.A. *et al.* (1995a) Neonatal excitotoxic hippocampal damage in rats causes postpubertal changes in prepulse inhibition of startle and its disruption by apomorphine. *Psychopharmacology* 122, 35–43.

Lipska, B.K., Chrapusta, S.J., Egan, M.F. & Weinberger, D.R. (1995b) Neonatal excitotoxic ventral hippocampal damage alters dopamine response to mild chronic stress and haloperidol treatment. *Synapse* 20, 125–130.

Lipska, B.K., Al-Amin, H.A. & Weinberger, D.R. (1998a) Excitotoxic lesions of the rat medial prefrontal cortex: effects on abnormal behaviors associated with neonatal hippocampal damage. *Neuropsychopharmacology* 19, 451–464.

Lipska, B.K., Khaing, Z.Z., Lerman, D.N. & Weinberger, D.R. (1998b) Neonatal damage of the rat ventral hippocampus reduces expression of a dopamine transporter. *Society of Neuroscience Abstract* 24, 365.

Lipska, B.K., Kolb, B., Halim, N. & Weinberger, D.R. (2001) Synaptic

abnormalities in prefrontal cortex and nucleus accumbens of adult rats with neonatal hippocampal damage. *Schizophrenia Research* 49, 47.

Liu, D., Diorio, J., Tannenbaum, B. *et al.* (1997) Maternal care, hippocampal glucocorticoid receptors, and hypothalamic–pituitary–adrenal responses to stress. *Science* 277, 1659–1662.

Liu, W.S., Pesold, C., Rodriguez, M.A. *et al.* (2001) Down-regulation of dendritic spine and glutamic acid decarboxylase 67 expressions in the reelin haploinsufficient heterozygous reeler mouse. *Proceedings of the National Academy of Sciences of the USA* 98, 3477–3482.

Lohr, J.B. & Bracha, S. (1989) Can schizophrenia be related to prenatal exposure to alcohol? Some speculations. *Schizophrenia Bulletin* 15, 595–603.

Loring, J.F., Paszty, C., Rose, A. *et al.* (1996) Rational design of an animal model for Alzheimer's disease: introduction of multiple human genomic transgenes to reproduce AD pathology in a rodent. *Neurobiological Aging* 17, 173–182.

McKinney, W.T. & Moran, E.C. (1981) Animal models of schizophrenia. *American Journal of Psychiatry* 138, 478–483.

McNiel, T.F. (1988) Obstetric factors and perinatal injuries. In: *Handbook of Schizophrenia*, Vol. 3. *Nosology, Epidemiology and Genetic* (eds M.T. Tsuang & J.C. Simpson), pp. 319–344. Elsevier, Amsterdam.

Mathe, J.M., Nomikos, G.G., Schilstrom, B. & Svensson, T.H. (1998) Non-NMDA excitatory amino acid receptors in the ventral tegmental area mediate systemic dizocilpine (MK-801) induced hyperlocomotion and dopamine release in the nucleus accumbens. *Journal of Neuroscience Research* 51, 583–592.

Mazer, C., Muneyyirci, J., Taheny, K. *et al.* (1997) Serotonin depletion during synaptogenesis leads to decreased synaptic density and learning deficits. I. The adult rat: a possible model of neurodevelopmental disorders with cognitive deficits. *Brain Research* 760, 68–73.

Mednick, S.A., Machon, R.A., Huttunen, M.O. & Bonett, D. (1988) Adult schizophrenia following prenatal exposure to influenza epidemic. *Archives of General Psychiatry* 45, 189–192.

Meng, Z.H., Feldpaush, D.L. & Merchant, K.M. (1998) Clozapine and haloperidol block the induction of behavioral sensitization to amphetamine and associated genomic responses in rats. *Brain Research Molecular Brain Research* 61, 39–50.

Mintz, M., Youval, G., Gigi, A. & Myslobodsky, M.S. (1997) Rats exposed to prenatal gamma-radiation at day 15 of gestation exhibit enhanced perseveration in T-maze. *Society of Neuroscience Abstract* 23, 1365.

Moghaddam, B. & Adams, B. (1998) Reversal of phencyclidine effects by group II metabotropic glutamate receptor agonist in rats. *Science* 281, 1349–1352.

Moghaddam, B., Adams, B., Verma, A. & Daly, D. (1997) Activation of glutamatergic neurotransmission by ketamine: a novel step in pathway from NMDA receptor blockade to dopaminergic and cognitive disruptions associated with the prefrontal cortex. *Journal of Neuroscience* 17, 2921–2927.

Mohn, A.R., Gainetdinov, R.R., Caron, M.G. & Koller, B.H. (1999) Mice with reduced NMDA receptor expression display behaviors related to schizophrenia. *Cell* 98, 427–436.

Montgomery, E.M., Bardgett, M.E., Lall, B., Csernansky, C.A. & Csernansky, J.G. (1999) Delayed neuronal loss after administration of intracerebroventricular kainic acid to preweanling rats. *Brain Research and Developmental Brain Research* 112, 107–116.

Moore, H., Ghajarnia, M. & Grace, A.A. (1998) Anatomy and function of prefrontal and limbic corticostriatal circuits in a rodent model of schizophrenia. *37th ACNP Annual Meeting Abstract* 37, 179.

Morgane, P.J., Austin-LaFrance, R., Bronzino, J. *et al.* (1993) Prenatal malnutrition and development of the brain. *Neuroscience and Biobehaviour Review* 17, 91–128.

Murase, S., Mathe, J.M., Grenhoff, J. & Svensson, T.H. (1993) Effects of dizocilpine (MK-801) on rat midbrain dopamine cell activity: differential actions on firing pattern related to anatomical localization. *Journal of Neural Transmission: General Section* **91**, 13–25.

Murray, R.M. & Lewis, S.W. (1987) Is schizophrenia a neurodevelopmental disorder? *British Medical Journal* **295**, 681–682.

Nestler, E.J. & Aghajanian, G.K. (1997) Molecular and cellular basis of addiction. *Science* **278**, 58–63.

O'Callaghan, E., Sham, P., Takei, N., Glover, G. & Murray, R.M. (1991) Schizophrenia after prenatal exposure to 1957, A2 influenza epidemic. *Lancet* **337**, 1248–1250.

O'Donnell, P. & Grace, A.A. (1998) Phencyclidine interferes with the hippocampal gating of nucleus accumbens neuronal activity *in vivo*. *Neuroscience* **87**, 823–830.

O'Donnell, P., Lewis, B.L., Lerman, D., Weinberger, D.R. & Lipska, B.K. (1999) Effects of neonatal hippocampal lesions on prefrontal cortical pyramidal cell responses to VTA stimulation. *Society of Neuroscience Abstract* **664.2**.

Ohnuma, T., Augood, S.J., Arai, H., McKenna, P.J. & Emson, P.C. (1998) Expression of the human excitatory amino acid transporter 2 and metabotropic glutamate receptors 3 and 5 in the prefrontal cortex from normal individuals and patients with schizophrenia. *Brain Research Molecular Brain Research* **56**, 207–217.

Ohshima, T., Ward, J.M., Huh, C.G. *et al.* (1996) Targeted disruption of the cyclin-dependent kinase 5 gene results in abnormal corticogenesis, neuronal pathology and perinatal death. *Proceedings of the National Academy of Sciences of the USA* **93**, 11173–11178.

Olney, J.W. & Farber, N.B. (1995) Glutamate receptor dysfunction and schizophrenia. *Archives of General Psychiatry* **52**, 998–1007.

Patel, V.B., Richardson, P.J. & Preedy, V.R. (2000) Non-cardiac nucleic acid composition and protein synthesis rates in hypertension: studies on the spontaneously hypertensive rat (SHR) model. *Clinical Chim Acta* **293**, 167–179.

Pearce, B.D., Steffensen, S.C., Paoletti, A.D., Henriksen, S.J. & Buchmeier, M.J. (1996) Persistent dentate granule cell hyperexcitability following neonatal infection with lymphocytic choriomeningitis virus. *Journal of Neuroscience* **16**, 220–228.

Pearce, B.D., Po, C.L., Pisell, T.L. & Miller, A.H. (1999) Lymphocytic responses and the gradual hippocampal neuron loss following infection with lymphocytic choriomeningitis virus (LCMV). *Journal of Neuroimmunology* **101**, 137–147.

Pellegrini, M., Mansouri, A., Simeone, A., Boncinelli, E. & Gruss, P. (1996) Dentate gyrus formation requires Emx2. *Development* **122**, 3893–3898.

Perrone-Bizzozero, N.I., Sower, A.C., Bird, E.D. *et al.* (1996) Levels of the growth-associated protein GAP-43 are selectively increased in association cortices in schizophrenia. *Proceedings of the National Academy of Sciences of the USA* **93**, 14182–14187.

Porter, F.D., Drago, J., Xu, Y. *et al.* (1997) Lhx2, a LIM homeobox gene, is required for eye, forebrain, and definitive erythrocyte development. *Development* **124**, 2935–2944.

Qin, Z.H., Zhang, S.P. & Weiss, B. (1994) Dopaminergic and glutamatergic blocking drugs differentially regulate glutamic acid decarboxylase mRNA in mouse brain. *Brain Research Molecular Brain Research* **21**, 293–302.

Rajakumar, N., Williamson, P.C., Stoessl, J.A. & Flumerfelt, B.A. (1996) Neurodevelopmental pathogenesis of schizophrenia. *Society of Neuroscience Abstract* **22**, 1187.

Rakic, P. (1996) Experimental deletion of specific cortical neurons: relevance to schizophrenia. *35th ACNP Annual Meeting Abstract* **35**, 91.

Robinson, T.E. & Kolb, B. (1997) Persistent structural modifications in nucleus accumbens and prefrontal cortex neurons produced by previous experience with amphetamine. *Journal of Neuroscience* **17**, 8491–8497.

Roffman, J.L., Lipska, B.K., Bertolino, A. *et al.* (2000) Local and downstream effects of excitotoxic lesions in the rat medial prefrontal cortex on *in vivo* ^{1}H-MRS signals. *Neuropsychopharmacology* **22**, 430–439.

Rott, R., Herzog, S., Fleischer, B. *et al.* (1985) Detection of serum antibodies to Borna disease virus in patients with psychiatric disorders. *Science* **228**, 755–756.

Rupniak, N.M.J. & Iversen, S.D. (1993) Cognitive impairment in schizophrenia: how experimental models using nonhuman primates may assist improved drug therapy for negative symptoms. *Neuropsychologia* **31**, 1133–1146.

Sams-Dodd, F., Lipska, B.K. & Weinberger, D.R. (1997) Neonatal lesions of the rat ventral hippocampus result in hyperlocomotion and deficits in social behaviour in adulthood. *Psychopharmacology* **132**, 303–310.

Saunders, R.C., Kolachana, B.S., Bachevalier, J. & Weinberger, D.R. (1998) Neonatal lesions of the temporal lobe disrupt prefrontal cortical regulation of striatal dopamine. *Nature* **393**, 169–171.

Scheibel, A.B. & Kovelman, J.A. (1981) Disorientation of the hippocampal pyramidal cell and its processes in the schizophrenic patient. *Biological Psychiatry* **16**, 101–102.

Schroeder, H., Grecksch, G., Becker, A., Bogerts, B. & Höllt, V. (1999) Alterations of the dopaminergic and glutamatergic neurotransmission in adult rats with postnatal ibotenic acid hippocampal lesion. *Psychopharmacology* **145**, 61–66.

Selemon, L.D., Castner, S.A., Algan, O., Goldman-Rakic, P.S. & Rakic, P. (2000) Selective deletion of thalamic neurons in early gestation as a primate model of schizophrenia (abstract). *39th ACNP Annual Meeting, Puerto Rico*, p. 44.

Sheldon, M., Rice, D.S., D'Arcangelo, G. *et al.* (1997) Scrambler and yotari disrupt the disabled gene and produce a reeler-like phenotype in mice. *Nature* **389**, 730–733.

Sibley, D.R. (1999) New insights into dopaminergic receptor function using antisense and genetically altered animals. *Annual Review of Pharmacological Toxicology* **39**, 313–341.

Solbrig, M.V., Koob, G.F., Fallon, J.H. & Lipkin, W.I. (1994) Tardive dyskinetic syndrome in rats infected with Borna disease virus. *Neurobiological Disease* **1**, 111–119.

Solbrig, M.V., Koob, G.F., Joyce, J.N. & Lipkin, W.I. (1996a) A neural substrate of hyperactivity in Borna disease: changes in brain dopamine receptors. *Virology* **222**, 332–338.

Solbrig, M.V., Koob, G.F., Fallon, J.H., Reid, S. & Lipkin, W.I. (1996b) Prefrontal cortex dysfunction in Borna disease virus (BDV)-infected rats. *Biological Psychiatry* **40**, 629–636.

Spanagel, R. & Weiss, F. (1999) The dopamine hypothesis of reward: past and current status. *Trends in Neuroscience* **22**, 521–527.

Steiner, H. & Gerfen, C.R. (1998) Role of dynorphin and enkephalin in the regulation of striatal output pathways and behavior. *Experimental Brain Research* **123**, 60–76.

Stevens, K.E., Kem, W.R., Mahnir, V.M. & Freedman, R. (1998) Selective α7-nicotinic agonists normalize inhibition of auditory response in DBA mice. *Psychopharmacology* **136**, 320–327.

Suddath, R.L., Christisin, G.W., Torrey, E.F., Casanova, M. & Weinberger, D.R. (1990) Anatomical abnormalities in the brains of monozygotic twins discordant for schizophrenia. *New England Journal of Medicine* **322**, 789–794.

Susser, E.S. & Lin, S.P. (1992) Schizophrenia after prenatal exposure to the Dutch Hunger Winter of 1944–45. *Archives of General Psychiatry* **49**, 983–988.

Talamini, L.M., Koch, T., Ter Horst, G.J. & Korf, J. (1998) Methylazoxymethanol acetate-induced abnormalities in the entorhinal cortex of the rat; parallels with morphological findings in schizophrenia. *Brain Research* **789**, 293–306.

Tomasiewicz, H., Ono, K., Yee, D. *et al.* (1993) Genetic deletion of a neural cell adhesion molecule variant (N-CAM-180) produces distinct defects in the central nervous system. *Neuron* **11**, 1163–1174.

Tonkiss, J. & Galler, J.R. (1990) Prenatal protein malnutrition and working memory performance in adult rats. *Behavioral Brain Research* **40**, 95–107.

Vanderschuren, L.J., Schmidt, E.D., De Vries, T.J. *et al.* (1999) A single exposure to amphetamine is sufficient to induce long-term behavioral, neuroendocrine, and neurochemical sensitization in rats. *Journal of Neuroscience* **19**, 9579–9586.

Varty, G.B. & Higgins, G.A. (1995) Examination of drug-induced and isolation-induced disruptions of prepulse inhibition as models to screen antipsychotic drugs. *Psychopharmacology* **122**, 15–26.

Vawter, M.P., Hemperly, J.J., Hyde, T.M. *et al.* (1998) VASE-containing N-CAM isoforms are increased in the hippocampus in bipolar disorder but not schizophrenia. *Experimental Neurology* **154**, 1–11.

Verma, A. & Moghaddam, B. (1996) NMDA receptor antagonists impair prefrontal cortex function as assessed via spatial delayed alternation performance in rats: modulation by dopamine. *Journal of Neuroscience* **16**, 373–379.

Waltrip, R.W. II, Buchanan, R.W., Summerfeld, A. *et al.* (1995) Borna disease virus and schizophrenia. *Psychiatrics Research* **56**, 33–44.

Wan, R.Q. & Corbett, R. (1997) Enhancement of postsynaptic sensitivity to dopaminergic agonists induced by neonatal hippocampal lesions. *Neuropsychopharmacology* **16**, 259–268.

Wan, R.-Q., Giovanni, A., Kafka, S.H. & Corbett, R. (1996) Neonatal hippocampal lesions induced hyperresponsiveness to amphetamine: behavioral and *in vivo* microdialysis studies. *Behavioral Brain Research* **78**, 211–223.

Wan, R.Q., Hartman, H. & Corbett, R. (1998) Alteration of dopamine metabolites in CSF and behavioral impairments induced by neonatal hippocampal lesions. *Physiological Behavior* **65**, 429–436.

Weickert, C.S. & Weinberger, D.R. (1998) A candidate molecule approach to defining developmental pathology in schizophrenia. *Schizophrenia Bulletin* **24**, 303–316.

Weinberger, D.R. (1986) The pathogenesis of schizophrenia: a neurodevelopmental theory. In: *The Neurology of Schizophrenia* (eds H.A. Nasrallah & D.R. Weinberger), pp. 397–406. Elsevier, Amsterdam.

Weinberger, D.R. (1987) Implications of normal brain development for the pathogenesis of schizophrenia. *Archives of General Psychiatry* **44**, 660–669.

Weinberger, D.R. (1999) Cell biology of the hippocampal formation in schizophrenia. *Biological Psychiatry* **45**, 395–402.

Weinberger, D.R. & Lipska, B.K. (1995) Cortical maldevleopment, anti-psychotic drugs, and schizophrenia: in search of common ground. *Schizophrenia Research* **16**, 87–110.

Wilkinson, L.S., Killcross, S.S., Humby, T. *et al.* (1994) Social isolation in the rat produces developmentally specific deficits in prepulse inhibition of the acoustic startle response without disrupting latent inhibition. *Neuropsychopharmacology* **10**, 61–72.

Woerner, M.G., Pollack, M. & Klein, D.F. (1973) Pregnancy and birth complications in psychiatric patients: a comparison of schizophrenic and personality disorder patients with their siblings. *Acta Psychiatrica Scandinavica* **49**, 712–721.

Wolf, M.E., White, F.J. & Hu, X.-T. (1993) Behavioral sensitization to MK-801 (dizocilpine): neurochemical and electrophysiological correlates in the mesoaccumbens dopamine system. *Behavioral Pharmacology* **4**, 429–442.

Wood, G.K., Tomasiewicz, H., Rutishauser, U. *et al.* (1998) NCAM-180 knockout mice display increased lateral ventricle size and reduced prepulse inhibition of startle. *Neuroreport* **9**, 461–466.

Wu, C.L. & Melton, D.W. (1993) Production of a model for Lesch–Nyhan syndrome in hypoxanthine phosphoribosyltransferase-deficient mice. *Nature Genetics* **3**, 235–240.

Yonezawa, Y., Kuroki, T., Kawahara, T., Tashiro, N. & Uchimura, H. (1998) Involvement of gamma-aminobutyric acid neurotransmission in phencyclidine-induced dopamine release in the medial prefrontal cortex. *European Journal of Pharmacology* **341**, 45–56.

Young, C.E., Arima, K., Xie, J. *et al.* (1998) SNAP-25 deficit and hippocampal connectivity in schizophrenia. *Cerebral Cortex* **8**, 261–268.

Zaharia, M.D., Kulczycki, J., Shanks, N., Meaney, M.J. & Anisman, H. (1996) The effects of early postnatal stimulation on Morris watermaze acquisition in adult mice: genetic and maternal factors. *Psychopharmacology* **128**, 227–239.

Zhao, Y., Sheng, H.Z., Amini, R. *et al.* (1999) Control of hippocampal morphogenesis and neuronal differentiation by the LIM homeobox gene Lhx5. *Science* **284**, 1155–1158.

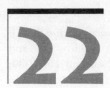

Brain imaging in schizophrenia

P. Liddle and C. Pantelis

Historical overview, 403
Imaging techniques, 404
    Structural imaging techniques, 404
    Functional imaging techniques, 405
Whole brain volume and cerebrospinal fluid spaces, 406
    Intracranial and whole brain changes, 406
    Ventricular and sulcal cerebrospinal fluid spaces, 406
Brain regions implicated in schizophrenia, 406
    Frontal neocortex, 406
    Temporal neocortex, 408
    Parietal cortex, 409
    Cingulate cortex, 409
    Hippocampus and amygdala, 410

Subcortical structures, 411
    Basal ganglia, 411
    Thalamus, 412
    Cerebellum, 412
Schizophrenia as a disorder of connectivity, 412
    Correlations between abnormalities at separate sites, 412
    Abnormal correlation between cerebral activity at spatially remote sites, 412
    Assessment of connectivity using structural imaging, 413
Conclusions, 413
Acknowledgements, 414
References, 414

In vivo images of the structure and function of the human brain not only confirm that there are demonstrable brain abnormalities in schizophrenia, but also offer the tantalizing prospect of providing information that could inform diagnosis and guide treatment in individual patients. However, abnormalities of macroscopic structure are small, and often difficult to identify in individuals. For example, although enlargement of the cerebral ventricles is one of the most robust abnormalities in schizophrenia, in the majority of patients ventricular size lies within the normal range (Raz & Raz 1990). In general, abnormalities of function are more substantial, but techniques for imaging brain function present a kaleidoscope of activity that is exquisitely sensitive to a myriad of influences on the external and internal milieu. After a brief review of imaging techniques, we examine the evidence for abnormalities of structure and function in various different brain regions. Finally, we examine the evidence suggesting that the cardinal abnormality in schizophrenia is a disruption of connections between neurones leading to impaired co-ordination of neural activity at spatially remote sites.

Historical overview

The first evidence of abnormal brain structure in schizophrenia, provided by *in vivo* imaging techniques, was the demonstration using pneumoencephalography that the cerebral ventricles, especially the third ventricle, are enlarged in at least some cases (Huber 1964). With the advent of the less invasive technique of X-ray computerized tomography (CT), Johnstone *et al.* (1976) confirmed that patients with severe persistent illness have ventricular enlargement. Subsequent studies using patients who were more representative of the natural range of illness severity have confirmed the existence of ventricular enlargement, but

meta-analyses reveal a somewhat smaller effect size than that found in severe chronic cases. Raz and Raz (1990) identified a moderate effect size for both lateral and third ventricular size of 0.7 and 0.66, respectively, while a smaller effect for cortical sulcal cerebrospinal fluid (CSF) space enlargement was also found.

The first functional imaging studies employed techniques involving the injection or inhalation of radioactive xenon to assess local cerebral perfusion, which is an indirect indicator of local neural activity. Using the xenon injection technique, Ingvar and Franzen (1974) demonstrated that medicated patients with chronic schizophrenia have an abnormally low ratio of activity in frontal cortex to that in posterior brain areas, compared with the ratio observed in healthy subjects. However, not all studies have confirmed this hypofrontality. In a study using positron emission tomography (PET) to measure resting state regional oxygen metabolism in a small group of predominantly unmedicated first episode cases, Sheppard *et al.* (1983) failed to find any evidence of reduced frontal metabolism. Subsequent studies, considered in greater detail below, show that resting state blood flow and metabolism depend on phase of illness and symptom profile.

While studies of the resting state blood flow or metabolism are potentially informative about current clinical state, studies of the cerebral activity during the performance of a specific cognitive task can provide information about brain activity associated with task performance. In a seminal study, Weinberger *et al.* (1986) demonstrated that schizophrenic patients produce less activation of the frontal cortex than healthy controls during performance of the Wisconsin Card Sorting Test (WCST), a complex test of executive function. Despite the difficulties of interpretation of cognitive activation studies, because it is not easy to distinguish failure to activate the brain because of failure to engage in the task from a failure to activate a specific region despite adequate engagement in the task, the cognitive activation procedure has proven to be very fruitful in exploring brain function in schizophrenia. The fact that deoxyhaemoglobin is paramagnetic has allowed the development of functional magnetic resonance imaging (fMRI) for the assessment of regional cerebral function without the need to administer radioactive tracer substances, leading to a rapid growth in the use of functional imaging techniques.

Imaging techniques

Structural imaging techniques

The technique of X-ray CT, which was widely employed for studies of brain in schizophrenia in the 15 years following the initial study by Johnstone *et al.* (1976), has now largely been superseded by magnetic resonance imaging (MRI) techniques, which provide better delineation of tissue types. MRI provides images based on the phenomenon of nuclear magnetic resonance (NMR). NMR depends on the fact that atomic nuclei containing unpaired protons or neutrons (e.g. the proton in a hydrogen atom) have a magnetic moment that causes them to precess like spinning tops in an applied magnetic field. If a radiofrequency pulse with frequency matching the rotation frequency is applied, the nuclear particles absorb energy in a way that raises them to a higher energy level and brings the precession into phase. When the radiofrequency pulse is removed they return to the ground state by transferring energy to the environment. This is known as spin–lattice or T1 relaxation. In addition they also lose phase coherence in a process known as spin–spin or T2 relaxation. The T1 and T2 relaxation times differ depending on the tissue type, meaning that they can be used for the generation of contrast in images. Various different protocols for delivering the radiofrequency excitation pulses and for detecting the emitted radiation allow measurement of various aspects of brain structure and function.

Volumetric and morphological measurements using MRI

T1-weighted images, which provide thin slices encompassing the whole brain and extracerebral tissue, provide good contrast between grey and white matter, delineate sulci and gyri and permit the measurement of the volume of specific cortical and subcortical structures. Dual echo sequences provide simultaneous T2-weighted and proton-density images, which allow better differentiation of CSF, grey and white matter and volumetric analysis of these regions, and have been used for semiautomated and automated analyses.

Magnetic resonance spectroscopy

Magnetic resonance spectroscopy (MRS) requires a radiofrequency transmitter and receiver coil focused on a particular nucleus of interest (e.g. ^{31}P, ^{1}H, ^{19}F, ^{13}C), which allows different aspects of *in vivo* neurochemistry to be assessed. A number of reviews examine the methods involved in spectroscopy and summarize the literature in schizophrenia (Keshavan *et al.* 2000; Vance *et al.* 2000). While most MRS studies have had to define a volume of interest (VOI) from which the signal is generated, thereby limiting the areas that can be examined, more recent multislice or chemical shift spectroscopic imaging techniques may be more useful in assessing the relationship between different brain regions (Bertolino *et al.* 1996).

The spectra derived from proton (^{1}H) spectroscopy provide information about N-acetylaspartate (NAA), which exists intraneuronally and assesses neuronal mass and integrity, while choline metabolites provide indices of myelin composition and phospholipid metabolism. Other metabolites include: creatine (including phosphocreatine), a general marker of energy metabolism; glutamine, localized mainly in glial cells; and glutamate, an excitatory neurotransmitter found primarily within glutaminergic neurones.

In contrast, phosphorus-31 (^{31}P) MRS provides information about membrane phospholipid metabolism and energy metabolism, and is relevant to assessing the integrity of cell membranes. ^{31}P-MRS allows *in vivo* investigation of phosphomonoesters (PMEs: phospholipid precursors) and phosphodiesters (PDEs: phospholipid breakdown products) which indirectly reflect the rates of cell membrane synthesis and degradation, while phosphocreatine (PCr) and inorganic phosphate (Pi) are indirect indicators of energy metabolism.

T2-relaxometry

T2-relaxometry, which entails the measurement of T2 relaxation time, provides objective (rater-independent) information about brain tissue integrity. For example, increased hydration (e.g. oedema) lengthens T2, while iron deposition reduces T2. T2 relaxation is also prolonged in dysplastic conditions with a neurodevelopmental basis, providing a potentially important method to examine the neurodevelopmental hypothesis of schizophrenia. It has not been extensively used in schizophrenia to date. Hitherto, all studies have been in patients with chronic illness and have generally produced inconsistent findings. However, evidence for frontotemporal abnormalities in schizophrenia (Williamson *et al.* 1992) is consistent with the other recent findings discussed below.

Techniques to assess white matter

The technique of diffusion tensor/weighted imaging (DTI/DWI) assesses the anisotropy of water diffusion and allows the integrity of white matter tracts to be examined, thereby providing a novel means to examine fibre pathways and brain connectivity directly. Initial studies using this technique have identified abnormal fibre pathways in frontostriatal regions diffusely across the brain (Lim *et al.* 1999) and in the corpus callosum (Foong *et al.* 2000). While promising, DTI needs refinement and application in studies of larger samples of patients.

Magnetization transfer imaging (MTI) is another novel technique, which allows the visualization of protons tightly bound to macromolecular structures, such as myelin and cell membranes in white matter. Foong *et al.* (2001) recently used MTI in schizophrenia and identified abnormalities in frontotemporal regions, consistent with other structural and functional imaging literature discussed below. Because myelin content of tissue affects relaxation times, abnormalities of myelination can also be detected by relaxometry.

Novel analysis techniques in structural imaging

Recent innovations in analysis of structural imaging data include semiautomated and automated analysis methods, rather than more laborious manual tracing techniques. These include voxel-based analyses (e.g. Paillere-Martinot *et al.* 2001; Sigmundsson *et al.* 2001; Pantelis *et al.* 2002). While these recent innovations require further validation, they are particularly helpful in examining all brain structures simultaneously, compared with manual tracing techniques which usually target a limited number of regions. However, automated voxel-based methods of estimating tissue volumes may give misleading results if the sulcal/gyral pattern is abnormal. Studies so far have not allowed for this possibility, although there is evidence of anomalous cortical gyrification in schizophrenia (Vogeley *et al.* 2001; Yücel *et al.* 2002a).

Functional imaging techniques

Several techniques, including PET, single photon emission computerized tomography (SPECT) and fMRI provide indirect measurements of the spatial variation in neural activity associated with mental activity. To understand the information provided by these techniques, it is necessary to summarize some features of neural activity and the way regional cerebral blood flow (rCBF) is regulated to support that activity.

The resting state

In the resting state, neural firing is not random and grey matter is not uniformly active. Blood flow and metabolism in healthy subjects are greatest in frontal cortex and medial parietal cortex, regions that are engaged during internally generated mental activity. Abnormalities of self-generated mental activity play an important part in schizophrenia, and studies of resting state brain activity are informative, provided that the clinical state of the patients is assessed with sufficient care. Many studies of the resting state (reviewed by Andreasen *et al.* 1992) reveal underactivity of the frontal cortex, especially in chronic cases, but other studies, especially those of acutely ill patients, reveal resting-state hyperfrontality. At least some of this variability between patients in the patterns of resting state cerebral activity can be attributed to differences in symptom profile. Liddle *et al.* (1992) demonstrated that each of three major groups of persistent schizophrenic symptoms is associated with a distinct pattern of abnormal function of brain regions normally engaged in the types of mental process implicated in the relevant symptoms. In particular, they found that reality distortion (delusions and hallucinations) and disorganization symptoms were associated with overactivity at different frontal loci, while psychomotor poverty (comprising core negative symptoms) was associated with frontal underactivity. Subsequent studies (reviewed by Liddle 2000) have confirmed all the major features of these findings, although it should be noted that some studies of acutely psychotic patients (Erkwoh *et al.* 1997) provide a more complex picture, presumably because of additional mental processes in acute psychosis. Antipsychotic medication also produces changes in resting brain activity. Ngan *et al.* (2002) found that a single dose of risperidone produced decreases in lateral and medial frontal lobe activity, but that the changes in medial frontal activity were associated with subsequent reduction in severity of psychotic symptoms.

Haemodynamic response to neural stimulation

Increased neural firing during mental activity produces an increase in local perfusion that exceeds the immediate need for oxygen. Consequently, measurement of changes in rCBF, using either PET or SPECT with a radioactive tracer that accumulates in brain tissue in proportion to local perfusion, provides a sensitive index of neural activity. Unfortunately, the use of radioactive tracers limits the number of scans that can be performed in a single subject. However, paramagnetic properties of deoxyhaemoglobin provide a non-invasive way to detect local neural activity, using fMRI. Following a magnetizing pulse that aligns the protons in tissue, the magnetic resonance signal decays rapidly owing to processes that cause dephasing of the spinning protons. The dephasing of protons arises not only from interactions with other nuclei (the spin–spin interactions responsible for T2 relaxation) but also from the effects of local magnetic field inhomogeneities (T2* relaxation). One source of inhomogeneity is paramagnetic deoxyhaemoglobin in capillaries. In the vicinity of active neurones, increased perfusion removes deoxyhaemoglobin, and the strength of the magnetic resonance signal decays less rapidly. This enhancement of signal in the vicinity of active neurones is known as the blood oxygen level-dependent (BOLD) effect.

This haemodynamic response can be imaged using various 'single-shot' techniques, in which the information required to construct an image is obtained following application of a single pulse of magnetization. Using the technique known as echoplanar imaging, a slice of brain can be imaged in 40 ms, and the entire brain can be imaged within 2–3 s. In a typical fMRI study, several hundred brain images are collected during 10–20 min. In block-design studies, the mental state of interest is maintained for 20–30 s. Blocks of the mental state of interest alternate with blocks in which an appropriate baseline mental state is maintained. In event-related designs, the haemodynamic response to individual mental events is compared with a sustained baseline state.

Whole brain volume and cerebrospinal fluid spaces

Intracranial and whole brain changes

Assessment of intracranial volume (ICV) and whole brain volume (WBV) provides information about the impact of premorbid and morbid factors on overall brain structure in schizophrenia. Because cranial vault size is determined by age 6, comparison of abnormalities in ICV with abnormalities in WBV provides an indication of the developmental stage at which the abnormalities might have arisen (for discussion see Woods 1998). Also, accounting for global measures provides information about whether changes in particular brain structures are local or part of a more global change.

Meta-analyses indicate that WBV is smaller (by about 2%) in schizophrenia compared with controls (Ward *et al.* 1996; Wright *et al.* 2000), while intracranial volume (ICV) may show a smaller reduction (Ward *et al.* 1996). These differences are more consistently seen in chronic patients. The majority of studies that have examined grey and white matter compartments separately have found that it is grey matter volume that is reduced, although some studies of regional brain volume have reported white matter deficits (Breier *et al.* 1992; Cannon *et al.* 1998). Reduced brain volume is observed from the outset of illness (Zipursky *et al.* 1998; Rapoport *et al.* 1999) and, in particular, has been reported in neuroleptic-naïve first episode patients (Gur *et al.* 1999).

Twin and sibling studies also provide information about familial/genetic contributions to structural abnormalities identified. Thus, results from a recent twin study (Baaré *et al.* 2001) suggested that smaller ICV may be a genetically determined vulnerability to schizophrenia, while WBV may have both genetic and environmental determinants. In this context, it is of interest that the Edinburgh study of individuals at high risk for schizophrenia on account of having at least two affected family members found that the patients developing psychosis had smaller WBV (Lawrie *et al.* 2001).

Longitudinal follow-up studies of brain volume provide the most important means to assess the issue of progression of brain structural abnormalities in schizophrenia (Velakoulis *et al.* 2000b). DeLisi *et al.* (1997) identified reduction in hemispheric volume over a 4-year follow-up period in 50 first episode schizophrenia patients compared with 20 controls. More recently, Wood *et al.* (2001) followed 30 first episode psychosis patients, 12 patients with chronic schizophrenia and 26 control subjects with repeated MRI scans. There were no differences between first episode patients and controls in ICV or WBV at initial assessment; however, there was progressive loss of WBV over the 2- to 4-year follow-up period. Taken together with the twin and sibling studies, these studies confirm that WBV is reduced in schizophrenia, and also indicate that these changes are progressive.

Ventricular and sulcal cerebrospinal fluid spaces

There is a more consistent literature demonstrating enlarged ventricles in schizophrenia, particularly involving lateral and third ventricles (Shenton *et al.* 2001). However, it should be noted that such changes may not be specific to schizophrenia as they have also been noted in depressed patients (Elkis *et al.* 1995). Several studies have reported ventricular enlargement, predominantly in non-familial rather than familial cases (Cannon *et al.* 1998; Baaré *et al.* 2001), which is consistent with the observed association with obstetric complications (McNeil *et al.* 2000). Nevertheless, there is evidence that genetic factors also contribute to ventricular enlargement. Sharma *et al.* (1998) found that unaffected family members, whose position within the family indicated that they were obligate carriers of the predisposition to schizophrenia, had enlarged left lateral ventricles. Furthermore, there is substantial evidence that third ventricular enlargement may be genetically determined (Staal *et al.* 2000), consistent with the findings from the Edinburgh high-risk study in which high-risk individuals had abnormally enlarged third ventricles (Lawrie *et al.* 2001). Regionally specific CSF abnormalities include left temporal horn enlargement (for discussion see Shenton *et al.* 2001), which is consistent with left temporal structural abnormalities discussed below.

Recent longitudinal studies have also provided evidence for progressive ventricular and sulcal enlargement in schizophrenia from illness onset (Giedd *et al.* 1999; Mathalon *et al.* 2001). Further, in at least some studies, ventricular enlargement has been associated with poor outcome (Staal *et al.* 1999) and with duration of untreated psychosis (Madsen *et al.* 1999).

Brain regions implicated in schizophrenia

Frontal neocortex

Grey matter volume in frontal cortex and subregions

Both manual and automated or semiautomated techniques have been used to segment the brain into grey and white matter and CSF compartments. A number of studies have variously defined prefrontal subregions to assess whether abnormalities are widespread or regionally specific. The results from the majority of the published studies suggest that the volumetric differences in prefrontal cortex in schizophrenia result from selective loss of grey matter in heteromodal dorsolateral prefrontal cortex (Schlaepfer *et al.* 1994; Goldstein *et al.* 1999; Gur *et al.* 2000a). This is associated with grey matter volume reduction in other heteromodal association cortical regions in schizophrenia. It is not observed in patients with bipolar disorder (Schlaepfer *et al.* 1994). These studies suggest that structural abnormalities are apparent in a region consistently implicated by functional imaging studies (see below).

Other studies have also identified structural abnormalities in inferior frontal regions, including the orbitofrontal cortex, in treated (Szeszko *et al.* 1999) and drug-naïve patients (Crespo-Facorro *et al.* 2000; Gur *et al.* 2000a). In the large study by Gur *et al.* (2000a), comparing neuroleptic-naïve and chronic patients with schizophrenia with healthy controls, gender-related differences were found. While both males and females had reduced grey matter in dorsolateral prefrontal cortex, only males had smaller dorsomedial prefrontal cortex. In contrast, only women had smaller orbitofrontal regions. These latter abnormalities were associated with negative symptoms, depression and poorer premorbid functioning. While these findings demonstrate that involvement of the dorsal prefrontal cortex is a consistent feature of schizophrenia, there may be gender differences for orbitofrontal cortex, which may be related to a greater degree of affective disturbance in females. Further, these frontal abnormalities are observed early in the course of illness.

Evidence for frontal involvement from *in vivo* neurochemistry (MRS)

The findings from ^{31}P-MRS in the prefrontal cortex have been summarized elsewhere (Keshavan *et al.* 2000; Vance *et al.* 2000). Although there are some inconsistencies between studies, several studies have identified reduced PMEs in first- and multi-episode patients. In contrast, PDEs are elevated mainly in first episode patients, suggesting an increased membrane turnover at the onset of illness. These findings may reflect abnormal synaptic pruning in schizophrenia (Keshavan *et al.* 2000). Recent interest in phosphorus MRS has centred on the role of fatty acids as possible treatments for schizophrenia (Berger *et al.* 2002).

The findings from proton (^{1}H) MRS of prefrontal cortex suggest that there are reductions in NAA and NAA/Cr ratio in schizophrenia, including first episode neuroleptic-naïve patients, and in schizophrenia spectrum disorders (Vance *et al.* 2000). These findings are consistent with the volumetric studies described above, and indicate that prefrontal cortical volume reduction is caused by deficits in neuronal number or in neuronal integrity. While many of these studies strongly implicate the dorsolateral prefrontal region in schizophrenia, few MRS studies have examined other prefrontal areas such as the orbitofrontal cortex.

Staging of frontal cortical structural abnormalities

While it remains unclear at what stage in neurodevelopment the changes occur in schizophrenia, the studies that can inform this question include: those examining genetic vs. environmental influences on brain structural abnormalities; studies that assess ICV (as discussed earlier); studies assessing gyral and fissural morphology; and longitudinal investigations. Woods *et al.* (1996), in their tissue segmentation study in chronic schizophrenia, found reduced ICV in the frontal region while tissue/ICV ratios were lower in frontal, temporal and parietal regions, suggesting that frontal abnormalities occurred early in life before brain growth was complete, and generalized changes in the

brain occurred later after brain growth had occurred. These findings are consistent with data showing that frontal abnormalities are apparent in first episode patients (Shenton *et al.* 2001) as well as with preliminary data in premorbid high-risk individuals (Lawrie *et al.* 2001; Pantelis *et al.* 2002). Further, twin and sibling studies provide evidence that there is a genetic effect on frontal lobe volumes in schizophrenia.

While these data suggest that frontal abnormalities are apparent premorbidly in schizophrenia, the few available follow-up studies provide evidence that there is further progression of abnormalities in frontal regions (Gur *et al.* 1998; Madsen *et al.* 1999), particularly on the left. Decreases in both frontal and temporal regions were also observed in a study of childhood-onset schizophrenia (Rapoport *et al.* 1999). Further, such changes have been associated with symptom severity, including an association of prefrontal and temporal lobe grey matter decline and greater negative symptoms (Mathalon *et al.* 2001).

Associations have been found between reduced grey matter volume and neuropsychological tests of memory and executive function (Baaré *et al.* 1999). More recently, studies using both ^{1}H-MRS together with functional imaging (PET and fMRI) have identified relationships between decreased NAA in dorsolateral prefrontal cortex and impaired function of the neuronal network for working memory (Callicott *et al.* 2000).

The available data from these studies indicate that frontal grey matter abnormalities are present from illness onset, may be apparent premorbidly and that further progressive changes occur following illness onset. Further, they are associated particularly with negative symptoms and with neuropsychological deficits.

Function of prefrontal cortex

The demonstration by Weinberger *et al.* (1986) that schizophrenic patients produce less activation of the frontal cortex than healthy controls during performance of the WCST has been replicated many times, with various tests of executive function (Weinberger & Berman 1996). Unfortunately, in many studies employing complex tasks, it is difficult to rule out the possibility that the patients were not as engaged in the task as the healthy controls. However, Weinberger and Berman (1996) have demonstrated that even when patients are matched with controls for performance, the schizophrenic patients exhibit less activation of frontal cortex during performance of the WCST.

Nevertheless, the relationship between diminished activation and task performance remains a vexed question. Fletcher *et al.* (1998) demonstrated that during a word learning task, frontal activation was only diminished under circumstances where the processing load was high and performance was impaired. Similarly, Carter *et al.* (1998) and Perlstein *et al.* (2001), using the N-back working memory task, in which the participant is required to respond when a presented item matches the previous N item presented, found that schizophrenic patients only exhibited a deficit in frontal activation when memory load was high and performance was impaired.

In contrast to the evidence for hypofrontality, several studies have reported that schizophrenic patients exhibit greater activation of frontal cortex than healthy subjects during working memory tasks (Callicott *et al.* 2000; Manoach *et al.* 2000). A potential clue to understanding why frontal activation is low under some circumstances and increased under others is provided by the observation that in some of the studies reporting diminished frontal activation in patients during executive tasks the diminished activation could be attributed partly to excessive activity in the less demanding baseline comparison condition. Mendrek (2001) found that acutely ill first episode patients failed to activate lateral frontal cortex during the 2-back working memory task, relative to a baseline 0-back task that placed little demand on working memory. This failure of activation was attributable both to excessive activity in lateral frontal cortex during the baseline 0-back task and to diminished activity during the 2-back task. After 6 weeks' antipsychotic treatment, the activation in the 2-back condition relative to the 0-back condition had improved greatly, mainly because of resolution of the previously excessive activation in the 0-back condition. Thus, in acute first episode schizophrenia, diminished frontal activation can be attributed to two abnormalities: excessive activation during the low-load baseline task, and a reduced activation during more demanding tasks. The former abnormality resolves during treatment, while the latter is an enduring feature.

One of the roles of the dorsolateral prefrontal cortex is the resolution of conflict between competing responses (MacDonald *et al.* 2000). A possible explanation for the complex relationship between processing load and lateral frontal activation in acute schizophrenia is that an externally specified task must compete with abnormal self-generated mental activity, associated with psychotic symptoms. When the externally specified task entails only a low load, this competition leads to excessive dorsolateral frontal activation. However, when the externally specified task entails a higher processing load, the lateral prefrontal cortex is unable to meet the demand, resulting in both defective performance and less activation than occurs in healthy subjects.

Substantial evidence indicates that reduced dopaminergic activity contributes to impaired frontal lobe function in schizophrenia. Weinberger *et al.* (1988) demonstrated that diminished activation during the WCST was correlated with low levels of the dopamine metabolite homovanillic acid in cerebrospinal fluid. The indirect dopaminergic agonist amphetamine can partially ameliorate the failure to activate frontal cortex during the WCST (Daniel *et al.* 1991). Furthermore, using fMRI, Egan *et al.* (2001) demonstrated that individuals with a tendency to slower degradation of dopamine by virtue of genetically determined variation in function of the enzyme catechol-O-methyl-transferase (COMT) exhibited a more efficient physiological response in prefrontal cortex. It is probable that neurotransmitters other than dopamine also modulate frontal function. Honey *et al.* (1999) demonstrated that the atypical antipsychotic risperidone, which blocks serotonin 5-HT$_2$ receptors in addition to dopamine D$_2$ receptors, produced enhancement of frontal function compared with that seen during treatment with typical antipsychotics, which block mainly D$_2$ receptors.

Temporal neocortex

Structure of temporal neocortex

The available evidence suggests that the whole of the temporal lobe may be smaller in patients with schizophrenia (for review see Shenton *et al.* 2001), most likely resulting from reduced volume of grey matter (Gur *et al.* 2000b). However, like the situation in frontal cortex, the volumetric defects may differ in its various gyri. Particularly implicated in schizophrenia is the posterior part of superior temporal gyrus that includes the planum temporale, an area specialized for the processing of language (Shapleske *et al.* 1999). However, there is also structural imaging evidence for reduced volume of parahippocampal gyrus (Wright *et al.* 2000) and more recent evidence that the fusiform gyrus is smaller (Paillere-Martinot *et al.* 2001) and may show progressive change during the early phase of the illness (Pantelis *et al.* 2002). Studies also report abnormalities in the sulcal and gyral pattern of the temporal lobe (Kikinis *et al.* 1994), suggestive of developmental abnormalities.

Longitudinal studies of the whole temporal lobe have generally not found progressive loss of volume (DeLisi *et al.* 1995; Wood *et al.* 2001), or the change in schizophrenia has been similar to normals (Gur *et al.* 1998). However, this may depend on the neurodevelopmental stage at which patients are assessed, as data from childhood-onset schizophrenia indicate progressive loss of volume (Rapoport *et al.* 1999).

Superior temporal gyrus

The temporal lobe region most consistently implicated in schizophrenia is the superior temporal gyrus (STG), including the planum temporale. While in the review by Shenton *et al.* (2001) 67% of studies examining volume of the whole STG (including grey and white matter) show reduced volume, 100% of studies examining grey matter of STG demonstrate reduced volume, indicating remarkable consistency. This abnormality is observed in first episode patients and appears to be specific to schizophrenia rather than affective psychosis (Hirayasu *et al.* 1998).

In a meta-analysis of studies examining the planum temporale, patients with schizophrenia showed a reduction in the normal pattern of leftward asymmetry as a result of a relatively larger right planum than in normal controls (Shapleske *et al.* 1999). However, because of the variable methodologies used to measure this structure, the findings have been variable between studies and include reversal of asymmetry and reduced volume in left planum temporale (for discussion see Shenton *et al.* 2001). Abnormalities in STG and planum temporale have been associated with positive symptoms (Kwon *et al.* 1999) and with thought disorder (Petty *et al.* 1995).

Symptom expression and the superior temporal gyrus

The role of the STG in auditory processing, particularly in processing of language, suggests that it is likely to have a role in the expression of symptoms such as auditory hallucinations. To test the hypothesis that impaired ability to monitor the source of internally generated mental activity might be involved in the generation of hallucinations, McGuire et al. (1995) used PET to assess cerebral activity while the participants imagined hearing a stranger's voice completing sentences in schizophrenic patients prone to hallucinations and two control groups: non-hallucinating patients and healthy subjects. The healthy subjects and the non-hallucinating patients exhibited activation in the STG, but this activation was significantly diminished in the patients prone to hallucinations.

The evidence that abnormal structure of the superior temporal gyrus is associated with formal thought disorder (Petty et al. 1995) suggests that abnormal function of the STG might also have a role in formal thought disorder. Using PET to examine cerebral activity while patients produced speech in response to presented pictures, McGuire et al. (1998) demonstrated that severity of positive formal thought disorder was correlated inversely with amount of activity in the left STG. This finding was subsequently confirmed by Kircher et al. (2001) using fMRI.

Parietal cortex

Structural abnormalities of parietal cortex

While the parietal lobe has not been the focus of many structural imaging studies, there is evidence for its involvement structurally in schizophrenia (for review see Shenton et al. 2001), in line with the notion that heteromodal association cortex is especially affected in schizophrenia (Ross & Pearlson 1996). A number of studies have found structural abnormalities in heteromodal regions, including parietal regions (Schlaepfer et al. 1994; Goldstein et al. 1999). Niznikiewicz et al. (2000) have undertaken the most comprehensive study of the various gyri of the parietal lobe to date, although the sample consisted of only 15 male patients with chronic schizophrenia and 15 male control subjects. These authors identified a reversal of the normal left greater than right asymmetry in patients with schizophrenia, particularly in the angular gyrus of the inferior parietal lobule, consistent with involvement of the semantic–lexical network. They also reported correlations between the volumes of inferior parietal lobule and regions in prefrontal and temporal cortex, consistent with the notion of an interconnected network involving these regions.

Parietal lobe and symptom expression

Underactivity of the parietal lobe has been implicated in several classes of schizophrenic symptoms. In particular, parietal underactivity is correlated with severity of psychomotor poverty symptoms (Liddle et al. 1992) and with severity of disorganiza-

tion symptoms (Liddle et al. 1992; Kaplan et al. 1993). The association with disorganization is consistent with the evidence that formal thought disorder is associated with reduced volume of temporoparietal language areas (Niznikiewicz et al. 2000). In addition, patients who exhibit delusions of control exhibit decreased ability to activate parietal cortex during the selection of motor activity (Spence et al. 1997). This is supported by a preliminary finding of reduced volume of parietal cortex in patients with passivity delusions compared with those not having these phenomena (Velakoulis et al. 2000).

Cingulate cortex

Structural abnormalities of the cingulate cortex

There are few published structural imaging studies of the cingulate, despite evidence for its involvement from neuropathology and functional imaging studies. Volumetric studies are limited by difficulties in delineating the boundaries of this structure, which has led to inconsistent findings, including those of recent studies using parcellation methods. Two studies in first episode schizophreniform patients did not identify abnormalities in cingulate volume (Hirayasu et al. 1999; Szeszko et al. 1999), although Hirayasu et al. (1999) found reduced volume of subgenual cingulate in affective psychosis patients with a family history of affective disorder. These findings contrast with those of Goldstein et al. (1999), who found reduced volume in cingulate and paracingulate gyri in schizophrenia.

Because of the difficulties defining the boundaries of the cingulate, automated methods of analysis using voxel-based morphometry (VBM) may be advantageous. In contrast to the manual tracing studies, these recent VBM investigations have identified cingulate abnormalities in chronic schizophrenia (Sigmundsson et al. 2001) and in childhood onset schizophrenia (Sowell et al. 2000). However, because these techniques rely on the accuracy of the coregistration method used, morphological anomalies in cingulate surface anatomy in patients compared with controls may masquerade as volumetric differences.

Using ^{1}H-MRS, Deicken et al. (1997) found lower NAA bilaterally in anterior cingulate regions, which was not associated with duration of illness or medication dosage, suggesting that neuronal integrity or function of the cingulate is impaired in schizophrenia. However, other studies have not found abnormality of NAA in the anterior cingulate cortex (Bertolino et al. 1998).

Abnormal cingulate gyrification

Yücel et al. (2002b) provide a detailed examination of the degree of fissurization of the cingulate and paracingulate in normal subjects and in patients with chronic schizophrenia. Patients had reduced cingulate fissurization in the left hemisphere, and manifested a relative absence of the paracingulate sulcus compared with normal subjects. Future studies assessing the volume of the cingulate cortex will need to control for such differences in gross surface anatomy.

Selective attention and response competition

An extensive body of evidence indicates that the dorsal part of the anterior cingulate cortex and adjacent medial frontal cortex are involved in selective attention and in the identification of conflict between competing responses (MacDonald *et al.* 2000). Schizophrenic patients exhibit less activation of anterior cingulate cortex than healthy subjects during the Stroop task, which entails competition between competing responses (Carter *et al.* 1997), and which has been related to cingulate morphology (Yücel *et al.* 2002a).

Cingulate cortex and disorganization symptoms

Disorganization symptoms, such as formal thought disorder and inappropriate affect, are associated with impairment in tasks that entail selection between competing responses. Several studies have demonstrated that the severity of disorganization symptoms is significantly correlated with increased rCBF in the anterior cingulate and adjacent medial frontal cortex (Liddle *et al.* 1992; Ebmeier *et al.* 1993; Yuasa *et al.* 1995). While this excessive activity might reflect pathological overactivity of the anterior cingulate, it is also possible that it reflects an appropriate response to the intrusion of irrelevant material into current mental processing, arising from a defect elsewhere in the brain. It should be noted that the evidence indicating a tendency for excessive activity in the anterior cingulate in the resting (but symptomatic) state in schizophrenia might explain, at least in part, the diminished activation relative to baseline of this brain region during the Stroop task, reported by Carter *et al.* (1997).

Hippocampus and amygdala

Structural abnormalities of the hippocampal formation and amygdala

With the introduction of improved MRI methodologies in recent years, providing higher image resolution, studies have consistently identified abnormalities in the hippocampus or the amygdalo–hippocampal complex in patients with schizophrenia, particularly affecting the left side (Nelson *et al.* 1998; Wright *et al.* 2000). In their meta-analysis of hippocampal and amygdala volumes in schizophrenia, Nelson *et al.* (1998) found significant mean effect sizes for left (0.37) and right hippocampus (0.39), corresponding to a bilateral reduction of 4%. In a second meta-analysis of studies measuring the amygdalo–hippocampal complex, the effect sizes rose to 0.67 and 0.72 respectively. No left–right differences were identified and there was no effect of duration of illness identified in this study. Similarly, Wright *et al.* (2000) identified significant volume reductions for studies assessing the amygdala alone (6%

bilaterally), a similar magnitude in those assessing the amygdalo–hippocampal complex, while smaller reductions of around 3% bilaterally were found in studies assessing the hippocampus separately. However, these studies did not contrast first episode and chronic patients, and could not assess the effects of handedness or gender, as most studies were of right-handed males.

Investigations in first episode schizophrenia suggest that hippocampal volume reduction is apparent at illness onset, and is predominantly left-sided (Hirayasu *et al.* 1998; Velakoulis *et al.* 1999), while patients with established schizophrenia show bilateral hippocampal volume reduction (Velakoulis *et al.* 1999). Velakoulis *et al.* (1999) identified similar changes in both first episode schizophreniform and affective psychosis patients, suggesting that these findings may not be specific to schizophrenia, while the results from Hirayasu *et al.* (1998) suggested a similar pattern but were not significant. While the former investigators separated the hippocampus from the amygdala, the latter measured the amygdalo–hippocampal complex. Future studies need to separate these structures as they may be differentially affected in these disorders, because there is evidence that the amygdala is larger in affective psychosis (Altshuler *et al.* 2000), so that combining these structures would confound the assessment of diagnostic specificity.

In a study of monozygotic twins discordant for schizophrenia, Suddath *et al.* (1990) demonstrated that the affected twin almost invariably has a smaller hippocampal volume than the unaffected cotwin, even though in many cases for both twins the volume was in the normal range. This finding not only indicates that in most cases of schizophrenia hippocampal volume is probably decreased, compared with what it might have been in the absence of schizophrenia, but also suggests that environmental factors contribute to the decrease. In the Edinburgh study of individuals with multiply affected family members there was no identified genetic contribution to the observed hippocampal volume reduction (Lawrie *et al.* 2001). Two studies identified a specific effect of perinatal birth complications in causing the smaller hippocampi observed in schizophrenia (Stefanis *et al.* 1999; McNeil *et al.* 2000). This is consistent with the notion that neurochemical (e.g. glutamate) or hormonal effects (e.g. cortisol) can reduce hippocampal volume, and supports the view that hippocampal volume reduction is not specific to psychotic disorders. Despite the evidence that environmental factors contribute to the reduction in hippocampal volume reported in schizophrenia, there is also evidence that genes have a role. For example, Seidman *et al.* (1999) found significant volume reductions bilaterally in the amygdalo–hippocampal region and thalamus in first-degree relatives.

The question of whether or not there are progressive changes specific to the hippocampus after the onset of schizophrenia remains controversial. Longitudinal studies using manual tracing to measure the hippocampus have generally not identified changes during the course of the illness (Lieberman *et al.* 2001; Wood *et al.* 2001), but some cross-sectional studies have reported relationships between the volume of medial temporal lobe structures and the duration of illness (Matsumoto *et al.*

2001; Velakoulis *et al.* 2001). Data from childhood-onset schizophrenia suggests that changes may occur during adolescence (Giedd *et al.* 1999).

MRS abnormalities of the hippocampal formation

Studies of the hippocampus–amygdala using ^{1}H-MRS, including the more recent ones (Bertolino *et al.* 1998), are reasonably consistent in finding reduction of intraneuronal NAA in the hippocampus (Vance *et al.* 2000). Callicot *et al.* (1998) found reduced hippocampal NAA in a large sample of healthy siblings. However, to date there have been no longitudinal studies using MRS in high-risk populations.

Hippocampal formation and symptom expression

While the evidence from structural studies indicates that the volume of medial temporal structures is decreased in schizophrenia, the majority of the evidence from functional imaging studies suggests that positive psychotic symptoms, especially hallucinations, are associated with overactivity of medial temporal lobe structures. Liddle *et al.* (1992) found that severity of reality distortion (delusions and hallucinations) was positively correlated with rCBF in the hippocampal formation and parahippocampal gyrus. Subsequently, Silbersweig *et al.* (1995) and Shergil *et al.* (2000) demonstrated overactivity of the hippocampus and other medial temporal lobe structures during the occurrence of auditory hallucinations. It should be noted that all of these studies reported that positive symptoms were associated with activation in a distributed network of frontal, temporal and subcortical sites. None the less, the observation by Liddle *et al.* (2000) that the reduction in hippocampal metabolism produced by the first dose of risperidone in previously unmedicated first episode schizophrenic patients was strongly predictive of the subsequent decrease in severity of reality distortion symptoms supports the hypothesis that hippocampal overactivity plays a primary part in reality distortion.

Hippocampal activation during memory tasks

In a PET study designed to determine whether memory impairment in schizophrenia is more strongly associated with malfunction of frontal cortex or of temporal cortex, Heckers *et al.* (1998) found that schizophrenic patients exhibited reduced hippocampal activation, relative to baseline, during conscious recollection of studied words, but robust activation of the lateral frontal cortex during the effort to retrieve poorly encoded material. It should be noted that the reduced hippocampal activation during conscious recollection was accounted for by increased activity in the baseline state.

Function of the amygdala

During a study of the induction of sad mood, Schneider *et al.* (1998) found that schizophrenic patients exhibited less activa-

tion of the amygdala than healthy controls, despite a similar severity of induced negative affect. In contrast, in an fMRI study of the processing of facial expressions, Phillips *et al.* (1999) found that a small group of non-paranoid schizophrenic patients exhibited excessive activation of the amygdala while processing expressions of disgust, associated with the misperception of disgust as fear.

Subcortical structures

Basal ganglia

The basal ganglia have a cardinal role in the regulation of cortical activity by virtue of their involvement in the corticostriatal–thalamic loops that provide feedback to frontal cortex. Several studies have demonstrated that overactivity of the ventral striatum is associated with the production of delusions and/or hallucinations (Liddle *et al.* 1992; Silbersweig *et al.* 1995). Furthermore, antipsychotic treatment is associated with reduction in activity in the corticostriatal–thalamic loops (Holcomb *et al.* 1996; Liddle *et al.* 2000).

The feedback provided by the corticostriatal–thalamic loops is modulated by dopaminergic input from the midbrain. Blockade of D_2 receptors in the striatum has long been regarded as a potentially crucial aspect of the action of antipsychotic medication. Using either SPECT or PET, it is possible to measure the displacement of labelled D_2 ligands, such as iodobenzamide or [^{11}C]raclopride, from striatal receptors, following procedures that promote dopamine release. Several studies have shown that the amount of displacement of D_2 ligands following the administration of amphetamine is increased in schizophrenia (Laruelle *et al.* 1996; Breier *et al.* 1997), implying excessive release of endogenous dopamine. Furthermore Laruelle *et al.* (1996) demonstrated that the amount of ligand displacement was correlated with the severity of transient positive symptoms induced by the amphetamine.

By measuring the D_2 receptor availability before and after pharmacological depletion of endogenous dopamine, it is possible to estimate the level of endogenous dopamine in striatal synapses and, in addition, to measure the total density of D_2 receptors. Using this technique, Abi-Dargham *et al.* (2000) demonstrated that schizophrenic patients have higher levels of intrasynaptic dopamine than healthy subjects and, furthermore, after removing endogenous dopamine, the number of available D_2 receptors was greater than in healthy controls. Overall, these studies indicate that the dopamine system is over-responsive in schizophrenia, leading to increased levels of intrasynaptic dopamine at baseline and also to excessive release following procedures such as administration of amphetamine yet, paradoxically, D_2 receptors appear to be increased rather than downregulated. One explanation of these findings is that there is excessive phasic release of dopamine, together with a diminished level of tonic dopaminergic activity leading to D_2 receptor upregulation.

Thalamus

Although reliable assessment of the volume of the thalamus is difficult, the evidence indicates that the volume of the thalamus is decreased in schizophrenia. In a meta-analysis, Konick and Friedman (2001) found that the effect size for differences between patients and controls was −0.29, although the magnitude of the effect size increased to −0.41 when outliers were removed. Gilbert *et al.* (2001) reported that thalamic volume is reduced even in first episode cases. Lawrie *et al.* (1999) reported reduced thalamic volume in individuals at risk for schizophrenia, with multiply affected family members.

Functional imaging studies reveal reduced thalamic activation in schizophrenic patients in a variety of tasks that engage association cortex (Andreasen *et al.* 1996; Kiehl & Liddle 2001). Despite the evidence for diminished thalamic volume and diminished activation during cognitive tasks, there is substantial evidence that the thalamus is overactive during the occurrence of symptoms such as hallucinations (Silbersweig *et al.* 1995) and disorganization symptoms (Liddle *et al.* 1992), consistent with the hypothesis that psychotic symptoms entail excessive feedback via corticostriatal–thalamic circuits.

Cerebellum

The cerebellum receives input from most areas of association cortex via the midbrain, and sends reciprocal projections back to association cortex via the thalamus. Consistent with these connections, reduced activation of the cerebellum is often observed in schizophrenia during tasks that normally engage association cortex, particularly the frontal cortex (Andreasen *et al.* 1996; Kiehl & Liddle 2001; Mendrek 2001). Furthermore, MRI studies provide some evidence for a reduction in the volume of the cerebellar vermis (Ichimiya *et al.* 2001).

Schizophrenia as a disorder of connectivity

The evidence indicating structural and functional abnormalities in distributed brain systems suggests that the core abnormality in schizophrenia is unlikely to be a focal abnormality at a single cerebral location. Furthermore, the evidence that a particular brain region, such as the prefrontal cortex or the hippocampus, can be either under- or overactive in different circumstances indicates that the core abnormality is dynamic in nature. Taken together, these observations suggest that the core problem might be an abnormality of the connections between neurones, rather than a loss of neural cell bodies. Such a disturbance of connectivity might arise from an abnormality of the myelinated axons that make up white matter, or from an abnormality of the synapses and/or dendrites that are a major component of the neuropil surrounding cell bodies in grey matter.

There are several approaches to testing the hypothesis of abnormal connectivity. The first strategy is to measure the relationship between measurements of brain structure or function in separate brain areas. The demonstration that abnormalities in one area are correlated with abnormalities measured in another area indicates that the pathophysiology of schizophrenia involves pathological influence that is exerted at a distance, but does not directly demonstrate that the connections between the areas are abnormal. The second approach compares the patterns of correlation between physiological activity at spatially remote cerebral sites in patients with that in healthy individuals. The term functional connectivity is used to describe such correlations between cerebral activity at spatially remote sites (Friston *et al.* 1993). While correlated cerebral activity does not necessarily imply a direct anatomical connection between the sites involved, it nevertheless provides an index of the coordination of cerebral activity at distant sites. The third approach entails direct assessment of structural features that are indicative of intracerebral connections, such as the assessment of white matter tracts using diffusion tensor imaging. In this section we review functional imaging studies that illustrate these three different approaches to assessing connectivity in schizophrenia.

Correlations between abnormalities at separate sites

In a study of monozygotic twins discordant for schizophrenia, Weinberger *et al.* (1992) found that hippocampal volume, measured using MRI, predicted prefrontal rCBF activation during the WCST. This finding suggests that prefrontal malfunction is secondary to hippocampal structural abnormality. However, more recent studies have pointed to microstructural abnormality in the prefrontal cortex itself. Bertolino *et al.* (2000a) found that NAA in dorsolateral prefrontal cortex, measured with MRS, selectively predicted amphetamine-induced displacement of [^{11}C]raclopride from dopamine D_2 receptors in the striatum, implying that prefrontal cellular abnormality was associated with excessive endogenous dopamine levels in the striatum. Furthermore, in two separate studies, Bertolino *et al.* (2000b) found that NAA level in the dorsolateral prefrontal cortex was correlated with activation of the distributed working memory network, including the dorsolateral prefrontal, temporal and inferior parietal cortices, during performance of working memory tasks.

Abnormal correlation between cerebral activity at spatially remote sites

Several PET studies have focused on the question of whether or not schizophrenia is characterized by an abnormal correlation between the activity in the frontal and temporal lobes. Frith *et al.* (1995) observed that activation of frontal cortex during paced word generation (relative to a baseline measured during word repetition) was accompanied by suppression of activity in the superior temporal gyrus in healthy subjects. In patients with severe persistent illness, the magnitude of frontal activation was normal, but there was an aberrant increase in activity in the superior temporal gyrus. This observation was confirmed by Fletcher *et al.* (1996) in a study of medication-naïve first episode cases, raising the possibility that it is a characteristic feature of schizophrenia at all phases of the illness. Neither Frith *et al.* (1995) nor Fletcher *et al.* (1996) directly computed the correlation between activity in frontal and temporal cortex, but in a subsequent reanalysis of the data of Frith *et al.*, Liddle (2000) demonstrated that there was indeed a negative correlation in healthy controls and a positive correlation in patients, indicating aberrant functional connectivity. Furthermore, Liddle (2000) demonstrated abnormal connectivity between frontal cortex and a range of other cerebral sites including thalamus, cingulate cortex and precuneus.

To test the hypothesis that abnormal frontotemporal connectivity is a trait marker for schizophrenia, Spence *et al.* (2000) performed a similar study of word generation in remitted patients with minimal symptoms, and also in obligate carriers of the predisposition to schizophrenia. They found that neither the remitted patients nor obligate carriers had abnormal frontotemporal connectivity. Thus, this anomaly appears to be a state marker, characteristic of symptomatic cases. None the less, Spence *et al.* (2000) did observe that the remitted patients had decreased connectivity between lateral prefrontal cortex and anterior cingulate cortex.

Consistent with the evidence for abnormal connectivity between frontal cortex and diverse cerebral sites, Josin and Liddle (2001) demonstrated that chronic schizophrenic patients could be distinguished from healthy controls with 100% reliability using data regarding functional connectivity between prefrontal cortex and 11 other cerebral sites. Similarly, Meyer-Lindenberg *et al.* (2001) achieved 94% success in the diagnosis of schizophrenia on the basis of abnormal patterns of connectivity during both 2-back and 0-back conditions of an *N*-back working memory task in a comparison between medication-free patients and healthy controls. In particular, the patients did not exhibit the normal connectivity between dorsolateral prefrontal cortex and anterior cingulate. Overall, there is strong evidence for abnormal functional connectivity between lateral frontal cortex and other brain regions in schizophrenia. The question of whether or not any of these abnormalities might be a trait marker remains a subject of debate. The current evidence points towards an abnormality of functional connectivity between lateral prefrontal cortex and anterior cingulate cortex in all phases of the illness.

When reporting correlations as evidence of functional connectivity, no assumptions are made about the causal influence of one cerebral area on another. The strength of the causal influence that activity in one area has on activity in the other area is known as the effective connectivity between those areas. Deductions about effective connectivity can only be drawn from functional imaging data if assumptions are made a priori about the connections that exist between cerebral areas. The technique of path analysis or structural equation modelling can be employed to test the plausibility of a priori models in which the direction of the connections between a set of cerebral areas are specified. As an illustration of such an approach, Jennings *et al.* (1998) demonstrated abnormal connectivity between frontal cortex and temporal cortex and also between lateral frontal cortex and anterior cingulate cortex in schizophrenia during semantic processing. Similarly, Fletcher *et al.* (1999) used path analysis to demonstrate a disruption of the normal modulation of prefrontal–temporal interactions by the anterior cingulate cortex in schizophrenic patients during word generation.

Assessment of connectivity using structural imaging

The majority of the evidence for reduced cerebral tissue volume in schizophrenia indicates that the reduction in grey matter exceeds that in white matter. Futhermore, despite some reports from postmortem studies of decreased cell numbers in grey matter, the balance of evidence indicates no widespread decrease in numbers of neurones in neocortex (Pakkenberg 1993). Thus, it is plausible that the diminution of cerebral tissue in schizophrenia might largely reflect a diminution of neurophil as a result of diminished volume of the synapses and dendrites that constitute the connections between neurones. Because the development of connections reflects usage during the period of development, the correlations between grey matter volume in different regions provide an indirect index of the connectivity between those areas during development. Woodruff *et al.* (1997) observed that the correlation between frontal and temporal lobe volumes was significantly reduced in a group of schizophrenic patients compared with healthy controls. They interpreted this as evidence for frontal–temporal dissociation during development.

While the evidence for grey matter abnormality points towards a possible abnormality of dendrites and synapses, preliminary studies using diffusion tensor imaging also provide evidence of abnormality of the myelinated axons that constitute white matter. Buchsbaum *et al.* (1998) found abnormality of frontal–striatal connections, while Lim *et al.* (1999) reported abnormalities extending across much of the brain. Foong *et al.* (2000) found abnormality of white fibres in the splenium of the corpus callosum, suggesting a specific abnormality of interhemispheric connectivity.

Conclusions

The evidence indicates subtle diminution of cerebral tissue volume in diverse brain areas in schizophrenia. Features such as abnormal gyrification suggest that the primary abnormality arises early in development. On the other hand, there is some evidence from longitudinal studies for progression of abnormalities during the course of the illness. Consistent with the widespread abnormalities of brain structure, there are also widespread abnormalities of function. In some areas, such as frontal lobes, medial temporal lobe, basal ganglia and thalamus, both abnormal increases and decreases in activity have been reported, indicating that the core problem is dynamic in nature.

Preliminary evidence points to a disorder of the development of connections between cerebral areas, which might entail abnormality of long myelinated axons, and of synapses and dendrites. However, despite the fact that a substantial number of imaging findings in schizophrenia have been replicated, there are also many inconsistencies between studies. These inconsistencies probably arise from a variety of sources, including the heterogeneity of schizophrenia, the sensitivity of brain function to subtle variations in circumstances, and the evolving nature of imaging technology. Therefore, the findings of individual studies should be interpreted with caution.

Acknowledgements

We thank Dr Stephen Wood for commenting on various drafts of the chapter. Dr Pantelis' imaging work was supported by the National Health and Medical Research Council (grant numbers 145737, 145627, 114253, 981112, 970598) and grants from the Ian Potter and Stanley Foundations.

References

Abi-Dargham, A., Rodenhiser, J., Printz, D. *et al.* (2000) From the cover: increased baseline occupancy of D_2 receptors by dopamine in schizophrenia. *Proceedings of the National Academy of Sciences of the USA* **97**, 8104–8109.

Altshuler, L.L., Bartzokis, G., Grieder, T. *et al.* (2000) An MRI study of temporal lobe structures in men with bipolar disorder or schizophrenia. *Biological Psychiatry* **48**, 147–162.

Andreasen, N.C., Rezai, K., Alliger, R. *et al.* (1992) Hypofrontality in neuroleptic-naive patients and in patients with chronic schizophrenia: assessment with xenon-133 single photon emission computed tomography and the Tower of London. *Archives of General Psychiatry* **49**, 943–958.

Andreasen, N.C., O'Leary, D.S., Cizadlo, T. *et al.* (1996) Schizophrenia and cognitive dysmetria: a positron emission tomography study of dysfunctional prefrontothalamic–cerebellar circuitry. *Proceedings of the National Academy of Sciences of the USA* **93**, 9985–9990.

Baaré, W.F., Hulshoff Pol, H.E., Hijman, R. *et al.* (1999) Volumetric analysis of frontal lobe regions in schizophrenia: relation to cognitive function and symptomatology. *Biological Psychiatry* **45**, 1597–1605.

Baaré, W.F., van Oel, C.J., Hulshoff Pol, H.E. *et al.* (2001) Volumes of brain structures in twins discordant for schizophrenia. *Archives of General Psychiatry* **58**, 33–40.

Berger, G.E., Wood, S.J., Pantelis, C. *et al.* (2002) Implications of lipid biology for the pathogenesis of schizophrenia. *Australian & New Zealand Journal of Psychiatry* **36**, 355–366.

Bertolino, A., Nawroz, S., Mattay, V.S. *et al.* (1996) Regionally specific pattern of neurochemical pathology in schizophrenia as assessed by multislice proton magnetic resonance spectroscopic imaging. *American Journal of Psychiatry* **153**, 1554–1563.

Bertolino, A., Callicott, J.H., Elman, I. *et al.* (1998) Regionally specific neuronal pathology in untreated patients with schizophrenia: a proton magnetic resonance spectroscopic imaging study. *Biological Psychiatry* **43**, 641–648.

Bertolino, A., Breier, A., Callicott, J.H. *et al.* (2000a) The relationship between dorsolateral prefrontal neuronal N-acetylaspartate and evoked release of striatal dopamine in schizophrenia. *Neuropsychopharmacology* **22**, 125–132.

Bertolino, A., Esposito, G., Callicott, J.H. *et al.* (2000b) Specific relationship between prefrontal neuronal N-acetylaspartate and activation of the working memory cortical network in schizophrenia. *American Journal of Psychiatry* **157**, 26–33.

Breier, A., Buchanan, R.W., Elkashef, A. *et al.* (1992) Brain morphology and schizophrenia: a magnetic resonance imaging study of limbic, prefrontal cortex, and caudate structures. *Archives of General Psychiatry* **49**, 921–926.

Breier, A., Su, T.P., Saunders, R. *et al.* (1997) Schizophrenia is associated with elevated amphetamine-induced synaptic dopamine concentrations: evidence from a novel positron emission tomography method. *Proceedings of the National Academy of Sciences of the USA* **94**, 2569–2574.

Buchsbaum, M.S., Tang, C.Y., Peled, S. *et al.* (1998) MRI white matter diffusion anisotropy and PET metabolic rate in schizophrenia. *Neuroreport* **9**, 425–430.

Callicott, J.H., Egan, M.F., Bertolino, A. *et al.* (1998) Hippocampal N-acetyl aspartate in unaffected siblings of patients with schizophrenia: a possible intermediate neurobiological phenotype. *Biological Psychiatry* **44**, 941–950.

Callicott, J.H., Bertolino, A., Mattay, V.S. *et al.* (2000) Physiological dysfunction of the dorsolateral prefrontal cortex in schizophrenia revisited. *Cerebral Cortex* **10**, 1078–1092.

Cannon, T.D., van Erp, T.G., Huttunen, M. *et al.* (1998) Regional gray matter, white matter, and cerebrospinal fluid distributions in schizophrenic patients, their siblings, and controls. *Archives of General Psychiatry* **55**, 1084–1091.

Carter, C.S., Mintun, M., Nichols, T. & Cohen, J.D. (1997) Anterior cingulate gyrus dysfunction and selective attention deficits in schizophrenia: $[^{15}O]H_2O$ PET study during single-trial Stroop task performance. *American Journal of Psychiatry* **154**, 1670–1675.

Carter, C.S., Perlstein, W., Ganguli, R. *et al.* (1998) Functional hypofrontality and working memory dysfunction in schizophrenia. *American Journal of Psychiatry* **155**, 1285–1287.

Crespo-Facorro, B., Kim, J., Andreasen, N.C., O'Leary, D.S. & Magnotta, V. (2000) Regional frontal abnormalities in schizophrenia: a quantitative gray matter volume and cortical surface size study. *Biological Psychiatry* **48**, 110–119.

Daniel, D.G., Weinberger, D.R., Jones, D.W. *et al.* (1991) The effect of amphetamine on regional cerebral blood flow during cognitive activation in schizophrenia. *Journal of Neuroscience* **11**, 1907–1917.

Deicken, R.F., Zhou, L., Schuff, N. & Weiner, M.W. (1997) Proton magnetic resonance spectroscopy of the anterior cingulate region in schizophrenia. *Schizophrenia Research* **27**, 65–71.

DeLisi, L.E., Tew, W., Xie, S. *et al.* (1995) A prospective follow-up study of brain morphology and cognition in first-episode schizophrenic patients: preliminary findings. *Biological Psychiatry* **38**, 349–360.

DeLisi, L.E., Sakuma, M., Tew, W. *et al.* (1997) Schizophrenia as a chronic active brain process: a study of progressive brain structural change subsequent to the onset of schizophrenia. *Psychiatry Research* **74**, 129–140.

Ebmeier, K.P., Blackwood, D.H.R., Murray, C. *et al.* (1993) Single photon emission tomography with ^{99m}Tc-exametazime in unmedicated schizophrenic patients. *Biological Psychiatry* **33**, 487–495.

Egan, M.F., Goldberg, T.E. & Kolachana, B.S. (2001) Effect of COMT Val108/158 Met genotype on frontal lobe function and risk for schizophrenia. *Proceedings of the National Academy of Sciences of the USA* **98**, 6917–6922.

Elkis, H., Friedman, L., Wise, A. & Meltzer, H.Y. (1995) Meta-analyses of studies of ventricular enlargement and cortical sulcal prominence in mood disorders: comparisons with controls or patients with schizophrenia. *Archives of General Psychiatry* **52**, 735–746.

Erkwoh, R., Sabri, O., Steinmeyer, E.M. *et al.* (1997) Psychopathological and SPET findings in never-treated schizophrenia. *Acta Psychiatrica Scandinavica* **96**, 51–57.

Fletcher, P.C., Frith, C.D., Grasby, P.M. *et al.* (1996) Local and distributed effects of apomorphine on fronto-temporal function in acute unmedicated schizophrenia. *Journal of Neuroscience* **16**, 7055–7062.

Fletcher, P.C., McKenna, P.J., Frith, C.D. *et al.* (1998) Brain activations in schizophrenia during a graded memory task studied with functional neuroimaging. *Archives of General Psychiatry* **55**, 1001–1008.

Fletcher, P., McKenna, P.J., Friston, K.J., Frith, C.D. & Dolan, R.J. (1999) Abnormal cingulate modulation of fronto-temporal connectivity in schizophrenia. *Neuroimage* **9**, 337–342.

Foong, J., Maier, M., Clark, C.A. *et al.* (2000) Neuropathological abnormalities of the corpus callosum in schizophrenia: a diffusion tensor imaging study. *Journal of Neurology, Neurosurgery and Psychiatry* **68**, 242–244.

Foong, J., Symms, M.R., Barker, G.J. *et al.* (2001) Neuropathological abnormalities in schizophrenia: evidence from magnetization transfer imaging. *Brain* **124**, 882–892.

Friston, K.J., Liddle, P.F., Frith, C.D. & Frackowiak, R.S.J. (1993) Functional connectivity: the principal component analysis of large (PET) data sets. *Journal of Cerebral Blood Flow and Metabolism* **13**, 5–14.

Frith, C.D., Friston, K.J., Herold, S. *et al.* (1995) Regional brain activity in chronic schizophrenic patients during the performance of a verbal fluency task. *British Journal of Psychiatry* **167**, 343–349.

Giedd, J.N., Jeffries, N.O., Blumenthal, J. *et al.* (1999) Childhood-onset schizophrenia: progressive brain changes during adolescence. *Biological Psychiatry* **46**, 892–898.

Gilbert, A.R., Rosenberg, D.R., Harenski, K. *et al.* (2001) Thalamic volumes in patients with first-episode schizophrenia. *American Journal of Psychiatry* **158**, 618–224.

Goldstein, J.M., Goodman, J.M., Seidman, L.J. *et al.* (1999) Cortical abnormalities in schizophrenia identified by structural magnetic resonance imaging. *Archives of General Psychiatry* **56**, 537–547.

Gur, R.E., Cowell, P., Turetsky, B.I. *et al.* (1998) A follow-up magnetic resonance imaging study of schizophrenia: relationship of neuroanatomical changes to clinical and neurobehavioral measures. *Archives of General Psychiatry* **55**, 145–152.

Gur, R.E., Turetsky, B.I., Bilker, W.B. & Gur, R.C. (1999) Reduced gray matter volume in schizophrenia. *Archives of General Psychiatry* **56**, 905–911.

Gur, R.E., Cowell, P.E., Latshaw, A. *et al.* (2000a) Reduced dorsal and orbital prefrontal gray matter volumes in schizophrenia. *Archives of General Psychiatry* **57**, 761–768.

Gur, R.E., Turetsky, B.I., Cowell, P.E. *et al.* (2000b) Temporolimbic volume reductions in schizophrenia. *Archives of General Psychiatry* **57**, 769–775.

Heckers, S., Rauch, S.L., Goff, D. *et al.* (1998) Impaired recruitment of the hippocampus during conscious recollection in schizophrenia. *Nature Neuroscience* **1**, 318–323.

Hirayasu, Y., Shenton, M.E., Salisbury, D.F. *et al.* (1998) Lower left temporal lobe MRI volumes in patients with first-episode schizophrenia compared with psychotic patients with first-episode affective disorder and normal subjects. *American Journal of Psychiatry* **155**, 1384–1391.

Hirayasu, Y., Shenton, M.E., Salisbury, D.F. *et al.* (1999) Subgenual cingulate cortex volume in first-episode psychosis. *American Journal of Psychiatry* **156**, 1091–1093.

Holcomb, H.H., Cascella, N.G., Thakur, G.K. *et al.* (1996) Functional sites of neuroleptic action in the human brain: PET/FDG studies

with and without haloperidol. *American Journal of Psychiatry* **153**, 41–49.

Honey, G.D., Bullmore, E.T., Soni, W. *et al.* (1999) Differences in frontal cortical activation by a working memory task after substitution of risperidone for typical antipsychotic drugs in patients with schizophrenia. *Proceedings of the National Academy of Sciences of the USA* **96**, 13432–13437.

Huber, G. (1964) Neuroradiologie und Psychiatrie. In: *Psychiatrie der Gegenwart, Forschung und Praxis*, Vol. 1 *Grundlagenforschung Zur Psychiatrie* Part B. (eds H.W. Gruhle, R. Jung, W. Mayer-Gross & M. Muller), pp. 253–290. Springer-Verlag, Berlin.

Ichimiya, T., Okubo, Y., Suhara, T. & Sudo, Y. (2001) Reduced volume of the cerebellar vermis in neuroleptic-naive schizophrenia. *Biological Psychiatry* **49**, 20–27.

Ingvar, D.H. & Franzen, G. (1974) Anomalies of cerebral blood flow distribution in patients with chronic schizophrenia. *Acta Psychiatrica Scandinavica* **50**, 425–462.

Jennings, J.M., McIntosh, A.R., Kapur, S., Zipursky, R.B. & Houle, S. (1998) Functional network differences in schizophrenia: an rCBF study of semantic processing. *Neuroreport* **9**, 1697–1700.

Johnstone, E.C., Crow, T.J., Frith, C.D., Husband, J. & Kreel, L. (1976) Cerebral ventricular size and cognitive impairment in chronic schizophrenia. *Lancet* **2**, 924–926.

Josin, G.M. & Liddle, P.F. (2001) Neural network analysis of the pattern of functional connectivity between cerebral areas in schizophrenia. *Biological Cybernetics* **884**, 117–122.

Kaplan, R.D., Szechtman, H., Franco, S. *et al.* (1993) Three clinical syndromes of schizophrenia in untreated subjects: relation to brain glucose activity measured by positron emission tomography (PET). *Schizophrenia Research* **11**, 47–54.

Keshavan, M.S., Stanley, J.A. & Pettegrew, J.W. (2000) Magnetic resonance spectroscopy in schizophrenia: methodological issues and findings. II. *Biological Psychiatry* **48**, 369–380.

Kiehl, K.A. & Liddle, P.F. (2001) An event-related functional magnetic resonance imaging study of an auditory oddball task in schizophrenia. *Schizophrenia Research* **48**, 159–171.

Kikinis, R., Shenton, M.E., Gerig, G. *et al.* (1994) Temporal lobe sulco-gyral pattern anomalies in schizophrenia: an *in vivo* MR three-dimensional surface rendering study. *Neuroscience Letters* **182**, 7–12.

Kircher, T.J., Liddle, P.F., Brammer, M.J. *et al.* (2001) Patterns of brain activation and formal thought disorder in schizophrenia. *Archives of General Psychiatry* **58**, 769–774.

Konick, L.C. & Friedman, L. (2001) Meta-analysis of thalamic size in schizophrenia. *Biological Psychiatry* **49**, 28–38.

Kwon, J.S., McCarley, R.W., Hirayasu, Y. *et al.* (1999) Left planum temporale volume reduction in schizophrenia. *Archives of General Psychiatry* **56**, 142–148.

Laruelle, M., Abi-Dargham, A., van Dyck, C.H. *et al.* (1996) Single photon emission computerized tomography imaging of amphetamine-induced dopamine release in drug-free schizophrenic subjects. *Proceedings of the National Academy of Sciences of the USA* **93**, 9235–9240.

Lawrie, S.M., Whalley, H., Kestelman, J.N. *et al.* (1999) Magnetic resonance imaging of brain in people at high risk of developing schizophrenia. *Lancet* **353**, 30–33.

Lawrie, S.M., Whalley, H.C., Abukmeil, S.S. *et al.* (2001) Brain structure, genetic liability, and psychotic symptoms in subjects at high risk of developing schizophrenia. *Biological Psychiatry* **49**, 811–823.

Liddle, P.F. (2000) Functional brain imaging of schizophrenia. In: *The Psychopharmacology of Schizophrenia* (eds M. Reveley & W. Deakin), pp. 109–130. Arnold, London.

Liddle, P.F., Friston, K.J., Frith, C.D. *et al.* (1992) Patterns of cerebral blood flow in schizophrenia. *British Journal of Psychiatry* **160**, 179–186.

Liddle, P.F., Lane, C.M.J. & Ngan, E.T.C. (2000) Immediate effects of risperidone on cortico-striato-thalamic loops and the hippocampus. *British Journal of Psychiatry* **177**, 402–407.

Lieberman, J., Chakos, M., Wu, H. *et al.* (2001) Longitudinal study of brain morphology in first episode schizophrenia. *Biological Psychiatry* **49**, 487–499.

Lim, K.O., Hedehus, M., Moseley, M. *et al.* (1999) Compromised white matter tract integrity in schizophrenia inferred from diffusion tensor imaging. *Archives of General Psychiatry* **56**, 367–374.

MacDonald, A.W. III, Cohen, J.D., Stenger, V.A. & Carter, C.S. (2000) Dissociating the role of the dorsolateral prefrontal and anterior cingulate cortex in cognitive control. *Science* **288**, 1835–1838.

McGuire, P.K., Silbersweig, D.A., Wright, I. *et al.* (1995) Abnormal monitoring of inner speech: a physiological basis for auditory hallucinations. *Lancet* **346**, 596–600.

McGuire, P.K., Quested, D., Spence, S. *et al.* (1998) Pathophysiology of 'positive' thought disorder in schizophrenia. *British Journal of Psychiatry* **173**, 231–235.

McNeil, T.F., Cantor-Graae, E. & Weinberger, D.R. (2000) Relationship of obstetric complications and differences in size of brain structures in monozygotic twin pairs discordant for schizophrenia. *American Journal of Psychiatry* **157**, 203–212.

Madsen, A.L., Karle, A., Rubin, P. *et al.* (1999) Progressive atrophy of the frontal lobes in first-episode schizophrenia: interaction with clinical course and neuroleptic treatment. *Acta Psychiatrica Scandinavica* **100**, 367–374.

Manoach, D.S., Gollub, R.L., Benson, E.S.*et al.* (2000) Schizophrenic subjects show aberrant fMRI activation of dorsolateral prefrontal cortex and basal ganglia during working memory performance. *Biological Psychiatry* **48**, 99–109.

Mathalon, D.H., Sullivan, E.V., Lim, K.O. & Pfefferbaum, A. (2001) Progressive brain volume changes and the clinical course of schizophrenia in men: a longitudinal magnetic resonance imaging study. *Archives of General Psychiatry* **58**, 148–157.

Matsumoto, H., Simmons, A., Williams, S. *et al.* (2001) Structural magnetic imaging of the hippocampus in early onset schizophrenia. *Biological Psychiatry* **49**, 824–831.

Mendrek, A. (2001) *An fMRI study of state and trait abnormalities in schizophrenia*. PhD thesis, University of British Columbia.

Meyer-Lindenberg, A., Poline, J.B., Kohn, P.D. *et al.* (2001) Evidence for abnormal cortical functional connectivity during working memory in schizophrenia. *American Journal of Psychiatry* **158**, 1809–1817.

Nelson, M.D., Saykin, A.J., Flashman, L.A. & Riordan, H.J. (1998) Hippocampal volume reduction in schizophrenia as assessed by magnetic resonance imaging: a meta-analytic study. *Archives of General Psychiatry* **55**, 433–440.

Ngan, T.C., Lane, C.M.J., Ruth, T.J. *et al.* (2002) Immediate and delayed effects of risperidone on cerebral metabolism: correlations with symptom change. *Journal of Neurosurgery, Neurology and Psychiatry* **72**, 106–110.

Niznikiewicz, M., Donnino, R., McCarley, R.W. *et al.* (2000) Abnormal angular gyrus asymmetry in schizophrenia. *American Journal of Psychiatry* **157**, 428–437.

Paillere-Martinot, M., Caclin, A. *et al.* (2001) Cerebral gray and white matter reductions and clinical correlates in patients with early onset schizophrenia. *Schizophrenia Research* **50**, 19–26.

Pakkenberg, B. (1993) Total nerve cell numbers in neocortex in chronic schizophrenics and controls using optical dissectors. *Biological Psychiatry* **34**, 786–772.

Pantelis, C., Velaloukis, D. McGorry, P.D. *et al.* (2002) Neuroanatomical abnormalities in people who develop psychosis. *Lancet* (in press).

Perlstein, W.M., Carter, C.S., Noll, D.C. & Cohen, J.D. (2001) Relation of prefrontal cortex dysfunction to working memory and symptoms in schizophrenia. *Amercian Journal of Psychiatry* **158**, 1105–1113.

Petty, R.G., Barta, P.E., Pearlson, G.D. *et al.* (1995) Reversal of asymmetry of the planum temporale in schizophrenia. *American Journal of Psychiatry* **152**, 715–721.

Phillips, M.L., Williams, L., Senior, C. *et al.* (1999) A differential neural response to threatening and non-threatening negative facial expressions in paranoid and non-paranoid schizophrenics. *Psychiatry Research* **92**, 11–31.

Rapoport, J.L., Giedd, J.N., Blumenthal, J. *et al.* (1999) Progressive cortical change during adolescence in childhood-onset schizophrenia: a longitudinal magnetic resonance imaging study. *Archives of General Psychiatry* **56**, 649–654.

Raz, S. & Raz, N. (1990) Structural brain abnormalities in the major psychoses: a quantitative review of the evidence from computerized imaging. *Psychological Bulletin* **108**, 93–108.

Ross, C.A. & Pearlson, G.D. (1996) Schizophrenia, the heteromodal association neocortex and development: potential for a neurogenetic approach. *Trends in Neuroscience* **19**, 171–176.

Schlaepfer, T.E., Harris, G.J., Tien, A.Y. *et al.* (1994) Decreased regional cortical gray matter volume in schizophrenia. *American Journal of Psychiatry* **151**, 842–848.

Schneider, F., Weiss, U., Kessler, C. *et al.* (1998) Differential amygdala activation in schizophrenia during sadness. *Schizophrenia Research* **34**, 133–142.

Seidman, L.J., Faraone, S.V., Goldstein, J.M. *et al.* (1999) Thalamic and amygdala–hippocampal volume reductions in first-degree relatives of patients with schizophrenia: an MRI-based morphometric analysis. *Biological Psychiatry* **46**, 941–954.

Shapleske, J., Rossell, S.L., Woodruff, P.W. & David, A.S. (1999) The planum temporale: a systematic, quantitative review of its structural, functional and clinical significance. *Brain Research Reviews* **29**, 26–49.

Sharma, T., Lancaster, E., Lee, D. *et al.* (1998) Brain changes in schizophrenia: volumetric MRI study of families multiply affected with schizophrenia – the Maudsley Family Study 5. *British Journal of Psychiatry* **173**, 132–138.

Shenton, M.E., Dickey, C.C., Frumin, M. & McCarley, R.W. (2001) A review of MRI findings in schizophrenia. *Schizophrenia Research* **49**, 1–52.

Sheppard, G., Gruzelier, J., Manchanda, R. *et al.* (1983) ^{15}O positron emission tomographic scanning of predominantly never-treated acute schizophrenic patients. *Lancet* **ii**, 1448–1452.

Shergill, S.S., Brammer, M.J., Williams, S.C., Murray, R.M. & McGuire, P.K. (2000) Mapping auditory hallucinations in schizophrenia using functional magnetic resonance imaging. *Archives of General Psychiatry* **57**, 1033–1038.

Sigmundsson, T., Suckling, J., Maier, M. *et al.* (2001) Structural abnormalities in frontal, temporal, and limbic regions and interconnecting white matter tracts in schizophrenic patients with prominent negative symptoms. *American Journal of Psychiatry* **158**, 234–243.

Silbersweig, D.A., Stern, E., Frith, C. *et al.* (1995) A functional neuroanatomy of hallucinations in schizophrenia. *Nature* **378**, 176–179.

Sowell, E.R., Levitt, J., Thompson, P.M. *et al.* (2000) Brain abnormalities in early-onset schizophrenia spectrum disorder observed with statistical parametric mapping of structural magnetic resonance images. *American Journal of Psychiatry* **157**, 1475–1484.

Spence, S.A., Brooks, D.J., Hirsch, S.R. *et al.* (1997) A PET study of voluntary movement in schizophrenic patients experiencing passivity phenomena (delusions of alien control). *Brain* **120**, 1997–2011.

Spence, S.A., Liddle, P.F., Stefan, M.D. *et al.* (2000) Functional anatomy of verbal fluency in people with schizophrenia and those at genetic risk. *British Journal of Psychiatry* **176**, 52–60.

Staal, W.G., Hulshoff Pol, H.E. & Kahn, R.S. (1999) Outcome of schizophrenia in relation to brain abnormalities. *Schizophrenia Bulletin* **25**, 337–348.

Staal, W.G., Hulshoff Pol, H.E., Schnack, H.G. et al. (2000) Structural brain abnormalities in patients with schizophrenia and their healthy siblings. *American Journal of Psychiatry* **157**, 416–421.

Stefanis, N., Frangou, S., Yakeley, J. et al. (1999) Hippocampal volume reduction in schizophrenia: effects of genetic risk and pregnancy and birth complications. *Biological Psychiatry* **46**, 697–702.

Suddath, R.L., Christison, G.W., Torrey, E.F., Casanova, M.F. & Weinberger, D.R. (1990) Anatomical abnormalities in the brains of monozygotic twins discordant for schizophrenia. *New England Journal of Medicine* **322**, 789–794.

Szeszko, P.R., Bilder, R.M., Lencz, T. et al. (1999) Investigation of frontal lobe subregions in first-episode schizophrenia. *Psychiatric Research and Neuroimaging* **90**, 1–15.

Vance, A.L., Velakoulis, D., Maruff, P. et al. (2000) Magnetic resonance spectroscopy and schizophrenia: what have we learnt? *Australian and New Zealand Journal of Psychiatry* **34**, 14–25.

Velakoulis, D., Pantelis, C., McGorry, P.D. et al. (1999) Hippocampal volume in first-episode psychoses and chronic schizophrenia: a high-resolution magnetic resonance imaging study. *Archives of General Psychiatry* **56**, 133–141.

Velakoulis, D., Maruff, P., Suckling, J. et al. (2000a) Reduced volume of inferior parietal lobe in chronic schizophrenia patients with delusions. *Schizophrenia Research* **41**, 118.

Velakoulis, D., Wood, S.J., McGorry, P.D. & Pantelis, C. (2000b) Evidence for progression of brain structural abnormalities in schizophrenia: beyond the neurodevelopmental model. *Australian and New Zealand Journal of Psychiatry* **34**, S113–S126.

Velakoulis, D., Wood, S.J., Smith, D.J. et al. (2002) Increased duration of illness is associated with reduced volume in right medial temporal/anterior cingulate grey matter in patients with chronic schizophrenia. *Schizophrenia Research* **57**, 43–49.

Vogeley, K., Tepest, R., Pfeiffer, U. et al. (2001) Right frontal hypergyria differentiation in affected and unaffected siblings from families multiply affected with schizophrenia: a morphometric MRI study. *American Journal of Psychiatry* **158**, 494–496.

Ward, K.E., Friedman, L., Wise, A. & Schulz, S.C. (1996) Meta-analysis of brain and cranial size in schizophrenia. *Schizophrenia Research* **22**, 197–213.

Weinberger, D.R. & Berman, K.F. (1996) Prefrontal function in schizophrenia: confounds and controversies. *Philosophical Transactions of the Royal Society of London B, Biological Science* **351**, 1495–1503.

Weinberger, D.R., Berman, K.F. & Zec, R.F. (1986) Physiologic dysfunction of dorsolateral prefrontal cortex in schizophrenia. I. Regional cerebral blood flow evidence. *Archives of General Psychiatry* **43**, 114–124.

Weinberger, D.R., Berman, K.F. & Illowsky, B.P. (1988) Physiologic dysfunction of dorsolateral prefrontal cortex in schizophrenia. III. A new cohort and evidence for a monoaminergic mechanism. *Archives of General Psychiatry* **45**, 609–615.

Weinberger, D.R., Berman, K.F., Suddath, R. et al. (1992) Evidence of dysfunction of a prefrontal–limbic network in schizophrenia: a magnetic resonance imaging and regional cerebral blood flow study of discordant monozygotic twins. *American Journal of Psychiatry* **149**, 890–897.

Williamson, P., Pelz, D., Merskey, H. et al. (1992) Frontal, temporal, and striatal proton relaxation times in schizophrenic patients and normal comparison subjects. *American Journal of Psychiatry* **149**, 549–551.

Wood, S.J., Velakoulis, D., Smith, D.J. et al. (2001) A longitudinal study of hippocampal volume in first episode psychosis and chronic schizophrenia. *Schizophrenia Research* **52**, 37–46.

Woodruff, P.W.R., Wright, I.C., Shurique, N. et al. (1997) Structural brain abnormalities in male schizophrenics reflect frontotemporal dissociation. *Psychological Medicine* **27**, 1257–1263.

Woods, B.T. (1998) Is schizophrenia a progressive neurodevelopmental disorder? Toward a unitary pathogenetic mechanism. *American Journal of Psychiatry* **155**, 1661–1670.

Woods, B.T., Yurgelun-Todd, D., Goldstein, J.M., Seidman, L.J. & Tsuang, M.T. (1996) MRI brain abnormalities in chronic schizophrenia: one process or more? *Biological Psychiatry* **40**, 585–596.

Wright, I.C., Rabe-Hesketh, S., Woodruff, P.W.R. et al. (2000) Meta-analysis of regional brain volumes in schizophrenia. *American Journal of Psychiatry* **157**, 16–25.

Yuasa, S., Kurachi, M., Suzuki, M. et al. (1995) Clinical symptoms and regional cerebral blood flow in schizophrenia. *European Archives of Psychiatry and Clinical Neuroscience* **246**, 7–12.

Yücel, M., Pantelis, C., Stuart, G.W. et al. (2002a) Anterior cingulate activation during Stroop task performance: a PET to MRI coregistration study of individual patients with schizophrenia. *American Journal of Psychiatry* **159**, 251–254.

Yücel, M., Stuart, G.W., Maruff, P. et al. (2002b) Paracingulate morphologic differences in males with established schizophrenia: a maynetic resonance imaging morplometic study. *Biological Psychiatry* **52**, 15–23.

Zipursky, R.B., Lambe, E.K., Kapur, S. & Mikulis, D.J. (1998) Cerebral gray matter volume deficits in first episode psychosis. *Archives of General Psychiatry* **55**, 540–546.

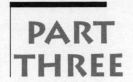

PART THREE

Physical Treatments

23

The neuroscience and clinical psychopharmacology of first- and second-generation antipsychotic drugs

J.L. Waddington, S. Kapur and G.J. Remington

Origins of contemporary concepts, 421
Evolution of the D_2-dopamine receptor blockade
 hypothesis, 422
 Dopamine receptor antagonism, 422
 Initial concepts of dopamine receptor typology,
 422
 Current concepts of dopamine receptor typology,
 422
Contemporary variants of the D_2-receptor blockade
 hypothesis, 423
 Current status of selective D_3 antagonists, 423
 Current status of selective D_4 antagonists, 423
 Current status of selective D_1-like antagonists, 423
 From indirect to direct examination of the
 D_2-receptor blockade hypothesis, 424
Reappraisal of the D_2-dopamine receptor blockade
 hypothesis by PET and SPECT, 424
 Concepts of striatal D_2 occupancy threshold, 424
 Striatal D_2 occupancy in relation to 5-HT_2 and
 extrastriatal D_2 occupancy, 424
Impact of clozapine as the prototype second-
 generation antipsychotic, 425
 Evolving concepts of the antipsychotic action of
 clozapine, 425
 Clozapine and dopamine receptor subtypes, 425

Clozapine and non-dopaminergic receptors, 426
New cellular and behavioural models of
 antipsychotic drug action and schizophrenia,
 426
Reappraisal of clozapine by PET and SPECT, 427
 Striatal D_2 vs. 5-HT_2 occupancy, 427
 Variant D_2 occupancy threshold models, 427
 Synthesis, 427
The 'atypicality' controversy, 428
 Clinical issues, 428
 Mechanistic issues, 428
Second-generation antipsychotic drugs subsequent to
 clozapine, 428
 Amisulpride, 428
 Olanzapine, 429
 Quetiapine, 430
 Risperidone, 430
 Sertindole, 431
 Ziprasidone, 432
 Zotepine, 432
Emergent agents and pharmacogenomics, 433
New directions: mechanisms and third-generation
 antipsychotics?, 433
Acknowledgements, 434
References, 434

Origins of contemporary concepts

Although the discovery and introduction of neuroleptic drugs in the 1950s has been of profound significance (for a uniquely personal memoire of these early events see Deniker 1983), we are entering the sixth decade of an incremental search for the basis of their antipsychotic activity. However, over the past several years we have witnessed a greater rate of advance than occurred over preceding decades, as a result of two complementary developments: the emergence of deeper insights into brain function fostered by new investigatory tools, including neuroimaging techniques for the direct exploration of drug action in living subjects, and the introduction of a still evolving tranche of new antipsychotic agents whose actions can be better probed using such technology and interpreted in the light of these insights. Yet these remain challenging times. What is the contemporary role of conventional (first-generation) antipsychotics and what can we learn from their neuronal effects? How are we to synthesize

the preclinical and clinical profiles of these new (second-generation) agents and assimilate them into clinical practice to best patient advantage (Kane 1999; Waddington & Quinn 2000)?

Enthusiasm engendered by recent developments must be tempered by recognition that the concept that still underpins much contemporary theorizing, namely the dopamine (DA) receptor blockade hypothesis, is now some 40 years old. It remains a chastening fact that *all* known antipsychotic drugs evidencing clinical efficacy in appropriately controlled clinical trials exert, *inter alia*, at least some competitive antagonism of brain DA receptors. However, only recently has this notion been given material pathophysiological relevance by neuroimaging findings that indicate increased subcortical release of DA in schizophrenia, at least during phases of exacerbation of psychosis (Laruelle & Abi-Dargham 1999; Abi-Dargham *et al.* 2000). Equally, in relation to new antipsychotics, the term 'atypical' enjoys considerably greater currency than the descriptor 'second-generation' favoured here; yet the theoretical, biological and clinical underpinings of 'atypicality' are poorly defined and engender considerable controversy (Kane 1999; Remington & Kapur 2000; Waddington & Casey 2000). This chapter seeks to document these advances and controversies. It focuses on challenges presented by the second-generation agents, as typified by clozapine and elaborated subsequently by amisulpride, olanzapine, quetiapine, risperidone, sertindole, ziprasidone and zotepine; yet it is mindful of what we have learned and have still to learn from their first-generation counterparts.

Evolution of the D_2-dopamine receptor blockade hypothesis

Dopamine receptor antagonism

The common action of first- (and second-) generation antipsychotic drugs to block brain DA receptors was posited initially from neurochemical observations (Carlsson & Lindqvist 1963), which were subsequently elaborated by a wealth of behavioural findings (Niemegeers & Janssen 1978). The relationship of these properties to therapeutic efficacy in schizophrenia received strong but indirect support from data indicating the *in vitro* affinities of a wide range of antipsychotic drugs for brain DA antagonist binding sites to correlate highly with their clinical potencies to control psychotic symptoms (Seeman 1980). However, one particularly important study for giving clinical embodiment to these laboratory findings was the critical demonstration that the antipsychotic activity of flupentixol resided in its α (i.e. *cis* (Z) and DA receptor blocking) rather than its β (i.e. *trans* (E) and non-DA receptor-blocking) geometric isomer (Johnstone *et al.* 1978).

Initial concepts of dopamine receptor typology

In conceptual terms, these now classical (although at the time heuristic and radical) notions remain, but have required material modification in their detail as our knowledge base in the neurosciences has expanded. In particular, our concepts of DA receptor typology and function have undergone substantial revision. Specifically, it was recognized subsequently that DA receptors existed as two major subtypes: D_1 and D_2 (Kebabian & Calne 1979). Re-evaluation of the above relationship in terms of this D_1/D_2 schema indicated the clinical potencies of antipsychotics to be correlated highly with their affinities for the D_2 but not for the D_1 receptor. Furthermore, this relationship held not just for rat striatal but also for postmortem human putaminal tissue and, importantly, no differences were apparent between the affinities of such drugs for D_2 receptors in caudate or putamen (the mesostriatal DAergic system, presumed to mediate extrapyramidal side-effects) vs. nucleus accumbens (the mesocorticolimbic system, presumed to mediate antipsychotic efficacy) of human postmortem brain (Seeman 1980; Reynolds *et al.* 1982; Seeman & Ulpian 1983; Richelson & Nelson 1984; Waddington 1993; Lidsky 1995). Similarly, selective or prefer-

ential D_2 antagonists, such as the substituted benzamide sulpiride or the butyrophenone haloperidol, respectively, appeared to reproduce the essential clinical activity of non-selective antipsychotics such as the phenothiazines (e.g. fluphenazine) and thioxanthenes (e.g. flupentixol) which block both D_1 and D_2 receptors (Ehman *et al.* 1987). On this basis, D_2-receptor blockade was ascribed a prepotent or even exclusive role in mediating antipsychotic activity (Seeman 1980).

Current concepts of dopamine receptor typology

Over the past decade, molecular biological/gene cloning techniques have indicated the number of DA receptor subtypes to be yet larger than envisaged originally. Until very recently, theory has encompassed six DA receptor protein sequences which, on the basis of structural and pharmacological characteristics, are best subsumed under the umbrella of two *families* of D_1-like (D_1 and D_5 according to primate-based nomenclature) and D_2-like ($D_{2long/short}$, D_3 and D_4) receptors (Waddington 1993; Missale *et al.* 1998). Within the D_1-like family, the D_1 receptor evidences a general mesostriatal–corticolimbic localization, while its D_5 counterpart evidences primarily a characteristic low-density localization within particular corticolimbic regions (Waddington *et al.* 1998, 2001; Niznik *et al.* 2002). Conversely, within the D_2-like family, the D_2 receptor, having a general mesostriatal–limbic localization, exists in both 'long' and 'short' isoforms generated by alternate splicing and whose functional distinctions are only now being clarified; the D_3 and D_4 receptor evidence low-density localizations within distinct corticolimbic regions (Levant 1997; Tarazi & Baldessarini 1999; Waddington *et al.* 2001).

On this basis, previous studies of the correlation between clinical antipsychotic potencies and affinities for the 'D_2' receptor actually reflected generic affinities for all members of the D_2-like family, because of the inability of the ligands utilized to distinguish between them. However, subsequent studies using cloned cell lines have indicated both clinical antipsychotic potencies and the free concentrations of antipsychotics in patient plasma to correlate generally with their affinities for the D_2 receptor when expressed independently of its D_3 and D_4 siblings (Seeman 1992; Waddington 1993). It has been argued recently that this prepotent binding to D_2 receptors also varies along a dimension additional to conventional affinity, namely 'tightness' relative to that of DA; thus, those antipsychotics binding more tightly may be more likely, while those binding less tightly may be less likely, to induce extrapyramidal side-effects despite similar extents of occupancy of those D_2 receptors (Seeman & Tallerico 1998).

Very recently, a variant D_2-like receptor, $D_{2longer}$, with a unique TG splice site has been identified in some (but not all) postmortem brains from both control subjects and patients with schizophrenia (Liu *et al.* 2000; Seeman *et al.* 2000). However, given its variable prevalence in human brain, occurrence at about 2–3% of the total population of D_2 transcripts therein, unknown regional distribution, no known functional characteristics other than high affinity for antipsychotics and linkage to inhibition of adenylyl cyclase, and no known selective agonists or antagonists for more incisive studies, any relevance for antipsychotic drug action remains to be clarified.

Contemporary variants of the D_2-receptor blockade hypothesis

Current status of selective D_3 antagonists

Its high affinity for most antipsychotics and predominantly 'peri-striatal' limbic localization have generated much interest in the D_3 receptor as a potentially novel therapeutic target for antipsychotic activity (Sokoloff *et al.* 1992). However, no known antipsychotic drug shows more than a modest preference for D_3 over D_2 receptors, and clinical antipsychotic potencies appear to correlate less strongly with affinities for the D_3 than for the D_2 receptor (Seeman 1992; Waddington 1993). Additionally, it has proved difficult to identify specific functional roles for the D_3 receptor in the absence of antagonists showing material selectivity over its D_2 and D_4 counterparts (Levant 1997). Indeed, using mice with targeted gene deletion ('knockout') of the D_3 receptor as an alternative approach, those functions putatively ascribed to the D_3 receptor have been shown to be conserved in D_3 'knockouts' and, rather, to be absent in their D_2 'knockout' counterparts (Boulay *et al.* 1999a,b; Xu *et al.* 1999; Waddington *et al.* 2001; McNamara *et al.* 2002). Furthermore, the most recent preclinical studies with new selective D_3 antagonists (e.g. S33084: Millan *et al.* 2000) do not indicate them to be active in at least traditional models of antipsychotic activity in ther manner of (selective or non-selective) D_2 antagonists. On this basis, the role of D_3 antagonism in antipsychotic activity remains uncertain, and only controlled clinical trials with selective D_3 antagonists will ultimately clarify this long-standing conundrum.

Current status of selective D_4 antagonists

Similarly, the D_4 receptor has also been offered as a potential novel therapeutic target on the basis of its high affinity for many antipsychotics and its predominantly corticolimbic localization (Van Tol *et al.* 1991; Tarazi & Baldessarini 1999). However, no known antipsychotics evidence more than a modest preference for D_4 over D_2 receptors, and clinical antipsychotic potencies appear to correlate less strongly with affinities for the D_4 than for the D_2 receptor (Seeman 1992; Waddington 1993). Additionally, the recent availability of a wide range of selective D_4 agonists and, particularly, of D_4 antagonists for preclinical studies has not indicated potential in at least traditional models of antipsychotic activity; indeed, it has proved difficult to identify any consistent psychopharmacological signature for such agents (Tarazi & Baldessarini 1999; Clifford & Waddington 2000; Waddington *et al.* 2001).

Nevertheless, on the basis of the above profile and controversial evidence suggesting *inter alia* abnormalities of the D_4 receptor in schizophrenia (Tarazi & Baldessarini 1999), clinical trials

with selective D_4 antagonists have proceeded. In the first such study (Kramer *et al.* 1997), the D_4 antagonist L 745 870 was found to be without either antipsychotic activity or extrapyramidal side-effects in schizophrenia; indeed, it was associated with some worsening of psychotic symptoms relative to placebo. However, subsequent studies have indicated L 745 870 to evidence partial agonist activity at the D_4 receptor (Gazi *et al.* 1999); hence its capacity to reveal any antipsychotic activity of D_4 antagonists may be compromised. In a subsequent study (Truffinet *et al.* 1999), the mixed D_4–$5\text{-}HT_{2A}$ antagonist fananserin was also found to be without antipsychotic activity; although it was not associated with exacerbation of psychosis, there appeared to be some worsening of akathisia.

Despite these cautionary initial observations, some other selective D_4 antagonists (Tarazi & Baldessarini 1999; Clifford & Waddington 2000; Hrib 2000) continue to attract clinical attention, while others have not proved candidates for clinical development as a result of pharmacokinetic or toxicological issues. Recent studies in non-human primates indicate the selective D_4 antagonists NGD94-1 to reverse cognitive deficits following repeated exposure to the N-methyl-D-aspartate (NMDA) receptor-mediated psychotomimetic phencyclidine (PCP) while increasing levels of the DA metabolite homovanillic acid in cerebrospinal fluid (Jentsch *et al.* 1999), and PNU-101387 to prevent stress-induced cognitive deficits (Arnsten *et al.* 2000). Such findings raise the possibilty of therapeutic effects at the level of cognitive impairment which contributes materially to functional impairment in schizophrenia (Green *et al.* 2000).

Current status of selective D_1-like antagonists

Given the above weight of evidence indicating a primary role for D_2 receptor antagonism in antipsychotic drug action, it engendered some initial surprise that studies with selective D_1-like antagonists indicated them to be active in essentially all traditional functional models held to predict antipsychotic activity (Waddington 1993); however, this unexpected profile might have a basis in D_1-like–D_2-like interactions which have a critical role in regulating the totality of DAergic neurotransmission (Waddington *et al.* 1994). Although subsequent clinical trials have indicated each of the selective D_1-like antagonists SCH 39166 (de Beaurepaire *et al.* 1995; Den Boer *et al.* 1995; Karlsson *et al.* 1995) and NNC 01-0687 (Karle *et al.* 1995) to be without antipsychotic activity, these limited trials have been conducted generally in small numbers of patients with varying degrees of experimental rigour. Unexpectedly, two of these (Den Boer *et al.* 1995; Karle *et al.* 1995) have suggested some activity to ameliorate negative symptoms. Also, no known agent is able to distinguish meaningfully between D_1 and D_5 receptors (Sugamori *et al.* 1998).

This area has subsequently experienced some considerable neglect, but recently renewed interest in the antipsychotic potential of NNC 01-0687 may provide additional information. Furthermore, it should be noted that cortical D_1-like receptor-mediated processes play an important part in regulating aspects of cognitive function that are known to be impaired in schizophrenia, and antipsychotics downregulate D_1 and D_5 receptors in the prefrontal cortex of non-human primates, perhaps via cortical D_2 antagonism (Lidow *et al.* 1998). Thus, as for D_4 receptors, such findings raise the possibilty of D_1-like receptor-mediated therapeutic effects at the level of cognitive impairment.

From indirect to direct examination of the D_2-receptor blockade hypothesis

In the course of their evolution, the above notions of receptor action have proved heuristic over some two decades. However, it must be emphasized that, in the main, they derive from indirect lines of investigation. One of the major advances of the past decade has been the emergence of functional neuroimaging techniques for the direct visualization and quantification of drug–receptor interactions in living patients: positron emission tomography (PET) and single photon emission computed tomography (SPECT). These techniques cannot yet directly address all of the issues raised by indirect approaches, but they are a powerful new approach to determining both their validity and, critically, their specific relationship to clinical phenomena on an individual patient as well as a population basis.

Reappraisal of the D_2-dopamine receptor blockade hypothesis by PET and SPECT

Concepts of striatal D_2 occupancy threshold

With techniques such as PET and SPECT now available, there has arisen the opportunity to provide *in vivo* evidence to better delineate parameters of D_2 (actually, D_2-like) receptor occupancy in relation to both clinical efficacy and D_2-related side-effects. In addition, they have been used to examine the *in vivo* relationship between D_2 and 5-HT$_2$ (actually, 5-HT$_{2A/C}$) blockade for second-generation antipsychotics, a fundamental premise in the proposed advantageous profiles of these compounds.

Critical to our understanding regarding the relationship between D_2 occupancy and antipsychotic efficacy has been the proposal that there is a 'threshold', in the range of 65–70% (Farde *et al.* 1992; Nordstrom *et al.* 1993; Kapur *et al.* 2000a). This is not absolute; individuals can respond below this threshold and, conversely, lack of response can be seen in individuals with D_2 blockade exceeding this threshold (Wolkin *et al.* 1989; Coppens *et al.* 1991; Kapur *et al.* 2000a). However, administering an antipsychotic dose that exceeds this threshold appears to optimize the chance of clinical response. This has been clearly demonstrated in a recent study in which low-dose haloperidol (1 or 2.5 mg/day) was administered to 22 patients with first episode schizophrenia (Kapur *et al.* 2000a). A threshold of 65% occupancy optimally separated responders and non-responders: 80% of responders were above this threshold, whereas 67% of non-responders were below it. Of the 11 non-responders, all could tolerate a dose increase to 5 mg/day. Six of seven individuals with previous D_2 occupancies below 65% demonstrated clinical improvement, in contrast to only one of four individuals who had previous D_2 occupancies above 65%. This finding is thus in keeping with other reports indicating that, although response may be optimized by exceeding a threshold of 65–70%, non-response exists in the face of adequate D_2 blockade.

Added to this information have been data indicating that exceeding a threshold of 80% D_2 occupancy markedly increases the risk of eptrapyamidal side-effects (EPSs) (Farde *et al.* 1992; Nordstrom *et al.* 1993; Kapur *et al.* 2000a). This also indicates that there is a relatively narrow therapeutic window, as defined by D_2 occupancy. The optimal chance of clinical response occurs with D_2 blockade above 65%, but EPS risk is greatest with 80% or greater occupancy (Kapur *et al.* 2000a). How does this translate into actual clinical doses? Using haloperidol as the reference, 2 mg/day has been reported to result in a mean D_2 occupancy of 67% (Kapur *et al.* 1996); therefore, it represents the minimal dose that would be associated with the best chance of clinical efficacy. Haloperidol in the range of 5 mg results in D_2 occupancy in the range of 80% (Nyberg *et al.* 1996), and one would expect a substantial increase in risk for EPSs with doses at or above this level. Saturation of D_2 receptors is approached at 10–20 mg haloperidol (Coppens *et al.* 1991). These data dovetail with clinical evidence, including several large reviews and meta-analyses, indicating that optimal dosage is in the range of 2–12 mg haloperidol equivalents daily (Baldessarini *et al.* 1988; Bollini *et al.* 1994).

It is necessary to acknowledge that optimal dosage may vary as a function of both phase (acute vs. stabilized) and stage (first or early episode vs. chronic) of illness. It has been suggested, for example, that first-episode patients may require lower doses of antipsychotic medication, and clinical studies suggest that patients who have been previously treated may need higher doses than first episode patients (McEvoy *et al.* 1991; Remington *et al.* 1998). More recent PET data offer indirect support for this, with a 34% increase in D_2 receptors after long-term antipsychotic exposure having been reported (Silvestri *et al.* 1999). Theoretically, upregulation in D_2 receptors could require increments in dose to obtain the same effect on DAergic transmission (Kapur 2000). This being said, such a finding is unlikely to account for or justify the megadoses that have been documented in relation to antipsychotic use, and does not feature in the receptor changes seen as a function of age that likely contribute to the lower doses required in geriatric populations (Fitzgerald & Seeman 1999).

Striatal D_2 occupancy in relation to 5-HT$_2$ and extrastriatal D_2 occupancy

A pharmacological feature that characterizes all second-generation antipsychotics reviewed here, with the exception of amisulpride, is greater 5-HT$_2$ vs. D_2 blockade, and this has been postulated to account for the diminished risk of EPSs with these agents. This line of thinking is based on evidence that 5-HT can modulate DAergic function at the level of the nigrostriatal pathway, as well as reports indicating that administration of selective $5-HT_2$ antagonists can diminish antipsychotic-induced EPSs (Kapur & Remington 1996). The net result is a wider therapeutic window between those doses that maximize chance of clinical response and those that induce EPSs. While this may be the case, it is not without limitations, as will be considered further in relation to specific second-generation agents; it should be noted that 600 mg chlorpromazine is associated with almost complete occupancy of both D_2 and $5-HT_2$ receptors (Trichard *et al.* 1998).

A second adverse event that has been linked to D_2 blockade, and one that certainly characterizes all first-generation antipsychotics, is hyperprolactinaemia. As with other D_2-related processes, neuroimaging has been able to illuminate the nature of this relationship. For example, D_2 occupancy significantly predicted risk for elevated prolactin: the likelihood was 15% with D_2 occupancy below 72% but that likelihood rose to 86% with higher D_2 occupancies (Kapur *et al.* 2000a). A second report, in this case using raclopride, reported a lower threshold for hyperprolactinaemia of 50% (Nordstrom & Farde 1998). This difference may be accounted for, at least in part, by pharmacodynamic differences between blood–brain barrier permeability; in addition, a number of factors are known to influence prolactin levels (Molitch 1995). Both reports suggest that a threshold for hyperprolactinaemia exists but, as with other D_2 thresholds discussed, this is not an all-or-none phenomenon.

Finally, some comment is warranted regarding reported D_2 occupancy values. Various factors may influence these, including the scanner itself, the ligands employed, time at scanning in relation to last administered dose and other technical variables. Differences between reports may be partly explained thereby and, in comparing results, it is important to consider such factors. It should also be noted that the values reported here reflect striatal D_2 occupancy levels. However, antipsychotic response has been linked to mesocorticolimbic D_2 blockade (Davis *et al.* 1991; see *Initial concepts of dopamine receptor typology* above), while prolactin levels are mediated through D_2 blockade in the pituitary (Moore *et al.* 1999). That results from striatal D_2 binding can be extrapolated to reflect D_2 occupancy in extrastriatal regions garners support from PET studies showing no significant differences between striatal and extrastriatal D_2 occupancy in patients treated with haloperidol (Farde *et al.* 1997), although SPECT studies to the contrary also exist (Pilowsky *et al.* 1997b; Bigliani *et al.* 2000).

Impact of clozapine as the prototype second-generation antipsychotic

Evolving concepts of the antipsychotic action of clozapine

We are now traversing the 15th anniversary of the pivotal North American trial (Kane *et al.* 1988) which established the antipsy-

chotic efficacy of clozapine in a material minority of patients refractory to conventional antipsychotics, in the essential absence of extrapyramidal side-effects. However, it should be emphasized that clozapine, even at that time, was not a new drug; rather, it had been synthesized and investigated pharmacologically in the early 1960s and enjoyed long appreciation in Europe for its high therapeutic efficacy with low extrapyramidal side-effect liability before diminishing utilization because of concern over its propensity to induce potentially fatal agranulocytosis (for a personal memoire of these early events see Hippius 1989).

Nevertheless, such historical completeness cannot detract from the status of clozapine as an agent which has, over the past decade, influenced materially our perspectives on antipsychotic drug action (Waddington *et al.* 1997). Recent meta-analysis has sustained the superior clinical efficacy and EPS profile of clozapine, although the extent to which this might relate particularly to negative symptoms, manifestation of the deficit syndrome and cognitive impairment, or refractoriness *per se*, and might be reflected in levels of functioning, may have been somewhat overestimated (Keefe *et al.* 1999; Rosenheck *et al.* 1999; Simpson *et al.* 1999; Wahlbeck *et al.* 1999). However, its agranulocytosis liability and mandatory blood count monitoring programme, together with its liability to induce seizures, sedation, hypotension, hypersalivation and weight gain, mean that this important agent is unlikely to attain widespread use as a 'frontline' antipsychotic, although it still appears underutilized for patients unresponsive to or intolerant of other agents (Waddington *et al.* 1997; Kane 1999). Uniquely, however, it indicates that our clinical expectations for new antipsychotics can be revised upwards (Waddington & O'Callaghan 1997) and suggests that our pharmacological efforts be directed towards identifying the basis of its advantageous therapeutic profile and resolving the mechanisms of its numerous non-motoric side-effect liabilities with a view to identifying more utilitarian agents.

This mission is far from straightforward. Clozapine is a highly non-selective compound which demonstrates an extensive range of actions at multiple levels of neuronal function associated with numerous neurotransmitter systems (Ashby & Wang 1996; Waddington *et al.* 1997; Leysen 2000; Waddington & Casey 2000). Indeed, in seriously confounding any such goal, the breadth of these actions means that clozapine can be considered either as a rich reservoir for theorizing on or, alternatively, extremely muddy waters in which to fish for the substrate of a new generation of improved antipsychotic agents.

Clozapine and dopamine receptor subtypes

While clozapine evidences modest *in vitro* affinity both for D_2-like ($D_4 > D_{2L/S} \approx D_3$) and for D_1-like ($D_1 \approx D_5$) receptors, particular attention has focused on a purported selectivity for the D_4 receptor (Van Tol *et al.* 1991; Seeman *et al.* 1997) which might be better described as a limited preference of uncertain functional significance (Waddington *et al.* 1997; Tarazi & Baldessarini 1999; Waddington & Casey 2000). While some of the pharmacological actions of clozapine are attenuated modestly in D_4 receptor 'knockout' mice (Rubinstein *et al.* 1997), no other antipsychotics or selective D_4 antagonists were examined in the same manner, and the importance of its D_4 antagonist affinity (Seeman *et al.* 1997) has recently been revised downwards by a major proponent in favour of mechanisms based on the nature of its actions at the D_2 receptor (Seeman & Tallerico 1998). More specifically, it has been argued that the ability of clozapine (a drug with a high dissociation constant, i.e. 'loose' binding) to occupy the D_2 receptor appears reduced using a ligand of lower dissociation constant (i.e. 'tight' binding), particularly in the presence of higher levels of endogenous DA in competition therewith.

Thus, on taking into account the characteristics of the ligand used, competition from endogenous DA, and antipsychotic cerebrospinal fluid concentrations of free drug, including active metabolites, the relationship between affinity for the D_2 receptor and clinical antipsychotic potency appears sustained, in a manner that resolves for clozapine a previously described deviation from this relationship (Seeman *et al.* 1997; Seeman & Tallerico 1998). There are also clinical implications to this complex but heuristic pharmacodynamic analysis, in that 'loose'-binding antipsychotics such as clozapine should, in competition with endogenous DA in basal ganglia vs. corticolimbic regions: (i) induce less extrapyramidal side-effects than 'tight'-binding antipsychotics such as haloperidol; and (ii) may lead to more rapid relapse after discontinuation, as a result of rapid dissociation from D_2 receptors; indeed, essentially 'all' aspects of antipsychotic efficacy and EPS liability for clozapine are purported to be explicable in terms of D_2 receptor-mediated effects (Seeman & Tallerico 1999). It will be important to clarify through further preclinical and clinical experimentation the extent to which these putative pharmacodynamic effects and their predictions are sustained.

Clozapine and non-dopaminergic receptors

This dibenzodiazepine evidences considerably higher *in vitro* antagonist affinity for numerous non-DAergic than for DA receptor subtypes, particularly α ($\alpha_1 > \alpha_2$), H ($H_1 > H_3$), M ($M_1 > M_5 > M_{4(agonist)} > M_3 > M_2$) and 5-HT (5-HT$_{2A}$ = 5-HT$_6$ > 5-HT$_{2C}$ > 5-HT$_7$ > 5-HT$_3$ > 5-HT$_{1A(partial agonist)-F}$), together with actions at other levels of synaptic transmission (Waddington *et al.* 1997; Leysen 2000). These diverse non-DAergic effects of clozapine have engendered many alternative formulations for its clinical profile in terms of antipsychotic efficacy with low EPS liability but propensity for numerous other adverse effects.

Among the more prominent formulations at a conventional level, a combination of high 5-HT$_{2A}$ with D_2-like antagonism has been long posited to underpin the clinical advantages not only of clozapine but also of other second-generation antipsychotics (Meltzer *et al.* 1989). This could derive from enhanced release of DA to mitigate EPSs caused by D_2 blockade in the basal ganglia, and to ameliorate negative symptoms and cogni-

tive dysfunction as a result of putative DAergic deficits in the prefrontal cortex (Meltzer 1999; but see Carpenter *et al.* 2000a); indeed clozapine, but not haloperidol, has been shown to preferentially augment DA release in prefrontal cortex relative to caudate in non-human primates (Youngren *et al.* 1999). However, some anomalies are evident: the second-generation agent amisulpride is essentially devoid of 5-HT$_{2A}$ antagonism, while the first-generation agent chlorpromazine is a potent antagonist of 5-HT$_{2A}$ as well as D_2-like receptors (Trichard *et al.* 1998). Furthermore, preclinical studies examining the effects of 5-HT$_{2A}$ antagonism on antipsychotic-induced catalepsy are not in overall accordance with such a model (Wadenberg 1996; Seeman *et al.* 1997). Nevertheless, this proposition has proved influential and heuristic to the field. The high affinity of clozapine for 5-HT$_6$ receptors has prompted consideration of this site also as contributing to an advantageous antipsychotic profile (Meltzer 1999); however, this has received less systematic evaluation.

Among alternative formulations, one variant posits 5-HT$_{1A}$ partial agonism with D_2-like antagonism (Newman-Tancredi *et al.* 1996). This may contribute not only to mitigation of EPSs (Wadenberg 1996) but also to enhancement of prefrontal DA release and putative therapeutic effects (Rollema *et al.* 1997). Another variant posits α_2 antagonism (Blake *et al.* 1998; Leysen 2000) also to augment prefrontal DA release and D_2-like antagonist-induced suppression of conditioned avoidance responding in a traditional model of antipsychotic activity (Hertel *et al.* 1999). The α_2 antagonist idazoxan may augment the clinical efficacy of the first-generation antipsychotic fluphenazine so that it approaches, but does not attain, the profile of clozapine (Litman *et al.* 1996).

Although heterogeneous, each of these formulations encompasses, in addition to D_2-like antagonism, an action associated putatively with enhancement of DA release in the prefrontal cortex, in accordance with contemporary perspectives on the pathophysiology of schizophrenia (Waddington & Morgan 2001). An important challenge is to confirm whether second-generation agents as a class manifest one of these actions, or whether second-generation antipsychotic activity can be mediated by diverse mechanisms.

New cellular and behavioural models of antipsychotic drug action and schizophrenia

At a cellular level, a classical model has related prediction of antipsychotic efficacy vs. EPS liability to development of depolarization block in DA cells of the mesocorticolimbic vs. mesostriatal systems (Grace *et al.* 1997). However, among conceptually novel models, expression of the intermediate–early gene *c-fos* is induced by numerous physiological and pharmacological stimuli, including antipsychotic drugs, in a manner that might reveal neuroanatomical sites and functional pathways of drug action. As do first-generation antipsychotics, clozapine induces *c-fos* in the shell region of the nucleus accumbens; however, relative to such agents, which particularly induce *c-fos* in the striatum as a correlate of EPS liability, clozapine and its desmethyl metabolite induce *c-fos* preferentially in the thalamic paraventricular nucleus and selectively in the prefrontal cortex (Young *et al.* 1998), brain regions which are congruent with contemporary formulations of fronto–striato–pallido–thalamo–frontal network dysfunction in schizophrenia (Waddington & Morgan 2001). As above, the extent to which 'all' as opposed to 'some' second-generation agents might share this profile is not yet clear.

Over the past several years a new generation of behavioural models with face and possible construct validity for schizophrenia have been introduced, informed by increased understanding of the psychology and pathobiology of this disorder (Higgins 1998; Ellenbroek & Cools 2000). These allow us to go beyond more traditional models whereby attenuation of DA agonist-induced hyperactivity and of conditioned avoidance responding are held to indicate antipsychotic efficacy, while attenuation of DA agonist-induced stereotypy and induction of catalepsy are held to indicate EPS liability (Kinon & Lieberman 1996; Arnt & Skarsfeldt 1998). These newer models include prepulse inhibition of acoustic startle (Swerdlow *et al.* 1998), PCP-induced social withdrawal (Sams-Dodd 1999) and neonatal ventral hippocampal lesions (Lipska & Weinberger 2000). The extent to which these new models meaningfully reproduce negative and cognitive as well as positive aspects of psychopathology, and reflect the therapeutic profile of clozapine and other second-generation antipsychotics, presents a considerable challenge.

Reappraisal of clozapine by PET and SPECT

Striatal D_2 vs. 5-HT_2 occupancy

Although the precise scope of the clinical advantages of clozapine remains open to debate, *in vitro* work points to at least two mechanisms of action that might account for these features and which can be addressed using PET and SPECT: greater 5-HT_2 vs. D_2 activity (Coward *et al.* 1989; Meltzer *et al.* 1989) and low 'loose'-binding affinity for the D_2 receptor. Neuroimaging data in patients with schizophrenia have offered support for both of these models. Reports have now confirmed low D_2 occupancy for clozapine, even at the highest therapeutic dose of 900 mg; in contrast, 5-HT_2 blockade is consistently higher, with occupancy approaching saturation (Farde *et al.* 1992, 1994; Kapur *et al.* 1999). At this level, it accords with the 5-HT_2 : D_2 ratio model proposed by Meltzer *et al.* (1989) based on *in vitro* work.

Variant D_2 occupancy threshold models

These *in vivo* D_2 occupancy data for clozapine constitute a fundamental finding. Neuroimaging studies have led to the notion that optimal clinical response is achieved when D_2 blockade exceeds a 65–70% threshold (Farde *et al.* 1992; Nordstrom *et al.*

1993; Kapur *et al.* 1999); yet data now indicate clozapine, an antipsychotic with at least comparable and likely greater efficacy than all other antipsychotics, to achieve that efficacy at D_2 occupancies below this proposed threshold. How can this apparent anomaly be reconciled? One explanation is that the model of a 65–70% threshold is incorrect. However, this finding has been confirmed at several centres, using different antipsychotics (Farde *et al.* 1992; Nordstrom *et al.* 1993; Kapur *et al.* 1999). An alternative explanation is that antipsychotic efficacy can be achieved through mechanisms that are not exclusively dependent on D_2 activity. Indeed, in the case of clozapine, might D_2 activity be a 'red herring', without material relation to its antipsychotic effect and distinguishing it from a class of antipsychotics that are dependent on D_2 antagonism to effect antipsychotic activity?

An answer to this conundrum appears to evolve through an integration of both *in vitro* and *in vivo* evidence. Based on the *in vitro* work described above, suggesting that antipsychotic compounds may differ in the nature of their binding to the D_2 receptor, first-generation antipsychotics such as haloperidol bind 'tightly' and dissociate slowly, while clozapine binds 'loosely' and dissociates rapidly (Seeman & Tallerico 1999; Kapur & Seeman 2000). More recent *in vivo* data involving PET complements this line of thinking. It appears that clozapine is characterized by transient D_2 occupancy, such that levels measured 12–24 h after the last administered dose are markedly lower than those evident within the first several hours (Kapur *et al.* 2000b,c). Thus, the apparently low D_2 occupancy of antipsychotic agents such as clozapine can be accounted for, at least in part, by transient D_2 blockade, and their clinical efficacy does not contradict a model predicated on D_2 antagonism.

Synthesis

What are the implications of these data? First, they further support the notion that while most second-generation antipsychotics (amisulpride excepted) share in common the pharmacological profile of greater 5-HT_2 vs. D_2 antagonism *in vitro*, there are aspects to these same dimensions that differentiate these agents *in vivo*. Neuroimaging data have thus provided us with key information indicating that, at the very least, these differences offer a conceptual framework for classifying second-generation antipsychotics and evaluating potential similarities and differences within the clinical setting (Kapur 1998; Remington & Kapur 2000). In addition, these results support the position that sustained D_2 occupancy is not required for antipsychotic efficacy. For example, it has been demonstrated with haloperidol decanoate, administered monthly, that antipsychotic efficacy can be maintained when mean D_2 occupancy decreases from 73% (60–82%) at week 1 to 52% (20–74%) at week 4 (Nyberg *et al.* 1995). The question remains as to how long an antipsychotic must bind to the D_2 receptor in order to optimize the likelihood of clinical response while minimizing risk of D_2-related adverse events.

The 'atypicality' controversy

Clinical issues

Over the past decade the term 'atypical' has emerged to enjoy widespread use for the appelation of clozapine and, subsequently, of the still expanding array of newer antipsychotics for which it has served as progenitor. The most widely espoused core feature is antipsychotic efficacy at doses that cause materially fewer or no EPSs (Meltzer 2000), and such a monotheistic definition confers operational advantage. Yet it engenders practical and conceptual problems in the absence of clear theoretical underpinnings (Gerlach 2000). Waddington and O'Callaghan (1997) and Remington and Kapur (2000) have raised the issue as to whether yet further factors should be considered. Clozapine teaches us that it is realistic to set yet higher standards for new antipsychotics, to encompass the following: superior efficacy, including negative symptoms and otherwise refractory psychopathology and cognitive dysfunction; reduced neuroendocrine sequelae, such as elevation of prolactin secretion; lack of subjective dysphoria; reduced sedative effects; reduced autonomic/cardiovascular effects, such as prolongation of QTc interval; lack of sexual dysfunction; lack of weight gain; advantages such as freedom from tardive dyskinesia. Rare idiosyncratic reactions and liabilities relating to unexpected sudden death might also be considered, but are yet more difficult to estimate.

However, it will emphasized below that these agents are diverse in these regards, and it should be considered (Waddington & O'Callaghan 1997) whether it might be preferable to apply polytheistic criteria, such as are used for schizophrenia itself, whereby satisfying any combination of several of the above might be deemed to constitute material advantage in a manner that does not imply generic characteristics; these would encompass efficacy, non-motoric side-effect and quality-of-life domains. Among alternative descriptors are 'new', 'novel' and 'second-generation' antipsychotics; it is this last term that has been preferred by some (Kane 1999; Waddington & Quinn 2000) and adopted here, in accordance with World Psychiatric Association guidelines.

Mechanistic issues

An alternative level of analysis of 'atypicality' is in mechanistic terms. The diverse pharmacological properties of clozapine have prompted exploration as to which combination(s) of these might underpin its advantageous and disadvantageous features, and whether any such combination generalizes to some or indeed all second-generation antipsychotics (Kinon & Lieberman 1996; Arnt & Skarsfeldt 1998; Waddington & Casey 2000). In overall terms, second-generation agents evidence generally similar properties in traditional animal models which predict antipsychotic efficacy with low EPS liability, although not all have yet been examined in the newer models of putatively greater homology. However, at a clinical level, the appelation

'atypical' may mislead as to any unitary pharmacological basis for their superior profiles; they are mechanistically as well as clinically diverse, as will be reviewed individually below.

Second-generation antipsychotic drugs subsequent to clozapine

Amisulpride

This substituted benzamide analogue of sulpiride is *in vitro* a low affinity, selective antagonist of D_2-like ($D_{2L/S} = D_3 \gg D_4$) with little or no affinity for D_1-like or non-DAergic receptors (Coukell *et al.* 1996; Schoemaker *et al.* 1997; Waddington *et al.* 1997). In patients with schizophrenia, PET studies indicate lower doses of amisulpride (50–100 mg) to occupy only 4–26% of striatal D_2 receptors, while higher doses (200–800 mg) occupy 38–76% thereof (Martinot *et al.* 1996). More recently, it has been confirmed that such occupancy of D_2 receptors by 200–1200 mg amisulpride occurs in the absence of cortical 5-HT_2 receptor occupancy (Trichard *et al.* 1998). Its congener, sulpiride, evidences a generally similar pharmacological profile, but its earlier origins have resulted in less extensive contemporary investigation by PET or SPECT.

It has been argued on the basis of preclinical studies using conventional models that lower doses of amisulpride (and possibly sulpiride) preferentially block presynaptic D_2-like autoreceptors to give a relative *enhancement* of DAergic function, which may confer clinical effectiveness against 'negative' symptoms, while higher doses antagonize certain postsynaptic DA receptor-mediated functions, perhaps particularly in corticolimbic regions, to exert antipsychotic efficacy but with little or no induction of catalepsy to predict low EPS liability (Coukell *et al.* 1996; Perrault *et al.* 1997). However, there are few data examining the properties of amisulpride (or sulpiride) in the new generation of preclinical models noted above (Depoortere *et al.* 1997; Waddington & Casey 2000).

Initial clinical studies suggested that lower doses of amisulpride (50–300 mg) reduce negative symptom scores relative to placebo without any elevation of positive symptoms and with little or no induction of EPSs. Subsequently, more extensive trials have confirmed 100 mg amisulpride to produce a sustained reduction in negative symptom scores without EPSs, relative to placebo, although with a high drop-out rate because of recrudescence of psychosis. Conversely, 400–800 mg amisulpride was at least as effective as 16–20 mg haloperidol in reducing total psychopathology and positive symptom scores, and was more effective in reducing negative symptom scores with fewer EPSs. In patients with predominantly negative symptoms, low-dose amisulpride was more effective than placebo over a 6-month period, while over a 1-year period it showed little advantage over low-dose haloperidol in reducing these symptoms. In terms of adverse effects, amisulpride can induce some dose-related EPSs, prolactin elevation with associated endocrine effects, insomnia, agitation, dry mouth and weight gain, but few cardiovascular events (Coukell *et al.* 1996; Loo *et al.* 1997; Speller *et al.* 1997).

In comparative studies for acute exacerbations of schizophrenia, the efficacy of 1000 mg amisulpride against positive and negative symptom scores was similar to that of 25 mg flupentixol, with fewer EPSs but larger increases in prolactin (Wetzel *et al.* 1998), while the efficacy and adverse effect profile of 800 mg amisulpride differed little from that of 8 mg risperidone, other than weight gain being significantly less among patients receiving amisulpride (Coulouvrat & Dondey-Nouvel 1999; Peuskens *et al.* 1999). In a 1-year study of chronic illness comparing 200–800 mg amisulpride with 5–20 mg haloperidol, amisulpride was associated with greater reductions in negative symptom, overall function and quality of life scores, but not in positive symptom scores, with fewer EPSs but comparable incidence of endocrine events (Colonna *et al.* 2000).

However, as for most second-generation antipsychotics, particular attention focuses on any purported advantage in terms of reducing negative symptom scores, and whether this has its basis in a direct action against enduring primary/'deficit' features or an indirect effect secondary to reduced EPSs and alleviation of positive and depressive psychopathology (Kirkpatrick *et al.* 2000). While this challenge can be addressed statistically using path analysis (Moller *et al.* 1995), the interpretation of variance in negative symptom scores that is unexplained by EPSs and positive or depressive symptoms as a 'direct' effect is uncertain. Hence studies which involve patients identified as having enduring primary/'deficit' features are to be preferred (Kirkpatrick *et al.* 2000). A recent study (Danion *et al.* 1999) has reported 50–100 mg amisulpride to be more effective than placebo in reducing negative symptom scores in chronically ill patients selected for high baseline scores, in the face of modest effects on positive and depressive symptoms with no difference in EPSs from placebo. However, proposed criteria for the specification of primary negative symptoms/'deficit' features of schizophrenia were not utilized. Amisulpride is now available in Europe and some other countries but not yet in North America. As for pharmacological studies, the early origins of sulpiride have resulted in a considerably less extensive body of contemporary clinical trials; thus, it is not possible to define or compare its therapeutic profile in the same terms, other than a reduced liability to induce EPSs.

Olanzapine

Olanzapine, a thienobenzodiazepine with a pharmacological profile overlapping with but not identical to that of clozapine, is a broad, high affinity *in vitro* antagonist of 5-HT $(5\text{-HT}_{2A/C} = 5\text{-HT}_6 > 5\text{-HT}_3) = M_{1\text{-}4} = H_1 > D_2\text{-like}$ $(D_{2L/S} = D_3 = D_4) > D_1\text{-like} = \alpha (\alpha_1 > \alpha_2)$ receptors (Bymaster *et al.* 1996; Schotte *et al.* 1996; Waddington *et al.* 1997). Like clozapine, it demonstrates greater 5-HT$_2$ vs. D$_2$ activity *in vitro*, and this has subsequently been confirmed *in vivo* using neuroimaging techniques. Both PET and SPECT studies in patients with schizophrenia have demonstrated that at therapeutic doses its

D$_2$ occupancy ($\sim$ 40–80%) appears greater than for clozapine, but less than for risperidone (Pilowsky *et al.* 1996; Kapur *et al.* 1998, 1999). PET studies have indicated that at currently recommended therapeutic doses (5–20 mg/day), the profile of greater 5-HT$_2$ vs. D$_2$ blockade can be shown. As dosage is increased, however, 5-HT$_2$ occupancy approaches saturation, while D$_2$ occupancy continues to rise. Ultimately, the 5-HT$_2$: D$_2$ ratio purported to account for atypical features such as reduced EPSs is lost (Kapur *et al.* 1998). As many clinicians would agree, this agent appears to have a wider than expected therapeutic dose range before EPSs are evident clinically; one possible explanation for this is the inherent muscarinic activity that has been identified for olanzapine, at least *in vitro* (Bymaster *et al.* 1996), a feature not shared by risperidone (Janssen *et al.* 1988). The extent to which this might translate to reduced liability for tardive dyskinesia (Beasley *et al.* 1999) requires further long-term systematic study.

Preclinical models have supported a favourable profile for olanzapine on a number of dimensions. This holds true for conventional indices of antipsychotic activity, e.g. inhibition of conditioned avoidance responding and reversal of DA agonist-induced effects vis-à-vis limited induction of catalepsy (Moore *et al.* 1992), but it also evidences a favourable, sometimes clozapine-like, profile in newer models (Waddington *et al.* 1997), including reversal of PCP-related behaviours (Bakshi & Geyer 1995) and drug-discrimination responding (Porter & Strong 1996).

There are now numerous controlled trials evaluating olanzapine in schizophrenia (Beasley *et al.* 1996; Dellva *et al.* 1997; Tollefson *et al.* 1997; Tran *et al.* 1997; Hamilton *et al.* 1998). The optimal dose range appears to be 5–20 mg/day, although there are some anecdotal reports indicating that higher doses, i.e. up to 30–40 mg/day, may effect a further response in individuals who have not demonstrated optimal response at lower doses (Reich 1999; Sheitman *et al.* 1997). It is, perhaps, easier to employ higher doses with this compound, because from the standpoint of side-effects it is generally well tolerated. One investigation found olanzapine superior to haloperidol in 'first episode' patients, although the definition included individuals who had been ill as long as 5 years (Sanger *et al.* 1999). When compared to conventional antipsychotics in more chronic populations, it appears to be as effective, if not more so, for positive symptoms and possibly superior for negative symptoms (Beasley *et al.* 1997b). Again, issues arise as to whether this effect is through primary or secondary negative symptom change. It may be efficacious also against depressive symptoms in the context of individuals being treated for psychosis (Tollefson *et al.* 1998) and, like other second-generation antipsychotics, improvements in aspects of neurocognitive testing have been documented in some studies (Purdon *et al.* 2000). Several reports have addressed whether it might be as effective as clozapine in refractory schizophrenia (Dursun *et al.* 1999; Weiss *et al.* 1999), but there are no conclusive data in this regard.

The most problematic side-effect linked to olanzapine has been weight gain (Allison *et al.* 1999; Ganguli 1999; Wirshing *et al.* 1999), which is not necessarily dose-dependent. Elevated triglycerides have been reported (Sheitman *et al.* 1999), as has diabetes (Wirshing *et al.* 1998; Goldstein *et al.* 1999; Lindenmayer & Patel 1999) which is not seen only in those who have gained weight. Other adverse events include somnolence, constipation and dry mouth, with transient increases in prolactin and in liver enzymes, specifically the transaminases (Beasley *et al.* 1997a). While structurally related to clozapine, olanzapine has not been associated with the same risk of agranulocytosis. However, there are several anecdotal reports suggesting that it is not entirely without risk in this regard (Finkel *et al.* 1998; Benedetti *et al.* 1999; Naumann *et al.* 1999).

Quetiapine

The dibenzothiazepine quetiapine demonstrates *in vitro* broad lower affinity antagonism of $H_1 > 5\text{-HT}$ ($5\text{-HT}_{2A} > 5\text{-HT}_7$) $= \alpha_{1/2} > D_2$-like ($D_{2L/S} = D_3 > D_4$) $> D_1$-like $= M$ receptors (Fulton & Goa 1995; Goldstein & Arvanitis 1995; Schotte *et al.* 1996; Waddington *et al.* 1997); it has an active 7-hydroxy metabolite (Pullen *et al.* 1992). PET data in patients with schizophrenia are particularly interesting on several levels. Like clozapine, D_2 occupancy is quite low and while 5-HT_2 blockade is consistently higher, it does not approach saturation across the recommended therapeutic dosage range up to 750 mg/day (Kapur *et al.* 2000c). An important additional finding is its transient D_2 occupancy; it is like clozapine in this respect and, in fact, evidences yet 'looser' binding. Furthermore, while *in vivo* data indicate high 5-HT_2 blockade with clozapine, even at the lowest therapeutic dosage, this is not the case for quetiapine, where doses of 300–600 mg have been associated with blockade of 78% of 5-HT_2 receptors (Kapur *et al.* 2000c). In general, data relating to efficacy at this point would favour clozapine (Remington & Kapur 2000); whether this is a function of their different capacities for 5-HT_2 blockade remains an unanswered question. By the same token, clinical differences between these two agents, if confirmed, could reflect differences either in 'tightness' of binding or in one of the many other pharmacological properties that distinguish them (Fleischhacker & Hummer 1997; Waddington *et al.* 1997).

In both conventional and new preclinical models, quetiapine evidences a profile predictive of antipsychotic activity with low EPS liability; this includes activity in some models thought to reflect negative symptoms, e.g. amphetamine-induced social isolation (Migler *et al.* 1993; Ellenbroek *et al.* 1996; Waddington *et al.* 1997).

To date, there have been a limited number of published controlled trials involving quetiapine (Borison *et al.* 1996; Arvanitis & Miller 1997; Peuskens & Link 1997; Small *et al.* 1997; Emsley *et al.* 2000). In dosages of up to 750 mg/day, it has been shown to be superior to placebo and comparable to conventional antipsychotics in treating positive and negative symptoms. Its EPS profile is comparable to placebo, even at higher dosage, and it is not associated with sustained prolactin elevation. There are at least preliminary data that it can positively influence other clinical features such as depression (Arvanitis & Miller 1997; Small *et al.* 1997) and cognition (Sax *et al.* 1998).

The side-effect that has raised the greatest concern with quetiapine has been a potential risk for cataracts, a finding identified in preclinical work with dogs. Recommendations regarding ophthalmic evaluation have been put in place, and it is reassuring that early follow-up data have not confirmed this finding in humans exposed to quetiapine (Smith *et al.* 1997; Nasrallah *et al.* 1999). Non-significant QTc prolongation has been noted, as has weight gain, although this seems less than that reported for clozapine and olanzapine. There does not appear to be the risk of agranulocytosis seen with clozapine but, as for clozapine and olanzapine, transient increases in liver enzymes have been reported. Other side-effects include somnolence, dizziness, dry mouth, constipation, dyspepsia and postural hypotension (Fulton & Goa 1995; Hirsch *et al.* 1996; Kasper 2000). In general, however, the incidence of these adverse events is relatively low.

Risperidone

Risperidone, a benzisoxazole, patterns itself after clozapine and most of the second-generation antipsychotics in terms of combined $5\text{-HT}_2/D_2$ activity. Indeed, it has very high *in vitro* affinity for 5-HT ($5\text{-HT}_{2A} > 5\text{-HT}_7 \gg 5\text{-HT}_{1A\text{-F/2C/3/6}}$) and high affinity for D_2-like ($D_{2L/S} > D_3 = D_4$), α ($\alpha_1 > \alpha_2$) and H_1 receptors (Schotte *et al.* 1996; Waddington *et al.* 1997); the metabolite 9-OH-risperidone appears to be as potent as the parent compound (He & Richardson 1995).

PET data in patients with schizophrenia have confirmed *in vivo* risperidone's profile of generally greater 5-HT_2 vs. D_2 occupancy. Lower doses are now being advocated, an argument given yet more strength by the lack of compelling evidence from phase III trials to indicate that doses exceeding 6–8 mg/day offer superior clinical efficacy, although they produce EPSs in a dose-related fashion (Chouinard *et al.* 1993; Marder & Meibach 1994; Peuskens 1995; Simpson & Lindenmayer 1997). PET studies have indicated that at the currently recommended therapeutic dose range (2–6 mg/day) a profile of greater 5-HT_2 vs. D_2 blockade can be shown (Kapur *et al.* 1995). As dosage is increased, however, 5-HT_2 occupancy approaches saturation while D_2 occupancy continues to rise. Ultimately, the $5\text{-HT}_2/D_2$ ratio purported to account for features such as reduced EPSs is lost and from this standpoint risperidone begins to look like a first-generation antipsychotic (Kapur *et al.* 1995). Whether the benefits of decreased acute EPSs might translate into a diminished risk for tardive dyskinesia when compared to first-generation antipsychotics (Jeste *et al.* 2000) requires further long-term systematic study.

To summarize, both risperidone and olanzapine are characterized by higher D_2 blockade even at lower therapeutic doses when compared to clozapine, and by gradual increases in D_2 occupancy with increasing dosage. Unlike clozapine, where greater 5-HT_2 vs. D_2 antagonism is seen across all doses, this differential gradually diminishes for risperidone and olanzapine as 5-HT_2 receptors are saturated and D_2 blockade continues to rise

(Kapur *et al.* 1999). What are the implications of these data? They further support the notion that while most second-generation antipsychotics share the pharmacological profile of greater 5-HT$_2$ vs. D$_2$ antagonism *in vitro*, there are aspects to these same dimensions that differentiate these agents. Clozapine and quetiapine, for example, are more transient in their D$_2$ blockade than either risperidone or olanzapine, both of which are more transient than haloperidol (Seeman & Tallerico 1999; Kapur & Seeman 2000; Kapur *et al.* 2000b,c). The low risk of EPS with clozapine and quetiapine may reflect their transient D$_2$ binding, and dose increments of either may not incur the same dose-related increase in risk of EPS.

Preclinical data from traditional models (He & Richardson 1995; Waddington *et al.* 1997) provide support for risperidone's antipsychotic potential as well as reduced risk of EPSs. Results involving newer models, e.g. prepulse inhibition and reversal of PCP-induced social withdrawal, have produced variable results (Kitaichi *et al.* 1994; Corbett *et al.* 1995; Varty & Higgins 1995; Waddington *et al.* 1997).

There are now numerous double-blind trials demonstrating the efficacy of risperidone in various stages and phases of psychosis (Chouinard *et al.* 1993; Marder & Meibach 1994; Curtis & Kerwin 1995; Peuskens 1995; Lemmens *et al.* 1999). The need to distinguish specific patient populations appears to be an important one for the interpretation of results. For example, in patients with first episode psychosis, risperidone has not been shown to be clinically superior to haloperidol, although it is significantly better from the standpoint of EPSs and side-effects in general. Indeed, there are few data to support a general clinical superiority for second-generation antipsychotics in first episode psychosis. The high response rate in these individuals may account for the lack of differences between first- and second-generation agents. Also, it remains to be determined whether the newer antipsychotics may yet claim superiority on measures over and above global or psycho-pathological outcome, such as cognition and quality of life.

For other aspects of psychosis, e.g. chronic/partial responders, refractory and acute exacerbation, if there is any advantage for risperidone it is rather modest, and often the data are not consistent (Mattes 1997; Lemmens *et al.* 1999; Remington & Kapur 2000). Claims for improvement in negative symptoms certainly generate considerable attention, because first-generation antipsychotics can be helpful but their utility in this respect seems quite limited. Once again, any purported advantages are limited and inconsistent across studies; moreover, any such changes may reflect improvement in secondary negative symptoms rather than the more enduring deficit state (Mattes 1997). Cognitive improvement has been documented (Gallhofer *et al.* 1996; Green *et al.* 1997), but the same qualifications regarding interpretation of these data hold true.

In terms of side-effects other than EPSs, elevated prolactin with risperidone in at least some individuals distinguishes it from other 5-HT$_2$/D$_2$ antagonists (Chung & Eun 1998; Dickson & Glazer 1999), and poses another dilemma in the link between D$_2$ occupancy and side-effects. The same argument made for its risk of EPSs, that it is simply a dose-related phenomenon, does not seem sufficient as elevated prolactin occurs even at lower therapeutic doses. Moreover, the recorded elevations are as high as is seen with a first-generation antipsychotic such as haloperidol, and perhaps higher. Two possible explanations may account for why risperidone distinguishes itself from other second-generation antipsychotics on this dimension. First, it binds 'tightly' to the D$_2$ receptor, in the manner of a first-generation antipsychotic and unlike other newer agents such as clozapine and quetiapine (Kapur & Seeman 2000). Secondly, its pharmacological profile includes the active metabolite 9-OH-risperidone, thought to be as potent as the parent compound (He & Richardson 1995), with poorer permeability at the level of the blood–brain barrier. Because the tuberoinfundibular system is located outside the blood–brain barrier, one result might be sustained and prolonged D$_2$ occupancy therein, associated in turn with high prolactin levels. Headache and nausea have been noted, as have insomnia and anxiety/agitation (Chouinard *et al.* 1993; Marder & Meibach 1994). The latter may reflect akathisia, as this too seems dose-related. QTc prolongation has been noted, but not found to be clinically significant.

Sertindole

This indole derivative is a high affinity *in vitro* antagonist of 5-HT (5-HT$_{2A/C}$ > 5-HT$_7$) > α_1 > D$_2$-like (D$_{2L/S}$ = D$_3$ = D$_4$) receptors (Sanchez *et al.* 1991; Dunn & Fitton 1996; Waddington *et al.* 1997). Sertindole has yet to receive extensive study using PET. In patients with schizophrenia, initial SPECT studies indicated 20–24 mg sertindole to evidence 'high' occupancy both of striatal D$_2$ receptors and of cortical 5-HT$_2$ receptors (Pilowsky *et al.* 1997a; Travis *et al.* 1998). More recently, however, quantitative SPECT studies have indicated 8–24 mg sertindole to occupy 47–74% of basal ganglia D$_2$ receptors, and suggest that previous higher estimates may have been influenced by prior treatment with depot antipsychotics (Kasper *et al.* 1998; Bigliani *et al.* 2000). In relation to the controversy as to whether some second-generation antipsychotics might evidence preferential occupancy of extrastriatal DA receptors, 12–24 mg sertindole has been reported using SPECT to occupy 52–67% of D$_2$ receptors in the striatum but 76–91% of those in the temporal cortex (Bigliani *et al.* 2000).

In traditional preclinical models, the profile of sertindole is one that would predict antipsychotic efficacy with low EPS liability (Sanchez *et al.* 1991; Dunn & Fitton 1996). In non-human primates, sertindole induces EPS only at doses 5- to 10-fold higher than those associated with antipsychotic activity (Casey 1996). Regarding new preclinical models, it exerts some reversal of PCP-induced social isolation (Sams-Dodd 1999), but otherwise it has received less extensive evaluation (Waddington & Casey 2000).

Extensive clinical trials (Dunn & Fitton 1996; Zimbroff *et al.* 1997) have shown 12–24 mg sertindole to be superior to placebo and indistinguishable from 4–16 mg haloperidol in reducing both positive and negative symptom scores; although reduction in negative symptom scores with sertindole was significant relative to placebo while that with haloperidol was not, the reductions effected by sertindole and haloperidol did not differ materially from one another. In a 1-year study of chronic illness, 24 mg sertindole did not significantly delay time to broadly defined 'treatment failure' in comparison with 10 mg haloperidol, and overall reductions in both positive and negative symptom scores did not differ materially. However, patients treated with sertindole did remain free of hospitalization and remained compliant longer than did their haloperidol counterparts, and significant differences in negative symptom scores at variable time points over the year were in favour of sertindole (Daniel et al. 1998).

Overall, sertindole appears indistinguishable from placebo and materially superior to haloperidol in terms of EPS liability during acute treatment and induces significantly fewer EPSs than does haloperidol over long-term treatment, with prolactin levels being little altered. However, it can induce nasal congestion, decreased ejaculatory volume, weight gain and prolongation of cardiac QT and QTc intervals (Dunn & Fitton 1996; Zimbroff et al. 1997; Daniel et al. 1998). It is this prolongation of cardiac QTc interval which has engendered the greatest controversy in relation to sertindole; indeed, after becoming available in Europe, although not marketed in the USA, it was then withdrawn from use because of regulatory concerns over the clinical significance of such prolongation, particularly liability for potentially fatal ventricular arrhythmias. Findings suggest that sertindole may be a pseudo-irreversible α_1 antagonist (Ipsen et al. 1997) and a high-affinity antagonist of human cardiac potassium HERG channels (Rampe et al. 1998), and that this latter effect in particular may contribute to prolongation of QTc interval. However, while sertindole may prolong QTc interval to a somewhat greater extent than other second-generation antipsychotics, such prolongation does occur with other antipsychotics, both first- and second-generation; indeed, the first-generation antipsychotic thioridazine has a particular liability in this regard which appears to exceed that of sertindole (Reilly et al. 2000), and this has attracted the concern of regulatory authorities.

The challenge is how to interpret these findings eclectically. In general terms, prolongation of QTc interval during long-term treatment with first-generation antipsychotics, including thioridazine, does not appear to be associated with ventricular tachyarrhythmias in patients with schizophrenia in the absence of cardiac disease, although these may occur as a rare side-effect of such antipsychotics, particularly if a patient has additional risk factors (Kitayama et al. 1999). Furthermore, drug surveillance data, which are inevitably limited as a result of its withdrawal, confirm prolongation of QTc interval by sertindole in the absence of clinical or electrocardiographic evidence of cardiac arrhythmias or of other clinical evidence of cardiac abnormalities (Pezawas et al. 2000). This still unresolved saga appears to have sensitized regulatory authorities to these issues such that some newer compounds have received increased scrutiny;

yet sertindole has become the subject of regulatory reappraisal in Europe.

Ziprasidone

Ziprasidone, an indolone derivative, has in vitro antagonist properties as follows: high 5-HT (5-HT$_{2A}$ = 5-HT$_{1D/7}$ > 5-HT$_{1A(agonist)/2C}$) > D$_2$-like (D$_{2L/S}$ = D$_3$ > D$_4$) > α (α_1 > α_2) > H$_1$ receptors. In addition, it inhibits reuptake of both noradrenaline (NA) and 5-HT (Seeger et al. 1995; Schotte et al. 1996; Waddington et al. 1997). Initial PET data involving control subjects confirm the profile of greater 5-HT$_2$ vs. D$_2$ occupancy in vivo (Fischman et al. 1996), but systematic studies in patients are awaited. The pattern of 5-HT$_2$ occupancy is similar to that seen with clozapine, olanzapine and risperidone, in that levels approximating saturation are seen even at the lower end of the therapeutic dosage range, i.e. > 95% within 4 h following 40 mg. Its pattern of D$_2$ occupancy is more in keeping with risperidone and olanzapine, with levels in excess of 65% at doses of 20–40 mg (Bench et al. 1996). Although the issue of D$_2$ transience has yet to be formally assessed, initial time–activity curves, in conjunction with evidence indicating only short-term prolactin elevation, would suggest that its occupancy may be more transient than would be seen with first-generation antipsychotics (Bench et al. 1996).

In preclinical studies using traditional models, its antipsychotic activity with low EPS liability has been supported (Seeger et al. 1995; Waddington et al. 1997); it has been studied less extensively in newer models (Waddington & Casey 2000).

Published data relating to clinical efficacy for ziprasidone are as yet limited. In doses ranging from 40 to 160 mg/day, it has been shown to be superior to placebo and similar to haloperidol in terms of global outcome, as well as positive and negative symptom reduction (Goff et al. 1998; Keck et al. 1998). Greater improvement in affective symptoms vs. placebo has also been noted (Keck et al. 1998).

Its EPS profile is superior to a first-generation antipsychotic such as haloperidol, and it appears to cause only transient prolactin elevation which returns to baseline (Goff et al. 1998). While second-generation antipsychotics appear generally more prone to induce weight gain, evidence to date with ziprasidone suggests that it is comparable to placebo in this regard (Keck et al. 1998; Allison et al. 1999). Pooled data from placebo-controlled trials indicate the three most commonly noted adverse events for ziprasidone to be somnolence, nausea and constipation, although overall it appears relatively well tolerated (Davis & Markham 1997). The most significant issue with ziprasidone has focused on its propensity for QTc prolongation. Although final approval for its release in the USA was delayed by a request for additional information in this regard, it has now been fully approved for first-line usage.

Zotepine

This dibenzothiazepine analogue of clozapine is a high-affinity *in vitro* antagonist of 5-HT $(5\text{-HT}_{2A/C} = 5\text{-HT}_{6/7}) = \alpha_1 = H_1 > D_2$-like $(D_{2L/S} = D_3 = D_4) > D_1$-like $(D_{1A} > D_{1B})$ receptors which also inhibits reuptake of NA (Waddington *et al.* 1997; Prakash & Lamb 1998); like some other second-generation antipsychotics, but not their first-generation counterparts, this agent causes an acute increase in cortical DA release (Rowley *et al.* 2000). Zotepine has yet to receive extensive investigation using PET. However, in preliminary SPECT studies, 150–200 mg zotepine was associated with 57–61% occupancy of D_2 receptors (Barnas *et al.* 1997); there are as yet no such studies of 5-HT$_2$ or other receptor occupancies.

In traditional preclinical models, the profile of zotepine is one that would predict antipsychotic efficacy with low EPS liability (Needham *et al.* 1996; Prakash & Lamb 1998); however, there are few data examining the properties of this agent in the new generation of preclinical models noted above or in non-human primates (Waddington & Casey 2000).

Clinical studies indicate 150–300 mg zotepine to be superior to placebo and 300–600 mg chlorpromazine, and indistinguishable from 10–20 mg haloperidol in reducing total psychopathology and positive symptom scores during acute exacerbation, but superior to haloperidol in reducing negative symptom scores. Zotepine induced fewer EPSs than chlorpromazine or haloperidol and a degree of sedation comparable to chlorpromazine, with greater weight gain and uricosuric activity (Prakash & Lamb 1998; Cooper *et al.* 2000a). In a 6-month study of patients with chronic illness (Cooper *et al.* 2000b), 150–300 mg zotepine was more effective than placebo in preventing recurrence of psychosis, with greater overall improvement and reduction in positive but not negative symptom scores. Zotepine did not differ from placebo in EPS liability, but was associated with greater sedation, weight gain and uricosuric activity (Cooper *et al.* 2000b). Zotepine is available in many European and other countries worldwide, but not in North America.

Emergent agents and pharmacogenomics

Although these second-generation antipsychotics constitute material progress in the treatment of schizophrenia, it is important that their profiles are not overinterpreted. While several recent reviews and meta-analyses have, in general terms, attested their advantages, at least for those agents available for sufficient time to have generated meaningful bodies of data, they also indicate their limitations (Kasper *et al.* 1999; Leucht *et al.* 1999; Wahlbeck *et al.* 1999; Geddes *et al.* 2000). Thus, they are perhaps best conceptualized as more of an incremental advance rather than any radical shift in our therapeutic armamentarium. Furthermore, as clinical experience has accrued, further liabilities associated with these second-generation antipsychotics have become apparent, or putative associations identified as causes of concern which require clarification: for example, progressive weight gain has become recognized as a material problem with some such agents (Allison *et al.* 1999), and has

been termed 'the new tardive dyskinesia of atypical antipsychotics'. Additionally, now substantial clinical experience with clozapine has engendered concern over its association with rare but potentially fatal instances of myocarditis, cardiomyopathy and thromboembolism (Kilian *et al.* 1999; Hagg *et al.* 2000). Such issues reinforce the necessity of continuing to search for yet more effective and benign treatment modalities.

One approach to this challenge seeks to identify improved agents within our current understanding (or presumption) of putative mechanisms. These include the partial D_2 presynaptic agonist and postsynaptic antagonist aripiprazole (Lawler *et al.* 1999), which at 15–30 mg/day appears to exert antipsychotic activity superior to placebo and equivalent to 10 mg haloperidol, with EPS and prolactin profiles indistinguishable from placebo, no clinically meaningful QTc prolongation and less weight gain than for haloperidol (Carson *et al.* 2001). In preliminary reports, the variant 5-HT$_{2A}$/D$_2$ and particularly $\alpha_{1/2}$ antagonist iloperidone (Szewczak *et al.* 1995) at 4–12 mg appear to exert antipsychotic efficacy on comparison with placebo and 15 mg haloperidol, with a favourable side-effect profile (Cucchiaro *et al.* 2001). These agents are still in clinical development; thus, it is not yet possible to define or compare their therapeutic profiles vis-à-vis those second-generation agents reviewed above, other than apparently reduced liability to induce EPS. There are also compounds in preclinical development with various combinations of partial agonist/antagonist activities at 5-HT$_{1A}$, D$_2$-like and other receptors, such as S 16924 (Millan *et al.* 1998) and PD 158771 (Akunne *et al.* 2000).

Recently, the DAergic agent mazindol was found to be without effect against primary and/or secondary negative symptoms thought to have a basis in reduced cortical DAergic function (Carpenter *et al.* 2000b). It should be noted that, to date, clinical trials with novel drugs lacking D$_2$ antagonist properties have not revealed material antipsychotic activity, e.g. the 5-HT$_{2A}$ antagonist M100 907 (formerly MDL 100 907: Kehne *et al.* 1996; Talvik-Lofti *et al.* 2000). Conversely, the non-D$_2$ antagonist, putative σ ligand EMD 57445 (panamesine), which may have antipsychotic activity, has been shown to give rise to a D$_2$ antagonist metabolite (Muller *et al.* 1999).

An alternative approach is to improve treatment with existing agents, in terms of pharmacogenetic prediction of optimal responsivity to individual agents. This strategy, now generic to clinical pharmacology in all medical specialities, is a developing area in antipsychotic therapy, with a particular current focus on genomic prediction of responsivity to clozapine (Arranz *et al.* 2000).

New directions: mechanisms and third-generation antipsychotics?

A more intellectually satisfying approach seeks to target alternative non-DAergic systems implicated in the pathophysiology of schizophrenia, some of which may interact with DAergic function (Waddington & Morgan 2001).

In association with evidence indicating abnormalities in schizophrenia of membrane phospholipids and/or their polyunsaturated (essential) fatty acid constituents (Fenton *et al.* 1999; Peet *et al.* 1999), the effects of administering n-3 (ω-3) and n-6 (ω-6) fatty acids have been studied. Initial controlled studies, while provocative for n-3 (ω-3) fatty acids as adjuncts to antipsychotic therapy or as sole treatment, were characterized by limited data from small trials; hence they are difficult to analyse and interpret with confidence (Fenton *et al.* 1999; Joy *et al.* 2002). More recent studies continue to generate both provocative (Peet *et al.* 2001) and negative (Fenton *et al.* 2001) findings in diverse patient populations, hence consideration of duration and severity of illness in large-scale controlled trials may be necessary to further these issues. The low level of side-effects encountered with these 'natural' substances would facilitate such studies.

Fuelled by the more homologous psychotomimetic activity of the non-competitive NMDA–glutamate antagonist PCP and evidence for glutamatergic deficits in the brain in schizophrenia, the interaction of antipsychotics with NMDA–glutamatergic function and the clinical effects of NMDA–glutamatergic modulators now constitutes a major and provocative research front (Duncan *et al.* 1999; Jentsch & Roth 1999; Heresco-Levy 2000).

Another approach seeks novel mechanisms of antipsychotic activity through either serendipitous findings or tangential extrapolation from current themes. Identification of a preclinical profile predictive of antipsychotic activity with low EPS liability for xanomeline, an M_1/M_4-preferring muscarinic agonist (Shannon *et al.* 2000), typifies this approach. Yet more intellectually fulfilling, and theoretically capable of generating fundamental therapeutic advances, are ongoing attempts to identify new therapeutic targets in terms of increased understanding of the cellular and molecular pathology of schizophrenia, including avenues such as modifiers of gene expression.

A problem that faces these different approaches is one of nonspecificity. While agents selective for certain systems and/or receptors are often the focus of preclinical investigations, there has been a more recent trend to develop putative antipsychotics that are pharmacologically 'rich', impacting on a variety of neurotransmitters and their receptors. This has been partially driven by the belief that schizophrenia reflects a number of different symptom clusters that are mediated by different mechanisms. Having the 'ideal' antipsychotic, one that is pharmacologically designed to meet each of these requirements, is appealing but unlikely. Indeed, this approach is problematic on several levels (Remington & Kapur 2000; Waddington & Morgan 2001). For example, our current understanding regarding mediating factors in different syndrome clusters is at best superficial. Employing an agent with multiple actions that then effects a clinical response makes it very difficult to distinguish the precise pharmacological features that led to the observed changes. In addition, there is the risk of incorporating features that are clinically insignificant but of importance from the standpoint of side-effects. Finally, a 'one size fits all' medication precludes the possibility of shaping treatment to the specific features of the illness that predominate in a given individual. A more sophisticated pharmacological approach would be to define the different dimensions, develop targeted treatments for each, and combine these drugs in a flexible manner that addresses each patient's unique requirements along those diverse dimensions. This requires that we better understand the pathophysiologies that appear to underlay different symptom clusters.

Acknowledgements

The authors' studies are supported by the Stanley Medical Research Institute, a Galen Fellowship from the Irish Brain Research Foundation, the Royal College of Surgeons in Ireland, and the Institute of Biopharmaceutical Sciences under the Higher Education Authority's Programme for Research in Third Level Institutions (JLW), a Canadian Research Chair in Schizophrenia, the Canadian Institute of Health Research and the Ian Douglas Bebensee Foundation (S.K. and G.J.R.).

References

Abi-Dargham, A., Rodenhiser, J., Printz, D. *et al.* (2000) Increased baseline occupancy of D_2 receptors by dopamine in schizophrenia. *Proceedings of the National Academy of Sciences of the USA* 97, 8104–8109.

Akunne, H.C., Zoski, K.T., Davis, M.D. *et al.* (2000) PD 158771, a potential antipsychotic agent with D2/D3 partial agonist and 5-HT1A agonist actions. I. Neurochemical effects. *Neuropharmacology* 39, 1197–1210.

Allison, D.B., Mentore, J.L., Heo, M. *et al.* (1999) Antipsychotic-induced weight gain: a comprehensive research synthesis. *American Journal of Psychiatry* 156, 1686–1696.

Arnsten, A.F.T., Murphy, B. & Merchant, K. (2000) The selective dopamine D_4 receptor antagonist, PNU-101387G, prevents stress-induced cognitive deficits in monkeys. *Neuropsychopharmacology* 23, 405–410.

Arnt, J. & Skarsfeldt, D. (1998) Do novel antipsychotics have similar pharmacological characteristics? A review of the evidence. *Neuropsychopharmacology* 18, 63–101.

Arranz, M.J., Munro, J., Birkett, J. *et al.* (2000) Pharmacogenetic prediction of clozapine response. *Lancet* 355, 1615–1616.

Arvanitis, L.A. & Miller, B.G. (1997) Multiple fixed doses of 'Seroquel' (quetiapine) in patients with acute exacerbation of schizophrenia: a comparison with haloperidol and placebo. *Biological Psychiatry* 42, 233–246.

Ashby, C.R. & Wang, R.Y. (1996) Pharmacological actions of the atypical antipsychotic drug clozapine: a review. *Synapse* 24, 349–394.

Bakshi, V.P. & Geyer, M.A. (1995) Antagonism of phencyclidine-induced deficits in prepulse inhibition by the putative atypical antipsychotic olanzapine. *Psychopharmacology* 122, 198–201.

Baldessarini, R.J., Cohen, B.M. & Teicher, M.H. (1988) Significance of neuroleptic dose and plasma level in the pharmacological treatment of psychoses. *Archives of General Psychiatry* 45, 79–91.

Barnas, C., Tauscher, J., Kufferle, B. *et al.* (1997) I IBZM SPECT imaging of dopamine-2 receptors in psychotic patients treated with zotepine. *European Neuropsychopharmacology* 7 (Suppl. 2), S215.

Beasley, C.M., Tollefson, G., Tran, P. et al. (1996) Olanzapine versus placebo and haloperidol: acute phase results of the North American double-blind olanzapine trial. Neuropsychopharmacology 14, 111–123.

Beasley, C.M., Tollefson, G.D. & Tran, P.V. (1997a) Safety of olanzapine. Journal of Clinical Psychiatry 58, 13–17.

Beasley, C.M., Tollefson, G.D. & Tran, P.V. (1997b) Efficacy of olanzapine: an overview of pivotal clinical trials. Journal of Clinical Psychiatry 58, 7–12.

Beasley, C.M., Dellva, M.A., Tamura, R.N. et al. (1999) Randomised double-blind comparison of the incidence of tardive dyskinesia in patients with schizophrenia during long-term treatment with olanzapine or haloperidol. British Journal of Psychiatry 174, 23–30.

Bench, C.J., Lammertsma, A.A., Grasby, P.M. et al. (1996) The time course of binding to striatal dopamine D_2 receptors by the neuroleptic ziprasidone (CP-88,059-01) determined by positron emission tomography. Psychopharmacology 124, 141–147.

Benedetti, F., Cavallaro, R. & Smeraldi, E. (1999) Olanzapine-induced neutropenia after clozapine-induced neutropenia. Lancet 354, 567.

Bigliani, V., Mulligan, R.S., Acton, P.D. et al. (2000) Striatal and temporal cortical D_2/D_3 receptor occupancy by olanzapine and sertindole in vivo: a (^{125}I) epidepride single photon emission tomography (SPECT) study. Psychopharmacology 150, 132–140.

Blake, T.-J., Tillery, C.E. & Reynolds, G.P. (1998) Antipsychotic drug affinities at α2-adrenoceptor subtypes in postmortem human brain. Journal of Psychopharmacology 12, 151–154.

Bollini, P., Pampallona, S., Orza, M.J., Adams, M.E. & Chalmers, T.C. (1994) Antipsychotic drugs: is more worse? A meta-analysis of the published randomized control trials. Psychological Medicine 24, 307–316.

Borison, R.L., Arvanitis, L.A. & Miller, B.G. (1996) ICI 204,636, an atypical antipsychotic: efficacy and safety in a multicenter, placebo-controlled trial in patients with schizophrenia. Journal of Clinical Psychopharmacology 16, 158–169.

Boulay, D., Depoortere, R., Perrault, G. et al. (1999a) Dopamine D_2 receptor knock-out mice are insensitive to the hypolocomotor and hypothermic effects of dopamine D_2/D_3 receptor agonists. Neuropharmacology 38, 1389–1393.

Boulay, D., Depoortere, R., Rosstene, W. et al. (1999b) Dopamine D_3 receptor agonists produce similar decreases in body temperature and locomotor activity in D_3 knock-out and wild type mice. Neuropharmacology 38, 555–565.

Bymaster, F.P., Calligaro, D.O., Falcone, J.F. et al. (1996) Radioreceptor binding profile of the atypical antipsychotic olanzapine. Neuropsychopharmacology 14, 87–96.

Carlsson, A. & Lindqvist, A. (1963) Effect of chlorpromazine or haloperidol on formation of 3-methoxytyramine in mouse brain. Acta Pharmacologica et Toxicologica 20, 140–144.

Carpenter, W.T., Conley, R. & Kirkpatrick, B. (2000a) On schizophrenia and new generation drugs. Neuropsychopharmacology 22, 660–661.

Carpenter, W.T., Breier, A., Buchanan, R.W. et al. (2000b) Mazindol treatment of negative symptoms. Neuropsychopharmacology 23, 365–374.

Carson, W.H., Ali, M., Dunbar, G., Ingenito, A. & Saha, A.R. (2001) A double-blind, placebo-controlled trial of aripiprazole and haloperidol. Schizophrenia Research 49, 221–222.

Casey, D.E. (1996) Behavioral effects of sertindole, risperidone, clozapine and haloperidol in cebus monkeys. Psychopharmacology 124, 134–140.

Chouinard, G., Jones, B., Remington, G. et al. (1993) A Canadian multicenter placebo-controlled study of fixed doses of risperidone and haloperidol in the treatment of chronic schizophrenic patients. Journal of Clinical Psychopharmacology 13, 25–40.

Chung, Y.-C. & Eun, H.-B. (1998) Hyperprolactinemia induced by risperidone. International Journal of Neuropsychopharmacology 1, 93–94.

Clifford, J.J. & Waddington, J.L. (2000) Topographically based search for an 'ethogram' among a series of novel D_4 dopamine receptor agonists and antagonists. Neuropsychopharmacology 22, 538–544.

Colonna, L., Saleem, P., Dondey-Nouvel, L.D. & Rein, W. (2000) Long-term safety and efficacy of amisulpride in subchronic or chronic schizophrenia. International Clinical Psychopharmacology 15, 13–22.

Cooper, S.J., Tweed, J., Raniwalla, J., Butler, A. & Welch, C. (2000a) A placebo-controlled comparison of zotepine versus chlorpromazine in patients with acute exacerbation of schizophrenia. Acta Psychiatrica Scandinavica 101, 218–225.

Cooper, S.J., Butler, A., Tweed, J., Welch, C. & Raniwalla, J. (2000b) Zotepine in the prevention of recurrence: a randomised, double-blind placebo-controlled study for chronic schizophrenia. Psychopharmacology 150, 237–243.

Coppens, H.J., Slooff, C.J., Paans, A.M. et al. (1991) High central D_2-dopamine receptor occupancy as assessed with positron emission tomography in medicated but therapy-resistant schizophrenic patients. Biological Psychiatry 29, 629–634.

Corbett, R., Camacho, F., Woods, A.T. et al. (1995) Antipsychotic agents antagonize non-competitive N-methyl-D-aspartate antagonist-induced behaviors. Psychopharmacology 120, 67–74.

Coukell, A.J., Spencer, C.M. & Benfield, P. (1996) Amisulpride: a review of its pharmacodynamic and pharmacokinetic properties and therapeutic efficacy in the management of schizophrenia. CNS Drugs 6, 237–256.

Coulouvrat, D. & Dondey-Nouvel, L. (1999) Safety of amisulpride (Solian): a review of 11 clinical studies. International Clinical Psychopharmacology 14, 209–218.

Coward, D.M., Imperato, A., Urwyler, S. & White, T.G. (1989) Biochemical and behavioural properties of clozapine. Psychopharmacology 99, S6–S12.

Cucchiaro, J., Nann-Vernotica, R., Lasser, T. et al. (2001) A randomised, double-blind multicenter phase III study of iloperidone versus haloperidol and placebo in patients with schizophrenia or schizoaffective disorder. Schizophrenia Research 49, 223–224.

Curtis, V.A. & Kerwin, R.W. (1995) A risk–benefit assessment of risperidone in schizophrenia. Drug Safety 12, 139–145.

Daniel, D.G., Wozniak, P., Mack, R.J. & McCarthy, B.G. (1998) Long-term efficacy and safety comparison of sertindole and haloperidol in the treatment of schizophrenia. Psychopharmacology Bulletin 34, 61–69.

Danion, J.M., Rein, W. & Fleurot, O. (1999) Improvement of schizophrenic patients with primary negative symptoms treated with amisulpride. American Journal of Psychiatry 156, 610–616.

Davis, K.L., Kahn, R.S., Ko, G. & Davidson, M. (1991) Dopamine in schizophrenia: a review and reconceptualization. American Journal of Psychiatry 148, 1474–1486.

Davis, R. & Markham, A. (1997) Ziprasidone. CNS Drugs 8, 153–162.

De Beaurepaire, R., Labelle, Naber, D. et al. (1995) An open trial of the D_1 antagonist SCH 39166 in six cases of acute psychotic states. Psychopharmacology 121, 323–327.

Dellva, M.A., Tran, P., Tollefson, G.D., Wentley, A.L. & Beasley, C.M. (1997) Standard olanzapine versus placebo and ineffective-dose olanzapine in the maintenance treatment of schizophrenia. Psychiatric Services 48, 1571–1577.

Den Boer, J.A., van Megen, H.J.G.M., Fleischhacker, W.W. et al. (1995)

Differential effects of the D_1-DA receptor antagonist SCH 39166 on positive and negative symptoms of schizophrenia. *Psychopharmacology* **121**, 317–322.

Deniker, P. (1983) Discovery of the clinical uses of neuroleptics. In: *Discoveries in Pharmacology*, Vol. 1 (eds M.J. Parnham & J. Bruinvels), pp. 163–180. Elsevier, Amsterdam.

Depoortere, R., Perrault, G. & Sanger, D.J. (1997) Potentiation of pre-pulse inhibition of the startle reflex in rats: pharmacological evaluation of the procedure as a model for detecting antipsychotic activity. *Psychopharmacology* **132**, 366–374.

Dickson, R.A. & Glazer, W.M. (1999) Hyperprolactinemia and male sexual dysfunction. *Journal of Clinical Psychiatry* **60**, 125.

Duncan, G.E., Zorn, S. & Lieberman, J.A. (1999) Mechanisms of typical and atypical antipsychotic drug actions in relation to dopamine and NMDA receptor hypofunction hypotheses of schizophrenia. *Molecular Psychiatry* **4**, 418–428.

Dunn, C.J. & Fitton, A. (1996) Sertindole. *CNS Drugs* **5**, 224–230.

Dursun, S.M., Gardner, D.M., Bird, D.C. & Flinn, J. (1999) Olanzapine for patients with treatment-resistant schizophrenia: a naturalistic case-series outcome study. *Canadian Journal of Psychiatry* **44**, 701–704.

Ehmann, T.S., Delva, J.J. & Beninger. R.J. (1987) Flupenthixol in chronic schizophrenic inpatients: a controlled comparison with haloperidol. *Journal of Clinical Psychopharmacology* **3**, 173–175.

Ellenbroek, B.A. & Cools, A.R. (2000) Animal models for the negative symptoms of schizophrenia. *Behavioural Pharmacology* **11**, 223–233.

Ellenbroek, B.A., Lubbers, L.J. & Cools, A.R. (1996) Activity of 'Seroquel' (ICI 204,636) in animal models for atypical properties of antipsychotics: a comparison with clozapine. *Neuropsychopharmacology* **15**, 406–416.

Emsley, R.A., Raniwalla, J., Bailey, P.J. & Jones, A.M. (2000) A comparison of the effects of quetiapine ('Seroquel') and haloperidol in schizophrenic patients with a history of and a demonstrated, partial response to conventional antipsychotic treatment. *International Clinical Psychopharmacology* **15**, 121–131.

Farde, L. Nordstrom, A.L., Wiesel, F.A. et al. (1992) Positron emission tomographic analysis of central D_1 and D_2 dopamine receptor occupancy in patients treated with classical neuroleptics and clozapine. Relation to extrapyramidal side-effects. *Archives of General Psychiatry* **49**, 538–544.

Farde, L., Nordstrom, A.L., Nyberg, S., Halldin, C. & Sedvall, G. (1994) D_1-, D_2-, and 5-HT$_2$-receptor occupancy in clozapine-treated patients. *Journal of Clinical Psychiatry* **55** (Suppl. B), 67–69.

Farde, L., Suhara, T., Nyberg, S. et al. (1997) A PET-study of (^{11}C)FLB 457 binding to extrastriatal D_2-dopamine receptors in healthy subjects and antipsychotic drug-treated patients. *Psychopharmacology* **133**, 396–404.

Fenton, W.S., Hibbeln, J. & Knable, M. (1999) Essential fatty acids, lipid membrane abnormalities, and the diagnosis and treatment of schizophrenia. *Biological Psychiatry* **47**, 8–21.

Fenton, W.S., Dickerson, F., Boronow, J., Hibbeln, J.R. & Knable, M. (2001) A placebo-controlled trial of omega-3 fatty acid (ethyl eicosapentaenoic acid) supplementation for residual symptoms and cognitive impairment in schizophrenia. *American Journal of Psychiatry* **158**, 2071–2074.

Finkel, B., Lerner, A., Oyffe, I. et al. (1998) Olanzapine treatment in patients with typical and atypical neuroleptic-associated agranulocytosis. *International Clinical Psychopharmacology* **13**, 133–135.

Fischman, A.J., Bonab, A.A., Babich, J.W. et al. (1996) Positron emission tomographic analysis of central 5-hydroxytryptamine$_2$ receptor occupancy in healthy volunteers treated with the novel antipsychotic agent, ziprasidone. *Journal of Pharmacology and Experimental Therapeutics* **279**, 939–947.

Fitzgerald, P. & Seeman, P. (1999) Neuroreceptor studies in the elderly: potential for understanding. In: *Late-Onset Schizophrenia* (eds R. Howard & D. Castle), pp. 205–216. Biomedical Publishing, Wrightson, Philadelphia.

Fleischhacker, W.W. & Hummer, M. (1997) Drug treatment of schizophrenia in the 1990s: achievements and future possibilities in optimising outcomes. *Drugs* **53**, 915–929.

Fulton, B. & Goa, K.L. (1995) ICI-204,636: an initial appraisal of its pharmacological properties and clinical potential in the treatment of schizophrenia. *CNS Drugs* **4**, 68–78.

Gallhofer, B., Bauer, U., Lis, S., Krieger, S. & Gruppe, H. (1996) Cognitive dysfunction in schizophrenia: comparison of treatment with atypical antipsychotic agents and conventional neuroleptic drugs. *European Neuropsychopharmacology Supplement* **6**, 13–20.

Ganguli, R. (1999) Weight gain associated with antipsychotic drugs. *Journal of Clinical Psychiatry* **60**, 20–24.

Gazi, L., Bobirnac, I., Danzeisen, M. et al. (1999) Receptor density as a factor governing the efficacy of the dopamine D_4 receptor ligands, L-745,870 and U-101958 at human recombinant $D_{4.4}$ receptors expressed in CHO cells. *British Journal of Pharmacology* **128**, 613–620.

Geddes, J., Freemantle, N., Harrison, P. & Bebbington, P. (2000) Atypical antipsychotics in the treatment of schizophrenia: systematic overview and meta-regression analysis. *British Medical Journal* **321**, 1371–1376.

Gerlach, J. (2000) Atypical antipsychotics: an inspiring but confusing concept. *Psychopharmacology* **148**, 1–2.

Goff, D.C., Posever, T., Herz, L. et al. (1998) An exploratory haloperidol-controlled dose-finding study of ziprasidone in hospitalized patients with schizophrenia or schizoaffective disorder. *Journal of Clinical Psychopharmacology* **18**, 296–304.

Goldstein, J.M. & Arvanitis, L.A. (1995) ICI 204,636 (Seroquel): a dibenzothiazepine atypical antipsychotic: review of preclinical pharmacology and highlights of phase II clinical trials. *CNS Drug Reviews* **1**, 50–73.

Goldstein, L.E., Sporn, J., Brown, S. et al. (1999) New-onset diabetes mellitus and diabetic ketoacidosis associated with olanzapine treatment. *Psychosomatics* **40**, 438–443.

Grace, A.A., Bunney, B.S., Moore, H. & Todd, C.L. (1997) Dopamine-cell depolarization block as a model for the therapeutic actions of antipsychotic drugs. *Trends in Neurosciences* **20**, 31–37.

Green, M.F., Marshall, B.D., Wirshing, W.C. et al. (1997) Does risperidone improve verbal working memory in treatment-resistant schizophrenia? *American Journal of Psychiatry* **154**, 799–804.

Green, M.F., Kern, R.S., Braff, D.L. & Mintz, J. (2000) Neurocognitive deficits and functional outcome in schizophrenia: are we measuring the 'right stuff'? *Schizophrenia Bulletin* **26**, 119–136.

Hagg, S., Spigset, O. & Soderstrom, T.G. (2000) Association of venous thromboembolism and clozapine. *Lancet* **355**, 1155–1156.

Hamilton, S.H., Revicki, D.A., Genduso, L.A. & Beasley, C.M. (1998) Olanzapine versus placebo and haloperidol: quality of life and efficacy results of the North American double-blind trial. *Neuropsychopharmacology* **18**, 41–49.

He, H. & Richardson, J.S. (1995) A pharmacological, pharmacokinetic and clinical overview of risperidone, a new antipsychotic that blocks serotonin 5-HT$_2$ and dopamine D_2 receptors. *International Clinical Psychopharmacology* **10**, 19–30.

Heresco-Levy, U. (2000) N-Methyl-D-asparate (NMDA) receptor-based treatment approaches in schizophrenia: the first decade. *International Journal of Neuropsychopharmacology* **3**, 243–258.

Hertel, P., Fagerquist, M.V. & Svensson, T.H. (1999) Enhanced cortical dopamine output and antipsychotic-like effects of raclopride by α_2 adrenoceptor blockade. *Science* **286**, 105–107.

Higgins, G.A. (1998) From rodents to recovery: development of animal models of schizophrenia. *CNS Drugs* **9**, 59–68.

Hippius, H. (1989) The history of clozapine. *Psychopharmacology* **99**, S3–S5.

Hirsch, S.R., Link, C.G.G., Goldstein, J.M. & Arvanitis, L.A. (1996) ICI 204,636: a new atypical antipsychotic drug. *British Journal of Psychiatry* **168** (Suppl. 29), 45–56.

Hrib, N.J. (2000) The dopamine D_4 receptor: a controversial therapeutic target. *Drugs of the Future* **25**, 587–611.

Ipsen, M., Zhang, Y., Dragsted, J., Han, C. & Mulvany, M.J. (1997) The antipsychotic drug sertindole is a specific inhibitor of alpha 1A-adrenoceptors in rat mesenteric small arteries. *European Journal of Pharmacology* **336**, 29–35.

Janssen, P.A., Niemegeers, C.J., Awouters, F. *et al.* (1988) Pharmacology of risperidone (R 64,766), a new antipsychotic with serotonin-S2 and dopamine-D_2 antagonistic properties. *Journal of Pharmacology and Experimental Therapeutics* **244**, 685–693.

Jentsch, J.D. & Roth, R.H. (1999) The neuropsychopharmacology of phencyclidine: from NMDA receptor hypofunction to the dopamine hypothesis of schizophrenia. *Neuropsychopharmacology* **20**, 201–225.

Jentsch, J.D., Taylor, J.R., Redmond, D.E. *et al.* (1999) Dopamine D_4 receptor antagonist reversal of subchronic phencyclidine-induced object retrieval/detour deficits in monkeys. *Psychopharmacology* **142**, 78–84.

Jeste, D.V., Okamoto, A., Napolitano, J., Kane, J.M. & Martinez, R.A. (2000) Low incidence of persistent tardive dyskinesia in elderly patients with dementia treated with risperidone. *American Journal of Psychiatry* **157**, 1150–1155.

Johnstone, E.C., Crow, T.J., Frith, C.D., Carney, M.W. & Price, J.S. (1978) Mechanism of the antipsychotic effect in the treatment of acute schizophrenia. *Lancet* **1**, 848–851.

Joy, C.B., Mumby-Croft, R. & Joy, L.A. (2002) Polyunsaturated fatty acid (fish or evening primrose oil) for schizophrenia (Cochrane Review). In: *The Cochrane Library, Issue 2*. Update Software, Oxford.

Kane, J.M. (1999) Pharmacologic treatment of schizophrenia. *Biological Psychiatry* **46**, 1396–1408.

Kane, J., Honigfeld, G., Singer, J. *et al.* (1988) Clozapine for the treatment-resistant schizophrenic. *Archives of General Psychiatry* **45**, 789–796.

Kapur, S. (1998) A new framework for investigating antipsychotic action in humans: lessons from PET imaging. *Molecular Psychiatry* **3**, 135–140.

Kapur, S. (2000) Receptor occupancy by antipsychotics: concepts and findings. In: *Neurotransmitter Receptors in Actions of Antipsychotics* (ed. M.S. Lidow), pp. 163–176. CRC Press, London.

Kapur, S. & Remington, G. (1996) Serotonin–dopamine interaction and its relevance to schizophrenia. *American Journal of Psychiatry* **153**, 466–476.

Kapur, S. & Seeman, P. (2000) Antipsychotic agents differ in how fast they come off the dopamine D_2 receptors: implications for atypical antipsychotic action. *Journal of Psychiatry and Neuroscience* **25**, 161–166.

Kapur, S., Remington, G., Zipursky, R.B., Wilson, A.A. & Houle, S. (1995) The D_2 dopamine receptor occupancy of risperidone and its relationship to extrapyramidal symptoms: a PET study. *Life Sciences* **57**, L103–L107.

Kapur, S., Remington, G., Jones, C. *et al.* (1996) High levels of dopamine D_2 receptor occupancy with low-dose haloperidol treatment: a PET study. *American Journal of Psychiatry* **153**, 948–950.

Kapur, S., Zipursky, R.B., Remington, G. *et al.* (1998) 5-HT$_2$ and D_2 receptor occupancy of olanzapine in schizophrenia: a PET investigation. *American Journal of Psychiatry* **55**, 921–928.

Kapur, S., Zipursky, R.B. & Remington, G. (1999) Clinical and theoretical implications of 5-HT$_2$ and D_2 receptor occupancy of clozapine, risperidone, and olanzapine in schizophrenia. *American Journal of Psychiatry* **156**, 286–293.

Kapur, S., Zipursky, R., Jones, C., Remington, G. & Houle, S. (2000a) Relationship between dopamine D_2 occupancy, clinical response, and side effects: a double-blind PET study of first-episode schizophrenia. *American Journal of Psychiatry* **157**, 514–520.

Kapur, S., Zipursky, R., Remington, G. & Seeman, P. (2000b) Fast koff at the dopamine D_2 receptor (not high affinity at other receptors) is the key to clozapine's uniqueness and atypical antipsychotic activity. *International Journal of Neuropsychopharmacology* **3** (Suppl. 1), S95.

Kapur, S., Zipursky, R., Jones, C. *et al.* (2000c) A positron emission tomography study of quetiapine in schizophrenia: a preliminary finding of an antipsychotic effect with only transiently high dopamine D_2 receptor occupancy. *Archives of General Psychiatry* **57**, 553–559.

Karle, J., Clemmesen, L., Hansen, L. *et al.* (1995) NNC 01-0687, a selective dopamine D_1 receptor antagonist, in the treatment of schizophrenia. *Psychopharmacology* **121**, 328–329.

Karlsson, P., Smith, L., Farde, L. *et al.* (1995) Lack of apparent antipsychotic effect of the D_1-dopamine receptor antagonist SCH 39166 in acutely ill schizophrenic patients. *Psychopharmacology* **121**, 309–316.

Kasper, S. (2000) Review of quetiapine and its clinical applications in schizophrenia. *Expert Opinion on Pharmacotherapy* **1**, 783–801.

Kasper, S., Tauscher, J., Kufferle, B. *et al.* (1998) Sertindole and dopamine D_2 receptor occupancy in comparison to risperidone, clozapine and haloperidol: a ^{123}I-IBZM SPECT study. *Psychopharmacology* **136**, 367–373.

Kasper, S., Hale, A., Azorin, J.M. & Moller, H.J. (1999) Benefit-risk evaluation of olanzapine, risperidone and sertindole in the treatment of schizophrenia. *European Archives of Psychiatry and Clinical Neuroscience* **249** (Suppl. 2), 12–14.

Kebabian, J.W. & Calne, D.B. (1979) Multiple receptors for dopamine. *Nature* **277**, 93–96.

Keck, P., Buffenstein, A., Ferguson, J. *et al.* (1998) Ziprasidone 40 and 120 mg/day in the acute exacerbation of schizophrenia and schizoaffective disorder: a 4-week placebo-controlled trial. *Psychopharmacology* **140**, 173–184.

Keefe, R.S.E., Silva, S.G., Perkins, D.O. & Lieberman, J.A. (1999) The effects of atypical antipsychotc drugs on neurocognitive impairment in schizophrenia: a review and meta-analysis. *Schizophrenia Bulletin* **25**, 201–222.

Kehne, J.H., Baron, B.M., Carr, A.A. *et al.* (1996) Preclinical characterization of the potential of the putative atypical antipsychotic MDL 100,907 as a potent 5-HT$_{2A}$ antagonist with a favorable CNS safety profile. *Journal of Pharmacology and Experimental Therapeutics* **277**, 968–981.

Kilian, J.G., Kerr, K., Lawrence, C. & Celermajer, D.S. (1999) Myocarditis and cardiomyopathy associated with clozapine. *Lancet* **354**, 1841–1845.

Kinon, B.J. & Lieberman, J.A. (1996) Mechanisms of action of atypical antipsychotic drugs: a critical analysis. *Psychopharmacology* **124**, 2–34.

Kirkpatrick, B., Kopelowicz, A., Buchanan, R.W. & Carpenter, W.T. (2000) Assessing the efficacy of treatments for the deficit syndrome of schizophrenia. *Neuropsychopharmacology* **22**, 303–310.

Kitaichi, K., Yamada, K., Hasegawa, T., Furukawa, H. & Nabeshima, T. (1994) Effects of risperidone on phencyclidine-induced behaviors: comparison with haloperidol and ritanserin. *Japanese Journal of Pharmacology* 66, 181–189.

Kitayama, H., Kiuchi, K., Nejima, J. *et al.* (1999) Long-term treatment with antipsychotic drugs in conventional doses prolonged QTc dispersion, but did not increase ventricular tachyarrhythmias in patients with schizophrenia in the absence of cardiac disease. *European Journal of Clinical Pharmacology* 55, 259–262.

Kramer, M.S., Last, B., Getson, A. & Reines, S.A. (1997) The effects of a selective D_4 dopamine receptor antagonist (L-745,870) in acutely psychotic inpatients with schizophrenia. *Archives of General Psychiatry* 54, 567–572.

Laruelle, M. & Abi-Dargham, A. (1999) Dopamine as the wind of the psychotic fire: new evidence from brain imaging studies. *Journal of Psychopharmacology* 13, 358–371.

Lawler, C.P., Prioleau, C., Lewis, M.M. *et al.* (1999) Interactions of the novel antipsychotic aripiprazole (OPC-14597) with dopamine and serotonin receptor subtypes. *Neuropsychopharmacology* 20, 612–627.

Lemmens, P., Brecher, M. & Van Baelen, B. (1999) A combined analysis of double-blind studies with risperidone vs. placebo and other antipsychotic agents: factors associated with extrapyramidal symptoms. *Acta Psychiatrica Scandinavica* 99, 160–170.

Leucht, S., Pitschel-Walz, G., Abraham, D. & Kissling, W. (1999) Efficacy and extrapyramidal side-effects of the new antipsychotics olanzapine, quetiapine, risperidone and sertindole compared to conventional antipsychotics and placebo: a meta-analysis of randomized controlled trials. *Schizophrenia Research* 35, 51–68.

Levant, B. (1997) The D_3 dopamine receptor: neurobiology and potential clinical relevance. *Pharmacological Reviews* 49, 231–252.

Leysen, J.E. (2000) Receptor profile of antipsychotics. In: *Atypical Antipsychotics* (eds B.A. Ellenbroek & A.R. Cools), pp. 57–81. Birkhauser, Basle.

Lidow, M.S., Williams, G.V. & Goldman-Rakic, P.S. (1998) The cerebral cortex: a case for a common site of action of antipsychotics. *Trends in Pharmacological Sciences* 19, 136–140.

Lidsky, T.I. (1995) Re-evaluation of the mesolimbic hypothesis of antipsychotic drug action. *Schizophrenia Bulletin* 21, 67–74.

Lindenmayer, J.P. & Patel, R. (1999) Olanzapine-induced ketoacidosis with diabetes mellitus. *American Journal of Psychiatry* 156, 1471.

Lipska, B.K. & Weinberger, D.R. (2000) To model a psychiatric disorder in animals: schizophrenia as a reality test. *Neuropsychopharmacology* 23, 223–239.

Litman, R.E., Su, T.P., Potter, W.Z., Hong, W.W. & Pickar, D. (1996) Idazoxan and response to typical neuroleptics in treatment-resistant schizophrenia. *British Journal of Psychiatry* 168, 571–579.

Liu, I.S.C., George, S.R. & Seeman, P. (2000) The human $D_{2Longer}$ receptor has a high-affinity state and inhibits adenylyl cyclase. *Molecular Brain Research* 77, 281–284.

Loo, H., Poirier-Littre, M.-F., Theron, M., Rein, W. & Fleurot, O. (1997) Amisulpride versus placebo in the medium-term treatment of the negative symptoms of schizophrenia. *British Journal of Psychiatry* 170, 18–22.

McEvoy, J.P., Hogarty, G.E. & Steingard, S. (1991) Optimal dose of neuroleptic in acute schizophrenia: a controlled study of the neuroleptic threshold and higher haloperidol dose. *Archives of General Psychiatry* 48, 739–745.

McNamara, F., Clifford, J. Tigh, O. *et al.* (2002) Phenotypic ethologically-based resolution of spoutaneous and D_2-like vs. D_1-like agonist-induced behavioural topography in mice with congenic D_3 dopamine receptor 'knockout'. *Synapse* 46, 19–31.

Marder, S.R. & Meibach, R.C. (1994) Risperidone in the treatment of schizophrenia. *American Journal of Psychiatry* 151, 825–835.

Martinot, J.L., Pailliere-Martinot, M.L., Poirier, M.F. *et al.* (1996) *In vivo* characteristics of dopamine D_2 receptor occupancy by amisulpride in schizophrenia. *Psychopharmacology* 124, 154–158.

Mattes, J.A. (1997) Risperidone: how good is the evidence for efficacy? *Schizophrenia Bulletin* 23, 155–161.

Meltzer, H.Y. (1999) The role of serotonin in antipsychotic drug action. *Neuropsychopharmacology* 21, 106S–115S.

Meltzer, H.Y. (2000) An atypical compound by any other name is still a . . . *Psychopharmacology* 148, 16–19.

Meltzer, H.Y., Matsubara, S. & Lee, J.-C. (1989) Classification of typical and atypical antipsychotic drugs on the basis of dopamine D_1, D_2 and serotonin$_2$ pKi values. *Journal of Pharmacology and Experimental Therapeutics* 251, 238–246.

Migler, B.M., Warawa, E.J. & Malick, J.B. (1993) Seroquel: behavioral effects in conventional and novel tests for atypical antipsychotic drug. *Psychopharmacology* 112, 299–307.

Millan, M.J., Gobert, A., Newman-Tancredi, A. *et al.* (1998) S 16924 (R)-2-{1-[2-(2,3-dihydro-benzol[1,4]dioxin-5-yloxy)-ethyl]-pyrrolidin-3yl}-1-(4-fluoro-phenyl)-ethanone), a novel, potential antipsychotic with marked serotonin $(5-HT)_{1A}$ agonist properties. I. Receptorial and neurochemical profile in comparison with clozapine and haloperidol. *Journal of Pharmacology and Experimental Therapeutics* 286, 1341–1355.

Millan, M.J., Dekeyne, A., Rivet, J.-M. *et al.* (2000) S33084, a novel, potent, selective, and competitive antagonist at dopamine D_3-receptors. II. Functional and behavioral profile compared with GR218,231 and L741,626. *Journal of Pharmacology and Experimental Therapeutics* 293, 1063–1073.

Missale, C., Nash, S.R., Robinson, S.W., Jaber, M. & Caron, M.G. (1998) Dopamine receptors: from structure to function. *Physiological Reviews* 78, 189–225.

Molitch, M. (1995) Prolactin. In: *The Pituitary* (ed. M. Molitch), pp. 136–183. Blackwell, Oxford.

Moller, H.-J., Muller, H., Borison, R.L., Schooler, N.R. & Chouinard, G. (1995) A path-analytical approach to differentiate between direct and indirect drug effects on negative symptoms in schizophrenic patients: a re-evaluation of the North American risperidone study. *European Archives of Psychiatry and Clinical Neuroscience* 245, 45–49.

Moore, H., West, A.R. & Grace, A.A. (1999) The regulation of forebrain dopamine transmission: relevance to the pathophysiology and psychopathology of schizophrenia. *Biological Psychiatry* 46, 40–55.

Moore, N.A., Tye, N.C., Axton, M.S. & Risius, F.C. (1992) The behavioral pharmacology of olanzapine, a novel 'atypical' antipsychotic agent. *Journal of Pharmacology and Experimental Therapeutics* 262, 545–551.

Muller, M.J., Grunder, G., Wetzel, H. *et al.* (1999) Antipsychotic effects and tolerability of the sigma ligand EMD 57445 (panamesine) and its metabolites in acute schizophrenia: an open clinical trial. *Psychiatry Research* 89, 275–280.

Naumann, R., Felber, W., Heilemann, H. & Reuster, T. (1999) Olanzapine-induced agranulocytosis. *Lancet* 354, 566–567.

Needham, P.L., Atkinson, J., Skill, M.J. & Heal, D.J. (1996) Zotepine: preclinical tests predict antipsychotic efficacy and an atypical profile. *Psychopharmacology Bulletin* 32, 123–128.

Newman-Tancredi, A., Chaput, C., Verriele, L. & Millan, J.J. (1996) Clozapine is a partial agonist at cloned, human serotonin $5-HT_{1A}$ receptors. *Neuropharmacology* 35, 119–121.

Niemegeers, C.J.E. & Janssen, P.A.J. (1978) A systematic study of the pharmacological activities of dopamine antagonists. *Life Sciences* 24, 2201–2216.

Niznik, H.B., Sugamori, K.S., Clifford, J.J. & Waddington, J.L. (2002) D_1-like dopamine receptors: molecular biology and pharmacology. In: *Handbook of Experimental Pharmacology: Dopamine in the CNS* (ed. G. Di Chiara), pp. 121–158. Springer, Heidelberg.

Nordstrom, A.L. & Farde, L. (1998) Plasma prolactin and central D_2 receptor occupancy in antipsychotic drug-treated patients. *Journal of Clinical Psychopharmacology* 18, 305–310.

Nordstrom, A.L., Farde, L., Wiesel, F.A. *et al.* (1993) Central D_2-dopamine receptor occupancy in relation to antipsychotic drug effects: a double-blind PET study of schizophrenic patients. *Biological Psychiatry* 33, 227–235.

Nyberg, S., Farde, L., Halldin, C., Dahl, M.L. & Bertilsson, L. (1995) D_2 dopamine receptor occupancy during low-dose treatment with haloperidol decanoate. *American Journal of Psychiatry* 152, 173–178.

Nyberg, S., Nakashima, Y., Nordstrom, A.-L., Halldin, C. & Farde, L. (1996) Positron emission tomography of *in vivo* binding characteristics of atypical antipsychotic drugs: review of D_2 and $5-HT_2$ receptor occupancy studies and clinical response. *British Journal of Psychiatry* 168 (Suppl. 29), 40–44.

Peet, M., Glen, I. & Horrobin, D. (1999) *Phospholipid Spectrum Disorder in Psychiatry*. Marius Press, Carnforth.

Peet, M., Brind, J., Ramchand, C.N., Shah, S. & Vankar, G.K. (2001) Two double-blind placebo-controlled pilot studies of eicosapentaenoic acid in the treatment of schizophrenia. *Schizophrenia Research* 49, 243–251.

Perrault, G.H., Depoortere, R., Morel, E., Sanger, D.J. & Scatton, B. (1997) Psychopharmacological profile of amisulpride: an antipsychotic drug with presynaptic D_2/D_3 dopamine receptor antagonist activity and limbic selectivity. *Journal of Pharmacology and Experimental Therapeutics* 280, 73–82.

Peuskens, J. (1995) Risperidone in the treatment of patients with chronic schizophrenia: a multi-national, multi-centre, double-blind, parallel-group study versus haloperidol. *British Journal of Psychiatry* 166, 712–726.

Peuskens, J. & Link, C.G. (1997) A comparison of quetiapine and chlorpromazine in the treatment of schizophrenia. *Acta Psychiatrics Scandinavica* 96, 265–273.

Peuskens, J., Bech, P., Moller, H.-J. *et al.* (1999) Amisulpride vs. risperidone in the treatment of acute exacerbations of schizophrenia. *Psychiatry Research* 88, 107–117.

Pezawas, L., Quiner, S., Moertl, D. *et al.* (2000) Efficacy, cardiac safety and tolerability of sertindole: a drug surveillance study. *International Clinical Psychopharmacology* 15, 207–214.

Pilowsky, L.S., Busatto, G.F., Taylor, M. *et al.* (1996) Dopamine D_2 receptor occupancy *in vivo* by the novel atypical antipsychotic olanzapine: a ^{123}I IBZM single photon emission tomography (SPET) study. *Psychopharmacology* 124, 148–153.

Pilowsky, L.S., O'Connell, P., Davies, N. *et al.* (1997a) *In vivo* effects on striatal dopamine D_2 receptor binding by the novel atypical antipsychotic drug sertindole: a ^{123}I IBZM single photon emission tomography (SPET) study. *Psychopharmacology* 130, 152–158.

Pilowsky, L.S., Mulligan, R.S., Acton, P.D. *et al.* (1997b) Limbic selectivity of clozapine. *Lancet* 350, 490–491.

Porter, J.H. & Strong, S.E. (1996) Discriminative stimulus control with olanzapine: generalization to the atypical antipsychotic clozapine. *Psychopharmacology* 128, 216–219.

Prakash, A. & Lamb, H.M. (1998) Zotepine: a review of its pharmacodynamic and pharmacokinetic properties and therapeutic efficacy in the management of schizophrenia. *CNS Drugs* 9, 153–175.

Pullen, R.H., Palermo, K.M. & Curtis, M.A. (1992) Determination of

an antipsychotic agent (ICI 204,636) and its 7-hydroxy metabolite in human plasma by high-performance liquid chromatography and gas chromatography-mass spectrometry. *Journal of Chromatography* 573, 49–57.

Purdon, S.E., Jones, B.D., Stip, E. *et al.* (2000) Neuropsychological change in early phase schizophrenia during 12 months of treatment with olanzapine, risperidone, or haloperidol. *Archives of General Psychiatry* 57, 249–258.

Rampe, D., Murawsky, M.K., Grau, J. & Lewis, E.W. (1998) The antipsychotic agent sertindole is a high affinity antagonist of the human cardiac potassium channel HERG. *Journal of Pharmacology and Experimental Therapeutics* 286, 788–793.

Reich, J. (1999) Use of high-dose olanzapine in refractory psychosis. *American Journal of Psychiatry* 156, 661.

Reilly, J.G., Ayis, S.A., Ferrier, I.N., Jones, S.J. & Thomas, S.H.L. (2000) QTc-interval abnormalities and psychotropic drug therapy in psychiatric patients. *Lancet* 355, 1048–1052.

Remington, G. & Kapur, S. (2000) Atypical antipsychotics: are some more atypical than others? *Psychopharmacology* 148, 3–15.

Remington, G., Kapur, S. & Zipursky, R.B. (1998) Pharmacotherapy of first-episode schizophrenia. *British Journal of Psychiatry* 172 (Suppl.), 66–70.

Reynolds, G.P., Cowey, L., Rossor, M.N. & Iversen, L.L. (1982) Thioridazine is not specific for limbic dopamine receptors. *Lancet* 2, 499–500.

Richelson, E. & Nelson, A. (1984) Antagonism by neuroleptics of neurotransmitter receptors of normal human brain *in vitro*. *European Journal of Pharmacology* 103, 197–204.

Rollema, H., Lu, Y., Schmidt, A.W. & Zorn, S.H. (1997) Clozapine increases dopamine release in prefrontal cortex by $5-HT_{1A}$ receptor activation. *European Journal of Pharmacology* 338, R3–R5.

Rosenheck, R., Dunn, L., Peszke, M. *et al.* (1999) Impact of clozapine on negative symptoms and on the deficit syndrome in refractory schizophrenia. *American Journal of Psychiatry* 156, 88–93.

Rowley, H.L., Needham, P.L., Kilpatrick, I.C. & Heal, D.J. (2000) A comparison of the acute effects of zotepine and other antipsychotics on rat cortical dopamine release, *in vivo*. *Naunyn-Schmiedeberg's Archives of Pharmacology* 361, 187–192.

Rubinstein, M., Phillips, T.J., Bunzow, J.R. *et al.* (1997) Mice lacking dopamine D_4 receptors are supersensitive to ethanol, cocaine, and methamphetamine. *Cell* 90, 991–1001.

Sams-Dodd, F. (1999) Phencyclidine in the social interaction test: an animal model of schizophrenia with face and predictive validity. *Reviews in the Neurosciences* 10, 59–90.

Sanchez, C., Arnt, J., Dragsted, N. *et al.* (1991) Neurochemical and *in vivo* pharmacological profile of sertindole, a limbic-selective neuroleptic compound. *Drug Development Research* 22, 239–250.

Sanger, T.M., Lieberman, J.A., Tohen, M. *et al.* (1999) Olanzapine versus haloperidol treatment in first-episode psychosis. *American Journal of Psychiatry* 156, 79–87.

Sax, K.W., Strakowski, S.M. & Keck, P.E. (1998) Attentional improvement following quetiapine fumarate treatment in schizophrenia. *Schizophrenia Research* 33, 151–155.

Schoemaker, H., Claustre, Y., Fage, D. *et al.* (1997) Neurochemical characteristics of amisulpride, an atypical dopamine D_2/D_3 receptor antagonist with both presynaptic and limbic selectivity. *Journal of Pharmacology and Experimental Therapeutics* 280, 83–97.

Schotte, A., Janssen, P.F., Gommeren, W. *et al.* (1996) Risperidone compared with new and reference antipsychotic drugs: *in vitro* and *in vivo* receptor binding. *Psychopharmacology* 124, 57–73.

Seeger, T.F., Seymour, P.A., Schmidt, A.W. *et al.* (1995) Ziprasidone (CP-88,059): a new antipsychotic with combined dopamine and serotonin receptor antagonist activity. *Journal of Pharmacology and Experimental Therapeutics* 275, 101–113.

Seeman, P. (1980) Brain dopamine receptors. *Pharmacological Reviews* 32, 229–313.

Seeman, P. (1992) Dopamine receptor sequences: therapeutic levels of neuroleptics occupy D_2 receptors, clozapine occupies D_4. *Neuropsychopharmacology* 7, 261–284.

Seeman, P. & Tallerico, T. (1998) Antipsychotic drugs which elicit little or no Parkinsonism bind more loosely than dopamine to brain D_2 receptors, yet occupy high levels of these receptors. *Molecular Psychiatry* 3, 123–134.

Seeman, P. & Tallerico, T. (1999) Rapid release of antipsychotic drugs from dopamine D_2 receptors: an explanation for low receptor occupancy and early clinical relapse upon withdrawal of clozapine or quetiapine. *American Journal of Psychiatry* 156, 876–884.

Seeman, P. & Ulpian, C. (1983) Neuroleptics have identical potencies in human brain limbic and putamen regions. *European Journal of Pharmacology* 94, 145–148.

Seeman, P., Corbett, R. & Van Tol, H.H.M. (1997) Atypical neuroleptics have low affinity for dopamine D_2 receptors or are selective for D_4 receptors. *Neuropsychopharmacology* 16, 93–110.

Seeman, P., Nam, D., Ulpian, C., Liu, I.S.C. & Tallerico, T. (2000) New dopamine receptor, $D_{2Longer}$, with unique TG splice site, in human brain. *Molecular Brain Research* 76, 132–141.

Shannon, H.E., Rasmussen, K., Bymaster, F.P. *et al.* (2000) Xanomeline, an M_1/M_4 preferring muscarinic cholinergic receptor agonist, produces antipsychotic-like activity in rats and mice. *Schizophrenia Research* 42, 249–259.

Sheitman, B.B., Lindgren, J.C., Early, J. & Sved, M. (1997) High-dose olanzapine for treatment-refractory schizophrenia. *American Journal of Psychiatry* 154, 1626.

Sheitman, B.B., Bird, P.M., Binz, W., Akinli, L. & Sanchez, C. (1999) Olanzapine-induced elevation of plasma triglyceride levels. *American Journal of Psychiatry* 156, 1471–1472.

Silvestri, S., Seeman, J.C., Negrte, S. *et al.* (1999) Dopamine D_2 upregulation and 5-HT_2 downregulation measured after neuroleptic withdrawal using PET. *Schizophrenia Research* 36, 247.

Simpson, G.M. & Lindenmayer, J.P. (1997) Extrapyramidal symptoms in patients treated with risperidone. *Journal of Clinical Psychopharmacology* 17, 194–201.

Simpson, G.M., Josiassen, R.C., Stanilla, J.K. *et al.* (1999) Double-blind study of clozapine dose–response in chronic schizophrenia. *American Journal of Psychiatry* 156, 1744–1750.

Small, J.G., Hirsch, S.R., Arvanitis, L.A., Miller, B.G. & Link, C.G. (1997) Quetiapine in patients with schizophrenia: a high- and low-dose double-blind comparison with placebo. *Archives of General Psychiatry* 54, 549–557.

Smith, D., Pantelis, C., McGrath, J., Tangas, C. & Copolov, D. (1997) Ocular abnormalities in chronic schizophrenia: clinical implications. *Australia and New Zealand Journal of Psychiatry* 31, 252–256.

Sokoloff, P., Martres, M.-P., Giros, B., Bouthenet, J.-L. & Schwartz, J.-C. (1992) The third dopamine receptor (D_3) as a novel target for antipsychotics. *Biochemical Pharmacology* 43, 659–666.

Speller, J.C., Barnes, T.R.E., Curson, D.A., Pantelis, C. & Alberts, J.L. (1997) One-year, low-dose neuroleptic study of in-patients with chronic schizophrenia characterised by persistent negative symptoms: amisulpride vs haloperidol. *British Journal of Psychiatry* 171, 564–568.

Sugamori, K.S., Hamadanizadeh, S.A., Scheideler, M.A. *et al.* (1998) Functional differentiation of multiple dopamine D_1-like receptors by NNC 01-0012. *Journal of Neurochemistry* 71, 1685–1693.

Swerdlow, N.R., Varty, G.B. & Geyer, M.A. (1998) Discrepant findings of clozapine effects on prepulse inhibition of startle: is it the route or the rat? *Neuropsychopharmacology* 18, 50–56.

Szewczak, M.R., Corbett, R., Rush, D.K. *et al.* (1995) The pharmacological profile of iloperidone, a novel atypical antipsychotic agent. *Journal of Pharmacology and Experimental Therapeutics* 274, 1404–1413.

Talvik-Lofti, M., Nyberg, S., Nordstrom, A.L. *et al.* (2000) High 5-HT_{2A} receptor occupancy in M100907-treated schizophrenic patients. *Psychopharmacology* 148, 400–403.

Tarazi, F.I. & Baldessarini, R.J. (1999) Dopamine D_4 receptors: significance for molecular psychiatry at the millennium. *Molecular Psychiatry* 4, 529–538.

Tollefson, G.D., Beasley, C.M., Tran, P.V. *et al.* (1997) Olanzapine versus haloperidol in the treatment of schizophrenia and schizoaffective and schizophreniform disorders: results of an international collaborative trial. *American Journal of Psychiatry* 154, 457–465.

Tollefson, G.D., Sanger, T.M., Lu, Y. & Thieme, M.E. (1998) Depressive signs and symptoms in schizophrenia: a prospective blinded trial of olanzapine and haloperidol. *Archives of General Psychiatry* 55, 250–258.

Tran, P.V., Hamilton, S.H., Kuntz, A.J. *et al.* (1997) Double-blind comparison of olanzapine versus risperidone in the treatment of schizophrenia and other psychotic disorders. *Journal of Clinical Psychopharmacology* 17, 407–418.

Travis, M.J., Busatto, G.F., Pilowsky, L.S. *et al.* (1998) Serotonin: 5-HT_{2A} receptor occupancy *in vivo* and response to the new antipsychotics olanzapine and sertindole. *British Journal of Psychiatry* 173, 290–291.

Trichard, C., Paillere-Martinot, M.L., Attar-Levy, D. *et al.* (1998) Binding of antipsychotic drugs to cortical 5-HT_{2A} receptors: a PET study of chlorpromazine, clozapine, and amisulpride in schizophrenic patients. *American Journal of Psychiatry* 155, 505–508.

Truffinet, P., Tamminga, C.A., Fabre, L.F. *et al.* (1999) Placebo-controlled study of the D_4/5-HT_{2A} antagonist fananserin in the treatment of schizophrenia. *American Journal of Psychiatry* 156, 419–425.

Van Tol, H.H.M., Bunzow, J.R., Guan, H.-C. *et al.* (1991) Cloning of the gene for a human dopamine D_4 receptor with high affinity for the antipsychotic clozapine. *Nature* 350, 610–614.

Varty, G.B. & Higgins, G.A. (1995) Examination of drug-induced and isolation-induced disruptions of prepulse inhibition as models to screen antipsychotic drugs. *Psychopharmacology* 122, 15–26.

Waddington, J.L. (1993) Pre- and postsynaptic D_1 to D_5 dopamine receptor mechanisms in relation to antipsychotic activity. In: *Antipsychotic Drugs and Their Side Effects* (ed. T.R.E. Barnes), pp. 65–85. Academic Press, London.

Waddington, J.L. & Casey, D.E. (2000) Comparative pharmacology of classical and novel (second-generation) antipsychotics. In: *Schizophrenia and Mood Disorders: the New Drug Therapies in Clinical Practice* (eds P.F. Buckley & J.L. Waddington), pp. 3–13. Butterworth Heinemann, Oxford.

Waddington, J.L. & Morgan, M.G. (2001) Pathobiology of schizophrenia: implications for clinical management and treatment. In: *Comprehensive Care of Schizophrenia: a Textbook of Clinical Management* (eds J.A. Lieberman & R.M. Murray), pp. 27–35. Martin Dunitz, London.

Waddington, J.L. & O'Callaghan, E. (1997) What makes an antipsychotic 'atypical'? *CNS Drugs* 7, 341–346.

Waddington, J.L. & Quinn, J.F. (2000) From first to second generation antipsychotics. In: *Atypical Antipsychotics* (eds B.A. Ellenbroek & A.R. Cools), pp. 19–33. Birkhauser-Verlag, Basel.

Waddington, J.L., Daly, S.A., McCauley, P.G. & O'Boyle, K.M. (1994) Levels of functional interaction between 'D-1-like' and 'D-2-like' dopamine receptor systems. In: *Dopamine Receptors* (ed. H.B. Niznik), pp. 511–537. Marcel Dekker, New York.

Waddington, J.L., Scully, P.J. & O'Callaghan, E. (1997) The new antipsychotics, and their potential for early intervention in schizophrenia. *Schizophrenia Research* **28**, 207–222.

Waddington, J.L., Deveney, A.M., Clifford, J.J. *et al.* (1998) D_1-like dopamine receptors: regulation of psychomotor behavior, D_1-like: D_2-like interactions and effects of D_{1A} targeted gene deletion. In: *Dopamine Receptor Subtypes* (eds P. Jenner & R. Demirdamar), pp. 45–63. IOS Press, Amsterdam.

Waddington, J.L., Clifford, J.J., McNamara, F.N. *et al.* (2001) The psychopharmacology–molecular biology interface: exploring the behavioural roles of dopamine receptor subtypes using targeted gene deletion ('knockout'). *Progress in Neuro-Psychopharmacology and Biological Psychiatry* **25**, 925–964.

Wadenberg, M.L. (1996) Serotonergic mechanisms in neuroleptic-induced catalepsy in the rat. *Neuroscience and Biobehavioral Reviews* **20**, 325–339.

Wahlbeck, K., Cheine, M., Essali, A. & Adams, C. (1999) Evidence of clozapine's effectiveness in schizophrenia: a systematic review and meta-analysis of randomized trials. *American Journal of Psychiatry* **156**, 990–999.

Weiss, E.L., Longhurst, J.G., Bowers, M.B. & Mazure, C.M. (1999) Olanzapine for treatment-refractory psychosis in patients responsive to, but intolerant of, clozapine. *Journal of Clinical Psychopharmacology* **19**, 378–380.

Wetzel, H., Grunder, G., Hillert, A. *et al.* (1998) Amisulpride versus flupentixol in schizophrenia with predominantly positive symptomatology: a double-blind controlled study comparing a selective D_2-like antagonist to a mixed D_1-/D_2-like antagonist. *Psychopharmacology* **137**, 223–232.

Wirshing, D.A., Spellberg, B.J., Erhart, S.M., Marder, S.R. & Wirshing, W.C. (1998) Novel antipsychotics and new onset diabetes. *Biological Psychiatry* **44**, 778–783.

Wirshing, D.A., Wirshing, W.C., Kysar, L. *et al.* (1999) Novel antipsychotics: comparison of weight gain liabilities. *Journal of Clinical Psychiatry* **60**, 358–363.

Wolkin, A., Barouche, F., Wolf, A.P. *et al.* (1989) Dopamine blockade and clinical response: evidence for two biological subgroups of schizophrenia. *American Journal of Psychiatry* **146**, 905–908.

Xu, M., Koeltzow, T.E., Cooper, D.C., Tonegawa, S, & White, F.J. (1999) Dopamine receptor mutant and wild-type mice exhibit identical responses to putative D_3 receptor-selective agonists and antagonists. *Synapse* **31**, 210–215.

Young, C.D., Meltzer, H.Y. & Deutch, A.Y. (1998) Effects of desmethylclozapine on fos protein expression in the forebrain: *in vivo* biological activity of the clozapine metabolite. *Neuropsychopharmacology* **19**, 99–103.

Youngren, K.D., Inglis, F.M., Pivirotto, P.J. *et al.* (1999) Clozapine preferentially increases dopamine release in the Rhesus monkey prefrontal cortex compared with the caudate nucleus. *Neuropsychopharmacology* **20**, 403–412.

Zimbroff, D.L., Ane, J.M., Tamminga, C.A. *et al.* (1997) Controlled, dose–response study of sertindole and haloperidol in the treatment of schizophrenia. *American Journal of Psychiatry* **154**, 782–791.

24 Acute pharmacological treatment of schizophrenia

S. Miyamoto, T.S. Stroup, G.E. Duncan, A. Aoba and J.A. Lieberman

Introduction, 442
Therapeutic goals of acute treatment, 442
    Suppression of symptoms, 442
    Treatment of behavioural disturbances, 443
    Determination of treatment regimen and drug dosages, 443
    Remission of episode, 443
Pharmacological agents, 444
    Antipsychotics, 444
    Adjunctive treatments, 447
    Experimental treatments, 449
Practical clinical issues, 456

Who to treat? 456
Predictors of treatment response, 456
Early intervention, 457
Which drugs to use in acute emergency? 457
Dose–response relationships, 458
Treatment of different stages of illness, 459
    First episode, 459
    Exacerbation of chronic schizophrenia, 460
    Chronic/residual, 460
Conclusions, 462
References, 462

Introduction

The goals and strategies of acute treatment of schizophrenia vary according to the phase and severity of the illness. Pharmacological treatment is the most important element of the acute management of different stages of the illness, and clinicians are faced with a number of considerations and decisions about drug treatment. Adequate treatment during the acute stage of the illness could set the stage for subsequent long-term treatment. Currently available conventional antipsychotics are suboptimal, however, because a substantial proportion of patients with schizophrenia fail to respond to these drugs and because they cause undesirable acute and chronic side-effects (for review see Miyamoto *et al*. 2000a). Consequently, there has been an intensive search for more effective and safer antipsychotic agents. The reintroduction of clozapine, because of its efficacy in treatment-refractory patients and in spite of its risk of agranulocytosis, represented a major step forward. Newer atypical antipsychotic drugs may have significant advantages over typical drugs in terms of side-effect profile and efficacy. In addition, novel potential antipsychotic compounds based on specific neurochemical hypotheses are currently under development (for review see Miyamoto *et al*. 2002). This chapter provides a comprehensive overview of acute pharmacological treatment of schizophrenia, and offers current information with respect to the atypical antipsychotic therapies for acute schizophrenia and ongoing experimental treatments.

Therapeutic goals of acute treatment

The acute phase of schizophrenia often requires intensive inpatient treatment. To allow for effective treatment, clinicians should select and 'titrate' the doses of both pharmacological and psychosocial interventions on the basis of an evaluation of the symptoms and sociobehavioural functioning of the patient (Kopelowicz & Liberman 1995). If a trusting relationship between a patient and a clinician is established during the acute treatment, that relationship can be further enhanced as the patient improves (Gaebel & Marder 1996).

Suppression of symptoms

During the acute phase, patients demonstrate active symptoms of schizophrenia. This can occur during a first episode or as a relapse in a patient who had previously been stable (Mardey 1996). The primary treatment goal during this phase is to alleviate or reduce the most severe symptoms of the illness, particularly pathological excitement/agitation, hostility and exacerbated psychotic symptoms (Marder 1996; Sharif 1998; Feifel 2000). Agitation and hostility, which are often associated with positive symptoms, are commonly identified as high-priority targets for patients hospitalized for acute schizophrenia, especially in the first days of inpatient treatment (Feifel 2000). Special attention should be paid to the presence of suicidal ideation. Cohen *et al*. (1994) reported that as many as 81% of first-admission psychotic patients who attempted suicide had histories of hallucinations. Patients experiencing command auditory hallucinations telling them to engage in dangerous behaviours should be evaluated and treated as soon as possible (Marder 1996). In addition, those who have a history of violent acts while psychotic should be considered dangerous until the psychosis is well controlled (Marder 1996). In most situations hospitalization is necessary for patients who are felt to pose a serious threat of harm to themselves or others, who are unable to care for themselves, or who have general medical or psychiatric problems that are not safely or effectively treated in a less intensive setting (American Psychiatric Association 2000). Family members and friends are often helpful in determining the risk of a patient's harming self or others, and in assessing the individual's ability to care for himself or herself. The therapeutic goal of hospitalization is suppression of these active symptoms to a level compatible with safe discharge (Sharif 1998).

Treatment of behavioural disturbances

In the acute phase, a second treatment goal is to control acutely disturbed behaviours such as agitated behaviour, violence and pathological excitement. Patients have a substantial risk of self-injury or suicide, and other unpredictable dangerous behaviours to themselves or others. Among patients with schizophrenia, 40% report suicidal thoughts, 20–40% attempt suicide and 9–13% die by suicide (Meltzer 1998). Violent or aggressive behaviour can be associated with various pathogenic mechanisms. For example, pathological cognitive misinterpretations (e.g. delusions and hallucinations) may produce aberrant aggression; pathological arousal (e.g. mania, catatonic excitement and drug/alcohol abuse) may lead directly to aggression; or frustration may arise when social goals and desires are blocked, or when patients are repeatedly admitted to units (for review see Hyde & Harrower-Wilson 1996). Rapid treatment is essential to reduce the risk of violence or self-harm. Prior to discharge, clinicians should ensure that the patient does not represent an acute danger to self or others (Sharif 1998).

Determination of treatment regimen and drug dosages

A third important goal of acute treatment is to formulate short-term treatment plans, and to lay the foundation for long-term maintenance treatment after discharge (Sharif 1998; American Psychiatric Association 2000; Feifel 2000). Nearly all acute episodes of schizophrenia should be treated with antipsychotic medications (American Psychiatric Association 2000). Once patients are diagnosed, pharmacotherapy should be applied as early in this phase as possible (Marder 1996; Lieberman & Fenton 2000). If patients experience clinical improvement from pharmacological treatment with minimal adverse effects, they will be more likely to continue medications after they recover from the acute episode. Therefore, the initial selection of an appropriate antipsychotic drug at a reasonable dosage is critical. The antipsychotic drug and dosage that appropriately balance side-effects and efficacy should be used (Marder 1996).

Patients' preferences appear to be a particularly important factor in determining the course of treatment. If a patient reports a favourable subjective response to a particular medication in the past, this drug may be the best choice because this increases the chance of good compliance (Van Putten *et al.* 1984). Once the drug at an adequate dosage is selected, the trial should last at least 3 weeks before the medication is changed (American Psychiatric Association 2000), while a full antipsychotic response will not occur until after discharge in most cases (Sharif 1998). Decisions made in the inpatient service should be made collaboratively with the patient and outpatient providers so that they will likely be continued in the outpatient setting. Careful management of drug side-effects is also essential, because patients may experience uncomfortable side-effects of an antipsychotic before they experience clinical improvement. Side-effects can affect a patient's attitude toward maintenance drug treatment and in subsequent acute episodes (Marder 1996).

If a patient fails to respond after an adequate trial, it is reasonable for clinicians to ensure that the patient was receiving an adequate dosage and that the patient was compliant by monitoring a plasma concentration of the drug (Marder 1996). If the plasma level is adequate, the clinician is faced with the following alternatives:

1 wait longer for a response;
2 change drugs;
3 add an additional drug; or
4 initiate a high-dose trial (Marder 1996).

However, because a review of studies failed to find any advantage of high-dose treatment over conventional dosage of an antipsychotic drug, this should be a rare strategy (Thompson 1994). Because of short inpatient stays, the challenge for clinicians appears to be to provide an adequate treatment period without aggressively escalating the dosage (Sharif 1998).

Remission of episode

The fourth therapeutic goal of acute treatment is to achieve full remission of the episode. At present, there is little doubt that schizophrenia has a chronic and progressive course in the majority of patients (for review see Lieberman 1999). It has been suggested that antipsychotic drug treatment can interrupt and ameliorate the pathophysiological process that causes psychotic symptoms and leads to clinical deterioration (Lieberman *et al.* 1990a, 1997; Wyatt 1991; Lieberman 1999). Supporting this notion in part, preclinical studies have demonstrated that both typical and atypical antipsychotic drugs can prevent N-methyl-D-aspartate receptor (NMDA-R) antagonist-induced neurodegenerative changes in the brain (for review see Olney & Farber 1995). Studies of maintenance antipsychotic treatment have demonstrated the prophylactic effect of antipsychotics in preventing relapse (Davis & Andriukaitis 1986). Taken together, adequate acute pharmacological treatment can not only suppress the symptoms of schizophrenia, but also mitigate the following course of the illness and produce more favourable outcomes, although associated negative and cognitive symptoms may persist (Lieberman *et al.* 1997; Sheitman *et al.* 1997; Lieberman 1999; Robinson *et al.* 1999).

In addition to the drug treatment, psychosocial issues must also be addressed. These interventions should be combined with pharmacotherapy and must be properly adapted to the particular phase and stage of schizophrenia to effect a rapid return to the best level of functioning (Gaebel & Marder 1996; American Psychiatric Association 2000). For example, it is important to address issues such as housing and financial problems as early as possible, as these will surely threaten therapeutic gains of antipsychotic treatment if they are not resolved (Sharif 1998). Other stressors that might have contributed to the relapse need to be identified and addressed. Along similar lines, a thorough assessment should be made of family dynamics, the family's (or other caregiver's) understanding of the patient's illness and the need for ongoing family psychoeducation/therapy (Sharif 1998). To develop an alliance between clinicians, institutions, the patient and family, a relationship based on co-operation and trust is essential to achieving successful remission of the episode (Liberman & Kopelowicz 1995). The clinician should provide information to the patient and family on the nature and treatment of the illness, as well as factors that influence the course and outcome, including medication compliance, in a manner that is appropriate to the patient's ability to understand them (American Psychiatric Association 2000). It seems likely that the quality of life during first years of illness will be better when full remission of an episode is achieved. The ultimate goal of acute treatment appears to be a patient who understands his or her illness and can voluntarily accept indicated therapeutic measures (Gaebel & Marder 1996).

Pharmacological agents

Antipsychotics

Typicals

Efficacy of typical antipsychotics

Typical antipsychotic drugs (phenothiazines, butyrophenones and thioxanthenes), which are also referred to as conventional, standard, classical, traditional or first-generation antipsychotic drugs, have had a profound impact on neuroscience research and, until recently, they have been the core treatment of schizophrenia (Schulz & McGorry 2000). The typical antipsychotics are effective for alleviating positive symptoms of schizophrenia and in preventing their recurrence in many patients (for review see Miyamoto *et al.* 2000a, 2002). Approximately 30% of patients with acutely exacerbated psychotic symptoms, however, have little or no response to conventional antipsychotics, and up to 50% of patients have only a partial response to medication (Kane 1989; Fleischhacker 1995). The typical antipsychotic drugs have only limited therapeutic effects on negative symptoms, mood symptoms and cognitive deficits. In particular, primary negative symptoms are resistant to the typical drugs (Fleischhacker 1995; Hawkins *et al.* 1999). The presence of negative symptoms and cognitive impairment often leads to poor social and vocational function (Green 1996; Keefe *et al.* 1999). Thus, clinicians seem to have reached a consensus that atypical antipsychotics are preferable to the typical drugs in most situations (McEvoy *et al.* 1999). At this time, the only groups of patients in which the typical agents are clearly preferable are those

for whom there is a clear indication for short- or long-acting injectable preparations, or who have a history of excellent response to an older agent with minimal side-effects (Sharif 1998; Schulz & McGorry 2000).

Safety of typical antipsychotics

Both conventional and atypical antipsychotics are associated with a wide range and a variable degree of discomforting acute and long-term adverse effects, including extrapyramidal side-effects (EPSs), sedation, anticholinergic, autonomic and cardiovascular effects, weight gain, sexual dysfunction, hyperprolactinaemia and neuroleptic malignant syndrome, a condition that is potentially life-threatening (Fleischhacker 1995; Barnes & McPhillips 1999; see Chapters 23, 28 and 29). However, in contradiction to atypical antipsychotics, up to 70% of patients given recommended therapeutic dosages of conventional antipsychotics develop acute EPSs (Chakos *et al.* 1992). There are four types of EPS: parkinsonian symptoms, akathisia, dystonia and tardive dyskinesia (TD). Severe akathisia can cause patients to feel anxious or irritable and can result in aggressive or suicidal acts (Marder 1996). Thus, akathisia can be frequently misdiagnosed by the psychiatrist as anxiety or agitation rather than as a drug side-effect (Van Putten & Marder 1987). The most troublesome neurological side-effect, TD, can be irreversible, and incidence rates have been estimated at about 5% per year in the non-elderly and as high as 30% per year in the elderly (Woerner *et al.* 1998; Kane 1999a). The risk of TD has been a major rationale for preferences of atypical over typical drugs (Schulz & McGorry 2000). Further, the anticholinergic drugs that are often used to reduce EPSs can also produce serious side-effects (e.g. dry mouth, constipation, delirium and memory deficits) (Fleischhacker & Hummer 1997), and the drugs may worsen TD (Beaumont 2000). All these adverse effects can contribute to treatment non-compliance, and hence increase rates of relapse and rehospitalization during the course of the chronic illness (Fleischhacker 1995; Barnes & McPhillips 1999).

Atypicals

Since the reintroduction of clozapine in 1990, a series of atypical antipsychotic agents have been developed (for review see Blin 1999; Miyamoto *et al.* 2000a; Waddington & Casey 2000). Each of the new agents was designed to try to capture the unique efficacy profile of clozapine, while avoiding agranulocytosis (Kinon & Lieberman 1996; Lieberman 1996). Although there is currently no uniform definition of the term 'atypical', in its broadest sense it is used to refer to drugs that have at least equal antipsychotic efficacy and produce fewer EPSs or prolactin elevation than conventional drugs (Lieberman 1996). A more restrictive definition would require that atypical drugs have superior antipsychotic efficacy (i.e. they are effective in treatment-resistant schizophrenic patients, or in reducing negative symptoms and/or neurocognitive deficits; Miyamoto *et al.* 2002).

The atypical antipsychotics include amisulpride, aripiprazole, clozapine, iloperidone, olanzapine, quetiapine, risperidone, sulpiride and ziprasidone. In late 2001 aripiprazole and iloperidone were in late Phase III trials. Sulpiride and amisulpiride are not marketed in the USA, but they are widely used in European and other countries. The others are all approved by the US Food and Drug Administration (FDA). These atypical agents represent the first significant advances in the pharmacological treatment of schizophrenia in the past four decades. A risk–benefit analysis of the typical versus the newer atypical antipsychotics favours the use of the newer agents as first-line drugs (Lieberman 1996). They are at least as effective as typical antipsychotics in the treatment of exacerbated psychotic symptoms and are superior with regard to EPSs, which may translate into increased patient acceptability and compliance, with possible reduction in relapse rates (Sharif 1998).

Efficacy of atypical antipsychotics

Although the proportion of patients who improve and the magnitude of therapeutic effects vary greatly, atypical antipsychotics appear to be at least as effective for psychotic symptoms as conventional drugs (for review see Markowitz *et al.* 1999; Remington & Kapur 2000). There have been a number of double-blind studies comparing the efficacy and tolerability of atypical antipsychotic drugs with typical agents in chronic schizophrenic patients with acute exacerbations.

Nine double-blind clinical trials have demonstrated that clozapine is at least as effective as conventional antipsychotics for positive symptoms in acutely psychotic patients with schizophrenia (for review see Buchanan 1995; Buchanan & McKenna 2000). Chakos *et al.* (2001), in a review and meta-analysis of seven controlled trials comparing clozapine to a typical antipsychotic in treatment-resistant schizophrenia, found that clozapine is superior to typical antipsychotics in terms of overall psychopathology, EPSs and compliance rate.

Four double-blind trials of risperidone have reported that the antipsychotic effect size favours risperidone over typical antipsychotics, including haloperidol, perphenazine, zuclopenthixol and levomepromazine (methotrimeprazine), in patients with acute exacerbations of schizophrenia (Borison *et al.* 1992; Hoyberg *et al.* 1993; Huttunen *et al.* 1995; Blin *et al.* 1996). At selected dosage, risperidone appears to be as effective as haloperidol in treating positive symptoms (Borison *et al.* 1992; Claus *et al.* 1992; Marder & Meibach 1994), more effective in treating negative symptoms (Borison *et al.* 1992; Claus *et al.* 1992; Marder & Meibach 1994) and faster in onset of action (Borison *et al.* 1992; Claus *et al.* 1992; Chouinard *et al.* 1993b).

The efficacy of olanzapine in comparison to haloperidol was evaluated in two large double-blind clinical trials in acutely exacerbated patients with chronic schizophrenia. In the North American clinical trials of 335 patients, the high dose ranges of olanzapine (12.5–17.5 mg/day) were superior to haloperidol (10–20 mg/day) for overall symptomatology, as measured by the Brief Psychiatric Rating Scale (BPRS) total score (Beasley *et al.*

1996). With regard to negative symptoms, the high dose of olanzapine was significantly more effective than haloperidol. However, in the Eastern hemisphere clinical trial of 431 patients, response to three dosage ranges of olanzapine (5, 10 or 15 ± 2.5 mg/day) did not significantly differ from haloperidol (15 ± 5 mg/day), as measured by the BPRS, the Positive and Negative Syndrome Scale (PANSS) and the Clinical Global Impression (CGI) score (Beasley *et al.* 1997). With respect to side-effect profile, olanzapine showed less acute EPSs, especially dystonias, than haloperidol in both trials (Beasley *et al.* 1996, 1997).

In an international trial comparing olanzapine (5–20 mg/day) with haloperidol (5–20 mg/day) over 6 weeks in 1996 patients with schizophrenia, schizophreniform disorder or schizoaffective disorder, olanzapine demonstrated significantly greater overall efficacy than haloperidol in the BPRS total score, the PANSS negative subscale, arid CGI severity score (Tollefson *et al.* 1997). Furthermore, olanzapine was more effective than haloperidol in reducing depressive symptoms. Duggan *et al.* (2000) reviewed the data from nine published and unpublished studies of olanzapine versus typical antipsychotics, and found that olanzapine has advantages in positive, negative and depressive symptoms in short-term studies.

Two double-blind studies compared the efficacy of quetiapine to a typical antipsychotic in patients with an acute exacerbation of chronic schizophrenia. In a 6-week double-blind placebo-controlled multicentre trial in 361 patients, quetiapine was comparable to haloperidol (12 mg/day) in reducing positive symptoms at doses ranging from 150 to 750 mg/day, and in reducing negative symptoms at doses ranging from 75 to 750 mg/day (Arvanitis *et al.* 1997). Results of a double-blind quetiapine (mean dose, 407 mg/day) vs. chlorpromazine (mean dose, 384 mg/day) trial among 201 patients also demonstrated equiefficacy in the treatment of both positive and negative symptoms (Peuskens & Link 1997). In both studies, quetiapine showed more favourable side-effect profiles than the conventional antipsychotics (Arvanitis *et al.* 1997; Peuskens & Link 1997).

There has been only one study published comparing ziprasidone to a typical antipsychotic. Goff *et al.* (1998) found that ziprasidone (160 mg/day) was superior to placebo and comparable to haloperidol (15 mg/day) in alleviating overall psychopathology and positive symptoms in 90 patients with an acute exacerbation of schizophrenia or schizoaffective disorder, but ziprasidone had a lower potential to induce EPSs than haloperidol. In a 6-week double-blind trial of 302 acutely ill patients, ziprasidone (80 and 160 mg/day) was more effective than placebo in improving the PANSS total, BPRS total, BPRS core items, CGI-S, and PANSS negative subscale scores (Daniel *et al.* 1999). Ziprasidone at 160 mg/day significantly improved depressive symptoms as compared with placebo (Daniel *et al.* 1999).

Amisulpride appears to be as effective as haloperidol and flupentixol in treating positive symptoms associated with acute exacerbations of schizophrenia (Moller *et al.* 1997; Puech *et al.* 1998; Wetzel *et al.* 1998) and superior to haloperidol in improving negative symptoms in acutely ill patients (Moller *et al.* 1997). The optimal dosage of amisulpride in this indication was found to be 400–800 mg/day (Moller *et al.* 1997; Puech *et al.* 1998). At low dosage (50–300 mg/day), amisulpride has been shown to be effective in ameliorating predominant negative symptoms in chronic schizophrenic patients (Boyer *et al.* 1995; Paillere-Martinot *et al.* 1995; Loo *et al.* 1997).

Geddes *et al.* (2000) recently carried out a systematic overview and meta-analyses of 52 randomized trials comparing atypicals (clozapine, olanzapine, risperidone, quetiapine, sertindole and amisulpride) with conventional drugs (haloperidol or chlorpromazine). There was no difference in efficacy and overall tolerability between typical and atypical antipsychotics if adequate dosage adjustments are made. For example, the advantages of atypical antipsychotics in terms of efficacy and drop-out rates were not seen if haloperidol is used at a dosage of 12 mg/day or less, although atypicals still caused fewer EPSs (Geddes *et al.* 2000). There is therefore a growing need to consider the comparator dose of drugs in order to evaluate the relative efficacy and tolerability of typical and atypical antipsychotics.

Atypical antipsychotics are not effective in all patients and against all symptom dimensions of psychotic disorders (Table 24.1). It is clear that for many patients the atypical drugs are unable to fully reverse already established impairment in cognition, negative symptoms and social disability (Meltzer 1999b). Thus, the possible use of these agents in the prodromal period of schizophrenia, before the emergence of psychosis, is an important issue in need of research and clarification (Meltzer 1999b).

Efficacy against negative and cognitive symptoms

Studies of the early course of illness have shown that about 70% of schizophrenics develop negative symptoms before the onset of positive symptoms (Häfner *et al.* 1992). However, there is a continuing debate as to whether atypical antipsychotics are effective in treating primary negative symptoms (Remington & Kapur 2000). Thus, the possible advantages of atypical drugs for patients with predominantly negative symptoms are unclear (Campbell *et al.* 1999).

In addition, the effectiveness of atypical antipsychotics in improving cognitive impairment has not yet been clearly proved. A meta-analysis of 15 studies (only three of which were double-blind) of atypical antipsychotics for cognitive impairment in patients with schizophrenia suggests that they may improve attention and executive function (Keefe *et al.* 1999). However, available results are relatively inconsistent and modest in effect size. Furthermore, there are statistical limitations and a lack of standard conventions in the studies of cognition (Dawkins *et al.* 1999). It appears that there could be significant differences among the atypical drugs in terms of what types of cognition they improve.

Antidepressant effects

Atypical antipsychotics have been associated with a reduction in the incidence of suicidality, which may be caused, at least in part, by antidepressant effects of these agents (Meltzer 1998, 1999a). Clozapine, risperidone and olanzapine, in particular, appear to have greater efficacy than typical antipsychotics for depressive symptoms (Marder *et al.* 1997; Tollefson *et al.* 1998; Meltzer 1999a; Conley *et al.* 2000; Table 24.1). Antidepressant activity

Table 24.1 Clinical and side-effect profile of atypical antipsychotic drugs (after Dawkins *et al.* 1999).

Drug	Clozapine	Risperidone	Olanzapine	Quetiapine	Ziprasidone
Clinical effect					
Psychotic symptoms	+++	+++?	+++?	++	++
Negative symptoms	+	+	+	+	+
Cognitive symptoms	++?	++?	++?	+?	?
Mood symptoms	+++	++	+++?	++?	++?
Refractory symptoms	+++	+++?	+++?	++?	++?
Side-effect					
EPSs	–––	++*	+*	–––	+*
TD	–––	+	?	?	?
Prolactin elevation	–––	+++	–	––	–––
Weight gain	++	+	++	+	––

EPSs, extrapyramidal side-effects; TD, tardive dyskinesia.
+ to +++, weakly (for clinical effect) or active (for side-effect) to strongly active; – to –––, weak to little activity; ?, questionable to unknown activity.
* Dose dependent.

of the atypical agents may have important clinical consequences because perceived improvement in anxiety and depression is a strong predictor of compliance and emergence of depressive symptoms often accompanies relapse (Miyamoto *et al.* 2002).

Comparison between atypical antipsychotics

Tran *et al.* (1997) carried out the first randomized double-blind head-to-head study comparing olanzapine (10–20 mg/day; mean dose = 17.2 mg/day) with risperidone (4–12 mg/day; mean dose = 17.2 mg/day) in the treatment of 339 patients with schizophrenia and other psychotic disorders over 28 weeks. They demonstrated that olanzapine was superior to risperidone in effects on some measures of negative and depressive symptoms as well as long-term efficacy (Tran *et al.* 1997). However, this study has received several criticisms including the relatively high dosages of risperidone used and the statistical methods (Lieberman 2001).

Recently, Conley and Mahmoud (2001) compared risperidone (2–6 mg/day; mean modal dose = 4.8 mg/day) with olanzapine (5–20 mg/day; mean modal dose = 12.4 mg/day) in a randomized double-blind treatment trial of 377 patients with schizophrenia or schizoaffective disorder over 8 weeks. The study found significantly greater efficacy of risperidone than olanzapine in reducing anxiety/depression and positive symptoms at week 8, but not at end-point (Conley & Mahmoud 2001). It has been suggested that higher olanzapine dosage may be optimal (Stahl 1999).

Peuskens *et al.* (1999) compared amisulpride (800 mg/day) with risperidone (8 mg/day) in a double-blind study of 228 patients with acute exacerbations of schizophrenia for 8 weeks. The investigators found that both treatments were equally effective against positive symptoms, and there was a trend in favour of greater improvement in negative symptoms assessed on the PANSS negative subscale in patients receiving amisulpride.

Parenteral forms

Many of the antipsychotics are available in a short-acting parenteral form. Intramuscular (i.m.) preparations are particularly useful in the management of acute pathological excitement and agitation (Buckley 1999). The main indication for the use of a short-acting parenteral form in the acute situation is to treat severely disturbed patients who cannot be verbally redirected, who may be violent and who may have to be medicated over objection (Sharif 1998). A single intramuscular injection of a high potency conventional drug such as haloperidol or fluphenazine can result in rapid calming without an excess of sedation. However, for younger patients (adolescents and young adults), high doses of high potency drugs can lead to dystonia, which may increase the patient's agitation (Marder 1996).

Among atypical antipsychotics, a short-acting intramuscular parenteral form of olanzapine is currently available in some countries, and ziprasidone is in late-stage clinical development in the USA (Breier *et al.* 2000; Potkin & Cooper 2000). In a ran-

domized open-label trial, ziprasidone i.m. appears to be at least as effective as haloperidol i.m. in reducing the symptoms of acute agitation associated with psychosis (Swift *et al.* 1999). Furthermore, ziprasidone i.m. may be rapidly effective with significantly less liability for EPSs than haloperidol (Swift *et al.* 1999; Potkin & Cooper 2000; Lesem *et al.* 2001). In a recent large double-blind study, olanzapine (10 mg) i.m. rapidly and effectively produced a sustained and safe alleviation of acute agitation in patients with schizophrenia (Wright *et al.* 2001).

Several typical antipsychotic drugs (e.g. haloperidol or fluphenazine) are available in long-acting depot formulations (see Chapter 25). Long-acting depot medications are not usually prescribed for acute psychotic episodes, because they take months to reach a stable steady state and are eliminated very slowly (Marder *et al.* 1989). However, they are especially advantageous in patients with a clear history of non-compliance not related to drug side-effects, those with a history of severe relapses upon medication discontinuation, and patients with active substance abuse, who are more likely to be non-compliant with oral medications (Sharif 1998). In addition, depot preparations have lowered relapse rates by an average of 15% compared to oral neuroleptics in six double-blind randomized trials (Glazer & Kane 1992).

Adjunctive treatments

Various adjunctive treatments have been used to enhance the response to antipsychotic medications. In addition, ancillary medications are commonly prescribed for comorbid conditions in schizophrenia (American Psychiatric Association 2000).

Benzodiazepines

As adjunctive treatment, benzodiazepines have been advocated partly because of the potential role of GABAergic agents in modulating dopamine transmission, although the evidence for efficacy is not compelling (for review see Wolkowitz & Pickar 1991; Wassef *et al.* 1999). Short-term acute treatment with high-dose benzodiazepines may reduce anxiety, agitation and psychotic symptoms in as many as 50% of patients (Arana *et al.* 1986b; Wolkowitz & Pickar 1991). Double-blind controlled studies, however, have not conclusively established a beneficial effect of longer-term treatment with benzodiazepines on psychotic symptoms in schizophrenia (Wolkowitz *et al.* 1988, 1992; Wolkowitz & Pickar 1991). The studies have found a marked interindividual variability in response to adjunctive benzodiazepines, and any positive effects reported have generally been transient (Wolkowitz *et al.* 1992; Wassef *et al.* 1999). In a double-blind comparison of alprazolam, diazepam and placebo for the treatment of negative symptoms in 55 outpatients with schizophrenia who had been maintained on antipsychotics, Csernansky *et al.* (1998) found no significant sustained effect on negative symptoms in patients who received a benzodiazepine.

Benzodiazepines are often used adjunctively in the emergency treatment of patients who are acutely psychotic (see below). The combination of lorazepam in doses up to 10 mg/day with a high potency antipsychotic has been found to be safer and more effective than large doses of antipsychotics alone in controlling agitated behaviour and pathological excitement (Salzman *et al.* 1986; Sharif 1998). Lorazepam has the advantage of reliable absorption when it is administered either orally or parenterally (Janicak *et al.* 1993). However, adequate doses of adjunctive benzodiazepines are probably underutilized, in large part because of an exaggerated fear of the potential for dependence or drug-seeking behaviour (Sharif 1998). Nevertheless, once behavioural control is achieved (usually within the first few hours to days), the benzodiazepine dose should be gradually decreased and eventually discontinued (Sharif 1998). This is especially true for patients with a history of a substance use disorder. Dependence and abuse are potential problems that require a critical look at benzodiazepines as a practical option for use by outpatients on a long-term basis (Wassef *et al.* 1999).

Lithium

Lithium has been studied both as monotherapy as well as an adjunctive agent in schizophrenia (for review see Atre-Vaidya & Taylor 1989; Christison *et al.* 1991; Siris 1993). As the sole drug used to treat psychotic symptoms, lithium appears to have limited efficacy and may worsen symptoms in some patients (Atre-Vaidya & Taylor 1989). Early small studies using lithium as an adjunct in treatment-resistant patients have suggested that it may enhance the efficacy of antipsychotic medication (Small *et al.* 1975; Growe *et al.* 1979; Carman *et al.* 1981; see Chapter 26). Two recent placebo-controlled studies, however, found no benefit when well-characterized neuroleptic-resistant patients were treated with lithium (approximately 1.0 mEq/L) added to haloperidol or fluphenazine decanoate (Wilson 1993; Schulz *et al.* 1999). Augmentation with lithium may be beneficial for affective symptoms, impulsivity or excitement (Christison *et al.* 1991; Hogarty *et al.* 1995; Terao *et al.* 1995). Terao *et al.* (1995), in a study of 21 treatment-resistant schizophrenias treated in an 8-week randomized double-blind cross-over design with lithium or placebo, in addition to a typical antipsychotic, reported that the addition of lithium improved anxiety and depression but there was no benefit for negative symptoms. Improvement in hostility and aggression by the addition of lithium may be mediated through an improvement in manic-like symptoms (Christison *et al.* 1991). Treatment-emergent problems associated with lithium include worsening of pre-existing EPSs, additive cognitive side-effects and, possibly, increased risk of irreversible neurotoxicity (Siris 1993; Freeman & Stoll 1998).

Anticonvulsants

Anticonvulsants have been considered a useful adjunctive treatment for specific subgroups of schizophrenic patients (for review see Johns & Thompson 1995). Patients with manic, impulsive and violent behaviour or with abnormal EEGs may be more likely to show a beneficial response to the addition of carbamazepine or valproic acid (for review see Simhandl & Meszaros 1992; Siris 1993). Patients who have had a clozapine-related seizure may also benefit from the addition of an anticonvulsant (Lieberman 1998).

Carbamazepine

Carbamazepine augmentation of conventional neuroleptics has been associated with modest reductions in persistent symptoms, including tension, aggression and paranoia, in several controlled trials (Neppe 1983; Luchins 1984; Okuma *et al.* 1989). Okuma *et al.* (1989) conducted a 4-week multi-institutional double-blind study comparing the effects of adjunctive carbamazepine and placebo with typical antipsychotics in 162 patients with schizophrenia or schizoaffective disorders who were described as treatment-resistant with 'excited psychotic states'. Carbamazepine augmentation was found superior to placebo plus neuroleptics in patients with 'violence, aggression, and paranoia'; however, the overall differences between groups were small.

Side-effects and interactions may limit the use of carbamazepine. Carbamazepine and haloperidol in combination have been reported to induce disorientation and ataxia (Kanter *et al.* 1984; Yerevanian & Hodgman 1985). In addition, induction of hepatic microsomal enzymes by carbamazepine can substantially lower blood levels of certain antipsychotic agents (Kidron *et al.* 1985; Kahn *et al.* 1990; Goff & Baldessarini 1995) and, in one report, resulted in clinical deterioration (Arana *et al.* 1986a). Leucht *et al.* (2000) have recently reviewed eight studies comparing carbamazepine plus antipsychotics and placebo plus antipsychotics in the treatment of schizophrenia, and concluded that carbamazepine should not be recommended for routine clinical use for treatment of schizophrenia or augmentation of antipsychotic treatment of schizophrenia.

Valproic acid (sodium valproate)

Valproic acid (sodium valproate) does not significantly affect serum concentrations of most antipsychotic drugs, but results from three small controlled augmentation trials have been inconsistent (for review see Wassef *et al.* 1999). Linnoila *et al.* (1976) conducted a double-blind crossover study of 32 chronic psychiatric patients with dyskinesias, with each phase lasting 14 days. At study end, the combination of valproic acid with a typical antipsychotic was superior to an antipsychotic alone in reducing global psychopathology in 14 of 32 patients. In a placebo-controlled 12-week trial in 12 hospitalized patients with acute exacerbation of chronic schizophrenia, addition of divalproex sodium to haloperidol has demonstrated efficacy for negative symptoms and global psychopathology (Wassef *et al.* 2000). In contrast, addition of valproic acid to conventional neuroleptics did not produce any benefit in six treatment-resistant patients in a 4-week placebo-controlled crossover trial (Ko *et al.* 1985). Because of the limited data available, definitive conclusions on the therapeutic efficacy of valproic acid for the treatment of schizophrenia cannot be drawn.

Antidepressants

Efficacy against depressive symptoms

The value of adjunctive antidepressants for depressive symptoms in schizophrenia was initially demonstrated in 1987 (Siris et al. 1987; see also Chapter 9). However, in a placebo-controlled trial reported in 1989, Kramer et al. (1989) found that addition of desipramine or amitriptyline after initiating haloperidol to actively psychotic schizophrenic inpatients showed worsening of psychosis as well as no significant therapeutic advantage for depressive symptoms. Subsequently, Siris et al. (1994) have demonstrated that imipramine added to conventional agents in stable outpatients significantly improved depression without adversely affecting psychotic symptoms. Similarly, desipramine improved symptoms of depression, anxiety and psychosis when added to fluphenazine decanoate in a double-blind placebo-controlled trial of 33 depressed stable schizophrenic patients (Hogarty et al. 1995). Benefits of desipramine were only significant in female patients and did not achieve significance until week 12 (Hogarty et al. 1995). The investigators noted that improvement of psychotic symptoms may have resulted from successful prophylaxis against depressive episodes, which were associated with worsening of psychosis. Several trials of tricyclic antidepressants added to conventional agents have suggested their use for acute and maintenance treatment of depressive symptoms in stable schizophrenic patients (Plasky 1991; Siris et al. 1991). In an analysis of double-blind studies, Plasky (1991) suggested that adjunctive antidepressant treatment may be successful for the treatment of depression in schizophrenia only when the acute psychotic episode has stabilized. The use of selective serotonin reuptake inhibitor (SSRI) antidepressants in schizophrenic patients with depression is not well studied. Similarly, addition of antidepressants to second-generation atypical antipsychotics has not been reported in schizophrenia patients with comorbid depression.

Efficacy against negative symptoms

Siris et al. (1991) carried out a randomized placebo-controlled study to assess the therapeutic efficacy of adjunctive imipramine when added to fluphenazine decanoate and benztropine, among 27 well-stabilized patients with schizophrenia and schizoaffective disorder with negative symptoms, who also met the criteria for postpsychotic depression. They found that the imipramine-treated group had superior global and negative-symptom ratings at 6–9 weeks. Siris et al. further confirmed the efficacy of imipramine as an adjunctive treatment against negative symptoms in a more heterogeneous sample of 72 patients with postpsychotic depression in schizophrenia, but the effects were somewhat smaller (Siris et al. 2000).

There is considerable evidence that augmentation with SSRIs improves negative symptoms of chronic schizophrenia (for review see Evins & Goff 1996). Fluoxetine and fluvoxamine significantly improved negative symptoms when added to conventional antipsychotics in four controlled trials, producing generally modest effects (Silver & Nassar 1992; Goff et al. 1995a; Silver & Shmugliakov 1998; Silver et al. 2000). In one study, fluoxetine (20 mg/day) added to depot neuroleptics decreased ratings of negative symptoms by 23% compared to a 12% reduction with placebo; this improvement occurred despite a mean 20% elevation in haloperidol serum concentrations and a 65% increase in fluphenazine levels (Goff et al. 1995a). However, addition of sertraline (50 mg/day) to haloperidol produced no symptomatic change in an 8-week placebo-controlled trial in 36 chronic schizophrenic inpatients (Lee et al. 1998). In the only reported controlled trial of SSRI augmentation of an atypical agent, fluoxetine (mean dose 49 mg/day) produced no improvement in negative symptoms when added to clozapine in 33 patients (Buchanan et al. 1996).

β-Blockers

Adrenergic β-receptor antagonists (β-blockers) may be a valuable adjunct in the treatment of neuroleptic-induced EPSs (akathisia) (for review see Siris 1993). In addition, they appear to be effective in decreasing aggression in schizophrenia (Haspel 1995). The use of β-blockers (e.g. propranolol) as an adjunct to antipsychotic medication has also been proposed previously as potentially useful in the treatment of treatment-refractory schizophrenia (for review see Berlant 1987). However, a recent meta-analysis of five randomized controlled studies with 117 participants does not show evidence for any effect of β-blockers as an adjunctive to conventional antipsychotic medication (Wahlbeck et al. 2000). At present, available data on the use of β-blockers as adjunctive medication to antipsychotics for schizophrenia appear to be too weak to allow precise conclusions regarding the effect of this treatment or the need for further trials.

Experimental treatments

Subtype selective dopamine antagonists

It has been suggested that selective dopamine D_4 receptor antagonists may be potential novel antipsychotic drugs. Clozapine has a relatively higher affinity for the D_4 vs. D_2 or D_3 receptors (Van Tol et al. 1991; Table 24.2). Not only clozapine, but also a number of clinically efficacious antipsychotics have relatively high affinity for this receptor site (Table 24.2). In addition, an increase in D_4 receptors has been reported in the brains of patients with schizophrenia (Seeman et al. 1993). Furthermore, the D_4 receptor, enriched in the prefrontal cortex and hippocampus, is located in dopamine terminal fields potentially associated with emotion and cognition, but not with movement, underscoring the potential of this receptor as a target. The selective D_4 antagonist sonepiprazole (U-101387) increases dopamine release in the frontal cortex but decreases dopamine release in the nu-

Table 24.2 Affinity of antipsychotic drugs for human neurotransmitter receptors (K_i, nM) (after Miyamoto *et al.* 2002).

Receptor	Clozapine	Risperidone	Olanzapine	Quetiapine	Ziprasidone	Aripiprazole[¶]	Iloperidone**	Haloperidol
D_1	290	580	52	1300	130	410[‡]	320	120
D_2	130	2.2	20	180	3.1	0.52[‡]	6.3	1.4
D_3	240	9.6	50	940	7.2	9.1[‡]	7.1	2.5
D_4	47	8.5	50	2200	32	260[‡]	25	3.3
$5\text{-}HT_{1A}$	140	210	2100	230	2.5		93	3600
$5\text{-}HT_{1D}$*	1700	170	530	>5100	2			>5000
$5\text{-}HT_{2A}$	8.9	0.29	3.3	220	0.39	20[†]	5.6	120
$5\text{-}HT_{2C}$	17	10	10	1400	0.72		43	4700
$5\text{-}HT_6$	11	2000	10	4100	76	160[§]	63	6000
$5\text{-}HT_7$	66	3	250	1800	9.3	15[§]	110	1100
α_1	4	1.4	54	15	13	57[†]	1.4[†]	4.7
α_2	33	5.1	170	1000	310		160	1200
H_1	1.8	19	2.8	8.7	47		470[†]	440
m_1	1.8	2800	4.7	100	5100			1600

Values are geometric means of at least three determinations.

* Bovine.
[†] Rat.
[‡] CHO cells.
[§] HEK cells.
[¶] Affinity data from Lawler *et al.* (1999).
** Affinity data from Kongsamut *et al.* (1996).

cleus accumbens in rats (Danysz 2000). Sonepiprazole attenuates apomorphine-induced impairment of prepulse inhibition in rats (Mansbach *et al.* 1998a). It also antagonized the decrease in *c-fos* expression in the medial prefrontal cortex and neurotensin mRNA in the nucleus accumbens produced by repetitive amphetamine administration in rats, suggesting possible antipsychotic action of the agent (Feldpausch *et al.* 1998). Sonepiprazole is currently in Phase II clinical trials in patients with schizophrenia (Danysz 2000). An initial clinical trial with another highly selective D_4 antagonist, L-745,870, failed to demonstrate any antipsychotic activity in the treatment of schizophrenia (Bristow *et al.* 1997; Kramer *et al.* 1997). While the single dose tested makes it difficult to draw firm conclusions regarding the potential efficacy of D_4 antagonists as antipsychotic agents (Mansbach *et al.* 1998b), this drug actually caused a worsening of symptoms (Bristow *et al.* 1997). Similarly, NGD-94-1 also did not show clinical efficacy in limited trials in schizophrenics (Danysz 2000). More extensive testing of D_4 antagonists in patients with schizophrenia will be necessary to assess the therapeutic potential of such drugs.

Dopamine agonists

Partial D_2 agonist

Partial dopamine agonists are agents with good affinity for one or more dopamine receptors, but with intrinsic activity less than dopamine (Miyamoto *et al.* 2000a). Thus, such drugs may antagonize the actions of dopamine yet, by agonistic actions, acti-

vate other dopamine-related functions (Coward *et al.* 1989). It has been proposed that some D_2-like dopamine agonists have a greater affinity for autoreceptors than for heteroreceptors. The action of these agonists at autoreceptors would induce a receptor-mediated inhibition of both the synthesis and release of dopamine from nerve terminals, without producing significant activation of heteroreceptors on target cells (Kinon & Lieberman 1996). Such partial dopamine agonists are therefore proposed to act as dopaminergic 'buffers', reducing dopaminergic transmission without completely blocking it when dopaminergic activity is excessive or, conversely, stimulating it when it is reduced (Coward *et al.* 1989; Fleischhacker 1995).

The first of this class to show consistent and robust efficacy comparable to clinically used antipsychotic drugs, both conventional and atypical, is aripiprazole (Ozdemir 2000). Aripiprazole (OPC-14597) is a dual dopamine autoreceptor partial agonist and postsynaptic D_2 receptor antagonist (Kikuchi *et al.* 1995; Semba *et al.* 1995). It has a modest affinity for $5\text{-}HT_2$ receptors, but no appreciable affinity for D_1 receptors (Lawler *et al.* 1999; Table 24.2). Aripiprazole decreased striatal dopamine release (Semba *et al.* 1995) and inhibited the activity of dopamine neurones when applied locally to the ventral tegmental area in rats (Momiyama *et al.* 1996). Animal behavioural studies showed that the compound exhibited weak cataleptogenic effects compared to haloperidol and chlorpromazine despite the fact that it has almost identical D_2 receptor antagonistic activity (Kikuchi *et al.* 1995). The potency of aripiprazole to upregulate striatal D_2 receptors in response to chronic treatment was much smaller than that of haloperidol, suggesting lower potential for EPSs, including tardive dyskinesia (Inoue *et al.* 1997). Aripiprazole is currently undergoing worldwide Phase III development. Preliminary clinical studies have shown its efficacy in alleviating both positive and negative symptoms of schizophrenia. Although current dogma suggests that such a D_2-selective agent would cause profound EPSs and high sustained prolactin elevation, neither side-effect has been seen clinically with aripiprazole (Toru *et al.* 1994; Petrie *et al.* 1998; Saha *et al.* 1999). It has been proposed that aripiprazole induces 'functionally selective' activation of D_2 receptors coupled to diverse G proteins (and hence different functions), thereby explaining its unique clinical effects (Lawler *et al.* 1999). Based on available data, it would appear that aripiprazole is the first compound with partial D_2 agonist properties to be a clinically effective antipsychotic agent. Similar to aripiprazole, S-33592, a benzopyranopyrrole partial agonist at dopamine D_2/D_3 receptors, has shown a promising antipsychotic profile in the preliminary studies (Gobert *et al.* 2000; Rivet *et al.* 2000).

CI-1007 (R-(+)-1,2,3,6-tetrahydro-4-phenyl-1 [(3-phenyl-3-cyclohexen-1-yl)methyl]pyridine maleate) is a new dopamine autoreceptor agonist and partial dopamine D_2/D_3 receptor agonist that is currently under development for the treatment of schizophrenia (Wright *et al.* 1994; Pugsley *et al.* 1995; Sramek *et al.* 1998). In preclinical studies, CI-1007 demonstrated that it inhibited the firing of dopamine neurones and reduced the synthesis, metabolism, utilization and release of dopamine in the brain (Pugsley *et al.* 1995; Iyer *et al.* 1998). In addition, it produced behavioural effects predictive of antipsychotic efficacy and indicated a low liability for EPSs and TD (Meltzer *et al.* 1995). The results of initial clinical study suggest that patients with schizophrenia tolerate slightly higher initial doses of CI-1007 than do healthy subjects (Sramek *et al.* 1998).

Full D_1 agonist

Evidence has accumulated to suggest an important role for D_1-like dopamine receptors in the pathophysiology and management of schizophrenia (Goldman-Rakic 1999; Sedvall & Karlsson 1999; Miyamoto *et al.* 2001). Okubo *et al.* (1997) found decreased D_1-like receptor binding using positron emission tomography (PET) in the frontal cortex and basal ganglia of drug-naïve schizophrenics, and correlation between the reduction in prefrontal D_1-like receptors and the severity of negative symptoms and cognitive disturbance. Such data are consistent with the fact that pyramidal neurones in the prefrontal cortex postulated to be involved in working memory express a high degree of D_1-like dopamine receptors (Goldman-Rakic 1999; Goldman-Rakic *et al.* 2000). Recent evidence in monkeys indicates that chronic neuroleptic exposure for 6 months results in decreased prefrontal cortical D_1-like receptor density (Lidow *et al.* 1997). In addition, treatment with a full D_1-like receptor agonist, ABT 431, reversed neuroleptic-associated deficits in working memory (Castner *et al.* 2000). Low doses of selective full D_1-like receptor agonists, such as dihydrexidine, A77636 and SKF81297, have been reported to have

cognitive-enhancing actions in non-human primates (Arnsten *et al.* 1994; Schneider *et al.* 1994; Cai & Arnsten 1997). It is proposed that either insufficient or excessive D_1-like receptor stimulation is deleterious to cognitive function of the prefrontal cortex, thus an 'optimal' level of D_1-like receptor activation is necessary for normal cognitive function (Williams & Goldman-Rakic 1995; Goldman-Rakic *et al.* 2000). The finding that full D_1-like receptor agonists can improve working memory suggests that such classes of drugs might be novel potential treatments for cognitive symptoms of schizophrenia (Nichols & Mailman 1995, 1999; Ghosh *et al.* 1996; Castner *et al.* 2000; Miyamoto *et al.* 2000a).

5-HT agents

5-HT_{2A} antagonist

The 5-HT_{2A} receptor subtype has received considerable attention because of its potential roles in the therapeutic action of atypical antipsychotic drugs (Schmidt *et al.* 1995; Lieberman *et al.* 1998); it is involved in perception, mood regulation and motor control (Meltzer 1996). Available evidence indicates that 5-HT_{2A} receptor stimulation has a role in promoting the synthesis and release of dopamine, either by effects on firing rates of neurones, or via heteroreceptors on dopamine nerve terminals, or both (Ugedo *et al.* 1989; Schmidt *et al.* 1992, 1995; Meltzer 1996). 5-HT_{2A} receptor blockade may therefore contribute to 'normalizing' levels of dopamine release (O'Neill *et al.* 1999) and theoretically possess antipsychotic activity, especially for negative symptoms of schizophrenia (for review see Lieberman *et al.* 1998). In fact, 5-HT_{2A} blockade can increase firing of midbrain dopamine neurones and reverse the effects of NMDA antagonism (Svensson *et al.* 1995) and hypofrontality (Svensson *et al.* 1989) on A10 dopamine neuronal firing. Three placebo-controlled double-blind trials have demonstrated that addition of ritanserin, a relatively selective 5-HT_{2A} and 5-HT_{2C} antagonist, to a classical antipsychotic agent produced significant reductions in negative symptoms (primarily affective expression and social withdrawal) and depressed mood in chronic schizophrenia (Reynetjens *et al.* 1986; Gelders 1989; Duinkerke *et al.* 1993).

M-100907 (formerly MDL-100,907) is a selective 5-HT_{2A} receptor antagonist devoid of affinity to dopamine receptors (Lieberman *et al.* 1998). Like the atypical antipsychotics, it decreases the firing rate of A10, but not A9, neurones after chronic treatment (Sorensen *et al.* 1993) and it induces 5-HT_{2A} receptor internalization *in vitro* (Willins *et al.* 1999). M-100907 inhibited the behavioural response not only to amphetamine and cocaine (Sorensen *et al.* 1993; Arnt 1995; O'Neill *et al.* 1999), but also to NMDA-R antagonists at doses that did not affect spontaneous activity given alone in rodents (Maurel-Remy *et al.* 1995; Gleason & Shannon 1997; Carlsson *et al.* 1999). M-100907, like clozapine, markedly increases dopamine release in the medial prefrontal cortex in rats (Schmidt & Fadayel 1995), suggesting that the agent may have efficacy for negative symptoms. In contrast, it attenuates dopamine release in the nucleus accumbens induced by the NMDA-R antagonist MK-801 (Schmidt & Fadayel 1996). M-100907 also antagonized MK-801-induced prepulse inhibition deficit in rats (Varty *et al.* 1999). Further, in electrophysiological studies, it prevented phencyclidine (PCP)-induced blockade of NMDA responses (Wang & Liang 1998). These preclinical results suggest that M-100907 can attenuate variable responses to NMDA-R antagonists *in vivo* and modulate NMDA-R-mediated neurotransmission. However, M-100907 exhibited lower antipsychotic efficacy compared with haloperidol in Phase III clinical trials (Carlsson 2000), and the drug is no longer being actively developed. Insufficient data are currently published to judge adequately the efficacy of the drug, but the unpublished data from the Phase III trial indicate that monotherapy with a $5HT_{2A}$ antagonist is not a viable treatment strategy.

5-HT$_{1A}$ agonist

It has been suggested that the partial agonist activity of clozapine at 5-HT$_{1A}$ receptors may contribute to its therapeutic action (Meltzer 1996; Newman-Tancredi *et al.* 1996). Preclinical studies have suggested that serotonin 5-HT$_{1A}$ agonists may potentiate the antipsychotic activity of dopaminergic antagonists (Evenden 1992). Activation of inhibitory 5-HT$_{1A}$ autoreceptors may also counteract the induction of EPSs as a result of striatal D_2 receptor blockade (Lucas *et al.* 1997). Further, in schizophrenic patients, increased 5-HT$_{1A}$ receptor binding was seen in the prefrontal cortex (Burnet *et al.* 1996; Simpson *et al.* 1996). Based on these preclinical data, compounds that act as serotonin 5-HT$_{1A}$ agonists are being developed as potential antipsychotic compounds.

The novel benzopyranopyrrolidine and potential antipsychotic S-16924 ((+)-2-[[1-[2-(2,3-dihydrobenzo[1,4]dioxin-5-yloxy)ethyl]-pyrrolidin-3yl]]-1-(4-fluorophenyl)ethanone), displays high affinity for dopamine $D_{2/4}$, α_1-adrenergic and serotonin 5-HT$_{2A/2C}$ receptors, similar to that of clozapine, in addition to being a potent partial 5-HT$_{1A}$ agonist (Millan *et al.* 1998b; Cussac *et al.* 2000). Reflecting its partial agonist actions at 5-HT$_{1A}$ receptors, it attenuates cerebral serotonergic transmission, and preferentially facilitates dopaminergic transmission in mesocortical as compared to mesolimbic and nigrostriatal pathways (Bengtsson *et al.* 1998; Millan *et al.* 1998a). S-16924 exhibited a profile of potential antipsychotic activity and low EPS liability in animal behavioural models, similar to clozapine (Millan *et al.* 1998b; Cussac *et al.* 2000).

BSF 190555 (BTS 79018), a mixed dopamine D_2/D_3 antagonist and a partial 5-HT$_{1A}$ agonist, has been developed as a potential new antipsychotic agent (Birch *et al.* 1999; Wicke & Gross 2000). BSF 190555 shows significantly less affinity for α_1 adrenoceptors, H_1 and muscarinic receptors. After oral dosage, the agent showed good activity in rodent antipsychotic tests and very little potential to cause EPSs, as measured by its ability to induce catalepsy in rats (Birch *et al.* 1999). In the light of this promising profile of activity, BSF 190555 has potential as a novel antipsychotic agent with a predicted low propensity to cause EPSs (Wicke & Gross 2000).

Muscarinic agents

It has been postulated that neurochemical alterations in the dopaminergic–cholinergic balance may be central to psychotic symptoms in both Alzheimer's disease and schizophrenia (for review see White & Cummings 1996). The hypothesis suggests that psychotic symptoms may be related, at least in part, to either a relative hyperdopaminergia and/or a hypocholinergia, and thus might be treated by either dopaminergic antagonists or cholinergic agonists (White & Cummings 1996; Bymaster *et al.* 1999). Recent findings that partial agonists of M_2/M_4 muscarinic receptors are active in animal models that predict antipsychotic activity suggest the potential usefulness of muscarinic agonists in the treatment of schizophrenia (Sauerberg *et al.* 1998).

PTAC [(5R,6R)-6-(3-propylthio-1,2,5-thiadiazol-4-yl)-1-azabicyclo[3.2.1]octane] is a muscarinic partial agonist at muscarinic M_2/M_4 receptor subtypes and $M_1/M_3/M_5$ antagonist (Bymaster *et al.* 1998; Sauerberg *et al.* 1998). Although PTAC has minimal or no affinity for central dopamine receptors, the drug acts as a functional dopamine antagonist in many paradigms (consistent with known dopamine–acetylcholine interactions). PTAC blocks apomorphine-induced climbing in mice (Bymaster *et al.* 1999), inhibits the effects of D_1 and D_2 dopamine receptors agonists in 6-hydroxydopamine-lesioned rats and antagonizes amphetamine-induced *Fos* induction and hyperactivity (Bymaster *et al.* 1998). In addition, after chronic administration, PTAC selectively reduced the number of spontaneously active A10, but not A9, dopamine cells (Bymaster *et al.* 1998). Such selective effects on the mesocorticolimbic dopamine projection neurones are similar to those observed for the atypical antipsychotics clozapine and olanzapine (Chiodo & Bunney 1983; Skarsfeldt 1995). The notable preclinical data of the effects of PTAC provide strong encouragement to examine the potential therapeutic effects of M_2/M_4 muscarinic agonists in schizophrenic patients.

Xanomeline is a direct muscarinic receptor agonist which preferentially acts at M_1 and M_4 receptors with little or no affinity for dopamine receptors (Bymaster *et al.* 1994; Shannon *et al.* 1994). Xanomeline has been demonstrated to have positive effects on cognitive and psychotic-like symptoms (e.g. hallucinations and delusions) in Alzheimer's disease (Bodick *et al.* 1997). Both electrophysiologically and behaviourally, xanomeline produces antipsychotic-like effects in rats and mice, which are similar to those produced by clozapine and olanzapine as well as PTAC (Shannon *et al.* 2000). In addition, one preliminary report suggests that xanomeline has the potential to enhance prefrontal cortical function (Perry *et al.* 1999). These data suggest that xanomeline might be efficacious in treating not only positive, but also negative and cognitive symptoms in schizophrenia (Perry *et al.* 1999; Shannon *et al.* 2000). Among the agents developed for the treatment of Alzheimer's disease that are being examined in schizophrenia are donepezil, metrifonate, glantamine and xanomeline (Miyamoto *et al.* 2002).

Adrenergic agents

α_2 Agonist

It is generally believed that the dysfunction of the prefrontal cortex (PFC) contributes to the cognitive deficits seen in schizophrenia (for review see Arnsten *et al.* 1996; Friedman *et al.* 1999b). In addition to dopaminergic inputs, noradrenergic inputs from the locus ceruleus to the PFC have an important role in cognitive function (for review see Friedman *et al.* 1999a). A high density of α_2 receptors has been observed in the area of the principal sulcus of the PFC (Goldman-Rakic *et al.* 1990) and α_2 receptor activity may be the most important mechanism of noradrenergic neurotransmission in this region (Friedman *et al.* 1999b). Indeed, the α_2 agonist clonidine has been shown to improve performance on working memory tasks in young monkeys with noradrenergic depleting lesions of the PFC, presumably through its drug actions at postsynaptic α_2 receptors in the PFC (Arnsten & Goldman-Rakic 1985). Clonidine also improves PFC-mediated cognitive dysfunction in schizophrenia (Fields *et al.* 1988). In addition, guanfacine, a selective α_{2A} agonist (Uhlen *et al.* 1995), improves PFC-mediated working memory in aged non-human primates, but without the significant adverse effects associated with clonidine (e.g. sedation, hypotension) (Arnsten *et al.* 1988). A recent placebo-controlled double-blind study, albeit only preliminarily reported, demonstrated the efficacy and safety of guanfacine as adjunctive treatment of cognitive impairment in schizophrenia (Friedman *et al.* 2000). Those patients receiving guanfacine plus risperidone showed significant improvement on tasks of working memory and attention compared with patients receiving typical neuroleptics plus guanfacine (Friedman *et al.* 2000). The potential ability of α_2 agonists to improve cognitive performance on tasks dependent on PFC function appears to be of great importance in the search for a new pharmacological approach for schizophrenia.

α_1 and α_2 antagonists

Clozapine and risperidone have potent antagonist properties at α_1 and α_2 adrenergic receptors (ARs) (Table 24.2). Millan *et al.* (2000a,b) have recently postulated the significance of the α_1 and α_2 AR antagonistic activity for the antipsychotic effects of neuroleptics. Blockade of α_1-ARs preferentially suppresses mesolimbic vs. nigrostriatal dopaminergic transmission (Svensson *et al.* 1995). Prazosin, a selective α_1 AR antagonist, increases dopamine output in the shell of the nucleus accumbens in rats, similar to clozapine, olanzapine and quetiapine (Marcus *et al.* 2000). Interestingly, prazosin can inhibit MK-801-induced hyperlocomotion and dopamine release in the nucleus accumbens (Mathe *et al.* 1996). Bakshi and Geyer (1997) previously suggested that antagonism of α_1 ARs may have a major role in

mediating the blockade of PCP-induced deficits in prepulse inhibition by certain antipsychotics. In addition, blockade of inhibitory α_2 AR heteroceptors on terminals of dopaminergic fibres can enhance frontocortical dopaminergic transmission compared with subcortical dopaminergic pathways (Gobert *et al.* 1998). Litman *et al.* (1996) reported that combined treatment with the α_2 AR antagonist idazoxan and the typical neuroleptic fluphenazine can produce a 'clozapine-like' profile of antipsychotic activity. Finally, antagonist properties of α_2 ARs appear to be implicated in the functional actions of clozapine in humans (Elman *et al.* 1999) and contribute to an improvement in mood (Millan *et al.* 2000b).

The novel compound S-18327 (1-[2-[4-(6-fluoro-1,2-benzisoxazol-3-yl)piperid-1-yl]ethyl]3-phenylimidazolin-2-one) displays marked antagonist properties at α_1- and α_2-ARs (Millan *et al.* 2000b). S-18327 has modest affinity for D_1, D_2 and D_3 receptors, and high affinity for D_4 and 5-HT_{2A} receptors like clopazine, but it is chemically distinct and displays weak affinity for histaminic and muscarinic receptors (Millan *et al.* 2000b). S-18327 displays a broad-based pattern of potential antipsychotic activity at doses appreciably lower than those eliciting EPSs (Millan *et al.* 2000a). Moreover, S-18327 potently blocked NMDA antagonist-induced hyperlocomotion in rats (Millan *et al.* 2000a). Antagonism by S-18327 of α_2 ARs enhances adrenergic transmission and reinforces frontocortical dopaminergic transmission, whereas blockade of α_1 ARs inhibits dorsal raphe-derived serotonergic pathways (Millan *et al.* 2000b). These unique profiles of activity may contribute to the potential antipsychotic properties of S-18327, although the putative therapeutic significance of the α_1 and α_2 AR antagonistic activity remains unknown.

Glutamatergic agents

Antipsychotic drug actions in relation to the NMDA-R hypofunction hypothesis of schizophrenia

Since the late 1950s, the anaesthetics phencyclidine (PCP) and ketamine have been known to induce a psychotomimetic state that closely resembles some features of schizophrenia (Javitt & Zukin 1991). Recent clinical studies have demonstrated that subanaesthetic doses of ketamine can induce behavioural effects in healthy humans that resemble positive, negative and cognitive symptoms of schizophrenia (Krystal *et al.* 1994; Malhotra *et al.* 1996). In chronic stabilized schizophrenic patients, ketamine can also exacerbate cognitive impairment and, in some cases, reproduce specific psychotic symptoms that are remarkably similar to those experienced during active phases of their illness (Lahti *et al.* 1995a,b; Malhotra *et al.* 1997). Both ketamine and PCP are potent non-competitive NMDA-R antagonists. These drugs bind to a site within the calcium channel of the NMDA-R complex, and thereby interfere with calcium flux through the channel. The ability of NMDA antagonists to induce a spectrum of schizophrenia-like symptoms has led to the hypothesis that decreased NMDA-R function may be a predisposing or causative factor in schizophrenia (Deutsch *et al.* 1989; Javitt & Zukin 1991; Olney & Farber 1995; Coyle 1996).

The well-documented psychotomimetic effects of NMDA antagonist in humans suggest that effects of the drugs in experimental animals could present useful pharmacological models of schizophrenia (for review see Duncan *et al.* 1999c). In our recent studies, striking effects of subanaesthetic doses of ketamine were observed on regional brain patterns of ^{14}C-2-deoxyglucose (2-DG) uptake in both rats (Duncan *et al.* 1998b, 1999a) and mice (Miyamoto *et al.* 2000b, 2001). Ketamine induces robust and neuroanatomically selective patterns of brain metabolic activation, with especially large effects observed in the hippocampus, nucleus accumbens and medial prefrontal cortex (Duncan *et al.* 1998b, 1999a). Pretreatment of rats with clozapine, olanzapine and ziprasidone, but not haloperidol or risperidone, can block these effects of ketamine (Duncan *et al.* 1998a, 2000a,b). Similarly, clozapine and olanzapine, but not haloperidol, effectively block NMDA antagonist-induced electrophysiological responses (Wang & Liang 1998), deficits in prepulse inhibition (Bakshi *et al.* 1994; Bakshi & Geyer 1995) and deficits in social interactions (Corbett *et al.* 1995). Thus, in a wide range of experimental paradigms, atypical antipsychotic drugs selectively antagonize the consequences of experimentally induced NMDA-R hypofunction, raising the possibility that the therapeutic effects of these agents may be associated with a similar neurochemical action (Duncan *et al.* 1999b).

Therapeutic potential of glycine site agonists

If reduced NMDA-R function is involved in the pathophysiology of schizophrenia, then drugs that enhance NMDA-R function could be therapeutic agents and potentially improve upon, or supplement, current antipsychotic treatments (for review see Duncan *et al.* 1999c). Direct agonists of the NMDA-R may not be feasible candidates in this regard, because of the propensity of such drugs to produce excessive excitation and seizures.

Glycine is a positive allosteric modulator and obligatory co-agonist at the NMDA-R (Johnson & Ascher 1987; Leeson & Iversen 1994) and this allosteric regulatory site represents a potential target for drugs to augment NMDA-mediated neurotransmission. Preclinical studies have demonstrated that glycine-site agonists reverse the effects of non-competitive NMDA-R antagonists (Javitt *et al.* 1997). There have been several clinical studies to test effects of different glycine site agonists in patients with schizophrenia. The earliest open-label studies in this regard used glycine in doses of 5–15 g/day and obtained inconsistent results (Rosse *et al.* 1989; Costa *et al.* 1990). In more recent double-blind studies with glycine, higher doses were administered (30–60 g/day) and more robust and consistent effects were found, primarily in the improvement of negative symptoms (Javitt *et al.* 1994; Heresco-Levy *et al.* 1996, 1999). Glycine at a dosage of 60 g/day produced a 30% mean reduction in negative symptoms and also improved a qualitative measure of cognitive functioning in schizophrenic patients resistant to typical antipsychotics ($n = 15$) or clozapine ($n = 7$) (Heresco-

Levy *et al.* 1999). However, in two double-blind placebo-controlled studies of glycine (30–60 g/day) added to clozapine in schizophrenia, glycine as an adjunct to clozapine produced no significant change in positive or negative symptoms or cognitive functioning (Potkin *et al.* 1999; Evins *et al.* 2000). Glycine has a poor central nervous system bioavailability and the doses needed to effect clinical benefit (30–60 g/day) are very difficult to administer.

D-Cycloserine is a partial agonist at the glycine regulatory site on the NMDA-R. Thus, at low levels, D-Cycloserine can act in synchrony with the full agonist glycine to stimulate responses, but at higher doses D-cycloserine would block the effects of endogenous glycine (Henderson *et al.* 1990). D-Cycloserine has been tested in schizophrenia and, in a very narrow dosage range, the agent was shown to improve negative symptoms when administered alone (van Berckel *et al.* 1996), and when added to conventional antipsychotic agents such as haloperidol (Goff *et al.* 1995b, 1999d). Interestingly, when D-cycloserine was administered in conjunction with clozapine, the negative symptoms of the patients worsened (Goff *et al.* 1996, 1999c). These results parallel the recent preclinical study of the effect of D-Cycloserine in rats, which shows that D-Cycloserine (1 mg/kg) can enhance *c-fos* induction after treatment with haloperidol (0.3 mg/kg), but not clozapine (20 mg/kg) (Leveque *et al.* 2000). A ready explanation for these effects is not available, but understanding the mechanisms involved in the worsening of negative symptoms after administration of D-Cycloserine to clozapine-treated patients may be an important clue in understanding the actions of both of these drugs. D-Cycloserine did not improve cognitive functioning when added to conventional agents in a study that utilized formal cognitive testing (Goff *et al.* 1999d). The poor penetration of the blood–brain barrier by glycine, and the partial agonistic properties of D-Cycloserine, appear to make these agents less than optimal for providing pharmacological agonism of the glycine regulatory site on the NMDA-R (Duncan *et al.* 1999c).

D-Serine is a full agonist on the strychnine-insensitive glycine site of NMDA-R (Hashimoto & Oka 1997) and is more permeable than glycine at the blood–brain barrier, thus requiring a lower dosage. In an 8-week clinical trial of treatment-resistant patients with schizophrenia, D-serine (30 mg/kg/day) added to typical antipsychotics ($n = 25$) or risperidone ($n = 4$) demonstrated significant improvements not only in negative and cognitive symptoms but also positive symptoms, which is different from glycine (Tsai *et al.* 1998). Consistent with the findings with glycine and D-cycloserine, D-serine (30 mg/kg/day) in addition to clozapine did not improve any symptoms (Tsai *et al.* 1999).

Although most of the studies on glycine site agonists involved very small numbers of patients, and dosing challenges with glycine and D-cycloserine may make them impractical for clinical use, studies on these compounds provide strong support for a role of NMDA-R function in the pathophysiology and pharmacotherapy of schizophrenia. Recently, Wolosker *et al.* (1999) have purified an enzyme from type II astrocytes that converts L-serine to D-serine. It may be that effectors of this enzyme (directly or through possible receptor-mediated regulation) can provide a mechanism to modulate NMDA-R function. Examining the effects of synthetic compounds with greater potency and full agonistic activity at the glycine regulatory site could be an intriguing line of future research. However there are no such compounds available for testing at present.

Potentiation of NMDA-R function by inhibition of glycine uptake

Glycine transporters have been identified on both neuronal and glial cells in the central nervous system. A function of these transporters has been suggested to control the extracellular glycine concentration (Bergeron et al. 1998). Although there is some controversy as to whether the glycine regulatory site on the NMDA-R is saturated under physiological conditions, recent data demonstrate that inhibition of glycine transport by glycine transporter type 1 antagonist can potentiate electrophysiological effects of NMDA (Berger et al. 1998; Bergeron et al. 1998). Furthermore, the glycine uptake inhibitor glycyldodecylamide attenuated PCP-induced hyperactivity more potently than glycine (Javitt & Frusciante 1997; Javitt et al. 1997). These preclinical data suggest that inhibition of glycine uptake could represent a feasible approach to potentiate NMDA-R-mediated neurotransmission and, possibly, treat schizophrenic patients.

Glutamate release-inhibiting drugs

A number of studies have indicated that administration of relatively low (subanaesthetic) doses of NMDA antagonists induces behavioural and brain metabolic activation in experimental animals and humans (Duncan et al. 1999b). Consistent with these data, NMDA antagonists increase glutamate release in rats (Moghaddam et al. 1997). In contrast to the increase in glutamate release by subanaesthetic doses of ketamine, anaesthetic doses of the drug decreased glutamate levels (Moghaddam et al. 1997). The effect of different doses of ketamine on glutamate levels is consistent with our observations of increased 2-DG uptake in response to a subanaesthetic dose, and reduction in 2-DG uptake in response to an anaesthetic dose of ketamine (Duncan et al. 1998b).

The stimulatory effect of NMDA-R antagonism presumably results from disinhibitory actions, perhaps by reducing excitatory input to inhibitory interneurones (Duncan et al. 1999b). In hippocampal formation, GABAergic interneurones are more sensitive to the effects of NMDA antagonists than the glutamate-containing pyramidal cells (Grunze et al. 1996), providing support for the hypothesis that NMDA antagonism could result in excitatory effects by disrupting recurrent inhibitory circuits (Duncan et al. 1999b).

If behavioural activation induced by NMDA antagonists is related to increased glutamate release, pharmacological agents that decrease glutamate release should block the effects of the drugs. Glutamate release can be inhibited by Na^+-channel blockers, Ca^{2+}-channel blockers, K^+-decreasing agents, toxins that prevent fusion of vesicles with the presynaptic membrane, and presynaptic group II metabotropic glutamate autoreceptor agonists (Battaglia et al. 1997a; Attwell et al. 1998; Anand et al. 2000).

Administration of LY-354740, a group II metabotropic glutamate receptor agonist, blocked both behavioural activation and increased glutamate release induced by PCP in rats (Moghaddam & Adams 1998). In humans, Anand et al. (2000) found that lamotrigine, a new anticonvulsant agent that inhibits glutamate release, can reduce the ketamine-induced neuropsychiatric effects. These data suggest the possibility that glutamate release-inhibiting drugs (e.g. LY-354740 and lamotrigine) could be useful in the treatment of schizophrenia. The use of such drugs as therapeutic agents in the treatment of schizophrenia may seem contradictory to the above discussion of the potential utility of indirect glutamate antagonists. However, it is possible that both hyper- and hypoglutamatergic function may occur in schizophrenia during different phases of the illness, with acute psychotic episodes associated with a hyperglutamatergic state, and chronic illness related more to a hypoglutamatergic state, that could effectively produce a sensitization of glutamate receptors. Although clearly speculative, such a scenario could explain the apparent incongruities in hypotheses of potential efficacy of positive modulators and negative modulators of glutamate systems.

AMPA/kainate receptor antagonists

The increased release of glutamate observed in response to NMDA antagonist could mediate some of the behavioural actions of the drugs by activation of non-NMDA receptors, including α-amino-3-hydroxy-5-methyl-isoxazole-4-propionic acid (AMPA) and kainate receptors (Moghaddam et al. 1997). In support of the hypothesis that behavioural effects of N7MDA antagonists relate to increased glutamate release, administration of an AMPA/kainate receptor antagonist, LY-293558, partially reversed impairment of working memory induced by subanaesthetic doses of ketamine in rats (Moghaddam et al. 1997). Furthermore, AMPA/kainate receptor antagonists (e.g. GYKI 52466) reduce NMDA antagonist-induced hyperlocomotion (Bubser et al. 1992; Hauber & Andersen 1993; Willins et al. 1993) and neurodegeneration (Sharp et al. 1995). These data suggest that AMPA/kainate receptor antagonists may have utility for treatment of cognitive deficits in which NMDA-R hypofunction is suspect (Moghaddam et al. 1997).

Potential of positive modulators of AMPA receptors

In apparent contrast to the postulated utility of AMPA/kainate receptor antagonists as antipsychotics, ampakines, a class of compounds that allosterically enhance AMPA receptor function, have also been suggested to represent potential adjunctive treatments for schizophrenia. Ampakines enhance excitatory (glutamatergic) transmission, facilitate long-term potentiation, learning and memory in rodents (Hampson *et al.* 1998a,b), and have synergistic effects with typical and atypical antipsychotics on blocking behavioural effects of methamphetamine (Johnson *et al.* 1999). In addition, preliminary results suggest that chronic administration of an ampakine (CX-516) can improve negative and cognitive symptoms in schizophrenia patients who also receive clozapine (Goff *et al.* 1999a). Effect sizes favouring CX-516 over placebo were moderate to large (0.5–1.2) on tests of cognitive performance (Goff *et al.* 1999a). Such findings appear to be paradoxical with regard to the foregoing discussion of the hypothesis that AMPA antagonists can reduce the effects induced by NMDA-R hypofunction in some preclinical models. Further clinical experience with the effects of positive and negative modulators of non-NMDA glutamate receptors are needed to clarify the potential of these compounds for treatment of schizophrenia (Miyamoto *et al.* 2002).

Practical clinical issues

Who to treat?

Antipsychotics can significantly reduce the risk of relapse in first episode schizophrenic patients, at least for the first year or two (Kane 1999b). For example, the 1-year randomized placebo-controlled study conducted by Kane *et al.* (1982) of 28 first episode schizophrenic patients found that none of patients receiving active fluphenazine decanoate relapsed within 1 year, compared with 41% of those who received placebo. Similarly, a randomized placebo-controlled trial conducted by Crow *et al.* (1986) on 120 patients with first episode schizophrenia reported that 46% of the patients on active medication relapsed within 2 years, compared with 62% of those on placebo. However, it is noteworthy that 38–59% of patients who received placebo were free from relapse for the first year or two in these studies. In an early double-blind study on over 400 acutely ill schizophrenic patients, 23% of placebo-treated subjects demonstrated marked or moderate improvement within 6 weeks (National Institute of Mental Health Psychopharmacology Service Center Collaborative Study Group 1964). Moreover, on average among multiepisode schizophrenic patients, 24% of the patients who have been in remission with medication for long periods of time are unchanged within a year or two of discontinuing treatment (Kane 1999b). These studies suggest that a considerable proportion of schizophrenic patients may remit without medication or with a placebo effect. In theory, it would be reasonable to withhold antipsychotic medications from patients who will recover without them or those who will not improve with them. Unfortunately, the literature is not particularly helpful in supplying reliable predictors of drug response (Marder 1997). Moreover, in the practical treatment setting of acute schizophrenia, it is impossible to identify reliably patients who will recover spontaneously unless they are first tried without medication (Hirsch & Barnes 1995). In addition, the initial treatment without medication appears to be impractical, be-cause a delay in the treatment of acute exacerbations may be associated with poorer clinical outcomes (May *et al.* 1976; Wyatt 1995) and rapid management and discharge are frequently required in day-to-day clinical practice situations (Hirsch & Barnes 1995). Unfortunately, even if first episode patients do respond to treatment with typical antipsychotics, 70–80% of patients will experience a second episode within the following 5 years (Prudo & Blum 1987; Wiersma *et al.* 1998). This high rate may be because patients are administered maintenance treatment for an insufficient duration or because of early treatment withdrawal (Kane 1999b).

It has been proposed that schizophrenic patients might be better treated in the long term by offering them a period off medication when they are feeling well and only reinstitutional treatment if they experience early signs of relapse. This so-called 'targeted' or 'intermittent' strategy would allegedly reduce the long-term risks and subjective discomfort associated with adverse effects of medication (Carpenter *et al.* 1987; Hirsch & Barnes 1995). This strategy has been tested in a number of large-scale controlled studies (for review see Gaebel 1995; Kane 1999b), all of which demonstrated that relapse rates with intermittent treatment were approximately twice as high as those with continuous treatment. Continuous treatment is thus preferred. The earlier ambivalence regarding continuous treatment was partly because of the risk of developing TD with the typical antipsychotics (Kane 1999b). Studies using clozapine treatment, however, demonstrated that it is associated with little or no incidence of TD, and may have therapeutic value in a proportion of established cases of TD (Kane *et al.* 1988). Moreover, studies have shown that newer atypical antipsychotics such as olanzapine have a lower risk of developing TD than conventional agents (Beasley *et al.* 1999). Therefore, continuous treatment with an atypical antipsychotic may be the best strategy to prevent relapse, while minimizing the risk of TD, in patients who consistently take oral medications (Kane 1999b; see Chapter 25).

Predictors of treatment response

To choose an optimal treatment strategy that will lead to the best response from the patients while minimizing side-effects, significant efforts are underway to identify the factors that contribute to the outcome of acute treatment with antipsychotics (Gaebel 1996). Lieberman and colleagues have examined the potential predictors of acute treatment response of first episode patients with schizophrenia or schizoaffective disorder since 1986. They found that patients with spontaneous EPSs prior to antipsychotic exposure (Chatterjee *et al.* 1995) and patients who later develop TD (Chakos *et al.* 1996) are less likely to respond to treatment. They also demonstrated that male gender, a history of obstetric complications, worse attention at baseline, more severe positive symptoms and the development of parkinsonism during acute antipsychotic treatment were associated with a significantly lower likelihood of response to treatment (Robinson *et al.* 1999).

Early intervention

Renewed attention has focused on treatment response of first episode patients because of the widely held belief that early intervention with antipsychotic medications after the onset of psychosis may favourably alter the subsequent course of the illness (for review see Wyatt 1991, 1995; Lieberman 1996). This notion, which often invokes the 'toxic psychosis hypothesis' as a mechanism (for review see Lieberman *et al.* 1996b; Lieberman 1999), is largely based on one naturalistic study (Loebel *et al.* 1992). Lieberman (1999) has hypothesized that a limited neurodegenerative process is involved in the pathophysiology of schizophrenia, and that the pathological process is reflected by the psychotic symptoms and is most active in the early stages of the illness. In addition, the duration and number of periods of active positive symptoms during the first episode of illness, prior to receiving antipsychotic medication, appear to be a significant predictor of the time to treatment response, relapse and long-term outcome (Huber *et al.* 1980; May *et al.* 1981; Crow *et al.* 1986; Lieberman *et al.* 1990b; Wyatt 1991; Loebel *et al.* 1992). Specifically, the treatment response and outcome are diminished with longer duration of psychosis before treatment is started (for review see McGlashan 1996; Lieberman *et al.* 1997). These findings have important consequences for the development of early detection and intervention strategies for acute episodes (Gaebel & Marder 1996; McGlashan 1996; Lieberman 1999).

Other naturalistic studies, however, have found no significant association between the duration of prior or untreated psychosis and clinical outcome (Robinson *et al.* 1999; Craig *et al.* 2000; Ho *et al.* 2000). Larsen *et al.* (2001) have recently reviewed the literature on early intervention programmes in schizophrenia. They conclude that the existence of a causal relationship between longer duration of untreated psychosis and poorer outcome is not yet perfectly established. Thus, prospective controlled trials are necessary to determine whether early intervention with specific antipsychotic agents improves the early course of the illness in first episode patients (Lieberman & Fenton 2000).

Which drugs to use in acute emergency?

In emergency settings, selection of an agent for the management of the gross agitation, excitement and violent behaviour sometimes associated with psychosis can be based on clinical symptoms, differences in efficacy or side-effects of candidate drugs or, more pragmatically, the formulation of a drug as it affects route of administration, onset and duration (Hirsch & Barnes 1995; Allen 2000). Currier (2000) has recently found that most agitated patients will assent to oral medication and, in a survey of 51 psychiatric emergency services, the medical doctors estimated that only 10% of emergency patients require injectable medications. The US Health Care Finance Administration's (HCFA) regulations regarding so-called 'chemical restraint' call for it to be a last resort, which would suggest that oral medication should be offered whenever it is possible to speak with the patient (Allen 2000). Nevertheless, intramuscular treatments remain necessary for some agitated or aggressive patients who refuse oral medications of any kind. In these situations, many clinicians avoid high doses of antipsychotic medications in favour of a combination of an antipsychotic and a benzodiazepine, as discussed below.

Typical antipsychotics

The use of high doses of typical antipsychotics during the first days of treatment ('rapid neuroleptization') should be avoided because of lack of efficacy and risk of adverse effects, as described in more detail below (Hirsch & Barnes 1995; American Psychiatric Association 2000). The use of intravenous typical antipsychotics may be associated with rapid onset, yet intravenous care is available in a small minority of psychiatric settings, because of the risk of cardiac arrythmias and other autonomic complications (Hirsch & Barnes 1995; Allen 2000). Prior to the development of atypical antipsychotics, many clinicians favoured intramuscular preparations of high-potency typical antipsychotics because of the perceived benefits of reliable drug delivery (Hillard 1998). They were generally viewed as much safer than low-potency typical antipsychotics and barbiturates (Allen 2000). The onset of action of intramuscular administration is generally slower than that of intravenous. However, droperidol i.m. is absorbed so rapidly that there is little difference between intramuscular and intravenous administration (Cressman *et al.* 1973). In a randomized double-blind prospective study in 68 violent or agitated patients, Thomas *et al.* found droperidol i.m. (5 mg) to have a faster onset of efficacy for agitation than haloperidol (5 mg), but the two agents were equivalent at 1 h (Thomas *et al.* 1992).

Benzodiazepines

Recently, benzodiazepines have achieved popularity in acute psychiatric emergencies because of their efficacy, safety and tolerability (for review see Allen 2000). In clinical practice, 'cocktails' consisting typically of haloperidol i.m., a benzodiazepine, and an anticholinergic agent have been routinely administered (Binder & McNiel 1999; Currier 2000). The use of benzodiazepines may allow a more rapid sedative effect and reduce the amount of antipsychotic drugs that are needed to control agitated psychotic patients (Hyde & Harrower-Wilson 1996; Marder 1996). All available evidence suggests that benzodiazepines, including lorazepam (Salzman *et al.* 1991; Battaglia *et al.* 1997b; Foster *et al.* 1997), midazolam (Wyant *et al.* 1990), clonazepam (Chouinard *et al.* 1993a) and flunitrazepam (Dorevitch *et al.* 1999), are at least as effective as haloperidol alone for controlling agitation. In addition, Battaglia *et al.* found lorazepam (2 mg) alone more sedative than haloperidol (5 mg) alone (Battaglia *et al.* 1997b). Intramuscular absorption of lorazepam and midazolam is rapid and complete, with onset at 15–30 min (Allen 2000). In general, oral benzodiazepines are also rapidly effective (Allen 2000). These medications appear to be an effective method for eliminating the unnecessary restraints or seclusion (Dubin & Feld 1989). However, no dose-finding studies of benzodiazepines have been performed for agitation (Allen 2000).

Atypical antipsychotics

First-line treatments for behavioural emergencies have changed significantly with the advent of atypical antipsychotics. In 1996, conventional antipsychotics were still regarded as first-line agents in the management of schizophrenia (McEvoy et al. 1996); however, by 1999, the newer atypical antipsychotics were recommended as first-line treatment for schizophrenia by the medication experts in the USA in most clinical situations, including in an acute episode (McEvoy et al. 1999).

It is possible to combine oral atypical antipsychotics and benzodiazepines in a manner that safely achieves good behavioural control and initiates superior long-term care for schizophrenia (Currier 2000). It would be best to avoid combining antipsychotics in favour of sequential trials of monotherapy with different antipsychotics (Feifel 2000). It is also possible to safely escalate the dose of atypical antipsychotics more rapidly than is usual in outpatient settings to achieve target doses typically utilized for the treatment of schizophrenia (Feifel 2000; Karagianis et al. 2001). Once behavioural control is achieved, benzodiazepines should be discontinued and the patient should be maintained on the atypical antipsychotics alone (Sharif 1998).

One of the major advantages of atypical antipsychotics is a lower rate of the worrisome side-effects such as akathisia that may worsen agitation. Although the antiaggressive characteristics of clozapine are well established in chronically psychotic patients (for review see Glazer & Dickson 1998; Buckley 1999), clozapine initiation is contraindicated at sedative doses in the psychiatric emergency service, because of its serious potential side-effects, including seizures and agranulocytosis (Currier 2000). Czobor et al. (1995), in a subanalysis of the US multicentre comparative trial between risperidone and haloperidol, noted a greater selective effect of risperidone (2–16 mg/day) on hostility than haloperidol (20 mg/day) in 139 patients with schizophrenia. Moreover, risperidone (5–15 mg/day) has been shown to be more effective than perphenazine (16–48 mg/day) in controlling hostility associated with psychosis in a double-blind study in 107 chronic schizophrenics with acute exacerbations (Hoyberg et al. 1993). In a subanalysis conducted on the results of a large international randomized double-blind trial, Kinon et al. demonstrated that olanzapine (5–20 mg/day) is superior to haloperidol (5–20 mg/day) in reducing agitation and positive symptoms in 1996 patients in the acute phase of schizophrenia (Kinon et al. 2001b). Quetiapine was preliminarily found to be superior to haloperidol (12.5 mg/day) in reducing agitation at a dose of 600 mg/day in two 6-week double-blind randomized studies (Goldstein 1998; Hellewell et al. 1998).

A final concern is the patient who appears to accept oral medication but does not swallow it, so-called 'cheeking or spitting' (Allen 2000). Currier and Simpson (2001) have recently found that the combination of oral risperidone liquid concentrate (2 mg) and oral lorazepam (2 mg) was equivalent in efficacy to haloperidol i.m. (5 mg) and lorazepam i.m. (2 mg) in agitated psychotic patients who accept oral medications. More recently, Kinon et al. (2001a) preliminarily reported a prospective open-label study, assessing the efficacy and safety of the orally disintegrating tablet formulation of olanzapine that dissolves shortly after contact with saliva, for up to 6 weeks in 85 acutely ill non-compliant schizophrenic patients (Kinon et al. 2001a). Orally disintegrating olanzapine (10–20 mg/day) demonstrated significant efficacy in improving overall psychopathology and reducing non-compliant attitudes and behaviours. The unique oral formulation of olanzapine was well-tolerated (Kinon et al. 2001a).

Clinicians can now choose between the available formulations of several atypical antipsychotic agents when treating agitated patients with schizophrenia. Because the usefulness of these drugs in acute emergency situations has been largely unexplored, and there has been less clinical experience with them compared with conventional agents, clinicians must determine how to use the new agents most effectively and safely. Moreover, several differentiating factors should be considered when selecting among atypical antipsychotics that may be used for extended periods of time. For example, significantly more weight gain and incidences of hyperglycaemia and diabetic ketoacidosis are associated with clozapine and olanzapine than with the other atypical agents (Wirshing et al. 1998, 1999; Allison et al. 1999; see Chapter 29).

Dose–response relationships

Rapid neuroleptization

Rapid neuroleptization has been proposed as a strategy for providing rapid and effective control of excitement and agitation in acute psychotic patients (for review see Donlon et al. 1979). This practice involves the use of high doses of high-potency typical antipsychotic drugs, usually haloperidol, administered intramuscularly over brief intervals of time within a 24-h period, until the patient demonstrates obvious sedation or side-effects (Polak & Laycob 1971; Donlon et al. 1979). A number of well-controlled double-blind studies comparing high-dose strategies with standard regimens revealed no significant superiority for high dosage in either degree or rapidity of response in acute psychotic patients (Neborsky et al. 1981; Escobar et al. 1983; Coffman et al. 1987). Moreover, higher doses of neuroleptic medication produced a significantly higher incidence of EPSs (Neborsky et al. 1981; Escobar et al. 1983; Coffman et al. 1987). Thus, the rapid neuroleptization technique has largely been discontinued as a therapeutic strategy.

Effective doses of typical antipsychotics

The goal of pharmacotherapy is to maximize efficacy and minimize adverse effects with the lowest effective dose (Janicak &

Davis 1996). The neuroleptic threshold hypothesis, first considered by Haase (1961) and subsequently revised by McEvoy *et al.* (1991), states that fine motor as opposed to classic BPS signal the minimum effective dose for many acutely psychotic patients (Haase 1961; McEvoy *et al.* 1991; for review see Janicak & Davis 1996). Determining the optimal dose of typical antipsychotics for an acute schizophrenic episode, however, has been an elusive goal, with the possible exception of chlorpromazine or haloperidol (for review see Hirsch & Barnes 1995; Janicak & Davis 1996). Patients are likely to demonstrate an optimal therapeutic response at 300–1000 mg/day of chlorpromazine equivalents (Baldessarini *et al.* 1988; American Psychiatric Association 2000). Raising the dosage above this range is unlikely to lead to more rapid response or greater improvement, and lower dosage may be insufficient for many acutely psychotic patients (Baldessarini *et al.* 1988; Gaebel & Marder 1996; Marder 1996). A number of dosage comparison studies have failed to support the routine use of higher doses of typical antipsychotics (Levinson *et al.* 1990; Van Putten *et al.* 1990; McEvoy *et al.* 1991; Volavka *et al.* 1992; Janicak *et al.* 1993). When groups of patients are assigned to higher doses such as more than 2000 mg chlorpromazine or 40 mg haloperidol, the rate and amount of improvement are no greater than for those assigned to more moderate doses (Marder 1996). Moreover, these higher doses are frequently associated with neurological side-effects, particularly akathisia and akinesia, that can cause discomfort and worsen the outcome of treatment (Levinson *et al.* 1990; Van Putten *et al.* 1990; Gaebel & Marder 1996).

Accumulating data from imaging studies have provided some new guidance for antipsychotic dosing strategies in acute schizophrenia. The findings from PET studies demonstrate that low doses (e.g. 2 mg) of haloperidol induce high levels of striatal D_2 receptor occupancy (53–74%) with substantial clinical improvement (Kapur *et al.* 1996). The data may support the efficacy of lower doses of conventional drugs, particularly for first episode schizophrenic patients (Kapur *et al.* 2000).

Effective doses of atypical antipsychotics

Although clinical trial data show that atypical antipsychotics are efficacious and cause fewer BPS than the conventional agents, optimal dosing constitutes a critical issue in their effective use. When risperidone was first released, a final dosage of 6 mg/day was recommended on the basis of data from large fixed dose trials, particularly the North American trials (Chouinard *et al.* 1993b; Marder & Meibach 1994), which demonstrated that 6 mg/day was associated with the greatest improvement and similar EPSs to placebo. However, Kasper (1998) reviewed clinical trials and market research with risperidone and concluded that the most effective dosage with minimal side-effects is 4–6 mg/day (Kasper 1998). Brain imaging studies have provided a scientific rationale in support of the clinical observations relating to those of lower doses of risperidone. A PET study by Nyberg *et al.* (1999) demonstrated that mean D_2 occupancy in

eight first episode or drug-free schizophrenic patients who received 6 mg/day of risperidone was 82%, which is probably higher than necessary for achieving optimal clinical effects without EPSs. After dosage reduction to 3 mg/day mean D_2 occupancy was 72%, suggesting that 3–4 mg/day may be the optimal dosage (Nyberg *et al.* 1999). On the basis of naturalistic trials, clinical audit, Phase IV trials, PET data and 5 years of practical experience, Williams (2001) has suggested that the currently recommended target dosage with respect to efficacy and tolerability of risperidone is 4 mg/day for most schizophrenic patients (Williams 2001).

The recommended starting dosage of olanzapine is 5–10 mg/day (for review see Bhana *et al.* 2001). The effective dosage of olanzapine in clinical trials may be between 10 and 20 mg/day for most schizophrenic patients (Beasley *et al.* 1996, 1997; Nemeroff 1997; Tollefson *et al.* 1997; Tran *et al.* 1997; Sacristan *et al.* 2000). However, these data do not indicate whether higher doses of olanzapine are more efficacious. Kapur *et al.* (1998) demonstrated in PET studies that striatal D_2 occupancy in schizophrenic patients treated with olanzapine varied from 71 to 80% in the dosage range of 10–20 mg/day. At dosage above 20 mg/day, which led to higher than 80% D_2 occupancy, EPSs and prolactin elevation were observed in the patients (Kapur *et al.* 1998).

Treatment of different stages of illness

First episode

First episode patients as a group may differ from chronic patients in several aspects of treatment responses. First, patients with first episode schizophrenia have relatively high rates of response to antipsychotic treatment, and lower rates of relapse during maintenance treatment (Lieberman *et al.* 1993, 1996b; Robinson *et al.* 1999). Two first-episode studies found very large remission rates (83%, Lieberman *et al.* 1993 or 87%, Robinson *et al.* 1999) after 1 year of treatment with a standardized antipsychotic drug regimen. Surprisingly, remission did not occur until a median of 9 weeks (Robinson *et al.* 1999) or 11 weeks of treatment (Lieberman *et al.* 1993). Despite the apparent heightened responsiveness of first episode patients, residual cognitive deficits and poor psychosocial adjustment are common (Gupta *et al.* 1997; Bilder *et al.* 2000). Secondly, first episode patients may require a lower mean dose of antipsychotic medication, and may be more sensitive to drug side-effects compared to more chronic patients (McEvoy *et al.* 1991; Lieberman 1996; Lieberman *et al.* 1996b). One study found that lower doses of risperidone (2–4 mg/day) were more efficacious than higher doses (5–8 mg/day) in ameliorating both positive and negative symptoms, suggesting that patients with first episode schizophrenia may require lower doses of risperidone (Kopala *et al.* 1997). In addition, the lower dose group exhibited no EPSs, whereas 32% of the higher dose group developed akathisia or parkinsonism (Kopala *et al.* 1997). However, conclusions regarding dose–response relationships must be considered preliminary, because this study was not a fixed-dose design.

Several double-blind controlled studies have been reported that address the question of whether first episode patients respond better to atypical antipsychotic drugs. Sanger *et al.* (1999) analysed results from the 83 first episode patients (out of a total of 1996 subjects) who participated in a double-blind 6-week comparison of olanzapine and haloperidol. First episode patients who received olanzapine had significantly better clinical response and fewer EPSs than the haloperidol group. Interestingly, first episode patients treated with olanzapine achieved a significantly higher response rate than chronic patients treated with olanzapine. In addition, chronic patients treated with haloperidol developed significantly fewer EPSs than first episode patients treated with haloperidol. Mean doses of haloperidol and olanzapine were similar between first episode and chronic patient groups (10.8 vs. 11.0 mg/day and 11.6 vs. 12.0 mg/day, respectively; Sanger *et al.* 1999). This study suggests that the relative benefits of olanzapine compared to haloperidol may be greater in first episode patients than in chronic patients. However, issues of non-equivalent dosing between drugs may be of particular concern in light of recent work indicating that optimal D_2 receptor blockade may be achieved in first episode patients with haloperidol 0.25–2 mg/day (Kapur *et al.* 2000). Thus, a relatively high dose of haloperidol used in the study may have biased the results in favour of olanzapine in terms of EPSs and efficacy. The recent study comparing the efficacy of olanzapine and haloperidol for 104 weeks in 262 patients with first episode psychotic disorder have provided another opportunity to compare these agents (Lieberman *et al.* 2000a). The patients treated with olanzapine (mean dose, 9.1 mg/day) demonstrated a higher response rate (55% vs. 46%) and greater cognitive improvement than the patients treated with haloperidol (mean dose, 4.4 mg/day).

Lieberman *et al.* (2000b) have also preliminarily reported a 52-week study of clozapine versus chlorpromazine in 164 first episode treatment-naïve schizophrenia patients in China. The cumulative response rates of patients at 12 and 52 weeks were 81.2% and 96.3%, respectively, for clozapine (mean dose, 292 mg/day), and 68.3 and 97.7% for chlorpromazine (mean dose, 319 mg/day). The first episode patients treated with clozapine had more rapid response, fewer EPSs and higher treatment retention and relapse prevention than the chlorpromazine group (Lieberman *et al.* 2000b). Taken together, these results are consistent with the suggestion that atypical antipsychotics should be considered as a first-line medication for first episode patients (Lieberman 1996).

Exacerbation of chronic schizophrenia

As a group, chronic patients have greater morbidity on most clinical and biological dimensions of the illness (Lieberman 1999). Lieberman (1993, 1996) reported a 'deterioration' in the neuroleptic response over recurrent episodes in first-episode patients with schizophrenia. With each recurring episode there

seems to be, possibly as a result of hypothesized illness-related toxic influences or sensitization mechanisms, an aggravating effect on further episodes (Lieberman *et al.* 1996b, 1997). Consequently, there is a pattern of decreasing responsiveness to treatment over subsequent episodes of psychotic exacerbation, either as a result of progression of the illness itself, or the development of tolerance to antipsychotic treatment effects (Wyatt 1991; Lieberman *et al.* 1996a,b). Studies that followed patients over successive episodes of illness found that some of the patients took longer to recover or, in some cases, failed to recover as they had in their previous episode (Wyatt 1991; Lieberman *et al.* 1996a). These findings suggest that longer pretreatment duration may be associated with longer time to remission (Wyatt 1991; Loebel *et al.* 1992, 1996a). Thus, early detection and intervention with antipsychotic medications appear to be the essential strategies for the treatment of acute exacerbations of chronic schizophrenia (Wyatt 1995; Gaebel & Marder 1996; McGlashan 1996).

The results of double-blind clinical trials suggest that atypical antipsychotic drugs could be used as a first-line agent in the treatment of chronic schizophrenic patients with acute exacerbations, and their favourable adverse effects profile could help to enhance compliance from the onset of intervention. However, there are currently few data on comparisons of these drugs with respect to efficacy and outcome over the chronic phase of the illness, making recommendations for choosing among them difficult.

Chronic/residual

Residual impairment following active phases of illness often increases between episodes during the initial years of the illness (Lieberman *et al.* 1996b). The clinical feature of this phase is similar to that of the prodromal phase, except that negative symptoms (e.g. emotional blunting and social withdrawal) and impairment in role functioning tend to be more common in the residual stage (American Psychiatric Association 1994). During the residual phase, some of the positive symptoms (e.g. delusions or hallucinations) may persist, but may no longer be accompanied by strong affect. In addition to negative symptoms, eccentric behaviour, illogical thinking and mild loosening of associations are often seen (American Psychiatric Association 1994). In the residual phase, the specific treatment goals are to reduce negative symptoms and cognitive impairment and to improve role functioning.

Atypicals for negative symptoms

Although atypical antipsychotics have generally demonstrated superior efficacy for negative symptoms compared to high-potency conventional agents, the degree of improvement is usually quite modest (for review see Goff & Evins 1998). For example, across several studies, the effect size of risperidone (6 mg/day) compared to placebo on negative symptoms was small (0.27) (Marder *et al.* 1997). Path analysis has suggested that both risperidone and olanzapine exert direct effects upon negative symptoms independent of differences in psychotic, depressive or EPSs (Moller 1993; Tollefson & Sanger 1997). Recently, Volavka *et al.* (1999) preliminarily reported a prospective double-blind randomized study, comparing the effects of clozapine, olanzapine, risperidone and haloperidol, for 14 weeks in 157 treatment-resistant inpatients. Clozapine (mean dose, 527 mg/day) and olanzapine (mean dose, 30 mg/day), but not risperidone (mean dose, 12 mg/day), demonstrated significantly greater efficacy than haloperidol (mean dose, 26 mg/day) in reducing negative symptoms (Volavka *et al.* 1999). However, it is debated whether the efficacy of clozapine for negative symptoms extends to the treatment of primary negative symptoms of the deficit syndrome (Conley *et al.* 1994; Carpenter *et al.* 1995; Meltzer 1995). Few data are available from controlled trials to guide treatment of negative symptoms that persist despite optimal treatment with atypical antipsychotics (Goff & Evins 1998). Augmentation strategies are commonly employed by clinicians to treat residual negative symptoms of chronic schizophrenia, but evidence supporting this practice is derived mostly from an older literature describing combinations of augmenting agents added to conventional agents (Miyamoto *et al.* 2002).

Several adjunctive treatments, including $5-HT_{2A}$ antagonists, SSRIs and glycine site agonists, may be useful for the treatment of negative symptoms during the residual phase. However, with regard to the adjunctive treatment of atypical antipsychotics with $5-HT_{2A}$ antagonists, it is unlikely that augmentation with $5-HT_{2A}$ antagonists (e.g. nefazadone) will further improve the response of negative symptoms, because the available atypical agents can achieve maximal occupation of $5-HT_{2A}$ receptors at usual therapeutic doses (Kapur *et al.* 1999). Of interest, in contrast to the effectiveness of the combinations of the glycine site agonists with conventional agents on negative symptoms, all of these agonists, including glycine, D-cycloserine and D-serine, failed to improve, or even worsened, negative symptoms when added to clozapine (Tsai *et al.* 1991; Goff *et al.* 1999c; Potkin *et al.* 1999; Evins *et al.* 2000). Whether strategies that enhance NMDA-R activation will improve response to other second-generation agents remains uncertain, although both olanzapine and ziprasidone resemble clozapine in certain models of NMDA-R responsivity (Duncan *et al.* 2000a,b).

Anticholinergics

Addition of anticholinergic agents to conventional agents, which are commonly added to conventional antipsychotics for control of EPSs (McEvoy 1983), was associated with reductions in negative symptoms in one study (Tandon *et al.* 1988), but not in others (Gerlach *et al.* 1977; Johnstone *et al.* 1983; Goff *et al.* 1991; Hogarty *et al.* 1995). As suggested by Tandon and Greden (1989), whether primary negative symptoms are improved by anticholinergics cannot be answered by studies in which subjects are treated with conventional agents; by attenuating psychomotor side-effects of the neuroleptic the anticholinergic may be improving secondary negative symptoms only. To address this issue, two small placebo-controlled trials have administered anticholinergic agents to medication-free patients. Negative symptoms were improved by biperiden in one study (Tandon *et al.* 1990) and were unchanged with trihexyphenidyl in the other (Goff *et al.* 1994). While the efficacy of augmentation with muscarinic anticholinergic agents for negative symptoms remains poorly established, the potential cognitive impairment that these agents can produce is well-described (Baker *et al.* 1983; Strauss *et al.* 1990).

Dopamine agonists

Dopamine agonists have also been studied as augmenting agents for negative symptoms. Three of four placebo-controlled trials demonstrated improvement of negative symptoms following a single dose of amphetamine given orally or intravenously (Wolkin *et al.* 1987; Van Kammen & Boronow 1988; Mathew & Wilson 1989; Sanfilipo *et al.* 1996); in one study efficacy for negative symptoms was not affected by coadministration with pimozide (Van Kammen & Boronow 1988). However, Casey *et al.* (1961) found no clinical benefit in an extended 20-week placebo-controlled trial of amphetamine augmentation of chlorpromazine. Augmentation trials of psychostimulants added to atypical agents have not been reported.

Cognitive functioning

A wide range of cognitive deficits are usually present at the time of the first psychotic episode (Mohamed *et al.* 1999) and remain stable or only slowly progressive during the course of the illness, independent of psychotic symptoms (Aleman *et al.* 1999; Gold *et al.* 1999; Harvey *et al.* 1999). Cognitive deficits are particularly prominent in patients meeting criteria for the deficit syndrome (Buchanan *et al.* 1994) and in patients with tardive dyskinesia (Waddington *et al.* 1990). Because cognitive deficits are powerful determinants of vocational and social functioning and may, more than psychotic symptoms, influence quality of life (Green 1996), targeting cognitive impairments appears to be a major focus of treatment at the residual phase of schizophrenia.

The conventional neuroleptics produce small and inconsistent effects upon cognitive functioning; sustained attention improved in some studies, whereas motor control (finger tapping) worsened, and memory and executive functioning were minimally affected (King 1990). Studies in patients with schizophrenia have found either no effect following a switch to clozapine (Goldberg *et al.* 1993), or improvements in a wide range of cognitive functions, including verbal fluency, attention and reaction time (Keefe *et al.* 1999; Meltzer & McGurk 1999). In general, clozapine, olanzapine and risperidone have demonstrated superior efficacy compared to conventional agents on tests of verbal fluency, digit–symbol substitution, fine motor function and executive function (Keefe *et al.* 1999; Meltzer & McGurk 1999). Measures of learning and memory were least affected by atypical agents (Keefe *et al.* 1999). Because these tests all measure performance during a timed trial, enhanced performance with atypical agents could result, in part, from reduced parkinsonian side-effects (Keefe *et al.* 1999). Although methodological issues limit comparisons between atypical agents, preliminary evidence suggests that risperidone may be more effective for visual and working memory than clozapine (Meltzer & McGurk 1999).

In a recent double-blind trial in the treatment of cognitive impairment in early phase schizophrenia, risperidone (mean dose, 6 mg/day) and olanzapine (mean dose, 11 mg/day) produced significantly greater improvement in verbal fluency compared to haloperidol (mean dose, 10 mg/day), and olanzapine was superior to both haloperidol and risperidone in effects upon motor skills, non-verbal fluency and immediate recall (Purdon *et al.* 2000). However, this finding is complicated by the high incidence of anticholinergic administration prior to the final cognitive assessment. As in efficacy studies for negative symptoms, dose equivalency is an important factor in trials comparing cognitive effects of atypical agents, particularly because excessive dosing can impair performance on time-sensitive tasks and can increase anticholinergic exposure.

Augmentation with a full D_1 agonist (Castner *et al.* 2000) or glutamatergic agents, including glycine, D-serine and ampakines, may have promise for cognitive deficits that are seen during the residual phase of schizophrenia (Goff *et al.* 1999b; Miyamoto *et al.* 2002).

Conclusions

It is likely that atypical antipsychotic agents have advantages over conventional drugs in terms of side-effects, compliance and efficacy. However, the full extent of their clinical profiles and the appropriate first choice among these agents at different stages of the illness remain to be determined by extensive clinical observation and additional controlled studies comparing their efficacy and effectiveness. Yet there is a hope that greater use of newer drugs and numerous augmentation and experimental strategies could not only improve the outcome in schizophrenia but also add to our understanding of the neurobiological basis of the illness.

References

Aleman, A., Hijman, R., de Hann, E.H. *et al.* (1999) Memory impairment in schizophrenia: a meta-analysis. *American Journal of Psychiatry* 156, 1358–1366.

Allen, M.H. (2000) Managing the agitated psychotic patient: a reappraisal of the evidence. *Journal of Clinical Psychiatry*, 61 (Suppl. 14), 11–20.

Allison, D.B., Mentore, J.L., Heo, M. *et al.* (1999) Antipsychotic-induced weight gain: a comprehensive research synthesis. *American Journal of Psychiatry* 156, 1686–1696.

American Psychiatric Association (1994) *Diagnostic and Statistical Manual of Mental Disorders. Fourth Edition (DSM-IV)*. American Psychiatric Association, Washington, DC.

American Psychiatric Association (2000) *Practice guideline for the treatment of patients with schizophrenia. In Practice Guidelines for the Treatment of Psychiatric Disorders*, pp. 299–412. American Psychiatric Association, Washington, DC.

Anand, A., Charney, D.S., Oren, D.A. *et al.* (2000) Attenuation of the neuropsychiatric effects of ketamine with lamotrigine: support for hyperglutamatergic effects of N-methyl-D-aspartate receptor antagonists. *Archives of General Psychiatry* 57, 270–276.

Arana, G.W., Goff, D.C., Friedman, H. *et al.* (1986a) Does carbamazepine-induced reduction of plasma haloperidol levels worsen psychotic symptoms? *American Journal of Psychiatry* 143, 650–651.

Arana, G.W., Ornsteen, M.L., Kanter, F. *et al.* (1986b) The use of benzodiazepines for psychotic disorders: a literature review and preliminary clinical findings. *Psychopharmacology Bulletin* 22, 77–87.

Arnsten, A.F. & Goldman-Rakic, P.S. (1985) Alpha 2-adrenergic mechanisms in prefrontal cortex associated with cognitive decline in aged nonhuman primates. *Science* 230, 1273–1276.

Arnsten, A.F., Cai, J.X. & Goldman-Rakic, P.S. (1988) The alpha-2 adrenergic agonist guanfacine improves memory in aged monkeys without sedative or hypotensive side effects: evidence for alpha-2 receptor subtypes. *Journal of Neuroscience* 8, 4287–4298.

Arnsten, A.F., Cai, J.X., Murphy, B.L. *et al.* (1994) Dopamine D_1 receptor mechanisms in the cognitive performance of young adult and aged monkeys. *Psychopharmacology (Berl)* 116, 143–151.

Arnsten, A.F., Steere, J.C. & Hunt, R.D. (1996) The contribution of alpha 2-noradrenergic mechanisms of prefrontal cortical cognitive function: potential significance for attention-deficit hyperactivity disorder. *Archives of General Psychiatry* 53, 448–455.

Arnt, J. (1995) Differential effects of classical and newer antipsychotics on the hypermotility induced by two dose levels of D-amphetamine. *European Journal of Pharmacology* 283, 55–62.

Arvanitis, L.A., Miller, B.G. & the Seroquel Trial 13 Study Group (1997) Multiple fixed doses of 'Seroquel' (quetiapine) in patients with acute exacerbation of schizophrenia: a comparison with haloperidol and placebo. *Biological Psychiatry* 42, 233–246.

Atre-Vaidya, N. & Taylor, M.A. (1989) Effectiveness of lithium in schizophrenia: do we really have an answer? *Journal of Clinical Psychiatry* 50, 170–173.

Attwell, P.J., Singh, K.N., Sane, D.E. *et al.* (1998) Anticonvulsant and glutamate release-inhibiting properties of the highly potent metabotropic glutamate receptor agonist (2S, 2′R, 3′R)-2-(2′,3′ dicarboxycyclopropyl)glycine (DCG-IV). *Brain Research* 805, 138–143.

Baker, L.A., Cheng, L.Y. & Amara, I.B. (1983) The withdrawal of benztropine mesylate in chronic schizophrenic patients. *British Journal of Psychiatry* 143, 584–590.

Bakshi, V.P. & Geyer, M.A. (1995) Antagonism of phencyclidine-induced deficits in prepulse inhibition by the putative atypical antipsychotic olanzapine. *Psychopharmacology (Berl)* 122, 198–201.

Bakshi, V.P. & Geyer, M.A. (1997) Phenyclidine-induced deficits in prepulse inhibition of startle are blocked by prazosin, an alpha-1 noradrenergic antagonist. *Journal of Pharmacology and Experimental Therapeutics* 283, 666–674.

Bakshi, V.P., Swerdlow, N.R. & Geyer, M.A. (1994) Clozapine antagonizes phencyclidine-induced deficits in sensorimotor gating of the startle response. *Journal of Pharmacology and Experimental Therapeutics* 271, 787–794.

Baldessarini, R.J., Cohen, B.M. & Teicher, M.H. (1988) Significance of neuroleptic dose and plasma level in the pharmacological treatment of psychoses. *Archives of General Psychiatry* 45, 79–91.

Barnes, T.R.E. & McPhillips, M.A. (1999) Critical analysis and comparison of the side-effect and safety profiles of the new antipsychotics. *British Journal of Psychiatry* 174 (Suppl. 38), 34–43.

Battaglia, G., Monn, J.A. & Schoepp, D.D. (1997a) *In vivo* inhibition of veratridine-evoked release of striatal excitatory amino acids by the group II metabotropic glutamate receptor agonist LY354740 in rats. *Neuroscience Letter* **229**, 161–164.

Battaglia, J., Moss, S., Rush, J. *et al.* (1997b) Haloperidol, lorazepam, or both for psychotic agitation? A multicenter, prospective, double-blind, emergency department study. *American Journal of Emergency Medicine* **15**, 335–340.

Beasley, C.M.J., Tollefson, G., Tran, P. *et al.* (1996) Olanzapine versus placebo and haloperidol: acute phase results of the North American double-blind olanzapine trial. *Neuropsychopharmacology* **14**, 111–123.

Beasley, C.M.J., Hamilton, S.H., Crawford, A.M. *et al.* (1997) Olanzapine versus haloperidol: acute phase results of the international double-blind olanzapine trial. *European Journal of Neuropsychopharmacology* **7**, 125–137.

Beasley, C.M., Dellva, M.A., Tamura, R.N. *et al.* (1999) Randomised double-blind comparison of the incidence of tardive dyskinesia in patients with schizophrenia during long-term treatment with olanzapine or haloperidol. *British Journal of Psychiatry* **174**, 23–30.

Beaumont, G. (2000) Antipsychotics: the future of schizrenia treatment. *Current Medical Research and Opinion* **16**, 37–42.

Bengtsson, H.J., Kullberg, A., Millan, M.J. *et al.* (1998) The role of 5-HT_{1A} autoreceptors and alpha$_1$-adrenoceptors in the modulation of 5-HT release. III. Clozapine and the novel putative antipsychotic S 16924. *Neuropharmacology* **37**, 349–356.

Berger, A.J., Dieudonne, S. & Ascher P. (1998) Glycine uptake governs glycine site occupancy at NMDA receptors of excitatory synapses. *Journal of Neurophysiology* **80**, 3336–3340.

Bergeron, R., Meyer, T.M., Coyle, J.T. *et al.* (1998) Modulation of N-methyl-D-aspartate receptor function by glycine transport. *Proceedings of the National Academy of Sciences of the USA* **95**, 15730–15734.

Berlant, J.L. (1987) One more look at propranolol for the treatment of refractory schizophrenia. *Schizophrenia Bulletin* **13**, 705–714.

Bhana, N., Foster, R.H., Olney, R. *et al.* (2001) Olanzapine: an updated review of its use in the management of schizophrenia. *Drugs* **61**, 111–161.

Bilder, R.M., Goldman, R.S., Robinson, D. *et al.* (2000) Neuropsychology of first-episode schizophrenia: initial characterization and clinical correlates. *American Journal of Psychiatry* **157**, 549–559.

Binder, R.L. & McNiel, D.E. (1999) Emergency psychiatry: contemporary practices in managing acutely violent patients in 20 psychiatric emergency rooms. *Psychiatric Services* **50**, 1553–1554.

Birch, A.M., Bradley, P.A., Gill, J.C. *et al.* (1999) N-Substituted (2,3-dihydro-1,4-benzodioxin-2-yl)methylamine derivatives as D$_2$ antagonists/5-HT_{1A} partial agonists with potential as atypical antipsychotic agents. *Journal of Medicinal Chemistry* **42**, 3342–3355.

Bhin, O., Azorin, J.M. & Bouhours, P. (1996) Antipsychotic and anxiolytic properties of risperidone, haloperidol, and methotrimeprazine in schizophrenic patients. *Journal of Clinical Psychopharmacology* **16**, 38–44.

Blin, O. (1999) A comparative review of new antipsychotics. *Canadian Journal of Psychiatry* **44**, 235–244.

Bodick, N.C., Offen, W.W., Levey, A.I. *et al.* (1997) Effects of xanomeline, a selective muscarinic receptor agonist, on cognitive function and behavioral symptoms in Alzheimer disease. *Archives of Neurology* **54**, 465–473.

Borison, R.L., Pathiraja, A.P., Diamond, B.I. *et al.* (1992) Risperidone: clinical safety and efficacy in schizophrenia. *Psychopharmacology Bulletin* **28**, 213–218.

Boyer, P., Lecrubier, Y., Puech, A.J. *et al.* (1995) Treatment of negative symptoms in schizophrenia with amisulpride. *British Journal of Psychiatry* **166**, 8–72.

Breier, A., Wright, P., Birkett, M. *et al.* (2000) A double-blind dose response study comparing intramuscular olanzapine, haloperidol and placebo in acutely agitated schizophrenic patients. In ACNP 39th Annual Meeting Abstract, Puerto Rico, p. 348.

Bristow, L.J., Kramer, M.S., Kulagowski, J. *et al.* (1997) Schizophrenia and L-745,870, a novel doparnine D$_4$ receptor antagonist. *Trends in Pharmacological Sciences* **18**, 186–188.

Bubser, M., Keseberg, U., Notz, P.K. *et al.* (1992) Differential behavioral and neurochemical effects of competitive and non-competitive NMDA receptor antagonists in rats. *European Journal of Pharmacology* **229**, 75–82.

Buchanan, R.W. (1995) Clozapine: efficacy and safety. *Schizophrenia Bulletin* **21**, 579–591.

Buchanan, R. & McKenna, P. (2000) Clozapine: clinical use and experience. In: *Schizophrenia and Mood Disorders: the New Drug Therapies in Clinical Practice* (eds P.F. Buckley & J.L. Waddington), pp. 21–31.

Buchanan, R.W., Strauss, M.E., Kirkpatrick, B. *et al.* (1994) Neuropsychological impairments in deficit vs. nondeficit forms of schizophrenia. *Archives of General Psychiatry* **51**, 804–811.

Buchanan, R.W., Kirkpatrick, B., Bryant, N. *et al.* (1996) Fluoxetine augmentation of clozapine treatment in patients with schizophrenia. *American Journal of Psychiatry* **153**, 1625–1627.

Buckley, P.F. (1999) The role of typical and atypical antipsychotic medications in the management of agitation and aggression. *Journal of Clinical Psychiatry*, **60** (Suppl. 10) 52–60.

Burnet, P.W., Eastwood, S.L. & Harrison, P.J. (1996) 5-HT_{1A} and 5-HT_{2A} receptor mRNAs and binding site densities are differentially altered in schizophrenia. *Neuropsychopharmacology* **15**, 442–455.

Bymaster, F.P., Wong, D.T., Mitch, C.H. *et al.* (1994) Neurochemical effects of the M$_1$ muscarinic agonist xanomeline (LY246708/NNC11-0232). *Journal of Pharmacology and Experimental Therapeutics* **269**, 282–289.

Bymaster, F.P., Shannon, H.E., Rasmussen, K. *et al.* (1998) Unexpected antipsychotic-like activity with the muscarinic receptor ligand (5R,6R)6-(3-propylthio-1,2,5-thiadiazol-4-yl)-l-azabicyclo[3.2.1]octane. *European Journal of Pharmacology* **356**, 109–119.

Bymaster, F.P., Shannon, H.E., Rasmussen, K. *et al.* (1999) Potential role of muscarinic receptors in schizophrenia. *Life Sciences* **64**, 527–534.

Cai, J.X. & Arnsten, A.F. (1997) Dose-dependent effects of the dopamine D$_1$ receptor agonists A77636 or SKF81297 on spatial working memory in aged monkeys. *Journal of Pharmacology and Experimental Therapeutics* **283**, 183–189.

Campbell, M., Young, P.I., Bateman, D.N. *et al.* (1999) The use of atypical antipsychotics in the management of schizophrenia. *British Journal of Clinical Pharmacology* **47**, 13–22.

Carlsson, A. (2000) Focusing on dopaminergic stabilizers and 5-HT_{2A} receptor antagonists. *Current Opinion in CPNS and Investigative Drugs* **2**, 22–24.

Carlsson, M.L., Martin, P., Nilsson, M. *et al.* (1999) The 5-HT_{2A} receptor antagonist M100907 is more effective in counteracting NMDA antagonist- than dopamine agonist-induced hyperactivity in mice. *Journal of Neural Transmission* **106**, 123–129.

Carman, J.S., Bigelow, L.B. & Wyatt, R.J. (1981) Lithium combined with neuroleptics in chronic schizophrenic and schizoafffective patients. *Journal of Clinical Psychiatry* **42**, 124–128.

Carpenter, W.T., Jr., Heinrichs, D.W. & Hanlon, T.E. (1987) A comparative trial of pharmacologic strategies in schizophrenia. *American Journal of Psychiatry* 144, 1466–1470.

Carpenter, W.T., Jr., Conley, R.R., Buchanan, R.W. *et al.* (1995) Patient response and resource management; another view of clozapine treatment of schizophrenia. *American Journal of Psychiatry* 152, 827–832.

Casey, J.F., Hollister, L.E., Klett, C.J. *et al.* (1961) Combined drug therapy of chronic schizophrenics: controlled evaluation of placebo, dextoamphetamine, imipramine, isocarboxazid and trifluoperazine added to maintenance doses of chlorpromazine. *American Journal of Psychiatry* 117, 997–1003.

Castner, S.A., Williams, G.V. & Goldman-Rakic, P.S. (2000) Reversal of antipsychotic-induced working memory deficits by short-term dopamine D_1 receptor stimulation. *Science* 287, 2020–2022.

Chakos, M.H., Mayerhoff, D.I., Loebel, A.D. *et al.* (1992) Incidence and correlates of acute extrapyramidal symptoms in first episode of schizophrenia. *Psychopharmacology Bulletin* 28, 81–86.

Chakos, M.H., Alvir, J.M., Woerner, M.G. *et al.* (1996) Incidence and correlates of tardive dyskinesia in first episode of schizophrenia. *Archives of General Psychiatry* 53, 313–319.

Chakos, M., Lieberman, J., Hoffman, E. *et al.* (2001) Effectiveness of second-generation antipsychotics in patients with treatment-resistant schizophrenia: a review and meta-analysis of randomized trials. *American Journal of Psychiatry* 158, 518–526.

Chatterjee, A., Chakos, M., Koreen, A. *et al.* (1995) Prevalence and clinical correlates of extrapyramidal signs and spontaneous dyskinesia in never-medicated schizophrenic patients. *American Journal of Psychiatry* 152, 1724–1729.

Chiodo, L.A. & Bunney, B.S. (1983) Typical and atypical neuroleptics: differential effects of chronic administration on the activity of A_9 and A_{10} midbrain dopaminergic neurons. *Journal of Neuroscience* 3, 1607–1619.

Chouinard, G., Annable, L., Turnier, L. *et al.* (1993a) A double-blind randomized clinical trial of rapid tranquilization with i.m. clonazepam and i.m. haloperidol in agitated psychotic patients with manic symptoms. *Canadian Journal of Psychiatry* 38 (Suppl. 4), S114–S121.

Chouinard, G., Jones, B., Remington, G. *et al.* (1993b) A Canadian multicenter placebo-controlled study of fixed doses of risperidone and haloperidol in the treatment of chronic schizophrenic patients. *Journal of Clinical Psychopharmacology* 13, 25–40.

Christison, G.w., Kirch, D.G. & Wyatt, R.J. (1991) When symptoms persist: choosing among alternative somatic treatments for schizophrenia. *Schizophrenia Bulletin* 17, 217–245.

Claus, A., Bollen, J., De Cuyper, H. *et al.* (1992) Risperidone versus haloperidol in the treatment of chronic schizophrenic inpatients: a multicentre double-blind comparative study. *Acta Psychiatrica Scandinavica* 85, 295–305.

Coffman, J.A., Nasrallah, H.A., Lyskowski, J. *et al.* (1987) Clinical effectiveness of oral and parenteral rapid neuroleptization. *Journal of Clinical Psychiatry* 48, 20–24.

Cohen, S., Lavelle, J., Rich, C.L. *et al.* (1994) Rates and correlates of suicide attempts in first-admission psychotic patients. *Acta Psychiatrica Scandinavica* 90, 167–171.

Conley, R.R. & Mahmoud, R. (2001) A randomized double-blind study of risperidone and olanzapine in the treatment of schizophrenia or schizoaffective disorder. *American Journal of Psychiatry* 158, 765–774.

Conley, R., Gounaris, C. & Tamminga, C. (1994) Clozapine response varies in deficit versus non-deficit schizophrenic subjects. *Biological Psychiatry* 35, 746–747.

Conley, R.R., Mahmoud, R. & the Risperidone Study Group (2000) Efficacy of risperidone vs. olanzapine in the treatment of patients with schizophrenia or schizoaffective disorder. *International Journal of Neuropsychopharmacology* 3 (Suppl. 1), S151 (P.01.219).

Corbett, R., Camacho, F., Woods, A.T. *et al.* (1995) Antipsychotic agents antagonize non-competitive N-methyl-D-aspartate antagonist-induced behaviors. *Psychopharmacology (Berl)* 120, 67–74.

Costa, J., Khaled, E., Sramek, J. *et al.* (1990) An open trial of glycine as an adjunct to neuroleptics in chronic treatment-refractory schizophrenics. *Journal of Clinical Psychopharmacology* 10, 71–72.

Coward, D., Dixon, K., Enz, A. *et al.* (1989) Partial brain dopamine D_2 receptor agonists in the treatment of schizophrenia. *Psychopharmacology Bulletin* 25, 393–397.

Coyle, J.T. (1996) The glutamatergic dysfunction hypothesis for schizophrenia. *Harvard Review of Psychiatry* 3, 241–253.

Craig, T.J., Bromet, E.J., Fennig, S. *et al.* (2000) Is there an association between duration of untreated psychosis and 24-month clinical outcome in a first-admission series? *American Journal of Psychiatry* 157, 60–66.

Cressman, W.A., Plostnieks, J. & Johnson, P.C. (1973) Absorption, metabolism and excretion of droperidol by human subjects following intramuscular and intravenous administration. *Anesthesiology* 38, 363–369.

Crow, T.J., MacMillan, J.F., Johnson, A.L. *et al.* (1986) A randomised controlled trial of prophylactic neuroleptic treatment. *British Journal of Psychiatry* 148, 120–127.

Csernansky, J.G., Riney, S.J., Lombrozo, L. *et al.* (1988) Double-blind comparison of alprazolam, diazepam, and placebo for the treatment of negative schizophrenic symptoms. *Archives of General Psychiatry* 45, 655–659.

Currier, G.W. (2000) Atypical antipsychotic medications in the psychiatric emergency service. *Journal of Clinical Psychiatry* 61 (Suppl. 14), 21–26.

Currier, G.W. & Simpson, G.M. (2001) Risperidone liquid concentrate and oral lorazepam versus intramuscular haloperidol and intramuscular lorazepam for treatment of psychotic agitation. *Journal of Clinical Psychiatry* 62, 153–157.

Cussac, D., Newman-Tancredi, A., Nicolas, J.P. *et al.* (2000) Antagonist properties of the novel antipsychotic, S16924, at cloned, human serotonin $5\text{-}HT_{2C}$ receptors: a parallel phosphatidylinositol and calcium accumulation comparison with clozapine and haloperidol. *Naunyn-Schmiedeberg's Archives of Pharmacology* 363, 549–554.

Czobor, P., Volavka, J. & Meibach, R.C. (1995) Effect of risperidone on hostility in schizophrenia. *Journal of Clinical Psychopharmacology* 15, 243–249.

Daniel, D.G., Zimbroff, D.L., Potkin, S.G. *et al.* (1999) Ziprasidone 80 mg/day and 160 mg/day in the acute exacerbation of schizophrenia and schizoaffective disorder: a 6-week placebo-controlled trial. *Neuropsychopharmacology* 20, 491–505.

Danysz, W. (2000) Sonepiprazole. *Current Opinion in CPNS and Investigative Drugs* 2, 97–104.

Davis, J.M. & Andriukaitis, S. (1986) The natural course of schizophrenia and effective maintenance drug treatment. *Journal of Clinical Psychopharmacology* 6, 2S–10S.

Dawkins, K., Lieberman, J.A., Lebowitz, B.D. *et al.* (1999) Antipsychotics: past and future – National Institute of Mental Health Division of Services and Intervention Research Workshop, July 14, 1998. *Schizophrenia Bulletin* 25, 395–404.

Deutsch, S.I., Mastropaolo, J., Schwartx, B.L. *et al.* (1989) A 'glutamatergic hypothesis' of schizophrenia: rationale for pharmacotherapy with glycine. *Clinical Neuropharmacology* 12, 1–13.

Donlon, P.T., Hopkin, J. & Tupin, J.P. (1979) Overview: efficacy and safety of the rapid neuroleptization method with injectable haloperidol. *American Journal of Psychiatry* 136, 273–278.

Dorevitch, A., Katz, N., Zemishlany, Z. et al. (1999) Intramuscular flunitrazepam versus intramuscular haloperidol in the emegency treatment of aggressive psychotic behavior. American Journal of Psychiatry 156, 142–144.

Dubin, W.R. & Feld, J.A. (1989) Rapid tranquilization of the violent patient. American Journal of Emergency Medicine 7, 313–320.

Duggan, L., Fenton, M., Dardennes, R.M. et al. (2000) Olanzapine for schizophrenia. Cochrane Database Syst Rev CD001359.

Duinkerke, S.J., Botter, P.A., Jansen, A.A. et al. (1993) Ritanserin, a selective 5-HT$_{2/1C}$ antagonist, and negative symptoms in schizophrenia: a placebo-controlled double-blind trial [see comments]. British Journal of Psychiatry 163, 451–455.

Duncan, G.E., Leipzig, J.N., Mailman, R.B. et al. (1998a) Differential effects of clozapine and haloperidol on ketamine-induced brain metabolic activation. Brain Research 812, 65–75.

Duncan, G.E., Moy, S.S., Knapp, D.J. et al. (1998b) Metabolic mapping of the rat brain after subanesthetic doses of ketamine: potential relevance to schizophrenia. Brain Research 787, 181–190.

Duncan, G.E., Miyamoto, S., Leipzig, J.N. et al. (1999a) Comparison of brain metabolic activity patterns induced by ketamine, MK-801 and amphetamine in rats: support for NMDA receptor involvement in responses to subanesthetic dose of ketamine. Brain Research 843, 171–183.

Duncan, G.E., Sheitman, B.B. & Lieberman, J.A. (1999b) An integrated view of pathophysiological models of schizophrenia. Brain Research Review 29, 250–264.

Duncan, G.E., Zorn, S. & Lieberman, J.A. (1999c) Mechanisms of typical and atypical antipsychotic drug action in relation to dopamine and NMDA receptor hypofunction hypotheses of schizophrenia. Molecular Psychiatry 4, 418–428.

Duncan, G.E., Miyamoto, S., Leipzig, J.N. et al. (2000a) Comparison of the effects of clozapine, risperidone, and olanzapine on ketamine-induced alterations in regional brain metabolism. Journal of Pharmacology and Experimental Therapeutics 293, 8–14.

Duncan, G.E., Miyamoto, S. & Lieberman, J.A. (2000b) Ziprasidone blocks ketamine-induced brain metabolic activation. Biological Psychiatry 47, 15S.

Elman, I., Goldstein, D.S., Eisenhofer, G. et al. (1999) Mechanism of peripheral noradrenergic stimulation by clozapine. Neuropsychopharmacology 20, 29–34.

Escobar, J.I., Barron, A. & Kiriakos, R. (1983) A controlled study of neuroleptization with fluphenazine hydrochloride injections. Journal of Clinical Psychopharmacology 3, 359–362.

Evenden, J.L. (1992) Effects of 8-hydroxy-2-(di-N-propylamino) tetralin (8-OH-DPAT) after repeated administration on a conditioned avoidance response (CAR) in the rat. Psychopharmacology (Berl) 109, 134–144.

Evins, A. & Goff, D. (1996) Adjunctive antidepressant drug therapies in the treatment of negative symptoms of schizophrenia. CNS Drugs 6, 130–147.

Evins, A.E., Fitzgerald, S.M., Wine, L. et al. (2000) Placebo-controlled trial of glycine added to clozapine in schizophrenia. American Journal of Psychiatry 157, 826–828.

Feifel, D. (2000) Rationale and guidelines for the inpatient treatment of acute psychosis. Journal of Clinical Psychiatry 61 (Suppl. 14), 27–32.

Feldpausch, D.L., Needham, L.M., Stone, M.P. et al. (1998) The role of dopamine D$_4$ receptor in the induction of behavioral sensitization to amphetamine and accompanying biochemical and molecular adaptations. Journal of Pharmacology and Experimental Therapeutics 286, 497–508.

Fields, R.B., Van Kammen, D.P., Peters, J.L. et al. (1988) Clonidine improves memory function in schizophrenia independently from change in psychosis: preliminary findings. Schizophrenia Research 1, 417–423.

Fleischhacker, W.W. (1995) New drugs for the treatment of schizophrenic patients. Acta Psychiatrica Scandinavica (Suppl.), 388, 24–30.

Fleischhacker, W.W. & Hummer, M. (1997) Drug treatment of schizophrenia in the 1990s: achievements and future possibilities in optimising outcomes. Drugs 53, 915–929.

Foster, S., Kessel, J., Berman, M.E. et al. (1997) Efficacy of lorazepam and haloperidol for rapid tranquilization in a psychiatric emergency room setting. International Clinical Psychopharmacology 12, 175–179.

Freeman, M.P. & Stoll, A.L. (1998) Mood stabilizer combinations: a review of safety and efficacy. American Journal of Psychiatry 155, 12–21.

Friedman, J.I., Adler, D.N. & Davis, K.L. (1999a) The role of norepinephrine in the pathophysiology of cognitive disorders: potential applications to the treatment of cognitive dysfunction in schizophrenia and Alzheimer's disease. Biological Psychiatry 46, 1243–1252.

Friedman, J.I., Temporini, H. & Davis, K.L. (1999b) Pharmacologic strategies for augmenting cognitive performance in schizophrenia. Biological Psychiatry 45, 1–16.

Friedman, J., Adler, D., Temporini, H. et al. (2000) Alpha-2 agonists enhance cognition of schizophrenic patients in combination with atypical but not typical neuroleptics. In 22nd CINP Congress Brussels, Belgium.

Gaebel, W. (1995) Is intermittent, early intervention medication an alternative for neuroleptic maintenance treatment? International Clinical Psychopharmacology 9 (Suppl. 5), 11–16.

Gaebel, W. (1996) Prediction of response to acute neuroleptic treatment in schizophrenia. International Clinical Psychopharmacology 11 (Suppl. 2), 47–54.

Gaebel, W. & Marder, S. (1996) Conclusions and treatment recommendations for the acute episode in schizophrenia. International Clinical Psychopharmacology 11 (Suppl. 2), 93–100.

Geddes, J., Freemantle, N., Harrison, P. et al. (2000) Atypical antipsychotics in the treatment of schizophrenia: systematic overview and meta-regression analysis. British Medical Journal 321, 1371–1376.

Gelders, Y.G. (1989) Thymosthenic agents, a novel approach in the treatment of schizophrenia. British Journal of Psychiatry (Suppl.), 33–36.

Gerlach, J., Rasmussen, P.T., Hansen, L. et al. (1977) Antiparkinsonian agents and long-term neuroleptic treatment: effect of G 31.406, orphenadrine, and placebo on parkinsonism, schizophrenic symptoms, depression and anxiety. Acta Psychiatrica Scandinavica 55, 251–260.

Ghosh, D., Snyder, S.E., Watts, V.J. et al. (1996) 9-Dihydroxy-2,3,7,11b-tetrahydro-1H-naph[1,2,3-de]isoquinoline: a potent full dopamine D$_1$ agonist containing a rigid-beta-phenyldopamine pharmacophore. Journal of Medical Chemistry 39, 549–555.

Glazer, W.M. & Dickson, R.A. (1998) Clozapine reduces violence and persistent aggression in schizophrenia. Journal of Clinical Psychiatry 59 (Suppl. 3), 8–14.

Glazer, W.M. & Kane, J.M. (1992) Depot neuroleptic therapy: an underutilized treatment option. Journal of Clinical Psychiatry 53, 426–433.

Gleason, S.D. & Shannon, H.E. (1997) Blockade of phencyclidine-induced hyperlocomotion by olanzapine, clozapine and serotonin receptor subtype selective antagonists in mice. Psychopharmacology (Berl) 129, 79–84.

Gobert, A., Rivet, J.M., Audinot, V. et al. (1998) Simultaneous quantification of serotonin, dopamine and noradrenaline levels in single frontal cortex dialysates of freely-moving rats reveals a complex pattern of reciprocal auto- and heteroreceptor-mediated control of release. *Neuroscience* **84**, 413–429.

Gobert, A., Rivet, J.M., Cussac, D. *et al.* (2000) S33592, a benzopyranopyrrole partial agonist at dopamine D_2/D_3 receptors and potential antipsychotic agent. I. modulation of dopaminergic transmission in comparison to aripiprazole, preclamol and raclopride. *Society for Neuroscience Abstracts* **26**, 274.

Goff, D. & Baldessarini, R. (1995) Antipsychotics. In: *Drug Interactions in Psychiatry* (eds D. Ciraulo, R. Shader, D. Greenblatt & W. Creelman), pp. 129–174. Baltimore, MA.

Goff, D.C. & Evins, A.E. (1998) Negative symptoms in schizophrenia: neurobiological models and treatment response. *Harvard Review of Psychiatry* **6**, 59–77.

Goff, D.C., Arana, G.W., Greenblatt, D.J. *et al.* (1991) The effect of benztropine on haloperidol-induced dystonia, clinical efficacy and pharmacokinetics: a prospective, double-blind trial. *Journal of Clinical Psychopharmacology* **11**, 106–112.

Goff, D.C., Amico, E., Dreyfuss, D. *et al.* (1994) A placebo-controlled trial of trihexyphenidyl in unmedicated patients with schizophrenia. *American Journal of Psychiatry* **151**, 429–431.

Goff, D.C., Midha, K.K., Sarid-Segal, O. *et al.* (1995a) A placebo-controlled trial of fluoxetine added to neuroleptic in patients with schizophrenia. *Psychopharmacology (Berl)* **117**, 417–423.

Goff, D.C., Tsai, G., Manoach, D.S. *et al.* (1995b) Dose-finding trial of D-cycloserine added to neuroleptics for negative symptoms in schizophrenia. *American Journal of Psychiatry* **152**, 1213–1215.

Goff, D.C., Tsai, G., Manoach, D.S. *et al.* (1996) D-cycloserine added to clozapine for patients with schizophrenia. *American Journal of Psychiatry* **153**, 1628–1630.

Goff, D.C., Posever, T., Hertz, L. *et al.* (1998) An exploratory haloperidol-controlled dose-finding study of ziprasidone in hospitalized patients with schizophrenia or schizoaffective disorder. *Journal of Clinical Psychopharmacology* **18**, 296–304.

Goff, D., Berman, I., Posever, T. *et al.* (1999a) A preliminary dose-escalation trial of CX 516 (ampakine) added to clozapine in schizophrenia. *Schizophrenia Research* **36**, 280.

Goff, D.C., Bagnell, A.L. & Perlis, R.H. (1999b) Glutamatergic strategies for cognitive impairment in schizophrenia. *Psychiatry Annals* **29**, 649–654.

Goff, D.C., Henderson, D.C., Evins, A.E. *et al.* (1999c) A placebo-controlled crossover trial of D-cycloserine added to clozapine in patients with schizophrenia. *Biological Psychiatry* **45**, 512–514.

Goff, D.C., Tsai, G., Levitt, J. *et al.* (1999d) A placebo-controlled trial of D-cycloserine added to conventional neuroleptics in patients with schizophrenia. *Archives of General Psychiatry* **56**, 21–27.

Gold, S., Arndt, S., Nopoulos, P. *et al.* (1999) Longitudinal study of cognitive function in first-episode and recent-onset schizophrenia. *American Journal of Psychiatry* **156**, 1342–1348.

Goldberg, T.E., Greenberg, R.D., Griffin, S.J. *et al.* (1993) The effect of clozapine on cognition and psychiatric symptoms in patients with schizophrenia. *British Journal of Psychiatry* **162**, 43–48.

Goldman-Rakic, P.S. (1999) The relevance of the dopamine-D_1 receptor in the cognitive symptoms of schizophrenia. *Neuropsychopharmacology* **21**, S170–S180.

Goldman-Rakic, P.S., Lidow, M.S. & Gallager, D.W. (1990) Overlap of dopaminergic, adrenergic, and serotoninergic receptors and complementarity of their subtypes in primate prefrontal cortex. *Journal of Neuroscience* **10**, 2125–2138.

Goldman-Rakic, P.S., Muly III, E.C. & Williams, G.V. (2000) D_1 receptors in prefrontal cells and circuits. *Brain Research Review* **31**, 295–301.

Goldstein, J.M. (1998) 'Seroquel' (quetiapine fumarate) reduces hostility and aggression in patients with acute schizophrenia. Presented at the 151st Annual Meeting of the American Psychiatric Association Toronto, Canada.

Green, M.F. (1996) What are the functional consequences of neurocognitive deficits in schizophrenia? *American Journal of Psychiatry* **153**, 321–330.

Growe, G.A., Crayton, J.W., Klass, D.B. *et al.* (1979) Lithium in chronic schizophrenia. *American Journal of Psychiatry* **136**, 454–455.

Grunze, H.C., Rainnie, D.G., Hasselmo, M.E. *et al.* (1996) NMDA-dependent modulation of CA1 local circuit inhibition. *Journal of Neuroscience* **16**, 2034–2043.

Gupta, S., Andreasen, N.C., Arndt, S. *et al.* (1997) The Iowa Longitudinal Study of Recent Onset Psychosis: one-year follow-up of first episode patients. *Schizophrenia Research* **23**, 1–13.

Haase, H.J. (1961) Extrapyramidal modification of fine movements: a 'conditio sine qua non' of the fundamental therapeutic action of neuroleptic drugs. In: *Systeme Extrapyramidal et Neuroleptique* (ed. J.M. Bordeleau), pp. 329–353. Editions Psychiatriques, Montreal.

Häfner, H., Riecher-Rossler, A., Maurer, K. *et al.* (1992) First onset and early symptomatology of schizophrenia: a chapter of epidemiological and neurobiological research into age and sex differences. *European Archives of Psychiatry and Clinical Neuroscience* **242**, 109–118.

Hampson, R.E., Rogers, G., Lynch, G. *et al.* (1998a) Facilitative effects of the ampakine CX516 on short-term memory in rats: correlations with hippocampal neuronal activity. *Journal of Neuroscience* **18**, 2748–2763.

Hampson, R.E., Rogers, G., Lynch, G. *et al.* (1998b) Facilitative effects of the ampakine CX516 on short-term memory in rats; enhancement of delayed-nonmatch-to-sample performance. *Journal of Neuroscience* **18**, 2740–2747.

Harvey, P.D., Silverman, J.M., Mohs, R.C. *et al.* (1999) Cognitive decline in late-life schizophrenia: a longitudinal study of geriatric chronically hospitalized patients. *Biological Psychiatry* **45**, 32–40.

Hashimoto, A. & Oka, T. (1997) Free D-aspartate and D-serine in the mammalian brain and periphery. *Progress in Neurobiology* **52**, 325–353.

Haspel, T. (1995) Beta-blockers and the treatment of aggression. *Harvard Review of Psychiatry* **2**, 274–281.

Hauber, W. & Andersen, R. (1993) The non-NMDA glutamate receptor antagonist GYKI 52466 counteracts locomotor stimulation and anti-cataleptic activity induced by the NMDA antagonist dizocilpine. *Naunyn-Schmeideberg's Archives of Pharmacology* **348**, 486–490.

Hawkins, K.A., Mohamed, S. & Woods, S.W. (1999) Will the novel antipsychotics significantly ameliorate neuropsychological deficits and improve adaptive functioning in schizophrenia? *Psychological Medicine* **29**, 1–8.

Hellewell, J.S.E., Cameron-Hands, D. & Cantillon, M. (1998) Seroquel: evidence for efficacy in the treatment of hostility and aggression. *Schizophrenia Research* **29**, 154–155.

Henderson, G., Johnson, J.W. & Ascher, P. (1990) Competitive antagonists and partial agonists at the glycine modulatory site of the mouse N-methyl-D-aspartate receptor. *Journal of Physiology* **430**, 189–212.

Heresco-Levy, U., Javitt, D.C., Ermilov, M. *et al.* (1996) Double-blind, placebo-controlled, crossover trial of glycine adjuvant therapy for treatment-resistant schizophrenia. *British Journal of Psychiatry* **169**, 610–617.

Heresco-Levy, U., Javitt, D.C., Ermilov, M. *et al.* (1999) Efficacy of high-dose glycine in the treatment of enduring negative symptoms of schizophrenia. *Archives of General Psychiatry* **56**, 29–36.

Hillard, J.R. (1998) Emergency treatment of acute psychosis. *Journal of Clinical Psychiatry* **59** (Suppl. 1), 57–60.

Hirsch, S.R. & Barnes, T.R.E. (1995) The clinical treatment of schizophrenia with antipsychotic medication. In: *Schizophrenia* (eds S.R.

Hirsch & D.R. Weinberger), pp. 443–468. Blackwell Science, Oxford.

Ho, B.C., Andreasen, N.C., Flaum, M. et al. (2000) Untreated initial psychosis: its relation to quality of life and symptom remission in first-episode schizophrenia. American Journal of Psychiatry 157, 808–815.

Hogarty, G.E., McEvoy, J.P., Ulrich, R.F. et al. (1995) Pharmacotherapy of impaired affect in recovering schizophrenic patients. Archives of General Psychiatry 52, 29.

Hoyberg, O.J., Fensbo, C., Remvig, J. et al. (1993) Risperidone versus perphenazine in the treatment of chronic schizophrenic patients with acute exacerbations. Acta Psychiatrica Scandinavica 88, 395–402.

Huber, G., Gross, G., Schuttler, R. et al. (1980) Longitudinal studies of schizophrenic patients. Schizophrenia Bulletin 6, 592–605.

Huttunen, M.O., Piepponen, T., Rantanen, H. et al. (1995) Risperidone versus zuclopenthixol in the treatment of acute schizophrenic episodes: a double-blind parallel-group trial. Acta Psychiatrica Scandinavica 91, 271–277.

Hyde, C.E. & Harrower-Wilson, C. (1996) Psychiatric intensive care in acute psychosis. International Clinical Psychopharmacology 11 (Suppl. 2), 61–65.

Inoue, A., Miki, S., Seto, M. et al. (1997) Aripiprazole, a novel antipsychotic drug, inhibits quinpirole-evoked GTPase activity but does not up-regulate dopamine D_2 receptor following repeated treatment in the rat striatum. European Journal of Pharmacology 321, 105–111.

Iyer, R.N., Davis, M.D., Juneau, P.L. et al. (1998) Brain extracellular levels of the putative antipsychotic CI-1007 and its effects on striatal and nucleus accumbens dopamine overflow in the awake rat. Journal of Pharmacy and Pharmacology 50, 1147–1153.

Janicak, P.G. & Davis, J.M. (1996) Antipsychotic dosing strategies in acute schizophrenia. International Clinical Psychopharmacology 11 (Suppl. 2), 35–40.

Janicak, P.G., Davis, J.M., Preskorn, S.H. et al. (1993) Principles and Practice of Psychopharmacology. Williams and Wilkins, Baltimore.

Javitt, D.C. & Frusciante, M. (1997) Glycyldodecylamide, a phencyclidine behavioral antagonist, blocks cortical glycine uptake: implications for schizophrenia and substance abuse. Psychopharmacology (Berl) 129, 96–98.

Javitt, D.C. & Zukin, S.R. (1991) Recent advances in the phencyclidine model of schizophrenia. American Journal of Psychiatry 148, 1301–1308.

Javitt, D.C., Zylberman, I., Zukin, S.R. et al. (1994) Amelioration of negative symptoms in schizophrenia by glycine. American Journal of Psychiatry 151, 1234–1236.

Javitt, D.C., Sershen, H., Hashim, A. et al. (1997) Reversal of phencyclidine-induced hyperactivity by glycine and the glycine uptake inhibitor glycyldodecylamide. Neuropsychopharmacology 17, 202–204.

Johns, C.A. & Thompson, J.W. (1995) Adjunctive treatments in schizophrenia: pharmacotherapies and electroconvulsive therapy. Schizophrenia Bulletin 21, 607–619.

Johnson, J.W. & Ascher, P. (1987) Glycine potentiates the NMDA response in cultured mouse brain neurons. Nature 325, 529–531.

Johnson, S.A., Luu, N.T., Herbst, T.A. et al. (1999) Synergistic interactions between ampakines and antipsychotic drugs. Journal of Pharmacology and Experimental Therapeutics 289, 392–397.

Johnstone, E.C., Crow, T.J., Ferrier, I.N. et al. (1983) Adverse effects of anticholinergic medication on positive schizophrenic symptoms. Psychological Medicine 13, 513–527.

Kahn, E.M., Schulz, S.C., Perel, J.M. et al. (1990) Change in haloperidol level due to carbamazepine: a complicating factor in combined medication for schizophrenia. Journal of Clinical Psychopharmacology 10, 54–57.

Kane, J.M. (1989) The current status of neuroleptic therapy. Journal of Clinical Psychiatry 50, 322–328.

Kane, J. (1999a) Olanzapine in the long-term treatment of schizophrenia. British Journal of Psychiatry 174, 26–29.

Kane, J.M. (1999b) Management strategies for the treatment of schizophrenia. Journal of Clinical Psychiatry 60, 13–17.

Kane, J.M., Rifkin, A., Quitkin, F. et al. (1982) Fluphenazine vs placebo in patients with remitted, acute first-episode schizophrenia. Archives of General Psychiatry 39, 70–73.

Kane, J., Honigfeld, G., Singer, J. et al. (1988) Clozapine for the treatment-resistant schizophrenic: a double-blind comparison with chlorpromazine. Archives of General Psychiatry 45, 789–796.

Kanter, G.L., Yerevanian, B.I. & Ciccone, J.R. (1984) Case report of a possible interaction between neuroleptics and carbamazepine. American Journal of Psychiatry 141, 1101–1102.

Kapur, S., Remington, G., Jones, C. et al. (1996) High levels of dopamine D_2 receptor occupancy with low-dose haloperidol treatment: a PET study. American Journal of Psychiatry 153, 948–950.

Kapur, S., Zipursky, R.B., Remington, G. et al. (1998) 5-HT$_2$ and D_2 receptor occupancy of olanzapine in schizophrenia: a PET investigation. American Journal of Psychiatry 155, 921–928.

Kapur, S., Zipursky, R.B. & Remington, G. (1999) Clinical and theoretical implications of 5-HT$_2$ and D_2 receptor occupancy of clozapine, risperidone, and olanzapine in schizophrenia. American Journal of Psychiatry 156, 286–293.

Kapur, S., Zipursky, R., Jones, C. et al. (2000) Relationship between dopamine D_2 occupancy, clinical response, and side effects: a double-blind PET study of first-episode schizophrenia. American Journal of Psychiatry 157, 514–520.

Karagianis, J.L., Dawe, I.C., Thakur, A. et al. (2001) Rapid tranquilization with olanzapine in acute psychosis: a case series. Journal of Clinical Psychiatry 62 (Suppl. 2), 12–16.

Kasper, S. (1998) Risperidone and olanzapine: optimal dosing for efficacy and tolerability in patients with schizophrenia. International Clinical Psychopharmacology 13, 253–262.

Keefe, R.S.E., Silva, S.G., Perkins, D.O. et al. (1999) The effects of atypical antipsychotic drugs on neurocognitive impairment in schizophrenia: a review and meta-analysis. Schizophrenia Bulletin 25, 201–222.

Kidron, R., Averbuch, I., Klein, E. et al. (1985) Carbamazepine-induced reduction of blood levels of haloperidol in chronic schizophrenia. Biological Psychiatry 20, 219–222.

Kikuchi, T., Tottori, K., Uwahodo, Y. et al. (1995) 7-(4-[4-(2,3-Dichlorophenyl)-1-piperazinyl]butyloxy)-3,4-dihydro-2(1H)-quinolinone (OPC-14597), a new putative antipsychotic drug with both presynaptic dopamine autoreceptor agonistic activity and postsynaptic D_2 receptor antagonistic activity. Journal of Pharmacology and Experimental Therapeutics 274, 329–336.

King, D.J. (1990) The effect of neuroleptics on cognitive and psychomotor function. British Journal of Psychiatry 157, 799–811.

Kinon, B.J. & Lieberman, J.A. (1996) Mechanisms of action of atypical antipsychotic drugs: a critical analysis. Psychopharmacology (Berl) 124, 2–34.

Kinon, B.J., Milton, D.R. & Hill, A.L. (2001a) Efficacy of olanzapine orally-disintegrating tablet in the treatment of acutely ill noncompliant schizophrenic patients. Biological Psychiatry 49, 171S.

Kinon, B.J., Roychowdhury, S.M., Milton, D.R. et al. (2001b) Effective resolution with olanzapine of acute presentation of behavioral agitation and positive psychotic symptoms in schizophrenia. Journal of Clinical Psychiatry 62 (Suppl. 2), 17–21.

Ko, G.N., Korpi, E.R., Freed, W.J. et al. (1985) Effect of valproic acid on behavior and plasma amino acid concentrations in chronic schizophrenic patients. Biological Psychiatry 20, 209–215.

Kongsamut S., Roehr, J.E., Cai, J. *et al.* (1996) Iloperidone binding to human and rat dopamine and 5-HT receptors. *European Journal of Pharmacology* 317, 417–423.

Kopala, L.C., Good, K.P. & Honer, W.G. (1997) Extrapyramidal signs and clinical symptoms in first-episode schizophrenia: response to low-dose risperidone. *Journal of Clinical Psychopharmacology* 17, 308–313.

Kopelowicz, A. & Liberman, R.P. (1995) Biobehavioral treatment and rehabilitation of schizophrenia. *Harard Review of Psychiatry* 3, 55–64.

Kramer, M.S., Vogel, W.H. DiJohnson, C. *et al.* (1989) Antidepressants in 'depressed' schizophrenic inpatients. A controlled trial. *Archives of General Psychiatry* 46, 922–928.

Kramer, M.S., Last, B., Getson, A. *et al.* (1997) The effects of a selective D_4 dopamine receptor antagonist (L-745,870) in acutely psychotic inpatients with schizophrenia. D_4 Dopamine Antagonist Group. *Archives of General Psychiatry* 54, 567–572.

Krystal, J.H., Karper, L.P., Seibyl, J.P. *et al.* (1994) Subanesthetic effects of the noncompetitive NMDA antagonist, ketamine, in humans: Psychotomimetic, perceptual, cognitive, and neuroendocrine responses. *Archives of General Psychiatry* 51, 199–214.

Lahti, A.C., Holcomb, H.H., Medoff, D.R. *et al.* (1995a) Ketamine activates psychosis and alters limbic blood flow in schizophrenia. *Neuroreport* 6, 869–872.

Lahti, A.C., Koffel, B., LaPorte, D. *et al.* (1995b) Subanesthetic doses of ketamine stimulate psychosis in schizophrenia. *Neuropsychopharmacology* 13, 9–19.

Larsen, T.K., Friis, S., Haahr, U. *et al.* (2001) Early detection and intervention in first-episode schizophrenia: a critical review. *Acta Psychiatrica Scandinavica* 103, 323–334.

Lawler, C.P., Prioleau, C., Lewis, M.M. *et al.* (1999) Interactions of the novel antipsychotic aripiprazole (OPC-14597) with dopamine and serotonin receptor subtypes. *Neuropsychopharmacology* 20, 612–627.

Lee, M.S., Kim, Y.K. Lee, S.K. *et al.* (1998) A double-blind study of adjunctive sertraline in haloperidol-stabilized patients with chronic schizophrenia. *Journal of Clinical Psychopharmacology* 18, 399–403.

Leeson, P.D. & Iversen, L.L. (1994) The glycine site on the NMDA receptor: structure-activity relationships and therapeutic potential. *Journal of Medicinal Chemistry* 37, 4053–4067.

Lesem, M.D., Zajecka, J.M., Swift, R.H. *et al.* (2001) Intramuscular ziprasidone, 2 mg versus 10 mg, in the short-term management of agitated psychotic patients. *Journal of Clinical Psychiatry* 62, 12–18.

Leucht, S., McGrath, J., White, P. *et al.* (2000) Carbamazepine for schizophrenia and schizoaffective psychoses. *Cochrane Database System Review* CD001258.

Leveque, J.C., Macias, W., Rajadhyaksha, A. *et al.* (2000) Intracellular modulation of NMDA receptor function by antipsychotic drugs. *Journal of Neuroscience* 20, 4011–4020.

Levinson, D.F., Simpson, G.M., Singh, H. *et al.* (1990) Fluphenazine dose, clinical response, and extrapyramidal symptoms during acute treatment. *Archives of General Psychiatry* 47, 761–768.

Liberman, R.P. & Kopelowicz, A. (1995) Basic elements in biobehavioral treatment and rehabilitation of schizophrenia. *International Clinical Psychopharmacology* 9 (Suppl. 5), 51–58.

Lidow, M.S., Elsworth, J.D. & Goldman-Rakic, P.S. (1997) Down-regulation of the D_1 and D_5 dopamine receptors in the primate prefrontal cortex by chronic treatment with antipsychotic drugs. *Journal of Pharmacology and Experimental Therapeutics* 281, 597–603.

Lieberman, J.A. (1993) Prediction of outcome in first-episode schizophrenia. *Journal of Clinical Psychiatry* 54 (Suppl.), 13–17.

Lieberman, J.A. (1996) Atypical antipsychotic drugs as a first-line treatment of schizophrenia: a rationale and hypothesis. *Journal of Clinical Psychiatry* 57 (Suppl. 11), 68–71.

Lieberman, J.A. (1998) Maximizing clozapine therapy: managing side effects. *Journal of Clinical Psychiatry* 59 (Suppl. 3), 38–43.

Lieberman, J.A. (1999) Is schizophrenia a neurodegenerative disorder?: a clinical and pathophysiological perspective. *Biological Psychiatry* 46, 729–739.

Lieberman, J.A. (2001) Hypothesis and hypothesis testing in the clinical trial. *Journal of Clinical Psychiatry* 62 (Suppl. 9), 5–8.

Lieberman, J.A. & Fenton, W.S. (2000) Delayed detection of psychosis: causes, consequences, and effect on public health. *American Journal of Psychiatry* 157, 1727–1730.

Lieberman, J., Kane, J., Woerner, M. *et al.* (1990a) Prediction of relapse in schizophrenia. *Clinical Neuropharmacology* 13, 434–435.

Lieberman, J.A., Kinon, B.J. & Loebel, A.D. (1990b) Dopaminergic mechanisms in idiopathic and drug-induced psychoses. *Schizophrenia Bulletin* 16, 97–109.

Lieberman, J. A., Jody, D., Geisler, S. *et al.* (1993) Time course and biologic correlates of treatment response in first-episode schizophrenia. *Archives of General Psychiatry* 50, 369–376.

Lieberman, J.A., Alvir, J.M., Koreen, A. *et al.* (1996a) Psychobiologic correlates of treatment response in schizophrenia. *Neuropsychopharmacology* 14, 13S–21S.

Lieberman, J.A., Koreen, A., Chakos, M. *et al.* (1996b) Factors influencing treatment response and outcome of first-episode schizophrenia implications for understanding the pathophysiology of schizophrenia. *Journal of Clinical Psychiatry* 57, 5–9.

Lieberman, J.A., Sheitman, B.B. & Kinon, B.J. (1997) Neurochemical sensitization in the pathophysiology of schizophrenia deficits and dysfunction in neuronal regulation and plasticity. *Neuropsychopharmacology* 17, 205–229.

Lieberman, J.A., Mailman, R.B., Duncan, G. *et al.* (1998) Serotonergic basis of antipsychotic drug effects in schizophrenia. *Biological Psychiatry* 44, 1099–1117.

Lieberman, J.A., Tohen, M., McEvoy, J. *et al.* (2000a) Olanzapine versus haloperidol in the treatment of first episode psychosis. In 39th ACNP Annual Meeting San Juan, Puerto Rico.

Lieberman, J.A., Phillips, M., Kong, L. *et al.* (2000b) Efficacy and safety of clozapine versus chlorpromazine in first-episode psychosis: results of a 52 week randomized double blind trial. In 39th ACNP Annual Meeting San Juan, Puerto Rico.

Linnoila, M., Viukari, M. & Kietala, O. (1976) Effect of sodium valproate on tradive dyskinesia. *British Journal of Psychiatry* 129, 114–119.

Litman, R.E., Su, T.P., Potter, W.Z. *et al.* (1996) Idazoxan and response to typical neuroleptics in treatment-resistant schizophrenia. Comparison with the atypical neuroleptic, clozapine. *British Journal of Psychiatry* 168, 571–579.

Loebel, A.D., Lieberman, J.A., Alvir, J.M.J. *et al.* (1992) Duration of psychosis and outcome in first-episode schizophrenia. *American Journal of Psychiatry* 149, 1183–1188.

Loo, H., Poirier-Littre, M.F., Theron, M. *et al.* (1997) Amisulpride versus placebo in the medium-term treatment of the negative symptoms of schizophrenia. *British Journal of Psychiatry* 170, 18–22.

Lucas, G., Bonhomme, N., De Deurwaerdere, P. *et al.* (1997) 8-OH-DPAt, a 5-HT_{1A} agonist and ritanserin, a $5\text{-HT}_{2A/C}$ antagonist, reverse haloperidol-induced catalepsy in rats independently of striatal dopamine release. *Psychopharmacology (Berl)* 131, 57–63.

Luchins, D.J. (1984) Carbamazepine in violent non-epileptic schizophrenics. *Psychopharmacology Bulletin* 20, 569–571.

McEvoy, J.P. (1983) The clinical use of anticholinergic drugs as treatment for extrapyramidal side effects of neuroleptic drugs. *Journal of Clinical Psychopharmacology* 3, 288–302.

McEvoy, J.P., Hogarty, G.E. & Steingard, S. (1991) Optimal dose of neuroleptic in acute schizophrenia. A controlled study of the neuroleptic threshold and higher haloperidol dose. *Archives of General Psychiatry* 48, 739–745.

McEvoy, J.P., Weiden, P.J., Smith, T.E. *et al.* (1996) The expert consensus guideline series: treatment of schizophrenia. *Journal of Clinical Psychiatry* 57, 1–58.

McEvoy, J.P., Scheifler, P.L. & Frances, A. (1999) The expert consensus guideline series: treatment of schizophrenia 1999. *Journal of Clinical Psychiatry* 60, 1–80.

McGlashan, T.H. (1996) Early detection and intervention in schizophrenia: research. *Schizophrenia Bulletin* 22, 327–345.

Malhotra, A.K., Pinals, D.A., Weingartner, H. *et al.* (1996) NMDA receptor function and human cognition: the effects of ketamine in healthy volunteers. *Neuropsychopharmacology* 14, 301–307.

Malhotra, A.K., Pinals, D.A., Adler, C.M. *et al.* (1997) Ketamine-induced exacerbation of psychotic symptoms and cognitive impairment in neuroleptic-free schizophrenics. *Neuropsychopharmacology* 17, 141–150.

Mansbach, R.S., Brooks, E.W., Sanner, M.A. *et al.* (1998a) Selective dopamine D_4 receptor antagonists reverse apomorphine-induced blockade of prepulse inhibition. *Psychopharmacology (Berl)* 135, 194–200.

Mansbach, R.S., Brooks, E.W., Sanner, M.A. *et al.* (1998b) Selective dopamine D_4 receptor antagonists reverse apomorphine-induced blockade of prepulse inhibition. *Psychopharmacology (Berl)* 135, 194–200.

Marcus, M.M., Nomikos, G.G. & Svensson, T.H. (2000) Effects of atypical antipsychotic drugs on dopamine output in the shell and core of the nucleus accumbens: role of $5-HT_{2A}$ and alpha$_1$-adrenoceptor antagonism. *European Neuropsychopharmacology* 10, 245–253.

Marder, S.R. (1996) Pharmacological treatment strategies in acute schizophrenia. *International Clinical Psychopharmacology* 11 (Suppl. 2), 29–34.

Marder, S.R. (1997) Antipsychotic drugs. In: *Psychiatry* (eds A. Tasman, J. Kay & J.A. Lieberman), pp. 1569–1585. W.B. Saunders, Philadelphia.

Marder, S.R. & Meibach, R.C. (1994) Risperidone in the treatment of schizophrenia. *American Journal of Psychiatry* 151, 825–835.

Marder, S.R., Hubbard, J.W., Van Putten, T. *et al.* (1989) Pharmacokinetics of long-acting injectable neuroleptic drugs: clinical implications. *Psychopharmacology (Berl)* 98, 433–439.

Marder, S.R., Davis, J.M. & Chouinard, G. (1997) The effects of risperidone on the five dimensions of schizophrenia derived by factor analysis: combined results of the North American trials. *Journal of Clinical Psychiatry* 58, 538–546.

Markowitz, J.S., Brown, C.S. & Moore, T.R. (1999) Atypical antipsychotics. Pharmacology, pharmacokinetics, and efficacy. *Annals of Pharmacotherapy* 33, 73–85.

Mathe, J.M., Nomikos, G.G., Hildebrand, B.E. *et al.* (1996) Prazosin inhibits MK-801-induced hyperlocomotion and dopamine release in the nucleus accumbens. *European Journal of Pharmacology* 309, 1–11.

Mathew, R.J. & Wilson, W.H. (1989) Changes in cerebral blood flow and mental state after amphetamine challenge in schizophrenic patients. *Neuropsychobiology* 21, 117–123.

Maurel-Remy, S., Bervoets, K. & Millan, M.J. (1995) Blockade of phencyclidine-induced hyperlocomotion by clozapine and MDL 100,907 in rats reflects antagonism of $5-HT_{2A}$ receptors. *European Journal of Pharmacology* 280, R9–11.

May, P.R., Tuma, A.H., Yale, C. *et al.* (1976) Schizophrenia: a follow-up study of results of treatment. *Archives of General Psychiatry* 33, 481–486.

May, P.R., Tuma, A.H. & Dixon, W.J. (1981) Schizophrenia: a follow-up study of the results of five forms of treatment. *Archives of General Psychiatry* 38, 776–784.

Meltzer, H.Y. (1995) Clozapine: is another view valid? *American Journal of Psychiatry* 152, 821–825.

Meltzer, H.Y. (1996) Pre-clinical pharmacology of atypical antipsychotic drugs: a selective review. *British Journal of Psychiatry* 29 (Suppl), 23–31.

Meltzer, H.Y. (1998) Suicide in schizophrenia: risk factors and clozapine treatment. *Journal of Clinical Psychiatry* 59 (Suppl. 3), 15–20.

Meltzer, H.Y. (1999a) Outcome in schizophrenia: beyond symptom reduction. *Journal of Clinical Psychiatry* 60 (Suppl. 3), 3–7.

Meltzer, H.Y. (1999b) Treatment of schizophrenia and spectrum disorders: pharmacotherapy, psychosocial treatments, and neurotransmitter interactions. *Biological Psychiatry* 46, 1321–1327.

Meltzer, H.Y. & McGurk, S.R. (1999) The effects of clozapine, risperidone, and olanzapine on cognitive function in schizophrenia. *Schizophrenia Bulletin* 25, 233–255.

Meltzer, L.T., Christoffersen, C.L., Corbin, A.E. *et al.* (1995) CI-1007, a dopamine partial agonist and potential antipsychotic agent. II. Neurophysiological and behavioral effects. *Journal of Pharmacology and Experimental Therapeutics* 274, 912–920.

Millan, M.J., Gobert, A., Newman-Tancredi, A. *et al.* (1998a) S 16924 ((R)-2-[1-[2-(2,3-dihydro-benzo[1,4]dioxin-5-yloxy)-ethyl]-pyrrolidin-3yl]-1-(4-fluoro-phenyl)-ethanone), a novel, potential antipsychotic with marked serotonin (5-HT)1A agonist properties. I. Receptorial and neurochemical profile in comparison with clozapine and haloperidol. *Journal of Pharmacology and Experimental Therapeutics* 286, 1341–1355.

Millan, M.J., Schreiber, R., Dekeyne, A. *et al.* (1998b) S 16924 ((R)-2-[1-[2-(2,3-dihydro-benzo[1,4]dioxin-5-yloxy)-ethyl]-pyrrolidin-3yl]-1-(4-fluoro-phenyl)-ethanone), a novel, potential antipsychotic with marked serotonin (5-HT)1A agonist properties. II. Functional profile in comparison to clozapine and haloperidol. *Journal of Pharmacology and Experimental Therapeutics* 286, 1356–1373.

Millan, M.J., Brocco, M., Rivet, J.M. *et al.* (2000a) S18327 (1-[2-[4-(6-fluoro-1,2-benzisoxazol-3-yl)piperid-1-yl]ethyl]3-phenyl imidazolin-2-one), a novel, potential antipsychotic displaying marked antagonist properties at alpha(1)- and alpha(2)-adrenergic receptors. II. Functional profile and a multiparametric comparison with haloperidol, clozapine, and 11 other antipsychotic agents. *Journal of Pharmacology and Experimental Therapeutics* 292, 54–66.

Millan, M.J., Gobert, A., Newman-Tancredi, A. *et al* (2000b) S18327 (1-[2-[4-(6-fluoro-1,2-benzisoxazol-3-yl)piperid-l-yl]ethyl]3-phenyl imidazolin-2-one), a novel, potential anttipsychotic displaying marked antagonist properties at alpha(1)- and alpha(2)-adrenergic receptors. I. Receptorial, neurochemical, and electrophysiological profile. *Journal of Pharmacology and Experimental Therapeutics* 292, 38–53.

Miyamoto, S., Duncan, G.E., Mailman, R.B. *et al.* (2000a) Developing novel antipsychotic drugs: strategies and goals. *Current Opinion in CPNS and Investigative Drugs* 2, 25–39.

Miyamoto, S., Leipzig, J.N., Lieberman, J.A. *et al.* (2000b) Effects of ketamine, MK-801, and amphetamine on regional brain 2-deoxyglucose uptake in freely moving mice. *Neuropsychopharmacology* 22, 400–412.

Miyamoto, S., Mailman, R.B., Lieberman, J.A. *et al.* (2001) Blunted brain metabolic response to ketamine in mice lacking D_{1A} dopamine receptors. *Brain Research* 894, 167–180.

Miyamoto, S., Duncan, G.E., Goff, D.C. *et al.* (2002) Therapeutics of schizophrenia. In: *Neuropsychopharmacology: The Fifth Generation of Progress* (eds D. Charney, J. Coyle, K. Davis & C. Nemeroff), pp. 775–807. Raven Press, New York.

Moghaddam, B. & Adams, B.W. (1998) Reversal of phencyclidine effects by a group II metabotrophic glutamate receptor agonist in rats. *Science* 281, 1349–1352.

Moghaddam, B., Adams, B., Verman, A. *et al.* (1997) Activation of glutamatergic neurotransmission by ketamine: a novel step in the pathway from NMDA receptor blockade to dopaminergic and cognitive disruptions associated with the prefrontal cortex. *Journal of Neuroscience* 17, 2921–2927.

Mohamed, S., Paulsen, J.S., O'Leary, D. *et al.* (1999) Generalized cognitive deficits in schizophrenia: a study of first-episode patients. *Archives of General Psychiatry* 56, 749–754.

Moller, H.J. (1993) Neuroleptic treatment of negative symptoms in schizophrenic patients: efficacy problems and methodological difficulties. *European Neuropsychopharmacology* 3, 1–11.

Moller, H.J., Boyer, P., Fleurot, O. *et al.* (1997) Improvement of acute exacerbations of schizophrenia with amisulpride: a comparison with haloperidol: PROD-ASLP Study Group. *Psychopharmacology (Berl)* 132, 396–401.

Momiyama, T., Amano, T., Todo, N. *et al.* (1996) Inhibition by a putative antipsychotic quinolinone derivative (OPC-14597) of dopaminergic neurons in the ventral tegmental area. *European Journal of Pharmacology* 310, 1–8.

National Institute of Mental Health Psychopharmacology Service Center Collaborative Study Group (1964) Phenothiazine treatment in acute schizophrenia. *Archives of General Psychiatry* 10, 246–261.

Neborsky, R., Janowsky, D., Munson, E. *et al.* (1981) Rapid treatment of acute psychotic symptoms with high- and low-dose haloperidol: behavioral considerations. *Archives of General Psychiatry* 38, 195–199.

Nemeroff, C.B. (1997) Dosing the antipsychotic medication olanzapine. *Journal of Clinical Psychiatry* 58 (Suppl. 10), 45–49.

Neppe, V.M. (1983) Carbamazepine as adjunctive treatment in nonepileptic chronic inpatients with EEG temporal lobe abnormalities. *Journal of Clinical Psychiatry* 44, 326–331.

Newman-Tancredi, A., Chaput, C., Verriele, L. *et al.* (1996) Clozapine is a partial agonist at cloned, human serotonin 5-HT$_{1A}$ receptors. *Neuropharmacology* 35, 119–121.

Nichols, D.E. & Mailman, R.B. (1995) Substituted hexahydro[a]phenanthridines. *US Patent* 5, 134.

Nichols, D.E. & Mailman, R.B. (1999) Fused isoquinolines as dopamine receptor ligands. *US Patent* 5, 110.

Nyberg, S., Eriksson, B., Oxenstierna, G. *et al.* (1999) Suggested minimal effective dose of risperidone based on PEt-measured D$_2$ and 5-HT$_{2A}$ receptor occupancy in schizophrenic patients. *American Journal of Psychiatry* 156, 869–875.

Okubo, Y., Suhara, T., Suzuki, K. *et al.*(1997) Decreased prefrontal dopamine D1 receptors in schizophrenia revealed by PET. *Nature* 385, 634–636.

Okuma, T., Yamashita, I., Takahashi, R. *et al.* (1989) A double-blind study of adjunctive carbamazepine versus placebo on excited states of schizophrenic and schizoaffective disorders. *Acta Psychiatrica Scandinavica* 80, 250–259.

Olney, J.W. & Farber, N.B. (1995) Glutamate receptor dysfunction and schizophrenia. *Archives of General Psychiatry* 52, 998–1007.

O'Neill, M.F., Heron-Maxwell, C.L. & Shaw, G (1999) 5-HT$_2$ receptor antagonism reduces hyperactivity induced by amphetamine, cocaine, and MK-801 but not D$_1$ agonist C-APB. *Pharmacology, Biochemistry and Behavior* 63, 237–243.

Ozdemir, V. (2000) Aripiprazole. *Current Opinion in CPNS Investigative Drugs* 2, 105–111.

Paillere-Martinot, M.L., Lecrubier, Y., Martinot, J.L. *et al.* (1995) Improvement of some schizophrenic deficit symptoms with low doses of amisulpride. *American Journal of Psychiatry* 152, 130–134.

Perry, K.W., Bymaster, F.P., Shannon, H.E. *et al.* (1999) The muscarinic agonist xanomeline has antipsychotic-like activity in animals and in man. *Schizophrenia Research* 36, 117–118.

Petrie, J.L., Saha, A.R. & McEvoy, J.P. (1998) Acute and long-term efficacy and safety of aripiprazole: a new atypical antipsychotic. *Schizophrenia Research* 29, 155.

Peuskens, J. & Link, C.G. (1997) A comparison of quetiapine and chlorpromazine in the treatment of schizophrenia. *Acta Psychiatrica Scandinavica* 96, 265–273.

Peuskens, J., Bech, P., Moller, H.J. *et al.* (1999) Amisulpride vs. risperidone in the treatment of acute exacerbations of schizophrenia. Amisulpride study group. *Psychiatry Research* 88, 107–117.

Plasky, P. (1991) Antidepressant usage in schizophrenia. *Schizophrenia Bulletin* 17, 649–657.

Polak, P. & Laycob, L. (1971) Rapid tranquilization. *American Journal of Psychiatry* 128, 640–643.

Potkin, S. & Cooper, S. (2000) Ziprasidone and zotepine: clinical use and experience. In: *Schizophrenia and Mood Disorders: The New Drug Therapies in Clinical Practice* (eds P.F. Buckley & J.L. Waddington), pp. 49–58. Butterworth-Heinemann, Woburn, MA.

Potkin, S.G., Jin, Y., Bunney, B.G. *et al.* (1999) Effect of clozapine and adjunctive high-dose glycine in treatment-resistant schizophrenia. *American Journal of Psychiatry* 156, 145–147.

Prudo, R. & Blum, H.M. (1987) Five-year outcome and prognosis in schizophrenia: a report from the London field research centre of the international pilot study of schizophrenia. *British Journal of Psychiatry* 150, 345–354.

Puech, A., Fleurot, O. & Rein, W. (1998) Amisulpride, and atypical antipsychotic, in the treatment of acute episodes of schizophrenia: a dose-ranging study vs. haloperidol. The Amisulpride Study Group. *Acta Psychiatrica Scandinavica* 98, 65–72.

Pugsley, T.A., Davis, M.D., Akunne, H.C. *et al.* (1995) Cl-1007, a dopamine partial agonist and potential antipsychotic agent. I. Neurochemical effects. *Journal of Pharmacology and Experimental Therapeutics* 274, 898–911.

Purdon, S.E., Jones, B.D., Stip, E. *et al.* (2000) Neuropsychological change in early phase schizophrenia during 12 months of treatment with olanzapine, risperidone, or haloperidol. The Canadian Collaborative Group for research in schizophrenia. *Archives of General Psychiatry* 57, 249–258.

Remington, G. & Kapur, S. (2000) Atypical antipsychotics: are some more atypical than others? *Psychopharmacology (Berl)* 148, 3–15.

Reynetjens, A., Gelders, M.L., Hoppenbrouwers, J.A. *et al.* (1986) Thymosthenic effects of ritanserin (R 55667), a centrally acting serotonin-S2 receptor blocker. *Drug Development Research* 8, 205–211.

Rivet, J.M., Brocco, M., Dekeyne, A. *et al.* (2000) S33592, a benzopyranopyrrole partial agonist at dopamine D$_2$/D$_3$ receptors and potential antipsychotic agent. II. Functional profile in comparison to aripiprazole, preclamol and raclopride. *Society for Neuroscience Abstracts* 26, 273.

Robinson, D.G., Woerner, M.G., Alvir, J.M. *et al.* (1999) Predictors of treatment response from a first episode of schizophrenia or schizoaffective disorder. *American Journal of Psychiatry* 156, 544–549.

Rosse, R.B., Theut, S.K., Banay-Schwartz, M. *et al.* (1989) Glycine adjuvant therapy to conventional neuroleptic treatment in schizophrenia: an open-label, pilot study. *Clinical Neuropharmacology* 12, 416–424.

Sacristan, J.A., Gomez, J.C., Montejo, A.L. *et al.* (2000) Doses of olanzapine, risperidone, and haloperidol used in clinical practice: results of a prospective pharmacoepidemiologic study. EFESO Study Group. Estudio Farmacoepidemiologico en la Esquizofrenia con Olanzapina. *Clinical Therapy* 22, 583–599.

Saha, A.R., Petrie, J.L. & Ali, M.W. (1999) Safety and efficacy profile of aripiprazole, a novel antipsychotic. *Schizophrenia Research* 36, 295.

Salzman, C., Green, A.I., Rodriguez-Villa, F. *et al.* (1986) Benzodiazepines combined with neuroleptics for management of severe disruptive behavior. *Psychosomatics* 27, 17–22.

Salzman, C., Solomon, D., Miyawaki, E. *et al.* (1991) Parenteral lorazepam versus parenteral haloperidol for the control of psychotic disruptive behavior. *Journal of Clinical Psychiatry* 52, 177–180.

Sanfilipo, M., Wolkin, A., Angrist, B. *et al.* (1996) Amphetamine and negative symptoms of schizophrenia. *Psychopharmacology (Berl)* 123, 211–214.

Sanger, T.M., Lieberman, J.A., Tohen, M. *et al.* (1999) Olanzapine versus haloperidol treatment in first-episode psychosis. *American Journal of Psychiatry* 156, 79–87.

Sauerberg, P., Jeppesen, L., Olesen, P.H. *et al.* (1998) Muscarinic agonists with antipsychotic-like activity: structure-activity relationships of 1,2,5-thiadiazole analogues with functional dopamine antagonist activity. *Journal of Medicinal Chemistry* 41, 4378–4384.

Schmidt, C.J. & Fadayel, G.M. (1995) The selective 5-HT$_{2A}$ receptor antagonist, MDL 100,907, increases dopamine efflux in the prefrontal cortex of the rat. *European Journal of Pharmacology* 273, 273–279.

Schmidt, C.J. & Fadayel, G.M. (1996) Regional effects of MK-801 on dopamine relase effects of competitive NMDA or 5-HT$_{2A}$ receptor blocade. *Journal of Pharmacology and Experimental Therapeutics* 277, 1541–1549.

Schmidt, C.J., Fadayel, G.M. Sullivan, C.K. *et al.* (1992) 5-HT$_2$ receptors exert a state-dependent regulation of dopaminergic function: studies with MDL 100,907 and the amphetamine analogue, 3,4-methylenedioxymethamphetamine. *European Journal of Pharmacology* 223, 65–74.

Schmidt, C.J., Sorensen, S.M., Kehne, J.H. *et al.* (1995) The role of 5-HT$_{2A}$ receptors in antipsychotic activity. *Life Sciences* 56, 2209–2222.

Schneider, J.S., Sun, Z.Q. & Roeltgen, D.P. (1994) Effects of dihydrexidine, a full dopamine D$_1$ receptor agonist, on delayed response performance in chronic low dose MPTP-treated monkeys. *Brain Research* 663, 140–144.

Schulz, C. & McGorry, P. (2000) Traditional antipsychotic medications: contemporary clinical use. In: *Schizophrenia and Mood Disorders: the New Drug Therapies in Clinical Practice* (eds P.F. Buckley & J.L. Waddington), pp. 14–20. Butterworth-Heinemann, Woburn, MA.

Schulz, S.C., Thompson, P.A., Jacobs, M. *et al.* (1999) Lithium augmentation fails to reduce symptoms in poorly responsive schizophrenic outpatients. *Journal of Clinical Psychiatry* 60, 366–372.

Sedvall, G.C. & Karlsson, P. (1999) Pharmacological manipulation of D$_1$-dopamine receptor function in schizophrenia. *Neuropsychopharmacology* 22, S181–S188.

Seeman, P., Guan, H.C. & Van Tol, H.H. (1993) Dopamine D$_4$ receptors elevated in schizophrenia. *Nature* 365, 441–445.

Semba, J., Watanabe, A., Kito, S. *et al.* (1995) Behavioural and neurochemical effects of OPC-14957, a novel antipsychotic drug, on dopaminergic mechanisms in rat brain. *Neuropharmacology* 34, 785–791.

Shannon, H.E. Bymaster, F.P., Calligaro, D.O. *et al.* (1994) Xanomeline: a novel muscarinic receptor agonist with functional selectivity for Ml receptors. *Journal of Pharmacology and Experimental Therapeutics* 269, 271–281.

Shannon, H.E., Rasmussen, K., Bymaster, F.P. *et al.* (2000) Xanomeline, an M$_1$/M$_4$ preferring muscarinic cholinergic receptor agonist, pro-

duces antipsychotic-like activity in rats and mice. *Schizophrenia Research* 42, 249–259.

Sharif, Z.A. (1998) Common treatment goals of antipsychotics: acute treatment. *Journal of Clinical Psychiatry* 59 (Supp. 19), 5–8.

Sharp, J.W., Petersen, D.L. & Langford, M.T. (1995) DNQX inhibits phencyclidine (PCP) and ketamine induction of the hsp 70 heat shock gene in the rat cingulate and retrosplenial cortex. *Brain Research* 687, 114–124.

Sheitman, B.B., Lee, H., Strauss, R. *et al.* (1997) The evaluation and treatment of first-episode psychosis. *Schizophrenia Bulletin* 23, 653–661.

Silver, H. & Nassar, A. (1992) Fluvoxamine improves negative symptoms in treated chronic schizophrenia: an add-on double-blind, placebo-controlled study. *Biological Psychiatry* 31, 698–704.

Silver, H. & Shmugliakov, N. (1998) Augmentation with fluvoxamine but not maprotiline improves negative symptoms in treated schizophrenia: evidence for a specific serotonergic effect from a double-blind study. *Journal of Clinical Psychopharmacology* 18, 208–211.

Silver, H., Barash, I., Aharon, N. *et al.* (2000) Fluvoxamine augmentation of antipsychotics improves negative symptoms in psychotic chronic schizophrenic patients: a placebo-controlled study. *International Clinical Psychopharmacology* 15, 257–261.

Simhandl, C. & Meszaros, K. (1992) The use of carbamazepine in the treatment of schizophrenic and schizoaffective psychoses: a review. *Journal of Psychiatry and Neuroscience* 17, 1–14.

Simpson, M.D., Lubman, D.I., Slater, P. *et al.* (1996) Autoradiography with [3H]8-OH-DPAt reveals increases in 5-HT$_{1A}$ receptors in ventral prefrontal cortex in schizophrenia. *Biological Psychiatry* 39, 919–928.

Siris, S.G. (1993) Adjunctive medication in the maintenance treatment of schizophrenia and its conceptual implications. *British Journal of Psychiatry* 2 (Suppl.), 66–78.

Siris, S.G., Morgan, V., Fagerstrom, R. *et al.* (1987) Adjunctive imipramine in the treatment of postpsychotic depression: a controlled trial. *Archives of General Psychiatry* 44, 533–539.

Siris, S.G., Bermanzohn, P.C., Gonzalez, A. *et al.* (1991) The use of antidepressants for negative symptoms in a subset of schizophrenic patients. *Psychopharmacology Bulletin* 27, 331–335.

Siris, S., Pollack, S., Bermanzohn, P. *et al.* (2000) Adjunctive imipramine for a broader group of post-psychotic depressions in schizophrenia. *Schizophrenia Research* 44, 187–192.

Skarsfeldt, T. (1995) Differential effects of repeated administration of novel antipsychotic drugs on the activity of midbrain dopamine neurons in the rat. *European Journal of Pharmacology* 281, 289–294.

Small, J.G., Kellams, J.J., Milstein, V. *et al.* (1975) A placebo-controlled study of lithium combined with neuroleptics in chronic schizophrenic patients. *American Journal of Psychiatry* 132, 1315–1317.

Sorensen, S.M., Kehne, J.H., Fadayel, G.M. *et al.* (1993) Characterization of the 5-HT$_2$ receptor antagonist MDL 100907 as a putative atypical antipsychotic: behavioral, electrophysiological and neurochemical studies. *Journal of Pharmacology and Experimental Therapeutics* 266, 684–691.

Sramek, J.J., Eldon, M.A., Posvar, E. *et al.* (1998) Initial safety, tolerability pharmacodynamics, and pharmacokinetics of CI-1007 in patients with schizophrenia. *Psychopharmacology Bulletin* 34, 93–99.

Stahl, S.M. (1999) Selecting an atypical antipsychotic by combining clinical experience with guidelines from clinical trials. *Journal of Clinical Psychiatry* 60, 31–41.

Strauss, M.E., Reynolds, K.S., Jayaram, G. *et al.* (1990) Effects of anticholinergic medication on memory in schizophrenia. *Schizophrenia Research* 3, 127–129.

Svensson, T.H., Tung, C.S. & Grenhoff, J. (1989) The 5-HT$_2$ antagonist ritanserin blocks the effect of prefrontal cortex inactivation on rat

A10 dopamine neurons *in vivo*. *Acta Physiologica Scandinavica* **136**, 497–498.

Svensson, T.H., Mathe, J.M., Andersson, J.L. *et al.* (1995) Mode of action of atypical neuroleptics in relation to the phencyclidine model of schizophrenia: role of 5-HT$_2$ receptor and alpha 1-adrenoceptor antagonism. *Journal of Clinical Psychopharmacology* **15**, 11S–18S.

Swift, R.H., Harrigan, E.P. & Van Kammen, D.P. (1999) A comparison of intramuscular ziprasidone with im haloperidol. *Schizophrenia Research* **36**, 298.

Tandon, R. & Greden, J.F. (1989) Cholinergic hyperactivity and negative schizophrenic symptoms. A model of cholinergic/dopaminergic interactions in schizophrenia. *Archives of General Psychiatry* **46**, 745–753.

Tandon, R., Greden, J.F. & Silk, K.R. (1988) Treatment of negative schizophrenic symptoms with trihexyphenidyl. *Journal of Clinical Psychopharmacology* **8**, 212–215.

Tandon, R., Mann, N.A., Eisner, W.H. *et al.* (1990) Effect of anticholinergic medication on positive and negative symptoms in medication-free schizophrenic patients. *Psychiatry Research* **31**, 235–241.

Terao, T., Oga, T., Nozaki, S. *et al.* (1995) Lithium addition to neuroleptic treatment in chronic schizophrenia: a randomized, double-blind, placebo-controlled, cross-over study. *Acta Psychiatrica Scandinavica* **92**, 220–224.

Thomas, H., Jr., Schwartz, E. & Petrilli, R. (1992) Droperidol versus haloperidol for chemical restraint of agitated and combative patients. *Annals of Emergency Medicine* **21**, 407–413.

Thompson, C. (1994) The use of high-dose antipsychotic medication. *British Journal of Psychiatry* **164**, 448–458.

Tollefson, G.D. & Sanger, T.M. (1997) Negative symptoms: a path analytic approach to a double-blind, placebo- and haloperidol-controlled clinical trial with olanzapine. *American Journal of Psychiatry* **154**, 466–474.

Tollefson, G.D., Beasley, C.M.J., Tran, P.V. *et al.* (1997) Olanzapine versus haloperidol in the treatment of schizophrenia and schizoaffective and schizophreniform disorders: results of an international collaborative trial. *American Journal of Psychiatry* **154**, 457–465.

Tollefson, G.D., Sanger, T.M., Lu, Y. *et al.* (1998) Depressive signs and symptoms in schizophrenia: a prospective blinded trial of olanzapine and haloperidol. *Archives of General Psychiatry* **55**, 250–258.

Toru, M., Miura, S. & Kudo, Y. (1994) Clinical experiences of OPC-14597, a dopamine autoreceptor agonist in schizophrenic patients. *Neuropsychopharmacology* **10**, 122S.

Tran, P.V., Hamilton, S.H., Kuntz, A.J. *et al.* (1997) Double-blind comparison of olanzapine versus risperidone in the treatment of schizophrenia and other psychotic disorders. *Journal of Clinical Psychopharmacology* **17**, 407–418.

Tsai, G., Yang, P., Chung, L.C. *et al.* (1998) D-Serine added to antipsychotics for the treatment of schizophrenia. *Biological Psychiatry* **44**, 1081–1089.

Tsai, G.E., Yang, P., Chung, L.C. *et al.* (1999) D-Serine added to clozapine for the treatment of schizophrenia. *American Journal of Psychiatry* **156**, 1822–1825.

Ugedo, L., Grenhoff, J. & Svensson, T.H. (1989) Ritanserin, a 5-HT$_2$ receptor antagonist, activates midbrain dopamine neurons by blocking serotonergic inhibition. *Psychopharmacology (Berl)* **98**, 45–50.

Uhlen, S., Muceniece, R., Rangel, N. *et al.* (1995) Comparison of the binding activities of some drugs on alpha 2A, alpha 2B and alpha 2C-adrenoceptors and non-adrenergic imidazoline sites in the guinea pig. *Pharmacology and Toxicology* **76**, 353–364.

van Berckel, B.N., Hijman, R., van der Linden, J.A. *et al.* (1996) Efficacy and tolerance of D-cycloserine in drug-free schizophrenic patients. *Biological Psychiatry* **40**, 1298–1300.

Van Kammen, D.P. & Boronow, J.J. (1988) Dextro-amphetamine diminishes negative symptoms in schizophrenia. *International Clinical Psychopharmacology* **3**, 111–121.

Van Putten, T. & Marder, S.R. (1987) Behavioral toxicity of antipsychotic drugs. *Journal of Clinical Psychiatry* **48** (Suppl.), 13–19.

Van Putten, T., May, P.R. & Marder, S.R. (1984) Response to antipsychotic medication: the doctor's and the consumer's view. *American Journal of Psychiatry* **141**, 16–19.

Van Putten, T., Marder, S.R. & Mintz, J. (1990) A controlled dose comparison of haloperidol in newly admitted schizophrenic patients. *Archives of General Psychiatry* **47**, 754–758.

Van Tol, H.H., Bunzow, J.R., Guan, H.C. *et al.* (1991) Cloning of the gene for a human dopamine D$_4$ receptor with high affinity for the antipsychotic clozapine. *Nature* **350**, 610–614.

Varty, G.B., Bakshi, V.P. & Geyer, M.A. (1999) M100907, a serotonin 5-HT$_{2A}$ receptor antagonist and putative antipsychotic, blocks dizocilpine-induced prepulse inhibition deficits in Sprague-Dawley and Wistar rats. *Neuropsychopharmacology* **20**, 311–321.

Volavka, J., Cooper, T., Czobor, P. *et al.* (1992) Haloperidol blood levels and clinical effects. *Archives of General Psychiatry* **49**, 354–361.

Volavka, J., Czobor, P, Sheitman, B. *et al.* (1999) Clozapine, olanzapine, risperidone, and haloperidol in treatment-resistant patients with schizophrenia and schizoaffective disorder. In 38th ACNP Annual Meeting Acapulco, Mexico.

Waddington, J. & Casey, D. (2000) Comparative pharmacology of classical and novel (second-generation) antipsychotics. In: *Schizophrenia and Mood Disorders: the New Drug Therapies in Clinical Practice* (eds P.F. Buckley, & J.L. Waddington), pp. 3–13. Butterworth-Heinemann, Woburn, MA.

Waddington, J.L., Youssef, H.A. & Kinsella, A. (1990) Cognitive dysfunction in schizophrenia followed up over 5 years, and its longitudinal relationship to the emergence of tardive dyskinesia. *Psychological Medicine* **20**, 835–842.

Wahlbeck, K., Cheine, M.V., Gilbody, S. *et al.* (2000) Efficacy of beta-blocker supplementation for schizophrenia: a systematic review of randomized trials. *Schizophrenia Research* **41**, 341–347.

Wang, R.Y. & Liang, X. (1998) M100907 and clozapine, but not haloperidol or raclopride, prevent phencyclidine-induced blockade of NMDA responses in pyramidal neurons of the rat medial prefrontal cortical slice. *Neuropsychopharmacology* **19**, 74–85.

Wassef, A.A., Dott, S.G., Harris, A. *et al.* (1999) Critical review of GABA-ergic drugs in the treatment of schizophrenia. *Journal of Clinical Psychopharmacology* **19**, 222–232.

Wassef, A.A., Dott, S.G., Harris, A. *et al.* (2000) Randomized, placebo-controlled pilot study of divalproex sodium in the treatment of acute exacerbations of chronic schizophrenia. *Journal of Clinical Psychopharmacology* **20**, 357–361.

Wetzel, H., Grunder, G., Hillert, A. *et al.* (1998) Amisulpride versus flupentixol in schizophrenia with predominantly positive symptomatology: a double-blind controlled study comparing a selective D$_2$-like antagonist to a mixed D$_1$/D$_2$-like antagonist. The Amisulpride Study Group. *Psychopharmacology (Berl)* **137**, 223–232.

White, K.E. & Cummings, J.L. (1996) Schizophrenia and Alzheimer's disease: clinical and pathophysiologic analogies. *Comprehensive Psychiatry* **37**, 188–195.

Wicke, K.M. & Gross, G. (2000) The potential antipsychotic BSF 190555 shows 5-HT$_{1A}$ agonism in two rat in vivo models. *Society for Neuroscience Abstracts* **26**, 276.

Wiersma, D., Nienhuis, F.J., Slooff, C.J. *et al.* (1998) Natural course of schizophrenic disorders: a 15-year followup of a Dutch incidence cohort. *Schizophrenia Bulletin* **24**, 75–85.

Williams, G.V. & Goldman-Rakic, P.S. (1995) Modulation of memory fields by dopamine D_1 receptors in prefrontal cortex. *Nature* **376**, 572–575.

Williams, R. (2001) Optimal dosing with risperidone: updated recommendations. *Journal of Clinical Psychiatry* **62**, 282–289.

Willins, D.L., Narayanan, S., Wallace, L.J. *et al.* (1993) The role of dopamine and AMPA/kainate receptors in the nucleus accumbens in the hypermotility response to MK801. *Pharmacology, Biochemistry and Behavior* **46**, 881–887.

Willins, D.L., Berry, S.A., Alsayegh, L. *et al.* (1999) Clozapine and other 5-hydroxytryptamine-$_{2A}$ receptor antagonists alter the subcellular distribution of 5-hydroxytryptamine-2A receptors *in vitro* and *in vivo*. *Neuroscience* **91**, 599–606.

Wilson, W.H. (1993) Addition of lithium to haloperidol in non-affective, antipsychotic non-responsive schizophrenia: a double blind, placebo controlled, parallel design clinical trial. *Psychopharmacology (Berl)* **111**, 359–366.

Wirshing, D.A., Spellberg, B.J., Erhart, S.M. *et al.* (1998) Novel antipsychotics and new onset diabetes. *Biological Psychiatry* **44**, 778–783.

Wirshing, D.A., Wirshing, W.C., Kysar, L. *et al.* (1999) Novel antipsychotics: comparison of weight gain liabilities. *Journal of Clinical Psychiatry* **60**, 358–363.

Woerner, M.G., Alvir, J.M., Saltz, B.L. *et al.* (1998) Prospective study of tardive dyskinesia in the elderly: rates and risk factors. *American Journal of Psychiatry* **155**, 1521–1528.

Wolkin, A., Angrist, B., Wolf, A. *et al.* (1987) Effects of amphetamine on local cerebral metabolism in normal and schizophrenic subjects as determined by positron emission tomography. *Psychopharmacology (Berl)* **92**, 241–246.

Wolkowitz, O.M. & Pickar, D. (1991) Benzodiazepines in the treatment of schizophrenia: a review and reappraisal. *American Journal of Psychiatry* **148**, 714–726.

Wolkowitz, O.M., Breier, A., Doran, A. *et al.* (1988) Alprazolam augmentation of the antipsychotic effects of fluphenazine in schizophrenic patients: preliminary results. *Archives of General Psychiatry* **45**, 664–671.

Wolkowitz, O.M., Turetsky, N., Reus, V.I. *et al.* (1992) Benzodiazepine augmentation of neuroleptics in treatment-resistant schizophrenia. *Psychopharmacology Bulletin* **28**, 291–295.

Wolosker, H., Sheth, K.N., Takahashi, M. *et al.* (1999) Purification of serine racemase: biosynthesis of the neuromodulator D-serine. *Proceedings of the National Academy of Sciences of the USA* **96**, 721–725.

Wright, J.L., Caprathe, B.W., Downing, D.M. *et al.* (1994) The discovery and structure–activity relationships of 1,2,3,6-tetrahydro-4-phenyl-1-[(arylcyclohexenyl)alkyl]pyridines: dopamine autoreceptor agonists and potential antipsychotic agents. *Journal of Medicinal Chemistry* **37**, 3523–3533.

Wright, P., Birkett, M., David, S.R. *et al.* (2001) Double-blind, placebo-controlled comparison of intramuscular olanzapine and intramuscular haloperidol in the treatment of acute agitation in schizophrenia. *American Journal of Psychiatry* **158**, 1149–1151.

Wyant, M., Diamond, B.I., O'Neal, E. *et al.* (1990) The use of midazolam in acutely agitated psychiatric patients. *Psychopharmacology Bulletin* **26**, 126–129.

Wyatt, R.J. (1991) Neuroleptics and the natural course of schizophrenia. *Schizophrenia Bulletin* **17**, 325–351.

Wyatt, R.J. (1995) Early intervention for schizophrenia: can the course of the illness be altered? *Biological Psychiatry* **38**, 1–3.

Yerevanian, B.I. & Hodgman, C.H. (1985) A haloperidol–carbamazepine interaction in a patient with rapid-cycling bipolar disorder. *American Journal of Psychiatry* **142**, 785–786.

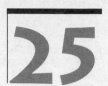

Maintenance treatment

S.R. Marder and D.A. Wirshing

Introduction, 474
Phases of treatment, 474
Relapse in schizophrenia, 474
   Factors affecting relapse, 474
   Impact of psychotic relapse, 476
Effectiveness of long-term maintenance
   pharmacotherapy, 476
Treatment adherence in schizophrenia, 476
   Treatment adherence and relapse, 476
   Strategies for improving adherence, 477
Duration of maintenance treatment: first episode and
   multiepisode patients, 477
Drug selection for maintenance treatment, 475
   Depot vs. oral drugs, 477
   Prescribing long-acting depot antipsychotics, 478
   Newer vs. older drugs, 479

Maintenance therapy strategies, 479
   Dose reduction strategies, 479
   Monitoring of prodromal symptoms, 480
Effects of maintenance medication on functional
   outcome, 481
Management of comorbid conditions during
   maintenance, 481
   Negative symptoms, 481
   Neurocognitive symptoms, 482
   Depression, 482
   Unstable mood, 483
   Anxiety, 483
   Substance abuse, 484
Interactions of pharmacological and psychosocial
   treatments during maintenance, 484
References, 485

Introduction

The separation of treatment into acute and maintenance phases is instructive for developing principles of treatment. However, in the real world of patient care, individuals may not fit comfortably in either category. Some patients have illnesses that are partially refractory to medications and, as a result, never adequately recover from psychosis. Others appear to be in a state of remission, but these individuals cannot be considered stable because they relapse abruptly when they are stressed. Patients who have recovered from psychotic symptoms, but have symptoms in other dimensions, including depression, anxiety, negative symptoms and substance abuse, may be inadequately managed if they are considered stable (Emsley *et al.* 1999).

Phases of treatment

A number of approaches have been taken to define clinical states in schizophrenia. The American Psychiatric Association Treatment Guidelines for Schizophrenia (American Psychiatric Association 1997) proposes three stages. The *acute phase* – described in prior chapters – begins when patients experience a psychotic episode and ends when psychotic symptoms remit. As these symptoms remit, patients enter a stage where they improve, but are more vulnerable to relapse under certain circumstances such as environmental stress or a change in pharmacological treatment. This stage is the *stabilization phase* and may last for several months until patients enter the *stable phase*. This is the phase that is usually associated with maintenance treatment. Other researchers have defined greater numbers of clinical states which include information about multiple symptom dimensions

as well as illness severity (Revicki *et al.* 1996; Shumway *et al.* 1997).

A perspective on the frequency of these states can be gained from a study of a cohort of patients from the Netherlands who had broadly defined schizophrenia (Wiersma *et al.* 1998). Only 24.8% of the patients experienced complete remissions between episodes. The most common outcome was two or more episodes followed by a negative symptom syndrome. Seventeen per cent of patients had episodes followed by partial remissions with anxiety and depression. Eleven per cent of patients were chronically psychotic. In other words, individuals who are being treated during the maintenance phase of treatment are usually patients with chronic persistent psychopathology rather than those who have fully recovered from psychosis. Management requires the clinical team to minimize the risk of psychosis and to manage persisting psychopathology.

In this chapter we define *maintenance treatment* broadly and include patients who meet criteria for being stable as well as those who continue to have persistent symptoms. The focus will be on patients who have recovered from a psychotic episode and where the main focus is not on decreasing psychotic symptoms but on preventing another relapse and improving overall social adjustment and quality of life.

Relapse in schizophrenia

Factors affecting relapse

In developing a plan for relapse prevention it is important to understand the environmental and biological factors that influence psychotic relapse in schizophrenia. A number of models

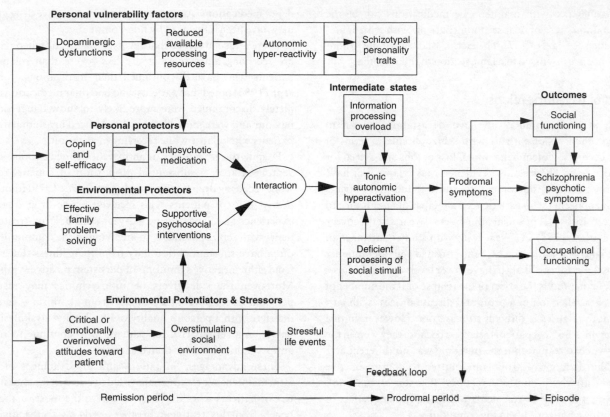

Fig 25.1 Framework for describing environmental and psychobiological factors that influence the course of schizophrenia.

have been proposed for explaining their interaction. Figure 25.1 displays one such model which includes both personal and environmental factors that can affect relapse and outcome (Nuechterlein *et al.* 1992). Either can be protective of the patient and thereby make relapse less likely, whereas others tend to promote psychotic relapse either by protecting against relapse or by a tendency to provoke a psychotic relapse. A number of these factors are particularly important and should be highlighted. Antipsychotic medications are personal protective factors for preventing relapse whereas illness-related factors such as dopaminergic dysfunctions are viewed as vulnerability factors. Environmental factors such as stressful life events can contribute to relapse while certain psychosocial interventions can be effective for relapse prevention. This model demonstrates that there are multiple factors that should be considered in developing a treatment plan that minimizes the risk of relapse.

A substantial amount of research supports parts of this model. A number of studies indicate that environmental stress can increase the risk of relapse (Vaillant 1964; Hirsch *et al.* 1996). This stress may be manifest in life events or levels of stress (Das *et al.* 1997) or in environments that are inherently stressful. Stressful family environments can be associated with a greater risk of psychotic relapse. Studies carried out in the 1970s (Wynne 1981) reported that disordered communication within a family can be stressful for individuals with schizophrenia. A larger body of work from the UK found that a family climate that was characterized by hostility and criticism – termed high

expressed emotion (EE) – was associated with higher rates of psychotic relapse (Vaughn & Leff 1976). In one of the original studies of EE in families, 76% of patients returning to a home characterized by high EE relapsed while only 28% relapsed from low EE families (Brown *et al.* 1972). The relationship between high EE and relapse has been replicated by a number of groups and has served as the target for family orientated interventions. The evidence that environmental factors influence the course of schizophrenia is reviewed in Chapters 31 and 12. It is important to note that these studies have been criticized by family members who view these studies as suggesting that families have responsibility when patients do poorly. More sophisticated studies (Hahlweg & Wiedemann 1999) indicate that the attitudes of relatives may be responses to patients' behaviours. The importance of these studies is that they suggest that individuals with schizophrenia are sensitive to stresses in their environments and may be particularly sensitive to hostility and criticism in their homes.

Substance abuse is a consistent predictor of relapse (LeDuc & Mittleman 1995; Ayuso-Gutiérrez and del Río Vega 1997). This is likely to result, in part, from the direct biological effects of the substances that are taken. Stimulant drugs, alcohol, cocaine and other drugs can provoke relapses in patients who are stable. In addition, patients who abuse substances are also likely to be those who are non-compliant with medications, those who are living in stressful urban environments and those who may be homeless.

Non-adherence with maintenance medications can be the most common cause of relapse among patients with schizophrenia (Weiden & Glazer 1997). The factors that contribute to non-compliance are discussed in a later section of this chapter.

Impact of psychotic relapse

Relapse in schizophrenia can have devastating short-term effects on the lives of patients with schizophrenia in terms of suicide attempts, violent behaviours, loss of jobs and a need for hospitalization. There is also evidence that relapse can have long-term effects on outcome. One study found that patients with schizophrenia who experienced a relapse did not return to their prerelapse level of social adjustment 1 year after recovery (Johnson *et al*. 1983). A 7-year follow-up study (Curson *et al*. 1985) found that patients who demonstrated a greater number of relapses were more likely to have lower levels of social adjustment. Whether this is the effect of the relapse or if the number of relapses is a reflection of a profound disease process with *pari passu* more relapses is difficult to tease out. However, in one study in which 66% of patients relapsed because they were in the group switched to placebo, the outcome was no different at 7 years than the control group randomized to continue active treatment of whom only 6% relapsed (Curson *et al*. 1986). Moreover, it is difficult to calculate the demoralizing effect of interrupting a patient's life in the community.

Effectiveness of long-term maintenance pharmacotherapy

This chapter refers to the newer or atypical antipsychotics as second-generation antipsychotics. The older agents will be referred to as the conventional agents. The reason for not using the term atypical is that the increasing use of these agents has made that term misleading.

A substantial literature indicates that conventional and – to a lesser extent – second-generation antipsychotic medications are effective for preventing relapse in stabilized patients with schizophrenia. The most definitive studies in this area consisted of double-blind comparisons of patients who continued to receive an antipsychotic and patients who were assigned to a placebo. Davis *et al*. (1989) reviewed studies that included 3720 patients and found that, within time periods of mostly 1 year or less, 55% relapsed on placebo whereas 21% relapsed on an antipsychotic. This difference was highly significant ($\chi^2 = 483$; d.f. = 1; $P < 10^{-10}$). Baldessarini *et al*. (1988) found similar results. Fifty-five per cent of patients relapsed on placebo and 14% on active antipsychotic. The body of work reviewed by these authors strongly supports the practice of continuing an antipsychotic even after patients have recovered from psychosis. Both reviews focused on studies conducted before second-generation antipsychotics were introduced. There are indications, discussed below, suggesting that relapse rates may be even lower on newer drugs. In addition, most of these studies did not utilize long-acting depot medications. As a result, relapse in the active drug groups may have been influenced by non-compliance.

There is also evidence that relapses that occur when patients are receiving antipsychotics are less severe than relapses in patients who have discontinued their medications. Johnson *et al*. (1983) noted that patients who had their medications completely discontinued were more likely to show dangerous behaviour and were more likely to be admitted involuntarily than patients who relapse while receiving medication.

Despite the advantages of antipsychotic medications in preventing relapse, a substantial proportion of patients relapse while receiving drug treatment. Hogarty *et al*. (1979) found that nearly 48% of patients who received active drug treatment experienced a relapse during a 2-year period. Drug-treated patients with schizophrenia who are living in the community will often have substantial disability from their illness that results from either negative symptoms or persistent positive symptoms. Moreover, the side-effects of antipsychotics may result in personal discomfort – particularly from akathisia – and may interfere with a person's quality of life. Tardive dyskinesia (see below) is a serious risk for patients who continue to receive antipsychotics for more than 6 months.

These advantages, limitations and disadvantages of long-term maintenance treatment have led to a search for characteristics of patients who are likely to derive the most or the least benefit from this treatment. In other words, are there individuals who can safely have their medications discontinued? Clinicians are often faced with patients who have been stable for years and who are asking to have their medications discontinued. It is tempting to give these individuals a trial without antipsychotics. However, controlled studies have found that these patients also have high relapse rates when their medications are discontinued (Hogarty *et al*. 1976). Kane (1987) reviewed six such studies and found that patients who bad been in remission for 1–5 years had a relapse rate of 75% over a 15-month period. Others have evaluated whether there are characteristics of individuals who do well without maintenance medications. Unfortunately, there are no reliable criteria for selecting patients who are good candidates for management without maintenance medications (Johnstone & Geddes 1994).

These observations – when taken together – indicate that there are no reliable predictors that can lead a clinician to discontinue medications safely. There may be individuals who have mild psychotic episodes that respond quickly to medications who are reasonable risks, but these patients are uncommon. As will be noted in a later section on prodromal symptoms, there are signs which indicate points in time when patients are at a greater risk of relapse.

Treatment adherence in schizophrenia

Treatment adherence and relapse

Treatment adherence can refer to adherence to taking prescribed medications, participating in psychosocial treatments or making appointments with the treatment team. Medication adherence has received the most thorough study. As many as 30% – and perhaps an even higher proportion of patients with schizophrenia – have serious problems with medication compliance (Kane 1985). Weiden and Glazer (1997) studied patients who were frequently readmitted to an inpatient unit in New York. Non-compliance with medication regimen was the most common reason for rehospitalization followed by non-response to medications. Relatively little has been published about adherence to treatments other than medication.

It is probably inaccurate to categorize patients as simply adherent or non-adherent to medication; rather, there is a continuum from outright drug refusal to partial adherence with a physician's recommendations. It is also likely that clinicians underestimate the amount of treatment non-adherence. One study found that occasional patients develop methods to avoid ingesting their medications, even in a hospital setting (Van Putten et al. 1990). Others may become less reliable pill-takers over time, resulting in falling blood levels and decreased protection against relapse.

Non-adherence is related to a number of factors. Patients who experience medication side-effects are more likely to fail to comply with their medication regimen. Van Putten (1974) found that patients who experienced side-effects were less likely to take their medications as prescribed. Although all forms of extrapyramidal side-effects (EPSs) were related to poor compliance, akathisia was particularly prominent. Severe psychopathology, substance abuse and a poor relationship with one's treating clinician can be factors which impair adherence (Fenton et al. 1997). Others have pointed out that patients who are more thought disordered (Irwin et al. 1985) are more likely to be non-compliant. This relationship to thought disorder is troubling because it suggests that the most severely impaired patients may be among the most vulnerable to not taking their medication.

Strategies for improving adherence

Managing treatment adherence is an important part of maintenance therapy treatment plans. A number of strategies have been developed to improve adherence in outpatients with schizophrenia. Regarding medication adherence. Blackwell (1973) has suggested that clinicians regularly monitor compliance in patients. He recommends that this be carried out in a manner that is unlikely to induce a defensive response. For example, the clinician can enquire as to how difficult it is for the patient to remember to take medications on a regular basis. This query can lead to a useful dialogue regarding compliance.

Special programmes have been developed for improving treatment adherence in clinical settings. Having patients communicate with their outpatient treatment team prior to discharge can improve attendence at outpatient appointments as well as clinical outcome (Olfson et al. 1998). Psychoeducational programmes for patients can also improve treatment

adherence (Hornung et al. 1998). A recent study by Herz et al. (2000) found that patients who received a treatment programme that included psychoeducation, family treatment and monitoring of prodromal symptoms decreased relapse rates. Other studies have found that social skills training that directly focuses on issues of treatment adherence can be effective (Smith et al. 1997).

If side-effects are the cause of treatment adherence in some individuals, then treating patients with a newer antipsychotic or treating side-effects more aggressively is likely to be helpful. In addition, there is some evidence that newer agents are more effective for managing the cognitive disturbances and the resultant lack of illness awareness that contributes to non-adherence (Marder 1998). Although these advantages of newer drugs suggest that they may improve compliance, this has not been demonstrated in well-controlled studies.

Duration of maintenance treatment: first episode and multiepisode patients

The management of patients who are recovering from their first episode of schizophrenia can be particularly difficult. Many of these patients – along with their families – want to believe that the first episode is not the beginning of a chronic illness. These patients often resist the notion that they maintain a vulnerability to subsequent psychotic episodes and, as a result, many will pressure to have their medications discontinued as soon as possible. These younger patients are more likely to return to work or school. As a result, many perceive medications as slowing them down or interfering with their community life. However, the pressure to withdraw medications should be balanced against the reality that 40–60% of these individuals will suffer a psychotic relapse in a year if their medications are discontinued (Kane et al. 1982; Crow et al. 1986).

These issues were addressed by a group who developed consensus guidelines for the duration of long-term maintenance therapy for relapse prevention (Kissling et al. 1991). The guidelines recommend that first episode patients receive 1–2 years of antipsychotic maintenance and that patients who have had multiple episodes receive at least 5 years of maintenance. Patients with severe or dangerous episodes should probably receive antipsychotics for an indefinite period of time.

Drug selection for maintenance treatment

Depot vs. oral drugs

Antipsychotics can be administered in long-acting injectable forms. The most common form is the decanoate ester. The drug is administered intramuscularly as a decanoate ester in an oily vehicle such as sesame oil. The drug gradually diffuses from the oily vehicle into the surrounding tissues. The rate limiting step appears to be the rate of diffusion because once the drug enters the tissue it is rapidly hydrolysed and the parent compound is released (Marder *et al.* 1989). When injections are administered at intervals of every 2–6 weeks – depending on the pharmacological characteristics of the compound – patients maintain a relatively stable plasma concentration. Also, because the maximum plasma concentration peak is lower than the peak with oral compounds, side-effects may be milder. This potential side-effect advantage for long-acting agents has not been clearly demonstrated in controlled studies. In addition, depot drugs may have earned a reputation for causing a higher incidence of side-effects because they have frequently been prescribed at relatively high doses. Nevertheless, it is reasonable to expect that the relatively low doses of depot drugs that are frequently effective will result in very low rates of side-effects. This low rate of side-effects was recently demonstrated in a multicentre study by Kane *et al.* (2002) who found that patients treated with doses of haloperidol decanoate as high as 200 mg/month had strikingly low rates of EPSs.

Clinicians in the USA have only two long-acting depots available: fluphenazine, which is available as an enanthate or a decanoate, and haloperidol decanoate. Other agents including flupentixol decanoate, perphenazine decanoate and enanthate, zuclopentixol decanoate, fluspirilene decanoate and bromperidol decanoate are available in Canada and many European countries. Zuclopentixol acetate is an intermediate agent that maintains plasma levels for 72 h. At this time none of the second-generation (or atypical) antipsychotics are available as long-acting agents although formulations of some of these agents have been developed and are under investigation.

Long-acting depot are nearly always prescribed during the maintenance phase of treatment. They are a reasonable therapeutic choice for patients who fail to comply with taking their medications and for those who have difficulty remembering to take their pills. A number of both controlled and uncontrolled studies have compared the rates of relapse on depot and oral antipsychotics. The uncontrolled studies have shown substantial advantages for depots (Karson *et al.* 1982). The results have been less clear in well-designed double-blind studies. This is probably because patients who enter well-controlled studies tend to be compliant and co-operative. In addition, the additional resources available in research settings may improve the treatment adherence and the outcomes for patients who receive oral drugs. Nevertheless, Davis *et al.* (1989) reviewed six well-controlled studies comparing oral and depot medication and found that relapse rates were significantly lower in the depot-treated patients. In contrast, a Cochrane Collaboration review looked at each of the comparisons and concluded that the advantage of depot over oral drugs had not been proven (Adams & Eisenbruch 2000). However, in our opinion, the Cochrane review was overly conservative and did not adequately weigh the studies by their quality. Perhaps the best comparison was a double-blind multisite study which compared oral fluphenazine and fluphenazine decanoate (FD) for 2 years (Hogarty *et al.* 1979). Patients who received FD demonstrated a lower risk of relapse than those assigned to oral fluphenazine. Moreover, the best outcomes were found for patients who received FD supple-

mented by a form of social therapy. These results – when taken together – suggest that depot antipsychotics probably have advantages over oral drugs for patients who are reasonably reliable as well as for patients who have a history of poor medication compliance.

Despite the advantages of depot compounds, there is a reluctance of many psychiatrists to prescribe them and by many patients to take them. This is less of a problem in many settings in Europe – particularly the UK – where long-acting antipsychotics are prescribed far more often than they are in the USA. Some of the reluctance to prescribe newer agents is based on very understandable factors. Many patients dislike injections and clinicians in many settings find themselves poorly equipped for administering shots. Another explanation for the low utilization of depots in the USA and other countries is that these agents have been commonly prescribed at excessive doses leading to high rates of EPSs. As a result, many patients are reluctant to take these agents. It will be interesting to learn how this reluctance may be changed by the introduction of long-acting forms of risperidone and olanzapine as well as other agents.

Prescribing long-acting depot antipsychotics

There are important differences in the pharmacokinetics of long-acting compounds which should guide how they are prescribed (Marder *et al.* 1989). Short-acting oral or intramuscular compounds usually reach a peak plasma concentration relatively rapidly. This is followed by a slower excretion. The kinetics of these agents is determined by their elimination half-lives. In contrast, long-acting drugs are absorbed continually during the interval between injections. The kinetics of long-acting injectable antipsychotics are determined by their absorption from multiple injection sites. As a result, it takes long-acting compounds much longer to reach steady state and they are eliminated much more slowly. Whereas most oral antipsychotics reach a stable steady state within about 5 days, long-acting agents may require as much as 3 or even 6 months to reach steady state. For example, the decanoate forms of haloperidol and fluphenazine require about 3 months to reach steady state, and substantial plasma concentrations can be detected months after therapy has been discontinued. As a result, long-acting drugs are poorly suited for acute treatment because the clinician needs to wait months for the patient to reach steady state. Moreover, if the dose is too high, it may take months for the plasma concentration to reach a well-tolerated level.

Another important difference between oral and depot compounds is that depots, because they are administered intramuscularly, are much more bioavailable. Orally administered drugs undergo extensive first-pass metabolism in liver and gut. As a result, the amount of circulating active drug may be substantially reduced. Drugs that are administered intramuscularly or intravenously are much more bioavailable because they do not undergo first-pass metabolism. This is important in converting patients from oral to depot drugs. If a clinician attempts to convert a patient using a formula for converting oral to depot drugs, he or she may find that a patient who was an extensive metabolizer of their antipsychotic required much more drug to reach an adequate dosage. When this patient is converted to a depot drug, first-pass metabolism will no longer be relevant and the direct conversion may lead to an excessive depot dose.

These observations suggest some important principles for conversion from depot to oral compounds. The first principle is that patients should be started on a modest dose of the depot compound, even if they did well on a high oral dose. This recommendation is based on the greater bioavailability of depot compounds. For example, fluphenazine decanoate 12.5 mg every 2 weeks or haloperidol decanoate 100 mg every 2 weeks are reasonable choices for many patients. Another important principle is that patients should gradually be changed from oral to depot drugs. Because it takes 3 or more months to reach a stable steady state on depots, patients should be maintained on their oral medications until they reach an adequate plasma level of depot. For example, if a patient is receiving oral haloperidol 10 mg/day, it is reasonable to start with haloperidol decanoate 100 mg every 2 weeks and to gradually decrease the oral dose over the next 3 months. The patient could eventually be converted to 100–200 mg every 4 weeks.

Newer vs. older drugs

Nearly all of the well-controlled studies of relapse prevention assigned patients to conventional antipsychotics. There are a number of reasons to believe that outcomes with newer antipsychotics may be better than outcomes with older agents. The newer agents have side-effect profiles that are usually more acceptable to patients and may lead to better compliance. In addition, the lower liability for causing EPSs could lead clinicians to prescribe optimal doses of these agents. In contrast, conventional antipsychotics can cause EPSs at doses that are very close to the optimal clinical dose. As a result, clinicians are often forced to reduce the maintenance dose to a level that is considerably lower than the dose that is effective for acute treatment.

A number of studies support the advantages of newer agents for long-term treatment. A study in the state hospitals in Connecticut compared treatment-refractory patients who were assigned to clozapine with individuals who were maintained on their usual antipsychotics (Essock et al. 2000). Although clozapine did not result in a greater likelihood of hospital discharge, patients taking clozapine had a higher likelihood of remaining in days in the community following discharge. In the year following hospital discharge, 83% of patients taking clozapine remained in the community compared to 59% of patients receiving conventional drugs. Clozapine patients also accrued more days in the community (average 330) than patients on conventional drugs (average 263 days; $P < 0.05$). A recent VA Cooperative Study compared haloperidol and clozapine in treatment-refractory patients (Rosenheck et al. 1997). This study was not designed as a relapse prevention trial, but rather as a comparison of the two agents in individuals who were poor responders to conventional therapy. An analysis of patients who completed the trial is somewhat informative about the usefulness of the two drugs in patients living in the community. Clozapine-treated patients had fewer mean days of hospitalization (143.8 days) than haloperidol-treated patients (168.1 days; $P = 0.03$), suggesting an advantage of clozapine in preventing relapse. Although these studies focused on chronically psychotic rather than well-stabilized patients, they suggest an advantage for clozapine.

Other data suggest that risperidone and olanzapine also reduce relapse rates compared to older agents. Conley et al. (1999) calculated the rehospitalization rates of all patients who were discharged from the Maryland State Hospital System on clozapine or risperidone. (Because many patients who have relapses can be managed without rehospitalization, rates of rehospitalization tend to be considerably lower than relapse rates.) At 2 years, 87% of the patients receiving clozapine and 66% of the patients receiving risperidone did not require rehospitalization, suggesting that both agents were preferable to older drugs. Tran et al. (1998) combined data from three double-blind extensions of acute studies comparing olanzapine and haloperidol. The estimated 1-year risk of relapse was 19.7% with olanzapine and 28% with haloperidol. These results cannot be directly compared with data from relapse prevention studies because both studies monitored patients who were already perceived as being responders to their medication regimen.

These findings suggest that the newer antipsychotics may have advantages during maintenance therapy in that they are associated with a reduced risk of psychotic relapse. Unfortunately, there are no studies comparing newer agents with long-acting depot drugs. This is important because these later agents – described in an earlier section – have been associated with a substantially reduced risk of relapse when compared with orally administered conventional drugs.

Maintenance therapy strategies

Dose reduction strategies

Making decisions about the optimal drug dosage during the maintenance phase of treatment can be particularly difficult because the patient is usually clinically stable. As a result, drug dosage cannot be titrated against clinical response. If the dosage is too low, this may not be apparent until the patient relapses. If the dosage is higher than necessary, the patient may be exposed to unnecessary side-effects. In addition, there are data suggesting that higher doses may expose patients to a greater risk of developing tardive dyskinesia. For these reasons, strategies have been proposed for decreasing the maintenance dosage of antipsychotics. These strategies are usually reserved for patients who have been reasonably stable for periods of 6 months or more.

One strategy proposes treating patients with much lower doses of a conventional antipsychotic than are usually prescribed. Studies by three groups (Marder et al. 1987; Hogarty et al. 1988; Kane 1995) indicate that a substantial number (but by no means all) of 'maintenance' patients do well on doses of fluphenazine decanoate that are only 20% of the usual doses. These doses were in the range of 5–10 mg of fluphenazine decanoate every 14 days. Much lower doses in the range of 1.25–2 mg were associated with substantially higher relapse rates. Although the Marder and Hogarty studies reported a greater risk of mild psychotic exacerbations with doses in the 20% range, these episodes were usually rather mild and were seldom associated with a need for rehospitalization. These minor exacerbations were usually easily controlled by a small dosage adjustment. In addition, patients receiving the lower dose had fewer side-effects and in the Marder study complained less of anxiety and depression and had a lower drop-out rate. Kane (1995) reported that patients on lower doses also had lower dyskinesia ratings, suggesting that the low-dose strategy may reduce vulnerability to tardive dyskinesia. These findings suggest that there are likely to be benefits associated with the use of the lowest effective dose of maintenance neuroleptic.

Dosage reduction strategies have not been studied with newer agents. This is in part because these strategies were largely based on concerns about EPSs. As second-generation compounds cause fewer EPSs, these are less of a concern. As a result, patients will tolerate similar doses of the newer agents to those used for acute treatment. Moreover, at the optimal dosage for relapse prevention, patients will not need to endure the discomforting effects of EPSs. It is unclear if dosage reduction is important for maintenance treatment with these agents. Because newer agents have side-effects such as sedation, hypotension and weight gain, it is possible that some dosage reduction during maintenance may be helpful.

Another dosage reduction strategy, targeted treatment, is discussed below in the section on prodromal symptoms.

Monitoring of prodromal symptoms

Individuals with schizophrenia seldom relapse abruptly. Rather, there is commonly a period during which patients move from their stable state to a more psychotic state. It is reasonable to assume that intervening early in this process could prevent a full relapse or decrease the severity of a relapse. Observational studies found that patients appeared to move gradually from one state to another as they lost touch with reality. Retrospective studies found that patients and family members could frequently identify a period of several weeks prior to psychotic relapse during which patients demonstrated symptoms such as sleep loss, difficulty concentrating, feeling overwhelmed and demonstrating mood symptoms (Herz & Melville 1980; Herz et al. 1982). In these studies, patients frequently had dysphoric symptoms and mild psychotic symptoms before more severe psychosis emerged.

If prodromal symptoms are likely to be useful for triggering an intervention, it is important that they be identifiable in clinical situations. One study (Marder et al. 1994) found that only 45% of patients demonstrated prodromal episodes. This indicates that this form of early identification of episodes is only effective

in some patients. Moreover, fewer than half of prodromal episodes were followed by a psychotic relapse. This suggests that prodromal episodes are not a completely reliable indicator of relapse risk. Nevertheless, even if prodromal states do not invariably lead to relapse, they may still interfere with a patient's adjustment and may be reasonable targets for intervention.

A study by Herz et al. (2000) examined the effectiveness of a strategy that focused on early intervention when patients developed prodromal symptoms. Patients were randomly assigned to a strategy that focused on either treatment as usual or a special programme that included monitoring for prodromal symptoms and intervention – usually with additional antipsychotic medications – when they occurred. Patients in the experimental group also received psychoeducation that stressed early warning signs of relapse. The results indicated that the strategy for monitoring prodromal symptoms was effective in reducing both relapse and rehospitalization rates.

In another study (Marder et al. 1994), patients were treated with low doses of fluphenazine decanoate and monitored for prodromal symptoms. When prodromal symptoms were identified, oral fluphenazine or placebo was prescribed until the episode was adequately treated or the patients met criteria for a psychotic relapse. The decision to use oral supplementation was because oral medications increase plasma levels much more rapidly than depot formulations. The results of the study indicated that there was no difference between the active supplementation group and the placebo group during the first year. However, in the second year patients who received active supplementation spent a significantly lower proportion of time in an exacerbated state. This suggests that patients and their clinicians improve over time in their abilities to detect and manage prodromes. That is, both improved as they gain experience differentiating unimportant flucations in symptoms from important signs of impending relapse. In addition, the study supports the practice of monitoring patients for prodromal symptoms when patients are receiving depot compounds and intervening with additional oral medication when there is evidence of impending relapse.

Early intervention is also an important component of a proposed strategy for dosage reduction in patients in maintenance treatment. A number of investigators (Herz et al. 1982; Pietzcker 1985; Carpenter et al. 1987; Jolley et al. 1989) have studied targeted or intermittent therapy. Patients who are stable have their drug dosage gradually decreased until medications are completely discontinued. They are then followed very closely until there are signs that the individual is beginning to relapse. At the earliest sign of a recurrence, drugs are reinstituted. To make this strategy work, patients and their families are trained to detect prodromal signs. These studies differ from the prior studies of prodromes in that patients are drug-free. In the previously mentioned Marder and Herz studies, patients were receiving antipsychotics which were supplemented during prodromes.

All of the studies of intermittent treatment found that targeted treatment resulted in substantially higher relapses than in controls who received continuous treatment. Schooler (1991) reviewed these four studies and found that the 1-year relapse rate (using a sample-sized weighted mean) with continuous treatment was 17% compared to 37% with targeted treatment. Two-year rates were 24% for the continuous group and 50% for targeted. A review by Davis *et al.* (1989) also found a highly statistically significant difference favouring continuous treatment. Moreover, they reported that rehospitalization rates were significantly higher with targeted treatment. These effects of targeted treatment were confirmed by the National Institute of Mental Health Treatment Strategies in Schizophrenia study (Schooler *et al.* 1997). Patients with schizophrenia receiving fluphenazine decanoate were assigned to one of three groups: continuous moderate (12.5–50 mg every 2 weeks); continuous low dose (2.5–10 mg every 2 weeks); or a form of targeted treatment. Targeted treatment was associated with an increased risk of relapse as well as rehospitalization. Low-dose treatment resulted in a small increase in the risk of relapse, but not in an increased risk of rehospitalizations. Although most of the results from studies of targeted treatments are discouraging, it is conceivable that patients with insight and well-characterized prodromal symptoms may be effectively managed with targeted treatment.

Taken together these studies suggest that the routine monitoring of prodromal symptoms is a useful activity for many patients in long-term maintenance therapy. The Marder *et al.* study (Marder *et al.* 1994) found that the strategy tended to become more effective over time. This appeared to be a result of the regular prodromal rating occasions during which the patient and a nurse would review and revise the prodromal symptom rating list. These interactions may have led the patient and the clinician to become better at predicting when a patient was on the verge of an exacerbation. A number of instruments have been developed for monitoring prodromal symptoms. These include the Early Signs Questionnaire of Herz and Melville (1980) which focuses on common prodromal symptoms. Marder *et al.* (1994) took another approach. Patients and their families were interviewed regarding the signs and symptoms that preceded prior psychotic episodes. On each visit patients were queried about the presence or absence of these symptoms as well as their severity. The list was updated as patients and clinicians gained more experience in determining which symptoms were reliable predictors.

Effects of maintenance medication on functional outcome

One of the main goals of maintenance treatment is to improve social and vocational outcomes – also known as functional outcomes – for patients with schizophrenia. Although most evidence suggests that combinations of drugs and psychosocial treatments lead to the best outcomes, this chapter first considers the effects of drugs alone and then the integration of the two forms of treatment.

Some of the best evidence for the effects of antipsychotics on functional outcome does not come from well-controlled studies but from case reports and the experiences of clinicians when newer antipsychotics were introduced. A proportion of patients – probably a small proportion – demonstrated dramatic improvements when they were changed from older drugs to clozapine and other new drugs. Some of these patients, who appeared to be destined to a life of chronic mental illness, demonstrated remarkable recoveries and returned to work or school. These individuals experienced a drug-induced improvement that was more than just a decrease in positive symptoms. They reported an increase in motivation and a tendency to think more clearly.

Other studies with newer drugs also suggest that they are more effective for functional outcomes. Hamilton *et al.* (1998) evaluated quality of life in patients who received one of three dose ranges of olanzapine, placebo or haloperidol. Using the Quality of Life Scale (QLS) (Heinrichs *et al.* 1984) the authors found that total QLS was significantly improved on the medium ($P = 0.009$) and higher ($P = 0.037$) doses of olanzapine compared to placebo. Interestingly, patients in the olanzapine groups were more likely to be working. In contrast, haloperidol did not lead to significant improvement.

Management of comorbid conditions during maintenance

Negative symptoms

Negative symptoms of schizophrenia may be conceptualized as either primary or secondary. Primary negative symptoms are enduring symptoms that cannot be attributed to other sources such as drug side-effects or other symptom dimensions. They are an independent dimension of schizophrenia that was characterized by Kraepelin as a 'weakening of the wellsprings of volition' (Kraepelin 1971). Secondary negative symptoms may be caused by: psychotic symptoms (e.g. a person's paranoia prevents him or her from going outside his or her home, thus she is socially withdrawn); side-effects of drugs such as parkinsonism; depression; or environmental deprivation. Recent studies indicate that it can be useful to categorize individuals with enduring primary negative symptoms as having a 'deficit syndrome'. These patients have an illness that is often characterized by poor social functioning as well as impaired neurocognition (Buchanan *et al.* 1990). The two categories of negative symptoms can be difficult to distinguish from one another because both are characterized by symptoms that include blunted affect, alogia, anhedonia and social isolation and withdrawal.

Secondary negative symptoms are managed – whenever possible – by remedying the primary causes; e.g. diminishing the psychosis that caused the patient to be suspicious and isolated, or reversing drug-induced parkinsonism with anticholinergic treatment or by switching to a second-generation antipsychotic. The management of primary negative symptoms is a much greater clinical challenge. Although negative symptoms tend to improve with antipsychotic drugs, the effects are seldom as apparent as the effects on positive symptoms.

The new generation of antipsychotic medications including clozapine, risperidone, olanzapine and quetiapine have shown particular promise in treating the negative symptoms of schizophrenia. Controlled trials with newer antipsychotics have tended to show that patients on newer agents have greater improvements in negative symptoms than those on conventional agents. However, this improvement is difficult to interpret because patients also showed improvement in positive symptoms and EPSs. A meta-analysis by Leucht *et al.* (1999) found that the actual effect sizes for these differences in negative symptoms were small. Moreover, given the reduced EPSs associated with newer agents, the differences could have been related to effects on secondary negative symptoms. This issue has been addressed for studies of olanzapine (Tollefson *et al.* 1997) and risperidone (Moller 1995) using path analysis as a method for distinguishing primary and secondary negative symptoms. In both cases the data suggest that the newer agent was associated with reductions in primary negative symptoms. On the other band, the evidence from long-term trials does not support a negative symptom advantage for newer drugs (Buchanan *et al.* 1998).

Although the data supporting an advantage of second-generation agents for primary negative symptoms is ambiguous, it is our opinion that they can have a role in many patients with these symptoms. Clinicians continue to find patients who demonstrate substantial improvements when they are changed from older to newer drugs. For these individuals it is relatively unimportant to know whether this improvement results from improving primary or secondary symptoms. In some of these cases, EPSs can be relatively subtle and difficult to diagnose. Given the lack of other available treatment approaches for negative symptoms, changing to a newer drug is reasonable.

Another approach to the pharmacological treatment of negative symptoms is based on evidence that these symptoms can be controlled, at least in part, by affecting the *N*-methyl D-aspartate (NMDA)-type glutamate receptor (Javitt *et al.* 1994). This receptor is antagonized by phencyclidine (PCP), which can induce psychotic symptoms – both positive and negative – that mimic schizophrenia. Adjunctive NMDA agonists and partial agonists have thus been utilized to mitigate the symptoms of schizophrenia. There have been five published placebo-controlled studies of glycine (Javitt, *et al.* 1994; Heresco-Levy *et al.* 1996, 1999; Potkin *et al.* 1999) adjunctive treatment and four published studies of D-cycloserine adjunctive treatment (Goff *et al.* 1996, 1999; Heresco-Levy *et al.* 1999; Rosse *et al.* 1996) and one published paper on D-serine as an adjunct (Tsai *et al.* 1998). The major findings have been modest improvements in a range of symptoms: positive, negative, mood and cognitive. Generally, these studies have used small samples, and the effects were sometimes unconvincing. Studies with larger samples are necessary before the clinical usefulness of these drugs can be recommended.

Neurocognitive symptoms

Deficits in neurocognitive functions including memory, attention and executive function are an intrinsic feature of schizophrenia. The severity of these symptoms is relatively independent of the severity of positive and negative symptoms. Moreover, neurocognitive symptoms respond inconsistently to antipsychotic medications. Antipsychotics can improve some neurocognitive symptoms as acute schizophrenia is treated, but other functions may not improve or may worsen. These treatment effects are important during maintenance treatment because there is evidence that neurocognitive deficits are closely related to functional outcome (Green 1996). This suggests that if treatments improve cognitive functions they may, in turn, improve social and vocational outcomes.

A number of studies (reviewed by Keefe *et at.* 1999) have found that new antipsychotic agents have a beneficial effect on neurocognition compared with conventional agents. Several studies have demonstrated that clozapine has a beneficial effect on verbal fluency (Haggar *et al.* 1993; Buchanan *et al.* 1994; Hoff *et al.* 1996). Studies with risperidone suggest that this antipsychotic has a beneficial effect compared with conventional medications in such cognitive areas as working memory (Green *et al.* 1997), secondary memory (Kern *et al.* 1999) and motor speed and dexterity (Kern *et al.* 1998). A study from our Research Center has shown that risperidone also improves perception of emotion compared with haloperidol (Kee *et al.* 1998). One study (Purdon *et al.* 2000) found that treatment with olanzapine led to improvements in a number of cognitive areas including memory, attention, motor skills and executive functioning.

These apparent advantages of second-generation agents may be important in maintenance therapy, particularly if the treatment goal includes increased activities such as work or education which have higher cognitive demands. However, it has not been established that the differences that may be associated with the newer agents are clinically meaningful. On the other hand, clinicans, patients and families have reported that some individuals appear to have benefited substantially when they were changed to a newer agent.

Depression

Patients with schizophrenia commonly complain of depression. The subject of depression in schizophrenia is discussed in depth in Chapter 9. During the maintenance phase of treatment these episodes of depression can be secondary to drug-induced side-effects – particularly antipsychotic-induced akinesia – or they can be a component of a comorbid depression which is relatively common in schizophrenia. Another dilemma in evaluating depression in schizophrenia can occur when negative symptoms such as amotivation and anhedonia are difficult to discriminate from depressed mood.

There is evidence suggesting that adding antidepressants to antipsychotics can be effective in reducing depression in patients with schizophrenia who also have full depressive syndromes. These individuals will have the full depressive syndrome as defined in the criteria for major depressive disorder. Siris *et al.* (1994) studied the effects of adding imipramine or placebo to an antipsychotic medication in patients with comorbid schizophrenia and depression. Importantly, the protocol excluded any subjects whose symptom complex responded to a week's trial of adjunctive anticholinergics. This was an attempt to reduce the contribution and confound of an antipsychotic-induced 'akinetic' syndrome. The results showed that both depressive and negative symptoms, but not psychotic symptoms, improved in the imipramine-treated group.

Although selective serotonin reuptake inhibitors (SSRIs) are widely used for depression in schizophrenia, there is relatively little evidence from controlled studies supporting their use (Goff *et al.* 1990; Ames *et al.* 1993). Also, the addition of the 5-HT$_{1A}$ agonist buspirone has been shown to be of some benefit to small samples of patients (Brody *et al.* 1990). Considering that serotonergic antagonism is among the explanations posited for the enhanced efficacy of clozapine, it is theoretically curious that adjunctive putative serotonergic enhancing agents would improve some schizophrenic symptoms. Fluoxetine (or other SSRIs) may result in downregulation of postsynaptic serotonin receptors, thus causing the overall effect of the medication to be similar to serotonin blockade. Alternatively (or perhaps additionally), it may work by increasing the plasma level of the antipsychotic through competitive metabolism.

Despite the lack of controlled studies, most clinicians are likely to choose an SSRI for individuals with schizophrenia and depression. These agents are relatively safe and have much milder side-effects than heterocyclic agents. Given that this syndrome is relatively common, this area will obviously benefit from additional well-controlled studies.

There is also evidence that the newer antipsychotic medications may have some antidepressant activity themselves and that switching to these agents may be warranted. Both olanzapine and risperidone have demonstrated some improvement in depression compared to conventional antipsychotic agents (Marder *et al.* 1997; Tollefson *et al.* 1997). For both of these newer drugs, treatment with the second-generation agent resulted in greater improvement in depression than treatment with haloperidol. This improvement could have resulted from the reduced EPSs that is commonly associated with newer drugs. However, for both drugs there was some evidence that there was an antidepressant effect that was independent of EPSs. There is also evidence that clozapine treatment is associated with a decrease in suicide rate (Meltzer & Okayli 1995). This supports the view that newer drugs have antidepressant activity. At this stage these studies are only suggestive of a clinically meaningful effect. It is unclear if changing a patient with depression to a newer agent will be as effective as adding an antidepressant.

The studies cited in this section focused on the management of comorbid depression in individuals who are managed on an antipsychotic. These studies should be distinguished from those which focused on SSRIs – particularly fluoxetine – as adjunctive agents for improving core negative symptoms (Goff *et al.* 1995; Buchanan *et al.* 1996). The results from the later studies are ambiguous, whereas the effects of antidepressants on comorbid depression have substantial support.

Unstable mood

Patients with schizophrenia and schizoaffective illness are also vulnerable to mood instability. For stabilized patients who may have relapses of schizophrenia or excited or depressed moods, the goal of pharmacotherapy usually includes the prevention of mood and/or psychotic episodes. Patients with this combination of symptoms often benefit when a mood-stabilizing drug supplements their antipsychotic. Lithium is the most studied mood stabilizer for these patients. When combined with antipsychotics it has been reported to benefit patients with excited schizoaffective illness (Biederman *et al.* 1979) and schizophrenia (Hirschowitz *et al.* 1980).

Carbamazepine, another commonly used agent in bipolar disorder, is often prescribed to patients with schizoaffective illness. When used alone, carbamazepine has little to recommend it for stable but refractory schizophrenia. There is even some suggestion that it may destabilize some of these patients (Sramek *et al.* 1988). However, there is some controlled-study evidence that indicates that when combined with antipsychotics it may have benefit over antipsychotic alone in 'excited psychoses', including schizophrenia (Klein *et al.* 1984).

Although valproic acid, another anticonvulsant agent, is commonly used in the treatment of bipolar illness, there is relatively little empiric evidence supporting its use in schizophrenia. Keck *et al.* (1995) surveyed the concomitant use of risperidone with valproic acid and found the combination useful in schizoaffective disorder. The only published double-blind placebo-controlled study of this medication as an adjunct to antipsychotic medication in patients with schizophrenia suggested that patients on valproic acid required higher dosages of both haloperidol and biperiden. The study results suggest that valproic acid worsened psychotic symptoms but did cause some decrease in use of concomitant sedative medication consistent with its antimanic qualities (Dose *et al.* 1998).

Anxiety

It is estimated that up to 45% of patients with schizophrenia also have an anxiety disorder (Pallanti *et al.* 2000). The frequencies of specific anxiety disorders encountered amongst schizophrenia patients are panic disorder (32.1%) (Labbate *et al.* 1999) obsessive–compulsive disorder (17%), social phobia (20%), general anxiety disorder (15%) (Berman *et al.* 1995) and specific phobias (10%) (Jorgensen & Castle 1998). Anxiety symptoms in patients with schizophrenia are sometimes difficult to recognize and may be confused with akathisia. Evidence of *de novo* development of obsessive–compulsive symptoms has been accumulating amongst patients treated with atypical antipsychotic agents (Baker *et al.* 1997). Clozapine has been associated with *de novo* obsessive–compulsive symptoms in up to 10% of adults and adolescents.

It is important to ensure that anxiety symptoms in schizophrenia are not secondary to side-effects of antipsychotic medication treatment, side-effects of other medications such as bronchodilators, or other conditions such as withdrawal from CNS depressants, particularly benzodiazepines. Akathisia can be managed by reducing the antipsychotic dosage, β-blockers, benzodiazepines or anticholinergic medications. Managing withdrawal from benzodiazepines may require referral to a detoxification programme that includes treatment of substance abuse disorders.

Unfortunately, there are few empirical data to guide the management of patients with anxiety disorders and schizophrenia. The SSRIs have become first-line agents in the treatment of some anxiety symptoms. Although their effects in patients with schizophrenia have not been studied, it is reasonable to add these to antipsychotics as tools for managing anxiety symptoms. It should be noted that SSRIs can also be associated with akathisia, thus patients should be carefully monitored for this side-effect.

Benzodiazepines may be helpful for acute states of anxiety; however, the literature on the long-term use of benzodiazepines in schizophrenia is divided. Some studies have been mildly encouraging (Kellner *et al.* 1975; Lingjaerde 1982) but others have been frankly negative (Gundlach *et al.* 1966; Karson *et al.* 1982). The study by Karson *et al.* not only reported a lack of efficacy for adjunctive clonazepam in an acute treatment trial, but described the new development of violent behaviours in four of 13 patients during treatment. These findings suggest that benzodiazepines should probably be reserved for those cases that fail other adjunctive modalities.

Finally, effective non-pharmacological treatments should also be considered. Although cognitive–behavioural approaches to anxiety have not been studied in schizophrenia, they are worth considering for some patients with schizophrenia. These behavioural treatment approaches include exposure, anxiety management techniques, psychoeducation and cognitive restructuring (Arlow *et al.* 1997).

Substance abuse

The comorbidity of substance abuse among individuals with schizophrenia is surprisingly large, with 50–70% of patients with schizophrenia demonstrating abuse of one or more substances (Kosten & Ziedonis 1997). The odds that a given schizophrenic patient will meet the criteria for substance abuse is 4.6 times that of the normal population (Kirchner *et al.* 1998). Individuals with schizophrenia and comorbid substance abuse tend to have diminished functioning in a variety of domains when compared with individuals without comorbid substance abuse (Fischer *et al.* 1996). Moreover, as mentioned earlier in this chapter, substance abuse substantially increases the risk of psychotic relapse.

Treatment of the schizophrenia patient with comorbid substance abuse is problematic because substance abuse programmes commonly exclude patients with primary psychotic disorders and those programmes devoted to the treatment of schizophrenia often exclude patient with substance abuse. Individuals with schizophrenia and comorbid substance abuse are less likely to receive community-based services than individuals with schizophrenia alone (Fischer *et al.* 1996). Moreover, patients with comorbid substance abuse are more likely to be rehospitalized and are more likely to have poorer outcomes.

To address this duality, Ziedonis and Trudeau (1997) argue for a means to increase good outcomes through a motivation-based treatment model which sets appropriate goals for patients based on assignment to one of five motivational levels. This model also directs the pharmacotherapeutic strategy based on motivational level. It engages community outreach, guided reflection and therapy, and community reinforcement to help improve and maintain the motivation to stop abusing substances. More programmes around the country are beginning to target 'dual-diagnosis' patients. Even Alcoholics Anonymous groups are now held for 'double trudgers'.

The pharmacotherapy of comorbid substance abuse in schizophrenia is an area of growing interest, but with limited utility at this time. Several therapeutic agents may have a role in the treatment of substance abuse in schizophrenia, including naltrexone, disulfiram and desipramine (Krystal *et al.* 1999). Naltrexone has yet to demonstrate efficacy. While disulfiram may reduce both alcohol and cocaine consumption it is associated with difficult compliance issues. Based on pharmacological mechanisms, several other agents may be effective in the treatment of substance abuse, including amantadine, bromocriptine. carbamazepine, dextroamphetamine and risperidone for stimulant abuse, and carbamazepine and tiapride in preventing alcohol relapse (Wilkins 1997).

Importantly, many of the pharmacological therapies used to treat schizophrenia have significant interactions with substances of abuse. While antipsychotics help to diminish symptoms of intoxication of several substances, including cocaine, PCP and LSD, chronic administration of some antipsychotics may help to facilitate the abuse potential of some substances (Kosten & Ziedonis 1997). More specifically, chronic haloperidol administration can reinforce some of the effects of cocaine while substantially decreasing the amount necessary to produce a euphoric response by upregulating the postsynaptic receptor for dopamine. Of note, there has been some encouraging work with clozapine in dually diagnosed patients with schizophrenia, but further research with the other new agents is warranted (Buckley *et al.* 1994).

Interactions of pharmacological and psychosocial treatments during maintenance

In planning the management of patients during the maintenance or stable phase, clinicians should consider interactions between pharmacological and psychosocial treatments (see also Chapters 12 and 3l). As evidence indicates that there are complex interactions between these forms of treatments. An early study by May *et al.* (1981) randomly assigned recently diagnosed patients with schizophrenia to five conditions: milieu treatment, psychotherapy, electroconvulsive treatment (ECT), antipsychotic drugs and psychotherapy with antipsychotics. The patients who received drugs or ECT had the best outcomes during a 6-month period. Moreover, an analysis of outcomes after the trial indicated that the initial advantages of drugs were sustained 5 years later. This study provided strong evidence that drugs were relatively ineffective when patients were not treated with an antipsychotic.

A study by Hogarty *et al.* (1974) evaluated chlorpromazine or placebo and a form of individual psychotherapy or a control condition. The findings indicated that the psychosocial treatment was more effective in the presence of an antipsychotic. Also, patients who did not receive the antipsychotic tended to worsen when they received the psychosocial treatment. This study provides further support for the principle that psychosocial treatments should only be administered when patients have been treated with an antipsychotic. A later study by Hogarty *et al.* (1979) compared patients who received oral fluphenazine or long-acting fluphenazine decanoate in the context of a trial comparing patients who did and did not receive psychosocial treatment. Relapse rates were lowest in patients who received both fluphenazine decanoate and the psychosocial intervention. The results provide strong support for the principle that psychosocial treatments are more effective when patients take their medications reliably.

There is also evidence that psychosocial treatments can improve adherence with medications. One study (Falloon & Liberman 1983) found that patients who received family therapy demonstrated better compliance with drug-taking than those in a control group. This may explain why patients in family treatment appeared to require lower dosage of their antipsychotic medication. Hogarty *et al.* (1986, 1988) found an interesting interaction between antipsychotic dosage and family treatment. Patients who lived in a home environment that may have been stressful because of criticism and emotional overinvolvement (or high EE) demonstrated a greater tendency to relapse when they received reduced antipsychotic dosage. When family psychoeducation lowered the level of EE, relapse rates were reduced. Moreover, patients who received lower dosage had a better social adjustment. These interesting findings suggest that a psychosocial treatment that reduces stress will permit treatment with lower antipsychotic dosage.

Other evidence indicates that psychosocial and pharmacological treatments affect different outcome domains. Marder *et al.* (1996) developed psychosocial methods that focused on improving drug compliance and improving the relationship between patients and drug prescribers. Patients were randomly assigned to receive either behavioural skills training or supportive group therapy administered twice weekly for 2 years. The results indicated that the skills training improved areas of social adjustment whereas a drug strategy that used early intervention for patients who demonstrated early evidence of impending relapse was effective in reducing relapse. The study also found interactions indicating that patients who received skills training along with the early intervention strategy had the greatest improvements in social adjustment.

The recent introduction of newer antipsychotic drugs may also improve the effectiveness of psychosocial treatments. The best established characteristic of the newer drugs is their ability to diminish psychosis at dosage that leads to substantially less EPSs when compared to older agents. Since EPSs – particularly akathisia – can be discomforting for many patients, they can result in patients discontinuing their medications. In addition, patients who experience EPSs – particularly parkinsonian-induced akinesia – may appear lethargic and depressed. As a result, these patients may be less energetic in their participation in psychosocial treatments. In addition, there is evidence that the newer agents are more effective in treating the negative and neurocognitive symptoms in schizophrenia.

The hypothesis that patients who receive newer antipsychotics will be more receptive to psychosocial treatments is supported by a VA Cooperative Study that compared clozapine and haloperidol (Rosenheck *et al.* 1998). The investigators found that patients who received clozapine were more likely to participate in psychosocial treatments. Moreover, participation in these treatments led to improvements in quality of life.

The results from these studies of interactions are important because recent findings from the US Schizophrenia Patient Outcomes Research Team (PORT; Lehman & Steinwachs 1998) indicate that psychosocial treatments and rehabilitation are effective in schizophrenia but underutilized. Moreover, the introduction of newer antipsychotics has raised expectations regarding the goals of treatment for patients with chronic schizophrenia. Patients and their families are often not satisfied with treatment goals that focus solely on relapse prevention; these individuals are looking toward substantial improvements in social and vocational functioning. It is unlikely that these outcomes can be achieved without combining effective pharmacotherapy with well-selected and carefully timed psychosocial treatments.

References

Adams, C.E. & Eisenbruch, M. (2000) Depot fluphenazine for schizophrenia. *Cochrane Database System Review* 120, CD000307.

Ames, D., Wirshing, W., Marder, S., Yuwiler, A, & Brammer, G. (1993) Fluoxetine and haloperidol stabilized schizophrenics. APA 146th Meeting, San Francisco, New Research Program and Abstracts.

Arlow, P.B., Moran, M.E., Bermanzohn, P.C., Stronger, R. & Siris, S.G. (1997) Cognitive–behavioral treatment of panic attacks in chronic schizophrenia. *Journal of Psychotherapy Practice and Research* 6, 145–150.

American Psychiatric Association (1997) Practice guidelines for the treatment of patients with schizophrenia. *American Journal of Psychiatry* 154, 1–63.

Ayuso-Gutiérrez, J.L. & del Río Vega, J.M. (1997) Factors influencing relapse in the long-term course of schizophrenia. *Schizophrenia Research* 28, 199–206.

Baker. R., Bermanzohn, P., Wirshing, D. & Chengappa, K. (1997) Obsessions, compulsions, clozapine, and risperidone *CNS Spectrums* 2, 26–36.

Baldessarini, R.J., Cohen, B.M. & Teicher, M.H. (1988) Significance of neuroleptic dose and plasma level in the pharmacologic treatment of psychoses. *Archives of General Psychiatry* **45**, 79–91.

Berman, I., Kalinowski, A., Berman, S., Lengua, J. & Green, A. (1995) Obsessive and compulsive symptoms in chronic schizophrenia. *Comprehensive Psychiatry* **36**, 6–10.

Biederman, J., Lerner, Y. & Belmaker, R. (1979) Combination of lithium carbonate and haloperidol in schizo-affective disorder: a controlled study. *Archives of General Psychiatry* **36**, 327–333.

Blackwell, B. (1973) Drug therapy: patient compliance. *New England Journal of Medicine* **289**, 249–252.

Brody, D., Adler, L.A., Kim, T., Angrist, B. & Rotrosen, J. (1990) Effects of buspirone in seven schizophrenic subjects. *Journal of Clinical Psychopharmacology* **10**, 68–69.

Brown, G.W., Birley, J.L.T. & Wing, J.K. (1972) Influences of family life on the course of schizophrenic disorders. *British Journal of Psychiatry* **121**, 241-258.

Buchanan, R.W., Kirkpatrick, B., Heinrichs, D.W. & Carpenter, W.T (1990) Clinical correlates of the deficit syndrome of schizophrenia. *American Journal of Psychiatry* **147**, 290–294.

Buchanan, R., Holstein, C., Kirkpatrick, B., Ball, P. & Carpenter, W.T. (1994) The comparative efficacy and long-term effect of clozapine treatment on neuropsychological test performance. *Biological Psychiatry* **36**, 717–725.

Buchanan, R.W., Kirkpatrick, B., Bryant, N., Ball, P. & Breier, A. (1996) Fluoxetine augmentation of clozapine treatment in patients with schizophrenia. *American Journal of Psychiatry* **153**, 1625–1627.

Buchanan, R.W., Breier, A., Kirkpatrick, B., Ball, P. & Carpenter, W.T. (1998) Positive and negative symptom response to clozapine in deficit and nondeficit patients. *American Journal of Psychiatry* **155**, 751–760.

Buckley, P., Thompson, P., Way, L. & Meltzer, H. (1994) Substance abuse among patients with treatment-resistant schizophrenia: characteristics and implications for clozapine therapy. *American Journal of Psychiatry* **151**, 385–389.

Carpenter, W.T.J., Heinrichs, D.W., & Hanlon, T.E. (1987) A comparative trial of pharmacologic strategies in schizophrenia. *American Journal of Psychiatry* **144**, 1466–1470.

Conley, R.R., Love, R.C., Kelly, D.L. & Bartko, J.J. (1999) Rehospitalization rates of patients recently discharged on a regimen of risperidone or clozapine. *American Journal of Psychiatry* **156**, 863–868.

Crow, T.J., MacMillan, J.F., Johnson, A.L. & Johnstone, E.C. (1986) A randomised controlled trial of prophylactic neuroleptic treatment. *British Journal of Psychiatry* **148**, 120–127.

Curson, D.A., Barnes, T.R., Bamber, R.W. (1985) Long-term depot maintenance of chronic schizophrenic out-patients: the seven year follow-up of the Medical Research Council fluphenazine/placebo trial. III. Relapse postponement or relapse prevention? The implications for long-term outcome. *British Journal of Psychiatry* **146**, 474–480.

Curson, D.A., Hirsch, S.R., Platt, S.D., Bamber, R.W. & Barnes, T.R. (1986) Does short term placebo treatment of chronic schizophrenia produce long term harm? *British Medical Journal Clinical Research* **293**, 726–728.

Das, M.K., Kulhara, P.L. & Verma, S.K. (1997) Life events preceding relapse of schizophrenia. *International Journal of Social Psychiatry* **43**, 56–63.

Davis, J., Barter, J. & Kane, J.M. (1989) Antipsychotic drugs. In: *Comprehensive Textbook of Psychiatry*, Vol. 5. (eds H.I. Kaplan & B.J. Sadock), pp. 1591–1626. Williams and Wilkins; Baltimore.

Dose, M., Yassouridis, A,. Theison, M. & Emrich, H.M. (1998) Combined treatment of schizophrenia psychoses with haloperidol and valproate. *Pharmacopsychiatry* **4**, 122–125.

Emsley, R.A., Oosthuizen, P.P., Joubert, A.F., Roberts, M.C. & Stein, D.J. (1999) Depressive and anxiety symptoms in patients with schizophrenia and schizophreniform disorder. *Journal of Clinical Psychiatry* **60**, 747–751.

Essock, S.M., Frisman, L., Covell, N.H. & Hargreaves, W.A. (2000) Cost-effectiveness of clozapine compared with conventional antipsychotic medication for patients in state hospitals. *Archives of General Psychiatry* **57**, 987–994.

Falloon, I.R.H. & Liberman, R.P. (1983) Behavioral family interventions in the management of chronic schizophrenia. In: *Family Therapy in Schizophrenia* (ed. W.R. McFarlane), pp. 117–137. Guilford Press, New York.

Fenton, W.S., Blyler, C.R. & Heinssen, R.K. (1997) Determinants of medication compliance in schizophrenia: empirical and clinical findings. *Schizophrenia Bulletin* **23**, 637–651.

Fischer, E., Owen, R. & Cuffel, B. (1996) Substance abuse, community service use, and symptom severity of urban and rural residents with schizophrenia. *Psychiatric Services* **47**, 980–984.

Goff, D., Brotman, A.W., Waites, M. & McCormick, S. (1990) Trial of fluoxetine added to neuroleptics for treatment resistant schizophrenic patients. *American Journal of Psychiatry* **147**, 492–494.

Goff, D.C., Midha, K.K., Sarid-Segal, O., Hubbard, J.W. & Amico, E. (1995) A placebo-controlled trial of fluoxetine added to neuroleptic in patients with schizophrenia. *Psychopharmacology* **117**, 417–423.

Goff, D.,Tsai, G., Manoach, D.S. *et al.* (1996) D-cycloserine added to clozapine for patients with schizophrenia. *American Journal of Psychiatry* **24**, 512–514.

Goff, D.,Henderson, D.C., Evins, A.E. & Amico, E. (1999) A placebo-controlled crossover trial of D-cycloserine added to clozapine in patients with schizophrenia. *Biological Psychiatry* **24**, 512–514.

Green, M.F. (1996) What are the functional consequences of neurocognitive deficits in schizophrenia. *American Journal of Psychiatry* **153**, 321–330.

Green, M.F., Wirshing, W.C., Ames, D. *et al.* (1997) Does risperidone improve verbal working memory in treatment resistant schizophrenia? *American Journal of Psychiatry* **154**, 799–804.

Gundlach, R., Engelhardt, D.M.,Hankoff, L. (1966) A double-blind outpatient study of diazepam (Valium) and placebo. *Psychopharmacology (Berl)* **9**, 81–92.

Haggar, C., Kenny, J.T., Friedman, I., Ubogy, D. & Meltzer, H.Y. (1993) Improvement in cognitive functions and psychiatric symptoms in treatment-refractory schizophrenic patients receiving clozapine. *Biological Psychiatry* **34**, 702–712.

Hahlweg, K. & Wiedemann, G. (1999) Principles and results of family therapy in schizophrenia. *European Archives of Psychiatry and Clinical Neuroscience* **249** (Suppl. 4), 108–115.

Hamilton, S.H., Revicki, D.A., Genduso, L.A. *et al.* (1998) Olanzapine versus placebo and haloperidol: quality of life and efficacy results of the North American double-blind trial. *Neuropsychopharmacology* **18**, 41–49.

Heinrichs, D.W., Hanlon, E.T. & Carpenter, W.T.J. (1984) The Quality of Life Scale: an instrument for rating the schizophrenic deficit syndrome. *Schizophrenia Bulletin* **10**, 388–398.

Heresco-Levy, U. Javitt, D.C., Ermilov, M. *et al.* (1996) Double-blind, placebo-controlled, crossover trial of glycine adjuvant therapy for treatment-resistant schizophrenia. *British Journal of Psychiatry* **169**, 610–617.

Herz, M.I. & Melville, C. (1980) Relapse in schizophrenia. *American Journal of Psychiatry* **137**, 801–805.

Herz, M.I., Szymanski, H.V.,& Simon, J.C. (1982) Intermittent medication for stable schizophrenic outpatients: an alternative to maintenance medication. *American Journal of Psychiatry* **139**, 918–922.

Herz, M.I., Lamberti, J.S., Mintz, J. *et al.* (2000) A program for relapse prevention in schizophrenia: a controlled study. *Archives of General Psychiatry* 57, 277–283.

Hirsch, S., Bowen, J., Emami, J. *et al.* (1996) A one year prospective study of the effect of life events and medication in the aetiology of schizophrenic relapse. *British Journal of Psychiatry* 168, 49–56.

Hirschowitz, J., Casper, R. & Garver, D. (1980) Lithium response in good prognosis schizophrenia. *American Journal of Psychiatry* 137, 916–920.

Hoff, A., Faustman, W., Wieneke, M. *et al.* (1996) The effects of clozapine on symptom reduction, neurocognitive functioning, and clinical management in treatment refractory state hospital schizophrenic inpatients. *Neuropsychopharmacology* 15, 361–369.

Hogarty, G.E., Goldberg, S.C. & Schooler, N.R. (1974) Drug and sociotherapy in the aftercare of schizophrenic patients. *Archives of General Psychiatry* 31, 609–618.

Hogarty. G.E., Ulrich, R.F., Mussare, F. *et al.* (1976) Drug discontinuation among long term, successfully maintained schizophrenic outpatients. *Diseases of the Nervous System* 37, 494–500.

Hogarty, G.E., Schooler, N.R., R.F., U. *et al.* (1979) Fluphenazine and social therapy in the aftercare of schizophrenic patients: relapse analysis of two year controlled study of fluphenazine decanoate and fluphenazine hydrochloride. *Archives of General Psychiatry* 36, 1283–1294.

Hogarty, G.E., Anderson, C.M., Reiss, D.J. *et al.* (1986) Family psychoeducation, social skills training, and maintenance chemotherapy in the after-care treatment of schizophrenia. I. One year effects of a controlled study on relapse and expressed emotion. *Archives of General Psychiatry* 43, 633–642.

Hogart, G.E., McEvoy, J.P., Munetz, M. *et al.* (1988) Dose of fluphenazine, familial expressed emotion, and outcome in schizophrenia: results of a two-year controlled study. *Archives of General Psychiatry* 45, 797–805.

Hornung, W.P., Klingberg, S., Feldmann, R., Schonauer, K. & Schulze Monking, H. (1998) Collaboration with drug treatment by schizophrenic patients with and without psychoeducational training: results of a 1-year follow-up. *Acta Psychiatrica Scandinavica* 97, 213–219.

Irwin, M., Lovitz, A., Marder, S.R. *et al.* (1985) Psychotic patients' understanding of informed consent. *American Journal of Psychiatry* 142, 1351–1354.

Javitt, D.C., Zylberman, I., Zukin, S.R., Heresco-Levy, U. & Lindenmayer, J.-P. (1994) Amelioration of negative symptoms in schizophrenia by glycine. *American Journal of Psychiatry* 151, 1234–1236.

Johnson, D.A.W., Pasterski, J.M. Ludlow, J.M. *et al.* (1983) The discontinuance of maintenance neuroleptic therapy in chronic schizophrenic patients: drug and social consequences. *Acta Psychiatrica Scandinavica* 67, 339–352.

Johnstone, E.C. & Geddes, J. (1994) How high is the relapse rate in schizophrenia? *Acta Psychiatrica Scandinavica, Supplementum* 382, 6–10.

Jolley, A.G., Hirsch, S.R., McRink, A. & Manchanda, R. (1989) Trial of brief intermittent neuroleptic prophylaxis for selected schizophrenic outpatients: clinical outcome at one year. *British Medical Journal* 298, 985–990.

Jorgensen, L. & Castle, D. (1998) Anxiety and psychosis. *Australian and New Zealand Journal of Psychiatry* 32, 731.

Kane, J.M. (1985) Compliance issues in outpatient treatment. *Journal of Clinical Psychopharmacology* 5 (Suppl. 3), 22S–27S.

Kane, J.M. (1987) Treatment of schizophrenia. *Schizophrenia Bulletin* 13, 133–156.

Kane, J.M. (1995) Dosing issues and depot medication in the maintenance treatment of schizophrenia. *International Clinical Psychopharmacology* 10 (Suppl. 3), 65–71.

Kane, J.M., Rifkin, A., Quitkin, F., Nayak, D. & Ramos-Lorenzi, J. (1982) Fluphenazine vs. placebo in patients with remitted, acute first-episode schizophrenia. *Archives of General Psychiatry* 39, 70–73.

Kane, J.M., Davis, J.M., Schooler, N. *et al.* (2002) A multidose study of halperidol decanoate in the maintenance treatment of schizophrenia. *American Journal of Psychiatry* 159, 554–560.

Karson, C.N., Weinberger, D.R., Bigelow, L. & Wyatt, R.J. (1982) Clonazepam treatment of chronic schizophrenia: negative results in a double-blind, placebo-controlled trial. *American Journal of Psychiatry* 12, 1627–1628.

Keck, P.E., Jr., Strakowski, S.M. *et al.* (1995) Clinical predictors of acute risperidone response in schizophrenia, schizoaffective disorder, and psychotic mood disorders. *Journal of Clinical Psychiatry* 10, 466–470.

Kee, K.S., Kern, R.S., Marshall, B.D. & Green, M.F. (1998) Risperidone versus haloperidol for perception of emotion in treatment-resistant schizophrenia: preliminary findings. *Schizophrenia Research* 31, 159–165.

Keefe, R., Silva, S., Perkins, D. & Lieberman, J. (1999) The effects of atypical antipsychotic drugs on neurocognitive impairment in schizophrenia: a review and meta-analysis. *Schizophrenia Bulletin* 25, 201–222.

Kellner, R., Muldawer, M.D. & Pathak, D. (1975) Anxiety in schizophrenia: responses to chlordiazepoxide in an intensive design study. *Archives of General Psychiatry* 32, 1246–1254.

Kern, R.S., Green, M.F., Marshall, B.D. *et al.* (1998) Risperidone vs. haloperidol on reaction time, manual dexterity, and motor learning in treatment-resistant schizophrenic patients. *Biological Psychiatry* 44, 726–732.

Kern, R.S., Green, M.F., Marshall, B.D. *et al.* (1999) Risperidone vs. haloperidol on secondary memory: can new medications aid learning? *Schizophrenia Bulletin* 25, 223–232.

Kirchner, J., Owen, R.R., Nordquist, C. & Fischer, E.-P. (1998) Diagnosis and management of substance use disorder among inpatients with schizophrenia. *Psychiatric Services* 49, 82–85.

Kissling, W., Kane, J.M., Barnes, T.R.E., Dencker, S.J. & Fleischhacker, W.W. (1991) Guidelines for neuroleptic relapse prevention in schizophrenia: towards a consensus view. In: *Guidelines for Neuroleptic Relapse Prevention in Schizophrenia* (ed. W. Kissling), pp. 155–163. Springer-Verlag; Berlin.

Klein, E., Lerer, B. & Belmaker, R.H. (1984) Carbamazepine and haloperidol vs. placebo and haloperidol in excited psychoses. *Archives of General Psychiatry* 41, 165–170.

Kosten, T. & Ziedonis, D. (1997) Substance abuse and schizophrenia: editor's introduction. *Schizophrenia Bulletin* 23, 181–185.

Kraepelin, E. (1971) *Dementia Praecox and Paraphrenia*. Robert E. Krieger, New York.

Krystal, J., Madonick, S. & Petrakis, I.L. (1999) Towards a rational pharmacotherapy of comorbid substance abuse in schizophrenic patients. *Schizophrenia Bulletin* 35, S35–S49.

Labbate, L., Young, P. & Arana, G. (1999) Panic disorder in schizophrenia. *Canadian Journal of Psychiatry* 44, 480–490.

LeDuc, P.A. & Mittleman, G. (1995) Schizophrenia and psychostimulant abuse: a review and re-analysis of clinical evidence. *Psychopharmacology* 121, 407–427.

Lehman, A.F. & Steinwachs, D.M. (1998) Patterns of usual care for schizophrenia: initial results from the Schizophrenia Patient Outcomes Research Team (PORT) Client Survey. *Schizophrenia Bulletin* 24, 11–20.

Leucht, S., Pitschel-Walz, G., Abraham, D. & Kissling, W. (1999) Efficacy and extrapyramidal side-effects of the new antipsychotics olanzapine, quetiapine, risperidone, and sertindole compared to conventional antipsychotics and placebo: a meta-analysis of randomized controlled trials. *Schizophrenia Research* 35, 51–68.

Lingjaerde, O. (1982) Effect of the benzodiazepine derivative estazolam in patients with auditory hallucinations: a multicentre double-blind, cross-over study. *Acta Psychiatrica Scandinavica* 65, 339–354.

Marder, S.R. (1998) Facilitating compliance with antipsychotic medication. *Journal of Clinical Psychiatry* 59 (Suppl. 3), 21–25.

Marder, S.R., Van Putten, T., Mintz, J. *et al.* (1987) Low and conventional dose maintenance therapy with fluphenazine decanoate: two year outcome. *Archives of General Psychiatry* 44, 518–521.

Marder, S.R., Hubbard, J.W., Van Putten, T. & Midha, K.K. (1989) The pharmacokinetics of long-acting injectable neuroleptic drugs: clinical implications. *Psychopharmacology* 98, 433–439.

Marder, S.R., Wirshing, W.C., Van Putten, T. *et al.* (1994) Fluphenazine vs. placebo supplementation for prodromal signs of relapse in schizophrenia. *Archives of General Psychiatry* 51, 280–287.

Marder, S.R., Wirshing, W.C., Mintz, J. *et al.* (1996) Two-year outcome of social skills training and group psychotherapy for outpatients with schizophrenia. *American Journal of Psychiatry* 153, 1585–1592.

Marder, S.R., Davis, J.M., & Chouinard, G. (1997) The effects of risperidone on the five dimensions of schizophrenia derived by factor analysis: combined results of the North American trials. *Journal of Clinical Psychiatry* 58, 538–546.

May, P.R.A., Tuna, A.H., Tuma, A.H. & Dixon, W.J. (1981) Schizophrenia: a follow-up study of results of five forms of treatment. *Archives of General Psychiatry* 38, 776–784.

Meltzer, H.Y. & Okayli, G. (1995) Reduction of suicidality during clozapine treatment of neuroleptic-resistant schizophrenia: impact on risk–benefit assessment. *American Journal of Psychiatry* 152, 183–190.

Moller, H. (1995) The negative component in schizophrenia. *Acta Psychiatrica Scandinavica Supplementum* 388, 11–14.

Nuechterlein, K.H., Dawson, M.E., Gitlin, M. *et al.* (1992) Devleopmental processes in schizophrenic disorders: longitudinal studies of vulnerability and streess. *Schizophrenia Bulletin* 18, 387–425.

Olfson, M., Mechanic, D., Boyer, C.A. & Hansell, S. (1998) Linking inpatients with schizophrenia to outpatient care. *Psychiatric Services* 49, 911–917.

Pallanti, S., Quericioli, L. & Pazzagli, A. (2000) Social anxiety and premorbid personality disorders in paranoid schiophrenic patients treated with clozapine. *CNS Spectrums* 5, 29–43.

Pietzcker, A. (1985) A German multicentre study on the long-term treatment of schizophrenic outpatients. *Pharmacopsychiatry* 18, 333–338.

Potkin, S.G., Jin, Y. Bunney, B.G., Costa, J. & Gulasekaram, B. (1999) Effect of clozapine and adjunctive high-dose glycine in treatment-resistant schizophrenia. *American Journal of Psychiatry* 156, 145–147.

Purdon, S.E., Jones, B.D., Stip, E. *et al.* (2000) Neuropsychological change in early phase schizophrenia during 12 months of treatment with olanzapine, risperidone, or haloperidol. *Archives of General Psychiatry* 57, 249–258.

Revicki, D.A., Shakespeare, A. & Kind, P. (1996) Preferences for schizophrenia-related health states: a comparison of patients, caregivers, and psychiatrists. *International Clinical Psychopharmacology* 11, 101–108.

Rosenheck, R., Cramer, J., Xu, W. *et al.* (1997) A comparison of clozapine and haloperidol in hospitalized patients with refractory schizophrenia. Department of Veterans Affairs Cooperative Study Group on Clozapine in Refractory Schizophrenia. *New England Journal of Medicine* 337, 809–815.

Rosenheck, R., Tekell, J., Peters, J. *et al.* (1998) Does participation in psychosocial treatment augment the benefit of clozapine? *Archives of General Psychiatry* 55, 618–625.

Rosse, R., Fay-McCarthy M, Kendrick, K., Davis, R.E. & Deutsch, S.I. (1996) D-cycloserine adjuvant therapy to molindone in the treatment of schizophrenia. *Clinical Neuropharmacology* 19, 444–449.

Schooler, N.R. (1991) Maintenance medication for schizophrenia: strategies for dose reduction. *Schizophrenia Bulletin* 17, 311–324.

Schooler, N.R., Keith, S.J., Severe, J.B. *et al.* (1997) Relapse and rehospitalization during maintenance treatment of schizophrenia: the effects of dose reduction and family treatment [see comments]. *Archives of General Psychiatry* 54, 453–463.

Shumway, M., Chouljian, T. & Battle, C. (1997) Stakeholder preferences for schizophrenia outcomes: an evaluation of assessment methods. *Schizophrenia Research* 24, 258.

Siris, S.K., Bermanzohn, P.C., Mason, S.E. & Shuwall, M.A. (1994) Maintenance imipramine therapy for secondary depression in schizophrenia. *Archives of General Psychiatry* 51, 109–115.

Smith, T.E., Hull, J.W., Anthony, D.T. & Goodman, M. (1997) Posthospitalization treatment adherence of schizophrenic patients: gender differences in skill acquisition. *Psychiatry Research* 69, 123–129.

Sramek, J., Herrera, J., Costa, J. *et al.* (1988) A carbamazepine trial in chronic treatment-refractory schizophrenia. *American Journal of Psychiatry* 145, 748–750.

Tollefson, G., Beasley, C., Jr., Tran, P.V. *et al.* (1997) Olanzapine versus haloperidol in the treatment of schizophrenia and schizoaffective and schizophreniform disorders: results of an internation collaborative trial. *American Journal of Psychiatry* 154, 457–465.

Tran, P.V., Dellva, M.A., Tollefson, G.D., Wentley, A.L. & Beasley, C.M., Jr. (1998) Oral olanzapine versus oral haloperidol in the maintenance treatment of schizophrenia and related psychoses. *British Journal of Psychiatry* 172, 499–505.

Tsai, G., Yang, P., Chung, L.C., Lange, N. & Coyle, J.T. (1998) D-serine added to antipsychotics for the treatment of schizophrenia. *Biological Psychiatry* 44, 1081–1089.

Vaillant, G.E. (1964) Prospective prediction of schizophrenic remission. *Archives of General Psychiatry* 11, 509–518.

Van Putten, T. (1974) Why do schizophrenic patients refuse to take their drugs? *Archives of General Psychiatry* 31, 67–72.

Van Putten, T., Marder, S.R., Wirshing, W.C., Chabert, N. & Aravagiri, M. (1990) Surreptitious noncompliance with oral fluphenazine in a voluntary inpatient population [letter]. *Archives of General Psychiatry* 47, 786–787.

Vaughn, C.E. & Leff, J.P. (1976) The measurement of expressed emotion in the families of psychiatric patients. *British Journal of Clinical and Social Psychology* 15, 157–165.

Weiden, P. & Glazer, W. (1997) Assessment and treatment selection for 'revolving door' inpatients with schizophrenia. *Psychiatric Quarterly* 68, 377–392.

Wiersma, D., Nienhuis, F.J., Slooff, C.J. & Giel, R. (1998) Natural course of schizophrenic disorders: a 15-year followup of a Dutch incidence cohort. *Schizophrenia Bulletin* 24, 75–85.

Wilkins. J. (1997) Pharmacotherapy of schizophrenia patients with comorbid substance abuse. *Schizophrenia Bulletin* 23, 215–228.

Wynne, L.C. (1981) Current concepts about schizophrenics and family relationships. *Journal of Nervous and Mental Disease* 169, 82–89.

Ziedonis, D.M. & Trudeau, K. (1997) Motivation to quit using substances among individuals with schizophrenia: implications For a motivation-based treatment model. *Schizophrenia Bulletin* 23, 229–238.

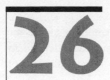

26 Treatment-resistant schizophrenia

T.R.E. Barnes, P. Buckley and S.C. Schulz

Definitions, 489
  Clinical criteria, 489
  Research criteria, 490
Clinical and neurobiological characteristics of
  response in treatment-refractory
  schizophrenia, 491
  Clinical and demographic variables, 491
  Neuroimaging, 493
  Neuroleptic plasma levels as a predictor of
    treatment response, 495
  Pharmacogenetics, 496
  Neurochemistry and neurophysiology, 496

Psychosocial approaches, 496
  Family psychoeducation and therapy, 497
  Cognitive–behavioural therapy, 497
  Cognitive rehabilitation or compensation
    strategies, 497
  Psychosocial programmes, 498
Pharmacological treatment, 498
  Antipsychotic drug strategies, 498
  Adjunctive pharmacological treatments, 503
Conclusions, 507
References, 507

While antipsychotic agents continue to be the mainstay of treatment of schizophrenia, there is a marked heterogeneity of response. A substantial minority of patients, between one-fifth and one-third, will derive little benefit from conventional antipsychotic drug therapy, although a smaller proportion would seem to be completely resistant (Brenner *et al.* 1990; Lieberman *et al.* 1992; Conley & Buchanan 1997). Studies of first-episode schizophrenia suggest that, even at an early stage of the illness, a small proportion of patients will show a lack of response, commonly leading to a protracted hospital admission (May 1968; MacMillan *et al.* 1986; Lieberman *et al.* 1989, 1992).

Broadening the definition of treatment resistance beyond psychopathology measures to include vocational, social and cognitive domains would classify a greater proportion of patients as treatment-resistant (Meltzer 1992). Present prevalence and incidence figures for treatment-refractory schizophrenia are largely based on stringent research criteria (Kane *et al.* 1988) and therefore may underestimate this problem by not including the many patients who manifest an incomplete and unsatisfactory response to antipsychotics (Osser & Albert 1990). This assertion is supported by the initial findings of a multicentre trial of treatment strategies involving 300 patients with schizophrenia (Schooler *et al.* 1997). By evaluating maintenance antipsychotic treatments and their interaction with family therapies, this study demonstrated that nearly 40% of the patients remained poorly stabilized at 6 months of treatment. Equally discouraging, a substantial number of those who showed initial treatment response were unable to sustain this through to the second year of observation.

These findings are in line with the notion that treatment resistance is not merely the result of institutionalization (Curson *et al.* 1992) or of acquired disabilities but, rather, represents a putative 'endogenous' trait that (regrettably) shows remarkable consistency over time. The seminal study of Kane *et al.* (1988) further supports this viewpoint. Here, 305 patients with current

evidence of a severe symptomatic schizophrenic illness were carefully determined as having a prior history of treatment resistance using stringent historical criteria (see Table 26.1). These patients were then enrolled in a 6-week prospective trial of haloperidol (60 mg/day) to confirm their apparent treatment non-responsivity. At the conclusion of this phase, only five patients emerged as treatment responders.

Definitions

Clinical criteria

Clinicians generally see treatment resistance as the presence of disability, encompassing functional and psychosocial dimensions, which continues despite trials of medication that have been adequate in terms of dose, duration and compliance. All of the elements of schizophrenia may contribute to poor community function including enduring positive and negative symptoms, affective symptoms, drug side-effects, cognitive dysfunction and disturbed behaviour. Between treatment-resistant individuals, the contribution of these various elements to overall function will vary markedly, prompting different treatment targets and strategies for different patients. The quality of the persistent psychotic experiences imports different functional significance, which will duly influence the extent of treatment responsiveness. This point is most readily illustrated by patients whose bizarre delusions are associated with marked social disruption and functional decline, in contrast with others experiencing similar intensity of delusions but of a less bizarre nature, for whom the impact on overall social functioning is far less.

Formal psychopathology scales for the clinical assessment of the persistently psychotic patient may fail to take due account of the impact of symptomatology on overall functioning, and fall short in appraising the qualitative nature and clinical ramifications of the disability which presents to the psychiatrist. Thus, on the basis of simple psychopathology scores, the treatment resistance of a patient with chronic delusions and hallucinations for which he/she retains (albeit partial) insight and functional capacity may be inappropriately equated with that of the patient whose apathy and lack of motivation result in severe social withdrawal and secondary deficits. Further, the application of such scales may contribute to a dichotomous view of treatment response, which assumes that patients who are deemed poor responders to antipsychotic therapy constitute a homogeneous group. While therapeutic trials have largely focused on overall group effects between responders and non-responders, it is nevertheless apparent (and in accord with clinical practice) that non-responders show considerable diversity in therapeutic response. Thus, within a group of non-responders, some may show only modest response to an experimental treatment, others a minimal change in symptoms and a few will deteriorate (Wolkowitz *et al.* 1988). Such differences may have fundamental implications for our understanding of treatment response but, largely because of inadequate sample sizes, this issue has yet to be subjected to appropriate scientific enquiry.

The alternative perspective posits that treatment resistance is not a marker for discrete response groups but, rather, is best conceptualized as a continuum (Brenner *et al.* 1990). This notion lends credence to the clinical observation that the majority of patients do not fall within a strictly defined responder/non-responder distinction, but are in fact suboptimal responders who continue to exhibit symptomatology and functional disability (Brenner *et al.* 1990; Kane *et al.* 1990; Osser & Albert 1990). Such 'partial responders' have now become an important focus of interest, particularly as we struggle to establish a valid and clinically meaningful classification of treatment resistance. Furthermore, with the demonstration that pharmacotherapy such as clozapine and psychological interventions such as cognitive–behavioural therapy are effective treatment options for severely ill patients, the characterization and management strategies for the partial responder have come under sharp review. Both patients and clinicians now have higher expectations for treatment response.

In addition to addressing the potential confounding variables of poor compliance (Weiden *et al.* 1991; Barnes *et al.* 1996), drug bioavailability (Van Putten *et al.* 1991) and a putative therapeutic window (Schulz *et al.* 1984; Baldessarini *et al.* 1988; Bitter *et al.* 1991), there has been greater recognition of a multidimensional perspective to treatment resistance and of the complexity of interrelationships between positive and negative symptomatology, functional deficits and behavioural disturbance (Brenner *et al.* 1990; Meltzer *et al.* 1990; Meltzer 1992). It has been acknowledged that improvement in cognitive function and psychopathology may, in some instances, occur independently of each other (Goldberg *et al.* 1987, 1993) and that such measures may exert different, yet equally pertinent, influences on eventual treatment outcome (Green *et al.* 2000; Liddle 2000). Recommendation that other facets of the illness receive particular attention in a manner similar to assessing symptomatology has led to the incorporation of instruments such as the quality of life scale (Heinrichs *et al.* 1984) and the independent living skill survey (Wallace 1986) into the routine evaluation of treatment response.

Research criteria

Historically, the concept of non-response to antipsychotic medication was ill defined and largely synonymous with chronic or frequent hospitalization (Conley & Buchanan 1997). In refining this to ensure methodological rigour and clear characterization of study samples, many researchers have sought explicit definitions of treatment resistance (see Table 26.1). Definitions have often been related to the purpose of the individual project, e.g. treatment of last resort (Kane *et al.* 1988) or neuropsychiatric differences between groups (Schulz *et al.* 1989). These definitions have not addressed clinical questions, such as when to change treatment.

The use of psychopathology rating scales has enhanced the reproducibility and consistency of the definition of poor response to neuroleptics. A threshold level of a 20% decrease in the total score on the Brief Psychiatric Rating Scale (BPRS) has been widely adopted as a measure of response to antipsychotics in clinical trials (Kane *et al.* 1988). However, this criterion is somewhat arbitrary, and was derived largely from earlier trials intended merely to demonstrate that antipsychotic medications were active. Thus, a 20% decrement in BPRS symptomatology is not an immutable benchmark and may, in some instances, confer the erroneous impression that substantial improvement or satisfactory clinical 'response' has been attained. A patient with an initial BPRS score of 48 may indeed achieve a 20% fall in BPRS with treatment (to a value of 38 or less) and yet still exhibit substantial impairment. Furthermore, if another patient at an initial BPRS rating of 38 fails to attain a similar 20% reduction in BPRS, then this subject will be designated a 'non-responder' and yet will likely possess an endpoint BPRS score that is broadly similar to that of the 'responder'. Quite apart from the selection of a particular definition of responsiveness, the use of this criterion threshold level has other related implications. For example, the acutely psychotic patient (e.g. BPRS of 58) may attain this 20% decrement more readily with treatment than another patient who, while not as floridly psychotic (e.g. BPRS of 38), may nevertheless experience disabling symptoms. In such circumstances, there is a differential effect through the range of BPRS rating with greater improvement at the lower range being necessary to be considered a 'responder' than at higher baseline points on the scale. This differential effect may underrepresent the true estimate of treatment resistance (Thompson *et al.* 1994).

The approach of Kane *et al.* (1988) and Schulz *et al.* (1989) stressed a specific level of symptomatology as the guideline for response. In both reports, a definite BPRS score was chosen as representing a mild level of symptoms. This is more like a medical approach to symptoms in that it aims at remission of symptoms or at least reduction to a low level. The criteria of

Table 26.1 Definition of response to antipsychotic medication treatment.

Definition	Purpose	Critique
20% decrease on BPRS total score (various authors)	To assess activity of a medication	Patients with initially high scores will still remain symptomatic
Threshold of rating response (e.g. < 35 on BPRS) (Kane *et al.* 1988)	An approach to defining remission, not just mild symptoms in 'treatment of last resort'	Still only focuses on rating scale symptoms, but does specifically assess antipsychotic activity
Core symptoms (Kane *et al.* 1988)	To determine whether a treatment has an effect on the main positive symptoms of schizophrenia	May lead to focus on positive symptoms
Threshold and medication blood level (Schulz *et al.* 1989)	To separate responders and non-responders while assuring appropriate medication concentration	Cross-sectional but does account for bioavailability of medications
Spectrum of response (Brenner *et al.* 1990)	To approach the wide range of poor response and specify treatment approaches	Perhaps more difficult to apply to research setting, but opens new avenues for the non-response category
Lack of stabilization despite medicine and family psychoeducation (Schooler *et al.* 1997)	To identify patients for study of long-term effects of medicine strategies and family therapy. Used as criteria for entry to lithium augmentation (Schulz *et al.* 1999)	Difficult to translate to the clinical arena

Kane *et al.* (1988) also included historical criteria, which are important for studies of treatments of last resort, while Schulz *et al.* (1989) included requirements of adequate medication levels before labelling a person treatment-resistant.

Clinical and neurobiological characteristics of response in treatment-refractory schizophrenia

Clinical and demographic variables

Beyond simply poor outcome itself, defining the clinical phenotype of treatment-refractory schizophrenia and any contributory factors thereof has proved elusive. Intuitively, one might expect that symptom presentation and persistence of positive or negative symptoms would predict subsequent treatment response and functional outcome. However, the strength of the relationship between initial symptoms and outcome is at best weak (McGlashan 1999).

Negative symptoms

The type I/type II model of schizophrenia (Crow 1980) considered the importance of symptomatology in response to antipsychotics in schizophrenic patients and suggested that positive symptoms were remediated by these drugs, while negative symptoms were persistent and refractory to conventional treatments. However, observations with conventional (Goldberg 1985; Meltzer *et al.* 1986) and atypical antipsychotic medica-

tion (Kane *et al.* 1988) challenge this notion. There have been claims for a beneficial effect on negative symptoms with certain conventional antipsychotics (pimozide, low-dose sulpiride) and several of the atypical drugs. Further, clinical trials with some of the atypical antipsychotics have shown superior efficacy in reducing negative symptoms ratings in acute schizophrenia. However, interpretation of these data should take account of the problems in distinguishing between secondary negative symptoms (caused by extrapyramidal side-effects (EPSs), particularly bradykinesia, or active avoidance and withdrawal secondary to delusional and paranoid thinking, or depressive features) from primary negative symptoms which represent a true absence of activity, drive and volition and a poverty of thought and flatness of affect (Barnes & McPhillips 1995; Kopelowicz *et al.* 2000). Thus, a key clinical issue is whether any observed benefit on negative symptoms in acute studies can be extrapolated to stable patients with persistent negative symptoms. To date, only amisulpride has been tested in such patients, with some evidence of benefit (Danion *et al.* 1999; Moller 2000; Muller *et al.* 2000).

Kirkpatrick *et al.* (2001) have made strong claims that the deficit syndrome – a pattern of illness characterized by primary enduring negative symptoms – is less treatment responsive and may even represent a different biological phenotype of schizophrenia. They have demonstrated that patients with the deficit syndrome have greater impairment of the frontal lobes (evidenced by smaller frontal lobes, lower frontal metabolism, dysfunctional eye movements, executive performance deficits). The dilemma herein, when considering the relationship of negative symptoms to treatment response, is that the deficit syndrome is far less common – even allowing for diagnostic imprecision – than the usual clinical pattern of fluctuating negative symptoms, which are at least in part of a secondary nature. It is this latter and more common clinical pattern that accounts for the variability in studies that have addressed the issue of negative symptoms and treatment response. Thus, while it appears that the deficit syndrome defines an inverse relationship between negative symptoms and treatment response, this is relevant to a small proportion of patients. This observation does not detract from the importance of the work and approach by Carpenter *et al.*, because their careful attempts to isolate a distinct phenotype contributes to our understanding of the pathophysiology of symptom expression and also provides a theoretical framework to the reduction of aetiological heterogeneity in this disorder(s) (Dalen & Hayes 1990; Kirkpatrick *et al.* 2001; for alternative viewpoint see Daniel & Weinberger 1991; see also Chapter 3).

Neurocognitive function

Subtyping of schizophrenia by diagnosis and predominant clinical features (e.g. paranoid, disorganized) to predict response appears to be of little heuristic merit (McGlashan *et al.* 1999). On the other hand, cognitive impairment has emerged as a key predictor of overall treatment response (Keefe *et al.* 1999; Harvey & Keefe 2001) and of functional outcome (Green 1996; Green *et al.* 2000; Velligan *et al.* 2000b). Cognitive impairment is observed to a substantial extent in first-episode schizophrenia (Bilder *et al.* 2001) and is persistent over the course of illness (Liddle & Crow 1984; Waddington *et al.* 2001). A recent review and meta-analysis has found that atypical antipsychotics can ameliorate cognitive impairments (Keefe *et al.* 1999) and this is of particular relevance to the heightened importance of cognition in assessing treatment response. It is observed that each of these drugs appears to have a different pattern of cognitive improvement (Purdon *et al.* 2000; Harvey & Keefe 2001) and these effects are independent of the EPS liability of each agent (Weiser *et al.* 2000). However, although cognition is now considered an important variable for treatment outcome, the effect of atypicals is modest and even those patients who show improvement still function at a level of cognitive performance below that of normal individuals (Galletly *et al.* 2000; see also Chapter 10).

Depressive features

Depression as a distinct syndrome within schizophrenia is common (Siris *et al.* 2001). It was originally conceptualized as a feature predicting positive outcome and treatment response (Siris 2000). However, outcome studies (Barnes *et al.* 1989; Birchwood *et al.* 2000) do not bear this out, particularly because comorbid depression is the single most salient predictor of suicide in schizophrenia. There have been attempts recently to examine the differential response of depressive symptoms beyond positive and negative symptoms (Tollefson *et al.* 1998; Siris 2000). This is driven by observations that atypical antipsychotics may have a direct antidepressant effect in patients with schizophrenia (Tollefson *et al.* 1998; Keck *et al.* 2000; see also Chapter 9).

Substance abuse

Depression is probably the most studied of the comorbid conditions that can impact on treatment outcome in schizophrenia. Substance abuse is another very common comorbid problem, but this has been appreciated only relatively recently (Seibyl & Lieberman 1993; Buckley *et al.* 1994; Duke *et al.* 1994, 2001). While it is unclear whether comorbid substance use causes an alteration in treatment responsivity so that patients become refractory to antipsychotic medications, it is clear that substance abuse has a profoundly deleterious impact on illness course and outcome (Buckley 1998). Patients who abuse illicit drugs or alcohol are more likely to have more prominent symptomatology, more frequent relapses and repeated hospitalizations (Seibyl & Lieberman 1993). The dynamic between persistent schizophrenic symptoms, antipsychotic side-effects and the potential for substance use as self-medication remains uncertain (Siris *et al.* 1987; Duke *et al.* 1994). Nevertheless, the potentially deleterious interaction of even modest substance abuse and psychosis in such individuals may (quite apart from interrelated adverse factors such as social deprivation and treatment compliance) confer a relative resistance to neuroleptic treatment. The neurochemical basis for such an effect, possibly acting through alteration of dopamine-receptor sensitivity, merits further attention because it may suggest more effective alternative treatment strategies for treatment-resistant schizophrenic patients who have comorbid substance use (Buckley *et al.* 1994). There is some evidence that atypical antipsychotics may reduce the pattern of substance use in this difficult-to-manage patient group (Buckley *et al.* 1994; Drake *et al.* 2000).

Physical illness

There is also evidence that physical illness is common in patients with schizophrenia (Phelan *et al.* 2001). Although the impact of physical comorbidity on treatment response in schizophrenia has not been well studied, intuitively one can expect this to confer a disadvantage in outcome. Moreover, this issue may be of even greater significance now that the adverse effect profile of endocrine and metabolic dysfunction with the atypicals comes into sharper relief (Buckley 1999).

Demographic and other clinical variables

Amongst all of the clinical and demographic predictors of treatment response in schizophrenia, an earlier age at onset has most consistently been associated with poor response and outcome (Kolakowska *et al.* 1985; Lieberman *et al.* 1993, 1996). On average, age of onset is approximately 5 years earlier in refractory patients (Meltzer 1997), although there is very wide variation in the onset of schizophrenia. The association between early illness onset and poor outcome is most pronounced in adolescent- and childhood-onset schizophrenia, which is generally poorly responsive to treatments (Schulz *et al.* 1998) and has a poor long-term outcome (Lay *et al.* 2000). Somewhat related is the insidious (?subclinical) pattern of poor premorbid personality, which manifests and antedates the expression of formal symptoms (Reichenberg *et al.* 2000; Waddington *et al.* 2001). Poorer premorbid personality is associated with poor outcome and is more pronounced in patients with treatment-refractory schizophrenia (Cannon *et al.* 1999; Robinson *et al.* 1999). It is at present unclear whether poor premorbid personality, insidious onset and early onset of illness coalesce – and confound – to generate the modern-day concept of duration of untreated psychosis (DUP) (McGlashan 1999; Beng-Choon & Andreasen 2000). However, DUP has been associated with a poorer response to treatment (Johnstone *et al.* 1990; Wyatt 1991; Loebel *et al.* 1992). This observation has served as a powerful impetus to conduct early intervention studies in schizophrenia with the presumed (and intuitive) expectation that such early intervention will realize a better treatment response and long-term outcome (McGlashan 1999; Waddington *et al.* 2001). The results of these studies will become available over the next 5 years and they will inform us on this important issue.

Gender is another robust predictor of treatment response (Leung & Chue 2000). It has been well established that female patients have a better response to treatment with conventional antipsychotic medications. It is, at present, less clear whether this also holds true for atypical antipsychotics. This is because most clinical trial samples predominantly consist of male patients (average distribution is 70% male and 30% female). Further, there is reason to suspect that female patients who are included in clinical trials tend to have more severe illnesses and may not be representative of female patients at large. It is proposed that this gender effect to modify the illness and to confer better treatment responsivity in female patients may be as a result of oestrogen regulation of dopaminergic tone (Leung & Chue 2000). This would accord with observations that oestrogen may enhance treatment response in postmenopausal female patients (Kulkarni *et al.* 2001) and, more speculatively, in partial responders in general. Alternatively, there are some data to suggest that the gender difference in treatment responsivity might be mediated through the effect of earlier age of onset in male vs. female patients (Meltzer 1997). This gender difference in age of onset appears to be obliterated in patient samples comprising both male and female treatment-refractory patients (Meltzer 1997).

Neurological soft signs have been associated with poor treatment response (Kolakowska *et al.* 1985). The literature in this regard, while not exhaustive with respect to treatment response, is consistent with this association.

In summary, poor premorbid function, early age of onset of illness, male gender and neurological soft signs (all of which are pronounced in male patients) are consistent predictors of poor response to treatment. Cognitive impairment is now emerging as an important predictor. Comorbid conditions also negatively influence treatment outcome. Duration of untreated psychosis is of heuristic importance but its real significance in terms of treatment response has yet to be clearly established. Other clinical variables have shown inconsistent or no predictive value in determining treatment response.

Neuroimaging

Although far from proven, the overrepresentation of structural brain abnormalities in patients with treatment-refractory schizophrenia is an enduring theme (Crow 1980; also see Chapter 22). Crow's original type I/type II model of schizophrenia (Crow 1980) proposed that poor response was associated with more brain abnormalities on neuroimaging. Early computerized tomography (CT) and magnetic resonance imaging (MRI) studies (meta-analysis/systematic review with respect to treatment response carried out by Friedman *et al.* 1992) reported greater ventricular enlargement (Weinberger *et al.* 1980; Schulz *et al.* 1983; Pandurangi *et al.* 1989; Kaplan *et al.* 1990; Lieberman *et al.* 1993; Davis *et al.* 1998), frontal (and to a lesser extent temporal) lobe sulcal prominence (Kolakowska *et al.* 1985; Kaiya *et al.* 1989; Friedman *et al.* 1991) and focal brain abnormalities (Lieberman *et al.* 1993). However, it should be pointed out that this literature is neither uniform nor consistent, despite the intuitive assertion that poor responder patients might have more 'damaged brains'. There are several studies that have not found associations between structural brain abnormalities and treatment response (Nasrallah *et al.* 1983; Schulz *et al.* 1989; Lieberman *et al.* 1996; Honey *et al.* 1999). Honey *et al.*, using similar methodology, were unable to replicate an earlier finding by Friedman *et al.* (1991) that clozapine response was inversely related to the amount of frontal cortex on CT imaging.

The majority of the studies cited above have evaluated actual treatment response to antipsychotic medication either by retrospective (Kolakowska *et al.* 1985) or prospective (Lieberman *et al.* 1996) design. However, there is another aspect of neuroimaging research that is directly relevant and overlaps substantially with the issue of treatment response. There is now a substantial literature suggesting that a proportion of patients show progressive brain changes when evaluated sequentially by either CT (Woods *et al.* 1990; Nair *et al.* 1997) or MRI (DeLisi *et al.* 1997; Jacobson *et al.* 1998; Mathalon *et al.* 2001). Although many of these studies lack sufficient clinical details to evoke cogent relationships between clinical characteristics (particularly treatment response) and progressive brain changes, there are several studies that have noted progressive brain pathomorphology (ventricular enlargement, global and selective predominantly frontotemporal decrements in grey matter) in association with the following indices of poor clinical outcome: worsening of clinical symptoms (Vita *et al.* 1988; Gur *et al.* 1994, 1998; Lieberman *et al.* 1996; Rapoport *et al.* 1997; Davis *et al.* 1998; Mathalon *et al.* 2001); prolonged and/or repeated hospitalization (DeLisi *et al.* 1992, 1997; Davis *et al.* 1998; Mathalon *et al.* 2001); protracted illness duration (Marsh *et al.* 1994; Davis *et al.* 1998); and greater overall functional impairment (Lieberman *et al.* 1996; DeLisi *et al.* 1997; Davis *et al.* 1998). There are, in counterbalance, several studies that show no progression of structural pathomorphology over time (Nasrallah *et al.* 1986; Illowsky *et al.* 1988; Sponheim *et al.* 1991; Jaskiw *et al.* 1994; Vita *et al.* 1994). However, on balance the literature now leans toward the interpretation that progressive brain changes are more pronounced in patients who have a more severe and clinically deteriorative form of illness. These findings, at least by inference, suggest that worsening clinical severity reflects progressive pathobiological processes in line with the notion of a neurodegenerative component to schizophrenia (Woods 1998; Lieberman 1999; Waddington *et al.* 2001). There is a need for additional prospective MRI studies that employ clinical trial methodology to the study of treatment response. Such studies could further evaluate this hypothesis and could integrate this within a neurobiological schema of treatment response. Additionally, it would be very useful to determine whether the pattern of brain dysmorphology differs across treatment with each of the atypical antipsychotics.

There is already a focused but nevertheless important published literature which addresses the latter issue (Jernigan *et al.* 1991; Chakos *et al.* 1994; Keshavan *et al.* 1994; Frazier *et al.* 1996; Westmoreland-Corson *et al.* 1999). Jernigan *et al.* (1991) reported that the caudate nucleus was bilaterally enlarged in patients with chronic schizophrenia who were receiving treatment with typical antipsychotic medications. Chakos *et al.* (1994) reported that the volume of the caudate nucleus decreased by approximately 10% when patients were changed from typical antipsychotic medications to clozapine. Other groups (Keshavan *et al.* 1994; Frazier *et al.* 1996) replicated these findings. More recently, Dr Andreasen's research group at the University of Iowa have noted a similar pattern for patients switching from typical antipsychotics to clozapine, risperidone or olanzapine. The extent to which such discrete structural changes reflect and/or predict treatment response to atypical antipsychotic medications remains to be clearly elucidated. Results from a study of treatment response to clozapine showed that nonresponders to clozapine had no change in the volume of the caudate nucleus (Scheepers *et al.* 2001). Similar work is needed in relation to the other atypical antipsychotics.

There is a substantial literature examining functional brain imaging parameters and treatment response (for review see Holcomb & Tamminga 2000). Recent work on symptom patterns and the localization of delusions, disorganization and hallucinations (Liddle *et al.* 1992; Tamminga *et al.* 1992; Silbersweig *et al.* 1998; Spence *et al.* 1998) offers a neural framework to bridge between knowledge of the functional neuroanatomy of schizophrenia and our understanding of the functional impact of antipsychotic medications. Buchsbaum *et al.* (1987) have shown that atypical antipsychotics increase metabolism in the basal ganglia, a finding that is well replicated (Wolkin *et al.* 1996). Buchsbaum *et al.* (1992) have also found that lower pretreatment metabolism in the basal ganglia is predictive of a good response, both to haloperidol and to clozapine. They also noted that poor responders showed lower frontal lobe metabolism. A similar but more generalized pattern of cortical hypometabolism was seen in non-responders in other studies (Wolkin *et al.*

1996; Bartlett *et al.* 1998). Cohen *et al.* (1997) showed a different pattern of brain metabolism in patients receiving clozapine vs. fluphenazine. Honey *et al.* (1999) reported a differential pattern of cerebral blood flow in patients receiving risperidone. Further studies are warranted to extend this work to examine the pattern of symptom response in relation to treatment with each of the atypical antipsychotics. Additionally, with the developments in cognitive neuroscience and with the potential for atypical antipsychotics to partly ameliorate cognitive deficits in patients with schizophrenia (Keefe *et al.* 1999), there is likely to be a substantial effort to understand the neural basis of enhanced cognitive functioning as a response to treatment with atypical antipsychotic medications.

Finally, there has been a long-standing interest in studying the extent to which antipsychotic medications that bind to neurotransmitter receptors can yield useful information to assist in predicting whether or not a patient will respond to treatment (Wolkin *et al.* 1989; Wolkin 1990; Holcomb & Tamminga 2000). The literature on typical antipsychotics and treatment response can be summarized as follows:

1 refractory patients have similar dopamine receptor occupancy rates during treatment with typical antipsychotic medications, as is seen with patients who are responders to these medications; and

2 saturating the dopamine receptors by using high doses of typical antipsychotics does not improve treatment response, either for responsive or refractory patients.

The literature on receptor occupancy with typical antipsychotics is more recent – and burgeoning – but focuses more on relationships between dosage, mechanism of action and motor side-effects (Kapur *et al.* 1997, 1999, 2000; Kapur & Seeman 2001). This literature provides an important theoretical framework for understanding our current dosing regimens with atypical antipsychotics and, accordingly, is of relevance with respect to refractory schizophrenia. For example, there is substantial evidence from PET studies (Nordstrom *et al.* 1995; Kapur *et al.* 1997) that even if the dosage of clozapine is increased to 900 mg/day, there is no corresponding increase and/or saturation of dopamine D_2 receptors. Indeed, mean D_2 receptor occupancy for clozapine is 47% and rises only to a ceiling of 80% with dosage escalation. This pattern is distinct from that observed from typical antipsychotics, wherein D_2 occupancy rates of 60–80% are commonplace with routine clinical doses and full saturation (and motor side-effects) is easily achieved when the dose of the typical antipsychotic is increased. The pattern of occupancy for each of the other atypical antipsychotics (risperidone, olanzapine, quetiapine and ziprasidone) is also different from that of the typical antipsychotics and is also different between each of the agents (Kapur *et al.* 1997, 1999, 2000). Risperidone at lower doses has moderate D_2 receptor occupancy and this increases toward saturation in a dose-dependent fashion. Olanzapine shows a similar general trend but it is less pronounced and saturation is not generally observed within the current recommended dosage range (maximum 20 mg/day). The pattern with ziprasidone appears even less pronounced and dose-influenced than with olanzapine, although there are fewer data for ziprasidone. Quetiapine appears similar to clozapine in its profile of dopamine receptor occupancy.

While such observations have provided information to advance the understanding of the receptor pharmacology of these drugs (with particular emphasis on efficacy, emergence of EPSs, D_2 and D_2/5-HT receptor relationships and the efficacy–EPS profile), these findings have a direct impact on the management of treatment-refractory schizophrenia. For example, the available data provide some rationale to suggest that risperidone at low doses of 1–2 mg/day is preferable to haloperidol or higher doses of risperidone (4–6 mg/day) when considering antipsychotic adjunctive therapy in treatment-resistant patients who have persistent positive symptoms despite an adequate trial of clozapine. Similarly, these data on receptor occupancy concur with clinical experience that olanzapine can be used at higher doses than 20 mg/day in treatment-refractory patients. There is ample opportunity for a large range of PET studies addressing the relationships between neurotransmitter receptor occupancy and treatment response to atypical antipsychotic medication. This work is likely to prove informative in providing dosage regimens for each atypical agent and for understanding their relative efficacy, dosing requirements and side-effect profile in patients with refractory schizophrenia.

Neuroleptic plasma levels as a predictor of treatment response

Plasma levels of antipsychotic medications (both typical and atypical) have been investigated as a potential factor in determining treatment resistance in schizophrenia (Baldessarini *et al.* 1988; Van Putten *et al.* 1991; Miller 1996). For typical antipsychotics there is wide interindividual variation, although overall levels of haloperidol (5 ng/mL and below; haloperidol is the least studied agent) are associated with poor treatment response, while high levels (20 ng/mL and above) are associated with neuroleptic toxicity and/or symptom exacerbation (Baldessarini *et al.* 1988; Van Putten *et al.* 1991; see also Chapter 23).

Therapeutic monitoring of clozapine plasma levels has also been reported to be useful as a guide to dosage with this drug. In an early study of 59 treatment-resistant schizophrenic patients, Hasegawa *et al.* (1993) observed that a clozapine concentration of 370 ng/mL discriminated clozapine responders from non-responders: 67% of responders and 72% of non-responders to clozapine were correctly classified using this cut-off point. It was noted that some patients responded well despite plasma clozapine levels considerably less than 370 ng/mL but poor responders had lower levels more frequently than good responders did. These results replicated those of Perry *et al.* (1991) and are consistent with subsequent studies (Miller *et al.* 1994; Potkin *et al.* 1994). There is evidence that increasing the plasma levels of clozapine to at least 370 ng/mL in patients who respond

poorly and who have clozapine levels less than this can produce further clinical improvement (Miller 1996).

In a naturalistic 2.5-year follow-up study of a previously reported sample, Miller *et al.* (1994) reported that 12 of the 14 patients who responded to clozapine showed a clozapine plasma level of 350 ng/mL. For seven patients who were non-responders and had clozapine plasma levels below 350 ng/mL, an increase in dosage to achieve a clozapine plasma level over 350 ng/mL was accompanied by a change in responder status in five of these seven patients. In another sample of 58 patients receiving clozapine, a clozapine plasma level of 420 ng/mL optimally classified patients as responders and non-responders at the fourth week of treatment (Potkin *et al.* 1994). By week 12 of clozapine therapy, 73% of those patients with an initially low plasma level which subsequently rose above 420 ng/mL were classified as responders, in contrast with the 29% response rate among patients with persistently low clozapine plasma levels. In another study of clozapine plasma levels during the first 6 weeks of treatment, a plasma level of 350 ng/mL discriminated between clozapine responders and non-responders with a sensitivity of 80% and a specificity of 22% (Kronig *et al.* 1995). In another study evaluating clozapine response at 12 weeks among 45 patients who received an average dosage of 306 mg/day, Spina *et al.* (2000) found that a cut-off clozapine concentration value of 350 ng/mL discriminated responders from non-responders at 72% sensitivity and 70% specificity. Side-effects were twice as common when the clozapine concentration exceeded 350 ng/mL. When a cut-off of 400 ng/mL was used, the sensitivity declined to 67%, while the specificity rose to 78%. The authors advocate the use of low doses of clozapine and to aim for clozapine plasma levels above 350–400 ng/mL in patients who, although tolerating clozapine well, have an inadequate symptomatic response.

The most methodologically rigorous study to date compared response to clozapine in three patient groups, randomized into a low, intermediate or moderate plasma level of clozapine (Van der Zwaag *et al.* 1996). Patients in the intermediate plasma range (350 ng/mL) fared best, in terms of both symptom response and side-effects. One observation of this study is that the plasma levels were set at an overall lower level and it would be helpful to have this study repeated with three plasma level groups which represented higher blood levels of clozapine. In this way the optimum therapeutic range could be evaluated, as could the notion of a therapeutic window. Buckley *et al.* (2001) examined the latter issue in a sample of 23 patients receiving 900 mg of clozapine. Eleven patients had plasma levels below 1000 g/mL and 12 had levels above this. Both groups showed a similar pattern of response to clozapine. These data are consistent with the proposition that, within its current dosage range, a therapeutic window does not exist for clozapine therapy.

The status – both clinical and research focus – of plasma levels as a predictor of response to clozapine and other atypical antipsychotics is unclear. Despite overall encouraging results, there has been a falling-off of research interest in plasma clozapine levels. There is as yet little evidence for the clinical utility of plasma levels in determining treatment response to risperidone, olanzapine, quetiapine or ziprasidone. There was some initial work on plasma levels of olanzapine (Perry *et al.* 1999) that was encouraging but there has been no subsequent work published on either olanzapine or any of the other atypical antipsychotics. This area may re-emerge as a research focus once the intramuscular (acute and long-acting) forms of atypical antipsychotics become more widely used and studied. Thus, the possibility that plasma levels of any or some of the atypical antipsychotics may prove clinically useful requires further study.

Pharmacogenetics

Pharmacogenetics is an emerging area of promise in determining antipsychotic treatment response in schizophrenia (Roth *et al.* 1999; Masellis *et al.* 2000; Otani & Aoshima 2000). The present focus is on the receptor affinity of atypical antipsychotics and is complementary to the functional neuroimaging of receptor profile of these agents (Kapur *et al.* 2000; Kapur & Seeman 2001). The pharmacogenetic approach seeks to determine whether polymorphism in key neurotransmitter receptors (especially dopamine and serotonin receptors) can explain the variability of treatment response among patients. To date, most studies have focused on clozapine treatment response and, utilizing the candidate gene approach, have sought associations between clinical measures of clozapine response and both serotonin receptor gene (CT 5-HT$_A$, 5-HT$_C$, 5-HT$_6$, 5-HT$_7$ receptors) and dopamine receptor gene (at D$_2$, D$_3$ and D$_4$ receptors) polymorphism. Some studies have shown positive associations and they highlight the potential of molecular receptor genetics to predict antipsychotic drug response with respect to serotonin receptors (Arranz *et al.* 1995, 2000; Yu *et al.* 1999). However, other groups have not found any association between serotonin receptor genes and treatment response (Malhotra *et al.* 1998; Schumacher 2000; Tsai *et al.* 2000). Despite the relevance of dopamine to antipsychotic mechanisms of action, the results of association studies thus far have not been encouraging (Rao *et al.* 1994; Marsellis *et al.* 2000). On the other hand, this is an encouraging line of enquiry and the studies published reflect variable methodology both in terms of molecular genetic techniques (receptor focus, statistics) and clinical characteristics (clozapine dosage, duration of treatment, retrospective vs. prospective definition of treatment response). Moreover, the focus has almost exclusively been on clozapine and it has yet to be determined whether this strategy may prove useful for other atypical antipsychotics.

There are two other aspects of molecular genetics that, although still in a nascent stage, may hold promise for the management of treatment refractory schizophrenia in the future. First, pharmacogenetics has to date centred on the prediction of treatment response and has not evaluated to the same extent the variability of occurrence of adverse effects during treatment with antipsychotic medications. At this time, side-effect profile seems to be the major discriminator between atypical antipsychotics and the receptor affinities of these agents appear to concur closer to side-effect profile than response profile (Richelson & Souder 2000). Accordingly, this is a potentially important area to explore further for treatment-resistant schizophrenia. Secondly, the application of genomics to the study of treatment refractory response offers considerable potential (Regalado 1999). A pharmacogenomic approach can examine the human genome to elucidate susceptibility loci for treatment response and for drug adverse effect profiles, in addition to determining the 'genetic' impact of clinical characteristics of the illness itself. This is likely to be an intense focus of research on treatment response over the coming years.

Neurochemistry and neurophysiology

There is also some literature, largely related to typical antipsychotic medications, that examines the use of neuroendocrine and neurochemical measures of dopamine–serotonin metabolism as predictors of treatment response (Bowers *et al.* 1984; Rao *et al.* 1994). These studies suggest that high pretreatment homovanillic acid (HVA), the metabolite of dopamine, and a decrease in HVA correlates with good response to treatment. This is consistent with other work showing that elevated prolactin is associated with good response (Kolakowska *et al.* 1985). The findings with respect to serotonin metabolites are less clear. There is no clear evidence for the role of dopamine–serotonin metabolites in predicting treatment response to atypical antipsychotics.

There is a substantial literature on the neurophysiological abnormalities (smooth eye pursuits, sensory gating and prepulse inhibition, backward masking, EEG rhythm) in patients with schizophrenia. There have been some attempts to discriminate response to treatment using these measures (Lieberman *et al.* 1993). In a first episode study by Lieberman *et al.* (1993), 12 of 70 patients did not respond to a treatment algorithm (of typical antipsychotic medications) at the end of 1 year. Elevated basal growth hormone and abnormal brain morphology were the two variables associated with poor response. Apomorphine or methylphenidate challenge, or eye-tracking dysfunction, were not associated with either time to or level of remission. This latter study is noteworthy because it applied a multivariate integrative approach to researching treatment response in schizophrenia. This approach is preferable to the single variable approach, because the single variable approach appears too insensitive to discriminate discrete pathobiological differences between treatment responsive and refractory patients (Csernansky *et al.* 1985; Garver *et al.* 2000). An integrative approach is more likely to delineate any putative subgroup of treatment-refractory patients.

Psychosocial approaches (see also Chapters 32 and 33)

The majority of reports concerning schizophrenic patients who have poor symptom reduction despite adequate trials of antipsychotic medications have focused on biological factors associated with poor response and on medication approaches. The treatment-unresponsive patient, it may be argued, may need more specific and/or more intensive psychosocial interventions than medication-responsive patients because of their disabilities. In addition, just as families may be burdened by having a family member with schizophrenia, families living with a person with treatment-refractory schizophrenia may need *extra* support. Therefore, a selection of the psychosocial approaches to schizophrenia are discussed in light of their possible contribution to refractory patients and the few reports of studies including such patients are described.

Family psychoeducation and therapy

In some ways, the concept of high expressed emotion (EE) could be said to have emerged from an enquiry into the cause(s) of poor outcome of schizophrenic patients who had been stabilized on antipsychotic medications, yet relapsed within months (Brown *et al.* 1972; Vaughn & Jeff 1976). Family assessments of this poor outcome, which may fall under the category of 'poor stabilization', indicated that high EE was associated with relapse. Various strategies to reduce relapse in schizophrenic patients, utilizing psychoeducational sessions and family therapy approaches to reduce high EE, improve problem solving and diminish isolation have been reported (Falloon *et al.* 1985; Schulz *et al.* 1986; Hogarty *et al.* 1991). Although many of these studies and reports have been aimed at reducing relapse in medication-stabilized patients, particular attention to how such approaches might be used for the severely ill and persistently ill patient have been slow to emerge. It is our impression that clinicians working in 'clozapine clinics' have developed programmes that include tenets of the family studies of the early 1980s. Such programmes generally involve substantial and ongoing psychoeducational programmes, family groups and staff collaboration with family and advocacy groups such as the National Alliance for the Mentally Ill (NAMI) in the USA. Clinics that have designed such programmes generally theorize that some or many treatment-refractory patients are especially sensitive to high EE and that families of such patients require more coping skills to deal successfully with their treatment-refractory family member.

Cognitive–behavioural therapy

Many clinicians have moved to more specific and structured talking therapy interventions for psychiatric patients with empirically demonstrated positive outcomes (Beck *et al.* 1979; Kingdon & Turkington 1991). This therapy had been adapted for application to schizophrenia with good outcome, as has been described elsewhere in this volume (see Chapter 33). Sensky *et al.* (2000) have specifically tested cognitive–behavioural therapy (CBT) in the treatment-refractory patient group. Patients not responsive to traditional antipsychotic medications were randomized to specific CBT treatment or a supportive approach labelled 'befriending'. Both groups showed improvement in the initial 9 months, with the CBT group demonstrating continuing improvement thereafter. Interestingly, there was a broad reduction of symptoms, including depression. That CBT can lead to further symptom reduction in persistently ill patients demonstrates that the synergy between medication and psychosocial programmes extends to this severely ill group. It could be hypothesized that if newer medications lead to better cognitive function – even in persistently ill patients (Green *et al.* 1997) – CBT may be even more useful than seen in trials with traditional medications. Clinically, it should be noted that the statistically significant effects of CBT did not emerge until the follow-up assessment; thus, programme design should focus on the long-term care of the patient.

Cognitive rehabilitation or compensation strategies

Although rehabilitation strategies have been the focus of some clinical research groups (Liberman *et al.* 1998), the neuropsychological investigations of more recent years have focused attention on the cognitive difficulties of schizophrenic patients (Green 1996). It is now well documented that a proportion of people with schizophrenia, at first episode and during the later stages of the illness, perform substantially below normal standards in a number of cognitive domains (Hutton *et al.* 1998; Harvey & Keefe 2001). Treatment-resistant patients may have even poorer function on the same tests, e.g. sustained attention, executive function, verbal memory and even mini-mental status examination (Kolakowska *et al.* 1985; Bartko *et al.* 1989). Perhaps those investigating or treating schizophrenia viewed cognitive function as a trait characteristic or were influenced by early reports of little change in executive function despite training but, for whatever reason, research reports of cognitive treatment strategies have been slow to emerge for the seriously ill patient.

For schizophrenic patients in general, that is to say patients not identified as non-responders, cognitive therapy or neuropsychological programmes have been reported to be helpful. Wykes *et al.* (1999) have pioneered cognitive remediation techniques, particularly targeting executive function deficits. In their randomized study comparing intensive cognitive remediation with intensive occupational therapy, a differential effect in favour of the former treatment was found for certain tests of cognitive flexibility and memory. These investigators concluded that cognitive remediation can reduce cognitive deficits and this may lead to improved social outcome, at least in the short term.

Velligan *et al.* (2000a) have postulated that a focus on compensation strategies rather than training patients to do the problem area functions better may lead to better outcomes. Their study, using compensatory or 'cognitive adaptation training', showed significantly better outcomes for schizophrenic patients not only in functioning, but also showed a reduction in psychotic symptoms. Although not a study of the treatment-resistant patient, this approach may have promise for this group of patients with significant cognitive problems.

Schulz *et al.* (1999) reported use of neuropsychology assess-

CHAPTER 26

ments in adolescent schizophrenic patients who are faced with the challenge of return to school (high school or college). By reviewing neuropsychological test results with families and teachers, the clinical team was able to devise an individualized treatment plan that accounted for a patient's strengths and/or weaknesses, e.g. audio taping classes to assist with poor sustained attention or working memory.

Can such approaches help the treatment-resistant patient? Clinicians and patients would certainly hope so and emerging evidence of plasticity of the nervous system would indicate that change can occur. The results of assessments of positive impact of new antipsychotic medications on neuropsychological test results (for a review see Meltzer & McGurk 1999) would lead to greater optimism for better outcomes with cognitive rehabilitation or compensation strategies.

Psychosocial programmes

While specific psychosocial approaches have been addressed, most clinical programmes offer a range of interventions, which include some or all of the above approaches as well as social skills training, group therapies and psychotherapies. Just as in many areas of medicine, individual types of programmes are addressed for efficacy, but they are then frequently combined in comprehensive programmes. Interventions such as social skills training are helpful for schizophrenia, but may lead to decreased relapses for patients when combined with family therapy (Hogarty et al. 1991).

Grace et al. (1996) reported on the impact of a psychosocial programme specifically for non-responders in reducing symptoms and improving outcomes in clozapine-treated patients. The programme was designed for patients defined as non-responsive by the same criteria used for the test of clozapine as treatment of last resort (Kane et al. 1988). The psychosocial interventions included a combination of psychosocial interventions including supportive psychotherapy, standard hospital programmes, weekly psychoeducation programmes and monthly support meetings for patients' family members. The authors report on long-term outcomes – up to 3 years – using objective rating scales. For example, BPRS scores were reduced from 55.5 to 31.5 over 3 years. There was also a significant improvement in cognitive function and negative symptoms. Even though there are reports of 6-month outcomes on quality of life as part of a comprehensive clozapine treatment programme (Meltzer et al. 1990), the Grace et al. (1996) report extends the length of study time and documents the usefulness of combined treatments in a substantially non-responsive group. Although not controlled, this report is a useful example of the impact of psychosocial interventions over a long period – exceeding the study period of many of the pivotal studies described earlier in this section.

Overall, the last 15 years have seen a number of reports of useful psychosocial interventions for schizophrenia in carefully controlled studies described here and reviewed in Chapter 33. However, studies which have prospectively identified the treat-

ment-refractory patient have been few. Further, as definitions of treatment resistance have been broadened to include partial responders, comorbid patients and poorly functioning patients, the psychosocial approaches will require further innovation and study.

Pharmacological treatment

Antipsychotic drug strategies

High-dose/megadose studies with conventional antipsychotics

Controlled studies comparing very high doses of conventional antipsychotics with standard dosage regimens in treatment-resistant patients have all failed to show a statistically significant advantage for the megadose regimen (Hirsch & Barnes 1994; Thompson 1994). However, there are methodological problems with these studies, including small sample sizes and the lack of a consistent valid definition of treatment resistance (Kane 1993). The latter problem is highlighted by the observation that in several of the studies a proportion of the patients on standard dose showed improvement, suggesting that their classification as treatment-resistant was premature.

Combining two or more antipsychotic medications when symptoms are persistent?

In clinical practice, the lack of a satisfactory response to a single antipsychotic often prompts the addition of another. A recent multicentre audit of prescribing of antipsychotic medication for inpatients in 47 mental health services in the UK (Harrington et al. 2002), involving 3132 inpatients, found that 48% were receiving more than one antipsychotic drug. In the majority of cases the reason for this polypharmacy was that a single antipsychotic had not been effective.

A combination of clozapine and a conventional antipsychotic has commonly been reported. There have been reports that conventional antipsychotics are used in up to 35% of patients receiving clozapine in some European countries (Leppig et al. 1989; Peacock & Gerlach 1994). McCarthy and Terkelsen (1995) reported that a conventional antipsychotic was added to clozapine in 30–35% of cases in Denmark. However, the research evidence to justify adding another antipsychotic in patients with only a partial response to clozapine monotherapy is limited to a few recent case reports, case series and small studies. Adjunctive antipsychotics tested include pimozide (Friedman et al. 1997), sulpiride (Stubbs et al. 2000), olanzapine (Gupta et al. 1998) and loxapine (Mowerman & Siris 1996), with reports of further clinical benefit. While the addition of risperidone in a couple of cases failed to produce any improvement (Koreen et al. 1995; Chong et al. 1996), the majority of reports involving this drug have been positive (McCarthy & Terkelsen 1995; Tyson et al. 1995; Henderson & Goff 1996; Morera et al. 1999; Raskin et al. 2000; Adesanya & Pantelis

498

2001). For example, in a 4-week open study, Henderson and Goff (1996) assessed the safety and efficacy of risperidone as an adjunct in 12 patients with schizophrenia who continued to exhibit positive and negative symptoms despite treatment with clozapine. Ten of the 12 patients had a 20% or greater reduction in their total BPRS scores, and the investigators considered that controlled trials of this adjunctive therapy were warranted.

Yuzda (2000) reviewed the evidence for efficacy with combined antipsychotics. She identified one randomized controlled trial (Shiloh et al. 1997), two open prospective trials (Henderson & Goff 1996; Mowerman & Siris 1996), one retrospective review (Friedman et al. 1997) and four anecdotal reports (McCarthy & Terkelsen 1995; Gupta et al. 1998; Takhar 1999). The bulk of the published data relate to combining conventional or atypical antipsychotics with clozapine. The RCT (Shiloh et al. 1997) involved 28 patients with a partial or unsatisfactory response to clozapine who were randomly allocated to clozapine plus sulpiride (600 mg/day) or clozapine plus placebo for 10 weeks. BPRS total score reductions were significantly greater ($P < 0.05$) in the sulpiride group, and there was a trend for more younger patients to have > 20% BPRS reduction. Yuzda (2000) identified several limitations of the study, including the small sample size and short duration, that the treatment groups were not matched for previous hospitalization and the exclusion of complete responders to clozapine. Overall, Yuzda (2000) concluded that the addition of a second antipsychotic to clozapine was an appropriate intervention, and the strongest evidence related to sulpiride. Otherwise, given the paucity of the published data, the addition of a conventional antipsychotic to an atypical could not be encouraged, particularly as there was potentially an increased risk of adverse effects and non-compliance. In relation to the former, Mujica and Weiden (2001) reported the development of neuroleptic malignant syndrome (NMS) in a patient after haloperidol was added to their atypical antipsychotic treatment.

Chong and Remington (2000) also reviewed adjunctive antipsychotics with clozapine. They considered that a limitation common to all the published studies was the lack of information regarding the previous exposure of study patients to the adjunctive antipsychotic. They argued that without such data, it remained an open question whether the responses observed could be attributed to the combination or simply to the second antipsychotic alone. Nevertheless, they concluded more positively that, despite the lack of controlled data, such combinations were safe and might be efficacious for those patients for whom clozapine had produced a less than optimal improvement. Raskin et al. (2000) questioned the safety of the combination of clozapine and risperidone, pointing to isolated references suggesting adverse reactions such as agranulocytosis (Godlesky & Sernyak 1996) and marked elevation of clozapine blood levels (Koreen et al. 1995).

Chong and Remington (2000) also addressed the possible mechanisms underlying any enhanced therapeutic effect of combined antipsychotics. Any pharmacodynamic synergy might be related to an increased level of D_2 dopamine receptor occupancy, above a threshold level. However, an increased risk of extrapyramidal side-effects might be expected to accompany such an increase. Other authors have postulated that an alteration of the interaction between 5-HT and D_2 activity might be relevant (Shiloh et al. 1997). Further, pharmacokinetic interactions might have a role, although the evidence for increased clozapine plasma levels with augmentation is uncertain (Shiloh et al. 1997; Procopio 1998). However, the mechanisms underlying this augmentation strategy have not been systematically studied (McCarthy & Terkelsen 1995).

Clozapine

Efficacy

Wahlbeck et al. (1999) evaluated the general effectiveness of clozapine in schizophrenia. They conducted a systematic review and meta-analysis of 31 randomized controlled clozapine trials involving over 2500 participants (average age 38 years), the majority of whom were men (74%). Twenty-six of the studies were less than 13 weeks in duration, with the remainder being longer term (6 months to 2 years in length). Only seven of the studies were limited to patients with treatment-resistant schizophrenia. In comparison with conventional drugs, clinical improvement was seen more frequently in those patients taking clozapine, both in the short- and the long-term. Also, in the relatively short-term, participants on clozapine had fewer relapses than those patients receiving conventional antipsychotic drugs. Wahlbeck et al. concluded that clozapine had convincing superiority in terms of clinical improvement, relapse prevention and acceptability as measured by the proportion of drop-outs. However, evidence that this superior clinical effect translated into better functioning was judged to be lacking. Examining particularly those studies in patients with treatment-resistant schizophrenia, clozapine was found to produce greater clinical improvement. The acceptability of treatment in such patients only favoured clozapine in the longer term studies. The authors noted the relative absence of functional and social outcomes, and called for an internationally recognized set of standard outcomes, including pragmatic assessments of functioning.

Critical review of trials of the pharmacological treatment of refractory schizophrenia confirms that clozapine remains the only antipsychotic of proven efficacy in the treatment of patients with such illnesses, the evidence for other atypicals, such as olanzapine and risperidone, being inconclusive (Cheine et al. 1999; Chakos et al. 2001). It was judged to be effective in a substantial proportion (30–60%) of those patients unresponsive to other drug treatment. However, using what they referred to as a 'non-stringent' criterion of 20–30% reduction in total psychopathology scores Chakos et al. (2001) found that fewer than half the patients responded in most studies. Thus, they conclude that a significant proportion of treatment-refractory patients will be left with persistent symptoms and substantial impairments.

The pivotal study (Kane et al. 1988) was a double-blind multicentre comparison of clozapine and chlorpromazine in

268 schizophrenic patients meeting stringent criteria for treatment resistance. These criteria included failure to respond to adequate trials with at least three antipsychotic drugs and a prospective single-blind trial of haloperidol, as well as no period of good functioning within the previous 5 years. By the end of the 6-week treatment period, clozapine treatment was associated with significantly greater improvement in both positive and negative symptoms. Using prospective clinically relevant criteria of improvement, 30% of the patients receiving clozapine could be classified as responders after 6 weeks, compared with only 4% of the chlorpromazine group. Subsequently, double-blind controlled studies in patients with treatment-resistant schizophrenia have confirmed the benefit with clozapine (Claghorn et al. 1987; Borison et al. 1988; Breier et al. 1994; Rosenheck et al. 1997). There is some evidence that relatively low doses may be sufficient to achieve a response in patients showing signs of resistance to conventional antipsychotic treatment early in their illness (Joffe et al. 1997). However, Grassi et al. (1999) raised the issue of possible loss of clinical efficacy with repeated trials of clozapine. They described three patients with schizophrenia who had shown a significant clinical improvement with clozapine and had maintained this benefit in the long term but relapsed after deciding to stop the drug. On restarting clozapine, all three patients failed to improve to the level of their initial clinical response.

There have also been claims that the drug has a specific positive effect on hostility and aggression in schizophrenia (Buchanan 1995; Buckley et al. 1995; Glazer & Dickson 1998; Volavka 1999) and symptoms of disorganization, and affective symptoms in patients with schizoaffective disorder (Meltzer 1995). In addition, there is evidence that clozapine, along with certain other atypical antipsychotics, is significantly more effective than conventional antipsychotics at improving cognitive function (Keefe et al. 1999; Lee & Yang 1999; Meltzer & McGurk 1999), one of the most consistent findings being that clozapine improves verbal fluency and attention.

The impact of clozapine on suicide has not been formally assessed. However, evidence from retrospective analyses of cohorts treated with clozapine, and projected suicide mortality rates, suggests that patients receiving this drug may have a lower rate of suicide than expected (Meltzer & Okayli 1995; Reid et al. 1998; Munro et al. 1999). The mechanism for any such an effect remains uncertain, although it has been postulated that improvement in symptoms, including depressive features, may be relevant, as might reduced extrapyramidal symptoms, better medication compliance, improved cognitive function and greater involvement and support from the clinical team, partly related to the regular blood testing (Meltzer 2000). Nevertheless, one study designed to assess the impact of clozapine on suicide (Sernyak et al. 2001) failed to demonstrate any positive effect. A cohort of 1415 patients started on clozapine as inpatients over a 4-year period was followed up for 3 years after discharge. When compared with a control group of 2830 patients with schizophrenia, the clozapine-treated patients were less likely to have died, but the investigators judged that this was entirely attributable to fewer deaths from respiratory disorders. There were no significant differences between the two groups in respect of suicide or accidental death. Further data relevant to this issue are awaited from the International Suicide Prevention Trial (InterSePT). This is a large prospective multicentre randomized controlled trial of suicide comparing clozapine and olanzapine in patients with a recent history of suicidality (Meltzer 1999).

Maintenance treatment

The Cochrane systematic review of clozapine studies (Wahlbeck et al. 2001) stated that, in the short term, participants in clozapine trials had fewer relapses than those patients receiving conventional drugs. The review concluded that 'this may be true for long-term treatment as well', reflecting the paucity of long-term controlled studies. For most studies, rehospitalization is taken as the main measure of relapse.

Retrospective observational studies of clozapine yield markedly lower readmission rates for clozapine in comparison with conventional drugs (Revicki et al. 1990; Reid et al. 1998). For example, observational retrospective mirror image studies have shown significant reductions in the number of hospitalizations in the 3 years or so following a switch to clozapine, compared with the same period before, when patients were receiving conventional antipsychotics (Pollack et al. 1998; Drew et al. 1999).

A randomized open trial compared the effectiveness of clozapine and conventional antipsychotics (Essock et al. 1996) in 227 long-term inpatients who were refractory to standard treatment. The two groups showed no difference in likelihood of discharge from hospital. For the clozapine patients ($n = 76$) and usual care group ($n = 48$) who did leave hospital, those receiving clozapine were more likely to survive out of hospital ($P < 0.05$) over a 2-year period. However, the difference between the two groups was more modest than in the non-randomized studies. The only relevant double-blind randomized study (Rosenheck et al. 1999) compared clozapine (100–900 mg/day) with haloperidol (5–30 mg/day) plus benztropine in 423 patients at 15 Veterans' Affairs Medical Centres. Significantly more (57%) clozapine-treated patients continued on the assigned treatment for the full year, compared with only 28% of the haloperidol group. Also, significantly more haloperidol patients discontinued because of worsening of symptoms or lack of efficacy (51%) in comparison to clozapine (15%). Overall, a higher proportion of patients on clozapine showed improvement (defined as reduction of 20% or more on key scales of mental state and quality of life) at 1 year, at a trend level. If relapse is defined as failure to maintain such improvement, then there was no difference in relapse between the two groups (see also Chapter 25).

Adverse effects

The side-effect profile of clozapine overlaps with the range of side-effects expected with conventional antipsychotic drugs, which include postural hypotension and sedation. The main advantage is the lower liability for EPSs such as parkinsonism and akathisia. In the study by Kane *et al.* (1988), EPSs were significantly lower in those patients treated with clozapine over 6 weeks. This was despite relatively high doses of clozapine, up to 900 mg/day, and the administration of a combination of chlorpromazine and an antiparkinsonian agent (benztropine) in the comparison group. Gerlach *et al.* (1996) found that patients with chronic schizophrenia treated with clozapine for an average of 5 years exhibited fewer parkinsonian signs, such as hypokinesia, rigidity and tremor, than patients receiving long-term treatment with conventional antipsychotics. Similarly, Kurz *et al.* (1995) reported on the EPSs developing in 92 patients receiving their initial 12 weeks of treatment with clozapine, and 59 patients receiving haloperidol. The cumulative incidence rates for both tremor and bradykinesia were lower in the clozapine-treated group (24% and 22% respectively) compared with the haloperidol group (39% and 48% respectively) although only the latter difference was statistically significant.

Clinical studies with clozapine have also found a lower liability for akathisia. The comparative study of clozapine and haloperidol by Kurz *et al.* (1995) found an incidence of 6% for akathisia in the clozapine-treated patients, compared with 32% for the haloperidol group. Wirshing *et al.* (1990) found that changing from a conventional antipsychotic to clozapine was effective in a case of apparently treatment-resistant akathisia. Nevertheless, some investigators have found the prevalence and severity of akathisia with clozapine to be similar to that of conventional antipsychotics (Claghorn *et al.* 1987; Cohen *et al.* 1991). Umbricht and Kane (1996) attribute these discrepant findings to a carry-over effect from previous medication, as the prevalence of akathisia appears to fall with continued clozapine treatment.

Side-effects more characteristic of clozapine include weight gain, tachycardia, sedation and daytime sleepiness, and seizures. Review of the full range of cardiovascular, endocrine and neurological side-effects associated with this drug are beyond the scope of this chapter, and the reader is referred to Chapters 29 and 30 and relevant reviews (Alvir *et al.* 1993; Umbricht & Kane 1996; Miller 2000; Ung Gu Kang *et al.* 2000; McIntyre *et al.* 2001).

Constipation is common, presumably related to the anticholinergic activity, and there is a risk of progress to signs of gastrointestinal obstruction with the additional administration of other medication with anticholinergic effects, such as tricyclic antidepressants and antiparkinsonian medication. Two potentially embarrassing problems for patients are hypersalivation and enuresis, although the latter is typically transitory (Warner *et al.* 1994). However, the most serious risk is the development of agranulocytosis (a reduction in the absolute neutrophil count to below 500/mm³), a problem that necessitates rigorous haematological monitoring. Compared with conventional antipsychotics, the cumulative incidence is greater with clozapine, generally found to be a little less than 0.8% (Atkin *et al.* 1996; Umbricht & Kane 1996; Munro *et al.* 1999). A detailed pharmacovigilance study of over 6000 patients treated with clozapine in the UK and Ireland found that 2.9% developed neutropenia and 0.8% developed agranulocytosis, with a peak incidence of both disorders in the first 6–18 weeks of treatment (Munro *et al.* 1999). The agranulocytosis proved to be reversible in all but two cases, giving a mortality rate of 0.016%. Honigfeld *et al.* (1998) examined US data from the Clozaril National Registry over the period of 1990–94. Out of 99 502 patients administered clozapine, a total of 382 had developed agranulocytosis, an incidence of 0.38%. On the basis of the expected agranulocytosis rate, these authors calculated that up to 149 deaths might have been anticipated, although the actual number was 12.

A Cochrane review by Wahlbeck *et al.* (2001) concluded that, within the context of clinical trials, the potentially dangerous blood white cell decline with clozapine seemed to be more frequent in children and adolescents and in the elderly than in young adults or middle-aged people. This is not entirely consistent with the findings of the UK database study (Munro *et al.* 1999), which identified increasing age and being Asian as key risk factors. Generally, more than 80% of cases occur in the first 3 months of treatment (Owens 1996), with the median length of time before the development of agranulocytosis being 60 days. Those patients developing agranulocytosis usually show recovery within 4–21 days of stopping clozapine.

Clozapine, like other antipsychotic medications, can reduce the seizure threshold, sometimes resulting in major motor seizures or myoclonus (Devinsky *et al.* 1991). The incidence of clozapine-related seizures has been variously estimated at between 0.8% and 20% (Welch *et al.* 1994). This variation probably reflects differences in the characteristics of the patient samples studied, the drug doses used, the duration of treatment and, possibly, the size of dosage increments. When Pacia and Devinsky (1994) monitored over 5000 patients treated with clozapine during the first 6 months after the drug was introduced in the USA, they found an incidence of seizures of 1.3%. Seizures tended to occur at a dosage around 600 mg/day during the maintenance phase, although patients with a history of seizures or epilepsy were at risk of fits even at the low dosage during the initial phase of treatment. Devinsky *et al.* (1991) estimated the cumulative incidence of seizures as 10% over 10 years of treatment. If fits develop, the Clozaril Monitoring Service in the UK advises that clozapine is stopped for 24 h and then restarted at 50% of the dose. Successful rechallenge with the drug is possible at a reduced dosage or with a more gradual dose increase. In a group of patients who had developed seizures while receiving clozapine, Welch *et al.* (1994) managed to avoid further seizures during rechallenge by titrating the dose against EEG findings. If the problem appears to be either one of individual patient susceptibility or related to a high maintenance dose, then anticonvulsant cover is probably indicated. Sodium valproate is the appropriate anticonvulsant in this situation. Carbamazepine is contraindicated because of its potential for causing agranulocytosis, and phenytoin induces the hepatic metabolism of clozapine (see also Chapter 28).

Other atypical antipsychotics (see also Chapters 23 and Chapter 24)

Risperidone

Preliminary findings suggest that risperidone might be of benefit in treatment-resistant schizophrenia (Marder & Meibach 1994; Cavallaro *et al.* 1995; Bondolfi *et al.* 1996; Warner *et al.* 1996). However, subsequent controlled studies (Bondolfi *et al.* 1998; Flynn *et al.* 1998; Wahlbeck *et al.* 2000; Azorin *et al.* 2001) have not provided convincing evidence of equivalence between risperidone and clozapine in treatment-resistant schizophrenia (Gilbody *et al.* 2002). However, the findings suggest that in a patient with poor response to conventional antipsychotics, a trial of risperidone may be worthwhile considering before embarking upon treatment with clozapine.

In a sample of 67 subjects with treatment-resistant schizophrenia, Wirshing *et al.* (1999) compared risperidone (6 mg/day) and haloperidol (15 mg/day) at fixed doses for 4 weeks, followed by flexible dosage for a further 4 weeks. Although risperidone showed some superior efficacy in the first 4 weeks, on the basis of BPRS scores, this was not maintained over the subsequent 4 weeks of blind treatment, during which time the dosage regimens were flexible. During this flexible-dose phase, mean daily dosage for risperidone and haloperidol increased to 7.5 and 19.4 mg respectively. Risperidone was better tolerated in that it was associated with significantly less akathisia and a lower use of anticholinergic medication. As the investigators note, the latter could have been a possible clue to treatment group, with the risk of compromising the blindness of the treatment.

Bouchard *et al.* (2000) examined the clinical effectiveness of risperidone over 12 months in a naturalistic study of 184 patients with chronic schizophrenia whose response to conventional antipsychotics was judged to be 'suboptimal' in that they had baseline total Positive and Negative Syndrome Scale (PANSS) score between 60 and 120. Patients were randomly assigned to be switched to risperidone or receive a conventional drug. On the basis of these findings, the investigators suggested that negative symptoms and general psychopathology, measured by PANSS subscales, may tend to improve early with risperidone, whereas the maximum improvement in positive symptoms occurs later.

In a controlled study by Bondolfi *et al.* (1998) 86 inpatients with chronic schizophrenia were assigned to treatment with either risperidone or clozapine for 8 weeks, in flexible dosage regimens. About two-thirds of the patients maintained doses of risperidone 6 mg/day or clozapine 300 mg/day. By the end of 6 weeks, the mean daily doses for risperidone and clozapine were 6.4 and 291 mg respectively. As the investigators noted, while the latter dose might be considered in line with European prescribing practice, it is low by US standards (Fleischhacker *et al.* 1994; Pollack *et al.* 1995). The criterion for clinical response was a 20% reduction in total PANSS score, and by the end of the study, 67% of risperidone-treated patients and 65% of those receiving clozapine were clinical responders according to this criterion. These figures are relatively high in comparison to similar clinical trials in treatment-resistant schizophrenia. This may be partly related to nature of the patient sample, which included patients who were intolerant of, rather than unresponsive to, conventional antipsychotics, and who therefore might be expected to show a better response to an atypical drug (Lieberman *et al.* 1994).

Azorin *et al.* (2001) noted that there were methodological problems with previous comparisons of risperidone and clozapine in patients with treatment refractory schizophrenia, such as small sample sizes and the use of suboptimal clozapine doses. They sought to overcome these deficiencies in their own prospective double-blind study comparing the two drugs. The criteria for treatment resistance set by these investigators were less rigorous than those used by Kane *et al.* (1988). The aim was to recruit a study sample that would be more representative of the patients treated with clozapine in clinical practice. Over the 12–week study period, the magnitude of response in the BPRS and Clinical Global Impression (CGI) scores was significantly greater in the clozapine group, with the proportion of responders (defined as those with a 20% or greater decrease in BPRS score) being 86% for clozapine patients and 70% for those treated with risperidone. Such response rates are higher than those seen in other treatment trials with treatment-resistant schizophrenia, and part of the explanation may lie in the broader criteria for treatment resistance that were used. For the patients completing the full 12 weeks of the study, the median final daily doses of clozapine and risperidone were 600 and 9 mg respectively. The latter, as the investigators discussed, may be seen as rather high in relation to current clinical practice. During the flexible dosage phase of the study, there was an increase in the dosage of risperidone while the clozapine dosage remained relatively steady. The reasons for this may include the guideline in the protocol that clinicians should increase the dosage for a patient if the response criterion had yet to be achieved.

Olanzapine

As with risperidone, early clinical reports suggested a possible role for high-dose olanzapine in the management of treatment-resistant schizophrenia (Martin *et al.* 1997; Sheitman *et al.* 1997; Baldacchino *et al.* 1998; Launer 1998) but the evidence from controlled studies (Conley *et al.* 1998; Tollefson *et al.* 2001) has not been entirely consistent. Whether, as Dursun *et al.* (1999) suggest, moderate to high dosages of olanzapine (up to 40 mg/day) offer an advantage over standard dosage for patients with treatment-resistant schizophrenia, remains to be determined.

Conley *et al.* (1998) tested the value of olanzapine in treatment-resistant schizophrenia in a fixed-dose double-blind trial using a study design almost identical to that of Kane *et al.* (1988). The criteria for treatment resistance differed from those applied by Kane *et al.* (1988) only in the stipulation that patients should have failed to respond to two, rather than three, defined trials of antipsychotic medication. Olanzapine 25 mg/day was compared with a combination of chlorpromazine 1200 mg/day and benztropine mesylate 4 mg/day over 6 weeks. No difference in efficacy between the two drug regimens emerged. The response criterion for significant clinical improvement was met by only 7% of the patients receiving olanzapine and none of the chlorpromazine patients. Thus, neither drug was associated with major symptomatic improvement, although olanzapine showed a better side-effect profile.

To examine response to clozapine after a lack of response to olanzapine, those patients in this study receiving olanzapine who failed to fulfil the response criterion of a 20% or greater improvement in total BPRS score were studied further (Conley et al. 1999). Thus, 27 treatment-refractory and olanzapine-unresponsive patients received a subsequent 8-week open trial of clozapine (mean dosage 693 mg/day). Eleven (41%) met the criteria for response with clozapine. The investigators concluded that a lack of response to olanzapine does not predict failure with clozapine.

More positive data on the efficacy of olanzapine in treatment-refractory schizophrenia come from a double-blind comparison (Tollefson et al. 2001) of flexible dose regimens of olanzapine (15–25 mg/day) and clozapine (200–600 mg/day) over 18 weeks. The study sample was 180 patients with schizophrenia who fulfilled criteria for treatment resistance (which included failure to respond to adequate trials of at least two oral antipsychotics of different chemical classes and a minimum score of 45 on the BPRS). The trial was designed as a 'non-inferiority' or therapeutic equivalence study. Using the response criteria adopted by Kane et al. (1988), the proportions of responders in the olanzapine (38%) and clozapine (34.5%) groups were similar. Overall, these investigators concluded that both agents were comparably effective in patients with treatment-refractory schizophrenia, and that olanzapine was better tolerated. The investigators discussed the apparent discrepancy between their results and those of Conley et al. (1998). They speculated that in the latter study the patient sample might have been especially refractory. They also discussed issues relating to dose selection. They considered the potential impact of the slow dose titration when initiating clozapine as against the relatively rapid dose increase possible with olanzapine. They also noted that in the majority of patients receiving olanzapine the dose was increased to the top of the authorized range. For clozapine, the mean daily dose was 303.6 mg, which might be considered low, at least by US standards.

Volavka et al. (2002) reported comparable efficacy between clozapine and olanzapine in a double-blind comparative study of olanzapine, clozaine, risperidone and haloperidol in treatment-refactory schizophrenia.

Quetiapine

The potential benefits offered to patients with treatment-refractory schizophrenia by quetiapine remain uncertain, but the indications from case reports (Baird 1999; Reznik et al. 2000; Brooks 2001) and published studies (Emsley et al. 2000; Buckley et al. 2001) warrant further controlled trials.

Emsley et al. (2000) screened a sample of patients with a history of partial response to antipsychotic medication with a prospective 4-week trial of fluphenazine 20 mg/day. The 288 subjects showing a poor response were then assigned to 8 weeks of treatment with either quetiapine 600 mg/day or what might be considered a relatively high dosage of haloperidol, 20 mg/day. In this international multicentre double-blind study, a criterion threshold for response of at least a 20% reduction in PANSS total score was used. On this basis, a significantly greater proportion (52%) of the quetiapine-treated patients were classified as responders compared with those receiving haloperidol (38%).

A recent subanalysis by Buckley et al. (2001) of the main quetiapine – haloperidol/study (Emsley et al. 2000) compared quetiapine 600 mg/day with haloperidol 20 mg/day over 8 weeks in treatment-resistant schizophrenic patients who had prospectively failed to respond to fluphenazine (20 mg/day) for 4 weeks. The criterion for response was a 20% reduction in PANSS score from baseline or a CGI score of less than 3. Of 95 patients failing to respond to fluphenazine, 54 were randomized to quetiapine and 41 to haloperidol. At 8 weeks, using the PANSS-based criterion, 59% of the quetiapine-treated patients were classified as responders compared with 38% of the haloperidol-treated patients. Using the CGI criterion, 51% and 25% of quetiapine and haloperidol patients, respectively, were classified as responders. The authors conclude that quetiapine 600 mg/day is significantly more effective than haloperidol 20 mg/day in treatment-resistant schizophrenia, but the absolute levels or change on the primary outcome variable, the PANSS total score, was modest. The principal benefit was seen in the CGI, which is based upon a subjective global clinical assessment.

Adjunctive pharmacological treatments

Mood stabilizers

Lithium

The use of adjunctive lithium in patients with treatment-refractory schizophrenia showed promise in early studies (Growe et al. 1979; Carmen et al. 1981; Small et al. 1975) but later studies tended not to find the same degree of improvement (Collins et al. 1991; Wilson 1993; Terao et al. 1995). Some of these studies are open to criticism regarding their small sample sizes and lack of rigorous criteria for treatment unresponsiveness. Overall, the findings of the published trials do not allow for confident statements about the potential value of adjunctive lithium (Conley & Buchanan 1997). There is some evidence that the combination is more likely to benefit those patients exhibiting affective symptoms (Wilson 1993). Improvement, when reported, has not been limited to such symptoms but, rather, has involved various areas of functioning, including thought disorder, social competence, irritability, hostility and psychotic excitement (Delva & Letemendia 1986; Christison *et al.* 1991). Specifically in respect of reports of lithium augmentation of clozapine (Bryois & Ferrero 1993), Chong and Remington (2000) noted the absence of controlled studies examining this combination.

Schulz *et al.* (1999) reported on a sample of 44 poor or partially responsive patients with schizophrenia who were unable to be stabilized despite 6 months of traditional antipsychotics and family treatment. They were randomly assigned to antipsychotic plus lithium or antipsychotic plus placebo for 8 weeks. This trial failed to show significant superiority for lithium as an adjunct, with no significant differences in response emerging between the two treatment groups. The authors noted that some patients went on to respond to clozapine – thus indicating their capacity to respond. Despite such disappointing results, the previous reports of success with lithium augmentation may tempt clinicians to use such a strategy. However, the strategy should be used with care, as there are potential adverse drug interactions. Delirium, encephalopathy and neurotoxicity have all been reported (Cohen & Cohen 1974; Miller & Menninger 1987; Lee & Yang 1999). Such complications are said to be unlikely to occur when the plasma lithium level is maintained below 0.5 mmol/L, and seem to reverse when the treatment is stopped. Chong and Remington (2000) cite reports of neurological symptoms, myoclonus, diabetic ketoacidosis and agranulocytosis in patients receiving both clozapine and lithium, but they note that the attribution of these adverse effects to the drug combination is uncertain as they have also been observed with clozapine monotherapy.

Carbamazepine and sodium valproate

Mood stabilizers such as sodium valproate and carbamazepine have been considered as useful adjunctive treatments for schizophrenic patients who have proved to be refractory to antipsychotics alone (Neppe 1988), although only the latter have been systematically assessed in clinical trials. The rationale for their use relates to their antiepileptic efficacy and the observation that patients with schizophrenia who manifest violent behaviour frequently exhibit EEG abnormalities. Neppe (1983) conducted a double-blind study of chronically psychotic patients with temporal lobe abnormalities on EEG, observed in the absence of any overt seizures. Nine out of the 11 patients benefited from concomitant carbamazepine treatment. The selection of patients for trials with carbamazepine may have been influenced by reports that carbamazepine is effective in treating patients with episodic dyscontrol (Stone *et al.* 1986). This is a syndrome characterized by unprovoked aggressive behaviour accompanied by quasi-epileptic phenomena and non-specific abnormalities on the EEG, usually involving the temporal lobe (Maletzky 1973).

Out of nine treatment studies reviewed by Schulz *et al.* (1990), four involved patients specifically labelled as violent. The conclusion was that those patients exhibiting symptoms such as excitement, impulsivity and aggression, and those showing abnormalities on EEG may be more likely to show a beneficial response (Schulz *et al.* 1990; Simhandl & Meszaros 1992). This may partly reflect the original assumptions about appropriate target symptoms. However, the nature of that response is commonly a non-specific improvement in behaviour and social adjustment. However, carbamazepine does not appear to be superior to lithium in its augmenting effect (Schulz *et al.* 1989, 1990), nor does it provide significant benefit when administered independently of neuroleptics (Carpenter *et al.* 1991). Careful serial monitoring of carbamazepine serum levels is advisable. Furthermore, plasma levels of antipsychotics may also require monitoring as carbamazepine is known to influence the metabolism of these drugs (Kahn *et al.* 1990).

Data collected between 1994 and 1996 on every adult inpatient within the facilities of the New York State Office of Mental Health revealed that the use of sodium valproate had more than doubled over the period (Citrome *et al.* 1998). The greatest percentage increase (134%) was in people with schizophrenia. This was not explained by the modest decrease in use of lithium or carbamazepine. A further study by the same authors (Citrome *et al.* 2000) reported additional data up to 1998. From 1994 to 1998 the adjunctive use of valproate nearly tripled in people with schizophrenia. As the authors noted, this use of valproate was outside the approved indications for the drug, and supported by only anecdotal evidence in the literature. They speculated that the popularity of the drug reflected a view that could effectively control irritability, hostility and aggression in such patients.

There is also evidence from case reports that valproate may be useful in the control of aggression in schizophrenia (Morinigo *et al.* 1989; Wassef *et al.* 1989). Further, Dose *et al.* (1998) found a statistically significant effect on 'hostile belligerence' when they tested the value of adjunctive valproate in a double-blind placebo-controlled study. In this study, acute inpatients with schizophrenia or schizoaffective disorder, but without EEG abnormalities or history of epilepsy, were randomly assigned to one of the two treatment regimens. Some evidence of symptom deterioration was reported on withdrawal of valproate after 4 weeks. However, no overall therapeutic benefit was seen for the combination of haloperidol (starting at 6 mg/day with the option of an increase of 3 mg/day every fifth day) and valproate (increased from 300 mg/day until plasma concentrations of 60–90 µg/mL were reached, with a dosage of 900–1200 mg/day) compared with haloperidol plus placebo. The authors concluded that the trend towards lower doses of sedative medication and the effect on hostile belligerence in the valproate-treated group might indicate that the drug has sedative properties and effects on psychomotor agitation and excitement.

Side-effects and interactions may limit the use of carbamazepine. For example, carbamazepine and haloperidol in combination have been reported to cause disorientation and ataxia (Kanter *et al.* 1984; Yerevanian & Hodgman 1985). Carbamazepine is contraindicated in patients receiving clozapine, because of its association with agranulocytosis. Further, carbamazepine is a powerful inducer of the hepatic microsomal enzyme oxidation system, and its introduction may cause a reduction of 50% or more in the plasma level of concurrent antipsychotic drugs (Arana *et al*. 1986; Jann *et al*. 1989; Kahn *et al*. 1990). Phenytoin, another possible option for seizure control, may also diminish clozapine plasma levels (Miller 1991). Valproate has proved to be the most useful anticonvulsant for this purpose (Haller & Binder 1990; Kando *et al*. 1994). However, the combination of clozapine and valproate is not without hazard. Side-effects such as sedation, enuresis, nausea and excessive salivation have been reported as well as hepatic dysfunction (Kando *et al*. 1994; Wirshing *et al*. 1997) and neurotoxicity (Costello & Suppes 1995).

Sodium valproate and lamotrigine as adjuncts to clozapine

Sodium valproate is used in combination with clozapine for two reasons. First, to increase the seizure threshold, and allow patients who have experienced seizures with clozapine to continue on the drug. Secondly, to improve the efficacy of the drug regimen, particularly in respect of disturbed aggressive behaviour. However, as discussed above, the research evidence to support such a strategy is limited.

Wilson (1995) performed a retrospective study of 100 patients receiving clozapine. Assessing 20 patients in whom anticonvulsants (including valproate) had been administered, he considered that they had a poorer outcome than those patients receiving clozapine alone. The explanation was thought to lie with pharmacodynamic or pharmacokinetic interactions between the drugs. However, the evidence for the effect of valproate on clozapine plasma levels is conflicting (Centorrino *et al*. 1994; Finlay & Warner 1994; Longo & Salzman 1995; Chong & Remington 2000).

Dursun *et al*. (1999) reported an open-label non-randomized case series of six outpatients with a 'partial response' to clozapine. Lamotrigine, an anticonvulsant and mood stabilizer, was added to the maximum tolerated dose of clozapine, the initial dose of 12.5 mg/day being subsequently titrated according to response. The consistent improvement in baseline BPRS scores led the investigators to conclude that clozapine plus lamotrigine might be a useful augmentation strategy for treatment-resistant schizophrenia, and warranted further study.

Benzodiazepines

Benzodiazepines are commonly prescribed in treatment-refractory schizophrenia to tackle symptoms of agitation, anxiety, irritability and distress. The majority of double-blind studies of adjunctive benzodiazepines in treatment-refractory patients have provided evidence for a positive treatment effect, but only in the short term (Lingjaerde *et al*. 1982; Wolkowitz *et al*. 1992), although the drugs are often used in the long term (Paton *et al*. 2000). The studies have generally reported improvement in symptoms such as anxiety, tension, hostility and excitement (Csernansky *et al*. 1988; Wolkowitz *et al*. 1988), with no convincing evidence for a specific antipsychotic effect. While no reliable clinical predictors of response have been identified, there is

some suggestion that prominent psychotic or anxiety symptoms, or high levels of motor tension, agitation or retardation are associated with a more favourable outcome (Wolkowitz & Pickar 1991; Johns & Thompson 1995). Although the use of adjunctive benzodiazepine treatment with clozapine is relatively common, according to Chong and Remington (2000) no studies have systematically examined the efficacy of this combination.

The potential hazards of benzodiazepines in treatment-resistant cases include disinhibition with aggressive impulsive behaviour (Pato *et al*. 1989), the risk of dependency and a rebound worsening of symptoms on drug withdrawal (Nestoros *et al*. 1983; Wolkowitz *et al*. 1990). Because of the reports of potentially fatal instances of orthostatic and cardiorespiratory dysregulation when benzodiazepines have been added to an existing clozapine regimen (Sassim & Grohmann 1988; Grohmann *et al*. 1989), it is recommended that such a strategy is used with caution (Conley & Buchanan 1997; Faisal *et al*. 1997). Chong and Remington (2000) cite reports of hypersalivation, lethargy, delirium, ataxia and loss of consciousness with this combination.

Antidepressants

Antidepressant medication can have a significant role in the treatment of the poorly responsive schizophrenic patient – especially as the concept of persistent illness has broadened in recent years. Augmentation strategies for refractory schizophrenia previously focused on a reduction of global or psychotic symptoms using agents such as lithium, carbamazepine or alprazolam. Building on studies of the use of tricyclic antidepressants, recent research in persistently ill schizophrenic patients has indicated there may be a role for the new *selective serotonin reuptake inhibitors (*SSRIs*)* for comorbid depression, negative symptoms, comorbid substance abuse and obsessive–compulsive symptoms. Evidence supporting the use of antidepressants for these indications and comments on safety are described.

Comorbid depression in schizophrenia

In years past, psychiatrists were not assertive in treating depression in schizophrenia with additional medication. Psychodynamic formulations pointed toward talking therapy as the appropriate treatment. Also, there was concern that psychosis could be reactivated by the administration of 'stimulating' antidepressants. Work by Siris *et al*. (1987) during the 1980s focused on the differential diagnoses of depression in schizophrenia – especially differentiation from drug-induced parkinsonism. This work demonstrated the usefulness of tricyclic antidepressants in this patient group – as well as the safety. Siris *et al*. (1993) suggested that where depressive symptoms are persistent, a 6-week trial of an adjunctive antidepressant is considered. Although the patients in these studies were not treatment-resistant by the criteria set by Kane *et al*. (1988), the presence of depression in a schizophrenic patient indicates the lack of a complete response and is associated with increased morbidity and even increased mortality. Building on the efficacy of antidepressant treatment for depressed schizophrenic patients, several groups of investigators have explored the use of SSRIs added to clozapine.

SSRIs and clozapine

When the new SSRIs were approved, their effects on negative symptoms when added to conventional antipsychotic regimens were examined (Goff *et al.* 1991; Silver & Nasser 1992). Evins and Goff (1996) concluded that substantial improvement in negative symptoms had been shown in the placebo-controlled studies involving fluoxetine and fluvoxamine. Examining the effects of fluoxetine to clozapine treatment in non-responders, Goff *et al.* (1991) noted that positive and negative symptoms as well as depression were improved. However, a double-blind placebo-controlled trial of fluoxetine augmentation (Buchanan *et al.* 1996) was not positive: no significant differences in symptoms emerged between the treatment groups.

Since then, other groups have examined the impact of other SSRIs added to clozapine to look for both behavioural and pharmacokinetic effects (Hiemke *et al.* 1994, 1996; Spina *et al.* 1998). Anghelescu *et al.* 1998) reported positive behavioural effects of paroxetine added to clozapine and noted no change in clozapine blood levels. In one case report, a fatality was noted in a person administered a combination of clozapine and fluoxetine (Ferslew *et al.* 1998). That fluoxetine may have an impact on clozapine and its metabolites is supported by a study by Spina *et al.* (1998) in which levels of clozapine, norclozapine and N-oxide were increased by 58%, 36% and 38% respectively. The same group went on to examine other SSRIs and found that paroxetine, but not sertraline, led to increased clozapine levels and again noted that, when using adjunctive SSRIs with clozapine, the monitoring of blood levels may be useful.

Comorbid obsessive–compulsive symptoms with schizophrenia

Obsessive–compulsive symptoms, comorbid with schizophrenia, may sustain the morbidity of the illness. As noted previously, comorbid symptoms are not synonymous with the 'treatment of last resort' category but can markedly diminish functioning. Some research groups have approached this problem in patients stabilized on conventional antipsychotics. In both open (Poyurovsky *et al.* 1999; Reznik & Sirota 2000a) and controlled studies (Reznik & Sirota 2000b), fluvoxamine has proved useful in reducing obsessive–compulsive disorder (OCD) symptoms. In the controlled trial by Reznik and Sirota (2000b), the combination reduced ratings of psychiatric and obsessive–compulsive symptoms by almost one-third.

The issue of OCD in schizophrenia is complicated further by the possibility that OCD symptoms may arise during clozapine treatment (Baker *et al.* 1992). For patients taking clozapine for refractory symptoms, there are often limited treatment alternatives for the prescribing clinician to consider, so the addition of an SSRI is commonly the first step. Given the pharmacokinetic interactions noted above, care should be taken in choosing an SSRI and clozapine blood levels should be monitored.

Comorbid substance abuse in patients with schizophrenia

In evaluating a person with schizophrenia, comorbid substance abuse can also lead to increased morbidity (Selzer & Lieberman 1993). The issues of dysphoric mood and breakthrough psychotic symptoms may lead clinicians to view such patients as 'treatment refractory'. One study by Siris *et al.* (1993) has indicated that antidepressants, added to antipsychotics, may reduce substance use. They note that this may be most useful in the dysphoric patient. As this review was written before front-line atypical antipsychotic medications were available, further studies in this area are warranted. As SSRIs have been shown to be useful for panic disorder, they may be helpful in this area.

In summary, as many researchers and clinicians have broadened their area of concern for the persistently ill patient, the potential for antidepressants to diminish symptoms of schizophrenia or comorbid symptoms has attracted attention. Although there are not many reports, the addition of SSRIs to clozapine may be helpful; however, the most carefully controlled trial was not positive (Buchanan *et al.* 1996). Perhaps more significantly, the antidepressant medications appear constructive for comorbid conditions: depression, OCD and substance abuse.

However, it should be noted that augmenting strategies are difficult to evaluate because of variables of time and potential medication interactions. In clinical practice, consideration should be given to re-evaluation of augmenting agents and an assessment of blood levels.

Electroconvulsive therapy (see also Chapter 27)

The value of electroconvulsive therapy (ECT) as an adjunct to antipsychotic medication in treatment-refractory schizophrenia is rather unclear. Several case reports have suggested that ECT can be helpful in refractory patients (Friedel 1986; Gujavarty *et al.* 1987; Milstein *et al.* 1990). In a retrospective study, Milstein *et al.* (1990) reported improvement in 60 (55%) of 110 treatment-refractory patients treated with ECT. In a prospective study, Chanpattana *et al.* 1999) treated 114 patients with treatment-resistant schizophrenia with ECT combined with flupenthixol 12–24 mg/day. Response criteria were met by 58 patients, 51 of whom entered a continuation phase of the study, being randomized to either flupenthixol alone, ECT alone or continuing on the combination for a further 6 months. Where either ECT or drug was discontinued, the relapse rate was significantly higher than among those who received the combination of ECT and flupenthixol. However, this study reinforces the concern that any beneficial effects of ECT are generally short-lived. Further, no reliable predictors of response have been identified. Nevertheless, the potential value of maintenance ECT in those refractory patients who have initially benefited from the treatment is probably worthy of further investigation.

Several case reports and case series have addressed specifically the augmentation of clozapine with ECT (Safferman & Munne 1992; Frankenburg *et al.* 1993; Bhatia *et al.* 1998; James & Gray 1999; Kales *et al.* 1999; Kupchik *et al.* 2000). In most cases, ECT was used where patients had proved to be unresponsive to clozapine. Generally, the combination was found to be safe and well tolerated, and effective in a proportion of the patients. However, these reports also suggested that any direct beneficial effects of the ECT may not be sustained (Kales *et al.* 1999). James and Gray (1999) used ECT to facilitate the initiation of clozapine in six patients with treatment-refractory schizophrenia who were refusing the blood tests and/or were non-compliant with the drug. A course of 12 ECTs was given over 6 weeks. These investigators considered that the strategy was successful in that the clinical improvement achieved was maintained after the ECT finished, by which time all the patients were compliant with both clozapine and the haematological monitoring.

Conclusions

The concept of treatment-refractory schizophrenia is a moving target. It has evolved substantially over the past 5 years, particularly with the outcomes of cognition, depression, suicidality and other comorbid conditions (such as substance abuse and persistent violence) coming into sharper focus. Other very meaningful outcomes such as work performance, lifetime aspirations and the notion of 'recovery' remain important to the consideration of treatment-refractory schizophrenia. However, our current advances in treatment have had less appreciable impact on these latter variables which, as yet, have not been operationalized as outcome measures. Related to this, while our field has made substantial progress in objectifying and quantifying treatment response among symptom domains, we still have only a rudimentary appreciation of the relative importance of each domain of response. For example, is a 40% reduction in symptoms equivalent to or more important than a 20% improvement in executive function? Defining the relative relationships between outcome measures and cogently articulating a hierarchy of response that has clinical face validity are key areas for further enquiry and debate.

While there are findings across a range of clinical and neurobiological investigations to allow discrimination between responders and non-responders, no single variable predominates as a reliable predictor of treatment response. It remains incumbent upon us, as researchers, to move towards a multivariate analysis of treatment response. Given the promise of genetics in this era, pharmacogenetics should be one constituent. Imaging, both structural and functional, will be another key component.

It is important to bear in mind that non-response to treatment with conventional antipsychotics is the cornerstone of the modern day definition of treatment-refractory schizophrenia. Available evidence suggests that the atypicals other than clozap-

ine are at least as effective as conventional drugs for refractory patients (Buckley *et al.* 2001). Therefore, one can conceptualize a second level or subgroup of refractory patients – those unresponsive to drugs such as risperidone, olanzapine, quetiapine, amisulpride or ziprasidone. Whether the proportion of refractory patients emanating from an individual trial with any of these agents differs to any great extent remains to be determined. In other words, the question of whether any of the atypical drugs, other than clozapine, is more efficacious than another in severe schizophrenia is still unanswered. Also, the sequence in which the drugs should be used in poorly responsive patients (for example, try drug A, then B, then C, or if A fails go directly to C) is a topic requiring further consideration. On current evidence, clozapine stands alone as the treatment of choice for refractory schizophrenia. When should one go to clozapine, how long should a patient who is not doing well on clozapine continue on this drug, and what is the best option to augment response to clozapine, are important questions in the management of patients with treatment refractory schizophrenia. The evidence available seems to suggest that a trial of risperidone or olanzapine may be worth trying before moving to clozapine. A third level or subgroup of refractory patients is now challenging psychiatrists in clinical practice. These are patients with schizophrenia that have proved to be unresponsive to clozapine. Whether the biology of schizophrenia differs across these three proposed levels of treatment refractoriness is another important question.

Finally, our focus on pharmacotherapy obfuscates the substantial developments in psychosocial therapies, particularly with the application of Assertive Community Treatment and CBT to the management of refractory schizophrenia. The challenge to optimizing treatment response in schizophrenia is to reconfigure (and fund) our mental systems to provide an integrated and comprehensive approach to the care of persons with severe schizophrenia.

References

Adesanya, A. & Pantelis, C. (2001) Adjunctive risperidone treatment in patients with 'clozapine-resistant schizophrenia' [letter]. *Australian and New Zealand Journal of Psychiatry* **34**, 533–534.

Alvir, J.M.J., Lieberman, J.A., Safferman, A.Z. *et al.* (1993) Clozapine-induced agranulocytosis: incidence and risk factors in the United States. *New England Journal of Medicine* **329**, 162–167.

Anghelescu, I., Szegedi, A., Schlegel, S. *et al.* (1998) Combination treatment with clozapine and paroxetine in schizophrenia: safety and tolerability data from a prospective clinical trial. *European Neuropsychopharmacology* **8**, 315–320.

Arana, G.W., Goff, D.C., Friedman, H. *et al.* (1986) Does carbamazepine-induced reduction of plasma haloperidol levels worsen psychotic symptoms? *American Journal of Psychiatry* **143**, 650–651.

Arranz, M., Collier, D., Sodhi, M. *et al.* (1995) Association between clozapine response and allelic variation in 5-HT$_A$ receptor gene. *Lancet* **346**, 281–282.

Arranz, M., Munro, J., Birkett, J. *et al.* (2000) Pharmacogenetic prediction of clozapine response. *Lancet* **355**, 1615–1616.

Atkin, K., Kendall, F., Gould, D. *et al.* (1996) Neutropenia and agranulocytosis in patients receiving clozapine in the UK and Ireland. *British Journal of Psychiatry* **169**, 483–488.

Azorin, J.-M., Spiegel, R., Remington, G. *et al.* (2001) A double-blind comparative study of clozapine and risperidone in the management of sever chronic schizophrenia. *American Journal of Psychiatry* **158**, 1305–1313.

Baird, J.W. (1999) The utility of quetiapine in a patient with a history of poor response to previous treatment. *Journal of Clinical Psychiatry* **60** (Suppl. 23), 15–16.

Baker, R.W., Chengappa, K.N., Baird, J.W. *et al.* (1992) Emergence of obsessive–compulsive symptoms during treatment with clozapine. *Journal of Clinical Psychiatry* **53**, 439–442.

Baldacchino, A.M., Stubbs, J.H. & Nevison-Andrews, D. (1998) The use of olanzapine in non-compliant or treatment-resistant clozapine populations in hospital. *Pharmaceutical Journal* **260**, 207–209.

Baldessarini, R.J., Cohen, B.M. & Teicher, M.H. (1988) Significance of neuroleptic dose and plasma level in the pharmacological treatment of psychosis. *Archives of General Psychiatry* **45**, 79–91.

Barnes, T.R.E., Curson, D.A. & Liddle, P.F. (1989) The nature and prevalence of depression in chronic schizophrenic in-patients. *British Journal of Psychiatry* **154**, 486–491.

Barnes, T.R.E. & McPhillips, M.A. (1995) How to distinguish between the neuroleptic-induced deficit syndrome, depression and disease-related negative symptoms in schizophrenia. *International Clinical Psychopharmacology* **10** (Suppl. 3), 115–121.

Barnes, T.R.E., McEvedy, C.J.B. & Nelson, H.E. (1996) Management of treatment resistant schizophrenia unresponsive to clozapine. *British Journal of Psychiatry* **169** (Suppl. 31), 31–40.

Bartko, G., Frecska, E., Zador, G. & Herczeg, I. (1989) Neurological features, cognitive impairment, and neuroleptic response in schizophrenic patients. *Schizophrenia Research* **2**, 311–313.

Bartlett, E.J., Brodie, J.D., Simkowitz, P. *et al.* (1998) Effects of haloperidol challenge on regional brain metabolism in neuroleptic-responsive and non-responsive schizophrenic patients. *American Journal of Psychiatry* **155**, 337–343.

Beck, A.T., Rush, A.J., Shaw, B.F. & Emery, G. (1979) *Cognitive Therapy of Depression*. Guilford Press, New York.

Beng-Choon, H., Andreasen, N.C. *et al.* (2000) Untreated initial psychosis: its relation to quality of life and symptom remission in first-episode schizophrenia. *American Journal of Psychiatry* **157**, 808–815.

Bhatia, S.C., Bhatia, S.K. & Gupta, S. (1998) Concurrent administration of clozapine and ECT: a successful therapeutic strategy for a patient with treatment resistant schizophrenia. *Journal of ECT* **14**, 280–283.

Bilder, R.M., Goldman, R.S., Robinson, D. *et al.* (2001) Neuropsychology of first-episode patients. *American Journal of Psychiatry* **155**, 337–343.

Birchwood, M., Iqbal, Z., Chadwick, P. *et al.* (2000) Cognitive approach to depression and suicidal thinking in psychosis. *British Journal of Psychiatry* **177**, 516–521.

Bitter, I., Volavka, J. & Scheurer, J. (1991) The concept of the neuroleptic threshold: an update. *Journal of Clinical Psychopharmacology* **11**, 28–33.

Bondolfi, G., Baumann, P. & Dufour, H. (1996) Treatment-resistant schziophrenia: clinical experience with new antipsychotics. *European Neuropsychopharmacology* **6**, S2–S25.

Bondolfi, G., Dufour, H., Patris, M. *et al.* on behalf of the Risperidone Study Group (1998) Risperidone versus clozapine in treatment-resistant chronic schizophrenia: a randomized double-blind study. *American Journal of Psychiatry* **155**, 499–504.

Borison, R.L., Diamond, B.I. & Sinha, D. (1988) Clozapine withdrawal rebound psychosis. *Psychopharmacology Bulletin* **24**, 260–263.

Bouchard, R.-H., Mérette, C., Pourcher, E. *et al.* & the Quebec Schizophrenia Study Group (2000) Longitudinal comparative study of risperidone and conventional neuroleptics for treating patients with schizophrenia. *Journal of Clinical Psychopharmacology* **20**, 295–304.

Bowers, M.B. Jr, Swigar, J.E. & Jatlow, P.I. (1984) Plasma catecholamine metabolites and early response to haloperidol. *Journal of Clinical Psychiatry* **45**, 249–251.

Breier, A., Buchanan, R.W., Kirkpatrick, B. *et al.* (1994) Effect of clozapine on positive and negative symptoms in outpatients with schizophrenia. *American Journal of Psychiatry* **151**, 20–26.

Brenner, H.D., Dencker, S.J., Goldstein, M.J. *et al.* (1990) Defining treatment refractoriness in schizophrenia. *Schizophrenia Bulletin* **16**, 551–562.

Brooks, J.O. III (2001) Successful outcome using quetiapine in a case of treatment-resistant schizophrenia with assaultive behaviour. *Schizophrenia Research* **50**, 133–134.

Brown, G.W., Birley, J.L.T. & Wing, J.K. (1972) Influences of family life on the course of schizophrenic disorders: a replication. *British Journal of Psychiatry* **121**, 241–258.

Bryois, C. & Ferrero, F. (1993) Clinical observation of 11 patients under clozapine–lithium association. *European Psychiatry* **8**, 213–218.

Buchanan, R.W. (1995) Clozapine: efficacy and safety. *Schizophrenia Bulletin* **21**, 579–591.

Buchanan, R.W., Kirkpatrick, B., Bryant, N., Ball, P. & Breier, A. (1996) Fluoxetine augmentation of clozapine treatment in patients with schizophrenia. *American Journal of Psychiatry* **153**, 1625–1627.

Buchsbaum, M.S., Wu, J.C., DeLisi, L.E. *et al.* (1987) Positron emission tomography studies of basal ganglia and somatosensory cortex neuroleptic drug effects: differences between normal controls and schizophrenic patients. *Biological Psychiatry* **22**, 479–494.

Buchsbaum, M.S., Potkin, S.G., Siegal, B.V. *et al.* (1992) Striatal metabolic rate and clinical response to neuroleptics in schizophrenia. *Archives of General Psychiatry* **49**, 966–974.

Buckley, P.F. (1998) Substance abuse and schizophrenia: a review. *Journal of Clinical Psychiatry* **59**, 26–30.

Buckley, P.F. (1999) Endocrine and metabolic effects of typical and atypical antipsychotics: contemporary clinical experience. In: *Managing the Side Effects of Drug Therapy in Schizophrenia* (ed. J.M. Kane), pp. 40–57. Scientific Press, London.

Buckley, P.F. (2001) Comparison of the effects of quetiapine and haloperidol in a cohort of patients with treatment resistant schizophrenia. *Schizophrenia Research* **49**, 221.

Buckley, P.F., Thompson, P., Way, L. *et al.* (1994) Substance use among patients with treatment resistant schizophrenia: characteristics and implications for clozapine therapy. *American Journal of Psychiatry* **151**, 385–389.

Buckley, P.F., Bartell, J., Donenwirth, K. *et al.* (1995) Violence and schizophrenia: clozapine as a specific antiaggressive agent. *Bulletin of the American Academy of Psychiatry and the Law* **23**, 607–611.

Buckley, P.F., Krowinski, A.C. & Miller, D.D. (2001) Clinical and biochemical correlates of 'high dose' clozapine therapy for treatment-refractory schizophrenia. *Schizophrenia Research* **49**, 223–229.

Cannon, M., Jones, P., Huttunen, M.O. *et al.* (1999) School performance in Finnish children and later development of schizophrenia: a population based longitudinal study. *Archives of General Psychiatry* **56**, 457–463.

Carmen, J.S., Bigelow, L.B. & Wyatt, R.J. (1981) Lithium combined with neuroleptics in chronic schizophrenic and schizoaffective patients. *Journal of Clinical Psychiatry* **42**, 124–128.

Carpenter, W.T., Kurz, R., Kirkpatrick, B. *et al.* (1991) Carbamazepine maintenance treatment in outpatient schizophrenics. *Archives of General Psychiatry* **48**, 69–72.

Cavallaro, R., Colombo, C. & Smeraldi, E. (1995) A pilot, open study on the treatment of refractory schizophrenia with risperidone and clozapine. *Human Psychopharmacology* 10, 231–234.

Centorrino, F., Baldessarini, R.J., Kando, J. *et al.* (1994) Serum concentrations of clozapine and its major metabolite effects of cotherapy with fluoxetine or valproate. *American Journal of Psychiatry* 151, 123–125.

Chakos, M.H., Lieberman, J.A., Bilder, R.M. *et al.* (1994) Increase in caudate nuclei volumes of first-episode schizophrenic patients taking antipsychotic drugs. *American Journal of Psychiatry* 151, 1430–1436.

Chakos, M.H., Lieberman, J.A., Hoffman, E. *et al.* (2001) Effectiveness of second generation antipsychotics in patients with treatment-resistant schizophrenia: a review and meta-analysis of randomized trials. *American Journal of Psychiatry* 158, 518–526.

Chanpattana, W., Chakrabhand, M.L., Sackeim, H.A. *et al.* (1999) Continuation ECT in treatment-resistant schizophrenia: a controlled study. *Journal of ECT* 15, 178–192.

Cheine, M.X., Wahlbeck, K. & Rimón, R. (1999) Pharmacological treatment of schizophrenia resistant to first-line treatment: a critical systematic review and meta-analysis. *International Journal of Psychiatry in Clinical Practice* 3, 159–169.

Chong, S.-A. & Remington, G. (2000) Clozapine augmentation. *Schizophrenia Bulletin* 26, 421–440.

Chong, S.-A., Tan, C.H. & Lee, H.S. (1996) Hoarding and clozapine-risperidone combination. *Canadian Journal of Psychiatry* 41, 315–316.

Christison, G.W., Kirch, D.G. & Wyatt, R.J. (1991) When symptoms persist: choosing among alternative somatic treatments for schizophrenia. *Schizophrenia Bulletin* 17, 217–245.

Citrome, L., Levine, J. & Allingham, B. (1998) Utilization of valproate: extent of inpatient use in the New York state office of mental health. *Psychiatric Quarterly* 4, 283–300.

Citrome, L., Levine, J. & Allingham, B. (2000) Changes in the use of valproate and other mood stabilizers for patients with schizophrenia from 1994 to 1998. *Psychiatric Services* 51, 634–638.

Claghorn, J., Honigfeld, G., Abuzzahab, F.S. *et al.* (1987) The risks and benefits of clozapine versus chlorpromazine. *Journal of Psychopharmacology* 7, 377–384.

Cohen, B.M., Keck, P.E., Satlin, A. & Cole, J.O. (1991) Prevalence and severity of akathisia in patents on clozapine. *Biological Psychiatry* 29, 1215–1219.

Cohen, B.M., Nordahl, T.E., Semple, W.E. *et al.* (1997) The brain metabolic patterns of clozapine- and fluphenazine-treated patients with schizophrenia during a continuous performance task. *Archives of General Psychiatry* 54, 481–486.

Cohen, W.J. & Cohen, N.H. (1974) Lithium carbonate, haloperidol and irreversible brain damage. *Journal of the American Medical Association* 230, 1283–1287.

Collins, P.J., Larkin, E.P. & Schubsachs, A.P.W. (1991) Lithium carbonate in chronic schizophrenia: a brief trial of lithium carbonate added to neuroleptics for treatment of resistant schizophrenic patients. *Acta Psychiatrica Scandinavica* 84, 150–154.

Conley, R.R. & Buchanan, R.W. (1997) Evaluation of treatment-resistant schizophrenia. *Schizophrenia Bulletin* 23, 663–674.

Conley, R.R., Tamminga, C.A., Bartko, J.J. *et al.* (1998) Olanzapine compared with chlorpromazine in treatment-resistant schizophrenia. *American Journal of Psychiatry* 155, 914–920.

Conley, R.R., Tamminga, C.A., Kelly, D.L. & Richardson, C.M. (1999) Treatment-resistant schizophrenic patients respond to clozapine after olanzapine non-response. *Biological Psychiatry* 46, 73–77.

Costello, L.E. & Suppes, T. (1995) A clinically significant interaction between clozapine and valproate [letter]. *Journal of Clinical Psychopharmacology* 15, 139–141.

Crow, T.J. (1980) Molecular pathology of schizophrenia: more than one disease process? *British Medical Journal* 1, 66–68.

Csernansky, J.G., Riney, S.J., Lombroso, L. *et al.* (1988) Double-blind comparison of alprazolam, diazepam and placebo for the treatment of negative schizophrenic symptoms. *Archives of General Psychiatry* 45, 65–659.

Curson, D.A., Pantelis, C., Ward, J. & Barnes, T.R.E. (1992) Institutionalism and schizophrenia thirty years on: clinical poverty and the social environment in three British mental hospitals in 1960 compared with a fourth in 1990. *British Journal of Psychiatry* 160, 230–241.

Dalen, P. & Hayes, P. (1990) The aetiological heterogeneity of schizophrenia: the problem and the evidence. *British Journal of Psychiatry* 157, 119–122.

Daniel, D.G. & Weinberger, D.R. (1991) *Ex multi uno*: a case for neurobiological homogeneity in schizophrenia. In: *Advances in Neuropsychiatry and Psychopharmacology, Schizophrenia Research*, Vol. 1 (eds. C.A. Tamminga & S.C. Schultz), pp. 227–235. Raven Press, New York.

Danion, J.-M., Rein, W., Fleurot, O. *et al.* (1999) Improvement of schizophrenic patients with primary negative symptoms treated with amisulpride. *American Journal of Psychiatry* 156, 610–616.

Davis, K.L., Buchsbaum, M.S., Shihabuddin, L. *et al.* (1998) Ventricular enlargement in poor-outcome schizophrenia. *Archives of General Psychiatry* 43, 783–793.

DeLisi, L.E., Stritzke, P., Riordan, H. *et al.* (1992) The timing of brain morphological changes in schizophrenia and their relationship to clinical outcome. *Biological Psychiatry* 31, 241–254.

DeLisi, L.E., Sakuma, M., Tew, W. *et al.* (1997) Schizophrenia as a chronic active brain process: a study of progressive brain structural change subsequent to the onset of schizophrenia. *Psychiatry Research* 74, 129–140.

Delva, N.J. & Letemendia, F.J. (1986) Lithium treatment in schizophrenia and schizoaffective disorders. In: *Contemporary Issues in Schizophrenia* (eds A. Kerr & P. Snaith), pp. 381–396. Royal College of Psychiatrists, Gaskell, London.

Devinsky, O., Honigfeld, G. & Patin, J. (1991) Clozapine-related seizures. *Neurology* 41, 369–371.

Dose, M., Hellweg, R., Yassourdis, A., Theison, M. & Emrich, H.M. (1998) Combined treatment of schizophrenic psychosis with haloperidol and valproate. *Pharmacopsychiatry* 31, 122–125.

Drake, R.E., Kie, H., McHugo, G.J. & Green, A.I. (2000) Effect of clozapine on alcohol and drug use disorders among patients with schizophrenia. *Schizophrenia Bulletin* 26, 441–449.

Drew, L.R.H., Hodgson, D.M. & Griffiths, K.M. (1999) Clozapine in community practice: a 3-year follow-up study in the Australian Capital Territory. *Australian and New Zealand Journal of Psychiatry* 33, 667–675.

Duke, P.J., Pantelis, C. & Barnes, T.R.E. (1994) South Westminster Schizophrenia Survey: alcohol use and its relationship to symptoms, tardive dyskinesia and illness onset. *British Journal of Psychiatry* 164, 630–636.

Duke, P.J., Pantelis, C., McPhillips, M.A. & Barnes, T.R.E. (2001) South Westminster Schizophrenia Survey: non-alcohol substance abuse. *British Journal of Psychiatry* 179, 501–513.

Dursun, S.M., McIntosh, D. & Milliken, H. (1999) Clozapine plus lamotrigine in treatment-resistant schizophrenia [letter]. *Archives of General Psychiatry* 56, 950.

Emsley, R., Raniwalla, J., Bailey, P.J. & Jones, A.M. (2000) A comparison of the effects of quetiapine ('seroquel') and haloperidol in schizophrenic patients with a history of and a demonstrated, partial response to conventional antipsychotic treatment: PRIZE Study Group. *International Clinical Psychopharmacology* 15, 121–131.

Essock, S.M., Hargreaves, W.A., Covell, N.H. & Goethe, J. (1996) Clozapine's effectiveness for patients in state hospitals: results from a randomized trial. *Psychopharmacology Bulletin* 32, 683–697.

Evins, A.E. & Goff, D.C. (1996) Adjunctive antidepressant drug therapies in the treatment of negative symptoms. *CNS Drugs* 6, 130–147.

Faisal, I., Lindenmayer, J.P., Taintor, Z. & Cancro, R. (1997) Clozapine–benzodiazepine interactions [letter]. *Journal of Clinical Psychiatry* 58, 547–548.

Falloon, I.R.H., Boyd, J.L., McGill, C.W. *et al.* (1985) Family management in the prevention of morbidity of schizophrenia: clinical outcome of a two year longitudinal study. *Archives of General Psychiatry* 42, 887–896.

Ferslew, K.E., Hagardorn, A.N., Harlan, G.C. & McCormick, W.F. (1998) A fatal drug interaction between clozapine and fluoxetine. *Journal of Forensic Science* 43, 1082–1085.

Finlay, P. & Warner, P. (1994) Potential impact of valproic acid therapy on clozapine disposition. *Biological Psychiatry* 36, 487–488.

Fleischhacker, W.W., Hummer, M., Kurz, M. *et al.* (1994) Clozapine dose in the United States and Europe: implications for therapeutic and adverse effects. *Journal of Clinical Psychiatry* 55 (Suppl. B), 78–81.

Flynn, S.W., MacEwan, G.W., Altman, S. *et al.* (1998) An open comparison of clozapine and risperidone in treatment-resistant schizophrenia. *Pharmacopsychiatry* 31, 25–29.

Frankenburg, F.R., Suppes, T. & McLean, P.E. (1993) Combined clozapine and electroconvulsive therapy. *Convulsive Therapy* 9, 176–180.

Frazier, J.A., Giedd, J.N., Kaysen, D. *et al.* (1996) Childhood-onset schizophrenia: brain MRI rescan after 2 years of clozapine maintenance treatment. *American Journal of Psychiatry* 153, 564–566.

Friedel, R.O. (1986) The combined use of neuroleptics and ECT in drug resistant schizophrenic patients. *Psychopharmacology Bulletin* 22, 928–930.

Friedman, J., Ault, K. & Powchik, P. (1997) Pimozide augmentation for the treatment of schizophrenic patients who are partial responders to clozapine. *Biological Psychiatry* 42, 522–523.

Friedman, L., Knutson, L., Shurell, M. *et al.* (1991) Prefrontal sulcal proiminence is inversely related to clozapine response. *Biological Psychiatry* 29, 865–877.

Friedman, L., Lys, C. & Schultz, S.C. (1992) The relationship of structural brain imaging parameters to antipsychotic treatment response: a review. *Journal of Psychiatry and Neuroscience* 17, 42–54.

Galletly, C. & Clark, R. & McFarlane, A. (2000) The effect of clozapine on the speed and accuracy of information processing in schizophrenia. *Progress in Neuropsychopharmacology and Biological Psychiatry* 24, 1329–1338.

Garver, D.L., Holcomb, J.A. & Christensen, J.D. (2000) Heterogeneity of response to antipsychotics from multiple disorders in the schizophrenia spectrum. *Journal of Clinical Psychiatry* 61, 964–972.

Gerlach, J. & Lublin, H. & Peacock, L. (1996) Extrapyramidal symptoms during long-term treatment with antipsychotics. special focus on clozapine and D_1 and D_2 dopamine antagonists. *Neuropsychopharmacology* 14 (Suppl. 3), 35–39.

Gilbody, S.M. & Bagnall, A.M. & Duggan, L. & Tuunainen, A. (2002) Risperidone versus other atypical antipsychotic medication for schizophrenia (Cochrane Review). In: *The Cochrane Library* 1, Update Software, Oxford.

Glazer, W.M. & Dickson, R.A. (1998) Clozapine reduces violence and persistent aggression in schizophrenia. *Journal of Clinical Psychiatry* 59 (Suppl. 3), 8–14.

Godlesky, L.S. & Sernyak, M.J. (1996) Agranulocytosis after addition of risperidone to clozapine treatment. *American Journal of Psychiatry* 153, 735–736.

Goff, D.C., Brotman, A.W., Waites, M. & McCormick, S. (1991) Trial of fluoxetine added to neuroleptics for treatment-resistant schizophrenic patients. *American Journal of Psychiatry* 148, 274.

Goldberg, S.C. (1985) Negative and deficit symptoms in schizophrenia do respond to neuroleptics. *Schizophrenia Bulletin* 11, 453–456.

Goldberg, T.E., Weinberger, D.R., Berman, K.F., Pliskin, N.H. & Podd, M.H. (1987) Further evidence for dementia of the prefrontal type in schizophrenia? A controlled study of teaching the Wisconsin Card Sorting Test. *Archives of General Psychiatry* 44, 1008–1014.

Goldberg, T.E., Greenberg, R.D., Griffith, S.J. *et al.* (1993) The effect of clozapine on cognitive and psychiatric symptoms in patients with schizophrenia. *British Journal of Psychiatry* 162, 73–78.

Grace, J., Bellus, S.B., Raulin, M.L. *et al.* (1996) Long-term impact of clozapine and psychosocial treatment of psychiatric symptoms and cognitive functioning. *Psychiatric Services* 47, 41–45.

Grassi, B., Ferrari, R., Epifani, M. *et al.* (1999) Clozapine lacks previous clinical efficacy when restarted after a period of discontinuation: a case series. *European Neuropharmacology* 9, 479–481.

Green, M.F. (1996) What are functional consequences of neurocognitive deficits in schizophrenia? *American Journal of Psychiatry* 53, 321–330.

Green, M.F., Marshall, B.D. Jr, Wirshing, W.C. *et al.* (1997) Does risperidone improve verbal working memory in treatment-resistant schizophrenia? *American Journal of Psychiatry* 154, 799–804.

Green, M.F., Kern, R.S., Braff, D.L. *et al.* (2000) Neurocognitive deficits and functional outcome in schizophrenia: are we measuring the 'right stuff'? *Schizophrenia Bulletin* 26, 119–136.

Grohmann, R., Ruther, E., Sassim, N. *et al.* (1989) Adverse effects of clozapine. *Psychopharmacology* 99, S101–S104.

Growe, G.A., Crayton, J.W., Klass, D.B. *et al.* (1979) Lithium in chronic schizophrenia. *American Journal of Psychiatry* 136, 454–455.

Gujavarty, K., Greenberg, L. & Fink, M. (1987) Electroconvulsive therapy and neuroleptic medication in therapy-resistant positive symptom psychosis. *Convulsive Therapy* 3, 185–195.

Gupta, S., Sonnenberg, S.J. & Frank, B. (1998) Olanzapine augmentation of clozapine. *Annals of Clinical Psychiatry* 10, 113–115.

Gur, R.E., Mozley, P.D., Shtasel, D.L. *et al.* (1994) Clinical subtypes of schizophrenia: differences in brain and CSF volume. *American Journal of Psychiatry* 151, 343–350.

Gur, R.E., Cowell, P., Turetsky, B.I. *et al.* (1998) A follow-up magnetic resonance imaging study of schizophrenia: relationship of neuroanatomical changes to clinical and neurobehavioral measures. *Archives of General Psychiatry* 55, 145–152.

Haller, E. & Binder, R.L. (1990) Clozapine seizures. *American Journal of Psychiatry* 147, 1067–1071.

Harrington, M., Lelliot, P., Paton, C. *et al.* (2002) The results of a multicentre audit of the prescribing of antipsychotic drugs for inpatients in the United Kingdom. *Psychiatric Bulletin* (in press).

Harvey, P.D. & Keefe, R.S. (2001) Studies of cognitive change in patients with schizophrenia following novel antipsychotic treatment. *American Journal of Psychiatry* 158, 176–184.

Hasegawa, M., Gutierrez-Esteinou, R., Way, L. & Meltzer, H.Y. (1993) Relationship between clinical efficacy and clozapine concentrations in plasma in schizophrenia: effect of smoking. *Journal of Clinical Psychopharmacology* 13, 383–390.

Heinrichs, D.W., Hanlon, E.T. & Carpenter, W.T. Jr (1984) The Quality of Life Scale: an instrument for rating the deficit syndrome. *Schizophrenia Bulletin* 10, 388–398.

Henderson, D.C. & Goff, D.C. (1996) Risperidone as an adjunct to clozapine therapy in chronic schizophrenics. *Journal of Clinical Psychiatry* 57, 395–397.

Hiemke, C., Weigmann, H., Dahmen, N. *et al.* (1994) Elevated serum levels of clozapine after addition of fluvoxamine. *Journal of Clinical Psychopharmacology* **14**, 279–281.

Hiemke, C., Weigmann, H., Härtter, S. *et al.* (1996) Combination of clozapine and SSRIs in schizophrenic patients. *European Neuropsychopharmacology* **6** (Suppl. 3), 217.

Hirsch, S.R. & Barnes, T.R.E. (1994) Clinical use of high-dose neuroleptics. *British Journal of Psychiatry* **164**, 94–96.

Hogarty, G.E., Anderson, C.M., Reiss, D.J. *et al.* (1991) Family psychoeducation, social skills training, and maintenance chemotherapy in the aftercare treatment of schizophrenia. II. Two-year effects of a controlled study on relapse and adjustment. Environmental-Personal indicators in the Course of Schizophrenia (EPICS) Research Group. *Archives of General Psychiatry* **48**, 340–347.

Holcomb, H.H. & Tamminga, C.A. (2000) Brian blood flow and metabolism in schizophrenia. In: *Schizophrenia in a Molecular Age* (ed. C.A. Tamminga). American Psychiatric Press, Washington, DC.

Honey, G.D., Bullmore, E.T., Soni, W. *et al.* (1999) Differences in frontal cortical activation by a working memory task asfter substitution of risperidone for typical antipsychotic drugs in patients with schizophrenia. Proceedings of the National Academy of Sciences of the USA **96**, 13432–13437.

Honigfeld, G., Arellano, F., Sethi, J., Bianchini, A. & Schein, J. (1998) Reducing clozapine-related morbidity and mortality: 5 years of experience with the Clozaril National Registry. *Journal of Clinical Psychiatry* **59** (Suppl. 3), 3–7.

Hutton, S.B., Puri, B.K., Duncan, L.-J. *et al.* (1998) Executive function in first-episode schizophrenia. *Psychological Medicine* **28**, 463–473.

Illowsky, B., Juliano, D.M., Bigelow, L.B. *et al.* (1988) Stability of CT scan findings in schizophrenia: results of a 8 year follow-up study. *Journal of Neurology, Neurosurgery and Psychiatry* **51**, 209–213.

Jacobson, L.K., Giedd, J.N., Castellanos, F.X. *et al.* (1998) Progressive reduction of temporal lobe structures in childhood-onset schizophrenia. *American Journal of Psychiatry* **155**, 678–685.

James, D.V. & Gray, N.S. (1999) Elective combined electroconvulsive and clozapine therapy. *International Clinical Psychopharmacology* **14**, 69–72.

Jann, M.W., Fidoen, G.S., Hernandez, J.M. *et al.* (1989) Clinical implications of increased antipsychotic plasma concentrations upon anticonvulsant cessation. *Psychiatry Research* **28**, 153–159.

Jaskiw, G.E., Juliano, D.M., Goldberg, T.E. *et al.* (1994) Cerebral ventricle enlargement in schizophreniform disorder does not progress: a seven year follow-up study. *Schizophrenia Research* **14**, 23–28.

Jernigan, T.L., Zisook, S., Heaton, R.K. *et al.* (1991) Magnetic resonance imaging abnormalities in lenticular nuclei and cerebral cortex in schizophrenia. *Archives of General Psychiatry* **48**, 881–890.

Joffe, G., Rybak, J., Burkin, M. *et al.* (1997) Clozapine response in early treatment-resistant schizophrenia. *International Journal of Psychiatry in Clinical Practice* **1**, 261–268.

Johns, C.A. & Thompson, J.W. (1995) Adjunctive treatments in schizophrenia: pharmacotherapies and electroconvulsive therapy. *Schizophrenia Bulletin* **21**, 607–619.

Johnstone, E.C., MacMillan, E.J. Frith, C.D. *et al.* (1990) Further investigation of the predictors of outcome following first schizophrenic episodes. *British Journal of Psychiatry* **157**, 182–189.

Kahn, E.M., Schulz, S.C., Perel, J.M. *et al.* (1990) Change in haloperidol level due to carbamazepine: a complicating factor in combined medication for schizophrenia. *Journal of Clinical Psychopharmacology* **10**, 54–57.

Kaiya, H., Uematsu, M., Ofuji, M. *et al.* (1989) Computerized tomography in schizophrenia: familial versus non-familial forms of illness. *British Journal of Psychiatry* **155**, 444–450.

Kales, H.C., Dequardo, J.R. & Tandon, R. (1999) Combined electroconvulsive therapy and clozapine in treatment-resistant schizophrenia. *Progress in Neuro-Psychopharmacology and Biological Psychiatry* **23**, 547–556.

Kando, J.C., Tohen, M., Castillo, J. & Centorrino, F. (1994) Concurrent use of clozapine and valproate in affective and psychotic disorders. *Journal of Clinical Psychiatry* **55**, 255–257.

Kane, J.M. (1993) Acute treatment. In: *Antipsychotic Drugs and Their Side-Effects* (ed. T.R.E. Barnes), pp. 169–181. Academic Press, London.

Kane, J.M., Honigfeld, G., Singer, J. *et al.* (1988) Clozapine for the treatment-resistant schizophrenic: a double blind comparison with chlorpromazine. *Archives of General Psychiatry* **45**, 789–796.

Kane, J.M., Honigfeld, G., Singer, J. & Meltzer, H.Y. (1990) Is clozapine response different in neuroleptic non-responders versus partial responders? *Archives of General Psychiatry* **47**, 189.

Kanter, G.L., Yerevsanian, B.I. & Ciccone, J.R. (1984) Case report of a possible interaction between neuroleptics and carbamazepine. *American Journal of Psychiatry* **141**, 1101–1102.

Kaplan, M.J., Laff, M., Kelly, K. *et al.* (1990) Enlargement of cerebral third ventricle in psychotic patients with delayed third response to neuroleptics. *Biological Psychiatry* **27**, 205–214.

Kapur, S. & Seeman, P. (2001) Does fast dissociation from the dopamine D receptor explain the action of atypical antipsychotics? A new hypothesis. *American Journal of Psychiatry* **158**, 360–369.

Kapur, S., Zipursky, R., Remingon, G. *et al.* (1997) PET evidence that loxapine is an equipotent blocker of 5-HT and D receptors: implications for the treatment of schizophrenia. *American Journal of Psychiatry* **154**, 1525–1529.

Kapur, S., Zipursky, R. & Remington, G. (1999) Clinical and theoretical implications of 5-HT and D receptor occupancy of clozapine, risperidone, and olanzapine in schizophrenia. *American Journal of Psychiatry* **156**, 286–293.

Kapur, S., Zipursky, R., Jones, C. *et al.* (2000) Relationship between dopamine D occupancy, clinical response, and side effects: a double-blind PET study of first-episode schizophrenia. *American Journal of Psychiatry* **157**, 514–520.

Keck, P.E., Strakowski, S.M. & McElroy, S.L. (2000) The efficacy of atypical antipsychotics in the treatment of depressive symptoms, hostility, and suicidality in patients with schizophrenia. *Journal of Clinical Psychiatry* **56**, 466–470.

Keefe, R., Silva, S., Perkins, D. *et al.* (1999) The effects of atypical antipsychotic drugs on neurocognitive impairment in schizophrenia: a review and meta-analysis. *Schizophrenia Bulletin* **25**, 201–222.

Keshavan, M.S., Bagwell, W.W., Haas, G.L. *et al.* (1994) Changes in caudate volume with neuroleptic treatment. *Lancet* **344**, 1434.

Kingdon, D.G. & Turkington, D. (1991) The use of cognitive behavior therapy with a normalizing rationale in schizophrenia: preliminary report. *Journal of Nervous and Mental Disease* **179**, 201–211.

Kirkpatrick, B., Buchanan, R.W., Ross, D.E. & Carpenter, W.T. Jr. (2001) Separate disease within the syndrome of schizophrenia. *Archives of General Psychiatry* **58**, 165–167.

Kolakowska, T., Williams, A.O., Arden, M. *et al.* (1985) Schizophrenia with good and poor outcome. *British Journal of Psychiatry* **146**, 229–246.

Kopelowicz, A., Zarate, R., Tripodis, K. *et al.* (2000) Differential efficacy of olanzapine for deficit and non-deficit negative symptoms in schizophrenia. *American Journal of Psychiatry* **157**, 987–993.

Koreen, A.R., Lieberman, J.A., Kronig, M. & Cooper, T.B. (1995) Cross-tapering clozapine and risperidone. *American Journal of Psychiatry* **152**, 1690.

Kronig, R.H., Munne, R.A., Szymanski, S. *et al.* (1995) Plasma clozapine levels and clinical response for treatment-refractory schizophrenic patients. *American Journal of Psychiatry* **152**, 179–182.

Kulkarni, J., Riedel, A., de Castella, A.R. *et al.* (2001) Estrogen: a potential treatment for schizophrenia. *Schizophrenia Research* **48**, 137–144.

Kupchik, M., Spivak, B., Mester, R. *et al.* (2000) Combined electroconvulsive–clozapine therapy. *Clinical Neuropharmacology* **23**, 14–16.

Kurz, M., Hummer, M., Oberbauer, H. *et al.* (1995) Extrapyramidal side effects of clozapine and haloperidol. *Psychopharmacolcogy* **118**, 52–56.

Launer, M.A. (1998) High dose olanzapine in treatment resistant schizophrenia. *Schizophrenia Research* **29**, 149–150.

Lay, B., Blanz, B., Hartman, M. *et al.* (2000) The psychosocial outcome of adolescent-onset schizophrenia: a 12-year follow-up. *Schizophrenia Bulletin* **26**, 801–816.

Lee, S.-H. & Yang, Y.-Y. (1999) Reversible neurotoxicity induced by a combination of clozapine and lithium: a case report. *Chinese Medical Journal* **62**, 184–187.

Leppig, M., Bosch, B., Naber, D. & Hippius, H. (1989) Clozapine in the treatment of 121 outpatients. *Psychopharmacology* **99**, S77–S79.

Leung, A. & Chue, P. (2000) Sex differnces in schizophrenia, a review of the literature. *Acta Psychiatrica Scandinavica* **101**, 3–38.

Liberman, R.P., Wallace, C.J., Blackwell, G. *et al.* (1998) Skills training versus psychosocial occupational therapy for persons with persistent schizophrenia. *American Journal of Psychiatry* **155**, 1087–1091.

Liddle, P.F. (2000) Cognitive impairment in schizophrenia: its impact on social functioning. *Acta Psychiatrica Scandinavica* **101**, 11–16.

Liddle, P.F. & Crow, T.J. (1984) Age disorientation in chronic schizophrenia is associated with global intellectual impairment. *British Journal of Psychiatry* **144**, 193–195.

Liddle, P.F., Friston, K.J., Frith, C.D. *et al.* (1992) Patterns of cerebral blood flow in schizophrenia. *British Journal of Psychiatry* **160**, 179–186.

Lieberman, J.A. (1999) Is schizophrenia a neurodegenerative disorder? A clinical and neurobiological perspective. *Biological Psychiatry* **46**, 729–739.

Lieberman, J.A., Jody, D., Geisler, S. *et al.* (1989) Treatment outcome of first-episode schizophrenia. *Psychopharmacology Bulletin* **25**, 92–96.

Lieberman, J.A., Alvir, J.M.J., Woerner, M. *et al.* (1992) Prospective study of psychobiology in first-episode schizophrenia at Hillside Hospital. *Schizophrenia Bulletin* **18**, 351–371.

Lieberman, J.A., Jody, D., Geisler, S. *et al.* (1993) Time course and biological predictors of treatment response in first-episode schizophrenia. *Archives of General Psychiatry* **50**, 369–376.

Lieberman, J.A., Safferman, A.Z., Pollack, S. *et al.* (1994) Clinical effects of clozapine in chronic schizophrenia: response to treatment and predictors of outcome. *American Journal of Psychiatry* **151**, 1744–1752.

Lieberman, J.A., Alvir, J.M., Koreen, A. *et al.* (1996) Psychobiological correlates of treatment response in schizophrenia. *Neuropsychopharmacology* **14**, S13–S21.

Lingjaerde, O. (1982) Effect of the benzodiazepine derivative estazolam in patients with auditory hallucinations. A multicentre double-blind, cross-over study. *Acta Psychiatrica Scandinavica* **65**, 339–354.

Loebel, A.D., Lieberman, J.A., Alvir, J.M.J. *et al.* (1992) Duration of psychosis and outcome in first-episode schizophrenia. *American Journal of Psychiatry* **149**, 1183–1188.

Longo, L.P. & Salzman, C. (1995) Valproic acid effects on serum concentrations of clozapine and norclozapine [letter]. *American Journal of Psychiatry* **152**, 650.

McCarthy, R.H. & Terkelsen, K.G. (1995) Risperidone augmentation of clozapine. *Pharmacopsychiatry* **28**, 61–63.

McGlashan, T.H. (1999) Duration of untreated psychosis in first episode schizophrenia: marker or determinant of course? *Biological Psychiatry* **46**, 899–907.

McIntyre, R.S., McCann, S.M. & Kennedy, S.H. (2001) Antipsychotic metabolic effects: weight gain, diabetes mellitus and lipid abnormalities. *Canadian Journal of Psychiatry* **46**, 273–281.

MacMillan, J.F., Crow, T.J., Johnson, A.L. *et al.* (1986) The Northwick Park study of first episodes of schizophrenia. III. Short-term outcome in trial entrants and trial eligible patients. *British Journal of Psychiatry* **148**, 128–133.

Maletzky, B.M. (1973) The episodic dyscontrol syndrome. *Diseases of the Nervous System* **34**, 178–185.

Malhotra, A.K., Goldman, D., Buchanan, R.W. *et al.* (1998) The dopamine D receptor (DRD) Ser9Gly polymorphism and schizophrenia: a haplotype relative risk study and association with clozapine response. *Molecular Psychiatry* **3**, 72–75.

Marder, S.R. & Meibach, R.C. (1994) Risperidone in the treatment of schizophrenia. *American Journal of Psychiatry* **152**, 825–835.

Marsh, L., Suddath, R.L., Higgins, N. *et al.* (1994) Medial temporal lobe structures in schizophrenia: relationship of size to duration of illness. *Schizophrenia Research* **11**, 225–238.

Martin, J., Gomez, J.C., Garcia-Bernardo, E. *et al.* (1997) Olanzapine in treatment-refractory schizophrenia: results of an open label study. *Journal of Clinical Psychiatry* **58**, 479–783.

Masellis, M., Basile, V., Ozdemir, V. *et al.* (2000) Pharmacogentics of antipsychotic treatment: lessons learned from clozapine. *Biological Psychiatry* **47**, 252–266.

Mathalon, D., Sullivan, E., Lim, K. *et al.* (2001) Progressive brain volume changes and the clinical course of schizophrenia in men: a longitudinal magnetic resonance imaging study. *Archives of General Psychiatry* **58**, 148–157.

May, P.R.A. (1968) *Treatment of Schizophrenia: a Comparative Study of Five Treatment Methods.* Science House, New York.

Meltzer, H.Y. (1992) Treatment of the neuroleptic non-responsive schizophrenic. *Schizophrenia Bulletin* **18**, 515–533.

Meltzer, H.Y. (1995) Atypical antipsychotic drug therapy for treatment-resistant schizophrenia. In: *Schizophrenia* (eds S.R. Hirsch & D.R. Weinberger), pp. 485–502. Blackwell Science, Oxford.

Meltzer, H.Y. (1997) Treatment-resistant schizophrenia: the role of clozapine. *Current Medical Research and Opinion* **141**, 1–20.

Meltzer, H.Y. (1999) Suicide and schizophrenia: clozapine and the InterSePT study. International Clozaril/Leponex Suicide Prevention Trial. *Journal of Clinical Psychiatry* **60** (Suppl. 12), 47–50.

Meltzer, H.Y. (2001) Treatment of suicidality in schizophrenia. *Annals of the New York Academy of Sciences* **932**, 44–58.

Meltzer, H.Y. & McGurk, S.R. (1999) The effects of clozapine, risperidone, and olanzapine on cognitive function in schizophrenia. *Schizophrenia Bulletin* **25**, 233–255.

Meltzer, H.Y. & Okayli, G. (1995) Reduction of suicidality during clozapine treatment of neuroleptic-resistant schizophrenics: impact on risk benefit assessment. *American Journal of Psychiatry* **152**, 183–190.

Meltzer, H.Y., Sommers, A.A. & Luchins, D.J. (1986) The effect of neuroleptics and other psychotropic drugs on negative symptoms in schizophrenia. *Journal of Clinical Psychopharmacology* **6**, 329–338.

Meltzer, H.Y., Burnett, S., Bastani, B. *et al.* (1990) Effects of six months of clozapine treatment on the quality of life of chronic schizophrenic patients. *Hospital and Community Psychiatry* **41**, 892–897.

Miller, D.D. (1991) Effect of phenytoin on plasma clozapine concentrations in two patients. *Journal of Clinical Psychiatry* 52, 23–35.

Miller, D.D. (1996) The clinical use of clozapine plasma concentrations in the management of treatment-refractory schizophrenia. *Annals of Clinical Psychiatry* 8, 99–109.

Miller, D.D. (2000) Review and management of clozapine side effects. *Journal of Clinical Psychiatry* 61 (Suppl. 8), 14–19.

Miller, D.D., Fleming, F., Holman, T.L. *et al.* (1994) Plasma clozapine concentrations as a predictor of clozapine response: a follow-up study. *Journal of Clinical Psychiatry* 55 (9 (Suppl. B), 117–121.

Miller, F. & Menninger, J. (1987) Lithium-neuroleptic neurotoxicity is dose-dependent. *Journal of Psychopharmacology* 7, 89–91.

Milstein, V., Small, J.G., Miller, M.J. *et al.* (1990) Mechanisms of action of ECT: schizophrenia and schizoaffective disorder. *Biological Psychiatry* 27, 1282–1292.

Moller, H.J. (2000) Amisulpride: a review of its efficacy in schizophrenia. *Acta Psychiatrica Scandinavica* 101, 17–22.

Morera, A.L., Barreiro, P. & Can-Munoz, J.L. (1999) Risperidone and clozapine combination for the treatment of refractory schizophrenia. *Acta Psychiatrica Scandinavica* 99, 305–307.

Morinigo, A., Martin, J., Gonzalez, S. *et al.* (1989) Treatment of resistant schizophrenia with valproate and neuroleptic drugs. *Hillside Journal of Clinical Psychiatry* 11, 199–207.

Mowerman, S. & Siris, S.G. (1996) Adjunctive loxapine in a clozapine-resistant cohort of schizophrenic patients. *Annals of Clinical Psychiatry* 8, 193–197.

Mujica, R. & Weiden, P. (2001) Neuroleptic malignant syndrome after the addition of haloperidol to atypical antipsychotic. *American Journal of Psychiatry* 158, 650–651.

Muller, N., Riedel, M. & Moller, H.-J. (2000) Therapy with amisulpride in schizophrenic negative symptoms. *Pharmakotherapie* 7, 111–116.

Munro, J., O'Sullivan, D., Andrews, C. *et al.* (1999) Active monitoring of 12 760 clozapine recipients in the UK and Ireland: beyond pharmacovigilance. *British Journal of Psychiatry* 175, 576–580.

Nair, T.R., Christensen, J.D., Kingsbury, S.J. *et al.* (1997) Progressive and cerebroventricular enlargement and the subtyping of schizophrenia. *Psychiatry Research* 74, 141–150.

Nasrallah, H.A., Kuperman, S. & Harma, B.J. (1983) Clinical differences between schizophrenia patients with and without enlarged ventricles. *Journal of Clinical Psychiatry* 44, 407–409.

Nasrallah, H.A., Olson, S.C., McCalley-Whitters, M. *et al.* (1986) Cerebral ventricular enlargement in schizophrenia: a preliminary follow-up study. *Archives of General Psychiatry* 43, 157–159.

Neppe, V.M. (1983) Carbamazepine as adjunctive treatment in nonepileptic chronic inpatients with EEG temporal lobe abnormalities. *Journal of Clinical Psychiatry* 44, 326–330.

Neppe, V.M. (1988) Carbamazepine in non-responsive psychosis. *Journal of Clinical Psychiatry* 49, 22–30.

Nestoros, J.N., Nair, N.P.V., Pulman, J.R. *et al.* (1983) High doses of diazepam improve neuroleptic resistant chronic schizophrenic patients. *Psychopathology* 81, 42–47.

Nordstrom, A., Farde, L., Nyberg, S. *et al.* (1995) D and 5-HT receptor occupancy in relation to clozapine serum concentrations in a PET study of schizophrenic patients. *American Journal of Psychiatry* 152, 1444–1449.

Osser, D.N. & Albert, L.G. (1990) Is clozapine response different in neuroleptic non-responders versus partial responders? *Archives of General Psychiatry* 47, 189.

Otani, K. & Aoshima, T. (2000) Pharmacogenetics of classical and new atypical antipsychotic drugs. *Therapeutic Drug Monitoring* 22, 118–121.

Owens, D.G.C. (1996) Adverse effects of antipsychotic agents: do newer agents offer advantages? *Drugs* 51, 895–930.

Pacia, S.V. & Devinsky, O. (1994) Clozapine-related seizures: experience with 5629 patients. *Neurology* 44, 2247–2249.

Pandurangi, A.K., Goldberg, S.C., Brink, D.D. *et al.* (1989) Amphetamine challenge test, response to treatment, and lateral ventricle size in schizophrenia. *Biological Psychiatry* 25, 207–214.

Pato, C.N., Wolkowitz, O.M., Rapaport, M., Schulz, S.C. & Pickar, D. (1989) Benzodiazepine augmentation of neuroleptic treatment in patients with schizophrenia. *Psychopharmacology Bulletin* 25, 263–266.

Paton, C., Banham, S. & Whitmore, J. (2000) Benzodiazepines in schizophrenia: is there a trend towards long-term prescribing? *Psychiatric Bulletin* 24, 113–114.

Peacock, L. & Gerlach, J. (1994) Clozapine treatment in Denmark: concomitant psychotropic medication and haematologic monitoring in a system with liberal usage practices. *Journal of Clinical Psychiatry* 55, 44–49.

Perry, P.J., Miller, D.D., Arndt, S.V. *et al.* (1991) Clozapine and norclozapine plasma concentrations and clinical response of treatment-refractory schizophrenic patients. *American Journal of Psychiatry* 148, 231–235.

Perry, P.J., Sanger, T. & Beasley, C.M. (1999) Plasma, olanzapine, and clinical response: reply. *Journal of Clinical Psychopharmacology* 19, 193–194.

Phelan, M., Stradins, L. & Morrison, S. (2001) Physical health of people with severe mental illness. *British Medical Journal* 322, 443–444.

Pollack, S., Lieberman, J.A., Fleischhacker, W.W. *et al.* (1995) A comparison of European and American dosing regimens of schizophrenic patients on clozapine: efficacy and side-effects. *Psychopharmacology Bulletin* 31, 315–320.

Pollack, S., Woerner, M.G., Howard, A., Fireworker, R.B. & Kane, J.M. (1998) Clozapine reduces rehospitalisation rates among schizophrenic patients. *Psychopharmacology Bulletin* 34, 89–92.

Potkin, S.G., Bera, R. & Gulasekaram, B. (1994) Plasma clozapine concentrations predict clinical response in treatment-resistant schizophrenia. *Journal of Clinical Psychiatry* 55 (9 Suppl. B), 133–136.

Poyurovsky, M., Isakov, V., Hromnikov, S. *et al.* (1999) Fluvoxamine treatment of obsessive–compulsive symptoms in schizophrenic patients. an add-on open study. *International Clinical Psychopharmacology* 14, 95–100.

Procopio, M. (1998) Sulpiride augmentation on schizophrenia. *British Journal of Psychiatry* 172, 449–450.

Purdon, S., Jones, B. & Stip, E. (2000) Neuropsychological change in early phase schizophrenia during 12 months of treatment with olanzapine, risperidone, or haloperidol. *Archives of General Psychiatry* 57, 249–258.

Rao, P.A., Pickar, D., Gejman, P.V. *et al.* (1994) Allelic variation in the D dopamine receptor (DRD) gene does not predict response to clozapine. *Archives of General Psychiatry* 51, 912–917.

Rapoport, J.L., Gield, J., Kumra, S. *et al.* (1997) Childhood onset schizophrenia: progressive ventricular change during adolescents. *Archives of General Psychiatry* 54, 897–903.

Raskin, S., Katz, G., Zislin, Z., Knobler, H.Y. & Durst, R. (2000) Clozapine and risperidone: combination/augmentation treatment of refractory schizophrenia: a preliminary observation. *Acta Psychiatrica Scandinavica* 101, 334–336.

Regalado, A. (1999) Inventing the pharmacogenomics business. *American Journal of Health System Pharmacy* 56, 40–50.

Reichenberg, A., Robinowitz, J., Weiser, M. *et al.* (2000) Premorbid functioning in a national population of male twins discordant for psychosis. *American Journal of Psychiatry* 157, 1514–1516.

Reid, W.H., Mason, M. & Hogan, T. (1998) Suicide prevention effects associated with clozapine therapy in schizophrenia and schizoaffective disorder. *Psychiatric Services* 49, 1029–1033.

Revicki, D.A., Luce, B.R., Weschler, J.M., Brown, R.E. & Adler, M.A. (1990) Cost-effectiveness of clozapine for treatment-resistant schizophrenic patients. *Hospital and Community Psychiatry* 41, 850–854.

Reznik, I. & Sirota, P. (2000a) An open study of fluvoxamine augmentation of neuroleptics in schizophrenia with obsessive and compulsive features. *Clinical Neuropharmacology* 23, 157–160.

Reznik, I. & Sirota, P. (2000b) Obsessive and compulsive symptoms in schizophrenia. a randomised controlled trial with fluvoxamine and neuroleptics. *Journal of Clinical Psychopharmacology* 20, 410–416.

Reznik, I., Benatov, R. & Sirota, P. (2000) Long-term efficacy and safety of quetiapine in treatment-refractory schizophrenia: a case report. *International Journal of Psychiatry in Clinical Practice* 4, 77–80.

Richelson, E. & Souder, T. (2000) Binding of antipsychotic drugs to human brain receptors. focus on newer generation compounds. *Life Sciences* 66, 29–39.

Robinson, D.G., Woerner, M.G., Alvir, J.M. *et al.* (1999) Predictors of treatment response from a first episode of schizophrenia or schizoaffective disorder. *American Journal of Psychiatry* 156, 544–549.

Rosenheck, R., Cramer, J., Xu, W. *et al.* (1997) A comparison of clozapine and haloperidol in hospitalised patients with refractory schizophrenia. *New England Journal of Medicine* 337, 809–815.

Rosenheck, R., Evans, D., Herz, L.*et al.* (1999) How long to wait for a response to clozapine: a comparison of time course of response to clozapine and conventional antipsychotic medication in refractory schizophrenia. *Schizophrenia Bulletin*, 25, 709–719.

Roth, B., Buckley, P.F. & Schulz, S.C. (1999) Molecular biology and antipsychotic medications. In: *Schizophrenia in a Molecular Age: Review of Psychiatry Series* (ed. C.A. Tamminga), (series eds. J. Oldham & M.B. Kiba). American Psychiatric Press, Washington, DC.

Safferman, A.Z. & Munne, R. (1992) Case report combining clozapine with ECT. *Convulsive Therapy* 8, 141–143.

Sassim, N. & Grohmann, R. (1988) Adverse drug reactions with clozapine and simultaneous application of benzodiazepines. *Pharmacopsychiatry* 21, 306–307.

Scheepers, F.E. & Gispen de Wed, C.C. & Hulshoff, H.E. & Kahn, R.S. (2001) Effect of clozapine on candate nucleus volume in relation to symptoms of schizophrenia. *American Journal of Psychiatry* 158, 644–645.

Schooler, N.R., Keith, S.J., Severe, J.B. *et al.* (1997) Relapse and rehospitalization during maintenance treatment of schizophrenia: the effects of dose reduction and family treatment. *Archives of General Psychiatry* 54, 453–463.

Schulz, S.C., Sinicrope, P., Kishore, P. *et al.* (1983) Treatment response and ventricular brain enlargement in young schizophrenic patients. *Psychopharmacology Bulletin* 19, 510–512.

Schulz, S.C., Butterfield, L., Garicano, M. *et al.* (1984) Beyond the therapeutic window: a case presentation. *Journal of Clinical Psychiatry* 45, 223–225.

Schulz, S.C. & House, J. & Andrews, M.B. (1986) Helping families in a schizophrenia program. In: *Family Involvement in the Treatment of Schizophrenia* (ed. M. Zucker Goldstein), pp. 19–34. American Psychiatric Press, Washington, DC.

Schulz, S.C., Conley, R.R., Kahn, E.M. & Alexander, J.E. (1989) Nonresponders to neuroleptics: a distinct subtype. In: *Schizophrenia: Scientific Progress* (eds S.C. Schulz & C.A. Tamminga), pp. 341–350. Oxford University Press, Oxford.

Schulz, S.C., Kahn, E.M., Baker, R.W. *et al.* (1990) Lithium and carbamazepine augmentation in treatment-refractory schizophrenia. In: *The Neuroleptic-Nonresponsive Patient: Characterisation and Treatment* (eds B. Angrist & S.C. Schulz), pp. 109–136. American Psychiatric Press, Washington, DC.

Schulz, S.C., Findling, R.L., Camlin, K. *et al.* (1998) Childhood and adolescent schizophrenia. In: *Schizophrenia* (ed. P.F. Buckley). Psychiatric Clinics of North America. WB Sanders: Philadelphia, PA.

Schulz, S.C., Thompson, P.A. & Jacobs, M. (1999) Lithium augmentation fails to reduce symptoms in poorly responsive schizophrenic outpatients. *Journal of Clinical Psychiatry* 60, 366–372.

Schumacher, J. (2000) Pharmacogenetics of clozapine response. *Lancet* 356, 506–507.

Seibyl, J.P. & Lieberman, J.A. (1993) Substance abuse and schizophrenia. In: *Psychiatric Clinica of North America* (eds P. Powchichk & S.C. Schulz), pp. 123–138. W.B. Sanders, Philadelphia.

Selzer, J.A. & Lieberman, J.A. (1993) Schizophrenia and substance abuse. *Psychiatric Clinics of North America* 16, 401–412.

Sensky, T., Turkington, D., Kingdon, D. *et al.* (2000) A randomized controlled trial of cognitive–behavioral therapy for persistent symptoms in schizophrenia resistant to medication. *Archives of General Psychiatry* 57, 165–172.

Sernyak, M.J., Desai, R., Stolar, M. & Rosenheck, R. (2001) Impact of clozapine on completed suicide. *American Journal of Psychiatry* 158, 931–937.

Sheitman, B.B., Lindgren, J.C., Early, J. *et al.* (1997) High-dose olanzapine for treatment-refractory schizophrenia. *American Journal of Psychiatry* 154, 1626.

Shiloh, R., Zemishlany, Z., Aizenberg, D. *et al.* (1997) Sulpiride augmentation in people with schizophrenia partially responsive to clozapine: a double-blind, placebo-controlled study. *British Journal of Psychiatry* 171, 569–573.

Silbersweig, D.A., Stern, E., Frith, C. *et al.* (1998) A functional neuroanatomy of hallucinations in schizophrenia. *Nature* 378, 176–179.

Silver, H. & Nasser, A. (1992) Fluvoxamine improves negative symptoms in treated chronic schizophrenia: an add-on double-blind, placebo-controlled study. *Biological Psychiatry* 31, 698–704.

Simhandl, C. & Meszaros, K. (1992) The use of carbamazepine in the treatment of schizophrenic and schizoaffective psychoses: a review. *Journal of Psychiatry and Neuroscience* 17, 1–14.

Siris, S.G. (2000) Depression in schizophrenia: perspectives in the era of 'atypical' antipsychotic agents. *American Journal of Psychiatry* 157, 1379–1389.

Siris, S.G., Morgan, V., Fagerstrom, R., Rifkin, A. & Cooper, T.B. (1987) Adjunctive imipramine in the treatment of postpsychotic depression: a controlled trial. *Archives of General Psychiatry* 44, 533–539.

Siris, S.G., Mason, S.E., Bermanzohn, P.C., Shuwall, M.A. & Aseniero, M.A. (1993) Adjunctive imipramine in substance-abusing dysphoric schizophrenic patients. *Psychopharmacological Bulletin* 29, 127–133.

Siris, S.G., Addington, D., Azorin, J.-M. *et al.* (2001) Depression in schizophrenia: recognition and management in the USA. *Schizophrenia Research* 47, 185–197.

Small, J.G., Kellans, J.J., Milstein, V. & Moore, J. (1975) A placebo-controlled study of lithium combined with neuroleptics in chronic schizophrenic patients. *American Journal of Psychiatry* 132, 1315–1317.

Spence, S.A., Hirsch, S.R., Brooks, D.J. *et al.* (1998) Prefrontal cortex activity in people with schizophrenia and control subjects: evidence from positive emission tomography for remission of 'hypofrontality' with recovery from acute schizophrenia. *British Journal of Psychiatry* 172, 316–323.

Spina, E., Avenoso, A., Facciola, G. *et al.* (1998) Effect of fluoxetine on the plasma concentrations of clozapine and its major metabolites in patients with schizophrenia. *International Clinical Psychopharmacology* **13**, 141–145.

Spina, E., Avenoso, A., Salemi, M. *et al.* (2000) Plasma concentrations of clozapine and its major metabolites during combined treatment with paroxetine or sertraline. *Pharmacopsychiatry* **33**, 213–217.

Sponheim, S.R., Iacono, W.G. & Beiser, M. (1991) Stability of ventricular size after the onset of psychosis in schizophrenia. *Psychiatry Research* **40**, 21–30.

Stone, J.L., McDaniel, K.D., Hughes, J.R. *et al.* (1986) Episodic dyscontrol disorder and paroxysmal EEG abnormalities: successful treatment with carbamazepine. *Biological Psychiatry* **21**, 208–212.

Stubbs, J.H., Haw, C.M., Staley, C.J. & Mountjoy, C.Q. (2000) Augmentation with sulpiride for a schizophrenic patients partially responsive to clozapine. *Acta Psychiatrica Scandinavica* **102**, 390–394.

Takhar, J. (1999) Pimozide augmentation in a patient with drug-resistant psychosis previously treated with olanzapine. *Journal of Psychiatry and Neuroscience* **24**, 248–249.

Tamminga, C.A., Thaker, G.K., Buchanan, R. *et al.* (1992) Limbic system abnormalities identified in schizophrenia using positron tomography with fluorodeoxygluclose and neocortical alterations with deficit syndrome. *Archives of General Psychiatry* **49**, 522–530.

Terao, T., Oga, T., Nozaki, S., Ohta, A. *et al.* (1995) Lithium addition to neuroleptic treatment in chronic schizophrenia: a randomized, double-blind, placebo-controlled, cross-over study. *Acta Psychiatrica Scandinavica* **92**, 220–224.

Thompson, C. (1994) The use of high-dose antipsychotic medication. *British Journal of Psychiatry* **164**, 448–458.

Thompson, P.A., Buckley, P.F. & Meltzer, H.Y. (1994) The brief psychiatric rating scale: effect of scaling system on clinical response assessment. *Journal of Clinical Pharmacology* **14**, 344–346.

Tollefson, G.D., Sanger, T.M., Lu, Y. *et al.* (1998) Depressive signs and symptoms in schizophrenia: a prospective blinded trial of olanzapine and haloperidol. *Archives of General Psychiatry* **55**, 250–258.

Tollefson, G.D., Birkett, M.A., Kiesler, G.M., Wood A.J. and the Lilly Resistant Schizophrenia Study Group (2001) Double-blind comparison of olanzapine versus clozapine in schizophrenic patients clinically eligible for treatment with clozapine. *Biological Psychiatry* **49**, 52–63.

Tsai, S., Hong, C., Yu, Y. *et al.* (2000) Association study of a functional serotonin transporter gene polymorphism with schizophrenia, psychopathology and clozapine response. *Schizophrenia Research* **44**, 177–181.

Tyson, S.C., Devane, C.L. & Risch, S.C. (1995) Pharmacokinetic interaction between risperidone and clozapine. *American Journal of Psychiatry* **152**, 1401–1402.

Umbricht, D. & Kane, J.M. (1996) Medical complications of new antipsychotic drugs. *Schizophrenia Bulletin* **22**, 475–483.

Ung Gu Kang, Jun Soo Kwon, Yong Min Ahn *et al.* (2000) Electrocardiographic abnormalities in patients treated with clozapine. *Journal of Clinical Psychiatry* **61**, 441–446.

Van der Zwagg, C., McGee, M., McEvoy, J.P. *et al.* (1996) Response of patients with treatment refractory schizophrenia to clozapine with three serum level ranges. *American Journal of Psychiatry* **153**, 1579–1584.

Van Putten, T., Marder, S.R., Wirshing, W.C. *et al.* (1991) Neuroleptic plasma levels. *Schizophrenia Bulletin* **17**, 197–216.

Vaughn, C. & Jeff, J. (1976) The influence of family and social factors in the course of psychiatric illness. *British Journal of Psychiatry* **129**, 125–137.

Velligan, D.I., Bow-Thomas, C.C., Huntzinger, C. *et al.* (2000a) Randomized controlled trial of the use of compensatory strategies to enhance adaptive functioning in outpatients with schizophrenia. *American Journal of Psychiatry* **157**, 1317–1323.

Velligan, D.I., Bow-Thomas, C.C., Mahurin, B.K., Miller, A.L. & Halgunseth, L.C. (2000b) Do specific neurocognitive deficits predict specific domains of community function in schizophrenia? *Journal of Nervous and Mental Disease* **188**, 518–524.

Vita, A., Sacchetti, E., Valvassori, G. *et al.* (1988) Brain morphology in schizophrenia: a 2- to 5-year CT scan follow-up study. *Acta Psychiatrica Scandinavica* **78**, 618–621.

Vita, A., Giobbio, G.M., Dieci, M. *et al.* (1994) Stability of cerebral ventricle size from the appearance of the first psychotic symptoms to the later diagnosis of schizophrenia. *Biological Psychiatry* **35**, 960–962.

Volavka, J. (1999) The effects of clozapine on aggression and substance use in schizophrenic patients. *Journal of Clinical Psychiatry* **60** (Suppl. 12), 43–46.

Volavka, J., Czobar, P., Sheitmen, B. *et al.* (2002) Clozapine, olanzapine, risperidone, and haloperidol in the treatment of patients with chronic schizophrenia and schizoaffective disorder. *American Journal of Psychiatry* **159**, 255–262.

Waddington, J.L., Scully, P.J., Quinn, J.F. *et al.* (2001) The origin and course of schizophrenia: implications for clinical practice. *Journal of Psychiatric Practice* **7**, 247–252.

Wahlbeck, K., Cheine, M., Essali, A. & Adams, C. (1999) Evidence of clozapine's effectiveness in schizophrenia: a systematic review and meta-analysis of randomised trials. *American Journal of Psychiatry* **156**, 990–999.

Wahlbeck, K., Cheine, M., Tuisku, K. *et al.* (2000) Risperidone versus clozapine in treatment-resistant schizophrenia: a randomized pilot study. *Progress in Neuropsychopharmacology and Biological Psychiatry* **24**, 911–922.

Wahlbeck, K., Cheine, M. & Essali, M.A. (2001) Clozapine versus typical neuroleptic medication for schizophrenia (Cochrane Review). In: *The Cochrane Library*, 4. Update Software, Oxford.

Wallace, C.J. (1986) Functional assessment in rehabilitation. *Schizophrenia Bulletin* **12**, 604–630.

Warner, J.P., Harvey, C.A. & Barnes, T.R.E. (1994) Clozapine and urinary incontinence. *International Clinical Psychopharmacology* **9**, 207–209.

Warner, J.P., Gledhill, J.A. & Wakeling, A. (1996) The use of risperidone in treatment-resistant schizophrenia: two case reports. *International Clinical Psychopharmacology* **11**, 65–66.

Wassef, A., Watson, D.J., Morrison, P. *et al.* (1989) Neuroleptic-valproic acid combination in treatment of psychotic symptoms: a three-case report. *Journal of Clinical Psychopharmacology* **9**, 45–48.

Weiden, P.J., Dixon, L., Frances, A. *et al.* (1991) Neuroleptic non-compliance in schziophrenia. In: *Advances in Neuropsychiatry and Psychopharmacology: Schizophrenia Research*, Vol. 1 (eds C.A. Tamminga & S.C. Schulz), pp. 285–296. Raven Press, New York.

Weinberger, D.R., Bigelow, L.B., Kleinman, J.E. *et al.* (1980) Cerebral ventricle enlargement in chronic schizophrenia: association with poor response to treatment. *Archives of General Psychiatry* **37**, 11–14.

Weiser, M., Schneider-Beeri, M., Nakash, N. *et al.* (2000) Improvement in cognition associated with novel antipsychotic drugs: a direct effect or reduction of EPS? *Schizophrenia Research* **46**, 81–89.

Welch, J., Manschrek, T. & Redmond, D. (1994) Clozapine-induced seizures and EEG changes. *Journal of Neuropsychiatry and Clinical Neuroscience* **6**, 250–256.

Westmoreland-Corson, P., Nopoulos, P., Miller, D.D., Arndt, S. & Andreasen, N.C.A. (1999) Change in basal ganglia volume over 2 years in patients with schizophrenia: typical versus atypical. *American Journal of Psychiatry* **156**, 1200–1204.

Wilson, W.H. (1993) Addition of lithium to haloperidol in non-affective, antipsychotic non-responsive schizophrenia: a double blind, placebo controlled, parallel design clinical trial. *Psychopharmacology* **111**, 359–366.

Wilson, W.H. (1995) Do anticonvulsants hinder clozapine treatment? *Biological Psychiatry* **37**, 132–133.

Wirshing, W.C., Phelan, C.K., van Putten, T., Marder, S.R. & Engel, J. (1990) Effects of clozapine on treatment-resistant akathisia and concomitant tardive dyskinesia. *Journal of Clinical Psychopharmacology* **10**, 371–373.

Wirshing, W.C., Ames, D., Bisheff, S. *et al.* (1997) Hepatic encephalopathy associated with combined clozapine and divalproex [letter]. *Journal of Clinical Psychopharmacology* **17**, 120–121.

Wirshing, D.A., Marshall, B.D., Green, M.F. *et al.* (1999) Risperidone in treatment-refractory schizophrenia. *American Journal of Psychiatry* **156**, 1374–1379.

Wolkin, A. (1990) Positron emission tomography and the study of neuroleptic response. In: *The Neuroleptic Nonresponsive Patient: Characterization and Treatment* (eds B. Angrist & S.C. Schultz), pp. 35–49. American Psychiatric Association, Washington DC.

Wolkin, A., Barouch, F., Wolf, A.P. *et al.* (1989) Dopamine blockade and clinical response: evidence for two biological subgroups of schizophrenia. *American Journal of Psychiatry* **146**, 905–908.

Wolkin, A., Sanfilipo, M., Duncan, E. *et al.* (1996) Blunted change in cerebral glucose utilization after haloperidol treatment in schizophrenic patients with prominent negative symptoms. *American Journal of Psychiatry* **153**, 346–354.

Wolkowitz, O.M. & Pickar, D. (1991) Benzodiazepines in the treatment of schizophrenia: a review and reappraisal. *American Journal of Psychiatry* **148**, 714–726.

Wolkowitz, O.M., Breier, A., Doran, A. *et al.* (1988) Alprazolam augmentation of the antipsychotic effects of fluphenazine in schizophrenic patients: preliminary results. *Archives of General Psychiatry* **45**, 664–671.

Wolkowitz, O.M., Rapaport, M.H. & Pickar, D. (1990) Benzodiazepine augmentation of neuroleptics. In: *The Neuroleptic-Nonresponsive Patient: Characterisation and Treatment* (eds B. Angrist & S.C. Schulz), pp. 89–108. American Psychiatric Press, Washington, DC.

Wolkowitz, O.M., Turetsky, N., Reus, V.I. *et al.* (1992) Benzodiazepine augmentation of neuroleptics in treatment-resistant schizophrenia. *Psychopharmacology Bulletin* **28**, 291–295.

Woods, B.T. (1998) Is schizophrenia a progressive neurodevelopmental disorder? Towards a unitary pathogenic mechanism. *American Journal of Psychiatry* **55**, 905–912.

Woods, B.T., Yurgelun-Todd, D. & Benes, F.M. (1990) Progressive ventricle enlargement in schizophrenia: comparison to bipolar and affective and correlation with clinical course. *Biological Psychiatry* **27**, 341–352.

Wyatt, R.J. (1991) Neuroleptics and the natural course of schizophrenia. *Schizophrenia Bulletin* **17**, 325–351.

Wykes, T., Reeder, C., Corner, J., Williams, C. & Everitt, B. (1999) The effects of neurocognitive remediation on executive processing in patients with schizophrenia. *Schizophrenia Bulletin* **25**, 291–307.

Yerevanian, B.I. & Hodgman, C.H. (1985) A haloperidol-carbamazepine interaction in a patient with rapid-cycling bipolar disorder [letter]. *American Journal of Psychiatry* **42**, 785–786.

Yu, Y.W., Tsai, S.J., Lin, C.H. *et al.* (1999) Serotonin-6 receptor variant (C267T) and clinical response to clozapine. *Neuroreport* **10**, 1231–1233.

Yuzda, M.S.K. (2000) Combination antipsychotics: what is the evidence? *Journal of Information Pharmacotherapy* **2**, 300–305.

Electroconvulsive therapy and schizophrenia

H.A. Sackeim

Current practice and recommendations, 517
Efficacy, 518
    Early studies, 518
    Studies of sham vs. real ECT in schizophrenia, 519
    Studies comparing ECT with neuroleptics or other therapies, 521
    Studies comparing combined ECT and medication treatment with medication alone or ECT alone, 525
    ECT and neuroleptic medication in medication-resistant schizophrenic patients, 528
    Atypical antipsychotics and electroconvulsive therapy, 532
Prediction of outcome, 533
    Demographic and clinical predictors, 533

Symptoms responsive to ECT, 533
    Special populations, 534
Treatment technique, 536
    Electrode placement, 536
    Stimulus intensity, 536
    Treatment duration and frequency, 536
    Continuation/maintenance ECT, 538
Side-effects, 538
    Cognition, 539
    Neuropathological effects, 539
    Movement disorders, 540
Mechanisms, 541
Conclusions, 542
Acknowledgements, 543
References, 544

Using intramuscular injection of camphor, Meduna (1935) was the first to deliberately induce seizures with the aim of treating schizophrenia. Cerletti and Bini (1938) introduced the use of electricity as a method of seizure induction, again with the intent of treating schizophrenia. During the 1940s and 1950s, electroconvulsive therapy (ECT) was widely adopted and its use extended to a number of disorders. In subsequent decades, particularly in the USA, the introduction of effective pharmacological treatments for schizophrenia and mood disorders led to a sharp drop in ECT utilization (Thompson & Blaine 1987). However, interest in ECT has increased in recent years and its use, after declining markedly from the levels in the 1950s, appears to be increasing (Thompson *et al.* 1994; Rosenbach *et al.* 1997; Olfson *et al.* 1998).

The efficacy of ECT in some disorders, such as major depression, is extremely well supported (Janicak *et al.* 1985; Sackeim 1989; Sackeim *et al.* 1995). Indeed, one can argue that the evidence regarding the efficacy of ECT is among the strongest in all of medicine in the treatment of major depression (Sackeim *et al.* 1993, 2000). However, the indications for the use of ECT and its efficacy in schizophrenia are less clear. Some authorities have dismissed or warned against the use of ECT in schizophrenia (Ottosson 1985; Hamilton 1986). More recently, the American Psychiatric Association (APA) Task Force on ECT stated that ECT is an effective treatment for 'psychotic schizophrenic exacerbations', particularly in the context of catatonia, when affective symptomatology is prominent, or when there is a history of a favourable response to ECT (American Psychiatric Association *et al.* 1990). The most recent APA Task Force Report emphasizes efficacy in psychotic exacerbations of short episode duration (American Psychiatric Association 2001). A number of experts have more decisively advocated that ECT is indicated

in schizophrenia or specific subtypes (Van Valkenburg & Clayton 1985; Abrams 1987; Kalinowsky 1988; Hertzman 1992; Fink & Sackeim 1996). However, others have noted that despite 'more than five decades of widespread clinical use, the administration of ECT to those with schizophrenia lacks a strong research base' (Tharyan 2000).

Here we review the literature on the use of ECT in schizophrenia and address many issues that confront the clinician. Is ECT useful in the treatment of schizophrenia? If so, for what types of schizophrenia or for what symptoms? At what point should ECT be considered? Should it be administered after neuroleptic medications have failed, or in combination with medications to enhance efficacy or to reduce neuroleptic dosage? Are there special risks in providing ECT to this population? How should ECT be administered? How many treatments should be given? How long do the beneficial and adverse effects last? Is there a place for maintenance ECT?

Current practice and recommendations

A number of surveys, in several countries, have examined the extent to which schizophrenic patients are represented among ECT recipients. The APA Task Force on ECT surveyed APA members in 1976 and estimated that 17% of patients who received ECT in the USA had diagnoses of schizophrenia (American Psychiatric Association 1978). Thompson and Blaine (1987), using medical record data collected by the National Institute of Mental Health, estimated that in 1980 16.6% of the patients who received ECT in public and private inpatient facilities in the USA carried the diagnosis of schizophrenia. These patients constituted only 2.1% of those admitted to these facilities with this diagnosis. Similarly, in a survey conducted at an American teaching hospital, Tancer *et al.* (1989) found that schizophrenic patients constituted 15% in 1970 and 11% in 1980–81 of those administered ECT.

In Great Britain, Pippard and Ellam (1981) sent a questionnaire to 3221 psychiatrists, of whom 1274 reported on the use of ECT. Of 2591 treatment series identified in this survey, 83% were for patients with depressive disorders and 13% were for patients with a diagnosis of schizophrenia. In Ireland, Latey and Fahy (1988) surveyed 49 psychiatrists and found that, of 391 treatment series given, most patients had depressive disorders, but 17% had schizophrenia. Malla (1986) retrospectively examined 5729 consecutive admissions between 1975 and 1978 to three general hospitals and the mental hospital in St John's, Newfoundland, Canada; 28.8% of the admissions that received ECT had a diagnosis of schizophrenia. In fact of all admissions of schizophrenic patients, 36.5% went on to receive ECT. Martin *et al.* (1984), in a study of ECT administered at the Clarke Institute in Toronto, Canada, found that patients with a primary discharge diagnosis of an affective disorder received 54.3% of the courses, whereas those with schizophrenia received 36.0%. Bland and Brintnell (1985) reviewed the use of ECT over an 11-year period, from 1972 to 1982, in the University of Alberta hospitals. Five per cent of patients received ECT, and approximately 75% of patients so treated had a discharge diagnosis of affective psychosis and 20% had a diagnosis of schizophrenia. Smith and Richman (1984) using Medicare data, hospital discharge statistics and questionnaires in selected Canadian hospitals found that during the years 1975–78 8.0% of females and 6.5% of males with schizophrenia and paranoid psychoses were treated with ECT. Shugar *et al.* (1984) reviewed data from 221 hospitals in Ontario during 1980–81 and observed that, of a total of 1977 courses of ECT administered, 24.3% were given to schizophrenic patients. They found great variation in the utilization of ECT between hospitals, with a range of 0.6–32.8%, with individuals with schizoaffective disorder having higher ECT rates.

Strömgren (1988), in a retrospective examination of all patients treated in 1984 with ECT at the Aarhus psychiatric hospital in Risskov, Denmark, found that only 2.9% had a diagnosis of schizophrenia. In contrast, Shukla (1981) described the use of ECT in an Indian rural teaching hospital between 1977 and 1980. Of the 503 cases reviewed, 75% of the patients had diagnoses of schizophrenia. In a recent national survey of psychiatrists in India, it was reported that 13.4% of psychiatric patients were administered ECT (Agarwal *et al.* 1992). Of this group, 43% had diagnoses of schizophrenia. In a recent survey in a hospital in Japan, over a 20-year period, 12% of patients who received ECT had a diagnosis of schizophrenia (Ishimoto *et al.* 2000). Thus, there appears to be marked variability both between and within countries in the representation of schizophrenic patients among those who receive ECT. Clearly, many prescribers consider schizophrenia an indication for ECT.

This diversity of practice is reflected in current recommendations of national medical and psychiatric organizations. The APA Task Force on ECT recently recommended the treatment for psychotic schizophrenic exacerbations when episode duration was short, when catatonic symptomatology was prominent or given a history of a favourable response to ECT (American Psychiatric Association 2001). This group suggested that ECT is also effective in related psychotic disorders, notably schizophreniform disorder and schizoaffective disorder, and in atypical psychosis when the clinical features were similar to those of other major diagnostic indications.

In contrast, a National Institutes of Health Consensus Development Panel (National Institutes of Health 1985) stated:

> Neuroleptics are the first line of treatment for schizophrenia. The evidence for the efficacy of ECT in schizophrenia is not compelling, but is strongest for those schizophrenic patients with a shorter duration of illness, a more acute onset, and more intense affective symptoms. It has not been useful in chronically ill schizophrenic patients. Although ECT is frequently advocated for treatment of patients with schizophreniform psychoses, schizoaffective disorders, and catatonia, there are no adequate controlled studies.

The Canadian Psychiatric Association stated that ECT was useful for some patients with schizophrenia (Pankratz 1980). Because it was felt that pharmacological agents were typically more effective, ECT should be reserved for the schizophrenic patient who had failed at least one adequate pharmacological trial. The British Royal College of Psychiatrists took a generally negative view of the efficacy of ECT in schizophrenia in its 1977 report (Royal College of Psychiatrists 1977), which it reversed in its 1995 report (Royal College of Psychiatrists 1995). Thus, among expert groups and national psychiatric associations, there is a lack of consensus regarding the role of ECT in schizophrenia.

Efficacy

Early studies

The efficacy of ECT in schizophrenia has been the subject of several critical reviews (Staudt & Zubin 1957; Riddell 1963; Turek & Hanlon 1977; Fink 1979; Salzman 1980; Scovern & Kilmann 1980; Kendell 1981; Taylor 1981; Small 1985; Fink & Sackeim 1996; Abrams 1997b). Many of the earlier reports on this use of ECT consisted of uncontrolled case material (Guttmann *et al.* 1939; Ross & Malzberg 1939; Zeifert 1941; Kalinowsky 1943; Kalinowsky & Worthing 1943; Danziger & Kindwall 1946; Kino & Thorpe 1946; Kennedy & Anchel 1948; Miller *et al.* 1953). Additionally, diagnostic practice preceded the introduction of operationalized criteria for schizophrenia and often patient samples and outcome criteria were poorly characterized. International differences in the rate of diagnosis of schizophrenia have been well described, with documentation that psychiatrists in the USA, compared with British colleagues, were overinclusive in diagnosing schizophrenia, often labelling patients with affective or schizoaffective disorder as schizophrenic. Thus, earlier American studies describing samples of schizophrenic patients may have contained substantial representation of mood disorder patients, who may be particularly likely to respond to ECT (Mowbray 1959; Kendell 1971; Abrams *et al.* 1974; Abrams & Taylor 1976b; Pope & Lipinski 1978; Pope *et al.* 1980).

Overall, the earlier reports on the use of ECT in schizophrenia were enthusiastic for patients with relatively recent onset of illness, with recovery or marked improvement noted in a large proportion of cases, typically on the order of 75% (Fink 1979; Small 1985). Historical comparisons (Ellison & Hamilton 1949; Gottlieb & Huston 1951; Currier *et al.* 1952; Bond 1954) and comparisons to psychotherapy or milieu therapy suggested that the introduction of ECT resulted in both superior short-term clinical outcome and more sustained remissions (Goldfarb & Kieve 1945; McKinnon 1948; Palmer *et al.* 1951; Wolff 1955; Rachlin *et al.* 1956). However, in this early era, the view was also expressed that ECT was considerably less effective in schizophrenic patients with insidious onset and long duration of illness (Cheney & Drewry 1938; Ross & Malzberg 1939; Zeifert 1941; Chafetz 1943; Kalinowsky 1943; Lowinger & Huddleson 1945; Danziger & Kindwall 1946; Shoor & Adams 1950; Herzberg 1954). In addition, it was suggested that schizophrenic patients often required intensive courses of ECT, involving more frequent and closely spaced treatments (Baker *et al.* 1960a; Kalinowsky 1943).

Studies of sham vs. real ECT in schizophrenia

ECT is a highly ritualized treatment, involving a repeated complex procedure. The sham vs. real ECT comparison is similar to the placebo-controlled trial in pharmacological research. With sham ECT, patients undergo the complete ECT procedure, including anaesthesia, but no electric current is applied. Superior response rates with 'real' ECT relative to sham conditions indicate that the passage of current and/or the production of a generalized seizure contribute to the efficacy of ECT. Sham ECT has been consistently found to be inferior to real ECT in the treatment of major depression (Sackeim 1989). Table 27.1 summarizes the sham vs. real ECT studies that have included schizophrenic patients.

Miller *et al.* (1953) selected 30 chronic patients who had been diagnosed with catatonic schizophrenia. The patients were randomized to three groups: unmodified (no anaesthetic agent) bilateral ECT; sham ECT with pentothal; or pentothal plus low-intensity non-convulsive stimulation for 5 min. All the treatment groups evidenced improvement in social performance, as evaluated by blind and non-blind raters, with no group differences.

Ulett *et al.* (1954, 1956) conducted a double-blind random assignment study involving 84 patients. Four treatment groups were contrasted: sham ECT involving seconal anaesthesia; ECT; subconvulsive photoshock; and convulsive photoshock. The photoshock therapy involved pretreating patients with an intravenous convulsant drug, hexazol, and then administering intermittent photic stimulation. In the subconvulsive condition,

photic stimulation resulted in a few minutes of generalized myoclonic activity without evidence of a generalized seizure or loss of consciousness. Patients received intravenous seconal to induce anaesthesia before each session. The two groups who experienced full convulsions (ECT or photoconvulsive) had significantly greater improvement in symptom ratings than the other two groups.

Brill *et al.* (1957, 1959a,b,c) studied a heterogeneous group of 97 patients, which included 67 patients diagnosed as having schizophrenic reactions, 14 with schizoaffective disorders and 16 with depressive reactions. The patients were randomized to one of five treatment groups: unmodified ECT; ECT plus succinylcholine; ECT plus thiopental; thiopental alone; and nitrous oxide alone. In this double-blind study, three different methods were used to evaluate clinical outcome 1 month following the end of treatment. There were no differences among the groups in ratings of therapeutic change. In particular, among the schizophrenic patients, the differences were slight between those who had received a form of ECT and those who had not.

Heath *et al.* (1964) selected 77 patients with a diagnosis of chronic schizophrenia. This randomized double-blind experiment was divided into two substudies. The first substudy compared the effects of four ECT treatments with four sham treatments in 45 patients. The second part involved 32 patients, divided into four groups. One group was administered eight real treatments; a second group was administered eight sham treatments; a third group constituted an 'untreated' control; and a fourth group was told that they would receive ECT, but their somatic treatment was left unchanged. In both substudies, a therapeutic advantage for real ECT was not identified. Heath *et al.* questioned whether 'the elaborate procedure involved in providing ECT was worth it' (Heath *et al.* 1964, p. 805).

Taylor and Fleminger (1980) conducted a randomized double-blind trial in a group of 20 schizophrenic patients. Of particular note, both patients with short duration of illness and patients with chronic conditions were excluded. All patients received standard doses of neuroleptics for at least 2 weeks before and throughout the ECT trial. Both groups improved in symptom scores, but the improvement with real ECT was significantly greater after six treatments and at the end of the treatment course. However, 3 months following the treatment course, the groups showed little difference.

Brandon *et al.* (1985) conducted a random assignment double-blind study with 17 patients, assigned to either real or sham ECT. Neuroleptics were restricted during the 4-week trial period in the following manner: patients were not permitted to commence a new course of neuroleptics, but if a patient was already stabilized on neuroleptic prior to starting the trial, this could be continued. At the end of the 4 weeks, the real ECT group showed significantly greater improvement in ratings of schizophrenic symptoms, depressive symptoms and global psychopathology. This difference was not maintained at 12- and 28-week assessment time points.

Abraham and Kulhara (1987) studied 22 schizophrenic patients. Patients were maintained on trifluoperazine (up to

Table 27.1 Prospective clinical trials comparing real and sham electroconvulsive therapy (ECT) in schizophrenia.

Study	Patients	Study design	Number of treatments	Results/comments
Miller *et al.* (1953)	30 chronic catatonic schizophrenics (average hospitalization was 10 years)	Sham vs. subconvulsive stimulation vs. ECT	ECT given 5 days per week for 3 weeks; subconvulsive and sham given 5 days per week for 4 weeks	All groups improved, with no differences among the groups
Ulett *et al.* (1954, 1956)	20 brief schizophrenic reactions included in sample of 84 patients	Sham vs. subconvulsive photic stimulation vs. convulsive photic stimulation vs. ECT	12–15 treatments, 3 times per week	Convulsive therapies superior to sham and subconvulsive stimulation. Study hampered by inhomogeneous groups, lack of diagnostic criteria, and lack of separate analysis for schizophrenia
Brill *et al.* (1957, 1959a,b,c)	67 of 97 patients had chronic schizophrenic reactions	Unmodified ECT vs. ECT and succinylcholine vs. ECT and tiopental vs. tiopental alone vs. nitrous oxide alone	Generally 20 treatments, three times per week	No difference in effectiveness among the 5 groups or in the pooled ECT vs. non-ECT groups; no difference in effectiveness for the 67 schizophrenics and the 30 depressives considered separately
Heath *et al.* (1964)	77 chronic schizophrenics with 5 years or greater hospitalization	Sham vs. ECT vs. 'untreated' control vs. group promised but not given ECT; many patients received phenothiazines during the trial	Sample divided into 45 patients who received real or sham ECT once a week for 4 weeks or no treatment and 32 patients who received real or sham ECT twice a week for 4 weeks, an 'untreated' control group, and a promised ECT but not delivered control group	The groups could not be distinguished in efficacy variables. Sample size was small for discrete treatment conditions
Taylor and Fleminger (1980)	20 schizophrenics by Present State Examination; both acute (<6 months) and chronic patients excluded	Sham vs. ECT; patients maintained on standard doses of neuroleptics (300 mg of CPZ/day or equivalent) for 2 weeks before entry into trial	8–12 treatments, three times per week, seven patients received bilateral ECT and three patients unilateral ECT	ECT superior to sham at 2, 4 and 8 weeks; no difference at 16 weeks
Brandon *et al.* (1985)	17 schizophrenics by Present State Examination	Sham vs. ECT; equivalent daily doses of neuroleptic in real and sham ECT groups	Eight treatments, twice weekly for 4 weeks	ECT superior to sham at 2 and 4 weeks; no difference at 12 and 28 weeks
Abraham and Kulhara (1987)	22 schizophrenic patients by the RDC with duration of illness <2 years	Sham vs. ECT; trifluoperazine held constant, no more than 20 mg/day	Eight treatments, twice weekly for 4 weeks	ECT group showed more rapid improvement than sham group; from 12 weeks to 6 months, no difference

CPZ, chlorpromazine; RDC, Research Diagnostic Criteria.

20 mg/day) and randomized to real or sham ECT. In this double-blind study, clinical outcome was superior with real ECT for up to 12 weeks after the start of treatment. Assessments conducted between 16 and 26 weeks yielded no group differences.

Summary

With the possible exception of Ulett et al. (1956), the early studies failed to demonstrate a therapeutic advantage for ECT relative to administration of general anaesthesia alone, i.e. sham ECT (Miller et al. 1953; Brill et al. 1959a,b,c; Heath et al. 1964). In contrast, at least in the short term, the three recent studies each found clinically significant therapeutic advantages for real ECT vs. sham ECT (Taylor & Fleminger 1980; Brandon et al. 1985; Abraham & Kulhara 1987). The source of this discrepancy is unknown. The recent studies had small samples, but this factor should have limited the possibility of obtaining statistically significant findings. It is noteworthy that Taylor and Fleminger (1980) explicitly focused on a 'middle-prognostic' group, and excluded patients with chronic conditions. The representation of patients with chronic schizophrenia in some of the early studies may have mitigated against establishing an ECT advantage (Heath et al. 1964). Another possibility is that in each of the recent studies, patients have been maintained on neuroleptic medications during the sham-ECT trial. There is reason to believe that the combination of ECT and neuroleptics is more effective than either form of monotherapy. Additive or synergistic ECT–neuroleptic interactions may have augmented the efficacy of real ECT conditions in the recent studies.

It is also noteworthy in recent work that the advantage of real ECT relative to sham conditions only pertained to the period of time during and immediately following administration of ECT. Within months, symptomatic differences between the groups were not evident. The importance of these negative findings is questionable. In each case, the treatment received following the randomized trial was uncontrolled. Indeed, in some cases, patients assigned to the sham condition went on to receive ECT. Without a better control over continuation therapy, it is impossible to determine whether the advantages observed in these studies for real ECT relative to sham conditions were truly short-lived.

Studies comparing ECT with neuroleptics or other therapies

From a clinical vantage point, determining that ECT is more effective than sham treatment is of limited utility. A more pressing question concerns the efficacy of ECT when compared with other somatic treatments, particularly the use of neuroleptic medication. Soon after the introduction of antipsychotic medications, a series of retrospective and prospective reports appeared that provided such comparisons. In general, the findings of the retrospective studies were inconclusive (DeWet 1957; Borowitz 1959; Ayres 1960; Rohde & Sargant 1961), although some contended that the combination of ECT and antipsychotic

medication was particularly effective (Ford & Jameson 1955; Rohde & Sargant 1961; Weinstein & Fischer 1971). Here we concentrate on the prospective investigations. This work is summarized in Table 27.2.

Baker et al. (1958) selected 48 chronically ill hospitalized female schizophrenics and assigned 18 to an ECT group, 15 to an insulin coma group, and 15 to a chlorpromazine (CPZ) group. The groups were treated for different treatment periods, ranging from 5 weeks for insulin coma to 8 weeks for CPZ. Improvement ratings were equivalent among the groups 1 week following the trial. However, relapse rates were significantly higher in the CPZ group than in the ECT or insulin coma group. This study was limited by use of low CPZ dosage. Additionally, the blindness of clinical ratings was not discussed, and the length of the follow-up for determining relapse was unspecified.

In a later report, Baker et al. (1960b) abandoned the CPZ group on the grounds of limited efficacy and added patients to the ECT and insulin coma conditions. The final sample of 37 ECT patients had a higher rate of treatment completion and hospital discharge than the final sample of 36 patients assigned to insulin coma.

Langsley et al. (1959) randomized 106 patients with 'acute schizophrenia' or manic reactions to ECT or CPZ conditions. Ratings by blind psychiatrists demonstrated that the groups were equivalent in short-term clinical improvement. However, there were indications that the CPZ group could be discharged earlier than the ECT group. Among other problems, the findings were not reported separately for patients with manic and schizophrenic diagnoses. In addition, the entry requirement of a maximum of 3 months of psychotic symptoms suggests that the schizophrenic group may have contained a large number of patients who would now be termed 'schizophreniform'. King (1960) studied 84 newly admitted women with schizophrenia. One group received unmodified ECT, followed by maintenance CPZ (300 mg/day). The other group received CPZ in rapidly increasing doses, with each patient receiving a maximum of 1200 mg/day by the seventh day. Rates of remission were found to be equivalent in the ECT and CPZ groups. However, the CPZ group had a shorter period to remission or discharge. In addition to the lack of clarity regarding the blindness of ratings, the study was compromised by the use of ECT in some patients who had insufficient response to CPZ and the use of CPZ in patients who did not respond to ECT, contaminating the group comparisons.

Ray (1962) assigned 60 consecutively admitted schizophrenic patients to one of three groups: unmodified bilateral ECT alone; CPZ alone; or combination ECT and CPZ. Outcome was grossly classified as no improvement, improvement with residual symptoms, and symptom-free. Ray (1962) reported that 50% of patients treated with ECT alone or CPZ showed no improvement. In contrast, this was observed in only 25% of the patients who received combination treatment. Perhaps because of the small sample size per treatment condition ($n = 20$), these differences in short-term response rate were not significant. Furthermore, it was unclear whether the assignment to treatment conditions was random and blindness of clinical evaluations was doubtful.

Table 27.2 Prospective clinical trials comparing ECT with neuroleptics or other treatments in schizophrenia.

Study	Patients	Study design	Nature of treatment	Results/comments
Baker *et al.* (1958)	48 'poor prognosis' schizophrenic females, aged 18–40	ECT vs. insulin coma therapy vs. CPZ; random assignment; blindness of evaluations uncertain	20 unmodified ECT at three per week; 30 insulin coma at six per week; 300 mg/day CPZ for 8 weeks	No differences among the groups in clinical outcome 1 week following acute trial; both ECT and insulin groups had lower relapse rates than medication group; medication dosage was low
Baker *et al.* (1960b)	73 'poor prognosis' schizophrenic females, aged 18–40; 33 patients had participated in Baker *et al.* (1958) in ECT or insulin conditions	ECT vs. insulin coma therapy; this study added patients to the ECT and insulin coma conditions reported by Baker *et al.* (1958)	ECT and insulin coma as in Baker *et al.* (1958)	ECT superior to insulin coma in percentage of patients who completed acute treatment and could be discharged
Langsley *et al.* (1959)	106 females (18–45) in psychotic manic or schizophrenic episode of short duration (<3 months)	ECT vs. CPZ; random assignment, single-blind	15–20 unmodified ECT at three per week; ~800 mg/day CPZ (range 200–2000 mg/day)	Clinical improvement was equivalent for ECT and CPZ, but the latter was associated with a shorter period to discharge
King (1960)	84 newly admitted female schizophrenic patients	ECT vs. CPZ; assigned alternately to treatments; blindness of evaluation uncertain	20 unmodified ECT at five per week; 900–1200 mg/day CPZ for 1 month	Rates of remission equivalent for ECT and CPZ; CPZ group had shorter period to remission or discharge; study contaminated by use of CPZ with some patients in the ECT group and vice versa; blindness unclear
Ray (1962)	60 schizophrenic patients with an average duration of illness between 1–2 years	ECT vs. CPZ vs. ECT plus CPZ; uncertain whether treatment assignment was random and evaluations blind	ECT group given ~15 unmodified treatments; 3 weekly for first 3 weeks and then tapered over 3 months; 250–300 mg/day CPZ for 10 weeks; combined group received both treatments	ECT alone and CPZ alone equivalent in rates of clinical improvement; combined treatment associated with the greatest rate of improvement. Improvement rated by clinical impression and medication dosage was low
Childers (1964)	80 newly admitted, schizophrenic females, 16–55 years of age	ECT vs. fluphenazine vs. CPZ vs. ECT plus CPZ; sequential assignment	12 ECT at three per week; fluphenazine 20 mg/day for 30 days; CPZ 1000 mg/day for 30 days; CPZ 1000 mg/day for 30 days plus 12 ECT	Improvement rates were: 55% ECT alone, 45% fluphenazine, 45% CPZ, and 80% CPZ and ECT; the combination treatment was most effective. Nature and blindness of outcome ratings not described
May (1968); May and Tuma (1965); May *et al.* (1976, 1981)	228 first-admission schizophrenic patients with middle prognosis by clinical judgement, 16–45 years of age	ECT vs. trifluoperazine vs. psychotherapy vs. psychotherapy plus trifluoperazine vs. milieu treatment alone; random assignment, single-blind, with long follow-up period	Averaged 19 ECT for males and 25 ECT for females at variable rate; trifluoperazine alone group had maximal dose of 25.5 mg/day	Short-term outcome was superior in groups that received medication relative to ECT and the ECT group had superior short-term outcome compared to psychotherapy or milieu treatment. Long-term outcome (up to 5 years) was statistically equivalent in somatic

Table 27.2 (cont.)

Study	Patients	Study design	Nature of treatment	Results/comments
				treatment groups and superior to psychotherapy or milieu treatment. However, ECT group showed trends for the best long-term outcome; dosage of medication was low by modern standards and treatment following the acute phase was uncontrolled
Bagadia *et al.* (1970)	300 schizophrenic patients, with varying prognosis scores	ECT vs. insulin coma vs. CPZ vs. trifluoperazine vs. trifluperidol vs. flupenthixol; groups matched for distributions of prognosis; unclear if assignment was random or whether evaluations were blind	Up to 10 unmodified ECT over 4 weeks; 20–30 insulin coma treatments at six treatments per week over 4 weeks; medications administered over a 3–4 week period: CPZ up to 2400 mg/day, trifluoperazine up to 60 mg/day, trifluperidol up to 6 mg/day, flupenthixol up to 15 mg/day	Relative to each of the other treatments, ECT resulted in the most rapid improvement and the highest rate of complete symptomatic remission. Ratings of symptomatic improvement were impressionistic; methodological details lacking
Murillo and Exner (1973a,b); Exner and Murillo (1973, 1977)	53 chronic 'process' schizophrenic patients	Regressive ECT vs. pharmacotherapy and psychotherapy; treatment assignment not randomized	Regressive treatment involved twice daily, bilateral ECT, 7 days per week, until regression occurred (helplessness, confusion, mutism and neurologic signs); medication group received haloperidol ($n = 11$), CPZ ($n = 6$) or CPZ plus trifluoperazine ($n = 4$) in unspecified doses; nature of concomitant psychotherapy not described	Regressive ECT superior to the medication and psychotherapy condition in extent of clinical improvement at discharge and 7–9 weeks following discharge; at 24–30 months postdischarge no differences between the groups in neuropsychological testing; study compromised by non-random assignment (medication group had refused regressive ECT) and lack of standardization of treatments
Bagadia *et al.* (1983)	38 schizophrenic patients, with positive symptoms but not depressive or manic features	ECT and placebo vs. 18 sham ECT and CPZ	Six modified bilateral ECT plus placebo; Six sham ECT with 400–900 mg/day CPZ over 2–3 weeks	Clinical improvement equivalent in the two groups; 40 patients dropped out of the trial and were not included in analyses

CPZ, chlorpromazine.

Childers (1964) sequentially assigned 80 newly admitted schizophrenic patients to bilateral ECT, fluphenazine, CPZ, or CPZ plus bilateral ECT. Global ratings were made of clinical improvement following the acute treatment phase and the blindness of ratings was not described. Impressionistically, the findings suggested that the combination treatment was more effective than ECT alone or neuroleptic alone (Table 27.2). However, with samples sizes of 20 per group, differences among the four treatment conditions in improvement rate were of marginal significance ($P = 0.08$), as was our explicit comparison of ECT alone and the combination treatment ($P = 0.09$).

May and colleagues conducted a landmark study in which

228 first-admission, 'middle prognosis' patients with schizophrenia were randomized to five treatment conditions: bilateral ECT; antipsychotic medication alone; psychotherapy alone; antipsychotic medication plus psychotherapy; or milieu therapy (May & Tuma 1965; May 1968; May *et al.* 1976, 1981). Diagnosis was based on independent interviews by six physicians. The characterization of middle prognosis was based on a clinical judgement that the patient was neither showing signs of rapid recovery during the evaluation period nor having little chance of recovering over a 2-year period.

Modified bilateral ECT (atropine, thiopental, succinylcholine) was administered at first at a rate of three treatments per week. The duration of the treatment course and the spacing of subsequent treatments were determined individually for each patient, based on response and side-effects. The main medication used was trifluoperazine, given orally, although intramuscular medication was also given and a few patients also received concomitant CPZ. Medication dosage was determined on an individual basis and an antiparkinsonian agent was also used (procyclidine). The medication groups had an average daily trifluoperazine dose of ~ 20 mg/day. Psychotherapy was given for an average of not less than 2 h/week. The therapists were residents or psychiatrists of limited experience, but each was supervised by a psychoanalyst. The content of the psychotherapy was uncontrolled, but was described as generally focusing on reality testing and as ego supportive.

Across a variety of objective outcome measures, the short-term findings favoured the medication conditions in terms of ratings of psychopathology, days hospitalized, discharge rate and costs. The short-term outcome results with ECT were intermediate between those of antipsychotic medications and psychological treatments (psychotherapy or milieu therapy). However, 2–5 year follow-up indicated that subsequent time spent in the hospital was equivalent for the medication and the ECT treated patients (May *et al.* 1976). Another follow-up study showed that, 3–5 years after discharge, the medication alone and the ECT groups tended to have the best outcome and the psychotherapy alone the worst outcome (May *et al.* 1981). Indeed, long-term outcome tended to be best in those initially assigned to ECT. May *et al.* (1981) concluded:

> Patients who had been treated with ECT fared, in the long run, at least as well as those given drug therapy, and in some respects even better, but not to a statistically significant extent. It seems that the status and role of ECT in the treatment of schizophrenia merit serious objective study. (p. 784)

A fundamental limitation in the interpretation of this work was the fact that the follow-up was naturalistic and treatment after the acute phase was uncontrolled. However, in a reanalysis of this study, Wyatt (1991) pointed out that during the follow-up period only the group treated with ECT had a statistically significant decrease in neuroleptic dosage. Despite lower neuroleptic dosage, the ECT group averaged 50 days of rehospitalization during the 2 years following discharge, compared with 70 days for neuroleptic alone, 55 days for neuroleptic and psychotherapy, 80 days for milieu therapy, and 120 days for psychotherapy alone (Wyatt 1991). Only the comparison between psychotherapy alone and ECT indicated a reliable difference.

Murillo and Exner (1973a,b; Exner & Murillo 1973, 1977) compared a group of 32 patients with process schizophrenia who were treated with 'regressive' ECT with a group of 21 similar patients treated with antipsychotic medications and psychotherapy. The patients were said to be characterized by a premorbid history of chronic disorganization, detachment, and chaotic and unpredictable behaviour. Assignment was not random, as the medication group comprised patients who had refused regressive ECT. Three different medications were used, haloperidol, CPZ and trifluoperazine, but dosage and duration were not specified. Analysis of 55 variables indicated that the groups were equivalent at study entry. At discharge, the ECT group differed significantly from the medication group in 28 of the 55 variables. All the differences favoured the ECT group, including symptomatic evaluations based on self-report and ratings by relatives and by referring physicians. Exner and Murillo (1977) conducted a long-term follow-up of a subgroup of these patients, with a minimum 24-month follow-up interval. Neuropsychological and projective testing revealed few, if any, differences between the groups. However, by family member and self-report, a significantly greater proportion of the ECT patients were working regularly in a full-time job, had taken a recent vacation, regularly drove a car and had terminated psychiatric treatment. In contrast, a higher proportion of the medication group were regularly taking medication and had recently visited physicians for problems not related to psychiatric causes. Lack of a standardized medication regimen, non-random assignment and uncertainty about the blindness of evaluations were clear limitations.

Bagadia *et al.* (1983) reported on 38 patients who were symptomatic for at least 1 month and manifested delusions, hallucinations or irrelevant verbal production in the context of clear consciousness and an absence of depressive or manic symptoms. Patients had not received antipsychotic medication within 3 weeks or ECT or insulin coma within 8 weeks of study entry. This double-blind random assignment study contrasted bilateral ECT and medication placebo with sham ECT and CPZ. Real and sham ECT involved administration of atropine, thiopental and succinylcholine. CPZ was started at 200 mg/day and increased gradually to 600 mg/day where it was maintained, increased or decreased after evaluation by a consultant psychiatrist, blind to the mode of treatment. An initial sample of 78 patients had been randomized, but 40 patients were excluded for irregular attendance, non-compliance or for discontinuation of treatment. Brief Psychiatric Rating Scale (BPRS) measures showed a trend for greater improvement in the real ECT group after 7 days, but no difference between the groups in total or subscale scores after 20 days. Both samples showed marked clinical improvement. In addition to a high drop-out rate, this study was limited by use of a fixed and low number of ECT treatments.

Summary

There has been a surprising paucity of prospective research contrasting ECT with pharmacological treatments of schizophrenia. The limitations of this literature in fundamental aspects of clinical trial methodology, particularly the reliability and validity of diagnosis, the nature of assignment to treatment groups and the blindness and reliability of clinical evaluations further underscore the need for caution in interpreting findings. Other limitations pertain to the adequacy of treatment delivery, both in terms of ECT administration and pharmacotherapy. With these caveats, it appears that generally short-term outcome was equivalent or superior with antipsychotic medication relative to ECT (Langsley *et al.* 1959; King 1960; Ray 1962; May & Tuma 1965; May 1968), although even here there were exceptions (Murillo & Exner 1973a). There is little indication from this literature about the clinical or treatment history features that might distinguish schizophrenics who preferentially respond to antipsychotic medications or ECT. In contrast, a seemingly consistent theme was the suggestion that patients who were administered ECT had superior long-term outcome compared with medication groups (Baker *et al.* 1958; May *et al.* 1971, 1981; Exner & Murillo 1977). Similarly, in a retrospective comparison of ECT, insulin coma, CPZ and reserpine, Ayres (1960) reported that schizophrenic patients treated with ECT were the least likely to require rehospitalization. This pattern is unexpected, given the perspective that virtually all the behavioural and physiological

effects of ECT are relatively short-lived (Snaith 1981; Sackeim 1988; Sackeim *et al.* 1990, 1993, 1995, 2000). Furthermore, most of these studies were conducted in an era when the importance of continuation and maintenance treatment was not appreciated and none controlled treatment following resolution of the schizophrenic episode. Nevertheless, the possibility that ECT may have beneficial long-term effects merits attention.

Studies comparing combined ECT and medication treatment with medication alone or ECT alone

Two of the studies described in Table 27.2 contained comparisons of ECT administered alone with ECT administered in combination with antipsychotic medication (Ray 1962; Childers 1964). Both studies produced suggestive evidence that combination treatment was more effective than monotherapy with ECT or antipsychotic medications. In the real vs. sham trial by Abraham and Kulhara (1987), all patients received 20 mg/day trifluoperazine, resulting in another comparison of combination treatment with medication alone (Table 27.1). This study found that in the short term real ECT (combination treatment) was more effective than sham ECT (antipsychotic medication alone). Table 27.3 summarizes all the prospective clinical

Table 27.3 Prospective clinical trials comparing combination treatment with ECT and antipsychotic medication with ECT alone or antipsychotic medication alone.

Study	Patients	Study design	Nature of treatment	Results/comments
Ray (1962)	60 schizophrenic patients with an average duration of illness between 1–2 years	ECT vs. CPZ vs. ECT plus CPZ; uncertain whether treatment assignment was random and evaluations blind	ECT group given ~15 unmodified treatments; 3 weekly for first 3 weeks and then tapered over 3 months; 250–300 mg/day CPZ for 10 weeks; combined group received both treatments	ECT alone and CPZ alone equivalent in rates of clinical improvement; combined treatment associated with the greatest rate of improvement. Improvement rated by clinical impression; medication dosage was low
Childers (1964)	80 newly admitted, schizophrenic females, 16–55 years of age	ECT vs. fluphenazine vs. CPZ vs. ECT plus CPZ; sequential assignment	12 ECT at three per week; fluphenazine 20 mg/day for 30 days; CPZ 1000 mg/day for 30 days; CPZ 1000 mg/day for 30 days plus 12 ECT	Improvement rates were: 55% ECT alone, 45% fluphenazine, 45% CPZ, and 80% CPZ and ECT; the combination treatment was most effective. Nature and blindness of outcome ratings not described
Smith *et al.* (1967)	54 schizophrenic patients, with average duration of 6 years since first episode and 20 previous admissions	ECT and CPZ vs. CPZ; every fifth white patient assigned to combination treatment, CPZ cell from a pharmacological study; study personnel blind to drug or placebo in CPZ cell	12 modified ECT at three per week plus an average of 400 mg/day CPZ; CPZ alone averaged 655 mg/day during 6-week acute trial	Various standardized ratings indicated that ECT and CPZ group had faster clinical response and superior outcome at end of 6-week acute trial. At 6 month and 1-year cross-sectional follow-up no differences observed. However, ECT and CPZ group had a higher discharge rate and a lower rehospitalization rate than CPZ only group

Table 27.3 (cont.)

Study	Patients	Study design	Nature of treatment	Results/comments
Small et al. (1982); Small (1985)	75 schizophrenic patients (Feighner criteria), with middle prognosis (>6 months and <2 years hospitalization)	ECT and tiotixene (n = 25) vs. tiotixene alone (n = 26) vs. ECT and placebo (n = 16) vs. placebo alone (n = 8); random assignment and modified double-blind design with standardized outcome measures	ECT groups received an average of 15 modified right unilateral treatments, at three per week; tiotixene alone group averaged 913 mg/day CPZ equivalents; tiotixene in combination group averaged 650 mg/day CPZ equivalents; considerable drop-out in ECT alone and placebo groups	Statistical findings never presented. Authors concluded that ECT and tiotixene was superior in clinical outcome to tiotixene alone, which in turn was superior to both ECT alone and placebo
Janakiramaiah et al. (1982)	60 schizophrenic or schizophreniform patients (RDC) with continuous illness between 2 months and 6 years	ECT and 300 mg/day CPZ vs. 300 mg/day CPZ alone vs. ECT and 500 mg/day CPZ vs. 500 mg/day CPZ alone; treatment free at study entry; random assignment; partial blindness in evaluations	Modified ECT administered at three per week; 300 mg CPZ group averaged 9.5 ECT and 500 mg CPZ group averaged 10.4 treatments; CPZ administered for 6 weeks	At completion of acute trial (6 weeks) inferior clinical outcome in the 300 mg/day CPZ group. ECT and 500 mg/day CPZ had earliest clinical response, but no advantage to combination treatment relative to 500 mg/day CPZ alone at 6 weeks
Ungvári and Pethö (1982)	75 recently admitted schizophrenic patients (RDC) with average duration of illness of ~7 years	ECT and low-dose haloperidol vs. high-dose haloperidol; study duration only 6 days; assignment to group random; blind evaluation	Two modified ECTs on each of three occasions over a period of 6 days plus an average of 6.5 mg/day haloperidol; high-dose haloperidol group averaged 72 mg/day (range 50–120 mg/day)	Analyses stratified by diagnostic distinction between systematic and unsystematic schizophrenia (similar to reactive/process distinction). Treatment groups equivalent among unsystematic schizophrenics; ECT and low-dose haloperidol superior to high-dose haloperidol among systematic schizophrenics. Short duration of trial and unusual ECT schedule limit clinical relevance
Abraham and Kulhara (1987)	22 schizophrenic patients by the RDC with duration of illness <2 years	Sham ECT vs. real ECT; trifluoperazine held constant during trial, 20 mg/day to all patients; random assignment, double-blind	Eight sham or real (modified) treatments, twice weekly for 4 weeks	ECT group showed more rapid improvement than sham group; from 12 weeks to 6 months, no difference
Das et al. (1991)	48 newly admitted schizophrenic patients; 30 described as chronic	Naturalistic comparison of patients treated with neuroleptics alone or neuroleptics and ECT; GAS completed at admission and discharge	Medications involved 500–900 mg/day CPZ, 15–45 mg/day trifluoperazine, or 15–45 mg/day haloperidol; adjunctive ECT used typically because of symptom severity, medication resistance or intolerance; ECT not described	Combined ECT and neuroleptic group more severely ill at baseline; both groups manifested strong improvement; extent of change in GAS scores greater in the combined ECT and neuroleptic group. Neuroleptic only group had half the length of stay. Non-blind naturalistic comparison

CPZ, chlorpromazine; GAS, Global Assessment Scale; RDC, Research Diagnostic Criteria.

trials that have compared ECT combined with antipsychotic medication with ECT alone or with antipsychotic medication alone.

The trials reported by Ray (1962) and Childers (1964) were described earlier. Smith *et al.* (1967) reported on a group of 54 largely chronic schizophrenic patients. Patients assigned to a combination ECT/CPZ group (*n* = 29) comprised every fifth white patient admission who met criteria for the NIMH-PSC Collaborative Study of Phenothiazines (NIMH-PSC Collaborative Study Group 1964). This treatment group was compared with one of the treatment conditions (*n* = 25) taken from a concurrent pharmacological trial (NIMH-PSC Collaborative Study Group 1964). The comparison group was treated only with CPZ. Clinical outcome was repeatedly evaluated with standardized scales during a 6-week acute treatment period and at 6-month and 1-year follow-up. Ratings were blind to type of neuroleptic medication or placebo, but presumably raters were not blind to status in the ECT group. On various global and symptomatic ratings, the combination condition showed more rapid clinical improvement and superior outcome at the end of the first 6 weeks. It was noted that the combination group displayed significantly less hostility and ideas of persecution at 6 weeks, but more confusion and memory deficits. Cross-sectional evaluation at the 6-month and 1-year follow-ups failed to distinguish the groups. However, the combination treatment was associated with significantly more rapid discharge, fewer days of hospitalization and fewer rehospitalizations during the year following admission. For example, 6 months after admission, 40% of the CPZ alone group had not been discharged compared with 14% in the group given combination treatment. The rehospitalization rates after discharge were 33% for CPZ alone and 10% for combination treatment. While limited by failing to use random assignment and fully blinded evaluations, this study suggested that ECT combined with antipsychotic medication may be superior to antipsychotic medication alone, both in the short and long term. As with previous studies, the lack of control over treatment received after the acute trial period was a critical limitation.

Small *et al.* (1982) and Small (1985) randomized 75 'middle prognosis' patients who met the Feighner *et al.* (1972) criteria for schizophrenia to one of four conditions: ECT combined with tiotixene, ECT and medication placebo, tiotixene alone, or medication placebo. A randomization scheme was used that resulted in small sample sizes for the ECT and placebo and placebo-only groups. Both the number of ECT treatments and medication dosages were titrated with the aim of achieving maximal clinical response. Tiotixene dosage was said to be equivalent in the two groups receiving active medication, but was reported as averaging 650 mg/day CPZ equivalents in the ECT and tiotixene group and 913 mg/day in the tiotixene alone group. Clinical outcome was assessed with a variety of standardized scales, with double-blind procedures. Across rating scales there was a hierarchy of clinical response. The best outcomes were observed with the combination of ECT and tiotixene, followed by tiotixene alone, ECT alone, and placebo alone. Scores on the Abnormal In-voluntary Movement Scale (AIMS) indicated that patients given only tiotixene had more orofacial movements that other treatment groups. ECT is known to exert an antiparkinsonian effect, both in some forms of idiopathic Parkinson's disease, as well as with neuroleptic-induced extrapyramidal side-effects (American Psychiatric Association 2001).

Janakiramaiah *et al.* (1982) studied 60 patients who fulfilled modified Research Diagnostic Criteria (RDC; Spitzer *et al.* 1978) for schizophrenia or schizophreniform illness. Patients were randomly assigned to one of four treatment groups: 300 mg/day CPZ; 300 mg/day CPZ with ECT; 500 mg/day CPZ; and 500 mg/day CPZ with ECT. Clinical assessments, conducted weekly for 6 weeks, were partially blind to treatment condition and involved global ratings, BPRS ratings and an evaluation of extrapyramidal symptoms. Consistently, from the second to the sixth week, the 300 mg/day CPZ only group had inferior clinical outcome compared with the other groups. After the first week of treatment, the combined 500 mg/day CPZ and ECT group had greater improvement than the other three groups. However, at the end of the trial there was no advantage to combining 500 mg/day CPZ with ECT relative to 500 mg/day CPZ alone.

In an unusual study, Ungvári and Pethö (1982) treated 75 recently admitted patients with schizophrenia, randomizing them to either a high-dosage haloperidol group (*n* = 39) or to a group that received ECT and low-dosage haloperidol (*n* = 36). The high-dosage group was administered between 50 and 120 mg/day of haloperidol, with an average dose of 72 mg/day. A total of six modified seizures were elicited with ECT, two seizures in each of three sessions over 6 days. Patients in the ECT group were also administered an average of 6.5 mg/day of haloperidol (range = 4.5–9 mg/day). The total duration of this trial was only 6 days, suggesting that patients in the ECT group were evaluated very shortly following a multiple seizure induction. Evaluations were blinded, using a modified version of the BPRS. Analyses of efficacy were stratified by the diagnostic distinction of Leonhard (1979), contrasting unsystematic and systematic schizophrenia. This distinction is similar to the process/reactive dichotomy. Both forms of treatment were efficacious in each patent subgroup. However, among systematic schizophrenic patients, the ECT/haloperidol treatment was notably superior to treatment with high-dosage haloperidol.

Das *et al.* (1991) reported a naturalistic prospective comparison of schizophrenic patients treated with medications alone or with medications combined with ECT. Over a 6-month period, 48 patients were identified who received CPZ, trifluoperazine or haloperidol. In this relatively young sample, 23 patients were administered concurrent ECT because of severe symptomatology, medication resistance or medication intolerance. The medication-alone group had half the hospital stay compared with the ECT group (17 vs. 34 days). Using the Global Assessment Scale (GAS), the ECT group was more impaired at admission. At discharge, the two groups had similar GAS scores, with the change significantly greater in the ECT group.

Summary

This literature is also characterized by a host of methodological difficulties. As in the comparisons of monotherapy with ECT or with antipsychotic medication, the adequacy of pharmacological monotherapy and combined antipsychotic/ECT treatment was often questionable. Relatively few of these studies involved random assignment, and fewer still involved fully blind outcome assessment. Nevertheless, it is noteworthy that in each of the three studies in which ECT alone was compared with ECT combined with antipsychotic medication there were suggestions that the combination was more effective (Ray 1962; Childers 1964; Small et al. 1982). A larger number of investigations have contrasted the combination treatment with monotherapy with an antipsychotic medication. With the exception of Janakiramaiah et al. (1982), in each instance there was evidence that treatment with an antipsychotic medication in combination with ECT was more effective than treatment with an antipsychotic medication alone (Ray 1962; Childers 1964; Smith et al. 1967; Small et al. 1982; Ungvári & Pethö 1982; Abraham & Kulhara 1987; Das et al. 1991). In some cases, a superior outcome was obtained despite an apparent lower average neuroleptic dose in the combination condition (Smith et al. 1967; Small et al. 1982; Ungvári & Pethö 1982). Few of these studies followed patients beyond the acute treatment period and in none was there standardization of continuation or maintenance treatments. Therefore, the relative persistence of any advantage for combination treatment is unknown. In this respect, the findings reported by Smith et al. (1967), suggesting a reduced rate of relapse in patients treated acutely with neuroleptics and ECT relative to neuroleptics alone, were particularly intriguing. When considered with the follow-up results of May et al. (1981) there is added reason to explore whether ECT, particularly in combination with antipsychotic medication, may exert a long-term beneficial effect in schizophrenia.

ECT and neuroleptic medication in medication-resistant schizophrenic patients

In general, the studies that used sham vs. real ECT designs and the studies that have contrasted ECT and traditional antipsychotic medications indicate that ECT has efficacy in the treatment of schizophrenia. In isolation, this fact is of limited clinical utility, because little has been identified about the patients most likely to benefit from ECT. Moreover, standard treatment of schizophrenia begins with trials of antipsychotic medication. A critical question is whether ECT is efficacious in patients who fail to respond to traditional neuroleptic medications. Such patients constitute between 5% and 25% of all individuals with this diagnosis (Meltzer 1992; Kane 1999). Few studies have explicitly examined the use of ECT in medication-resistant schizophrenic patients. This work is summarized in Table 27.4.

The earliest study was undertaken by Childers and Therrien (1961) and involved 48 schizophrenic patients. These patients were sequentially assigned to one of four groups: CPZ; trifluo-

perazine; placebo medication; or no treatment. At the end of 35 days, those patients who had not received active medication and had not improved were crossed over to one of the two active medication groups. This crossover occurred in all but one of the patients initially assigned to placebo or no treatment. Patients who failed to improve with CPZ or trifluoperazine alone (initial or crossover phase) were switched to the other medication and also received a concurrent course of ECT. Bilateral ECT was administered at a schedule of three per week for 5 weeks and patients also received concurrent CPZ or trifluoperazine. Eleven of 23 patients who had failed to respond to neuroleptic treatment were considered improved when switched to an alternative neuroleptic and ECT. In addition to non-blind evaluation, the significance of these findings was limited by the simultaneous use of an alternative neuroleptic with ECT.

Rahman (1968) reviewed the treatment of 176 schizophrenic patients admitted to a psychiatric hospital in East Pakistan during 1965. Patients were typically first treated with an antipsychotic medication (prochlorperazine, CPZ or trifluoperazine) and received ECT with antipsychotic medication only after they had failed to improve over a 2–3 month time period. Rahman (1968) concluded that ECT combined with one of the phenothiazines produced superior results than phenothiazines alone. All 50 patients that were treated with combination ECT and medication were rated as either improved (48%) or remitted (52%), rates that exceeded medication comparison groups.

In another impressionistic retrospective study, Lewis (1982) reviewed the charts of patients diagnosed as schizophrenic and who received ECT during a 4.5-year period (1974–78) at the Payne Whitney Clinic in New York. Of 29 patients identified, 23 had failed an adequate medication trial prior to receiving an average of 14 ECT treatments. This sample was relatively young, and presumably with relatively short duration of illness. In 24 of the 29 patients, outcome was rated as good or excellent. The significance of this observation was limited by the fact that clinical outcome was not rated at the termination of ECT, but rather at discharge from the hospital. In some cases, patients received other forms of treatment following ECT and prior to discharge.

Friedel (1986) prospectively identified 21 patients meeting DSM-III criteria for schizophrenia. These patients underwent a standardized trial with tiotixene. Neuroleptic dosage was increased until there was moderate to marked improvement, intolerable side-effects, or until tiotixene and desmethyltiotixene plasma levels exceeded 15 ng/mL. For 11 patients who showed no or slight improvement, dosage was increased further until plasma levels were greater than 15 ng/mL. These patients were non-responders and nine were administered ECT and were also continued on tiotixene at a dose of 30–60 mg/day. Eight of the nine patients had a complete remission and one patient was significantly improved. The extent of improvement in this open trial was impressive, particularly because the average patient had been continuously psychotic for over 3 years and had previously failed other neuroleptics and lithium. Friedel (1986) called for a randomized controlled trial of ECT combined with

Table 27.4 Clinical trials of ECT in medication-resistant schizophrenic patients.

Study	Patients	Study design	Nature of treatment	Results/comments
Childers and Therrien (1961)	48 newly admitted schizophrenic patients (26 chronic undifferentiated, 16 paranoid, 3 schizoaffective, 2 hebephrenic, and 1 simple)	Sequentially assigned to one of four groups: CPZ, trifluoperazine, placebo medication, or no treatment. Non-responders to placebo or no treatment crossed over to one of the active medication conditions. Medication non-responders given ECT and the alternative medication at reduced dosage	Initial treatment phase involved 1000 mg/day CPZ or 40 mg/day trifluoperazine for 35 days; medication failures received 15 ECT treatments at 3 per week plus either 500 mg/day CPZ or 20 mg/day trifluoperazine	23 of 48 patients failed to respond to medication alone; 11 of the 23 patients responded when ECT was combined with the alternative neuroleptic
Rahman (1968)	176 newly admitted schizophrenic patients. Average age of 28.9, with average 20 months duration of illness	Naturalistic, retrospective comparison of clinical outcome with one of three neuroleptics (prochlorperazine, CPZ, trifluoperazine) and ECT combined with neuroleptic. Patients typically received the combination after failing single neuroleptic treatment for 2–3 months	Typical neuroleptic treatment involved 75 mg/day prochlorperazine, 300 mg/day CPZ, or 15 mg/day trifluoperazine. Nature of ECT not described	All 50 patients who received combined ECT and neuroleptic treatment were considered improved (48%) or remitted (52%), rates superior to neuroleptic alone. Outcome criteria impressionistic and not blindly evaluated
Lewis (1982)	29 newly admitted schizophrenic (DSM-III) patients, with an average age of 27	Retrospective evaluation of outcome in medication-resistant patients; 23 of 29 rated as medication resistant, with most failing neuroleptic treatment equivalent to at least 1 gm/day CPZ for at least 3 weeks	Neuroleptic medication continued during ECT, but typically at reduced dosage; nature of ECT not described; average of 14 treatments administered	Outcome was rated as good or excellent in 24 of 29 patients. Outcome was assessed at time of discharge and other treatments intervened following ECT
Friedel (1986)	9 patients with DSM-III schizophrenia and moderate to severe psychotic symptoms	Larger group of 21 patients treated with thiothixene until plasma levels exceeded 15 ng/ml or were intolerant. Nine non-responders received ECT plus tiotixene	ECT ranged from 8 to 25 treatments with average of 13.6; 6 patients received unilateral and 3 patients received bilateral ECT. Tiotixene doses ranged from 30 to 60 mg/day during ECT	Eight of 9 patients achieved complete remission and one patient had mild symptoms following ECT. Open clinical trial that used strict standards for medication resistance
Gujavarty et al. (1987)	8 patients with DSM-III schizophrenia and moderate to severe symptoms	Retrospective chart review. Patients did not respond to 2 courses of neuroleptics, each in a generally accepted dose range for a least 6 weeks	Unilateral or bilateral ECT at 3 per week, with an average of 14.4 treatments; neuroleptic medication continued during ECT	Seven of the 8 patients improved, which was sustained in 5 patients after 6 and 12 months. Five of these 8 patients had a history of prominent affective symptoms

Table 27.4 (cont.)

Study	Patients	Study design	Nature of treatment	Results/comments
Konig and Glatter Gotz (1990)	13 patients with ICD-9 schizophrenia	Retrospective chart review. 11 of 13 patients referred for ECT due to medication resistance, typically failing in excess of 1 gm/day CPZ equivalents	Nature of ECT not described; patients received an average of 12.4 treatments; neuroleptic medication continued during ECT	Nine of the 13 patients judged to have good clinical outcome. In these patients, neuroleptic dosage was decreased by 72% following ECT
Milstein *et al.* (1990)	110 patients with DSM-IIIR schizophrenia (25 schizoaffective, 39 paranoid, 46 non-paranoid)	Patients were usually referred for ECT due to medication resistance or intolerance; clinical ratings prospectively collected with standardized instruments	Unilateral and bilateral ECT given, 3 per week, with an average of 16.8 treatments. Unilateral non-responders crossed over to bilateral ECT. 87 patients received concurrent neuroleptics	54% of sample rated as much improved or very much improved. Clinical response was independent of diagnostic subtype and categorization of concurrent neuroleptic treatment. Explicit criteria for medication resistance not used, nor internal analysis reported for resistant patients
Sajatovic and Meltzer (1993)	9 medication-resistant schizophrenic patients	Patients failed neuroleptic treatment prior to receiving ECT and loxapine; ECT responders administered continuation ECT. Open clinical trial	Details regarding ECT and medication dosage not provided; average of 8 ECT	Five of 9 patients had a good clinical response to combination ECT and loxapine. Of 5 patients given continuation ECT, 3 relapsed within 4 months
Chanpattana and Sackeim (2002) Chanpattana *et al.* (1999c,d)	253 DSM-IV schizophrenic patients who have not responded to at least two neuroleptic trials of different classes during the current episode	Open clinical trial involving combination bilateral ECT and flupenthixol. Initial remitters had to maintain clinical gains during a 3-week stabilization period, involving an ECT taper	Bilateral ECT given 3 times per week during the acute phase; flupentixol dose of 24 mg/day (1200 mg CPZ), depending on tolerability	54.5% of the 253 patients met remitter criteria after the stabilization phase; those randomized to single-blind continuation treatment with ECT and flupentixol had reduced relapse compared to those randomized to continuation ECT or flupentixol alone

CPZ, chlorpromazine.

neuroleptic medication vs. neuroleptic medication alone in a medication-resistant sample of schizophrenic patients.

Prompted by the Friedel (1986) report, Gujavarty *et al.* (1987) reviewed the records of 90 patients treated with ECT at their facility during a 2-year period. Eight patients with DSM-III diagnoses of schizophrenia were identified who had not improved after at least two trials of neuroleptic medication and had been continuously hospitalized for at least 90 days. These patients received an average of 14.4 ECT treatments. A variety of neuroleptic medications were also administered throughout the ECT course. Seven of the eight patients improved, with this improvement sustained in five patients at 6- and 12-month follow-ups. Gujavarty *et al.* (1987) noted, however, that five of the eight patients had manifested significant affective sympto-

matology in the past, raising the possibility that these were patients with schizoaffective disorder.

Konig and Glatter-Gotz (1990) conducted a retrospective survey of 13 schizophrenic patients who were treated with ECT at an Austrian hospital between 1979 and 1982. Eight cases were referred for ECT because of neuroleptic resistance. Three other patients also were considered treatment-resistant and had catatonic exacerbations while receiving neuroleptic treatment. Prior to ECT, these patients were treated with neuroleptics generally in excess of 1 g/day CPZ equivalents. One patient was medication intolerant. Nine of the 13 patients showed a good response to ECT. In these nine patients, neuroleptic dosage was reduced by 72% following ECT.

Milstein *et al.* (1990) reported on the treatment of 110 patients with DSM-IIIR diagnoses of schizoaffective disorder, paranoid schizophrenia or non-paranoid schizophrenia. Patients were referred for ECT because of failure to respond to medications or intolerable side-effects. Systematic criteria for medication resistance were not used. Standardized rating scales were administered prior to and following the ECT course, including the BPRS and the Clinical Global Impression (CGI). In this relatively young sample (average age of 26.4 years), 54% were rated as much improved or very much improved following ECT. Eighty-seven of the 110 patients received concurrent antipsychotic medications. Treatment outcome was independent of whether or not patients received neuroleptics during ECT or judgements of whether neuroleptic dosage was low or high. Clinical outcome was also independent of diagnostic subtyping as schizoaffective, paranoid or non-paranoid schizophrenia. Milstein et al. (1990) noted that the response rate was lower than that of patients with mood disorders treated at the facility. None the less, in a presumably largely medication-resistant sample, this study provided additional impressionistic evidence that ECT may be efficacious in schizophrenic patients resistant to traditional antipsychotic medications.

Sajatovic and Meltzer (1993) collected nine patients with schizophrenia or schizoaffective illness who had inadequate response to prior neuroleptic treatment. These patients then received ECT combined with loxapine. Five patients were regarded as manifesting significant clinical improvement, with the beneficial effects most marked for positive, relative to negative, symptoms. Of note, the presence of affective symptoms (schizoaffective disorder) was not associated with good ECT outcome. Five of the patients were administered continuation ECT, following the acute trial. While two patients maintained improvement, three relapsed within 4 months.

In perhaps the most important modern set of studies, Chanpattana and colleagues modified the criteria of Kane et al. (1988a) to select schizophrenic patients with established resistance to traditional antipsychotic medication (Chanpattana 1999, 2000; Chanpattana et al. 1999a,b,c,d; Chanpattana & Sackeim 2002). These studies used especially rigorous methodology in patient selection and treatment. During the current episode, patients with a DSM-IV diagnosis of schizophrenia had to fail at least two distinct periods of neuroleptic treatment from at least two different classes. The duration of each neuroleptic treatment period was at least 6 weeks, and did not result in significant symptomatic relief. To qualify as adequate, dosage of each neuroleptic trial had to be at least 750 mg/day CPZ equivalents. Duration of illness had to be more than 2 years. Other inclusion criteria required a baseline BPRS score (original 18 items, each item rated on a 0–6 scale) of 35 or greater and that the patient present with an acute psychotic exacerbation (chronic schizophrenia with acute exacerbation by DSM-IIIR criteria). There were 253 participants (157 male) across these studies.

Psychotropic medications were withdrawn at least 5 days before the start of ECT and flupenthixol was started immediately without a washout. Flupenthixol was started at 12 mg/day for the first week and then maintained at 24 mg/day (1200 mg CPZ equivalents), contingent on tolerability, until completion of the ECT course. All patients received benzhexol (4–15 mg/day) to prevent extrapyramidal symptoms. Modified bilateral ECT was administered three times per week, using a constant-current brief-pulse stimulus. At the first treatment session, seizure threshold was determined using the empirical titration procedure (Sackeim et al. 1987b). Electrical dosage was maintained at the threshold level unless seizure manifestations were inadequate. In such cases, charge was increased by 50%.

Patients who received 20 ECT treatments at the schedule of three per week and had final BPRS scores greater than 25 were classified as non-responders. Patients who had a BPRS score of 25 or less during the regular treatment course entered a 3-week stabilization period (Chanpattana 1999; Chanpattana et al. 1999a). During this period, ECT was given three times per week during the first week, and then once weekly during the second and third week. If the BPRS score was 25 or greater during this period and the total number of ECT treatments was less than 20, the patient returned to the regular schedule of three treatments per week. Responders were restricted to patients who completed the 3-week stabilization period, during which the BPRS score assessed prior to each treatment was consistently below 25.

Of the total of 253 participants, 138 patients (54.5%) met these fairly stringent criteria for response, including maintenance of clinical gains during the 3-week stabilization period (Chanpattana et al. 1999d; Chanpattana & Sackeim 2002). While this response rate compares favourably to those obtained in the original clozapine trial (Kane et al. 1988a) and other studies of treatment-resistant schizophrenia, the major limitation of this work was that it was open label, without blinding or a pharmacological comparison condition. Indeed, comparison to use of an atypical antipsychotic medication would be particularly instructive.

Several case series have been reported on the combined use of atypical antipsychotics and ECT in treatment-resistant patients with schizophrenia. They are discussed below.

Summary

We have yet to have a double-blind random assignment study contrasting the efficacy of ECT and neuroleptic treatment and continued neuroleptic treatment alone in medication-resistant schizophrenic patients. All the information we have on this issue comes largely from impressionistic observations or large case series. Nevertheless, it is evident that, starting with the report of Childers and Therrien (1961), there have been indications that some, if not many, medication-resistant schizophrenic patients may benefit substantially by the addition of ECT. These indications seemingly contradict the clinical tenet that ECT is of limited value in chronic schizophrenic patients with long durations of illness (Kalinowsky & Worthing 1943; Salzman 1980). Our own experience in treating chronically institutionalized schizophrenic patients with concurrent ECT and traditional neuroleptics has suggested that the combination may result in dramatic improvement in only a small minority of patients, and is without substantial benefit in most cases. We are left then with unanswered questions. It could be that the positive findings of Friedel (1986), Gujavarty *et al.* (1987), Milstein *et al.* (1990) and others reflect samples with high representation of patients with prominent affective symptomatology. It could be that, in the absence of affective symptoms, the combination of ECT and neuroleptic treatment is particularly valuable for medication-resistant patients who have relatively short duration of episode. Indeed, the impressive results obtained in the series reported by Chanpattana and colleagues (Chanpattana & Sackeim 2002) pertained in a sample selected for psychotic exacerbation. Whatever the source of these discrepant impressions, it is clear that we need better information, particularly about the clinical and historical features of those medication-resistant patients who may benefit from the combination treatment. As described below, duration of the current episode (as opposed to duration of illness) may be a potent predictor of response to ECT in medication-resistant schizophrenia (Chanpattana & Sackeim 2002).

Atypical antipsychotics and electroconvulsive therapy

Clozapine is an effective treatment for schizophrenic patients resistant to classical neuroleptics (Kane *et al.* 1988a; Lieberman *et al.* 1989). None the less, a substantial proportion of such patients do not respond to clozapine. There have been scattered case reports on the use of ECT in clozapine-resistant patients. Initially, there had been concern about the safety of combining ECT and clozapine, because of the risk of seizures with clozapine. The concern was that, with concurrent clozapine, ECT-induced seizures would be prolonged or result in status epilepticus (Bloch *et al.* 1996).

Masiar and Johns (1991) reported on a 26-year-old man with a 4-year history of chronic paranoid schizophrenia who received up to 800 mg/day of clozapine with limited response. The patient was administered bilateral ECT 4 days after discontinuing clozapine, which had been tapered over a 14-day period along with diazepam (20 mg/day to 5 mg/day). The patient had two spontaneous grand mal seizures, witnessed by staff on days four and six following the first and only ECT treatment. It was unknown whether the delayed seizures were caused by residual effects of the clozapine, the dosage reduction of the benzodiazepine, a delayed effect of ECT, or some combination.

Klapheke (1991a) reported on the safe use of ECT combined with clozapine in a 26-year-old woman with schizoaffective disorder who remained psychotic and combative while on clozapine (450 mg/day). Previously she had failed to respond to regimens involving molindone, mesoridazine, tiotixene, lithium, carbamazepine, clonazepam and imipramine. She was treated with two seizure inductions per ECT session for the first five sessions and then had four more treatments, with clozapine dosage increased from 450 to 600 mg/day during the ECT course. She tolerated ECT well and had a dramatic clinical response. A few months later the patient relapsed when clozapine

was stopped because of a drop in white blood cell count (Klapheke 1991b). She received a second course of ECT with concurrent loxapine, involving a total of nine bilateral treatments that produced only mild to moderate improvement.

Landy (1991) reported no difficulty in treating two delusionally depressed patients with ECT and clozapine. Both patients had failed to respond to a variety of somatic treatments, including ECT combined with a traditional neuroleptic, and exhibited marked response to the combination of ECT and clozapine.

Safferman and Munne (1992) summarized a case of a patient with schizophrenia who had had a response to clozapine alone, and while on clozapine was virtually symptom-free for 5 months. However, her psychosis recurred and did not improve despite continuation of clozapine (900 mg/day) for about 12 months and the addition of valproic acid, lithium and CPZ. With eight bilateral ECT treatments, concurrent with a reduced clozapine dose (400 mg/day), she manifested marked improvement.

In subsequent years there have been additional reports on the safe and effective use of combined clozapine/ECT (Frankenburg *et al.* 1993; Bhatia *et al.* 1998; James & Gay 1999). Benatov *et al.* (1996) noted that the combination of clozapine and ECT may be particularly valuable in patients who developed neuroleptic malignant syndrome (NMS) on traditional antipsychotics. Green *et al.* (1994) reported on two patients who could not or refused to take clozapine. After a course of ECT, clozapine was accepted and well tolerated.

In the most extensive case review to date, Kupchik *et al.* (2000) reported on 36 psychiatric patients treated with the combination of ECT and clozapine. Indications were resistance to classical antipsychotic agents, clozapine or ECT alone. Overall, 67% of the patients improved with the combined treatment. Adverse reactions occurred in 16.6% of patients and included prolonged ECT-induced seizures ($n = 1$), supraventricular ($n = 1$) and sinus tachycardia, and blood pressure elevation. Again, it appeared that combined ECT/clozapine treatment is effective and safe in treatment-resistant patients.

Summary

As yet, the published literature is relatively meagre on the use of ECT in schizophrenic patients resistant to clozapine and the more general use of combination ECT and clozapine in medication-resistant schizophrenia. Outside of what has been published, a few groups have additional experience with this combination and initial impressions have been salutary. Particularly because the schizophrenic patient who fails clozapine has very limited therapeutic options, having typically exhausted traditional pharmacological approaches, rigorous investigation of the combination of ECT and clozapine is needed.

To our knowledge, there has yet to be documentation of the safety or efficacy of ECT when combined with other newer atypical antipsychotics, such as olanzapine, quetiapine, risperidone, sertindole or ziprasidone. Clinical experience suggests that their combination with ECT is safe (American Psychiatric

Association 2001), but is uncertain that this combination is as effective as combined treatment with clozapine and ECT.

Prediction of outcome

With the introduction of the neuroleptics, the use of ECT in schizophrenia diminished sharply. In part, this resulted from the belief that ECT and antipsychotic medications overlapped in the patients most responsive to treatment. ECT was believed to be particularly effective in patients with short illness duration and acute onset (Kalinowsky 1943; Kalinowsky & Worthing 1943; Lowinger & Huddleson 1945; Herzberg 1954), and relatively ineffective in chronic patients. As described earlier, because neuroleptics were generally found to be as or more effective than ECT alone in the treatment of non-chronic patients, clinicians began to favour the use of neuroleptics. Relatively little attention was devoted to the issue of whether the symptoms most responsive to ECT and medications were comparable or whether there was equivalence in the quality of remission. The evidence suggesting that combination ECT and antipsychotic medication may be more efficacious than either form of treatment alone has had relatively little impact on practice. As we have seen, surprisingly little research has addressed the issue of whether medication-resistant patients may benefit from ECT.

Demographic and clinical predictors

This synopsis indicates that views concerning the predictors of clinical outcome have been critical in delimiting the use of ECT. Soon after the introduction of ECT, several investigators examined putative predictors. The features that were associated with positive clinical outcome in schizophrenia included being married (Herzberg 1954), having at least a skilled or clerical occupation (Herzberg 1954), an absence of premorbid personality disturbance and poor premorbid functioning (Wittman 1941), manifestation of catatonic symptoms (Kalinowsky & Worthing 1943; Hamilton & Wall 1948; Ellison & Hamilton 1949; Wells 1973), affective symptoms (Folstein et al. 1973; Wells 1973), and acute onset and short illness duration (Cheney & Drewry 1938; Ross & Malzberg 1939; Zeifert 1941; Kalinowsky 1943; Lowinger & Huddleson 1945; Danziger & Kindwall 1946; Herzberg 1954). It is noteworthy that many of these features have been found to predict outcome with pharmacological treatment (Leff & Wing 1971; World Health Organization 1979; Watt et al. 1983) and may be more general markers of prognosis. None the less, the meaningfulness of these findings is questionable given that these early studies often used assessment techniques of questionable reliability and lacked standardized diagnostic criteria. Unfortunately, very few recent studies have examined predictors of ECT response in schizophrenia.

Koehler and Sauer (1983) reviewed the records of 142 first admission schizophrenic patients treated only with ECT at the University of Heidelberg during 1948–50 and who were evaluated by Kurt Schneider. Presentation of first-rank (Schneiderian)

symptoms was associated with inferior ECT outcome. Landmark et al. (1987) retrospectively contrasted clinical outcome predictors for fluphenazine and bilateral ECT. A group of 120 patients were followed at an outpatient clinic and received fluphenazine decanoate; 65 of these patients had been treated earlier in their history with bilateral ECT at other facilities. Landmark et al. (1987) claimed that fluphenazine was associated with superior clinical outcome relative to ECT. Within the ECT group, preoccupation with delusions and hallucinations was a significant predictor of positive clinical outcome, while diagnosis of schizophrenia following first hospitalization predicted poorer outcome. The latter was interpreted as indicating poorer ECT outcome in chronic schizophrenic patients. Of note, the presence of catatonic symptoms was non-predictive.

In recent times, there have been only two prospective studies of predictors of ECT outcome in schizophrenia. Dodwell and Goldberg (1989) reported on 17 schizophrenic patients who were assessed with standardized instruments both before and following ECT. Of note, 12 of the 17 patients met the RDC for schizoaffective disorder, depressed type, and all patients were treated with concomitant neuroleptic medication. In this small sample, positive outcome was associated with short duration of illness (both historically and current episode), fewer schizoid and paranoid premorbid personality traits, and the presence of perplexity. Catatonic and depressive symptoms were not predictive.

By far the most comprehensive study in this area was reported by Chanpattana and Sackeim (2002). In the sample of 253 patients treated with bilateral ECT and flupenthixol (as described above), across the sample and independent of gender, duration of the current episode and severity of baseline negative symptoms were predictive of outcome. Shorter duration of current episode was associated with superior response, while greater negative symptoms was associated with inferior response. Duration of illness had weak relations with outcome and only among females. This is particularly consequential, as many had argued that long duration of illness was a negative predictive factor (American Psychiatric Association 1990), while it appears that the duration of current exacerbation is more critical.

There were marked sex differences in other clinical features and symptoms associated with response. Among males, more frequent psychiatric admissions and the paranoid subtype were associated with positive clinical outcome. Among females, shorter duration of illness, negative family history for schizophrenia, and higher baseline Mini-Mental State Examination (MMSE) scores were associated with response. Gender differences in the factors predictive of clinical outcome may not be surprising given established gender differences in the age of onset of schizophrenia, premorbid functioning, neurobiological and neuropsychological correlates, responsiveness to pharmacological treatment, and long-term course and functional outcome.

Symptoms responsive to ECT

As with patient features that predict outcome, in recent years little research has examined the symptoms of schizophrenia that

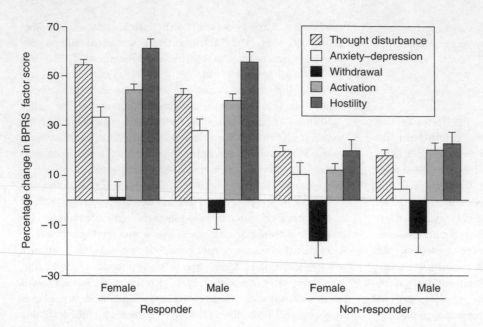

Fig 27.1 Percentage change in BPRS factor scores for responders and non-responders, as a function of gender. (After Chanpattana & Sackeim 2002.)

show most benefit from the use of ECT. Basic questions, such as the relative impact of ECT on positive and negative symptoms, have not been addressed in only one recent study (Chanpattana & Sackeim 2002).

The sham vs. real trials of Taylor and Fleminger (1980), Brandon *et al.* (1985) and Abraham and Kulhara (1987) generally found that while depressive symptoms in schizophrenic patients improved during an ECT course (combined with neuroleptic), they were not particularly responsive. Taylor and Fleminger (1980) reported that delusions of control, delusions of reference, delusional mood, thought interference and auditory hallucinations were particularly responsive. Similarly, Smith *et al.* (1967) had reported that combination ECT and CPZ resulted in particular improvement in symptoms of hostility and ideas of persecution relative to neuroleptic alone. Witton (1962) also claimed that ideas of persecution and auditory hallucinations showed an especially favourable response.

In the sample of 253 neuroleptic-resistant patients treated with ECT and flupenthixol, Chanpattana and Sackeim (2002) examined the BPRS symptoms and factor scores that were most and least sensitive to improvement. In contrast to prediction of final outcome, no gender differences were observed in the nature of symptomatic improvement over the treatment course (Fig. 27.1). Treatment resulted in marked improvement in specific positive symptoms, with an intermediate effect on affective symptoms, and no effect or worsening of specific negative symptoms. In particular, the BPRS factors of hostility, thought disturbance and activation showed robust improvement, anxiety–depression showed more moderate improvement, and the scores on the retardation factor were either unchanged or worsened. This suggests that the profile of clinical improvement following combined ECT/neuroleptic treatment is similar to that seen with traditional antipsychotic medications. Furthermore, despite the pronounced efficacy of ECT in the treatment of

major depression, affective symptoms are not especially responsive in patients with schizophrenia.

Special populations

Catatonia

It has long been contended that presentation of catatonic symptoms constitutes a special indication for the use of ECT (Kalinowsky & Worthing 1943; Hamilton & Wall 1948; Ellison & Hamilton 1949; Wells 1973; Fink 1989). Part of the difficulty in evaluating this claim is the recognition that catatonia may be manifested in a variety of psychiatric disorders or as a consequence of medical illness. Abrams and Taylor (1976a) examined 55 patients with catatonic symptoms who were admitted to an inpatient psychiatric unit and found that only four satisfied the research criteria for schizophrenia, with the others having a preponderance of affective disorders. Pataki *et al.* (1992) examined the records of admissions to an inpatient unit between 1985 and 1990. Of 43 cases with admission or discharge diagnoses of schizophrenia, catatonic subtype, 19 were felt to have records adequate for more detailed review. Only seven of these patients were identified as schizophrenic. Of the entire group of catatonic patients, 11 underwent ECT with excellent results in eight; 34 psychotropic medication trials were identified, with successful results in only two patients. Fink (1989) has advocated conceptualizing catatonia as a behavioural syndrome by itself, which can be associated with numerous disorders, not only schizophrenia, and for which ECT is the treatment of first choice. However, others (Fricchione 1989; Rosebush *et al.* 1992) have suggested use of benzodiazepines as the primary treatment for this syndrome. The small recent prospective study by Dodwell and Goldberg (1989) did not find catatonic symptoms to be predictive of ECT outcome. In an older sham vs. real ECT study conducted with catatonic schizophrenic patients, no effect of real ECT was discerned (Miller *et al*. 1953). A complication here is distinguishing between the treatment of catatonic manifestations and treatment of the underlying psychosis. In our experience, ECT results in rapid and often dramatic improvement in specific catatonic features, such as mutism and motility disturbance, but more variable effects on core psychotic phenomena. Catatonia may accompany or be a residual symptom of NMS, and there is evidence that ECT is rapidly effective in treating these catatonic manifestations (Caroff *et al*. 2000).

Lethal catatonia

Special consideration should be given to the syndrome of lethal catatonia. This is a life-threatening condition, characterized by stupor or excitement, hyperthermia, clouded consciousness, and autonomic dysregulation (Mann *et al*. 1986). Mann *et al*. (1986) identified 292 cases in the world literature published since 1960. In 256 (88%) cases, the lethal catatonia was believed to be an outgrowth of a functional psychotic disorder, with a primary diagnosis of schizophrenia in 117 cases. Of note, 176 (60%) of the 292 cases died. It has been suggested that the most common cause of death is pulmonary embolism (McCall *et al*. 1995). The literature on this syndrome, which consists solely of case series, suggests that neuroleptic treatment is of limited efficacy. Indeed, given the difficulty in distinguishing lethal catatonia from NMS, escalation of neuroleptic dosage may be counterproductive. In contrast, ECT, particularly when instituted prior to a comatose stage, appears to be particularly effective, and is favoured by many as the treatment of choice (Arnold & Stepan 1952; Tolsma 1967; Sedivec 1981; Gabris & Muller 1983; Mann *et al*. 1990; Rummans & Bassingthwaighte 1991; Singerman & Raheja 1994; McCall *et al*. 1995).

Schizoaffective disorder

Expert groups, such as the APA Task Force on ECT (American Psychiatric Association 1990), suggested that this form of treatment is particularly valuable when schizophrenic patients present with prominent affective symptoms. Some of the early investigators found that mood disturbance was a predictor of positive ECT outcome in schizophrenic patients (Folstein *et al*. 1973; Wells 1973). This may not be specific to ECT as affective features may portend a better prognosis in schizophrenia, regardless of treatment (World Health Organization 1979). Folstein *et al*. (1973) reviewed the charts of 118 consecutive patients who received ECT at a facility in New York. Regardless of diagnosis of schizophrenia, mood disorder or neurosis or personality disorder, the presence of a family history of mood disorder, suicide and symptoms of hopelessness, worthlessness and guilt were associated with favourable ECT outcome. Wells (1973) in a chart review of patients at the University of Rochester Medical Center identified 267 patients admitted between 1960 and 1969 with a diagnosis of schizophrenia and treated with

ECT. Schizoaffective and catatonic subtypes, patients in their first episode of illness and those with prominent depressive symptoms were each associated with superior outcome. Of note, however, in Chanpattana and Sackeim's (2002) study of patients with DSM-IV diagnoses of schizophrenia, affective symptoms did not have predictive value for final outcome.

The small prospective study by Dodwell and Goldberg (1989) did not observe predictive value for the quantitative evaluations of affective symptomatology or for RDC diagnosis as schizoaffective. On the other hand, these investigators reported that perplexity was a significant symptomatic predictor. Confusion or perplexity is a common feature of 'cycloid psychoses' (Leonhard 1961), which traditionally have been thought to be exquisitely responsive to ECT (Perris 1974). Ries *et al*. (1981) reported the only study restricted to the use of ECT in schizoaffective disorder. They identified nine patients who met the RDC for schizoaffective, depressed ($n = 5$) or manic subtype ($n = 4$), and who had failed two different antipsychotic medications prior to ECT. All patients were young (average age was 25.2 years), had paranoid delusions, and six of the nine patients had intermittent catatonic symptoms. Of note, confusion was moderate to severe in eight of the nine patients. All patients manifested a strong clinical response to ECT. This case series was in line with other reports suggesting that medication-resistant patients, characterized by marked psychotic and affective symptoms and by confusion, respond rapidly to ECT (Walinder 1972; Dempsey *et al*. 1975).

Neuroleptic malignant syndrome

Neuroleptic malignant syndrome shares clinical features with lethal catatonia and has been considered as an iatrogenic form of lethal catatonia induced by exposure to neuroleptics (Mann *et al*. 1990). When the clinical community became cognizant of NMS, there was reluctance to treat these patients with ECT. This reluctance was based on the fact that NMS has similar symptoms to malignant hyperthermia, a familial syndrome provoked by exposure to general anaesthesia and depolarizing muscle relaxants, such as succinylcholine (Liskow 1985). However, NMS and malignant hyperthermia have been shown to be unrelated syndromes (Addonizio & Susman 1987; Hermesh *et al*. 1988). Indeed, several reviews have documented that ECT is an effective treatment for NMS (Casey 1987; Devanand *et al*. 1987; Mann *et al*. 1990; Pearlman 1990; Davis *et al*. 1991), with only one case where the administration of anaesthesia or succinylcholine was associated with fever and raised creatine kinase levels and another case of hyperkalaemia (Trollor & Sachdev 1999). In one review, Davis *et al*. (1991) found that mortality rates in NMS patients were equivalent with ECT compared with bromocriptine, dantrolene, levodopa or amantidine, and averaged about half that of untreated patients. The complications and deaths that have been observed with the use of ECT have been tied to continued administration of neuroleptic medication and to cardiac dysregulation. Given the marked haemodynamic alterations associated with ECT, in the NMS patient it is advisable to first use medication strategies to stabilize autonomic function, before starting ECT. Because these patients must often be discontinued from antipsychotic medication, ECT has the unique properties of treating both the NMS and the underlying psychotic condition. Recent reviews continue to emphasize that ECT may be a preferred treatment in cases of severe NMS (Trollor & Sachdev 1999).

Treatment technique

Since the introduction of ECT, there have been a variety of improvements in treatment administration that have reduced morbidity, mortality and cognitive side-effects. These modifications include the use of general anaesthesia and muscle relaxants, more efficient electrical waveforms (i.e. brief pulse vs. sine wave stimuli), unilateral electrode placements, and the titration of electrical dosage to the needs of individual patients (American Psychiatric Association 1990, 2001). In the area of mood disorders, the introduction of some of these modifications of treatment technique has led to reconsideration of fundamental premises regarding the mode of action of ECT. It had long been contended that the production of a generalized seizure of adequate duration provided the necessary and sufficient conditions for antidepressant effects (Ottosson 1960; Fink 1979). Contradicting this view, it has been recently demonstrated that generalized seizures can be reliably produced that lack antidepressant effects (Sackeim et al. 1987a, 1993, 2000). Rather, for major depression, it appears that there are electrical dose–response relations and efficacy is contingent on the anatomic positioning of electrodes (electrode placement) and the extent to which electrical dosage exceeds seizure threshold (Sackeim et al. 1991, 1993, 2000; McCall et al. 2000). These findings in depression go beyond the sham vs. real ECT trial in demonstrating that physiological events over and above the production of a generalized seizure are critical to antidepressant response. These findings are also of obvious significance in designing optimal forms of ECT administration. Unfortunately, work refining ECT technique has concentrated almost exclusively on major depression.

Electrode placement

Whether electrodes are placed on one or both sides of the head can have marked effects on cognitive consequences (Sackeim 1992; Sackeim et al. 1993, 2000; Lisanby et al. 2000). Generally speaking, the traditional bifrontotemporal (bilateral placement) produces more extensive, severe and persistent amnestic effects than unilateral placements. Electrodes placed over the left hemisphere are associated with longer delay in return of orientation and greater verbal amnestic deficits than electrodes placed over the right hemisphere. In contrast, right unilateral ECT typically results in greater amnestic deficits for non-verbal material relative to left unilateral ECT (Daniel & Crovitz 1982, 1983; Weiner et al. 1986; Sackeim 1992). Left unilateral ECT is rarely used, although theories regarding lateralized disturbances in schizophrenia would support investigation of a thera-

peutic advantage (Gur 1978; Flor-Henry 1983). In mood disorders, there has been an ongoing debate about the relative efficacy of bilateral and right unilateral ECT, with over 40 comparative trials (Abrams 1986; Sackeim et al. 1993, 2000). This debate appears to be nearing resolution as the efficacy of right unilateral ECT is highly sensitive to the degree to which electrical dosage exceeds seizure threshold. At high stimulus intensity, right unilateral ECT appears to match the efficacy of bilateral ECT, but retains important cognitive advantages (Sackeim et al. 2000). Only four studies have compared unilateral and bilateral ECT in schizophrenia and these are summarized in Table 27.5.

Each of the four trials contrasting unilateral and bilateral ECT in schizophrenia failed to detect differences in efficacy. In each case, the patient samples had relatively short duration of illness and showed strong response to ECT. However, the conclusions that can be drawn from this work are limited. Two studies were conducted in outpatients and were characterized by inordinately high drop-out (Doongaji et al. 1973; Bagadia et al. 1988). El-Islam et al. (1970) determined the side of electrode placement (left or right) based on assessment of motoric lateralization (handedness, eyedness and footedness), an inappropriate procedure (American Psychiatric Association 2001). Wessels (1972) treated patients on a daily basis, using a fixed number of eight treatments. Therefore, at best, there are weak indications that right unilateral and bilateral ECT may be equivalent in efficacy when treating schizophrenia. These studies used inefficient electrical waveforms and high stimulus intensity (Wessels 1972; Doongaji et al. 1973). It is unknown whether the particular sensitivity of right unilateral ECT to electrical dosage, as seen in major depression, extends to schizophrenia (Sackeim et al. 1993, 2000; McCall et al. 2000).

Stimulus intensity

Regardless of electrode placement, in major depression there is evidence that higher electrical dosage above seizure threshold results in more rapid response (Robin & DeTissera 1982; Sackeim et al. 1993, 2000; Nobler et al. 1997). One study has examined this issue is patients with schizophrenia (Chanpattana et al. 2000). In the context of the studies examining the efficacy of combined treatment with flupenthixol and ECT, Chanpattana et al. randomized 62 patients to bilateral ECT conditions that were just above seizure threshold, twice the threshold, or four times the threshold. The groups did not differ in the number who met remitter criteria after the stabilization phase. However, the group treated just above threshold required more ECT treatments and more days to meet remitter status, while the other two groups did not differ. This initial study is in line with the findings in major depression, and suggests that higher stimulus intensity accelerates response in schizophrenia.

Treatment duration and frequency

Early in the history of ECT it was contended that schizophrenic

Table 27.5 Prospective clinical trials comparing unilateral and bilateral ECT in schizophrenia.

Study	Patients	Study design	Nature of treatment	Results/comments
el-Islam *et al.* (1970)	41 schizophrenic patients, aged 18–40 years, with delusions or hallucinations; schizoaffective and catatonic patients excluded	Sequential assignment to 'non-dominant' ($n = 20$) or bilateral ($n = 21$) conditions; double-blind evaluation	ECT at 2 per week; non-dominant hemisphere inappropriately determined; all patients received concomitant 15 mg/day trifluoperazine; unilateral patients averaged 7.0 treatments; bilateral averaged 7.3 treatments	Groups equivalent in clinical outcome, assessed as the number of treatments needed to relieve delusions and hallucinations, and in total number of treatments and time to discharge; slight non-significant advantage to unilateral ECT on a memory test
Wessels (1972)	100 South Sotho males, acute schizophrenia (Bleuler criteria), first admission	Sequential assignment to right unilateral ECT ($n = 51$) vs. bilateral ECT ($n = 49$). Double-blind evaluations 14 days following ECT with BPRS and NOSIE	ECT was unmodified and given daily for 8 treatments; Lancaster position for unilateral ECT; 200 mg/day CPZ during ECT course and increased to 300 mg/day until day 14 following ECT	Both forms of ECT resulted in substantial improvement, with no differences; 67% of patients rated as very much improved
Doongaji *et al.* (1973)	54 schizophrenic outpatients, aged 15–45 years; no treatment for at least 3 months prior to study; patients with illness <1 month or >2 year excluded	Randomized to left unilateral, right unilateral, and bilateral ECT. Randomization stratified by age and duration of illness; double-blind evaluation with BPRS and CGI; 32 patients initially randomized not analysed	Unmodified ECT given 3 per week for first 2 weeks and 2 per week for next 2 weeks (minimum 6 treatments); no concurrent medication other than chloral hydrate; both unilateral groups averaged 8 ECT, bilateral averaged 9.4	No efficacy differences among the treatment groups after 6 ECT, at the end of ECT, or after a 3 month follow-up; no difference in number of treatments; no explanation given for 32 patients being dropped from the sample prior to 6 ECT
Bagadia *et al.* (1988)	40 DSM-III schizophrenic outpatients, aged 18–65 years	Double-blind, random assignment to right unilateral ($n = 20$) vs. bilateral ($n = 20$) ECT; BPRS and CGI at baseline, after 3 treatments and after 6 treatments; 21 patients dropped due to non-compliance or discontinuation of treatment	Unmodified ECT given 3 per week for first 3 treatments and at 4-day intervals for next 3 treatments (only 6 treatments given); No concurrent medication other than chloral hydrate	Both groups showed substantial and equivalent clinical improvement; no attempt to account for the high drop-out rate

BPRS, Brief Psychiatric Rating Scale; CGI, Clinical Global Impression; CPZ, chlorpromazine; NOSIE, Nurse Observation Scale for Inpatient Evaluation.

patients required more closely spaced treatments and longer treatment courses than patients with other conditions (Kalinowsky 1943; Kennedy & Anchel 1948; Baker *et al.* 1960a). Kalinowsky (1943) argued that discontinuation of ECT after rapid improvement in acute schizophrenia almost invariably led to early relapse, which could be prevented by administering a more prolonged ECT course. Following this dictum, regressive forms of ECT were developed, in which multiple treatments were given on the same day, often 7 days per week, with the avowed aim of producing global disorientation and dissolution of the personality in schizophrenic patients (Glueck *et al.* 1957; Jacoby & van Houten 1960; Murillo & Exner 1973a; Exner & Murillo 1977). This view has continued into the modern era, as some experts contend that schizophrenic patients typically require 10–20 treatments, and that negative symptom manifestations (withdrawn, apathetic behaviour) may require even more treatments (Fink 1979). Empirical evidence bearing on this position is scant. Baker *et al.* (1960a) reported superior results in chronic schizophrenics after 20 treatments, relative to 12 treatments. King (1959) randomized 37 male chronic schizophrenic patients to ECT given three times per week or ECT given twice daily, six times per week. Both groups received 20 treatments, without discernible difference in outcome.

It should be noted that the recent trials of ECT in schizophrenia (e.g. sham vs. real ECT, comparisons of electrode placements) have used relatively small numbers of treatments, generally 6–12, with positive results. It is also noteworthy that early commentators on the treatment of acute mania often stated that a large number of ECT treatments were needed in this condition, at an intensive schedule (Kalinowsky & Hippius 1972). To the contrary, recent experience has been that, if anything, relative to depressed patients, manic patients show clinical response earlier in the treatment course and that daily treatment confers no advantage over more spaced treatment schedules (for review see Mukherjee *et al.* 1994). In the treatment of major depression, there had also been a belief that the administration of additional treatments after achieving symptomatic remission aided in delaying relapse. In the case of depression, this view was shown to be erroneous (Snaith 1981). Similarly, it is quite possible that beliefs that schizophrenic patients require particularly long courses of ECT to achieve response or to prevent relapse are without merit. In terms of practice, clinicians should be guided by manifestations of clinical improvement and side-effects when determining whether to continue with ECT. Prescribing a fixed number of treatments is not appropriate.

Trials in major depression have shown that a treatment frequency of twice per week generally results in less severe short-term cognitive side-effects than a treatment regimen of three times per week. However, the later schedule is associated with more rapid clinical improvement (Lerer *et al.* 1995; Shapira *et al.* 1998). A similar study in schizophrenia randomized 43 patients to twice- or thrice-weekly ECT combined with flupenthixol (Chanpattana *et al.* 1999b). The thrice-weekly group showed more rapid response. While there was no difference between the groups in a measure of global cognitive status, neurocognitive assessment was limited to the MMSE.

Continuation/maintenance ECT

ECT is the only somatic treatment in psychiatry that is typically stopped once shown to be effective. A minority of patients, most commonly individuals with affective disorders who relapse while receiving continuation or maintenance pharmacotherapy, receive ECT as a continuation or maintenance treatment (Decina *et al.* 1987; Kramer 1987; Thornton *et al.* 1990; Monroe 1991; Sackeim 1994). Interest in continuation/maintenance ECT in preventing relapse in mood disorders has increased markedly in recent years. In part, this may be a result of

preliminary evidence that standard pharmacological strategies are ineffective in preventing relapse following response to ECT, when patients have failed those strategies during treatment of the acute affective episode (Sackeim *et al.* 1990, 1993, 2000; Sackeim 1994). Similarly, ECT is often considered as an adjunctive treatment in schizophrenic patients who are resistant to traditional antipsychotic medications. In this specific population, little is known about the efficacy of traditional or atypical neuroleptics in preventing relapse.

Information on the use of ECT as a continuation or maintenance treatment in schizophrenia mainly comes from an older literature (Moore 1943; Weisz & Creel 1948; Karliner & Wehrheim 1965). Karliner and Wehrheim (1965) reported on maintenance convulsive treatment given to 57 patients, 12% of whom relapsed after up to 6 years of observation. Of 153 patients who refused such maintenance treatment, 79% relapsed. Diagnostically, both groups were heterogeneous consisting of schizophrenic, schizoaffective and manic-depressive patients. Asnis and Gabriel (1976) reported that maintenance ECT was successful in controlling symptoms in a number of patients with schizophrenia. Without question, difficulties in convincing patients of the need for maintenance ECT and with compliance have limited the use of this strategy in schizophrenia. None the less, particularly given its theoretical potential for medication-resistant patients and its potential for reducing concomitant neuroleptic dosage (Gardos *et al.* 1980), investigation in this area is needed. It is noteworthy that several reviews of maintenance therapy in schizophrenia do not mention ECT (Davis 1975; Carpenter *et al.* 1987; Schooler 1991).

Recently, there has been a controlled investigation of the efficacy of continuation ECT in schizophrenia. Chanpattana *et al.* (1999c) randomized 51 patients with schizophrenia who had remitted with the combination of ECT and flupenthixol into a controlled three-arm trial, of whom 45 patients were completers. In both the groups treated with continuation ECT alone or flupenthixol alone, 14 of the 15 completers (93%) relapsed over a 6-month period. In contrast, there was a significant advantage for the group treated with the combination of continuation ECT and flupenthixol in both intent-to-treat and completer analyses, with only 6 of 15 (40%) completers meeting relapse criteria. Eight patients received long-term maintenance treatment with the combination and none had a recurrence. Like the literature on the acute treatment of schizophrenia, this preliminary study suggests that combination continuation treatment with ECT and an antipsychotic medication may be more effective than either modality alone.

Side-effects

Modern ECT is associated with low rates of morbidity and mortality. It is estimated that mortality rates are about the same as with general anaesthesia for minor surgery, involving approximately one death per 10 000 patients treated (Abrams 1997a; American Psychiatric Association 2001). The low incidence of major complications is particularly impressive because ECT is often used in patients with pre-existing medical complications, given the belief that it is safer than antidepressant medications. The major source of morbidity and mortality with ECT is cardiovascular complication. The risk of serious complications is increased in the elderly, particularly the oldest age groups, in those with pre-existing medical conditions, particularly cardiac illness, and in those receiving concurrent medication for medical conditions (Alexopoulos *et al.* 1984; Burke *et al.* 1987; Cattan *et al.* 1990; Sackeim 1998). Consequently, the safety of ECT is expected to be particularly high among schizophrenic patients.

Cardiovascular collapse and respiratory depression may occur when reserpine is combined with ECT and this combination should be avoided (Bracha & Hess 1956; Foster & Gayle 1956; Kalinowsky 1956; Bross 1957). There were also suggestions after the introduction of neuroleptics that the combination of CPZ and ECT was associated with serious hypotensive crises (Weiss 1955; Gaitz *et al.* 1956; Kalinowsky 1956; Grinspoon & Greenblatt 1963). This concern has not been substantiated by subsequent experience (Gonzalez & Imahara 1964) and has not been raised for other antipsychotic medications.

Cognition

The cognitive effects of ECT are stereotyped and their magnitude is dependent on methods of treatment administration (Sackeim 1992, 2000). There is no reason to suspect that the nature of ECT-induced cognitive side-effects differs in schizophrenia, relative to other disorders. However, the presence of baseline cognitive deficits in schizophrenia is well documented (Heaton *et al.* 1978; Seidman 1983; Bilder *et al.* 1992; Saykin *et al.* 1994; Goldberg & Gold 1995) and there is evidence, in some patients, for progressive cognitive deterioration as part of the natural course of the disorder (Tsuang *et al.* 1979; Bilder *et al.* 1992). Given this, the question arises as to whether individuals with schizophrenia are at risk for more severe or persistent cognitive or other neuropsychiatric complications when treated with ECT.

Perlson (1945) conducted extensive psychological studies of a patient with chronic schizophrenia who received 248 ECT treatments over an approximately 3-year period, eventually being discharged in a remitted state. He concluded that the patient had no discernible intellectual or physical sequelae. In a long-term follow-up of schizophrenic patients treated with regressive ECT or with medications, Exner and Murillo (1977) could not detect differences in neuropsychological function or in projective test results. Buhrich *et al.* (1988) examined a group of 42 long-stay hospital patients with chronic schizophrenia. They divided this sample into two age- and sex-matched groups, based on temporal disorientation. A past history of ECT, among other physical treatment variables, did not distinguish patients with and without temporal disorientation. Gureje (1988) tested 70 individuals who met the Feighner criteria for definite schizophrenia, 56% of whom had received ECT treatments with the mean number of treatments being 10.8. He found that the number of ECT

treatments in the past was unrelated to objective measures of psychopathology, to performance on a variety of cognitive measures, or to neurological soft signs. Devanand *et al.* (1991) compared a group of eight patients (four with a diagnosis of schizophrenia), who each had received more than 100 bilateral modified sine wave ECT treatments, with a matched group of patients who had never received ECT. They found no difference between the groups in neuropsychological measures, suggesting that patients given many courses of ECT treatments do not manifest measurable cognitive impairment at long-term follow-up. Bagadia *et al.* (1983) randomized 38 schizophrenic patients to sham ECT plus CPZ or to real ECT and placebo. At trial completion, subjective forgetfulness was reported by 15% of the patients who received CPZ and by 40% of those who received ECT. However, no differences in objective cognitive measures were found. On the contrary, following ECT there was an improvement on almost all objective cognitive measures.

In contrast to these reports, Goldman *et al.* (1972) found that performance on the Bender–Gestalt and Benton Visual Retention Test was impaired in male chronic schizophrenic inpatients with a history of 50 or more ECT treatments, when compared with a control group of patients matched for age, education and race. Templer *et al.* (1973) replicated these findings in a sample of 44 hospitalized schizophrenic patients; the 22 patients in the index group had in the past received from 40 to 263 ECT treatments with a median number of 58.5. Both of these studies have been criticized as suffering from non-blind evaluations of ECT patients and controls, group differences in the degree of psychopathology, and for the use of inappropriate instruments for neuropsychological evaluation (Weiner 1984; Devanand *et al.* 1991). Overall, this is little reason to suspect that ECT results in more severe or extensive neuropsychological effects in schizophrenic patients than in other populations. There have been no recent studies using comprehensive neurocognitive batteries to examine effects of ECT in schizophrenia.

It is not uncommon to observe pronounced neuropsychological deterioration early in the course of schizophrenia (Bilder *et al.* 1992; Saykin *et al.* 1994). In our experience, when ECT is used as a treatment for acute psychotic episodes in young schizophrenic patients, occasionally patients or family members attribute the subsequent cognitive decline to this intervention. Despite similar progression in patients treated with neuroleptics, rarely are medications viewed as contributory. Perhaps sensitized by the acute cognitive effects of ECT, or by the mythology surrounding this treatment, some patients may be sensitized to attributing cognitive changes to ECT.

Neuropathological effects

It is generally contended that modern ECT, involving generalized seizures that last approximately 1 min, under conditions of general anaesthesia, muscle relaxation and continuous oxygenation does not provide the conditions necessary for neuronal death (Weiner 1984; Meldrum 1986; Siesjö *et al.* 1986; Devanand *et al.* 1994). Elegant animal studies have detailed the metabolic and molecular substrate for seizure-induced cell damage. During seizures, there are marked increases in cerebral glucose utilization and oxygen consumption. However, blood supply outstrips metabolic demand. When seizures are sustained for periods of hours, as in status epilepticus, supply may fall short of demand, with consequent cellular damage. The duration of the ECT-induced seizure is orders of magnitude below the threshold for this type of effect (Ingvar 1986; Meldrum 1986). Numerous studies of magnetic resonance imaging (MRI), cerebrospinal fluid and plasma markers of brain damage have reported negative findings following courses of ECT (Coffey et al. 1991; Zachrisson et al. 2000).

Weinberger et al. (1979) reported a significant correlation among schizophrenic patients between lateral ventricular size and previous ECT. A number of other computerized tomography (CT) and MRI studies have contrasted mood disorder or schizophrenic patients with positive and negative histories of ECT and found no differences with respect to measures of cerebral volume and sulcal widening (Nasrallah et al. 1982, 1984; Dolan et al. 1985; Pearlson et al. 1985; Kolbeinsson et al. 1986; Andreasen et al. 1990; Swayze et al. 1990). CT (Bergsholm et al. 1989) and MRI (Coffey et al. 1988, 1991; Scott et al. 1990) prospective longitudinal structural imaging studies of patients who have received ECT also have reported negative findings regarding treatment-associated changes. Importantly, Rabins et al. (1991) reported that depressed patients who were subsequently treated with ECT showed on MRI at pretreatment baseline greater temporal horn abnormality and generally had evidence of greater subcortical pathology than other depressed patients. This type of finding underscores the need for caution in interpreting retrospective associations between types of treatment and evidence of structural change.

Movement disorders

The potential for acute extrapyramidal syndromes (EPS), particularly neuroleptic-induced parkinsonism (NIP), and for persistent tardive dyskinesia (TD) is a major drawback of traditional neuroleptic treatment. EPS is a ubiquitous phenomenon, and estimates of the prevalence of tardive dyskinesia (TD) in individuals receiving traditional neuroleptic medication typically range from 25% to 50% (American Psychiatric Association 1980; Kane & Smith 1982; Lieberman et al. 1984; Jeste & Kaufman 1986). While EPS is generally considered to be reversible, prospective studies have suggested that NIP predicts the subsequent development of TD (Chouinard et al. 1988; Kane et al. 1988b). In elderly patients, NIP has been linked to greater cognitive impairment (Mukherjee et al. 1991) and to larger lateral ventricular size (Hoffman et al. 1987). NIP and akathisia may also persist following the discontinuation of neuroleptics (Melamed et al. 1991; Hermesh et al. 1992).

ECT has antiparkinsonian properties. In both open and sham-controlled trials, ECT has been found to improve clinical symptoms in idiopathic Parkinson's disease, at least on a short-term basis (Asnis 1977; Andersen et al. 1987; Douyon et al. 1989; for reviews see Faber & Trimble 1991; Kellner et al. 1994). Typically, levodopa requirements are sharply reduced when patients with idiopathic Parkinson's disease receive ECT. The clinical utility of ECT as a long-term treatment for medication-resistant Parkinson's disease has yet to be tested, as use of maintenance ECT has only been informally evaluated (Pridmore & Pollard 1996). ECT also has ameliorative effects on NIP (Gangadhar et al. 1983; Goswami et al. 1989). Goswami et al. (1989) studied nine schizophrenic inpatients with a longitudinal triphasic design, first using neuroleptics, then neuroleptics and ECT, and then neuroleptics. NIP was significantly reduced in step-wise fashion when patients were treated with ECT. Hermesh et al. (1992) reported a case in which NIP and akathisia continued for 3 months, despite two courses of anticholinergic treatment, a change to a low-potency neuroleptic and a neuroleptic-free period. These adverse effects responded dramatically to ECT and reemerged 3 months after discontinuation of ECT.

Mukherjee and Debsikdar (1994) introduced the notion that ECT may protect against the later development of NIP and TD. They examined 35 DSM-IIIR schizophrenic patients who were on neuroleptics for at least 2 weeks. All patients received 10 mg/day trifluoperazine, 28 patients received additional neuroleptic medications, and 24 patients were also receiving concurrent anticholinergic treatment. In addition, all patients were receiving ($n = 15$) or had received during the index episode ($n = 20$) a course of unmodified bilateral ECT. Standardized scales for evaluating EPS and TD were completed. None of the 35 patients had bradykinesia, rigidity or postural instability. Two patients had mild tremor of the upper extremities. Only one patient met the Research Diagnosis of Tardive Dyskinesia criteria (Schooler & Kane 1982) for probable TD (mild severity). The relative absence of signs of NIP and the low prevalence of TD were unexpected. Mukherjee and Debsikdar (1994) speculated that if NIP is a risk factor in the development of TD, ECT may ultimately protect against TD by preventing initial NIP. At the neurophysiological level, there is evidence that electroconvulsive shock (ECS) in rodents prevents the development of dopamine receptor supersensitivity with exposure to dopamine antagonists (Lerer et al. 1982). While intriguing, establishing such a protective role for ECT will require controlled prospective comparison of patients exposed to traditional neuroleptics with and without a prior history of ECT.

There is also case report literature that suggests that ECT may have some impact on manifestations of TD. Early reports suggested that ECT may contribute to manifestation of persistent TD (Uhrbrand & Faurbye 1960; Faurbye et al. 1964; Holcomb et al. 1983; Flaherty et al. 1984). A small series was also reported in which ECT produced no short-term change in TD severity (Asnis & Leopold 1978). More recently, a series of case studies have linked the use of ECT with often dramatic and long-term improvement in symptoms of TD (Price & Levin 1978; Rosenbaum et al. 1980; Chacko & Root 1983; Gosek & Weller 1988; Malek-Ahmadi & Weddige 1988; Hay et al. 1990). With one exception (Asnis & Leopold 1978), in the published reports the primary indication for use of ECT was the acute psychiatric condition, with effects on TD noted incidentally. In the absence of controlled prospective investigation, no firm conclusions can be offered regarding the value of ECT in the treatment of TD. The scattering of positive reports leave unanswered questions regarding possible effects of concomitant medications during the ECT course, improvement associated with neuroleptic withdrawal, and a host of other possibilities. None the less, our clinical experience suggests that the effects of ECT on manifestations of TD are variable. Some patients, often with severe forms of TD, show clinically meaningful improvement, with the diminution of TD symptoms typically occurring abruptly during the ECT course. Other patients, with seemingly similar conditions, show little benefit. It is our impression that ECT-related improvement is more likely in patients with severe TD manifestations. As in some of the positive case reports, we have observed sustained remission of TD manifestations following ECT. There are also two reports of linking ECT to amelioration of tardive dystonia, where other attempts at treatment are usually disappointing (Kwentus *et al.* 1984; Adityanjee *et al.* 1990).

Aside from these indications that ECT may alter manifestations of TD, there are suggestions that a history of ECT may be associated with a low prevalence or delayed development of TD. Gardos *et al.* (1980) evaluated 122 schizophrenic outpatients in Hungary and reported a striking absence of severe TD. They suggested that the low prevalence was a result of the avoidance of high dosage neuroleptic treatment. The bulk of these patients were treated with ECT during acute episodes and as a means of forestalling new episodes. According to Gardos *et al.* (1980), this use of ECT allowed for more moderate dosing of neuroleptics. In an American sample, Cole *et al.* (1992) reported that a history of previous ECT was associated with a lower risk and delayed appearance of TD. As noted, Mukherjee and Debsikdar (1994) found virtually no TD in an Indian sample, which they also attributed to the use of ECT. Schwartz *et al.* (1993), in an Israeli sample, reported a reduced incidence of TD among male schizophrenic patients with a history of ECT. If, in fact, ECT does offer long-term protection against the iatrogenic effects of later exposure to neuroleptics, this would contradict the general impression that the behavioural and physiological effects of ECT are typically transient (Sackeim 1988; Sackeim *et al.* 1995).

Mechanisms

With few exceptions (Milstein *et al.* 1990), there is little evidence that the biochemical and neurophysiological changes produced by ECT differ in schizophrenic patients compared with other psychiatric groups. Rather, the dilemma in accounting for the efficacy of ECT in schizophrenia is the same as that faced in other conditions. The application of an electrical stimulus to the brain and the production of a generalized seizure produce a remarkable diversity of short-term biochemical and neurophysiological changes. In animal models and humans, there has been little difficulty in demonstrating consistent effects on peptide, transmitter or hormone systems or in regional patterns of cerebral perfusion, metabolism and electrical activity (for reviews see Green & Nutt 1987; Sackeim 1988; Nutt *et al.* 1989; Fochtmann 1994; Sackeim *et al.* 1995). Rather, the problem has been in discerning which of these effects is linked to efficacy in particular disorders and which are epiphenomena.

Some have contended that the search for mechanisms of action of ECT is relatively hopeless given the plethora of physiological alterations that accompany and follow seizures (Kety 1974). However, in the case of major depression, we now know that seizures may be reliably produced that lack therapeutic properties (Sackeim *et al.* 1987a, 1993, 2000). This has created new optimism in the search for the physiological basis of antidepressant effects, by offering the opportunity to subtract the effects of therapeutic seizures from those that lack efficacy. Basic and clinical research along these lines has begun (Bhattacharya *et al.* 1991; Zis *et al.* 1991; Nobler *et al.* 1993, 1994, 2000; Sackeim *et al.* 1996). In addressing mechanisms of action in schizophrenia, it may also be helpful to better isolate the components of the ECT process that are necessary and sufficient for efficacy.

At this point, it is uncertain whether ECT exerts therapeutic action through the effects it shares with antipsychotic medication or through different means. Clinical research can aid in addressing this issue by more clearly establishing the extent to which resistance to antipsychotic medication predicts resistance to ECT (Prudic *et al.* 1990). In large part, a high degree of correlation has been assumed, with both classes of treatment generally thought to be more effective in schizophrenic patients with acute exacerbations and short duration of episode. Indeed, this overlap has led some to question whether ECT has much of a role in the treatment of schizophrenia (Royal College of Psychiatrists 1977, 1995; Abrams 1997b). This assumption is also reflected in the recent studies of ECT in medication-resistant schizophrenic patients. This work has examined the efficacy of ECT only when used in combination with neuroleptics (Friedel 1986; Gujavarty *et al.* 1987; Chanpattana *et al.* 1999c,d; Chanpattana & Sackeim 2002). Conceptually, this would suggest that the effects of the two approaches are additive or synergistic. In line with this view, the series of studies that contrasted combination treatment to neuroleptic treatment alone or ECT alone generally found the combination to be superior (Ray 1962; Childers 1964; Smith *et al.* 1967; Small *et al.* 1982).

One suggestion that has often been given for the apparent superiority of combination ECT and neuroleptic treatment to either of them alone is that ECT results in increased concentration of neuroleptic medication in neural tissue (Gujavarty *et al.* 1987). Specifically, it has been suggested that the transient disruption of the blood–brain barrier that occurs acutely with seizure induction (Bolwig *et al.* 1977) allows neuroleptics greater entry into brain. Aoba *et al.* (1983) found that plasma and red blood cell levels of haloperidol increased transiently by about 100% immediately after ECT in schizophrenic patients, indicating a redistribution phenomenon. However, Shibata *et al.* (1989) demonstrated a similar effect in rats, but did not find any changes in cerebral concentrations of haloperidol. They attributed the peripheral increase in plasma to a transient decrease in muscle storage during the convulsion. As reviewed here, one of the difficulties with this line of thinking is that there is substantial evidence that ECT is efficacious in the treatment of schizophrenia in the absence of concomitant neuroleptics (May 1968). Accounts of the utility of ECT that posit only an enhancement of medication effects are out of keeping with these clinical findings.

There is little doubt at both the physiological and behavioural levels that ECT and classical or atypical neuroleptics have distinct profiles. This is illustrated by the fact that ECT has powerful antipsychotic effects across a range of psychiatric and organic conditions, and yet ECT also has antiparkinsonian effects. This would suggest that ECT and classical antipsychotic medications differ in their alterations of dopaminergic transmission. Indeed, this is the case. Microdialysis studies in rodents indicate that ECS acutely results in increased concentrations of dopamine and dopamine metabolites in brain, with this effect showing a regional distribution (Nutt *et al.* 1989; Nomikos *et al.* 1991; Zis *et al.* 1991). Repeated treatment may produce enhanced tonic levels of dopamine or its metabolites in selective brain regions. Behavioural studies indicate that dopamine-mediated behaviours are enhanced following ECS. Locomotion and stereotypic behaviour provoked by apomorphine and amphetamine are increased following chronic ECS (Green & Deakin 1980; Costain *et al.* 1982; Chanpattana & Sackeim 2002). This increased dopaminergic tone is not mediated by changes at the D_2 receptor. Most studies have found that ECS has little effect on D_2 receptor density or second messenger function (Bergstrom & Kellar 1979; Atterwill 1980; Newman & Lerer 1989), while there is accumulating evidence that altered D_1 receptor function is responsible for enhanced behavioural responses to dopamine agonists following ECS (Newman & Lerer 1989; Barkai *et al.* 1990; Hao *et al.* 1990; Serra *et al.* 1990; Verma & Kulkarni 1991). This pattern of effects is quite distinct from the profile associated with traditional neuroleptics. Furthermore, ECT also differs in important ways from atypical neuroleptics, such as clozapine. It has been suggested that the therapeutic effects of clozapine are related to antagonist properties at both serotonin (5-HT_{1C}, 5-HT_2, 5-HT_3) and dopamine (D_2) receptors (Meltzer 1989; Meltzer *et al.* 1989; Owen *et al.* 1993). In contrast, it is well established that ECS leads to an enhancement of serotonin-mediated behaviour and, as opposed to classical antidepressant medications, to an increased density of 5-HT_2 receptors (Green *et al.* 1983; Kellar & Stockmeier 1986). Therefore, the biochemical effects of ECS on both dopamine and serotonin systems appear to be distinct from those of either typical or atypical neuroleptics. The fact that ECT is a powerful antipsychotic treatment presents a challenge for any unified theory regarding antipsychotic mechanisms.

Conclusions

There is a lack of consensus within the clinical community regarding the role of ECT in the treatment of schizophrenia. Expert groups differ in their recommendations and surveys indicate highly disparate rates of utilization between and within countries. Despite over 65 years of continuous use of convulsive therapy in schizophrenia, this lack of consensus is tied to an inadequate research base. ECT was introduced prior to the development of modern clinical trial methodology. Many of the clinical tenets regarding the use of ECT in schizophrenia derive from this era. Some of the best information we have came from studies conducted soon after the introduction of antipsychotic medications, where ECT was used as the gold standard against which to establish the efficacy of these new agents (Childers 1964; Smith *et al.* 1967; May 1968). However, since then the nature of pharmacological treatment of schizophrenia has advanced and the vast bulk of clinical research in ECT has concentrated on mood disorders.

There is little doubt that ECT is efficacious in the treatment of schizophrenia, at least in patients with acute exacerbations and short episode duration. However, even in this group, the short-term benefits of ECT are likely to be equivalent to or less than those of monotherapy with a traditional antipsychotic. In contrast, the available evidence suggests that combination treatment of ECT and neuroleptic is superior in short-term outcome to that of ECT alone or neuroleptic alone. The consistency of this observation is surprising, because it is usually difficult to establish the superiority of a treatment combination when a primary treatment – in this case, neuroleptic – exerts pronounced efficacy. The combination treatment of ECT and neuroleptic has advantages that may not be fully appreciated. In general, the work that suggested superior efficacy for the combination used lower neuroleptic doses for the combined treatment groups than for the neuroleptic alone groups. Furthermore, the antiparkinsonian effects of ECT may aid in limiting extrapyramidal side-effects and in offering greater flexibility in neuroleptic dosing. There are few concerns about the safety of this combination. Although the evidential base is less substantial, it also appears that ECT exerts additive or synergistic effects with atypical antipsychotic medications.

Close perusal of the literature on the use of ECT in schizophrenia produced the surprising suggestion that this treatment may exert long-term benefits. In several comparative studies, patients who received ECT, either alone or in combination with neuroleptics, had superior functioning at follow-up or were less subject to relapse than patients treated only with neuroleptics (Smith *et al.* 1967; Exner & Murillo 1977; May *et al.* 1981). This work was characterized by a variety of methodological limitations, the most important of which was lack of control over treatment following resolution of the acute episode. None the less, in these studies, patients who received antipsychotic medication during the acute episode typically continued with this treatment following discharge, while ECT samples may have received less aggressive maintenance treatment (Wyatt 1991).

Another, more tentative, suggestion that has emerged in recent work is that schizophrenic patients treated with ECT earlier in their history may be less likely or have delayed manifestation of NIP and tardive dyskinesia (Gardos *et al.* 1980; Cole *et al.* 1992; Mukherjee & Debsikdar, 1994). Among the possibilities here is a selection bias, whereby schizophrenic patients who receive ECT differ in vulnerability for these movement disorders relative to those not referred for this treatment. Alternatively, as suggested by Gardos *et al.* (1980), the use of ECT may have allowed more moderate exposure to traditional neuroleptics, thereby impacting on subsequent movement disorders. Mukherjee and Debsikdar (1994) offered the novel idea that manifestation of NIP is a prerequisite for later development of TD. The acute antiparkinsonian effects of ECT and its putative protective effects against later development of NIP may be related to a reduced prevalence of TD. Regardless, given their obvious clinical importance, these suggestions that ECT may have long-term clinical benefits and protective effects against movement disorders underscore the need for additional research.

At this point, there is little information to guide the clinician in determining which schizophrenic patient will benefit most from ECT or in optimizing specific aspects of treatment administration. The long-held view that protracted courses of ECT are required in schizophrenia has not been examined specifically in recent research, but is out of keeping with evidence that substantial response is often observed after 8–10 treatments (Taylor & Fleminger 1980; Brandon *et al.* 1985; Abraham & Kulhara 1987; Chanpattana *et al.* 1999b). It is noteworthy that the original sham vs. real ECT studies that failed to find a therapeutic effect for ECT concentrated on chronic samples (Miller *et al.* 1953; Brill *et al.* 1959a,b,c; Heath *et al.* 1964). In contrast, the more recent positive sham vs. real ECT studies (Taylor & Fleminger 1980; Brandon *et al.* 1985; Abraham & Kulhara 1987) sampled patients with shorter duration of episode and used concomitant antipsychotic medication. Recent research has not addressed the long-held view that ECT is of limited value in schizophrenic patients with insidious symptom onset and long illness duration (Kalinowsky 1943; Fink 1979; Salzman 1980; Kendell 1981). None the less, this accords with our experience that only a small minority of chronic institutionalized schizophrenic patients show palpable benefit from ECT, even when combined with neuroleptic treatment. However, in a small minority, ECT is associated with dramatic effects and can produce the first symptomatic remission to be observed in years. Among chronic patients, one can not predict who will benefit from ECT. It is our view that, regardless of chronicity, schizophrenic patients who have exhausted pharmacological alternatives deserve a course of ECT.

Recent reports have documented strong response to combination ECT and traditional neuroleptic treatment in patients with shorter illness duration, who have failed traditional neuroleptics (Friedel 1986; Gujavarty *et al.* 1987; Mukherjee & Debsikdar, 1994). Such patients may constitute the prime indication for the use of ECT in schizophrenia. This area requires considerable development. It is uncertain whether these positive reports pertain only to schizophrenic patients with prominent affective symptomatology (i.e. schizoaffective patients) or whether the positive effects are more general. There is only case series information on the utility of combining ECT with atypical neuroleptics such as clozapine, quetiapine, risperidone, etc. Because the clozapine (and other atypical neuroleptic)-resistant patient represents a distinctly difficult therapeutic dilemma, exploration of this combination would also seem worthwhile.

Acknowledgements

Preparation of this chapter was supported in part by grants MH35636, MH47739, MH57009, MH59069 and MH61609 from the National Institute of Mental Health, Bethesda, MD, USA.

References

Abraham, K.R. & Kulhara, P. (1987) The efficacy of electroconvulsive therapy in the treatment of schizophrenia: a comparative study. *British Journal of Psychiatry* **151**, 152–155.

Abrams, R. (1986) Is unilateral electroconvulsive therapy really the treatment of choice in endogenous depression? *Annals of the New York Academy of Sciences* **462**, 50–55.

Abrams, R. (1987) ECT in Schizophrenia [editorial]. *Convulsive Therapy* **3**, 169–170.

Abrams, R. (1997a) The mortality rate with ECT. *Convulsive Therapy* **13**, 125–127.

Abrams, R. (1997b) *Electroconvulsive Therapy*, 3rd edn. Oxford University Press, New York.

Abrams, R. & Taylor, M.A. (1976a) Catatonia: a prospective clinical study. *Archives of General Psychiatry* **33**, 579–581.

Abrams, R. & Taylor, M.A. (1976b) Mania and schizo-affective disorder, manic type: a comparison. *American Journal of Psychiatry* **133**, 1445–1447.

Abrams, R., Taylor, M.A. & Gastanaga, P. (1974) Manic-depressive illness and paranoid schizophrenia. *Archives of General Psychiatry* **31**, 640–642.

Addonizio, G. & Susman, V.L. (1987) ECT as a treatment alternative for patients with symptoms of neuroleptic malignant syndrome. *Journal of Clinical Psychiatry* **48**, 102–105.

Adityanjee, Jayaswal, S.K., Chan, T.M. & Subramanaim, M. (1990) Temporary remission of tardive dystonia following electroconvulsive therapy. *British Journal of Psychiatry* **156**, 433–435.

Agarwal, A.K., Andrade, C. & Reddy, M.V. (1992) The practice of ECT in India: issues relating to the administration of ECT. *Indian Journal of Psychiatry* **34**, 285–297.

Alexopoulos, G.S., Shamoian, C.J., Lucas, J., Weiser, N. & Berger, H. (1984) Medical problems of geriatric psychiatric patients and younger controls during electroconvulsive therapy. *Journal of the American Geriatric Society* **32**, 651–654.

American Psychiatric Association Task Force on ECT (1978) *Electroconvulsive Therapy. Task Force Report No. 14.* American Psychiatric Association, Washington, DC.

American Psychiatric Association Task Force on ECT (1990) *The Practice of ECT: Recommendations for Treatment, Training and Privileging.* American Psychiatric Press, Washington, DC.

American Psychiatric Association Task Force on ECT (2001) *The Practice of ECT: Recommendations for Treatment, Training and Privileging*. 2nd edn. American Psychiatric Press, Washington, DC.

American Psychiatric Association Task Force on Tardive Dyskinesia (1980) *Tardive Dyskinesia*. American Psychiatric Association, Washington, DC.

Andersen, K., Balldin, J., Gottfries, C.G. et al. (1987) A double-blind evaluation of electroconvulsive therapy in Parkinson's disease with 'on-off' phenomena. *Acta Neurologica Scandinavica* **76**, 191–199.

Andreasen, N.C., Swayze, V., Flaum, M., Alliger, R. & Cohen, G. (1990) Ventricular abnormalities in affective disorder: clinical and demographic correlates. *American Journal of Psychiatry* **147**, 893–900.

Aoba, A., Kakita, Y., Yamaguchi, N. et al. (1983) Electric convulsive therapy (ECT) increases plasma and red blood cell haloperidol neuroleptic activities. *Life Sciences* **33**, 1797–1803.

Arnold, O.H. & Stepan, H. (1952) Untersuchungen zur Frage der akuten todlichen Katatonie. *Wien Zeitscrift für Nervenheilkunde Deren Grenzgebiete* **4**, 235–258.

Asnis, G.M. (1977) Parkinson's disease, depression, and ECT: a review and case study. *American Journal of Psychiatry* **134**, 191–195.

Asnis, F. & Gabriel, A.N. (1976) ECT as maintence therapy in schizophrenia [letter]. *American Journal of Psychiatry* **133**, 858–859.

Asnis, G.M. & Leopold, M.A. (1978) A single-blind study of ECT in patients with tardive dyskinesia. *American Journal of Psychiatry* **135**, 1235–1237.

Atterwill, C.K. (1980) Lack of effect of repeated electroconvulsive shock on [^{3}H]spiroperidol and [^{2}H]5-hydroxytryptamine binding and cholinergic parameters in rat brain. *Journal of Neurochemistry* **35**, 729–734.

Ayres, C. (1960) The relative value of various somatic therapies in schizophrenia. *Journal of Neuropsychiatry* **1**, 154–162.

Bagadia, V.N., Dave, K.P. & Shah, L.P. (1970) A comparative study of physical treatments in schizophrenia. *Indian Journal of Psychiatry* **12**, 190–204.

Bagadia, V.N., Abhyankar, R.R., Doshi, J., Pradhan, P.V. & Shah, L.P. (1983) Report from a WHO collorabative center for psychopharmacology in India-1: re-evaluation of ECT in schizophrenia. *Psychopharmacology Bulletin* **19**, 550–555.

Bagadia, V.N., Abhyankar, R., Pradhan, P.V. & Shah, L.P. (1988) Re-evaluation of ECT in schizophrenia: right temporoparietal versus bitemporal electrode placement. *Convulsive Therapy* **4**, 215–220.

Baker, A.A., Game, J.A. & Thorpe, J.G. (1958) Physical treatment for schizophrenia. *Journal of Mental Science* **104**, 860–864.

Baker, A.A., Bird, G., Lavin, N.I. & Thorpe, J.G. (1960a) ECT in schizophrenia. *Journal of Mental Science* **106**, 1506–1511.

Baker, A.A., Game, J.A. & Thorpe, J.G. (1960b) Some research into the treatment of schizophrenia in the mental hospital. *Journal of Mental Science* **106**, 203–213.

Barkai, A.I., Durkin, M. & Nelson, H.D. (1990) Localized alterations of dopamine receptor binding in rat brain by repeated electroconvulsive shock: an autoradiographic study. *Brain Research* **529**, 208–213.

Benatov, R., Sirota, P. & Megged, S. (1996) Neuroleptic-resistant schizophrenia treated with clozapine and ECT. *Convulsive Therapy* **12**, 117–121.

Bergsholm, P., Larsen, J.L., Rosendahl, K. & Holsten, F. (1989) Electroconvulsive therapy and cerebral computed tomography: a prospective study. *Acta Psychiatrica Scandinavica* **80**, 566–572.

Bergstrom, D.A. & Kellar, K.J. (1979) Effect of electroconvulsive shock on monoaminergic receptor binding sites in rat brain. *Nature* **278**, 464–466.

Bhatia, S.C., Bhatia, S.K. & Gupta, S. (1998) Concurrent administration of clozapine and ECT: a successful therapeutic strategy for a patient with treatment-resistant schizophrenia. *Journal of ECT* **14**, 280–283.

Bhattacharya, S.K., Banerjee, P.K., Glover, V. & Sandler, M. (1991) Augmentation of rat brain endogenous monoamine oxidase inhibitory activity (tribulin) by electroconvulsive shock. *Neuroscience Letters* **125**, 65–68.

Bilder, R.M., Lipschutz-Broch, L., Reiter, G. et al. (1992) Intellectual deficits in first-episode schizophrenia: evidence for progressive deterioration. *Schizophrenia Bulletin* **18**, 437–448.

Bland, R.C. & Brintnell, S. (1985) Electroconvulsive therapy in a major teaching hospital: diagnoses and indications. *Canadian Journal of Psychiatry* **30**, 288–292.

Bloch, Y., Pollack, M. & Mor, I. (1996) Should the administration of ECT during clozapine therapy be contraindicated? *British Journal of Psychiatry* **169**, 253–254.

Bolwig, T.G., Hertz, M.M., Paulson, O.B., Spotoft, H. & Rafaelsen, O.J. (1977) The permeability of the blood–brain barrier during electrically induced seizures in man. *European Journal of Clinical Investigation* **7**, 87–93.

Bond, E.D. (1954) Results of psychiatric treatments with a control series. *American Journal of Psychiatry* **110**, 561–566.

Borowitz, A.H. (1959) An investigation into combined electroconvulsive and chlorpromazine therapy in the treatment of schizophrenia. *South African Medical Journal* **33**, 836–840.

Bracha, S. & Hess, J.P. (1956) Death occuring during combined reserpine–electroshock treatment. *American Journal of Psychiatry* **113**, 257.

Brandon, S., Cowley, P., McDonald, C. et al. (1985) Leicester ECT trial: results in schizophrenia. *British Journal of Psychiatry* **146**, 177–183.

Brill, N.Q., Crumpton, E., Eiduson, S. et al. (1957) Investigation of the therapeutic components and various factors associated with improvement with electroconvulsive treatment: a preliminary report. *American Journal of Psychiatry* **113**, 997–1008.

Brill, N.Q., Crumpton, E., Eiduson, S., Grayson, H.M. & Hellman, L.I. (1959a) Predictive and concomitant variables related to improvement with actual and simulated ECT. *Archives of General Psychiatry* **1**, 263–272.

Brill, N.Q., Crumpton, E., Eiduson, S. et al. (1959b) An experimental study of the relative effectiveness of various components of electroconvulsive therapy. *American Journal of Psychiatry* **115**, 734–735.

Brill, N.Q., Crumpton, E., Eiduson, S. et al. (1959c) Relative effectiveness of various components of electroconvulsive therapy. *Archives of Neurology and Psychiatry* **81**, 627–635.

Bross, R. (1957) Near fatality with combined ECT and resperine. *American Journal of Psychiatry* **113**, 933.

Buhrich, N., Crow, T.J., Johnstone, E.C. & Owens, D.G.C. (1988) Age disorientation in chronic schizophrenia is not associated with pre-morbid intellectual impairment or past physical treatment. *British Journal of Psychiatry* **152**, 466–469.

Burke, W.J., Rubin, E.H., Zorumski, C.F. & Wetzel, R.D. (1987) The safety of ECT in geriatric psychiatry. *Journal of the American Geriatric Society* **35**, 516–521.

Caroff, S.N., Mann, S.C., Keck, P.E. Jr & Francis, A. (2000) Residual catatonic state following neuroleptic malignant syndrome. *Journal of Clinical Psychopharmacology* **20**, 257–259.

Carpenter, W.T. (1987) A comparative trial of pharmacologic strategies in schizophrenia. *American Journal of Psychiatry* **144**, 1466–1470.

Carpenter, W.T., Heinrichs, D. W. & Hanlon, T.E. (1987) A comparative trial of pharmacologic strategies in schizophrenia. *American Journal of Psychiatry* **144**, 1466–1470.

Casey, D.A. (1987) Electroconvulsive therapy in the neuroleptic malignant syndrome. *Convulsive Therapy* **3**, 278–283.

Cattan, R.A., Barry, P.P., Mead, G. *et al.* (1990) Electroconvulsive therapy in octogenarians. *Journal of the American Geriatric Society* **38**, 753–758.

Cerletti, U. & Bini, L. (1938) Un neuvo metodo di shockterapie 'L'elettro-shock'. *Boll Acad Medica Roma* 136–138.

Chacko, R.C. & Root, L. (1983) ECT and tardive dyskinesia: two cases and a review. *Journal of Clinical Psychiatry* **44**, 265–266.

Chafetz, M.E. (1943) An active treatment for chronically ill patients. *Journal of Nervous and Mental Disease* **98**, 464–473.

Chanpattana, W. (1999) The use of the stabilization period in ECT research in schizophrenia. I. A pilot study. *Journal of the Medical Association of Thailand* **82**, 1193–1199.

Chanpattana, W. (2000) Maintenance ECT in treatment-resistant schizophrenia. *Journal of the Medical Association of Thailand* **83**, 657–662.

Chanpattana, W. & Sackeim, H.A. (2002) Electroconvulsive therapy in treatment-resistant schizophrenia: prediction of response and the nature of symptomatic improvement. *Schizophrenia Bulletin* (in press).

Chanpattana, W., Chakrabhand, M.L., Kirdcharoen, N. *et al.* (1999a) The use of the stabilization period in electroconvulsive therapy research in schizophrenia. II. Implementation. *Journal of the Medical Association of Thailand* **82**, 558–568.

Chanpattana, W., Chakrabhand, M.L., Kitaroonchai, W., Choovanichvong, S. & Prasertsuk, Y. (1999b) Effects of twice- versus thrice-weekly electroconvulsive therapy in schizophrenia. *Journal of the Medical Association of Thailand* **82**, 477–483.

Chanpattana, W., Chakrabhand, M.L., Sackeim, H.A. *et al.* (1999c) Continuation ECT in treatment-resistant schizophrenia: a controlled study. *Journal of ECT* **15**, 178–192.

Chanpattana, W., Somchai Chakrabhand, M.L., Kongsakon, R., Techakasem, P. & Buppanharun, W. (1999d) Short-term effect of combined ECT and neuroleptic therapy in tretment-resistant schizophrenia. *Journal of ECT* **15**, 129–139.

Chanpattana, W., Chakrabhand, M.L., Buppanharun, W. & Sackeim, H.A. (2000) Effects of stimulus intensity on the efficacy of bilateral ECT in schizophrenia: a preliminary study. *Biological Psychiatry* **48**, 222–228.

Cheney, C.O. & Drewry, P.H. (1938) Results of nonspecific treatment in dementia praecox. *American Journal of Psychiatry* **95**, 203–217.

Childers, R. (1964) Comparison of four regimens in newly admitted female schizophrenics. *American Journal of Psychiatry* **120**, 1010–1011.

Childers, R.T. & Therrien, R. (1961) A comparison of the effectiveness of trifluoperazine and chlorpromazine in schizophrenia. *American Journal of Psychiatry* **118**, 552–554.

Chouinard, G., Annable, L., Ross-Chouinard, A. & Mercier, P. (1988) A 5-year prospective longitudinal study of tardive dyskinesia: factors predicting appearance of new cases. *Journal of Clinical Psychopharmacology* **8** (Suppl.), 21S–26S.

Coffey, C.E., Figiel, G.S., Djang, W.T. *et al.* (1988) Effects of ECT on brain structure: a pilot prospective magnetic resonance imaging study. *American Journal of Psychiatry* **145**, 701–706.

Coffey, C.E., Weiner, R.D., Djang, W.T. *et al.* (1991) Brain anatomic effects of electroconvulsive therapy: a prospective magnetic resonance imaging study. *Archives of General Psychiatry* **48**, 1013–1021.

Cole, J.O., Gardos, G., Boling, L.A. *et al.* (1992) Early dyskinesia: vulnerability. *Psychopharmacology (Berlin)* **107**, 503–510.

Costain, D.W., Cowen, P.J., Gelder, M.G. & Grahame-Smith, D.G. (1982) Electroconvulsive therapy and the brain: evidence for increased dopamine-mediated responses. *Lancet* **2**, 400–404.

Currier, G.E., Cullinan, C. & Rothschild, D. (1952) Results of treatment of schizophrenia in a state hospital: changing trends since advent of electroshock therapy. *Archives of Neurology and Psychiatry* **67**, 80–82.

Daniel, W.F. & Crovitz, H.F. (1982) Recovery of orientation after electroconvulsive therapy. *Acta Psychiatrica Scandinavica* **66**, 421–428.

Daniel, W.F. & Crovitz, H.F. (1983) Acute memory impairment following electroconvulsive therapy. II. Effects of electrode placement. *Acta Psychiatrica Scandinavica* **67**, 57–68.

Danziger, L. & Kindwall, J.A. (1946) Prediction of the immediate outcome of shock therapy in dementia praecox. *Disease of the Nervous System* **7**, 299–303.

Das, P.S., Saxena, S., Mohan, D. & Sundaram, K.R. (1991) Adjunctive electroconvulsive therapy for schizophrenia. *National Medical Journal of India* **4**, 183–184.

Davis, J.M. (1975) Overview: maintenance therapy in psychiatry. I. Schizophrenia. *American Journal of Psychiatry* **132**, 1237–1245.

Davis, J.M., Janicak, P.G., Sakkas, P., Gilmore, C. & Wang, Z. (1991) Electroconvulsive therapy in the treatment of the neuroleptic malignant syndrme. *Convulsive Therapy* **7**, 111–120.

Decina, P., Guthrie, E.B., Sackeim, H.A., Kahn, D. & Malitz, S. (1987) Continuation ECT in the management of relapses of major affective episodes. *Acta Psychiatrica Scandinavica* **75**, 559–562.

Dempsey, G.M., Tsuang, M.T., Struss, A. & Dvoredsky-Wortsman, A. (1975) Treatment of schizo-affective disorder. *Comprehensive Psychiatry* **16**, 55–59.

Devanand, D.P., Sackeim, H.A. & Finck, A.D. (1987) Modified ECT using succinylcholine after remission of neuroleptic malignant syndrome. *Convulsive Therapy* **3**, 284–290.

Devanand, D.P., Verma, A.K., Tirumalasetti, F. & Sackeim, H.A. (1991) Absence of cognitive impairment after more than 100 lifetime ECT treatments. *American Journal of Psychiatry* **148**, 929–932.

Devanand, D.P., Dwork, A.J., Hutchinson, E.R., Bolwig, T.G. & Sackeim, H.A. (1994) Does ECT alter brain structure? *American Journal of Psychiatry* **151**, 957–970.

DeWet, J.S.T. (1957) Evaluation of a common method of convulsion therapy in Bantu schizophrenics. *Journal of Mental Science* **103**, 739–757.

Dodwell, D. & Goldberg, D. (1989) A study of factors associated with response to electroconvulsive therapy in patients with schizophrenic symptoms. *British Journal of Psychiatry* **154**, 635–639.

Dolan, R.J., Calloway, S.P. & Mann, A.H. (1985) Cerebral ventricular size in depressed subjects. *Psychological Medicine* **15**, 873–878.

Doongaji, D.R., Jeste, D.V., Saoji, N.J., Kane, P.V. & Ravindranath, S. (1973) Unilateral versus bilateral ECT in schizophrenia. *British Journal of Psychiatry* **123**, 73–79.

Douyon, R., Serby, M., Klutchko, B. & Rotrosen, J. (1989) ECT and Parkinson's disease revisited: a 'naturalistic study'. *American Journal of Psychiatry* **146**, 1451–1455.

Ellison, F.A. & Hamilton, D.M. (1949) The hospital treatment of dementia praecox: Part II. *American Journal of Psychiatry* **106**, 454–461.

Exner, J.E. Jr & Murillo, L.G. (1973) Effectiveness of regressive ECT with process schizophrenia. *Diseases of the Nervous System* **34**, 44–48.

Exner, J.E. Jr & Murillo, L.G. (1977) A long term follow-up of schizophrenics treated with regressive ECT. *Diseases of the Nervous System* **38**, 162–168.

Faber, R. & Trimble, M.R. (1991) Electroconvulsive therapy in Parkinson's disease and other movement disorders. *Movement Disorders* **6**, 293–303.

Faurbye, A., Rasch, P.J. & Peterson, P.B. (1964) Neurological symptoms in pharmacotherapy of psychoses. *Acta Psychiatrica Scandinavica* **40**, 10–27.

Feighner, J., Robins, E., Guze, S. *et al.* (1972) Diagnosis criteria for use in psychiatry research. *Archives of General Psychiatry* **26**, 57–63.

Fink, M. (1979) *Convulsive Therapy: Theory and Practice* Raven Press, New York.

Fink, M. (1989) Is catatonia a primary indication for ECT? [editorial]. *Convulsive Therapy* **5**, 1–4.

Fink, M. & Sackeim, H.A. (1996) Convulsive therapy in schizophrenia? *Schizophrenia Bulletin* **22**, 7–39.

Flaherty, J.A., Naidu, J. & Dysken, M. (1984) ECT, emergent dyskinesia, and depression. *American Journal of Psychiatry* **141**, 808–809.

Flor-Henry, P. (1983) *Cerebral Basis of Psychopathology*. John Wright, Boston.

Fochtmann, L.J. (1994) Animal studies of electroconvulsive therapy: foundations for future research. *Psychopharmacology Bulletin* **30**, 321–444.

Folstein, M., Folstein, S. & McHugh, P.R. (1973) Clinical predictors of improvement after electroconvulsive therapy of patients with schizophrenia, neurotic reactions, and affective disorders. *Biological Psychiatry* **7**, 147–152.

Ford, H. & Jameson, G.K. (1955) Chlorpromazine in conjunction with other psychiatric therapies: a clinical appraisal. *Diseases of the Nervous System* **16**, 179–185.

Foster, M.W.J. & Gayle, R.F.I. (1956) Chlorpromazine and reserpine as adjuncts in electroshock treatment. *Southern Medical Journal* **49**, 731–735.

Frankenburg, F.R., Suppes, T. & McLean, P.E. (1993) Combined clozapine and electroconvulsive therapy. *Convulsive Therapy* **9**, 176–180.

Fricchione, G.L. (1989) Catatonia: a new indication for benzodiazepenes? *Biological Psychiatry* **26**, 761–765.

Friedel, R.O. (1986) The combined use of neuroleptics and ECT in drug resistant schizophrenic patients. *Psychopharmacology Bulletin* **22**, 928–930.

Gabris, G. & Muller, C. (1983) La catatonie dite 'pernicieuse'. *Encephale* **9**, 365–385.

Gaitz, C.M., Pokorny, A.D. & Mills, M.J. (1956) Death following electroconvulsive therapy. *Archives of Neurology and Psychiatry* **75**, 493–499.

Gangadhar, B.N., Roychowdhury, J. & Channabasavanna, S. (1983) ECT and drug-induced parkinonism. *Indian Journal of Psychiatry* **25**, 212–213.

Gardos, G., Samu, I., Kallos, M. & Cole, J.O. (1980) Absence of severe tardive dyskinesia in Hungarian schizophrenic out-patients. *Psychopharmacology (Berlin)* **71**, 29–34.

Glueck, B., Reiss, B.B. & Bernard, L. (1957) Regressive electric shock therapy. *Psychiatric Quarterly* **31**, 117–136.

Goldberg, T.E. & Gold, J.M. (1995) *Neurocognitive Deficits in Schizophrenia*. In: *Schizophrenia* (eds S.R. Hirsch & D.R. Weinberger), pp. 146–162. Blackwell Science, Oxford.

Goldfarb, W. & Kieve, H. (1945) The treatment of psychotic like regressions of combat soldiers. *Psychiatric Quarterly* **19**, 555–565.

Goldman, H., Gomer, F.E. & Templer, D.I. (1972) Long-term effects of electroconvulsive therapy upon memory and perceptual-motor performance. *Journal of Clinical Psychology* **28**, 32–34.

Gonzalez, J.R. & Imahara, J. (1964) Electroshock therapy with the phenothiazine reserpine: a survey and report. *American Journal of Psychiatry* **121**, 253–256.

Gosek, E. & Weller, R.A. (1988) Improvement of tardive dyskinesia associated with electroconvulsive therapy. *Journal of Nervous and Mental Disease* **176**, 120–122.

Goswami, U., Dutta, S., Kuruvilla, K., Papp, E. & Perenyi, A. (1989)

Electroconvulsive therapy in neuroleptic-induced parkinsonism. *Biological Psychiatry* **26**, 234–238.

Gottlieb, J.S. & Huston, P.E. (1951) Treatment of schizophrenia. *Journal of Nervous and Mental Disease* **113**, 237–246.

Green, A.R. & Deakin, J.F. (1980) Brain noradrenaline depletion prevents ECS-induced enhancement of serotonin- and dopamine-mediated behaviour. *Nature* **285**, 232–233.

Green, A.R. & Nutt, D. (1987) Psychopharmacology of repeated seizures: possible relevance to the mechanisms of action of electroconvulsive therapy. In: *Handbook of Psychopharmacology*, Vol. 19 (eds L. Iversen, S. Iversen & S. Snyder), pp. 375–419. Plenum Press, New York.

Green, A.R., Heal, D.J., Johnson, P., Laurence, B.E. & Nimgaonkar, V.L. (1983) Antidepressant treatments: effects in rodents on dose–response curves of 5-hydroxytryptamine- and dopamine-mediated behaviours and 5-HT$_2$ receptor number in frontal cortex. *British Journal of Pharmacology* **80**, 377–385.

Green, A.I., Zalma, A., Berman, I., DuRand, C.J. & Salzman, C. (1994) Clozapine following ECT: a two-step treatment. *Journal of Clinical Psychiatry* **55**, 388–390.

Grinspoon, L. & Greenblatt, M. (1963) Pharmacotherapy combined with other treatment methods. *Comprehensive Psychiatry* **4**, 256–262.

Gujavarty, K., Greenberg, L.B. & Fink, M. (1987) Electroconvulsive therapy and neuroleptic medication in therapy-resistant positive-symptom psychosis. *Convulsive Therapy* **3**, 185–195.

Gur, R.E. (1978) Left hemisphere dysfunction and left hemisphere overactivation in schizophrenia. *Journal of Abnormal Psychology* **87**, 225–238.

Gureje, O. (1988) Schizophrenic patients treated with electroconvulsive therapy: their demographic, clinical and cognitive features. *East African Medical Journal* **65**, 379–386.

Guttmann, E., Mayer-Gross, W. & Slater, E.T.O. (1939) Short-distance prognosis of schizophrenia. *Journal of Neurology and Psychiatry* **2**, 25–34.

Hamilton, M. (1986) Electroconvulsive therapy. Indications and contraindications. *Annals of the New York Academy of Sciences* **462**, 5–11.

Hamilton, D.M. & Wall, J.H. (1948) The hospital treatment of dementia praecox. *American Journal of Psychiatry* **105**, 346–352.

Hao, X.Z., Mathë, A.A., Mathë, J.M. & Svensson, T.H. (1990) Electroconvulsive treatment attenuates behavioral response to SKF 38393 in reserpine-treated mice. *Psychopharmacology (Berlin)* **100**, 135–137.

Hay, D.P., Hay, L., Blackwell, B. & Spiro, H.R. (1990) ECT and tardive dyskinesia. *Journal of Geriatric Psychiatry and Neurology* **3**, 106–109.

Heath, E.S., Adams, A. & Wakeling, P.L. (1964) Short courses of ECT and simulated ECT in chronic schizophrenia. *British Journal of Psychiatry* **110**, 800–807.

Heaton, R.K., Baade, L.E. & Johnson, K.L. (1978) Neuropsychological test results associated with psychiatric disorders in adults. *Psychological Bulletin* **85**, 141–162.

Hermesh, H., Aizenberg, D., Lapidot, M. & Munitz, H. (1988) Risk of malignant hyperthermia among patients with neuroleptic malignant syndrome and their families. *American Journal of Psychiatry* **145**, 1431–1434.

Hermesh, H., Aizenberg, D., Friedberg, G., Lapidot, M. & Munitz, H. (1992) Electroconvulsive therapy for persistent neuroleptic-induced akathisia and parkinsonism: a case report. *Biological Psychiatry* **31**, 407–411.

Hertzman, M. (1992) ECT and neuroleptics as primary treatment for schizophrenia [editorial]. *Biological Psychiatry* **31**, 217–220.

Herzberg, F. (1954) Prognostic variables for electro-shock therapy. *Journal of General Psychology* 50, 79–86.

Hoffman, W.F., Laboratories, S.M. & Casey, D.E. (1987) Neuroleptic-induced parkinsonism in older schizophrenics. *Biological Psychiatry* 22, 427–439.

Holcomb, H.H., Sternberg, D.E. & Heninger, G.R. (1983) Effects of electroconvulsive therapy on mood, parkinsonism, and tardive dyskinesia in a depressed patient: ECT and dopamine systems. *Biological Psychiatry* 18, 865–873.

Ingvar, M. (1986) Cerebral blood flow and metabolic rate during seizures: relationship to epileptic brain damage. *Annals of the New York Academy of Sciences* 462, 194–206.

Ishimoto, Y., Imakura, A. & Nakayama, H. (2000) Practice of electroconvulsive therapy at University Hospital, the University of Tokushima School of Medicine from 1975 to 1997. *Journal of Medical Investigations* 47, 123–127.

el-Islam, M.F., Ahmed, S.A. & Erfan, M.E. (1970) The effect of unilateral ECT on schizophrenic delusions and hallucinations. *British Journal of Psychiatry* 117, 447–448.

Jacoby, M. & van Houten, Z. (1960) Regressive shock therapy. *Diseases of the Nervous System* 21, 582–583.

James, D.V. & Gray, N.S. (1999) Elective combined electroconvulsive and clozapine therapy. *International Clinical Psychopharmacology* 14, 69–72.

Janakiramaiah, N., Channabasavanna, S.M. & Murthy, N.S. (1982) ECT/chlorpromazine combination versus chlorpromazine alone in acutely schizophrenic patients. *Acta Psychiatrica Scandinavica* 66, 464–470.

Janicak, P.G., Davis, J.M., Gibbons, R.D. *et al.* (1985) Efficacy of ECT: a meta-analysis. *American Journal of Psychiatry* 142, 297–302.

Jeste, D.V. & Kaufman, C.A. (1986) Pathophysiology of tardive dyskinesia: evaluation of supersensitivity theory and alternative hypothesis. In: *Tardive Dyskinesia and Neuroleptics: from Dogma to Reason* (eds D.E. Casey & G. Gardos), pp. 32–38. American Psychiatric Association Press, Washington, DC.

Kalinowsky, L.B. (1943) Electric convulsion therapy with emphasis on importance of adequate treatment. *Archives of Neurology and Psychiatry* 50, 652–660.

Kalinowsky, L.B. (1956) The danger of various types of medication during electric convulsive therapy. *American Journal of Psychiatry* 112, 745–746.

Kalinowsky, L.B. (1988) Schizophrenia and ECT [letter]. *Convulsive Therapy* 4, 99.

Kalinowsky, L.B. & Hippius, H. (1972) *Pharmacological, Convulsive and Other Treatments in Psychiatry*. Grune & Stratton, New York.

Kalinowsky, L.B. & Worthing, H. (1943) Results with electric convulsive therapy in 200 cases of schizophrenia. *Psychiatric Quarterly* 17, 144–153.

Kane, J.M. (1999) Pharmacologic treatment of schizophrenia. *Biological Psychiatry* 46, 1396–1408.

Kane, J.M. & Smith, J.M. (1982) Tardive dyskinesia: prevalence and risk factors 1959–79. *Archives of General Psychiatry* 39, 473–481.

Kane, J.M., Honigfeld, G., Singer, J. & Meltzer, H.Y. (1988a) Clozapine for the treatment-resistant schizophrenic. *Archives of General Psychiatry* 45, 789–796.

Kane, J.M., Woerener, M. & Lieberman, J.A. (1988b) Tardive dyskinesia: prevalence, incidence, and risk factors. *Journal of Clinical Psychopharmacology* 8 (Suppl.), 52S–56S.

Karliner, W. & Wehrheim, H. (1965) Maintenance convulsive treatments. *American Journal of Psychiatry* 121, 1113–1115.

Kellar, K.J. & Stockmeier, C.A. (1986) Effects of electroconvulsive shock and serotonin axon lesions on beta-adrenergic and serotonin-2 receptors in rat brain. *Annals of the New York Academy of Sciences* 462, 76–90.

Kellner, C.H., Beale, M.D., Pritchett, J.T., Bernstein, H.J. & Burns, C.M. (1994) Electroconvulsive therapy and Parkinson's disease: the case for further study. *Psychopharmacology Bulletin* 30, 495–500.

Kendell, R.E. (1971) Psychiatric diagnosis in Britain and the United States. *British Journal of Hospital Medicine* 6, 147–155.

Kendell, R.E. (1981) The present status of electroconvulsive therapy. *British Journal of Psychiatry* 139, 265–283.

Kennedy, C.J. & Anchel, D. (1948) Regressive electric shock in schizophrenics refractory to other shock therapies. *Psychiatric Quarterly* 22, 317–320.

Kety, S.S. (1974) Biochemical and neurochemical effects of electroconvulsive shock. In: *Psychobiology of Convulsive Therapy* (eds M. Fink, S. Kety, J. McGaugh & T. Williams), pp. 285–294. V.H. Winton & Sons, Washington, DC.

King, P.D. (1959) A comparison of REST and ECT in the treatment of schizophrenics. *American Journal of Psychiatry* 116, 358–359.

King, P.D. (1960) Chlorpromazine and electroconvulsive therapy in the treatment of newly hospitalized schizophrenics. *Journal of Clinical and Experimental Psychopathology* 21, 101–105.

Kino, F.F. & Thorpe, T.F. (1946) Electrical convulsion therapy in 500 selected psychotics. *Journal of Mental Science* 92, 138–145.

Klapheke, M.M. (1991a) Clozapine, ECT, and schizoaffective disorder, bipolar type. *Convulsive Therapy* 7, 36–39.

Klapheke, M.M. (1991b) Follow-up on Clozapine and ECT [Letter]. *Convulsive Therapy* 7, 303–305.

Koehler, K. & Sauer, H. (1983) First rank symptoms as predictors of ECT response in schizophrenia. *British Journal of Psychiatry* 142, 280–283.

Kolbeinsson, H., Arnaldsson, O.S., Pëtursson, H. & Skúlason, S. (1986) Computed tomographic scans in ECT-patients. *Acta Psychiatrica Scandinavica* 73, 28–32.

Konig, P. & Glatter-Gotz, U. (1990) Combined electroconvulsive and neuroleptic therapy in schizophrenia refractory to neuroleptics. *Schizophrenia Research* 3, 351–354.

Kramer, B.A. (1987) Maintenance ECT: a survey of practice (1986). *Convulsive Therapy* 3, 260–268.

Kupchik, M., Spivak, B., Mester, R. *et al.* (2000) Combined electroconvulsive–clozapine therapy. *Clinical Neuropharmacology* 23, 14–16.

Kwentus, J.A., Schulz, S.C. & Hart, R.P. (1984) Tardive dystonia, catatonia, and electroconvulsive therapy. *Journal of Nervous and Mental Disease* 172, 171–173.

Landmark, J., Joseph, L. & Merskey, H. (1987) Characteristics of schizophrenic patients and the outcome of fluphenazine and of electroconvulsive treatments. *Canadian Journal of Psychiatry* 32, 425–428.

Landy, D.A. (1991) Combined use of clozapine and electroconvulsive therapy. *Convulsive Therapy* 7, 218–221.

Langsley, D.G., Enterline, J.D. & Hickerson, G.X.J. (1959) A comparison of chlorpromazine and EST in treatment of acute schizophrenic and manic reactions. *Archives of Neurology and Psychiatry* 81, 384–391.

Latey, R.H. & Fahy, T.J. (1988) Some influences on regional variation in frequency of prescription of electroconvulsive therapy. *British Journal of Psychiatry* 152, 196–200.

Leff, J.P. & Wing, J.K. (1971) Trial of maintenance therapy in schizophrenia. *British Medical Journal* 3, 599–604.

Leonhard, K. (1961) Cycloid psychoses. *Journal of Mental Science* 107, 633–648.

Leonhard, K. (1979) *The Classification of Endogenous Psychoses*. Irvington, New York.

Lerer, B., Jabotinsky-Rubin, K., Bannet, J., Ebstein, R.P. & Belmaker,

R.H. (1982) Electroconvulsive shock prevents dopamine receptor supersensitivity. *European Journal of Pharmacology* **80**, 131–134.

Lerer, B., Shapira, B., Calev, A. *et al.* (1995) Antidepressant and cognitive effects of twice- versus three-times-weekly ECT. *American Journal of Psychiatry* **152**, 564–570.

Lewis, A.B. (1982) ECT in drug-refractory schophrenics. *Hillside Journal of Clinical Psychiatry* **4**, 141–154.

Lieberman, J.A., Kane, J.M. & Woerner, M. (1984) Prevalence of tardive dyskinesia in elderly samples. *Psychopharmacology Bulletin* **20**, 22–26.

Lieberman, J.A., Kane, J.M. & Johns, C.A. (1989) Clozapine: guidelines for clinical management. *Journal of Clinical Psychiatry* **50**, 329–338.

Lisanby, S.H., Maddox, J.H., Prudic, J., Devanand, D.P. & Sackeim, H.A. (2000) The effects of electroconvulsive therapy on memory of autobiographical and public events. *Archives of General Psychiatry* **57**, 581–590.

Liskow, B.I. (1985) Relationship between neuroleptic malignant syndrome and malignant hyperthermia [letter]. *American Journal of Psychiatry* **142**, 390.

Lowinger, L. & Huddleson, J.H. (1945) Outcome on dementia praecox under electric shock therapy as related to mode of onset and to number of convulsions induced. *Journal of Nervous and Mental Disease* **102**, 243–246.

McCall, W.V., Mann, S.C., Shelp, F.E. & Caroff, S.N. (1995) Fatal pulmonary embolism in the catatonic syndrome: two case reports and a literature review. *Journal of Clinical Psychiatry* **56**, 21–25.

McCall, W.V., Reboussin, D.M., Weiner, R.D. & Sackeim, H.A. (2000) Titrated moderately suprathreshold vs fixed high-dose right unilateral electroconvulsive therapy: acute antidepressant and cognitive effects. *Archives of General Psychiatry* **57**, 438–444.

McKinnon, A.L. (1948) Electric shock therapy in a private psychiatric hospital. *Canadian Medical Association Journal* **58**, 478–483.

Malek-Ahmadi, P. & Weddige, R.L. (1988) Tardive dyskinesia and electroconvulsive therapy. *Convulsive Therapy* **4**, 328–331.

Malla, A. (1986) An epidemiological study of electroconvulsive therapy: rate and diagnosis. *Canadian Journal of Psychiatry* **31**, 824–830.

Mann, S.C., Caroff, S.N., Bleier, H.R. *et al.* (1986) Lethal catatonia. *American Journal of Psychiatry* **143**, 1374–1381.

Mann, S.C., Caroff, S.N., Bleier, H.R., Antelo, E. & Un, H. (1990) Electroconvulsive therapy of the lethal catatonia syndrome. *Convulsive Therapy* **6**, 239–247.

Martin, B.A., Kramer, P.M., Day, D., Peter, A.M. & Kedward, H.B. (1984) The Clarke Institute experience with electroconvulsive therapy. II. Treatment evaluation and standards of practice. *Canadian Journal of Psychiatry* **29**, 652–657.

Masiar, S.J. & Johns, C.A. (1991) ECT following clozapine. *British Journal of Psychiatry* **158**, 135–136.

May, P.R. (1968) *Treatment of Schizophrenia: A Comparative Study of Five Treatment Methods.* Science House, New York.

May, P.R. & Tuma, A.H. (1965) Treatment of schizophrenia: an experimental study of five treatment methods. *British Journal of Psychiatry* **111**, 503–510.

May, P.R., Tuma, A.H., Yale, C., Potepan, P. & Dixon, W. (1976) Schizophrenia: a follow-up study of results of treatment. II. Hospital stay over 2 to 5 years. *Archives of General Psychiatry* **33**, 481–486.

May, P.R., Tuma, A.H., Dixon, W.J. *et al.* (1981) Schizophrenia: a follow-up study of the results of five forms of treatment. *Archives of General Psychiatry* **38**, 776–784.

Meduna, L.J. (1935) Versuche uber die biologische Beeinflussung des Abaufes der Schizophrenia: Camphor und Cardiozolkrampfe. *Zeitschrift für die Gesellschäft der Neurologia und Psychiatrie* **152**, 235–262.

Melamed, E., Achiron, A., Shapira, A. & Davidoviez, S. (1991) Persis-

tent and progressive parkinsonism after discontinuation of chronic neuroleptic therapy: an additional tardive syndrome? *Clinical Neuropharmacology* **14**, 273–278.

Meldrum, B.S. (1986) Neuropathological consequences of chemically and electrically induced seizures. *Annals of the New York Academy of Sciences* **462**, 186–193.

Meltzer, H.Y. (1989) Clinical studies on the mechanism of action of clozapine: the dopamine-serotonin hypothesis of schizophrenia. *Psychopharmacology* **99** (Suppl.), S18–S27.

Meltzer, H.Y. (1992) Treatment of the neuroleptic-nonresponsive schizophrenic patient. *Schizophrenia Bulletin* **18**, 515–542.

Meltzer, H.Y., Matsubara, S. & Lee, J. (1989) Classifications of typical and atypical antipsychotic drugs on the basis of dopamine D_1, D_2, and serotonin$_2$ pK_i values. *Journal of Pharmacology and Experimental Therapuetics* **251**, 123–130.

Miller, D.H., Clancy, J. & Cumming, E. (1953) A comparison between unidirectional current nonconvulsive electrical stimulation given with Reiters machine, standard alternating current electroshock (Cerletti method), and Pentothal in chronic schizophrenia. *American Journal of Psychiatry* **109**, 617–620.

Milstein, V., Small, J.G., Miller, M.J., Sharpley, P.H. & Small, I.F. (1990) Mechanisms of action of ECT: schizophrenia and schizoaffective disorder. *Biological Psychiatry* **27**, 1282–1292.

Monroe, R.R.J. (1991) Maintenance electroconvulsive therapy. *Psychiatric Clinics of North America* **14**, 947–960.

Moore, M.P. (1943) The maintenance treatment of chronic psychotics by electrically induced convulsions. *Journal of Mental Science* **89**, 257–269.

Mowbray, R.M. (1959) Historical aspects of electric convulsant therapy. *Scottish Medical Journal* **4**, 373–378.

Mukherjee, S. & Debsikdar, V. (1994) Absence of neuroleptic-induced parkinsonism in psychotic patients receiving adjunctive electroconvulsive therapy. *Convulsive Therapy* **10**, 53–58.

Mukherjee, S., Decina, P., Scapicchio, P.L. & Caracci, G. (1991) Cognitive impairment in schizophrenic patients: relations to tardive dyskinesia and neurolpetic-induced parkinsonism. *Biological Psychiatry* **29**, 176A.

Mukherjee, S., Sackeim, H.A. & Schnur, D.B. (1994) Electroconvulsive therapy of acute manic episodes: a review of 50 years' experience. *American Journal of Psychiatry* **151**, 169–176.

Murillo, L.G. & Exner, J.E. Jr (1973a) The effect of regressive ECT with process schizophrenics. *American Journal of Psychiatry* **130**, 269–273.

Murillo, L.G. & Exner, J.E. Jr (1973b) Ataractic drugs versus ECT in schizophrenia [letter]. *American Journal of Psychiatry* **130**, 1162–1163.

Nasrallah, H.A., McCalley-Whitters, M. & Jacoby, C.G. (1982) Cerebral ventricular enlargement in young manic males: a controlled CT study. *Journal of Affective Disorders* **4**, 15–19.

Nasrallah, H.A., McCalley-Whitters, M. & Pfohl, B. (1984) Clinical significance of large cerebral ventricles in manic males. *Psychiatry Research* **13**, 151–156.

National Institutes of Health (1985) Consensus conference: electroconvulsive therapy. *Journal of the American Medical Association* **254**, 2103–2108.

National Institute of Mental Health (NIMH-PSC) Collaborative Study Group (1964) Phenothiazine treatment in acute schizophrenia. *Archives of General Psychiatry* **10**, 246–261.

Newman, M.E. & Lerer, B. (1989) Post-receptor-mediated increases in adenylate cyclase activity after chronic antidepressant treatment: relationship to receptor desensitization. *European Journal of Pharmacology* **162**, 345–352.

Nobler, M.S., Sackeim, H.A., Solomou, M. *et al.* (1993) EEG manifestations during ECT: effects of electrode placement and stimulus intensity. *Biological Psychiatry* **34**, 321–330.

Nobler, M.S., Sackeim, H.A., Prohovnik, I. *et al.* (1994) Regional cerebral blood flow in mood disorders. III. Treatment and clinical response. *Archives of General Psychiatry* **51**, 884–897.

Nobler, M.S., Sackeim, H.A., Moeller, J.R. *et al.* (1997) Quantifying the speed of symptomatic improvement with electroconvulsive therapy: comparison of alternative statistical methods. *Convulsive Therapy* **13**, 208–221.

Nobler, M.S., Luber, B., Moeller, J.R. *et al.* (2000) Quantitative EEG during seizures induced by electroconvulsive therapy: relations to treatment modality and clinical features. I. Global analyses. *Journal of ECT* **16**, 211–228.

Nomikos, G.G., Zis, A.P., Damsma, G. & Fibiger, H.C. (1991) Electroconvulsive shock produces large increases in interstitial concentrations of dopamine in the rat striatum: an *in vivo* microdialysis study. *Neuropsychopharmacology* **4**, 65–69.

Nutt, D.J., Gleiter, C.H. & Glue, P. (1989) Neuropharmacological aspects of ECT: in search of the primary mechanism of action. *Convulsive Therapy* **5**, 250–260.

Olfson, M., Marcus, S., Sackeim, H.A., Thompson, J. & Pincus, H.A. (1998) Use of ECT for the inpatient treatment of recurrent major depression. *American Journal of Psychiatry* **155**, 22–29.

Ottosson, J.-O. (1960) Experimental studies of the mode of action of electroconvulsive therapy. *Acta Psychiatrica Scandinavica Supplement* **145**, 1–141.

Ottosson, J.-O. (1985) Use and misuse of electroconvulsive treatment. *Biological Psychiatry* **20**, 933–946.

Owen, R.R.J., Gutierrez-Esteinou, R., Hsiao, J. *et al.* (1993) Effects of clozapine and fluphenazine treatment on responses to *m*-chlorophenylpiperazine infusions in schizophrenia. *Archives of General Psychiatry* **50**, 636–644.

Palmer, D.M., Sprang, H.E. & Hans, C.L. (1951) Electroshock therapy in schizophrenia: a statistical survey of 455 cases. *Journal of Nervous and Mental Disease* **114**, 162–171.

Pankratz, W.J. (1980) Electrtroconvulsive therapy: the position of the Canadian Psychiatric Association. *Canadian Journal of Psychiatry* **25**, 509–514.

Pataki, J., Zervas, I.M. & Jandorf, L. (1992) Catatonia in a university inpatient service (1985–90). *Convulsive Therapy* **8**, 163–173.

Pearlman, C. (1990) Neuroleptic malignant syndrome and electroconvulsive therapy [letter]. *Convulsive Therapy* **6**, 251–253.

Pearlson, G.D., Garbacz, D.J., Moberg, P.J., Ahn, H.S. & DePaulo, J.R. (1985) Symptomatic, familial, perinatal, and social correlates of computerized axial tomography (CAT) changes in schizophrenics and bipolars. *Journal of Nervous and Mental Disease* **173**, 42–50.

Perlson, J. (1945) Psychologic studies on a patient who received two hundred and forty-eight shock treatments. *Archives of Neurology and Psychiatry* **54**, 409–411.

Perris, C. (1974) A study of cycloid psychoses. *Acta Psychiatrica Scandinavica Supplement* **253**, 1–77.

Pippard, J. & Ellam, L. (1981) *Electroconvulsive Treatment in Great Britain*. Gaskell, London.

Pope, J.G. Jr & Lipinski, J.F. (1978) Diagnosis in schizophrenia and manic-depressive illness. *Archives of General Psychiatry* **35**, 811–827.

Pope, H.G. Jr, Lipinski, J.F., Cohen, B.M. & Axelrod, D.T. (1980) 'Schizoaffective disorder': an invalid diagnosis? A comparison of schizoaffective disorder, schizophrenia, and affective disorder. *American Journal of Psychiatry* **137**, 921–927.

Price, T.R. & Levin, R. (1978) The effects of electroconvulsive therapy on tardive dyskinesia. *American Journal of Psychiatry* **135**, 991–993.

Pridmore, S. & Pollard, C. (1996) Electroconvulsive therapy in Parkinson's disease: 30 month follow up. *Journal of Neurology, Neurosurgery and Psychiatry* **60**, 693.

Prudic, J., Sackeim, H.A. & Devanand, D.P. (1990) Medication resistance and clinical response to electroconvulsive therapy. *Psychiatry Research* **31**, 287–296.

Rabins, P.V., Pearlson, G.D., Aylward, E., Kumar, A.J. & Dowell, K. (1991) Cortical magnetic resonance imaging changes in elderly inpatients with major depression. *American Journal of Psychiatry* **148**, 617–620.

Rachlin, H.L., Goldman, G.S., Gurvitz, M., Lurie, A. & Rachlin, L. (1956) Follow-up study of 317 patients discharged from Hillside Hospital in 1950. *Journal of Hillside Hospital* **5**, 17–40.

Rahman, R. (1968) A review of treatment of 176 schizophrenic patients in the mental hospital Pabna. *British Journal of Psychiatry* **114**, 775–777.

Ray, S.D. (1962) Relative efficacy of ECT and CPZ in schizophrenia. *Journal of the Indian Medical Association* **38**, 332–333.

Riddell, S.A. (1963) The therapeutic efficacy of ECT. *Archives of General Psychiatry* **8**, 546–556.

Ries, R.K., Wilson, L., Bokan, J.A. & Chiles, J.A. (1981) ECT in medication resistant schizoaffective disorder. *Comprehensive Psychiatry* **22**, 167–173.

Robin, A. & De Tissera, S. (1982) A double-blind controlled comparison of the therapeutic effects of low and high energy electroconvulsive therapies. *British Journal of Psychiatry* **141**, 357–366.

Rohde, P. & Sargant, W. (1961) Treatment of schizophrenia in general hospitals. *British Medical Journal* **2**, 67–70.

Rosebush, P.I., Hildebrand, A.M. & Mazurek, M.F. (1992) The treatment of catatonia: benzodiazepines or ECT? [letter]. *American Journal of Psychiatry* **149**, 1279–1280.

Rosenbach, M.L., Hermann, R.C. & Dorwart, R.A. (1997) Use of electroconvulsive therapy in the Medicare population between 1987 and 1992. *Psychiatric Services* **48**, 1537–1542.

Rosenbaum, A.H., O'Connor, M.K., Duane, D.D. & Auger, R.G. (1980) Treatment of tardive dyskinesia in an agitated, depressed patient. *Psychosomatics* **21**, 765–766.

Ross, J.R. & Malzberg, B. (1939) A review of the results of the pharmacological shock therapy and the metrazol convulsive therapy in New York State. *American Journal of Psychiatry* **96**, 297–316.

Royal College of Psychiatrists (1977) The Royal College of Psychiatrists' Memorandum on the use of Electroconvulsive Therapy. I. Effectiveness of ECT: a review of the evidence. *British Journal of Psychiatry* **131**, 261–268.

Royal College of Psychiatrists (1995) *The ECT Handbook: The Second Report of the Royal College of Psychiatrists' Special Committee on ECT*. Royal College of Psychiatrists, London.

Rummans, T.A. & Bassingthwaighte, E. (1991) Severe medical and neurologic complications associated with near-lethal catatonia treated with electroconvulsive therapy. *Convulsive Therapy* **7**, 121–124.

Sackeim, H.A. (1988) Mechanisms of action of electroconvulsive therapy. In: *Annual Review of Psychiatry*, Vol. 7 (eds R.E. Hales & J. Frances), pp. 436–457. American Psychiatric Press, Washington, DC.

Sackeim, H.A. (1989) The efficacy of electroconvulsive therapy in treatment of major depressive disorder. In: *The Limits of Biological Treatments for Psychological Distress: Comparisons with Psychotherapy and Placebo* (eds S. Fisher & R.P. Greenberg), pp. 275–307. Erlbaum, Hillsdale, NJ.

Sackeim, H.A. (1992) The cognitive effects of electroconvulsive therapy. In: *Cognitive Disorders: Pathophysiology and Treatment* (eds W.H. Moos, E.R. Gamzu & L.J. Thal), pp. 183–228. Marcel Dekker, New York.

Sackeim, H.A. (1994) Continuation therapy following ECT: directions for future research. *Psychopharmacology Bulletin* **30**, 501–521.

Sackeim, H.A. (1998) The use of electroconvulsive therapy in late-life depression. In: *Geriatric Psychopharmacology*, 3rd edn (ed. C. Salzman), pp. 262–309. Williams & Wilkins, Baltimore, MD.

Sackeim, H.A. (2000) Memory and ECT: from polarization to reconciliation. *Journal of ECT* **16**, 87–96.

Sackeim, H.A., Decina, P., Kanzler, M., Kerr, B. & Malitz, S. (1987a) Effects of electrode placement on the efficacy of titrated, low-dose ECT. *American Journal of Psychiatry* **144**, 1449–1455.

Sackeim, H.A., Decina, P., Prohovnik, I. & Malitz, S. (1987b) Seizure threshold in electroconvulsive therapy: effects of sex, age, electrode placement, and number of treatments. *Archives of General Psychiatry* **44**, 355–360.

Sackeim, H.A., Prudic, J., Devanand, D.P. *et al.* (1990) The impact of medication resistance and continuation pharmacotherapy on relapse following response to electroconvulsive therapy in major depression. *Journal of Clinical Psychopharmacology* **10**, 96–104.

Sackeim, H.A., Devanand, D.P. & Prudic, J. (1991) Stimulus intensity, seizure threshold, and seizure duration: impact on the efficacy and safety of electroconvulsive therapy. *Psychiatric Clinics of North America* **14**, 803–843.

Sackeim, H.A., Prudic, J., Devanand, D.P. *et al.* (1993) Effects of stimulus intensity and electrode placement on the efficacy and cognitive effects of electroconvulsive therapy. *New England Journal of Medicine* **328**, 839–846.

Sackeim, H.A., Devanand, D.P. & Nobler, M.S. (1995) Electroconvulsive therapy. In: *Psychopharmacology: the Fourth Generation of Progress* (eds F. Bloom & D. Kupfer), pp. 1123–1142. Raven Press, New York.

Sackeim, H.A., Luber, B., Katzman, G.P. *et al.* (1996) The effects of electroconvulsive therapy on quantitative electroencephalograms: relationship to clinical outcome. *Archives of General Psychiatry* **53**, 814–824.

Sackeim, H.A., Prudic, J., Devanand, D.P. *et al.* (2000) A prospective, randomized, double-blind comparison of bilateral and right unilateral electroconvulsive therapy at different stimulus intensities. *Archives of General Psychiatry* **57**, 425–434.

Safferman, A.Z. & Munne, R. (1992) Combining clozapine with ECT. *Convulsive Therapy* **8**, 141–143.

Sajatovic, M. & Meltzer, H.Y. (1993) The effect of short-term electroconvulsive treatment plus neuroleptics in treatment-resistant schizophrenia and schizoaffective disorder. *Convulsive Therapy* **9**, 167–175.

Salzman, C. (1980) The use of ECT in the treatment of schizophrenia. *American Journal of Psychiatry* **137**, 1032–1041.

Saykin, A.J., Shtasel, D.L., Gur, R.E. *et al.* (1994) Neuropsychological deficits in neuroleptic naive patients with first-episode schizophrenia. *Archives of General Psychiatry* **51**, 124–131.

Schooler, N. (1991) Maintenance medication for schizophrenia: strategies for dose reduction. *Schizophrenia Bulletin* **17**, 311–324.

Schooler, N. & Kane, J.M. (1982) Research diagnoses for tardive dyskinesia. *Archives of General Psychiatry* **39**, 486–487.

Schwartz, M., Silver, H., Tal, I. & Sharf, B. (1993) Tardive dyskinesia in northern Israel: preliminary study. *European Neurology* **33**, 264–266.

Scott, A.I., Douglas, R.H., Whitfield, A. & Kendell, R.E. (1990) Time course of cerebra; magnetic resonance changes after electroconvulsive therapy. *British Journal of Psychiatry* **156**, 551–553.

Scovern, A.W. & Kilmann, P.R. (1980) Status of electroconvulsive therapy: review of the outcome literature. *Psychological Bulletin* **87**, 260–303.

Sedivec, V. (1981) Psychoses endangering life. *Ceskoslovenska Psychiatrie* **77**, 38–41.

Seidman, L.R. (1983) Schizophrenia and brain dysfunction: an integration of recent neurodiagnostic findings. *Psychological Bulletin* **94**, 195–238.

Serra, G., Collu, M., D'Aquila, P.S., De M.O.G. & Gessa, G.L. (1990) Possible role of dopamine D_1 receptor in the behavioural supersensitivity to dopamine agonists induced by chronic treatment with antidepressants. *Brain Research* **527**, 234–243.

Shapira, B., Tubi, N., Drexler, H. *et al.* (1998) Cost and benefit in the choice of ECT schedule: twice versus three times weekly ECT. *British Journal of Psychiatry* **172**, 44–48.

Shibata, M., Aoba, A., Kitani, K. *et al.* (1989) Redistribution of haloperidol after electroshock: experimental evidence. *Life Sciences* **44**, 749–753.

Shoor, M. & Adams, F.H. (1950) The intensive electric shock therapy of chronic disturbed psychotic patients. *American Journal of Psychiatry* **107**, 279–282.

Shugar, G., Hoffman, B.F. & Johnston, J.D. (1984) Electroconvulsive therapy for schizophrenia in Ontario: a report on therapeutic polymorphism. *Comprehensive Psychiatry* **25**, 509–520.

Shukla, G.D. (1981) Electroconvulsive therapy in a rural teaching general hospital in India. *British Journal of Psychiatry* **139**, 569–571.

Siesjö, B.K., Ingvar, M. & Wieloch, T. (1986) Cellular and molecular events underlying epileptic brain damage. *Annals of the New York Academy of Sciences* **462**, 207–223.

Singerman, B. & Raheja, R. (1994) Malignant catatonia: a continuing reality. *Annals of Clinical Psychiatry* **6**, 259–266.

Small, J.G. (1985) Efficacy of electroconvulsive therapy in schizophrenia, mania, and other disorders. I. Schizophrenia. *Convulsive Therapy* **1**, 263–270.

Small, J.G., Milstein, V., Klapper, M., Kellams, J.J. & Small, I.F. (1982) ECT combined with neuroleptics in the treatment of schizophrenia. *Psychopharmacology Bulletin* **18**, 34–35.

Smith, W.E. & Richman, A. (1984) Electroconvulsive therapy: a Canadian perspective. *Canadian Journal of Psychiatry* **29**, 693–699.

Smith, K., Surphlis, W.R., Gynther, M.D. & Shimkunas, A.M. (1967) ECT–chlorpromazine and chlorpromazine compared in the treatment of schizophrenia. *Journal of Nervous and Mental Disease* **144**, 284–290.

Snaith, R.P. (1981) How much ECT does the depressed patient need? In: *Electroconvulsive Therapy: an Appraisal* (ed. R.L. Palmer), pp. 61–64. Oxford University Press, New York.

Spitzer, R.L., Endicott, J. & Robins, E. (1978) Research diagnostic criteria: rationale and reliability. *Archives of General Psychiatry* **35**, 773–782.

Staudt, V.M. & Zubin, J. (1957) A biometric evaluation of the somatotherapies in schizophrenia. *Psychological Bulletin* **54**, 171–196.

Strömgren, L.S. (1988) Electroconvulsive therapy in Aarhus, Denmark, in 1984: its application in nondepressive disorders. *Convulsive Therapy* **4**, 306–313.

Swayze, V.W., Andreasen, N.C., Alliger, R.J., Ehrhardt, J.C. & Yuh, W.T. (1990) Structural brain abnormalities in bipolar affective disorder: ventricular enlargement and focal signal hyperintensities. *Archives of General Psychiatry* **47**, 1054–1059.

Tancer, M.E., Golden, R.N., Ekstrom, R.D. & Evans, D.L. (1989) Use of electroconvulsive therapy at a University hospital: 1970 and 1980–81. *Hospital and Community Psychiatry* **40**, 64–68.

Taylor, P.J. (1981) ECT in schizophrenia: a review. In: *Electroconvulsive Therapy: an Appraisal* (ed. R.L. Palmer), pp. 37–54. Oxford University Press, New York.

Taylor, P.J. & Fleminger, J.J. (1980) ECT for schizophrenia. *Lancet* **1**, 1380–1382.

Templer, D.I., Ruff, C.F. & Armstrong, G. (1973) Cognitive functioning and degree of psychosis in schizophrenics given many electroconvulsive treatments. *British Journal of Psychiatry* **123**, 441–443.

Tharyan, P. (2000) Electroconvulsive therapy for schizophrenia. *Cochrane Database System Review* **2**, 1469–1493.

Thompson, J.W. & Blaine, J.D. (1987) Use of ECT in the United States in 1975 and 1980. *American Journal of Psychiatry* **144**, 557–562.

Thompson, J.W., Weiner, R.D. & Myers, C.P. (1994) Use of ECT in the United States in 1975, 1980 and 1986. *American Journal of Psychiatry* **151**, 1657–1661.

Thornton, J.E., Mulsant, B.H., Dealy, R. & Reynolds, I.I.C. (1990) A retrospective study of maintenance electroconvulsive therapy in a university-based psychiatric practice. *Convulsive Therapy* **6**, 121–129.

Tolsma, F.J. (1967) The syndrome of acute pernicious psychosis. *Psychiatria Neurologia Neurochirurgia* **70**, 1–21.

Trollor, J.N. & Sachdev, P.S. (1999) Electroconvulsive treatment of neuroleptic malignant syndrome: a review and report of cases. *Australian and New Zealand Journal of Psychiatry* **33**, 650–659.

Tsuang, M.T., Woolson, R.F. & Fleming, J.A. (1979) Long-term outcome of major psychoses 1. schizophrenia and affective disorders compared with psychiatrically symptom-free surgical conditions. *Archives of General Psychiatry* **36**, 1295–1301.

Turek, I.S. & Hanlon, T.E. (1977) The effectiveness and safety of electroconvulsive therapy (ECT). *Journal of Nervous and Mental Disease* **164**, 419–431.

Uhrbrand, L. & Faurbye, A. (1960) Reversible and irreversible dyskinesia after treatment with perphenazine, chlorpromazine, reserpine, and ECT. *Psychopharmacologia* **1**, 408–418.

Ulett, G.A., Gleser, G.C., Caldwell, B.M. & Smith, K. (1954) The use of matched groups in the evaluation of convulsive and subconvulsive photoshock. *Bulletin of the Menninger Clinic* **18**, 138–146.

Ulett, G.A., Smith, K. & Gleser, G. (1956) Evaluation of convulsive and subconvulsive shock therapies utilizing a control group. *American Journal of Psychiatry* **112**, 795–802.

Ungvári, G. & Pethö, B. (1982) High-dose haloperidol therapy: its effectiveness and a comparison with electroconvulsive therapy. *Journal of Psychiatric Treatment and Evaluation* **4**, 279–283.

Van Valkenburg, C. & Clayton, P.J. (1985) Electroconvulsive therapy and schizophrenia. *Biological Psychiatry* **20**, 699–700.

Verma, A. & Kulkarni, S.K. (1991) Chronic electroconvulsive shock alters hypothermic response of B-HT 920 and SKF 38393 in rats. *Journal of Pharmacy and Pharmacology* **43**, 813–814.

Walinder, J. (1972) Recurrent familial psychosis of the schizo-affective type. *Acta Psychiatrica Scandinavica* **48**, 274–283.

Watt, D.C., Katz, K. & Shepherd, M. (1983) The natural history of schizophrenia: a 5 year prospective follow-up of a representative sample of schizophrenics by means of a standardized clinical and social assessment. *Psychological Medicine* **13**, 663–670.

Weinberger, D.R., Torrey, E.F., Neophytides, A.N. & Wyatt, R.J. (1979) Lateral cerebral ventricular enlargement in chronic schizophrenia. *Archives of General Psychiatry* **36**, 735–739.

Weiner, R.D. (1984) Does ECT cause brain damage? *Behavioral and Brain Sciences* **7**, 1–53.

Weiner, R.D., Rogers, H.J., Davidson, J.R. & Squire, L.R. (1986) Effects of stimulus parameters on cognitive side effects. *Annals of the New York Academy of Sciences* **462**, 315–325.

Weinstein, M.R. & Fischer, A. (1971) Combined treatment with ECT and antipsychotic drugs in schizophrenia. *Diseases of the Nervous System* **32**, 810–808.

Weiss, D.M. (1955) Changes in blood pressure with electroshock therapy in a patient receiving chlorpromazine hydrochloride (Thorazine). *American Journal of Psychiatry* **111**, 617–619.

Weisz, S. & Creel, J.N. (1948) Maintenance treatment in schizophrenia. *Diseases of the Nervous System* **9**, 10–14.

Wells, D.A. (1973) Electroconvulsive treatment for schizophrenia: a ten-year survey in a university hospital psychiatric department. *Comprehensive Psychiatry* **14**, 291–298.

Wessels, W.H. (1972) A comparative study of the efficacy of bilateral and unilateral electroconvulsive therapy with thioridazine in acute schizophrenia. *South African Medical Journal* **46**, 890–892.

Wittman, P. (1941) A scale for measuring prognosis in schizophrenic patients. *Elgin Papers* **4**, 20–33.

Witton, K. (1962) Efficacy of ECT following prolonged use of psychotropic drugs. *American Journal of Psychiatry* **119**, 79.

Wolff, G.E. (1955) Electric shock treatment. *American Journal of Psychiatry* **111**, 748–750.

World Health Organization (1979) *Schizophrenia: an International Follow-Up Study* John Wiley & Sons, New York.

Wyatt, R.J. (1991) Neuroleptics and the natural course of schizophrenia. *Schizophrenia Bulletin* **17**, 325–351.

Zachrisson, O.C., Balldin, J., Ekman, R. *et al.* (2000) No evident neuronal damage after electroconvulsive therapy. *Psychiatry Research* **96**, 157–165.

Zeifert, M. (1941) Results obtained from the administration of 12,000 doses of metrazol to mental patients. *Psychiatry Quarterly* **15**, 772–778.

Zis, A.P., Nomikos, G.G., Damsma, G. & Fibiger, H.C. (1991) *In vivo* neurochemical effects of electroconvulsive shock studied by microdialysis in the rat striatum. *Psychopharmacology (Berlin)* **103**, 343–350.

28 Neuroleptic-induced acute extrapyramidal syndromes and tardive dyskinesia

V.S. Mattay and D.E. Casey

Acute extrapyramidal syndromes, 552
    Clinical manifestations, 552
    Pathophysiology, 553
    Epidemiology, 554
    Treatment, 556
    Managing acute extrapyramidal syndromes, 556
Tardive dyskinesia, 558
    Clinical manifestations, 559
    Terminology, 559
    Differential diagnosis, 560
    Pathophysiology, 561

Neuroimaging and neuropathology, 562
Epidemiology, 562
Long-term outcome, 562
Complications, 563
Risk factors, 563
Managing tardive dyskinesia, 564
Treatment, 565
Conclusions, 567
Acknowledgements, 567
References, 567

Neuroleptic (antipsychotic) drugs are the mainstay of treatment for both acute and chronic psychoses. Since they were labelled 'neuroleptic' in the 1950s to encompass the concept of 'taking control of the neurone', this terminology has remained (Deniker 1984). Originally, it was believed that the antipsychotic and extrapyramidal motor side-effects of neuroleptic drugs developed at the same or very similar doses. Thus, this became identified as the neuroleptic threshold concept. This hypothesis was practically applied to indicate that when patients developed extrapyramidal syndromes (EPS), they were receiving an adequate antipsychotic dose. Eventually, the concept that antipsychotic and EPS effects were inextricably linked was gradually disproved. However, it is clear that traditional neuroleptic drugs have a very narrow therapeutic index, so that the majority of patients who do benefit from appropriate antipsychotic doses will also develop motor side-effects. While this is characteristic of traditional antipsychotics, it is not so for the newer generation of antipsychotics, popularly known as 'atypical antipsychotics' because of the significantly lower incidence of extrapyramidal side-effects associated with them, along with the minimal or absent effect on prolactin elevation.

Drug-induced disorders of motor function can develop along two separate general time courses. Acute EPS develop early in the course of treatment and may continue as long as neuroleptic drug therapy is prescribed. Tardive dyskinesia (TD) occurs much later during chronic neuroleptic therapy. While TD is often considered the most serious side-effect of neuroleptic drugs, acute EPS are considered as minor inconveniences to the patient. However, this perspective should be carefully reviewed because the majority (50–75%) of patients develop EPS, which may be an important cause of physical and mental impairment (Casey & Keepers 1988). Additionally, patients will often dis-

continue their neuroleptic drugs because of the mental and physical discomfort associated with acute EPS. In contrast, TD occurs in a minority of patients (approximately 20%) and is usually of mild severity, often not noticed by the patient and produces little or no disability or discomfort in most cases. Severe forms of TD are more rare, but can produce substantial impairment (Gardos *et al.* 1987; Casey & Keepers 1988).

This chapter reviews current knowledge about neuroleptic-induced acute EPS and TD. Information about clinical manifestations, pathophysiology, epidemiology, risk factors, outcome and treatment approaches is reviewed. Strategies for combining patient, drug and temporal information are used to develop clinical algorithms for maximizing the benefit and minimizing the short- and long-term detriments of these drugs.

Acute extrapyramidal syndromes

Since the initial use of neuroleptic drugs, the EPS of akathisia, dystonia and parkinsonism have been recognized. These disorders occur in most patients receiving typical neuroleptics and are often considered different manifestations of the same disorder with the same underlying pathophysiology. However, because there are several important distinctions between these different syndromes, it is important to consider them as separate entities.

Clinical manifestations

Akathisia

Akathisia is a syndrome of subjective feelings of restlessness or distress which may be accompanied by objective signs of these feelings. Patients may describe akathisia as anxiety, loss of internal calmness, an inability to relax, feeling uptight or internal jitteriness. Objective signs of restlessness are pacing, rocking back and forth while sitting or standing, lifting the feet as if marching in place, crossing and uncrossing the legs when sitting or other repetitive purposeless actions. There is some debate whether patients who deny inner feelings of restlessness, yet show objective signs of restlessness, should be diagnosed as having akathisia. A strict adherence to the originally proposed definition requires that subjective discomfort be present, and that the presence of only objective signs without subjective restlessness should be called pseudoakathisia (Barnes & Braude 1985). However, it is not clear that this distinction has either practical or heuristic value. Many patients appear to have classic objective signs of pacing and appear to be uncomfortably restless but do not admit to these subjective experiences. For some patients, it may be that their psychosis prevents them from giving accurate reports.

Akathisia can often be misdiagnosed as psychotic agitation, which leads to a further increase in neuroleptic dosage and greater aggravation of akathisia. It may begin within a few hours or days after starting an antipsychotic treatment (Adler *et al.* 1989). The core problem in this syndrome may be that psychotic patients often have great difficulty communicating their feelings of restlessness and discomfort, and may describe their feelings with bizarre and delusional statements.

Acute dystonia

Acute dystonia is characterized by involuntary muscle spasms that produce briefly sustained or fixed abnormal postures. These can include bizarre positions of the limbs and trunk, oculogyric crises, tongue protrusion, trismus, torticollis and laryngeal–pharyngeal constriction. If these symptoms occur within 7 days (usually within the first 24–48 h) of initiating or substantially increasing existing neuroleptic drug treatment, the patient should be given the benefit of the doubt and neuroleptic drug-induced dystonia should be the first item on the differential diagnosis. Because dystonia may often appear as isolated and fluctuating symptoms in the first few days, these unusual symptoms are often misdiagnosed as malingering, hysteria or seizures (Casey 1991a).

Parkinsonism

Drug-induced and idiopathic parkinsonism are phenomenologically identical. Drug-induced parkinsonism usually develops after several days to weeks of continuous neuroleptic treatment (Ayd 1961). The classic triad of tremor, rigidity and bradykinesia is present in both forms of the disorder. Tremor is a rhythmical to-and-fro motion that is usually worse at rest. Rigidity may be asymmetrical and is easily identified in the limbs as a ratchet-like or cogwheel resistance during passive motion. Bradykinesia, also referred to as akinesia, is the reduction in spontaneous activity. Usually, this is noticed as a mask-like facial expression, softening of the voice, decreased associated arm movements

during walking and reduced ability to initiate movement. Neuroleptic drug-induced parkinsonism can be diagnosed when any one or more of the triad of symptoms is present. As in idiopathic parkinsonism, symptoms may be unilateral, symmetrical or asymmetrically bilateral.

It is essential to distinguish bradykinesia from negative symptoms of psychosis, psychological withdrawal or depression. However, this is often very difficult to do and may not be fully achievable until neuroleptic drugs have been discontinued for several weeks or months. The rabbit syndrome is an uncommon side-effect characterized by perioral lip tremor (Villeneuve 1972; Casey 1992a). It can occur at any time during neuroleptic treatment and is most likely a variant of drug-induced parkinsonism because it has the characteristic tremor rate (3–6 Hz/cps) and responds to anti-EPS drugs, as does parkinsonism.

Pathophysiology

Current knowledge indicates that the pathophysiology of acute EPS involves a critical role for dopamine, a major role for acetylcholine, and a hypothetical role for serotonin.

Dopaminergic mechanisms

Because all commercially available effective neuroleptic drugs have in common the property of blocking dopamine D_2 receptors of the basal ganglia, reduced dopamine function is the most commonly proposed mechanism of acute EPS. Recent positron emission tomography (PET) studies suggest that EPS occur when D_2 occupancy exceeds a threshold somewhere in the range of 75–80% (Farde *et al.* 1992). However, not all data are supportive of the notion that D_2 receptor subtype mediates EPS. Animal models show that dopamine D_1 receptor antagonism can also produce dystonia and other acute EPS in monkeys (Gerlach *et al.* 1988; Casey 1992c). Although some neuroleptics, such as flupenthixol and clozapine, have both D_1 and D_2 antagonist properties, the lack of availability of pure D_1 antagonists precludes from delineating the relative contributions and interrelationships between D_1 and D_2 antagonism in neuroleptic-induced EPS. EPS were not observed in patients treated with clinically effective doses of clozapine that produce receptor occupancy rates of 55–65% for the D_1 receptor and just slightly higher rates for the D_2 receptor.

The ratio of D_4/D_2 occupancy may be another factor in contributing to lower EPS incidence with some of the novel antipsychotics. It is possible that D_4 receptors may have a role in dopamine-mediated modulation of GABAergic neuronal activity (Seeman *et al.* 1997).

Cholinergic mechanisms

The reciprocal balance between dopamine and acetylcholine in the basal ganglia and the high efficacy of anticholinergic drugs in reversing and mitigating EPS provide support for the proposed role for acetylcholine in mediating EPS. The high affinity of atypical antipsychotics with low EPS profile, such as clozapine and olanzapine, to muscarinic receptors lends further support to this mechanism.

Serotinergic mechanisms

Although the relationship between serotonin and dopamine antagonism with regard to EPS is still not completely clear, more recent hypotheses propose a high ratio of serotonin 5-HT$_2$/D$_2$ receptor blockade to be an important factor in the lower EPS incidence of the newer atypical neuroleptics. The significantly higher 5-HT$_{2A}$ than D$_2$ occupancy of many of the current atypical neuroleptics (risperidone, olanzapine, clozapine, quetiapine and ziprasidone) has been confirmed by several PET studies (Nyberg *et al.* 1996, 1997; Kapur 1998; Kapur *et al.* 1999). The reported association between 5-HT$_{2A}$ receptor blockade and attenuation of EPS (Bersani *et al.* 1990), combined with the associated improvement of cognitive function (Gallhofer *et al.* 1996) and negative symptoms (Davies & Janicak 1996), provide further support to the role of serotinergic mechanisms. Additionally, since 5-HT$_{2A}$ receptors are thought to interact directly with dopaminergic transmission, it is possible that restoration of striatal dopaminergic function by antagonism of these receptors may have a critical role in the amelioration of EPS and improvement of negative symptoms (Pehek 1996).

Akathisia is the least well-understood EPS. There are no neuroanatomical correlates to this disorder, and typical anti-EPS drug therapy is much less effective in akathisia than it is in other disorders (Casey & Keepers 1988; Adler *et al.* 1989). β-Adrenergic blockers, such as propranolol, effectively treat akathisia in many, but not all, patients (Lipinski *et al.* 1984). The exact mechanism of action of β-adrenergic blockers in the treatment of akathisia is still unclear.

Neuroleptic drug-induced dystonia has been hypothesized to be caused by either a hypo- or hyperdopaminergic state following the initiation of neuroleptic drug-induced blockade of dopamine receptors in the caudate, putamen and globus pallidus (Rupniak *et al.* 1986). However, the observation of dystonia on the second day of treatment following a single neuroleptic dose has been difficult to interpret. It appears that dystonia is associated with decreasing neuroleptic blood levels several hours after peak levels have been achieved (Garver *et al.* 1976). It is also possible that a higher than baseline level of the neuroleptic in the blood might produce dystonia. An additional difficulty with this model is that most patients do not just get a single dose of neuroleptic within the first 24–36 h of initiating treatment but, rather, they receive several doses within the first few days, often at 12- or 24-h intervals, so that dystonia is occurring sometime between the increasing blood levels following recent drug intake and the decreasing blood levels of the drug being metabolized throughout the subsequent 12–24 h. This complex situation indicates the importance of the possibility of a specific ratio between endogenous dopamine levels and the degree of receptor antagonism. Defining the relative balance of receptor blockade induced by the neuroleptic and high levels of endogenous dopamine, which are released by the dopamine feedback system after receptors have been blocked, will be critically important to understanding the pathophysiology of dystonia. Finally, as in akathisia, other neurotransmitter mechanisms may also be involved.

Neuroleptic drug-induced parkinsonism supposedly develops from blockade of nigrostriatal dopamine systems. The delay of several days before symptom onset after neuroleptics are initiated is not compatible with the mechanism of acute receptor blockade that takes place within hours after neuroleptics are administered. One more important temporal factor to account for is the partial or complete tolerance of neuroleptic drug-induced parkinsonism that may evolve over several months, even though neuroleptic treatment remains stable. This gradual development of tolerance also indicates the importance of compensatory processes which are not well understood and may be secondary consequences to dopamine receptor blockade (Casey 1987, 1991b).

The mechanisms determining individual susceptibility to drug-induced parkinsonism are still not clear. Some studies propose that women are at increased risk for the development of drug-induced parkinsonism along with other movement disorders such as tardive dyskinesia and suggest oestrogen-related dopamine receptor blockade as an explanation (Ayd 1961; Glazer *et al.* 1983). However, this gender predisposition has not been substantiated by other studies (Kennedy *et al.* 1971; Moleman *et al.* 1982). A genetic influence has been suggested, based on nearly twice the incidence of acute akathisia in schizophrenic patients homozygous for the Ser9Gly variant of the dopamine D$_3$ receptor gene (*DRD3*) as compared with patients non-homozygous for this allele (Eichhammer *et al.* 2000).

The possibility that increased susceptibility to drug-induced parkinsonism might be related to subclinical *Parkinson's disease* has also been suggested (Duvoisin 1977). In support of this notion are the findings of Rajput *et al.* (1982) showing pathological changes consistent with *Parkinson's disease* in two patients with drug-induced parkinsonism that had completely remitted following drug withdrawal. Likewise, using F18, Brooks (1991, 1993) reported reduced F18-dopa uptake in the putamen of individuals susceptible to drug-induced parkinsonism.

Epidemiology

Prevalence/incidence

EPS prevalence spans a wide range of 2–90% (Casey & Keepers 1988). Prevalence may approach 100% in highly vulnerable groups of patients (Ganzini *et al.* 1991b). The EPS risk is strongly influenced by patient, drug and time characteristics. There was a steady increase in the prevalence of acute EPS resulting from the widespread use of high doses of high potency neuroleptics in the 1970s and through the early 1990s (Casey 1996). However, as a result of the increasing usage of the newer atypical neuroleptics (clozapine, risperidone, olanzapine, quetiapine and ziprasidone) with lower EPS risk and the use of lower doses of high-potency compounds, the prevalence of neuroleptic-induced EPS is possibly decreasing. The incidence of dystonia gradually increased from 2.3% in the late 1950s (Ayd 1961) to approximately 10% in the 1980s (Keepers *et al.* 1983).

Patient variables

Age, gender and history of EPS all influence whether a patient will develop EPS with drug treatment. Young males receiving high doses of high-potency compounds are the most vulnerable to acute dystonia (Boyer *et al.* 1989; Casey 1992c), whereas drug-induced parkinsonism occurs more often in older patients, and akathisia is only slightly more common in middle-aged females (Ayd 1961; Keepers *et al.* 1983; Casey & Keepers 1988). Age undoubtedly has an important role in patient susceptibility to EPS. Adolescents and children are particularly vulnerable to acute dystonia, but this disorder seldom occurs in the elderly. Drugs that commonly cause dystonia in children, who present in emergency rooms when these drugs have been inadvertently taken, are the antiemetic compounds, such as prochlorperazine (Compazine), promethazine (Phenergan), metoclopramide (Reglan) or other drugs in this group, which function as dopamine receptor antagonists. A patient's history of prior EPS is a strong predictor of vulnerability to future EPS, if a similar drug and dosage are represcribed. The recurrence of these disorders can be reliably predicted with approximately 75–85% accuracy if prior history of EPS is known (Keepers & Casey 1987, 1991).

Drug characteristics

Correlating acute EPS with parameters of neuroleptic drug exposure is complex. The dose–response curve between typical neuroleptic drug dose and EPS is often an inverted U-shaped function. Therefore, lower doses produce fewer EPS than do moderate to high doses. However, very high doses or megadoses also produce fewer EPS than do moderate to high doses (Keepers *et al.* 1983; Casey & Keepers 1988). The fact that neuroleptics affect multiple neurotransmitters also greatly influences EPS rates. The relative balance between blockade of dopamine, acetylcholine, serotonin, histamine, norepinephrine and other receptors is undoubtedly important. Low-milligram, high-potency compounds (e.g. haloperidol (Haldol), fluphenazine (Prolixin)) have little anticholinergic activity and are more susceptible to produce EPS than high-milligram, low-potency compounds (e.g. chlorpromazine (Thorazine), thioridazine (Mellaril)), which have considerably more anticholinergic activity.

Atypical neuroleptics have lower incidence and severity of EPS than the typical neuroleptics. The atypical neuroleptics differ from each other and lie on some continuum of EPS liability. At the high end of the spectrum are haloperidol and the other classic high-potency neuroleptics, followed by risperidone, olanzapine, sertindole, ziprasidone and quetiapine. Clozapine

is at the lower end of the spectrum. The position of the low-potency antipsychotics on the EPS liability spectrum in relation to the novel antipsychotics is unclear, because of the lack of studies directly comparing these two groups.

Based on PET studies in several patients taking different antipsychotics, Farde *et al.* (1992) and Nordstrom *et al.* (1993) suggested that the threshold for clinical response and extrapyramidal side-effects could be separated, based on D_2 occupancy. In a more recent study, Kapur *et al.* (2000), using haloperidol, reported that patients with occupancy below 78% did not exhibit extrapyramidal symptoms, while the majority of patients with occupancy above 78% showed extrapyramidal side-effects. Based on these results they proposed that by optimizing D_2 occupancy, even with a typical antipsychotic such as haloperidol, it is possible to obtain an antipsychotic effect without extrapyramidal side-effects. This relationship between high D_2 occupancy and extrapyramidal side-effects is also supported by evidence from several studies that used single photon emission computerized tomographic techniques (Scherer *et al.* 1994; Schlegal *et al.* 1996; Knable *et al.* 1997; Schroder *et al.* 1998). All antipsychotics, typical or atypical, block a relevant number of D_2 receptors. However, these agents may differ in the kinetics of occupancy and the relationship of peak to trough occupancy.

EPS profiles of atypical neuroleptics

Clozapine appears to have the lowest potential for EPS and numerous studies have established EPS-free treatment with clozapine in the usual regimen (Kurz *et al.* 1995). The excellent EPS profile of clozapine is best explained on the basis of its low D_2 occupancy, which is less than 60% 12 h after administration (Kapur 1998; Kapur *et al.* 1999; Tauscher *et al.* 1999).

Risperidone is found to have an intermediate EPS profile, between that for classic antipsychotics and clozapine (Miller *et al.* 1998). In at least three multicentre controlled trials that compared several doses of risperidone with placebo and haloperidol, the incidence of EPS in patients treated with up to 6 mg/day of risperidone was not significantly different from that in the placebo group and was lower than that in patients treated with haloperidol (10–20 mg/day) (Marder 1992; Chouinard *et al.* 1993; Peuskens 1995). Therefore the occurrence of EPS can be prevented in most patients if the daily dosage is kept below 5 mg.

The incidence of EPS with olanzapine (17.2 mg/day) was found to be lower than that of risperidone (7.2 mg/day) in a double-blinded study (Tran *et al.* 1997a,b). The incidence of EPS is dose-dependent and is higher on 12.5–17.5 mg/day than with the medium dose range 7.5–12.5 mg/day (Beasley *et al.* 1996a,b). Both risperidone and olanzapine obtain a good antipsychotic response only at doses that occupy 65% or more of D_2 receptors (Scherer *et al.* 1994; Knable *et al.* 1997; Kapur 1998; Tauscher *et al.* 1999; Kapur *et al.* 2000).

Quetiapine is another atypical with lower liability to produce EPS in comparison to chlorpromazine (Peuskens 1995) and haloperidol (Fleischhacker *et al.* 1996). In two other studies it had an EPS profile similar to placebo (Arvanitis & Miller 1997; Small *et al.* 1997). The low EPS profile of quetiapine is more likely related to low D_2 affinity (which is similar to clozapine) and its antiadrenergic activity rather than to serotonergic mechanisms. Quetiapine also has significant activity at histaminic receptors.

Sertindole also has a very low EPS profile. In a double-blind placebo-controlled study the incidence of EPS was found to be similar to placebo (Van Kammen *et al.* 1996). Sertindole has a strong affinity for D_2, $5\text{-}HT_{2A}$ and α_1 receptors, and both serotinergic and adrenergic mechanisms could be implicated in its low EPS predilection.

Ziprasidone has a receptor profile similar to sertindole, but with slightly lower D_2 affinity. This drug has been well tolerated during clinical trials, both short- and long-term. Treatment emergent EPS were mild and infrequent during the clinical trials, with a notable absence of akathisia.

Until recently, the lower EPS profile of the atypical antipsychotics has been attributed to a variety of mechanisms including low D_2 occupancy, increased $5\text{-}HT_2$ receptor occupancy, α_1 adrenergic antagonism, involvement of D_4 receptor, antimuscarinic activity (M_1), etc. In a recent review article, Kapur and Seeman (2001a,b) propose that, in contrast to the multireceptor hypothesis, the atypical antipsychotic effect is more probably caused by appropriate modulation of the D_2 receptor alone. They propose that the blockade of other receptors is neither necessary nor sufficient. They suggest that all antipsychotics, typical or atypical, block a relevant number of D_2 receptors, although they may differ in the kinetics of occupancy and the relationship of peak to trough occupancy. All antipsychotics, typical or atypical, give rise to extrapyramidal side-effects only when they exceed 78–80% D_2 occupancy. As clozapine and quetiapine never exceed this threshold of D_2 occupancy, they never give rise to extrapyramidal side-effects. Olanzapine and risperidone, on the other hand, exceed this threshold in a dose-dependent fashion and give rise to extrapyramidal side-effects in a dose-dependent manner. Based on a thorough review of the literature they propose that fast dissociation from the dopamine D_2 receptor could better explain the low EPS profile of atypical antipsychotics.

Treatment

Treatment phase

Each EPS has a fairly characteristic temporal pattern. Akathisia may have its onset within a few hours to a few days of initiating neuroleptics. This best corresponds to the time course of brain blood drug levels, as studies have shown a correlation between peak D_2 receptor occupancy rates and akathisia (Farde 1992; Nordstrom *et al.* 1992). Acute dystonia, which has its onset within the first 96 h of beginning or rapidly increasing neuroleptic dosages, has not been consistently correlated with either blood levels or dopamine receptor occupancy in the brain. Parkinsonism may develop from a few days to a few weeks after initiating neuroleptic treatment (Ayd 1961). Because the acute EPS may spontaneously decrease or resolve over several weeks

or months of continuous neuroleptic treatment in many patients, extended anti-EPS drug therapy may not be necessary for all those patients who required it within the first few weeks of initiating neuroleptic treatment.

Treatment strategies

The management of neuroleptic drug-induced EPS falls into three separate treatment strategies:
1 initial prophylaxis;
2 therapy for treatment-emergent symptoms; and
3 extended prophylaxis.

Initial prophylaxis with anti-EPS drugs is controversial. Proponents argue that prophylaxis prevents dystonic episodes, which are potentially dangerous, and automatically treats subtle forms of bradykinesia or akathisia that may be unrecognized. Opponents argue that these drugs have their own side-effects, such as autonomic nervous system dysfunction, memory impairment and the risk of delirium. Therefore, prophylaxis unnecessarily exposes patients who would not develop acute EPS to these treatment side-effects. Dogmatically applying either approach to all patients fails to achieve the maximum benefits. Instead, a well-thought-out treatment strategy that incorporates knowledge about risk factors is the most useful approach.

Treating neuroleptic-induced emergent acute EPS with anti-EPS drugs is standard practice. All the anticholinergic and antihistaminic agents are more or less equally efficacious. Amantadine (Symmetrel), a prodopaminergic drug, is equally effective and has fewer anticholinergic side-effects. This agent must be used with caution in patients with renal disease, as it is primarily cleared through the kidneys.

Extended prophylaxis (arbitrarily defined as continued use of anti-EPS drugs for more than 3 months) is also controversial. This treatment approach can be initiated by either extending the initial prophylaxis or maintaining effective drug therapy for symptoms that were treatment-emergent. This strategy requires periodic review, as many patients who develop EPS at initiation of drug treatment may eventually develop tolerance to EPS and will no longer need all or some of the anti-EPS drug treatment.

Managing acute extrapyramidal syndromes

The algorithm (Fig. 28.1) identifies several essential points in managing acute EPS after a neuroleptic has been prescribed; careful consideration of the issues related to initial prophylaxis should be considered. Obtaining a careful psychiatric and neurological evaluation prior to starting neuroleptic therapy is critically important because it serves as a reference point for the patient at this time, as well as providing documentation for potential changes that may occur later. Initial prophylaxis is justified when there is:
1 a high risk of EPS;
2 documented predisposition to EPS; and
3 anticipated detrimental consequences of EPS (Casey & Keepers 1988).

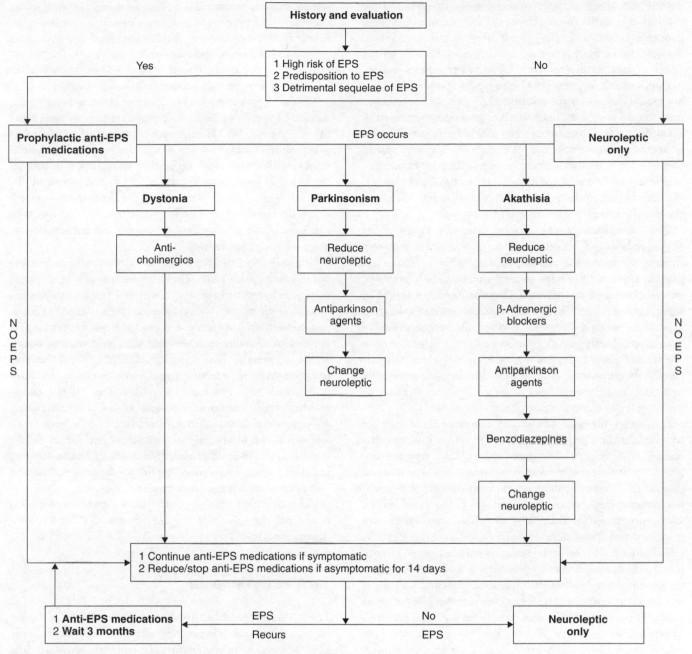

Fig 28.1 An algorithm for managing acute extrapyramidal syndromes (EPS). (From Casey 1995.)

By considering patient characteristics (age, gender, EPS history), drug characteristics (dosage, milligram potency, intrinsic anticholinergic action) and temporal aspects, the estimated risk of developing acute EPS can be closely approximated. Acute dystonic reactions can have important psychological consequences for future drug compliance. The paranoid patient who believes that external forces are controlling him/her may further solidify these beliefs when an acute dystonic reaction develops without warning and is beyond the patient's control.

Initial prophylaxis can be rationally employed for the first 7–10 days of neuroleptic treatment in high-risk patients. Then,

the anti-EPS drug may be gradually decreased and ultimately discontinued if no EPS develop. The efficacy for initial prophylaxis is well established. Several studies consistently show that anti-EPS agents reduce the rates of acute dystonia and other EPS (Keepers *et al.* 1983; Sramek *et al.* 1986; Casey & Keepers 1988; Boyer *et al.* 1989). In contrast, where there is a low risk of EPS, initial prophylaxis should not be initiated in conjunction with neuroleptics because the risk of anti-EPS drug side-effects greatly outweighs their potential benefit.

Managing treatment emergent EPS with anti-EPS agents is well-established standard care. Dystonia is treated with parenteral anticholinergic agents (benztropine (Cogentin), 2 mg every 30 min until symptom relief); or antihistaminic (diphenhydramine (Benadryl), 50–100 mg every 30 min until relief). Within 15 min, most symptoms improve on the first or second drug administration. If there is no improvement after a third injection, a search for other possible causes of dystonia should be initiated. Treatment with oral anticholinergics can be continued for a limited time if the diagnosis is confirmed by remission of symptoms. If symptoms recur when anticholinergic medication is tapered or discontinued despite attempts to lower the dose of the neuroleptic, then an alternative neuroleptic with a lower EPS profile should be used. In individuals at risk for anticholinergic side-effects, dopamine agonists such as amantidine have been shown to be effective (McEvoy *et al.* 1987).

There are several approaches for managing drug-induced parkinsonism and these follow a prioritized step-by-step strategy. Reducing the neuroleptic dose is the preferred approach. However, for many patients experiencing a psychotic exacerbation this is not practical. Therefore, adding an anti-EPS agent is the next and logical alternative. Changing to a different neuroleptic with a different side-effect profile, such as switching from a typical antipsychotic to an atypical antipsychotic or from one atypical agent to another is another option, although this is usually not necessary and can delay treatment while attempting to establish equipotent doses of drugs. Diphenhydramine or anticholinergic agents can be used acutely if needed.

Akathisia is the most difficult EPS to manage. That there are so many different drug approaches to akathisia indicates that none is truly effective for most patients. Like drug-induced parkinsonism, the preferred strategy is to reduce the neuroleptic dose. If this cannot be done on the basis of clinical grounds, β-adrenergic blockers which penetrate the blood–brain barrier, such as propranolol (Inderal) 30–120 mg/day, are often effective (Lipinski *et al.* 1984; Adler *et al.* 1989). If this is not effective, one could consider using the standard anticholinergic or antihistaminic agents. Eventually, switching to benzodiazepines may be necessary and helpful for some patients. Caution is warranted in adopting this strategy because this class of drugs used on an extended basis raises concern for potential problems of dependence and abuse. Finally, changing to a different neuroleptic with a lower EPS profile (e.g. sertindole, quetiapine, ziprasidone) may be a practical alternative.

Extending anti-EPS treatment on an open-ended basis will be necessary for a substantial subgroup of patients. Unfortunately, many patients improve but do not have their symptoms completely resolved. Therefore, patients will need to continue both their neuroleptic and anti-EPS drugs on an indefinite basis. However, if EPS are no longer present, drugs to control these symptoms should be reduced and discontinued. If EPS recur, then the antidote drug should be reinstituted. A review of extended prophylaxis studies published since 1980 found that 35–90% of patients benefited from this treatment strategy (Casey & Keepers 1988).

Much of the debate about the appropriate indications for anti-EPS drugs would be much less relevant if neuroleptic drugs were prescribed in lower doses. Because there is no compelling evidence that high neuroleptic doses routinely produce more benefit than standard doses (Baldessarini *et al.* 1988), a trend toward reduced neuroleptic dosage is encouraged. This would benefit the majority of patients, who would experience fewer acute EPS and would thus need fewer anti-EPS drugs.

The algorithm outlined in Fig. 28.1 for managing neuroleptic-induced EPS offers a balanced strategy to obtain the most benefit with the least risk. This approach encourages the practitioner to consider all the information available in making flexible decisions regarding treatment, rather than being locked into an inflexible all-or-none treatment approach. By considering all the information available, it is possible to predict with a reasonable degree of certainty who is likely to develop EPS and, thus, who may benefit from prophylaxis or from waiting until treatment-emergent symptoms develop.

Rates of EPS should not be the sole determinant in deciding which neuroleptic to use. These syndromes can be managed quite well in most patients with anti-EPS agents. In addition, other side-effects, such as hypotension, anticholinergic effects, photosensitivity, leucopenia and increased risk factors for cardiovascular mortality such as weight gain, impaired glucose tolerance and hyperlipidaemia (specifically triglycerides) must also be considered when selecting a neuroleptic. For example, clozapine, while it has a very low EPS profile (Casey 1989), is highly anticholinergic and causes agranulocytosis in approximately 1% of patients. Additionally, similar to some of the other atypicals such as olanzapine, risperidone, quetiapine and sertindole, it is considered to be an offender for increased weight gain and impaired glucose intolerance. The risk for diabetes mellitus and for impaired glucose tolerance may be at least twice as common in patients on atypical neuroleptics than in patients on typical neuroleptics (Hagg *et al.* 1998; Goldstein *et al.* 1999; Kapur & Remington 2001).

Tardive dyskinesia

TD is characterized by involuntary hyperkinetic abnormal movements that occur in predisposed patients during or shortly after (4–8 weeks) the termination of long-term neuroleptic drug treatment. The realistic concern about the potential irreversibility of TD has led to a careful reassessment about the appropriate indications for utilizing the highly efficacious neuroleptic drugs. The goal is to obtain the maximum benefits with the fewest risks. However, even when all precautions have been taken, some patients may develop TD.

TD was initially described in 1957 in the German literature (Schonecker 1957). Shortly thereafter, other cases were described in French literature (Sigwald *et al.* 1959). A Danish group published the first English language report in 1960 (Uhrbrand & Faurbye 1960). In the ensuing years, several other reports substantiated these original observations. Before the term 'tardive dyskinesia' was proposed in 1964 (Faurbye *et al.* 1964), descriptive terms such as 'buccolinguomasticatory syndrome' and 'terminal extrapyramidal insufficiency syndrome' appeared in the early literature.

Clinical manifestations

Repetitive involuntary hyperkinetic movements of the choreiform type typically characterize TD. Similar to EPS, external and internal stimuli strongly influence the clinical picture. The abnormal movements, in general, increase with stress, decrease with relaxation and disappear during sleep. They can be voluntarily suppressed for a short time (Baldessarini *et al.* 1980). While all parts of the body can be affected, the tongue and oral area are most frequently involved.

Typical abnormal movements in TD (Marsalek 2000)

1 Tongue: rolling, vermicular tongue motion, arrhythmic tongue protrusions (fly catching sign), tongue producing a bulge in the cheek (bon-bon sign).
2 Lips: pouting, smacking, puckering, sucking.
3 Chewing movements.
4 Facial and periorbital area: grimacing, paroxysms of rapid eye blinking.
5 Neck: arrhythmic head nodding.
6 Trunk: irregular rocking movements of the upper torso.
7 Upper extremities: abnormal stereotypic movements in the fingers may look as though the patient is playing an invisible piano or guitar.
8 Lower extremities: flexion/rotation of ankles, involuntary stamping movements, retroflexion of toes.
9 Laryngopharyngeal, diaphragmatic and intercostal musculature.
Although relatively uncommon, TD may involve the respiratory system with irregular breathing or swallowing that causes aerophagia, irregular respiratory rates, belching and grunting noises (Casey 1981).

Atypical forms of TD

Tardive dystonia

This is a syndrome of sustained abnormal postures or positions. Symptoms include torticollis, retrocollis, anterocollis, blepharospasm, grimacing and torsion of the trunk or limbs. These symptoms may persist for months or years after neuroleptics have been discontinued (Burke *et al.* 1982; Gardos *et al.* 1987). If a patient has received neuroleptic drugs, it is a particularly complex problem to discern whether abnormal dystonic symptoms are a result of neuroleptics or idiopathic dystonia. Occasionally, patients present to physicians with mild symptoms of dystonia or other motor dysfunction, and often receive neuroleptic drugs as potential treatments. When the histories of such patients are ambiguous as to when drug treatment began, it is very difficult to determine properly how much of the movement disorder should be attributed to drugs or to idiopathic

causes. One helpful point in making this distinction is the natural course of the symptoms. When neuroleptics are discontinued, tardive dystonia should remain stable or gradually improve. In contrast, idiopathic dystonias will usually slowly progress in severity, as well as have new symptoms develop over months and years. Unfortunately, the response of tardive dystonia to pharmacological interventions does not help to distinguish it from idiopathic dystonia because both syndromes do not respond well to any drug intervention. Some patients with either diagnosis may benefit from dopamine agonists, dopamine antagonists or cholinergic antagonists. At this time, it is not possible to identify in advance which patients, if any, will benefit from which medicines.

TD and tardive dystonia also occur in children. In some patients there may be few or none of the typical hyperkinetic orofacial dyskinesias but, rather, patients may express a predominance of limb and truncal symptoms. However, in other patients, classic TD symptoms are similar to those typically found in adults (Campbell *et al.* 1983; Gualtieri *et al.* 1984).

Tardive akathisia

This is a syndrome of persisting subjective and/or objective signs of restlessness (Barnes & Braude 1985). This disorder is symptomatically similar to acute akathisia but is differentiated by its persistence for months or years after neuroleptics have been discontinued.

Both tardive dystonia and tardive akathisia may occur alone or in combination with the typical orofacial and choreoathetoid signs of TD. Furthermore, they may persist for weeks or months after discontinuation of neuroleptics. An additional complication is that any of these disorders may also occur in combination with neuroleptic-induced acute EPS if patients are concurrently receiving these drugs. It is not yet clear whether these different tardive syndromes represent unique and different pathophysiological mechanisms, or are better explained by a unitary underlying pathophysiology that is phenomenologically expressed in different symptom clusters in different patients.

Terminology

Carefully classifying TD incorporates temporal aspects of this disorder. Covert TD describes TD that is unmasked when neuroleptic drug therapy is reduced or discontinued. Withdrawal TD appears when neuroleptics are reduced or discontinued but disappears spontaneously in 1–3 months. There is no uniformly agreed-upon definition of when TD should be characterized as irreversible. Twelve months has often been arbitrarily defined as the cut-off point for irreversible TD; however, there is no scientific basis for this arbitrary definition. Such a characterization fails to account for symptom change, which occurs in many patients over several years. Rather, a more useful concept utilizes a time-course continuum to characterize TD along the dimension of persisting vs. resolving (Casey 1987). Research criteria also exist for TD (Schooler & Kane 1982). These require at least 3 months of cumulative neuroleptic drug exposure, at least mild movements in two or more body areas or moderate symptoms in one body region for the diagnosis of presumed TD. Persisting TD requires that symptoms continue for 3 months or longer and that other conditions that might produce involuntary hyperkinetic dyskinesias have been ruled out. The Abnormal Involuntary Movement scale (AIMS) is the most commonly used rating tool for assessing TD (Guy 1976). It is useful to re-emphasize that rating scales have been developed to characterize the nature and severity of abnormal movements and are not diagnostic instruments. A diagnosis requires a thorough evaluation of epidemiological, aetiological, phenomenological and temporal aspects of symptom development, and is undertaken in conjunction with a thorough medical and neuropsychiatric evaluation.

Differential diagnosis

There are many causes of abnormal movements. These include idiopathic syndromes, other drug-induced movement disorders, hereditary diseases and dyskinesias that are secondary to systemic illnesses.

Idiopathic syndromes

Long before the introduction of neuroleptic drugs, Kraepelin and Bleuler described spontaneous dyskinesias in psychotic patients (Kraepelin 1907; Bleuler 1950; Casey 1985a). Both of these astute observers described 'grimacing' and 'irregular movements of the tongue and lips'. Unfortunately, comparative epidemiological studies cannot be carried out with current findings because Kraepelin and Bleuler did not record prevalence rates of these abnormalities at the turn of the twentieth century.

Stereotypic behaviour (seemingly purposeless and meaningless actions) and mannerisms (peculiar ways of completing normal actions) are frequently associated with psychoses and must be part of a differential diagnosis of TD. Several spontaneous hyperkinetic dyskinesias have been variously identified in the literature as 'spontaneous orofacial dyskinesia', 'senile dyskinesia' and 'blepharospasm–oromandibular dystonia' (Smith & Baldessarini 1980). These are all now generally classified as idiopathic focal dystonias. Both dyskinesias and dystonias occur with increasing age and are also more commonly seen in patients with concomitant neuromedical conditions (Lieberman et al. 1984). Tourette's syndrome, characterized by involuntary tics and vocalizations that begin before the age of 21, must also be considered. These can be differentiated by occurring early in life and by their waxing and waning course throughout a patient's lifetime. Simple tics or complex motor tics, as well as dental problems, must be carefully differentiated from TD (Casey 1981).

Neuroleptic drug-induced acute EPS

Neuroleptic drug-induced EPS coexists with TD in approximately one-third of patients who have TD and continue neuroleptic therapy (Casey 1981; Richardson & Craig 1982). Therefore, some patients may have more than one neuroleptic drug-induced movement disorder at the same time, and these must be distinguished from each other. The acute EPS respond to anti-EPS drugs, whereas TD usually remains unchanged or worsens with these agents. However, some patients with tardive dystonia may improve with anticholinergic anti-EPS drugs (Burke et al. 1982).

Other drug-induced dyskinesias

Several other drugs can produce symptoms similar to TD. There are a few compounds that, like neuroleptics, antagonize dopamine receptors but are not commonly known as neuroleptics, although they can produce TD with extended use. These include the dopamine antagonist antiemetic prochlorperazine (Compazine), the dyspeptic drug metoclopramide (Reglan) and the antidepressant amoxapine (Asendin). Dopamine agonists, such as bromocriptine (Parlodel) and pergolide (Permax), and the dopamine precursor L-dopa/carbidopa (Sinemet) can all produce hyperkinetic dyskinesias in patients with idiopathic parkinsonism. Chorea and stereotyped behaviour can be seen during both the acute phases of and withdrawal from amphetamine and other stimulant abuse. Chronic anticholinergic and antihistaminic use have rarely been associated with TD-like abnormal movements. Anticonvulsant agents at therapeutic or higher levels can produce hyperkinetic dyskinesias similar to TD. Oral contraceptives and chloroquine-based antimalarial agents also can produce chorea and hyperkinetic dyskinesias. Lithium carbonate and tricyclic antidepressants may aggravate existing TD, but there is no convincing evidence that these agents by themselves produce TD. However, they can produce rapid fine irregular tremors that may be superimposed on TD. There are a number of reports of TD associated with the use of serotonin-selective reuptake inhibitors, some of which were persistent even after discontinuation of the drug (Leo 1996). This list identifies only some of the more commonly prescribed drugs that may causes hyperkinetic involuntary movements.

Hereditary and systemic illnesses

Huntington's disease is characterized by choreoathetosis and dementia which may be preceded or accompanied by psychotic symptoms. If patients have received neuroleptics before the onset of chorea, the differential diagnosis becomes more complicated. A thorough family history, progression of symptoms and development of dementia can help to clarify the diagnosis. Since the identification of the Huntington disease gene in 1993, genetic testing using a highly sensitive and specific method for detecting the presence of the Huntington gene is now available. The gene is localized on the short arm of chromosome 4 and consists of unstable CAG trinucleotide repeat expansion. Huntington's disease occurs when there are more than 35 CAG repeats. Wilson's disease (hepatolenticular degeneration), a disorder of copper metabolism, can be distinguished from TD on the basis of clinical signs, laboratory tests and family history. The disease of iron metabolism, Hallervorden–Spatz disease, usually has its onset during childhood and is predominated by symptoms of dystonia and bradykinesia.

Endocrinopathies of hyperthyroidism, hypoparathyroidism or severe hyperglycemia have been infrequently associated with choreathetosis. Chorea of pregnancy (chorea gravidarum) may be pathophysiologically linked to mechanisms in common with oral contraceptive-induced chorea. Inflammatory or immune disorders, such as lupus erythematosus, Schonlein–Henoch purpura and Sydenham's chorea, can have dyskinesias as a component of the syndrome. Finally, inflammatory and space-occupying lesions of the central nervous system can produce dyskinesias that must be delineated from TD.

Pathophysiology

The pathophysiology of TD is still not completely understood. The dopamine supersensitivity hypothesis, proposed by Klawans and Rubovits in 1972, implicated an overactivity of the striatal dopaminergic system as being responsible for the hyperkinetic movements of TD. Klawans suggested that chemical denervation from neuroleptics led to denervation hypersensitivity of striatal dopamine receptors, which in turn led to increased numbers and affinity of D_2 receptors. This hypothesis, while compatible with many clinical and laboratory observations, has a number of limitations. For example, in animal studies, neuroleptic-induced receptor changes are observed within days (even after a single injection), whereas hyperkinetic movements of TD develop after months or years. Secondly, while supersensitivity in animals declines following 'desensitization' with DA agonists, these drugs are not effective in treating TD. Additionally, while supersensitivity in animals is almost invariable, TD develops in only a fraction of the patients. Postmortem studies, cerebrospinal fluid studies and radioligand imaging studies using PET also failed to demonstrate any direct evidence of DA supersensitivity in TD patients. The dopamine hypothesis also does not explain the spontaneous occurrence of dyskinesia in many schizophrenic patients as well as healthy subjects, and the increased risk with age. It is therefore possible that the dopamine hypothesis explains only some aspects of TD. Although evidence is lacking in humans, modifications to the dopamine hypothesis suggest that patients vulnerable to TD develop a greater and more persistent increase in DA turnover in response to DA blockade (Scatton 1977). An extension of the dopamine hypothesis suggests that TD is the result of an imbalance between D_1 and D_2 subtypes of D_2 receptors (Gerlach & Casey 1988).

The shortcomings of the dopamine hypothesis have led to other pathophysiological models of TD. Based on observations of similar changes in the GABA-synthesizing enzyme glutamic acid decarboxylase (GAD) in humans with TD and in animals treated with neuroleptics (Crane & Smeets 1974; Gunne et al. 1984; Andersson et al. 1989; Woerner et al. 1991), Gunne and Haggstrom (1985) proposed that TD was caused by an abnormality of GABA-related striatal neurones. Studies demon-

strating a reduction of GAD in the subthalamic nuclei of TD patients (Andersson et al. 1989), reduced levels of GABA in the cerebrospinal fluid of patients with TD (Thaker et al. 1987) and an increased saccadic distractibility (an eye movement controlled by GABA projections) in patients with TD lend further support to the GABA hypothesis. Alternatively, these GABA changes could also reflect increased dopaminergic activity, and thereby represent a secondary phenomenon.

More recent interest focuses on oxidative stress, production of free radicals and excitotoxic mechanisms leading to neurodegeneration. Support for the free radical hypothesis and increased oxidative stress comes from the following.

1 Neuroleptics increase catecholamine turnover which leads to excess production of free radicals, particularly in catecholamine-rich areas such as the basal ganglia. Basal ganglia neurones are especially vulnerable to membrane lipid peroxidation and cell death because of the high oxidative metabolism.

2 Neuroleptics can be neurotoxic because of the accumulation of iron in the basal ganglia and free radical mechanisms (Sachdev 1992).

3 Although not a consistent finding, a reduction in essential fatty acids in plasma phospholipids and increased cerebrospinal fluid indices of lipid peroxidation (Lohr et al. 1990) have been reported in patients with TD.

4 The role of age, diabetes, smoking and brain damage as risk factors for TD, the irreversibility of a proportion of TD, and the occurrence of spontaneous dyskinesias in schizophrenia.

Support for the excitotoxicity mechanism for neuroleptic-induced neurodegeneration comes from the following. Dopamine has an inhibitory effect on the release of excitatory neurotransmitters, and dopamine D_2 blockade leads to an increase of glutamate and aspartate release in the striatum (Carlsson & Carlsson 1990). The persistent activation of N-methyl-D-aspartate (NMDA) receptors and non-NMDA glutamate receptors leads to oxidative damage to cellular proteins, membranes and DNA, and ultimately to cell death. Secondary interaction of glutamatergic and free radical mechanisms may result in a vicious cycle that promotes oxidative damage in the striatum. The recently reported evidence of higher concentrations of N-acetylaspartate, N-aspartylglutamate and aspartate in the cerebrospinal fluid of patients with TD also lends support to the excitotoxicity mechanism (Tsai et al. 1998).

Sachdev (2000) proposes a model that encompasses all the above hypotheses. His model suggests that high levels of catecholamine turnover and oxidative metabolism in the striatum lead to neurotoxicity and cell death particularly in the GABAergic striatal neurones via free radical and excitatory mechanisms. This results in disinhibition of the lateral pallidal neurones and consequently functional disinhibition of the pallidothalamic outflow leading to the hyperkinetic state of TD. The prevalent dopaminergic tone influences its manifestation, with withdrawal of DA antagonism leading to the unmasking of the latent hyperkinetic state, while DA blockade produces the reverse. It appears that the dopamine receptor antagonism is crucial in the pathogenesis of TD. However, the mediating mechanisms for the antagonism are multiple, and DA receptor supersensitivity may only be one aspect although not the primary one. Many of these theories are undoubtedly oversimplified and no one theory or set of data offers a succinct explanation to understanding the complex disorder of TD.

Neuroimaging and neuropathology

A characteristic pathological finding in patients with TD is still elusive. Findings that neuroleptics interfere with normal mitochondrial function and produce mitochondrial ultrastructural changes in the basal ganglia of patients and animals suggest that mitochondrial dysfunction may have a role in TD. However, Eyles et al. (2000) demonstrated that these ultrastructural changes in the striatal mitochondria observed during neuroleptic therapy do not persist after drug withdrawal. Structural brain imaging studies have likewise been unyielding or inconsistent. Findings have ranged from decreased caudate volume (Mion et al. 1991), increased caudate volume (Brown et al. 1996) to no change in the volume of the caudate, putamen or globus pallidus (Elkashef et al. 1994).

Epidemiology

There is a wide variation in the prevalence (number of existing cases) of TD, ranging from 0.5% to more than 70% (Baldessarini et al. 1980; Kane & Smith 1982; Kane et al. 1984a,b, 1992; Casey 1985b, 1987). This is surely because of a wide range of characteristics unique to each study, such as differences in the types of patients studied, criteria for diagnosis and year of investigation. Most studies note that TD occurs at a prevalence of 15–20%. When this prevalence was corrected for the prevalence of spontaneous dyskinesia (5–6%) (Kane & Smith 1982; Casey & Hansen 1984) – dyskinesias that are clinically similar to TD but occur in patients who have never received neuroleptic treatment – the true average prevalence of TD was estimated to be about 15% (Gerlach & Casey 1988). In high-risk groups such as the elderly, the incidence may be as high as 70% in those chronically treated with neuroleptic drugs (Toenniessen et al. 1985; Casey 1987; Saltz et al. 1991). Because of the inherent limitations of retrospective studies, it has been much more revealing to examine the incidence of TD in newly medicated patients followed longitudinally. In two such prospective studies, Kane et al. (1986, 1988) found that the cumulative incidence of TD was 5%, 19% and 26% after 1, 4 and 6 years respectively. These studies showed that the incidence of TD increased linearly, at least for the first 5 years, with increasing duration of neuroleptic treatment. In high-risk subjects, the incidence increased dramatically. For example, in a cohort of older patients, the incidence was 26%, 52% and 60% after 1, 2 and 3 years respectively (Jeste et al. 1995). The incidence was similarly higher in subjects with very chronic psychosis (Chouinard et al. 1986; Waddington et al. 1990) and high-dose antipsychotic medication (Chouinard et al. 1986). Similar incidence rates after a 5-year follow-up were

reported in other studies (Yassa & Nair 1984; Morgenstern & Glazer 1993).

Studies with atypical neuroleptics suggest a lower risk of TD both in patients with existing TD and in patients at risk for developing TD with long-term treatment. In a study comparing clozapine and haloperidol in hospitalized patients with refractory schizophrenia, clozapine was associated with markedly greater reduction in TD over time (Rosenheck et al. 1997). Similarly, a lower incidence of TD was found in a double-blind placebo controlled study with risperidone (Chouinard 1995). A prospective study of patients with schizophrenia, schizophreniform disorder or schizoaffective disorder treated with olanzapine or haloperidol, who lacked evidence of TD at baseline, revealed that the incidence of newly emergent TD was significantly lower among olanzapine-treated patients than among haloperidol-treated patients (Tollefson et al. 1997).

Long-term outcome

TD improvement rates vary widely across studies from 0% to 92% (Casey 1985a,b, 1987, 1990; Casey & Gerlach 1986). The multiple contributions of patient, drug and temporal factors undoubtedly influence this outcome range. Age is negatively correlated with TD improvement. Younger patients are the most likely to improve, whereas elderly patients are the least likely to do so (Smith & Baldessarini 1980; Casey 1987; Kane et al. 1992). Nevertheless, this does not exclude any patient from the possibility of symptom improvement or resolution. Patients who have early therapeutic intervention (Quitkin et al. 1977) or those who have milder forms of dyskinesia are associated with a more favourable prognosis. Discontinuing neuroleptic drugs is positively correlated with a favourable outcome in most, but not all, studies (Quitkin et al. 1977; Casey 1985a,b, 1987; Casey & Gerlach 1986; Kane et al. 1986, 1992; Gardos et al. 1987). When neuroleptics can be discontinued, the signs of TD spontaneously resolve in some patients (Baldessarini et al. 1980), transiently worsen in others, and persist in some. The improvement is expected to continue for many years after cessation of the neuroleptics. Approximately one-third of patients with TD remit within 3 months of discontinuation of neuroleptics. Resolution of dyskinesias can also occur as long as 5 years after cessation of neuroleptics (Jeste & Wyatt 1982; Klawans & Tanner 1983). Some studies suggest that resolution of TD is more likely if neuroleptics are discontinued soon after onset of the dyskinesias and that remissions are less likely in patients over the age of 60.

TD may also improve when neuroleptic drugs are continued. In general, patients with TD rarely continue to worsen when low to moderate doses of neuroleptics are continued. Because this disorder tends to be a chronic long-term problem, the longer the follow-up, the more likely there is a chance to observe symptom change. Some patients show complete remission despite continued therapy (Gardos et al. 1994). Long-term follow-up studies have, in general, shown that the course of TD could be fluctuating, with spontaneous remissions (Gardos et al. 1988), if lower doses of neuroleptics were maintained for a long time.

Complications

The majority of TD patients have the milder form and may be unaware of its presence. In these cases TD is an aesthetic problem and may impair social relationships and impede employment. A small percentage of the patients (5–10%) suffer impairment from the dyskinesia. Orofacial dyskinesia may lead to dental problems, traumatic ulceration of the tongue and lips, difficulty in eating leading to weight loss and cachexia and, rarely, degenerative changes of temporomandibular joints. Pharyngeal involvement may sometimes cause aspiration pneumonia. Involvement of limbs and trunk may interfere with ambulation and falls, with consequent trauma. Respiratory dysfunction and speech abnormalities, although rare, may result from diaphragmatic involvement. Hypertrophy of the tongue and muscles of the trunk (Fann et al. 1977), increase in creatine kinase levels and fatal myoglobinuria (Lazarus & Toglia 1985), although extremely rare, have been reported in the most severe forms of TD. While there are some reports of a higher mortality rate in more severe forms of TD (McClelland et al. 1986; Youssef & Waddington 1987), there are also reports that do not confirm this (Kucharski et al. 1978).

Cognitive impairment also has been associated with TD (Casey 1997a). It is unclear, however, whether the cognitive dysfunction seen in some patients with TD is present before the onset of TD (Waddington et al. 1993).

Risk factors

Age and sex

TD prevalence is positively correlated with increasing age. Furthermore, TD develops more rapidly among elderly patients (Jeste et al. 1995). Approximately 5–10% of patients younger than 40 years develop TD, whereas elderly patients have prevalence rates of 50–70% for TD (Smith & Baldessarini 1980; Casey 1987, 1997b; Kane et al. 1992). Age is also negatively correlated with improvement of TD.

Women have a greater risk of TD compared with men at a ratio of 1.7:1 in most, but not all, studies (Casey 1987; Kane et al. 1992; Morgenstern & Glazer 1993). There may also be a female predominance in elderly TD sufferers, suggesting a gender and age interaction (Smith et al. 1978). While it is unclear why women are more susceptible to TD, risk factors such as oestrogen status, higher mg/kg body weight dosing and the greater prevalence of affective disorders (Owens 1999) have been suggested as potential contributing factors.

Psychiatric diagnosis

Vulnerability to TD is influenced by psychiatric diagnosis. Relatively brief exposure to neuroleptic drugs may cause TD in patients with affective disorders, particularly depression (Davis et al. 1976; Casey 1984, 1988a; Kane et al. 1984a). Depression may produce a state-dependent exacerbation of TD (Sachdev 1989) while mania may lead to the converse (Trelles et al. 1985). In schizophrenic patients, a family history of affective illness is reported to increase the risk. Schizophrenic patients with predominant negative symptoms, or evidence of cognitive impairment and neurological deficits, are reported to be more vulnerable (Waddington et al. 1987). Patients without psychotic diagnoses are also at risk for TD if they receive extended neuroleptic treatment.

Metabolic disorder

Diabetes mellitus

Diabetes mellitus (DM) is considered to be a risk factor for TD (Ganzini et al. 1991a, 1992). Both psychotic and non-psychotic patients receiving long-term neuroleptics have greater prevalence and more severe TD if they have DM. This is particularly important for elderly patients, as the risk of both TD and DM increases with age. While it needs to be verified, one explanation proposed by Mukherjee and Mahadik (1997) for the role of diabetes in increasing the risk of TD is the relationship between brain insulin resistance and oxyradical-mediated central microvascular abnormalities. Schultz et al. (1999) reported an association between abnormal movements and both hyperinsulinaemia and hyperglycaemia.

Phenylketonuria

While larger studies are needed to confirm these results, phenylketonuria is reported to be associated with a higher incidence of TD (Richardson et al. 1986). The ratio of plasma phenylalanine–neutral amino acid was also identified as a risk factor of dyskinesia in another study (Richardson et al. 1989).

Alcohol and drug abuse

An increased prevalence of dyskinetic movements in alcohol-abusing or drug-abusing schizophrenic patients (Dixon et al. 1992; Bailey et al. 1997; van Os et al. 1997) has been reported in both retrospective and prospective studies. However, the pathogenesis of this increased susceptibility is unclear.

Neuroleptic dose and duration of treatment

The degree of exposure (which includes both dose and duration of therapy) to neuroleptic drugs is directly associated with TD risk. The greater the total drug intake, the greater the likelihood of developing TD (Kane et al. 1984b; Casey 1997b). However, studies have not yet addressed the complex issue of teasing apart the relative risks of concomitantly increasing age and total drug exposure, because these two parameters often increase concomitantly in patients with chronic illness. There are no consistent data to show a relationship between neuroleptic blood level and the onset of TD (Fairbairn et al. 1983; Jeste et al. 1986). The probability that a patient who is receiving a typical neuroleptic will develop TD is about 5% per year, or 15% in 3 years (Kane 1995). Within elderly populations, the duration of exposure to neuroleptics appears to be a strong predictor of risk for TD; this risk increases rapidly during the first year of total lifetime neuroleptic use (Toenniessen *et al.* 1985; Saltz *et al.* 1991; Sweet *et al.* 1995).

Neuroleptic drug type

An analysis of the clinical literature indicates that any one of the traditional neuroleptic drugs is more or less likely to cause TD. Similarly, there is no convincing evidence that the depot neuroleptics carry a different TD risk. However, atypical neuroleptics have a considerably lower risk of producing TD both in patients with existing TD and in patients at risk for developing TD with long-term treatment (Casey 1999; Marsalek 2000). Except for one report (Dave 1994), no clear cases of TD were reported with clozapine. Risperidone, olanzapine, quetiapine and ziprasidone also produce fewer EPS, including TD, than typical neuroleptics (Chouinard 1995; Beasley *et al.* 1996a,b; Arvanitis & Miller 1997; Tandon *et al.* 1997; Tollefson *et al.* 1997).

Other drugs

The effect of anticholinergic or antihistaminic drugs in producing TD is controversial. There are data both for and against this hypothesis (Kane & Smith 1982; Casey 1987; Kane *et al.* 1992). These drugs will often temporarily aggravate existing TD, but TD symptoms return to baseline when these drugs are discontinued. Anticholinergic drugs may appear to be associated with TD because they are used in treating acute EPS. If acute EPS are the actual link to TD, then any treatment for acute EPS, such as antiEPS drugs, will also show a correlation with TD. Although tentative, data from clinical (Steen *et al.* 1997) and animal studies (Pert *et al.* 1979) supports the notion that concurrent administration of lithium in affective disorders may reduce the risk of TD.

Extrapyramidal syndromes

The occurrence of early acute drug-induced EPS as a risk factor for developing TD has been documented in several prospective studies (Barnes *et al.* 1983; Chouinard *et al.* 1986; Kane *et al.* 1986; Saltz *et al.* 1991; Jeste *et al.* 1995). These studies also support the hypothesis that patients with TD may have a vulnerability to developing extrapyramidal disorders.

Neuropsychiatric diagnosis

The evidence to date does not clearly support structural changes in the brain or the presence of brain damage (as evidenced by epilepsy, head trauma, dementia, etc.) as a risk factor for TD (Owens 1999). With respect to other psychiatric diagnosis, however, both retrospective (Casey 1988a; Gardos & Cole 1997) and prospective studies (Kane *et al.* 1986) suggest affec-

tive disorders, primarily unipolar depression, as a risk factor for TD. Changes in noradrenergic or sertonergic mechanisms (Marsalek 2000) have been implicated to explain these findings.

Genetic factors

Several recent studies support the notion of genetic predisposition to TD. Heterozygous carriers of mutated alleles of the metabolic enzyme CYP2D6 have been reported to show increased susceptibility to TD (Andreassen *et al.* 1997; Kapitany *et al.* 1998; Ellingrod *et al.* 2000). Similarly, a functional polymorphism in the promoter region of the metabolic enzyme CYP1A2 was found to be associated with TD (Basile *et al.* 2000). Several groups have also reported an association between Ser9Gly polymorphism in the D_3 receptor gene and TD (Steen *et al.* 1997; Williams *et al.* 1998; Segman *et al.* 1999; Liao *et al.* 2001). Likewise, Chen *et al.* (1997) report an association between Taq1 polymorphism of dopamine D_2 receptor gene and TD after long-term administration of antipsychotic treatment in patients with schizophrenia. While a positive association has been reported between serotonin 2C receptor gene and TD (Segman *et al.* 2001), studies looking for associations between serotonin 2A receptor genes and TD have yielded both positive (Segman *et al.* 2001; Tan *et al.* 2001) and negative results (Basile *et al.* 2001).

Racial difference

Ethnic differences, with higher rates in African Americans and people from the Dutch Antilles and lower rates in Chinese and other Asian populations in comparison to white patients have been reported (Morgenstern & Glazer 1993; Pandurangi & Aderibigbe 1995; Owens 1999). The basis of this racial difference is not clearly understood. While a thorough evaluation is warranted, differences in therapeutic strategies could possibly explain some of these observations.

Managing tardive dyskinesia

The clinical strategy for managing TD is presented in the algorithm shown in Fig. 28.2. The primary strategy in the management of TD is prevention. The goal is to provide appropriate neuroleptic drug treatment for those who benefit from it and at the same time minimize the TD risk. When neuroleptics are deemed necessary, patients should be given the smallest doses possible. Many physicians are adapting to the atypical neuroleptics as a first line of treatment. When long-term neuroleptic therapy is necessary, patients should be periodically evaluated (about every 3 months) for the early features of TD using standard assessments such as AIMS (Guy 1976).

Once TD becomes manifest, attempts are made to minimize the severity and to reduce the risk of worsening of the symptoms over time. After an initial evaluation of neuropsychiatric status, a thorough medical evaluation including a physical and neurological examination, laboratory testing and a review of the differential diagnosis should be performed. The next step should be

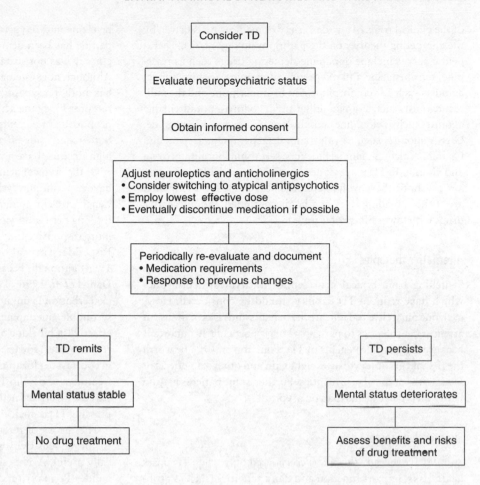

Fig 28.2 Clinical strategy for the management of TD. (From Casey 1999.)

evaluation of the antipsychotic therapy being implemented and adjusting the neuroleptic and anticholinergic drug regimen. The American Psychiatric Association Task Force on TD advocates using neuroleptic drugs in the lowest effective dose for those patients who benefit from this treatment (Kane *et al.* 1992). The primary indications for neuroleptics are acute and chronic schizophrenia and other psychoses, as well as some uncommon neurological disorders, such as Tourette's syndrome and Huntington's disease. Secondary indications include the treatment of acute mania, psychotic depression or unstable manic-depressive illness. Neuroleptics are not indicated for neuroses, personality disorders, insomnia or other non-psychotic conditions, although special circumstances may require considering these compounds. Switching to novel antipsychotics from typical antipsychotics should be strongly considered in all patients with TD, because these drugs have a lower potential for EPS and TD. Another issue is to assess the need for additional medications to suppress TD. Informed consent should be an important aspect of management and should include ongoing discussions of the risks and benefits of neuroleptic therapy, of no therapy and of alternative treatments for TD.

Prescribing neuroleptics is not a one-time decision. Regularly reviewing the benefits as well as the risks of neuroleptic and anti-EPS drugs is an important aspect of managing psychoses. Although a few patients may be able to discontinue these drugs,

patients with remitting and relapsing psychoses need to continue their drugs for symptom control. Documenting these re-evaluations and discussions with patients is essential. TD will either persist or remit. The mental status may remain stable or deteriorate with an exacerbation of psychosis. If such a relapse occurs, it will once again be necessary to re-evaluate the risks and benefits of treatment with neuroleptics, and adjust the neuroleptic dosage if indicated.

Data from several studies suggest that, with time, TD will either persist or remit. Adjustments in treatment should prioritize mental status as the primary concern for management. If mental status deteriorates, the risks and benefits of drug treatment should be reassessed and the neuroleptic dose adjusted if necessary.

Treatment

At present, there are no uniformly safe and effective treatments for TD. Benefit–risk analysis, potential side-effects of the suppressing agent, interactions with other medications and a history of success in prior studies in general guide selection of a therapeutic agent. For mild TD without functional impairment, therapeutic intervention is not indicated. Patients with moderate to severe TD are the usual candidates who need treatment aimed at controlling symptoms (Egan *et al.* 1997). The diversity of the clinical trials of a wide variety of medication is driven by the competing theories on the pathophysiology of TD. Therapeutic agents include dopamine-depleting drugs such as reserpine, tetrabenazine and oxypertine, dopamine agonists (direct agonists such as apomorphine and bromocriptine and the indirect agonists such as amantadine and levodopa), noradrenergic agonists such as clonidine, anticholinergics such as benztropine, GABA agonists such as valproate, diazepam, clonazepam and baclofen, calcium-channel blockers, serotonin, botulinum toxin and vitamin E. TD may not necessarily worsen with continuing antipsychotic therapy; however, the best chances for remission are if the offending drug can be discontinued and alternative drugs with lower EPS profile initiated.

Alternative therapies

Switching from typical neuroleptics to atypical neuroleptics which have reduced TD liability should be considered. However, one must clearly delineate the benefits and risks of the use of atypical neuroleptics to patients. This is particularly important because the possible benefits of TD reduction may not be worth the risk of agranulocytosis, weight gain and other side-effects of some of the atypical neuroleptics. Further, some patients may do better on typical agents than on atypicals.

Suppressive therapy

Suppressive therapy should be considered only when TD poses heath risks, impairs function and daily activities (such as problems with eating, breathing, walking or sleeping) or is bothersome to the patient. As suppressive drug therapy may not be worth the added risk, non-drug strategies to cope with the disabilities may be a viable alternative following an assessment of functional impairment by an occupational or physical therapist (Egan *et al.* 1997). If suppression with drug therapy is deemed necessary, because it is difficult to predict an individual's response to a particular drug, it may be necessary to have a systematic approach of trying different drug therapies to control TD symptoms. Several different treatment approaches are listed below.

Dopamine

Suppressing or masking TD is best achieved by reducing dopaminergic activity. However, this strategy is justified only in those uncommon cases where TD is severe, debilitating or life-threatening (Casey & Rabins 1978). Most cases of TD are not so severe that treatment with dopamine suppressants is justified solely on the basis of TD. However, many patients also have coexisting psychoses which will justify continuing neuroleptic therapy. Two strategies for reducing dopaminergic activity include presynaptic depletion with reserpine or by false neurotransmission with methyldopa (Aldomet), but these have not yielded consistently beneficial results (Jeste & Wyatt 1982; Kane *et al.* 1992). Other catecholamine depleters such as tetra-

benazine and oxypertine may also be considered. While oxypertine has been demonstrated to be effective in one study, its efficacy was not sustained over long periods (Soni *et al.* 1986) Although not systematically investigated, tetrabenazine, which has both presynaptic depleting and postsynaptic dopamine receptor blockade activity, has been shown to be effective in a proportion of patients. These drugs may have some potentially bothersome side-effects and the consequences of extended high-dose use have not been well explored.

Of the atypical neuroleptics, clozapine has been suggested to have a specific antidyskinetic effect. Extensive clinical trial experience with clozapine for managing TD suggests that treatment for long periods is warranted and that dystonic features may be more responsive than dyskinetic ones (Lieberman *et al.* 1991). Risperidone may also have an antidyskinetic effect (Chouinard 1995) although, because it may also induce TD (Buzan 1996; Daniel *et al.* 1996; Woerner *et al.* 1996), the risk of long-term exacerbation is unknown. Other atypicals such as olanzapine, sertindole, quetiapine and ziprasidone, like clozapine, are more effective in blocking 5-hydroxytryptamine (5-HT_2) than the D_2 receptor site. However, they are relatively potent D_2 antagonists in contrast to clozapine. While these agents are efficacious in the treatment of psychosis and have a lower EPS profile when compared with typical neuroleptics, the utility of these agents in suppressing TD is unclear.

The theory of resetting dopaminergic hypersensitivity back to normal sensitivity with dopamine agonists has not been clinically useful. Agents such as bromocriptine (Parlodel) and pergolide (Permax) or dopamine precursors, such as levodopa/carbidopa (Sinemet), have not yielded consistently beneficial results (Jeste & Wyatt 1982; Kane *et al.* 1992).

Serotonin

While the serotonin system has been implicated in modulating striatal dopamine release and could theoretically influence dyskinetic movements (Seibyl *et al.* 1989), the combined results of several studies using serotonergic drugs such as serotonin agonists (buspirone) and serotonin reuptake inhibitors (e.g. fluoxetine) and serotonin antagonists (e.g. cyproheptadine) have been inconclusive.

Acetylcholine

While anticholinergic agents can temporarily aggravate TD, they may be beneficial in high doses in some patients with tardive dystonia. The efficacy of clozapine may also be explained by its high anticholinergic properties. Loading the cholinergic system through precursor dietary supplements is an attractive but unsuccessful approach. Both choline and lecithin showed some initial promise, but later controlled trials were disappointing (Jeste & Wyatt 1982; Casey 1987; Kane *et al.* 1992). Results with physostigmine, an acetylcholinesterase inhibitor, have been inconsistent, and the lack of an oral form of this drug makes it impractical.

Botulinum toxin

Injection of this botulinum toxin (type A) primarily designed for idiopathic dystonia has been successfully applied in the treatment of tardive dystonia. It blocks acetylcholine release at the neurochemical junction and produces a chemical denervation with focal muscle paralysis that persists up to 3–4 months (Hughes 1994). Botulinum toxin injections have been used to treat blepharospasm, laryngeal dystonia, hemifacial spasm and torticollis. Patients who are responsive to botulinum toxin injections may also do well on a surgical procedure involving selective peripheral denervation of the involved musculature (Braun et al. 1994).

Free-radical reduction

One hypothesis proposes that TD is caused by structural damage from free-radical formation of catecholamine metabolism in the brain. While thus far clinical studies of the role of antioxidants have focused on treatment, more recent studies are exploring the use of these agents for both treatment and prevention. Clinical studies with α-tocopherol (vitamin E), however, have not yielded consistent results. An initial study showed some benefit (Lohr et al. 1987), but other studies have found variable or no benefit (Elkashef et al. 1990; Egan et al. 1992; Shriqui et al. 1992). Based on this evidence, Lohr and Lavori (1998) concluded that the effect of vitamin E was small and negligible, and it is not proven to be effective for TD in general. However, they add that a trial of vitamin E carried virtually no risk. Work with other antioxidants is still preliminary.

Other drugs

TD has been treated with many other drugs. Although GABA hypofunction has been proposed as part of the pathophysiology underlying TD, treatment with GABA agents has produced inconsistent results. Sodium valproate, clonazepam, diazepam, baclofen and progabide are the most commonly used drugs in this class. Benzodiazepines help some patients, although it is unclear whether this is a specific or a non-specific sedative effect. Long-term use of benzodiazepines carries the potential of dependence or abuse.

Other drugs with highly variable results include the serotonergic agents tryptophan or cyproheptadine (Periactin), lithium carbonate, the β-adrenergic blocker propranolol (Inderal) and the α-adrenergic agonist clonidine (Catapres). Also, studies with neuropeptides, such as metenkephalin, destyrosine, endorphin and vasopressin, as well as approaches through the opiate mechanisms with morphine and naloxone (Narcan), have all been ineffective. Compounds such as oestrogen, pyridoxine, manganese, phenytoin, ergoloid mesylates, papaverine and others have produced only sporadic benefit (Jeste & Wyatt 1982; Casey 1987; Kane et al. 1992). Trials with other drugs such as calcium-channel blockers (verapamil, diltiazem and nifedipine), manganese and niacin (Kunin 1976), lithium (Simpson et al.

1976), GM$_1$ ganglioside (Peselow et al. 1989) and ceruletide (a CCK analogue) (Egan et al. 1997) have had variable results.

Invasive measures

Invasive measures such as deep brain stimulation and pallidotomy have been shown to be useful (Wang et al. 1997; Weetman et al. 1997) in cases with severe and refractory TD. The effect of electroconvulsive therapy, although reported to be variable, has had a dramatic response in a few patients (Hay et al. 1990).

Conclusions

There are no psychotropic medications that are entirely free of side-effects. To maximize the therapeutic effects with minimal adverse effects, one must follow the basic principles of rational psychopharmacotherapy. A thorough knowledge of the risk factors and close monitoring for early signs of EPS along with early intervention will certainly enhance outcome. Continued efforts in developing newer atypical agents with more specific receptor profiles and low risk for adverse effects are encouraging. Further, exciting research advances in the field of genetics are now providing information on the contribution of gene mutations to individual variability in susceptibility to drug-induced EPS. Such studies will ultimately lead to pretreatment prediction of psychopharmacotherapeutic response and susceptibility to side-effects. It is very possible that over the next decade drugs could be chosen on the basis of individual genetic make-up.

Acknowledgements

The authors wish to thank Saumitra Das, MA and Sam Lee, BS (Clinical Brain Disorders Branch, NIMH, NIH) for their assistance in formatting and preparing the bibliography.

References

Adler, L., Angrist, B., Reiter, S. & Rotrosen, J. (1989) Neuroleptic-induced akathisia: a review. Psychopharmacology 97, 1–11.

Andersson, U., Haggstrom, J., Levin, E. et al. (1989) Reduced glutamate decarboxylase activity in the subthalamic nucleus in patients with tardive dyskinesia. Movement Disorder 4, 37–46.

Andreassen, O., MacEwan, T., Gulbrandsen, A., McCreadie, R. & Steen, V. et al. (1997) Non-functional CYP2D6 alleles and risk for neuroleptic-induced movement disorders in schizophrenic patients. Psychopharmacology 131, 174–179.

Arvanitis, L. & Miller, B. (1997) Multiple fixed dose of 'Seroquel' (quetiapine) in patients with acute exacerbation of schizophrenia: a comparison with haloperidol and placebo. Biological Psychiatry 42, 233–246.

Ayd, F. (1961) A survey of drug-induced extrapyramidal reactions. Journal of the American Medical Association 175, 1054–1060.

Bailey, L., Maxwell, S. & Brandabur, M. (1997) Substance abuse as a risk factor for tardive dyskinesia: a retrospective analysis of 1027 patients. *Psychopharmacological Bulletin* **33**, 177–181.

Baldessarini, R., Cole J., Davis, J. *et al.* (1980) Tardive dyskinesia: summary of a task force report of the American Psychiatric Association. *American Journal of Psychiatry* **137**, 1163–1172.

Baldessarini, R., Cohen, B. & Teicher, M. (1988) Significance of neuroleptic dose and plasma level in pharmacological treatment of psychosis. *Archives of General Psychiatry* **45**, 79–91.

Barnes, T. & Braude, W. (1985) Akathisia variants and tardive dyskinesia. *Archives of General Psychiatry* **42**, 874–878.

Barnes, T., Kidger, T. & Gore, S. (1983) Tardive dyskinesia: a 3-year follow-up study. *Psychological Medicine* **13**, 71–81.

Basile, V.S., Ozdemir, V., Masellis, M., *et al.* (2000). A functional polymorphism of the cytochrome P450 1A2 (*CYP1A2*) gene: association with tardive dyskinesia in schizophrenia. *Mol Psychiatry* **5**(4): 410–7.

Basile, V., Ozdemir, V., Masellis, M. *et al.* (2001) Lack of association between serotonin-2A receptor gene (*HTR2A*) polymorphisms and tardive dyskinesia in schizophrenia. *Molecular Psychiatry* **6**, 230–234.

Beasley, C.M. Jr, Sanger, T., Satterlee, W. *et al.* (1996a) Olanzapine versus placebo: results of a double-blind, fixed-dose olanzapine trial. *Psychopharmacology (Berlin)* **124**, 159–167.

Beasley, C.M. Jr, Tollefson, G., Tran, P. *et al.* (1996b) Olanzapine versus placebo and haloperidol: acute phase results of North American double-blind olanzapine trial. *Neuropsychopharmacology* **14**, 111–123.

Bersani, G., Grispini, A., Marini, S. *et al.* (1990) 5-HT$_2$ antagonist ritanserin in neuroleptic-induced parkinsonism: a double-blind comparison with orphenadrine and placebo. *Clinical Neuropharmacology* **13**, 125–137.

Bleuler, E. (1950) *Dementia Praecox or the Group of Schizophrenias.* International Universities Press, New York.

Boyer, W., Bakalar, N. & Lake, C. (1989) Anticholinergic prophylaxis of acute haloperidol-induced dystonic reactions. *Journal of Clinical Psychopharmacology* **7**, 164–166.

Braun, A., Fabbrini, G., Nouradian, M. (1994) Selective peripheral denervation for the treatment of spasmodic torticollis. *Neurosurgery* **35**, 58–62.

Brooks, D. (1991) Detection of preclinical Parkinson's disease with PET. *Neurology* **41** (Suppl. 2), 24–27.

Brooks, D.J. (1993) Functional imaging in relation to parkinsonian syndromes. *Journal of Neurological Science* **115**, 1–17.

Brown, K., Whit, T., Wardlaw, J., Walker, N. & Foley, D. (1996) Caudate nucleus morphology in tardive dyskinesia. *British Journal of Psychiatry* **169**, 631–636.

Burke, R.E., Fahn, S., Jankovic, J. (1982) Tardive dystonia: late-onset and persistent dystonia caused by antipsychotic drugs. *Neurology* **32**, 1335–1346.

Buzan, R. (1996) Risperidone-induced tardive dyskinesia. *American Journal of Psychiatry* **136**, 734–735.

Campbell, M., Grega, D. & Green, W. (1983) Neuroleptic-induced dyskinesias in children. *Clinical Neuropharmacology* **6**, 207–222.

Carlsson, M. & Carlsson, A. (1990) Interaction between glutamatergic and monoaminergic systems within the basal ganglia: implications for schizophrenia and Parkinson's disease. *Trends in Neurosciences* **13**, 272–276.

Casey, D. (1981) The differential diagnosis of tardive dyskinesia. *Acta Psychiatrica Scandinavica* **63** (Suppl. 291), 71–87.

Casey, D. (1984) Tardive dyskinesia and affective disorders. In: *Tardive Dyskinesia and Affective Disorders* (eds G. Gardos & D. Casey), pp. 1–20. American Psychiatric Press. Washington, DC.

Casey, D. (1985a) Spontaneous and tardive dyskinesias: clinical and laboratory studies. *Journal of Clincal Psychiatry* **46**, 42–47.

Casey, D. (1985b) Tardive dyskinesia: reversible and irreversible. In: *Dyskinesia, Research and Treatment* (eds D. Casey *et al.*), pp. 88–97. Springer-Verlag, Berlin.

Casey, D. (1987) Tardive dyskinesia. In: *Psychopharmacology: The Third Generation of Progress* (ed. H. Meltzer), pp. 1411–1419. Raven Press, New York.

Casey, D. (1988a) Affective disorders and tardive dyskinesia. *Encephale* **14**, 221–226.

Casey, D. (1988b) Dopamine D$_1$ and D$_2$ agonists and antagonists in cebus monkeys [Abstract]. *Proceedings of the Society of Biological Psychiatry* **13**.

Casey, D. (1989) Clozapine: neuroleptic-induced EPS and tardive dyskinesia. *Psychopharmacology* **99**, S47–S53.

Casey, D. (1990) Tardive dyskinesia. *Western Journal of Medicine* **153**, 535–541.

Casey, D. (1991a) Neuroleptic-induced acute dystonia. In: *Drug-Induced Movement Disorders* (ed. A. Lang & W. Weiner), pp. 21–40. Future Press, New York.

Casey, D. (1991b) Neuroleptic drug-induced extrapyramidal syndromes and tardive dyskinesia. *Schizophrenia Research* **4**, 109–120.

Casey, D. (1992a) The Rabbit Syndrome. In: *Disorders of Movement in Psychiatry and Neurology* (eds A. Joseph & R. Young), pp. 139–142. Blackwell Scientific Publications, Oxford.

Casey, D. (1992b) Dopamine D$_1$ (SCH 23390) and D$_2$ (haloperidol) antagonists in drug-naive monkeys. *Psychopharmacology* **107**, 18–22.

Casey, D. (1992c) Acute neuroleptic-induced dystonia. In: *Disorders of Movement in Psychiatry and Neurology* (ed. A. Joseph & R. Young), pp. 106–110. Blackwell Scientific Publications, Oxford.

Casey, D. (1995) Neuroleptic-induced acute extrapyramidal syndromes and tardive dyskinesia. *Schizophrenia*, 1st edn. (eds S.R. Hirsch & D.R. Weinberger), pp. 546–565. Blackwell Science, Oxford.

Casey, D. (1996) Extrapyramidal syndromes: epidemiology, pathophysiology and the diagnostic dilemma. *CNS Drugs* **5** (Suppl. 1), 1–12.

Casey, D. (1997a) The relationship of pharmacology to side effects. *Journal of Clinical Psychiatry* **58** (Suppl. 10), 55–62.

Casey, D. (1997b) Will the new antipsychotics bring hope of reducing the risk of developing extrapyramidal syndromes and tardive dyskinesia? *International Clinical Psychopharmacology* **12** (Suppl. 1), S19–S27.

Casey, D. (1999) Tardive dyskinesia and atypical antipsychotic drugs. *Schizophrenia Research* **35**, S61–S66.

Casey, D. & Gerlach, J. (1986) Tardive dyskinesia: what is the long-term outcome? In: *Tardive Dyskinesia and Neuroleptics: From Dogma to Reason* (ed. D. Casey & G. Gardos), pp. 76–97. American Psychiatric Press, Washington, DC.

Casey, D. & Hansen, T.E. (1984) *Neuropsychiatric Movement Disorders* (eds D. Jeste & R. Wyatt), Vol. 1, pp. 68–95. American Psychiatric Press, Washington DC.

Casey, D. & Keepers, G.A. (1988) Neuroleptic side effects: acute extrapyramidal syndromes and tardive dyskinesia. In: *Psychopharmacology: Current Trends* (eds D. Casey & A. Christensen), pp. 74–93. Springer-Verlag, Berlin.

Casey, D. & Rabins, P. (1978) Tardive dyskinesia as a life-threatening illness. *American Journal of Psychiatry* **135**, 969–971.

Chen, C., Wei, F., Koong, F. & Hsiao, K. (1997) Association of TaqI A polymorphism of dopamine D$_2$ receptor gene and dyskinesia in schizophrenia. *Biological Psychiatry* **41**, 827–829.

Chouinard, G. (1995) Effects of risperidone in tardive dyskinesia: an analysis of the Canadian multicenter risperidone study. *Journal of Clinical Psychopharmacology* **15**, 36S–44S.

Chouinard, G., Annable, L., Mercier, p. & Ross-Chouinard, A. (1986) A five year follow-up study of tardive dyskinesia. *Psychopharmacology Bulletin* 22, 259–263.

Chouinard, G., Jones, B., Remington, G. *et al.* (1993) A Canadian multicentre placebo-controlled study of fixed doses of risperidone and haloperidol in the treatment of chronic schizophrenic patients. *Clinical Psychopharmacology* 13, 25–40.

Crane, G.E. & Smeets, R.A. (1974) Tardive dyskinesia and drug therapy in geriatric patients. *Archives of General Psychiatry* 30, 341–343.

Daniel, D., Smith, K., Hyde, T. & Egan, M. (1996) Neuroleptic-induced tardive dyskinesia [letter]. *American Journal of Psychiatry* 153, 734.

Dave, M. (1994) Clozapine-related tardive dyskinesia. *Biological Psychiatry* 35, 886–887.

Davies, J. & Janicak, P. (1996) Risperidone: a new, novel (and better?) antipsychotic. *Psychiatry Annals* 26, 78–87.

Davis, K., Berger, P. & Hollister, L. (1976) Tardive dyskinesia and depressive illness. *Psychopharmacology Communications* 2, 125–130.

Deniker, P. (1984) Introduction of neuroleptic chemotherapy into psychiatry In: *Discoveries in Biological Psychiatry* (eds F. Ayd & B. Blackwell), pp. 155–164. Ayd Medical Communication, Baltimore.

Dixon, L., Weiden, P., Haag, G., Sweeney, J. & Frances, A. (1992) Increased tardive dyskinesia in alcohol-abusing schizophrenic patients. *Comparative Psychiatry* 33, 121–122.

Duvoisin, R. (1977) Problems in the treatment of parkinsonism. *Advances in Experimental Medical Biology* 90, 131–155.

Egan, M., Hyde, T.M., Albers, G.W. *et al.* (1992) Treatment of tardive dyskinesia with vitamin E. *American Journal of Psychiatry* 149, 773–777.

Egan, M., Apud, J. & Wyatt, R. (1997) Treatment of tardive dyskinesia. *Schizophrenia Bulletin* 23, 583–609.

Eichhammer, P., Albus, M., Borrmann-Hassenbach, M. *et al.* (2000) Association of dopamine D_3-receptor gene variants with neuroleptic induced akathisia in schizophrenic patients; a generalization of Steen's Study on *DRD3* and tardive dyskinesia. *American Journal of Medical Genetics* 96, 187–191.

Elkashef, A., Ruskin, P., Bacher, N. & Barrett, D. (1990) Vitamin E in the treatment of tardive dyskinesia. *American Journal of Psychiatry* 147, 505–506.

Elkashef, M., Buchanan, R., Gellad, F., Munson, R. & Breier, A. (1994) Basal ganglia pathology in schizophrenia and tardive dyskinesia: an MRI quantitative study. *American Journal of Psychiatry* 151, 752–755.

Ellingrod, V., Schultz, S.K. & Arndt, S. (2000) Association between cytochrome P4502D6 (CYP2D6) genotype, neuroleptic exposure and abnormal involuntary movement scale (AIMS) score. *Schizophrenia Research* 36, 1–3.

Eyles, D., Pond, S., Van der Schyf, C. & Halliday, G. (2000) Mitochondrial ultrastructure and density in a primate model of persistent tardive dyskinesia. *Life Science* 66, 1345–1350.

Fairbairn, A., Rowell, F., Hui, S. *et al.* (1983) Serum concentration of depot neuroleptics in tardive dyskinesia. *British Journal of Psychiatry* 142, 579–583.

Fann, W., Stafford, J. Malone, R., Frost, J. & Richman, B. (1977) Clinical research techniques in tardive dyskinesia. *American Journal of Psychiatry* 134, 759–762.

Farde, L. (1992) Selective D_1 or D_2 dopamine receptor blockade induces akathisia in humans: a PET Study with [^{11}C] SCH 23390 and [^{11}C] raclopride. *Psychopharmacology* 107, 23–29.

Farde, L., Nordstrom, A., Wiesel, F. *et al.* (1992) Positron emission tomographic analysis of central D_1-dopamine and D_2-dopamine receptor occupancy in patients treated with classical neuroleptics and clozapine: relation to extrapyramidal side-effects. *Archives of General Psychiatry* 49, 538–544.

Faurbye, A., Rasch, P., Bender Peterson, P., Brandenborg, G. & Pakken-

berg, H. (1964) Neurological symptoms in the pharmacotherapy of psychoses. *Acta Psychiatrica Scandinavica* 40, 10–26.

Fleischhacker, W., Link, C. & Hurst, B. (1996) ICL 204,636 (Seroquel): a putative new antipsychotic: results from Phase III trials. *Schizophrenia Research* 18, 132.

Gallhofer, B., Bauer, U., Lis, S., Krieger, S. & Gruppe, H. (1996) Cognitive dysfunction in schizophrenia: comparison of treatment with atypical antipsychotic agents and conventional neuroleptics drugs. *European Neuropsychopharmacology* 6, 2–13; 20.

Ganzini, L., Heintz, R., W., Keepers, G. & Casey, D. (1991a) Prevalence of tardive dyskinesia in neuroleptic-treated diabetics. *Archives of General Psychiatry* 48, 259–263.

Ganzini, L., Heintz, R., Hoffman, W. & Casey, D. (1991b) Acute extrapyramidal syndromes in neuroleptic-treated elders: a pilot study. *Journal of Geriatric Psychiatry and Neurology* 4, 222–225.

Ganzini, L., Casey, D., Hoffman, W. & Heintz, R. (1992) Tardive dyskinesia and diabetes mellitus. *Psychopharmacology Bulletin* 23, 281–286.

Gardos, G. & Cole. (1997) Tardive dyskinesia and affective disorder, In: *Neuroleptic-Induced Movement Disorders* (eds R. Yassa, N. Nair & D. Jeste), pp. 69–81. Cambridge University Press, Cambridge.

Gardos, G., Cole, J., Salomon, M. & Schniebolk, S. (1987) Clinical forms of severe tardive dyskinesia. *American Journal of Psychiatry* 144, 895–902.

Gardos, G., Cole, J., Haskell, D. *et al.* (1988) The natural history of tardive dyskinesia. *Journal of Clinical Psychopharmacology* 8 (Suppl. 4), 31S–37S.

Gardos, G., Casey, D.E., Cole, J.O. *et al.* (1994) Ten-year outcome of tardive dyskinesia. *American Journal of Psychiatry* 151, 836–841.

Garver, D., Davis, J., Dekirmenjian, H. *et al.* (1976) Dystonic reactions following neuroleptics: time course and proposed mechanisms. *Psychopharmacology* 47, 199–201.

Gerlach, J. & Casey, D. (1988) Tardive dyskinesia. *Acta Psychiatrica Scandinavica* 77, 369–378.

Gerlach, J., Casey, D., Kistrup, K. & Lublin, H. (1988) Dopamine D_1 and D_2 receptor functions in acute extrapyramidal syndromes and tardive dyskinesia. In: *Progress in Catecholamine Research. Part C. Clinical Aspects: Neurology and Neurobiology* (eds R. Belmaker, M. Sandler & A. Dahlstrom), 42C.

Glazer, W., Naftolin, F., Moore, D.C., Bowers, M.B. & MacLusky, N.J. (1983) The relationship of circulating estradiol to tardive dyskinesia in men and post-menopausal women. *Psychoneuroendocrinology* 8, 429–434.

Goldstein, L.E., Sporn, J., Brown, S. *et al.* (1999) New-onset diabetes mellitus and diabetic ketoacidosis associated with olanzapine treatment. *Psychosomatics* 40, 438–443.

Gualtieri, C., Quade, D., Hicks, R., Mayo, J. & Schroeder, S. (1984) Tardive dyskinesia and other clinical consequences of neuroleptic treatment in children and adolescents. *American Journal of Psychiatry* 141, 20–23.

Gunne, L. & Haggstrom, J. (1985) Pathophysiology of tardive dyskinesia. *Psychopharmacology* 232, 191–193.

Gunne, L., Haggstrom J. & Sjoquist, B. (1984) Association with persistent neuroleptic-induced dyskinesia of regional changes in brain: GABA synthesis. *Nature* 309, 347–349.

Guy, W. (1976) *ECDEU Assessment Manual for Psychopharmacology (revised 1976)*, pp. 534–537. United Staes Government Printing Office Washington, DC.

Hagg, S., Joelsson, L., Mjorndal, T. *et al.* (1998) Prevalence of diabetes and impaired glucose tolerance in patients treated with clozapine compared with patients treated with conventional depot neuroleptic medications. *Journal of Clinical Psychiatry* 59, 294–299.

Hay, D., Hay, L., Blackwell, B. & Spiro, H. (1990) ECT and tardive dyskinesia. *Journal of Geriatric Psychiatry and Neurology* 3, 106–109.

Hughes, A. (1994) Botulinum toxin in clinical practice. *Drugs* 48, 888–893.

Jeste, D. & Wyatt, R. (1982) *Understanding and Treating Tardive Dyskinesia*. Guilford Press, New York.

Jeste, D., Lohr, J., Kaufmann, C. & Wyatt, R. (1986) Pathophysiology of tardive dyskinesia: evaluation of supersensitivity theory and alternative hypothesis. In: *Tardive Dyskinesia and Neuroleptics: From Dogma to Reason.* (eds D. Casey & G. Gardos), pp. 15–32. American Psychiatric Press, Washington, DC.

Jeste, D., Caligiuri, M., Paulsen, J. *et al.* (1995) Risk of tardive dyskinesia in older patients. *Archives of General Psychiatry* 52, 756–765.

Kane, J. (1995) Tardive dyskinesia: epidemiological and clinical presentation. In: *Psychopharmacology: The Fourth Generation of Progress* (ed. D. Bloom), pp. 1485–1496. Kupfer, New York,

Kane, J. & Smith, J. (1982) Tardive dyskinesia: prevalence and risk factors, 1959–79. *Archives of General Psychiatry* 39, 473–481.

Kane, J., Woerner, M., Weinhold, P. *et al.* (1984a) Incidence and severity of tardive dyskinesia in affective illness. In: *Tardive Dyskinesia and Affective Illness*, pp. 22–28. American Psychiatric Press, Washington, DC.

Kane, J., Woerner, M., Weinhold, P. *et al.* (1984b) Incidence of tardive dyskinesia: five year data from a prospective study. *Psychopharmacology Bulletin* 20, 39–40.

Kane, J., Woerner, M., Borenstein, M., Wegner, J. & Lieberman, J. (1986) Integrating incidence and prevalence of tardive dyskinesia. *Psychopharmacological Bulletin* 22, 254–258.

Kane, J., Woerner, M. & Lieberman, J. (1988) Tardive dyskinesia: prevalence, incidence, and risk factors. *Journal of Clinical Psychopharmacology* 8 (Aug Suppl.), 52S–56S.

Kane, J., Jeste, D., Barnes, T. *et al.* (1992) *Tardive Dyskinesia: A Task Force: Report of the American Psychiatric Association.* American Psychiatric Association, Washington, DC.

Kapitany, T., Meszaros, K., Lenzinger, E. *et al.* (1998) Genetic polymorphisms for drug metabolism (CYP2D6) and tardive dyskinesia in schizophrenia. *Schizophrenia Research* 32, 101–106.

Kapur, S. (1998) A new framework for investigating antipsychotic action in humans: lessons from PET imaging. *Molecular Psychiatry* 3, 135–140.

Kapur, S. & Remington, G. (2001) Atypical antipsychotics: new directions and new challenges in the treatment of schizophrenia. *Annual Review of Medicine* 52, 503–517.

Kapur, S. & Seeman, P. (2001) Does fast dissociation from the dopamine D(2) receptor explain the action of atypical antipsychotics? A new hypothesis. *American Journal of Psychiatry* 158, 360–369.

Kapur, S., Zipurski, R. & Remington, G. (1999) Clinical and theoretical implications of 5-HT$_2$ and D$_2$ receptor occupancy of clozapine, risperidone, and olanzapine in schizophrenia. *American Journal of Psychiatry* 156, 286–293.

Kapur, S., Zipursky, R., Jones, C., Remington, G. & Houle, S. (2000) Relationship between dopamine D$_2$ occupancy, clinical response, and side effects: a double-blind PET study of first-episode schizophrenia. *American Journal of Psychiatry* 157, 514–520.

Keepers, G. & Casey, D. (1987) Prediction of neuroleptic-induced dystonia. *Journal of Clinical Psychopharmacology* 7, 342–344.

Keepers, G. & Casey, D. (1991) Use of neuroleptic-induced extrapyramidal symptoms to predict future vulnerability to side effects. *American Journal of Psychiatry* 148, 85–89.

Keepers, G., Clappison, V. & Casey, D. (1983) Initial anticholinergic prophylaxis for neuroleptic–induced extrapyramidal syndromes. *Archives of General Psychiatry* 40, 1113–1117.

Kennedy, P.H., Hershon, H.I. & McGuire, R. (1971) Extrapyramidal disorders after prolonged phenothiazine therapy. *British Journal of Psychiatry* 118, 509–518.

Klawans, H. & Rubovits, R. (1972) An experimental model of tardive dyskinesia. *Journal of Neural Transmission* 33, 235–246.

Klawans, H. & Tanner, C. (1983) The reversibility of permanent tardive dyskinesia. *Neurology* 33 (Suppl. 2), 163.

Knable, M., Heinz, A., Raedler, T. & Weinberger, D. (1997) Extrapyramidal side effects with risperidone and haloperidol at comparable D$_2$ receptor occupancy levels. *Psychiatry Research: Neuroimaging* 75, 91–101.

Kraepelin, E. (1907) *Clinical Psychiatry*. MacMillan, New York.

Kucharski, L., Smith, J. & Dunn, D. (1978) Morality and tardive dyskinesia. *American Journal of Psychiatry* 135, 1228.

Kunin, R. (1976) Manganese and niacin in the treatment of drug-induced dyskinesia. *Journal of Orthomolecular Psychiatry* 5, 4–27.

Kurz, M., Hummer, M., Oberbauer, H. & Fleischhacker, W. (1995) Efficacy of medium-dose clozapine for treatment-resistant schizophrenia. *American Journal of Psychiatry* 152, 1690–1691.

Lazarus, A. & Toglia, J. (1985) Fatal myoglobinuric renal failure in a patient with tardive dyskinesia. *Neurology* 35, 1055–1057.

Leo, R. (1996) Movement disorders associated with serotonin selective reuptake inhibitors. *Journal of Clinical Psychiatry* 57, 449–454.

Liao, D., Yeh, Y., Chen, H. (2001) Association between the Ser9Gly polymorphism of the dopamine D$_3$ receptor gene and tardive dyskinesia in Chinese schizophrenic patients. *Neuropsychobiology* 44, 95–98.

Lieberman, J., Kane, J. & Woerner, M. (1984) Prevalence of tardive dyskinesia in elderly samples. *Psychopharmacology Bulletin* 20, 22–26.

Lieberman, J.A., Saltz, B.L., Johns, C.A. (1991) The effects of clozapine on tardive dyskinesia. *British Journal of Psychiatry* 158, 503–510.

Lipinski, J., Zubenko, G., Cohen, B. & Barreira, P. (1984) Propranolol in the treatment of neuroleptic-induced akathisia. *American Journal of Psychiatry* 141, 412–415.

Lohr, J. & Lavori, P. (1998) Whither vitamin E and tardive dyskinesia? *Biological Psychiatry* 43, 861–862.

Lohr, J., Cadet, J., Lohr, M., Jeste, D. & Wyatt, R. (1987) Alphatocopherol in tardive dyskinesia. *Lancet* 1, 913–914.

Lohr, J., Kuczenski, R., Bracha, H.M.M. & Jeste, D. (1990) Increased indices of free radical activity in the cerebrospinal fluid of patients with tardive dyskinesia. *Biological Psychiatry* 28, 535–539.

McClelland, H., Dutta, D., Metcalf, A. & Kerr, T. (1986) Morality and facial dyskinesia. *British Journal of Psychiatry* 148, 310–316.

McEvoy, J., McCue, M. & Freter, S. (1987) Replacement of chronically administered anticholinergic drugs by amantadine in out-patient managment of chronic schizophrenia. *Current Therapy* 9, 429–433.

Marder, S. (1992) Risperidone: clinical development – North American results. *Clinical Neuropharmacology* 15 (Suppl. 1).

Marsalek, M. (2000) Tardive drug-induced extrapyramidal syndromes. *Pharmacopsychiatry* 33, 14–33.

Miller, C., Mohr, F., Umbrich, D. *et al.* (1998) The prevalence of acute extrapyramidal signs and symptoms in patients treated with clozapine, risperidone, and conventional antipsychotics. *Journal of Clinical Psychiatry* 59, 69–75.

Mion, C., Andreasen, N., Arndt, S., Swayze, V. & Cohen, G. (1991) MRI abnormalities in tardive dyskinesia. *Psychiatry Research* 40, 157–166.

Moleman, P., Schmitz, P. & Ladee, G. (1982) Extrapyramidal side-effects and oral haloperidol: an analysis of explanatory patient and treatment characteristics. *Journal of Clinical Psychiatry* 43, 492–496.

Morgenstern, H. & Glazer, W. (1993) Identifying risk factors for tardive dyskinesia among long-term outpatients maintained with neuroleptic medications. *Archives of General Psychiatry* 50, 723–733.

Mukherjee, S. & Mahadik, S. (1997) Diabetes mellitus and tardive dyskinesia. In: *Neuroleptic-induced Movement Disorders* (eds R. Yassa, N. Nair & D. Jeste), pp. 82–98. Cambridge University Press, Cambridge.

Nordstrom, A.-L., Farde, L. & Halldin, C. (1992) Time course of D_2 dopamine receptor occupancy examined by PET after single oral doses of haloperidol. *Psychopharmacology* 106, 433–438.

Nordstrom, A.-L., Farde, L., Wiesel, F.A. *et al.* (1993) Central D_2 dopamine receptor occupancy in relation to antipsychotic drug effects: a double-blind PET study of schizophrenic patients. *Biological Psychiatry* 33, 227–235.

Nyberg, S., Nakashima, Y., Nordstrom, A.L., Halldin, C. & Farde, L. (1996) Positron emission tomography of *in vivo* binding characteristics of atypical antopsychotic drugs: review of D_2 and $5\text{-}HT_2$ receptor occupancy studies and clinical response. *British Journal of Psychiatry* 168 (Suppl. 29), 40–44.

Nyberg, S., Farde, L. & Halldin, C. (1997) $5\text{-}HT_2$ and D_2 dopamine receptor occupancy induced by olanzapine in healthy subjects. *Neuropscyhopharmacology* 16, 1–7.

van Os, J., Fahy, T., Jones, P. *et al.* (1997) Tardive dyskinesia: who is at risk? *Acta Psychiatrica Scandinavica* 96, 206–216.

Owens, D. (1999) *A guide to the extrapyramidal side-effects of antipsychotic drugs.* Cambridge University Press, Cambridge.

Pandurangi, A. & Aderibigbe, Y. (1995) Tardive dyskinesia in non-western countries: a review. *European Archives of Psychiatry and Clinical Neuroscience* 246, 47–52.

Pehek, E. (1996) Local infusion of the serotonin antagonist ritanserin or ICS 205,930 increases *in vivo* dopamine release in the rat medial prefrontal cortex. *Synapse* 24, 12–18.

Pert, A., Rosenblatt, J., Sivit, C., Pert, C. & Bunney, W.J. (1979) Long-term treatment with lithium prevents the development of dopamine receptor supersensitivity. *Science* 135, 509–514.

Peselow, E., Irons, S., Rotrosen, J., Alonso, M. & Dorsey, F. (1989) GMI ganglioside as a potential treatment in tardive dyskinesia. *Psychopharmacology* 25, 277–280.

Peuskens, J. (1995) Risperidone in the treatment of patients with chronic schizophrenia: a multi-national, multi-centre, double blind, parallel group study versus haloperidol. *British Journal of Psychiatry* 166, 712–726.

Quitkin, F., Rifkin, A., Gochfeld, L. & Klein, D. (1977) Tardive dyskinesia: are first signs reversible? *American Journal of Psychiatry* 134, 84–87.

Rajput, A., Rozdilsky, B., Hornykiewicz, O. *et al.* (1982) Reversible drug-induced parkinsonism: clinicopathologic study of two cases. *Archives of Neurology* 39, 644–646.

Richardson, M. & Craig, T. (1982) The coexistence of parkinsonism-like symptoms and tardive dyskinesia. *American Journal of Psychiatry* 139, 341–343.

Richardson, M., Haugland, M., Pass, R. & Craig, T. (1986) The prevalence of tardive dyskinesia in a mentally retarded population. *Psychopharmacological Bulletin* 22, 243–249.

Richardson, M., Suckow, R., Whittaker, R. *et al.* (1989) The plasma phenylalanine/large neutral amino acid ratio: a risk factor for tardive dyskinesia. *Psychopharmacological Bulletin* 25, 47–51.

Rosenheck, R., Cramer, J., Xu, W. *et al.* (1997) A comparison of clozapine and haloperidol in hospitalized patients with refractory schizophrenia. *New England Journal of Medicine* 337, 809–815.

Rupniak, N., Jenner, P. & Marsden, C. (1986) Acute dystonia induced by neuroleptic drugs. *Psychopharmacology* 88, 403–419.

Sachdev, P. (1989) Depression-dependent exacerbation of tardive dyskinesia. *British Journal of Psychiatry* 155, 253–255.

Sachdev, P. (1992) Drug-induced movement disorders in institutionalized adults with mental retardation: clinical characteristics and risk factors. *Australian and New Zealand Journal of Psychiatry* 26, 242–248.

Sachdev, P. (2000) The current status of tardive dyskinesia. *Australian and New Zealand Journal of Psychiatry* 34, 355–369.

Saltz, B.L., Woerner, M.G., Kane, J.M. *et al.* (1991) Prospective study of tardive dyskinesia incidence in the elderly. *Journal of the American Medical Association* 266, 2402–2406.

Scatton, B. (1977) Differential regional development of tolerance to increase in dopamine turnover upon repeated neuroleptic. *European Journal of Pharmacology* 46, 363–369.

Scherer, J., Tatsch, K., Schwarz, J. *et al.* (1994) D_2-dopamine receptor occupancy differs between patients with and without extrapyramidal side effects. *Acta Psychiatrica Scandinavica* 90, 266–268.

Schlegel, S., Schlosser, R., Hiemke, C. *et al.* (1996) Prolactin plasma levels and D_2-dopamine receptor occupancy measured with IBZM-SPECT. *Psychopharmacology* 124, 285–287.

Schonecker, M. (1957) Ein eigentumliches Syndrom im oralen Bereich bei Megaphenapplikation. *Nervenaerzt* 28, 35–36.

Schooler, N. & Kane, J. (1982) Research diagnoses for tardive dyskinesia. *Archives of General Psychiatry* 39, 486–487.

Schroder, J., Silvestri, S., Bubeck, B. *et al.* (1998) D_2 dopamine receptor up-regulation, treatment response, neurological soft signs, and extrapyramidal side effects in schizophrenia: follow-up study with I-123-iodobenzamide single photon emission computed tomography in the drug-naive state and after neuroleptic treatment. *Biological Psychiatry* 43, 660–665.

Schultz, S., Arndt, S., Ho, B.-C., Oliver, S. & Andreasen, N. (1999) Impaired glucose tolerance and abnormal movements in patients with schizophrenia. *American Journal of Psychiatry* 156, 640–642.

Seeman, P.R., Corbett & Van Tol, H. (1997) Atypical neuroleptics have low affinity for dopamine D_2 receptors or are selective for D_4 receptors. *Neuropsychopharmacology* 16, 93–110.

Segman, R., Neeman, T., Heresco-Levy, U. *et al.* (1999) Genotypic association between the dopamine D_3 receptor and tardive dyskinesia in chronic schizophrenia. *Molecular Psychiatry* 4, 247–253.

Segman, R., Herseco-Levy, U., Finkel, B. *et al.* (2001) Association between the serotonin 2A receptor gene and tardive dykinesia in chronic schizophrenia. *Psychopharmacology (Berlin)* 152, 408–413.

Seibyl, J., Glazer, W. & Innis, R. (1989) Serotonin function in tardive dyskinesia. *Psychiatric Annals* 19, 310–314.

Shriqui, C., Bradwein, J., Annable, L. & Jones, B. (1992) Vitamin E in the treatment of tardive dyskinesia: a double-blind placebo-controlled study. *American Journal of Psychiatry* 149, 391–393.

Sigwald, J., Bouttier, D. & Raymondeaud, C. (1959) Quatre cas de dyskinesie facio-bucco-lingua-masticatrice a l'evolution prolongee secondaire a un traitment par les neuroleptiques. *Revue Neurologique* 100, 751–755.

Simpson, G., Branchey, M., Lee, J., Voitashevsky, A. & Zoubok, B. (1976) Lithium in tardive dyskinesia. *Pharmkopsychiatrics Neuropsychopharmakology* 9, 76–80.

Small, J., Hirsch, S.R., Arvanitis, L.A., Miller, B.G. & Link, C.G. (1997) Quetiapine in the patient with schizophrenia: a high- and low-dose double-blind comparison with placebo. *Archives of General Psychiatry* 54, 549–557.

Smith, J. & Baldessarini, R. (1980) Changes in prevalence, severity and recovery in tardive dyskinesia with age. *Archives of General Psychiatry* 37, 1368–1373.

Smith, J., Oswald, W., Kucharski, L. & Waterman, L. (1978) Tardive dyskinesia: age and sex differences in hospitalized schizophrenics. *Psychopharmacology* 58, 207–211.

Soni, S., Freeman, H. & Hussein, E. (1986) Oxypertine in tardive dyskinesia: an 8-week controlled study. *British Journal of Psychiatry* 144, 48–52.

Sramek, J., Simpson, G., Morrison, R. & Heiser, J. (1986) Anticholinergic agents for prophylaxis of neuroleptic-induced dystonic reactions: a prospective study. *Journal of Clinical Psychiatry* **47**, 305–309.

Steen, V.M., Lovlie, R., MacEwan, T. & McCreadie, R.G. (1997) Dopamine D_3-receptor gene variant and susceptibility to tardive dyskinesia in schizophrenic patients. *Molecular Psychiatry* **2**, 139–145.

Sweet, R., Mulsant, B., Gupta, B. *et al.* (1995) Duration of neuroleptic treatment and prevalence of tardive dyskinesia in late life. *Archives of General Psychiatry* **52**, 478–486.

Tan, E., Chong, S., Mahendran, R., Dong, F. & Tan, C. (2001) Susceptibility to neuroleptic-induced tardive dyskinesia and the T102C polymorphism in the serotonin type 2A receptor. *Biological Psychiatry* **50**, 144–147.

Tandon, R., Harrigan, E. & Zorn, S. (1997) Ziprasidone: a novel antipsychotic with unique pharmacology and therapeutic potential. *Journal of Serotonin Research* **4**, 159–177.

Tauscher, J., Kufferle, B., Asenbaum, S. *et al.* (1999) *In vivo* [123]I IBZM SPECT imaging of striatal dopamine-2 receptor occupancy in schizophrenic patients treated with olanzapine in comparison to clozapine and haloperidol. *Psychopharmacology (Berlin)* **141**, 175–181.

Thaker, G., Tamminga, C., Alphs, L. *et al.* (1987) Brain gamma-aminobutyric acid abnormality in tardive dyskinesia. *Archives of General Psychiatry* **44**, 522–529.

Toenniessen, L., Casey, D. & McFarland, B. (1985) Tardive dyskinesia in the aged: duration of treatment relationships. *Archives of General Psychiatry* **42**, 278–284.

Tollefson, G., Beasley, C.J., Tamura, R., Tran, P. & Potvin, J. *et al.* (1997) Blind, controlled, long-term study of the comparative incidence of treatment-emergent tardive dyskinesia with olanzapine or haloperidol. *American Journal of Psychiatry* **154**, 1248–1254.

Tran, P., Blin, O., *et al.* (1997a) Olanzapine versus haloperidol: acute phase of the international double-blind olanzapine trial. *European Neuropsychopharmacology* **7**, 125–137.

Tran, P., Hamilton, S., Kuntz, A. *et al.* (1997b) Double blind comparison of olanzapine versus risperidone in the treatment of schizophrenia and other psychotic disorders. *Journal of Clinical Psychopharmacology* **17**, 407–418.

Trelles, L., Trelles, J., Castaneda, C. & Castro, C. (1985) Disappearance of tardive dyskinesia in a manic attack [in French]. *Revue Neurologique* **5**, 415–416.

Tsai, G., Goff, D., Change, R. *et al.* (1998) Markers of glutamatergic neurotransmission and oxidative stress associated with tardive dyskinesia. *American Journal of Psychiatry* **155**, 1207–1213.

Uhrbrand, L. & Faurbye, A. (1960) Reversible and irreversible dyskinesia after treatment with perphenazine, chlorpromazine, reserpine, and electroconvulsive therapy. *Psychopharmacoligia* **1**, 408–418.

Van Kammen, D.P., McEvoy, J.P., Targum, S.D., Kardatzke, D. & Sebree, T.B. (1996) A randomized, controlled dose-ranging trial of sertindole in patients with schizophrenia. *Advances in Biochemical Psychopharmacology* **19**, 255–266.

Villeneuve, A. (1972) The Rabbit Syndrome: a peculiar extrapyramidal reaction. *Canadian Psychiatric Association Journal* **17**, 69–72.

Waddington, J., Youssef, H., Dolphin, C. & Kinsella, A. (1987) Cognitive dysfunction, negative symptoms, and tardive dyskinesia in schizophrenia. *Archives of General Psychiatry* **44**, 907–912.

Waddington, J., Youssef, H. & Kinsella, A. (1990) Cognitive dysfunction in schizophrenia followed up over 5 years, and its longitudinal relationship to the emergence of tardive dyskinesia. *Psychological Medicine* **20**, 835–842.

Waddington, J.L., O'Callaghan, E., Larkin, C. & Kinsella, A. (1993) Cognitive dysfunction in schizophrenia: organic vulnerability factor or state marker for tardive dyskinesia? *Brain and Cognition* **23**, 56–70.

Wang, Y., Turnbull, I., Calne, S., Stoessl, A. & Calne, D. (1997) Pallidotomy for tardive diskinesia. *Lancet* **349**, 777–778.

Weetman, J., Anderson, I., Gregory, R. & Gill, S. (1997) Bilateral posteroventral pallidotomy for severe antipsychotic induced tardive dyskinesia and dystonia [letter]. *Journal of Neurology, Neurosurgery, and Psychiatry* **63**, 554–556.

Williams, J., Spurlock, G., Holmans, P. *et al.* (1998) A meta-analysis and transmission disequilibrium study of association between the dopamine D_3 receptor gene and schizophrenia. *Molecular Psychiatry* **3**, 141–149.

Woerner, M., Kane, J. & Lieberman, J. (1991) The prevalance of tardive dyskinesia. *Journal of Clinical Psychopharmacology* **11**, 34–42.

Woerner, M., Sheitman, B., Lieberman, J. & Kane, J. (1996) Tardive dyskinesia induced by risperidone? *American Journal of Psychiatry* **153**, 843.

Yassa, R. & Nair, N. (1984) Incidence of tardive dyskinesia in an outpatients population. *Psychosomatics* **25**, 479–481.

Youssef, H. & Waddington, J. (1987) Mortality and morbidity in tardive dyskinesia: association in chronic schizophrenia. *Acta Psychiatrica Scandinavica* **75**, 74–77.

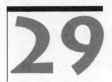

29 Non-neurological side-effects of antipsychotic drugs

D.C. Goff and R.I. Shader

Mood and behavioural effects, 573
  Akinetic depression, 574
  Postpsychotic depression, 574
Cognitive effects, 574
Endocrine effects, 575
  Hyperprolactinaemia, 575
  Thyroid effects, 576
  Syndrome of inappropriate antidiuretic hormone, 576
Weight gain, 576
Diabetes, 576
Sexual dysfunction, 577
Cardiovascular effects, 577

Cardiac conduction, 577
  Orthostatic hypotension, 578
Cutaneous effects, 578
  Allergic reactions, 578
  Photosensitivity, 578
Ocular effects, 579
Gastrointestinal and hepatic effects, 579
  Hepatic effects, 579
Haematological effects, 580
Seizures, 580
Neuroleptic malignant syndrome, 581
Conclusions, 581
References, 582

Non-neurological side-effects (NNSEs) of antipsychotic drugs may adversely affect compliance, quality of life and long-term health, but were largely overshadowed in the past by the attention paid to neurological side-effects. Because the newer atypical antipsychotics produce substantially fewer neurological side-effects, other side-effects increasingly have been brought to the forefront of clinical practice. In this chapter, the term 'neurological' refers to motor side-effects generally understood to involve extrapyramidal tracts.

The high-potency conventional neuroleptics (e.g. haloperidol, fluphenazine, pimozide) are relatively selective antagonists of dopamine D_2 receptors and so produce comparatively few non-neurological side-effects other than hyperprolactinaemia. The low-potency conventional neuroleptics (e.g. chlorpromazine, thioridazine) act on several other neurotransmitter systems, including muscarinic, adrenergic and histaminergic, thereby producing a wider range of side-effects. The atypical antipsychotics, while sharing D_2 and serotonin $5-HT_{2A}$ receptor antagonism, vary considerably in their affinity for additional receptors, thereby producing a diverse collection of NNSEs. In general, clozapine is the least selective for dopaminergic and serotonergic receptors and produces the greatest number and often the most severe NNSEs among the atypical antipsychotics. Olanzapine and quetiapine, while very well-tolerated, are intermediate in selectivity, and risperidone and ziprasidone are the most selective for D_2 and $5-HT_{2A}$ antagonism and, correspondingly, are expected to have a more limited number of NNSEs.

Cramer and Rosenheck (1998) surveyed the literature on antipsychotic medication and found that fewer than half of patients are compliant with treatment. When patients were asked to rate their experience with conventional antipsychotics, the negative impact of side-effects generally equalled or exceeded the perceived therapeutic benefit (Finn *et al.* 1990). Compliance can best be understood as the complex result of a patient's weighing of perceived therapeutic benefit against adverse effects (Adams & Howe 1993; Hogan *et al.* 1983). The improved compliance reported with several atypical agents has been attributed in part to the relative absence of neurological side-effects. However, in several studies patients rated sedation, weight gain, drooling and sexual dysfunction as even more distressing than neurological side-effects (Finn *et al.* 1990; Larsen & Gerlach 1996; Day *et al.* 1998). This suggests that the improved compliance associated with atypical agents may stem more from an appreciation of greater efficacy than a diminished concern about side-effects; the potential negative impact of NNSEs upon compliance should not be underestimated.

Mood and behavioural effects

The impact of mood upon compliance, therapeutic outcomes and suicide has received new attention as atypical agents have displayed pronounced antidepressant and anxiolytic effects compared with conventional neuroleptics (Kane *et al.* 1988; Marder & Meibach 1994; Tollefson *et al.* 1998). Soon after the introduction of chlorpromazine, the conventional antipsychotics were linked to dysphoric reactions (Fellner 1958). This emergence of dysphoric feelings may, in part, represent a direct effect of conventional antipsychotics, a consequence of extrapyramidal side-effects (EPSs) or the recognition of underlying depression previously obscured by psychotic symptoms. Acutely, conventional antipsychotics can produce dysphoria, anxiety and panic attacks which may be dose related (Sanberg & Norman 1989). Belmaker and Wald (1977) described apathy, profound inner restlessness, anergia and severe anxiety after they administered haloperidol 5 mg intravenously to themselves. Neither investigator was able to return to work for 36 h after this experiment. Caine and Polinsky (1979) reported dysphoria in six of 72 patients with Tourette's syndrome who received haloperidol 2.5–4.0 mg/day. These symptoms were not associated with EPSs and were alleviated with dose reduction. Van Putten *et al.* (1984) reported a 23% incidence of dysphoria following a single oral dose of haloperidol 5 mg, and a 25% incidence following a dose of tiotixine (thiothixene) 0.22 mg/kg. Onset of dysphoria did not correlate with plasma concentrations of haloperidol but did appear to correspond with emergence of akathisia.

Acute dysphoric reactions to antipsychotic agents can be quite distressing. In one study, six of 14 schizophrenia patients attributed their refusal of treatment to prior experiences of neuroleptic-associated dysphoria (Van Putten *et al.* 1981). An early dysphoric response, which may include feelings of listlessness or tension, has also been associated with a poor antipsychotic response in several studies of conventional agents (May *et al.* 1976, 1981; Van Putten & May 1978b; Singh & Kay 1979; Van Putten *et al.* 1981, 1989; Hogan & Awad 1992) and with subsequent poor compliance (Hogan *et al.* 1983; Van Putten 1983). This reaction is not restricted to high-potency agents; in one study, early dysphoria was associated with chlorpromazine at a slightly higher frequency than haloperidol and was not associated with akathisia (Hogan & Awad 1992). The incidence of acute dysphoric response to atypical agents has not been studied.

Akinetic depression

Neuroleptic-associated dysphoria may be a manifestation of parkinsonian akinesia in some patients. Van Putten and May (1978a) reported that more than half of akinetic patients developed a modest, although significant, worsening of dysphoric affect as their psychotic symptoms improved with conventional neuroleptics. Addition of the anticholinergic agent, trihexyphenidyl, improved depression and anxiety in these patients. Marder *et al.* (1984) found elevated levels of depression, interpersonal sensitivity and phobic anxiety in patients treated for 1 month with conventional doses of fluphenazine deconoate (25 mg biweekly) compared with low doses (5 mg biweekly). Ratings of anxiety and depression correlated with ratings of akathisia and retardation. However, Hogarty *et al.* (1995) reported that neither neuroleptic dose reduction nor addition of benztropine improved persistent dysphoria in most patients, whereas addition of thymoleptics improved diverse aspects of mood.

Postpsychotic depression

Although treatment with conventional neuroleptics may be associated with dysphoric response initially and development of EPSs may be linked to modest elevations of anxiety and depression, most depression experienced by patients with schizophrenia is probably unrelated to drug treatment (Barnes *et al.* 1989). Depressive symptoms were described following resolution of acute psychotic episodes long before the introduction of antipsychotic agents (Mayer-Gross 1920) and recently have been found to occur in up to 25% of patients early in the course of schizophrenia (Wassink *et al.* 1999). Robertson and Trimble (1982) reviewed 34 double-blind trials of conventional neuroleptics and concluded that depressive symptoms are more likely to improve than worsen with these agents. Early work attributing 'postpsychotic depression' to drug therapy has not been validated by controlled trials. Most evidence suggests that depressive symptoms are usually present at the time antipsychotic treatment is initiated and improve during the course of treatment, although they may become more prominent as psychotic symptoms recede (Knights & Hirsch 1981). However, in some patients postpsychotic depression may also represent a psychological response to illness, as patients are newly able to assess the impact of psychotic illness upon their lives (McGlashan & Carpenter 1976).

Cognitive effects

The demonstration of an association between tardive dyskinesia (TD) and cognitive impairment raised the concern that antipsychotic agents might produce persistent cognitive dysfunction (Struve & Willner 1983; Ganguli & Raghu 1985; Spohn *et al.* 1985; Waddington 1987; Sorokin *et al.* 1988). However, most evidence suggests that cognitive impairment is a pre-existent risk factor for TD, rather than the result of a shared neurotoxic process, although the mechanism of such an association remains unclear (Spohn & Strauss 1989). Castner *et al.* (2000) recently demonstrated in monkeys that administration of haloperidol for 1–4 months produced severe impairments in working memory and downregulation of D_1 receptors in the frontal cortex. Cognitive deficits were reversed with short-term administration of a D_1 agonist. At typical therapeutic dosage, treatment with conventional neuroleptics is most commonly associated with modest cognitive improvement, particularly in attention, vigilance, distractibility and idiosyncratic thinking (Spohn & Strauss 1989; Cassens & Inglis 1990; King 1990). Atypical antipsychotics have consistently demonstrated larger therapeutic effects upon cognitive functioning compared with conventional agents (Green *et al.* 1997; Keefe *et al.* 1999; Meltzer & McGurk 1999; Purdon *et al.* 2000), although these studies are limited by methodological problems (Harvey & Keefe 2001).

Trials of relatively low dosage of neuroleptics (e.g. chlorpromazine 60 mg/day) have failed to produce cognitive impairment in normal subjects (Liljequist *et al.* 1975, 1978; King 1990). However, cognitive dysfunction may occur at high dosage during clinical use, often associated with a worsening of psychotic symptoms (Tune *et al.* 1980; Cole 1982; Spohn & Strauss 1989). While cognitive impairment has been demonstrated in schizophrenia patients receiving a relatively high dosage of sedating phenothiazines, tolerance appears to develop to this effect (Kornetsky *et al.* 1959; Judson & MacCasland 1960; Latz & Kornetsky 1965). Kornetsky *et al.* (1959) also found that performance of normal subjects on psychomotor tests was more negatively affected by a single dose of phenothiazine (chlorpromazine 100 and 200 mg) than was performance of schizophrenia subjects.

Impairments of memory and the span of apprehension are common in schizophrenia patients prescribed anticholinergic agents for the control of parkinsonian side-effects of their antipsychotic medication. Tune *et al.* (1982) demonstrated that memory impairment in stabilized schizophrenia patients significantly correlated with serum anticholinergic activity and was unrelated to serum levels of antipsychotic medication as measured by radioreceptor assay. Of note, although olanzapine has high affinity *in vitro* for muscarinic acetylcholine receptors, olanzapine has demonstrated cognitive enhancement rather than impairment in animal and human studies, perhaps reflecting the differential effects of muscarinic receptor subtypes (Bymaster *et al.* 1999; Purdon *et al.* 2000).

Linnoila and colleagues (Linnoila 1973; Linnoila & Maki 1974) demonstrated significant impairment of driving-related psychomotor performance in normal subjects after a single 25 mg dose of thioridazine. The impact on simulated driving performance was greater than that produced by diazepam 10 mg or by haloperidol 5 mg. Although most evidence suggests that antipsychotic agents do not impair cognitive function at usual clinical dosage, clinicians should warn patients of the possible risks associated with driving, particularly early in the course of treatment with low-potency conventional antipsychotics. The addition of anticholinergic agents for control of EPSs represents a much more serious threat to cognitive functioning (Baker *et al.* 1983; Goff & Baldessarini 1993). The putative cognitive benefits associated with atypical agents, combined with the reduced need for anticholinergic coadministration, potentially are important advantages for the atypical agents in light of recent evidence indicating a strong correlation between cognitive function and quality of life in patients with schizophrenia (Green 1996).

Endocrine effects

Hyperprolactinaemia

Prolactin secretion from lactotroph cells of the pituitary is tonically inhibited by dopamine acting at D_2 receptors. Conventional neuroleptics elevate prolactin levels by blocking dopaminergic inhibition of the tuberoinfundibular system. In single dose trials, subtherapeutic doses of neuroleptics (i.e. haloperidol 0.5–1.5 mg) produce a maximal prolactin elevation within 1–2 h, which then returns to baseline over approximately 6 h (Gruen *et al.* 1978a,b). Although prolactin levels are generally normal in untreated schizophrenia patients (Nestores *et al.* 1980), Keks *et al.* (1987) demonstrated a blunted prolactin response to a single dose of haloperidol in medication-free men with schizophrenia. With repeated dosing, prolactin levels remain elevated and the degree of elevation tends to correlate with the percentage of D_2 receptor occupation above 50% (Nordstrom & Farde 1998). Six of 17 studies found a correla-

tion between prolactin levels and response to conventional neuroleptics, although these studies are complicated by methological problems (Green & Brown 1988). Additional evidence suggests that tolerance can develop to the prolactin-elevating effect of conventional agents, so that chronically treated patients may have prolactin serum concentrations within the normal range (Gruen *et al.* 1978a; Laughren *et al.* 1979; Kolakowski *et al.* 1981; Igarashi *et al.* 1985; Rubin & Meltzer 1987).

Antipsychotic-induced hyperprolactinaemia underlies several clinical side-effects, although the correlation between prolactin levels and symptoms is complex and estimations of their frequency have been quite variable. Elevated levels of prolactin stimulate breast tissue, which commonly results in breast tenderness, gynaecomastia and galactorrhoea. Galactorrhoea has been reported in as many as 57% of females treated with conventional agents, whereas gynaecomastia is an infrequent complication in men (Robinson 1957; Plante & Roy 1967; Windgassen *et al.* 1996). Hyperprolactaemia can also secondarily lower oestrogen and testosterone levels, which can affect menses and sexual function. As many as 90% of women treated with conventional neuroleptics report changes in their menstrual cycle and 50% report amenorrhoea (Sandison *et al.* 1960; Ghadirian *et al.* 1982; Sullivan & Lukoff 1990).

Hyperprolactinaemia resulting from pituitary tumours is associated with hypogonadism and the loss of up to 25% of trabecular bone density (Klibanski *et al.* 1988; Biller *et al.* 1992), although this potential adverse effect has not been well-studied in women taking antipsychotic agents. Osteopenia does not occur in hyperprolactinaemic women who maintain sufficient oestrogen levels to preserve menses (Klibanski *et al.* 1988), suggesting that oestrogen replacement therapy may be indicated in some cases of hyperprolactinaemia with secondary amenorrhoea. Haloperidol-treated psychiatric patients were found to have a 14% reduction in forearm bone mineral content compared with age- and sex-matched controls (Baastrup *et al.* 1976). Two studies that looked at pathological fractures in neuroleptic-treated patients reported elevated rates (20–25%), but these studies did not include control groups (Abraham *et al.* 1995; Halbreich *et al.* 1995). In addition, patients with schizophrenia are at increased risk for osteopenia on the basis of inadequate exercise, poor nutritional status, cigarette smoking and polydipsia. Hyperprolactinaemia also increases the risk for breast tumours in laboratory animals, but exposure to antipsychotic agents does not appear to increase the risk in humans (Overall 1978).

Kleinberg *et al.* (1999) reported that, despite hyperprolactinaemia comparable to levels produced by haloperidol 20 mg/day, risperidone at a typical clinical dosage of 4–6 mg/day was associated with very low rates of amenorrhoea (7%) and galactorrhoea (1%) in women; these rates did not differ from placebo. In contrast, risperidone 4–6 mg/day produced sexual dysfunction or gynaecomastia in 15% of male subjects compared with an 8% incidence with placebo. The degree of risperidone-induced elevation of prolactin did not correlate with any clinical side-effects. Olanzapine is associated with significantly less prolactin elevation at typical therapeutic doses than risperidone (Tran *et al.* 1997); ziprasidone, quetiapine and clozapine do not produce sustained hyperprolactinaemia (Kane *et al.* 1988; Arvanitis & Miller 1997; Crawford *et al.* 1997; Tran *et al.* 1997; Goff *et al.* 1998). Kapur *et al.* (2001) demonstrated that prolactin levels increase as D_2 receptor occupancy is increased from 55 to 79% with the addition of haloperidol to clozapine, suggesting that differences between agents in liability for hyperprolactinaemia can be accounted for, at least in part, by the relative degree of D_2 receptor blockade (Kapur *et al.* 1999).

Thyroid effects

Haloperidol and perphenazine are both reported to produce a toxic state resembling either thyroid storm or neuroleptic malignant syndrome when administered to patients with pre-existing hyperthyroidism (Weiner 1979; Jefferson & Marshal 1981). This neurotoxic reaction may include fever, rigidity, diaphoresis, dyspnoea and dysphagia. One fatality has been attributed to this combination (Weiner 1979). Although the frequency and mechanism of this adverse effect are unclear, animal studies have indicated that the combination of haloperidol and thyroxine may be toxic (Selye & Szabo 1972). In premarketing trials, quetiapine was found to elevate thyroid-stimulating hormone (TSH), although cases of frank hypothyroidism have not been reported, even when coadministered with lithium (Peuskens & Link 1997; Potkin *et al.* 1997).

Syndrome of inappropriate antidiuretic hormone

The syndrome of inappropriate antidiuretic hormone (SIADH) has been attributed to haloperidol or tiotixine (thiothixine) administration in individual case reports (Aljouni *et al.* 1974; Peck & Shenkman 1979). In an additional case, SIADH was associated with fluphenazine, tiotixine (thiothixine) and trifluoperazine, but resolved when the patient was treated with molindone (Glusac *et al.* 1990). Inappropriate release of antidiuretic hormone (vasopressin) may produce hyponatraemia and symptoms of water intoxication (confusion, lethargy, seizures), particularly in the presence of polydipsia. However, controlled studies in schizophrenia and normal subjects have not demonstrated an elevation of antidiuretic hormone associated with administration of antipsychotic agents (Kendler *et al.* 1978; Raskind *et al.* 1987; Sarai & Matsunaga 1989). In general, treatment with antipsychotic agents is more likely to normalize hyponatraemia in schizophrenia patients than to deregulate sodium metabolism (Illowsky & Kirch 1988). Several case reports have indicated that clozapine may be particularly effective in resolving hyponatraemia in patients with polydipsia (Henderson & Goff 1994).

Weight gain

Weight gain is a serious side-effect of antipsychotic treatment, potentially affecting self-esteem and compliance and placing pa-

tients at risk for cardiovascular disease, diabetes, hypertension, sleep apnoea and certain forms of cancer (National Institute of Health 1998). The long-term medical consequences of obesity are of particular concern given the higher rates of other cardiovascular risk factors in schizophrenia patients, including cigarette smoking (Goff *et al.* 1992) and diabetes (Mukherjee *et al.* 1996). Allison *et al.* (1999) performed a meta-analysis and meta-regression using data from controlled trials to estimate the mean weight gain after 10 weeks of treatment with antipsychotic agents. The effects of conventional agents ranged from a mean loss of 0.4 kg with molindone to a mean gain of 3.2 kg with thioridazine. Haloperidol produced a mean 1.1 kg weight gain. Among atypical agents, only ziprasidone produced no change in weight; the other atypicals were associated with the following estimates of weight gain at 10 weeks: risperidone 2.1 kg; olanazapine 4.15 kg; and clozapine 4.45 kg. Insufficient data were available to calculate mean weight gain with quetiapine. One naturalistic study of 82 patients found a mean weight gain with clozapine of 0.64 kg/week which did not plateau until about month 46 (Henderson *et al.* 2000). In contrast, in a study involving 1996 patients randomized to olanzapine, a mean weight gain of 0.32 kg/week was recorded during the first 6 weeks, which was then reduced to 0.11 kg/week after 30 weeks and reached a plateau after 52 weeks (Beasley *et al.* 2000). In a retrospective review of 92 male schizophrenia patients who had participated in randomized antipsychotic trials and were offered participation in a psychoeducational weight reduction program, Wirshing *et al.* (1999) found that patients treated with olanzapine, risperidone and quetiapine managed to lose more than 50% of the weight gained during the trial, whereas patients treated with clozapine did not lose weight. However, these results are complicated by relatively small numbers of patients and the brief duration of follow-up of clozapine-treated patients compared with olanzapine-treated patients (27 vs. 73 weeks). Risk factors for olanzapine-induced weight gain include increased appetite, male gender, youth and, inconsistently, low baseline weight. Weight gain does not appear to be dose-related. Of interest, some evidence has suggested that weight gain with olanzapine and clozapine may correlate with clinical response (Leadbetter *et al.* 1992; Beasley *et al.* 2000).

The mechanism of antipsychotic-induced weight gain is not fully understood. Weight gain with low-potency conventional agents and atypical agents has been proposed to result from serotonergic receptor blockade (Bernstein 1988; Wirshing *et al.* 1999), although histamine antagonism has also been associated with weight gain.

Diabetes

Type 2 diabetes mellitus has been reported in schizophrenia patients at rates considerably higher than in the general population (Keskiner *et al.* 1973; Mukherjee *et al.* 1996). This elevation in prevalence has been attributed in part to poor diet and lack of exercise. In addition, the phenothiazines have also been linked to elevated blood sugars in studies performed prior to current definitions of diabetes (Charatan & Bartlett 1955; Erle *et al.* 1977). More recently, several cases of new-onset diabetes have been reported following the initiation of clozapine and olanzapine (Popli *et al.* 1997; Wirshing *et al.* 1998; Goldstein *et al.* 1999). Henderson *et al.* (2000) studied 82 outpatients who were switched from conventional antipsychotics to clozapine and found that 37% were diagnosed with new-onset diabetes mellitus during the 5-year follow-up. Neither the clozapine dosage nor degree of weight gain was a significant predictor of treatment-emergent diabetes. Preliminary results from studies employing glucose tolerance tests have suggested that certain atypical agents may decrease insulin sensitivity, although these studies require replication in a prospective randomized trial design. Investigators at Eli Lilly examined non-fasting blood sugars obtained during randomized trials comparing olanzapine with haloperidol and placebo and did not find evidence of an increased rate of elevated blood sugars with olanzapine. Because non-fasting serum glucose measurements are not adequately sensitive or specific for diabetes, additional prospective controlled studies are needed to determine whether the atypicals increase the risk for diabetes.

Sexual dysfunction

Sexual side-effects are an important and under-recognized adverse effect of certain antipsychotic agents. Medication-free male schizophrenia patients report normal levels of sexual interest but decreased activity (Nestoros *et al.* 1981). As many as 60% of schizophrenia patients and 71% of non-schizophrenia patients report sexual dysfunction when treated with conventional neuroleptics. (Degen 1982; Mitchell & Popkin 1982; Bartholomew 1986). In one survey, 30% of women with schizophrenia treated with conventional agents complained of sexual dysfunction and 54% of men; changes in the quality of orgasm was the most common complaint (Ghadirian *et al.* 1982). Finn *et al.* (1990) found that men with schizophrenia rated impotence as bothering them more than any other drug side-effect and more than any symptom of their illness. Hyperprolactinaemia may be one mechanism responsible for sexual dysfunction, because secondary reduction of gonadal hormones can diminish libido in both sexes.

Erectile dysfunction often develops shortly after initiating conventional neuroleptic treatment, particularly with thioridazine. Kotin *et al.* (1976) found that 44% of men treated with thioridazine described difficulty in achieving an erection compared with 19% of men treated with other antipsychotic agents. In one case, chlorpromazine-induced ejaculatory dysfunction resolved after the daily dose was decreased from 1000 mg to 600 mg (Greenberg 1971). Erectile dysfunction usually resolves fairly quickly after the neuroleptic is discontinued (Mitchell & Popkin 1982). Thioridazine may also produce ejaculatory inhibition more frequently than other neuroleptics. Ejaculatory dysfunction is described by 30–50% of men treated with thiori-

dazine and may occur at a dosage as low as 30 mg/day (Heller 1961; Shader 1964; Blair & Simpson 1966; Kotin *et al.* 1976). Ejaculatory difficulties have also been reported with mesoridazine (Shader 1972) and occur infrequently with higher potency neuroleptics (Blair & Simpson 1966). Priapism or prolonged erection has been reported with phenothiazines, clozapine, risperidone and olanzapine (Dorman & Schmidt 1976; Rosen & Hanno 1992; Seftel *et al.* 1992; Emes & Millson 1994; Tekell *et al.* 1995; Deirmenjian *et al.* 1998; Heckers *et al.* 1998; Gordon & de Groot 1999). Mitchell and Popkin (1982) found 19 published reports of priapism with conventional neuroleptics; thioridazine or chlorpromazine were responsible in all but one case. α1-Adrenergic antagonism is probably the primary mechanism responsible for priapism (Compton & Miller 2001).

Cardiovascular effects

Cardiac conduction

Several reports of sudden death have been attributed to thioridazine or chlorpromazine therapy in young healthy patients (Aherwadker *et al.* 1964; Giles & Modlin 1968). Postmortem studies revealed intramyocardial lesions secondary to the accumulation of acid mucopolysaccharides believed to be related to chronic neuroleptic exposure (Richardson *et al.* 1966). The World Health Organization database of adverse drug reports recently linked myocarditis and cardiomyopathy to clozapine and less strongly to other antipsychotics as a group (Coulter *et al.* 2001). The frequency of fatal arrhythmias associated with antipsychotic treatment remains difficult to determine, because some cases may result from other causes such as aspiration or asphyxiation (Leestma & Koenig 1968; Moore & Book 1969). Efforts to determine whether the incidence of sudden death increased with the introduction of neuroleptic treatment produced conflicting results (Brill & Patton 1962; Richardson *et al.* 1966).

Thioridazine, and possibly certain metabolites, slows atrial and ventricular conduction and prolongs refractory periods (Descotes *et al.* 1979; Yoon *et al.* 1979; Hartigan-Go *et al.* 1996). Because the effect is concentration-dependent, thioridazine can be highly dangerous if taken in overdose or in combination with quinidine-like drugs (Risch *et al.* 1981). Chlorpromazine also prolongs the QT interval and atrial–ventricular conduction, even at relatively low dosage (150 mg/day) (Ban & St. Jean 1964). In addition, pimozide may produce significant changes in cardiac conduction as a result of its calcium-channel blocking properties (Opler & Feinberg 1991). It is recommended that serial electrocardiograms (ECGs) be performed when treatment with pimozide is started and the drug should be stopped if the QT interval exceeds 520 ms in adults or 470 ms in children (Baldessarini 1985). Extremely high doses of intravenous haloperidol (up to 1000 mg in 24 h) have been administered safely in patients with cardiac disease, although rare cases of *torsade de pointes* have been reported at these doses (Metzger & Friedman 1993; Hatta *et al.* 2001).

In materials submitted to the Psychopharmacological Drugs Advisory Committee of the Food and Drug Administration (FDA), Pfizer, Inc. reported results from a trial designed to examine ECG effects of atypical agents and thioridazine at maximum therapeutic serum concentrations and at the potentially higher concentrations that might occur in clinical practice if coprescribed with metabolic inhibitors. Using the Bazett correction, which adjusts the QT interval for heart rate, thioridazine produced the greatest mean delay in QTc (35.6 ms) followed by ziprasidone (20.3 ms), quetiapine (9.1 ms), olanzapine (6.8 ms) and haloperidol (4.7 ms). Quetiapine produced the greatest increase in heart rate (11 beats per minute) and so calculation of its effect on QTc was the most affected by the Bazett correction. Addition of metabolic inhibitors produced further increases in QTc when added to quetiapine (19.7 ms) and haloperidol (8.9 ms) only. The mean 39% increase in serum ziprasidone concentrations produced by ketaconazole coadministration did not result in an increase in the mean QTc duration. Although ziprasidone serum concentrations were found to correlate with QTc duration, the slope of the relationship was not steep (0.05 ms/ng/mL). In eight cases of overdose reported by the manufacturer and one published case (Burton *et al.* 2000), ziprasidone did not produce significant cardiac toxicity. Pfizer also reported to the FDA that only two of 3095 subjects (0.06%) in premarketing trials developed QTc intervals longer than 500 ms; participants in these trials were screened to exclude cardiac disease. In two reports of overdose with quetiapine, prolongation of the QT interval has been observed (Hustey 1999; Gajwani *et al.* 2000), whereas most reported cases of overdose with risperidone and olanzapine have described relatively benign ECG findings (Acri & Henretig 1998; Cohen *et al.* 1999). The cardiac effects of atypical agents in patients with underlying heart disease have not been adequately studied.

Orthostatic hypotension

Orthostatic hypotension is also commonly reported with low-potency neuroleptics and with some atypical agents; it is believed to result from α-adrenergic blockade (Richelson 1984). Oral administration of a moderate dosage of chlorpromazine (50–200 mg/day) generally does not produce significant changes in systolic blood pressure, whereas intravenous or intramuscular administration of moderate dosage is associated with a high frequency of hypotensive reactions (Bourgeois-Govardin *et al.* 1955; Blumberg *et al.* 1964; Korol *et al.* 1965). Silver *et al.* (1990) measured blood pressure at rest and standing in 196 schizophrenia patients chronically treated with conventional neuroleptics and found that 77% displayed postural hypotension after 1 min standing and 17% after 3 min. Although the mean systolic blood pressure drop at 1 min was 28 mmHg, patients did not report dizziness or light-headedness. The degree of blood pressure drop did not correlate with dose or with age of the patient. Thioridazine affected blood pressure significantly more than did chlorpromazine or haloperidol. Surprisingly, the drop in pressure did not correlate with α1 adrenergic receptor

binding activity. Clozapine and quetiapine also have potent α adrenergic antagonist effects and can produce orthostatic hypotension and resting tachycardia early in the course of treatment (Baldessarini & Frankenburg 1991; Arvanitis & Miller 1997; Small *et al.* 1997). Tolerance develops to the cardiovascular effects of both drugs and the use of low dosage at the initiation of treatment reduces the risks of hypotension (Ereshefsky *et al.* 1989). Despite gradual titration, quetiapine is associated with a 12–14% incidence of orthostatic hypotension in healthy non-elderly patients (Arvanitis & Miller 1997). Although hypotension has not been reported with risperidone in controlled trials in healthy subjects (Chouinard *et al.* 1993; Marder & Meibach 1994), in an uncontrolled naturalistic pharmacoepidemiological study of elderly patients treated with risperidone (mean dosage 1.6 mg/day), Zarate *et al.* (1997) reported hypotension in 29% of patients, symptomatic orthostasis in 10%, and cardiac arrest in 1.6%.

Cutaneous effects

Allergic reactions

Antipsychotic drugs can affect the skin as a result of allergic reactions, photosensitivity effects or pigmentary changes (Zelickson 1966; Kimyai-Asadi *et al.* 1999). Cutaneous allergic reactions to antipsychotic agents typically occur 2–10 weeks after the initiation of treatment and present with maculopapular rashes on the face, neck, chest or extremities. Discontinuation of the offending agent usually results in a clearing of skin lesions within a week. Cases of 'cross-allergy' to other antipsychotic drugs have been reported and should be monitored when switching to a new agent. Occasionally, antipsychotic agents can produce severe cutaneous reactions, such as exfoliative dermatitis, generalized urticaria and angioneurotic oedema. Discontinuation of the drug and treatment with antihistamines or topical steroids are usually sufficient for cutaneous reactions. Desensitization protocols have been developed for antibiotics, and recently fluoxetine, but have not been tested with antipsychotic agents (Leznoff & Binkley 1992).

Photosensitivity

Low-potency phenothiazines (e.g. chlorpromazine and thioridazine) produce enhanced sensitivity to sunlight in about 3% of patients. Photosensitivity reactions resemble sunburn and appear on areas of the body exposed to sunlight. Although the mechanism is not understood, photosensitivity may involve the formation of free radicals which can injure cells in the skin (Chignell *et al.* 1985). Patients treated with such agents should be warned about the risk of prolonged exposure to sunlight during summer months. Antipsychotic agents can also produce discoloration of exposed skin by affecting melatonin metabolism. Pigmentary changes may first appear like a dark tan and progress to blue or purple; they are frequently associated with pigmentary changes in the eye. The incidence of cutaneous pigmentation has been estimated at about 1–3% in patients treated with low-potency phenothiazines (Greiner & Berry 1964; Ban & Lehmann 1965; Ananth et al. 1972). Although it is generally believed that chlorpromazine is most likely to produce cutaneous pigmentation, Ban et al. (1985) reported similar rates with haloperidol in a multinational study. However, four cases have been reported of chlorpromazine-associated pigmentation which resolved when the patients were switched to haloperidol (Thompson et al. 1988).

Ocular effects

Ocular changes associated with pigmentation of the skin were first reported with chlorpromazine by Greiner and Berry (1964). As many as 79% of patients treated with chlorpromazine exhibit white or yellow–brown deposits on the cornea or lens (Siddall 1968). Epithelial keratopathy, presenting as clouding of the anterior cornea in the area of the palpebral fissure, has also been attributed to chlorpromazine exposure. Pigmentation of the retina is reported in about 20% of chlorpromazine-treated patients. Pigmentary changes in the eye, like cutaneous pigmentation, probably involve melanin metabolism and are related to the dose and duration of exposure to chlorpromazine. Fortunately, vision is rarely affected. Ocular pigmentation has also been reported with perphenazine, tiotixine (thiothixine) and trifluoperazine, but is believed to occur at a much lower frequency with these agents (Prien et al. 1970; Barron et al. 1972; Fraunfelder & Meyer 1982). Ulberg et al. (1970) reported the rare occurrence of ocular pigmentary changes in infants exposed in utero to phenothiazines.

Thioridazine appears to be unique in producing irreversible pigmentary retinopathy. While retinal toxicity has been reported at relatively low dosage, it usually results from dosage greater than 800 mg/day given for periods of several months or longer. Clinical manifestations include diminished visual acuity, loss of peripheral vision and scotoma. The mechanism of thioridazine-induced retinopathy remains unclear, although it may involve free-radical injury to the rods, resulting in part from a loss of the protective action of melanin. Cases of chromatopsia in which patients describe 'yellow vision' or 'red vision' have also been associated with thioridazine.

Two recent surveys of patients with schizophrenia have found lenticular opacities in 22 and 26% of patients – rates much higher than expected in the general population (Smith et al. 1997; McCarty et al. 1999). Several factors may increase risk for cataracts in patients with schizophrenia, including cigarette smoking, diabetes, trauma and ultraviolet exposure. In addition, patients treated for 2–5 years with phenothiazines were found to have a 3.5-fold higher rate of cataract extraction than a cohort matched for age and sex (Isaac et al. 1991). Haloperidol treatment was not associated with an increased incidence of cataracts. Quetiapine was found in preclinical toxicology studies performed in beagles to increase the frequency of cataracts; an increased rate of cataracts was not found in subsequent primate studies. Spontaneous clinician reports of lens opacities through June 1999, during which time an estimated 300 000 patients had been prescribed quetiapine, did not provide evidence of an increased rate compared with the expected rate in the general population (Nasrallah et al. 1999).

Gastrointestinal and hepatic effects

Xerostomia (dry mouth) is a common anticholinergic side-effect associated with low-potency neuroleptics and with antiparkinsonian agents (Sreebny & Schwartz 1986). Xerostomia may cause difficulties with chewing, swallowing and speaking, and increases vulnerability to dental caries and candidiasis. Attempts to alleviate a dry mouth by sucking on candy or drinking sweetened beverages can further increase the risk of dental infection and obesity. Although patients may cease to complain of a dry mouth over time, studies of salivary production in patients taking nortriptyline indicate that tolerance does not develop to this side-effect (Asberg et al. 1970; Bertram et al. 1979) and probably does not develop with antipsychotic-induced anticholinergic effects as well. Sialorrhoea occurs in approximately 23% of patients treated with clozapine (Baldessarini & Frankenburg 1991). Patients may report soaking their pillows at night and some experience a distressing sensation of choking on their saliva. The mechanism of clozapine-induced sialorrhoea remains unclear and is paradoxical in light of its strong anticholinergic effects. Impaired oesophageal motility may contribute to this side-effect, as demonstrated by barium swallow (Pearlman 1994).

In addition to the possible effects of clozapine upon oesophageal epistasis, anticholinergic effects of antipsychotic agents can impair the gag reflex, placing patients at risk for aspiration, particularly if swallowing is already impaired. The presence of TD may be an additional factor affecting the gag reflex; Craig et al. (1982) found an impaired gag reflex in 74% of schizophrenia patients with TD taking anticholinergic agents vs. 30% of the remainder of schizophrenia patients. However, in one study of drug-free schizophrenia patients, half displayed abnormalities in swallowing (Husser & Bragg 1969). Anticholinergic effects of low-potency neuroleptics and clozapine can also slow gastric emptying and impair intestinal and colonic motility, producing gastroesophageal reflux, anorexia, nausea, vomiting, constipation and abdominal distention or obstruction (Warnes et al. 1967; Davis & Nusbaum 1973; Giordano et al. 1975; Evans et al. 1979; Kemeny et al. 1980). Paralytic ileus has also been reported with haloperidol and clozapine (Maltbie et al. 1981; Erickson et al. 1995; Tang & Ungvari 1999).

Hepatic effects

Antipsychotic agents produce several effects on the liver, ranging from benign elevation of liver enzymes to cholestatic jaundice and hepatocellular toxicity (Leipzig 1992). Chlorpromazine is the best studied in relation to liver function, and may be the most likely to produce toxicity. Patients treated with chlorpromazine, clozapine and olanzapine commonly display mild elevation of liver enzymes during the first month of exposure, which appear to be benign and usually return to normal despite continued treatment (Dickes *et al.* 1957; Shay & Siplet 1957; Bartholomew *et al.* 1958; Lieberman *et al.* 1989; Tollefson *et al.* 1997). However, chlorpromazine has direct hepatotoxic effects which can result in subclinical cholecstasis and damage to liver cells (Sherlock 1979, 1989; Kaplowitz *et al.* 1986). Hydroxylated metabolites of chlorpromazine may be particularly hepatotoxic, possibly as a result of the production of free radicals (Samuels & Carey 1978; Watson *et al.* 1988). Patients who produce higher levels of these metabolites, because of reduced sulphoxidation of the parent compound, may be at greater risk for cholestatic jaundice. Approximately 1–2% of patients treated with chlorpromazine develop cholestatic jaundice within 1–5 weeks of starting to take the drug (Ishak & Irey 1972; Zimmerman & Ishak 1987). This appears to be a hypersensitivity reaction as it is usually accompanied by eosinophilia, fever and rash, and rapidly recurs when the patient is rechallenged. Fortunately, most patients recover within 1 year and tolerate other classes of antipsychotics without cross-reactivity. While haloperidol has also been associated with hepatotoxicity, the risk is estimated to be quite low (approximately 0.2%) (Crane 1959; Fuller *et al.* 1977; Dincsoy & Saelinger 1982; Leipzig 1992).

Haematological effects

Agranulocytosis caused by clozapine is the most serious haematological side-effect produced by antipsychotic agents. With weekly or biweekly monitoring, clozapine-induced agranulocytosis has been reduced to approximately 0.4% of exposed patients, with about 80% of cases occurring within the first 18 weeks of exposure (Krupp & Barnes 1989; Honigfeld *et al.* 1998). Ashkenazi Jews with histocompatibility antigen (HLA) types B38, DR4, DQW3 and patients of Finnish descent may be at increased risk (Amsler *et al.* 1977; Lieberman *et al.* 1990). The mechanism appears to be immune related, as sensitization is suggested by the more rapid relapse following rechallenge and by the presence of a distinct antibody in the immunoglobulin M (IgM) fraction of sera from patients who develop agranulocytosis (Lieberman *et al.* 1988; Claas 1989). Leucopenia is much more common with clozapine than agranulocytosis and is not associated with increased risk for agranulocytosis. Eosinophilia, leucocytosis and thrombocytopenia have also been reported with clozapine. Several cases have been reported of granulocytopenia occurring in patients treated with olanzapine following treatment with clozapine (Kraus *et al.* 2000; Teter *et al.* 2000). However, olanzapine has also been used safely during clozapine-induced agranulocytosis (Oyewumi & Al-Semaan 2000).

Earlier surveys of patients treated with relatively high doses of phenothiazines found an incidence of agranulocytosis of about 0.5% and benign leucopenia (white blood cell count

2.5–4.0 × 10⁹/L) in about 10% of patients (Pisciotta 1969, 1992; Litvak & Kaelblin 1971). Subsequent studies suggested that use of lower doses of chlorpromazine may have substantially reduced the risk of agranulocytosis, and that earlier studies may have included patients with complicating medical illnesses (Levinson & Simpson 1987). Phenothiazine-associated agranulocytosis generally occurs between 20 and 90 days after initiating treatment and may be more common in elderly women (Mandel & Gross 1968; Pisciotta 1969). Unlike clozapine, the phenothiazines are believed to produce agranulocytosis via direct bone marrow toxicity (Pisciotta 1971, 1973). Agranulocytosis secondary to both clozapine and phenothiazine exposure is generally reversible; with discontinuation of the drug and proper medical care, recovery is common (Lieberman *et al.* 1988). Granulocyte colony-stimulating factor may be effective in cases of severe granulocytopenia (Sperner-Unterweger *et al.* 1998).

Seizures

Chlorpromazine had been marketed for less than 1 year before a case of seizure was associated with its use (Anton-Stephens 1953). Logothetis (1967) studied 859 patients treated with phenothiazines over 5 years and found a 1.2% risk for seizures. The risk for seizures was strongly related to dosage, and approached 10% in patients treated with more than 1000 mg/day chlorpromazine. Rapid increases in dose and the presence of organic brain disease also increased the risk for seizures. Data from the Boston Collaborative Drug Surveillance Program indicated a 0.22% frequency of seizures in patients treated with chlorpromazine (Jick *et al.* 1970). Other surveys have supported the relationship between seizures and higher dosage of phenothiazines (Schlichther *et al.* 1956; Messing *et al.* 1984). The risk of seizures is greatest with clozapine, reaching an estimated frequency of 10% in patients receiving the drug for 3.8 years (Devinsky *et al.* 1991). The risk of clozapine-associated seizures is also increased with dosage and with rapid dose escalation. Most patients can continue treatment with clozapine after a seizure, with addition of an anticonvulsant or dose reduction (Devinsky *et al.* 1991). Prophylactic treatment with an anticonvulsant has been suggested for some patients treated with high-dose clozapine (Baldessarini & Frankenburg 1991). For antipsychotic agents other than clozapine, the risk of provoking seizures in patients with epilepsy appears to be quite small. One study found that the addition of psychotropic medication, including antipsychotics, was generally associated with improved seizure control (Ojemann *et al.* 1987).

The mechanism by which antipsychotic agents affect seizure threshold remains unclear. Animal studies suggest that the seizure threshold is elevated by dopamine agonists (McKenzie & Soroko 1972; Meldrum *et al.* 1975) and lowered by cholinergic agents (Millichap *et al.* 1968; Arnold *et al.* 1974). These observations led to the recommendation that highly anticholinergic agents such as thioridazine be selected for patients at risk for seizures (Remick & Fine 1979). However, seizures are probably quite infrequent with haloperidol, an agent without appreciable anticholinergic activity (Baldessarini & Lipinski 1976). In general, the least-sedating agents may be least likely to produce seizures (Itil & Soldatos 1980). In mice, chlorpromazine, promethazine and mepazine lower the seizure threshold, whereas trifluoperazine and prochloroperazine produce little or no effect (Tedeschi *et al.* 1958). Animal models and *in vitro* methods for assessing relative drug effects on seizure threshold have produced complex and often conflicting results (Tedeschi *et al.* 1958; Chen *et al.* 1968; Oliver *et al.* 1982). Effects on seizure threshold may follow curvilinear relationships with respect to brain concentrations for some conventional neuroleptics (Oliver *et al.* 1982). Olanzapine is reported to increase slowing on the EEG, but is not associated with epileptiform activity or seizures (Beasley *et al.* 2000; Pillmann *et al.* 2000).

Neuroleptic malignant syndrome

Neuroleptic malignant syndrome (NMS) is a potentially lethal complication of antipsychotic treatment, usually characterized by hyperthermia, rigidity, confusion, diaphoresis, autonomic instability, elevated creatinine phosphokinase (CPK) and leucocytosis. Most cases of NMS occur during the first 2 weeks of exposure, although it can occur at any time (Addonizio *et al.* 1987). NMS has been viewed as a spectrum disorder, with a full syndromal frequency estimated at 0.02–2.4% and with mild subsyndromal cases occurring at a rate of about 12% in patients treated with conventional neuroleptics (Addonizio *et al.* 1987; Keck *et al.* 1987, 1989; Adityanjee *et al.* 1988). Because of the relative infrequency of this adverse reaction, identification of risk factors and assessment of treatment efficacy remain quite preliminary. Possible risk factors for NMS include: male gender, the presence of organic brain disease or mental retardation, high dosage or rapid escalation of neuroleptic dose, concomitant lithium administration and intramuscular administration of high-potency antipsychotic agents (Addonizio *et al.* 1987; Keck *et al.* 1987, 1989). Cases of NMS have occurred most frequently with high-potency agents, but it remains unclear whether this association merely reflects the more widespread clinical use of these agents (Levenson 1985).

The mechanism of NMS also is uncertain. Parallels have been drawn between NMS and malignant hyperthermia, largely on the basis of common clinical characteristics (Addonizio *et al.* 1987). However, patients with a history of either NMS or malignant hyperthermia appear to be at no increased risk for developing the other syndrome, and analysis of muscle biopsies has not consistently demonstrated a physiological link between the two conditions (Addonizio *et al.* 1987). It has been observed that some patients with Parkinson's disease develop an NMS-like syndrome when dopamine agonists are abruptly discontinued, suggesting that dysregulation of dopaminergic function is involved in the aetiology of NMS (Friedman *et al.* 1985).

Neuroleptic-induced heatstroke may also present with fever and elevated CPK, but can usually be distinguished from NMS by the presence of agitation, muscle flaccidity and dry skin (Lazarus 1989). Heat intolerance has been demonstrated in patients treated with conventional neuroleptics, although whether this dysregulation in temperature control is entirely the result of medication or in part a characteristic of schizophrenia has not been clarified (Hermesh *et al.* 2000). Neuroleptic-induced heatstroke has been associated with mortality rates of 20–50% (Mann & Bolger 1978).

More difficult to rule out as part of the differential diagnosis of NMS is lethal catatonia, a febrile form of catatonia which occurs in medication-free patients and which often exhibits all the clinical signs of NMS (Weller 1992; White 1992). It is possible that some cases of NMS are actually lethal catatonia, or represent an interaction between lethal catatonia and dopamine-blocking drugs. White and Robins (1991) observed that in five consecutive cases of NMS, a catatonic state preceded the administration of a neuroleptic and the subsequent onset of NMS. These authors have suggested a 'neuroleptic-aggravated' form of catatonia (White & Robins 1991; White 1992).

If NMS develops, the offending agent should be immediately discontinued and the patient hospitalized for hydration, temperature control and monitoring of vital signs and renal function. Bromocriptine and dantrolene may facilitate recovery, although neither has been studied in controlled trials and data on efficacy remain unclear (Rosebush & Stewart 1989; Sakkas *et al.* 1991). Although a 15% mortality rate has been reported, patients with NMS usually recover within an average of 14 days, or approximately 30 days if treated with depot neuroleptic at the time of onset of NMS (Addonizio *et al.* 1987). Duration of time elapsed between the resolution of NMS and restarting antipsychotic medication appears to be an important determinant of the risk for relapse (Rosebush *et al.* 1989). Although cases have been reported of NMS occurring in patients treated with clozapine and the other atypical antipsychotics, the risk of NMS is thought to be lower (Anderson & Powers 1991; DasGupta & Young 1991; Miller *et al.* 1991; Meterissian 1996; Hasan & Buckley 1998; Johnson & Bruxner 1998; Levenson 1999; al-Waneen 2000). The relative frequency of NMS with atypical agents and the suggestion that some cases may be 'atypical' without rigidity remain controversial (Hasan & Buckley 1998).

Conclusions

Antipsychotic agents produce a diverse collection of NNSEs, reflecting the large number of neurotransmitter systems affected by the phenothiazines and atypical antipsychotics. Despite this wide range of side-effects, these agents have a very high therapeutic index and are relatively safe when taken in overdose. The most common side-effects are related to weight gain; the incidence of clinical side-effects related to hyperprolactinaemia in patients treated with conventional agents and risperidone remains unclear. The most serious side-effects include agranulocytosis with clozapine, cardiac arrhythmias which have been linked most convincingly to low-potency phenothiazines but remain a concern with certain atypical agents, and NMS, which can occur with any antipsychotic agent. As neurological side-effects become less pronounced with the new atypical agents, attention should increasingly be paid to the NNSEs which also significantly affect outcome and compliance. A broad understanding of many physiological systems is necessary to predict, diagnose and manage this wide range of adverse effects.

References

Abraham, G., Friedman, R., Verghese, C. & DeLeon, J. (1995) Osteoporosis and schizophrenia: can we limit known risk factors? *Biological Psychiatry* 38, 131–132.

Acri, A.A. & Henretig, F.M. (1998) Effects of risperidone in overdose. *American Journal of Emergency Medicine* 16, 498–501.

Adams, S.G. & Howe, J.T. (1993) Predicting medication compliance in a psychotic population. *Journal of Nervous and Mental Disease* 181, 558–560.

Addonizio, G., Susman, V.L. & Roth, S.D. (1987) Neuroleptic malignant syndrome: review and analysis of 115 cases. *Biological Psychiatry* 22, 1004–1020.

Adityanjee, Singh, S., Singh, G. & Ong, S. (1988) Spectrum concept of neuroleptic malignant syndrome. *British Journal of Psychiatry* 153, 107–111.

Aherwadker, S.J., Eferdigil, M.C. & Coulshed, N. (1964) Chlorpromazine therapy and associated acute disturbances of cardiac rhythm. *British Heart Journal* 36, 1251–1252.

Aljouni, K., Kern, M.W., Tures, J.F., Theil, G.B. & Hagan, T.C. (1974) Thiothixene induced hyponatraemia. *Archives of Internal Medicine* 134, 1103–1105.

Allison, D.B., Mentore, J.L., Heo, M. *et al.* (1999) Antipsychotic-induced weight gain: a comprehensive research synthesis. *American Journal of Psychiatry* 156, 1686–1696.

Amsler, H.A., Teerenhovi, L., Barth, E., Harjula, K. & Vuopio, P. (1977) Agranulocytosis in patients treated with clozapine: a study of the Finnish epidemic. *Acta Psychiatrica Scandinavica* 56, 241–248.

Ananth, J.V., Ban, T.A., Lehmann, H.E. & Rizvi, F.A. (1972) A survey of phenothiazine-induced skin pigmentation. *Indian Journal of Psychiatry* 14, 76–80.

Anderson, E.S. & Powers, P.S. (1991) Neuroleptic malignant syndrome associated with clozapine use. *Journal of Clinical Psychiatry* 52, 102–104.

Anton-Stephens, D. (1953) Preliminary observations on the psychiatric use of chlorpromazine. *Journal of Mental Science* 100, 543–547.

Arnold, P., Racine, R.J. & Wise, R. (1974) Effect of atropine, reserpine, 6-OHDA and handling on seizure development in the rat. *Experimental Neurology* 45, 355–363.

Arvanitis, L. & Miller, B. (1997) Multiple fixed doses of 'Seroquel' (quetiapine) in patients with acute exacerbation of schizophrenia: a comparison with haloperidol and placebo. *Biological Psychiatry* 42, 233–246.

Asberg, M., Cronholm, B., Sjooqvist, F. & Tuck, D. (1970) Correlation of subjective side effects with plasma concentrations of nortriptyline. *British Medical Journal* 4, 18–21.

Baastrup, P.C., Hollnagel, P., Sorensen, R. & Schou, M. (1976) Adverse reactions in treatment with lithium carbonate and haloperidol. *Journal of the American Medical Association* 236, 2645–2646.

Baker, L.A., Cheng, L.Y. & Amara, I.B. (1983) The withdrawal of benztropine mesylate in chronic schizophrenic patients. *British Journal of Psychiatry* 143, 584–590.

Baldessarini, R. (1985) *Chemotherapy in Psychiatry: Principles and Practice*, 2nd edn. Harvard University Press, Cambridge, MA.

Baldessarini, R.J. & Frankenburg, R. (1991) Clozapine: a novel antipsychotic agent. *New England Journal of Medicine* 324, 746–754.

Baldessarini, R.J. & Lipinski, J.F. (1976) Toxicity and side effects of antipsychotic, antimanic and antidepressant medications. *Psychiatry Annuals* 6, 484–493.

Ban, T.A. & Lehmann, H.E. (1965) Skin pigmentation, a rare side effect of chlorpromazine. *Canadian Psychiatric Association Journal* 10, 112–124.

Ban, T.A. & St. Jean, A. (1964) The effects of phenothiazines on the electrocardiogram. *Canadian Medical Association Journal* 91, 537–540.

Ban, T.A., Guy, W. & Wilson, W.H. (1985) Neuroleptic-induced skin pigmentation in chronic hospitalized schizophrenic patients. *Canadian Journal of Psychiatry* 30, 406–408.

Barnes, T.R.E., Curson, D.A., Liddle, P.F. & Patel, M. (1989) The nature and prevalence of depression in chronic schizophrenic in-patients. *British Journal of Psychiatry* 154, 486–491.

Barron, C.N., Murchison, T.E., Rubin, M.L. *et al.* (1972) Chlorpromazine and the eye of the dog. VI. A comparison of phenothiazine tranquilizers. *Experimental and Molecular Pathology* 16, 172–179.

Bartholomew, A.A. (1986) A long acting phenothiazine as a possible agent to control deviant sexual behavior. *American Journal of Psychiatry* 124, 77–83.

Bartholomew, L.G., Cain, J.G., Frazier, S. *et al.* (1958) Effect of chlorpromazine on the liver. *Gastroenterology* 34, 1096–1107.

Beasley, C.M.J., Grundy, S.L., Gannon, K.S. & Berg P.H. (2000) Overview of the safety of olanzapine. In: *Olanzapine (Zyprexa): a Novel Antipsychotic* (eds P.V. Tran, F.P. Bymaster, N. Tye *et al.*), pp. 280–199. Lippincott, Williams & Wilkins Healthcare, Philadelphia.

Belmaker, R.H. & Wald, D. (1977) Haloperidol in normals. *British Journal of Psychiatry* 131, 222–223.

Bernstein, J.G. (1988) Psychotropic drug induced weight gain: mechanisms and management. *Clinical Neuropharmacolology* 11, S194–S206.

Bertram, U., Kragh-Sorenson, P., Rafaelson, O.J. & Larsen, N. (1979) Saliva secretion following long term antidepressant treatment with nortriptyline controlled by plasma levels. *Scandinavian Journal of Dental Research* 87, 58–64.

Biller, B., Baum, H., Rosenthal, D. *et al.* (1992) Progressive trabecular osteopenia in women with hyperprolactinaemic amenorrhoea. *Journal of Clinical Endocrinology and Metabolism* 75, 692–697.

Blair, J. & Simpson, G. (1966) Effect of antipsychotic drugs on reproductive functions. *Dieases of the Nervous System* 27, 645–647.

Blumberg, A.G., Klein, D.F. & Pollack, M. (1964) Effects of chlorpromazine amd imipramine on systolic blood pressure in psychiatric patients: relationship to age, diagnosis and initial blood pressure. *Journal of Psychiatic Research* 2, 51–60.

Bourgeois-Govardin, M., Nowill, W.K., Margolis, G. & Stephen, C.R. (1955) Chlorpromazine: a laboratory and clinical investigation. *Anesthesiology* 16, 829–847.

Brill, M. & Patton, R.E. (1962) Clinical-statistical analysis of population changes in New York state mental hospitals since the introduction of psychotropic drugs. *American Journal of Psychiatry* 119, 20–33.

Burton, S., Heslop, K., Harrison, K. & Barnes, M. (2000) Ziprasidone overdose [letter]. *American Journal of Psychiatry* 157, 835.

Bymaster, F.P., Perry, K.W., Nelson, D.L. *et al.* (1999) Olanzapine: a basic science update. *British Journal of Psychiatry* 174 (Suppl. 37), 36–40.

Caine, E.D. & Polinsky, R.J. (1979) Haloperidol-induced dysphoria in patients with Tourette syndrome. *American Journal of Psychiatry* 136, 1216–1217.

Cassens, G., Inglis, A.K., Appelbaum P.S. & Gutheil T.G.. (1990) Neuroleptics: effects on neuropsychological function in chronic schizophrenic patients. *Schizophrenia Bulletin* **16**, 477–499.

Castner, S.A., Williams, G.V. & Goldman-Rakic, P.S. (2000) Reversal of working memory deficits by short-term dopamine D$_1$ receptor stimulation. *Science* **287**, 2020–2022.

Charatan, F.B.E. & Bartlett, N.G. (1955) The effect of chlorpromazine ('Largactil') on glucose tolerance. *Journal of Mental Scieince* **101**, 351–353.

Chen, G., Ensor, C.R. & Bohner, B. (1968) Studies of drug effects on electrically induced extensor seizures and clinical implications. *Archives of International Pharmacodynics* **172**, 183–218.

Chignell, C.F., Motten, A.G. & Buettner, G.R. (1985) Photoinduced free radicals from chlorpromazine and related phenothiazines: relationship to phenothiazine-induced photosensitization. *Environmental Health Perspective* **64**, 103–110.

Chouinard, G., Jones, B., Remington, G. *et al.* (1993) A Canadian multicenter placebo-controlled study of fixed doses of risperidone and haloperidol in the treatment of chronic schizophrenic patients. *Journal of Clinical Psychopharmacology* **13**, 25–40.

Claas, F.H.J. (1989) Drug-induced agranulocytosis: review of possible mechanisms, and prospects for clozapine studies. *Psychopharmacology* **99** (Suppl.), 113–117.

Cohen, L.G., Fatalo, A., Thompson, B.T. *et al.* (1999) Olanzapine overdose with serum concentrations. *Annuals of Emergency Medicine* **34**, 275–278.

Cole, J.O. (1982) Psychopharmacology update: antipsychotic drugs – is more better? *McLean Hospital Journal* **7**, 61–87.

Compton, M.T. & Miller, A.H. (2001) Priapism associated with conventional and atypical antipsychotic medications: a review. *Journal of Clinical Psychiatry* **62**, 362–366.

Coulter, D.M., Bate, A., Meyboom, R.H.B., Lindquist, M. & Edwards, I.R. (2001) Antipsychotic drugs and heart muscle disorder in international pharmacovigilance: data mining study. *British Medical Journal* **322**, 1207–1209.

Craig, T.J., Richardson, M.A., Bark, N.J. & Klebanov, R. (1982) Impairment of swallowing, tardive dyskinesia, and anticholinergic use. *Psychopharmacology (Berl)* **18**, 84–86.

Cramer, J.A. & Rosenheck, R. (1998) Compliance with medication regimens for psychiatric and medical disorders. *Psychiatric Services* **49**, 196–210.

Crane, G.E. (1959) Cycloserine as an antidepressant agent. *American Journal of Psychiatry* **115**, 1025–1026.

Crawford, A., Beasley, C. Jr & Tollefson, G. (1997) The acute and long-term effect of olanzapine compared with placebo and haloperidol on serum prolactin concentrations. *Schizophrenia Research* **26**, 41–54.

DasGupta, K. & Young, A. (1991) Clozapine-induced neuroleptic malignant syndrome. *Journal of Clinical Psychiatry* **52**, 105–107.

Davis, J.T. & Nusbaum, M. (1973) Chlorpromazine therapy and functional large bowel obstruction. *American Journal of Gastroenterology* **60**, 635–639.

Day, J.C., Kinderman, P. & Bentall, R. (1998) A comparison of patients' and prescribers' beliefs about neuroleptic side effects: prevalence, distress and causation. *Acta Psychiatrica Scandinavica* **97**, 93–97.

Degen, K. (1982) Sexual dysfunction in women using major tranquilizers. *Psychosomatics* **23**, 959–961.

Deirmenjian, J.M., Erhart, S.M., Wirshing, D.A., Spellberg, B.J. & Wirshing, W.C. (1998) Olanzapine-induced reversible priapism: a case report. *Journal of Clinical Psychopharmacology* **18**, 351–353.

Descotes, J., Lievre, M., Ollagnier, M., Faucon, G. & Evreux, J.C. (1979) Study of thioridazine cardiotoxic effects by means of His bundle activity recording. *Acta Pharmacologica Toxicologica (Copenhagen)* **44**, 370–376.

Devinsky, O., Honigfeld, G. & Patin, J. (1991) Clozapine-related seizures. *Neurology* **41**, 369–371.

Dickes, R., Schenker, V. & Deutsch, L. (1957) Serial liver-function and blood studies in patients receiving chlorpromazine. *New England Journal of Medicine* **256**, 1–7.

Dincsoy, H. & Saelinger, D.A. (1982) Haloperidol-induced chronic cholestatic liver disease. *Gastroenterology* **83**, 694–700.

Dorman, B.W. & Schmidt, J.D. (1976) Association of priapism in phenothiazine therapy. *Journal of Urology* **116**, 51–53.

Emes, C.E. & Millson, R.C. (1994) Risperidone-induced priapism. *Canadian Journal of Psychiatry* **39**, 315–316.

Ereshefsky, M.D., Watanabe, M.D. & Tran-Johnson, T.K. (1989) Clozapine: an atypical antipsychotic agent. *Clinical Pharmacy* **8**, 691–709.

Erickson, B., Morris, D.M. & Reeve, A. (1995) Clozapine-associated postoperative ileus: case report and review of the literature. *Archives of General Psychiatry* **52**, 508–509.

Erle, G., Basso, M., Federspil, G., Sicolo, N. & Scandellari, C. (1977) Effect of chlorpromazine on blood glucose and plasma insulin in man. *European Journal of Clinical Pharmacology* **11**, 15–18.

Evans, D.L., Rogers, J.F. & Peiper, S.C. (1979) Intestinal dilatation associated with phenothiazine therapy: a case report and literature review. *Journal of Psychiatry* **136**, 970–972.

Fellner, C.H. (1958) A clinical note on drug induced depression. *American Journal of Psychiatry* **115**, 547–548.

Finn, S.E., Bailey, J.M., Schultz, R.T. & Faber, R. (1990) Subjective utility ratings of neuroleptics in treating schizophrenia. *Psychological Medicine* **20**, 843–848.

Fraunfelder, F.T. & Meyer, S.M. (1982) *Drug-Induced Ocular Side Effects and Drug Interactions*, 2nd edn. Lea & Febiger, Philadelphia.

Friedman, J.H., Feinberg, S.S. & Feldman, R.G. (1985) A neuroleptic malignant-like syndrome due to levodopa therapy withdrawal. *Journal of the American Medical Association* **254**, 2792–2795.

Fuller, C.M., Yassinger, S., Donlon, P., Imperato, T.J. & Ruebner, B. (1977) Haloperidol-induced liver disease. *Western Journal of Medicine* **127**, 515–518.

Gajwani, P., Pozuelo, L. & Tesar, G.E. (2000) QT interval prolongation with quetiapine (Seroquel) overdose. *Psychosomatics* **41**, 63–65.

Ganguli, R. & Raghu, U. (1985) Tardive dyskinesia, impaired recall, and informal consent. *Journal of Clinical Psychiatry* **46**, 434–435.

Ghadirian, A.M., Chouinard, G. & Annable, L. (1982) Sexual dysfunction and plasma prolactin levels in neuroleptic-treated schizophrenic outpatients. *Journal of Nervous and Mental Disease* **170**, 463–467.

Giles, T.O. & Modlin, R.K. (1968) Death associated with ventricular arrhythmias and thioridazine hydrochloride. *Journal of the American Medical Association* **205**, 108–110.

Giordano, J., Huang, A. & Canter, J.W. (1975) Fatal paralytic ileus complicating phenothiazine therapy. *Southern Medical Journal* **68**, 351–353.

Glusac, E., Patel, H., Josef, N.C. & Yeragani, V.K. (1990) Polydipsia and hyponatraemia induced by multiple neuroleptics but not molindone. *Canadian Journal of Psychiatry* **35**, 268–269.

Goff, D. & Baldessarini, R. (1993) Drug interactions with antipsychotic agents. *Journal of Clinical Psychopharmacology* **13**, 57–67.

Goff, D.C., Henderson, D.C. & Amico, E. (1992) Cigarette smoking in schizophrenia: relationship to psychopathology and medication side effects. *American Journal of Psychiatry* **149**, 1189–1194.

Goff, D., Posever, T. & Herz, L. (1998) An exploratory haloperidol-controlled dose-finding study of ziprasidone in hospitalized patients with schizophrenia or schizoaffective disorder. *Journal of Clinical Psychopharmacology* **18**, 296–304.

Goldstein, L.E., Sporn, J., Brown, S. *et al.* (1999) New-onset diabetes mellitus and diabetic ketoacidosis associated with olanzapine treatment. *Psychosomatics* **40**, 438–443.

Gordon, M. & de Groot, C.M. (1999) Olanzapine-associated priapism. *Journal of Clinical Psychopharmacology* **19**, 192.

Green, M. (1996) What are the functional consequences of neuro-cognitive deficits in schizophrenia? *American Journal of Psychiatry* **153**, 321–330.

Green, A.I. & Brown, W.A. (1988) Prolactin and neuroleptic drugs. *Endocrinology and Metabolism Clinics of North America* **17**, 213–223.

Green, M., Marshall, B. & Wirshing, W. (1997) Does risperidone improve verbal working memory in treatment-resistant schizophrenia? *American Journal of Psychiatry* **154**, 799–804.

Greenberg, H. (1971) Inhibition of ejaculation by chlorpromazine. *Journal of Nervous and Mental Disease* **152**, 364–366.

Greiner, A.C. & Berry, K. (1964) Skin pigmentation and corneal and lens opacities with prolonged chlorpromazine therapy. *Canadian Medical Association Journal* **90**, 663–664.

Gruen, P.H., Sacher, E.J., Altman, N. *et al.* (1978a) Relation of plasma prolactin to clinical response in schizophrenic patients. *Archives of General Psychiatry* **35**, 1222–1227.

Gruen, P.H., Sacher, E.J., Langer, G. *et al.* (1978b) Prolactin responses to neuroleptics in normal and schizophrenics subjects. *Archives of General Psychiatry* **35**, 108–116.

Halbreich, U., Rojansky, N. & Palter, S. (1995) Decreased bone mineral density in medicated psychiatric patients. *Psychosomatic Medicine* **57**, 485–491.

Hartigan-Go, K., Bateman, N., Nyberg, G., Martensson, E. & Thomas, S.H.L. (1996) Concentration-related pharmacodynamic effects of thiordazine and its metabolites in humans. *Clinical Pharmacology and Therapeutics* **60**, 543–553.

Harvey, P.D. & Keefe, R.S.E. (2001) Studies of cognitive change in patients with schizophrenia following novel antipsychotic treatment. *American Journal of Psychiatry* **158**, 176–184.

Hasan, S. & Buckley, P. (1998) Novel antipsychotics and the neuroleptic malignant syndrome. a review and critique. *American Journal of Psychiatry* **155**, 1113–1116.

Hatta, K., Takahashi, T., Nakamura, H. *et al.* (2001) The association between intravenous haloperidol and prolonged QT interval. *Journal of Clinical Psychopharmacology* **21**, 257–261.

Heckers, S., Anick, D., Boverman, J.F. & Stern, T.A. (1998) Priapism following olanzapine administration in a patient with multiple sclerosis. *Psychosomatics* **39**, 288–290.

Heller, J. (1961) Another case of inhibition of ejaculation as a side effect of mellaril. *American Journal of Psychiatry* **118**, 173.

Henderson, D.C. & Goff, D.C. (1994) Clozapine for polydipsia and hyponatraemia in chronic schizophrenics. *Biological Psychiatry* **36**, 768–770.

Henderson, D., Cagliero, E., Gray, C. *et al.* (2000) Clozapine, diabetes mellitus, weight gain, and lipid abnormalities: a five year naturalistic study. *American Journal of Psychiatry* **157**, 975–981.

Hermesh, H., Shiloh, R., Epstein, Y. *et al.* (2000) Heat intolerance in patients with chronic schizophrenia maintained with antipsychotic drugs. *American Journal of Psychiatry* **157**, 1327–1329.

Hogan, T.P. & Awad, A.G. (1992) Subjective response to neuroleptics and outcome in schizophrenia: a re-examination comparing two measures. *Psychological Medicine* **22**, 347–352.

Hogan, T.P., Awad, A.G. & Eastwood, M.R. (1983) A self-report scale predictive of drug compliance in schizophrenics: reliability and discriminative validity. *Psychological Medicine* **13**, 177–183.

Hogarty, G.E., McEvoy, J.P., Ulrich, R.F. *et al.* (1995) Pharmacotherapy of impaired affect in recovering schizophrenic patients. *Archives of General Psychiatry* **52**, 29–41.

Honigfeld, G., Arellano, F., Sethi, J., Bianchini, A. & Schein, J. (1998) Reducing clozapine-related morbidity and mortality: 5 years experience with the Clozaril National Registry. *Journal of Clinical Psychiatry* **59** (Suppl. 3), 3–7.

Husser, A.E. & Bragg, D.G. (1969) The effect of chlorpromazine on the swallowing function in chronic schizophrenic patients. *American Journal of Psychiatry* **126**, 570–573.

Hustey, F.M. (1999) Acute quetiapine poisoning. *Journal of Emergency Medicine* **17**, 995–997.

Igarashi, Y., Higuchi, T., Toyoshima, R., Noguchi, T. & Moroji, T. (1985) Tolerance to prolactin secretion in the long-term treatment with neuroleptics in schizophrenia. *Advances in Biochemistry and Psychopharmacology* **40**, 95–98.

Illowsky, B.P. & Kirch, D.G. (1988) Polydipsia and hyponatraemia in psychiatric patients. *American Journal of Psychiatry* **145**, 675–683.

Isaac, N., Walker, A., Jick, H. & Gorman, M. (1991) Exposure to phenothiazine drugs and risk of cataract. *Archives of Ophthalmology* **109**, 256–260.

Ishak, K.G. & Irey, N.S. (1972) Hepatic injury associated with the phenothiazines. *Archives of Pathology* **93**, 283–304.

Itil, T. & Soldatos, C. (1980) Epileptogenic side effects of psychotropic drugs. *Journal of the American Medical Association* **244**, 1460–1463.

Jefferson, J.J. & Marshal, J.R. (1981) *Neuropsychiatric Features of Medical Disorders.* Plenum, New York.

Jick, O., Miettinen, O.S., Shapiro, S. *et al.* (1970) Comprehensive drug surveillance. *Journal of the American Medical Association* **213**, 1455–1460.

Johnson, V. & Bruxner, G. (1998) Neuroleptic malignant syndrome associated with olanzapine. *Australian and New Zealand Journal of Psychiatry* **32**, 884–886.

Judson, A.M. & MacCasland, B.W. (1960) The effects of chlorpromazine on psychological test scores. *Journal of Consulting Psychology* **24**, 192.

Kane, J., Honigfeld, G., Singer, J. & Meltzer, H. (1988) Clozapine for the treatment-resistant schizophrenic: a double-blind comparison with chlorpromazine. *Archives of General Psychiatry* **45**, 789–796.

Kaplowitz, N., Aw, T.Y., Simon, F.R. & Stolz, A. (1986) Drug-induced hepatotoxicity. *Annals of Internal Medicine* **104**, 826–839.

Kapur, S., Zipursky, R. & Remington, G. (1999) Clinical and theoretical implications of 5-HT$_2$ and D$_2$ occupancy of clozapine, risperidone and olanzapine in schizophrenia. *American Journal of Psychiatry* **156**, 286–293.

Kapur, S., Roy, P., Daskalakis, J., Remington, G. & Zipursky, R. (2001) Increased dopamine D$_2$ receptor occupancy and elevated prolactin level associated with addition of haloperidol to clozapine. *American Journal of Psychiatry* **158**, 311–314.

Keck, P.E.J., Pope, H.G.J. & McElroy, S.L. (1987) Frequency and presentation of neuroleptic malignant syndrome: a prospective study. *American Journal of Psychiatry* **144**, 1344–1346.

Keck, P.J., Pope, H., Cohen, B., McElroy, S. & Nierenberg, A. (1989) Risk factors for neuroleptic malignant syndrome: a case–control study. *Archives of General Psychiatry* **46**, 914–918.

Keefe, R., Silva, S., Perkins, D. & Lieberman, J. (1999) The effects of atypical antipsychotic drugs on neurocognitive impairment in schizophrenia: a review and meta-analysis. *Schizophrenia Bulletin* **25**, 201–222.

Keks, N.A., Copolov, D.L. & Singh, B.S. (1987) Abnormal prolactin response to haloperidol challenge in men with schizophrenia. *American Journal of Psychiatry* **144**, 1335–1337.

Kemeny, M.M., Martin, E.C., Lane, F.C. & Stillman, R.M. (1980) Abdominal distension and aortic obstruction associated with phenothiazines. *Journal of the American Medical Association* **243**, 683–684.

Kendler, K.S., Weitzman, R.E. & Rubin, R.T. (1978) Lack of arginine vasopressin response to central dopamine blockade in normal adults. *Journal of Clinical Endocrinology and Metabolism* **47**, 204–207.

Keskiner, A., Toumi, A.E. & Bousquet, T. (1973) Psychotropic drugs, diabetes and chronic mental patients. *Psychosomatics* **16**, 176–181.

Kimyai-Asadi, A., Harris, J.C. & Nousari, H.C. (1999) Critical overview: adverse cutaneous reactions to psychotropic medications. *Journal of Clinical Psychiatry* **60**, 714–725.

King, D.J. (1990) The effect of neuroleptics on cognitive and psychomotor function. *British Journal of Psychiatry* **157**, 799–811.

Kleinberg, D.L., Davis, J.M., de Coster, R., Van Baelen, B. & Brecher, M. (1999) Prolactin levels and adverse events in patients treated with risperidone. *Journal of Clinical Psychopharmacology* **19**, 57–61.

Klibanski, A., Biller, B., Rosenthal, D. & Saxe, V. (1988) Effects of prolactin and estrogen deficiency in amenorrhoeic bone loss. *Journal of Clinical Endocrinology and Metabolism* **67**, 124–130.

Knights, A. & Hirsch, S.R. (1981) 'Revealed' depression and drug treatment for schizophrenia. *Archives of General Psychiatry* **38**, 806–811.

Kolakowski, T., Braddock, L., Wiles, D., Franklin, M. & Gelder, M. (1981) Neuroendocrine tests during treatment with neuroleptic drugs. I. Plasma prolactin response to haloperidol challenge. *British Journal of Psychiatry* **139**, 400–412.

Kornetsky, C., Pettit, M., Wynne, R. & Evarts, E.V. (1959) A comparison of the psychological effects of acute and chronic administration of chlorpromazine and secobarbital (quinalbarbitone) in schizophrenic patients. *Journal of Mental Science* **105**, 190–198.

Korol, B., Lang, W.J., Brown, M.L. & Gershon, S. (1965) Effects of chronic chlorpromazine administration on systemic arterial pressure in schizophrenic patients: relationship of body position to blood pressure. *Clinical Pharmacology and Therapeutics* **6**, 587–591.

Kotin, J., Wilbert, D.E., Verburg, D. & Soldinger, S.M. (1976) Thioridazine and sexual dysfunction. *American Journal of Psychiatry* **133**, 82–85.

Kraus, S.A., Hinze-Selch, D., Haack, M. & Pollmacher, T. (2000) Granulocyte colony-stimulating factor plasma levels during clozapine- and olanzapine-induced granulocytopenia. *Acta Psychiatrica Scandinavica* **102**, 153–155.

Krupp, P. & Barnes, P. (1989) Leponex-associated granulocytopenia: a review of the situation. *Psychopharmacology* **99** (Suppl.), 118–121.

Larsen, E.B. & Gerlach, J. (1996) Subjective experience of treatment, side-effects, mental state and quality of life in chronic schizophrenic out-patients treated with depot neuroleptics. *Acta Psychiatrica Scandinavica* **93**, 381–388.

Latz, A. & Kornetsky, C. (1965) The effects of chlorpromazine and secobarbital under two conditions of reinforcement on the performance of chronic schizophrenic subjects. *Psychopharmacologia* **7**, 77–88.

Laughren, T.P., Brown, W.A. & Williams, B.W. (1979) Serum prolactin and clinical state during neuroleptic treatment and withdrawal. *American Journal of Psychiatry* **136**, 108–110.

Lazarus, A. (1989) Differentiating neuroleptic-related heatstroke from neuroleptic malignant syndrome. *Psychosomatics* **30**, 454–456.

Leadbetter, R., Shutty, M., Pavalonis, D. *et al.* (1992) Clozapine-induced weight gain: prevalence and clinical relevance. *American Journal of Psychiatry* **149**, 68–72.

Leestma, J.E. & Koenig, K.L. (1968) Sudden death and phenothiazines. *Archives of General Psychiatry* **18**, 137–148.

Leipzig, R.M. (1992) Gastrointestinal and hepatic effects of psychotropic drugs. In: *Advese Effects of Psychotropic Drugs* (eds J.M. Kane & J.A. Lieberman), pp. 408–430. Guilford New York.

Levenson, J.L. (1985) Neuroleptic malignant syndrome. *American Journal of Psychiatry* **142**, 1137–1145.

Levenson, J.L. (1999) Neuroleptic malignant syndrome associated after the initiation of olanzapine. *Journal of Clinical Psychopharmacology* **19**, 477–478.

Levinson, D.F. & Simpson, G.M. (1987) Serious non-extrapyramidal adverse effects of neuroleptics-sudden death, agranulocytosis and hepatotoxicity. In: *Psychopharmacology: the Third Generation of Progress* (eds H. Meltzer), pp. 1431–1436. Raven, New York.

Leznoff, A. & Binkley, K.E. (1992) Adverse cutaneous reactions associated with fluoxetine: strategy for reintroduction of this drug in selected patients. *Journal of Clinical Psychopharmacology* **12**, 355–357.

Lieberman, J.A., Johns, C.A., Kane, J.M. *et al.* (1988) Clozapine-induced agranulocytosis: non-cross reactivity with other psychotropic drugs. *Journal of Clinical Psychiatry* **49**, 271–277.

Lieberman, J.A., Kane, J.M. & Johns, C.A. (1989) Clozapine: guidelines for clinical management. *Journal of Clinical Psychiatry* **50**, 329–338.

Lieberman, J.A., Yunis, J., Egea, E. *et al.* (1990) HLA-B38, DR4, DQW 3 and clozapine-induced agranulocytosis in Jewish patients with schizophrenia. *Archives of General Psychiatry* **47**, 945–948.

Liljequist, R., Linnoila, A., Mattila, M.J., Saario, I. & Seppala, T. (1975) Effects of two weeks treatment with thioridazine, chlorpromazine, sulpiride, and bromazepam alone or in combination with alcohol. *Psychopharmacologia* **44**, 205–208.

Liljequist, R., Linnoila, M. & Mattila, M.J. (1978) Effect of diazepam and chlorpromazine on memory functions in man. *European Journal of Clinical Pharmacology* **14**, 339–343.

Linnoila, M. (1973) Effects of diazepam, chlorpromazine, thioridazine, haloperidol, flupenthixol, and alcohol on psychomotor skills related to driving. *Annals Medicinae Experimentacts et Biologiae Fenniae* **51**, 125–132.

Linnoila, M. & Maki, M. (1974) Acute effects of alcohol, diazepam, thioridazine, flupenthixol, and atropine on psychomotor performance profiles. *Arzneimittel-Forschung* **24**, 565–569.

Litvak, R. & Kaelblin, G. (1971) Agranulocytosis, leukopenia and psychotropic drugs. *Archives of General Psychiatry* **24**, 265–267.

Logothetis, J. (1967) Spontaneous epileptic seizures and electroencephalographic changes in the course of phenothiazine therapy. *Neurology* **17**, 869–877.

McCarty, C.A., Wood, C.A. & Fu, C.L. (1999) Schizophrenia, psychotropic medication, and cataract. *Opthalmology* **106**, 683–687.

McGlashan, T.H. & Carpenter, W.T.J. (1976) An investigation of the postpsychotic depressive syndrome. *American Journal of Psychiatry* **133**, 14–19.

McKenzie, G.M. & Soroko, F.E. (1972) The effects of apomorphine, (+) -amphetamine and L-dopa on maximal electroshock convulsions: a comparative study in the rat and mouse. *Journal of Pharmacy and Pharmacology* **24**, 696–701.

Maltbie, A.A., Varia, I.G. & Thomas, N.V. (1981) Ileus complicating haloperidol therapy. *Psychosomatics* **22**, 158–159.

Mandel, A. & Gross, M. (1968) Leukopenia and psychotropic drugs. *Archives of General Psychiatry* **24**, 265–267.

Mann, S.C. & Bolger, W.P. (1978) Psychotropic drugs, summer heat and humidity, and hyperpyrexia: a danger restated. *American Journal of Psychiatry* **135**, 1097–1100.

Marder, S.R. & Meibach, R.C. (1994) Risperidone in the treatment of schizophrenia. *American Journal of Psychiatry* **151**, 825–835.

Marder, S.R., VanPutten, T., Mintz, J. *et al.* (1984) Costs and benefits of two doses of fluphenazine. *Archives of General Psychiatry* **41**, 1025–1029.

May, P.R.A., Van Putten, T. & Yale, C. (1976) Predicting individual responses to drug treatment in schizophrenia: a test dose model. *Journal of Nervous and Mental Disease* **162**, 177–183.

May, P.R.A., Van Putten, T., Jenden, D.J. *et al.* (1981) Prognosis in schizophrenia: individual differences in psychological response to a test dose of antipsychotic drug and their relationship to blood and saliva levels and treatment outcome. *Comprehensive Psychiatry* 22, 147–152.

Mayer-Gross, W. (1920) Über die Stellungnahme zur abgelaufenen akuten Psychose: Eine Studie über verständliche Zusammenhange in der Schizophrenie. [The attitude towards past acute psychosis: a study on the intelligible context of schizophrenia.] *Zeitscrift für Gesamte Neurologie Psychiatrie* 60, 160–212.

Meldrum, B., Anlezark, G. & Trimble, M. (1975) Drugs modifying dopaminergic activity and behaviour, the EEG and epilepsy in *Papio papio*. *European Journal of Pharmacology* 32, 202–213.

Meltzer, H. & McGurk, S. (1999) The effect of clozapine, risperidone, and olanzapine on cognitive function in schizophrenia. *Schizophrenia Bulletin* 25, 233–255.

Messing, R.O., Closson, R.G. & Simon, R.P. (1984) Drug-induced seizures: a 10 year experience. *Neurology* 17, 869–877.

Meterissian, G.B. (1996) Risperidone-induced neuroleptic malignant syndrome: a case report and review. *Canadian Journal of Psychiatry* 41, 775–778.

Metzger, E. & Friedman, R. (1993) Prolongation of the corrected QT and Torsades de Pointes cardiac arrhythmia associated with intravenous haloperidol in the medically ill. *Journal of Clinical Psychopharmacology* 13, 128–132.

Miller, D.D., Sharafuddin, M.J.A. & Kathol, R.G. (1991) A case of clozapine-induced neuroleptic malignant syndrome. *Journal of Clinical Psychiatry* 52, 99–101.

Millichap, J.G., Pitchford, G.L. & Millichap, M.G. (1968) Anticonvulsant activity of antiparkinsonism agents. *Proceedings of the Society of Experimental Biological Medicine* 127, 1187–1190.

Mitchell, J.E. & Popkin, M.K. (1982) Antipsychotic drug therapy and sexual dysfunction in men. *American Journal of Psychiatry* 139, 633–637.

Moore, M.T. & Book, M.H. (1969) Sudden death in phenothiazine therapy. *Psychiatric Quarterly* 40, 389–402.

Mukherjee, S., Decina, P., Boccola, V., Saraceni, F. & Scapicchio, P. (1996) Diabetes mellitus in schizophrenic patients. *Comprehensive Psychiatry* 37, 68–73.

Nasrallah, H.A., Dev, V., Rak, I. & Raniwalla, J. (1999) Safety update with quetiapine and lenticular examinations: experience with 300 000 patients. Paper presented to the American College of Neuropsychopharmacology, Acapulco, Mexico.

National Institute of Health. (1998) Clinical guidelines on the identifcation, evaluation and treatment of overweight and obesity in adults: the evidence report. *Obesity Research* 6, 51S–209S.

Nestores, J.N., Lehmann, H.E. & Ben, T.A. (1980) Neuroleptic drugs and sexual function in schizophrenics. *Modern Problems in Pharmacopsychiatry* 15, 111–130.

Nestoros, J., Lehmann, H. & Ban, T. (1981) Sexual behavior of the male schizophrenic: the impact of illness and medications. *Archives of Sexual Behavior* 10, 421–442.

Nordstrom, A. & Farde, L. (1998) Plasma prolactin and central D_2 receptor occupancy in antipsychotic drug-treated patients. *Journal of Clinical Psychopharmacology* 18, 305–310.

Ojemann, L.M., Baugh-Bookman, C. & Dudley, D.L. (1987) Effect of psychotropic medications on seizure control in patients with epilepsy. *Neurology* 37, 1525–1527.

Oliver, A.P., Luchins, D.J. & Wyatt, R.J. (1982) Neuroleptic-induced seizures: an *in vitro* technique for assessing relative risk. *Archives of General Psychiatry* 39, 206–209.

Opler, L.A. & Feinberg, S.S. (1991) The role of pimozide in clinical psychiatry: a review. *Journal of Clinical Psychiatry* 52, 221–233.

Overall, J. (1978) Prior psychiatric treatment and the development of breast cancer. *Archives of General Psychiatry* 35, 898–899.

Oyewumi, L.K. & Al-Semaan, Y. (2000) Olanzapine: safe during clozapine-induced agranulocytosis. *Journal of Clinical Psychopharmacology* 20, 279–280.

Pearlman, C. (1994) Clozapine, nocturnal sialorrhoea and choking [letter]. *Journal of Clinical Psychopharmacology* 14, 283.

Peck, P. & Shenkman, L. (1979) Haloperidol induced syndrome of inappropriate secretion of antidiuretic hormone. *Clinical Pharmacology and Therapeutics* 26, 442–444.

Peuskens, J. & Link, C. (1997) A comparison of quetiapine and chlorpromazine in the treatment of schizophrenia. *Acta Psychiatrica Scandinavica* 96, 265–273.

Pillmann, F., Schlote, K., Broich, K. & Marnaros, A. (2000) Electroencephalogram alterations during treatment with olanzapine. *Psychopharmacology (Berl)* 150, 216–219.

Pisciotta, A.V. (1969) Agranulocytosis induced by certain phenothiazine derivatives. *Journal of the American Medical Association* 208, 1862–1868.

Pisciotta, A.V. (1971) Studies on agranulocytosis: a biochemical defect in chlorpromazine sensitive marrow cells. *Journal of Laboratory and Clinical Medicine* 78, 435–448.

Pisciotta, A.V. (1973) Immune and toxic mechanisms in drug-induced agranulocytosis. *Seminars in Hematology* 10, 279–310.

Pisciotta, A.V. (1992) Hematologic reactions associated with psychotropic drugs. In: *Adverse Effects of Psychotropic Drugs* (eds J.M. Kane & J.A. Lieberman), pp. 376–394. Guilford, New York.

Plante, N. & Roy, P. (1967) Galactorrhoea and neuroleptics. *Laval Medicine* 38, 103–107.

Popli, A.P., Konicki, P.E., Jurjus, G.J., Fuller, M.A. & Jaskiw, G.E. (1997) Clozapine and associated diabetes mellitus. *Journal of Clinical Psychiatry* 58, 108–111.

Potkin, S., Thyrum, P. & Bera, R. (1997) Pharmacokinetics and safety of lithium co-administered with 'seroquel' (quetiapine). *Schizophrenia Research* 24, 199.

Prien, R.F., DeLong, S.L., Cole, J.O. & Levine, J. (1970) Ocular changes occurring with prolonged high dose chlorpromazine therapy. *Archives of General Psychiatry* 23, 464–468.

Purdon, S.E., Jones, B.D.W., Stip, E. *et al.* (2000) Neuropsychological change in early phase schizophrenia during 12 months of treatment with olanzapine, risperidone, or haloperidol. *Archives of General Psychiatry* 57, 249–258.

Raskind, M.A., Courtney, N. & Mursburg, M.M. (1987) Antipsychotic drugs and plasma vasopressin in normals and acute schizophrenic patients. *Biological Psychiatry* 22, 453–462.

Remick, R.A. & Fine, S.H. (1979) Antipsychotic drugs and seizures. *Journal of Clinical Psychiatry* 40, 78–80.

Richardson, H.L., Graupner, K.I. & Richardson, M.E. (1966) Intramyocardial lesions in patients dying suddenly and unexpectedly. *Journal of the American Medical Association* 195, 254–260.

Richelson, E. (1984) Neuroleptic affinities for human brain receptors and their use in predicting adverse effects. *Journal of Clinical Psychiatry* 45, 331–336.

Risch, S.C., Groom, G.P. & Janowsky, D.S. (1981) Interfaces of psychopharmacology and cardiology: Part II. *Journal of Clinical Psychiatry* 42, 47–57.

Robertson, M.M. & Trimble, M.R. (1982) Major tranquillizers used as antidepressants: a review. *Journal of Affective Disorders* 4, 173–193.

Robinson, B. (1957) Breast changes in the male and female with chlorpromazine or reserpine therapy. *Medical Journal of Australia* 44, 239–241.

Rosebush, P. & Stewart, T. (1989) A prospective analysis of 24 episodes of neuroleptic malignant syndrome. *American Journal of Psychiatry* 146, 717–725.

Rosebush, P.I., Stewart, T.D. & Gelenberg, A.J. (1989) Twenty neuroleptic rechallenges after neuroleptic malignant syndrome in 15 patients. *Journal of Clinical Psychiatry* 50, 295–298.

Rosen, S.I. & Hanno, P.M. (1992) Clozapine-induced priapism. *Journal of Urology* 148, 876–877.

Rubin, R.T. & Meltzer, H.Y. (1987) Prolactin and schizophrenia. In: *Psychopharmacology: The Third Generation of Progress*. Raven, New York.

Sakkas, P., Davis, J.M., Janicak, P.G. & Wang, Z. (1991) Drug treatment of the neuroleptic malignant syndrome. *Psychopharmacology Bulletin* 27, 381–384.

Samuels, A.M. & Carey, M.C. (1978) Effects of chlorpromazine hydrochloride and its metabolites on Mg^2 and Na^+, K^+-ATPase activities of canalicular-enriched rat liver plasma membranes. *Gastroenterology* 74, 1183–1190.

Sanberg, P.R. & Norman, A.B. (1989) Underrecognized and underresearched side effects of neuroleptics. *American Journal of Psychiatry* 146, 411–412.

Sandison, R.A., Whitelaw, E. & Currie, J.D. (1960) Clinical trials with Mellaril in the treatment of schizophrenia. *Journal of Mental Science* 106, 732–741.

Sarai, M. & Matsunaga, H. (1989) ADH secretion in schizophrenic patients on antipsychotic drugs. *Biological Psychiatry* 26, 576–580.

Schlichther, W., Bristow, M.E., Schultz, S. & Henderson, A.C. (1956) Seizures occurring during intensive chlorpromazine therapy. *Canadian Medical Association Journal* 74, 364–366.

Seftel, A.D., Saenz de Tejada, I., Szetela, B., Cole, J. & Goldstein, I. (1992) Clozapine-associated priapism: a case report. *Journal of Urology* 147, 146–148.

Selye, H. & Szabo, S. (1972) Protection against haloperidol by catatoxic steroids. *Psychopharmacologica* 24, 430–434.

Shader, R.I. (1964) Sexual dysfunction associated with thioridazine hydrochloride. *Journal of the American Medical Association* 188, 1007–1009.

Shader, R. (1972) Sexual dyfunction associated with mesoridazine besylate (Serentil). *Psychopharmacologia* 27, 293–294.

Shay, H. & Siplet, H. (1957) Study of chlorpromazine jaundice, its mechanism and prevention; special reference to serum alkaline phosphatase and glutamic oxalacetic transaminase. *Gastroenterology* 32, 571–591.

Sherlock, S. (1979) Progress report: hepatic reactions to drugs. *Gut* 20, 634–648.

Sherlock, S. (1989) Drugs and the liver. In: *Diseases of Liver and Biliary System*, 8th edn (eds S. Sherlock), pp. 372–409. Blackwell Science, Oxford.

Siddall, J.R. (1968) Ocular complications related to phenothiazines. *Diseases of the Nervous System* 29 (Suppl.), 10–13.

Silver, H., Kogan, H. & Zlotogorski, D. (1990) Postural hypotension in chronically medicated schizophrenics. *Journal of Clinical Psychiatry* 51, 459–462.

Singh, M.M. & Kay, S.R. (1979) Dysphoric response to neuroleptic treatment in schizophrenia: its relationship to autonomic arousal and prognosis. *Biological Psychiatry* 14, 277–294.

Small, J., Hirsch, S., Arvanitis, L., Miller, B. & Link, C. (1997) Quetiapine in patients with schizophrenia. *Archives of General Psychiatry* 54, 549–557.

Smith, D., Pantelis, C., McGrath, J., Tangas, C. & Copolov, D. (1997) Ocular abnormalities in chronic schizophrenia: clinical implications. *Australian and New Zealand Journal of Psychiatry* 31, 252–256.

Sorokin, J.E., Giordani, B., Mohs, R.C. *et al.* (1988) Memory impairment in schizophrenic patients with tardive dyskinesia. *Biological Psychiatry* 23, 129–135.

Sperner-Unterweger, B., Czeipek, I., Gaggl, S. *et al.* (1998) Treatment of severe clozapine-induced neutropenia with granulocyte colony-stimulating factor (G-CSF): remission despite continuous treatment with clozapine. *British Journal of Psychiatry* 172, 82–84.

Spohn, H.E. & Strauss, M.E. (1989) Relation of neuroleptic and anticholinergic medication to cognitive functions in schizophrenia. *Journal of Abnormal Psychology* 98, 367–380.

Spohn, H.E., Coyne, L., Lacoursiere, R., Mazur, D. & Hayes, K. (1985) Relation of neuroleptic dose and tardive dyskinesia to attention, information-processing, and psychophysiology in medicated schizophrenics. *Archives of General Psychiatry* 42, 849–859.

Sreebny, L.M. & Schwartz, S.S. (1986) A reference guide to drugs and dry mouth. *Gerontology* 5, 75–99.

Struve, F.A. & Willner, A.E. (1983) Cognitive dysfunction of tardive dyskinesia. *British Journal of Psychiatry* 143, 597–600.

Sullivan, G. & Lukoff, D. (1990) Sexual side effects of antipsychotic medication: evaluation and interventions. *Hospital and Community Psychiatry* 41, 1238–1241.

Tang, W.K. & Ungvari, G.S. (1999) Clozapine-induced intestinal obstruction [letter]. *Austalia and New Zealand Journal of Medicine* 29, 560.

Tedeschi, D.H., Benigni, J.P., Elder, C.J., Yeager, J.C. & Flanigan, J.V. (1958) Effects of various phenothiazines on minimal electroshock seizure threshold and spontaneous motor activity of mice. *Journal of Pharmacology and Experimental Therapeutics* 123, 35–38.

Tekell, J.L., Smith, E.A. & Silva, J.A. (1995) Prolonged erection associated with risperidone treatment. *American Journal of Psychiatry* 152, 1097.

Teter, C.J., Early, J.J. & Frachtling, R.J. (2000) Olanzapine-induced neutropenia in patients with history of clozapine treatment: two case reports from a state psychiatric institution [letter]. *Journal of Clinical Psychiatry* 61, 872–873.

Thompson, T.R., Lal, S., Yassa, R. & Gerstein, W. (1988) Resolution of chlorpromazine-induced pigmentation with haloperidol substitution. *Acta Psychiatrica Scandinavica* 78, 763–765.

Tollefson, G., Beasley, C. Jr, Tran, P. *et al.* (1997) Olanzapine versus haloperidol in the treatment of schizophrenia and schizoaffective and schizophreniform disorders: results of an international collaborative trial. *American Journal of Psychiatry* 154, 457–465.

Tollefson, G.D., Sanger, T.M., Lu, Y. & Thieme, M.E. (1998) Depressive signs and symptoms in schizophrenia: a prospective blinded trial of olanzapine and haloperidol. *Archives of General Psychiatry* 55, 250–258.

Tran, P., Hamilton, S., Kuntz, A. *et al.* (1997) Double-blind comparison of olanzapine versus risperidone in the treatment of schizophrenia and other psychotic disorders. *Journal of Clinical Psychopharmacology* 17, 407–418.

Tune, L.E., Creese, I., DePaulo, J.R. *et al.* (1980) Clinical state and serum neuroleptic levels measured by radioreceptor assay in schizophrenia. *American Journal of Psychiatry* 137, 187–190.

Tune, L.E., Strauss, M.E., Lew, M.F., Breitlinger, E. & Coyle, J.T. (1982) Serum levels of anticholinergic drugs and impaired recent memory in chronic schizophrenic patients. *American Journal of Psychiatry* 139, 1460–1462.

Ulberg, S., Linquist, N. & Sjostrand, S. (1970) Accumulation of chorio-retinotoxic drugs in the foetal eye. *Nature* 225, 1257.

Van Putten, T. (1983) The clinical management of non-compliance. In: *The Chronic Psychiatric Patient in the Community: Principles of Treatment* (eds. I. Barofsky & R.D. Budson), pp. 383–395. Spectrum Publications, Jamaica, New York.

Van Putten, T. & May, P.R.A. (1978a) 'Akinetic depression' in schizophrenia. *Archives of General Psychiatry* 35, 1101–1107.

Van Putten, T. & May, P.R.A. (1978b) Subjective response as a predictor of outcome in pharmacotherapy. *Archives of General Psychiatry* **35**, 477–480.

Van Putten, T., May, P.R.A., Marder, S.R. & Wittam, L. (1981) Subjective response to antipsychotic drugs. *Archives of General Psychiatry* **38**, 187–190.

Van Putten, T., May, P.R.A. & Marder, S.R. (1984) Akathisia with haloperidol and thiothixene. *Archives of General Psychiatry* **41**, 1036–1039.

Van Putten, T., Marder, S.R., Aravagiri, M., Chabert, N. & Mintz, J. (1989) Plasma homovanillic acid as a predictor of response to fluphenazine treatment. *Psychopharmacology Bulletin* **25**, 89–91.

Waddington, J.L. (1987) Tardive dyskinesia in schizophrenia and other disorders: associations with ageing, cognitive dysfunction, and structural brain pathology in relation to neuroleptic exposure. *Psychopharmacology* **2**, 11–22.

al-Waneen, R. (2000) Neuroleptic malignant sydnrome associated with quetiapine. *Canadian Journal of Psychiatry* **45**, 764–765.

Warnes, H., Lehmann, H.E. & Ban, T.A. (1967) Adynamic ileus during psychoactive medication. *Canadian Medical Association Journal* **96**, 1112–1113.

Wassink, T.H., Flaum, M., Nopoulos, P. & Andreasen, N.C. (1999) Prevalence of depressive symptoms early in the course of schizophrenia. *American Journal of Psychiatry* **156**, 315–316.

Watson, R.G.P., Olomu, A., Clements, D. *et al.* (1988) A proposed mechanism for chlorpomazine jaundice-defective hepatic sulphoxidation combined with rapid hydroxylation. *Journal of Hepatology* **7**, 72–78.

Weiner, M. (1979) Haloperidol, hyperthyroidism, and sudden death. *American Journal of Psychiatry* **16**, 717–718.

Weller, M. (1992) NMS and lethal catatonia. *Journal of Clinical Psychiatry* **53**, 294.

White, D.A.C. (1992) Catatonia and the neuroleptic malignant syndrome: a single entitity? *British Journal of Psychiatry* **161**, 558–560.

White, D.A.C. & Robins, A.H. (1991) Catatonia: harbinger of the neuroleptic syndrome. *British Journal of Psychiatry* **158**, 419–421.

Windgassen, K., Wesselmann, U. & Monking, H. (1996) Galactorrhoea and hyperprolactinaemia in schizophrenic patients on neuroleptics: frequency and etiology. *Neuropsychobiology* **33**, 142–146.

Wirshing, D., Spellberg, B., Erhart, S., Marder, S. & Wirshing, W. (1998) Novel antipsychotics and new onset diabetes. *Biological Psychiatry* **44**, 778–783.

Wirshing, D.A., Wirshing, W.C., Kysar, L. *et al.* (1999) Novel antipsychotics: comparison of weight gain liabilities. *Journal of Clinical Psychiatry* **60**, 358–363.

Yoon, M.S., Han, J., Dersham, G.H. & Jones, S.A. (1979) Effects of thioridazine (Mellaril) on ventricular electrophysiologic properties. *American Journal of Cardiology* **43**, 1155–1158.

Zarate, C. Jr, Baldessarini, R., Siegel, A. *et al.* (1997) Risperidone in the elderly: a pharmacoepidemiologic study. *Journal of Clinical Psychiatry* **58**, 311–317.

Zelickson, A.S. (1966) Skin changes and chlorpromazine: some hazards of long-term drug therapy. *Journal of the American Medical Association* **198**, 341–344.

Zimmerman, H.J. & Ishak, K.G. (1987) Hepatic injury due to drugs and toxins. In: *Pathology of the Liver*, 2nd edn. (eds R.N.M. McSween, P.P. Anthony & P.J. Schever), pp. 503–576. Churchill Livingstone, Edinburgh.

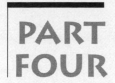

PART FOUR

Psychosocial Aspects

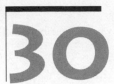

Schizophrenia and violence

P.J. Taylor and S.E. Estroff

Social attitudes and climate, 591
Is there a greater than chance association between
    violence and schizophrenia? 592
    Schizophrenia and homicide, 592
    Non-fatal violence and schizophrenia, 593
Psychopathology and violence, 595
    Critical timings: life course and illness and violence
        careers compared, 595
    Evidence for a possible relationship between
        symptoms of schizophrenia and violence, 596
    Some apparent causal links between symptoms
        and violence, 597
Violence and schizophrenia in social context, 598
    Social network influences on violence and
        schizophrenia, 598
Violence risk assessment and schizophrenia, 599

Risk assessment: the principles, 599
Clinical judgement vs. actuarial prediction debate,
    600
Relevant risk assessment tools and limits to
    application in practice, 601
Prevention rather than prediction? 602
Violence management and prevention in the context
    of schizophrenia, 602
Basic management strategies, 602
Role of medication, 605
Psychological treatments, 606
Social supports and therapies, 606
The place of coercion and security, 607
Conclusions, 608
References, 608

In this chapter, we critically review research that has been reported, mainly in the 1990s, on violence towards other people by individuals with schizophrenia. We take into account the social, service and scientific contexts within which the studies have been generated, and provide a concise and selective overview, rather than an exhaustive review, of the main approaches and findings relevant to the topic. In particular, we summarize and attempt to integrate current perspectives and investigations of the clinical, epidemiological, risk prediction and prevention, and social influences on violence and schizophrenia.

The current generation of studies of violence in relation to schizophrenia represent promising methodological and conceptual advances over earlier work. The conceptual frames are increasingly multidimensional, and the methods more precise. Still, a brief, reliably predictive rating scheme for use in the emergency room or on site in a volatile residential situation eludes the field. No quick and clean means for unravelling the complexities that attend interpersonal violence among people with schizophrenia is at hand. At the same time, we are closer to grasping the dimensions of illness, biography, relationships and circumstance that undoubtedly contribute to violent acts and threats by people with schizophrenia. Controversy about whether schizophrenia directly or indirectly causes violence, about whether people with schizophrenia are more prone to violence than others, about how best to treat those who have been violent and the extent to which such treatment is preventative of (further) violence will no doubt continue well past the next similar review. We will not settle all these questions here, but we seek to sharpen some and to inform with sound evidence where possible.

Social attitudes and climate

Interpersonal violence holds an enduring fascination for many people which is often laced with revulsion and fear. Brutal crime is a recurring theme in our imaginations and in daily life, in various forms of fiction and in the news media. In England and Wales, violent crime is still unusual, but constitutes the majority of newspaper coverage of crime (Howitt 1998). There, throughout the 1990s, violence to the person constituted about 6% of crimes reported to the police (Home Office 1991–2000), while for at least part of the period it constituted 65% of crime reported in the press (Williams & Dickinson 1993). There is a mismatch between media representations of violence and its actual occurrence. Within this context, the often rehearsed observation that people with schizophrenia are disproportionately likely to be presented in the media as violent creates an unwelcome commonality with the rest of us. It is arguable that it is even more troubling that governments seem to prefer the drama of violence and its public portrayal to the facts about people with mental disorder in relation to violence. In Britain, mental health care, treatment and legislation were matters for the government Department of Health – until December 2000. Then, the Secretary of State at the Home Office (the government department for law and order in England and Wales) became a cosignatory with his counterpart at the Department of Health on a White Paper on reform of mental health legislation. This was the precursor of the Bill in 2002, similarly co-signed, which, if passed by parliament, could become statute. Radical reform is necessary, they said, because 'as the tragic toll of homicides and suicides involving such patients has made clear . . . current legislation has failed to protect the public' (Department of Health, Home Office 2000). Contrary to this suggestion, analysis of figures published annually by the Home Office for England and Wales would suggest that the contribution of people with mental disorders to the national homicide figures has been declining (Taylor & Gunn 1999).

There is no evidence to suggest that the existing mental health law had influenced this progress, but there is some evidence that legislation that focuses primarily on public protection may have an unwanted effect. That is, such laws and the processes and service development associated with them may inaccurately and needlessly increase public fear of violence from people with psychiatric disorders. Phelan and Link (1998) found that, in the USA, public perception that people with mental illness are violent had increased significantly between 1950 and 1996. The change in public ratings was mainly in terms of the use of 'dangerousness' terminology instead of other descriptions of violence in legislation and in the public debate. Phelan and Link argued that the revised views of mentally ill people as, by and large, prone to violence probably reflects the widespread adoption of the dangerousness criterion in mental health law in support of compulsory detention and forced treatment in inpatient and outpatient settings.

Is there a greater than chance association between violence and schizophrenia?

At the start of the 1980s, the evidence for any kind of association between violence and schizophrenia (and other psychosis) was equivocal. Indeed, it was possible to find evidence to support each of the principal positions that: (i) people with schizophrenia were less likely; (ii) as likely; and (iii) more likely to be violent than people in the general population (Taylor 1982). Monahan and Steadman (1983) illustrated one of the main reasons for this muddle when they classified and analysed the sort of studies published up to that time. Studies were more or less equally divided between those that studied true rates of crime or violence among 'treated' disorder groups (i.e. enrolled in psychiatric facilities, often as inpatients), and true rates of mental disorder among 'treated' criminals (generally people in prison). There was, at that time, no research that allowed testing of the relationship between true rates of psychiatric disorder and true rates of violence. Some of the work in the 1990s has remedied this and, collectively, establishes a significant, if modest, relationship between schizophrenia and violence (Brennan *et al.* 2000). Brennan's meta-analysis, however, included studies which were representative of the older type (confusing or mixing treated and untreated sample types). The 'MacArthur' violence risk assessment study (Steadman *et al.* 1998), for example, was included, but it fits within the class of 'true rates of violence among treated disorder' research, and the results for Brennan's epidemiological purpose were thus biased by the nature of the treated sample. Wessely and Taylor (1991) explored other possible sources of bias against detecting true associations between mental disorder and violence, and also drew out the extent to which the different approaches from criminology and from clinical practice may have contributed to contradictory findings.

Schizophrenia and homicide

Studies of homicide have an inherent appeal for testing a hypothesis that mental disorder and violence are related. Homicide is unequivocal evidence of violence. There are no messy problems with differing perceptions about the nature and severity of the assault. There is a high rate of reporting and clear-up, so it is relatively straightforward to study a near complete sample of such violence for a given community, and commonly there is a wealth of data on record. Homicide is probably the sort of violence most likely to drive public policy, as indicated by the quote above from the proposals for mental health legislative reform for England and Wales. This is not unique to the UK. In California, for example, one homicide resulted in a civil case (*Tarasoff* v *Regents of Univerity of California*) which became known worldwide. In encoding a 'duty to warn' the putative victim in the event of specific threats of violence, *Tarasoff* profoundly affected provider–patient relationships and treatment for people with mental disorder in the USA, and threatened to do so in other jurisdictions as well.

From a scientific point of view, it is important to keep attempts to understand relationships between homicide and mental disorder separate from attempts to do so for non-fatal violence and mental disorder. Homicide is rarely a recidivist crime and, on a population basis, not clearly related to other forms of violence. Langan and Farrington (1998) drew attention to a major difference between the USA and England and Wales in crime rates according to victim surveys. The USA had a homicide rate six times higher than that in England, but a lower rate of other violence. Within the UK, too, there are differences. For men, the homicide rate in Scotland is twice that in England, although it is similar for women. Other sorts of personal violence occur at three times the rate in England than in Scotland for men, and at over twice the rate for women (Soothill *et al.* 1999).

Role of special inquiries into homicides by people with mental disorder

Among people with mental illness, homicide is more likely to be against people known to the perpetrator than against strangers (I. Johnston & P.J. Taylor, submitted), but it is the much rarer homicide against a stranger, particularly a middle income and educated stranger, that tends to attract dramatic media attention and drive the public agenda. A press conference on the evidence that mentally disordered homicides were becoming fewer in England and Wales prompted one tabloid to publish a short column on the facts, but to search the world for an apparently conflicting 'human interest' case. 'Every commuter's worst nightmare . . . a *deranged* man pushed her into the pathway of a subway train' (*Evening Standard*, 5 January 1999; our italics). This event, in New York, also produced one of the more informative and sensitive media reports on perpetrators of homicide who have a mental illness (Winerip 1999). Following this kind of homicide in England and Wales, to date the independent or public inquiry has been favoured over recourse to civil law suit.

In England, in December 1992, a young man with schizophrenia stabbed and killed another young man who he did not know, and who had been doing nothing more provocative than waiting for a train. This event was followed by an independent public inquiry (Ritchie *et al*. 1994). The investigation, in turn, resulted in a statement by the Department of Health (1994) that, for those who have had contact with the mental health services, 'In cases of homicide, it will always be necessary to hold an inquiry which is independent of the providers involved'. From the numbers of inquiries published since then, it seems likely that this mandate has not invariably been followed. Peay (1996) has admirably set out the pros and cons of such an approach. Concerns include the substantial cost, and the problem that 'their case-by-case focus largely undermines any more general lessons that might be learnt about risk management' (Peay 1997).

Reiss (2001) calls the value of these public spectacles into question from the perspective of counterfactual theory. This postulates that certain rules governing thought processes (mutability rules) tend to restrict or distort the outcome of deliberations. In pursuing an inquiry, these rules determine which features or events are selected for change to improve on reality; the choice tends to be of the most obvious or accessible features. With respect to homicide inquiries, this can give rise to two lines of potential error or distortion. The first is in the focus of the inquiry – on the most obvious event, the homicide – rather than the less obvious but more desirable – its absence. Thus, the inquiry team is trapped into a paradox: in seeking the better outcome it must focus on what led to the worse. Secondly, these cognitive limitations also affect the choice of factors. It is not necessarily the case, however, that the more obvious events and accessible events provide the critical shift between being safe and killing.

Risk of homicides

The National Confidential Inquiry (NCI 2001) into homicide and suicide provides a broader perspective than individual inquiries, although not immune from the limitations just discussed. Data collection began in 1996, and now extends through the UK (NCI 2001). For the homicide part of the study, there are three stages to data collection.
1 Identification of a comprehensive national sample of homicides, irrespective of mental health history of the perpetrator.
2 Identification of those individuals within this sample who have been in contact with mental health services.
3 Collection of clinical data about this last group.
During the 3 years covered by the 2001 report (April 1996–March 1999), the Inquiry was notified of 1579 homicides in England and Wales: 766 cases of murder, 801 of manslaughter and 12 of infanticide. Fifteen people accused were found unfit to plead. Of the 1594 convictions, 34% were found to have a lifetime diagnosis of mental disorder, but just 5% to have a diagnosis in their lifetime of schizophrenia. Findings were similar

overall for Scotland (April 1997–March 2000), with 39% of those cases with a psychiatric report (196 of 227 convicted) having some kind of mental disorder, but only five people (3%) with schizophrenia. Too few reports were available for analysis in Northern Ireland.

It has been shown consistently that the order of association between schizophrenia and homicide is affected by the overall rates of homicide for the community (Schipkowensky 1973; Coid 1983; Reiss & Roth 1993–94). This provides indirect confirmation that previous estimates of association between homicide and psychiatric disorder are likely to be fairly accurate, because rates of schizophrenia in the population are relatively constant between nations. In those countries or regions with more or less comparable homicide rates, the proportion of people who have been convicted of homicide who also have schizophrenia is remarkably similar, at about 5–10% (former West Germany, Häfner & Böker 1973; Iceland, Petursson & Gudjonsson 1981; Greater London and Home Counties, Taylor & Gunn 1984; Contra Costa County, California, Wilcox 1985; Sweden, Lindqvist 1989; Finland, Eronen *et al*. 1996). At the time of the data collection, over 1 year, for the London study, the 1-year prevalence for schizophrenia for the area was about 0.4%, placing the risk of homicide by a man with schizophrenia about 12 times higher than that for the general population. Grove and Meehl (1996) were able to calculate the relative risk in Finland for women as well as men for the period 1984–91. Assuming here 0.7% prevalence of schizophrenia among the general population, the age adjusted odds ratio for women was 6.5 (CI 2.6–16.0) and for men was 8 (95% CI 6.1–10.4). However, Hafner and Boker (1973) also emphasized the other important statistic – that the risk of a person with schizophrenia committing a homicidal attack would be no greater than 0.05%, and at least 100 times less than their risk of suicide.

Non-fatal violence and schizophrenia

Swanson *et al*. (1990) drew on the Epidemiologic Catchment Area (ECA) surveys of over 10 000 people in three different communities in the USA. One strength of the study was its community base and avoidance of selection for mental illness. However, some people were excluded, such as those in institutions and those who were homeless at the time of the survey. As people with mental disorder and challenging behaviours might be particularly likely to fall into these groups, even this measure of selection could have resulted in biasing the findings towards an underestimate of association. Another valuable feature of the Swanson study, given the underestimation of violence likely with reliance on official records (Mulvey *et al*. 1994), was that violence was rated according to self-report of occurrence during the 12 months prior to interview. People with schizophrenia alone were four times more likely to have reported violence than those without mental disorder, but if the schizophrenia was complicated by other diagnoses, and particularly by substance misuse, then the rate was much higher. Link *et al*. (1992) identified a community sample in New York and added a subset of people using inpatient and outpatient services, but excluded people in correctional institutions. People with psychosis, not further specified, were significantly more likely over their lifetime to the point of study to have been involved in incidents of hitting, fighting and weapon use than any others.

Both of these groups of researchers added important riders to their findings, emphasizing the relatively low rate of violence by people with schizophrenia or other psychiatric disorders. Swanson *et al.* pointed out that people with schizophrenia still only accounted for 3% of the total violence in the sample, while Link and his group were even more pointed: 'If higher rates of violence/illegal behaviour are a "rational" justification for the exclusion of mental patients and former patients one might as well advocate exclusion of men or high school graduates in preference for women or college graduates.'

Another group of studies draws on the combination of identification by birth cohort, which provides a sound basis for selection, and tests for disorder–violence relationships exclusively by subsequent linkage between health and criminal records of the cohort. The latter may introduce bias because of the limitations of such archival data, particularly in the underestimate of the target problems – violence (Mulvey *et al.* 1994), and also mental disorder, given that its recognition depends on the existence of hospital records, generally inpatient records. The base samples are very large, ranging from 11 540 (Ortmann 1981; in Denmark) to over 350 000 in another Danish study by Hodgins *et al.* (1996). The subsamples with the disorders of interest, however, are much more modest in size, and the ultimate subgroup with disorder and criminal convictions smaller still. This is an inevitable problem with all community-based studies, but it is important to be clear that it exists, because the sample sizes given are almost invariably for the birth cohort itself. Hodgins (1992), in her study of a Swedish birth cohort, found that people with 'major mental disorder' (cited as more or less equivalent to psychosis) identified on this basis had four times the level of violence as people without mental disorder. Her subsequent similar work with a Danish birth cohort (Hodgins *et al.* 1996) found a similar elevation in rate. Tiihonen *et al.* (1997) did a comparable study with a birth cohort from northern Finland. He offered figures to show how unlikely it would be that people with schizophrenia in that area had not had a hospital registration. He found a sevenfold increase in association between violence and schizophrenia compared with people without disorder.

A related group of studies has relied on official record linkage in complete cohorts identified by other means. Wessely *et al.* (1994) used a psychiatric case register which captured all contacts with psychiatric services in one south London borough between 1965 and 1984. Five hundred and thirty-eight people were identified with a confirmed diagnosis of schizophrenia, and a same size control sample was generated of cases from the same register matched by age band, gender and year of entry onto the case register. For women in the schizophrenia group, there was an increased rate of offending across all categories. For men, the nearly fourfold increase associated specifically with the diagnosis of schizophrenia was confined to violent offending. In

Australia, Wallace *et al.* (1998) had access to an even more substantial register of contacts with psychiatric services, the Victoria case register, established in 1961, which covers the whole of the state's population of 4.5 million. This database was linked with the higher courts' database, recording convictions for more serious offences. An association between schizophrenia and various forms of violence was established; as with other studies the associations were much higher in the event of co-occurring substance abuse. For the 3 years studied (1993–95) 0.09% of men and 0.01% of women with schizophrenia were convicted of homicide.

One study has combined all the advantages of selection as a birth cohort with near complete data collection over a 21-year period (Arseneault *et al.* 2000). Nine hundred and sixty-one people, representing 94% of a total city birth cohort (Dunedin), were interviewed at regular intervals through their lives and at age 21, no matter where they were residing a the time – inside or outside the country, or inside or outside institutions. A range of independent data from official records and from associates were also available. Three hundred and eighty-nine in the cohort had developed psychiatric disorder, 39 of them within the schizophrenia spectrum. Ninety-two people had court convictions and/or self-reported acts of significant violence. Allowing for comorbidity, three disorders held a significant relationship with violence: those in the schizophrenia spectrum, cannabis dependence and alcohol dependence. People with at least one of these three disorders constituted one-fifth of the sample, but accounted for over half of the violent crime. Ten per cent of the violence overall was uniquely attributable to the people in the schizophrenia group.

Changes following community care

Perhaps the greatest value of the Australian study (Wallace *et al.* 1998) lies in its extension to test the relationship between violence and schizophrenia – and other mental disorders too – over time. Specifically, the registers were used to test a public fear, converted into a hypothesis, that violence by people with schizophrenia has become more likely since the shift of service provision to a predominantly community care model (Mullen *et al.* 2000). Deinstitutionalization occurred rather later in Victoria than in some other parts of the world. Accordingly, two cohorts of patients with schizophrenia were identified from the case register: the first admitted in 1975, and the second in 1985. Each subject was followed for 10 years following first admission for schizophrenia. Each was then matched on age, gender and area of residence to a control subject from the electoral roll who did not appear on the case register. Across all categories of offending except sexual offending, and in both periods, people with schizophrenia were significantly more frequently convicted than the healthy controls. For the men with schizophrenia, there was a 40% increase in offending between the 1975 and 1985 cohorts. However, there was also an increase of 50% in comparable offending between the control cohorts. This suggested that the increase in violence among the people with schizophrenia was more likely to reflect a general change in society than an increase as a result of giving them ordinary freedoms.

Psychopathology and violence

Given the statistical association between antisocial violence and schizophrenia, it is important to know how they may be linked and, in turn, what may be helpful in preventing such violence. Effective strategies for doing so will, as indicated, have little effect in the community as a whole, but may limit much harm to those people with schizophrenia who could become violent, to their families and associates, and to their relationships with them. It may be that schizophrenia and violence are linked only through some common aetiological factor. As the root of neither schizophrenia nor violence is yet clear, a hypothesis of common causation, or at least some causative factors in common, remains plausible. One cluster of studies using adoption cohorts principally served to underscore the complexity of social, genetic and developmental relationships, and that no simple explanatory model is likely to be substantiated. Brennan *et al.* (1996), reworking earlier work by Moffitt (1984), found no intergenerational link from violent crime to violent crime, but evidence that there was an increased rate of schizophrenia in the offspring of men who had been convicted of violent crimes. A partial explanation was sought in assortative mating, with mental illness in the mother accounting for the finding. This could not, however, explain all the variance; nor could any other potential confounders when tested individually, including socioeconomic status, or coincident illness in the father. Could this, asked the authors, indicate some inherited deficit in information processing which might account for a propensity to both problems? Whether or not this is the case, inquiry into phenomenology as the possible mediator between illness and violence, when they occur together, seems a promising route to understanding how this co-occurrence may arise.

The main themes in formulating questions are on relative timing of illness and violence careers, and whether and how symptoms may trigger violence. Are some symptoms more likely than others to be associated with violence? Are they more likely to be coincident in time with a violent act? Is violence more likely than not to be reported as consequent upon symptoms? Are some symptom combinations more potent than single symptoms in inciting violent acts? Is there anything in the nature of relevant symptoms – perhaps their impact on the individual or their social context – which makes violent action due to them more likely?

Critical timings: life course and illness and violence careers compared

By definition, the manifestations of schizophrenia are not always evident in any given individual; there is usually a period of normal development, followed by a clear, if sometimes insidious, break in health. In the early 1970s, a number of studies provided evidence that people who had schizophrenia and were convicted of a particular act of violence were significantly older than either those with similar convictions or those in the general population treated for the illness (Hafner & Boker 1973; Walker & McCabe 1973). This suggested that, for these people, perhaps the illness had to reach a certain developmental stage before antisocial violence emerged.

In an English study of pretrial prisoners, 40 men were identified who had schizophrenia and who had inflicted actual physical harm on others (Taylor 1993). Data were collected retrospectively, but in most cases contemporaneous school or social records were available to supplement the man's account. Just one man had started to be excessively violent in his childhood, long before any of the symptoms of illness were evident. Five had been violent before the illness was clearly identified, but possibly within a prodromal phase. In all the other cases (34) violence was only established well after the onset of the illness.

Four other studies have taken a view of relative times of onset of violent and illness careers using retrospective or case record data. Three studies – two in Sweden (Lindqvist & Allebeck 1990; Hodgins 1992) and one in the UK (Wessely *et al.* 1994) – found distinctive patterns of offending among people with schizophrenia, compared with the general population in the first two cases, and a sample of people without psychosis but in contact with psychiatric services for the UK study. In each study, women with schizophrenia tended to be older than women in the general population at the onset of any kind of criminality, while for the men there were two peaks. In Hodgin's (1992) study, early-onset offending was between 15 and 18 and later onset after 21; the rate of violence in the latter group exceeded that of the early-start group. Coid *et al.* (1993; in Taylor & Hodgins 1994) interviewed and searched the records of 280 psychotic probands and 210 cotwins from the Maudsley twin register. Among the people with psychosis, 21% had a criminal record, compared with 11% of the cotwins. Overall, there was a significant correlation ($r = 0.66$) between offending generally and onset of illness, with offending postdating onset of illness in 60% of cases. Only 20 people from the series had been convicted of a violent offence; of these 14 men and two women had schizophrenia. For 12 of these men and both women the violence started after the onset of the illness.

Tengstrom *et al.* (2001) have proposed another frame, that of early and late starters in terms of offending among men with schizophrenia. Among a sample of violent male offenders with schizophrenia in Sweden, there were significant differences in family history, behavioural and academic problems in school, age of first report of substance misuse, and age of contact with social welfare agencies such as foster care. The early starters are represented as having a 'lifelong pattern of antisocial behaviour' which predates symptoms of schizophrenia, while the late starters are described as less functional socially, later life substance abusers and with fewer and less violent crimes. The authors argue that the early starters pose different challenges for treatment and violence risk assessment, particularly because of the apparently robust roles of 'psychopathy' and substance abuse in their modus operandi.

When schizophrenia clearly emerges before the onset of significant violence this does suggest that in some way the illness may have a direct role in the violence. The Dunedin birth cohort, with emphasis on prospective data collection from birth, should provide a further opportunity for testing this suggested relationship (Arseneault *et al.* 2000). Preliminary analysis of mechanisms to explain links between disorders and violence showed that predisposition to perceive excessive threat in the environment accounted for 19% of the association between each of the substance misuse disorders to be significantly associated with violence. Perceived threat accounted for 32% of the association between schizophrenia spectrum disorders and violence, at least from the age of 18. While other factors better explained the association between substance misuse and violence, early perceived threats remained an important if incomplete explanation of the violence among the schizophrenia group.

Evidence for a possible relationship between symptoms of schizophrenia and violence

From well-documented individual cases, such as Daniel McNaughton (West & Walk 1977), through historical studies of samples unselected for violence (Wilkins 1993) to studies in the 1970s both of criminal (Hafner & Boker 1973) and clinical samples (Rofman *et al.* 1980), delusions, or predominantly delusional forms of schizophrenia, have consistently emerged as likely to be related to violence. The detailed account of McNaughton's pathology leading up to his attempted assassination of the then British prime minister in 1842 provides one of the best examples there is of how the symptoms may exert their effect (West & Walk 1977).

> In reply to the questions put to him, the prisoner said he was persecuted by a system or crew at Glasgow, Edinburgh, Liverpool, London, and Boulogne. That this crew preceded or followed him wherever he went; that he had no peace of mind, and he was sure it would kill him; that physicians could be of no service to him . . . . They had followed him to Boulogne on two occasions; they would never allow him to learn French, and wanted to murder him . . . . He mentioned having applied to Mr A. Johnston, M.P. for Kilmarnock, for protection; Mr Johnston had told him that he [the prisoner] was labouring under a delusion, but that he was sure he was not . . . ; the person at whom he fired at Charing Cross to be one of the crew . . . . He observed that when he saw this person . . . every feeling of suffering which he had endured for months and years rose up at once in his mind, and he conceived that he should obtain peace by killing him.

Hallucinations, by contrast, have not generally been found to have any special relationship to violence in criminal samples (Hafner & Boker 1973; Taylor 1985), although they may be more relevant in clinical samples (Depp 1983; Werner *et al.* 1984; Juninger 1990) or more mixed samples (Janofsky *et al.* 1988; Lowenstein *et al.* 1990).

Rudrick (1999) completed a computerized study of the literature, specifically on command hallucinations. While there was agreement about compliance with commands and the benevolence and familiarity of the commanding voice, most agreed that there was no immediate relationship between a commanding voice and violence to self or others. One subsequent study of violence in a 3-month period prior to hospitalization did find an association between violence to others and command hallucinations (McNiel *et al.* 2000); another, focusing on inpatients, found no such relationship, but did confirm an association between content of command hallucinations and self-harm (Rogers *et al.* 2002). The fact that command hallucinations nevertheless tend to be construed as potentially worrying may, however, preclude demonstration of any association, at least within a hospital setting. Hellerstein *et al.* (1987) found no relationship between either self- or other-directed violence and command hallucinations, but noted that such hallucinating patients were more likely to have been placed in seclusion or under special nursing than those without.

McNiel (1994) noted that, where hallucinations had been shown to occur with violence, this was generally in association with other symptoms. This was also the case for the index offences of a high security hospital population of patients convicted of very serious offences (Taylor *et al.* 1998).

Most of the data linking delusions and violence do only that, requiring neither that the delusions should be close in time to the violence, nor that there should be any attribution of the violence to them. Thus, Link and Stueve (1994) studied symptoms over 1 year and a combination of self- and officially reported violence over 5 years in 386 never-treated community controls and 362 patients attending mental health services in New York. A cluster of symptoms identified by the Psychiatric Epidemiology Interview Schedule (PERI), labelled threat/control-override symptoms, proved important. They were experiences of: (i) mind dominated by forces beyond your control; (ii) thoughts put into your head that are not your own; (iii) people who wished to do you harm. The association was so strong that when entered into models that included the more traditionally accepted risk indicators of gender, age and ethnic group, none of the latter held any independent relationship with violence. Swanson *et al.* (1996) revisited the Epidemiologic Catchment Area (ECA) data, applying this measure of the symptomatology. A higher proportion of people who reported symptoms of any kind also reported at least one violent episode in the year prior to interview than those without symptoms, but threat/control-override symptoms at any stage were very significantly more strongly associated with violence in the period. A second national replication of the relationship was attempted in Israel (Link *et al.* 1998). The sampling process in this study was complex, to take account of socioeconomic status, gender, ethnicity and exposure to the Holocaust. The final sample included all people from a large (19 000) Israeli national population register sample who had screened positive for mental disorder, and an 18% sample of those screening negative. The measure of threat and the measures of control-override over

1 year were associated independently and together with violence reported for a 5-year period.

Some apparent causal links between symptoms and violence

One hundred and twenty men with psychosis and 91 men without such illnesses were selected from a large London, UK, pretrial prisoner cohort and interviewed within 6 weeks of their index offence in over 80% of cases (Taylor 1985). It was evident both from the reports of the men and from contemporaneous police and prison entry records that over 90% of those diagnosed with psychosis had been psychotic at the time of the index offence. Each man was asked to give a free account of the offence and his reasons for it. Although not necessarily recognizing their motives as delusional, about half of these men attributed their offence to their delusions, but only half. If violence is to be attributed to symptoms of disorder it seems therefore that at least three conditions should be met. An overarching relationship between symptoms having occurred at some time and violence having occurred at some time seems the weakest, but concurrence in time, and some specific reference to the symptoms as causative makes a much stronger case. In the pretrial prisoner study there was also a requirement for some evidence of acting on symptoms other than in the criminal frame.

A strong association between delusional drive and serious offending was replicated from a record study of a complete (English) national sample of high-security hospital patients with psychosis (Taylor et al. 1998). Hallucinations had little effect on their own, but an additive effect with the delusions. In this series, about one-fifth of the people with psychosis had evidence of preillness personality disorders, deriving from conduct and emotional disorders of childhood. Such direct symptom effect was mainly among those with 'pure' psychosis. In the group with comorbid personality disorder, nearly half had no such evidence of symptom influence. For them, affective disturbances, including flatness or incongruity of affect, were of significance.

Possible dissent on the relevance of delusions to violence arises in the USA MacArthur violence risk assessment study (Appelbaum et al. 2000). Over 1000 patients completed a baseline interview, and over 70% of these some follow-up interviews. Compared with what one would expect from a predominantly public-funded health service, the sample is very unusual, with only 17% suffering from schizophrenia or schizoaffective disorder and a further 13% bipolar disorder. The relationship between violence and delusions appears to have been tested across all diagnostic groups rather than exclusively within the psychotic samples. In brief, a finding of the presence of delusions at one point in time was not related to the occurrence of violence during the following 10-week period. The subjects were people in treatment for their disorder, but it is not clear whether the symptoms had been relieved or whether they persisted during those 10 weeks. People with self-reported threat/control-override symptoms at baseline had had significantly higher rates of violence in the previous 10 weeks than those without. The apparent lack of prospective association between delusions and violence in this study is probably illustrative of methodological challenges. In particular, it illustrates the difficulty in constructing appropriate models for testing the predictive value of remediable/treatable factors previously shown to correlate with violence, rather than providing evidence against their association or potential predictive value. There may also be real differences in the relevance of delusions according to seriousness of violence, other antecedents of the individuals under study, and even wider community or international differences.

However the literature on delusions and violence is construed, one further thing is evident, that most people with schizophrenia or any other psychotic illness have delusions at some stage, and most are not unusually aggressive or violent. This means that other factors must come into play in association with a particular delusion, or that delusions which lead to violence have some special qualities. Delusional content has, to a large extent, been addressed by the threat/control-override studies. The pretrial prisoner study mentioned above had also identified passivity delusions, and the perhaps related religious delusions and delusions of paranormal influence as significantly associated with offences attributed to delusional drive (Taylor 1987). There is also evidence from a series of Bulgarian offenders which further supports the influence of delusional content (Taylor 1999). In the former study, paranoid delusions, while not uncommonly associated in this way, did not distinguish between the men who said they were acting on delusions and those who described other motives for their offence. Such classifications of content are, however, unlikely to be sufficient for a useful understanding of when dangerous action may occur. Gilligan's (1992) formulation, while difficult to fit into a research schedule, is vital for good clinical practice:

> But even the most apparently 'insane' violence has a rational meaning to the person who commits it . . . and even the most apparently rational, self-interested, selfish, or 'evil' violence is caused by motives that are utterly irrational and ultimately self-destructive . . . Violent behaviour, whether it is labelled as 'bad' or 'mad', is psychologically meaningful.

Content aside, in order to investigate further what special features of delusions may lead to action on them, a semistructured interview – the Maudsley Assessment of Delusions Schedule (MADS) – was devised for rating delusions along nine dimensions (Taylor et al. 1994). An individual is asked to identify a belief which he or she regards as most important at the time, and all the questions are structured about that belief. The dimensions are: conviction; belief maintenance; affective impact; positive action on the belief; negative actions such as withdrawal, idiosyncrasy, preoccupation, systematization and insight. In a sample of 83 general psychiatric patients with at least one delusion, nearly two-thirds said that they had acted in some way on their belief within the 28 days prior to interview (Wessely et al. 1993). Features of the belief which were significantly associated with acting on it in some harmful way (including harm to self as well as to others) were seeking information to support the belief, a belief in having found it, being depressed or frightened by it, and making adjustments to it on contradiction (Buchanan *et al.* 1993). This last feature raises a possible route by which delusions may lead to violence against close associates of the sufferer. Contradiction of an expressed belief which seems strange or disruptive is quite a natural response from someone who does not share the belief. Such concern is most likely to come from family or others close to the individual concerned, including professional mental health staff. Cycles of contradiction, modification, further contradiction and modification, all in the context of rising tension, could well lead to violent action.

Violence and schizophrenia in social context

Increased and enhanced application of social science methods and concepts to the study of schizophrenia and violence is emergent in the 'new generation' of research. To a large extent, earlier work included primarily demographic variables as the social factors of interest (Monahan & Steadman 1983). When included in analyses, gender, age, ethnicity, and sometimes social class, challenged single causal hypotheses about the connections between schizophrenia and violence, but offered few alternative explanations or avenues of research (Monahan 1992).

At present, more complex questions are being posed regarding the influence of social and cultural factors on the occurrence, meaning and responses to violence by people with schizophrenia. Estroff *et al.* (1998), among others, suggested redirecting attention to determining: who is at risk for violence from whom, under what circumstances, and at what stage of life and illness? This approach requires a multidimensional view of violence and illness that includes relationships, living situations, biographical experiences, and familial customs regarding conflict and illness, along with clinical variables. The goals are to position violence by people with schizophrenia within their biographical and daily lives in order to deepen and perhaps complicate our understanding of the contributing factors.

An exemplar of this approach is the MacArthur Risk Assessment study. Steadman *et al.* (1998) compared the violent acts and threats of the discharged psychiatric patients in their study with others who lived in the same neighbourhoods. In addition, they scrutinized the types and locations of violence, and identified the targets when possible. In this way, violence is properly situated within the interpersonal and social context within which it occurs (Steadmand & Silver 2000).

There is some cross-cultural work suggesting that rates of violence among people with schizophrenia vary between industrialized and developing countries. (Volavka *et al.* 1997). Violent incidents among first contact patients with schizophrenia in the WHO Determinants of Outcome study were three times higher in developing compared with industrialized countries – a finding which must qualify repeated demonstrations that outcome for schizophrenia is better in developing compared with industrialized countries. Whatever the explanation, the point is

that illness or disorder presentations, definitions of acceptable vs. unacceptable violence, and response to this violence and to people with schizophrenia are culturally constructed.

Social network influences on violence and schizophrenia

A variety of social relationship factors have been shown to have significant roles in the occurrence of violent acts and threats by people with schizophrenia (Estroff & Zimmer 1994; Estroff *et al.* 1994; Swanson *et al.* 1998). Relatively recently in the study of violence, researchers have begun to identify towards whom threats and acts were directed – with an eye not only to understanding who might be at risk of being a target, but also considering the provocative role that others might have in violent incidents. One approach has been to situate violence within a relational context rather than to assume a priori that it is a symptom or derivative of schizophrenia *per se*. In the absence of information about the other participants in violent incidents, we are left with unidimensional, illness-based hypotheses.

Tardiff *et al.* (1997), Steadman *et al.* (1998) and Vaddadi *et al.* (1997) all identified the targets of violent acts and threats, and in each case the nuclear family, particularly household members and close relatives, predominated. While this information represents an advance, none of these studies investigated or reported the temporal dimension of conflict with or hostility from the targets. Much of the research on the familial context of violence in schizophrenia is framed by a presumption of 'family burden', an approach that by its presumption precludes empirical investigation of multiple parties to the violent acts and of threats ascribed to the person with schizophrenia. If we reconceive of violence associated with schizophrenia as largely domestic violence (see Bergman & Ericsson 1996), it is necessary to expand data collection beyond the symptoms, behaviours and characteristics of the diagnosed family member.

Boye *et al.* (2001) took an innovative tack, examining the relationship between relatives' distress and patients' symptoms and behaviours. They found that a cluster of anxiety–depressive symptoms and behaviours of the person with schizophrenia was most highly correlated with the distress of relatives – more so than positive symptoms and threatening behaviours. In another analysis of the same cohort, Bentsen *et al.* (1998) replicated a finding of Estroff *et al.* (1998) that financial dependence on the family or lack of employment were related to the hostility of the relatives toward the patients.

In a series of analyses of a cohort of severely mentally ill persons, Estroff and colleagues (Estroff & Zimmer 1994; Estroff *et al.* 1994; Swanson *et al.* 1997; Estroff *et al.* 1998) found that:

Both patients with schizophrenia who committed violent acts and threats and their closest relatives felt mutual threat and hostility, and the relatives who reported themselves to be most hostile toward the patient were most likely to be a target of violence by the patient.

Overall social network members are at relatively low risk for being a target of violence by a person with a psychiatric disorder.

Immediate family members are at a higher risk than others in the social network; living in a household with the respondent, and for a longer time, also increase the risk of being a target.

Mothers are the social network member at most risk for being a target, and a repeat target of violent acts and threats, particularly when the adult child lives with the mother, is financially dependent, and has a diagnosis of schizophrenia. Social network members of a person with a diagnosis of schizophrenia have a higher risk for being a target of violence than social network members of those with other diagnoses.

The patterns of violence within these social networks parallel those within the general population with one exception: there is an excess of child to parent violence.

A recent investigation by Tengstrom *et al.* (2001) suggests that parental discord and conflict, along with parental substance abuse, are significant factors in the family histories of early starter offenders with schizophrenia.

Taken together, these few but evocative investigations suggest that the social histories and current contexts of people with schizophrenia deserve considerably more attention than has been paid in the past. Research and interventions that are directed at an individual with a psychiatric disorder without placing that individual in social and interpersonal context are incomplete (Hyde 1997), and will be ineffective in relation to understanding co-occurrence of violence and schizophrenia.

Violence risk assessment and schizophrenia

Risk assessment: the principles

Depending on the individual, risk can be both an exciting and a worrying prospect. This duality immediately leads to a problem that confounds agreement in policy and precision in research. Similar risks viewed by different people in different circumstances can be assessed very differently, and adjustments immediately made accordingly. A child might, for example, view sliding on ice on a footpath/sidewalk as a very enticing prospect, and start to move in a way that would maximize the chance of this happening. An elderly woman with fragile bones would view the prospect with horror, and take all actions possible to minimize it. Either way, it becomes apparent that the concept of assessing and managing risk is familiar in principle to almost everyone.

A further problem, pertinent for the discussion here, is that, once identified, risk is often redistributed rather than reduced. Adams (1995), a geographer who has specialized in transport planning, provides essential reading. On redistribution of risk, he describes how introduction of the miner's lamp, a device generally considered to have improved safety in the mines, was actually followed by an *increase* in explosions and fatalities. Its

advantages were counterbalanced by its permitting extension of mining into methane-rich areas where the risks for explosion were even higher. After his wide ranging review Adams concludes:

So, can we manage risk better?

With each chapter, hopes and expectations become more modest.

They are all guessing; if they knew for certain, they would not be dealing with risk.

Human behaviour will always be unpredictable because it will always be responsive to human behaviour – including your behaviour.

In matters of health and behaviour, such as schizophrenia and violence, these observations seem particularly apt. For example, while older neuroleptics such as phenothiazines provided relief from psychotic symptoms, they have been associated with and also sometimes caused irreversible side-effects such as tardive dyskinesia. While deinstitutionalization reduced the deterioration and degradation of confinement, these moves often increased challenges for families, mental health providers and newly freed individuals with few community coping skills. Conner and Norman (1996) provide a comprehensive overview of further confounders of risk assessment in the field of health. The health belief model, perhaps especially pertinent to persuading people to give up smoking or other drugs, requires that in order to act to limit risks to health, the individual concerned has to believe in the connection between a particular piece of behaviour and the desired outcome or feared cost. A person with schizophrenia, whose symptoms may be well controlled by prescribed medication but who may become violent as a consequence of some of the symptoms if they are uncontrolled, must hold a complex set of health beliefs in order to be able to make real consent to such treatment and to comply with it. He or she must believe that the symptoms are part of a disorder of health, that it is desirable to control them, that the medication achieves that control and that better control would not be achieved by more direct means, such as attacking perceived persecutors. That is quite a long list of causal connections that the person must make in order to accept voluntarily the prescribed health regimen. In addition, there is the issue of locus of control. Does the person concerned think that he or she can influence health, or rather that his or her influence is insignificant relative to all the other forces in play. Self-control is an especially important issue for a person with passivity delusions. Adoption, unconsciously, of a third model – protection motivation theory – might lead a patient with paranoid delusions to a violent act rather than behaviour likely to lead to health or amelioration of symptoms.

This brief introduction to risk assessment and management may elicit despair about the potential for improvements, but is intended to promote realism. Not all risk can be identified or managed, nor is it possible always to agree on *acceptable* risks and *acceptable* management measures. Risk assessment and management are dynamic processes, and effective work in this area requires constant reference to the feedback loop. The National Health Service Management Executive (1993), in

England, acknowledged this clearly and set out a template for the tasks. First, it is suggested, the risk(s) must be identified, and then a more detailed analysis can take place. A decision can then be taken as to whether the risk can be controlled or not. A transparent process will follow, of accepting the risk and moving to eliminate or reduce it, or avoiding the risk within the service and moving to transfer it somewhere more appropriate. Some risks may be so high that a principal management strategy will be to set up arrangements to lower the cost of the problem when it occurs. Whatever the chosen action, the management phase sets off a process of reanalysis – has the risk changed as a result of the action? To what extent, then, do management strategies need adjustment – because the first actions proved insufficient, or maintenance activity is now called for, or because the original action has become more than would now be necessary.

Application of such dynamic and context dependent principles in clinical practice requires a broad view of the range of risks of adverse events which face a person with schizophrenia – and of their own assessments as well as those of mental health professionals. The nature of the risk(s) needs clarification and a separate assessment completing for each. Apart from the risk of physical violence to others, firesetting would be considered separately, reckless harm and/or omission errors may be as dangerous as any deliberate acts, while accusations, threats and provocation may inflict psychological harm. No risk assessment in these circumstances is complete without considering the additional risks of self-harm, self-neglect, exploitation by others, or even of injustice.

It has been established that people with mental disorder are much more likely to be arrested at the scene of their presumed crime than those who do not have mental disorder (Robertson 1988). The vulnerability of people with some mental disorders at police interview, including vulnerability to false confessions, is well recognized in England and Wales, with attendant guidance on minimizing such risk (Irving & Hilgendorf 1980; Gudjonsson et al. 1993; Pearse et al. 1998). For people with schizophrenia, delusional memories of offences may contribute to this. One man with schizophrenia had been excluded from the pretrial prisoner sample mentioned earlier, because, after he had served 18 months or so in prison on a charge for a murder to which he had confessed in some detail, it was subsequently established that he could not have done it. Three other men with mental illness were convicted of criminal damage to property, on the evidence of witnesses, but had themselves apparently recalled, and confessed to, offences which were far more serious (Taylor & Kopelman 1984). It is known also that people with psychiatric disorders may be at greater risk of becoming victims of crime more generally (Lehman & Linn 1984; Meuser et al. 1998). Prurient media interest has already been mentioned. As if this list were not enough, the more ordinary clinical risks must be considered too: poor treatment compliance, substance misuse or absconding. The process of risk assessment is lengthy and complex, one risk often impinging on another. The notion that a standard risk assessment schedule can adequately encompass all this is unlikely, if attractive.

The US-based MacArthur risk assessment project has nevertheless provided a very useful template for a systematic consideration of the factors likely to be relevant to lowering or raising the risk for violence (Steadman et al. 1994). Four principal domains are suggested. Two cover relatively fixed factors. The first of these is the dispositional domain, which includes demographic characteristics, personality and cognition; the second covers historical data, inclusive of social and family history, education, work, psychiatric history, and criminal and violence history. The other two domains, contextual and clinical, offer more prospect of short- to medium-term change and intervention. The contextual domain incorporates perceived stress, social supports and means for violence; the clinical domain covers diagnosis, symptoms, substance misuse and function.

Clinical judgement vs. actuarial prediction debate

Actuarial assessment is founded on probabilities derived from statistical tables and, even in this difficult field, offers some prospect of predicting the group likelihood of events for a collection of people with similar characteristics. Alone, this model rarely, if ever, translates well to assessment of an individual. Clinical judgement, however, has rarely been well defined in clinical practice. In research comparisons of clinical and actuarial methods of risk assessment, it is unusual to see clinical judgement defined at all. Contemporary responses to this problem seem to result primarily in attempts to draw up checklists or scales. This is not in itself a bad practice, but amounts to a substitution of clinical judgement with quasi actuarial methods, without resolving the conundrum of what constitutes clinical judgement.

Greenhalgh and Plsek (2001) have offered a series of articles in the application of complexity science to health care, and the first two (Plsek & Greenhalgh 2001; Wilson & Holt 2001) seem particularly pertinent here. The essence of complexity science is recognition of the multiplicity of interacting and self-regulating systems within the body and behaviour of any individual, and between that person and his or her wider environment, social and political cultures, with each system being dynamic and fluid. A small change in any one part of this web of interacting systems may lead to much larger changes in another. 'For all these reasons neither illness nor human behaviour is predictable and neither can safely be "modelled" in a simple cause and effect system' (Wilson & Holt 2001). This, in turn, leads to their perspective on clinical judgement '[which] in these circumstances involves an irreducible element of factual uncertainty and relies to a greater or lesser extent on intuition . . . uncritical adherence to rules, guidelines or protocols may do more harm than good.' 'Health can only be maintained (or re-established) through a holistic approach that accepts unpredictability'. They recommend solutions which include observation and reflection, building on subtle emergent forces, multiple actions and or 'experiment and tune' systems.

Comparative studies of clinical and actuarial predictions are often presented as favouring actuarial methods of risk assessment, but in an area so heavily dependent on statistical analyses, the final interpretation often seems to depend on the nature of the statistics. Grove and Meehl (1996) are exceptionally steadfast in their position. They assert that 136 'studies over a wide range of predictands' favour 'mechanical' algorithmic prediction procedures over the clinical, and:

> We conclude that this literature is almost 100% consistent . . . [with] results obtained by Meehl in 1954. Forty years of additional research . . . has not altered the conclusion . . . It has only strengthened that conclusion.

Some authors have come to different conclusions using different statistical approaches, working with the same data. Lidz *et al.* (1993) found clearly in favour of clinical over actuarial predictions of violence for men, although not women, attending for emergency psychiatric assessments. Ironically, it may have been a reading of actuarial data on the likely effect of gender on risk of violence in the general population, incorporated into the assessment of a group with mental disorder, that led to the error about the women. Gardner *et al.* (1996a,b), applying different statistical methods of analysis, found clearly in favour of the actuarial assessment on these same data. Mossman (1994) provides perhaps the most valuable assessment of the analytical difficulties specific to the clinical field (with an advanced version for those with a higher knowledge and understanding of maths; Mossman 1995). With the one caveat that past behaviour alone may be a better predictor of future violence than clinical judgements, Mossman's interpretation of the collective data up to that point is that mental health professionals are at least better than chance in their violence predictions. An additional problem for research on violence prediction is that evaluation of risk assessment in the clinical setting has never yet been adequate to the task of allowing for interventions informed by the clinical assessment. It is arguable that the usual clinician response to a prediction of violence by a presenting patient is to introduce a management or treatment strategy with a prospect of minimizing the chance that the prediction will be borne out in fact. It is essential that evaluation of clinician prediction strategies should take this into account, but they do not.

Relevant risk assessment tools and limits to application in practice

A twenty-first century holy grail is the idea that there is, or can be, a clinical tool which would provide a reliable and valid risk of violence score for each individual, based on sufficient knowledge about factors which increase or decrease the likelihood of violence by someone with a mental disorder. The tool could be computerized for widespread use. There are numerous grounds for questioning this as anything but fantasy, as already indicated (Adams 1995; Conner & Norman 1996). Monahan and Steadman (1996) have used a meteorology model to show how often predictions can be wrong, even within a field which has a wealth of data on which to base predictions, high technology for making further measures and a long history of adjusting techniques according to experience. So, 'weather derivatives' are available to limit the impact of not being able to control

weather, or getting the predictions wrong (Surowiecki 2001). While people may want such financial cushioning in the event of being attacked by someone with a mental illness, the emphasis seems to be much more on an expectation of control – by locking away indefinitely or enforcing compliance with management plans, including prescribed drugs.

Most assessment tools that purport to be of potential value in this field depend heavily on two things – the one following from the other. They rely on the concept of past behaviour being a good predictor of future behaviour, and thus they use factors which are not susceptible to change. Once an individual has attained a high-risk score on the Psychopathy Check List – Revised (PCL-R) (Hare 1991), for example, or the Violence Risk Appraisal Guide (VRAG) (Quinsey *et al.* 1998), which incorporate past behaviour ratings, it is unlikely that the score can ever change. The individual may change in ways that, in reality, reduce the risk he or she poses, but that will make little difference to their actuarial rating. These scales do not necessarily translate outside the cultures in which they were validated. With respect to the PCL-R, Cooke and Michie (1999) found that both the prevalence and expression of the disorder so defined may vary between North America and the UK. Its value for predicting violence is generally presented as high (Hare *et al.* 1999), although again there may need to be more caution in this respect outside North America (Reiss *et al.* 2000). The PCL-R has been applied to people with schizophrenia (Monahan *et al.* 2000), but its appropriateness to this group is even less clear.

The HCR-20 (Webster *et al.* 1995) contains a core of 10 historical items, which inevitably have considerable overlap with other history-based scales such as the PCL-R and the VRAG. To these, five dynamic clinical items and five dynamic risk variables have been added. The clinical items cover lack of insight, negative attitudes, active symptoms of mental illness, impulsivity, and unresponsiveness to treatment; the dynamic risk variables are: plans lack feasibility, exposure to destabilizers, lack of personal support, non-compliance with remediation attempts, and stress. It appears that the subscales may perform differently according to context. In an intensive care unit, for example, the clinical variables have been shown to perform better than the other two, while the dynamic risk variables perform best for a sample in the community (Webster *et al.* 1997, 2000). The possibility that different variables may be needed to predict violent behaviour in hospital than in the community receives indirect validation from the study of Tardiff *et al.* (1997). None of the 1068 consecutively admitted patients who were violent in the hospital were subsequently violent in the community, but there was a strong relationship between pre- and posthospitalization violence.

There are very few sound studies of the capacity of various instruments or methods to predict risk. The MacArthur violence risk assessment study was designed to identify variables of potential value for a risk assessment tool that could be useful in clinical practice with people with a mental disorder. It is, however, essentially a correlational study, although one founded on prospectively collected data. Monahan *et al.* (2000) introduced the resulting new tool to be tested for its value in clinical practice. Their 'decision tree' approach has a face validity and apparently sound, if complex, mathematical properties. The idea is that subgroups of ever-decreasing size (and greater specificity) would be identified on a hierarchical basis. A χ-squared automatic interaction detector (CHAID) algorithm was used to assess the statistical significance of the bivariate association between each of the 106 eligible risk factors and violence in the community/no violence in the community during the 12 months of follow-up after a hospital admission. The sample of nearly 1000 psychiatric patients, discharged after a brief hospital admission, was partitioned according to the value of the risk factor with the strongest association, and the procedure was repeated until no more partition was possible. Further steps, or iterations, were then created by pooling all those individuals who had not been partitioned in this way, and repeating the process through two further iterations. At that point, the process had classified just over 70% of the sample as low (half the 18% base rate of violence for the sample) or high (twice the base rate) risk.

In the first iteration, seriousness of previous arrest separated the groups, such that only 9% of those without such an arrest were violent, but 36% of those with such a history were violent in the 12 months after first interview. After this primary cut, for the latter group, violent fantasies showed potential for further refining the classification, with 53% of the group with serious arrest histories who had violent fantasies having been violent during follow-up, compared with 27% who did not. Variables other than violent fantasies were better secondary classifiers for the moderate and low seriousness of arrest groups; most of these were fixed variables, such as paternal drug use. People with schizophrenia, as noted earlier, were in a minority in this sample, so it is difficult to know how generalizable the results may be outside a managed care sample in the USA. In the second iteration for this highly selected group, schizophrenia appeared as a protective factor against physical violence in the following 12 months, a finding which is at odds with those from the major epidemiological studies.

Few other researchers are as candid about the stage reached in their research as the MacArthur team, and many studies purporting to be of risk prediction do not start with a clearly defined prediction and then test it over time. Buchanan and Leese (2001) identified just 21 studies of this kind since 1970, based on original data in peer-reviewed journals, and from which figures for sensitivity and specificity could be obtained. The studies were heterogeneous in sensitivity and specificity, with overall estimates of 0.52 and 0.68 respectively; an index of effectiveness ranged from − 0.10 to 1.1, with an overall mean of 0.58, and a rather better effect for actuarial than clinical predictions. It should also be noted that the studies were heterogeneous for sample type, with seven of them conducted with prisoners, and 14 in a variety of hospital (including high-security) to community settings, each differing in prevalence and nature of mental disorder. The authors interpret the results with reference to the new concept of 'dangerous severe personality disorder', which the British government has introduced, but the findings are relevant to schizophrenia too. The overall estimate for sensitivity would suggest that for every 10 people who would be violent, five would be identified and detained and five would be missed. For every 10 people who would not be violent, six would be identified and released, and four would be detained.

Prevention rather than prediction?

The National Confidential Inquiry (1999) raised a further problem for would-be risk assessors. Only a very small proportion of those who had killed – 28% of those with mental disorder and 8% of those without it – had been in any contact with psychiatric services in the 12 months prior to the killing, and thus few had presented the opportunity for risk assessment or preventive intervention. Perhaps more important than expending resources on more and better risk assessment tools would be to consider whether it is possible to make mental health services more attractive and, in turn, more effective for potential users. Munro and Rumgay's (2000) analysis of all 40 independent inquiry after homicide reports published in England and Wales between 1988 and 1997 would suggest these as meaningful goals. Even with the advantage of hindsight, and access to a range of data unlikely to be paralleled in routine clinical practice, the inquiry teams concluded that the homicides could have been predicted *in only* 11 (28%) of cases. However, they considered that 26 (65%) of them could have been prevented, and gave examples. One young man, for example, had given no indication whatsoever of his capacity for killing his mother, but had his symptoms of schizophrenia been adequately treated, the inquiry team concluded that the homicide would not have happened.

Violence management and prevention in the context of schizophrenia

Basic management strategies

Principles

An abiding principle of violence management and prevention in the context of schizophrenia is that not only should everyone *be* as safe as possible, but they should also *feel* safe. If the person with the schizophrenia *feels* safe, it is likely that the first important step to real safety has been achieved. Indeed, the Royal College of Psychiatrists (1996) puts this as one of the core general principles in the management of risk.

A management plan should change the balance between risk and safety, following the principle of negotiating safety.
When seeing a patient who presents a risk of dangerous behaviour, the clinician should aim to make the patient feel safer and less distressed as a result of the interview.
A patient's account of perceived problems may or may not fit with that of other observers, but it is important that his or her views be heard and understood if a potentially dangerous situation is to be managed. A patient needs to feel respected as a person, as more than 'just a case' or 'a schizophrenic', and to

become engaged in a process of assessment which may merge almost imperceptibly into treatment. Beauford *et al.* (1997) report a novel investigation of the role of therapeutic alliance in evaluating the risk for violence that supports this contention. In their study, patients with a poor initial therapeutic relationship were significantly more likely to threaten or carry out violent acts than patients with a more positive therapeutic alliance.

In order to deliver the kind of genuinely calm, warm and positive acceptance of the individual necessary to this process, the assessor too must feel safe. In a hospital setting this may include ensuring that the physical setting of the assessment is appropriate – clean, quiet and comfortable, without 'accidental' weapons (such as heavy ashtrays) and giving a sense of privacy. Availability of other supporting staff is vital. In inpatient, outpatient or community settings, it is important that support staff are at least aware of the starting time, location and expected completion time of any interview, and that they know what to do in the event of overrun or any clear crisis. A session which has already been judged as at high risk of violence occurring might call for more than one member of staff to be physically present, or support staff designated to specific observation duties, with good sight lines maintained at all times. Nothing in the way of advance practical preparation, however, can cover every eventuality, and the skill to adjust to the ever-changing circumstances and interactions is what is ultimately required. Stanko (1993) has emphasized this outside the mental health care setting, but it is as important within it. The capacity to negotiate with patients – for safety as well as for other desired goals – is at the core of successful management, and likely to require specific training together with ongoing support and supervision to maintain and develop it. McGauley (1997) has written of the role of psychodynamic psychotherapy in such circumstances – not especially for its direct treatment potential, but rather for adding an extra dimension to the understanding of risky qualities in relationships, and to provide support and supervision, as necessary.

Much serious violence is likely to follow directly from symptomatology, in which case specific treatment of the illness would follow and relieve risk of violence together with the symptoms. Even in this context, the nature and quality of immediate social relationships are likely to be relevant, and those relationships are likely to need assessment, support and, occasionally, distance. Some serious violence, and a good deal of lesser antisocial behaviour, is likely to be associated more indirectly with the illness, through the secondary disabilities, disadvantage and dependency that it can bring, or with premorbid relationship styles and experiences. Perhaps about one-fifth of people who become seriously violent in the context of schizophrenia have had seriously adverse experiences, including abuse, throughout childhood (Heads *et al.* 1997), and such social support systems and networks as they have may still carry similar qualities. A particular need for comprehensive care packages in this field should be beginning to become apparent.

Those close to the person with schizophrenia are most likely to become victims of violence (Estroff *et al.* 1998; I. Johnston & R.J. Taylor, submitted). Relationships with people who have

schizophrenia are not easy, and the attitudes and understanding of close associates, including long-term professional therapists, supervisors or key workers, are likely to need assessment from time to time. Some of the former may be unable to imagine or perceive a possibility of violence by their loved one, and be incapable of taking steps to diffuse a volatile situation or protect themselves. Others may have developed a tense and critical manner which could exacerbate aggression on the part of the person with schizophrenia, again a problem not confined to family or lay carers (Moore & Kuipers 1999). If violence is considered to be a risk therefore, it is not just the patient who must be managed, but also the potential victims and the environment. Decent affordable residences must be available so that people with schizophrenia are not forced by lack of alternatives to live with their relatives or in other highly charged, combative or threatening surroundings. Similarly, adequate income supports would relieve some of the financial stresses that plague patients and their families and often provoke disputes (Estroff *et al.* 1998).

Changing the environment

If factors thought to increase the risk of a violent act, such as alcohol or illicit drugs, or factors likely to increase its seriousness, such as availability of weapons, cannot be managed in one environment, then a change of environment may be a fundamental part of the management strategy. If the potential victim is known, but not capable of self-protection, or unknown, then the same may apply, but a different kind of case management might serve as well. People with schizophrenia unwilling or unable to co-operate with management and treatment strategies, and in this context who then put their own health or safety or the safety of others at risk, will be liable, in most jurisdictions, to coercion or compulsion in treatment. If the risk is considered to be of serious harm, then this may have to be under conditions of physical security. The guiding principle is that if security is necessary, it should always be at the lowest possible level compatible with the safety of all parties, including the patient.

Existing literature on the management of violence or potential violence by people with schizophrenia or other mental disorders rightly falls into the two rather separate categories of inpatient and outpatient work. The two situations are clearly different and Tardiff *et al.* (1997) have shown that risk factors for the community are likely to be different.

Management of inpatient violence

The Royal College of Psychiatrists Research Unit (1998) conducted a systematic review of the management of imminent violence in the inpatient setting. Even in the area of psychopharmacology, where one might have expected research methodology to be at its most straightforward, there were very few clinical trials of any substance, and even fewer of a randomized controlled type. As a result, the College group was forced to base many of its recommendations on consensus rather than evidence. It is arguable that some of the research gaps could be easily remediable, such as evidence on whether substance misuse has a significant role in inpatient violence, the value of specific treatment for pertinent disorders and the importance of qualities in staff communication. Nevertheless, the difficulties of designing and implementing research in the inpatient setting when people are feeling under threat are not to be minimized (Taylor & Schanda 2000). This latter review sets out some of the natural limits to research methodology in this field, but shows some impressive progress too. Carmel and Hunter (1991) were able to demonstrate in a longitudinal study the importance of specific training in the management of violence. Phillips and Rudestam 1995) conducted a randomized controlled trial of didactic training in violence management, didactive training coupled with practical skills training for the same period, and no training. The groups were small, but there was a clear advantage for the doubly trained group. Smoot and Gonzales (1995) emphasized the beneficial effect on staff of a training programme in accurate empathy. The staff on the experimental unit showed a decrease in staff turnover, less sick leave, fewer incidents of restraint and seclusion and a reduction in financial costs than the unit without such training. Lancee *et al.* (1995) studied styles of limit setting among nurses, showing that, at least in a role-playing situation between nurses and consenting patients, affective involvement with patients coupled with clearly given options for resolving a particular problem resulted in significantly less anger and aggression. Other styles, including sharing or belittlement, unsurprisingly, generated significantly more anger than other styles.

Work which was more environmentally focused serves to underscore the importance of monitoring the effect of change. Clinical experience and literature have both suggested that overcrowding in inpatient units may be a source of provocation, and that people with a propensity for violence may have a particular need for substantial personal space (Dietz & Wilder 1982). However, Palmstierna and Wistedt (1995), studying a psychiatric intensive care unit, found that after the number of beds was halved to 10, without other obvious changes in patient type or regime, there was a fourfold, although non-significant, increase in the number of incidents. They suggested that the accompanying increase in privacy for patients may, for this aspect of their behaviour, have fostered greater covert aggression or violence.

When attempts to prevent or diffuse violence fail, then the essence of any general management strategy is containment or removal, at least until treatment can be effective. Within hospital, this can only mean intensification of care in some way. This may be achieved by increasing staff supervision, possibly through continuous one-to-one care, possibly by specified frequency of observations. Apart from the increased attention possible under these arrangements, the provision may allow for more active management of the patient within the space available; e.g. separating from potential antagonists, or implementing specific behavioural treatments. Dialectical behaviour therapy has a growing popularity and potential value in this area (Low *et al.* 2001). It has been shown to reduce rates of self-harm among women detained in an English high-security hospital because of

their perceived threat to others, and might with benefit be evaluated in other groups and for repeated violence against others.

Rarely, a patient may have to be restrained physically by staff, who should have received specific training in techniques for doing so with safety. Physical restraints are almost never maintained in the UK, but appear more popular in the state hospitals in the USA. Seclusion, the locked isolation of a patient from others on the unit, is another measure that may occasionally prove necessary. However, this is a very serious step and requires explicit policies that will incorporate documentation practice and specified periods for formal review (Royal College of Psychiatrists 1990). Even if these more extreme management techniques become necessary, it is as well to keep in mind Lion and Soloff's (1984) injunction:

> The staff restraining the patient today will be seeking a therapeutic alliance tomorrow. The patient remains a vulnerable human being and, even when it appears that there is little rapport with the patient, every effort must be made to continue talking to him or her, explaining what is happening and why and reassuring.

Care planning for community patients

Patient care must be attuned to level of need, and in this and the importance of a clearly documented treatment and care plan, inpatient and outpatient care do have a major principle in common. In order to achieve a good match between need and service, the quality of assessment must be high and a wide range of clinical and other support services available. In England and Wales, the process was formalized by government guidance in 1990 under the title 'Care Programme Approach' (Department of Health 1990). Designed originally for people preparing for discharge from hospital inpatient care, clarifications in the courts over time mean that it should apply to anyone in, or about to be in, the community. Prisoners with mental health problems, for example, are entitled to assessment under the Care Programme Approach. The approach recognizes the importance of clear allocation of responsibility, and nomination of a key worker or case manager, who may be of any discipline, but is commonly a community psychiatric nurse. The key worker is involved in a detailed multidisciplinary assessment of need, including risk, and then ensures that the plan is carried out, carries out those aspects appropriate to his or her skills, and organizes regular review and monitoring. As a consequence, the plan is adjusted from time to time. A key goal is continuity of good and directly relevant care.

Similar models have been implemented elsewhere in the world, with slight variations, both in the details of implementation and in the position designation. Marshall and colleagues, in conducting a systematic Cochrane review of such treatments, took a decision to separate case management from assertive community treatment (ACT). Randomized controlled trials of case management compared with 'standard care' showed little advantage for it other than keeping patients in contact with services, and there was little to indicate that there was any specific effect with respect to violence (Marshall & Lockwood 2001). Rather larger numbers of trials of ACT, almost all US-based, showed general advantages for ACT but only one study showed an advantage in respect of imprisonment rate (Marshall *et al.* 1999). Walsh and colleagues, in a subsequent substantial randomized controlled trial of intensive case management compared with standard care in the UK, specifically for people with established psychotic illness, failed to show an advantage for intensive case management either in reduction of suicidal behaviour (Walsh *et al.* 2001a) or violence to others (Walsh *et al.* 2001b). Standard care and intensive case management were comparable save for the case load. Intensive case managers had only half the case load of regular case managers and, overall, made twice as many contacts of various kinds within the patient therapeutic context. Nothing is known about the nature or quality of these relationships, the content or tone of the contacts or the skills of the manager. These factors should be the focus for future research, particularly because there are indications that remaining in treatment does have an influence on decreasing the occurrence of interpersonal violence (Swanson *et al.* 2000; Swartz & Monahan 2001).

Role of medication

This is discussed at length in Chapters 24, 25 and 26 but here we give special emphasis on the role of medication in relation to treating and preventing violence. Because the illness itself, and not uncommonly specific symptoms of the illness, seems to have some direct relationship with violence when the two occur together, it follows that specific treatments may be as important in the management of violence as of the illness. Medication is now generally accepted as the most effective of specific treatments for the disorder among most people with schizophrenia, although a substantial minority of the people find little benefit from it. It is less clear whether the impact of illness on violence is similar inside and outside hospital, but it may be that the impact of delusions is more important outside hospital (Taylor 1985; Taylor *et al.* 1998), and other features of the disorder, such as hallucinations (Hellerstein *et al.* 1987) or thought disorder (Janofsky *et al.* 1988), more important in hospital. Steinert *et al.* (2000) found that aggressive incidents in hospital decreased significantly after neuroleptic treatment was started. The effect of negative symptoms within a hospital setting may be similar to those described in a sample of people with dementia by Nillson *et al.* (1988), for whom aggression was particularly likely to arise around activities of daily living. Arango *et al.* (1999) evaluated violent incidents among 63 inpatients with schizophrenia and found that three factors correctly classified those with incidents and those without. The three factors were: (i) higher score on the Positive and Negative Syndrome Scale (PANSS) general psychopathology scale; (ii) lack of insight into symptoms; and (iii) violence in the previous week. Whether or not there is a symptomatic distinction, it is clear that there is a distinction between treating disorder with a prospect of imminent violence and the longer term treatment of disorder and lifetime risk. On this

point, Krakowski *et al.* 1999) investigated the heterogeneity of violent behaviours among psychiatric inpatients. They found significant differences between patients who were persistently assaultive and those who engaged in transient violence, and between patients who were violent and those who were not. The patients whose violence persisted were more hostile, suspicious, neurologically impaired and irritable than those with transient incidents.

The Royal College of Psychiatrists' (1998) systematic review identified only one trial of medication that satisfied all the design criteria specified including randomization, clinician blind, patient blind, more than 20 subjects in each group, and follow-up achieved for at least 80% of the study group. This was a study, in essence, of chemical restraint (Thomas *et al.* 1992). Taylor and Buckley (2000) reviewed the range of medications that have been applied. There appeared to be international differences in favoured medication; e.g. in the acute presentation of violence in schizophrenia (and with other conditions) in the USA, benzodiazepines are favoured (Fava 1997), but they are rarely used alone in England. Typical antipsychotics remain a mainstay of treatment, but increasingly clozapine or the newer antipsychotics are favoured. The latter, however, are unlikely to be useful in acute crisis. The Schizophrenia Patient Outcomes Research Team (PORT) treatment guidelines recommended clozapine for people with schizophrenia who are also persistently violent (Lehman *et al.* 1998). Work among high-security hospital patients in England would suggest that those with schizophrenia show improvement in illness features, and expressions of violence too, with much the same frequency as one would expect in general psychiatric populations (Dalal *et al.* 1999). Swinton and Haddock (2000) showed a particularly favourable effect on the discharge of very long-stay violent patients. Several studies have suggested that clozapine possesses a specific antiaggressive effect (Volavka *et al.* 1993; Buckley *et al.* 1995; Rabinowitz *et al.* 1996). This seems to be largely founded on an observation that resort to violence may lessen with little apparent improvement in psychotic symptoms. What has not yet been tested is the extent to which clozapine may relieve the affective impact of the psychotic symptoms even if the latter are not alleviated.

Newer antipsychotics have been less well-researched in this respect, but risperidone (Buckley 1998) and olanzapine (Beesley *et al.* 1998) are showing some promise. For the longer term, the possible advantages for clozapine or the newer antipsychotics in treating schizophrenia have to be set beside the risks of noncompliance, given the fact that no depot preparation is available, or in the case of clozapine could be available, and the possible risks of rebound into psychosis and possibly violence on abrupt cessation of the drugs (Special Hospitals' Treatment Resistant Schizophrenia Research Group 1996).

Combinations of drugs have also been tried for the purpose of reducing violence and its risks. Lithium, carbamazepine, sodium valproate and β-blockers have each been proposed for augmentation strategies in patients with schizophrenia and persistent violence, and there are a number of useful reviews and studies (Christison *et al.* 1991; Ratey *et al.* 1992; Volavka 1995; Fava 1997). An important consideration, particularly for those patients in the community, is that combinations of drugs other than those prescribed may have to be taken into consideration. Tiihonen and Schwartz (2000) consider the risks and benefits of pharmacological intervention for preventing violence among people with mental illness who also use alcohol and illicit drugs.

Additional research is necessary to fine tune different medication and treatment regimens for different types of patients in inpatient and community settings, in view of both environmental differences and the likely variations among patients in either setting. The well-worn but still pertinent goal of finding the right drugs and dosage for the right person in their current context should not be obscured by the cascade of new drugs *per se.*

Psychological treatments

Surprisingly little in the way of research has been reported regarding psychological or psychodynamic treatment modalities for preventing or decreasing violence. The psychoeducation approach is perhaps the most well known and promising because it focuses directly on hostility, criticism and overinvolvement in the familial context of patients with schizophrenia. It is logical to assume that the consistent findings of decreased relapse and readmission rates for people with schizophrenia in these studies (Pekkala & Merinder 2001) reflects, at least in part, a decrease in threats and acts of violence within the family which usually precipitate an admission. Unfortunately, violent acts and threats have not been considered as primary outcome indicators in psychoeducation outcome research, so we are left with logical surmise. In view of the family context of much violence by and around people with schizophrenia (see below), this approach would seem to be a prime candidate for further investigation of violence reduction and prevention.

Cognitive–behaviour therapy (CBT) has recently been 'imported' from its original application in treating depression to treatment in schizophrenia. Carefully designed and controlled studies remain to be reported, but initial results are encouraging with regard to reduction of relapse rates (Jones *et al.* 2001). CBT is problematic in that it is not widely available, requires well-trained and experienced therapists, and can be unfeasible financially for un- or underinsured patients or financially lean public treatment systems.

Within the maturation of the psychiatric consumer movement has come the development of consumer–provider-run treatment programmes. There are several pilot efforts in the USA that involve mediation between the patient and family or household in the event of violent conflict that could lead to hospitalization. The approach assumes that violent conflict involves contributions from all parties, not just the identified patient, and seeks to negotiate a truce or separation of the parties – somewhat short of a hospitalization for one of them. Consumer–providers and traditional mental health profession-

als team up to deliver this intervention in most of the pilots. Needless to say, rigorous research on the efficacy of this approach is awaited.

Social supports and therapies

While intensive case management and assertive case treatment as complete packages may not have been found to have a convincing effect on violence reduction among people with schizophrenia in community settings, there are indications that some of the elements or benefits of such management *can* reduce violence. Several studies have found that patients who used more services, had access to more and better services, and who formed closer relationships with staff were less likely to commit violent acts or threats or need involuntary treatment than those who used few if any services and did not report close relations with staff (Estroff & Zimmer 1994; Swanson *et al.* 1997; Swartz *et al.* 1999; Ridgley *et al.* 2001). It is unlikely that the primary mechanism by which this occurs is the demonstrated increased contact with services and staff for patients in these types of programmes.

Estroff (2000) suggests that the development of therapeutic and instrumental alliances between patients and staff in community programmes is a promising basis for preventing violence. When these relationships are based on trust, and when they endure, there are opportunities to intervene before conflict turns assaultive, and increased likelihood that staff will be aware of a patient's distress, experienced threat or decompensation (see also Beauford *et al.* 1997). Patient–staff ratios and adequacy of community resources are, however, seldom at optimal levels for this kind of dynamic work. Thus, the failure to find significant advantages for case management (Marshall & Lockwood 2001) and community treatment teams (Tyrer *et al.* 2001) may be more reflective of inadequate funding and dysfunctional mental health policy than of the effectiveness of the treatment models. At the same time, few outcome studies of these modalities have paid adequate attention to the prevention and occurrence of violence. Johnson and Hickey (1999) report an uncontrolled study of arrests and incarcerations among psychosocial clubhouse members showing substantial decline in criminal justice system involvement during clubhouse membership. We await rigorous targeted research on community programmes designed to reduce violence among people with schizophrenia.

Substance misuse in combination with schizophrenia substantially increases the risk for violence. It is notoriously difficult to field, fund and maintain well-designed and implemented programmes for this population of patients. Yet, in a comprehensive review of substance misuse and violent behaviour among people with serious psychiatric disorders, Soyka (2000) concludes a discussion of psychosocial interventions by declaring, 'this is where the future for these patients lies'. This considered optimism is based on decidedly thin evidence from randomized controlled trials (Ley *et al.* 2001). Despite their ironic paucity and underuse in the USA, there is reasoned enthusiasm for specialized integrated psychiatric and substance abuse treatment programmes (Watkins *et al.* 2001).

The place of coercion and security

The latter part of the twentieth century saw legislation in many countries that enshrined the principle that, as far as possible, the treatment and management of mental disorder should follow the same principles as treatment and management of any other disorder of health; that is, it should be entirely voluntary and in the least restrictive manner and setting, whether delivered as an inpatient or an outpatient. Prior to the Mental Health Act (MHA) 1959 for England and Wales, almost all inpatient treatment there had to be conducted under a compulsory treatment order. Ironically, subsequent large-scale closure of mental hospitals and reduction in use of inpatient beds seems to have been associated in the US and UK with a return to increased reliance on compulsory treatment and/or a wish to coerce people into treatment in the community (Appelbaum 2001).

In the UK, under the MHA 1983, still extant in 2001, there are two routes into compulsory treatment for mental disorder. If the disorder is schizophrenia, then the usual route would be that two doctors, one with special experience in psychiatry, would make independent recommendations that, on grounds of mental illness, an individual needs to be detained in hospital in the interests of his or her own health or safety or the safety of others, and a social worker, having consulted with the nearest relative, agrees that no alternative is possible. The managers of the hospital where the person is to be detained must then formally accept the patient and the detention. The detention is subject to review at prescribed intervals. Various alternatives for emergencies exist, but this is the usual route. The smaller number of people who offend and who are convicted of an imprisonable criminal offence may have sentences set aside, and be detained by the court on the evidence of two doctors. In the case of people thought likely to pose a serious risk of harm to the public, a higher court may impose an order restricting discharge. Patients who fall into this last group may only be discharged with the consent of the Home Secretary or a tribunal chaired by a judge. Mental health legislation is under review in the UK, and may be extended by, for example, broadening the definition of mental disorder; a tribunal may be called on to decide the case for detention as well as to review it.

Most attention in the last decade of the twentieth century has been directed at ideas of compulsory or mandatory outpatient treatment. In the UK, there are already a number of provisions that have been insufficiently tested as to feasibility or efficacy. Within the civil part of the MHA, for example, there is a provision for guardianship which would allow a so-called 'guardian' to be appointed, usually a social worker, and for that guardian to determine the place of residence of the individual and to be able to require that the individual attends a centre or hospital for treatment or review. There is no provision for enforcement of a specific treatment. There is very little use of guardianship, cynics would say because it requires commitment of services to the pa-

tient concerned. A similar provision, the guardianship order, could be made by any criminal court on conviction for an imprisonable criminal offence. For those people who have offended seriously, and had a restriction order imposed, on finally leaving hospital the discharge is more likely than not to be conditional. The usual conditions of the discharge are supervision by a named psychiatrist, a named social worker, and residence at a place they agree. The Mental Health (Patients in the Community) Act 1995 was implemented with the idea of extending compulsory care in the community, but offered little if anything that was not already available under guardianship, and has similarly been little used. One of the goals in the British government's proposed legislative reform is to extend compulsory care and treatment in the community. Is there any evidence that this would have advantages for anyone? A review of outpatient commitment in the USA (Ridgley *et al.* 2001) concluded: 'No randomized clinical trials have examined the relative efficacy of involuntary outpatient treatment and assertive community treatment. Thus the empirical literature does not tell us whether a court order is necessary to achieve good outcomes.' Further, we do not know 'whether court orders without intensive treatment have any effect. In the USA there has been widespread experience of mandatory outpatient treatment, and very few states are without some such law (American Psychiatric Association 1999). The so-called first-generation outcome studies in the USA were perhaps limited by naturalistic designs. Generalization from results has to be made with caution, because of differences in methodology and definitions of success. Taken together, they suggested improved outcome for patients under managed care, in some cases specifically in relation to violence in the community. There are two randomized controlled trials. Swanson *et al.* (2000) studied 262 people who had been involuntarily hospitalized and then ordered to undergo a period of outpatient commitment on discharge. Many had schizophrenia or schizophrenia spectrum disorders. With the agreement of the court, the order was rescinded on a random basis, except in the case of subjects with a history of serious assault. This last group, together with one random half of the others, received an initial period of outpatient commitment of 90 days, with renewal or not following standard practice. The other half did not have the 90-day commitment. Extended outpatient commitment, lasting longer than the initial 90 days, was associated with a variety of advantages in attendance and outcome, including lower incidence of violence behaviour.

By contrast, Steadman *et al.* (2001) found no such advantage in their smaller series of 142 people, none of whom had a history of violence, and who were randomly assigned to court-ordered treatment (78) including enhanced services, and an enhanced service package alone (64). Over the same period of follow-up (12 months), no one was arrested for violent crime, and an equivalent minority of each group were arrested at least once for a non-violent crime.

There are no such studies specifically of offender patients. In the UK, a number of naturalistic studies of people leaving high-security hospital are consistent in showing that reoffending is less common in the groups under compulsory supervision in the community than in the groups without, regardless of diagnosis (Walker & McCabe 1973; Acres 1975; Bailey & McCullogh 1992; Davison *et al.* 1999). It seems unlikely that anyone will have the courage, or regard it as ethically sound, formally to randomize compulsory supervision for serious offender patients. It may be that we simply have to accept that there is little evidence of advantage of compulsory treatment in the community for the generality of people with schizophrenia, but there is a suggestion of advantage for those with schizophrenia who have a history of violence.

Conclusions

True community and birth cohort studies conducted since 1990 have consistently shown a small but significant association between violence and schizophrenia. We note that none of them take account of socially sanctioned violence such as war, death or harm caused by motor vehicles, and it might be expected that people with schizophrenia would be under-represented in these latter areas. There is considerable evidence from various perspectives that the disease itself is directly relevant to committing violence, perhaps particularly in relation to more serious violence. Symptoms, particularly delusions and perceived threat from others, seem to have important roles, each with implications for treatment (Estroff *et al.* 1994; Taylor *et al.* 1998; Krakowski *et al.* 1999; Arseneault *et al.* 2000).

Violence to others, however, is also a social phenomenon. By definition it cannot occur unless others are present, so it is perhaps unsurprising that many of the social factors known to be important among people without psychiatric illness who are violent are important also for those who are ill. It is likely that the illness affects relationships, and it is also known that much of the most serious violence occurs within the family or within relationships that at least the person with schizophrenia may perceive to be close. Risk assessment tools that are reliable and useful in an individual case still elude us, but much can be learned about the process of assessment from the efforts that have been made to devise such tools. Such assessment is only ethical if transparent and combined with appropriate limits on the extent of management interventions. The evidence base for the efficacy of a variety of treatment and management strategies remains weak. In spite of these limitations, and in spite of occasional terrible tragedies, gloom is unjustified.

Contrary to popular fears, there has been little change in the amount and severity of violence among people with schizophrenia since the move to community care, and that which does occur is entirely in line with others in society (Mullen *et al.* 2000). Indeed, in England and Wales, there is a suggestion that the contribution of people with mental illness in national homicide figures is actually falling (Taylor & Gunn 1999).

Because so much is at stake for the person with schizophrenia who may lose basic freedoms, and for those who might come to harm, informed efforts to improve both assessment and inter-

ventions are urgently needed. The research community has made laudable progress toward conceptual sophistication and methodological rigour in the quest to make the schizophrenia–violence connections transparent. Continued efforts to build on these advances will assist policy makers and governments to make rational responses to sometimes volatile circumstances, and will benefit those to whom more considered programmes and effective services are provided – and which they richly deserve.

References

Acres, D.I. (1975) *The After-Care of Special Hospital Patients.* Appendix 3 in the Report of the Committee on Mentally Abnormal Offenders. Home Office, DHSS. HMSO Cmnd. 6244: London, pp. 704–707.

Adams, J. (1995) *Risk.* UCL Press, London.

American Psychiatric Association (1999) *Mandatory Outpatient Treatment.* American Psychiatric Association, Washington DC.

Appelbaum, P.S. (2001) Thinking carefully about outpatient commitment. *Psychiatric Services* **52**, 347–350.

Appelbaum, P.S., Robbins, T.C. & Monahan, J. (2000) Violence and delusions: data from the MacArthur Violence Risk Assessment Study. *American Journal of Psychiatry* **157**, 566–572.

Arango, C., Calcedo Barba, A. & Gonzalez-Salvador, C.O.A. (1999) Violence in inpatients with schizophrenia: a prospective study. *Schizophrenia Bulletin* **25**, 493–503.

Arseneault, L., Caspi, A., Moffitt, T.E., Taylor, P.J. & Silva, P.A. (2000) Mental disorders and violence in a total birth cohort: *Archives of General Psychiatry* **57**, 979–986.

Bailey, J. & MacCulloch, M. (1992) Patterns of reconviction in patients discharged from a special hospital: implications for aftercare. *Journal of Forensic Psychiatry* **3**, 445–461.

Beauford, J.E., McNeil, D.E. & Binder, R.L. (1997) Utility of the initial therapeutic alliance in evaluating psychiatric patients' risk of violence. *American Journal of Psychiatry* **154**, 1272–1276.

Beesley, C.M., Taylor, M.E., Kiester, S.*et al.* (1998) The influence of pharmacotherapy on self-directed and externally-directed aggression in schizophrenia. *Schizophrenia Research* **29**, 28.

Bentsen, H., Notland, T.H., Boye, B., *et al.* (1998) Criticism and hostility in relatives of patients with schizophrenia or related psychoses: demographic and clinical predictors. *Act Psychiatrica Scandinavica* **97**, 76–85.

Bergman, B. & Ericsson, E. (1996) Family violence among psychiatric in-patients as measured by the Conflict Tactics Scale (CTS). *Acta Psychiatrica Scandinavica* **94**, 168–174.

Boye, B., Bentsen, H., Ulstein, I. *et al.* (2001) Relatives, distress and patients, symptoms and behaviours: a prospective study of patients with schizophrenia and their relatives. *Acta Psychiatrica Scandinavica* **104**, 42–50.

Brennan, P.A., Mednick, S.A. & Jacobson, B. (1996) Assessing the role of genetics in crime using adoption cohorts. In: *Genetics of Criminal and Antisocial Behaviour: Ciba Foundation Symposium 194* (eds G.R. Bock & J.A. Goode), pp. 115–123. John Wiley and Sons, Chichester.

Brennan, P.A., Grekin, E.R. & Vanman, E.J. (2000) Major mental disorders and crime in the community. In: *Violence Among the Mentally Ill* (ed. S. Hodgins), pp. 3–18. Kluwer Academic, Dordrecht.

Buchanan, A. & Leese, M. (2001) Detention of the 'dangerous severely personality disordered': some data. *Lancet* **358**, 1955–1959.

Buchanan, A., Reed, A., Wessely, S. *et al.* (1993) Acting on delusions.

II. The phenomenological correlates of acting on delusions. *British Journal of Psychiatry* **163**, 77–82.

Buckley, P.F. (1998) The management of aggression in schizophrenia. *Schizophrenia Monitor* **8**, 19–22.

Buckley, P., Bartell, J., Donerworth, K. *et al.* (1995) Violence and schizophrenia: clozapine as a specific antiaggression agent. *Bulletin of the American Academy of Psychiatry and the Law* **23**, 607–611.

Carmel, H. & Hunter, M. (1991) Psychiatrists injured by patient attack. *Bulletin of the American Academy of Psychiatry and the Law* **19**, 309–316.

Christison, G.W., Kirch, D.G. & Wyatt, R.J. (1991) When symptoms persist: choosing among alternative somatic treatment for schizophrenia. *Schizophrenia Bulletin* **17**, 217–245.

Coid, J. (1983) The epidemiology of abnormal homicide and murder followed by suicide. *Psychological Medicine* **13**, 855–860.

Coid, B., Lewis, S.W. & Reveley, A.M. (1993) A twin study of psychosis and criminality. *British Journal of Psychiatry* **162**, 87–92.

Conner, M. & Norman, P. (1996) *Predicting Health Behaviour*. Open University Press, Buckingham.

Cooke, D.J. & Michie, C. (1999) Psychopathy across cultures: North America and Scotland compared. *Journal of Abnormal Psychology* **108**, 55–68.

Dalal, B., Larkin, E., Leese, M. & Taylor, P.J. (1999) Clozapine treatment of long-standing schizophrenia and serious violence. *Criminal Behaviour and Mental Health* **9**, 168–178.

Davison, S.E., Jamieson, E. & Taylor, P.J. (1999) Route of discharge for special (high security) hospital patients with personality disorders: its relationship with reconviction. *British Journal of Psychiatry* **174**, 224–227.

Department of Health (1990) Caring for People. The Care Programme Approach (CPA) for people with a Mental Illness Referred to the Specialist Psychiatric Services. Circular HC(90)23/LASSL(90)11. Department of Health, London.

Department of Health (1994) *Guidance on the Discharge of Mentally Disordered People and Their Continuing Care in the Community*. NHS Executive HSG (94) 27 and LASSL (94) 4.

Department of Health, Home Office (2000) *Reforming the Mental Health Act*. The Stationery Office, Norwich. Cm5016-I and 5016-II.

Depp, F.C. (1983) Assaults in a public mental hospital. In: *Assaults Within Psychiatric Facilities* (eds J.R. Lion & W.H. Reid), pp. 21–45. Grune & Stratton, New York.

Dietz, P.E. & Rada, R.T. (1982) Battery incidents and batterers in a maximum security hospital. *Archives of General Psychiatry* **39**, 31–34.

Eronen, M., Hakola, P. & Tiihonen, J. (1996) Mental disorders and homicidal behavior in Finland. *Archives of General Psychiatry* **53**, 497–501.

Estroff, S.E. (2000) Social and Community Services and the risk for violence among people with serious psychiatric disorders: in search of mechanisms. In: *Violence Among the Mentally Ill* (ed. S.Hodgins), pp. 383–388. Kluwer Academic, the Netherlands.

Estroff, S.E. & Zimmer, C. (1994) Social networks, social support and the risk for violence among persons with severe, persistent mental illness. In: *Violence and Mental Illness: Developments in Risk Assessment* (eds J. Monahan & H. Steadman), pp. 259–293. University of Chicago Press, Chicago.

Estroff, S.E., Zimmer, C.R., Lachicotte, W.S. & Benoit, J. (1994) The influence of social networks and social support on violence by persons with serious mental illness. *Hospital and Community Psychiatry* **45**, 669–679.

Estroff, S.E., Swanson, J.W., Lachicotte, W.S., Swartz, M. & Bolduc, M. (1998) Risk reconsidered: targets of violence in the social networks of people with serious psychiatric disorders. *Social Psychiatry and Psychiatric Epidemiology*, **33** (Suppl. 1), 95–101.

Fava, M., ed. (1997) Psychopharmacologic treatment of pathological aggression. In: *Psychiatric Clinics of North America*. pp. 427–452. W.B. Saunders, Philadelphia.

Gardner, W., Lidz, C.W., Mulvey, E.P. & Shaw, E.C. (1996a) A comparison of actuarial methods for identifying repetitively violent patients with mental illnesses. *Law and Human Behavior* **20**, 35–48.

Gardner, W., Lidz, C.W., Mulvey, E.P. & Shaw, E.C. (1996b) Clinical versus actuarial predictions of violence by patients with mental illnesses. *Journal of Consulting and Clinical Psychology* **64**, 602–609.

Gilligan, J. (1992) *Violence: Reflections on our Deadliest Epidemic*. Jessica Kingsley, London.

Greenhalgh, T. & Plsek, P.E. (2001) The challenge of complexity in healthcare. *British Medical Journal* **323**, 625–628.

Grove, W.M. & Meehl, P.E. (1996) Comparative efficiency of informal (subjective, impressionistic) and formal (mechanical, alogorithmic) prediction procedures: the clinical–statistical controversy. *Psychology, Public Policy and Law* **2**, 293–323.

Gudjonsson, G.H., Clare, I., Rutters, S. & Pearse, J. (1993) *Persons At Risk During Interviews in Police Custody: The Identification of Vulnerabilities*. Royal Commission on Criminal Justice Research Report. HMSO, London.

Häfner, H. & Böker, W. (1973) *Crimes of Violence by Mentally Abnormal Offenders* (translated by H. Marshall, 1982). Cambridge University Press, Cambridge.

Hare, R.D. (1991) *The Hare Psychopathy Checklist: Revised*. Multi Health Systems, Toronto, Ontario.

Hare, R.D., Cooke, D.J. & Hart, S.D. (1999) Psychopathy and sadistic personality disorder. In: *Oxford Textbook of Psychopathology* (eds T. Millon, P.H. Blaney & R.D. Davies), pp. 555–584. Oxford University Press, Oxford.

Heads, T.C., Leese, M. & Taylor, P.J. (1997) Social integration, aspects of illness and offending/violent behaviour among people with schizophrenia regarded as seriously dangerous to others: patterns of social isolation and dysfunction and correlates with symptomatology. *Criminal Behaviour and Mental Health* **7**, 117–130.

Hellerstein, D., Frosch, W. & Koenigsberg, H.W. (1987) The clinical significance of command hallucinations. *American Journal of Psychiatry* **144**, 219–221.

Hodgins, S. (1992) Mental disorder, intellectual deficiency and crime. *Archives of General Psychiatry* **49**, 476–483.

Hodgins, S., Mednick, S.A., Brennan, P.A., Schulsinger, F. & Engberg, M. (1996) Mental disorder and crime: evidence from a Danish birth cohort. *Archives of General Psychiatry* **54**, 489–496.

Home Office (1991–2000) *Notifiable Offences*. Home Office Statistical Bulletin, published annually. Home Office Research and Statistics Department, London, SW1H 9AT.

Howitt, D. (1998) *Crime, the Media and the Law*. John Wiley, Chichester.

Hyde, A.P. (1997) Coping with the threatening, intimidating, violent behaviors of people with psychiatric disabilities living at home: guidelines for family caregivers. *Psychiatric Rehabilitation Journal* **21**, 144–149.

Irving, B. & Hilgendorf, L. (1980) *Police Interrogation Research Study No 1*. The Psychological Approach Royal Commission on Criminal Procedure. HMSO, London.

Janofsky, J.S., Spears, S. & Neubauer, D.N. (1988) Psychiatrists' accuracy in predicting violent behaviour on an inpatient unit. *Hospital and Community Psychiatry* **39**, 1090–1094.

Johnson, J. & Hickey, S. 1999) Arrests and incarcerations after psychosocial programme involvement: clubhouse vs. jailhouse. *Psychiatric Rehabilitation Journal* **23**, 66–69.

Jones, C., Carmac, I., Mota, J. & Campbell, C. (2001) Cognitive behavior therapy for schizophrenia (Cochrane Review). In: *The Cochrane Library* **3**. Update Software, Oxford.

Junginger, J. (1990) Predicting compliance with command hallucinations. *American Journal of Psyphiatry* **147**, 245–247.

Krakowski, M., Czobor, P. & Chou, J.C. (1999) Course of violence in patients with schizophrenia: relationship to clinical symptoms. *Schizophrenia Bulletin* **25**, 505–517.

Lancee, W.J., Gallop, R. & McCaye Toner, B. (1995) The relationship between nurses' limit-setting styles and anger in psychiatric inpatients. *Psychiatric Services* **6**, 609–613.

Langhan, P.A. & Farrington, D.P. (1998) *Crime and Justice in the United States and in England and Wales, 1981–96*. US Department of Justice, Office of Justice Programs, Bureau of Justice Statistics, Washington, DC.

Lehman, A.F. & Linn, L.S. (1984) Crimes against discharged mental patients in board and care homes. *American Journal of Psychiatry* **141**, 271–274.

Lehman, A.F. & Steinwachs, D.M. & the PORT Co-Investigators (1998) Translating research into practice: the schziophrenia PORT Treatment Recommendations. *Schizophrenia Bulletin* **24**, 1–10.

Ley, A., Jeffery, D.P., McLaren, S. & Siegfried, N. (2001) Treatment programmes for people with both severe mental illness and substance misuse (Cochrane Review). In: *The Cochrane Library*, **3**. Update Software, Oxford.

Lidz, C.W., Mulvey, E.P. & Gardner, W. (1993) The accuracy of predictions of violence to others. *Journal of the American Medical Association* **269**, 1007–1011.

Lindqvist, P. (1989) Criminal homicide in Northern Sweden 1970–81: alcohol intoxication, alcohol abuse and mental disease. *International Journal of Law and Psychiatry* **8**, 19–37.

Lindqvist, P. & Allebeck, P. (1990) Schizophrenia and crime: a longitudinal follow-up of 644 schizophrenics in Stockholm. *British Journal of Psychiatry* **157**, 345–350.

Link, B.G. & Stueve, A. (1994) Psychotic symptoms and the violent/illegal behavior of mental patients compared to community controls in violence and mental disorder. In: *Developments and Risk Assessment* (eds J. Monahan and H.J. Steadman), pp. 137–155. University of Chicago Press, Chicago.

Link, B.G., Andrews, H.A. & Cullen, F.T. (1992) The violent and illegal behaviour of mental patients reconsidered. *American Sociological Review* **57**, 175–292.

Link, B.G., Stueve, A. & Phelan, J. (1998) Psychotic symptoms and violent behaviors: probing the component of 'threat/control-override' symptoms. *Social Psychiatry and Psychiatric Epidemiology* **33**, S55–S60.

Lion, J.R. & Soloff, P.H. (1984) Implementation of seclusion and restraint. In: *The Psychiatric Uses of Seclusion and Restraint* (ed. K. Tardiff), pp. 19–34. American Psychiatric Press, Washington, DC.

Low, G., Jones, D., Duggan, C., Power, M. & MacLeod, A. (2001) The treatment of deliberate self-harm in borderline personality disorder using dialectical behaviour therapy: a pilot study in a high security hospital. *Behavioural and Cognitive Psychotherapy* **29**, 85–92.

Lowenstein, M., Binder, R.L. & McNiel, D.E. (1990) The relationship between admission symptoms and hospital assaults. *Hospital and Community Psychiatry* **41**, 311–313.

McGauley, G.A. (1997) The actor, the act and the environment: forensic psychotherapy and risk. *International Review of Psychiatry* **9**, 257–264.

McNiel, D.E. (1994) Hallucinations and violence. In: *Violence and Mental Disorder Developments in Risk Assessment* (eds J. Monahan & H. Steadman), pp. 183–202. University of Chicago Press, Chicago.

McNiel, D.E., Eisner, J.P. & Binder, R.L. (2000) The relationship between command hallucinations and violence. *Psychiatric Services* **51**, 1288–1292.

Marshall, M. & Lockwood, A. (2001) Assertive community treatments for people with severe mental disorders (Cochrane Review). In: *The Cochrane Library* **3**. Update Software, Oxford.

Marshall, M., Gray, A., Lockwood, A. & Green, R. (1999) Case management for people with severe mental disorders (Cochrane Review). In: *The Cochrance Library, Issue 1*. Update Software, Oxford.

Meuser, K.T., Goodman, L.B., Trumbetta, S.L. *et al.* (1998) Trauma and posttraumatic stress disorder in severe mental illness. *Journal of Consulting and Clinical Psychology* **66**, 493–499.

Moffitt, T.E. (1984) *Genetic influences of parental psychiatric illness on violent and recidivistic criminal behaviour*. PhD thesis, University of Southern California, Los Angeles, CA, USA.

Monahan, J. (1992) Violence and mental disorder: perceptions and evidence. *American Psychologist* **47**, 511–521.

Monahan, J. & Steadman, H. (1983) Crime and mental disorder: an epidemiological approach. In: *Crime and Justice: an Annual Review of Research*, Vol. 3 (eds N. Morris & M. Tonry), pp. 145–189. University of Chicago Press, Chicago.

Monahan, J. & Steadman, H.J. (1996) Violent storms and violent people: how meteorology can inform risk communication in mental health law. *American Psychologist* **51**, 931–938.

Monahan, J., Steadman, H.J., Applebaum, P.S. *et al.* (2000) Developing a clinically useful actuarial tool for assessing violence risk. *British Journal of Psychiatry* **176**, 312–319.

Moore, E. & Kuipers, E. (1999) The measurement of expressed emotion in relationships between staff and service users: the use of short speech samples. *British Journal of Clinical Psychology* **38**, 345–356.

Mossman, D. (1994) Assessing predictions of violence: being accurate about accuracy. *Journal of Consulting and Clinical Psychology* **62**, 783–779.

Mossman, D. (1995) Dangerous decisions: an essay on the mathematics of clinical violence prediction and involuntary hospitalization. *University of Chicago Law School Roundtable* **2**, 95–138.

Mullen, P.E., Burgess, P., Wallace, C., Palmer, S. & Ruschena, D. (2000) Community care and criminal offending in schizophrenia. *Lancet* **355**, 614–617.

Mulvey, E.P., Shaw, E. & Lidz, C.W. (1994) Why use multiple sources in research on patient violence in the community? *Criminal Behaviour and Mental Health* **4**, 253–258.

Munro, E. & Rumgay, J. (2000) Role of risk assessment in reducing homicides by people with mental illness. *British Journal of Psychiatry* **176**, 116–120.

National Confidential Inquiry (2001) *Safety first: Five-year report of the National Confidential Inquiry into Suicide and Homicide by People with Mental Illness*. Department of Health, London SE1 6XH.

National Confidential Inquiry into Suicide and Homicide by People with Mental Illness (1999) *Safer Services*. Department of Health, London.

National Health Service (NHS) Management Executive (1993) *Risk Management in the NHS*. Department of Health, London.

Nillson, K., Palmstierna, T. & Wistedt, B. (1988) Aggressive behaviour in hospitalised psychogeriatric patients. *Acta Psychiatrica Scandinavica* **55**, 65–73.

Ortmann, J. (1981) Psykisk Afvigelse og kriminel adfaerd. *Under En Søgelse Af 11533 Maend Født* i, 1953. I det metropolitane omrde københavn. Forksningsrapport 17. Justitminsteriet: Copenhagen, Denmark.

Palmstierna, T. & Wistedt, B. (1995) Changes in the pattern of aggressive behaviour among inpatients with changed ward organisation. *Acta Psychiatrica Scandinavica* **91**, 32–35.

Pearse, J., Gudjonsson, G.H., Clare, I.C.H. & Rutter, S. (1998) Police interviewing and psychological vulnerabilities: predicting the likelihood of a confession. *Journal of Community and Applied Social Psychology* **8**, 1–21.

Peay, J., ed. (1996) *Inquiries After Homicide*. Duckworth, London.

Peay, J. (1997) Clinicians and inquiries: demons, drones or demigods? *International Review of Psychiatry* **9**, 171–177.

Pekkala, E. & Merinder, L. (2001) Psychoeducational for schizophrenia (Cochrane Review). In: *The Cochrane Library*, **3**. Update Software, Oxford.

Petursson, H. & Gudjonsson, G.H. (1981) Psychiatric aspects of homicide. *Acta Psychiatrica Scandinavica* **64**, 363–372.

Phelan, J.C. & Link, B.G. (1998) The growing belief that people with mental illnesses are violent: the role of the dangerousness criterion for civil commitment. *Social Psychiatry and Psychiatric Epidemiology* **33**, s7–s12.

Phillips, D. & Rudestam, K.E. (1995) Effect of non-violence self-defense training on male psychiatric staff members' aggression and fear. *Psychiatric Services* **46**, 164–168.

Quinsey, V.I., Harris, G.T., Rice, M.E. & Cormier, C.A. (1998) *Violent Offenders: Appraising and Managing the Risk*. American Psychological Association, Washington.

Rabinowitz, J., Avnon, M. & Rosenberg, V. (1996) Effect of clozapine on physical and verbal aggression. *Schizophrenia Research* **22**, 249–255.

Ratey, J.J., Sårgi, P. & O'Driscoll, G.A. (1992) Nadolol to treat aggression and psychiatric symptomatology in chronic psychiatric inpatients: a double-blind, placebo-controlled study. *Journal of Clinical Psychiatry* **53**, 41–46.

Reiss, D. (2001) Counterfactuals and inquiries after homicide. *Journal of Forensic Psychiatry* **12**, 169–181.

Reiss, A.J. & Roth, J.A., eds. (1993–94). *Understanding and Preventing Violence*, Vols 1–4. National Academy Press, Washington, DC.

Reiss, D., Meux, C. & Grubin, D. (2000) The effect of psychopathy on outcome in high security patients. *Journal of the American Academy of Psychiatry and the Law* **28**, 309–314.

Ridgely, M.S., Borum, R. & Petrila, J. (2001) *The Effectiveness of Involuntary Outpatient Treatment: Empirical Evidence and the Experience of Eight States*. RAND Publication MR-1340-CSCR. http:/www.rand.org/publications/MR/MR1340.

Ritchie, J.H., Dick, D. & Lingham, R. (1994) *The Report of the Inquiry into the Care and Treatment of Christopher Clunis*. HMSO, London.

Robertson, G. (1988) Arrest patterns among mentally disordered offenders. *British Journal of Psychiatry* **153**, 313–316.

Rofman, E.S., Askinazi, C. & Fant, E. (1980) The prediction of dangerous behavior in emergency civil commitment. *American Journal of Psychiatry* **137**, 1061–1064.

Rogers, P., Watt, A., Gray, N.S., MacCulloch, M. & Gournay, K. (2002) Content of command hallucinations predicts self-harm but not violence in a medium secure hospital. *Journal of Forensic Psychiatry* **13**, 245–256.

Royal College of Psychiatrists (1990) The seclusion of psychiatric patients. *Psychiatric Bulletin* **14**, 754–756.

Royal College of Psychiatrists (1996) *Assessment and Clinical Management of Risk of Harm to Other People*. Council Report CR53. Royal College of Psychiatrists, London.

Royal College of Psychiatrists Research Unit (1998) *Management of Imminent Violence Clinical Practice Guidelines to Support Mental Health Services* Occasional paper OP41. Royal College of Psychiatrists, London.

Rudrick, A. (1999) Relation between command hallucinations and dangerous behaviour. *Journal of the American Academy of Psychiatry and the Law* **27**, 253–257.

Schipkowensky, N. (1973) Epidemiological aspects of homicide. In: *World Biennial of Psychiatry and Psychotherapy* Vol. 2 (ed. S. Arieti), pp. 192–215.

Smoot, S.L. & Gonzales, J.L. (1995) Cost-effective communication skills training for state hospital empoyees. *Psychiatric Services* **46**, 819–822.

Soothill, K., Francis, B., Ackerley, E. & Colletts, S. (1999) *Homicide in Britain: A Comparative Study of Rates in Scotland and England and Wales*. Scottish Executive, Edinburgh.

Soyka, M. (2000) Substance misuse, psychiatric disorder, and violent and disturbed behaviour. *British Journal of Psychiatry* **176**, 345–350.

Special Hospitals' Treatment Resistant Schizophrenia Group (1996) Schizophrenia, violence, clozapine and risperidone: a review. *British Journal of Psychiatry* **169**, 21–30.

Stanko, E.A. (1993) Everyday violence and experience of crime. In: *Violence In Society* (ed. P.J. Taylor), pp. 169–180. Royal College of Physicians, London.

Steadman, H.J. & Silver, E. (2000) Immediate precursors of violence among persons with mental illness: a return to a situational perspective. In: *Violence Among the Mentally Ill* (ed. S. Hodgins), Kluwer Academic, the Netherlands.

Steadman, H.J., Monahan, J., Appelbaum, P.S. *et al.* (1994) Designing a new generation of risk assessment research. In: *Violence and Mental Disorder Developments in Risk Assessment* (eds J. Monahan & H. Steadman), pp. 297–318. Chicago University Press, Chicago.

Steadman, H.J., Mulvey, E.P., Monahan, J. *et al.* (1998) Violence by people discharged from acute psychiatric inpatient facilities and by others in the same neighborhoods. *Archives of General Psychiatry* **55**, 393–401.

Steadman, H.J., Silver, E., Monahan, J. *et al.* (2000) A classification tree approach to the development of actuarial violence risk assessment tools. *Law and Human Behavior* **24**, 83–100.

Steadman, H.J., Gounis, K., Dennis, D. *et al.* (2001) Assessing the New York City and voluntary outpatients commitment pilot program. *Psychiatric Services* **52**, 330–336.

Steinert, T., Sippach, T. & Gebhardt, R.P. (2000) How common is violence in schizophrenia despite neuroleptic treatment? *Pharmacopsychiatry* **33**, 98–102.

Surowiecki, J. (2001) What weather costs. *The New Yorker* 23 July 2001, p. 29.

Swanson, J.W., Holzer, C.F., Ganju, V.K. & Jono, R.T. (1990) Violence and psychiatric disorder in the community: evidence from the Epidemiologic Catchment Area Surveys. *Hospital and Community Psychiatry* **41**, 761–770.

Swanson, J., Borum, R., Swartz, M. & Monahan, J. (1996) Psychotic symptoms and disorders and the risk of violent behavior in the community. *Criminal Behaviour and Mental Health* **6**, 309–329.

Swanson, J.W., Estroff, S.E., Swartz, M. *et al.* (1997) Violence and severe mental disorder in clinical and community populations: the effects of psychotic symptoms, comorbidity, and disaffiliation from treatment. *Psychiatry* **60**, 1–22.

Swanson, J.W., Estroff, S.E., Swartz, M.S. *et al.* (1998) Psychiatric impairment, social contact, and violent behavior. *Social Psychiatry and Pshchiatric Epidemiology* **33**, 86–94.

Swanson, J.W., Swartz, M.S., Borum, R. *et al.* (2000) Involuntary outpatient commitment and reduction of violent behaviour in persons with severe mental illness. *British Journal of Psychiatry* **176**, 324–331.

Swartz, M.S. & Monahan, J. (2001) Special section on involuntary outpatient commitment: introduction. *Psychiatric Services* **52**, 323–324; the whole section 323–350.

Swartz, M.S., Swanison, J.W., Wagner, H.R., *et al.* (1999) Can involuntary outpatient treatment reduce hospital recidivism? Findings from a randomized trial with severely mentally ill individuals. *American Journal of Psychiatry* **156**, 1968–1975.

Swinton, M. & Haddock, A. (2000) Clozapine in special hospital: a retrospective case–control study. *Journal of Forensic Psychiatry* **2**, 587–596.

Tarasoff *v* Regents of University of California 1178 Cal Rptr 129 529 P(2d) 553 (1974).

Tarafsoff *v* Regents of California 551 P(2d) 333 1312 Cal Rptr 14 (1976).

Tardiff, K., Marzuk, P.M., Leon, A.C. & Portera, L. (1997) A prospective study of violence by psychiatric patients after hospital discharge. *Psychiatric Services* **48**, 678–681.

Taylor, P.J. (1982) Schizophrenia and violence. In: *Abnormal Offenders Delinquency and the Criminal Justice System* (eds J. Gunn & D.P. Farrington), pp. 269–284. Wiley, Chichester.

Taylor, P.J. (1985) Motives for offending among violent and psychotic men. *British Journal of Psychiatry* **147**, 491–498.

Taylor, P.J. (1987) The schizophrenic offender. In: *Psychiatric Disorders and the Criminal Process*. Proceedings of the 2nd Annual Leicester Symposium. Schering Health Care, Burgess Hill.

Taylor, P.J. (1993) Schizophrenia and crime: distinctive patterns in association. In: *Crime and Mental Disorder* (ed. S. Hodgins), , pp. 63–85. Sage, Newbury Park, CA.

Taylor, P.J. (1999) Disorders of volition: forensic aspects. In: *Disorders of Volition and Action in Psychiatry* (eds C. Williams & A. Sims), pp. 66–84. University of Leeds, Leeds.

Taylor, P.J. & Buckley, P. (2000) *Treating Violence in the Context of Psychosis*. In: *Schizophrenia and Mood Disorders. The New Drug Therapies in Clinical Practice* (eds P. J. Buckley & J. L. Waddington), pp. 297–316. Butterworth-Heinemann, Oxford.

Taylor, P.J. & Gunn, J.C. (1984) Violence and psychosis. *British Medical Journal* **288**, 1945–1949; **289**, 9–12.

Taylor, P.J. & Gunn, J. (1999) Homicides of people with mental illness: myth and reality. *British Journal of Psychiatry* **174**, 9–14.

Taylor, P.J. & Hodgins, S. (1994) Violence and psychosis: critical timings. *Criminal Behaviour and Mental Health* **4**, 267–289.

Taylor, P.J. & Kopelman, M. (1984) Amnesia for criminal offences. *Psychological Medicine* **14**, 581–588.

Taylor, P.J. & Schanda, H. (2000) Violence against others by psychiatric hospital inpatients with psychosis. In: *Violence Among the Mentally Ill* (ed. S. Hodgins), pp. 251–275. Kluwer Academic, the Netherlands.

Taylor, P.J., Garety, P., Buchanan, A. *et al.* (1994) Delusions and violence. In: *Violence and Mental Disorder Developments in Risk Assessment* (eds J. Monahan & H. Steadman), pp. 161–182. University of Chicago Press, Chicago.

Taylor, P.J., Leese, M., Williams, D. *et al.* (1998) Mental disorder and violence: a special (high security) hospital study. *British Journal of Psychiatry* **172**, 218–226.

Tengstrom, A., Hodgins, S. & Kullgren, G. (2001) Men with schizophrenia who behave violently: the usefulness of an early- versus late-start offender typology. *Schizophrenia Bulletin* **27**, 205–218.

Thomas, H.J., Schwartz, E. & Petrelli, R. (1992) Droperidol versus haloperidol for clinical restraint of agitated and combative patients. *Annals of Emergency Medicine* **21**, 407–413.

Tiihonen, J. & Swartz, M.S. (2000) Pharmacological intervention for preventing violence among the mentally ill with secondary alcohol- and drug-use disorders. In: *Violence Among the Mentally Ill* (ed. S. Hodgins), pp. 193–212. Kluwer Academic, the Netherlands.

Tiihonen, J., Isohanni, M., Räsänen, P., Koiranen, M. & Moring, J. (1997) Specific major mental disorders and criminality: a 26-year prospective study of the 1966 Finland birth cohort. *American Journal of Psychiatry* **154**, 840–845.

Tyrer, P., Coid, J., Simmonds, S., Joseph, P. & Marriott, S. (2001) Community treatment teams for people with severe mental illness and disordered personality. In: *The Cochrane Library* 3. Update Software, Oxford.

Vaddadi, K.S., Soosai, E., Gilleard, C.J. & Adlard, S. (1997) Mental illness, physical abuse and burden of care on relatives: a study of acute psychiatric admission patients. *Acta Psychiatrica Scandinavica* **95**, 313–317.

Volavka, J. (1995) Neurochemistry of violence. In: *Neurobiology of Violence* (ed. J. Volavka), pp. 49–76. American Psychiatric Press, Washington, DC.

Volavka, J., Zito, J., Vitral, J. *et al.* (1993) Clozapine effects on hostility and aggression in schizophrenia. *Journal of Clinical Psychopharmacology* **13**, 287–289.

Volavka, J., Laska, E., Baker, S. *et al.* (1997) History of violent behavior and schizophrenia in different cultures: analyses based on the WHO Study on Determinants of Outcomes of Severe Mental Disorders. *British Journal of Psychiatry* **171**, 9–14.

Walker, N. & McCabe, S. (1973) *Crime and Insanity in England*, Vol. 2. *New Solutions and New Problems*. Edinburgh University Press, Edinburgh.

Wallace, C., Mullen, P., Burgess, P. *et al.* (1998) Serious criminal offending and mental disorder. *British Journal of Psychiatry* **172**, 477–484.

Walsh, E., Harvey, K., White, I. *et al.* (2001a) Suicidal behaviour in psychosis: prevalence and predictors from a randomised controlled trial of case management: report from the UK 700 Trial. *British Journal of Psychiatry* **178**, 255–260.

Walsh, E., Gilvarry, C., Samele, C. *et al.* for the UK 700 Group (2001b) Reducing violence in severe mental illness: randomised controlled trial of intensive case management compared with standard care. *British Medical Journal* **323**, 1093–1096.

Watkins, K.E., Burnam, A., Kung, F.-Y. & Paddock, S. (2001) A national survey of care for persons with co-occurring mental and substance use disorders. *Psychiatric Services* **52**, 1062–1068.

Webster, C.D., Eaves, D., Douglas, K.S. & Winthrup, A. (1995) *The HCR-20 Scheme: the Assessment of Dangerousness and Risk*. Simon Fraser University and Forensic Psychiatric Services Commission of British Columbia, Vancouver.

Webster, C.D., Douglas, K.S., Eaves, D. & Hart, S.D. (1997) *The HCR-20: Assessing Risk for Violence*, Version 2. Mental Health, Law and Policy Institute, Simon Fraser University, Vancouver.

Webster, C.D., Douglas, K.S., Belfrage, H. & Link, B.G. (2000) Capturing change. In: *Violence Among the Mentally Ill* (ed. S. Hodgins), pp. 119–144. Kluwer Academic, the Netherlands.

Werner, P.D., Rose, T.L., Yesavage, J.A. & Seeman, K. (1984) Psychiatrists' judgements of dangerousness in patients on an acute care unit. *American Journal of Psychiatry* **141**, 263–266.

Wessely, S. & Taylor, P.J. (1991) Madness and crime: criminology versus psychiatry. *Criminal Behaviour and Mental Health* **1**, 193–228.

Wessely, S., Buchanan, A., Reed, A. *et al.* (1993) Acting on delusions. I. Prevalence. *British Journal of Psychiatry* **163**, 69–76.

Wessely, S., Castle, D., Douglas, A.J. & Taylor, P.J. (1994) The criminal careers of incident cases of schizophrenia. *Psychological Medicine* **24**, 483–502.

West, D.J. & Walk, A. (1977) *Daniel McNaughton, His Trial and the Aftermath*. Gaskell, London.

Wilcox, D.E. (1985) The relationship of mental illness to homicide. *American Journal of Forensic Psychiatry* **6**, 3–15.

Wilkins, R. (1993) Delusions in children and teenagers admitted to Bethlem Royal Hospital in the 19th century. *British Journal of Psychiatry* **162**, 487–492.

Williams, P. & Dickinson, J. (1993) Fear of crime: read all about it? The relationship between newspaper crime reporting and the fear of crime. *British Journal of Criminology* **33**, 33–56.

Wilson, T. & Holt, T. (2001) Complexity and clinical care. *British Medical Journal* **323**, 685–688.

Winerip, M. (1999) Bedlam on the streets. *The New York Times Magazine* 23 May 1999.

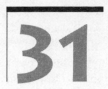

31 Schizophrenia and psychosocial stresses

P.E. Bebbington and E. Kuipers

Domains of psychosocial stress, 613
Reactive psychoses, 614
Setting the agenda for a social aetiology, 614
Expressed emotion and relapse in schizophrenia, 615
    Alternatives to the use of the EE measure, 615
    EE and the prediction of relapse, 615
    New studies of the predictive capacity of EE, 616
    Inferences from family intervention in
        schizophrenia, 617
    The meaning of EE (construct validity), 618
    The origins of EE, 620
    EE as an attribute of professional carers, 621
    EE and burden, 621

EE studies: conclusions, 622
Life event studies, 622
    The concept of triggering, 623
    Life event studies in schizophrenia, 623
    Increased sensitivity to events, 625
Post-traumatic stress disorder and schizophrenia,
    625
Early social environment in people who develop
    schizophrenia, 626
Interplay of stress, medication and relapse in
    schizophrenia, 627
Conclusions, 627
References, 629

Our previous chapter on this topic (Bebbington *et al.* 1995) focused on research into factors reflecting directly on the potential psychosocial causation of schizophrenia. Thus, we covered in detail methodological issues and empirical results of studies linking the emergence of schizophrenic symptoms with: (i) antecedent life events, and (ii) family atmosphere, as detected by the expressed emotion (EE) measure.

In the current revision of the chapter, we have updated these sections, but we have also shortened them. This enables us to broaden the type of evidence used to explore the psychosocial reactivity of psychotic symptoms. This includes the issues of psychogenic psychosis and of schizophrenic symptoms in the context of post-traumatic stress disorder.

It is timely to broaden the debate for three reasons. The first concerns emerging evidence of the effectiveness of cognitive–behaviour therapy in the treatment of schizophrenia (Kuipers *et al.* 1997, 1998; Tarrier *et al.* 1999; Sensky *et al.* 2000; systematically reviewed by Pilling *et al.* 2002). The establishment of the meaning of clients' symptoms in terms of their experiences and circumstances is often an important element in this treatment. Thus, the impact of the psychosocial environment over the whole life span is likely to be explored.

The second reason is that no predominant causes of schizophrenia have yet been identified. Thus, it might be argued that the genetic project in schizophrenia has been, relatively speaking, a failure, at least in so far as major genes are concerned. The total investment in the search for the genetic basis for schizophrenia is now estimated to have exceeded $400 million, and the conclusion is that major genes for schizophrenia are not widespread, even if they exist in particular families, and that no generally distributed contributory gene is likely to increase the risk of schizophrenia in siblings by more than threefold (Owen 2000).

Finally, the argument for the importance of psychosocial causation gains strength from the identification of groups of people with undeniable symptoms of schizophrenia, but with few of the traditional biological markers of the condition. Black Britons of Caribbean origin or ancestry form such a group despite having high rates of schizophrenia (Bhugra *et al.* 1997; Hutchinson *et al.* 1997; McDonald & Murray 2000).

Domains of psychosocial stress

Psychiatric classification is still primarily based on the clinical features of individual disorders. Attempts to base classification on aetiological principles have been successful in relatively few conditions. Perhaps because of the medical basis of psychiatry, favoured aetiological hypotheses have tended to involve organic causes, although the attempt to identify such causes has gone relatively unrewarded. However, it has resulted in deliberate refinements of classification. Thus, in order to further the search for organic causation, early psychiatrists attempted to separate off those cases of symptom-defined disorder which appeared to have a social aetiological origin.

The psychogenic element in psychiatric disorders was recognized by psychiatrists, certainly by the mid-nineteenth century (Griesinger 1861). Having made the decision to do so, it was easy to distinguish conditions such as bereavement responses from depressive disorders 'proper', but by the early twentieth century similar attempts to separate off so-called 'reactive psychoses' were being made. This strategy results in a core group of disorders that are covertly defined by not having an intimate relationship to a social causation.

Oddly, this has not prevented researchers from continuing to tease out social influences on these ring-fenced disorders, and they have, perhaps ironically, been rather successful in this. This is particularly so in the case of depressive disorder, although the relation of stressful life events to the onset of depressive disorders, defined by the exclusion of cases immediately and intimately related to social causes, tends to mean that the social causation in the remaining disorders is more subtle.

A similar pattern is apparent in the case of psychosis. The search for a social aetiology of psychosis has tended to follow the exclusion of those cases in which social causes appear paramount. These disorders have been characterized as reactive psychoses. These days, this is predominantly a Scandinavian diagnosis. Nevertheless, the development of the idea of reactive psychosis had the inevitable result that cases where social reactivity was not completely salient came to be regarded as essentially biological in origin. Much of the evidence in this chapter is focused on the social reactivity of schizophrenic psychoses following definitions that essentially exclude immediate and salient social causes.

The idea that schizophrenia is a socially reactive condition has become virtually the accepted view in clinical psychiatry over the last 40 years or so, as we emphasized in the original version of this chapter (Bebbington *et al.* 1995). Since then, our knowledge about the influence of psychosocial stress on schizophrenia has certainly been extended, although not revolutionized. The study of the impact of events has broadened to considerations of early trauma, the investigation of links between post-traumatic stress disorder and schizophrenic symptoms, and attempts to demonstrate specificity in the relationship between events and the onset of schizophrenic episodes.

In the 6 years since our last edition, the number of papers on aspects of EE has proliferated. Some studies have added to the already strong consensus that EE does indeed predict relapse. Others have sought to understand more about what a high EE rating means for the family environment of the person with schizophrenia. Yet others have examined the potential origins of high EE environments. Finally, alternative measures have been suggested, given the high level of training required to rate EE accurately.

Reactive psychoses

If we consider psychosis as a psychological process rather than a set of diagnostic categories, the study of reactive psychoses may illuminate this process. Nearly half the cases of psychosis in Scandinavia are diagnosed as reactive (Retterstøl 1986; Lindvall *et al.* 1993), and Scandinavian psychiatrists, at any rate, appear to be capable of making this diagnosis with acceptable reliability (Hansen *et al.* 1992).

Reactive psychosis has characteristic symptoms and a characteristic course (Ungvari & Mullen 2000). It seems to be typified by perplexity, a pleomorphic clinical picture and an acute onset. It also has a relatively benign and episodic course, but is not synonymous with schizoaffective disorder (Brockington *et al.* 1982). It does overlap somewhat with the concept of cycloid psychosis (Brockington *et al.* 1982; Jonsson *et al.* 1991).

Kapur and Pandurangi (1979; Pandurangi & Kapur 1980) suggest that people suffering from reactive psychosis showed more affective symptoms and more vulnerable personalities than those with non-reactive conditions. Mahendra (1977) reported similar findings. In a long-term follow-up study of 91 patients with reactive psychosis at Johns Hopkins Hospital in Baltimore, Stephens *et al.* (1982) found more precipitating stress in comparison with process schizophrenia, as well as the clinical features described by the Scandinavian authors.

Separating off a diagnosis of reactive psychosis would reduce the association of the left-over group of psychoses with antecedent stressful events. One would thus expect non-reactive psychosis in Scandinavian countries to be less associated with stress than in countries where the diagnosis of reactive psychosis is less often made. However, the assessment of the social context of reactive psychosis has almost invariably been made clinically and is therefore likely to be associated with a higher error rate than more rigorous social investigations. Reactive psychosis has been defined in the American Diagnostic and Statistical Manual (DSM) (American Psychiatric Association 1987, 1994) in a manner so strict as to virtually eliminate the possibility of diagnosing it (Munoz *et al.* 1987; Hansen *et al.* 1992; Jauch & Carpenter 1998a,b). The consequence of this may be to increase the social reactivity of schizophrenia in countries using DSM.

Overall, reactive psychosis does seem to be distinguishable from nuclear schizophrenia both by its close relationship to an antecedent stress, and by its clinical features: specifically a greater admixture of affective symptoms and a more benign course. This has an interesting parallel in the work of van Os *et al.* (1994); among subjects with Research Diagnostic Criteria (RDC) schizophrenia, episodes that followed stressful events showed less typical symptoms than those that did not.

Setting the agenda for a social aetiology

The earliest scientific demonstrations of the social reactivity of schizophrenia using modern standards of methodology lean heavily on the work of George Brown and John Wing. They first established a relationship between the poverty of the social environment and the prevalence of negative symptoms in schizophrenia (Wing & Freudenberg 1961; Brown *et al.* 1966; Wing 1966; Wing & Brown 1970; Drake & Sederer 1986). However, it must be acknowledged parenthetically that the relationship was weaker in a replication carried out some 30 years later by Curson *et al.* (1992).

These early writers were also aware that trying to overcome negative symptoms by providing a more stimulating environment carried the opposite risk: too much pressure placed on patients in rehabilitation programmes sometimes led to the re-emergence of positive florid symptoms of schizophrenia (Wing *et al.* 1964; Stevens 1973; Goldberg *et al.* 1977; Drake & Sederer 1986).

It was against this background that Brown and Birley (1968) carried out their seminal study into the effects of life events in schizophrenia. The same group also developed the idea that stresses within the families of patients may provoke relapse, testing it tangentially through the expressed emotion (EE) measure. This too dates back a long way (Brown *et al.* 1958, 1962; Brown 1959), and derives some of its impetus from contemporaneous but untested (and now discredited) ideas about the origins of this condition in family dynamics (Bateson *et al.* 1956; Laing & Esterson 1964).

The importance of these early empirical studies should not be underestimated. While authors may flirt with the idea that *none* of the non-genetic aetiological component in schizophrenia is socioenvironmental (McGuffin *et al.* 1994), the social reactivity of the condition is nowadays generally accepted. That was not the case in the 1950s.

There has been an explosion of EE research in the last 15 years, and this has provided some of the strongest evidence for the social reactivity of schizophrenia. In contrast, the findings concerning life events remain less robust. Most recent studies have not directly examined the relationship between life events and schizophrenia episodes, but have added to our knowledge in more indirect ways.

Expressed emotion and relapse in schizophrenia

One of the most compelling indications of the social reactivity of schizophrenia is the large body of work detailing the impact of family atmosphere on its course. The main impetus for this has been the elaboration of the measure Expressed Emotion (EE) over the last 40 years. The measure was developed by Brown (Brown & Rutter 1966; Brown *et al.* 1972) and its history has been reviewed extensively.

In the previous version of this chapter (Bebbington *et al.* 1995), we covered the existing literature concerning the predictive capacity of EE in schizophrenia and the evidence for family influence on its course that arises from therapeutic interventions. We also discussed the links between EE and the processes that are presumed to be reflected in the measure. We are now in a position to update this review.

EE is rated from an audio tape of an interview with a carer, the Camberwell Family Interview (CFI) of Brown and Rutter (1966), subsequently modified by Vaughn and Leff (1976). The ratings are based on the content and, more importantly, the prosodic aspects of speech such as pitch and emphasis. This is intended to allow the rating of emotional aspects of communication regardless of specific content. Five scales are rated from the interview: frequency ratings of the numbers of critical comments (CCs) and of positive remarks, and global ratings of hostility, warmth and emotional overinvolvement (EOI). Critical comments, hostility and overinvolvement have turned out to be the most predictive of relapse, and are incorporated in an overall rating of EE. EE is probably dimorphic, because hostility and criticism are clearly related to each other but less so to overinvolvement. In the research literature, the cut-off points have tended to vary somewhat. This causes problems of comparability although, as Kavanagh (1992) points out, 'The data do not

support the contention that EE results are significantly affected by changing criteria.' Relative insensitivity to changes in sampling and criteria is an indication of robust findings. However, critics have pointed out that the variation of criteria has been carried out *post hoc* in some cases, in order to ensure a significant result, thus risking spuriously positive findings.

Alternatives to the use of the EE measure

The CFI is a long interview and the assessment of EE involves specific skills. Even experienced clinicians are unable to estimate EE with better than chance success without training (King *et al.* 1994). Thus, there has been an impetus to find an alternative measure. One development has been the Five Minute Speech Sample (FMSS) which, as its name implies, involves assessment of a very short period of the relatives' speech. Several authors have now reported on the use of the FMSS as a substitute for the full CFI (Shimodera *et al.* 1999). It is generally found that people identified as high EE on the FMSS are almost invariably rated so from the CFI, but low scores on the FMSS are sometimes rated high by the classical procedure. This tendency of the FMS to under-rate EE was confirmed by Uehara *et al.* (1997). It is seen in the relatively small proportions of people identified as high EE. In one small study, Stark and Siol (1994) rated the EE of patients' relatives and therapists using the FMSS. A third of both relatives and therapists were rated as high EE. This contrasts with the approximately median split seen worldwide in EE studies based on the CFI (Bebbington & Kuipers 1994; see below). Nevertheless, Moore and Kuipers (1999) found that the FMSS identified criticism in staff carers adequately.

Lenior *et al.* (1997, 1998a,b) have used the FMSS to construct composite scales: six items covered criticism/dissatisfaction, while two concerned emotional overinvolvement. In a follow-up study, the six-item scale was significantly predictive whereas the simple EE dichotomy was not. A score combining the individual scores of family members was particularly predictive.

Kavanagh *et al.* (1997) have developed another measure: a 30-item self-completion questionnaire for relatives, the Family Attitude Scale (FAS), which they claim is capable of predicting high levels of criticism and hostility on the CFI.

EE and the prediction of relapse

The literature using EE as a measure predictive of relapse in schizophrenia tends to rely on rather similar research designs. Typically, a sample of patients is followed up following recovery from an episode of florid symptoms of schizophrenia. Before they are discharged, although usually well on the way to recovery, their carers are interviewed with the CFI to establish levels of EE. The interview focuses on the 3 months before the admission. Patients are followed-up prospectively for a period of 9 months or 1 year, and evaluated for signs of relapse. The definition of relapse has typically varied, in some cases being based on symptomatic criteria, and in others merely on readmission to hospital. Patients are divided into high and low EE groups. This may be

Table 31.1 Predictive studies of expressed emotion in schizophrenia.

Study	Location	n
Brown et al. (1962)	England	97
Brown et al. (1972)	England	91
Leff & Vaughn (1976)	England	37
Leff et al. (1982)	England	12
Vaughn et al. (1984)	California	36
Moline et al. (1985)	Illinois	16
MacMillan et al. (1986)	England	73
Nuechterlein et al. (1986)	California	36
Karno et al. (1987)	California	43
Leff et al. (1987); Wig et al. (1987)	India	77
McCreadie & Phillips (1988); McCreadie et al. (1991)	Scotland	59
Parker et al. (1988)	Australia	57
Bertrando et al. (1992)	Italy	9
Gutiérrez et al. 1988)	Spain	32
Tarrier et al. (1988a)	England	37
Budzyna-Dawidowski et al. (1989)	Poland	36
Arévalo & Vizcaro 1989)	Spain	31
Barrelet et al. (1990)	Switzerland	42
Buchkremer et al. (1991)	Germany	99
Stirling et al. (1991)	England	33
Možný & Votpkova (1992)	Czechoslovakia	82
Montero et al. (1992)	Spain	60
Vaughan et al. (1992)	Australia	89
Niedermeier et al. (1992)	Germany	48
Ivanović et al. 1994)	Yugoslavia	60
Tanaka et al. (1995)	Japan	52
Linszen et al. (1996)	Netherlands	76
King & Dixon (1999)	Canada	69

defined either in terms of the attributes of a designated 'key' relative, or on the basis that at least one relative in the immediate family is rated as high EE. Case definition has varied between different studies, in some instances being operationally defined in terms of nuclear schizophrenia, while others include schizoaffective cases.

There are now nearly 30 prospective studies of the role of EE as a risk factor for relapse in schizophrenia (summarized in Table 31.1). We carried out an aggregate analysis of the 25 studies of EE available at the time (Bebbington & Kuipers 1994). Where possible, data on individual cases were obtained from the original authors (17 studies). In the remaining eight, published results were used to reconstruct data on individual cases as completely as possible. One study (Dulz & Hand 1986) was omitted because a substantial proportion of subjects were not living with their EE-rated relative, and it was impossible to work out which. In the other studies, we were able to exclude subjects in this category, resulting in a reduction in numbers. As a result, the relationship between EE and relapse was different from that quoted in the published reports. Altogether 15 studies showed an association beyond the 5% level, two just failed to reach this level,

five showed a non-significant trend, and three either no trend or a small trend in the reverse direction. Based on these 25 studies, the total number of cases was 1346. The numbers were less than this in some analyses because of the problem of missing variables, particularly where the analysis involved several variables.

Worldwide, the proportion of high EE cases was 52%. This is striking in view of the fact that the original cut-off for EE was chosen because it was a median value. The lowest rates have been detected in developing countries, notably India (Wig et al. 1987), China, where high EE was found in only 28% of relatives in Chengdu (Maosheng et al. 1998), and in Bali (Kurihara et al. 2000). In those studies where gender information was provided (n = 855), 60% of cases were male. Of those cases where medication status was reported (n = 884), two-thirds were receiving medication. Sixty-two per cent of patients were in high contact with their relatives. The overall relapse rate for high EE cases was 50%, whereas that in low EE cases was 21%. This result was overwhelmingly significant. The aggregate analysis found that the effect of EE was actually stronger than that of medication. The strength of the association of relapse with EE was virtually identical in the medicated and non-medicated groups.

Hogarty (1985) suggested that the evidence for the predictive capacity of EE was relatively meagre for females. Our aggregate analysis suggested that although the outcome in terms of relapse was better overall in females, the strength of the association between relapse and high EE was virtually identical in the two genders (Bebbington & Kuipers 1995).

Face-to-face contact was found to be a significant variable in the original British studies (Leff & Vaughn 1976). However, studies from elsewhere in the world have shown this less consistently. In our aggregate analysis, we were able to examine the relationship between contact, EE and relapse in over 800 subjects. The strength of association between high EE and relapse was greater where contact was high, while living in high contact with a low EE relative was, if anything, protective.

Multivariate analyses of this data set confirmed that the association of relapse with high EE was highly significant and unaffected by the location of the study. There had been speculation that patients with schizophrenia living with low EE relatives would not require the protection of medication (Brown et al. 1972). However, in our analysis, medication and EE were independently related to relapse, confirming that EE status should have no bearing on the decision to prescribe medication. The basic data on which the multivariate analysis was based are shown in Fig. 31.1, which emphasizes the very high rate of relapse in patients unprotected by medication who live in high contact with high EE relatives. These conclusions were essentially confirmed by a further meta-analysis by Butzlaff and Hooley (1998), in this instance based on 27 studies.

New studies of the predictive capacity of EE

There was a plethora of predictive studies of EE in schizophrenia in the early 1990s, since when they have become somewhat less

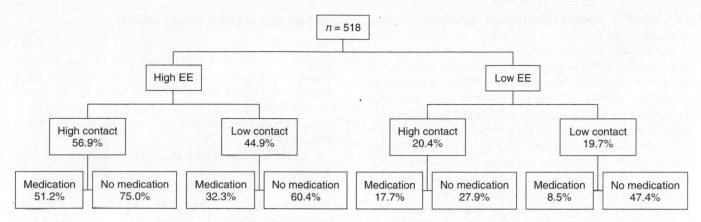

Fig 31.1 Relapse rates according to expressed emotion (EE), contact and medication status. (From Bebbington & Kuipers 1994.)

frequent, probably indicating that the predictive capacity of the measure is now established beyond doubt. The newer studies are nevertheless worth reviewing for a variety of reasons.

A Japanese study is of considerable interest because there is a widespread Western stereotype that there are considerable social constraints on the expression of emotion and dissent in that country. The 9-month relapse odds ratio in relation to the EE dichotomy was 2.7 (Tanaka *et al.* 1995) and at 2-year follow-up it was still as high as 1.9 (Mino *et al.* 1997).

Among these more recent studies, it should be noted that King and Dixon (1999) found significant effects of EE on relapse at 9 months, but not at 6 and 18 months. This team found that relapse was not associated with compliance, nor was there an effect of the amount of contact with high EE relatives. Mino *et al.* (1998) also claim that EE was associated with greater emotional withdrawal in patients at follow-up.

Schulze-Monking and Buchkremer (1995) argue that EE is more predictive of relapse than of rehospitalization. They also found in their follow-up study that the predictive capacity of EE only became significant after 4 years of illness.

Two studies have examined the predictive value of EE after controlling for other variables. Interestingly, this has the effect of increasing it. Thus, in the Japanese 2-year follow-up, after controlling for other confounding variables, the odds ratio increased to 4.6 (Mino *et al.* 1997). Linszen *et al.* (1997, 1998) studied the prognostic value of EE in their Dutch treatment study. EE was assessed in the context of 13 other predictor variables. Relapse was operationalized in terms of symptoms. Six variables were predictive, but the major predictor was EE with a hazard ratio of 4.9. The effect was maintained when patients in their first episode were examined separately. Interestingly, within the group of subjects from high EE families, cannabis use was also a major predictor of poor outcome.

The interval between the last version of this chapter has allowed the publication of long-term follow-up studies. It is of interest that in one study EE was quite stable over 5 years (Huguelet *et al.* 1995). Tarrier *et al.* (1994) have reported the predictive capacity of EE over 5 and 8 years in patients who had not relapsed 2 years after family intervention. Even in this atten-

uated group, they still found fewer relapses in patients from low EE backgrounds.

Schulze-Monking *et al.* (1997a) rated EE at outset and 20 months later in the relatives of patients with schizophrenia. Patients from a persistently high EE background had particularly bad 2- and 8-year outcomes. High EE was associated with more frequent rehospitalization, more symptoms and poorer psychosocial adjustment. A fluctuatingly high level of EE seemed less disadvantageous than a persistently high level. Schulze-Monking *et al.* (1997b) found that persistent effects of EE on relapse rates and hospital bed days over an 8-year period were more marked for parents than other relatives, and particularly so if the patients had already been ill for several years.

Huguelet *et al.* (1995) carried out a 5-year follow-up of patients with first admissions for schizophrenia. Relapse rates, rehospitalization and social outcome over the whole period were worse in patients from high EE homes.

There is some evidence of an effect of EE on social outcome (King & Dixon 1995). Inoue *et al.* (1997) found small but significant differences in patients' social functioning in relation to EE at 9-month follow-up. Sufferers from high EE families deteriorated slightly, while those from a low EE background improved somewhat. In their study in Valencia, Montero *et al.* (1998) reported that low EE did not predict improved social adjustment in schizophrenia at 2-year follow-up.

Inferences from family intervention in schizophrenia

The acknowledgement that the family atmosphere has a role in relapse in schizophrenia led to a number of intervention studies (Falloon *et al.* 1982, 1985; Leff *et al.* 1982, 1985, 1989, 1990; Hogarty *et al.* 1986; Tarrier *et al.* 1988a; Kuipers *et al.* 1989; McCreadie *et al.* 1991; Vaughan *et al.* 1992; Linszen *et al.* 1997, 1998). Overall, these interventions have been successful, indicating that it is possible to modify family atmosphere and thus to reduce relapse rates. However, this is probably dependent upon the timing of intervention, the techniques used and the expertise of the therapists using them. Moreover, the changes leading to a reduction in EE may be a sufficient but not a necessary component of intervention (Hogarty *et al.* 1986).

The Amsterdam study of family treatment in schizophrenia (Linszen *et al.* 1996) was generally unsuccessful, although it is not exactly clear why. There was an overall low rate of relapse, but this was actually slightly greater in low EE families in receipt of family treatment, raising the possibility that the intervention paradoxically increased stress levels in these families.

A meta-analysis of these treatments has recently been carried out by the British National Schizophrenia Guideline Group (Kuipers *et al.* 1999; Pilling *et al.* 2002). In the process, a number of related issues have been clarified. Nineteen randomized controlled trials comparing family therapy with some other treatment were identified. They were conducted in a wide range of cultural and service contexts. The early studies of intervention (Falloon *et al.* 1982, 1985; Leff *et al.* 1982, 1985; Hogarty *et al.* 1986) showed excellent outcomes. Overall, the literature confirms these good results. However, in their review, Mari and Streiner (1994) suggested that intervention in the more recent studies appears less effective. The apparent decline in effectiveness was attributed to the enthusiasm and charisma of the people conducting the earlier studies. However, the diminishing effect of family intervention with time may also be explained by the fact that the later studies involved *group* treatments of the families, whereas the earlier studies consistently relied on the treatment of individual families. Thus, for single family therapy the 'number needed to treat' (NNT) to prevent relapse in the first year of treatment is 6.3, while to prevent readmission it is 5.7. In other words, around six people must be treated in order to prevent one bad outcome. In the second year of treatment the equivalent values are 3.9 and 3.5. Values in these ranges are generally taken to indicate a clinically worthwhile effect. The NNT to prevent a relapse in the *follow-up period* after the end of treatment is 7.1 for individual family treatment, although this falls to 20.8 for readmission.

It was only possible to calculate a general figure for relapse for group treatments. This resulted in an NNT of –32. The negative figure indicates that group-based family treatment is marginally (but non-significantly) *worse* than the comparison treatment. It seems inherently unlikely that group treatments are entirely ineffective, given that social comparison can be a powerfully reassuring group process. However, when the chosen outcome variable is the re-emergence of psychotic symptoms, or readmission to hospital, it is clear that single family interventions are much more effective, and must be considered the first choice of therapists. Finally, it is worth noting that there was little evidence to support the contention that the effects of family therapy might be mediated through improved compliance with medication.

These studies thus provide useful support for arguing that the elements of family atmosphere detected by the EE measure are causally related to relapse in schizophrenia.

The meaning of EE (construct validity)

The EE measure uses an individual relative's behaviour in the artificial conditions of the CFI to predict the likelihood of subsequent relapse in the patient with whom the relative lives. It is presumed that it is able to do this because it reflects some significant and enduring aspect of the interplay between the patient and the relatives, or the relatives' ability to cope with crises (Kuipers 1979).

A number of studies have addressed the question of what the EE measure means in practice for relationships between carers and their relatives with schizophrenia. This has potentially important implications for the origins of EE and the mechanisms that underlie its predictive capacity.

It has long been known that relatives who make frequent critical comments when alone behave similarly in the presence of the patient, albeit usually with more restraint (Brown & Rutter 1966; Rutter & Brown 1966). This view is supported by the work on Negative Affective Style. This is a coding system which can be used to assess families taking part in a standardized task designed to recreate everyday interaction in a laboratory setting (Goldstein *et al.* 1968; Doane *et al.* 1981). Negative Affective Style in these direct interactions is consistently highly correlated with EE measured in the usual way (Strachan *et al.* 1986; Miklowitz *et al.* 1989).

However, we now have considerably more information about how high ratings on the EE measure are related to aspects of the patients' and the relatives' behaviour in psychosis and in other conditions (Table 31.2). It can be seen from this that EE is picking up a number of different attributes of interpersonal behaviour. Some of these are not closely related conceptually, although they may well occur together in given relatives and families.

Some of these studies have returned to the old idea that relationships within the families of people with schizophrenia were characterized by communication deviance (Wynne & Singer 1963). Demonstrable communication deviance in the parents of people with schizophrenia is associated with high EE. Docherty (1995) has suggested that the association of the latter with outcome arises spuriously because the communication deviance arises from a genetic vulnerability to schizophrenia. However, communication deviance appeared to change at a different rate from EE in one psychoeducational treatment programme (Rund *et al.* 1995). In this particular study, communication deviance was more predictive of outcome than EE.

Among other attributes of families, high EE relatives of people with schizophrenia were found to be more competitive than low EE families (Wuerker 1996). The author concluded that high EE families have a family system characterized both by over-responsiveness and conflict overdominance.

Rosenfarb *et al.* (1995) used a direct interaction task and not only demonstrated that people with schizophrenia who had high EE relatives exhibited more subclinical odd behaviours, but that the relatives responded very quickly to specific instances in a way that let to further odd behaviour. This suggests strongly that a bidirectional interaction underlies the predictive capacity

Table 31.2 Behaviour and attitudes characteristic of high EE families.

Carers

Fears and anxieties (Greenley 1986)
Negative affective style (Strachan *et al.* 1986; Miklowitz *et al.* 1989)
Poor listening (Kuipers *et al.* 1983)
Non-illness attributions (Brewin *et al.* 1991)
Attribution of negative outcomes to patient (Brewin *et al.* 1991; Barrowclough *et al.* 1994)
Maladaptive coping (Kuipers 1983; Bledin *et al.* 1990)
More burdened (Smith *et al.* 1993; Scazufca & Kuipers 1996)
Communication deviance (Rund *et al.* 1995)
Overcompetitive (Wuerker 1996)
Overalertness to odd behaviour (Rosenfarb *et al.* 1995)
Feeling themselves unable to control patients' symptoms (Barrowclough & Parle 1997)
Less empathic (Harrison *et al.* 1998)
Inflexibility, intolerance (Hooley & Hiller 2000)
Self-critical (Docherty *et al.* 1998)
Guilt prone (Bentsen *et al.* 1998a)
Internal locus of control (Hooley 1998)
Lack of knowledge about the disorder (Harrison *et al.* 1998)
Feeling patients were able to control their symptoms (Weisman *et al.* 1998; Lopez *et al.* 1999)
More conventional and less satisfied (Hooley & Hiller 2000)

Patients

More critical (Brown & Rutter 1966; Strachan *et al.* 1989; Scazufca *et al.* 2001)
Less autonomous (Strachan *et al.* 1989)
Ready to perceive relatives as inscrutable (Stark & Siol 1994)
More subclinical odd behaviours (Rosenfarb *et al.* 1995)
Perceive relatives as critical (Tompson *et al.* 1995)
More negative autobiographical memories (Cutting & Docherty 2000)

Interaction

Negative (Hooley & Hahlweg 1986; Hubschmid & Zemp 1989)
Rigid conflict-prone structure (Hubschmid & Zemp 1989)

of EE. Woo *et al.* (1997) reported highly significant differences from the same study, with patients from high EE families showing relatively more hostile and unusual behaviour. Bentsen *et al.* (1996) reported that EOI was characteristic of those relatives who spent a lot of time with the patients. Patients who lived with EOI relatives actually showed less difficult behaviour, but tended to be anxious and depressed.

Other characteristics of carers and sufferers are of possible importance. In one small study, high EE carers were rejected and perceived as inscrutable by their relatives with schizophrenia (Stark & Siol 1994). People with schizophrenia are poorer judges of affect in experimental tests (Bell *et al.* 1997). However, in a different study, patients living with critical relatives were quite able to perceive their criticality (Tompson *et al.* 1995); moreover, such perceptions were associated with outcome. This may work in both directions. Bad memories of the interaction with relatives may be connected with the perception of criticism. Thus, Cutting and Docherty (2000) found that schizophrenia patients with high EE relatives recounted fewer happy memories and more stressful memories that those with low EE relatives.

Giron and Gomez-Beneyto (1998) showed that relatives' ability to judge the patients' mood state was inversely associated with relapse, and this appeared to be independent of the relatives' levels of criticism. Low EE parents of people with schizophrenia showed higher levels of differentiation and integration than high EE parents. They were also rated lower on self-criticism (Docherty *et al.* 1998). Bentsen *et al.* (1998a) found guilt proneness particularly high in relatives also rated high on EOI.

A number of recent studies have addressed themselves to the idea that high EE relatives make attributions that distinguish them from low EE relatives, and which may be linked to higher relapse rates. Barrowclough *et al.* (1994) found that high EE relatives made relatively more attributions about illness. Relatives rated high on criticism attributed more causes as internal to the patient and those rated on hostility also thought the causes were controllable by the patient.

Harrison *et al.* (1998) found that critical attitudes on the part of carers towards people with schizophrenia were associated with relative ignorance about the disorder and a tendency to attribute negative symptoms to the patient's personality. Interestingly, they also found that criticism was more marked when negative symptoms were a less salient feature of the illness. Weisman *et al.* (1998) have also found that carers rated high on EE tend to attribute more control over symptoms to their relatives with schizophrenia. These authors have now extended this work to show that it applies to high and low EE relatives within the same household (Weisman *et al.* 2000). Lopez *et al.* (1999) found that attributions by relatives that patients' behaviour and symptoms were under their control were related both to levels of criticism and to outcome.

Barrowclough and Parle (1997) showed that relatives' EE and distress levels were associated with their appraisal of symptom threat and of their ability to control the symptoms. Raune (unpublished data) provided similar data indicating that relatives of people with first episodes of schizophrenia who were rated as high EE appear to be responding to a high level of perceived threat in their social environment. Bentsen *et al.* (1997) found that there were relationships between aspects of carers' locus of control, criticism and overinvolvement. Attributing outcomes to chance was strongly associated with overinvolvement, while attributing them to the actions of powerful others was more characteristic of critical relatives. High EE carers themselves actually have a more internal locus of control, as well as attributing internal control to their relatives with schizophrenia (Hooley 1998). Illness attributions increased as criticism and overinvolvement were reduced in the course of family treatment (Brewin 1994).

Hooley and Hiller (2000) have provided information on the personality characteristics of relatives of people with schizophrenia. High EE relatives were found to be more conventional and less satisfied with themselves and their lives. They were also less flexible, less tolerant and less empathic. The finding of relative inflexibility remained after controlling for potentially confounding demographic variables.

Kuipers (1992) has likened the EE measure to blood pressure. The latter is an indirect way of measuring cardiovascular function which is extremely predictive of certain outcomes. We now know that blood pressure is related to a variety of pathophysiological processes, and this increased knowledge has enhanced the range of potential palliatives and treatments. In the same way, EE has justified its use as a predictor. This does not preclude the use of other measures, not does it prevent the emergence of richer and more sophisticated explanations of its predictiveness (Table 31.2).

The origins of EE

Quite early on in the history of EE research, there were concerns about the origins of the behaviours it measures. This has a theoretical implication. Could it be that the EE measure is predictive merely because relatives respond in a characteristic way to sufferers whose illness has a poor prognosis for other reasons? In the first fully worked out study of EE (Brown et al. 1972), the authors did control for the extent of positive symptoms in the patients, but found that EE was still predictive.

Birchwood and Smith (1987) have argued that high EE and the behaviours associated with it develop as the response of some relatives to the burden of living with a person with schizophrenia. They base their argument on the fact that high EE is less apparent in relatives of patients experiencing first rather than subsequent admissions for schizophrenia.

It has generally been found that there are no differences in terms of prior levels of positive symptoms in patients whose relatives are rated high or low EE. However, other work has suggested that at least some components of high EE are associated with abnormalities of various sorts in the patient (Miklowitz et al. 1983; Mavreas et al. 1992). This is particularly so in relation to social deficits. Dingemans et al. (1996) found that EE was related to pre-existing social deficits, but not to symptom levels. This was essentially because of relatives who scored high on EOI. Likewise, Huguelet et al. (1995) found that high EE in this group was associated with worse premorbid functioning.

Boye et al. (1999) studied variables that predicted changes in EE ratings in carers reinterviewed 4 months after their relatives had been discharged from hospital. Although the findings were complicated, high or unstable levels of EE were associated with variables indicative of increased contact. However, patients with consistently low EE relatives were actually more ill at admission, perhaps indicating a greater tolerance of disordered behaviour and a longer period before a crisis.

It is unclear whether the interactions that seem to characterize these families predate the onset of schizophrenia. McCreadie et al. (1994) have data at least suggesting the possibility that parental hostility ratings relate to an earlier rejecting style of parental rearing. However, Schreiber et al. (1995) conducted an interesting experiment, interviewing parents with the CFI separately with regard to a child with schizophrenia and to a well sibling. EOI was less and warmth was greater towards the well child. The authors took this to mean that EE was reactive and

thus a state rather than a trait. However, the opposite causal direction remains a possibility. Bean et al. (1996) found that patients with first episodes of schizophrenia were negatively labelled by people they designated as significant others. Negative labelling was greater in those with later onsets, with a long period of deterioration and poorer occupational functioning.

Bentsen et al. (1998b) found that the strongest predictors of high EE included the number of admissions and a lack of paid employment on the part of the patient. Although Davis et al. (1996) found some differences in the pattern of relationships between relatives and patients with schizophrenia related to the sex of each member of the dyad, the differences were few.

Birchwood and Smith (1987) put forward a model whereby families' coping style develops over time. There is little to argue with in this. It is difficult to see how the characteristics of high EE might arise except from an interaction between the relative and the patient. However, this does not mean that particular responses on the part of the relatives have no influence on the subsequent course of the disorder. This is why intervention studies have been useful whatever the origins of EE-related behaviours. Nevertheless, there is evidence that relatives may exhibit high EE attitudes even at first episode, suggesting that its development is often rapid (Kuipers & Raune 2000).

Reports of 'troublesome' symptoms do tend to be predictive of high EE but may reflect subjective burden on the part of relatives (Bentsen et al. 1998b). In a Japanese study, criticism was most often directed towards positive symptoms (one-third in all; Shimodera et al. 1998). Moreover, although difficult behaviour on the part of the patients may cause distress to their relatives and thus lead to suboptimal responses, it is clear that these responses are not uniform: two relatives of the same patient may differ in their EE ratings. Beltz et al. (1991) have also shown that there is no consistent relationship between staff and family carers' levels of EE.

It is thus virtually certain that the pattern of high EE-related behaviours and frequent relapses represents a vicious cycle rather than linear causality. It seems that if this cycle is entered, high EE can be an extremely persistent characteristic of relatives. Favre et al. (1989) found considerable stability of EE over a 9-month period, while McCreadie et al. (1993) have reported that this stability extends to 5 years. In both of these studies there was an intermediate minority of relatives who moved between high and low EE status. Although few of the changes observed seemed to depend on the clinical state of patients, it is possible that there is a subgroup of relatives who typically become high EE under stress. It is of interest that the frequency of relapse in this fluctuating group in McCreadie's study resembled that in patients living with relatives rated persistently high in EE, and that they were noticeably different from the consistently low EE group.

It is our view that the EE measure taps into the quality and style of interactions within family systems which are necessarily complex. Living with a high EE relative must represent a chronic stress. However, it is very likely that low EE relationships are not merely neutral, in the sense of representing an absence of stress, but actually have positive and beneficial effects on patients. Thus, Hubschmid and Zemp (1989) found that low EE relatives made significantly more emotionally positive and supportive statements in interaction with patients. This has parallels with the results of our aggregate analysis, suggesting that high contact with low EE relatives is actually protective for patients who are not on medication; in other words, vulnerable patients do better with a bigger dose of their relatives. There is some corroboration from electrophysiological studies suggesting that the presence of low EE relatives actually serves to reduce arousal (Tarrier *et al.* 1988b; Tarrier 1989; Hegerl *et al.* 1990).

However, work by Dixon *et al.* (2000) goes against this. They attempted to test directly the idea that high EE relatives provide a stressful environment for people with schizophrenia. They argued that memory-loaded vigilance tests are stress-sensitive and that the presence of a high EE relative would therefore reduce the patient's performance. In fact the reverse was true, leading them to conclude that patients in the presence of low EE relatives were in fact underaroused. These results could, however, also be interpreted in terms of the role of anxiety in improving performance, and may therefore not reflect an adverse level of underarousal. Finally, patients themselves are well able to perceive critical environments, confirming that such relationships can have direct effects (Scazufca *et al.* 2001).

EE as an attribute of professional carers

The ideas developed in the research into family burden, relationships and interventions have been extended. After all, relatives are not the only carers, and many of the features of informal caring have their counterpart in formal therapeutic relationships. If therapeutic relationships can also have high EE characteristics and this too can be shown to have an adverse effect on outcome, the argument for psychosocial reactivity is strengthened.

Of particular interest are the important relationships developed in key working. Kuipers and colleagues (Kuipers & Moore 1995) hypothesized that key workers were likely to share some of the attitudes seen in informal carers. Prior work had already suggested this possibility (Watts 1988; Herzog 1992), and detailed examination revealed it to be the case. Staff carers showed a range of relationships, with around 40% being critical with at least one client. They also found the same behaviour difficult: social withdrawal and embarrassing or disruptive behaviour (Moore *et al.* 1992a). A hostel characterized by staff who were rated high on EE had a more rapid throughput of clients for negative reasons than a hostel with low EE staff (Ball *et al.* 1992). If they had been rated as high on EE, staff in direct interaction with clients showed more 'benign criticism' and were less supportive (Moore *et al.* 1992b). Similar findings were reported in relation to key workers in community mental health teams (Oliver & Kuipers 1996). Staff in low EE relationships were better able to tolerate the slow pace of change, to appreciate the clients' perspective and to be positive about at least one aspect of the client even if they had very difficult behaviour. High EE relationships with clients were unrelated to satisfaction at work, which appeared to be mediated by other factors. Others have produced

similar findings, for instance that patients in hostels with critical staff rate themselves as having poorer quality of life (Snyder *et al.* 1994).

Tattan and Tarrier (2000) investigated case managers from the UK 700 study of the effects of intensive case management (UK 700 group 1999). They used the FMSS to assess levels of EE, albeit in an idiosyncratic way. On this basis, 27% of staff–patient relationships were rated as high EE. The EE level of case managers was not related to patient characteristics, nor indeed to outcome. However, it was predictive of the overall quality of the relationship with patients and this in turn was linked to various outcomes. Sixty-one per cent of those rated high in EE had a poor relationship with the corresponding client, compared with none of the low EE group. Positive relationships were associated at 12-month follow-up with lower positive and negative symptoms and with less disability. As we have suggested above, the FMSS may have problems in rating EE effectively, but it is clear from those results that some characteristic of the relationship was affecting outcome despite the relatively short time the staff and clients were in contact.

There are clear implications in this research for staff training. Willetts and Leff (1997) developed a training programme designed to increase the knowledge of staff of social factors affecting schizophrenia, and their access to strategies for managing their relationships with clients. However, this failed to reduce staff EE levels, and this is clearly an area where effective interventions need to be developed.

EE and burden

Another approach has been to use measures of burden as a proxy for EE. In objective terms, living with someone who has developed schizophrenia is likely to be stressful and upsetting. Indeed, Davis and Schultz (1998) have established that grief symptoms are common long after the event in people whose children have developed schizophrenia, and are unrelated to the amount of current contact time. However, it is the level of *perceived* burden that is most characteristic of relatives who are rated high on EE. Thus, Bentsen *et al.* (1996) found that patients who lived with overinvolved relatives actually showed less difficult behaviour.

There is now considerable evidence that high EE relatives are overwhelmed by the difficulties occasioned by living with a schizophrenic relative. Bogren (1997), in a small Swedish study, found high EE associated with subjectively poorer quality of life and subjective and objective burden. Boye *et al.* (1998) found higher General Health Questionnaire (GHQ) scores in a Norwegian sample of relatives with high or fluctuating ratings of emotional overinvolvement, but not in those expressing hostility or making critical comments. This coheres with the clinical view of emotionally overinvolved relatives. Barrowclough *et al.* (1996) found that self-blaming beliefs in relatives at a time of acute relapse had the effect of increasing distress. In one study, perceived family burden was found to be more predictive of relapse than EE (Levene *et al.* 1996).

Some studies of relatives have focused on the relationship between EE, burden and coping style. Scazufca and Kuipers (1999) found that relatives typically used problem-focused coping, but subjective burden, distress and high EE were associated with avoidant coping, usually regarded as maladaptive. Scazufca and Kuipers (1996) carried out a follow-up study of EE, relatives' burden and patient social functioning, which were strongly related to each other but not to positive and negative symptoms. Scazufca and Kuipers (1998) found that burden declined in tandem with EE. Reductions in EE level at follow-up were most clearly associated with reduction in burden and in the amount of contact with the patient. They concluded that EE was a measure of the relative's *appraisal* of difficulties (Scazufca & Kuipers 1996). Finally, Budd *et al.* (1998) reported that the coping styles of 'collusion', 'criticism/coercion', 'overprotectiveness', 'emotional overinvolvement' and 'resignation' were associated with high subjective burden, while the opposite was true of 'warmth'.

EE studies: conclusions

The more recent research on EE has confirmed its predictive value and developed ideas about mechanisms. EE has been found in staff carers as in relatives, and in a range of other conditions. The usefulness of alternative measures is becoming clearer.

Probably the most productive areas are in the development of EE in identifying therapeutic (or otherwise) relationships as well as therapeutic environments. Overall, the evidence of the impact of social factors on psychosis has been corroborated by these studies, and continues to confirm that such factors, while powerful, are amenable to change.

Life event studies

In our previous version, we dealt with methodological issues at length, and readers who are interested, particularly in the measurement of life events, should refer to it (Bebbington *et al.* 1995). There are a number of strategies that might be used to establish a link between life events and schizophrenia.

1 *Reaction to a single type of event.* Steinberg and Durell (1968) showed that the frequency of schizophrenic breakdown was significantly higher in the few months immediately after conscription into the army.

2 *Reaction to a wide range of life events.* This strategy brings up issues of measurement, as events are not equivalent, and their relative impact must be assessed.

While it might seem obvious to assess the impact of events by asking subjects how they were actually affected, these subjective accounts may be biased. There have been two basic attempts to deal with this problem, the so-called 'inventory approach', exemplified by the work of Holmes and Rahe (1967), and a semi-structured interview organized around role areas (Brown 1974; Brown & Harris 1978). In the former, events recorded by checking them against an inventory are scored by a *rating sample*, the scores then being averaged to give a stress rating. In the interview approach, recent experiences elicited through the Life Events and Difficulties Schedule (LEDS) are presented to a *rating panel*, which ascribes a severity rating to them (Brown & Harris 1978). As the interviewer is able to provide a considerable amount of context, this means that the individual circumstances of the event can be taken into account, in a way that is not feasible with the simple inventory approach. Thus, some degree of individuality of response is retained, while the subjects' own evaluation is removed from consideration. This represents a reasonable compromise between uncontrolled subjectivity and the crudeness of attributing the same impact to all events of a given type.

In order to evaluate the temporal relationship between events and any kind of psychiatric disorder, both the event and the disorder must be dated, and this can be difficult. As a way of strengthening the inference of causality, Brown and Harris (1978) developed a rating of independence, i.e. the degree to which events could be regarded as independent of behaviour altered by impending breakdown.

If we are to examine a wide range of events, rather than a single type of event, there are several different ways in which the association between life events and relapse in schizophrenia might be tested.

1 *Retrospective within-patient designs* comparing the experience of life events between a defined period immediately prior to the onset of illness and a more distant period.

2 *Retrospective case–control designs* in which the life event experience of the cases prior to onset is compared with an equivalent period in controls, usually the period immediately preceding interview.

These approaches can actually be combined in a single study. A difficulty with the case–control design is that people with schizophrenia may be abnormally sensitive to the impact of stress; the possible reasons for this are dealt with below. They may thus respond adversely to relatively minor disturbances in their social world. In consequence, their experience of life events may be no more than would be expected. This is a reason why within-case comparisons are a necessary part of the evidence.

3 *Prospective designs.* These are prospective in the sense that the life event history is established prior to an episode of recurrence. Thus, patients may be interviewed, say, every 2 months, at which time life events and symptom worsening are evaluated for the intervening period. The evaluations themselves inevitably have to be retrospective. A continuous series of periods is defined in which life events or exacerbations, or both, may have occurred. The experience of life events in the period *immediately preceding* that in which an exacerbation occurred can then be compared with dissimilar periods in the same subject, or in other subjects who did not experience exacerbations. Thus, this design also has within-subject and case–control variants. The controls by definition are people with a prior episode of schizophrenia who have not relapsed. This is quite a powerful design, but depends crucially on evaluating patients sufficiently

frequently for events in one period to be reasonably close in time to an exacerbation in the next period.

The strategy of monitoring events and onsets prospectively can be used to produce analyses based on case–control comparisons, or on event–no event comparisons. Examples of the latter include the study of Hardesty et al. (1985), who made a forward count of relapse or of increased morbidity from event onset. This allowed them to demonstrate an increased relapse rate in proximity to events. Day (1989) has also provided an analysis of this type.

The concept of triggering

Several authors have claimed that life events 'trigger' episodes of schizophrenia. This term has two separate and unconnected meanings. One is that the life events' stress merely adds the final impetus toward illness in somebody who was already strongly predisposed because of an underlying diathesis (Brown et al. 1973). This is another way of saying that, in comparison with other factors, the role of life events is not very important. This can be tested out by examining the strength of the association between events and onset or relapse.

The other meaning of the 'triggering' hypothesis concerns the length of the causal period in which life events are thought to operate. This has a methodological implication, as it is important that the antecedent period chosen for canvassing a life event history should be at least as long as the causal period. Events would be seen as having a triggering role in this sense if they occurred in close proximity to the onset of relapse of disorder. It has generally been held that a 6-month period of study should be sufficient to cover all events that might have a role in engendering relapse, although this has been queried (Bebbington et al. 1993; Hirsch et al. 1996).

Life event studies in schizophrenia

Seventeen systematic studies have specifically examined the effect of life events on the aetiology or course of schizophrenia (see Table 31.3). The seminal early study of this type found a significantly raised rate of life events limited to the 3 weeks before the onset or relapse of schizophrenic illness (Brown & Birley 1968). Many subsequent studies from a wide range of cultural settings have been carried out, but they provide inconsistent support for these initial findings. Most have used retrospective designs, although prospective studies have been reported more recently. Some have found a statistically significant excess of independent events in the 3 or 4 weeks before relapse compared with control periods. Thus, the multicentre World Health Organization (WHO) study (Day et al. 1987) demonstrated, in five of six centres, results similar to those of Brown and Birley (1968). Ventura et al. (1989) examined patients on regular neuroleptic medication and again obtained positive results. Hultman et al. (1997) also found an excess of events in the 3 weeks before relapse.

Other studies, using widely varying methods, have found sig-

nificantly increased rates of independent events during longer periods of time, up to 6 months or 1 year preceding relapse or illness onset (Dohrenwend et al. 1987; Bebbington et al. 1993; Hirsch et al. 1996). The latter two of these were reviewed in detail in the earlier version of this chapter (Bebbington et al. 1995). In a further analysis of the Camberwell Collaborative Psychosis study, Bebbington et al. (1996) found that the association between life events and psychosis was not affected by type of onset or by number of prior episodes. Not was it diminished by allowing for social class, ethnicity or marital status.

In contrast, other studies yielded negative results (Jacobs & Myers 1976; Malzacher et al. 1981; Al Khani et al. 1986; Chung et al. 1986; Gureje & Adewumni 1988; Malla et al. 1990). Some of these negative studies did find non-significant patterns of elevation of life event rates preceding illness onset (e.g. for Japan and for two of three developing countries in the WHO study; Day et al. 1987).

Prospective life event studies in the field of schizophrenia suffer from few of the important methodological problems of retrospective studies but, to date, have not offered consistent support for the triggering hypothesis. One study in California found no significant change in positive symptoms in the 3 weeks after major independent events occurred (Hardesty et al. 1985). The analysis in this study was limited by the small numbers of cases and the small numbers of major independent events that occurred (3% of the total number of life events occurring, so the negative findings might represent a type II error). Two studies in California found a significant association of events preceding illness in patients on regular neuroleptics, but not in patients who had recently come off medication (Ventura et al. 1989, 1992). Prospective studies in Canada and in London, UK, could find no increase in independent major events in the 4 weeks preceding relapse (Malla et al. 1990; Hirsch et al. 1996). However, Hirsch et al. (1996) did find that the life events over the whole of the study did significantly distinguish outcome groups. Data from this well-conducted study are shown in Fig. 31.2.

Because the impact of most life events is likely eventually to dissipate, it could be hypothesized that episodes provoked by events would be relatively benign. There is some evidence for this from the follow-up element in the Camberwell Collaborative Psychosis Study. Patients with event-associated episodes required less antipsychotic medication, but nevertheless spent more time in remission that those with unassociated episodes (van Os et al. 1994). Ventura et al. (2000) have recently demonstrated that the recurrence of psychotic symptoms is not the only response to stressful life events of people who have experienced prior episodes of schizophrenia. In many instances, the response is the development of non-psychotic depressive symptoms. This links into the literature on affective prodromes of relapse (Birchwood et al. 1992), not all of which lead to the re-emergence of psychotic symptoms (Yung & McGorry 1996). It also raises questions about the specificity of diagnosis and the idea of a continuum with more normal reactions, for instance, to loss (Table 31.3).

Table 31.3 Studies of independent life events in schizophrenic illness.

Study	Country	Period/method	Patient sample	Number	Significant results for time period 3–5 weeks	> 3/12
Retrospective						
Brown & Birley (1968)	UK	12/52	Broad group: 30% first onset	50	Yes, for 3 weeks	Not addressed
Jacobs & Myers (1976)	UK	12/52	Broad group: 30% first onset	50	Yes, for 3 weeks	NS
Malzacher et al. (1981)	UK	1 year: not LEDS	Narrow definition: all first onset	62	Not addressed	NS
Canton & Fraccon (1985)	Germany	6/12	First onset	90	Not addressed	Possible support
Chung et al. (1986)	Italy	6/12: not LEDS	24 first onset	54	Not addressed	NS
Al Khani et al. (1986)	USA	6/12	Narrow definition: some first onset	15	NS	NS
Day et al. (1987) WHO	Saudi Arabia	1 year	Narrow definition: recent onset	48	Small subgroups only	Not addressed
	10 centres world-wide	12/52	Broad definition: some first onset	13–67	Yes for 5 of 6 analysed fully	Yes, for 'non-fateful' events
Dohrenwend et al. (1987)	USA	6/12: not LEDS	21 first onset	66	NS	Yes, for up to 6 months
Gureje & Adewumni (1988)	Nigeria	6/12: not LEDS	All first onset: RDC definition	42	NS	NS
Bebbington et al. (1993)	UK	6/12	Narrow definition	52	Not addressed	Not addressed
Hultman et al. (1997)	Sweden	9/12 after discharge or at relapse	DSM-III schizophrenia	25	Excess of life events 3 weeks before relapse	NS
Prospective						
Leff et al. (1973)	UK	Clinical trial	9 on medication relapsed	116	For medicated only (5 weeks)	Not addressed
	UK	Clinical trial	9 on medication relapsed	116	For medicated only (5 weeks)	NS
Hardesty et al. (1985)	USA	1 year	2–3 years in remission	36	NS (morbidity 3/52 post LE)	NS unless trivial events included
Ventura et al. (1989)	USA	1 year on medication (see 1992*)	Recent onset: 11/30 relapsers		Yes for 4 weeks	NS
Malla et al. (1990)	Canada	1 year	7 relapsed	22	Not addressed	Yes, for up to 1 year
Ventura et al. (1992)	USA	1 year off medication (see 1989*)	Recent onset: off medication	13	NS for those off medication status	
Hirsch et al. (1996)	UK	1 year on/off medication	Narrow. Relapses: off medication 21/35; on medication 5/36	71	NS for both on and off medication groups	

Recent onset: illness history < 2 years.
DSM: Diagnostic and Statistical Manual; LEDS: Life Events and Difficulties Schedule; RDC: Research Diagnostic Criteria.

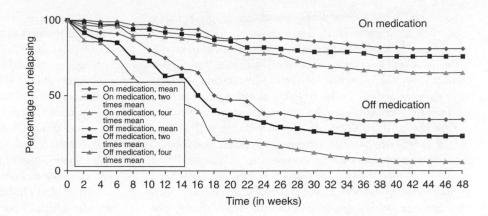

Fig 31.2 Estimates of survival function for different life event rates. (Modified with permission from Hirsch *et al.* 1996.)

Increased sensitivity to events

As we suggested earlier, people with schizophrenia may be abnormally sensitive to events. If this were so, it would make it difficult to demonstrate event–relapse relationships using the methods we have described. What evidence is there for increased sensitivity and what form might it take?

Some authors have claimed (MacDonald *et al.* 1998) that people with schizophrenia may have less effective strategies for coping with stress. Pallanti *et al.* (1997) provide evidence of sensitivity to events in terms of coping deficits. They assessed 41 patients with schizophrenia at 2-week intervals. Patients whose relapse did not follow a life event in the month before relapse showed less effective coping and poorer information processing capacity, at least as indicated by the P300 auditory event-related potential. The implication is that patients who have good coping resources will only be unsettled by events of considerable threat, in contrast to those without.

There is an extensive literature in the study of depression directed at the stress-buffering function of social support (Alloway & Bebbington 1987). Hultman *et al.* (1997) have investigated schizophrenia in similar terms, and made the interesting finding that the time between events and relapse was increased in people with better social support and a coping strategy characterized by active support seeking. The psychological mediation of vulnerability to stress may also involve hopelessness. This is very common in people who have newly developed schizophrenia, and appears to be linked to poor outcome (Aguilar *et al.* 1997).

There are also indications of a reduction in the normal biological mechanisms for dealing with stress in people with schizophrenia (Jansen *et al.* 1998; Sumiyoshi *et al.* 1999). Finlay and Zigmond (1997) have provided some evidence that stress leads to the release of dopamine, more marked in the prefrontal cortex than in subcortical sites. This mechanism might explain the way in which stress operates to exacerbate positive symptoms in schizophrenia. Others have speculated that gene–environment interactions in this condition actually take the form of sensitization to environmental stress (van Os & Marcelis 1998).

In bipolar disorder, it has been suggested that life events may only be in excess in early episodes, and that the apparent independence of events of later episodes arises through the process of kindling (Ramana & Bebbington 1995). There has been little examination of this possibility in schizophrenia; in a small study (*n* = 32) of American veterans, life events were more likely to be associated with earlier episodes of schizophrenia (Castine *et al.* 1998) while Bebbington *et al.* (1996) did not find this association.

Post-traumatic stress disorder and schizophrenia

Evidence is accumulating to show that there is a close relationship between post-traumatic stress disorder (PTSD) and psychotic symptoms. As yet, its nature remains obscure, but if any such relationship exists, it would have obvious links with the role of stress in the aetiology of schizophrenia.

What evidence is there that people suffering from PTSD have an increased likelihood of developing psychotic symptoms, and what might it mean? PTSD is a condition defined essentially by an intimate relationship between the content of symptoms and the experience of strongly traumatic events, in particular, the phenomenon of re-experiencing. One possibility is that some people who have been exposed to extreme trauma develop psychotic symptoms (delusions, hallucinations) whose content is also closely related to the details of the traumatic experience. If this happens, it may come about by a totally different process from the genesis of symptoms in disorders forming the majority of cases of schizophrenia, or it may not. The situation is analogous to the relationship between depressive bereavement reactions – in which the event is clearly in the forefront of the thinking of sufferers – and the generality of depressive disorders – where the link between a depressogenic event and the mood disorder may be much less apparent to sufferers. Most authorities from Freud (1917) onwards have tended to think that the psychosocial processes involved in depression and bereavement responses are quite similar.

Some might argue that florid symptoms in PTSD merely mimic psychotic symptoms. Thus, re-experiencing may have a compelling visual or auditory quality that might be mistaken for hallucinations. However, even in veterans exposed to extreme combat stress, the distinction between flashbacks and psychotic symptoms can be clearly made (Ivezic *et al.* 1999). Some authors have reported series of cases where the psychotic phenomena are obviously related in a meaningful way to the trauma. Thus, Ivezic *et al.* (1999) emphasize the strong symbolic relationship, the meaningful connection with the experience. Likewise, David *et al.* (1999) reported that in Vietnam veterans, the psychotic symptoms were related to aspects of combat and to guilt, averring that the relationship was 'non-bizarre'. However, the level of psychotic symptoms was not related to the severity of PTSD.

Psychotic symptoms in response to combat experiences are not uncommon. Forty per cent of one sample of Vietnam veterans had experienced psychotic symptoms in the 6 months before assessment (David *et al.* 1999). In all but one case, these included auditory hallucinations. The role of affect in their production is clear, and a majority of such cases met criteria for major depressive disorder (David *et al.* 1999; Hamner *et al.* 1999); anxiety is also likely to be an important link. It is of interest that people with PTSD and those with schizophrenia both display abnormal startle responses (Howard & Ford 1992).

In another study, veterans comorbid for PTSD and psychosis showed far more disturbance than those with either condition alone (Sautter *et al.* 1999). However, in some studies the meaningful connection between the characteristics of trauma and the content of symptoms is not always so apparent. Thus, Butler *et al.* (1996) have suggested that, in their series, the psychotic symptoms associated with PTSD did not seem to be linked to re-experiencing the trauma. Likewise, in another study, the severity of psychotic symptoms associated with combat-related PTSD was correlated with the severity of PTSD symptoms, but there seemed to be no link between psychotic symptoms and re-experiencing the traumatic event (Hamner *et al.* 1999). It appeared almost as though the psychotic symptoms were an alternative way of re-experiencing. It is of interest that patients with PTSD who also have psychotic symptoms may display reduced plasma dopamine hydroxylase, a biological marker indicative of increased vulnerability to stress (Hamner & Gold 1998).

Hamner *et al.* (2000) compared veterans with long-standing PTSD and psychotic features with a sample of patients with schizophrenia who did not meet criteria for PTSD. They found very few differences in the form and intensity of the psychotic features, both positive and negative.

The alternative strategy of investigating levels of PTSD in people diagnosed as suffering from schizophrenia has also been used. In some cases this arose from a concern that the experiences of treatment were themselves traumatic. Thus, in an Australian study, half of 45 psychotic patients met criteria for PTSD in relation to their psychotic and treatment experiences (Shaw *et al.* 1997). Meyer *et al.* (1999) have examined the experience of hospitalization and treatment as a source of trauma and PTSD in people with schizophrenia. However, three-quarters of

the PTSD symptoms were related to the symptoms of psychosis, not to the traumas of treatment. It is not clear what is meant when PTSD symptoms are attributed to the experience of psychotic symptoms – PTSD is traditionally defined against an external rather than an internal reference.

Mueser *et al.* (1998) studied 275 patients with a range of severe mental disorders. Forty-three per cent had PTSD as a result of a severe trauma at some stage of their lives, often in childhood, However, only 2% of these had the diagnosis recorded in their notes. Ninety-eight per cent of the sample had been exposed to at least one severe trauma.

Priebe *et al.* (1998) found that over half (51%) of community patients with schizophrenia also met criteria for PTSD, and this did not appear to be related to treatment traumas. However, it was related to levels of neurotic symptoms.

Early social environment in people who develop schizophrenia

The stress–vulnerability paradigm in schizophrenia is usually applied with the implicit view that the vulnerability is genetic, or perhaps related to the early physical environment. This is reflected in a reluctance to attribute to social factors significant effects that cannot easily be subsumed under mere triggering. However, biological indicators of vulnerability are by no means universal in individuals with schizophrenia. There is therefore no logical reason why vulnerability should not in some cases be psychological, arising from early social experiences. Thus, in a recent case–control study, early parental loss was found to be more common in people with psychiatric diagnoses (Agid *et al.* 1999). This applied to people with schizophrenia ($n = 76$) as much as to those with bipolar disorder and major depressive disorder. The odds ratio comparing patients with schizophrenia with controls was 3.8. Fuchs (1999) compared patients with late paraphrenia and with severe late onset depression. He found more discriminatory, humiliating or threatening experiences in early life in the first group, and more early loss in the second.

Ellason and Ross (1997) found a significant association of child physical and sexual abuse with psychotic symptoms, confirming the work by Mueser *et al.* (1998) described in the previous section. There are concerns about the reliability of such reports in people whose mental state is affected by schizophrenia. However, Goodman *et al.* (1999) have demonstrated that accounts of abuse are consistent over time, and conclude that the information obtained is sufficiently reliable to allow research in this area.

The most striking evidence for the impact of adverse environment in childhood may come from the prospective study of Myhrman *et al.* (1994). These authors used the Finnish 1966 birth cohort: in this mothers were asked before the birth if the child was wanted, wanted but mistimed, or unwanted. At follow-up, the prevalence of schizophrenia was twice as high (1.5% vs. 0.7%) in those offspring who had been unwanted babies. After correction for sociodemographic variables the odds ratio was 2.4. Unwantedness could act as a prenatal stress, or as a marker associated with behaviours associated with risk either in mother or child.

Another Finnish study (Tienari et al. 1994) compared adopted children of mothers with a diagnosis of schizophrenia with a group of adopted children of control mothers. As expected, the first group was found to contain more people with severe mental illness, including schizophrenia. However, all children did well in 'healthy' adoptive families. Differences were only found where the adoptive families were rated as 'disturbed'. One interpretation of this is that the family environment was playing a crucial part in moderating genetic risk (Kinderman & Cooke 2000), although the adoptive families might equally have been disturbed in response to odd presymptomatic behaviour on the part of the adopted child. Nevertheless, both of these Finnish studies suggest a role for distal social factors.

It is also possible that the early environment may create dispositions that lead to chronicity and poor outcome. In a German multivariate study of schizophrenia, traumatic experiences and adverse circumstances in childhood were related to relapse and rehospitalization (Doering et al. 1998). Fowler (1999) found that severe distal trauma histories are common in those with chronic psychosis, but not those in their first episode (who include many heading for a good outcome).

The effect of a stressful early environment is quite likely to be mediated through enduring cognitive predispositions, that is to say, a mechanism at the psychological level. However, even this is not a necessary assumption. Thus, it has been suggested that early stress may be responsible for 'miswiring' dopaminergic inputs to GABAergic cortical neurones: these projections continue to mature into early adulthood and may be responsible in part for vulnerability to the development of schizophrenic symptoms (Benes 1997).

Interplay of stress, medication and relapse in schizophrenia

The role of medication in preventing relapse in schizophrenia may be to modify overall vulnerability to stress. This obviously has a bearing on the question of whether people with schizophrenia have an increased sensitivity to the social environment. We have already had evidence from our aggregate analysis of EE studies that medication can have an effect in protecting patients from the adverse effects of living with high EE relatives. There is some evidence that medication has a similar role in protecting people with schizophrenia from the effects of life event stress. A number of studies have addressed this issue. Birley and Brown (1970) found that the relationship between life events and relapse was weakest in those patients who had been off medication for less than 1 year. The relationship was stronger both in patients who had not taken medication for more than 1 year and for those who remained on medication. Leff et al. (1973) used data from a double-blind placebo-controlled trial to examine the effect of medication on the life event–relapse relationship. In

a post hoc analysis, life events appeared to precede relapse in patients on active medication but not those on placebo. Bartko et al. (1987) reports similar findings from a non-randomized design. The implication is that those patients who are on medication require an event before they will relapse, while patients without medication may be so sensitive to small changes in their environment that the sort of life event picked up in the research studies are not necessary.

However, for methodological reasons these studies are inconclusive. More weight can be placed on the prospective studies of Ventura et al. (1992) and Hirsch et al. (1996). Ventura et al. (1992), investigating patients with short histories of illness, found an excess of events in those on regular medication compared with those not receiving any. Nuechterlein et al. (1994) used a longitudinal design to assess the effects of life events and expressed emotion on schizophrenic relapse. Their results indicate that life events are more important when patients are on medication, a further suggestion that medication may raise the threshold for stress vulnerability. Hirsch et al. (1996) studied a population with more long-standing illness. They failed to find any differences in the experience of event prerelapse in medicated and unmedicated groups. This is possibly a type II error, as only five of 36 patients on medication relapsed during the 1-year follow-up. This study is interesting because it compares the relative size of the effect of medication with that of the cumulative event rate and found that the former was much the greater. This is an interesting contrast to the results from the meta-analysis of EE studies described above. However, within the medicated and unmedicated groups, the cumulative effect of life events on the risk of relapse was the same, correlating with the number of life events experienced (see Fig. 31.2).

Other links with the EE research have been postulated. Leff and Vaughn (1980) found that there was a much stronger event–relapse relationship in schizophrenic patients who came from low EE families than those who came from high EE families. These patients were largely off medication. It seems from this as though patients required one sort of stress or the other, but that either would do. People living with a high EE relative may be so vulnerable in consequence that very small perturbations in the social environment can precipitate relapse. Leff et al. (1983) used results from their family intervention study to explore this issue further. They concluded that for patients off medication, relapse can be provoked by either life event or contact with a high EE relative. However, for patients on medication relapse appeared to require the presence of the two factors in combination.

Conclusions

The findings surveyed in this chapter are wide-ranging and complex. What can be made of them? The EE studies suggest a large and robust effect of a predictor that is now known to reflect stressful aspects of the home environment. On this basis social factors appear to be important. Why is it that the life event research does not corroborate the EE research in a more convincing manner? One possibility is that the relatively abrupt changes represented by life events may not be so important in producing relapse as continuing, albeit perhaps relatively low, levels of stress occasioned by living with a high EE family member. Another explanation is that the rating of life events is essentially derived from research concerned mainly with depressive disorders. In consequence, the ratings may be set at the wrong threshold for picking up the life events important in schizophrenia. If people with schizophrenia are unnaturally sensitive to life events, it is possible that the relapse is brought about by events that on the surface would seem incapable of provoking an emotional response. One study (Malla et al. 1990) only found a significant effect of events on relapse if trivial events or 'hassles' were included in the analysis. The study of Bebbington et al. (1993) described above also suggested that events of mild threat were in excess in schizophrenia, as in other psychoses. This would certainly tie in with the experience of many clinicians, who in managing people with long-standing schizophrenia work quite hard to protect them from even minor changes in their daily routines.

It is also possible that events are rated along dimensions of reduced relevance for schizophrenia, and there is preliminary evidence that intrusiveness may be an important concept in this context (Harris 1987). Likewise, Rooke and Birchwood (1998) have examined the relationship between humiliating, entrapping and defeating life events and depression in schizophrenia.

In our view, the evidence concerning the psychosocial reactivity of schizophrenia is important because it reflects on the nature of the condition. If we take psychotic experience as a whole, it is clear there is a spectrum of reactivity: the most reactive conditions tend to have a notable admixture of affective symptoms in the clinical picture. This is true whether we define schizophrenia quite narrowly, or whether we also include schizoaffective disorder and affective psychosis. It is also true of psychotic conditions defined closely in relation to psychosocial stress, that is, reactive psychosis and the psychotic features associated with PTSD.

However, affective symptoms are less rare in schizophrenia than once thought – they are quite widespread and are often linked with prodromes of psychotic relapse (Birchwood & Iqbal 1998). It appears that both life events and high EE may be associated with an increase in affective symptoms in people with schizophrenia, and one could postulate that the emergence of psychotic symptoms in response to psychosocial stress represents a further stage in a continuous process that is initially restricted to symptoms of anxiety and depression. It is apparent that this final stage is not necessarily reached in all circumstances (Yung & McGorry 1996).

Obviously not every member of the general population responds to stress by developing psychotic symptoms. Thus, there must be something unusual about the people who do react in this way, either in their biogenetic make-up, or in their circumstances, or both. The concept of psychosis has drawn its strength from a sense that the mental experiences it expresses are so bizarre and unusual that they represent a categorical separation from the normal. This was very much the position of the influential psychopathologist Karl Jaspers (1913) who used it to argue for biological causation.

However, in recent years this view has been changing, at least in some quarters. Around 4% of the general population admit to hallucinatory experiences (Johns et al. 2002), and it is possible that the capacity for psychotic experience of this sort is not at all uncommon. Moreover, intensive studies of delusional thinking suggest that it cannot be categorically separated from the illogicalities of most normal thinking, and that it is best distinguished in dimensional terms (Garety & Hemsley 1994; Appelbaum et al. 1999). As David Hume said, rationality is a coat we wear for special occasions.

The effect of these developments has been to normalize our conceptualizations of psychotic experience, and this in turn suggests that 'normal' psychosocial processes have more of a part to play in its origins. Few adherents of psychosocial explanations would go so far as to exclude all possibility of genetic or physical environmental causes; most argue only for a shift in balance.

Cognitive therapy has implications for the psychosocial reactivity of schizophrenia in that apparently intractable delusions can be modified. In the process, the conceptualization of delusions as categorically distinct is weakened. Moreover, this comes about by changing the social context of the person with schizophrenia. This is done by introducing a new social relationship – the therapist uses his or her relationship with the patient to offer alternative views of their experiences in a way that normalizes them (Sensky et al. 2000). In the process, not only are delusions modified, but also hallucinations (Kuipers et al. 1998). Our own cognitive model of psychosis, which was developed in relation both to the practice and to the practical experience of cognitive therapy, incorporates psychosocial elements (Garety et al. 2001). The model is new, in that it incorporates disruptions in automatic cognitive processes and maladaptive conscious appraisals; it covers delusions and hallucinations in one framework; and it accords a central role to emotion. However, an integral part of the model is the consideration of how social factors may contribute to the origins, maintenance and recurrence of symptoms. The work on the impact of early loss and trauma on the later development of schizophrenia can certainly be interpreted in this way. We suggest that early adverse experience such as social trauma may create an enduring cognitive vulnerability reflected in negative schemata of the self and the world that facilitate external attributions and low self-esteem. Evidence consistent with a role for such negative schemata in the development of psychosis has been found by van Os (personal communication) in a cohort of 7000 people in the Netherlands. Birchwood et al. (2000) have argued similarly that childhood adversity may fuel voices and persecutory ideas through schemata like this.

Pre-existing schemata also affect the content of psychotic attributions (Bowins & Sugar 1998). Implicit in these ideas is the possibility that social circumstances may influence both the content and the fact of psychotic experience.

Life events can be seen as having a dual role. They may act as a priming agent by inculcating characteristic patterns of interpretation. Events of this sort are quite likely to occur at a young age, but may happen in adulthood, particularly if the associated trauma is both overwhelming and difficult to process within existing schemata (e.g. rape). Many asylum seekers with psychosis have had experiences of this type. The second role of life events is as a triggering agent. Events are particularly likely to do this if they have characteristics ('demand characteristics') that tend to elicit the typical responses of schizophrenic thinking. It is clear that some events are particularly likely to elicit ideas of persecution. Kaffman (1984) demonstrated that the delusional symptoms of 34 patients with paranoid disorder had a basis in truth. Harris (1987) used this idea in her elaborations of the concept of intrusiveness, arguing that this was a characteristic of events associated with psychotic relapse. Raune (unpublished data) has obtained some corroboration of this. The review of life circumstances undertaken in cognitive–behaviour therapy affords compelling examples of life events fulfilling both priming and triggering functions, but the idea of paranoia-inducing events has yet to be subject to adequate empirical investigation, and poses considerable methodological difficulties.

The final social element in the model concerns the role of isolation. We propose that isolation contributes to the patient's acceptance of psychotic appraisal by reducing access to other, more normalizing, explanations. The idea is that exposure to people with alternative views is important, particularly at crucial stages in the development of delusional thinking. Exposure to therapists in the course of cognitive–behaviour therapy is a special example of this. White et al. (2000) found that insight in schizophrenia is greater in people with larger social networks.

These ideas linking social factors with cognitive models of schizophrenia are clearly speculative at present. They will require sophisticated methods of research to substantiate them. Nevertheless, this kind of research should enhance our understanding of the social reactivity of psychosis, and improve both the treatment and long-term management of schizophrenia.

References

Agid, O., Shapira, B., Zislin, J. et al. (1999) Environment and vulnerability to major psychiatric illness: a case–control study of early parental loss in major depression, bipolar disorder and schizophrenia. Molecular Psychiatry 4, 163–172.

Aguilar, E.J., Haas, G., Manzanera, F.J. et al. (1997) Hopelessness and first-episode psychosis: a longitudinal study. Acta Psychiatrica Scandinavica 96, 25–30.

Al Khani, M.A.F., Bebbington, P.E., Watson, J.P. & House, F. (1986) Life events and schizophrenia: a Saudi Arabian study. British Journal of Psychiatry 148, 12–22.

Alloway, R. & Bebbington, P.E. (1987) The buffer theory of social support: a review of the literature. Psychological Medicine 17, 91–108.

American Psychiatric Association (1987) Diagnostic and Statistical Manual of Mental Disorders, 3rd Edn. Revised. American Psychiatric Association, Washington, DC.

American Psychiatric Association (1994) Diagnostic and Statistical Manual of Mental Disorders, 4th Edn. American Psychiatric Association, Washington, DC.

Appelbaum, P.S., Robbins, P.C. & Roth, L.H. (1999) Dimensional approach to delusions: comparison across types and diagnoses. Americal Journal of Psychiatry 156, 1938–1943.

Arévalo, J. & Vizcaro, C. (1989) 'Emocion expresada' y curso de la esquizofrenia en una muestra espanola. Analisis Y Modificacion de Conducta 15, 3–23.

Ball, A., Moore, E. & Kuipers, L. (1992) Expressed Emotion in community care staff: a comparison of patient outcome in a nine month follow-up of two hostels. Social Psychiatry and Psychiatric Epidemiology 27, 35–39.

Barrelet, L., Ferrero, F., Szigetty, L., Giddey, C. & Pellizzer, G. (1990) Expressed Emotion and first admission schizophrenia: nine month follow-up in a French cultural environment. British Journal of Psychiatry 156, 357–362.

Barrowclough, C. & Parle, M. (1997) Appraisal, psychological adjustment and expressed emotion in relatives of patients suffering from schizophrenia. British Journal of Psychiatry 170, 26–30.

Barrowclough, C., Johnston, M. & Tarrier, N. (1994) Attributions, expressed emotion, and patient relapse: an attributional model of relatives' response to schizophrenic illness. Behavior Therapy 25, 67–88.

Barrowclough, C., Tarrier, N. & Johnston, M. (1996) Distress, expressed emotion, and attributions in relatives of schizophrenia patients. Schizophrenia Bulletin 22, 691–702.

Bartko, G., Maylath, E. & Herczeg, I. (1987) Comparative study of schizophrenic patients relapsed on and off medication. Psychiatry Research 22, 221–227.

Bateson, G., Jackson, D.D., Hally, J. & Weakland, J.H. (1956) Towards a theory of schizophrenia. Behavioural Science 1, 251–264.

Bean, G., Beiser, M., Zhang-Wong, J. & Iacono, W. (1996) Negative labelling of individuals with first episode schizophrenia: the effect of premorbid functioning. Schizophrenia Research 22, 111–118.

Bebbington, P. & Kuipers, L. (1994) The predictive utility of expressed emotion in schizophrenia: an aggregate analysis. Psychological Medicine 24, 707–718.

Bebbington, P.E. & Kuipers, E. (1995) Predicting relapse in schizophrenia: gender and expressed emotion. International Journal of Mental Health 24, 7–22.

Bebbington, P.E., Wilkins, S., Jones, P. et al. (1993) Life events and psychosis: initial results from the Camberwell Collaborative Psychosis study. British Journal of Psychiatry. 162, 72–79.

Bebbington, P.E., Bowen, J., Hirsch, S.R. & Kuipers, L. (1995) Schizophrenia and psychosocial stressors. In: Schizophrenia (eds S.R. Hirsch & D. Weinberger), pp. 587–604. Blackwell Science, Oxford.

Bebbington, P.E., Wilkins, S., Sham, P. et al. (1996) Life events before psychotic episodes: do clinical and social variables affect the relationship? Social Psychiatry and Psychiatric Epidemiology 31, 122–128.

Bell, M., Bryson, G. & Lysaker, P. (1997) Positive and negative affect recognition in schizophrenia: a comparison with substance abuse and normal control subjects. Psychiatry Research 73, 73–82.

Beltz, J., Bertrando, P., Clerici, M. et al. (1991) Emotive Espresso e schizophrenia: dai familiari agli operatori psichiatrici. Symposium on Expressed Emotion in Latin Based Languages, Barcelona, Spain.

Benes, F.M. (1997) The role of stress and dopamine–GABA interactions in the vulnerability for schizophrenia. Journal of Psychiatric Research 31, 257–275.

Bentsen, H., Boye, B., Munkvold, O.G. et al. (1996) Emotional over-involvement in parents of patients with schizophrenia or related psychosis: demographic and clinical predictors. British Journal of Psychiatry 169, 622–630.

Bentsen, H., Munkvold, O.G., Notland, T.H. et al. (1997) Relatives' locus of control and expressed emotion in schizophrenia and related psychoses. *British Journal of Clinical Psychology* 36, 555–567.

Bentsen, H., Notland, T.H., Munkvold, O.G. *et al.* (1998a) Guilt proneness and expressed emotion in relatives of patients with schizophrenia or related psychoses. *British Journal of Medical Psychology* 71, 125–138.

Bentsen, H., Notland, T.H., Boye, B. *et al.* (1998b) Criticism and hostility in relatives of patients with schizophrenia or related psychoses: demographic and clinical predictors. *Acta Psychiatrica Scandinavica* 97, 76–85.

Bertrando, P., Beltz, J., Bressi, C. *et al.* (1992) Expressed emotion and schizophrenia in Italy: a study of an urban population. *British Journal of Psychiatry* 161, 223–229.

Bhugra, D., Leff, J., Der Mallett, R.G., Corridan, B. & Rudge, S. (1997) Incidence and outcome of schizophrenia in whites, African-Caribbeans and Asians in London. *Psychological Medicine* 27, 791–798.

Birchwood, M. & Iqbal, Z. (1998) *Depression and Suicidal Thinking in Psychosis: a Cognitive Approach.* In: . *Outcome and Innovation in Psychological Treatment of Schizophrenia* (eds T. Wykes, N. Tarrier & S. Lewis), pp. 81–100. Wiley, Chichester.

Birchwood, M. & Smith, J. (1987) Schizophrenia in the family. In: *Coping with Disorder in the Family* (ed. J. Orford), pp. 7–38. Croom-Helm, London.

Birchwood, M., McMillan, F. & Smith, J. (1992) Early intervention. In: *Innovations in the Psychological Managment of Schizophrenia* (eds M. Birckwood & N. Tarrier), pp. 115–146. Wiley, Chichester.

Birchwood, M., Meaden, A., Trower, P., Gilbert, P. & Plaistow, J. (2000) The power and omnipotence of coices: subordination and entrapment by voices and by significant others. *Psychological Medicine* 30, 337–344.

Birley, J.L.T. & Brown, G.W. (1970) Crises and life changes preceding the onset or relapse of acute schizophrenia: clinical aspects. *British Journal of Psychiatry* 116, 327–333.

Bledin, K., MacCarthy, B., Kuipers, L. & Woods, B. (1990) Expressed emotion in the daughters of people with dementia. *British Journal of Psychiatry* 157, 221–227.

Bogren, L.Y. (1997) Expressed emotion, family burden, and quality of life in parents with schizophrenic children. *Nordic Journal of Psychiatry* 51, 229–233.

Bowins, B. & Sugar, G. (1998) Delusions and self-esteem. *Canadian Journal of Psychiatry* 43, 154–158.

Boye, B., Munkvold, O.G., Bentsen, H. *et al.* (1998) Pattern of emotional over-involvement in relatives of patients with schizophrenia: a stress syndrome analogue? *Nordic Journal of Psychiatry* 52, 493–500.

Boye, B., Bentsen, H., Notland, T.H. *et al.* (1999) What predicts the course of expressed emotion in relatives of patients with schizophrenia or related psychoses? *Social Psychiatry and Psychiatric Epidemiology* 34, 35–43.

Brewin, C.R. (1994) Changes in attribution and expressed emotion among the relatives of patients with schizophrenia. *Psychological Medicine* 24, 905–911.

Brewin, C.R., MacCarthy, B., Duda, K. & Vaughn, C.E. (1991) Attribution and Expressed Emotion in the relatives of patients with schizophrenia. *Journal of Abnormal Psychology* 100, 546–554.

Brockington, I.F., Altman, E., Hillier, V., Meltzer, H.V. & Nand, S. (1982) The clinical picture of bipolar affective disorder in its depressed phase: a report from London and Chicago. *British Journal of Psychiatry* 141, 558–562.

Brown, G.W. (1959) Experiences of discharged chronic schizophrenic mental hospital patients in various types of living group. *Millbank Memorial Fund Quarterly* 37, 105–131.

Brown, G.W. (1974) Meaning measurement and stress of life events. In: *Stressful Life Events: Their Nature and Effects* (eds B.S. Dohrenwend & B.P. Dohrenwend), pp. 217–243. John Wiley, New York.

Brown, G.W. & Birley, J.L.T. (1968) Crises and life changes and the onset of schizophrenia. *Journal of Health and Social Behaviour* 9, 203–214.

Brown, G.W. & Harris, T.O. (1978) *Social Origins of Depression.* Tavistock, London.

Brown, G.W. & Rutter, M.L. (1966) The measurement of family activities and relationships. *Human Relations* 19, 241–263.

Brown, G.W., Carstairs, G.M. & Topping, G.C. (1958) The post hospital adjustment of chronic mental patients. *Lancet* ii, 685–689.

Brown, G.W., Monck, E.M., Carstairs, G.M. & Wing, J.K. (1962) Influence of family life on the course of schizophrenic illness. *British Journal of Preventive and Social Medicine* 16, 55–68.

Brown, G., Bone, M., Dalison, B. & Wing, J. (1966) *Schizophrenia and Social Care.* Oxford University Press, London.

Brown, G.W., Birley, J.L.T. & Wing, J.K. (1972) Influence of family life on the course of schizophrenic disorders: a replication. *British Journal of Psychiatry* 121, 241–258.

Brown, G.W., Harris, T.O. & Peto, J. (1973) Life events and psychiatric disorders. II. Nature of causal link. *Psychological Medicine* 3, 159–176.

Buchkremer, G., Stricker, K., Holle, R. & Kuhs, H. (1991) The predictability of relapses in schizophrenic patients. *European Archives of Psychiatry and Clinical Neuroscience* 240, 292–300.

Budd, R.J., Oles, G. & Hughes, I.C.T. (1998) The relationship between coping style and burden in the carers of relatives with schizophrenia. *Acta Psychiatrica Scandinavica* 98, 304–309.

Budzyna-Dawidowski, P., Rostworowska, M. & de Barbaro, B. (1989) Stability of Expressed Emotion: a 3 year follow-up study of schizophrenic patients. Paper presented at the 19th Annual Congress of the European Association of Behaviour Therapy, Vienna, September 10–24.

Butler, R.W., Mueser, K.T., Sprock, J. & Braff, D.L. (1996) Positive symptoms of psychosis in post-traumatic stress disorder. *Biological Psychiatry* 39, 839–844.

Butzlaff, R.L. & Hooley, J.M. (1998) Expressed emotion and psychiatric relapse: a meta-analysis. *Archives of General Psychiatry* 55, 547–552.

Canton, G. & Fraccon, I.G. (1985) Life events and schizophrenia: a replication. *Acta Psychiatrica Scandinavica* 71, 211–216.

Castine, M.R., Meador-Woodruff, J.H. & Dalack, G.W. (1998) The role of life events in onset and recurrent episodes of schizophrenia and schizoaffective disorder. *Journal of Psychiatric Research* 32, 283–288.

Chung, R.K., Langeluddecke, P. & Tennant, C. (1986) Threatening life events in the onset of schizophrenia, schizophreniform psychosis and hypomania. *British Journal of Psychiatry* 148, 680–686.

Curson, D.A., Pantelis, C., Ward, J. & Barnes, T.R.E. (1992) Institutionalism and schizophrenia 30 years on: clinical poverty and the social environment in three British mental hospitals in 1960 compared with a fourth in 1990. *British Journal of Psychiatry* 160, 230–241.

Cutting, L.P. & Docherty, N.M. (2000) Schizophrenia outpatients' perceptions of their parents: is expressed emotion a factor? *Journal of Abnormal Psychology* 109, 266–272.

David, D., Kutcher, G.S., Jackson, E.I. & Mellman, T.A. (1999) Psychotic symptoms in combat-related post-traumatic stress disorder. *Journal of Clinical Psychiatry* 60, 29–32.

Davis, D.J. & Schultz, C.L. (1998) Grief, parenting, and schizophrenia. *Social Science and Medicine* 46, 369–379.

Davis, J.A., Goldstein, M.J. & Nuechterlein, K.H. (1996) Gender differences in family attitudes about schizophrenia. *Psychological Medicine* **26**, 689–696.

Day, R. (1989) Schizophrenia. In: *Innovations in the Psychological Managment of Schizophrenia* (eds G.W. Brown & T.O. Harris), pp. 113–137. Unwin Hyman, London.

Day, R., Neilsen, J.A., Korten, A. *et al.* (1987) Stressful life events preceding the acute onset of schizophrenia: a cross national study from the World Health Organization. *Culture, Medicine and Psychiatry* **11**, 123–206.

Dingemans, P.M., Lenior, M.E. & Linszen, D.H. (1996) Patient psychopathology and parental expressed emotion. *Tijdshrift Voor Psychiatrie* **38**, 660–667.

Dixon, M.J., King, S., Stip, E. & Cormier, H. (2000) Continuous performance test differences among schizophrenic out-patients living in high and low expressed emotion environments. *Psychological Medicine* **30**, 1141–1153.

Doane, J.A., West, K.L., Goldstein, M.J., Rodnick, E.H. & Jones, J.E. (1981) Parental communication deviance and affective style: predictors of subsequent schizophrenia spectrum disorders in vulnerable adolescents. *Archives of General Psychiatry* **38**, 679–685.

Docherty, N.M. (1995) Expressed emotion and language disturbances in parents of stable schizophrenia patients. *Schizophrenia Bulletin* **31**, 411–418.

Docherty, N.M., Cutting, L.P. & Bers, S.A. (1998) Expressed emotion and differentiation of self in the relatives of stable schizophrenia outpatients. *Psychiatry* **61**, 269–278.

Doering, S., Muller, E., Kopcke, W. *et al.* (1998) Predictors of relapse and rehospitalization in schizophrenia and schizoafective disorder. *Schizophrenia Bulletin* **24**, 87–98.

Dohrenwend, B.P., Levav, I., Shrout, P.E. *et al.* (1987) Life stress and psychopathology: progress with research begun with Barbara Snell Dohrenwend. *American Journal of Community Psychology* **15**, 677–713.

Drake, R.E. & Sederer, L.I. (1986) The adverse effects of intensive treatment of chronic schizophrenia. *Comprehensive Psychiatry* **27**, 313–326.

Dulz, B. & Hand, I. (1986) Short-term relapse in young schizophrenics: can it be predicted and affected by family (CFI), patient, and treatment variables? An experimental study. In: *Treatment of Schizophrenia: Family Assessment and Intervention* (eds M.J. Goldstein, I. Hand & K. Hahlweg). Springer, Berlin.

Ellason, J.E. & Ross, C.A. (1997) Childhood trauma and psychiatric symptoms. *Psychological Reports* **80**, 447–450.

Falloon, I.R.H., Boyd, J.L., McGill, C.W. *et al.* (1982) Family management in the prevention of exacerbations of schizophrenia: a controlled study. *New England Journal of Medicine* **306**, 1437–1440.

Falloon, I.R.H., Boyd, J.L., McGill, C.W. *et al.* (1985) Family management in the prevention of morbidity of schizophrenia: clinical outcome of a two year longitudinal study. *Archives of General Psychiatry* **42**, 887–896.

Favre, S., Gonzales, C., Lendais, G. *et al.* (1989) Expressed Emotion (EE) of schizophrenic relatives. Poster presented at VIIIth World Congress of Psychiatry, Athens, 12–19 October.

Finlay, J.M. & Zigmond, M.J. (1997) The effects of stress on central dopaminergic neurons: possible clinical implications. *Neurochemical Research* **22**, 1387–1394.

Fowler, D. (1999) The relationship between trauma and psychosis. Paper Presented at the Merseyside Psychotherapy Institute, Liverpool, May 1999.

Freud, S. (1917) Mourning and melancholia. In: *Collected Papers*, Vol. IV. Hogarth, London.

Fuchs, T. (1999) Life events in late paraphrenia and depression. *Psychopathology* **32**, 60–69.

Garety, P.A. & Hemsley, D.R. (1994) *Delusions: Investigations Into the Psychology of Delusional Reasoning*. Oxford University Press, Oxford.

Garety, P., Kuipers, E., Fowler, D., Freeman, D. & Bebbington, P. (2001) Theoretical paper: a cognitive model of the positive symptoms of psychosis. *Psychological Medicine* **31**, 189–195.

Giron, M. & Gomez-Beneyto, M. (1998) Relationship between empathic family attitude and relapse in schizophrenia: a 2-year follow-up prospective study. *Schizophrenia Bulletin* **24**, 619–627.

Goldberg, S.C., Schooler, N.R., Hogarty, G.E. & Roper, M. (1977) Prediction of relapse in schizophrenic outpatients treated by drug and sociotherapy. *Archives of General Psychiatry* **34**, 171–184.

Goldstein, M., Judd, L.L., Rodnick, E.H., Alkire, A. & Gould, E. (1968) A method for studying social influence and coping patterns within families of disturbed adolescents. *Journal of Nervous and Mental Disease* **147**, 233–251.

Goodman, L.A., Thompson, K.M., Weinfurt, K. *et al.* (1999) Reliability of reports of violent victimization and posttraumatic stress disorder among men and women with serious mental health. *Journal of Trauma and Stress.* **12**, 587–599.

Greenley, J.R. (1986) Social control and EE. *Journal of Nervous and Mental Disorders* **174**, 24–30.

Griesinger, W. (1861) *Die Pathologie und Therapie der Psychischen Krankheiten.*, 2nd edn. Braunschweig. Wreden. Translated as *Mental Pathology and Therapeutics* by C.L. Robertson & J. Rutherford). New Sydenham Society, London.

Gureje, O. & Adewumni, A. (1988) Life events in schizophrenia in Nigerians: a controlled investigation. *British Journal of Psychiatry* **153**, 367–375.

Gutiérrez, E., Escudero, V., Valero, J.A. *et al.* (1988) Expresión de emociones y curso de la esquizofrenia. II. Expresión de emociones y curso de la esquizofrenia en pacientes en remisión, *Análisisy Modificación de Conducta* **14**, 275–316.

Hamner, M.B. & Gold, P.B. (1998) Plasma dopamine β-hydroxylase activity in psychotic and non-psychotic post-traumatic stress disorder. *Psychiatry Research* **77**, 174–181.

Hamner, M.B., Fruech, B.C., Ulmer, H.G. & Arana, G.W. (1999) Psychotic features and illness severity in combat veterans with chronic post-traumatic stress disorder. *Biological Psychiatry* **45**, 846–852.

Hamner, M.D., Frueh, B.C., Ulmer, H.G. *et al.* (2000) Psychotic features in chronic posttraumatic stress disorder and schizophrenia: comparative severity. *Journal of Nervous and Mental Disease* **188**, 217–221.

Hansen, H., Dahl, A.A., Bertelsen, A. *et al.* (1992) The Nordic concept of reactive psychosis: a multicenter reliability study. *Acta Psychiatrica Scandinavica* **86**, 55–59.

Hardesty, J., Falloon, I.R.H. & Shirin, K. (1985) The impact of life events, stress and coping on the morbidity of schizophrenia. In: *Family Management of Schizophrenia* (ed. I.R. Falloon). Johns Hopkins University Press, Baltimore.

Harris, T.O. (1987) Recent developments in the study of life events in relation to psychiatric and physical disorders. In: *Psychiatric Epidemiology: Progress and Prospects* (ed. B. Cooper), pp. 81–100. Croom-Helm, London.

Harrison, C.A., Dadds, M.R. & Smith, G. (1998) Family caregivers' criticism of patients with schizophrenia. *Psychiatric Services* **49**, 918–924.

Hegerl, U., Priebe, S., Wildgrube, C. & Muller-Oerlinghausen, B. (1990) Expressed Emotion and auditory evoked potentials. *Psychiatry* **53**, 108–114.

Herzog, T. (1992) Nurses, patients and relatives: a study of family patterns on psychiatric wards. In: *Family Intervention in Schizophrenia:*

Experiences and Orientations in Europe (eds C.L. Cazzullo & G. Invernizzi). ARS, Milan.

Hirsch, S., Bowen, J., Emami, J. *et al.* (1996) A one year prospective study of the effects of life events and medication in the aetiology of schizophrenic relapse. *British Journal of Psychiatry* **168**, 49–56.

Hogarty, G.E. (1985) Expressed Emotion and schizophrenic relapse: implications from the Pittsburg Study. In: *Controversies in Schizophrenia* (ed. M. Alpert), pp. 354–365. Guilford, New York.

Hogarty, G.E., Anderson, C.M., Reiss, D.J. *et al.* (1986) Family psychoeducation, social skills training and maintenance chemotherapy in the aftercare treatment of schizophrenia. I. One year effects of a controlled study on relapse and Expressed Emotion. *Archives of General Psychiatry* **43**, 633–642.

Holmes, T.H. & Rahe, R.H. (1967) The Social Readjustment Rating Scale. *Journal of Psychosomatic Research* **11**, 213–218.

Hooley, J.M. (1998) Expressed emotion and locus of control. *Journal of Nervous and Mental Disease* **186**, 374–378.

Hooley, J.M. & Hiller, J.B. (2000) Personality and expressed emotion. *Journal of Abnormal Psychology* **109**, 40–44.

Hooley, J.M. & Hahlweg, K. (1986) The marriages and interaction patterns of depressed patients and their spouses: comparison of high and low ee dyads. In: *Treatment of Schizophrenia: Family Assessment and Intervention* (eds M.J. Goldstein, I. Hand & K. Hahlweg). Springer, Berlin.

Howard, R. & Ford, R. (1992) From the jumping Frenchmen of Maine to post-traumatic stress disorder: the startle response in neuropsychiatry. *Psychological Medicine* **22**, 695–707.

Hubschmid, T. & Zemp, M. (1989) Interactions in high- and low-EE families. *Social Psychiatry and Psychiatric Epidemiology* **24**, 113–119.

Huguelet, P., Favre, S., Binyet, S., Gonzalez, C. & Zabala, I. (1995) The use of the Expressed Emotion Index as a predictor of outcome in first admitted schizophrenic patients in a French speaking area of Switzerland. *Acta Psychiatrica Scandinavica* **92**, 447–452.

Hultman, C.M., Wieselgren, I.M. & Ohman, A. (1997) Relationships between social support, social coping and life events in the relapse of schizophrenic patients. *Scandinavian Journal of Psychology.* **38**, 3–13.

Hutchinson, G., Takei, N., Bhugra, D. *et al.* (1997) Increased rate of psychosis among African-Caribbeans in Britain is not due to an excess of pregnancy and birth complications. *British Journal of Psychiatry* **171**, 145–147.

Inoue, S., Tanaka, S., Shimodera, S. & Mino. Y. (1997) Expressed emotion and social function. *Psychiatry Research* **72**, 33–39.

Ivanović, M., Vuletić, Z. & Bebbington, P.E. (1994) Expressed Emotion in the families of patients with schizophrenia and its influence on the course of illness. *Social Psychiatry and Psychiatric Epidemiology* **29**, 61–65.

Ivezić, S., Oruć, L. & Bell, P. (1999) Psychotic symptoms in post-traumatic stress disorder. *Military Medicine* **164**, 73–75.

Jacobs, S. & Myers, J. (1976) Recent life events and acute schizophrenic psychosis: a controlled study. *Journal of Nervous and Mental Disease* **162**, 75–87.

Jansen, L.M.C., Gispen-De-Wied, C.C., Gademan, P.J. *et al.* (1998) Blunted cortisol response to a psychosocial stressor in schizophrenia. *Schizophrenia Research* **33**, 87–94.

Jaspers, K. (1913) Kausale and verständliche Zusammenhänge zwischen Schicksal und Psychose bei der Dementia Praecox (Schizophrenia). *Zeitschrift Neurologie* **14**, 158–263.

Jauch, D.A. & Carpenter, W.T. Jr (1998a) Reactive psychosis I. Does the pre-DSM-III concept define a third psychosis? *Journal of Nervous and Mental Disease* **176**, 72–81.

Jauch, D.A. & Carpenter, W.T. Jr (1998b) Reactive psychosis I. Does the pre-DSM-IIIR concept define a third psychosis? *Journal of Nervous and Mental Disease* **176**, 82–86.

Johns, L.C., Nazroo, J.Y., Bebbington, P. & Kuipers, E. (2002) Occurrence of hallucinatory experiences in a community sample and ethnic variations. *British Journal of Psychiatry* **180**, 174–178.

Jonsson, S.A., Jonsson, H., Nyman, A.K., Nyman, G. & E. (1991) The concept of cycloid psychosis: sensitivity and specificity of syndromes derived by multivariate clustering techniques. *Acta Psychiatrica Scandinavica* **85**, 353–362.

Kaffman, M. (1984) Paranoid disorders: the core of truth behind the delusional system. *International Journal of Family Therapy* **6**, 220–232.

Kapur, R.L. & Pandurangi, A.K. (1979) A comparative study of reactive psychosis and acute psychosis without precipitating stress. *British Journal of Psychiatry* **135**, 544–550.

Karno, M., Jenkins, J.H., de la Selva, A. *et al.* (1987) Expressed Emotion and schizophrenic outcome among Mexican-American families. *Journal of Nervous and Mental Disease* **175**, 143–151.

Kavanagh, D.J. (1992) Interventions for families and social networks. In: *Schizophrenia: an Overview and Practical Handbook* (ed. D.J. Kavanagh). Chapman & Hall, London.

Kavanagh, D.J., O'Halloran, P., Manicavasagar, V. *et al.* (1997) The Family Attitude Scale: reliability and validity of a new scale for measuring the emotional climate of families. *Psychiatry Research* **70**, 185–195.

Kinderman, P. & Cooke, A. (2000) *Recent Advances in Understanding Mental Illness and Psychotic Experiences*. A report by the British Psychological Society Division of Clinical Psychology. British Psychological Society, Leicester.

King, S. & Dixon, M.J. (1995) Expressed emotion, family dynamics and symptom severity in a predictive model of social adjustment for schizophrenic young adults. *Schizophrenia Research* **14**, 121–132.

King, S. & Dixon, M.J. (1999) Expressed emotion and relapse in young schizophrenia outpatients. *Schizophrenia Bulletin* **25**, 377–386.

King, S., Lesage, A.D. & Lalonde, P. (1994) Psychiatrists' ratings of expressed emotion. *Canadian Journal of Psychiatry* **39**, 358–360.

Kuipers, E. & Moore, E. (1995) Expressed Emotion and staff–client relationships: implications for community care of the severely mentally ill. *International Journal of Mental Health* **24**, 13–26.

Kuipers, E. & Raune, D. (2000) The early development of expressed emotion and burden in the families of first onset psychosis. In: *Early Intervention in Psychosis* (eds M. Birchwood, D. Fowler & C. Jackson), pp. 128–140. Wiley, Chichester.

Kuipers, E., Garety, P., Fowler, D. *et al.* (1997) London–East Anglia randomised controlled trial of cognitive–behavioural therapy for psychosis. I. Effects of the treatment phase. *British Journal of Psychiatry* **171**, 319–327.

Kuipers, E., Fowler, D., Garety, G. *et al.* (1998) The London–East Anglia randomised controlled trial of cognitive behaviour therapy for psychosis. III. Follow up and economic evaluation at 18 months. *British Journal of Psychiatry.* **173**, 61–61–68.

Kuipers, E., Bebbington, P., Pilling, S. & Orbach, G. (1999) Family intervention in psychosis: who needs it. *Epidemiologin E Psichiatria Sociale* **8**, 169–173.

Kuipers, L. (1979) Expressed Emotion: a review. *British Journal of Social and Clinical Psychology* **18**, 237–243.

Kuipers, L. (1983) *Family factors in schizophrenia: an intervention study*. PhD thesis, University of London.

Kuipers, L. (1992) Expressed Emotion research in Europe. *British Journal of Psychology* **31**, 429–443.

Kuipers, L., Sturgeon, D., Berkowitz, R. & Leff, J.P. (1983) Characteristics of Expressed Emotion: its relationship to speech and looking in schizophrenic patients and their relatives. *British Journal of Clinical Psychology* 22, 257–264.

Kuipers, L., MacCarthy, B., Hurry, J. & Harper, R. (1989) A low cost supportive model for relatives of the long term adult mentally ill. *British Journal of Psychiatry*. 154, 775–782.

Kurihara, T., Kato, M., Tsukahara, T., Takano, Y. & Reverger, R. (2000) The low prevalence of high levels of expressed emotion in Bali. *Psychiatry Research* 17, 229–238.

Laing, R.D. & Esterson, A. (1964) *Sanity, Madness and the Family*. Penguin, Harmondsworth.

Leff, J.P. & Vaughn, C. (1976) Schizophrenia and family life. *Psychology Today* 10, 13–18.

Leff, J.P. & Vaughn, C.E. (1980) The interaction of life events and relative's Expressed Emotion in schizophrenia and depressive neurosis. *British Journal of Psychiatry* 136, 146–153.

Leff, J.P., Hirsch, S.R., Gaind, R., Rohde, P.D. & Stevens, B.C. (1973) Life events and maintenance therapy in schizophrenic relapse. *British Journal of Psychiatry* 123, 659–660.

Leff, J.P., Kuipers, L., Berkowitz, R., Eberlein-Fries, R. & Sturgeon, D. (1982) A controlled trial of intervention in the families of schizophrenic patients. *British Journal of Psychiatry* 141, 121–134.

Leff, J.P., Kuipers, L., Berkowitz, R., Vaughn, C.E. & Sturgeon, D. (1983) Life events, relatives' Expressed Emotion and maintenance neuroleptics in schizophrenic relapse. *Psychological Medicine* 13, 799–806.

Leff, J.P., Kuipers, L., Berkowitz, R. & Sturgeon, D. (1985) A controlled trial of social intervention in the families of schizophrenic patients: two year follow up. *British Journal of Psychiatry* 146, 594–600.

Leff, J.P., Wig, N., Ghosh, A. *et al.* (1987) Influence of relatives' Expressed Emotion on the course of schizophrenia in Chandigarh. *British Journal of Psychiatry* 151, 166–173.

Leff, J.P., Berkowitz, R., Sharit, N. *et al.* (1989) A trial of family therapy vs. a relatives' group for schizophrenia. *British Journal of Psychiatry* 154, 58–66.

Leff, J.P., Berkowitz, R., Shavit, N. *et al.* (1990) A trial of family therapy vs. a relatives group for schizophrenia: two-year follow-up. *British Journal of Psychiatry* 157, 571–577.

Lenior, M.E., Dingermans, P.M.A.J. & Linszen, D.H. (1997) A quantitative measure for expressed emotion. *Psychiatry Research* 69, 53–65.

Lenior, M.E., Dingemans, P.M.A.J. & Linszen, D.H. (1998a) Expressed emotion and psychotic relapse: scalability of the items of the five minute speech sample. *Tijdschrift Voor Psychiatrie* 40, 14–26.

Lenior, M.E., Linszen, D.H. & Dingemans, P.M.A.J. (1998b) The association between parental expressed emotion and psychotic relapse: applying a quantitative measure for expressed emotion. *International Clinical Psychopharmacology* 13 (Suppl. 1), 81–87.

Levene, J.E., Lancee, W.J. & Seeman, M.V. (1996) The perceived family burden scale: measurement and validation. *Schizophrenia Research* 22, 151–157.

Lindvall, M., Axelsson, R. & Ohman, R. (1993) Incidence of cycloid psychosis: a clinical study of first-admission psychotic patients. *European Archives of Psychiatry and Clinical Neuroscience* 242, 197–202.

Linszen, D., Dingemans, P., Van-der-Does, J.W. *et al.* (1996) Treatment, expressed emotion and relapse in recent onset schizophrenic disorders. *Psychological Medicine* 26, 333–342.

Linszen, D.H., Dingemans, P.M., Nugter, M.A. *et al.* (1997) Patient attributes and expressed emotion as risk factors for psychotic relapse. *Schizophrenia Bulletin* 23, 119–130.

Linszen, D.H., Dingemans, P.M.A.J., Scholte, W.F., Lenior, M.W. & Goldstein, M. (1998) Early recognition, intensive intervention and other protective and risk factors for psychotic relapse in patients with first psychotic episodes in schizophrenia. *International Clinical Psychopharmacology* 13 (Suppl. 1), 7–12.

Lopez, S.R., Nelson, K.A., Snyder, K.S. & Mintz, J. (1999) Attributions and affective reactions of family members and course of schizophrenia. *Journal of Abnormal Psychology* 108, 307–314.

McCreadie, R.G. & Phillips, K. (1988) The Nithsdale Schizophrenia Survey. VII. Does relatives' high Expressed Emotion predict relapse? *British Journal of Psychiatry* 152, 477–481.

McCreadie, R.G., Phillips, K., Harvey, J.A. *et al.* (1991) The Nithsdale Schizophrenia Surveys. VIII. Do relatives want family intervention and does it help? *British Journal of Psychiatry* 158, 110–113.

McCreadie, R.G., Robertson, L.J., Hall, D.J. & Berry, I. (1993) The Nithsdale Schizophrenia Surveys. XI. Relatives' expressed emotion: stability over five years and its relations to relapse. *British Journal of Psychiatry* 162, 393–397.

McCreadie, R.G., Williamson, D.J., Athawes, R.W.B. *et al.* (1994) The Nithersdale schizophrenia surveys. XIII. Parental rearing patterns, current symptomatology and relatives' expressed emotion. *British Journal of Psychiatry* 165, 247–352.

McDonald, C. & Murray, R.M. (2000) Early and late environmental risk factors for schizophrenia. *Brain Research, Brain Research Review* 31, 130–137.

MacDonald, E.M., Pica, S., McDonald, S., Hayes, R.L. & Baglioni, A.J. Jr (1998) Stress and coping in early psychosis: role of symptoms, self-efficacy, and social support in coping with stress. *British Journal of Psychiatry* 172 (Suppl. 33), 122–127.

McGuffin, P., Asherson, P., Owen, M. & Farmer, A. (1994) The strength of the genetic effect: is there room for an environmental influence in the aetiology of schizophrenia? *British Journal of Psychiatry* 164, 593–599.

MacMillan, J.F., Gold, A., Crow, T.J., Johnson, A.L. & Johnstone, E.C. (1986) The Northwick Park study of first episodes of schizophrenia. IV. Expressed Emotion and relapse. *British Journal of Psychiatry* 148, 133–143.

Mahendra, B. (1977) Stress and the major psychiatric illnesses. *Acta Psychiatrica Scandinavica* 56, 161–167.

Malla, A.K., Cortese, L., Shaw, T.S. & Ginsberg, B. (1990) Life events and relapse in schizophrenia: a one year prospective study. *Social Psychiatry and Psychiatric Epidemiology* 25, 221–224.

Malzacher, M., Merz, J. & Ebnother, D. (1981) Einschneidende Lebensereignisse im Vorfeld akuter schizophrener Episoden: Erstmals erkrankte Patienten im Vergleich mit einer Normalstichprobe. *Archiv Fur Psychiatrie und Nervenkrankheiten* 230, 227–242.

Maosheng, R., Zaijin, H. & Mengze, S. (1998) Emotional expression among relatives of schizophrenic patients. *Chinese Journal of Psychiatry* 31, 237–239.

Mari, D.J.J. & Streiner, D.L. (1994) An overview of family interventions and relapse on schizophrenia: meta-analysis of research findings. *Psychological Medicine* 24, 565–578.

Mavreas, V.G., Tomaras, V., Karydi, V., Economon, M. & Stefanis, C. (1992) Expressed Emotion in families of chronic schizophrenics and its association with clinical measures. *Social Psychiatry and Psychiatric Epidemiology*. 27, 4–9.

Meyer, H., Taiminen, T., Vuori, T., Aijala, A. & Helenius, H. (1999) Post-traumatic stress disorder symptoms related to psychosis and acute involuntary hospitalization in schizophrenic and delusional patients. *Journal of Nervous and Mental Disease* 187, 343–352.

Miklowitz, D.J., Goldstein, M.J. & Falloon, I.R.H. (1983) Premorbid and symptomatic characteristics of schizophrenics from families with high and low levels of Expressed Emotion. *Journal of Abnormal Psychology* 3, 359–367.

Miklowitz, D.J., Goldstein, M.J., Doane, J.A. *et al.* (1989) Is Expressed

Emotion an index of a transactional process. I. Parent's affective style. *Family Process* **28**, 153–167.

Mino, Y., Inoue, S., Tanaka, S. & Tsuda, T. (1997) Expressed emotion among families and course of schizophrenia in Japan: a 2-year cohort study. *Schizophrenia Research* **24**, 333–339.

Mino, Y., Inoue, S., Shimodera, S. *et al.* (1998) Expressed emotion of families and negative–depressive symptoms in schizophrenia: a cohort study in Japan. *Schizophrenia Research* **34**, 159–168.

Možný, N.P. & Votpkova, P. (1992) Expressed Emotion, relapse rate and utilisation of psychiatric inpatient care in schizophrenia: a study from Czechoslovakia. *Social Psychiatry and Psychiatric Epidemiology* **27**, 174–179.

Moline, R.A., Singh, S., Morris, A. & Meltzer, H.Y. (1985) Family expressed emotion and relapse in schizophrenia in 24 urban American patients. *American Journal of Psychiatry* **142**, 1078–1081.

Montero, I., Gomez-Beneyto, M., Ruiz, I., Puche, E. & Adam, A. (1992) The influence of family Expressed Emotion on the course of schizophrenia in a sample of Spanish patients: a two year follow-up study. *British Journal of Psychiatry* **161**, 217–222.

Montero, I., Perez, I.R. & Gomez-Beneyto, M. (1998) Social adjustment in schizophrenia: factors predictive of short-term social adjustment in a sample of schizophrenic patients. *Acta Psychiatrica Scandinavica* **97**, 116–121.

Moore, E. & Kuipers, E. (1999) The measurement of expressed emotion in relationships between staff and service users: the use of short speech samples. *British Journal of Clinical Psychology* **38**, 345–356.

Moore, E., Ball, R.A. & Kuipers, L. (1992a) Expressed Emotion in staff working with the long-term adult mentally ill. *British Journal of Psychiatry* **161**, 802–808.

Moore, E., Kuipers, L. & Ball, R. (1992b) Staff patient relationships in the case of the long-term mentall ill: a content analysis of EE interviews. *Social Psychiatry and Psychiatric Epidemiology* **27**, 28–34.

Mueser, K.T., Goodman, L.B., Trumbetta, S.L. *et al.* (1998) Trauma and post-traumatic stress disorder in severe mental illness. *Journal of Consulting and Clinical Psychology.* **66**, 493–499.

Munoz, R.A., Amado, H. & Hyatt, S. (1987) Brief reactive psychosis. *Journal of Clinical Psychiatry* **48**, 324–327.

Myhrman, A., Rantakallio, P., Isohanni, M., Jones, P. & Partanen, U. (1994) Unwantedness of a pregnancy and schizophrenia in the child. *British Journal of Psychiatry* **169**, 637–640.

Niedermeier, T., Watzl, H. & Cohen, R. (1992) Prediction of relapse of schizophrenic patients: Camberwell Family Interview versus content anlysis of verbal behavior. *Psychiatry Research* **41**, 275–282.

Nuechterlein, K.H., Snyder, K.S., Dawson, M.E. *et al.* (1986) Expressed Emotion, fixed-dose fluphenazine decanoate maintenance, and relapse in recent onset schizophrenia. *Psychopharmacology Bulletin* **22**, 633–639.

Nuechterlein, K.H., Dawson, M.E., Ventura, J. *et al.* (1994) The vulnerability–stress model of schizophrenia relapse: a longitudinal study, *Acta Psychiatrica Scandinavica Suppl.* **89**, 58–64.

Oliver, N. & Kuipers, E. (1996) Stress and its relationship to expressed emotion in community mental health workers. *International Journal of Social Psychiatry* **42**, 150–159.

van Os, J., Fahy, T.A., Bebbington, P. *et al.* (1994) The influence of life events on the subsequent course of psychotic illness: a prospective follow-up of the Camberwell Collaborative Psychosis Study. *Psychological Medicine* **24**, 503–513.

Vaughan, K., Doyle, M., McConathy, N. *et al.* (1992) The relationship between relatives' EE and schizophrenic relapse: an Australian replication. *Social Psychiatry and Psychiatric Epidemiology* **27**, 10–15.

Owen, M.J. (2000) Molecular genetic studies of schizophrenia. *Brain Research, Brain Research Review* **31**, 179–186.

Pallanti, S., Quercioli, L. & Pazzagli, A. (1997) Relapse in young paranoid schizophrenic patients: a prospective study of stressful life events. *American Journal of Psychiatry* **154**, 792–298.

Pandurangi, A.K. & Kapur, R.L. (1980) Reactive psychosis: a prospective study. *Acta Psychiatrica Scandinavica* **61**, 89–95.

Parker, G., Johnston, P. & Hayward, L. (1988) Parental 'Expressed Emotion' as a predictor of schizophrenic relapse. *Archives of General Psychiatry* **45**, 806–813.

Pilling, S., Bebbington, P., Kuipers, E. *et al.* (2002) Psychological treatments in schizophrenia. I. Meta-analysis of family intervention and cognitive behaviour therapy. *Psychological Medicine* **32**, 763–782.

Priebe, S., Broker, M. & Gunkel, S. (1998) Involuntary admission and post-traumatic stress disorder symptoms in schizophrenia patients. *Comprehensive Psychiatry* **39**, 220–224.

Ramana, R. & Bebbington, P. (1995) Social influences on bipolar affective disorders. *Social Psychiatry and Psychiatric Epidemiology* **30**, 152–160.

Retterst, N. (1986) Classification of functional psychoses with special reference to follow-up studies. *Psychopathology* **19**, 5–15.

Rooke, O. & Birchwood, M. (1998) Loss, humiliation and entrapment as appraisals of schizophrenic illness: a prospective study of depressed and non-depressed patients. *British Journal of Clinical Psychology* **37**, 259–268.

Rosenfarb, I.S., Goldstein, M.J., Mintz, J. & Nuechterlein, K.H. (1995) Expressed emotion and subclinical psychopathology observable within the transactions between schizophrenic patients and their family members. *Journal of Abnormal Psychology* **142**, 259–267.

Rund, B.R., Oie, M., Borchgrevink, T.S. & Fjell, A. (1995) Expressed Emotion, communication deviance and schizophrenia: an exploratory study of the relationship between two family variables and the course and outcome of a psychoeducational treatment programme. *Psychopathology* **28**, 220–228.

Rutter, M.L. & Brown, G.W. (1966) The reliability and validity of measures of family life and relationships in families containing a psychiatric patient. *Social Psychiatry* **1**, 38–53.

Sautter, F.J., Brailey, K., Uddo, M.M. *et al.* (1999) PTSD and comorbid psychotic disorder: comparison with veterans diagnosed with PTSD or psychotic disorder. *Journal of Traumatic Stress* **12**, 73–88.

Scazufca, M. & Kuipers, E. (1996) Links between expressed emotion and burden of care in relatives of patients with schizophrenia. *British Journal of Psychiatry* **168**, 580–587.

Scazufca. M. & Kuipers, E. (1998) Stability of expressed emotion in relatives of those with schizophrenia and it relationship with burden of care and perception of patients' social functioning. *Psychological Medicine* **28**, 453–461.

Scazufca, M. & Kuipers, E. (1999) Coping strategies in relatives of people with schizophrenia before and after psychiatric admission. *British Journal of Psychiatry* **174**, 154–158.

Scazufca, M., Kuipers, E. & Menezes, P. (2001) Perception of negative emotions in close relatives by patients with schizophrenia. *British Journal of Clinical Psychology* **40**, 167–175.

Schreiber, J.L., Breier, A. & Pickar, D. (1995) Expressed emotion: trait or state? *British Journal of Psychiatry* **166**, 647–649.

Schulze-Monking, H. & Buchkremer, G. (1995) Emotional family atmosphere and relapse: investigations on the role of relapse definition, duration of illness and resignation of relatives. *European Psychiatry* **10**, 85–91.

Schulze-Monking, H., Hornung, W.P., Stricker, K. & Buchkremer, G. (1997a) Expressed emotion development and course of schizophrenic illness: considerations based on results of a CFI replication. *European Archives of Psychiatry and Clinical Neuroscience* **247**, 31–34.

Schulze-Monking, H., Hornung, W.P., Stricker, K. & Buchkremer, G.

(1997b) Expressed emotion in an 8 year follow-up. *European Psychiatry* **12**, 105–110.

Sensky, T., Turkington, D., Kingdon, D. *et al.* (2000) A randomized controlled trial of cognitive behavioural therapy for persistent symptoms in schizophrenia resistant to medication. *Archives of General Psychiatry* **57**, 165–172.

Shaw, K., McFarlane, A. & Bookless, C. (1997) The phenomenology of traumatic reactions to psychotic illness. *Journal of Nervous and Mental Disorder* **185**, 434–441.

Shimodera, S., Inoue, S., Tanaka, S. & Mino, Y. (1998) Critical comments made to schizophrenic patients by their families in Japan. *Comprehensive Psychiatry* **39**, 85–90.

Shimodera, S., Mino, Y., Inoue, S. *et al.* (1999) Validity of a five-minute speech sample in measuring expressed emotion in the families of patients with schizophrenia in Japan. *Comprehensive Psychiatry* **40**, 372–376.

Smith, J., Birchwood, M., Cochrane, R. & George, S. (1993) The needs of high and low expressed emotion families: a normative approach. *Social Psychiatry and Psychiatric Epidemiology* **28**, 11–16.

Snyder, K.S., Wallace, C.J., Moe, K. & Liberman, R.P. (1994) Expressed emotion by residential care operators and residents' symptoms and quality of life. *Hospital and Community Psychiatry* **45**, 1141–1143.

Stark, F.M. & Siol, T. (1994) Expressed emotion in the therapeutic relationship with schizophrenic patients. *European Psychiatry* **9**, 299–303.

Steinberg, H. & Durell, J. (1968) A stressful situation as a precipitant of schizophrenic symptoms: an epidemiological study. *British Journal of Psychiatry* **114**, 1097–1105.

Stephens, J.H., Shaffer, J.W. & Carpenter, W.T. (1982) Reactive psychoses. *Journal of Nervous Mental Disorder* **170**, 657–663.

Stevens, B.C. (1973) Evaluation of rehabilitation for psychotic patients in the community. *Acta Psychiatica Scandinavica* **46**, 136–140.

Stirling, J., Tantam, D., Thomas, P., Newby, D. & Montague, L. (1991) EE and early onset schizophrenia: a one year follow-up. *Psychological Medicine* **21**, 675–685.

Strachan, A.M., Leff, J.P., Goldstein, M.J., Doane, A. & Burrt, C. (1986) Emotional attitudes and direct communication in the families of schizophrenics: a cross-national replication. *British Journal of Psychiatry* **149**, 279–287.

Strachan, A.M., Feingold, D., Goldstein, M.J., Miklowitz, D.J. & Nuechterlein, K.H. (1989) Is Expressed Emotion an index of a transactional process. II. Patient's coping style. *Family Process* **28**, 169–181.

Sumiyoshi, T., Saitoh, T., Yotsutsuji, T. *et al.* (1999) Differential effects of mental stress on plasma homovanillic acid in schizophrenia and normal controls. *Neuropsychopharmacology* **20**, 365–369.

Tanaka, S., Mino, Y. & Inoue, S. (1995) Expressed emotion and the course of schizophrenia in Japan. *British Journal of Psychiatry* **167**, 794–798.

Tarrier, N. (1989) Electrodermal activity, expressed emotion and outcome in schizophrenia. *British Journal of Psychiatry* **155** (Suppl. 5), 51–56.

Tarrier, N., Barrowclough, C., Vaughan, C. *et al.* (1988a) The community management of schizophrenia: a controlled trial of a behavioural intervention with families to reduce relapse. *British Journal of Psychiatry* **153**, 532–542.

Tarrier, N., Barrowclough, C., Porceddu, K. & Watts, S. (1988b) The assessment of psychophysiological reactivity to the expressed emotion of the relatives of schizophrenic patients. *British Journal of Psychiatry* **152**, 618–624.

Tarrier, N., Barrowclough, C., Porceddu, K. & Fitzpatrick, E. (1994) The Salford Family Intervention Project: relapse rates of schizophrenia at five and eight years. *British Journal of Psychiatry* **165**, 829–832.

Tarrier, N., Wittkowski, A., Kinney, C. *et al.* (1999) Durability of the effects of cognitive–behaviour therapy in the treatment of chronic schizophrenia: 12-month follow-up. *British Journal of Psychiatry* **174**, 500–504.

Tattan, T. & Tarrier, N. (2000) The expressed emotion of case managers of the seriously mentally ill: the influence of expressed emotion on clinical outcomes. *Psychological Medicine* **30**, 195–204.

Tienari, P., Wynne, L.C., Moring, J. *et al.* (1994) The Finnish adoptive family study of schizophrenia: implications for family research. *British Journal of Psychiatry Supplement* **23**, 20–26.

Tompson, M.C., Goldstein, M.J., Lebell, M.B. *et al.* (1995) Schizophrenic patients' perceptions of their relatives' attitudes. *Psychiatry Research* **57**, 155–167.

Uehara, T., Yokoyama, T., Goto, M. *et al.* (1997) Expressed emotion from the five-minute speech sample and relapse of outpatients with schizophrenia. *Acta Psychiatrica Scandinavica* **95**, 454–456.

UK 700 Group (1999) Comparison of intensive and standard case management for patients with psychosis: rationale of the trial. *British Journal of Psychiatry* **174**, 74–78.

Ungvari, G.S. & Mullens, P.E. (2000) Reactive psychosis revisited. *Australian and New Zealand Journal of Psychiatry* **34**, 458–467.

van Os, J. & Marcelis, M. (1998) The ecogenetics of schizophrenia. *Schizophrenia Research* **23**, 127–135.

Vaughn, C. & Leff, J.P. (1976) The influence of family and social factors on the course of psychiatric illness: a comparison of schizophrenic and depressed neurotic patients. *British Journal of Psychiatry* **129**, 125–137.

Vaughn, C.E., Snyder, K.S., Jones, S., Freeman, W.B. & Falloon, I.R.H. (1984) Family factors in schizophrenic relapse: replication in California of British research in Expressed Emotion. *Archives of General Psychiatry* **41**, 1169–1177.

Ventura, J., Nuechterlein, K.H., Lukoff, D. & Hardisty, J.P. (1989) A prospective study of stressful life events and schizophrenic relapse. *Journal of Abnormal Psychology* **98**, 407–404.

Ventura, J., Nuechterlein, K.H., Hardisty, J.P. & Gitlin, M. (1992) Life events and schizophrenic relapse after withdrawal of medication: a prospective study. *British Journal of Psychiatry.* **161**, 615–620.

Ventura, J., Nuechterlein, K.H., Subotnik, K.L., Hardesty, J.P. & Mintz, J. (2000) Live events can trigger depressive exacerbation in the early course of schizophrenia. *Journal of Abnormal Psychology* **109**, 139–144.

Watts, S. (1988) *A descriptive investigation of the incidence of high EE in staff working with schizophrenic patients in a hospital setting.* Unpublished dissertation, Diploma in Clinical Psychology, British Psychological Society.

Weisman, A.G., Nuechterlein, K.H., Goldstein, M.J. & Snyder, K.S. (1998) Expressed emotion, attributions, and schizophrenia symptom dimensions. *Journal of Abnormal Psychology* **107**, 355–359.

Weisman, A.G., Nuechterlein, K.H., Goldstein, M.J. & Snyder, K.S. (2000) Controllability perceptions and reactions to symptoms of schizophrenia: a within-family comparison of relatives with high andlow expressed emotion. *Journal of Abnormal Psychology* **109**, 167–171.

White, R., Bebbington, P., Pearson, J., Johnson, S. & Ellis, D. (2000) The social context of insight in schizophrenia. *Social Psychiatry and Psychiatric Epidemiology* **35**, 500–507.

Wig, N.N., Menon, D.K., Bedi, H. *et al.* (1987) The distribution of Expressed Emotion components among relatives of schizophrenic patients in Aarhus and Chandigarh. *British Journal of Psychiatry* **151**, 160–165.

Willetts, L.E. & Leff, J. (1997) Expressed emotion and schizophrenia: the efficacy of a staff training programme. *Journal of Advanced Nursing* **26**, 1125–1133.

Wing, J.K. (1966) Social and psychological changes in a rehabilitation unit. *Social Psychiatry*. **1**, 21–28.

Wing, J.K. & Brown, G.W. (1970) *Institutionalism and Schizophrenia. A Comparative Study of Three Mental Hospitals 1960–68*. Cambridge University Press, Cambridge.

Wing, J.K. & Freudenberg, R.K. (1961) The response of severely ill chronic schizophrenic patients to social stimulation. *American Journal of Psychiatry* **118**, 311–322.

Wing, J.K., Monck, E., Brown, G.W. & Carstairs, G.M. (1964) Morbidity in the community of schizophrenic patients discharged from London mental hospitals in 1959. *British Journal of Psychiatry* **110**, 10–21.

Woo, S.M., Goldstein, M.J. & Nuechterlein, K.H. (1997) Relatives' expressed emotion and non-verbal signs of subclinical psychopathology in schizophrenia patients. *British Journal of Psychiatry* **170**, 58–61.

Wuerker, A.M. (1996) Communication patterns and expressed emotion in families of persons with mental disorders. *Schizophrenia Bulletin* **22**, 671–690.

Wynne, L.C. & Singer, M. (1963) Thought disorder and family relations of schizophrenics. I. *Archives of General Psychiatry* **9**, 191–206.

Yung, A.R. & McGorry, P.D. (1996) The initial prodrome in psychosis: descriptive and qualitative aspects. *Australian and New Zealand Journal of Psychiatry* **30**, 587–599.

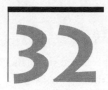

32 Psychiatric rehabilitation

T.K.J. Craig, R.P. Liberman, M. Browne, M.J. Robertson and D. O'Flynn

Conceptual framework, 638
General principles of rehabilitation, 638
Organization and delivery of services, 639
    Assertive Community Treatment, 640
    Token economy and social learning programmes, 640

Specific interventions, 641
    Enhancing skills, 641
    Modifying environments, 646
Conclusions, 651
References, 651

Despite advances in the treatment of schizophrenia, a significant number of patients experience a chronic or intermittent illness with enduring difficulty in managing everyday activities. Stigma, inadequate or inaccessible treatment services, unemployment, poor quality housing and lack of leisure opportunities all complicate the social disablement that arises from the disease itself. Researchers and practitioners alike have increasingly acknowledged the necessity of indefinite continuous maintenance treatment of persons with schizophrenia and other mental disabilities, using psychosocial as well as drug therapies. Just as individuals with schizophrenia are more likely to relapse when withdrawn from antipsychotic drugs, so susceptibility to stress-induced relapse increases when effective psychosocial treatments are terminated. Moreover, regular ongoing psychosocial services, flexibly available according to patients' changing needs, assure higher levels of community functioning and quality of life. The realization that the continuous application of biopsychosocial therapies can reduce the long-term disability and persisting or relapsing psychotic symptoms inherent in disabling mental disorders such as schizophrenia has given birth to the field of *psychiatric rehabilitation* (Anthony & Liberman 1986; Liberman 1992; Liberman *et al.* 1999).

While early and effective intervention for acute psychotic episodes is important for minimizing long-term disability, psychiatric rehabilitation emphasizes continuous comprehensive services for symptom control, prevention or mitigation of relapses, and optimizing the chronically ill patient's performance in social, vocational, educational and familial roles. Treatment should be linked to the phase of the person's illness and provide the least amount of support necessary from the helping professionals. The clinical practice of psychiatric rehabilitation joins together three approaches.

1 Pharmacotherapy judiciously keyed to the type and severity of psychopathology with dosage that does not produce sedation, neuromotor and other toxic side-effects that interfere with positive and active engagement in rehabilitation.

2 Development of skills in the patient that are linked to stressors and life situations, as well as personal assets and deficits, which challenge the individual's adaptation and independence.

3 A range of supportive social services, such as case management, which offer a decent quality of life, even to individuals whose symptoms and functional disabilities persist despite best efforts at treatment and rehabilitation.

In addition, a pillar of psychiatric rehabilitation is based on the assumption that disabled persons need empowerment to be actively involved in treatment decisions and to achieve the highest possible quality of life in the community (Anthony *et al.* 1988). Empowerment can develop from teaching disabled persons the skills they need for self-advocacy, self-help and also by public health efforts at destigmatization (Kommana *et al.* 1997; Liberman, 2003).

The challenge to psychiatric rehabilitation is of public health proportions. With the fragmented mental health service system in the USA, thousands of homeless mentally ill people live wretchedly and even more are warehoused in prisons and locked residential facilities in the community. These regressive trends, eerily reminiscent of the dark ages of prenineteenth century indifference to the mentally ill, come just at the time when internationally replicated studies have shown that substantial symptomatic and social recoveries can be achieved with more than half of individuals with chronic schizophrenia when continuous rehabilitative services are available over a 20–40-year period (Harding *et al.* 1987).

The failure to provide high-quality continuous psychiatric treatment is brought into bold relief by the availability of new rehabilitative technologies which, when systematically organized and delivered, have the potential for accelerating recovery by reducing morbidity, disability and handicaps (Kopelowicz & Liberman, 2003). Psychosocial treatments have been widely found to engender positive outcomes in a number of areas, including reduced relapse rates, treatment compliance and increased social and independent living skills. Cognitive–behavioural therapies have also been found to have significant positive effects on other areas of functioning, including improved cognitive functioning, amelioration of psychotic symptoms refractory to medications, and lowered rates of risky behaviours, such as unprotected sex and smoking (Heinssen *et al.* 2000; see also Chapter 33).

In summary, the emphasis of psychiatric rehabilitation is on providing continuous, comprehensive and co-ordinated services to control symptoms, prevent relapse and optimize performance in social, vocational, educational and familial roles. A rehabilitation programme may include educational activities, supported employment, social and life skills training, creative therapies and recreation (Glynn *et al.* 1994; Hume & Pullen 1995; Wallace *et al.* 2001b). Social and life skills programmes are a core element in rehabilitation, addressing the multiplicity of needs associated with independent functioning in the community, including making friends, managing one's illness, establishing independent recreation, managing money, self-care and domestic skills (Wallace *et al.* 2001b). By designing special programmes that can compensate for patients' deficits, rehabilitation practitioners can offer supports in work, housing and community life that may offer normalizing experiences. Thus, enhancing skills and modifying environments to be more supportive of adaptive functioning are the twin features of psychiatric rehabilitation.

Conceptual framework

The consequences of enduring mental health problems are social as well as personal and have been defined as follows.

1 *Impairments*: the positive and negative, affective and cognitive symptoms and signs of the disorder.

2 *Disabilities*: the difficulties in fully performing tasks, consequent on persistent impairments (e.g. in the areas of self-care, social relationships and work).

3 *Handicap*: the disadvantage and exclusion from social roles, consequent on impairments and disabilities, principally stigma, alienation from friends and family, unemployment, homelessness and poverty.

As social factors have a major role in disabilities and handicaps, diagnosis and cross-sectional severity of symptoms are poor predictors of outcome, especially in the functional domains (Strauss & Carpenter 1977). The often fluctuating course of mental disorder is best conceptualized by the *vulnerability–stress–coping–competence model* (Anthony & Liberman 1986). In this model, biological vulnerabilities predispose a person to schizophrenia when he or she is exposed to environmental stress (e.g. a life event, change in life phase or use of some illicit drugs). These stresses can be mitigated by interventions that enhance coping and competence, such as medication, social support and skill building. Symptoms and disabilities emerge when these protective factors are overwhelmed by stress, or when they 'atrophy as a result of disease, reinforcement of the sick role or loss of motivation' (Anthony & Liberman 1986, p. 547). Even in the absence of major life events or the noxious effects of illicit drugs and alcohol, vulnerable individuals can succumb to ambient levels of tension or conflict in their environment, or microstressors if they lack the protection conferred by medication, coping abilities and social support.

General principles of rehabilitation

Psychiatric rehabilitation aims to reduce exposure to stress and to optimize protective factors through the best use of medication and social skills training. However, protective services must be delivered in the context of a therapeutic alliance infused with empathy, enthusiasm, warmth and respect for the views, strengths and needs of persons with schizophrenia and their families (Strauss 1994). While this chapter concentrates on describing specific rehabilitation techniques, we cannot emphasize enough the importance of embedding services within a comprehensive, co-ordinated, collaborative, consumer-orientated and supportive framework. Some salient principles of psychiatric rehabilitation are depicted in Table 32.1.

Foremost for psychiatric rehabilitation is the necessity for a collaborative relationship. Patients who are active participants in their care are more likely to co-operate with treatment, less likely to default from care and more likely to achieve success in their personal goals. A comprehensive assessment is essential, not least because patients typically come to rehabilitation services after many years of 'revolving door' treatment from discontinuous sources and unreliable accounts of past treatment.

A newly validated tool for integrating assessment with rehabilitative interventions is the Client's Assessment of Strengths, Interests and Goals (CASIG), the first method for assessment that can be embedded in the clinical process of planning and evaluating treatment in an ongoing fashion (Wallace *et al.* 2001a). Based on CASIG's comprehensive assessment of symptoms, personal goals, instrumental skills and deficits, environmental resources available to the individual (including the family and community-based services), attitudes toward and use of medication, and quality of life, a treatment plan can be tailored to that individual. The same functional domains can be periodically administered to evaluate progress toward goals and the need to change the treatment plan. CASIGs can also be aggregated across patients to conduct programme-wide evaluations and compare programmes.

An assessment of symptoms and functional status – repeatedly checked and monitored – drives the clinician's decision-making regarding the timing, intensity, form and comprehensiveness of treatments that need to be provided. If remissions of psychotic symptoms and social recoveries are to be accelerated and sustained, the treatment decisions must be guided by ongoing periodic assessment of the individual's psychopathology, functional assets and deficits, deviant behaviours and personal and environmental resources that can be mobilized for community support. Assessment and intervention are inextricably interwoven in the pursuit of realistic goals and removal of obstacles to rehabilitation. Moreover, the individual patient and his or her relatives or caregivers must be engaged collaboratively in the assessment, goal setting and treatment process from the very start. When patients and their natural support network are active partners in the clinical process, progress in rehabilitation is greatly facilitated.

Table 32.1 Some key principles of psychiatric rehabilitation.

- Services must be comprehensive, continuous, co-ordinated, collaborative, consumer orientated and delivered with respect and positive attitudes reflecting the belief that patients – given their biological endowments, biobehavioural vulnerabilities, learning experiences and resources – are always doing the best they can. It is the task of treaters to organize and deliver services that will enable patients to function better.
- Services should be individualized and keyed to the phase and type of the person's disorder: acute, stabilizing, stable, recovering or refractory.
- Outreach and engagement of the patient is predicated on the understanding that motivation for treatment is not an intrinsic trait but rather can be generated by the way in which services are provided and the quality of the therapeutic relationship.
- Motivation for participating in the full array of services – from pharmacological to psychosocial – should be developed by matching treatments to the personally relevant goals of each patient.
- Patients, family members and other natural supporters should become active participants on an extended treatment and rehabilitation team.
- Treatment (e.g. medications) and rehabilitation (e.g. skills training) are inextricably interwoven – they are two sides of the same coin.
- Rehabilitation services should be linked to individualized needs assessments, deficits and strengths, neurocognitive functioning and personal goals of patients.
- The mainstay of psychiatric rehabilitation is creating learning environments wherein patients may acquire knowledge and skill that will empower them to function at higher levels with better quality of life.
- Wrapping social supports around patients can compensate for their behavioural deficits, instrumental role disabilities, and neurocognitive and symptomatic impairments, thereby enabling patients to function in acceptable and normalizing social and community roles.
- Cognitive remediation – or 'training the brain' – may provide a higher platform or point of departure for skills training and other rehabilitation services.
- Generalization of behaviour does not take place automatically; rather, it requires planning and programming for opportunities, encouragement and reinforcement from the natural environment for patients' use of the skills they have learned in a clinic or mental health setting. Thus, it is advisable to involve the patient's natural support system in the rehabilitation enterprise from the very start.

A key aspect of rehabilitation is the recognition that peoples' behaviour varies substantially from one situation to another. In general, task performance is more stable than social behaviour and simple skills are more transferable than complex ones. Many of the improvements seen in a narrow rehabilitation setting are responses dependent upon the particular characteristics of that environment and do not readily transfer or generalize to other more complex settings and situations. Therefore, care must be given to preparing people for the environments in which they will be expected to function and, in a reciprocal manner, preparing the environments so that patients receive encouragement, reinforcement and support to consolidate their progress. In general, it is probably better to rehabilitate *in vivo* than in the contrived setting of the hospital clinic, psychosocial clubhouse or mental health centre.

Most rehabilitation programmes draw heavily upon cognitive–behavioural principles and strategies. The two major strategies are:

1 teaching skills for coping with the challenges of community life; and

2 engineering psychosocial services and environments to be supportive in assisting the individual to compensate for symptoms, cognitive impairments and role deficiencies.

Principles inherent in skills training derive from the field of social learning, including motivational enhancements, modelling, coaching, shaping, positive reinforcement and programming for generalization (Liberman 1988). When these behavioural learning principles are used consistently and contingently upon small increments of adaptive behaviour exhibited by the patient, they can overcome persistent psychotic symptoms and neurocogni-

tive deficits in improving role functioning (Eckman *et al.* 1992b; Liberman *et al.* 2001).

Long-term goals are typically comprehensive, dealing with the relevant domains of life function – social, familial, interpersonal, medical, vocational, recreational and spiritual. Short-term goals, which may involve weeks or a few months, are the stepping stones towards the long-term goals and need to be 'SMART' (specific, measurable, achievable, realistic and time-limited) – set in collaboration with the patient, relatives and other natural supporters (Tauber *et al.* 2000). Specific interventions and treatments are devised with the aim of producing a series of consistent, if modest, achievements, backed up by frequent praise, encouragement and support.

Organization and delivery of services

There are two prototypes for the organization and delivery of rehabilitative services to persons with schizophrenia and other severe and persistent mental disorders. The model currently receiving most attention is a community-based team approach termed Assertive Community Treatment (Test 1992; Phillips *et al.* 2001). It was originally developed by an interdisciplinary team of clinicians at the University of Wisconsin (Stein & Test 1980; Stein & Santos 1998) as an alternative to mental hospitalization and as a means of improving patients' quality of lives by maintaining their tenure in the community. The second evidence-based mode for organizing and delivering services is primarily, but not exclusively, hospital-based and has been termed the token economy or social learning programme

(Ayllon & Azrin 1968; Liberman 1972; Paul & Lentz 1977; Kazdin 1982; Liberman & Corrigan 1994).

Assertive Community Treatment

At the present time, when lengths of stay in hospital are necessarily brief, there is the need to wrap the multiple components of rehabilitation services in a comprehensive community-based system of care. In both Britain and America, clinical case management provides the most popular vehicle for continuing care in the community. Several alternative models have emerged (see Chapter 34) and there have been a number of comprehensive reviews (Mueser et al. 1998; Latimer 1999; Phillips et al. 2001). These suggest that the Assertive Community Treatment model, and possibly other forms of intensive clinical case management, substantially reduce psychiatric hospital use, contribute to longer tenure in the community, and have modest effects on symptoms and subjective quality of life, although little impact on social functioning. It is not surprising that social functioning is not significantly improved by an outreach system that does not formally or systematically teach social and independent living skills to patients. British studies have failed to replicate the American findings of reductions in hospitalization or of improved outcomes over 'standard' care (Holloway & Carson 1998; Thornicroft et al. 1998; Burns et al. 1999), possibly reflecting differences in the implementation of Assertive Community Treatment or differences in the extent of resources and networks for community care available in 'standard' services in Britain.

Assertive Community Treatment provides a continuum of psychiatric, medical and social services to persons with schizophrenia in the community through the operation of mobile outreach teams of clinicians doing whatever is necessary to keep patients in the community and out of hospitals (Test 1992). This framework for delivering services is also referred to as 'intensive case management' or 'training in community living'. As the needs of patients change with different phases of their illness, the continuous treatment team must offer varying degrees of case management support and appropriate forms of pharmacotherapy, family education, social service entitlements, housing, skills training, vocational rehabilitation, financial support, health care, crisis intervention, rehabilitation, and advocacy. Case management has a central role in co-ordinating services and in assuring that quality and continuity of care remain. Specific duties of case managers include discharge planning from the inpatient setting, establishing linkages with community programmes, networking with these programmes to confirm that linkages have occurred, assuring that quality community care is offered, and advocating for services when they are insufficient, of poor quality or not provided at all (Kanter 1989).

Token economy and social learning programmes

Token economies rely on laws of operant conditioning to establish contingencies of reinforcement that increase the frequency of targeted desirable behaviours (Skinner 1953). Handing out tokens (e.g. points on a patient's 'credit' card, or poker chips) contingent on adaptive behaviour, which can be exchanged for snacks, beverages and privileges, make tokens rewarding in themselves. Using tokens to manage behavioural contingencies provides several benefits.

1 Tokens permit more immediate reinforcement of spontaneous skills by bridging the delay between target responses and back-up reinforcement.

2 Distribution of reinforcers is more flexible with behaviours being able to be rewarded at any time.

3 Intermittent reinforcement enables new behaviours to be maintained over extended periods when immediate token or back-up reinforcement is unavailable.

4 Learning to improve one's functioning in a token economy may prepare patients for living in the economy outside the hospital (Ayllon & Azrin 1968; Kazdin & Bootzin 1972).

The technique can be used to modify any behaviour and it has been suggested that it is particularly beneficial for people suffering from schizophrenia, as they may be less responsive to everyday social rewards (Layne & Wallace 1982).

Several steps must be accomplished to implement a successful token economy. First, behaviours to be targeted in the token economy must be identified. These include self-care and appropriate social behaviours, for which all patients receive tokens, and overly aggressive or hostile behaviours, which result in token 'fines'. Each behaviour needs to be sufficiently described and operationalized so that it can be reliably recognized by patients and staff.

Next, contingencies must be created that govern the consequences of these behaviours. Contingencies describe 'if–then' rules connecting a target behaviour with a reinforcer or fine. When setting up a token economy, payments and fines should be determined on an individual basis by a staff team familiar with the patient's behavioural level of functioning. Individualization will increase the likelihood that patients will achieve a positive balance of tokens each day, which is desirable for motivating patients, as rewards must not be too difficult to obtain. As the token economy progresses, specific contingencies can be adjusted, depending on the frequency with which the behaviours are performed by the patient group and the fluctuating rate of commodity purchases.

Token economies provide several advantages for the management of the inpatient behavioural milieu (Kazdin 1982). The token economy is not affected by satiation, a common problem when specific reinforcers, such as food or ward privileges, are used. In fact, research has shown that tokens by themselves may assume a greater and more generalized incentive value than any single primary reward.

Token economies have been extensively studied in the treatment of chronic institutionalized psychiatric patients. The token economy approach has been used to increase self-care skills and reduce the expression of symptoms, aggression and bizarre behaviour (Atthowe & Krasner 1968; Ayllon & Azrin 1968; Maley et al. 1973; Hall et al. 1977; Glynn & Mueser 1992).

Results have shown that symptoms and self-care skills of subjects in these studies have significantly improved, even after other treatments were unsuccessful. In an early study, Wincze *et al.* (1972) compared a token economy with verbal feedback as a means of reducing delusional speech of 10 patients suffering from chronic paranoid schizophrenia. Patients received tokens at fixed intervals for not expressing delusional ideas. Verbal feedback involved challenging and correcting delusional statements. The frequency of delusional statements decreased for seven of 10 patients in the token condition. In another early study, Liberman *et al.* (1973) reported on four controlled case studies in which a multiple baseline was used. Patients were paired with a favourite staff member each evening to share pleasant banter and snacks. After several non-contingent meetings, patients were told that the length of the evening chat would be proportional to the number of tokens earned for delusion-free talk during four daily intervals. After only 18 days, the frequency of delusional speech fell by 200–600%. Three of the four patients maintained their improvement after the social contingencies were slowly faded.

In a classic study by Paul and Lentz (1977), 84 chronic patients were randomly assigned to token economy, milieu therapy or traditional custodial care. After 14 weeks of treatment, every resident in the social learning (token economy) programme showed dramatic improvements in overall functioning. The average patient increased interpersonal and communication skills by over 1200% of entry level. Patients in the milieu therapy group also improved. By the end of the second year, fewer than one-quarter of the patients in either experimental condition were on maintenance medication and 97% of the token economy patients, 71% of the milieu group, but only 45% of the custodial care group had been discharged and were living in the community. The social learning programme was the most cost effective when the costs of hospitalization were included.

The token economy approach has been successfully employed in many settings around the world. Li and Wang (1994) in China randomized 52 chronic schizophrenia patients to a token economy programme or to a treatment-as-usual condition in which they did not receive training or reinforcement but were individually asked to perform the same daily tasks and activity programme as the experimental subjects. After 3 months, the severity of negative symptoms, assessed by an independent researcher, had declined in both groups but the effect was much greater in the experimental group.

Despite evidence in its favour, the approach has waned in popularity. There are several reasons for this decline. First, it is widely believed that the results may have more to do with changes in the way staff interact with patients than with the use of tokens *per se* (Baker *et al.* 1977; Liberman *et al.* 1977). Secondly, these programmes are expensive, requiring relatively high staffing levels, high-calibre nursing staff and intensive training. Finally, there are concerns about the ethics of a programme in which patients must 'earn' rewards that some see as their right. Nevertheless, the principles of contingency management are probably an important aspect of all treatment pro-grammes and the method may still have something to offer, particularly in residential units that deal with severe disability and challenging behaviours (Silverstein *et al.* 1999).

Specific interventions

Enhancing skills

There are three approaches to building skills in individuals with schizophrenia and other serious mental disorders; one has been already described, the token economy, which requires the systematic application of behavioural learning principles and contingent reinforcement in the context of a living environment. The other two approaches also require application of precision teaching techniques based on social learning theory: social skills training and cognitive remediation. In the former, the social and independent living skills of the individual are targeted for enhancement, whereas in the latter the therapeutic targets are the cognitive functions of the individual (e.g. memory, verbal learning, sustained attention and reaction time).

Social skills training

Social skills training, used to improve social and daily living skills for independence in the community, is the most widely utilized psychosocial intervention in the rehabilitation of severely mentally ill people (Liberman *et al.* 1986, 1989, 1993; Bellack *et al.* 1997). Three broad models underpin most approaches (Corrigan *et al.* 1992). The *response topography* model suggests that complex skills can be decomposed into a number of discrete 'micro' skills. For example, conversation comprises non-verbal signals such as eye contact, facial expression and gestures as well as appropriate verbal responses. The *content-related behaviour model*, in contrast, emphasizes the content of behaviours such as how to ask for information. In both models, participants learn the expressive components of social skills – for example, how to introduce themselves, paying attention to non-verbal expression as well as to appropriate content. These approaches have been criticized for failing to produce flexible responses in more complex situations (Trower *et al.* 1978) and they have been largely overtaken by *cognitive problem-solving* models which describe the skill deficit in terms of impaired information processing characteristics of schizophrenia (Liberman *et al.* 1980; Wallace *et al.* 1985; Mueser *et al.* 1991).

The social problem-solving approach teaches social norms and rules to improve the patient's ability to interpret cues from the social environment and generate appropriate responses to these cues. Support for this model comes from studies showing associations between poor performance in skills training and difficulties comprehending interpersonal problems (Donahoe *et al.* 1991; Liberman *et al.* 2001), a lack of comprehension of the rules and goals of interpersonal situations (Corrigan & Green 1993) and an unawareness of the linguistic rules that underlie conversation (Trower *et al.* 1978).

In practice, these variants of social skills training are usually combined and integrated by a step-by-step method of instruction. Complex interpersonal behaviours are broken down into smaller steps which can be addressed through a variety of teaching methods including motivational interviewing, didactic and Socratic instruction, shaping, modelling, corrective feedback and *in vivo* and homework exercises. Functional assessment is carried out to determine the patient's assets, deficits and resources available for strengthening skills, a process which should be carried out periodically to evaluate progress and suggest changes in the goals and training pace and techniques. Attempts are made to identify barriers to learning and the system of natural reinforcers that may be acting to strengthen or weaken adaptive behaviours. This information is used to build up a profile of the patient's strengths and difficulties, to identify the aspects of skill training that may be needed and to negotiate goals that are realistic and acceptable to the patient (Heinssen *et al*. 1995).

Skills training can be delivered in an individual, family or group format. Group-based approaches typically use a structured programme comprising a number of discrete skill sets such as conversational skills, job skills and symptom monitoring. One popular approach is the modular programme for training social and independent living skills developed by Wallace, Liberman and their colleagues at the UCLA Clinical Research Center for Schizophrenia and Psychiatric Rehabilitation. This programme teaches a range of skills including medication self-management, basic conversation skills, grooming and self-care, workplace skills and interpersonal problem-solving. The approach uses didactic and Socratic instruction, videotape demonstrations, role-play, problem-solving exercises, *in vivo* exercises and homework practice (Wallace *et al*. 1985; Liberman & Corrigan 1993; Liberman *et al*. 1993).

Each module has a trainer's manual, participant's workbook and demonstration videotape. It is specified in the manual exactly what the trainer is to say and do to teach all the module's skills. Once familiar with the structure and learning activities of the modules, trainers can use their own clinical style to teach the skills and 'deconstruct' a module to individualize its use. Clinicians can learn to use the system and implement these learning activities with a high level of fidelity (Eckman *et al*. 1992a; Wallace *et al*. 1992; Liberman & Corrigan 1993). Numerous empirical trials have documented the efficacy, durability, generalizability and cross-cultural applicability of the modules (Liberman *et al*. 1998; Kopelowicz *et al*. 1999; Wallace *et al*. 1999; Heinssen *et al*. 2000).

There have been many clinical trials of psychosocial skills training showing benefits over standard care in terms of improved conversational skills, assertiveness, recreational skills, grooming, job finding and medication management (Wong *et al*. 1988; Scott & Dixon 1995; Dilk & Bond 1996; Penn & Mueser 1996; Heinssen *et al*. 2000; Tsang & Pearson 2001). As would be predicted by treatment-specific outcomes, social skills training has only modest impact on symptoms, relapse and hospitalization, with some studies finding no significant advantage over more traditional occupational therapy or group-based supportive psychotherapy (Dobson *et al*. 1995; Hayes *et al*. 1995; Liberman *et al*. 1998; Bustillo *et al*. 2001).

In one randomized controlled trial in which patients with schizophrenia were trained in medication and symptom management while receiving low-dose fluphenazine decanoate, relapse rates were kept very low when incipient exacerbations were treated with placebo supplements, as compared with patients who received supportive group therapy and supplemental fluphenazine at prodromal periods (Marder *et al*. 1996). While having only a modest impact on symptoms, it also appears that neither positive nor negative symptoms, other than severe thought disorder, predict the level of participation, acquisition of skills or overall response (Eckman *et al*. 1992b; Corrigan *et al*. 1994; Lysaker *et al*. 1995; McKee *et al*. 1997; Smith *et al*. 1999), although enduring psychotic symptoms may reduce the retention of skills after brief training (Mueser *et al*. 1992).

Data on the extent to which new skills generalize across settings or fade with time are sparse, but growing in recent years. There is some evidence for the benefit of including 'booster' sessions and for carrying out *in vivo* training exercises away from the initial treatment setting. In one study at the UCLA Clinical Research Center, 80 stable DSM-IIIR schizophrenia outpatients were randomly assigned to receive either skills training or supportive group psychotherapy. Skills training involved twice-weekly sessions over 6 months with continuing weekly group meetings for 12 months. Symptomatic improvement occurred in both groups but patients who received the modular training showed greater increases in knowledge and living skills that were maintained across the 12-month follow-up. Only a single booster session was needed to maintain performance at post-training levels. In that study, the experimental group achieved significantly better outcomes on measures of social adjustment over the study period (Marder *et al*. 1996).

Two recent studies have explored the addition of social skills training to case management. In one study, 84 schizophrenic men with persistent, largely treatment resistant symptoms were randomly assigned to either social skills training or occupational therapy (Liberman *et al*. 1998). Each group of patients received intensive clinic-based treatment for 6 months followed by 18 months of assertive case management. The social skills training was carried out by an occupational therapist and three assistants, focusing on four modules taken from the UCLA Social and Independent Living Skills Program: basic conversation, recreation for leisure, medication management and symptom management. Case managers encouraged patients to use the skills they had learned in their everyday community living. Patients were followed up over 2 years, during which time those receiving social skills training showed significantly greater knowledge and performance of independent living skills, including improved function in areas not explicitly dealt with in the training sessions. Only the social skills group reported significant improvements in the use of transportation, job seeking and job maintenance.

In another controlled trial, individuals with schizophrenia were randomly assigned to receive risperidone or haloperidol and again to clinic-based social skills training or to clinic-based skills training augmented by *in vivo* booster training sessions joined with advocacy by a case manager who aimed to generate opportunities, encouragement and reinforcement from the patients' natural support network for employing their skills in everyday life. Regardless of medication condition, those patients who obtained *in vivo* amplified skills training exhibited significantly better social adjustment in their community life over a 1-year follow-up period (Glynn *et al.* 2002). When patients were living with an immediate family member or live-in partner, the advocacy and consultation by the case manager resulted in continued improvements in community functioning over a 2-year follow-up period.

At the Santa Barbara Community Mental Health Center, a controlled effectiveness trial with severely mentally ill patients introduced a programme termed 'partners in autonomous living' in which friends, relatives or staff from group homes were nominated by patients to assist them in using the social and independent living skills acquired at the mental health centre. The skills training at the mental health centre included twice weekly participation in the medication management, symptom management, recreation for leisure, and basic conversation skills modules. The natural supporters received orientation skills training and how it could be generalized and met with their patients for an average of 30 min per week over a 6-month period. Those patients who were randomly assigned to 'partners in autonomous living' revealed significantly greater interpersonal skills at the completion of the project (Tauber *et al.* 2000).

Skills training methods have been successfully employed with acute inpatients (Kopelowicz *et al.* 1998; Smith *et al.* 1999), persons with residual symptoms (Dobson *et al.* 1995; Hayes *et al.* 1995) and those with severe and persistent illness (Wallace *et al.* 1992; Liberman *et al.* 1994, 1998; Silverstein *et al.* 1999; Spaulding *et al.* 1999). Finally, successful attempts have been made to employ brief interventions to enhance compliance with medication (Kemp *et al.* 1996, 1998). From these studies it appears that most patients can benefit if procedures for skills training are adapted to their particular deficits, symptom profiles and cognitive impairments. Because there is so much overlap in learning principles and training techniques, it is impractical to compare the relative superiority of different social skills training approaches.

Cognitive remediation

While the types and extent of cognitive dysfunctions vary greatly among persons with schizophrenia, recent evidence has accumulated that abnormalities in verbal learning, verbal recall, secondary verbal memory, spatial and verbal working memory, sustained attention and executive functions (e.g. planning and initiating activities, changing response strategies as external conditions change) are correlated with psychosocial functioning in work, self-care and interpersonal domains (Mueser *et al.* 1991; Kern *et al.* 1992; Bowen *et al.* 1994; Corrigan *et al.*

1994; Green 1996; Storzbach & Corrigan 1996; Green & Nuechterlein 1999). Prospective studies have indicated that poorer neurocognition at baseline predicts the amount of learning of community living skills that takes place subsequently (Kopelowicz *et al.* 2001). It is therefore a very appealing idea that remediation of these neurocognitive impairments might lead to improved personal and social functioning. In essence, cognitive remediation aims to retrain and improve basic processes of memory, attention, speed of information processing and abstraction. Another strategy, to bypass neurocognitive abnormalities through creating supportive and prosthetic environments for the individual with schizophrenia, will be described below in the section on Modifying environments.

Early efforts to treat cognition in schizophrenia directly were carried out using self-instructional approaches (Meichenbaum & Cameron 1973). These involved the rehearsal of self-instructions aimed at maintaining attention to tasks and inhibiting impulsive responses. The self-instruction was initially rehearsed while performing simple laboratory tasks and then gradually introduced to more complex *in vivo* social or work tasks. The original study (Meichenbaum & Cameron 1973) demonstrated improvement on psychological tests, interview performance and social behaviour. However, while improvements on specific tasks were observed, there was little generalization to areas that had not been the focus of the intervention (Spaulding *et al.* 1986; Bentall *et al.* 1987).

From this early work, the development of remediation strategies has proceeded from the systematic exploration of the efficacy of particular 'laboratory-based' interventions to the gradual incorporation of these findings into broader clinic-based interventions. Perhaps the most widely reported studies concern the development of interventions designed to remediate the specific deficits of individual patients. In these *individualized* approaches, patients receive a neuropsychological assessment, the results of which are then used to devise an intervention comprising a series of exercises of increasing complexity. The extent to which the initial neuropsychological assessment 'drives' the intervention or is a basic underpinning for wider strategies varies somewhat between studies. For example, Spaulding and colleagues base the programme explicitly on the patient's deficit profile (Spaulding & Sullivan 1991). They describe a patient with moderate problems with executive function and socially inappropriate behaviour. Over a course of 10 sessions, the patient was taught how to generate alternative precepts and cognitive flexibility in social situations. After training, the patient was retested and showed improvements on the Wisconsin Card Sorting Test and on measures of irritability and attitude. People with schizophrenia have been shown to be able to remember verbal and visual information more effectively when it was organized into meaningful categories or when items were placed on a continuum (Storzbach & Corrigan 1996).

There have also been reports of interventions based on cognitive exercise programmes borrowed from neuropsychological rehabilitation, some of which can be administered by computer. In one of the more recent of these studies Medalia *et al.* (1998)

used the Orientation-Remedial Module from a computerized program originally developed for people with brain injury and compared this with a control intervention that involved watching National Geographic documentaries. Experimental and control conditions each involved three 20-min sessions spread over a 6-week period. The experimental intervention included instructions in how to complete tasks that were also the outcome measure. One test required participants to press the space bar on the keyboard whenever the letter A appeared on the screen. Scores were obtained for the number of letter presses and the percentage of correct responses. Subjects in the experimental condition showed improved performance on the training task but it is impossible to say whether this would generalize to clinically relevant tasks and settings. There was no immediate effect on mental state. Regarding the shaping of attending behaviours, Silverstein et al. (1998, 1999) have tested this method in league with social skills training. In one study, they found that severely attentionally impaired subjects were able to increase their attention spans from <5 to 45 min in a skills training class (Silverstein et al. 1998).

In a clinically relevant study, patients with chronic schizophrenia were randomly assigned to intensive cognitive remediation (CR) or to an 'intensive occupational therapy' control condition (Wykes et al. 1999). Patients receiving the intensive CR attended for individual daily 1-h sessions that focused on executive functioning deficits (cognitive flexibility, working memory and planning). The intervention drew heavily on behavioural and learning techniques: procedural learning, targeted reinforcement, massed practice and errorless learning. Some improvement in cognitive function was seen with both therapies, but a differential effect in favour of CR was found for tests of cognitive flexibility and memory subgroups. There was an interesting trend for patients receiving atypical antipsychotic medication to benefit more from CR. Social functioning, which was not addressed directly, also tended to improve in those patients whose cognitive flexibility scores improved with treatment.

One approach to direct remediation is undertaken in a dyadic format after a relationship is established between patient and therapist. Specific cognitive deficits are identified through laboratory tasks, analysis of the patient's symptoms and observation of behaviour. The impairments are addressed in a series of exercises, starting with simple laboratory tasks and gradually progressing to complex in vivo performance of tasks that demand more effective use of the impaired processes. Reports of successful cases include patients from the entire spectrum of rehabilitation candidates, from mildly to severely cognitively impaired, in settings ranging from outpatient clinics to public institutions. An accumulation of reports over the years provides substantial evidence for effectiveness, but conclusive verification will require large-scale highly controlled outcome studies (Olbrich & Mussgay 1990; Burda et al. 1991; Stuve et al. 1991; Green 1993; Spaulding 1993; Goldberg 1994).

In contrast to these patient-specific interventions are training courses designed around broad deficits found in most persons with schizophrenia. Individual deficits are acknowledged and are used to make some adjustments to the programme although the primary emphasis remains on a training model and not on cognitive deficit profiles of the individual members. The approach has grown from the basic rehabilitation principle that has long recognized the importance of tackling complex tasks in small steps. The Integrated Psychological Therapy (IPT) model, developed at the University of Bern by Brenner, Hodel and their colleagues (Brenner et al. 1992), comprises five subcomponents arranged hierarchically so that simple cognitive processes are addressed first, followed by increasingly complex tasks: cognitive differentiation, social perception, verbal communication, social skills and problem-solving. The training is delivered in a group format of 60–75-min sessions, delivered daily over approximately 3 months. Patients without impairments in a particular area are encouraged to help those who have them on the grounds that this will help to generalize skills and increase self-esteem. Cognitive remediation is theoretically achieved through the repeated practice of the training exercises although is not directly addressed in the sort of detail described in the more ideographical approaches described earlier. Two of the subcomponents – social skills and problem solving – bear a close resemblance to social skills training programmes.

Controlled studies have shown IPT to be superior to standard hospital treatment (Brenner et al. 1992) and to a non-specific group treatment (Spaulding et al. 1999). Spaulding et al. randomly allocated 90 long-term inpatients from a state hospital with treatment-resistant schizophrenia to receive either IPT or supportive group therapy. Cohorts received their respective treatments for 1 h, three times weekly over a 6-month period. At 3 months, a 12-week course of social skills training was introduced to both groups. All patients also received the same structured psychosocial inpatient programme comprising close attention to optimizing medication, milieu-based behavioural treatment (token economy), patient and family psychoeducation and occupational therapy.

Subjects in both groups showed significant improvements in several measures of neurocognition, positive symptoms and social skills, but those in the IPT group showed greater improvements in conceptual disorganization, attentional processing, knowledge and skills concerning medication management and social competence as measured by the Assessment of Interpersonal Problem-Solving Skills Task (Donahoe et al. 1991). Greatest gains were seen in terms of the patients' ability to apprehend details of social situations, to incorporate these details into a more complete understanding of the situation and to match solutions to this situation. The IPT treatment effect on these measures was nearly double that of the standard inpatient rehabilitation programme. In terms of outcome, the effect of adding IPT to a comprehensive rehabilitation programme was comparable in size to the superiority of clozapine over typical antipsychotics in reducing symptoms of treatment refractory schizophrenia. The effect size of IPT also compared favourably with family interventions in the area of expressed emotion and emotional overinvolvement, and with social skills training on social competence, hospital discharge and relapse rate (Spaulding *et al.* 1999).

A similar retraining programme has been described by Van der Gaag *et al.* (1992, 1994, 2002) in the Netherlands. Three main training strategies were used: self-instruction, mnemonics and inductive reasoning. The programme was compared with an attention–placebo intervention over a 22-week study period. Patients in the experimental condition attended short 15–25 min training sessions twice weekly over a 3-month period. The first 12 sessions included visual, auditory, tactile and proprioceptive perception tasks; sessions 13–15 focused on integrating perceptual and language processing; and sessions 16–22 dealt with more complex exercises of social perception. At the end of training, the experimental group had improved performance on measures of social perception and memory, but was no better on measures of attention or problem solving.

Heinssen and Victor (1994) also developed a treatment modality to increase patients' vocational functioning through cognitive remediation. In this procedure, graduated steps working towards a final task were developed in order to ensure success while enhancing the cognitive processes that would facilitate appropriate task behaviour. For example, to teach participants how to water plants, an explanation of the task and the skills sequence to be followed was given. Next, a sorting task was implemented, where patients sorted plants into wet and dry categories. This type of gradual progression continued until the patients were watering the plants effectively on their own. Environmental manipulations were also used to decrease distractions and compensate for impaired memory and executive functioning. This type of training was effective in improving job interest, work activity and the accuracy of behavioural performance (Heinssen & Victor 1994).

Despite the focal success of these interventions and the clear demonstrations that it is possible to 'train the brain' (Liberman 2002), more research must be done to provide satisfactory understanding of exactly what is being measured by neuropsychological tests of cognitive impairment in schizophrenia and, hence, how cognitive remediation may contribute to real-life benefits for persons with schizophrenia (Hayes & McGrath 2000). Some steps in this direction are being taken by Kern and Liberman at the UCLA Clinical Research Center for Schizophrenia and Psychiatric Rehabilitation, where errorless learning methods, utilizing functions in the parietal association cortex that are not impaired in schizophrenia, have been shown to improve performance on entry-level job tasks that were validated by employers, work foremen and vocational counsellors (Liberman 2002).

Goal-orientated therapeutic contracting

This pragmatic approach, initially developed and validated for persons with schizophrenia by Liberman and colleagues at the Oxnard (California) Community Mental Health Center, engages patients in an active process of setting realistic goals that are incremental steps toward their long-term 'dreams' in life (Austin *et al.* 1976; Liberman & Bryan 1977). For example, a man may express the wish for having a girlfriend with whom to share emotional and sexual intimacy. To achieve this goal, many intervening steps are necessary, each with reinforcers associated with their attainment. The step-wise progression to a long-term goal is depicted in Table 32.2 for this individual. The reinforcers associated with the attainment of each behavioural goal often combine tangible social and intrapersonal rewards. For example, after successfully meeting a young woman on a scenic hike and getting a date with her, the consequences were praise from his therapist and a gift certificate for a department store from his mother so he could purchase new clothes and shoes. By the time the individual achieves his or her long-term goal, the frequency

Table 32.2 An example of one patient's step-wise programme in his goal-orientated therapeutic contract aimed at achieving the long-term goal to meet a girlfriend. For each step along the continuum, the patient and clinician negotiate a 'contract' which specifies the goal and the consequences of achieving that goal. Reinforcement Surveys (Lecomte *et al.* 2000) can be used to help identify relevant rewards to be used as consequences and the emphasis is on abundant 'pay offs' for achieving goals so that motivation can be maximized.

- Go to shopping mall and make three different enquiries regarding merchandise with female sales clerks who are your age and attractive. Smile, make eye contact, ask the sales clerk to show you the merchandise so you can examine it close-up, then thank the clerk for her time and effort.
- At a local coffee shop, ask the woman at the counter how she likes her job, what she enjoys most and least about the work, and thank her for the coffee.
- Go to the city's Park and Recreation Department and obtain information on the various social and recreational activities that are sponsored.
- Participate and complete the Recreation for Leisure Module in the UCLA Social and Independent Living Skills Programme (including generalization assignments).
- Participate and complete the Basic Conversation Skills Module (including generalization or 'homework' assignments).
- Attend your local hiking club meeting and introduce yourself to three women and three men.
- Participate in a hike and find out three pieces of information about four of the hikers, disclosing similar information about yourself at low levels of self-disclosure.
- Participate and complete the Friendship and Intimacy Module.
- Invite one of the women on the hike to have coffee with you after the hike.
- Ask the woman out for a date.

of tangible and social reinforcers is faded and replaced by natural reinforcers (e.g. enjoying a heterosocial and heterosexual relationship), self-efficacy and enhanced self-esteem.

Therapeutic contracting explicitly removes patients from a passive role in treatment as they work collaboratively with therapists and natural supporters (e.g. family members) to achieve goal-directed autonomous behaviour. In this modality, patients progress sequentially through more complex stages after meeting criteria for successfully achieving prior less complex stages. Each stage entails specific responsibilities from both patient and clinician. The four stages, as outlined by Heinssen and colleagues, are as follows:

1 *Problem definition*, during which a model of illness and recovery is established, presenting problems are clarified and treatment priorities are defined.

2 *Reframing presenting problems*, when adaptive self-concepts are established through reformulating problems as long-term goals to be accomplished.

3 *Behavioural experimentation*, during which optimal learning conditions are established to avoid overstimulation and boredom, the performance of adaptive skills is encouraged daily, and the patient's feelings of self-control and personal efficacy are established.

4 *Sustaining long-term growth*, when the self-control, self-evaluative and self-corrective skills that have been learned are internalized.

Therapeutic contracting has been found to be effective in a wide range of areas, including increased treatment compliance, positive therapeutic outcomes, patient satisfaction and cost-effectiveness of long-term treatment. These results have also been shown to be generalizable, as they have been replicated in public and private psychiatric hospitals and in an outpatient facility (Heinssen *et al*. 1995). Therapeutic contracting can be implemented during inpatient hospitalization and used as a bridge to outpatient services to further treatment gains and facilitate continuity of care.

Modifying environments

Specific interventions employed in rehabilitation, besides enhancing skills, aim to help people manage the demands of everyday life by modifying the environment and providing supports that can make tangible contributions to greater personal satisfaction and acceptance by the community.

Vocational rehabilitation

Employment is central to human health, providing financial, social and psychological benefits to people with mental health problems: an income without depending on social service benefit, social contacts, a social role other than that of psychiatric patient, psychological recovery and even prolonged symptom remission and freedom from relapses (Liberman & Kopelowicz 1994; Lysaker & Bell 1995; Bell *et al*. 1996). Many persons with schizophrenia want jobs, alternatives to welfare dependency

and traditional day centres (Shepherd *et al*. 1994). The right to work is enshrined in the Universal Declaration of Human Rights (1948) and the United Nations Standard Rules (1994). Employment is a core component of social policy across Europe and America, where governments want to improve health and to reduce welfare spending and social exclusion.

Most people with severe mental illness now live in the community but few have jobs and many are socially isolated. Unemployment rates for people with serious mental health problems range from 60% to nearly 100% and are particularly high if they have additional disadvantages in the labour market: ethnic minority group membership, poor educational and employment history or a criminal record (Lehman 1995; Meltzer *et al*. 1995). These high unemployment rates are as much a product of social factors – the economy, discrimination, organizational policies and welfare regulations – as of the personal consequences of mental illness (Warner 1994). Most employers and employees are not yet ready to work alongside mentally ill people, and modern organizations may be technologically demanding and stressful, and themselves a cause of ill health. Coping strategies that may be helpful in some circumstances can be problematic in the workplace. For example, a person may find that taking frequent breaks from a task helps to reduce the intensity of anxiety or psychotic symptoms but such practices may not be acceptable to an employer (Cook & Razzano 2000). To compound these difficulties, mental health professionals may ignore or even discourage employment. One recent American survey of 719 people diagnosed with schizophrenia found that only one-quarter were receiving vocational rehabilitation or had such services included in their treatment plan (Lehman & Steinwachs 1998).

The presence of acute symptoms, neurocognitive dysfunctions, medication side-effects, residual negative symptoms, poor social skills and instrumental role deficits can all disrupt employability or job performance (Johnstone *et al*. 1990; Massel *et al*. 1990; Fenton & McGlashan 1991; Van Os *et al*. 1995; Green 1996). All these factors need to be taken into account in helping people back to work. On the other hand, when there is a good match or fit between a person and his or her job, engagement in tasks that can be mastered can both displace symptoms and facilitate job tenure (Massel *et al*. 1990; Wallace *et al*. 1999).

Prediction of successful vocational rehabilitation is difficult because employment depends on the local labour market, the national economy and welfare system as well as on personal resources and choices (Anthony 1994). Assessment is best carried out in work settings, rather than with interviews or tests. Successful job searching or placement may involve helping the person develop coping strategies or seek an 'ecological niche' – a job where the employer and coworkers collaborate with the rehabilitation team to adjust the demands of the job to better fit the person's abilities and tolerance (Jacobs *et al*. 1984; Drake *et al*. 1999; Tsang & Pearson 2001).

There has been burgeoning interest in helping people with severe mental illness obtain meaningful employment and a corresponding proliferation of approaches. Most approaches aim to enable people to work productively for wages within social security or welfare regulations. The earliest models in the post-asylum era involved the transfer of the hospital farm, workshop or work crew into community-based sheltered workshops or enclaves that provided part-time, low or unpaid occupation in segregated settings. The rationale of these early models was to give patients experience in 'work hardening' so as to prepare them to enter competitive employment in the open labour market, although their success in achieving this goal was severely limited (Baronet & Gerber 1998). Sheltered employment has fallen out of favour, partly because of its poor performance in achieving open employment, and partly because the segregation involved in this approach encourages dependence and institutionalization. In Europe, the sheltered workshop evolved into small businesses or 'social firms' that operate as commercial businesses in the open market, although they receive some governmental subsidy. These social firms sell quality products and provide equal and full pay to both disabled and non-disabled employees. Some firms have attained commercial viability, high user satisfaction and reduced use of mental health services (Grove *et al.* 1997). Similar operations appear as consumer-run businesses in the USA (Schwartz 1998).

Another internationally popular model has been the 'Clubhouse', which emerged in the USA in the 1950s as an alternative to the traditional sheltered workshop. The Clubhouse provides a setting for friendships, support, social activity and lengthy preparation for employment. Members participate in all aspects of running the organization and are expected to arrive on time, complete tasks and share responsibility for all aspects of Clubhouse life. This phase leads to 'transitional employment' in which members are placed in a series of paid but temporary jobs with mainstream employers, a process that is intended to help the members acquire the skills and experience needed to cope with open employment (Beard *et al.* 1982). The Clubhouse model has been criticized on the grounds that such prevocational training undermines confidence and may actually deter people from finding competitive employment; that it has not proven effective in helping members develop work skills; and that it limits patients to unskilled employment (Bond *et al.* 1997). The Clubhouse model is slowly being overtaken in the USA by behaviourally orientated strategies of vocational rehabilitation: supported employment and job-finding training.

Supported employment

Following its extraordinary success in securing normal employment for the developmentally disabled, supported employment has become the most important new development in the vocational rehabilitation of the severely mentally ill (Anthony & Blanch 1987). Although the implementation of supported work programmes may vary, several common components have been identified (Bond *et al.* 1997):

1 a goal of permanent, competitive employment;
2 minimal screening for employability;
3 avoidance of prevocational training;
4 individualized placement (rather than in an enclave or work crew);
5 time-unlimited support by an employment specialist or job coach and liaison between the vocational staff member and other clinicians on the patient's mental health team; and
6 consideration of patient preferences for type of job.

Supportive employment uses a 'place-then-train' approach, instead of the traditional 'train-then-place' method that had failed to obtain competitive employment for the vast majority of the seriously mentally ill in the era of the sheltered workshop (Bond 1992). Rather than spending lengthy periods in preparatory prevocational settings, participants are matched with existing jobs in the local community and are provided with on-the-job training in work skills, instruction in work habits and supportive counselling by a job coach whose goal is to sustain the productive involvement of the mentally ill person at the work site.

Much emphasis is placed on helping the individual maintain the job. When the programme participant must acquire a new work or social skill, the job coach or employment specialist provides assistance, usually through verbal instruction, encouragement, liaison with the individual's supervisor or employer and real-time demonstrations. The behavioural requirements of any job are broken down by a 'task analysis' into small chunks, which are then taught to the participant, moving at the participant's own rate of learning. Because a key element in supported employment is integration of the job coach with the mental health team responsible for the patient's comprehensive and continuing care, specialized services are always available to sustain the individual on the job. These may include attendance at social skills training sessions (Mueser & Liberman 1988), medication regulated by a psychiatrist, or crisis intervention at or away from the job site. Thus, co-ordination of a wide array of mental health services, as well as consultation and liaison with the employer or supervisor at the worksite, are essential components in the performance standards for job coaches and employment specialists (Drake & Becker 1996).

Most studies of supported employment have found superior vocational outcomes as compared with more traditional mental health treatment or conventional vocational counselling (Mueser & Bond 2000). An 'accelerated' approach, defined as immediate placement in competitive employment, as opposed to a gradual approach, which included a minimum of 4 months of prevocational training before placement, was more effective in terms of employment outcomes in a sample of 86 patients with severe mental illness (Bond *et al.* 1995). In a review of the literature, Bond *et al.* (1997) found that people in the supported work programmes had a higher rate of obtaining competitive employment. Drake *et al.* (1994) also found that supportive employment that was closely co-ordinated with clinical care increased the rate of competitive employment. In three recent controlled studies (Bond *et al.* 1995; Drake *et al.* 1996, 1999), an average of 65% of severely mentally ill subjects who received supported employment obtained competitive employment, compared with 26% of subjects in the control conditions (Bustillo *et al.* 2001).

Positive findings in other areas of outcome have also been reported for supported employment: lower hospital admissions, better medication compliance, less abuse of alcohol, better familial role performance, higher self-esteem and more social activity (Kuldau & Dirks 1977; Bond & Dincin 1986; Bond 1992). Research on supported employment raises a number of questions that require further study, including how to increase the retention rate of patients in these programmes, how to effectively place and maintain employment for those with skills beyond entry-level, the extent of support needed, and what patient characteristics are most suited to success in these programmes.

An element that would likely buttress supported employment but is rarely used is the addition of social skills training. Social skills training could equip the mentally ill person with the conversational and problem-solving skills to meet the interpersonal expectations and demands of the work culture and setting (Mueser & Liberman 1988). Mentally ill individuals often find the person–person interactions in the work setting (e.g. conversation with coworkers during breaks, asking a supervisor for assistance on a task) more stressful than the actual job tasks; thus, skills training *in vivo* might protect schizophrenic individuals from stress-induced relapse. Necessary skills and social supports are developed for the individual, in consultation with the employer, to assist the mentally ill individual to meet the specific requirements of the work environment.

In one programme that integrated skills training with supported employment in Hong Kong, a succession of social skills were taught, including basic conversational skills, general skills for succeeding on the job (e.g. maintaining a good relationship with a supervisor) and specific skills for dealing with one's job (e.g. receptionist would learn how to field enquiries from visitors and on the phone). A controlled study of the programme discovered 47% of those who received skills training and follow-up support were employed at 3 months after training ended. This contrasted with 23% employed of those who received skills training alone and nil employed who were in the control group (Tsang & Pearson 2001).

A user-friendly manualized Workplace Fundamentals Module has been designed and tested for use in concert with supported employment. The module contains a trainer's manual, participant's workbook, demonstration video and user's guide. It is readily implemented in a wide variety of supported or transitional employment programmes and has been shown to result in improved vocational outcomes for those learning the skills in the context of supported employment (Wallace *et al*. 1999). Multisite controlled studies are underway in the USA to evaluate the degree to which the Workplace Fundamentals Module can increase tenure on the job for mentally ill individuals who obtain employment, but so often fail to maintain their jobs beyond 6 months.

Job-finding clubs

Because some patients prefer to find their own jobs without the intercession of an employment specialist or job developer, some supported work programmes utilize skills training, job-finding clubs and/or career planning before actual job placement. Patients may need training in job-finding skills, which can be conducted in club-like settings (Azrin & Besalel 1979; Azrin & Philip 1979; Jacobs *et al*. 1984). Basic skills taught during job-finding seminars include identifying job leads, writing résumés, filling out job applications, rehearsing interviewing skills and using public transportation. Patients who demonstrate mastery of these skills are encouraged to look for work. During the job-seeking phase, the club offers resources to support the arduous search, e.g. counsellors, buddy-system of mutual aid, newspapers, phones and maps.

Research on job-finding clubs has shown them to be an effective means of helping patients obtain employment. Controlled studies have found employment rates of 42–90% for participants in job-finding clubs, compared with 10–33% employment outcome for individuals participating in control programmes (Keith *et al*. 1977; Azrin & Philip 1979; Eisenberg & Cole 1986). In another evaluative study of the job club, 66% of the participants found work or were enrolled full-time in job training programmes, requiring on average 22 days of participation in the club. Six-month follow-up data revealed that 68% of those employed were still working (Jacobs *et al*. 1984). More recent evaluations of the job club programme have found lower employment rates, with individuals suffering from schizophrenia or bipolar disorder doing more poorly than those with anxiety or substance abuse disorders. Thus, the job-finding club may be utilitarian for only a subset of persons with schizophrenia. Interestingly, while fewer persons with schizophrenia were successful in obtaining employment, of those who succeeded, the job-retention rates were as high as for individuals from other diagnostic categories (Jacobs *et al*. 1990).

Supported housing

Affordable, accessible and acceptable housing is a cornerstone of modern rehabilitation services. We are rapidly moving from an era in which the mental hospital provided all the necessities of daily living on one site, to one in which a spectrum of provisions is aimed at enabling as many individuals as possible to live in ordinary housing, albeit with support. The first step along this road was the development of transitional housing, from the 24-h highly staffed residential care or board and care home (Goldberg *et al*. 1985), through staffed group homes, to progressively less intensively supervised, more normalized community settings.

This spectrum of housing alternatives was particularly influential during hospital closures. One study of the fate of persons living in a spectrum of community-based housing was the longitudinal follow-up of patients discharged from Friern Barnet hospital in North London (O'Driscoll *et al*. 1993; Leff *et al*. 1994, 1996). This research was unique in its coverage of a large population of ex-asylum patients using a prospective design and including an economic analysis (Knapp *et al*. 1990). Nearly 80% of all long-stay patients were discharged to staffed accommodations in the community where the majority continued to reside over a 5-year follow-up period. Of the 671 patients discharged to community homes, 126 died in the subsequent 5 years – a death rate that, although higher than the general population, was comparable to other samples of severely mentally ill people. Only nine patients could not be traced at follow-up, of which only three were known to have become homeless. Just over one-third of patients were readmitted to hospitals during the follow-up, the majority having relatively brief admissions (Leff *et al.* 1994, 1996).

The community homes were much less restrictive than the hospital wards and provided a comfortable atmosphere, which was favoured by patients. Patients made more friends, a majority of whom were ordinary members of the community. While individual patients showed large fluctuations in symptoms, there was no overall change in psychiatric state for the sample as a whole during the follow-up period. Problems with social behaviour also remained stable (Anderson *et al.* 1993; Leff *et al.* 1994, 1996). A comprehensive analysis of health and social care costs suggested that once the relatively high cost of caring for the difficult-to-place patients was taken into account, there was little difference between hospital and community care. Indeed, considering the improved outcomes suggested that community-based care was more cost-effective than the hospital (Knapp *et al.* 1990).

While similar findings for these '*trans*-institutional' residential models have been reported from several countries (Goldberg *et al.* 1985; Gibbons & Butler 1987; Okin & Pearsall 1993; Farragher *et al.* 1996; Donnelly *et al.* 1997), the approach has not been without its critics. The best programmes have worked hard to enable consumer choice, easy access and unhampered movement between levels of care. However, all too many schemes have been run with convenience for agencies and staff rather than consumer choice in mind, imposed unrealistic targets for residents to 'move on', and generally forced residents to meet service needs rather than providing care tailored to the waxing and waning needs of the residents (Hogan & Carling 1992; Carling 1995).

In the face of such criticism, there has been the emergence of supported housing models which rely less on having a range of facilities into which to 'slot' patients, and more on a partnership between the providers of ordinary housing and mental health services, the latter providing a range of flexible mobile case management, consultation, training and treatment services which enable patients to manage in housing of their choice (Carling 1993; Ogilvie 1997). This approach is often preferred by patients and their care-providers (Carling 1993; Hatfield 1993) and may be associated with improved quality of life and reduced time in hospital.

There have been several large-scale evaluations of supported housing in the USA. The Programme of Chronic Mental Illness, sponsored by the Robert Wood Johnson Foundation and the US Department of Housing and Urban Development, for example, brought together housing and health authorities in nine cities to target services for severely mentally ill people. This comprehen-sive system of support and housing subsidy had a beneficial impact on the quality of life of many people, although the results varied from city to city and there was little effect on clinical outcomes (Goldman *et al.* 1994; Lehman *et al.* 1994). In a study of 74 mentally ill persons living in community integrated residences, the level of their satisfaction with their housing arrangements – with flexible amounts of staff support and supervision – was as high as individuals living independently. Moreover, residents' hospital use decreased from a mean of 47.7 days during the year before programme placement to 5.3 days during their first year in the programme (Hanrahan *et al.* 2001).

More recently, the US Department of Health and Human Services and the Department of Housing and Urban Development funded experimental programmes targeted at the homeless mentally ill, placing many in appropriate community-based housing and demonstrating reductions in symptoms, reduced hospitalization and some improvement of social functioning and quality of life (Dickey *et al.* 1996; Shern *et al.* 1997). Tsemberis and Eisenberg (2000) examined the effectiveness of the Pathways to Housing programme in New York City over a 5-year period. The programme, which provided immediate access to independent apartments for homeless mentally ill individuals and provided support services in the context of a modified assertive community treatment model, was compared with a more traditional linear residential treatment approach. After 5 years, 88% of the programme's tenants remained housed, compared with only 47% of the patients in the traditional treatment system. These studies demonstrated that even patients with severe psychiatric disabilities and addictions are capable of maintaining independent housing when provided with the necessary supportive services.

Compensating for deficits: cognitive adaptive therapy

There is mounting evidence that neurocognitive impairments are central to the difficulties in instrumental and role functioning often experienced by persons with schizophrenia (Green 1996; Velligan *et al.* 1997) and that cognitive deficits may serve as 'rate-limiting factors' in the ability of individuals with this disorder to benefit from psychosocial rehabilitation (Green 1993). Despite the improvements in neurocognition that may be conferred by treatment with atypical antipsychotic medications (Meltzer 1992; Green *et al.* 1997; Velligan *et al.* 1999), significant deficits remain. Velligan and colleagues at the University of Texas have developed and tested a strategy called *cognitive adaptation training*, which involves environmental modifications in patients' homes to compensate for their residual cognitive impairments and improve their daily functioning. The compensatory strategies include the use of signs, labels and electronic devices designed to cue and sequence appropriate behaviours. Four types of assessments are conducted prior to implementing cognitive adaptation training:

1 behavioural assessment of apathy and disinhibition;
2 neurocognitive assessment of executive functioning, attention and memory;

3 functional needs assessment in activities of daily living; and
4 environmental assessment in the home to identify triggers of maladaptive behaviour, safety hazards and availability of needed equipment.

Apathetic behaviours can be altered by providing prompting and cueing that help the patient initiate each step in a sequenced task. Checklists may be used for complex tasks, signs and labels may be placed in front of the patient along with needed equipment, or electronic devices such as tape recorders may provide cues and instructions. For disinhibited behaviour, distracting stimuli and triggers are removed, patients are redirected and supplies are organized. Patients with impairment in executive functioning are provided with a greater amount of structure and more obvious environmental cues. Interventions are altered as necessary during weekly visits to the home by cognitive adaptation training therapists.

In a randomized, controlled study (Velligan *et al.* 2000), 45 outpatients with schizophrenia or schizoaffective disorder were randomly assigned to 9 months of either:
1 standard medication treatment;
2 standard medication plus cognitive adaptation training; or
3 standard medication plus a condition designed to control for therapist time and environmental changes unrelated to cognitive deficits.
Significant differences were found between the groups in levels of psychotic symptoms, motivation, and global functioning at the end of the 9-month period. Relapse rates were also significantly lower in the cognitive adaptation training group (13% vs. 33% for the medication only group and 69% for the control condition). The results of this study are encouraging, demonstrating that compensatory strategies may improve outcomes for persons with schizophrenia. Additional research will be needed to explore whether such strategies are as effective as other available treatments, and the added benefits that may accrue from combining compensatory strategies with other treatments (e.g. assertive community treatment).

Family psychoeducation

Because the family is typically an important part of the patient's natural support system and living environment, improving family attitudes, knowledge and coping skills regarding mental illness can result in better opportunities, encouragement and reinforcement for the generalization of social and independent living skills. Family interventions have been shown to have significant benefits for both patient outcome and family adjustment. On average, relapse rates among patients with schizophrenia with family therapy are 24% vs. 64% for those receiving standard care (Bustillo *et al.* 2001).

In psychoeducational programmes, relatives are engaged as essential allies in treatment and rehabilitation. The psychoeducational model has five major aims:
1 to develop collegial relationships among the treatment team, family members, and other support persons;
2 to educate the family about the patient's particular mental

disorder, and to direct them to locally available treatment and rehabilitation resources;
3 to strengthen treatment alliances by acknowledging the efforts and basic good intentions of family members;
4 to develop step-by-step communication and problem-solving skills; and
5 to develop a network of like-thinking people to serve as support persons and provide resources.

A typical psychoeducational session begins with information about the nature of schizophrenia and the medication and psychosocial interventions available for its treatment. Topics include positive and negative symptoms, effects of psychotropic medications and treatment options in psychiatric rehabilitation. Material is presented didactically, followed by guided discussion. Patients and relatives alike are considered the 'experts' at these meetings and are invited to discuss various points about symptoms and treatments in terms of their own experiences. To varying degrees, education programmes are enhanced with basic skills training of the patients and relatives in interpersonal communication, problem-solving and contingency management. One approach that emphasizes these traditional cognitive–behavioural techniques is called *behavioural family management* (Falloon *et al.* 1985).

Several well-controlled studies (Goldstein *et al.* 1978; Falloon *et al.* 1982, 1985; Hogarty & Anderson 1986; Tarrier *et al.* 1988) have shown that the rate of relapse and subsequent hospitalization for patients whose families participate in psychoeducation and skills training is significantly less than for customary treatments. While it is clear that patients benefit from having their families involved in treatment, the mechanisms of the treatment effects are unknown and the critical components of the various approaches have not been identified. Acquiring communication and problem-solving skills has been shown to be important, but affective and socioecological factors may also be crucial. For example, family members are typically distressed by the patient's bizarre or asocial behaviour, anxious about increased financial burden for the patient's treatment, uncertain about future plans and isolated from their own social supports as a result of caregiving responsibilities, stigma and embarrassment (Creer & Wing 1974). In some families, these stressors produce high levels of expressed emotion (criticism, disappointment, hostility and overprotectiveness).

Patients who return to families with high expressed emotion are more likely to relapse than those whose families are low in expressed emotion (Brown *et al.* 1972; Vaughn & Leff 1976; Vaughn *et al.* 1982; Leff & Vaughn 1985). Changes in expressed emotion may thus be part of the beneficial effect of family education and treatment. One outcome study that showed better social and independent functioning and improved quality of life for patients in the family treatment group also showed lower expressed emotion and emotional burden in the family members (Falloon *et al.* 1985). These effects have also been found to be maintained in the majority of patients and their families for as long as 8 years (Tarrier *et al.* 1994). Similar relationships between the emotional climate of group homes and the clinical outcomes of patients residing there have also been demonstrated (Snyder *et al.* 1994).

Conclusions

While the arrival of a new generation of antipsychotic medications during the past decade has captivated practitioners and consumers alike, actual advances in the treatment and rehabilitation of persons with schizophrenia have been more substantial in the arena of psychosocial services (Geddes & Carney 2001; Wallace *et al.* 2001b; Kopelowicz *et al.* 2002). A number of recent innovations can be expected to improve the prospects for psychiatric rehabilitation:

1 Illness self-management techniques, such as those found in the UCLA social and independent living skills programme, which will permit patients to assume more responsibility for monitoring their symptoms and seek early and flexible levels of intervention.

2 Functional assessment that is more individualized and better linked to prescriptions for rehabilitation.

3 The integration of social learning and assertive community treatment techniques and procedures, so that cognitive–behaviour therapy can be used to teach patients how to adapt to community living.

4 Continued investigation in the cognitive sciences to further inform professionals on how to compensate for or overcome cognitive impairments.

5 Family involvement in treatment and rehabilitation, as well as in advocacy for the needed services and research; and the provision of services by professionals, including education, skills training and social support, to family caregivers.

There continues to be a great discrepancy between what is known from research and demonstration studies about effective psychosocial treatments and rehabilitation, and what is actually implemented at the clinical level. This discrepancy between available technology and common practice prevents thousands of persons with schizophrenia from achieving more optimal states of functioning. A number of obstacles are often encountered when attempting to develop and implement a rehabilitation programme, especially in treatment settings where 'traditional' treatment has long been the norm (e.g. state hospitals). Financial concerns and reluctance of administrative and direct care staff are only some of the barriers that need to be overcome if a sound and effective programme is to be put into place (Stuve & Menditto 1999). This is also true regarding outpatient treatment, which also must address the complications of integrating treatment from a variety of care providers in different settings and from different disciplines, including psychiatric, case management and vocational services (Monroe-DeVita & Mohatt 1999). Effective data-collection and management systems must be developed and utilized to track the progress of patients and to facilitate well-informed treatment decisions (Buican *et al.* 1999).

Administrative, financial, organizational and systems' obsta-

cles confound the best efforts of practitioners and researchers to apply state-of-the-art treatments. In addition, reliance on publications and conferences to disseminate innovations can never succeed in producing knowledge and technology transfer from research into practice. Much more active brokering models of dissemination must be used to overcome the professional inertia in systems of mental health care (Backer *et al.* 1986).

The following caveats can help to bridge the gap between research and practice:

1 Increase the number of accessible services through active outreach and mobile case management services.

2 Provide continuous and indefinite treatment and rehabilitation in the context of reliable and mutually respectful therapeutic relationships.

3 Engage the patient's and family's self-help and active participation in rehabilitation.

4 Assist the patient and caregivers in achieving the delicate balance between risk-taking and protective measures to reduce stress-related relapses.

5 Galvanize administrative and programme support for comprehensive and co-ordinated services.

Bringing innovative techniques and approaches into the realistic arena of clinical practice will maximize recovery and rehabilitation for persons with schizophrenia. With this in mind, there needs to be greater insistence by consumer advocacy groups (e.g. the National Alliance for the Mentally Ill) and policymakers that health care providers deliver the more proven or evidence-based psychosocial interventions and that the training of professionals and their licensure and certification include the skills to deliver these treatments. Consumers and their families can help by insisting that practitioners and agency administrators provide flexible, individually tailored care and demand access to information about the empirical basis for the care they receive.

Acknowledgement

We are grateful to Dr William Spaulding of the University of Nebraska–Lincoln for his helpful comments on an early draft of this chapter.

References

Anderson, J., Dayson, D., Wills, W. *et al.* (1993) The TAPS Project 13: clinical and social outcomes of long-stay psychiatric patients after 1 year in the community. *British Journal of Psychiatry* 162, 45–56.

Anthony, W. (1994) Characteristics of people with psychiatric disabilities that are predictive of entry into the rehabilitation process and successful employment. *Psychosocial Rehabilitation Journal* 17, 3–13.

Anthony, W. & Blanch, A.K. (1987) Supported employment for persons who are psychiatrically disabled: an historical and conceptual perspective. *Psychosocial Rehabilitation Journal* 11, 5–23.

Anthony, W. & Liberman, R.P. (1986) The practice of psychiatric rehabilitation: historical, conceptual and research base. *Schizophrenia Bulletin* 12, 542–559.

Anthony, W.A., Cohen, M., Farkas, M. & Cohen, F. (1988) Case management: more than a response to a dysfunctional system. *Community Mental Health Journal* 24, 219–228.

Atthowe, J.M. & Krasner, L. (1968) Preliminary report on the application of contingent reinforcement procedures (token economy) on a chronic psychiatric ward. *Journal of Abnormal Psychology* 73, 37–43.

Austin, N.K., Liberman, R.P., King, L.W. & DeRisi, W.J. (1976) A comparative evaluation of two day hospitals: behavior therapy vs. milieu therapy. *Journal of Nervous and Mental Disease* 163, 253–261.

Ayllon, T. & Azrin, N. (1968) *The Token Economy: A Motivational System for Therapy and Rehabilitation.* Appleton Century Crofts, New York.

Azrin, N.H. & Besalel, V.B. (1979) *Job Club Counselor's Manual: a Behavioral Approach to Vocational Counseling.* University Park Press, Baltimore.

Azrin, N.H. & Philip, R.A. (1979) Job club method for the job handicapped: comparative outcome study. *Rehabilitation Counseling Bulletin* 23, 144–155.

Backer, T.E., Liberman, R.P. & Kuehnel, T.G. (1986) Dissemination and adoption of innovative psychosocial interventions. *Journal of Consulting and Clinical Psychology* 54, 111–118.

Baker, R., Hall, J.N., Hutchinson, K. & Bridge, G. (1977) Symptom changes in chronic schizophrenic patients on a token economy ward: a controlled experiment. *British Journal of Psychiatry* 131, 381–393.

Baronet, A. & Gerber, G. (1998) Psychiatric rehabilitation: efficacy of four models. *Clinical Psychology Review* 18, 189–228.

Beard, J.H., Propst, R.N. & Malamud, T.J. (1982) The Fountain House model of rehabilitation. *Psychosocial Rehabilitation Journal* 5, 47–53.

Bell, M.D., Lysaker, P.H. & Milstein, R.M. (1996) Clinical benefits of paid work activity in schizophrenia. *Schizophrenia Bulletin* 22, 51–67.

Bellack, A.S., Mueser, K.T., Gingerich, S. & Agresta, J. (1997) *Social Skills Training for Schizophrenia: a Step-by-Step Guide.* Guilford, New York.

Bentall, R., Higson, P. & Lowe, C.F. (1987) Teaching self instructions to chronic schizophrenic patients: efficacy and generalization. *Behavioural Psychotherapy* 15, 58–76.

Bond, G.R. (1992) *Handbook of Psychiatric Rehabilitation* (ed. R.P. Liberman), pp. 244–275. Macmillan, New York.

Bond, G.R. & Dincin, J. (1986) Accelerating entry into transitional employment in a psychosocial rehabilitation agency. *Rehabilitation Psychology* 31, 143–155.

Bond, G.R., Dietzen, L.L., McGrew, J.H. & Miller, L.D. (1995) Accelerating entry into supported employment for persons with severe psychiatric disabilities. *Rehabilitation Psychology* 40, 75–94.

Bond, G.R., Drake, R.E., Mueser, K.T. & Becker, D.R. (1997) An update on supported employment for people with severe mental illness. *Psychiatric Services* 48, 335–346.

Bowen, L., Wallace, C.J., Glynn, S.M. *et al.* (1994) Schizophrenics' cognitive functioning and performance in interpersonal interactions and skills training procedures. *Journal of Psychiatric Research* 28, 289–301.

Brenner, H.D., Hodel, B., Roder, V. & Corrigan, P. (1992) Treatment of cognitive dysfunctions and behavioral deficits in schizophrenia. *Schizophrenia Bulletin* 18, 21–26.

Brown, G.W., Birley, J.L.T. & Wing, J.K. (1972) Influence of family life on the course of schizophrenic disorders: a replication. *British Journal of Psychiatry* 121, 241–258.

Buican, B., Spaulding, W.D., Gordon, B. & Hindman, T. (1999) Clinical decision support systems in state hospitals. *New Directions in Mental Health Services* 84, 99–112.

Burda, P.C., Starkey, T.W. & Dominguez, F. (1991) Computer administered treatment of psychiatric inpatients. *Computers in Human Behavior* 7, 1–5.

Burns, T., Creed, F., Fahy, T. *et al.* (1999) Intensive versus standard case management for severe psychotic illness: a randomised trial. *Lancet* 353, 2185–2189.

Bustillo, J.R., Lauriello, J., Horan, W.P. & Keith, S.J. (2001) The psychosocial treatment of schizophrenia: an update. *American Journal of Psychiatry* 158, 163–175.

Carling, P. (1993) Housing and supports for persons with mental illness: emerging approaches to research and practice. *Hospital and Community Psychiatry* 44, 439–449.

Carling, P. (1995) *Returning to Community, Building Support Systems for People with Psychiatric Disabilities.* Guilford, New York.

Cook, J.A. & Razzano, L. (2000) Vocational rehabilitation for persons with schizophrenia: recent research and implications for practice. *Schizophrenia Bulletin* 26, 87–103.

Corrigan, P.W. & Green, M.F. (1993) Schizophrenic patients' sensitivity to social cues: the role of abstraction. *American Journal of Psychiatry* 150, 589–594.

Corrigan, P.W., Schade, M. & Liberman, R.P. (1992) *Handbook of Psychiatric Rehabilitation* (ed. R.P. Liberman), pp. 95–126. Macmillan, New York.

Corrigan, P.W., Wallace, C.J., Schade, M.L. & Green, M.F. (1994) Learning medication self-management skills in schizophrenia: relationships with cognitive deficits and psychiatric symptoms. *Behavior Therapy* 25, 5–15.

Creer, C. & Wing, J. (1974) *Schizophrenia at Home.* Institute of Psychiatry, London.

Dickey, B., Gonzalez, O., Latimer, E. *et al.* (1996) Use of mental health services by formerly homeless adults residing in group and independent housing. *Psychiatric Services* 47, 152–158.

Dilk, M.N. & Bond, G.R. (1996) Meta-analytic evaluation of skills training research for individuals with severe mental illness. *Journal of Consulting and Clinical Psychology* 64, 1337–1346.

Dobson, D.J., McDougall, G., Busheikn, J. & Aldous, J. (1995) Effects of social skills training and social milieu treatment on symptoms of schizophrenia. *Psychiatric Services* 46, 376–380.

Donahoe, C.P., Carter, M.J., Bloem, W.D. *et al.* (1991) Assessment of interpersonal problem-solving skills. *Psychiatry* 53, 329–339.

Donnelly, M., McGilloway, S., Mays, N., Perry, S. & Lavery, C. (1997) A 3–6 year follow-up of former long-stay psychiatric patients in Northern Ireland. *Social Psychiatry and Psychiatric Epidemiology* 32, 451–458.

Drake, R.E. & Becker, D.R. (1996) The individual placement and support model of supported employment. *Psychiatric Services* 47, 473–475.

Drake, R.E., Becker, D., Biesanz, J.C. *et al.* (1994) Rehabilitative day treatments vs. supported employment. I. Vocational outcomes. *Community Mental Health Journal* 30, 519–532.

Drake, R.E., McHugo, G.J., Becker, D.R., Anthony, W.A. & Clark, R.E. (1996) The New Hampshire study of supported employment for people with severe mental illness. *Journal of Consulting and Clinical Psychology* 64, 391–399.

Drake, R.E., McHugo, G., Bebout, R.R. *et al.* (1999) A randomized clinical trial of supported employment for inner-city patients with severe mental illness. *Archives of General Psychiatry* 56, 627–633.

Eckman, T.A., Tucker, D.E. *et al.* (1992a) *Schizophrenia and Affective Psychoses* (eds F. Ferrero & R. Salvati), pp. 64–77. John Libbey, Rome.

Eckman, T.A., Wirshing, W.C., Marder, S.R. *et al.* (1992b) Technique for training schizophrenic patients in illness self-management: a controlled trial. *American Journal of Psychiatry* 149, 1549–1555.

Eisenberg, M.G. & Cole, H.W. (1986) A behavioral approach to job seeking for psychiatrically impaired persons. *Journal of Rehabilitation* 27, 46–49.

Falloon, I.R.H., Boyd, J.L., McGill, C.W. *et al.* (1982) Family management in the prevention of exacerbations of schizophrenia: a controlled study. *New England Journal of Medicine* 306, 1437–1440.

Falloon, I.R.H., Boyd, J.L., McGill, C.W. *et al.* (1985) Family management in the prevention of morbidity of schizophrenia: clinical outcome of a 2-year longitudinal study. *Archives of General Psychiatry* 42, 887–896.

Farragher, B., Carey, T. & Owens, J. (1996) Long-term follow-up care of rehabilitated patients with chronic psychiatric illness in Ireland. *Psychiatric Services* 47, 1120–1122.

Fenton, W. & McGlashan, T. (1991) Natural history of schizophrenia subtypes: positive and negative symptoms. *Archives of General Psychiatry* 48, 978–986.

Geddes, J. & Carney, S. (2001) Recent advances in evidence-based psychiatry. *Canadian Journal of Psychiatry* 46, 403–406.

Gibbons, J.S. & Butler, J.P. (1987) Quality of life for new long-stay psychiatric inpatients: the effects of moving to a hostel. *British Journal of Psychiatry* 151, 347–354.

Glynn, S.M. & Mueser, K.T. (1992) Social–learning programmes. In: *Handbook of Psychiatric Rehabilitation* (ed. R.P. Liberman), pp. 127–152. Macmillan, New York.

Glynn, S.M., Liberman, R.P., Bowen, L. *et al.* (1994) *Behavior Therapy in Psychiatric Hospitals* (eds P.W. Corrigan & R.P. Liberman), pp. 39–59. Springer, New York.

Glynn, S.M., Marder, S.R., Liberman, R.P. *et al.* (2002) Supplementing clinic-based skills training for schizophrenia with manualized community support: effects on social adjustment. *American Journal of Psychiatry* 159, 829–837.

Goldberg, J. (1994) Cognitive retraining in a community psychiatric rehabilitation program. In: *Cognitive Technology in Psychiatric Rehabilitation* (ed. W. Spaulding), pp. 67–86. University of Nebraska Press, Lincoln, NE.

Goldberg, D.P., Bridges, K., Cooper, W. *et al.* (1985) Douglas House: a new type of hostel ward for chronic psychotic patients. *British Journal of Psychiatry* 147, 383–388.

Goldman, H.H., Morrissey, J.P. & Ridgely, M.S. (1994) Evaluating the Robert Wood Johnson Foundation program on chronic mental illness. *Milbank Quarterly* 72, 37–47.

Goldstein, M., Rodnick, E., Evans, J., May, P. & Steinberg, M. (1978) Drug and family therapy in the aftercare of acute schizophrenics. *Archives of General Psychiatry* 35, 1169–1177.

Green, M.F. (1993) Cognitive remediation in schizophrenia: is it time yet? *American Journal of Psychiatry* 150, 178–187.

Green, M.F. (1996) What are the functional consequences of neurocognitive deficits in schizophrenia. *American Journal of Psychiatry* 153, 321–330.

Green, M.F. & Nuechterlein, K.H. (1999) Should schizophrenia be treated as a neurocognitive disorder? *Schizophrenia Bulletin* 25, 309–318.

Green, M.F., Marshall, B.D., Wirshing, W.C. *et al.* (1997) Does risperidone improve verbal working memory in treatment-resistant schizophrenia. *American Journal of Psychiatry* 154, 799–804.

Grove, B., Freudenberg, M. *et al.* (1997) *The Social Firm Handbook: New Directions in the Employment, Rehabilitation and Integration of People with Mental Health Problems.* Pavilion, Brighton.

Hall, J.N., Baker, R.D. & Hutchinson, K. (1977) A controlled evaluation of token economy procedures with chronic schizophrenic patients. *Behavioural Research and Therapy* 15, 261–283.

Hanrahan, P., Luchins, D.J., Savage, C. & Goldman, H.H. (2001) Housing satisfaction and service use by mentally ill persons in community integrated living arrangements. *Psychiatric Services* 52, 1206–1209.

Harding, C.M., Brooks, G.W., Ashikaga, T. *et al.* (1987) The Vermont longitudinal study of persons with severe mental illness. I. Methodology, study sample, and overall status 32 years later. *American Journal of Psychiatry* 144, 718–726.

Hatfield, A.B. (1993) A family perspective on supported housing. *Hospital and Community Psychiatry* 44, 496–497.

Hayes, R.L. & McGrath, J.J. (2000) *Cognitive Rehabilitation for People with Schizophrenia and Related Conditions.* Cochrane Library, Oxford.

Hayes, R.L., Halford, W.K. & Varghese, F.T. (1995) Social skills training with chronic schizophrenic patients: effects on negative symptoms and community functioning. *Behavior Therapy* 26, 433–449.

Heinssen, R. & Victor, B. (1994) *Cognitive Technology in Psychiatric Rehabilitation* (ed. W. Spaulding), pp. 159–182. University of Nebraska Press, Lincoln, NE.

Heinssen, R., Levendusky, P. & Hunter, R. (1995) Client as colleague: therapeutic contracting with the seriously mentally ill. *American Psychologist* 50, 522–532.

Heinssen, R.K., Liberman, R.P. & Kopelowicz, A. (2000) Psychosocial skills training for schizophrenia: lessons from the laboratory. *Schizophrenia Bulletin* 26, 21–46.

Hogan, M. & Carling, P. (1992) Normal housing: a key element of a supported housing approach for people with psychiatric disabilities. *Community Mental Health Journal* 26, 221–225.

Hogarty, G.E. & Anderson, C.M. (1986) Medication, family psychoeducation, and social skills training: first year relapse results of a controlled study. *Psychopharmacology Bulletin* 22, 860–862.

Holloway, F. & Carson, J. (1998) Intensive case management for the severely mentally ill: a controlled trial. *British Journal of Psychiatry* 172, 19–22.

Hume, C. & Pullen, I. (1995) *Rehabilitation in Psychiatry.* Churchill Livingstone, Edinburgh.

Jacobs, H.E., Kardashian, S., Kreinbring, R.K., Ponder, R. & Simpson, A.S. (1984) A skills oriented model facilitating employment among psychiatrically disabled persons. *Rehabilitation Counseling Bulletin* 28, 87–96.

Jacobs, H.E., Liberman, R.P. *et al.* (1990) The job-finding club: predictors of outcome. Paper presented at the 143rd Annual Meeting of the American Psychiatric Association, New York, NY.

Johnstone, E., Macmillan, J., Frith, C.D., Benn, D.K. & Crow, T.J. (1990) Further investigation of the predictors of outcome following first schizophrenic episodes. *British Journal of Psychiatry* 157, 182–189.

Kanter, J. (1989) Clinical case management: definition, principles, components. *Hospital and Community Psychiatry* 40, 361–368.

Kazdin, A.E. (1982) The token economy: a decade later. *Journal of Applied Behavior Analysis* 15, 431–445.

Kazdin, A.E. & Bootzin, R.R. (1972) The token economy: an evaluative review. *Journal of Applied Behavior Analysis* 5, 343–372.

Keith, R.D., Engelkes, J.R. & Winborn, B.B. (1977) Employment-seeking preparation and activity: experimental job placement training model for rehabilitation clients. *Rehabilitation Counseling Bulletin* 21, 159–165.

Kemp, R., Hayward, P., Applewhaite, G., Everitt, B. & David, A. (1996) Compliance therapy in psychotic disorders: randomised controlled trial. *British Medical Journal* 312, 345–349.

Kemp, R., Kirov, G., Everitt, B., Hayward, P. & David, A. (1998) Randomised controlled trial of compliance therapy: 18 month follow-up. *British Journal of Psychiatry* 172, 413–419.

Kern, R.S., Green, M.F. & Satz, P. (1992) Neuropsychological predictors of skills training for chronic psychiatric patients. *Psychiatry Research* **43**, 223–230.

Knapp, M., Beecham, J., Anderson, J. et al. (1990) The TAPS Project III: predicting the community costs of closing psychiatric hospitals. *British Journal of Psychiatry* **157**, 661–670.

Kommana, S., Mansfield, M. & Penn, D.L. (1997) Dispelling the stigma of schizophrenia. *Psychiatric Services* **48**, 1393–1395.

Kopelowicz, A. & Liberman, R.P. (2003) Recovery from schizophrenia. *Directions in Psychiatry* (in press).

Kopelowicz, A., Wallace, C.J. & Zarate, R. (1998) Teaching psychiatric inpatients to re-enter the community: a brief method of improving the continuity of care. *Psychiatric Services* **49**, 1313–1316.

Kopelowicz, A., Zarate, R., Gonzalez, V. & Tripodis, K. (1999) Social skills training for Latinos with schizophrenia. *Schizophrenia Research* **36**, 327–328.

Kopelowicz, A., Liberman, R.P. & Ventura, J. (2001) Neurocognitive correlates of recovery from schizophrenia. In: *Understanding and Treating Schizophrenia* (eds H.D. Brenner & R. Genner). Hogrefe & Huber, Toronto.

Kopelowicz, A., Liberman, R.P. & Zarate, R. (2002) Psychosocial treatments for schizophrenia. In: *A Guide to Treatments That Work* (eds P.E. Nathan & J.M. Gorman). pp. 201–208. Oxford University Press, New York.

Kuldau, J.M. & Dirks, S.J. (1977) Controlled evaluation of a hospital-originated community transitional system. *Archives of General Psychiatry* **34**, 1331–1340.

Latimer, E. (1999) Economic impacts of assertive community treatment: a review of the literature. *Canadian Journal of Psychiatry* **44**, 443–454.

Layne, C. & Wallace, L.T. (1982) Impaired preferences for praise in schizophrenic adolescents. *Journal of Clinical Psychology* **38**, 51–55.

Lecomte, T., Liberman, R.P. & Wallace, C.J. (2000) Identifying and using reinforcers to enhance treatment of pesons with serious mental illness. *Psychiatric Services* **51**, 1312–1314.

Leff, J. & Vaughn, C. (1985) *Expressed Emotion in Families: Its Significance for Mental Illness*. Guilford, New York.

Leff, J., Thornicroft, G., Coxhead, N. & Crawford, C. (1994) The TAPS Project 22: a five-year follow-up of long-stay psychiatric patients discharged to the community. *British Journal of Psychiatry* **165**, 13–17.

Leff, J., Trieman, N. & Gooch, C. (1996) Team for the assessment of psychiatric services (TAPS) Project 33: prospective follow-up study of long-stay patients discharged from two psychiatric hospitals. *American Journal of Psychiatry* **153**, 1318–1324.

Lehman, A.F. (1995) Vocational rehabilitation in schizophrenia. *Schizophrenia Bulletin* **21**, 645–656.

Lehman, A.F. & Steinwachs, D. (1998) Patterns of usual care for schizophrenia: initial results from the Schizophrenia Patient Outcomes Research Team (PORT) survey. *Schizophrenia Bulletin* **24**, 11–20.

Lehman, A.F., Postrado, L.T., Roth, D., McNary, S.W. & Goldman, H.H. (1994) Continuity of care and client outcomes in the Robert Wood Johnson Foundation program on chronic mental illness. *Milbank Quarterly* **72**, 105–122.

Li, F. & Wang, M. (1994) A behavioural training programme for chronic schizophrenic patients: a 3 month randomised controlled trial in Beijing. *British Journal of Psychiatry* **165**, 32–37.

Liberman, R.P. (1972) Behavioral modification of schizophrenia: a review. *Schizophrenia Bulletin* **Fall**, 37–48.

Liberman, R.P. (1988) Coping with chronic mental disorders. In: *Psychiatric Rehabilitation for Chronic Mental Patients* (ed. R.P. Liberman), pp. 147–198. American Psychiatric Press, Washington, DC.

Liberman, R.P., ed. (1992) *Handbook of Psychiatric Rehabilitation*. MacMillan, New York.

Liberman, R.P. (2002) Cognitive remediation. In: *Comprehensive Treatment of Schizophrenia* (eds H. Kashima, I.R.H. Falloon, M. Mizuno & M. Asai), pp. 254–278. Springer-Verlag, Tokyo.

Liberman, R.P. (2003) Teaching mentally disabled persons to be their own case managers. *Psychiatric Services* in press.

Liberman, R.P. & Bryan, E. (1977) Behavior therapy in a community mental health center. *American Journal of Psychiatry* **134**, 401–406.

Liberman, R.P. & Corrigan, P.W. (1993) Designing new psychosocial treatments for schizophrenia. *Psychiatry* **56**, 238–249.

Liberman, R.P. & Corrigan, P.W. (1994) Implementing and maintaining behavior therapy programs. In: *Behavior Therapy in Psychiatric Hospitals* (eds P.W. Corrigan & R.P. Liberman), pp. 201–219. Springer, New York.

Liberman, R.P. & Kopelowicz, A. (1994) Recovery from schizophrenia: is the time right? *Journal of the California Alliance for the Mentally Ill* **5**, 67–69.

Liberman, R.P., Teigan, J. et al. (1973) Reducing delusional speech in chronic paranoid schizophrenics. *Journal of Applied Behavioral Analysis* **6**, 57–64.

Liberman, R.P., Fearn, C.H., DeRisi, W., Roberts, J. & Carmona, M. (1977) The credit incentive system: motivating the participation of patients in a day hospital. *British Journal of Social and Clinical Psychology* **16**, 85–94.

Liberman, R.P., Wallace, C.J., Vaughn, C.E., Snyder, K.S. & Rust, C. (1980) Social and family factors in the course of schizophrenia: toward an interpersonal problem-solving therapy for schizophrenics and their relatives. In: *Psychotherapy of Schizophrenia: Current Status and Future Directions* (eds J. Strauss, J. Fleck & M. Bowers), pp. 21–54. Plenum, New York.

Liberman, R.P., Mueser, K.T., Wallace, C.J. et al. (1986) Training skills in the psychiatrically disabled: learning coping and competence. *Schizophrenia Bulletin* **12**, 631–647.

Liberman, R.P., De Risi, W.J. & Mueser, K. (1989) *Social Skills Training for Psychiatric Patients*. Pergamon Press, New York.

Liberman, R.P., Wallace, C.J., Blackwell, G. et al. (1993) Innovations in skills training for the seriously mentally ill: the UCLA Social and Independent Living Skills Modules. *Innovations and Research* **2**, 43–60.

Liberman, R.P., Kopelowicz, A. & Young, A.S. (1994) Biobehavioral treatment and rehabilitation of schizophrenia. *Behavior Therapy* **25**, 89–107.

Liberman, R.P., Wallace, C.J., Blackwell, G. et al. (1998) Skills training versus psychosocial occupational therapy for persons with persistent schizophrenia. *American Journal of Psychiatry* **155**, 1087–1091.

Liberman, R.P., Kopelowicz, A. & Smith, T.E. (1999) Psychiatric rehabilitation. In: *Comprehensive Textbook of Psychiatry*, 7th edn (eds B.J. Sadock & V. Sadock), pp. 3218–3245. Lippincott: Williams & Wilkins, Baltimore.

Liberman, R.P., Eckman, T.A. & Marder, S.R. (2001) Training in social problem-solving among person with schizophrenia. *Psychiatric Services* **52**, 31–33.

Lysaker, P.H. & Bell, M. (1995) Work rehabilitation and improvements in insight in schizophrenia. *Journal of Nervous and Mental Disease* **183**, 103–106.

Lysaker, P.H., Bell, M., Zito, W.S. & Bioty, S.M. (1995) Social skills at work: deficits and predictors of improvement in schizophrenia. *Journal of Nervous and Mental Disease* **183**, 688–692.

McKee, M., Hull, J.W. & Smith, T.E. (1997) Cognitive and symptom correlates of participation in social skills training groups. *Schizophrenia Research* **23**, 223–229.

Maley, R.F., Feldman, G.L. & Ruskin, R.S. (1973) Evaluation of patient improvement in a token economy treatment program. *Journal of Abnormal Psychology* **82**, 141–144.

Marder, S.R., Wirshing, W.C., Mintz, J. *et al.* (1996) Two-year outcome of social skills training and group psychotherapy for outpatients with schizophrenia. *American Journal of Psychiatry* **153**, 1585–1592.

Massel, H.K., Liberman, R.P., Mintz, J. *et al.* (1990) Evaluating the capacity to work of the mentally ill. *Psychiatry* **53**, 31–44.

Medalia, A., Aluma, M., Tryon, W. & Merriam, A.E. (1998) Effectiveness of attention training in schizophrenia. *Schizophrenia Bulletin* **24**, 147–152.

Meichenbaum, D.M. & Cameron, R. (1973) Training schizophrenics to talk to themselves: a means of developing attentional controls. *Behavior Therapy* **4**, 515–534.

Meltzer, H.Y. (1992) Dimensions of outcome with clozapine. *British Journal of Psychiatry* **160**, 46–53.

Meltzer, H., Gill, B., Petticrew, M. *et al.* (1995) OPCS surveys of psychiatric morbidity in Great Britain. Report 1: the prevalence of psychotic morbidity among adults living in private house holds. HMSO, London.

Monroe-DeVita, M.B. & Mohatt, D.F. (1999) The state hospital and the community: an essential continuum for persons with severe and persistent mental illness. *New Directions in Mental Health Services* **84**, 85–97.

Mueser, K.T. & Bond, G.R. (2000) Psychosocial treatment approaches for schizophrenia. *Current Opinion in Psychiatry* **13**, 27–35.

Mueser, K.T. & Liberman, R.P. (1988) Skills training in vocational rehabilitation. In: *Vocational Rehabilitation of Persons with Prolonged Mental Illness* (eds J.A. Ciardello & M.D. Bell), pp. 81–103. Johns Hopkins University Press, Baltimore.

Mueser, K.T., Bellack, A.S., Douglas, M.S. & Wade, J.H. (1991) Predictions of social skill acquisition in schizophrenia and major affective disorder patients from memory and symptomatology. *Psychiatry Research* **37**, 381–396.

Mueser, K.T., Kosmidis, M.H. & Sayers, M.D. (1992) Symptomatology and the prediction of social skills acquisition in schizophrenia. *Schizophrenia Research* **8**, 59–68.

Mueser, K.T., Bond, G.R., Drake, R.E. & Resnick, S.G. (1998) Models of community care for severe mental illness: a review of research on case management. *Schizophrenia Bulletin* **24**, 37–74.

O'Driscoll, C., Wills, W., Leff, J. & Margolius, O. (1993) The TAPS Project 10: the long-stay populations of Friern and Claybury hospitals – the baseline survey. *British Journal of Psychiatry* **162**, 30–35.

Ogilvie, R.J. (1997) The state of supported housing for mental health consumers: a literature review. *Psychiatric Rehabilitation Journal* **21**, 122–131.

Okin, R.L. & Pearsall, D. (1993) Patients perceptions of their quality of life 11 years after discharge from a state hospital. *Hospital and Community Psychiatry* **44**, 236–240.

Olbrich, R. & Mussgay, L. (1990) Reduction of schizophrenic deficits by cognitive training: an evaluative study. *European Archives of Psychiatry and Clinical Neuroscience* **239**, 366–369.

van Os, J., Fahy, T., Jones, P. *et al.* (1995) Increased intracerebral cerebrospinal fluid spaces predict unemployment and negative symptoms of psychotic illness: a prospective study. *British Journal of Psychiatry* **166**, 750–758.

Paul, G.L. & Lentz, R.J. (1977) *Psychosocial Treatments of Chronic Mental Patients: Milieu Versus Social-Learning Programs.* Harvard University Press, Cambridge, MA.

Penn, D.L. & Mueser, K.T. (1996) Research update on the psychosocial treatment of schizophrenia. *American Journal of Psychiatry* **153**, 607–617.

Phillips, S.D., Burns, B.J., Edgar, E.R. *et al.* (2001) Moving assertive community treatment into standard practice. *Psychiatric Services* **52**, 771–779.

Schwartz, G. (1998) Incube Inc. & the TAP Program: an innovative program for consumer-run business development in New York City. *Life in the Day* **2**, 6–11.

Scott, J.E. & Dixon, L.B. (1995) Psychological interventions for schizophrenia. *Schizophrenia Bulletin* **21**, 621–630.

Shepherd, G., Murray, A. & Muijen, M. (1994) Relative values: the differing views of users, family carers and professionals on services for people with schizophrenia in the community. Sainsbury Centre for Mental Health, London.

Shern, D.L., Felton, C.J., Hough, R.L. *et al.* (1997) Housing outcomes for homeless adults with mental illness: results from the second-round McKinney program. *Psychiatric Services* **48**, 239–241.

Silverstein, S.M., Pierce, D.L., Saytes, M. *et al.* (1998) Behavioral treatment of attentional dysfunction in chronic, treatment-refractory schizophrenia. *Psychiatric Quarterly* **69**, 95–105.

Silverstein, S., Menditto, A., Stuvey, P. *et al.* (1999) Shaping procedures as cognitive retraining techniques in individuals with severe and persistent mental illness. *Psychiatric Rehabilitation Skills* **3**, 59–76.

Skinner, B.F. (1953) *Science and Human Behavior.* Macmillan, New York.

Smith, T.E., Hull, J.W., Romanelli, S., Fertuck, E. & Weiss, K.A. (1999) Symptoms and neurocognition as rate limiters in skills training for psychotic patients. *American Journal of Psychiatry* **156**, 1817–1818.

Snyder, K.S., Wallace, C.J., Moe, K. & Liberman, R.P. (1994) Expressed emotion by residential care operators and residents symptoms and quality of life. *Hospital and Community Psychiatry* **45**, 1141–1143.

Spaulding, W.D. (1993) Schizophrenia: origins, processes, treatment, and outcome. In: *Contemporary Psychology*, Vol. 38 (eds R.L. Cromwell & C.R. Snyder), pp. 299–312. Oxford University Press, New York.

Spaulding, W.D. & Sullivan, M. (1991) From the laboratory to the clinic: psychological methods and principles in psychiatric rehabilitation. In: *Handbook of Psychiatric Rehabilitation* (ed. R.P. Liberman), pp. 30–55. MacMillan, New York.

Spaulding, W.D., Storms, L., Goodrich, V. & Sullivan, M. (1986) Applications of experimental psychopathology in psychiatric rehabilitation. *Schizophrenia Bulletin* **12**, 560–577.

Spaulding, W.D., Reed, D.R., Sullivan, M., Richardson, C. & Weiler, M. (1999) Effects of cognitive treatment in psychiatric rehabilitation. *Schizophrenia Bulletin* **25**, 657–676.

Stein, L.I. & Santos, A.B. (1998) *Assertive Community Treatment of Persons with Severe Mental Illness.* W.W. Norton, New York.

Stein, L.I. & Test, M.A. (1980) Alternative to mental hospital treatment. I. Conceptual model, treatment program and clinical evaluation. *Archives of General Psychiatry* **37**, 392–397.

Storzbach, D.M. & Corrigan, P.W. (1996) Cognitive rehabilitation for schizophrenia. In: *Cognitive Rehabilitation for Neuropsychiatric Disorders* (eds P.W. Corrigan & S.C. Yudofsky), pp. 299–328. American Psychiatric Press, Washington, DC.

Strauss, J. (1994) The person with schizophrenia as a person. II. Approaches to the subjective and complex. *British Journal of Psychiatry* **164**, 103–107.

Strauss, J. & Carpenter, W.T. (1977) The prediction of outcome in schizophrenia. III. Five-year outcome and its predictors. *Archives of General Psychiatry* **34**, 159–163.

Stuve, P. & Menditto, A.A. (1999) State hospitals in the new millenium: rehabilitating the 'not ready for rehab' players. *New Directions in Mental Health Services* **84**, 35–46.

Stuve, P., Erickson, R.C. & Spaulding, W. (1991) Cognitive rehabilitation: the next step in psychiatric rehabilitation. *Psychosocial Rehabilitation Journal* **15**, 9–26.

Tarrier, N., Barrowclough, C., Vaughn, C. *et al.* (1988) The community managment of schizophrenia: a controlled trial of a behavioral intervention with families to reduce relapse. *British Journal of Psychiatry* **153**, 532–542.

Tarrier, N., Barrowclough, C., Porceddu, K. & Fitzpatrick, E. (1994) The Salford Family Intervention Project: relapse rates of schizophrenia at 5 and 8 years. *British Journal of Psychiatry* **165**, 829–832.

Tauber, R., Wallace, C.J. & Lecomte, T. (2000) Enlisting indigenous community supporters in skills training programs for persons with severe mental illness. *Psychiatric Services* **51**, 1428–1432.

Test, M.A. (1992) Training in community living. In: *Handbook of Psychiatric Rehabilitation* (ed. R.P. Liberman), pp. 153–170. Macmillan, New York.

Thornicroft, G., Wykes, T., Holloway, F., Johnson, S. & Szmukler, G. (1998) From efficacy to effectiveness in community mental health services: PRISM Psychosis Study. *British Journal of Psychiatry* **173**, 423–427.

Trower, P., Bryant, B. & Argyle, M. (1978) *Social Skills and Mental Health*. Methuen, London.

Tsang, H.W.H. & Pearson, V. (2001) Work-related social skills training for people with schizophrenia in Hong Kong. *Schizophrenia Bulletin* **27**, 139–148.

Tsemberis, S. & Eisenberg, R.F. (2000) Pathways to housing: supported housing for street-dwelling homeless individuals with psychiatric disabilities. *Psychiatric Services* **51**, 487–493.

Van der Gaag, M. (1992) *The Results of Cognitive Training in Schizophrenic Patients*. Eburon, Delft.

Van der Gaag, M., Woonings, F., van den Bosch, R.J. *et al.* (1994) Cognitive training of schizophrenic patients: a behavioral approach based on experimental psychopathology. In: *Cognitive Technology in Psychiatric Rehabilitation* (ed. W. Spaulding), pp. 139–158. University of Nebraska Press, Lincoln.

Van der Gaag, M., Kern, R.S., Van den Bosch, R.J. & Liberman, R.P. (2002) A controlled trial of cognitive remediation in schizophrenia. *Schizophrenia Bulletin* **28**, 167–176.

Vaughn, C.E. & Leff, J.P. (1976) The influence of family and social factors on the course of psychiatric illness: a comparison of schizophrenic and depressed neurotic patients. *British Journal of Psychiatry* **129**, 125–137.

Vaughn, C.E., Snyder, K.S., Freeman, W. *et al.* (1982) Family factors in schizophrenic relapse: a replication. *Schizophrenia Bulletin* **8**, 425–426.

Velligan, D.I., Mahurin, R.K., Diamond, P.L. *et al.* (1997) The functional significance of symptomatology and cognitive function in schizophrenia. *Schizophrenia Research* **25**, 21–31.

Velligan, D.I., Newcomer, J.W., Pultz, J. *et al.* (1999) Changes in cognitive function with quetiapine fumarate versus haloperidol. In: *1999 Annual Meeting New Research Program Abstracts*, p. 247. American Psychiatric Association, Washington, DC.

Velligan, D.I., Bow-Thomas, C.C., Huntzinger, C. *et al.* (2000) Randomized controlled trial of the use of compensatory strategies to enhance adaptive functioning in outpatients with schizophrenia. *American Journal of Psychiatry* **157**, 1317–1323.

Wallace, C.J., Boone, S.E., Donahoe, C.P. & Foy, D.W. (1985) The chronic mentally disabled: indpendent living skills training. In: *Clinical Handbook of Psychological Disorders: a Step-by-Step Treatment Manual* (ed. D. Barlow), pp. 147–168. Guilford, New York.

Wallace, C.J., Liberman, R.P., MacKain, S.J., Blackwell, G. & Eckman, T.A. (1992) Effectiveness and replicability of modules for teaching social instrumental skills to the severely mentally ill. *American Journal of Psychiatry* **149**, 654–658.

Wallace, C.J., Tauber, R. & Wilde, J. (1999) Teaching fundamental workplace skills to persons with serious mental illness. *Psychiatric Services* **50**, 1147–1153.

Wallace, C.J., Lecomte, T., Wilde, J. & Liberman, R.P. (2001a) CASIG: a consumer-centered assessment for planning individualized treatment and evaluating program outcomes. *Schizophrenia Research* **50**, 105–119.

Wallace, C.J., Liberman, R.P., Kopelowicz, A. & Yaeger, D. (2001b) Psychiatric rehabilitation. In: *Treatments of Psychiatric Disorders: the DSM IV Edition* (ed. G.O. Gabbard), pp. 1093–1112. American Psychiatric Press, Washington, DC.

Warner, R. (1994) *Recovery from Schizophrenia: Psychiatry and Political Economy,* .Routledge & Kegan Paul, London.

Wincze, J.P., Leitenberg, H. *et al.* (1972) The effect of token reinforcement and feedback on delusional verbal behavior of chronic paranoid schizophrenics. *Journal of Applied Behavior Analysis* **5**, 247–262.

Wong, S.E., Flanagan, S.G., Kuehnel, T.G. *et al.* (1988) Training chronic mental patients to independently practice personal grooming skills. *Hospital and Community Psychiatry* **39**, 874–879.

Wykes, T., Reeder, C., Corner, J., Williams, C. & Everitt, B. (1999) The effects of neurocognitive remediation on executive processing in patients with schizophrenia. *Schizophrenia Bulletin* **25**, 291–307.

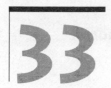

33 Psychological treatments for schizophrenia

B.V. Martindale, K.T. Mueser, E. Kuipers, T. Sensky and L. Green

General principles of psychosocial treatment
   strategies, 658
   Psychological therapies and psychosis, 658
   Special needs and considerations, 659
   Early interventions in psychosis, 663

Specific types of therapy for schizophrenia, 664
   Family interventions, 664
   Individual and group psychotherapies, 667
Future directions of psychological treatments, 678
References, 679

The very idea of psychological interventions having a role in the treatment of schizophrenia has a long complex history of acceptance and rejection which has mirrored to some extent the prevailing theories of the nature of the disorder. It also has to be recognized that even when there is solid empirical evidence for the effectiveness of a psychological intervention, there appear to be considerable obstacles to be overcome in making such interventions more available (Lehman *et al.* 1998; Leff 2000). This contrasts considerably with the rush to implementation that greets an advance in the pharmacological treatment of schizophrenia.

Whereas Kraepelin (1919/1971) and his predecessors made few recommendations on psychological treatments, Bleuler (1911/1950), on the other hand, devoted a significant part of the chapter on 'Therapy' in his book *Dementia Praecox or The Group of Schizophrenias* to discussion of the influence of psychosocial factors on the illness and its treatment. Bleuler wrote: 'At the present time, the only type of therapy that can seriously be considered for schizophrenia as a whole is the psychic method.' It is clear from Bleuler's writings that he believed that psychotherapy for schizophrenia could be clinically effective, although this optimism was tempered by his frank acknowledgement that little was known as to how the treatment should be conducted.

Following Bleuler's writings, a split emerged in the academic psychiatry community as to whether schizophrenia could be treated with psychotherapy. Freud did not rule out the possibility of therapy for schizophrenia in his early writings, but over time he grew more pessimistic and adamant that successful therapy could not be carried out on the basis of: 'The incapacity of these patients for transference (so far as the pathological process extends), their consequent inaccessibility to therapeutic efforts' (Freud 1915, p. 197).

Despite Freud's influence, many psychoanalysts disagreed and found that it was possible to develop therapeutic relationships with persons with psychosis. Sullivan was particularly influential. In the 1920s he developed an inpatient treatment unit specializing in the intensive treatment of young men with schizophrenia (Sullivan 1962). He viewed schizophrenia as a return to earlier childhood forms of communication resulting from problematic relationships, and he developed psychotherapeutic interventions designed to correct these relationships. In 1927, Sullivan (1994) anticipated the modern focus on early interventions. Like Sullivan, Fromm-Reichman (1950) also strongly maintained that patients with schizophrenia retain some capacity to relate to others interpersonally, setting the stage for therapeutic work based on psychodynamic principles, but differing from traditional psychoanalysis in technique.

Although early controlled trials challenged the use of therapy based on the psychoanalytic approach of the time, many ideas stemming from psychoanalysis permeate contemporary psychological approaches such as cognitive–behavioural therapy (CBT) that show promising signs of being useful in treatment approaches (Martindale 1998; Furlan 1999; Bateman 2000) and are also an important feature in understanding patients' problems in the need-adapted approach (Alanen 1997a), some group approaches (Schermer & Pines 1999; Kanas 2000) and in linking with contemporary family interventions (Migone 1995).

Although classical psychoanalytic technique is very rarely used in persons with psychosis, psychoanalysts have made considerable contributions to further understanding the unconscious mental processes in psychosis and have treated patients with psychotic problems, sometimes with apparent therapeutic success (Rosenfeld 1965; Searles 1965; Bion 1967; Robbins 1993). These clinicians and others have also raised awareness of the very difficult emotional and other psychological states that therapists will encounter in themselves when they work primarily within the relationship established with the patients. These understandings have helped other clinicians' attempts to maintain empathic relationships with patients with psychotic conditions. Some of their work has formed a basis for the view that early relationships have an important role in increasing later vulnerability to psychosis (Winnicott 1965). Sadly, these latter theories were also used to attribute blame to families

(Appleton 1974; Terkelsen 1983), which impeded formal research and therapeutic endeavours with families. However, these ideas have regained renewed support from the work of researchers such as Tienari *et al.* (1994), who have studied the relative contributions of nature and nurture to schizophrenia. Their findings offer support to contemporary views concerning the place of interventions in prodromal phases. This is well discussed by McGorry (2000b).

Psychoanalysts working in public and institutional settings have modified the traditional psychoanalytic techniques; e.g. those of Rosen (1953) and Searles (1965); and more radical approaches such as those of Sechehaye (1956) and Laing (1960). These were based partly on the ability of the individual therapist or those in therapeutic community settings to share the patient's psychotic experience while maintaining a supportive relationship with the patient. Pullen (1999) has described the strengths and weaknesses of these approaches, especially when used in a therapeutic community setting.

Following the advent of neuroleptic medications, a number of controlled trials compared the use of neuroleptics with psychotherapeutic treatments based on the psychoanalytic ideas and techniques of the time. These are discussed below. With few exceptions, the conclusion of these trials was that there did not seem to be demonstrable benefit from psychotherapy. In spite of the fact that there were serious limitations in all of the trials (Karon 1989), the prevailing climate in psychiatry changed, especially in the USA where psychoanalysis had had dominance over other approaches. The rapid advances in neuroscience and neuropharmacology in the last three decades led to a strong swing of emphasis from psychological to biological approaches. For some decades, the main focus of treatment has been on medication for a narrow aspect of schizophrenia (its positive symptoms). The idea of the relationship as having therapeutic potential in itself has been ignored.

In recent years the pendulum has started to swing again. Clinical trials of formal psychological treatments, which have used counselling or non-specific befriending as a further control group alongside the 'treatment as usual, mainly medication' control group (Tarrier *et al.* 1998, 1999; Sensky *et al.* 2000), have reported surprisingly good results leading to interest in the importance of the non-specific therapeutic powers of the treatment relationship and the importance of forming a good working alliance with the patient (Paley & Shapiro 2002).

Related to these changes in awareness, some centres – particularly in Scandinavia – have reversed the emphasis that regards other therapies as subsidiary or supplementary to medication. In the Scandinavian need-adapted approach, neuroleptics are important agents used in moderation when there is need for additional support for psychotherapeutically and psychosocially orientated therapy (Alanen 1997a).

This chapter examines a range of contemporary psychological approaches to patients with psychosis.

General principles of psychosocial treatment strategies

Psychological therapies and psychosis

The therapeutic alliance

Whatever the therapeutic goals, be they biological, social or psychological, we would argue that a high degree of psychological sensitivity is necessary for all professionals if they are to be successfully involved in the treatment of persons with psychosis and their families. Recent guidelines stress the importance of staff attitudes and state that the effectiveness of any treatment depends on a good, trusting and collaborative relationship between the service user and the clinician (British Psychological Society 2000).

User and carer dissatisfaction is often related to a lack of sensitivity of staff to the needs and distress of the user and the family. Ball *et al.* (1992) found poorer outcome for clients in a naturalistic study of a hostel characterized by a high expressed emotion style of management compared with a low expressed emotion hostel. Snyder *et al.* (1994) found that critical attitudes in staff were associated with a poorer quality of life for residents.

Some research trials have compared a specific psychological treatment modality for psychosis with control groups that include both 'simple' befriending or supportive counselling controls as well as 'treatment as usual'. They have found that patients improved on a number of scales in the first two groups and outcomes were not greatly distinguishable from one another in many aspects but they were both statistically better improved than the 'treatment as usual' control (Tarrier *et al.* 1998; Sensky *et al.* 2000). This would indicate that 'treatment as usual' lacks a sufficiently empathic and supportive relationship and that these factors can have ameliorative power.

Other studies also point to the quality of the helping alliance being associated with a more favourable outcome with severely disturbed patients in both psychiatric inpatient treatment (Clarkin *et al.* 1987) and in community care treatments (Priebe & Gruyters 1993). Patients with schizophrenia who are dissatisfied with their treatment are more likely to drop out from treatment and to be rehospitalized (Priebe & Bröker 1999).

A psychological attitude

Cullberg (2000) succinctly addressed the importance of a humanistic approach when he stated:

How fruitful and essential it is to keep (both) the humanistic and biological perspectives alive in the understanding of, and the work with, psychotic conditions.
Important human experiences can easily be depreciated and slip through our fingers if approval is only given to knowledge that is built on evidence-based, controlled research. Conversely, there is the danger that the personal notions of professionals are accepted in an uncritical way.

McGorry (2000) echoes the importance of a psychological perspective in writing: While the potential quality of psychopharmacological treatment of psychosis has improved substantially over the past decade, and the systems for providing treatment and care have also been enhanced in many countries, the loss of a psychological and personal perspective has meant that mental health professionals have become deskilled and ill-equipped to properly understand their patients and to respond with skill to their human and developmental needs.

Cultural issues

Psychological attitudes should include the careful consideration of culturally sensitive issues that may have an important role in psychotic conditions.

Case example

An unmarried Asian woman admitted to a Western hemisphere hospital in a severe suicidal and psychotic state was discovered to be pregnant. Although she was not conscious of her pregnancy, she spoke of an alien that she was trying to kill. After some time it transpired that this alien referred not only to the shame in her family both from her pregnancy and extramarital sexuality, but also the identity of the father of the child, which would cause additional unbearable shame and disappointment, especially to her own elderly and caring father and his immediate family who maintained values of a traditional Hindu caste. The patient had long struggled with her dual but conflicting loyalties to the cultural codes of her parents and the very different codes of younger persons in her adoptive country.

A culturally sensitive approach may also allow for greater recognition of the traditional cultural healing means and the dangers of assuming that the recommendations of the mental health professional are acceptable and understood in the culture of the disturbed person and their family (Jablensky et al. 1992; Rosen 1994).

Range of psychological therapy modalities and goals in psychosis

The loss of psychological skills, which McGorry (2000) refers to, has come about partly because of the overly optimistic expectation that neuroscience would find pharmacological solutions to the numerous and multifaceted problems characteristic of schizophrenia. There is now a resurgence of interest in psychosocial approaches. They have potential relevance to many aspects of care and treatment and the research base is slowly accumulating. Below is a list of a few of the areas in which psychological approaches are relevant:

Attaining and sustaining a therapeutic relationship
Making an (ongoing) assessment and formulation of the current major psychological issues at each stage of the course of the disturbance
Identifying psychological strengths and potential assets
Working alongside the family (many different methods)
Targeting expressed emotion
Early psychological intervention
  (i) prodromal states
  (ii) psychotic states
Reducing the duration of untreated psychosis in the community
Medication compliance
Relapse prevention
Reducing the severity of enduring psychotic states
Specific focus on hallucinations and delusions
Decoding the unconscious meaning of psychotic symptoms
Retaining/recovering other skills and capacities
Helping young people to re-engage with developmental trajectories
Substance misuse programmes
Working on traumas that have preceded the psychosis, and ushered in the psychosis, and/or the traumatic effects of a psychotic breakdown
Helping with personality difficulties existent prior to the psychosis, including low self-esteem and relationship difficulties
Providing a supportive relationship
Attending to cognitive defects

The following are just some of the psychological methods and/or theoretical frameworks likely to be useful in some persons with psychosis:

Cognitive–behavioural approaches
Psychoeducational approaches
Interpersonal therapy
Psychodynamic and psychoanalytic theories and treatments
Need-adapted therapy
Problem-solving therapies
Art and music therapy
Systemic approaches
Motivational interviewing (linked with CBT)

Many of these approaches can be offered in individual, group, therapeutic community and family contexts. It is important to acknowledge that there may be profound differences between professionals as to what they see as treatment even if they all espouse a psychological approach. To put things at their most extreme: on the one hand there are professionals who see schizophrenia as a disorder with defined symptoms and the focus of treatment is on removing or reducing the symptoms by whatever treatment works for the patient. At the other extreme are professionals whose main long-term focus is improving the capacities and personality of the person vulnerable to psychosis. Despite differences in approaches and foci of treatment, a common element of all psychotherapies for schizophrenia, as with other disorders, is helping patients to achieve personal goals, whether directly illness-related or not. The beneficial role of medication is reviewed elsewhere in this book.

Special needs and considerations

Researchers, clinicians and family members are often disappointed by the relatively modest gains achieved by patients with schizophrenia in psychotherapy. On the one hand, small gains may reflect the limitations of currently available treatments. On the other hand, a poor understanding of the deficits and special needs of patients with schizophrenia may lead to unrealistic expectations for success, and disappointment when expectations are not met. Five particular factors need to be taken into account when providing psychotherapy for schizophrenia and evaluating the results:

1 the importance of comprehensive and long-term treatment;
2 individual differences in treatment needs;
3 the role of the patient;
4 the limitations imposed by cognitive deficits; and
5 therapist variables.

Comprehensive and long-term treatment

Since the earliest descriptions of schizophrenia, its pervasive and chronic nature has been understood to be an integral part of the illness. Similar conceptualizations of schizophrenia persist in modern diagnostic systems for the disorder. According to the DSM-IV (American Psychiatric Association 1994), schizophrenia is defined not only by the presence of specific negative, positive and cognitive symptoms, but also in terms of impaired psychosocial functioning, including problems establishing and maintaining social relationships, capacity for competitive work, and self-care and independent living skills *with impaired functioning lasting at least 6 months*. Although longitudinal data have challenged the assumption that schizophrenia necessarily has a deteriorating course (Harding *et al.* 1987a,b), the illness, when defined by a disturbance that has already lasted 6 months, is one that can be life-long in its severity for about 50% (Bleuler 1972; Ciompi & Müller 1976; Tsuang *et al.* 1979). The net result is that patients often need assistance in meeting a wide variety of needs, ranging from learning how to handle the tasks of day-to-day living, to engaging in social interactions, coping with depression and the management of psychotic symptoms.

The need for extended comprehensive treatment of schizophrenia for a significant percentage of patients has long been recognized (Ciompi 1987b; Wing 1987). In recent years, the importance of comprehensive treatment has become even more apparent as recognition has grown of common associated problems in persons with schizophrenia. For example, persons with schizophrenia and other severe mental illnesses are more likely to have problems related to substance abuse (Regier *et al.* 1990), housing instability and homelessness (Susser *et al.* 1989), trauma and post-traumatic stress disorder (Mueser *et al.* 1998) and infectious diseases such as the hepatitis C virus (Rosenberg *et al.* 2001). For those in whom the illness has become relatively established, psychotherapy has the best chance of being effective if patients' external circumstances are relatively stable and in the context of comprehensive treatment that addresses housing, medical factors and other comorbid disorders that can have a profound impact on the course of the illness.

While the treatment for schizophrenia needs to be compre-

hensive and long-term for many, the duration of psychotherapy may vary, depending on the focus of therapy. Some patients may benefit from long-term psychosocial interventions throughout their lives, while others may require more limited therapy. Clinical expectations need to take into account the limitations of brief psychotherapy.

Individual differences in treatment needs

The heterogeneity of schizophrenia has often been interpreted as reflecting either multiple aetiologies or multiple disease entities (Carpenter *et al.* 1993; Tsuang & Faraone 1995). Despite this heterogeneity, the search has continued for a unitary model of psychotherapy for all patients. One negative consequence of this search has been that many individuals' needs go unmet. Another consequence is that interventions that are effective for some patients may be prematurely abandoned because their effects are not sufficiently robust for the whole group. Only some of the differences are described below.

Cognitive functioning

Evidence of heterogeneity in areas commonly assumed to be impaired in schizophrenia underscores the importance of individual differences. Significant variability has been found on the Wisconsin Card Sorting Test (WCST; Heaton 1991) which reflects prefrontal cortical functioning. Although patients with schizophrenia have repeatedly been found to perform more poorly on the WCST (Berman *et al.* 1986; Weinberger *et al.* 1986), the performance of many patients is in the normal range (Bellack *et al.* 1990a; Braff *et al.* 1991). Also, among patients with impairments on the WCST, there is considerable variety in the extent to which they can be taught to improve their performance (Goldberg *et al.* 1987; Bellack *et al.* 1990b).

Social skills

Similar evidence of heterogeneity exists in social skills. Mueser *et al.* (1991a) found that 50% of schizophrenia patients had persistent deficits in social skills over a 1-year period, while 11% did not differ from non-patient controls, and the remainder showed variable performance. Thus, the common assumption that patients with schizophrenia have deficits in their social skills is true for many but not for all patients.

Changes over time

In addition to the variability between patients, significant changes occur within patients over time and these have a bearing on their treatment needs. Young patients need special help in dealing with the fact that they have a serious illness which may interfere with their personal goals and their ability to achieve independence (Jackson *et al.* 2001), a problem which may contribute to their high vulnerability to suicide and substance abuse (Test *et al.* 1989; Caldwell & Gottesman 1990). Because of a reluctance to accept having a mental illness, young patients often have the most problems with adhering to treatment recommendations (Amador *et al.* 1991; Amador & Gorman 1998) such as taking medication regularly (McEvoy *et al.* 1989) and are therefore most prone to frequent relapses and rehospitalizations.

Older patients may adjust to the difficulties of the illness through withdrawal or positive coping strategies (Wing 1987; Strauss 1989) but they face unique problems of their own. For example, parents are unable to continue caring for an offspring with schizophrenia as the patient grows older, necessitating a shift in caretaking responsibility to either siblings (Horwitz *et al.* 1992) or the mental health system (Bartels *et al.* 1997). A survey of the needs of schizophrenia patients in regular contact with their families indicated that concern over what happens when a parent dies was ranked fourth highest out of 45 topics (parents ranked this concern fifth) (Mueser *et al.* 1992). These concerns are justified as increased support services are required to help elders with schizophrenia continue to live in the community as they lose their natural support systems (Bartels & Levine 1998; Bartels *et al.* 1999).

Consequences of trauma and abuse

It is often overlooked that patients with psychotic disorders have a much higher likelihood of having experienced physical and sexual abuse and trauma than the general population (Ross *et al.* 1994; Read 1997; Mueser *et al.* 2002). Mueser *et al.* (2002) point out that post-traumatic stress disorder (PTSD) is therefore likely to be common but, in fact, it is rarely diagnosed. As controlled research indicates that PTSD can be effectively treated in the general population, the possibility of this group of patients with PTSD should be considered and the likelihood of treatment benefits certainly should be carefully evaluated.

In order for psychotherapy to meet the real needs of patients, interpatient differences and changes over time need to be taken into account. Clinical practice must attempt to distinguish between shared and individual needs in the provision of psychotherapy. Research is sorely needed that addresses which patients will profit from which interventions.

Role of the patient

The problems of psychosis experienced by patients with schizophrenia, combined with negative symptoms (e.g. apathy, anhedonia) have often led to the false assumption that patients are not capable of actively participating in their own treatment. Indeed, many patients seem unmotivated and are unco-operative with their treatment. However, such apparent disinterest and passivity should not be interpreted as immutable traits.

Negative symptoms are not always stable over time and may be secondary to demoralization, psychotic symptoms, medication side-effects and other factors that vary with time. McGlashan and Fenton (1992), Carpenter *et al.* (1988) and Paul and Lentz (1977) have shown that even extremely withdrawn

chronic schizophrenia patients can be motivated by a systematic incentive programme. In addition, there is a growing body of evidence that schizophrenia patients actively employ coping strategies to manage persistent symptoms and share these strategies with one another (Wiedl & Schottner 1991; Mueser *et al.* 1997b).

Strauss (1989) has argued that it is important to view schizophrenia patients as having an active 'will', and that their behaviour is goal-directed and reflects an attempt to cope with the illness as best they can. Several implications follow from this assumption. First, if patients are actively trying to cope, they may benefit from learning basic information about their illness and factors that may influence their vulnerability to relapse. Educating patients about schizophrenia and its management can enable them to become more active participants in the treatment of their own illness (Ascher-Svanum & Krause 1991; Schaub 1998; Klingberg *et al.* 1999). Nevertheless, patient education is far from the norm and little research has addressed the question of what should be taught and when and how.

A second implication of Strauss's suggestion (Strauss 1989) is that patients are capable of learning specific strategies for coping with psychotic symptoms. Persistent psychotic symptoms are present in a substantial proportion of patients in the postacute stage of their illness (Harrow & Silverstein 1977; Silverstein & Harrow 1978) and are associated with high levels of distress (Falloon & Talbot 1981; Mueser *et al.* 1991c). There are numerous case reports describing the successful use of behaviour modification techniques to control psychotic symptoms (Bellack 1986), and one controlled trial (Tarrier *et al.* 1993a,b). Although these techniques are not likely to produce enduring fundamental changes in the illness, they may reduce the subjective distress associated with chronic psychotic symptoms and better enable patients to pursue personal goals.

A third implication of viewing the patient as actively coping with the illness is the need to involve him or her in goal setting and treatment planning. Treatments are too often imposed on patients by the treatment team and family. As a consequence, patients often fail to adhere to treatment recommendations, increasing their risk of relapse and creating tensions in their relationships with family members and treatment providers. To be sure, engaging the patient to establish treatment goals can be a long arduous process. Failure to do so, however, courts the larger risk of undermining the very purpose of treatment.

Engaging patients as partners in the treatment process is critical to addressing the concerns of many patients who have expressed dissatisfaction with the traditional hierarchical relationship between patients and psychiatric treatment providers (Chamberlin 1978; Segal *et al.* 1993). In addition to the lack of attention to patients' own perceived needs, specific concerns expressed by patients about mental health practices include the use of coercive interventions, lack of respect, overpathologizing normal reactions, and encouraging them to passively accept the 'patient' role (Chamberlin & Rogers 1990; Deegan 1990; Carling 1995). Psychotherapy needs to take place in a context of a mutual understanding and respect for the patient's ultimate right to make decisions concerning his or her own treatment.

Limitations imposed by cognitive deficits

Schizophrenia is characterized by a wide variety of impairments in information processing, including memory, attention, speed of processing, abstract reasoning and sensorimotor integration (Sharma & Harvey 2000). These impairments in cognitive functioning are associated with impairments in functioning, including self-care skills, capacity for independent living and social relationships (Penn *et al.* 1995; Green 1996; Green *et al.* 2000). Despite the voluminous literature on cognitive deficits in schizophrenia, psychosocial treatments rarely take these deficits into account beyond presenting information more slowly and repeatedly. This single strategy is insufficient to address the range of cognitive impairments that affect how information is acquired and utilized by these patients. Effective techniques need to be incorporated into psychosocial programmes.

Two issues need to be addressed in order to improve existing psychotherapy technologies that take into account the cognitive impairments of the illness. First, the influence of cognitive deficits on learning and retention in treatment must be determined so that treatments can be modified accordingly. For example, poor memory has been shown to be associated with a slower rate of skill acquisition in social skills training, while pretreatment psychotic symptoms tend to be unrelated to skills acquisition (Silverstein *et al.* 1998; Mueser *et al.* 1991b; Kern *et al.* 1992). These findings suggest that longer or more intensive training may be necessary to produce positive outcomes.

The second issue is the impact of cognitive deficits on the generalization of treatment effects. A basic pretext of all psychotherapy is that information learned in the session must be generalized to the patient's natural environment. Yet, such generalization is contingent upon cognitive processes that are often disrupted in schizophrenia. Research has begun to focus more closely on the enhancement of cognitive functioning as a critical treatment goal (Sharma & Harvey 2000). However, cognitive impairment remains a reality in the treatment of most patients with schizophrenia, and strategies are needed to promote the generalization of targeted skills into patients' natural environments. Until effective cognitive rehabilitation methods have been demonstrated, the generalization of skills may need to be facilitated through the prompting of these skills by clinicians or natural supports in the community (Tauber *et al.* 2000). Cognitive rehabilitation techniques are reviewed later in this chapter.

In addition to the limitations imposed by cognitive impairment on the retention and generalization skills, problems with abstract thinking and concept formation in schizophrenia can limit the ability of patients to participate in some insight-orientated interventions. When providing supportive humanistic treatment, the pace of psychotherapy must be slow and comfortable, with frequent pauses to evaluate patient comprehension and clarify questions. In addition, patients may need to be helped to remember the role of therapy in making steps towards their desired goals.

Therapist variables

The outcome research literature on the psychological treatments of schizophrenia is less well advanced than in the wider psychotherapy literature. Phenomena such as 'equivalent outcomes paradox' and 'investigator allegiance' have been insufficiently investigated or acknowledged in this field (Paley & Shapiro 2002). 'Equivalent outcomes paradox' refers to the fact that different methods of psychotherapy tend to produce similar outcomes despite variations in technical and theoretical orientation (Luborsky *et al.* 1975; Wampold *et al.* 1997). 'Investigator allegiance' refers to the fact that results of comparative studies can be subtly but seriously distorted as a result of the researcher's allegiance to one of the treatments being compared (Luborsky *et al.* 1999).

Although it seems clear that family interventions and CBT can improve clinical outcomes in psychosis, there is little evidence yet for their clear superiority compared with therapies matched for therapist attention (Dickerson 2000; Huxley *et al.* 2000). It is not yet clear how much these different therapies achieve similar outcomes through different processes, or through common factors not recognized in the model of therapy, or whether the research designs are insensitive to differences.

It is important to emphasize that relatives cite as helpful the non-specific aspects of interventions, such as support and reassurance, more commonly than the specific (Budd & Hughes 1997). Lambert and Bergin (1994) estimated that specific factors accounted for only 12% of the variance across therapies.

Lambert and Bergin (1994) suggest that such factors as warmth, attention, instillation of hope, feeling of being supported and the regularity of therapy may be amongst the largest mediators of outcome in all therapies and should not be regarded as trivial. Therapist variables in these characteristics may account for much success or failure in schizophrenia psychotherapy and supportive counselling may well prove to have considerable benefits if made more widely available. However, those staff offering it will themselves need appropriate support and supervision as relationships may be particularly difficult to maintain because of organizational constraints and interpersonal emotional stress resulting from contact with persons with psychosis (Hinshelwood 1987; Leff 2000; Martindale 2001).

In some parts of Scandinavia, clinical policies are implemented that recognize that stable external relationships over time are needed to help minimize the chances of destabilizing again a thinly re-established healthier mental structure in patients. Primary staff are not allocated if they will be leaving the service within a year and patients are informed of their entitlement to longer term regular supportive psychotherapy (Johannessen *et al.* 2000).

According to Luborsky *et al.* (1999), investigator allegiance accounts for some 69% of the variance in outcome comparative studies in the wider field of psychotherapy. Paley and Shapiro

(2002) 'unpacked' this phenomena and showed how unwittingly inadequate and non-robust descriptions of standard care or comparison control groups were created. Researchers often do not follow Wampold *et al*.'s (1997) stricture that only bona fide therapies (i.e. intended to be therapeutic) should be included in order to reduce investigator allegiance to the active treatment. For example, in Sensky *et al*. (2000) the comparison befriending group only discussed neutral topics and it is not known what would have been different if symptoms had been discussed as in the active group.

Reports counter to authors' allegiance are very rarely published. It is clear that far more research is needed into numerous therapist variables that may play a crucial part in determining the long-term outcome of schizophrenia independent of treatment modality. The limits of available research should not interfere with the pressing need for all mental health staff to be trained to ensure that their basic attitudes to fellow human beings with problems related to psychosis do not add to their already considerable burden.

Early interventions in psychosis

Early psychological treatment intervention in psychosis is currently a topic that is arousing a great deal of interest and cautious optimism. The schizophrenia spectrum disorders currently often run a chronic course with pervasive consequences and the question is being keenly asked as to whether early diagnosis and a range of early psychological, social and pharmacological interventions directed at various aspects of the disorder can improve the long-term outcome, as does early intervention in some cancers and vascular disease (Larsen & Opjordsmoen 1996).

It is now more widely accepted that schizophrenia is a heterogeneous condition that describes similar phenomena that may be the manifestation of late phases of several biological and psychological processes (Ciompi 1987a). 'Wait and see' diagnostic policies may be overlooking major opportunities for secondary prevention in persons already suffering considerably (Birchwood 2000). The concept of early intervention, the health system issues and the research base are well described by McGorry (2000b) and Birchwood (2000) and will be summarized below.

The future development of realistic preventive measures in early psychosis will need to attend to the following phases:
1 the prepsychotic phase;
2 early detection of psychosis and intensive treatment; and
3 recovery during the critical period.
The logic of early detection and intensive treatment is that there are critical periods in which effective interventions at particular times may alter the long-term course of the illness (Birchwood 2000).

Prepsychotic phase

The current interest in prepsychotic interventions marks a return to the 1927 observations of Harry Stack Sullivan (1994):
'the psychiatrist sees too many end states and deals professionally with too few of the prepsychotic'.

The prepsychotic phase is complex to consider, partly because – although all persons will be affected in varying ways, both qualitatively and quantitatively, by mental disorder or 'disease' – only some will go on to develop psychosis without treatment. The term 'prodromal' is misleading because it implies inevitability about the future course.

McGorry (2000b) emphasized that several reviews of prepsychotic states indicate that most of the disabling consequences of the subsequent psychosis are manifest prior to the latter's onset, especially the deficits in social functioning. Häfner *et al*. (1995) demonstrated that the social status lost during the prodromal or prepsychotic phase is the main factor determining long-term social outcome. At this point in time, there has been little research evidence that demonstrates that interventions for a range of disordered mental states with a high risk of transition to psychosis will reduce the risk of that transition. The short-term study of Phillips *et al*. (1999) with a group of 88 such young people is a favourable pointer. In this a combination of medication and active psychological intervention is compared with supportive case management. This is an area deserving of a great deal of further careful evaluation of many types of intervention.

Early detection and phase-specific treatment in first-episode psychosis

It is necessary to stress the need to refer to 'psychosis' and not 'schizophrenia' because diagnostic systems tend to dictate a diagnosis of schizophrenia only if certain psychotic symptoms have been present for certain periods of time – 6 months in the case of DSM-IV (American Psychiatric Association 1994). This is far too long for early detection and treatment. The key elements of one combination of psychological and pharmacological approaches have been well laid out by McGorry and Jackson (1999). They stress the importance of the mindset of the treating clinicians: 'the focus on recovery rather than rehabilitation, quality of life and health in a positive sense, not merely abolition of symptoms in the shortest possible time'. McGorry (2000b) also addresses the importance of implementing interventions with proven track records: 'It is the failure to follow through with treatments of proved effectiveness which constitutes the greatest failure of modern psychiatry'.

Linszen *et al*. (1998) noted the rapid relapse rate when high-quality treatments offered in a research trial were withdrawn after 15 months, during which there had been low relapse rates. However, the important question of how long effective treatments should be maintained remains unclear from research. Birchwood (2000) presents evidence for the critical period being the first 5 years after first onset of psychosis.

Aims of psychological treatments in the early phases
(adapted from Birchwood 2000)

1 Because psychotic symptoms and social functioning do not strictly mirror one another, each require independent attention.

2 Reduce relapse rate and the duration and severity of relapses. Impending relapse varies considerably in its manifestations between persons; one aim is therefore to try to clarify the personal relapse 'signature'.

3 To treat PTSD in relation to the psychosis and/or to any traumatic events that may have preceded the psychosis.

4 To improve patients appraisals about their 'self' that result from the psychosis. This may well include depression and suicidal vulnerability, loss of personal sense or of valued goals.

5 To attend to ideas about the psychosis (such as it being an uncontrollable force) and to the power and malevolence of hallucinations.

6 To develop a strategy to prevent harmful criticism and hostility.

7 To attend to premorbid psychological and social functioning problems of the individual, sometimes attending to the family context.

There is now accruing evidence that the duration of untreated psychosis in the community can be reduced by community-wide education and antistigma programmes (Johannessen *et al.* 2000). Education and training need to be conducted with mental health professionals to reduce interventions that are themselves unnecessarily harmful and militate against psychotherapeutic stances (McGorry 2000b). Accruing evidence supports the feasibility of introducing more optimal initial management of psychosis that addresses many of the above concerns (McGorry *et al.* 1996; Power *et al.* 1998). There is also the more specific need-adapted approach that is specifically organized to be initiated with the first onset of psychosis and is described in a later section of this chapter. Specialized early intervention services are being set up in several countries and the UK Government intends to fund 50 such services by the year 2004, especially targeting young persons who have often fallen in between adult and child services (Department of Health 1999).

Relapse prevention has a long history in terms of maintenance of medication and of altering expressed emotion in families (this history is discussed in the family therapy section that follows later in this chapter). There is now a considerable focus on assisting individuals to identify relapse signs and symptoms in order to develop preventive strategies. These strategies have been well reviewed by Spencer *et al.* (2000). Most psychosocial interventions are only effective during the period when they are being delivered and research has not yet clarified whether relapse prevention provides tools for patients that allow for relinquishment of high degrees of monitoring by mental health professionals.

Specific types of therapy for schizophrenia

Family interventions

In the last 20 years, the mental health profession has undergone an evolution in its attitude toward relatives of people with schizophrenia. Until the early 1980s, carers, who were often the main providers of support, were often blamed, stigmatized or ignored by mental health services. The confluence of several factors has resulted in a shift to the current view of families as being important allies of professionals in the management of schizophrenia. These include:

1 research documenting that negative family affect is predictive of symptom relapses;

2 recognition of the impact of care on a relative – in the UK, carers have more recently been seen as individuals with needs of their own in Standard 6 of the UK National Service Framework (Department of Health 1999); and

3 the strong dissatisfaction expressed by some family members over their treatment by professionals.

Expressed Emotion (EE) research

In a series of now classic studies, Brown, Vaughn, Leff and their colleagues showed that high levels of criticism, hostility or emotional overinvolvement (e.g. extreme self-sacrificing behaviour, dramatic displays of emotion) in the relatives of schizophrenia patients, referred to as high EE, predicted psychotic relapses during the 9 months following a symptom remission (Vaughn & Leff 1976). Since this early research, nearly 30 studies conducted on more than 1400 people with schizophrenia have replicated the essential findings that EE, assessed in individual interviews with each relative, is associated with a higher risk of relapse (Bebbington & Kuipers 1994; Butzlaff & Hooley 1998; see also Chapter 31). The importance of these findings is amplified by the fact that similar results have been found across different cultures; that EE ratings appear to be independent of patient psychopathology and chronicity; and that behavioural observation research of family interactions supports the construct validity of EE (Miklowitz *et al.* 1984; Mueser *et al.* 1993; Rosenfarb *et al.* 1995; Woo *et al.* 1997; see also Chapter 31).

Although many studies have replicated the finding that patients living with high EE families are at increased risk of relapse, a few studies have not found these results (Stirling *et al.* 1991). A variety of factors can be identified which may account for different findings across studies, such as whether all relatives were interviewed, patient selection criteria (e.g. not selecting patients with persistent psychotic symptoms) and the stage of the illness in which EE was assessed (e.g. following an acute exacerbation or during symptom stabilization). Furthermore, many EE studies have been conducted on relatively small sample sizes, which have low statistical power to detect effects of moderate magnitude. The positive effects of family therapy provide additional support for the validity of EE assessments for families containing high EE relatives of people with schizophrenia (reviewed below).

Impact of care

The family members of patients with schizophrenia often report significant levels of subjective distress, economic burden, risks to their personal safety and social isolation (Noh & Turner 1987; Lefley 1989). In response to the burden, some family members attempt to exert greater control over their ill relative's disruptive behaviour through critical or intrusive interactions (Greenley 1986). It has now been found that family burden is correlated with EE (Smith *et al.* 1993; Scazufca & Kuipers 1996). High EE relatives were more likely to find social withdrawal and poor role performance difficult to deal with. This in turn can be shown to activate further disturbed behaviour (Rosenfarb *et al.* 1995). This escalating cycle, which may also be worsened by relatives' attributions about difficult behaviour (Brewin *et al.* 1991; Barrowclough & Parle 1997), seems likely to add to the overall stress in the family and contribute to a deteriorating cycle (Mueser & Glynn 1999).

In contrast, low EE families may be better able to recognize and de-escalate conflict (Hubschmid & Zemp 1989). These more tolerant families seem likely to both promote more adaptive behaviour and to maintain it. These are also goals of therapy.

Family advocacy and consumer movement

In addition to EE research and recognition of the impact of caring for someone with psychosis, the family advocacy movement and mental health consumerism have played a vital part in establishing a more collaborative relationship between families and professionals. Family members of patients with schizophrenia have articulated their dissatisfaction with how they are treated by mental health professionals and the quality of their relative's treatment (Lefley & Johnson 1990). Families have protested about the stigma of mental illness in the general public and the negative attitudes of professionals towards relatives. To overcome these problems, families have begun to educate the public, dispel myths about mental illness and demand more information, respect and co-operation from professionals. Regrettably, despite these efforts, stigma still remains a key issue for those with severe mental health problems (May 2000).

The vitality of the consumer movement is evident from the numerous organizations of family members and consumers that have formed in recent years to advocate for the needs of the mentally ill and their relatives: in the UK, the National Schizophrenia Fellowship (NSF); Schizophrenia – A National Emergency (SANE); National Association for Mental Health (MIND); in the USA, National Alliance for the Mentally Ill (NAMI). Their message has been loud and clear: (i) families are not to blame for mental illness; (ii) relatives and patients have the right to basic information about psychiatric illness and its treatment; and (iii) resources and treatment standards for the mentally ill are inadequate. One consequence of this movement has been the increase in books about psychiatric illness published for families (Torrey 1988) and for professionals about working with families of the mentally ill (Kuipers *et al.* 1992; Marsh 1992). Thus, family advocacy and recognition of the interaction between family stress and patient functioning have helped to fuel the development of family interventions and, in turn, improve the outcome for schizophrenia.

Short-term family therapy

Among empirical trials of short-term family interventions, several approaches have focused primarily on providing education to relatives alone (Birchwood *et al.* 1992; Vaughan *et al.* 1992), while others have included the patient in the family sessions and broadened the scope of therapy objectives to include both education and improved family functioning (Mills & Hansen 1991).

The controlled research on short-term family therapy for schizophrenia indicates that these programmes: (i) improve the understanding of family members about their relative's illness and that this knowledge is maintained for at least brief follow-up periods; (ii) produce modest improvements in family burden, although it is unclear how long these improvements last; and (iii) have limited effects on the social adjustment, symptomatology or relapse of patients. These studies support the feasibility of brief interventions for families with a schizophrenia patient, but also suggest that longer treatment durations are necessary for patients to achieve significant clinical change (Pitsschel-Walz *et al.* 2001).

Long-term family therapy

In contrast to short-term family therapy programmes, controlled research on most long-term programmes lasting at least 9 months has provided strong support for their clinical efficacy. An early exception to this trend was the only study to examine the efficacy of a psychodynamically orientated intervention (Kottgen *et al.* 1984). This study found no differences in relapse rates between patients who were assigned to the family treatment and patients who received customary treatment. However, the interpretation of these findings is limited by the small sample size and the fact that the therapy groups were poorly attended (e.g. less than half the relatives and patients attended at least 75% of the scheduled sessions).

Several long-term family therapy models have been developed, empirically tested and found to produce beneficial clinical effects at 2-year follow-ups. These models include: Falloon's behavioural family therapy model (Falloon *et al.* 1985; Cardin *et al.* 1986), Tarrier and Barrowclough's behavioural approach (Barrowclough & Tarrier 1992; Tarrier *et al.* 1999); Leff *et al.* and Anderson *et al.*'s psychoeducational method (Leff *et al.* 1985, 1989; Anderson *et al.* 1986; Hogarty *et al.* 1991; Schooler *et al.* 1997); and McFarlane's multiple family group support model (McFarlane *et al.* 1993, 1996). More recently, studies have been extended to non-Western settings, e.g. China (Xiong *et al.* 1994; Zhang *et al.* 1994), Hispanic America (Telles *et al.* 1995) and first episodes (Linszen *et al.* 1996).

Although the specific clinical strategies employed across different family therapy models are not identical, they share more in common than they differ. Lam (1991) identified seven common ingredients of effective family interventions for schizophrenia:

1 A positive approach and genuine working relationship between the therapist and family.

2 The provision of family therapy in a stable, structured format with additional contacts with therapists if necessary.

3 A focus on improving stress and coping in the 'here and now' rather than dwelling on the past.

4 Encouragement of respect for interpersonal boundaries within the family.

5 The provision of information about the biological nature of schizophrenia, so as to reduce blaming the patient and family guilt.

6 The use of behavioural techniques, such as breaking down goals into manageable steps.

7 Improving communication between family members.

Control studies have been conducted comparing customary treatment with long-term family therapy using the models of Falloon *et al.* (1985), Leff *et al.* (1985), Tarrier *et al.* (1989) and Hogarty *et al.* (1991). In addition, Randolph *et al.* (1994) replicated the effects of family therapy (vs. customary treatment) using the model of Falloon *et al.* These studies indicate that family therapy has a significant effect on reducing relapse rates to an average of about 50% of standard (no family therapy) treatment. Furthermore, those studies which have assessed other dimensions of functioning have generally reported positive effects of treatment on patient social adjustment and reduced family 'burden' (Falloon & Pederson 1985; Falloon *et al.* 1987; Tarrier *et al.* 1989). There is also some evidence that long-term family intervention for schizophrenia may be cost effective because it reduces the number of days that patients spend in hospital (Cardin *et al.* 1986; Tarrier *et al.* 1991). These studies indicate that family therapy is one of the most potent interventions known for schizophrenia.

Two controlled studies have also been conducted that compared the efficacy of individual family therapy with therapy provided in multiple family groups (Leff *et al.* 1990; McFarlane *et al.* 1993, 1996). Two trends are notable from these two studies. First, relapse rates over 2 years are relatively low for both individual and multiple family group formats, compared with the relapse rates of other studies that used customary care as a control group. Secondly, the differences in relapse rates between the individual and multiple family group formats are small, although the difference approached significance (*P* < 0.06) for the McFarlane *et al.* (1993) study. A further study by McFarlane *et al.* (1996) compared 83 families with multifamily treatment with 89 who received single family treatment, but no significant differences were found at 2-year follow-up on relapse rates.

Nevertheless, a more recent meta-analysis of all available randomized controlled trials (RCTs) of family therapy for schizophrenia suggests that multifamily group studies may account for the apparent reductions in efficacy of more recent family intervention studies (as described by Pharoah *et al.* 2000). Our review (of 19 RCTs) carried out for a guidelines group of the Royal College of Psychiatrists and the British Psychological Society showed that single family interventions were more efficacious than multiple family group interventions (Pilling *et al.* 2002).

Treatment strategies for schizophrenia study

Treatment strategies for schizophrenia (TSS) was a large (over 300 patients) multisite study – involving five hospitals – of pharmacological and family treatment strategies for schizophrenia that was completed by the National Institute of Mental Health (Keith *et al.* 1989; Schooler *et al.* 1989, 1993, 1997). This study examined three different pharmacological management strategies: standard-dose fluphenazine decanoate, low dose, and 'targeted' dose, i.e. medication was given only when symptoms worsened; and two different family treatment strategies – 'supportive' vs. 'applied' treatment – in a factorial design. Patients were randomized to one of the three medication groups after a 4–6-month stabilization period, with medication provided in a double-blind fashion for an additional 2 years. Psychiatrists were free to medicate with open-label medication if early warning signs appeared or a symptom exacerbation occurred. For the supportive family treatment condition, relatives were provided with an educational workshop patterned after the 'survival skills workshop', developed by Anderson *et al.* (1986), followed by multiple family support education groups held monthly for the approximate 2.5 years of the study, and case management as needed. For the applied family treatment condition, families received all the treatments provided to the supportive condition (i.e. the educational workshop, monthly multiple family groups and case management) as well as approximately 1.5 years of home-based behavioural family therapy (initiated at the beginning of the study), based on the behavioural family therapy model of Falloon *et al.* (1985).

Several clear effects emerged from the TSS study (Schooler *et al.* 1997; Mueser *et al.* 2001). First, patients in families who received the supportive treatment did as well over the study as did patients in families who received the applied treatment, suggesting little added effect for behavioural family therapy to the supportive family treatment condition. Secondly, rehospitalization rates were low for both family interventions (41% cumulative rehospitalization rate over 2 years for the applied treatment, 43% for the supportive treatment), suggesting that combined family and pharmacological treatments were beneficial. Thirdly, there were no interactions between pharmacological and family treatment conditions. Fourthly, families who participated in the behavioural family therapy programme reported decreased tension in the home, and relatives indicated lower levels of rejecting attitudes towards the patient.

The results of this study appear to be in line with the studies of Leff *et al.* (1990) and McFarlane *et al.* (1993), who found similar effects for single and multiple family interventions for schizophrenia. Falloon *et al.* (1985) and Randolph *et al.* (1994) both reported that behavioural family therapy reduced relapse rates when compared with a standard treatment which involved no family intervention. The TSS study did not include a no-family intervention group, so it is unclear whether both interventions were effective. In addition, the TSS study design precluded the measurement of relapse rates across all patients. As the beneficial effects of family intervention are most evident in the reduction of relapse rates, the lack of relapse data as opposed to rehospitalization rates in the TSS study has made it difficult to compare with other studies.

Future directions for family therapy

Recent meta-analytic reviews confirm the encouraging results of research on family therapy for schizophrenia (Pharoah *et al.* 2000; Bustillo *et al.* 2001; Pitsschel-Walz *et al.* 2001). A key question remains about implementation (Fadden 1997). It would also be useful to know whether any family or patient characteristics are predictive of a differential response to treatment. The recent research by Linszen suggested that in early episodes intensive 'Falloon' style interventions for low EE families led to worse outcome (Linszen *et al.* 1996). It may be the case that not all families need intensive sessions, and that monthly support over the longer term would be more appropriate (Bustillo *et al.* 2001).

The issue of the durability of family therapy now has some answers. The intervention study of Tarrier *et al.* (1989) lasted for 9 months, and assessments at 2 years indicated some maintenance of effects; many studies provided family therapy for 2 years. McFarlane (1990) has argued against limiting the duration of family therapy. Pilling *et al.* (2002) also argue for longer term interventions. As we have discussed previously in this chapter, the expectation that time-limited psychosocial interventions will have long-lasting effects on schizophrenia may be inconsistent with the chronic nature of the illness, yet there are often practical limitations to how much therapy can be offered. The ultimate resolution probably lies somewhere between the two poles of time-limited or indefinite family therapy. Some families who either are living with a severely ill relative or face multiple hardships (e.g. poverty, substance abuse) may require ongoing family therapy as a social prosthesis against high levels of stress. Other families may need therapy for only a limited period, provided that they have access to a therapist for booster sessions. At present it seems clear that sustained intervention is more successful than a brief one (less than 3 months), and that for frequent relapsers who live with carers the families may benefit from relatively simple ongoing interventions (Bustillo *et al.* 2001). Future research can usefully confirm this.

Remaining questions about family therapy pertain to the timing of the intervention. Tarrier *et al.* (1991) have suggested that families are more amenable to intervention when the patient is in the acute stage of the illness, and most studies have initiated therapy at this time. There are obvious engagement issues when families are offered therapy at non-crisis times (McCreadie 1996; G. Szmukler, E. Kuipers, W. Mahposa *et al.* submitted). A related issue is whether the provision of family therapy during early episodes might improve an otherwise chronic trajectory. Research conducted to date on family therapy has focused mainly on patients who have had the illness for many years.

Family treatment provided at an earlier stage might prevent relatives and patients from adopting maladaptive strategies for coping with stress (e.g. high-EE behaviours, social withdrawal), strategies that have negative long-term consequences. Some of these coping styles may account for the worsening in negative symptoms found during the first few years after schizophrenia has developed (Fenton & McGlashan 1992).

Some resent research in first episodes suggests that EE and 'burden' are already well established and that many families are triggered into high EE responses (Kuipers & Raune 2000). Interest in early intervention is widespread, but as yet no published family or individual studies exist to confirm this optimism.

Individual and group psychotherapies

Cognitive therapy

Evidence has been accumulating for some years in the literature on the efficacy of cognitive–behavioural therapy (CBT) as an adjunctive treatment in the management of schizophrenia. CBT focuses on altering the content of thoughts, including beliefs, attitudes and interpretations of events, through rational disputation and consideration of alternative perspectives. CBT interventions are distinguished from cognitive rehabilitation or cognitive remediation approaches, which focus on changing neurocognitive processes that are frequently impaired in schizophrenia, such as memory, attention and concentration, speed of information processing and executive functions. This section reviews and comments on some of this evidence, before considering briefly some clinical aspects of CBT in schizophrenia. The focus is exclusively on CBT with patients. Cognitive approaches have also been developed for work with families and carers but are not considered further here.

Efficacy of CBT: published evidence

The first reports of psychological interventions in schizophrenia using cognitive techniques were published 50 years ago. Beck (1952) reported a case study in which cognitive techniques were used to treat delusional beliefs. Other early case studies focused predominantly on the application of CBT to the management of delusions or hallucinations (Watt *et al.* 1973; Alford *et al.* 1982). Later studies started to extend the focus of cognitive interventions from exclusively positive psychotic symptoms to include affective symptoms (Fowler & Morley 1989; Chadwick & Lowe 1990). More recent studies have further widened the range of outcomes, to include social functioning (Tarrier *et al.* 1993; Garety *et al.* 1994), adherence with treatment (Hayward *et al.* 1995), coping (Tarrier *et al.* 1993), understanding of the illness (Hayward *et al.* 1995) and self-esteem (Garety *et al.* 1994; Haddock *et al.* 1996).

In the last decade, published results have started to appear of randomized controlled trials of CBT in schizophrenia, several of which have now been included in a systematic review in the Cochrane Library (Jones *et al.* 2000). Table 33.1 summarizes some features of these trials. The table includes studies which used individual CBT; several further studies have been published of group interventions (Eckman *et al.* 1992; Bradshaw 1993; Haddock *et al.* 1998; Hornung *et al.* 1999).

The majority of these studies have focused on patients with positive psychotic symptoms that have endured despite adequate drug treatment (Table 33.1). The drug treatments involved have included standard as well as atypical antipsychotic drugs, but no study has yet compared cognitive therapy with clozapine, which would be of great interest in terms of cost-effectiveness as well as efficacy. Other studies have been less selective in the patients recruited, and two have had wide inclusion criteria, each recruiting acutely psychotic inpatients (Drury *et al.* 1996a,b; Kemp *et al.* 1996).

All of these randomized controlled trials have shown CBT to be more effective than the comparison intervention for at least some of their chosen outcome measures. Some have reported outcomes favouring CBT over longer term follow-up (Kemp *et al.* 1998; Kuipers *et al.* 1998; Drury *et al.* 2000; Tarrier *et al.* 2000).

Only limited meta-analyses are possible of data from these trials, mainly because of the different outcomes assessed. However, the Cochrane review reported that, compared with routine clinical care, CBT reduced significantly the odds of relapse or readmission at 18-month follow-up (the odds ratio favouring CBT was 0.46, 95% CI 0.16–0.83). For this outcome, the reviewers calculated the number needed to treat as six (i.e. six patients would need to be treated with CBT to prevent one relapse over and above the rate in routine clinical care). A more recent meta-analysis, including seven studies and 340 patients, found a post-treatment effect size of 0.65, and an effect size of 0.93 for the four studies reporting follow-up, indicating robust effects of CBT (Gould *et al.* 2001). Given the likely costs of a relapse, and particularly of inpatient admission or intensive follow-up, these data begin to make a good case for the cost-effectiveness of CBT as an adjunctive treatment in schizophrenia. The results above refer particularly to positive symptoms, but there is also now evidence for the efficacy of CBT in reducing negative symptoms, at least over a 9-month follow-up (Sensky *et al.* 2000).

Interpreting the published research evidence

Taken together, the studies reviewed above provide strong support for the effectiveness as well as efficacy of CBT for schizophrenia. Individually, each study has methodological limitations, but most of these limitations are not common to all the studies cited. Those studies that have focused on specific symptoms, such as delusions or hallucinations, have not necessarily confined their samples to people diagnosed as having schizophrenia, and caution is therefore required in attempting to generalize their results to samples with schizophrenia. Nevertheless, results have been fairly consistent across the published reports.

A major problem in the studies cited above, as in trials of psychological interventions generally, is the choice of an appropriate intervention with which to compare CBT. Several studies have included 'usual clinical treatment' as a comparison condition, but this has the disadvantage that treatment group allocation cannot easily be concealed from the clinicians treating the study participants. This problem is compounded by the fact that some studies have not established that the CBT and control groups were comparable in terms of their antipsychotic medications before and after the intervention.

More generally, it is difficult to show that the improvements of patients receiving CBT are attributable to the specific effects of CBT. This has been well reviewed by Paley and Shapiro (2002). A striking example of this is the befriending intervention used in the recent trial by Sensky *et al.* (2000). This intervention aimed to be non-directive and entirely non-specific. Audiotapes of the intervention sessions confirmed that the therapists were using general therapeutic techniques but not cognitive ones. Nevertheless, at the end of the 9-month intervention, both CBT and befriending had resulted in significant (and clinically substantial) reductions in positive symptoms, negative symptoms and affective disturbance. It was only at 9-months' follow-up that the two treatments showed divergent results, with the CBT group showing continuing improvements and the befriending group showing overall deterioration towards their preintervention symptomatology. Anecdotally, factors contributing to the

Table 33.1 Randomized controlled trials of cognitive–behaviour therapy in schizophrenia. (As with the earlier case studies and open trials, the randomized trials have varied as to their main focus of intervention.)

Study	*n*	Focus	Comparison interventions
Tarrier *et al.* (1993a)	27	Drug-resistant symptoms	Problem-solving
Drury *et al.* (1996a,b)	40	Acute psychosis	Structured activities and support
Kemp *et al.* (1996)	47	Compliance	Non-specific counselling
Lecompte & Pelc (1996)	64	Compliance	'Unstructured interviews'
Kuipers *et al.* (1997)	60	Drug-resistant symptoms	Usual clinical treatment
Tarrier *et al.* (1998)	87	Drug-resistant symptoms	Supportive counselling or routine care
Sensky *et al.* (2000)	90	Drug-resistant symptoms	Befriending

success of the befriending intervention appear to include the experience and enthusiasm of the therapists coupled with the patients' experience of participating in a research trial. Clearly, these factors are common to most if not all psychological interventions.

Such non-specific effects are probably much less important with increasing length of follow-up, and enduring effects of CBT are likely to be brought about by specific benefits attributable to CBT itself. It might also be helpful for researchers to gather data to demonstrate that changes in their chosen outcomes are likely to have been brought about by mechanisms predicted by the cognitive model and targeted in the therapeutic intervention. However, examining outcomes and explanatory processes concurrently has been discouraged by the customary dichotomy between pragmatic and explanatory study designs.

Some of the outcome measures used in the published studies reflect overall psychopathology (the Brief Psychopathological Rating Scale is one example). If the published evidence relied exclusively on such generic outcomes, it could possibly be argued that CBT was exerting its effects not on psychotic symptoms but on depression, anxiety and other features that CBT is known to be effective in treating, and which are commonly found in schizophrenia. It is important to note that the studies cited above have included outcome measures specific for psychotic symptoms, and thus the efficacy of CBT in these studies cannot be attributed to improvements in depressive or anxiety symptoms. Tarrier and colleagues used as their main outcome measures the frequency and severity of psychotic symptoms, initially elicited using the Present State Examination (Tarrier et al. 1993b, 1998). Garety et al. (1994) also used the Present State Examination to identify psychotic symptoms that were targeted in assessing outcomes and used additional outcome measures that are specific to psychosis, such as the Maudsley Assessment of Delusions Scale (Buchanan et al. 1993). Sensky et al. (2000) chose to use the Comprehensive Psychopathology Rating Scale (CPRS; Asberg et al. 1978) as their main outcome measure, because this has been widely used in pharmacological interventions in schizophrenia. However, in their study, CBT not only led to significantly greater reductions than befriending in *total* CPRS scores, but also in ratings of the Schizophrenia Change Scale, a validated subscale of the CPRS specifically developed to measure change in psychotic symptoms (Montgomery et al. 1978). It is therefore clear that CBT is effective in treating directly the psychotic symptoms in schizophrenia, rather than exerting its benefits in treating features of depression or anxiety that may be present in patients with schizophrenia.

Therapy

Several treatment manuals are now available (Kingdon & Turkington 1994; Fowler et al, 1995; Chadwick et al. 1996; Nelson 1997). Among these, there are differences of detail in conceptualization and focus. However, the interventions have much in common, and can clearly be recognized as having developed from the cognitive model. As in other applications of the model, conceptualization of the individual's problems is a crucial element, with negotiation of an understanding of the problems and the therapeutic tasks shared as far as possible between patient and therapist. Engaging the patient in therapy initially can be more challenging than with depression or anxiety, and benefits from experience and skill. Once the therapeutic relationship has been well established, many of the cognitive and behavioural techniques commonly used in cognitive therapy can be applied to working with people with schizophrenia.

In schizophrenia, as in other disorders, an important factor that has encouraged the application of CBT has been the development of effective methods to understand and quantify the phenomena that are often the focus of therapy, and therefore crucial to the assessment of outcomes. Helping patients to see their experiences as quantifiable and multidimensional rather than 'all or nothing' phenomena is a task common to cognitive interventions generally. Shifting from seeing delusions or hallucinations merely as present or absent to effectively disaggregating their properties and characterizing them in a multidimensional way (Garety et al. 1998) is arguably a prerequisite for the application of CBT. Later work has given rise to increasingly sophisticated cognitive models (Nuechterlein & Subotnik 1998) and associated methods of assessment.

A further example of multidimensional conceptualization, which is particularly applicable to working with people who are psychotic, is the concept of 'normalization' (Kingdon & Turkington 1994). This involves helping the patient to understand his or her experiences as falling along continua which include normal everyday experiences, and explaining shifts along these continua using a stress–vulnerability model, which is again very commonly applied in CBT more generally.

Further developments

Most studies to date have not included data on health economic outcomes, which will clearly be necessary to support the provision of CBT in routine clinical practice. Given that group interventions are likely to be more cost-effective than individual therapy, it is not surprising that these have been the focus of recent investigation (Wykes et al. 1999; Chadwick et al. 2000). Some preliminary information is already available on factors which could predict the likelihood of favourable outcomes (Chadwick & Lowe 1990; Garety et al. 1997, 2000), but more data are needed to allow specialist interventions to be targeted towards those individuals likely to benefit from them. To date, CBT interventions in schizophrenia have been undertaken by specialist clinicians. Such experts will continue to have a place alongside the clinical team in contributing to the management of individual patients. However, another challenge is to identify cognitive interventions that can effectively be incorporated into routine practice by members of the clinical team. Over time, such interventions are likely to be refined for application in particular situations, such as early intervention (Birchwood 1995), assertive outreach and the management of comorbid substance abuse.

One of the strengths of the cognitive approach, illustrated well by the instruments mentioned above (which were developed to assess delusions or hallucinations), is the reciprocal relationship between clinical practice and cognitive psychology. Just as empirical observations giving rise to testable hypotheses form the cornerstone of cognitive therapy, so such empirical observations have been influential in guiding research to further basic understanding of cognitive processes. Importantly, this is a reciprocal relationship, with developments in cognitive psychology also informing therapy.

Psychodynamic[1] theories and therapies

It is important to distinguish between: (i) psychodynamic theories and psychodynamic knowledge about psychosis; and (ii) psychodynamic methods and techniques of treatment. The validity of an aspect of theory and the effectiveness of a particular technique are not necessarily correlated.

Psychodynamic theories and knowledge of psychosis are a complex mixture of: (i) descriptions of psychological phenomena that are close to clinical experience usually derived from prolonged therapy relationships with persons who have had psychosis and their families; and (ii) more inferential ideas about unconscious functioning in psychosis. However, the ideas are derived from the clinical phenomena and usually tested out with the patient using interpretation over time.

Psychodynamic methods in psychosis are the particular techniques used to try to be therapeutically useful to such persons, but using combinations of psychodynamic theory of the psychotic mind, theory of technique and the current theory of the effective agents of psychological change.

Psychodynamic theories offer some contributions to the understanding of:

1 the antecedent psychodynamics, psychological capacities and personal vulnerabilities that may contribute to a particular person's mind being more readily overwhelmed;
2 the mental mechanisms resorted to in the face of unbearable affects or knowledge;
3 the disguised personal meaning or significance of the content of psychotic phenomena (both the positive and negative symptoms of psychosis); and
4 the sometimes disturbing impact of psychosis on family members and mental health professionals that can, in turn, alter the quality of both their own functioning and their relationship with the person with the psychosis.

Useful but highly summarized accounts of some theories can be found in the following texts: Bateman and Holmes (1995), Alanen (1997a) and Etchegoyen (2001). Good detailed accounts of case material that illustrate engaging patients in the psychodynamic approach and making sense of psychotic clinical material can be found in Lotterman (1996), Robbins (1993) and Jackson and Williams (1994).

[1] For the purpose of this chapter, the word psychodynamic will be used to cover related words such as psychoanalytic.

Psychoanalysts have been trained to manage and observe defence mechanisms that humans resort to in order to avoid too much painful reality. Observations of staff groups in institutions involved in treating persons with psychosis can be particularly informative about the emotional difficulty for staff in sustaining contact with much mental illness. These observations reveal the psychological defences and the disturbed feelings evoked in 'normal' persons working in such settings with the resulting barriers to improving services (Obholzer & Roberts 1994; Hinshelwood & Skogstad 2000).

Psychodynamic methods and outcome research

Psychodynamic methods with psychotic patients have undergone radical changes over the years. Historically, Freud did not think that psychotic patients were treatable with analytic methods because he thought that their 'self-absorption' made them incapable of forming a transference relationship with the analyst (Freud 1932). However, in the subsequent 40 years, many psychoanalysts adapted treatment techniques and were able to remain therapeutically engaged with persons vulnerable to psychosis, especially in the USA. Harry Stack Sullivan (1962), Frieda Fromm-Reichmann (1950), Harold Searles (1965) and Ping-Nie Pao (1979) are just a few of the more distinguished clinicians and authors from this period who adapted techniques different from the classical methods used for non-psychotic patients. These pioneers stood out from the rest of the field by their insistence that through psychotherapeutic means patients could be understood and that some persons could be helped to improve the quality of their lives.

With the advent of neuroleptic medication, influential research trials were undertaken. These trials were believed by many not to have shown additional benefits from psychodynamically based approaches over the comparison treatments, such as medication and 'reality adaptive supportive psychotherapy'. As a result of these conclusions and a number of other factors in the prevailing culture, psychodynamic treatment and understanding for persons with psychosis became marginalized and even actively discouraged in the USA (Lehman & Steinwachs 1998). All studies have methodological limitations and these certainly did. For very contrasting and more detailed commentaries on these studies, the reader is referred to Mueser and Berenbaum (1990) and Karon (1989). There are several issues that argue to the conclusion that the value of psychoanalytically orientated therapies has not yet been properly evaluated.

In the influential California study of May (1968), the experience of the therapists in the psychodynamic treatment of psychosis was usually minimal and the research treatment was discontinued on discharge from hospital. If there is one thing that has been learned over the years, it is that psychodynamic work with persons with psychosis is very difficult to learn and to practice. One cannot imagine heart surgeons allowing the future of heart surgery to be determined by outcome studies on the effectiveness of surgery by residents who have only just learned to take out an appendix! Furthermore, there is no acknowledgement in these relatively crude research methods that a particular treatment method may suit one patient or professional and be ill suited to others.

In recent years it has become increasingly clear that longer term therapeutic relationships tend to have increasing benefits. Certainly, a psychodynamic therapy that was discontinued on leaving hospital and not continued for a long time into the patient's normal living circumstances would not nowadays be regarded as therapeutic (Thorsen *et al.* 1999).

The study by Grinspoon *et al.* (1972) was conducted with a chronic population. The Michigan study (Karon & Vandenbos 1972, 1981) showed markedly positive outcome for the group treated by the most experienced psychotherapists but the benefits could have had other explanations as the numbers were small for the effect factor.

The study of Gunderson *et al.* (1984) was a comparison between 'reality adaptive supportive therapy' (RAS) and 'exploratory insight orientated' (EIO) therapy. In the former, the therapy focused on problems in the current living situation of the patient. In contrast to EIO therapy, in RAS there was little attempt either to explore the past or to seek correlates between past experience and the present. Rather, the exploration of the present was intended to identify problems that could be solved or that could be expected to recur in the future so that more effective coping strategies could be mapped out. In EIO, there was a focus on exploring the past and seeking correlates with the present to increase insight. There was a very large drop-out rate in both groups, but the results inclined towards greater ego strength in the EIO group and reduced hospitalization and higher employment rates in the RAS group.

Especially in the USA, mainstream psychoanalysis lost its way in the early postwar decades by an excessive emphasis on both the detachment of the analyst and the focus on interpretation and insight being the crucial, if not only, factors in bringing about psychic change. The popularity of Kohut (1971, 1977) and his followers can be seen as a balancing reaction to this with his focus on accurate empathy rather than detached insight and his rethinking of other features of the therapeutic relationship which allowed serious disordered narcissistic phenomena to be better treated. Wallerstein (1995) eloquently describes the findings from the Menninger study that supportive and other elements in psychoanalytic therapy led to enduring structural psychic change that surprised many analysts. Wallerstein gives a detailed account of the changes in techniques from those of classical psychoanalysis for use in the psychoanalytically informed supportive therapies for persons with conditions such as psychosis. Some of these techniques would correspond to many aspects of RAS.

We make these points to emphasize that for the more disturbed hospitalized patients, contemporary psychoanalytic practitioners may not regard a predominant focus on interpretation and reconstruction of earlier relationships (EIO) as good technique, especially in highly medicated patients. The early research in the USA was probably based on practitioners using this outdated technique, yet is often quoted to show the lack of evidence for the effectiveness of psychodynamic approaches. It is therefore important that these studies should not lead to the conclusion that contemporary psychodynamic approaches and psychoanalytic knowledge do not have a contribution to therapeutic work with psychotic patients.

In Europe, similar developments in psychoanalysis had been going on:

1 The psychoanalytic method was extended to include a much more careful monitoring, understanding and digestion of the countertransference experience as a therapeutic tool.
2 A much greater focus was placed on the 'here and now' of the relationship and on emotional containment, with a much reduced emphasis on reconstruction.
3 Supportive psychodynamic casework with the severely ill by social workers was highly valued by psychiatrists.

These changes in psychoanalysis were little noticed in the public institutions working with persons with psychosis in the Western World outside of Scandinavia, except through the work of a few individuals. It was overshadowed by the tremendous growth of brain research and the hope that schizophrenia and related disorders could be exclusively understood as brain disorders that would be 'cured' when the 'single' biological abnormality or the right pharmacological agent was found. Other changes in the pattern of provision of care also contributed to the decreasing interest in the mental health field in seeing the therapeutic *relationship* as primary and the increasingly reductionistic approach to psychosis, as had been the case to some extent within psychoanalysis and psychosis in previous decades (Robbins 1993).

Eisenberg recently stated: 'Neuroscience is prospering, but the very pace and elegance of discovery in the neurosciences is reinforcing reductionism. The integration of brain science with mind science remains elusive' (Eisenberg 1999). Fifteen years ago Eisenberg wrote: 'Mindlessness in psychiatry is beginning to replace brainlessness.' In his 1999 review he states:

> Were I to be writing that paper today [his article of 15 years ago] I would be more generous in acknowledging the contribution of psychoanalysis. [Psychoanalysis] taught trainees to listen to patients, and to try to understand their distress, not simply to classify them . . . . [Those] tasks are being squeezed out of clinical practice and residency training.

In Scandinavia, the need-adapted approach (see below) has evolved by modifying psychoanalytic theories and practice, integrating these with appropriate support and very carefully phased therapy that acknowledges the very real fragility of the psychotic mind. Systemic models of interpersonal functioning have also found their place, often combined with individual psychodynamic approaches or in sequence.

Need-adapted therapy

This approach was pioneered in Finland some 30 years ago; it is increasingly widely practiced in Scandinavian countries and is beginning to influence practice in other Western European countries.

Practitioners, while accepting the evidence for a range of biological factors that may contribute to the risk an individual has to psychosis, attribute much greater emphasis to vulnerability being determined, to varying degrees, by the interaction of these factors during developmental periods with psychosocial and family environments (Alanen 1997a; Cullberg 2001).

Evidence for this view comes from the work of Tienari *et al.* (1994) in Finland. This is the only long-term study in the world that has carefully studied both the genetic factors and the psychological environment in the same individuals. Adopted-away children of mothers with schizophrenia and their adopting families have been followed for many years and compared with a control group of adopted-away children with biological parents without a history of psychosis. The findings have reconfirmed the mother's genetic contribution to a range of mental health disorders in the offspring, including psychosis. Just as importantly, the researchers concluded from their findings that disturbed mental health in the adopting parents and in the adoptive rearing environment (including disturbed communication, parental conflict and lack of empathy) was the major contributing factor to the increased risk. Conversely, a healthy family environment seemed to significantly protect the genetically vulnerable child from disturbances.

These findings have given strong support to those Scandinavian professionals who have long thought that skilled psychologically based individual and family approaches have a great deal to contribute to the understanding, therapy, rehabilitation and overall welfare of many persons with psychotic vulnerability.

Essence of the approach

The following is a summary based on a number of descriptions. The fullest exposition and discussion is to be found in Alanen's book (1997a) and in Alanen (1997b). Yrjö Alanen, working with colleagues in Turku and then with the Finnish National Schizophrenia Project, has been the leading proponent over several decades. Others have provided their own descriptions (Cullberg *et al.* 2000; Johannessen *et al.* 2000) and discussed variations (Bechgaard & Rosenbaum 1994).

It is essential *that the whole team, especially the nursing staff, shares the basic approach* and works closely together with the patient and his or her family to formulate an understanding of the problems. A capacity of the staff team to utilize systemic, psychodynamic and medical understanding is necessary. Out of this shared understanding a therapeutic focus evolves and is modified with progress; *need-adapted* therapy refers to the fact that the therapy is adapted to match the patients' most important and evolving therapeutic issues. Depending on the focus, the therapeutic setting will be family, individual or therapeutic milieu (or combinations). Alanen stressed the importance of both the personality and training of the therapist members of the team so that patients' evolving therapeutic needs can be adequately met (Alanen 1997a, p. 190). The interested reader is referred to three case illustrations given in the chapter on therapeutic experiences in Alanen's book (1997a) as well as the following composite picture.

Case illustration

Illa, a 27-year-old single woman, was seen by two members of the need-adapted team in her own home within 24 h of referral. The immediate members of her family were involved in the initial meeting. The need-adapted team members covered a range of core disciplines including those with training in family, cognitive and psychodynamic work relevant to psychosis.

Illa had been disturbed for at least 6 months, had disengaged from most of her previous activities and was contrary in manner. She was hallucinating, paranoid and disorganized in her thinking. She had been using illicit drugs occasionally.

The main focus in the two home meetings that took place that first week was gaining rapport with Illa and her family and paying close attention to what each member found most stressful. Minor tranquillizers were prescribed to improve sleep.

One member of the team offered to be the primary therapist for Alla and the other member made it clear that she was available as the primary resource for the family.

The team had available a low-staffed low-stimulus home-like house for six persons if Illa needed this. A hospital bed could be used if there was acute danger not contained by frequent visits or recourse to the house. If symptoms did not settle quickly they would prescribe 50 mg chlorpromazine equivalents (e.g. 1 mg risperidone), increasing weekly to no more than 150 mg equivalents over 3 weeks. The main focus in the early weeks was creating conditions to allow a reduction of the crisis and stresses that had been building up over recent months. In Illa's case this meant that over 6 months all members of the family were helped to both continue to support Illa but also to enjoy increasing amounts of time recovering some of the important and pleasurable areas of their lives. These had been lost as they had responded to the anxiety about Illa by spending more and more time with her. Prior to referral, their increasing involvement had not led to improvement in Illa's health and their own had deteriorated. The team generated an atmosphere of anticipation that the psychosis would settle and that they were available on a longer term basis to help Illa, at a pace she could manage, to lead as full a life as possible.

After 2 months Illa's psychotic symptoms had nearly disappeared. During this time her primary worker had slowly gathered an increasingly clearer picture of Illa and her capacities and the areas of adult life that prior to the psychosis she had been finding difficult and the private difficulties, worries and events that had preceded her deterioration.

From now on, the help for Illa was increasingly individually focused. Illa realized that her therapist was not only available to help her when she had psychotic symptoms, but was there to help with problems that had been preoccupying her prior to the psychotic deterioration. By the end of a year after the referral she was taking on some part-time voluntary work. She was wondering whether to get further help for problems related to her self-esteem or see how much further she could get with the ongoing support of the same primary worker, who would continue to be available. She was thinking about getting her own accommodation. For brief periods when she was working, considering accommodation or in certain social situations, she could be overcome with anxiety and have troublesome suspicious thoughts, but she was becoming more familiar with these and developing better coping strategies and had a small supply of medication.

A great emphasis is placed on the importance of *continuity and quality of the therapeutic relationships*. In Stavanger, in Western Norway, the patient's rights include right of access twice a week to psychotherapeutic contact with an experienced therapist for a period of 5 years if necessary. Furthermore, the primary nurse or key worker with such persons must not be expecting to move on within a year. (Thorsen *et al.* 1999). Alanen's view was that making provision for the therapeutic relationship to continue into years 3–5 leads to progressive gains and continuing development for those individuals who have the ability to make use of longer term individual psychotherapy (Alanen *et al.* 1986, 1994).

Active early engagement of the family. At first referral, relevant members of the team actively engage not only with the individual but also with his or her family and other key persons as soon as possible – preferably prior to admission – if this proves necessary.

The three main aims of early engagement are:
1 to gather a shared understanding of the context (*informative*);
2 by seeing the family network *in vivo*, it is possible to begin to formulate strengths and vulnerabilities of the family (*diagnostic*); and
3 to offer early support to all involved (*therapeutic*).

The consequences of early engagement are:
1 reduced likelihood that the disturbance will be seen as something permanent;
2 the possibility of attending to any emotionally traumatic attributes given to hospitalization; and
3 the psychotic state is often reduced as a consequence of the meeting.

A Hermeneutic approach is at the core. The therapeutic intervention is based on a mutual search for psychological understanding of the patient and the family's ongoing situation. The therapeutic aim is to arrive at shared images of the predicaments and to use these images to guide the treatment process.

Medication is regarded as treatment that supports psychotherapy; neuroleptics are given in small or moderate doses, the minimum necessary to maintain psychotherapeutic engagement (starting with 50 mg equivalent doses of chlorpromazine, e.g. risperidone 1 mg). In the initial phase of the treatment, with its focus on family and individual centred investigation and establishment of the therapeutic relationships, the use of neuroleptics is postponed; minor tranquillizers are used in the first instance for poorly contained anxiety states and to assist disturbed sleep. Especially with acutely ill first admission patients, neuroleptic use may not be needed in later phases of treatment.

Outcome studies *

A number of outcome studies have now been reported. Because the very essence of the treatment approach is both an individualized one and a changing one, as the treatment focus evolves for each person and their family, it is not easily subject to randomized controlled trials. Persons with schizophrenia are heterogeneous and have different capacities and suitability for different interventions. Furthermore, the need-adapted approach has been developed for use by whole services. Two persons with, for example, similar forms of hallucinations and delusions will vary enormously in their motivation and in the life situation in which they have developed a psychosis. Need-adapted treatment decisions will centre on these individual differences and contexts. Many other approaches (and RCT research) would tend towards focusing on a particular treatment and evaluating outcome of the symptoms that were *common to* a group of patients. The RCT design, by its nature, draws inferences from groups the membership of which is determined by randomization between two (or more) alternatives which can be described as in 'equipoise' (i.e. there is a plausible case for either option being superior). By contrast, the 'need-adapted approach' is based on the competing principle that informed choice based on an idiographic assessment of need for *each individual* is paramount. This makes controlled trials of need-adapted approaches very difficult to design. The problem is further exacerbated by the fact that the need-adapted approach is an integrated one, with the therapy being dependent on several interventions over time rather than a single one.

Although each element, such as family intervention, could be evaluated, the design really needs to test whether the '*need-adapted approach*' itself is effective, rather than each component. To do this, we would need to construct a viable alternative to a treatment being 'need-adapted'. This is not a problem with the RCT design as such, but with the conceptualization of what is being tested. Possibly, an ethically acceptable model would be to use cluster randomization (between treatment centres), some of which were randomly assigned to a 'need-adapted' approach and others to a 'strict protocol' condition. In the latter, the adaptation to individual need is strictly defined by a protocol derived from the best evidence available. Although, in principle, this could be done, there would clearly be huge logistical difficulties in gathering sufficient centres in which all staff members would agree to be randomized about a 'philosophy of care'.

* The comments in the next two paragraphs are adapted from a personal communication from Dr Frank Margison of Gaskell House, Manchester.

Outcome has therefore tended to be measured by comparing cohorts of patients. Numbers of patients have been quite large. In the successive cohorts of new patients in the schizophrenia subgroup treated in Turku, where Professor Yrjö Alanen conducted treatment and research, increasing percentages of successive cohorts are without disability pensions and in active work at 5-year follow-up, the latest cohort of 30 patients at 5 years had 82% without pensions and 57% in active work and 61% were without psychotic symptoms (Alanen 1997a).

Pooled results from 65 patients in their first admissions and treated in four Scandinavian centres were reported by Alanen *et al.* (1994) and compared with other 5-year follow-up studies. The findings were favourable whether one looks at those with a definite diagnosis of schizophrenia or those with schizophreniform disorders. Of the former, 46% were not on medication, 39% were in a full remission and 59% had good social relationships.

The Parachute study is an ongoing 17-centre study in Sweden investigating outcome in intensive psychosocial need-adapted therapy and low-dose neuroleptic treatment. A pilot study for a catchment area in Stockholm, with 3-year follow-up, found that this approach was feasible. Very few inpatient beds were needed with consequent considerable cost reduction. This was made feasible through the introduction of a home-like small crisis house that could be used for the large majority of first episode patients. Much lower doses of medication were used than in the comparison group. For those who had neuroleptics, the average dose at 12 months was 84 mg, compared with 198 mg in the control group, and this gap widened with increasing time. Good clinical results were obtained in terms of symptom reduction and patients being without disability pensions (Cullberg 2000).

The 17-centre extension of the pilot study has involved 253 first episode cases compared with both a historical and prospective control group – the latter being first episode cases treated in a high-quality inpatient service. The 1-year results confirm the feasibility of this approach on a large scale in the community and that outcomes are at the least comparable with controls (Cullberg 2001). The satisfaction of the patients and their families with the care provided is high.

These favourable clinical outcomes (using a high-quality need-adapted approach with low-dose medication) raise questions as to what degree and for which subgroups neuroleptics contribute to outcome (i) when intensive psychosocial support is available for first episode psychosis and (ii) when too high doses of neuroleptics or even unnecessary medication have negative effects. The advocacy of neuroleptics is based on many control trials showing superior symptomatic outcome where intensive psychosocial treatment was *not* provided.

In a recent multicentre trial in Finland, an experimental group of consecutive newly diagnosed psychotic patients in three localities ($n = 107$) were treated by staff who had considerable experience of the need-adapted approach and who did not use neuroleptics where possible. These patients were compared with a consecutively diagnosed control group also treated by the need-adapted approach but using medication as usual (Lehtinen *et al.* 2000). At 2-year follow-up 43% of the experimental group had not been prescribed neuroleptics at all (control group 5.9%) and only 3% had had daily dosages at any time in excess of 450 mg chlorpromazine. The clinical outcomes were relatively good using the Global Assessment Scale (GAS; Endicott *et al.* 1976) and Grip on Life assessments (Salakongas *et al.* 1989). Forty-nine per cent of the experimental group had a GAS score of 7 or more (25% in the control group) and 58% had had no psychotic symptoms in the second year (41% in the control group). Fifty-one per cent had had less than 2 weeks in hospital during the 2 years (26% in the control group) and 66% retained 'grip on life' (55% in control group). The experimental group had more severe diagnoses but received a greater amount of family therapy. Although the study does have methodological limitations, the findings indicate that neuroleptic treatment is not essential in all cases and support the possibility that psychosocial interventions can be effective alternatives in first episode psychosis.

Social skills training

This intervention is dealt with at length in Chapter 32. For completeness we give a brief overview of this approach.

Social dysfunction is a defining characteristic of schizophrenia that is semi-independent of other domains of the illness (Strauss *et al.* 1974; Lenzenweger *et al.* 1991; Brekke *et al.* 1997). Patients with schizophrenia often have poor premorbid social functioning (Langfeldt 1937; Zigler & Glick 1986), which is related to impaired social functioning after the onset of the illness (Mueser *et al.* 1990). Furthermore, social functioning after people have developed schizophrenia is predictive of the course and outcome of the disorder (Rajkumar & Thara 1989; Perlick *et al.* 1992; Harrison *et al.* 1996a). According to the expanded stress–vulnerability–coping skills model of schizophrenia (Liberman *et al.* 1986a), both social support and coping skills mediate the noxious effects of stress on patients, protecting them from stress-induced relapses.

Improving social functioning is an important treatment priority in schizophrenia, because it is a valued dimension of quality of life, and because poor social functioning appears to contribute to a worse course of illness. Social skills training is a widely used treatment approach for improving social functioning in schizophrenia. Social skills are specific response capabilities necessary for effective performance. These skills tend to be stable over time and make a unique contribution to the performance of social roles and quality of life (Bellack *et al.* 1990a; Mueser 1991a). Over the past several decades an extensive technology of skills training has been developed and empirically tested as a strategy for teaching social skills to psychiatric patients and improving their social adjustment (Liberman *et al.* 1989; Bellack *et al.* 1997).

A vast literature on social skills training has emerged since the first systematic applications of the methods to patients with schizophrenia in the 1960s. The research on skills training has been periodically reviewed (Dilk & Bond 1996; Smith *et al.* 1996; Heinssen *et al.* 2000). Several conclusions have been reached based on both single case studies and controlled trials. First, patients with schizophrenia are capable of acquiring and maintaining new social skills, including conversational skills, assertiveness and medication management. Secondly, some generalization of new skills to patients' natural environments occurs, with the extent of generalization limited by the complexity of the skill and the severity of cognitive deficits in the patients. Thirdly, the primary impact of skills training is on improving social functioning, with less impact on symptom severity, relapse rates or rehospitalization rates.

Early controlled research on social skills training for schizophrenia was limited by the tendency to employ shorter term interventions of less than 6 months (Bellack *et al.* 1984; Liberman *et al.* 1986b; Dobson *et al.* 1995; Hayes *et al.* 1995), or to conduct follow-up assessments only on patients who did not relapse (Hogarty *et al.* 1986, 1991). More recent controlled research has shown that longer term skills training programmes have a robust effect on improving social functioning (Marder *et al.* 1996; Liberman *et al.* 1998).

Future research questions

Research provides support for the effects of skills training on social functioning in schizophrenia, but many questions persist regarding its clinical utility. What is the optimal frequency of training sessions? For how long should treatments be provided? At what stage of the illness should skills training be initiated? Which patients benefit the most from skills training? What strategies can be used to promote the generalization of skills for patients with the most severe cognitive deficits? While the timing and sequencing of skills training remain unclear, the widespread availability of social skills training, and the positive results of controlled trials suggest that it will continue to be an important treatment strategy for improving social functioning in schizophrenia.

Group therapy and therapeutic milieu treatments

Deterioration in social relationships and social involvement commonly precede psychotic episodes and are conspicuous features of their aftermath. Therefore it is not surprising that there is a long history of exposing selected patients with psychosis to special group situations as a setting for clarification of social difficulties and for therapeutic endeavours towards improvement of interpersonal relating. Group therapy for persons with psychotic vulnerabilities cover a wide spectrum of settings, from small group settings to larger therapeutic communities, and a wide range of therapeutic objectives and theoretical models underpinning the endeavours. Schermer and Pines (1999) and González de Chávez Menéndez and García-Ordás Alvarez (1992) give excellent complementary overviews of these approaches, which are distinct from the more behavioural model used in much of social skills training discussed separately in

this chapter and in Chapter 32. González de Chávez Menéndez and García-Ordás Alvarez particularly focus on how group therapies differ and can complement individual and family therapies and provide an important frame of reference for psychotic patients to anchor themselves and gain a sense of time and progress and provide a slow socializing influence. They also point out how group therapy can improve the relations between the patients and the members of the therapy team.

Small group therapies

Kanas (1986) has reviewed 40 years of outcome research literature of small group treatments for patients with psychosis where there is a control condition. Although the research is variable in quality, he found that the overall evidence available indicates that group therapies were more effective than 'no group' controls but with considerable variation according to the main theoretical approach (educational, interpersonal and psychodynamic). As a consequence, Kanas developed a new model that combines the most useful aspects of previous approaches according to his research review. He calls this the *integrative* approach. The focus and goals of this model vary depending on the phase of illness and whether the patients are inpatients or outpatients. In the former and in more disturbed patients, the group work involves enabling the members to work together on better managing psychotic symptoms, whereas for patients in a less disturbed state the focus is more on difficulties in interpersonal relationships. In both, the technique involves focusing on patient-generated topics relating to difficulties in their current lives with minimal emphasis on reconstructing the past. It also involves an actively supportive stance by the therapists. Therapists should be quick to set boundaries well within the emotional limits of what the patients can tolerate, e.g. of anger and silence. The results of the initial investigations seem to indicate that the integrative approach is very acceptable to patients and is experienced as helpful, with few drop-outs (Kanas 2000). Larger controlled studies are needed with longer term follow-up and clarification as to which patients benefit from short- and longer term groups.

The therapeutic community

A therapeutic community approach for persons with psychotic disorders has a long history stemming back to reformers such as Pinel (1806), Tuke (1813) and Conolly (1856) who believed that the course of mental illness could be determined by the patient's environment. Asylums were built and intended to be peaceful and pleasant, offering the opportunity to engage in purposeful activities. Wing and Brown (1970) demonstrated a clear inverse correlation between the quality of the hospital's social environment and the extent of the signs and symptoms of patients.

Pullen (1999) provided an excellent overview of the characteristics considered to be therapeutic in these communities and of the mixed vicissitudes of the endeavours in the USA and the

UK. He emphasizes, with examples, how vulnerable patients have been to the strengths and weaknesses of the leaders of therapeutic communities and that overall these communities illustrate the point that when liberal and democratic values flourish, so has the care of the mentally ill.

Extension of the group approach to national mental health policy

After a successful period of pilot studies in West Jerusalem with a population of 120 000, Litman (1997), while Director of Mental Health Services in Israel, instigated a community group therapy programme for the severely mentally ill throughout much of Israel. Thousands of patients with a range of severe psychiatric problems, especially schizophrenia, and relatives of persons with psychotic disorders became participants in stable community groups, some of which have been functioning for 20 years. This shift of emphasis obviously involved considerable training of staff in group processes and ongoing supervision for the complex issues, especially the countertransference manifestations, inevitable in group work of this nature. The shift from dyadic individual treatments led to an increase in the quality and quantity of therapeutic attention, especially as a result of multiprofessional involvement in the group work. These factors, together with a reduction in medication levels and the greater focus on interpersonal issues, facilitated the shift of attention from hospital to community and then to family orientated care, allowing for the possibility of personal and social growth and development. The stability of the group structure makes staff changes easier to accommodate.

This group programme has made a substantial contribution to reducing the number of psychiatric beds, as well as to greatly reducing the frequency and length of hospitalization, while the national population of Israel has grown exponentially. The quality of the patient's life is thought to have improved markedly.

Clearly, there is a great need for further qualitative and quantitative research work in these important treatment milieus.

Cognitive rehabilitation

We previously discussed the pervasiveness of cognitive impairment in schizophrenia, which is both related to psychosocial functioning and is predictive of less benefit from social skills training interventions. Traditional skills training approaches have attempted to circumvent these problems by minimizing cognitive demand and repeatedly practising simple response repertoires so that overlearned responses occur immediately in an automatic fashion. However, most social encounters do not follow a script that can be prepared in advance, and effective social interactions require accurate skills in social perception (Penn et al. 1997) and information processing to generate and evaluate appropriate response options (Trower et al. 1978; Wallace et al. 1980; McFall 1982). Several strategies have been developed to address the cognitive impairment that contributes to poor functioning, and limits response to social learning interventions in schizophrenia.

One strategy for overcoming the limiting effects of cognitive deficits in skills training has been to embed the training of specific behaviours within the broader training of social problem skills (Liberman 1989). Patients are taught the steps of problem solving identified by D'Zurilla and Goldfried (1971), which are then practised in anticipation of problems that could occur when attempting to manage a situation (e.g. medication management). The problem-solving approach to skills training has been used in several studies with generally favourable results (Liberman 1986; Marder 1996; Liberman et al. 1998). However, it is unclear whether the positive outcomes of the intervention were a result of the use of problem-solving strategies outside of the training setting (Bellack et al. 1989).

An alternative strategy to addressing the cognitive impairment characteristic of schizophrenia has been to attempt direct remediation of specific information processing deficits, such as attention, memory and abstract formation. These more 'molecular' approaches to improving cognitive functioning have been drawn from clinical work with patients with traumatic brain injury or stroke (Butler & Namerow 1988; Benedict 1989), and often include repeatedly practising computer-driven tasks that load on attention, memory and reasoning (Flesher 1990; Stuve et al. 1991; Medalia & Revheim 1999). Several controlled studies of cognitive rehabilitation methods targeting performance on specific cognitive functions have been completed (Olbrich & Mussgay 1990; Kern et al. 1995, 1996; Wexler et al. 1997; Medalia et al. 1998, 2000; Wykes et al. 1999). The general findings across studies are that cognitive rehabilitation strategies can improve performance on targeted cognitive tasks, with some generalization across different tasks but little demonstrated impact on social functioning.

Two comprehensive cognitive rehabilitation programmes have been developed and evaluated under controlled conditions: Brenner et al.'s (1990) Integrated Psychological Therapy (IPT) and Hogarty and Flesher's (1999a,b) Cognitive Enhancement Therapy (CET). The IPT programme first focuses on the remediation of basic cognitive capacities (e.g. concept formation, memory) before training in problem solving and social skills. Cognitive training proceeds on tasks adapted from neuropsychological test procedures (e.g. a card sorting task) and word games (e.g. finding synonyms and antonyms). Two early controlled trials of IPT reported modest gains in social skills but only minimal improvement in cognitive functioning (Brenner et al. 1990). A more recent controlled study compared the IPT programme with supportive group therapy in an inpatient programme that included careful pharmacological management and comprehensive social skills training (Spaulding et al. 1999). Patients who received IPT demonstrated greater improvement across a variety of cognitive tests and a laboratory measure of social problem solving, with minimal effects on clinical measures.

The CET approach is less molecular in its approach to improving cognitive functioning, and is based more on the hypothesis that problems in social functioning in schizophrenia are the result of a deficit in the ability of patients to get the 'gist' of social problems and situations. Based on a neurodevelopmental theory of cognitive development, accurate social perception is inferred when relatively small amounts of information are associated with specific social schemata about a situation that has been learned over the course of development. The CET approach is aimed at helping patients develop more accurate social perception through teaching how to capture the gist of social situations and interactions (Hogarty et al. 1999a,b). One controlled trial of CET is currently underway, with preliminary results indicating significant improvement in cognitive functioning, social cognition and cognitive disorganization (Hogarty et al. 1999b).

Research on cognitive rehabilitation suggests that it can be effective in improving some dimensions of cognitive performance, while its functional impact remains less clear. It may be unrealistic to expect molecular-based neurocognitive training programmes to have a major impact on social or independent living, even considering the evidence that cognitive impairment is related to functional capacity. Psychosocial rehabilitation programmes tend to have their greatest impact on the most proximate targets of intervention, with smaller effects on more 'downstream' correlated outcomes. For example, supported employment interventions for patients with severe mental illness tend to dramatically improve employment rates but have a negligible impact on other dimensions of functioning (Bond et al. 1997), despite evidence that work is associated with improvements in psychosocial functioning (Bell et al. 1996; Mueser et al. 1997a). Similarly, social skills training is effective at improving social competence in schizophrenia but does not have an established impact on the course of the illness (Heinssen et al. 2000), despite the fact that social functioning predicts outcome (Rajkumar & Thara 1989; Perlick 1992). Cognitive rehabilitation may have an important part to play in the treatment of selected patients with severe cognitive deficits, or with circumscribed cognitive impairments with known functional consequences. An alternative to the management of cognitive deficits is to focus on environmental change, compensatory strategies and coping skills, in which the functional significance of the intervention is easier to establish.

Arts therapies and psychosis

The arts therapies comprise art, music, dance, movement and drama specialists who have a history of contributing to the therapeutic activities offered to patients with psychotic disorders which dates back to the 1940s. Wood (2000) traces the development of art therapy from its first decades until, in the 1960s, it became allied to the humanistic schools of thought. In more recent decades it has developed its theoretical base with clear links with psychoanalytic ideas and other aspects of individual and group psychotherapy. It is only recently that the therapeutic contribution of art therapists has started to be evaluated in quantitative terms (Richardson & Jones 1997; P.

Richardson, K. Jones, C. Evans, P. Jenkins & Rowe, submitted). Qualitative and descriptive research is enabling these professionals to communicate better with colleagues and professionals from other disciplines (Killick & Greenwood 1995).

Not surprisingly, because symbolic expression is disturbed in psychosis, art therapists think about the images produced in individual and group art therapy in a different way from those produced by the non-psychotic aspects of the person. Art therapists pay particular attention to the expression of the psychosis in the use of the reliable and consistent boundaries and the space and structure provided, such as the folder in which the images are kept. They are aware of the extent to which representation of relatedness is depleted as a core feature of psychosis. By focusing carefully on his or her own ways of being alongside the patient with what is produced, the transference intensity can be reduced to a manageable level, especially persecutory anxiety. The overall aim of the arts therapies in psychotic disorders is to use the setting and particularly the means of expression to allow unbearable aspects of mental life to become 'representable'. Improvement would be gauged mainly by the extent to which affective interrelatedness is restored and sustained both in the imagery and in the therapy relationship.

Many art therapists find that the descriptions of the nature of relationships in psychosis by psychoanalysts, group and family experts and anthropologists best matches their own experiences of art therapy relationships (Killick & Greenwood 1995; Skaife & Huet 1998).

Music therapy, in some countries at least, does not aim to teach or perform music for patients, but allows them to express their emotional state and enter into an interactive dialogue with the therapist without needing any musical skills (Sloboda 1996). As in art therapy, verbal skills are not needed. Sloboda points out how music therapy can assist in assessment of mental state in psychotic patients and be a treatment method. She gives a case illustration of a man in a forensic unit who had killed his female partner and of the changes in mental state and in the therapeutic relationship during the therapy, which lasted more than a year. Appropriately trained dance, movement and drama therapists can use their own mediums in corresponding ways.

Personal and other therapies

Personal therapy (Hogarty et al. 1995) has been developed as a broad-based psychotherapeutic approach to schizophrenia which has the central goal of helping patients develop self-control strategies for the management of affect. Through the process of long-term individual therapy, personal therapy seeks to develop in patients an awareness of their subjective states in the context of their vulnerability to schizophrenia, including negative or unpleasant feelings, the possible choices for responding to these emotions, and the likely influences of their behaviours on others. Therapy is divided into three stages: the goals of the first stage (Basic) are to 'join' with the patient and stabilize the disorder; the goals of the second stage (Intermediate) are to develop self-awareness about affective, behavioural and cognitive states and to improve competence at self-regulation; and the goals of the third stage (Advanced) are to attend more to improving patients' life circumstances, including vocational functioning and interpersonal relationships. A wide range of strategies are incorporated into personal therapy, many drawn from behaviour therapy, including basic psychoeducation, social skills training, training in social perception and practising cognitive skills.

The results of one controlled study provide tentative support for the personal therapy approach in 151 patients, 97 of whom were living with family and 54 of whom were living independently (Hogarty et al. 1997a,b). Patients living with family were randomly assigned to receive either personal therapy or supportive therapy and family intervention. Patients living independently were randomly assigned to either personal therapy or supportive therapy. Patients who received personal therapy experienced significantly greater improvements in role functioning. However, among patients living independently personal therapy was also associated with higher relapse rates, whereas among patients living with family personal therapy resulted in lower relapse rates than the comparison intervention. Thus, results of this controlled trial of supportive therapy were encouraging, although they also suggest that the intervention was somewhat stressful for patients living independently.

Future directions of psychological treatments

Whatever advances accrue from genetic and neurobiological understanding and whatever improvements continue in antipsychotic medication, the focus on the psychological treatment aspects of psychotic disorders is likely to continue to grow considerably in importance in the coming years.

Much of this will result from continuing pressure from users and carer groups such as NAMI in the USA, RETHINK (formerly NSF) and MIND in the UK, and similar organizations in countries around the world campaigning for:

1 improved attitudes from health care professionals;

2 better standards of psychological care; and

3 improvements as a result of general trends towards greater expectations from health care.

The many campaigns for a reduction in stigma in schizophrenia, such as those of the World Psychiatric Association (Sartorius 1998), should potentiate these expectations. The crucial importance of stigma in exacerbating the plight of those vulnerable to psychosis has recently been well considered by a number of commentators in the same volume as the overview by Cancro and Meyerson (1999).

There is currently a great deal of interest in psychological interventions in the early stages of psychosis and the International Early Psychosis Association (IEPA) has been formed. Many studies have shown that on average there is a delay of between 1 and 2 years between the onset of psychosis and the initiation of treatment (Haas & Sweeney 1992; Loebel et al. 1992; Beiser

et al. 1993; Häfner et al. 1993) and an even longer period of prodromal illness – as much as a further 3 years – prior to frank psychosis (Loebel 1992). Research in this area, having clarified that it is possible to reduce the duration of untreated psychosis in a large community (Johannessen et al. 2000), is focusing on effective ways of offering early help to the individual and the family to minimize the chances of long-term disability. We anticipate that, in keeping with the multifaceted nature of schizophrenia, many types of interventions will prove to be worthwhile in these earlier phases.

The policy of waiting for diagnostic certainty, especially a duration of symptoms of 6 months or more as in the DSM-IV (American Psychiatric Association 1994), before specific treatment is offered should probably soon become a matter of history and regret. Many regard schizophrenia as a qualitative and quantitative spectrum of disorders (Pull 1999); certainly it is protean in its manifestations, therefore requiring a range of appropriate treatments. Individuals, whether or not they would have gone on to develop the full blown syndrome, are nevertheless suffering and have deteriorated in their psychosocial adjustment and are deserving of attention in their own right. Furthermore, a related factor meriting the development of early intervention is the evidence of 'neurotoxicity' during these early stages (Goldberg et al. 1993; Copolov et al. 2000).

In more than 40% of cases the prodromal phase has started before the age of 20 years and services are not often well organized around this age group – tending to be focused around the needs of either younger children or adults. Psychosis disrupts the normal developmental stages of this age group and psychological treatment services need to be better organized to make them more relevant and user friendly and geared to helping affected young persons regain psychologically important developmental trajectories.

The fact that it is possible to detect, years before, both individuals and families whose offspring are at greatly increased risk of later developing a psychosis means that the research focus will broaden even further. The question will be: what sort of psychological interventions will help which families (as well as teachers) to reduce that risk? It will be important that there is benefit for the difficulties that are already manifest. Gains will have to outweigh the burden to the family from the knowledge of being at increased risk.

One area clearly needing earlier attention and intervention is the psychological consequences of trauma and abuse that are almost ubiquitous in the history of persons with severe mental disorder; frequently this has occurred in childhood (Read 1997; Mueser et al. 1998). Evidence also exists for contributing risk factors that derive from parental mental illness and enduring communication disorders in families (Tienari 1994). Finding psychological interventions to reduce the impact of these factors are worthy of extensive research investigation. The fact that nearly half of all adults with schizophrenia have presented to child services during childhood (Zeitlin 2000) and that there is a high predictability of schizophrenia in certain childhood disorders (Hartmann et al. 1984; Zeitlin 2000) indicates the potential for future research on interventions in childhood. It is crucial that mental health professionals find ways of gaining the support of families in these endeavours and build on their existing strengths without repeating past tendencies to alienate families.

Comorbidity of substance abuse and dependence and psychosis is common and a serious contemporary problem, with a lifetime prevalence of approximately 50% (Regier *et al.* 1990). It is linked with an earlier age of onset of psychosis (Hambrecht & Häfner 1996; Addington & Addington 1998; Cantwell *et al.* 1999) and a wide range of negative outcomes (Drake & Brunette 1998). The future success of substance misuse preventative programmes in vulnerable young persons is of great importance (Mueser *et al.* 2002b).

Although the research emphasis is shifting towards early interventions, it is most important that the continuing needs of those whose problems are not ameliorated in the early stages are not relegated in importance, either in the provision of services or in researching their needs. Again the importance of partnership with long-term users of services is vital if effective developments are to continue, as Davidson *et al.* (2000) so vividly illustrate.

Many different types of psychological treatments have been covered in this chapter and pointers to future research have been given. It is vital that mental health professionals, now that we are beginning to see the end of a reductionistic approach to the problem of schizophrenia, will value the development of a plurality of psychological approaches that are likely to improve the quality of life of vulnerable persons. It is essential to respect the enormous difficulty of adequately researching multifaceted interventions, which often need to change in emphasis over the time and course of the disturbance. Without this respect, mental professionals may not hold onto the hard-won awareness of the unfortunate consequences for patients in recent decades resulting from reductionistic approaches of different kinds.

References

Addington, J. & Addington, D. (1998) Effect of substance misuse in early psychosis. *British Journal of Psychiatry* 172 (Suppl. 33), 134–136.

Alanen, Y.O. (1997a) *Schizophrenia: Its Origins and Need-Adapted Treatment.* Karnac Books, London.

Alanen, Y.O. (1997b) Vulnerability to schizophrenia and psychotherapeutic treatment of schizophrenic patients: towards an integrated view. *Psychiatry* 60, 142–157.

Alanen, Y.O., Räkköläinen, V., Laakso, J., Rasimus, R. & Kaljonen, A. (1986) *Towards Need-Specific Treatment of Schizophreniform Psychoses.* Springer-Verlag, Heidelberg.

Alanen, Y.O., Ugelstad, E., Armelius, B.-Å. *et al.* (1994) *Early Treatment for Schizophrenic Patients: Scandinavian Psychotherapeutic Approaches.* Scandinavian University Press, Norway.

Alford, G.S., Fleece, L. & Rothblum, E. (1982) Hallucinatory-delusional verbalizations: modification in a chronic schizophrenic by self-control and cognitive restructuring. *Behavior Modification* 6, 421–435.

Amador, X.F. & Gorman, J.M. (1998) Psychopathologic domains and insight in schizophrenia. *Psychiatric Clinics of North America* 21, 27–42.

Amador, X., Strauss, D., Yale, S. & Gorman, J.M. (1991) Awareness of illness in schizophrenia. *Schizophrenia Bulletin* 17, 113–132.

American Psychiatric Association (1994) *Diagnostic and Statistical Manual of Mental Disorders, DSM-IV.* American Psychiatric Association, Washington, DC.

Anderson, C.M., Reiss, D.J. & Hogarty, G.E. (1986) *Schizophrenia and the Family.* Guildford, New York.

Appleton, W.S. (1974) Mistreatment of patients' families by psychiatrists. *American Journal of Psychiatry* 131, 655–657.

Asberg, M., Montgomery, S.A., Perris, C., Shalling, D. & Sedvall, G. (1978) The comprehensive psychopathological rating scale. *Acta Psychiatrica Scandinavica Supplement* 271, 5–27.

Ascher-Svanum, H. & Krause, A.A. (1991) *Psychoeducational Groups for Patients with Schizophrenia: a Guide for Practitioners.* Aspen, Gaithersburg.

Ball, R.A., Moore, E. & Kuipers, L. (1992) EE in community care facilities: a comparison of patient outcome in a 9 month follow-up of two residential hostels. *Social Psychiatry and Psychiatric Epidemiology* 27, 35–39.

Barrowclough, C. & Parle, M. (1997) Appraisal, psychological adjustment and expressed emotion in relatives of patients suffering from schizophrenia. *British Journal of Psychiatry* 171, 26–30.

Barrowclough, C. & Tarrier, N. (1992) *Families of Schizophrenic Patients: Cognitive Behavioural Intervention.* Chapman & Hall, London.

Bartels, S.J. & Levine, K.J. (1998) Meeting the needs of older adults with severe and persistent mental illness: public policy in an era of managed and long-term care reform. *Public Policy and Aging Report* 9, 1–6.

Bartels, S.J., Mueser, K.T. & Miles, K.M. (1997) A comparative study of elderly patients with schizophrenia and bipolar disorder in nursing homes and the community. *Schizophrenia Research* 27, 181–190.

Bartels, S.J., Levine, K.J. & Shea, D. (1999) Community-based long-term care for older persons with severe and persistent mental illness in an era of managed care. *Psychiatric Services* 50, 1189–1197.

Bateman, A.W. (2000) Integration in psychotherapy: an evolving reality in personality disorder. *British Journal of Psychotherapy* 17, 147–156.

Bateman, A.W. & Holmes, J. (1995) *Introduction to Psychoanalysis: Contemporary Theory and Practice.* Routledge, London.

Bebbington, P.E. & Kuipers, L. (1994) The predictive utility in schizophrenia: an aggregate analysis. *Psychological Medicine* 24, 707–718.

Bechgaard, B. & Rosenbaum, B. (1994) Differences and similarities between the Nordic models. In: *Early Treatment for Schizophrenic Patients: Scandinavian Psychotherapeutic Approaches* (eds Y.O. Alanen, E. Ugelstad, B.-Å. Armelius *et al.*), pp. 77–82. Scandinavian University Press, Norway.

Beck, A.T. (1952) Successful outpatient psychotherapy of a chronic schizophrenic with a delusion based on borrowed guilt. *Psychiatry* 15, 305–312.

Beiser, M., Erickson, D., Fleming, J.A.E. & Iacono, W.G. (1993) Establishing the onset of psychotic illness. *American Journal of Psychiatry* 150, 1349–1354.

Bell, M.D., Lysaker, P.H. & Milstein, R.M. (1996) Clinical benefits of paid work activity in schizophrenia. *Schizophrenia Bulletin* 22, 51–67.

Bellack, A.S. (1986) Schizophrenia: behavior therapy's forgotten child. *Behavior Therapy* 17, 199–214.

Bellack, A.S., Turner, S.M., Hersen, M. & Luber, R.F. (1984) An examination of the efficacy of social skills training for chronic schizophrenic patients. *Hospital and Community Psychiatry* 35, 1023–1028.

Bellack, A.S., Morrison, R.L. & Mueser, K.T. (1989) Social problem solving in schizophrenia. *Schizophrenia Bulletin* 15, 101–116.

Bellack, A.S., Morrison, R.L., Wixted, J.T. & Mueser, K.T. (1990a) An analysis of social competence in schizophrenia. *British Journal of Psychiatry* **156**, 809–818.

Bellack, A.S., Mueser, K.T., Morrison, R.L., Tierney, A. & Podell, K. (1990b) Remediation of cognitive deficits in schizophrenia. *American Journal of Psychiatry* **147**, 1650–1655.

Bellack, A.S., Mueser, K.T., Gingerich, S. & Agresta, J. (1997) *Social Skills Training for Schizophrenia: a Step-by-Step Guide.* Guilford, New York.

Benedict, R.H.B. (1989) The effectiveness of cognitive remediation strategies for victims of traumatic head-injury: a review of the literature. *Clinical Psychology Review* **9**, 605–626.

Berman, K., Zec, R. & Weinberger, D. (1986) Physiologic dysfunction of dorsolateral prefrontal cortex in schizophrenia. *Archives of General Psychiatry* **43**, 126–135.

Bion, W.R. (1967) *Second Thoughts.* Heinemann, London.

Birchwood, M. (1995) Early intervention in psychotic relapse: cognitive approaches to detection and management. *Behaviour Change* **12**, 2–19.

Birchwood, M. (2000) The critical period for early intervention. In: *Early Intervention in Psychosis* (eds M. Birchwood, D. Fowler & C. Jackson), pp. 28–63. Wiley, Chichester.

Birchwood, M., Smith, J. & Cochrane, R. (1992) Specific and non-specific effects of educational intervention for families living with schizophrenia. *British Journal of Psychiatry* **160**, 806–814.

Bleuler, E. (1911/1950) *Dementia Praecox or the Group of Schizophrenias.* Translated by J. Zinkin. International Universities Press, New York.

Bleuler, M. (1972) *Die Schizophrenen Geistesstörungen Im Lichte Langjärigen Kranken-und Familiengeschichten.* Georg Thieme, Stuttgart.

Bond, G.R., Drake, R.E., Mueser, K.T. & Becker, D.R. (1997) An update on supported employment for people with severe mental illness. *Psychiatric Services* **48**, 335–346.

Bradshaw, W.H. (1993) Coping-skills training versus a problem-solving approach with schizophrenic patients. *Hospital and Community Psychiatry* **44**, 1102–1104.

Braff, D.L., Heaton, R., Kuck, J. *et al.* (1991) The generalized pattern of neuropsychological deficits in outpatients with chronic schizophrenia and heterogeneous Wisconsin card sorting test results. *Archives of General Psychiatry* **48**, 891–898.

Brekke, J.S., Raine, A., Ansel, M., Lencz, T. & Bird, L. (1997) Neuropsychological and psychophysiological correlates of psychosocial functioning in schizophrenia. *Schizophrenia Bulletin* **23**, 19–28.

Brenner, H.D., Kraemer, S., Hermanutz, M. & Hodel, B. (1990) Cognitive treatment in schizophrenia. In: *Schizophrenia: Concepts, Vulnerability and Intervention* (eds E.R. Straube & K. Hahlweg), pp. 161–192. Springer-Verlag, Berlin.

Brewin, C.R., MacCarthy, B., Duda, K. & Vaughn, C.E. (1991) Attribution and expressed emotion in the relatives of patients with schizophrenia. *Journal of Abnormal Psychology* **100**, 546–554.

British Psychological Society (2000) *Recent Advances in Understanding in Mental Illness and Psychotic Experiences.* Division of Clinical Psychology, British Psychological Society, Leicester.

Buchanan, A., Reed, A., Wessely, S. *et al.* (1993) Acting on delusions. II. The phenomenological correlates of acting on delusions. *British Journal of Psychiatry* **163**, 77–81.

Budd, R.J. & Hughes, I.C. (1997) What do relatives of people with schizophrenia find helpful about family intervention? *Schizophrenia Bulletin* **23**, 341–347.

Bustillo, J.R., Lauriello, J., Horan, W.P. & Keith, S.J. (2001) The psychosocial treatment of schizophrenia: an update. *American Journal of Psychiatry* **158**, 163–175.

Butler, R.W. & Namerow, N.S. (1988) Cognitive retraining in brain-injury rehabilitation: a critical review. *Journal of Neuropsychology and Rehabilitation* **2**, 97–101.

Butzlaff, R.L. & Hooley, J.M. (1998) Expressed emotion and psychiatric relapse: a meta-analysis. *Archives of General Psychiatry.* **55**, 547–552.

Caldwell, C.B. & Gottesman, I.I. (1990) Schizophrenics kill themselves too: a review of risk factors for suicide. *Schizophrenia Bulletin* **16**, 571–589.

Cancro, R. & Meyerson, A.T. (1999) Prevention of disability and stigma related to schizophrenia: a review. In: *Schizophrenia* (eds M. Maj & N. Sartorius), pp. 243–278. J. Wiley, Chichester.

Cantwell, R., Brewin, J., Glazebrook, C. *et al.* (1999) Prevalence of substance misuse in first-episode psychosis. *British Journal of Psychiatry* **174**, 150–153.

Cardin, V.A., McGill, C.W. & Falloon, I.R.H. (1986) An economic analysis: costs, benefits and effectiveness. In: *Family Management of Schizophrenia* (ed. I.R.H. Falloon), pp. 114–123. Johns Hopkins University Press, Baltimore.

Carling, P.J. (1995) *Return to Community: Building Support Systems for People with Psychiatric Disabilities.* Guilford, New York.

Carpenter, W.T., Heinrichs, D.W. & Wagman, A.M.I. (1988) Deficit and non-deficit forms of schizophrenia: the concept. *American Journal of Psychiatry* **145**, 578–583.

Carpenter, W.T., Buchanan, R.W., Kirkpatrick, B., Tamminga, C. & Wood, F. (1993) Strong interence, theory testing, and the neuroanatomy of schizophrenia. *Archives of General Psychiatry* **50**, 825–831.

Chadwick, P.D. & Lowe, C.F. (1990) The measurement and modification of delusional beliefs. *Journal of Consulting and Clinical Psychology* **58**, 225–232.

Chadwick, P.D., Birchwood, M. & Trower, P. (1996) *Cognitive Therapy for Delusions, Voices and Paranoia.* Wiley, Chichester.

Chadwick, P.D., Sambrooke, S., Rasch, S. & Davies, E. (2000) Challenging the omnipotence of voices: group cognitive behavior therapy for voices. *Behaviour Research and Therapy* **38**, 993–1003.

Chamberlin, J. (1978) *On Our Own: Patient-Controlled Alternatives to the Mental Health System.* Hawthorne, New York.

Chamberlin, J. & Rogers, J.A. (1990) Planning a community-based mental health system: perspectives of service recipients. *American Psychologist* **45**, 1241–1244.

Ciompi, L. (1987a) Review of follow-up studies on long-term evolution and aging in schizophrenia. In: *Schizophrenia and Aging* (eds N.E. Miller & G.D. Cohen), pp. 37–51. Guilford, New York.

Ciompi, L. (1987b) Toward a coherent multidimensional understanding and therapy of schizophrenia: converging new concepts. In: *Psychosocial Treatment of Schizophrenia: Multidimensional Concepts, Psychological, Family, and Self-Help Perspectives* (eds J.S. Strauss, W. Boker & H.D. Brenner), pp. 48–62. Hans Huber, Toronto.

Ciompi, L. & Müller, C. (1976) *Lebensweg und Alter der Schizophrenen. Eine Katamnestische Langzeitstudie Bis Ins Senium.* Springer Verlag, Berlin.

Clarkin, J.F., Hurt, S.W. & Crilly, J.L. (1987) Therapeutic alliance and hospital treatment outcome. *Hospital and Community Psychiatry* **40**, 641–643.

Conolly, J. (1856) *The Treatment of the Insane Without Mechanical Restraint.* Smith, Elder & Co, London.

Copolov, D., Velakoulis, D., McGorry, P. *et al.* (2000) Neurobiological findings in early phase schizophrenia. *Brain Research Reviews* **31**, 157–165.

Cullberg, J. (2000) *Psykoser: ett humanistiskt och biologiskt perspektiv.* Natur och Kultur. Stockholm.

Cullberg, J. (2001) The parachute project: first episode psychosis – background and treatment. In: *A Language for Psychosis: Psycho-*

analysis of Psychotic States (ed. P. Williams), pp. 115–125. Whurr Books, London.

Cullberg, J., Thorén, G., Åbb, S., Mesterton, A. & Svedberg, B. (2000) Integrating intensive psychosocial and low dose medical treatments for all first episode psychotic patients compared to 'treatment as usual': a three year follow-up. In: *Psychosis: Psychological Approaches and their Effectiveness* (eds B.V. Martindale, A. Bateman, M. Crowe & F. Margison), pp. 200–209. Gaskell, London.

Davidson, L., Stayner, D.A., Chinman, M.J., Lambert, S. & Sledge, W.H. (2000) Preventing relapse and re-admission in psychosis: using patients' subjective experience in designing clinical interventions. In: *Psychosis: Psychological Approaches and their Effectiveness* (eds B.V. Martindale, A. Bateman, M. Crowe & F. Margison), pp. 134–156. Gaskell, London.

Deegan, P.E. (1990) Spirit breaking: when the helping professionals hurt. *Humanistic Psychologist* 18, 301–313.

Department of Health (1999) *A National Service Framework for Mental Health: Modern Standards and Service Models*. NHS Executive, London.

Dickerson, F.B. (2000) Cognitive behavioural psychotherapy for schizophrenia: a review of recent empirical studies. *Schizophrenia Research* 43, 71–90.

Dilk, M.N. & Bond, G.R. (1996) Meta-analytic evaluation of skills training research for individuals with severe mental illness. *Journal of Consulting and Clinical Psychology Disorders* 64, 1337–1346.

Dobson, D.J.G., McDougall, G., Busheikin, J. & Aldous, J. (1995) Effects of social skills training and social milieu treatment on symptoms of schizophrenia. *Psychiatric Services* 46, 376–380.

Drake, R.E. & Brunette, M.F. (1998) Complications of severe mental illness related to alcohol and other drug use disorders. In: *Recent Developments in Alcoholism*, Vol. XIV *Consequences of Alcoholism* (ed. M. Galanter), pp. 285–299. Plenum, New York.

Drury, V., Birchwood, M., Cochrane, R. & Macmillan, F. (1996a) Cognitive therapy and recovery from acute psychosis: a controlled trial. I. Impact on psychotic symptoms. *British Journal of Psychiatry* 169, 593–601.

Drury, V., Birchwood, M., Cochrane, R. & Macmillan, F. (1996b) Cognitive therapy and recovery from acute psychosis: a controlled trial. II. Impact on recovery time. *British Journal of Psychiatry* 169, 602–607.

Drury, V., Birchwood, M. & Cochrane, R. (2000) Cognitive therapy and recovery from acute psychosis: a controlled trial. III. Five-year follow-up. *British Journal of Psychiatry* 177, 8–14.

D'Zurilla, T.J. & Goldfried, M.R. (1971) Problem solving and behavior modification. *Journal of Abnormal Psychology* 78, 107–126.

Eckman, T.A., Wirshing, W.C., Marder, S.R. *et al.* (1992) Technique for training schizophrenic patients in illness self-management: a controlled trial. *American Journal of Psychiatry* 149, 1549–1555.

Eisenberg, E. (1999) Psychiatry and neuroscience at the end of the century. *Current Opinion in Psychiatry* 12, 629–632.

Endicott, J., Spitzer, R.L., Fleiss, J.L. & Cohen, J. (1976) The Global Assessment Scale: a procedure for measuring overall severity of psychiatric disturbance. *Archives of General Psychiatry* 33, 766–771.

Etchegoyen, R.H. (2001) *The Fundamentals of Psychoanalytic Technique*. Karnac Books, London.

Fadden, G. (1997) Implementation of family interventions in routine clinical practice following staff training programmes: a major cause for concern. *Journal of Mental Health* 6, 599–612.

Falloon, I.R.H. & Pederson, J. (1985) Family management in the prevention of morbidity of schizophrenia: the adjustment of the family unit. *British Journal of Psychiatry* 147, 156–163.

Falloon, I.R.H. & Talbot, R.E. (1981) Persistent auditory hallucinations: coping mechanisms and implications for management. *Psychological Medicine* 11, 329–339.

Falloon, I.R.H., Boyd, J.L., McGill, C.W. *et al.* (1985) Family management in the prevention of morbidity of schizophrenia: clinical outcome of a two-year longitudinal study. *Archives of General Psychiatry* 49, 179–115l.

Falloon, I.R.H., McGill, C.W., Boyd, J.L. & Pederson, J. (1987) Family management in the prevention of morbidity of schizophrenia: social outcome of a two-year longtitudinal study. *Psychological Medicine* 17, 59–66.

Fenton, W.S. & McGlashan, T.H. (1992) Testing systems for assessment of negative symptoms in schizophrenia. *Archives of General Psychiatry* 49, 179–185.

Flesher, S. (1990) Cognitive rehabilitation in schizophrenia: a theoretical review and model of treatment. *Neuropsychology Review* 1, 223–246.

Fowler, D. & Morley, S. (1989) The cognitive–behavioural treatment of hallucinations and delusions: a preliminary study. *Behavioural Psychotherapy* 17, 267–282.

Fowler, D., Garety, P. & Kuipers, E. (1995) *Cognitive Behaviour Therapy for Psychosis*. .Wiley, Chichester.

Freud, S. (1915) *The Unconscious*. Standard Edition, Vol. 14. Hogarth Press, London.

Freud, S. (1932) *New Introductory Lectures on Psycho-Analysis*. Standard Edition, Vol. 22, p. 154. Hogarth Press, London.

Fromm-Reichmann, F. (1950) *Principles of Intensive Psychotherapy*. University of Chicago Press, Chicago.

Furlan, P.M. (1999) The effectiveness of cognitive–behavioural therapy in schizophrenia. In: *Schizophrenia*. (eds M. Maj & N.J. Sartorius), pp. 236–238. Wiley, Chichester.

Garety, P.A., Kuipers, L., Fowler, D., Chamberlain, F. & Dunn, G. (1994) Cognitive behavioural therapy for drug-resistant psychosis. *British Journal of Medical Psychology* 67, 259–271.

Garety, P.A., Fowler, D., Kuipers, E. *et al.* (1997) London–East Anglia randomised controlled trial of cognitive–behavioural therapy for psychosis. II. Predictors of outcome. *British Journal of Psychiatry* 171, 420–426.

Garety, P.A., Dunn, G., Fowler, D. & Kuipers, E. (1998) The evaluation of cognitive behavioural therapy for psychosis. In: *Outcome and Innovation in Psychological Treatment of Schizophrenia* (eds T. Wykes, N. Tarrier & S. Lewis), pp. 101–118. Wiley, Chichester.

Garety, P.A., Fowler, D. & Kuipers, E. (2000) Cognitive–behavioral therapy for medication-resistant symptoms. *Schizophrenia Bulletin* 26, 73–86.

Goldberg, T.E., Weinberger, D.R., Berman, K.F., Pliskin, N.H. & Podd, M.H. (1987) Further evidence for dementia of the prefrontal type in schizophrenia? A controlled study of teaching the Wisconsin Card Sorting Test. *Archives of General Psychiatry* 44, 1008–1014.

Goldberg, T.E., Hyde. T.M., Kleinman. J.E. & Weinberger, D.R. (1993) Course of schizophrenia: neuropsychological evidence for a static encephalopathy. *Schizophrenia Bulletin* 19, 797–804.

González de Chávez Menéndez, M. & García-Ordás Alvarez, A. (1992) Group therapy as a facilitating factor in the combined treatment approach to schizophrenia. In: *Psychotherapy of Schizophrenia: Facilitating and Obstructive Factors* (eds. A. Werbart & J. Cullberg), Scandinavian University Press, Oslo.

Gould, R.A., Mueser, K.T., Bolton, E., Mays, V. & Goff, D. (2001) Cognitive therapy for psychosis in schizophrenia: an effect size analysis. *Schizophrenia Research* 48, 335–342.

Green, M.F. (1996) What are the functional consequences of neurocognitive deficits in schizophrenia? *American Journal of Psychiatry* 153, 321–330.

Green, M.F., Kern, R.S., Braff, D.L. & Mintz, J. (2000) Neurocognitive deficits and functional outcome in schizophrenia: are we measuring the 'right stuff'? *Schizophrenia Bulletin* 26, 119–136.

Greenley, J.R. (1986) Social control and expressed emotion. *Journal of Nervous and Mental Disease* **174**, 24–30.

Grinspoon, L., Ewalt, J.R. & Shader, R.I. (1972) *Schizophrenia, Pharmacotherapy and Psychotherapy*. Williams & Wilkins, Baltimore.

Gunderson, J.G., Frank, A., Katz, H.M. *et al.* (1984) Effects of psychotherapy in schizophrenia. II. Comparative outcome of two forms of treatment. *Schizophrenia Bulletin* **10**, 564–598.

Haas, G.L. & Sweeney, J.A. (1992) Premorbid and onset features of first episode schizophrenia. *Schizophrenia Bulletin* **18**, 373–386.

Haddock, G., Bentall, R.P. & Slade, P.D. (1996) Psychological treatment of auditory hallucinations: focusing or distraction? In: *Cognitive–Behavioural Interventions with Psychotic Disorders* (eds G. Haddock & P.D. Slade), pp. 45–71. Routledge, London.

Haddock, G., Slade, P.D., Bentall, R.P., Reid, D. & Faragher, E.B. (1998) A comparison of the long-term effectiveness of distraction and focusing in the treatment of auditory hallucinations. *British Journal of Medical Psychology* **71**, 339–349.

Häfner, H., Maurer, K., Löffler, W. & Riecher-Rössler, A. (1993) The influence of age and sex on the onset of early course of schizophrenia. *British Journal of Psychiatry* **162**, 80–86.

Häfner, H., Nowotny, B., Löffler, W., van der Heiden, W. & Mauerer, K. (1995) When and how does schizophrenia produce social deficits? *European Archives of Psychiatry and Neuroscience* **246**, 17–28.

Hambrecht, M. & Häfner, H. (1996) Substance abuse and the onset of schizophrenia. *Biological Psychiatry* **39**, 1–9.

Harding, C.M., Brooks, G.W., Ashikaga, T., Strauss, J.S. & Breier, A. (1987a) The Vermont longitudinal study of persons with severe mental illness. I. Methodology, study sample and overall status 32 years later. *American Journal of Psychiatry* **144**, 718–726.

Harding, C.M., Brooks, G.W., Ashikaga, T., Strauss, J.S. & Breier, A. (1987b) The Vermont longitudinal study of persons with severe mental illness. II. Long-term outcome of subjects who retrospectively met DSM-III criteria for schizophrenia. *American Journal of Psychiatry* **144**, 727–735.

Harrison, G., Croudace, T., Mason, P., Glazebrook, C. & Medley, I. (1996) Predicting the long-term outcome of schizophrenia. *Psychological Medicine* **26**, 697–705.

Harrow, M. & Silverstein, M.L. (1977) Psychotic symptoms in s chizophrenia after the acute phase. *Schizophrenia Bulletin* **3**, 608–616.

Hartmann, E., Milofsky, E., Vaillant, G. *et al.* (1984) Vulnerability to schizophrenia: prediction of adult schizophrenia using childhood information. *Archives of General Psychiatry* **41**, 1050–1056.

Hayes, R.L., Halford, W.K. & Varghese, F.T. (1995) Social skills training with chronic schizophrenic patients: effects on negative symptoms and community functioning. *Behavior Therapy* **26**, 433–449.

Hayward, P., Chan, N., David, A., Kemp, R. & Youle, S. (1995) Medication self-management: a preliminary report on an intervention to improve medication compliance. *Journal of Mental Health* **4**, 511–517.

Heaton, R.K. (1991) *Wisconsin Card Sorting Test Manual*. Psychological Assessment Resources, Odessa, FL.

Heinssen, R.K., Liberman, R.P. & Kopelowicz, A. (2000) Psychosocial skills training for schizophrenia: lessons from the laboratory. *Schizophrenia Bulletin* **26**, 21–46.

Hinshelwood, R.D. (1987) The psychotherapist's role in a large psychiatric institution. *Psychoanalytic Psychotherapy* **2**, 207–215.

Hinshelwood, R.D. & Skogstad, W. (2000) *Observing Organisations. Anxiety, Defence and Culture in Health Care*. Routledge, London.

Hogarty, G.E. & Flesher, S. (1999a) Developmental theory for a cognitive enhancement therapy of schizophrenia. *Schizophrenia Bulletin* **25**, 677–692.

Hogarty, G.E. & Flesher, S. (1999b) Practice principles of cognitive enhancement therapy for schizophrenia. *Schizophrenia Bulletin* **25**, 693–708.

Hogarty, G.E., Anderson, C.M., Reiss, D.J.J.K.S. *et al.* (1986) Family psychoeducation, social skills training, and maintenance chemotherapy in the aftercare treatment of schizophrenia: one-year effects of a controlled study on relapse and expressed emotion. *Archives of General Psychiatry* **43**, 633–642.

Hogarty, G.E., Anderson, C.M., Reiss, D.J. *et al.* (1991) Family psychoeducation, social skills training, and maintenance chemotherapy in the aftercare treatment of schizophrenia. II. Two-year effects of a controlled study on relapse and adjustment. *Archives of General Psychiatry* **48**, 340–347.

Hogarty, G.E., Kornblith, S.J., Greenwald, D. *et al.* (1995) Personal therapy: a disorder-relevant psychotherapy for schizophrenia. *Schizophrenia Bulletin* **21**, 379–393.

Hogarty, G.E., Kornblith, S.J., Greenwald, D. *et al.* (1997a) Three year trials of personal therapy among schizophrenic patients living with or independent of family. I. Description of study and effects on relapse rates. *American Journal of Psychiatry* **154**, 1504–1513.

Hogarty, G.E., Greenwald, D., Ulrich, R.F. *et al.* (1997b) Three year trials of personal therapy among schizophrenic patients living with or independent of family. II. Effects of adjustment on patients. *American Journal of Psychiatry* **154**, 1514–1524.

Hornung, W.P., Feldmann, R., Klingberg, S., Buchkremer, G. & Reker, T. (1999) Long-term effects of a psychoeducational psychotherapeutic intervention for schizophrenic outpatients and their key-persons: results of a five-year follow-up. *European Archives of Psychiatry and Clinical Neurosciences* **249**, 162–167.

Horwitz, A.V., Tessler, R.C., Fisher, G.A. & Gamache, G.M. (1992) The role of adult siblings in providing social support to the severely mentally ill. *Journal of Marriage and the Family* **54**, 233–241.

Hubschmid, T. & Zemp, M. (1989) Interactions in high- and low-EE families. *Social Psychiatry and Psychiatric Epidemiology* **24**, 113–119.

Huxley, N.A., Rendall, M. & Sederer, L. (2000) Psychosocial treatments in schizophrenia: a review of the past 20 years. *Journal of Nervous and Mental Diseases* **188**, 187–201.

International Early Psychosis Association (IEPA). www.iepa.org.au.

Jablensky, A., Sartorius, N., Ernberg, G. *et al.* (1992) *Schizophrenia: Manifestation, Incidence and Course in Different Cultures*. Psychological Medicine Monographs (Suppl. 20). Cambridge University Press.

Jackson, H.J., McGorry, P.D. & Edwards, J. (2001) Cognitively oriented psychotherapy for early psychosis: theory, praxis, outcomes, and challenges. In: *Social Cognition in Schizophrenia* (eds P.W. Corrigan & D.L. Penn), pp. 249–284. American Psychological Association, Washington, DC.

Jackson, M. & Williams, P. (1994) *Unimaginable Storms: a Search for Meaning in Psychosis*. Karnac Books, London.

Johannessen, J.O., Larsen, T.K., McGlashan, T. & Vaglum, P. (2000) Early intervention in psychosis: the tips-project, a multi-centre study in Scandinavia. In: *Psychosis: Psychological Treatments and Their Effectiveness* (eds B.V. Martindale, A. Bateman, M. Crowe & F. Margison), pp. 210–234. Gaskell, London.

Jones, C., Cormac, I., Mota, J. & Campbell, C. (2000) Cognitive behaviour therapy for schizophrenia. *Cochrane Database of Systematic Reviews*, Issue 3.

Kanas, N. (1986) Group therapy with schizophrenics: a review of controlled studies. *International Journal of Group Psychotherapy* **36**, 339–351.

Kanas, N. (2000) Group psychotherapy and schizophrenia: an integrative model. In: *Psychosis: Psychological Approaches and their*

Effectiveness (eds. B.V. Martindale, A. Bateman, F. Margison & M. Crowe), pp. 120–133. Gaskell, London.

Karon, B.P. (1989) Psychotherapy versus medication for schizophrenia: empirical comparisons. In: *The Limits of Biological Treatments for Psychological Distress: Comparisons with Placebo* (eds S. Fisher & R.P. Greenberg), pp. 105–150. Lawrence Erlbaum, Hillsdale, NJ.

Karon, B.P. & Vandenbos, G.R. (1972) The consequences of psychotherapy for schizophrenic patients. *Psychotherapy: Theory, Research and Practice* 9, 111–119.

Karon, B.P. & Vandenbos, G.R. (1981) *Psychotherapy of Schizophrenia: The Treatment of Choice.* Aronson, New York.

Keith, S.J., Bellack, A., Frances, A., Mance, R. & Matthews, S. (1989) The influence of diagnosis and family treatment on acute treatment response and short-term outcome in schizophrenia. *Psychopharmacology Bulletin* 25, 336–339.

Kemp, R., Hayward, P., Applewhaite, G., Everitt, B. & David, A. (1996) Compliance therapy in psychotic patients: randomised controlled trial. *British Medical Journal* 312, 345–349.

Kemp, R., Hayward, P., Applewhaite, G., Everitt, B. & David, A. (1998) A randomised controlled trial of compliance therapy: 18 month follow-up. *British Journal of Psychiatry* 172, 413–419.

Kern, R.S., Green, M.F. & Satz, P. (1992) Neuropsychological predictors of skills training for chronic psychiatric patients. *Psychiatry Research* 43, 223–230.

Kern, R.S., Green, M.F. & Goldstein, M.J. (1995) Modification of performance on the Span of Apprehension, a putative marker of vulnerability to schizophrenia. *Journal of Abnormal Psychology* 104, 385–389.

Kern, R.S., Wallace, C.J., Hellman, S.G., Womack, L.M. & Green, M.F. (1996) A training procedure for remediating WCST deficits in chronic psychotic patients: an adaptation of errorless learning principles. *Journal of Psychiatric Research* 30, 283–294.

Killick, K. & Greenwood, H. (1995) Research in art therapy with people who have psychotic illnesses. In: *Art and Music: Therapy and Research* (eds A. Gilroy & C. Lee), pp. 101–116. Routledge, London.

Kingdon, D. & Turkington, D. (1994) *Cognitive–Behavioural Therapy of Schizophrenia.* Lawrence Erlbaum, Hove, Sussex.

Klingberg, S., Bachkremer, G., Holle, R., Monking, H.S. & Hornung, W.P. (1999) Differential therapy effects of psychoeducational psychotherapy for schizophrenic patients: results of a 2-year follow-up. *European Archives of Psychiatry and Clinical Neuroscience* 249, 66–72.

Kohut, H. (1971) *The Analysis of the Self: A Systematic Approach to the Psychoanalytic Treatment of the Narcissistic Personality Disorders.* International University Press, New York.

Kohut, H. (1977) *The Restoration of the Self.* International University Press, New York.

Kottgen, C., Sonnichsen, I., Mollenhauer, K. & Jurth, R. (1984) Group therapy with the families of schizophrenic patients: results of the Hamburg Camberwell Family Interview Study III. *International Journal of Family Psychiatry* 5, 83–94.

Kraepelin, E. (1919/1971) *Dementia Praecox and Paraphrenia.* Translated by R.M. Barclay. Robert E. Krieger, New York.

Kuipers, E. & Raune, D. (2000) The early development of expressed emotion and burden in the families of first onset psychosis. In: *Early Intervention in Psychosis* (eds M. Birchwood, D. Fowler & C. Jackson), pp. 128–142. Wiley, Chichester.

Kuipers, E., Garety, P., Fowler, D. *et al.* (1997) London–East Anglia randomised controlled trial of cognitive–behavioural therapy for psychosis. I. Effects of the treatment phase. *British Journal of Psychiatry* 171, 319–327.

Kuipers, E., Fowler, D., Garety, P. *et al.* (1998) London–East Anglia randomised controlled trial of cognitive–behavioural therapy for psy-

chosis. III. Follow-up and economic evaluation at 18 months. *British Journal of Psychiatry* 173, 61–68.

Kuipers, L., Leff, J. & Lam, D. (1992) *Family Work for Schizophrenia: a Practical Guide.* Gaskell, London.

Laing, R.D. (1960) *The Divided Self.* Tavistock, London.

Lam, D.H. (1991) Psychosocial family intervention in schixophrenia: a review of empirical studies. *Psychological Medicine* 21, 423–441.

Lambert, M.J. & Bergin, A.E. (1994) The effectiveness of psychotherapy. In: *Handbook of Psychotherapy and Behaviour Change*, 4th edn. (eds A.E. Bergin & S.L. Garfield), pp. 143–189. J. Wiley, New York.

Langfeldt, G. (1937) *The Prognosis in Schizophrenia and Factors Influencing the Course of the Disease.* Munksgaard, Copenhagen.

Larsen, T.K. & Opjordsmoen, S. (1996) Early identification and treatment of schizophrenia: conceptual and ethical considerations. *Psychiatry* 59, 371–380.

Lecompte, D. & Pelc, I. (1996) A cognitive–behavioral program to improve compliance with medication in patients with schizophrenia. *International Journal of Mental Health* 25, 51–56.

Leff, J. (2000) Commentary. *Advances in Psychiatric Treatment* 6, 250–251.

Leff, J., Kuipers, L., Berkowitz, R. & Sturgeon, D. (1985) A control trial of social intervention in the family of schizophrenic patients: two-year follow up. *British Journal of Psychiatry* 146, 594–600.

Leff, J., Berkowitz, R., Shavit, N. *et al.* (1989) A trial of family therapy vs. a relatives group for schizophrenia. *British Journal of Psychiatry* 154, 58–66.

Leff, J., Berkowitz, R., Shavit, N. *et al.* (1990) A trial of family therapy versus a relatives' group for schizophrenia: two-year follow-up. *British Journal of Psychiatry* 157, 571–577.

Lefley, H.P. (1989) Family burden and family stigma in major mental illness. *American Psychologist* 44, 556–560.

Lefley, H.P. & Johnson, D.L., eds. (1990) *Families as Allies in Treatment of the Mentally Ill. New Directions for Mental Health Professionals.* American Psychiatric Press, Washington, DC.

Lehman, A.F. & Steinwachs, D.M. (1998) Translating research into practice: the Schizophrenic Patient Outcome Research Team (PORT) treatment recommendations. *Schizophrenia Bulletin* 24, 1–10.

Lehman, A.F., Steinwachs, D.M. and the Schizophrenia PORT & Co-investigators of the Project (1998) Patterns of usual care for schizophrenia: initial results from the Schizophrenia Patient Outcomes Research Team (PORT) client survey. *Schizophrenia Bulletin* 24, 11–20.

Lehtinen, V., Aaltonen, J., Koffert, T., Räkköläinen, V. & Syvälahti, E. (2000) Two-year outcome in first episode psychosis treated according to an integrated model: is immediate neuroleptisation always needed? *European Psychiatry* 15, 312–320.

Lenzenweger, M.F., Dworkin, R.H. & Wethington, E. (1991) Examining the underlying structure of schizophrenic phenomenology: evidence for a three-process model. *Schizophrenia Bulletin* 17, 515–524.

Liberman, R.P., Mueser, K.T. & Wallace, C.J. (1986a) Social skills training for schizophrenic individuals at risk for relapse. *American Journal of Psychiatry* 143, 523–526.

Liberman, R.P., Mueser, K.T., Wallace, C.J. *et al.* (1986b) Training skills in the psychiatrically disabled: learning coping and competence. *Schizophrenia Bulletin* 12, 631–647.

Liberman, R.P., DeRisi, W.J. & Mueser, K.T. (1989) *Social Skills Training for Psychiatric Patients.* Allyn & Bacon, Needham Heights, MA.

Liberman, R.P., Wallace, C.J., Blackwell, G. *et al.* (1998) Skills training versus psychosocial occupational therapy for persons with persistent schizophrenia. *American Journal of Psychiatry* 155, 1087–1091.

Linszen, D., Dingemans, P., Van-der-Does, J.W. *et al.* (1996) Treatment, expressed emotion and relapse in recent onset schizophrenic disorders. *Psychological Medicine* 26, 333–342.

Linszen, D., Lenior, M., De Haan, L., Dingemans, P. & Gersons, B. (1998) Early intervention, untreated psychosis and the course of early schizophrenia. *British Journal of Psychiatry* **172** (Suppl. 33), 84–89.

Litman, S. (1997) Group therapy for the mentally ill: an effective treatment model in the community. Paper Presented to the 12th International Symposium for the Psychotherapy of Schizophrenia, London.

Loebel, A.D., Lieberman, J.A., Alvir, J.M.J. *et al.* (1992) Duration of psychosis and outcome in first-episode schizophrenia. *American Journal of Psychiatry* **149**, 1183–1188.

Lotterman, A. (1996) *Specific Techniques for the Psychotherapy of Schizophrenic Patients.* International Universities Press, CT.

Luborsky, L., Singer, B. & Luborsky, L. (1975) Comparative studies of psychotherapies: is it true that 'everyone has won and all have won prizes'? *Archives of General Psychiatry* **32**, 995–10008.

Luborsky, L., Diguer, L., Seligman, D.A. *et al.* (1999) The researcher's own therapy allegiances: a wild card in comparisons of treatment efficacy. *Clinical Psychology: Science and Practice* **6**, 95–106.

McCreadie, R.G. (1996) Managing the first episode of schizophrenia: the role of new therapies. *European Neuropsychopharmacology* **6** (Suppl. 2), S3–S5.

McEvoy, J.P., Freter, S., Everett, G. *et al.* (1989) Insight and the clinical outcome of schizophrenic patients. *Journal of Nervous and Mental Disease* **177**, 48–51.

McFall, R.M. (1982) A review and reformulation of the concept of social skills. *Behavioral Assessment* **4**, 1–33.

McFarlane, W.R. (1990) Multiple family groups and the treatment of schizophrenia. In: *Handbook of Schizophrenia*, Vol. 4 *Psychosocial Treatment of Schizophrenia* (eds M.I. Herz, S.J. Keith & J.P. Docherty), pp. 167–189. Elsevier, New York.

McFarlane, W.R., Dunne, E., Lukens, E. *et al.* (1993) From research to clinical practice: dissemination of New York State's family psychoeducation project. *Hospital and Community Psychiatry* **44**, 265–270.

McFarlane, W.R., Dushay, R.A., Stastny, P., Deakins, S.M. & Link, B.A. (1996) A comparison of two levels of family-aided assertive community treatment. *Psychiatric Services* **47**, 744–750.

McGlashan, W.H. & Fenton, W.S. (1992) The positive–negative distinction in schizophrenia: review of natural history validators. *Archives of General Psychiatry* **49**, 63–72.

McGorry, P.D. (2000a) Psychotherapy and recovery in early psychosis: a core clinical and research challenge. In: *Psychosis: Psychological Approaches and their Effectiveness* (eds B.V. Martindale, A. Bateman, F. Margison & M. Crowe), pp. 266–292. Gaskell, London.

McGorry, P.D. (2000b) The scope for preventive strategies in early psychosis: logic, evidence and momentum. In: *Early Intervention in Psychosis* (eds M. Birchwood, D. Fowler & C. Jackson), pp. 3–27. Wiley, Chichester.

McGorry, P.D. & Jackson, H. (1999) *The Recognition and Management of Early Psychosis: a Preventive Approach.* Cambridge University Press, Cambridge.

McGorry, P.D., Edwards, J., Mihalopoulos, C., Harrigan, S. & Jackson, H.J. (1996) The Early Psychosis Prevention and Intervention Centre (EPPIC): an evolving system of early detection and optimal management. *Schizophrenia Bulletin* **22**, 305–326.

Marder, S.R., Wirshing, W.C., Mintz, J. *et al.* (1996) Two-year outcome for social skills training and group psychotherapy for outpatients with schizophrenia. *American Journal of Psychiatry* **153**, 1585–1592.

Marsh, D.T. (1992) *Families and Mental Illness: New Directions in Professional Practice.* Praeger, New York.

Martindale, B.V. (1998) Commentary. *Advances in Psychiatric Treatment* **4**, 241–242.

Martindale, B.V. (2001) New discoveries concerning psychosis and their organisational fate. In: *A Language for Psychosis: Psychoanalysis of Psychotic States* (ed P. Williams), pp. 27–36. Whurr Books, London.

May, P.R.A. (1968) *Treatment of Schizophrenia: A Comparative Study of Five Treatment Methods.* Science House, New York.

May, R. (2000) Routes to recovery from psychosis: the roots of a clinical psychologist. *Clinical Psychology Forum* **146**, 6–10.

Medalia, A. & Revheim, N. (1999) Computer assisted learning in psychiatric rehabilitation. *Psychiatric Rehabilitation Skills* **3**, 77–98.

Medalia, A., Aluma, M., Tryon, W. & Merriam, A.E. (1998) Effectiveness of attention training in schizophrenia. *Schizophrenia Bulletin* **24**, 147–152.

Medalia, A., Revheim, N. & Casey, M. (2000) Remediation of memory disorders in schizophrenia. *Psychological Medicine* **30**, 1451–1459.

Migone, P. (1995) Expressed emotion and projective identification: a bridge between psychiatric and psychoanalytic concepts? *Contemporary Psychoanalysis* **31**, 617–639.

Miklowitz, D.J., Goldstein, M.J., Falloon, I.R.H. & Doane, J.A. (1984) Interactional correlates of expressed emotion in the families of schizophrenics. *British Journal of Psychiatry* **144**, 133–143.

Mills, P.D. & Hansen, J.C. (1991) Short-term group interventions for mentally ill young adults living in a community residence and their families. *Hospital and Community Psychiatry* **42**, 1144–1149.

Montgomery, S.A., Taylor, P. & Montgomery, D. (1978) Development of a schizophrenia scale sensitive to change. *Neuropharmacology* **17**, 1053–1071.

Mueser, K.T. & Berenbaum, H. (1990) Psychodynamic treatment of schizophrenia: is there a future? *Psychological Medicine* **20**, 253–262.

Mueser, K.T. & Glynn, S.M. (1999) *Behavioral Family Therapy for Psychiatric Disorders*, 2nd edn. New Harbinger Publications, Oakland, CA.

Mueser, K.T., Bellack, A.S., Morrison, R.L. & Wixted, J.T. (1990) Social competence in schizophrenia: premorbid adjustment, social skill, and domains of functioning. *Journal of Psychiatric Research* **24**, 51–63.

Mueser, K.T., Bellack, A.S., Douglas, M.S. & Morrison, R.L. (1991a) Prevalence and stability of social skill deficits in schizophrenia. *Schizophrenia Research* **5**, 167–176.

Mueser, K.T., Bellack, A.S., Douglas, M.S. & Wade, J.H. (1991b) Prediction of social skill acquisition in schizophrenic and major affective disorder patients from memory and symptomatology. *Psychiatry Research* **37**, 281–296.

Mueser, K.T., Douglas, M.S., Bellack, A.S. & Morrison, R.L. (1991c) Assessment of enduring deficit and negative symptom subtypes in schizophrenia. *Schizophrenia Bulletin* **17**, 565–582.

Mueser, K.T., Bellack, A.S., Wade, J.H., Sayers, S.L. & Rosenthal, C.K. (1992) An assessment of the educational needs of chronic psychiatric patients and their relatives. *British Journal of Psychiatry* **160**, 674–680.

Mueser, K.T., Bellack, A.S., Wade, J.H., Haas, G. & Sayers, S.L. (1993) Expressed emotion, social skill, and response to negative affect in schizophrenia. *Journal of Abnormal Psychology* **102**, 339–351.

Mueser, K.T., Becker, D.R., Torrey, W.C. *et al.* (1997a) Work and nonvocational domains of functioning in persons with severe mental illness: a longitudinal analysis. *Journal of Nervous and Mental Disease* **185**, 419–426.

Mueser, K.T., Valentiner, D.P. & Agresta, J. (1997b) Coping with negative symptoms of schizophrenia: patient and family perspectives. *Schizophrenia Bulletin* **23**, 329–339.

Mueser, K.T., Goodman, L.B., Trumbetta, S.L. *et al.* (1998) Trauma and posttraumatic stress disorder in severe mental illness. *Journal of Consulting and Clinical Psychology* **66**, 493–499.

Mueser, K.T., Sengupta, A., Schooler, N.R. *et al.* (2001) Family treatment and medication dosage reduction in schizophrenia: effects on patient social functioning, family attitudes, and burden. *Journal of Consulting and Clinical Psychology* **69**, 3–12.

Mueser, K.T., Rosenberg, S.D., Goodman, L.B. & Trumbetta, S.L. (2002a) Trauma, PTSD, and the course of severe mental illness: an interactive model. *Schizophrenia Research* **53**, 123–143.

Mueser, K.T., Fox, L. & Mercer, C. (2002b) Family intervention for severe mental illness and substance use disorder. In: *New Family Interventions and Associated Research in Psychosis* (ed. A. Schaub), pp. 205–227. Springer-Verlag, Vienna.

Nelson, H. (1997) *Cognitive Behavioural Therapy with Schizophrenia: a Practice Manual*. Stanley Thornes, Cheltenham.

Noh, S. & Turner, R.J. (1987) Living with psychiatric patients: implications for the mental health of family members. *Social Science and Medicine* **25**, 263–271.

Nuechterlein, K.H. & Subotnik, K.L. (1998) The cognitive origins of schizophrenia and prospects for intervention. In: *Outcome and Innovation in Psychological Treatment of Schizophrenia* (eds T. Wykes, N. Tarrier & S. Lewis), pp. 101–118. Wiley, Chichester.

Obholzer, A. & Roberts, V.A. (1994) *The Unconscious at Work*. Routledge, London.

Olbrich, R. & Mussgay, L. (1990) Reduction of schizophrenic deficits by cognitive training: an evaluative study. *European Archives of Psychiatry and Neurological Science* **239**, 366–369.

Paley, G. & Shapiro, D.A. (2002) Lessons from psychotherapy research for psychological interventions for people with schizophrenia. *Psychology and Psychotherapy: Theory, Research and Practice* **75**, 5–17.

Pao, P.-N. (1979) *Schizophrenic Disorders: Theory and Treatment from a Psychodynamic Point of View*. International Universities Press, New York.

Paul, G.L. & Lentz, R.J. (1977) *Psychosocial Treatment of Chronic Mental Patients: Milieu Versus Social-Learning Programs*. Harvard University Press, Cambridge, MA.

Penn, D.L., Mueser, K.T., Spaulding, W., Hope, D.A. & Reed, D. (1995) Information processing and social competence in chronic schizophrenia. *Schizophrenia Bulletin* **21**, 269–281.

Penn, D.L., Corrigan, P.W., Bentall, R.P., Racenstein, J.M. & Newman, L. (1997) Social cognition in schizophrenia. *Psychological Bulletin* **121**, 114–132.

Perlick, D., Stastny, P., Mattis, S. & Teresi, J. (1992) Contribution of family, cognitive and clinical dimensions to long-term outcome in schizophrenia. *Schizophrenia Research* **6**, 257–265.

Pharoah, F.M., Mari, J.J. & Streiner, D. (2000) Family intervention for schizophrenia (Cochrane Review). *Cochrane Library, Issue 2*. Update Software, Oxford.

Phillips, L.J., McGorry, P.D., Yung, A.R. *et al.* (1999) The development of preventive interventions for early psychosis: early findings and directions for the future. *Schizophrenia Research* **36**, 331.

Pilling, S. Bebbington, P. Kuipers, E. *et al.* (2002) Psychological treatments in schizophrenia. I. Meta-analysis of family intervention and CBT. *Psychological Medicine* **32**, 763–782.

Pinel, P. (1806) *A Treatise on Insanity*. Cadell & Davies, London.

Pitsschel-Walz, G., Leucht, S., Bauml, J., Kissling, W. & Engel, R.R. (2001) The effect of family interventions on relapse and rehospitalization in schizophrenia: a meta-analysis. *Schizophrenia Bulletin* **27**, 73–92.

Power, P., Elkins, K., Adlard, S. *et al.* (1998) Analysis of the initial treatment in the first episode psychosis. *British Journal of Psychiatry* **172** (Suppl. 33), 71–76.

Priebe, S. & Bröker, M. (1999) Prediction of hospitalizations by schizophrenia patients' assessment of treatment: an expanded study. *Journal of Psychiatric Research* **33**, 113–119.

Priebe, S. & Gruyters, T. (1993) The role of the helping alliance in psy-

chiatric community care: a prospective study. *Journal of Nervous and Mental Diseases* **181**, 552–557.

Pull, C.B. (1999) Diagnosis of schizophrenia: a review. In: *Schizophrenia* (eds M. Maj & N. Sartorius), pp. 1–37. J. Wiley, Chichester.

Pullen, G. (1999) The therapeutic community and schizophrenia. In: *Group Psychotherapy of the Psychoses: Concepts, Interventions and Contexts* (eds V. Schermer & M. Pines), pp. 359–387. International Library of Group Analysis, J. Kingsley, London.

Rajkumar, S. & Thara, R. (1989) Factors affecting relapse in schizophrenia. *Schizophrenia Research* **2**, 403–409.

Randolph, E.T., Eth, S., Glynn, S. *et al.* (1994) Behavioral family management in schizophrenia: outcome of a clinic-based intervention. *British Journal of Psychiatry* **64**, 501–506.

Read, J. (1997) Child abuse and psychosis: a literature review and implications for professional practice. *Professional Psychology: Research and Practice* **28**, 448–456.

Regier, D.A., Farmer, M.E., Rae, D.S. *et al.* (1990) Comorbidity of mental disorders with alcohol and other drug abuse: results from the Epidemiologic Catchment Area (ECA) study. *Journal of the American Medical Association* **264**, 2511–2518.

Richardson, P. & Jones, K. (1997–ongoing) *Art Therapy as an Adjunctive Treatment in Severe Mental Illness: A Randomised Controlled Evaluation*. National Research Register, DHSS, NRR Project N0466045336.

Robbins, M. (1993) *Experiences of Schizophrenia*. Guilford, New York.

Rosen, A. (1994) 100% Mabo: de-colonising people with mental illness and their families. *Australian and New Zealand Journal of Family Therapy* **15** (3), 128–142.

Rosen, J.N. (1953) *Direct Analysis: Selected Papers*. Grune & Stratton, New York.

Rosenberg, S.D., Goodman, L.A., Osher, F.C. *et al.* (2001) Prevalence of HIV, hepatitis B and hepatitis C in people with severe mental illness. *American Journal of Public Health* **91**, 31–37.

Rosenfarb, I.S., Goldstein, M.J., Mintz, J. & Nuechterlein, K.H. (1995) Expressed emotion and subclinical psychopathology observable within the transactions between schizophrenic patients and their family members. *Journal of Abnormal Psychology* **104**, 259–267.

Rosenfeld, H.A. (1965) *Psychotic States. A Psychoanalytical Approach*. Maresfield Reprints, London.

Ross, C., Anderson, G. & Clark, P. (1994) Childhood abuse and positive symptoms of schizophrenia. *Hospital and Community Psychiatry* **45**, 489–491.

Salakongas, R.K.R., Räkköläinen, V. & Alanen, Y.O. (1989) Maintenance of grip on life and goals of life: a valuable criterion for evaluating outcome in schizophrenia. *Acta Psychiatrica Scandinavica* **80**, 187–193.

Sartorius, N. (1998) Stigma: what can psychiatrists do about it? *Lancet* **352**, 1958–1959.

Scazufca, M. & Kuipers, E. (1996) Links between EE and burden of care in relatives of patients with schizophrenia. *British Journal of Psychiatry* **168**, 580–587.

Schaub, A. (1998) Cognitive–behavioural coping-orientated therapy for schizophrenia: a new treatment model for clinical service and research. In: *Cognitive Psychotherapy of Psychotic and Personality Disorders: Handbook of Theory and Practice* (eds C. Perris & P.D. McGorry), pp. 91–109. J. Wiley & Sons, Chichester.

Schermer, V.L. & Pines, M. (1999) *Group Psychotherapy of the Psychoses: Concepts, Interventions and Contexts*. International Library of Group Analysis, Jessica Kingsley, London.

Schooler, N.R., Keith, S.J., Severe, J.B. & Matthews, N.R. (1989) Acute treatment response and short-term outcome in schizophrenia. *Psychopharmacology Bulletin* **25**, 3331–3335.

Schooler, N.R., Keith, S.J., Severe, J.B. & Matthers, N.R. (1993) Treatment strategies in schizophrenia: effects of dosage reduction and family management on outcome. *Schizophrenia Research* 9, 260.

Schooler, N.R., Keith, S.J., Severe, J.B. *et al.* (1997) Relapse and rehospitalization during maintenance treatment of schizophrenia: the effects of dose reduction and family treatment. *Archives of General Psychiatry.* 54, 453–463.

Searles, H.F. (1965, Reprinted 1986) *Collected Papers on Schizophrenia and Related Subjects.* International Universities Press, Karnac Books, London.

Sechehaye, M.A. (1956) *A New Psychotherapy in Schizophrenia.* Grune & Stratton, New York.

Segal, S.P., Silverman, C. & Temkin, T. (1993) Empowerment and self-help agency practice for people with mental disabilities. *Social Work* 38, 705–712.

Sensky, T., Turkington, D., Kingdon, D. *et al.* (2000) A randomized controlled trial of cognitive–behavioral therapy for persistent symptoms in schizophrenia resistant to medication. *Archives of General Psychiatry* 57, 165–172.

Sharma, T. & Harvey, P., eds. (2000) *Cognition in Schizophrenia: Impairments, Importance and Treatment Strategies.* Oxford University Press, New York.

Silverstein, M.L. & Harrow, M. (1978) *American Journal of Psychiatry* 135, 1418–1426.

Silverstein, S.M., Schenkel, L.S., Valone, C. & Nuernberger, S.W. (1998) *Psychiatric Quarterly* 69, 169–191.

Skaife, S. & Huet, V. (1998) *Art Psychotherapy Groups: Between Picture and Words.* Routledge, London.

Sloboda, A. (1996) Music therapy and psychotic violence. In: *A Practical Guide to Forensic Psychotherapy* (eds E. Welldon & C. Van Velson), pp. 121–129. J. Kingsley, London.

Smith, J., Birchwood, M., Cochrane, R. & George, S. (1993) The needs of high and low expressed emotion families: a normative approach. *Social Psychiatry and Psychiatric Medicine* 28, 11–16.

Smith, T.E., Bellack, A.S. & Liberman, R.P. (1996) Social skills training for schizophrenia: review and future directions. *Clinical Psychology Review* 16, 599–617.

Snyder, K.S., Wallace, C.J., Moe, K. & Liberman, R.P. (1994) EE by residential care operators' and residents' symptoms and quality of life. *Hospital and Community Psychiatry* 45, 1141–1143.

Spaulding, W.D., Reed, D., Sullivan, M., Richardson, C. & Weiler, M. (1999) Effects of cognitive treatment in psychiatric rehabilitation. *Schizophrenia Bulletin* 25, 657–676.

Spencer, E., Murray, E. & Plaistow. J. (2000) Relapse prevention in early psychosis. In: *Early Intervention in Psychosis* (eds M. Birchwood, D. Fowler & C. Jackson), pp. 236–260. Wiley, Chichester.

Stirling, J., Tantam, D., Thomas, P. *et al.* (1991) Expressed emotion and early onset schizophrenia: a one-year follow-up. *Psychological Medicine* 21, 675–685.

Strauss, J.S. (1989) Subjective experiences of schizophrenia: toward a new dynamic psychiatry. II. *Schizophrenia Bulletin* 15, 179–187.

Strauss, J.S., Carpenter, W.T.J. & Bartko, J.J. (1974) The diagnosis and understanding of schizophrenia. III. Speculations on the processes that underlie schizophrenic symptoms and signs. *Schizophrenia Bulletin* 11, 61–69.

Stuve, P., Erickson, R.C. & Spaulding, W. (1991) Cognitive rehabilitation: the next step in psychiatric rehabilitation. *Psychosocial Rehabilitation Journal* 15, 9–26.

Sullivan, H.F. (1962) *Schizophrenia as a Human Process.* W.W. Norton, New York.

Sullivan, H.S. (1994) The onset of schizophrenia: classical articles 1927. *American Journal of Psychiatry* 151 (Suppl. 6), 135–139.

Susser, E., Struening, E.L. & Conover, S. (1989) Psychiatric problems in homeless men: lifetime psychosis, substance use, and current distress in new arrivals at New York City shelters. *Archives of General Psychiatry* 46, 845–850.

Szmukler, G., Kuipers, E., Mahposa, W. *et al.* (in press) Evaluation of a support programme for informal carers of the mentally ill, in press.

Tarrier, N., Barrowclough, C., Vaughan, C. *et al.* (1989) Community management of schizophrenia: a two-year follow-up of a behavioral intervention with families. *British Journal of Psychiatry* 154, 625–628.

Tarrier, N., Lowson, K. & Barrowcough, C. (1991) Some aspects of family interventions in schizophrenia. II. Financial considerations. *British Journal of Psychiatry* 159, 481–484.

Tarrier, N., Sharpe, L., Beckett, R. *et al.* (1993a) A trial of two cognitive behavioural methods of treating drug-resistant residual psychotic symptoms in schizophrenia patients. II. Treatment-specific changes in coping and problem-solving skills. *Psychiatry and Psychiatric Epidemiology* 28, 5–10.

Tarrier, N., Beckett, R., Harwood, S. *et al.* (1993b) A trial of two cognitive–behavioural methods of treating drug-resistant residual psychotic symptoms in schizophrenic patients. I. Outcome. *British Journal of Psychiatry* 162, 524–532.

Tarrier, N., Yusupoff, L., Kinney, C. *et al.* (1998) Randomised controlled trial of intensive cognitive behaviour therapy for patients with chronic schizophrenia. *British Medical Journal* 317, 303–307.

Tarrier, N., Wittkowki, A., Kinney, C. *et al.* (1999) Durability of the effects of cognitive–behavioural therapy in the treatment of chronic schizophrenia: 12 month follow-up. *British Journal of Psychiatry* 174, 500–504.

Tarrier, N., Kinney, C., McCarthy, E. *et al.* (2000) Two-year follow-up of cognitive– behavioural therapy and supportive counseling in the treatment of persistent symptoms in chronic schizophrenia. *Journal of Consulting and Clinical Psychology* 68, 917–922.

Tauber, R., Wallace, C.J. & Lecomte, T. (2000) Enlisting indigenous community supporters in skills training programs for persons with severe mental illness. *Psychiatric Services* 51, 1428–1432.

Telles, C., Karno, M., Mintz. J. *et al.* (1995) Immigrant families coping with schizophrenia: behavioral family intervention v. case management with a low-income Spanish-speaking population. *British Journal of Psychiatry* 167, 473–479.

Terkelsen, K.G. (1983) Schizophrenia and the family. II. Adverse effects of family therapy. *Family Process* 22, 191–200.

Test, M.A., Wallish, L.S., Allness, D.G. & Ripp, K. (1989) Substance use in young adults with schizophrenic disorders. *Schizophrenia Bulletin* 15, 465–476.

Thorsen, G.R.B.T., Haaland, T. & Johannessen, J.O. (1999) *Treatment of Schizophrenia; Patients Needs and Rights.* In: *The Psychosocial Treatment of Psychosis* (eds T.S. Borchgrevink, A. Fjell & B.R. Rund), pp. 192–204. Tano Aschehoug, Oslo.

Tienari, P., Wynne, L.C., Moring, I. *et al.* (1994) The Finnish adoptive family study of schizophrenia: implications for family research. *British Journal of Psychiatry* 164 (23), 20–26.

Torrey, E.F. (1988) *Surviving Schizophrenia: a Family Manual (Revised).* Harper & Row, New York.

Trower, P., Bryant, B. & Argyle, M. (1978) *Social Skills and Mental Health.* Methuen, London.

Tsuang, M.T. & Faraone, S.V. (1995) The case for heterogeneity in the etiology of schizophrenia. *Schizophrenia Research* 17, 161–175.

Tsuang, M.T., Woolson, R.F. & Fleming, J.A. (1979) Long-term outcome of major psychoses. I. Schizophrenia and affective disorders compared with psychiatrically symptom-free surgical conditions. *Archives of General Psychiatry* 39, 1295–1301.

Tuke, S. (1813) *Description of the Retreat.* W. Alexander, York.

Vaughan, K. *et al.* (1992) The Sydney intervention trial: a controlled trial of relatives' counselling to reduce schizophrenic relapse. *Social Psychiatry and Psychiatric Epidemiology* 27, 16–21.

Vaughn, C. & Leff, J. (1976) The influence of family and social factors on the course of psychiatric illness. *American Journal of Psychiatry* 129, 125–137.

Wallace, C.J., Nelson, C.J., Liberman, R.P. *et al.* (1980) A review and critique of social skills training with schizophrenic patients. *Schizophrenia Bulletin* 6, 42–63.

Wallerstein, R.S. (1995) *The Talking Cures*, pp. 139–142. Yale, New Haven.

Wampold, B.E., Mondin, G.W., Moody, M. *et al.* (1997) A meta-analysis of outcome studies comparing bona fide psychotherapies: empirically, 'all must have prizes'. *Psychological Bulletin* 122, 203–215.

Watts, F.N., Powell, G.E. & Austin, S.V. (1973) Modification of delusional beliefs. *British Journal of Medical Psychology* 46, 359–363.

Weinberger, D.R., Berman, K.F. & Zec, R.F. (1986) Physiologic dysfunction of dorsolateral prefrontal cortex in schizophrenia. I. Regional cerebral blood flow evidence. *Archives of General Psychiatry* 43, 114–124.

Wexler, B.E., Hawkins, K.A., Rounsaville, B. *et al.* (1997) Normal neurocognitive performance after extended practice in patients with schizophrenia. *Schizophrenia Research* 26, 173–180.

Wiedl, K.H. & Schottner, B. (1991) Coping with symptoms of schizophrenia. *Schizophrenia Bulletin* 17, 525–538.

Wing, J.K. (1987) Psychosocial factors affecting the long-term course of schizophrenia. In: *Psychosocial Treatment of Schizophrenia: Multidimensional Concepts, Psychological, Family, and Self-Help Perspectives* (eds J.S. Strauss, W. Boker & H.D. Brenner), pp. 13–29. Hans Huber, Toronto.

Wing, J.K. & Brown, G.W. (1970) *Institutionalism and Schizophrenia: a Comparative Study of Three Mental Hospitals, 1960–1968.* Cambridge University Press, Cambridge.

Winnicott, D.W. (1965) *The Maturational Processes and the Facilitating Environment.* .International Universities Press, New York.

Woo, S.M., Goldstein, M.J. & Nuechterlein, K.H. (1997) Relatives' expressed emotion and non-verbal signs of subclinical psychopathology in schizophrenic patients. *British Journal of Psychiatry* 170, 58–61.

Wood, C. (2000) *Art, psychotherapy and psychosis: the nature and politics of art therapy.* PhD thesis, University of Sheffield.

Wykes, T., Parr, A.M. & Landau, S. (1999a) Group treatment of auditory hallucinations: exploratory study of effectiveness. *British Journal of Psychiatry* 175, 180–185.

Wykes, T., Reeder, C., Corner, J., Williams, C. & Everitt, B. (1999b) The effects of neurocognitive remediation on executive processing in patients with schizophrenia. *Schizophrenia Bulletin* 25, 291–307.

Xiong, W., Phillips, M.R., Hu, X. *et al.* (1994) Family-based intervention for schizophrenic patients in China: a randomised controlled trial. *British Journal of Psychiatry* 165, 239–247.

Zeitlin, H. (2000) Continuities of childhood disorders into adulthood. In: *Interfaces between Child and Adult Mental Health* (eds P. Reder, M. McClure & A. Jolley), pp. 21–37. Family Matters, Routledge, London.

Zhang, M., Wang, M., Li, J. & Phillips, M.R. (1994) Randomised-control trial of family intervention for 78 first-episode male schizophrenic patients: an 18-month study in Suzhou, Jiangsu. *British Journal of Psychiatry* 165, 69–102.

Zigler, E. & Glick, M. (1986) *A Developmental Approach to Adult Psychopathology.* John Wiley & Sons, New York.

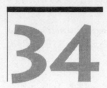

34 Mental health services

M. Muijen, F. Holloway and H. Goldman

The 'failure' of comunity care, 689
International challenges, 689
Core components of mental health, 689
Community mental health services, 690
  The Community Mental Health Team: the British model, 690
  Case management and assertive community treatment: the USA, 691
  Crisis intervention services, 692
  Early psychosis services, 692
Acute hospital care, 692
  Role, 692

Pressure, 693
Length of stay, 693
The inpatient unit as a therapeutic environment, 693
Day care/partial hospitalization, 694
  Day care/partial hospitalization as an alternative to admission, 694
  Day care and employment services, 695
Service integration, 696
Conclusions, 697
References, 697

Although the history of psychiatric thought can be traced back to the writings of Hippocrates, until the spectacular rise of the asylum in the nineteenth century mental health care in Europe and America depended largely on the family, almsgiving and generic provision for the indigent, either in institutions or as out-door relief. In 1403, the Bethlem in the City of London, sole specialist facility for the mentally ill in a country with a population of some 2.5 million, was recorded as containing six insane inmates (Scull 1979).

The asylum came to dominate practice and thought about mental health care in Europe during the eighteenth century (Bynum 1983) and in nineteenth century North America (Grob 1994). Over the past 200 years there have been cycles of renewal and reform within mental health services which have reflected changes in popular and professional attitudes towards mental illness, shifting institutional responses and changing patterns of funding and mental health legislation. A reform movement at the turn of the nineteenth century promoted 'moral treatment' within a rapidly expanding network of asylums. Moral treatment consisted of a range of approaches which emphasized kindness and minimizing coercion, the importance of activity and the development of self-control by the mentally ill amid scepticism about the then current physical treatments (Scull 1979). Mechanical restraint was abandoned. The aim was for patients to be admitted early in the course of their illness and discharged when their condition had recovered or improved. Adherents drew an optimistic distinction between incurable organic brain disease and functional disorders which might be amenable to moral treatment (Bynum 1983).

During the nineteenth century the asylums expanded. Conditions for patients deteriorated in overcrowded and underfunded institutions. Medicocultural perspectives on mental illness changed as degeneracy models of lunacy predominated. Discharge rates from the asylums declined and the mental health system entered its 'long sleep'. The 'long sleep' of the asylum lasted almost a hundred years and the awakening was initially painfully slow. In Britain the 1930 Mental Treatment Act endorsed voluntary inpatient treatment, outpatient clinics and aftercare, marking the beginning of a consistent policy favouring the development of community care. Therapeutic optimism returned following experiences of military psychiatry during World War II (Ramon 1988; Surgeon General 1999). Mental hospitals began literally both to open previously locked ward doors and metaphorically to become more permeable to the admission, discharge and readmission of patients. Rehabilitation and resettlement came to prominence in the 1950s, with the pioneers of the 'Open Door' movement (which predated the wide availability of antipsychotics) consciously drawing on the example of 'moral treatment' within the early nineteenth century asylum (Wykes & Holloway 2000).

Psychiatric bed numbers reached a peak across the industrialized Western World in 1954. The following decades have been characterized by deinstitutionalization and the lagging development of community mental health services. Significant reductions in bed numbers have occurred in all western European countries although, interestingly, bed numbers have very substantially increased in Japan over the past 40 years (Thornicroft & Goldberg 1999; Szmukler & Holloway 2001). These changes were associated with shifts in government policies towards community care, whereas in Japan growth in bed numbers was encouraged. Four examples are given of these policy shifts. France, following a ministerial circular issued in 1960, developed a model of 'sectorized psychiatry' with a sector of 70 000 population being provided for by a multidisciplinary team intended to provide preventative, curative and rehabilitative care (Kovess *et al.* 1995). In Italy, the radical reform introduced by Law 180 in 1978 led to a bold attempt to provide psychiatric care without recourse to a mental hospital (Tansella 1986). The British model of a comprehensive local psychiatric service organized around a general hospital base which evolved during the 1950s received official sanction in a White Paper of 1975 (Ramon 1988). In the USA, the 1963 Community Mental Health Centers (CMHC)

Act of 1963 instituted a federal policy of public services based on the CMHC. This was only to last for 18 years but led to an irrevocable shift from the previous system of care based on the state hospital (Bachrach 1991).

The 'failure' of community care

Radical critics have noted that deinstitutionalization was frequently in practice *trans*-institutionalization – the movement of vulnerable individuals from hospital settings to a range of poorly regulated community facilities (Scull 1977). The problem has not just been a shortage of beds and lack of support services in the community, but the uneven and unfocused development of community services. There are examples throughout the world of areas that have been well served for decades by excellent systems of care, such as South Verona in Italy and Madison, Wisconsin (see for example Sytema *et al.* 1996; Le Count 1998). In stark contrast, other areas, sometimes in close proximity to model services, have suffered serious neglect (Freeman 1999).

The perceived failure of the CMHC in the USA to meet the needs of people with severe mental illness (Mollica 1983) led to a reappraisal and a further cycle of reform, termed the 'community support' movement (Surgeon General 1999). Within this framework the social welfare needs of people with severe mental illness were at last fully recognized (Goldman 1998). Policy and practice in the industrialized world is now moving towards the provision of a seamless mental health service that addresses both the health and social care needs of individuals and carers and deploys advances in pharmacological and psychosocial treatments while actively addressing issues of poverty, isolation and social exclusion.

In many countries, community care was implemented without taking into account the severe disability associated with chronic mental illness, in the absence of effective treatments to address this disability and without a social welfare system attuned to the needs of people with disabling mental illness and their community carers. It is therefore understandable that community care has long attracted fierce criticism (Bassuk & Gerson 1978; Weller 1989; Blom-Cooper *et al.* 1995) to the extent that it was officially described in the UK as having 'failed' (Department of Health 1998). It has been observed that this alleged failure may merely reflect lack of implementation (Thornicroft & Goldberg 1999).

There has been a continuing debate between visionaries who have advocated models not yet implemented beyond local centres of excellence, and critics who have focused on the worst excesses of crude deinstitutionalization. The argument was never simply about the benefits of large asylums as the single provider of mental health care, or objections against the principle of community-based services. Rather, critics have rightly emphasized the neglect suffered in the community when hospitals were closed without the provision of a comprehensive range of community services. This has resulted in misery for some patients, carers and communities, transinstitutionalization into poor quality residential care and prisons and de-professionalization of staff (Mollica 1983). These failures have since been recognized by governments and professionals as unacceptable.

International challenges

Several countries have developed mental health strategies during the last few years in order to create homogeneous services, detailing to varying degrees the service models to be developed. This is reflected in recent policy documents from England, New Zealand, Australia and the USA (Australian Health Ministers 1998; Department of Health 1999, 2001; Mental Health Commission 1999; Surgeon General 1999). Many specify evidence, and most rely on the data on effectiveness and efficiency as published in the international literature. The English National Service Framework for Mental Health specifically grades the quality of the evidence base behind the seven standards that are set out (Department of Health 1999). The apparent agreement on preferred service models and absence of doubt about the feasibility of community-based mental health services in principle, if not in practice, is in strong contrast to the ambivalence of policies in the past.

However, this ostensible consensus regarding services is rather superficial, and hides deeper questions which need addressing if mental health care is to function effectively:

1 The nature of mental health problems.
2 The type and range of services required.
3 The effectiveness of the individual elements of care.
4 Structure and organization of care.

This book provides the best contemporary evidence about the nature of schizophrenia. The rest of this chapter will address the other questions.

Core components of mental health

There is now significant international consensus over the core principles, functions and components of a comprehensive system of mental health care. Central principles are that services should focus on the needs of people with mental health problems and be local, readily accessible and provided in the least restrictive setting possible. Detailed discussion of how need should be conceptualized is outside the scope of this chapter, but clarity over this issue is crucial in the design of effective services and in prioritizing the use of scarce resources (Holloway 2001). Competent services will combine the provision of social care and support with the delivery of effective treatments and an emphasis on the social recovery of the individual.

Core elements of the service system can be identified (see Table 34.1) and include both arrangements for undertaking key tasks (such as assessment of need and crisis response) and specific kinds of service (such as hospital beds and day care facilities). Some services, notably for the provision of specific psychological and medical treatments, can either be free-

Table 34.1 Core elements of a comprehensive mental health service system (adapted from Strathdee & Thornicroft 1996; Ramsay & Holloway 1998).

1 Systems for identification and assessment of individuals in need
2 Systems for consultation and liaison with primary care, general medical care and community agencies (including the criminal justice system)
3 Mechanisms for care planning and care co-ordination (in England the Care Programme Approach; (Department of Health 1999)
4 Systems of case management and assertive outreach
5 Systems for practical support with the tasks of daily living
6 Crisis response
7 Systems to support and educate carers and the community
8 Hospital beds
9 Day care, rehabilitation, education and work opportunities
10 Residential care and access to housing
11 Psychological treatment services

standing or located within other service elements such as the community mental health team (CMHT).

Community mental health services

Traditionally, psychiatric services were based on an inpatient unit supplemented by outpatient clinics, day hospitals and hostels and, as community care evolved, specialist community professionals such as community psychiatric nurses (CPNs) and social workers. Staff would work in professional isolation, rarely communicating with other disciplines, in a now-discredited fragmented and ill co-ordinated system of care (see Brown et al. 1966 for a detailed description of early patterns of community care for people with schizophrenia). Contemporary adult mental health services are increasingly based on the principle of sectorization, within which there is clear responsibility for a geographically defined catchment area and an emphasis on continuity of care (Johnson & Thornicroft 1993).

The Community Mental Health Team: the British model

The key element of a sectorized service in the UK has been the CMHT (Onyett et al. 1994; Strathdee & Thornicroft 1996). CMHT care involves assessment of need, monitoring and prescription of medication and provision of different forms of psychological intervention (including family intervention) (Tyrer et al. 2000). In the UK, some favour an integrated multidisciplinary health and social CMHT, supported by inpatient, residential and day care services (Strathdee & Thornicroft 1996; Ramsay & Holloway 1998, Tyrer et al. 2000). However, policy is increasingly moving towards the development of specialized services within the overall care system to undertake tasks such as crisis intervention, assertive community treatment and specific

early onset services (Department of Health 2001). There is also abundant opportunity for substitution between service components, e.g. replacing hospital beds by home treatment and domiciliary support services, day hospitals and community beds.

The development and running of a CMHT requires attention to a host of complex organizational and policy issues. Pathways into and out of care need to be defined: who makes decisions about eligibility for care by a CMHT and who decides about discharge from the caseload? Given the burden of demand for mental health care, prioritization of effort is essential (Holloway 2001). A crucial issue is the balance between the treatment of people with severe mental illnesses such as schizophrenia and people with non-psychotic disorders. Primary-care-based teams can increase the total numbers of people in contact with specialist services but may have no significant impact on those with psychotic illnesses (Jackson et al. 1993). CMHTs may evolve over time away from a focus on people with psychosis in response to demand from primary care (Shepherd et al. 1998). Alternatively, increased attention to people with a psychosis may result in less access to specialist care by other patient groups, and decreased satisfaction with the services by GPs (Harrison 2000), who in the UK have a major role in decisions over commissioning services.

Multidisciplinary and, increasingly, multiagency work within the CMHT raises questions of rivalries between staff groups, the definition of professional roles and core competencies, autonomy for staff and mechanisms of accountability (Royal College of Psychiatrists 2000). Work within CMHTs has been shown to be both rewarding and highly stressful (Oliver & Kuipers 1996; Wykes et al. 1997; Reid et al. 1999). Recruitment and retention of staff in CMHTs is particularly problematical for psychiatrists (Holloway et al. 2000). The relationship between a team and other services, notably the inpatient unit, also needs clarification. There is evidence that where community teams have control over admission and discharge decisions bed use is decreased (Marks et al. 1994; Mellsop et al. 1997).

Tyrer et al. (2000) carried out a meta-analysis of the efficacy of CMHTs for people with severe mental illness and disordered personality. Only five methodologically adequate studies were identified after a thorough search of the world literature. Each took place in a different context, offering a particular service model with varying commitment to targeting people with psychotic illnesses (Fenton et al. 1984; Hoult & Reynolds 1984; Merson et al. 1992; Burns et al. 1993; Tyrer et al. 1998). Tyrer et al. (1998) carried out their study in two quite distinct service settings with markedly differing levels of resources. Importantly, differences between the CMHT and control conditions were much less marked than those between the well-resourced and the poorly resourced catchment area. The meta-analysis concluded that the CMHT was 'not inferior to non-team standard care in any important respects and is superior in promoting greater acceptance of treatment. It may also be superior in reducing hospital admission and avoiding death by suicide' (Tyrer et al. 2000).

Reviewing the literature, Tyrer et al. (2000) concluded that the components of effective CMHT working remain unclear. Issues requiring further research include optimal case load sizes, the importance of clear operational policies, the necessary qualifications (and training) of staff, the impact of continuity of care and outcomes in relation to specific disorders. No study has adequately explored how expertise in specific complex treatments for psychosis of proven efficacy can be effectively deployed by staff working within a busy real-world CMHT or other vehicles for service delivery (Wykes & Holloway 2000).

Case management and assertive community treatment: the USA

Case management (CM) was initially introduced in the USA as a mechanism for co-ordinating community care in the era of deinstitutionalization (Intagliata 1982). There is no fully agreed typology of CM for the mentally ill. In addition to Assertive Community Treatment (ACT), the leading paradigm of CM, at least five other distinct models have been articulated (Mueser *et al.* 1998). These are 'brokerage' (arranging care); 'clinical' case management (working directly with the patient/client); intensive case management (ICM; characterized by low case-loads and an assertive approach); the 'strengths' model; and the 'rehabilitation' model. The common purpose shared by all forms of CM is 'to help patients survive and optimize their adjustment to the community' (Mueser *et al.* 1998).

Despite difficulties of definition, CM has been very actively researched. Thorough meta-analytic and structured reviews of the literature are available (Mueser *et al.* 1998; Marshall *et al.* 2000a,b; Ziguras & Stuart 2000). There are two unequivocal findings of controlled trials of CM teams: fewer people drop out of care and there is greater satisfaction with services compared with standard care. The principles of CM are increasingly adopted by mental health services (Holloway & Carson 1998). However, a large-scale recent study of ICM, the UK 700, found no substantive differences between CMHT care where case-loads of CPNs were 30 and enhanced care by case managers with case-loads of 15 (Burns *et al.* 1999).

The ACT team is the most extensively described and evaluated model of community treatment (Lehman & Steinwachs 1998). There is a substantial subsidiary literature describing and defining the ACT model (McGrew *et al.* 1994; Deci *et al.* 1995; Stein & Santos 1998; Teague *et al.* 1998). Its core features are:
1 low staff–patient ratios;
2 provision of services in the community;
3 shared rather than individual case-loads;
4 24 h coverage;
5 ACT team provides most services; and
6 service is time-unlimited (Mueser *et al.* 1998; see Table 34.2). Exploration of the active therapeutic ingredients of ACT is in its infancy. There is some evidence that the engagement process and consequent therapeutic relationship between the client and the team is a critical factor (Chinman *et al.* 1999, 2000).

Evidence from controlled trials suggests that, uniquely amongst forms of CM, ACT can reduce bed days (Marshall *et al.*

Table 34.2 Criteria for programme fidelity to the Act model (Teague *et al.* 1998).

Case-loads small – staff/patient ratio 10:1
Team share case-working
Regular team meetings to discuss work with case-load
Team leader practices
Continuity of staffing
Team fully recruited
Psychiatrist as team member (0.5 fte trained psychiatrists per 100 clients)
Nurse(s) as team member
Substance misuse specialist on staff
Vocational rehabilitation specialist on staff
Explicit admission criteria focused on severely mentally ill
Low admission rate to team case-load
Full responsibility for treatment services
Responsibility for crisis services
Responsibility for decision to admit to hospital
Responsibility for discharge planning
Time-unlimited services
Treatment *in vivo* rather than in the clinic
'No drop-out' policy
Assertive engagement
Intense services
Frequent client contact
Work with supporting community agencies and individuals
Substance misuse treatment provided by team

2000b) and hence the costs of care, at least in the short term for people who have had recent admissions. There is a suggestion that fidelity is associated with good outcome (Teague *et al.* 1998; Sashidharan *et al.* 1999). However, there is less strong evidence that clinical outcomes are improved with ACT (Mueser *et al.* 1998). This is surprising given the focus of ACT on providing support to people with psychotic illnesses in dealing with daily life difficulties and ensuring adherence to treatment. ACT has been shown to be effective in helping severely mentally ill homeless people to attain residential stability (Morse *et al.* 1997). Its efficacy is also increasingly established for dually diagnosed substance misusers (Drake *et al.* 1998; Ley *et al.* 2000) and forensic patients (Solomon & Draine 1995). Assertive outreach has strong face validity in the management of people who tend to drop out from mental health services (Sainsbury Centre for Mental Health 1988a) recommended as 'the predominant model for treatment of people suffering from…psychoses' in Denmark (Vendsborg *et al.* 1999). Under the English NHS National Plan outreach teams are to cover the whole country (Department of Health 2001). However, ACT or assertive outreach teams are labour-intensive and expensive. Such teams can only be justified on the basis of cost if targeted towards particularly high need/high demand groups of patients (Essock *et al.* 1998). The savings occur in the early years and are maintained as long as hospitalization rates remain at low levels. Effective strategies for transferring clients to lower intensity programmes as needs

Table 34.3 Features of an effective home treatment team (Smyth & Hoult 2000).

Available 24 h/day 7 days/week

Capable of rapid response – usually within the hour in urban areas

Able to spend time flexibly with the patient and their social network, including several visits daily if required

Addresses the social issues surrounding the crisis from the beginning

Medical staff accompany the team at assessment and are available round the clock

Is able to administer and supervise medication

Can provide practical, problem-solving help

Is able to provide explanation, advice and support for carers

Provides counselling

Acts as a gatekeeper to acute inpatient care

Remains involved throughout the crisis until its resolution

Ensures that patients are linked up to further continuing care

change must also be developed if teams are not to become saturated (Saylers *et al.* 1998).

Crisis intervention services

Hospital care accounts for the bulk of the costs of mental health services even in the era of deinstitutionalization. In an era when the priority is efficiency in health care, improving community services has relied upon substituting non-hospital care and reinvesting the resources that are released. Initially, the focus was on the long-stay patient. Home treatment has been described as offering a 'safe and feasible alternative to hospital care for patients with acute psychiatric disorder, and one that they and their carers generally prefer' (Smyth & Hoult 2000). It aims to save beds by active intervention until the presenting crisis has resolved, subsequently transferring care on to (or, more usually given that the majority of psychiatric admissions are readmissions, back to) the community services.

Smyth and Hoult (2000), who have direct experience in home treatment services in Australia and the UK, set out the 'features of an effective home treatment team' (Table 34.3) which they emphasize will be 'an integral part of the overall provision for psychiatric care'. The subject is one of intense debate, with opponents condemning supporters for drawing on unproven crisis intervention theory and an outdated evidence base (Pelosi & Jackson 2000). A meta-analysis of the crisis intervention literature came to the lukewarm conclusion that 'a pure form of crisis intervention policy…would be hard to justify . . . outside of a simple well-designed trial' (Joy *et al.* 2000). However, several studies illustrate the effectiveness of crisis care in reducing hospital use (Marks *et al.* 1994; Reding & Raphelson 1995; Wasylenki *et al.* 1997). There has been a lack of standardization of research and service implementation. Nevertheless, home treatment teams have become an integral part of the mental health system in Australia and are to be incorporated into the mainstream of UK services (Department of Health 2001).

Early psychosis services

The frequently excessive delay in people experiencing a first episode of psychosis receiving treatment and the importance of offering effective management of the first episode have been increasingly recognized (Frangou & Byrne 2000). In part, this is based on the concept of a 'critical period' for intervention during which potentially reversible cognitive and social decline may occur (Garety & Jolley 2000). The evidence for a relationship between outcome and duration of untreated psychosis is equivocal (Barnes *et al.* 2000). However, there is no doubt that first presentations represent a particular challenge of assessment (Power & McGorry 1999) and management (Kulkarni & Power 1999).

These considerations have led to trenchant calls for the development of specific services for the ascertainment, assessment and treatment of early psychosis (Frangou & Byrne 2000; Garety & Jolley 2000). The Early Psychosis Prevention and Intervention Centre (EPPIC) in Melbourne, Australia represents an influential and evolving service model (for an extended description of the service components see McGorry & Jackson 1999). However, at the time of writing we await data from controlled trials of early psychosis services against any form of standard care and trials comparing alternative arrangements for the provision of specialist early intervention care.

Acute hospital care

Role

The hospital has been increasingly marginalized in modern mental health care. Although some commentators have asserted that services could be run with very limited hospital beds (Polak & Kirby 1976; Mosher 1999), there is now a widespread agreement that a reasonable availability of some 24 h care is essential. Inpatient units are now perceived as settings to contain and resolve crises that cannot be safely or effectively managed in the community. Acute inpatient units therefore have to cope with a highly selected group of people who are a risk to themselves or others, mostly with very severe symptomatology and poor social functioning (Sederer & Dickey 1995) The aim of acute inpatient care is the rapid return of patients to their own place of residence. The success of this strategy relies on the effectiveness of community services to gate-keep hospital beds and support the early discharge people from hospital, the ability of hospitals to relieve problems rapidly and effectively and the ready availability of appropriately supportive accommodation for people with mental illness.

Despite a striking and sustained reduction in psychiatric bed numbers in most advanced countries (Szmukler & Holloway 2001), beds generally remain the most expensive single component of mental health services. In England, 66% of the mental health budget is committed to hospital care (Health Committee 2000). Although a lower proportion of spending in the USA, it is still disproportionately expensive considering the number of beds available (Mark *et al.* 1998). This can partly be attributed to loss of the economies of scale available in the traditional large mental hospital as bed numbers are reduced or the institutions are closed and replaced by small isolated units. A major additional factor in the increasing unit costs of inpatient care is the higher staff–patient ratio (Raftery 1992), necessary to compensate for past low standards of care and to cope with the increasing disability of inpatients and more rapid throughput.

Pressure

The experience of inpatient psychiatry in the UK, with its sustained decrease in psychiatric beds since 1955, suggests a system under enormous strain. Mean occupancy rates of 98% over several years have been reported (Greengross *et al.* 2000), and in many instances rates were over 100%. This increase in the intensity of the use of inpatient facilities has been fuelled not only by bed reductions, but also by significant increases in demand as reflected by voluntary and compulsory admissions. Between 1984 and 1994/95, the annual number of voluntary admissions to inpatient care increased by just over 10% and the number of compulsory admissions by almost 50% in England (Health Committee 2000). On average, 30% of inpatients in NHS acute adult psychiatric units in England and Wales are detained involuntarily (Ford *et al.* 1998). There is marked international variability in rates of voluntary and compulsory admission. The proportion of involuntary admissions in the USA is comparable to UK rates at 29% (Snowden & Cheung 1990). However, in Finland, between 1990 and 1993, when 35% of hospital beds were closed, rate of admissions remained stable and compulsory admissions declined by 14% (Korkeila *et al.* 1998). Across Scandinavian countries rates of compulsory admissions differed more than sevenfold (Hansson *et al.* 1999).

Inpatient and community services are interdependent. A major contributor to pressure on beds is any obstacle to discharge patients. A significant proportion of beds are 'blocked' by people who could be discharged if community or social care, or appropriate housing, were available (Beck *et al.* 1997; Shepherd *et al.* 1997). One study found that 30% of a sample of short-stay patients blocking beds could not be discharged because of a lack of suitable accommodation, and 19% because there was no domiciliary support available. In the same study, 33% of long-stay patients blocked beds because of a lack of move-on accommodation and 41% because no rehabilitation facilities were available (Shepherd *et al.* 1997).

The literature suggests that community services have surprisingly little impact on the rate of admission for people with schizophrenia. In Verona, reputed as a centre of excellence, 30% of patients with schizophrenia in contact with the service were admitted during a year (Gater *et al.* 1995). An international comparison of community- and hospital-based care suggested that rates of admissions did not differ across services, but that length of stay was shorter in the community-based services (Sytema & Burgess 1999). This is confirmed by data on

admissions in Madison, Wisconsin. Admissions almost doubled and mean length more than halved from 39 days to 14 days between 1981 and 1996, the time when Madison's mental health services were considered to be a model of good practice (Le Count 1998). This should not be read as a failure. A reduction in time in hospital results in major savings in beds, potentially lowers the risk of institutionalization and is undoubtedly preferred by patients. Nevertheless, the inability to prevent admissions is disappointing, suggesting a course of illness not simply responding to a change in service delivery model.

Length of stay

Few recent studies have used experimental designs to investigate the question of whether length of stay affects outcome (Johnstone & Zolese 1999). Earlier studies suggest that hospital duration can be shortened without any untoward impact on patient functioning, but several provisos need to be made. The definitions of 'brief' and 'standard' admission vary dramatically between studies, for example from 80 vs. 180 days (Mattes *et al.* 1977) to 22 vs. 28 days (Hirsch *et al.* 1979) and 11 vs. 60 days (Herz *et al.* 1977). As a result 'standard' care in some studies was substantially longer than 'brief admission' in others. This makes cross-study comparison problematical. Patient groups have differed, although studies have included a large proportion of patients with psychotic disorders. One project has addressed the issue of subgroups (Glick *et al.* 1976; Hargreaves *et al.* 1977). Results for patients with schizophrenia were inconclusive but there was persuasive evidence that patients with neurosis did not benefit from extended hospitalization. This reflects contemporary clinical practice.

More recent uncontrolled studies found no correlation between length of stay and outcome (Pfeiffer *et al.* 1996). However, there is some evidence that some clinical subgroups might be at higher risk of relapse following brief admission, especially young men with schizophrenia and multiple previous admissions (Appleby *et al.* 1996). The conclusion may be that length of stay is too crude a variable to predict outcome, especially because clinician and service factors may be stronger predictors than patient characteristics. For example, length of hospitalization on first admission for patients with similar clinical and social characteristics varied threefold in seven Nordic hospitals (Oiesvold *et al.* 1999). Interventions offered during admission are likely to be more important than stay in its own right.

The inpatient unit as a therapeutic environment

In contrast to the rich literature on community care, remarkably little research has been published in the last 25 years evaluating interventions in hospital settings for people with schizophrenia. This may be an indication of unquestioned habits based on tradition and routine but it more likely reflects the vagaries of research fashion and the lack of energy of practitioners working in a form of service perceiving itself as under constant pressure and out of favour. It may also reflect a shift in focus from research only on the effectiveness of services, to studies of the treatment provided in service settings (Lehman *et al.* 1998). However, in spite of a dearth of recent research on inpatient services, earlier research came up with findings of continuing relevance.

Studies have consistently found that any form of increased attention and motivation, irrelevant of ideological origin, application or therapist's expertise, produces better outcome (Erickson 1975). Outcome was mainly defined as functioning of the patients on the ward in these studies, and the effect of ward programmes on quality of life after discharge is largely unknown. However, there is evidence that hospital treatment and improved ward adjustment are not associated with better community functioning (Anthony *et al.* 1978). The then extant research on the effectiveness of ward programmes was succinctly summarized by Erickson (1975): 'There is little order and virtually no replication', and not much has changed since then.

The conclusion that any form of intervention and attention improves ward functioning needs to be put in perspective, because standard care as provided by these studies may well have been very basic. Although practice has changed considerably, this does not mean that quality of care has greatly improved. Disturbingly, recent evidence suggests that there has been little improvement in this area. In an observational study of eight randomly selected hospitals in the UK, 40% of patients did not take part in any social or recreational activity during their stay and 30% did not even participate in therapeutic activities; only 5% received psychological therapies (Sainsbury Centre for Mental Health 1998b). Appropriate early discharge policies may have contributed to this apparent impoverishment of the acute ward environment. However, early discharge may be caused by service pressures or financial constraints (Bezold *et al.* 1996) and, as a result, valuable assessments and treatments may not be taking place. The impression is that there is general confusion about what an acute ward should provide, apart from safety and medication, and that this is affecting staff morale and patient satisfaction (Moore 1998).

Commentators have repeatedly questioned whether contemporary inpatient care offers a therapeutic environment at all (Perring 1992; Sainsbury Centre for Mental Health 1998b). Accounts from patients about inpatient services are consistently negative (Perring 1992). It seems to be time to develop and evaluate approaches for hospital care that are compatible with its role within a community-based mental health service. Some descriptions of model services are provided in the literature (Jayaram *et al.* 1996), involving precise screening methods, frequent communication, immediate implementation of care programmes, highly skilled staff, involvement of carers and community services and early discharge planning.

Day care/partial hospitalization

Day care (referred to in the American literature as partial hospitalization) could be expected to fill the gap between home care and hospital. It offers greater structure and more intensive treatment than community services, but less restrictiveness and stigma than hospital wards. Its objectives vary and need to be differentiated between those that treat people with a severe and acute episode of mental illness who otherwise would have been treated in hospital, and those that offer rehabilitation to patients with a long-term mental illness (Rosie *et al.* 1995).

Day care/partial hospitalization as an alternative to admission

Day care/partial hospitalization as an alternative to inpatient care has consistently been found to be at least as good as inpatient care. Studies report little difference in outcome on measures such as psychopathology or social functioning between the two types of care after 12 months' follow-up (Wilder *et al.* 1966; Herz *et al.* 1977; Creed *et al.* 1990, 1997; Sledge *et al.* 1996). Both patients (Nienhuis *et al.* 1994) and their relatives (Nienhuis *et al.* 1994; Creed *et al.* 1997) preferred day care to hospital care. Furthermore, day treatment is considerably cheaper than hospital care (Creed *et al.* 1997), although costs to carers can be higher, including travel costs (Creed *et al.* 1997).

A proportion of acute patients cannot be treated in day care settings, at least initially. Day care/partial hospitalization may not be feasible because of behavioural, physical or social problems and patients admitted compulsorily have to be excluded from studies. Intriguingly, despite differences in place and time, studies have consistently reported that about 40% of all patients who would usually have been admitted could be cared for in a day hospital (Wilder *et al.* 1966; Herz *et al.* 1977; Creed *et al.* 1990, 1997; Nienhuis *et al.* 1994). Because, as argued earlier in this chapter, the threshold of admission to hospital has been raised over time, this suggests that the ability of day hospitals to care for patients with more severe pathology has increased (Creed *et al.* 1990, 1997).

Concerns expressed against day hospital programmes are (Hoge *et al.* 1992):
1 the longer length of treatment as compared with inpatient stays (Creed *et al.* 1990; Nienhuis *et al.* 1994), creating dependency;
2 the lack of continuity and increase in boundaries because of shifts in care from community services to wards and day care;
3 poor targeting of treatment; and
4 the high drop-out rate.

In defence of day care, one could argue that the few weeks of extended care are highly unlikely to create dependency, and may well be compensated for by the reduced stigma compared with admission. Moreover, the emphasis on continuity of care in community services makes this point less relevant. The introduction of case managers should alleviate concerns about boundaries. Poor targeting is a fair concern, and is the responsibility of good design. Finally, the high drop-out rate was mainly reported in earlier studies. In recent research evaluating day care for people with severe mental illness, typically including 40% of all people presenting with schizophrenia, the drop-out has been low (Nienhuis *et al.* 1994; Sledge *et al.* 1996; Creed et al. 1997). More important is an additional point about lack of opportunity to offer training in the patient's own environment, an objection shared with hospital care.

This leaves one with a dilemma. Acute day hospitals have been found to be equally effective and less expensive than hospitals for the care of at least 40% of patients potentially requiring admission, but they are not widely implemented for this purpose. An explanation may be the growing ability and availability of community services to cope with this population, and a reluctance to spend resources on a service that is perceived as a two-way compromise: not as safe as hospital but not as much in the community as home. It raises the need for studies testing the effectiveness of day care vs. or as an addition to home care services.

Day care and employment services

As part of the process of deinstitutionalization, the role of day care was to provide some activities to people leaving institutions. Facilities for this group were often poorly co-ordinated and lacking in provisions such as rehabilitation, leisure activities and support of relatives (Brewin et al. 1989). Individualized treatment programmes were difficult to implement because of poor staffing levels. The fit between patient need and provision was also often poor. Many day care facilities demanded either too much initiative or offered too little stimulation, resulting in demoralization. The likely consequence was a high drop-out rate and a risk of neglect. Some day centres allowed patients to use the centre as a social meeting place, and the patients' appreciation was expressed by an improvement in attendance. This conforms with research showing that attendees perceived the role of day centres as social rather than therapeutic (Holloway 1989).

The challenges for the younger psychiatric population who have not experienced long stays in hospital is different. They expect greater integration, and work is perceived as central in their lives (Mowbray et al. 1997). Increasingly, rehabilitation programmes concentrate on providing work opportunities, and these suggest that many people with schizophrenia can benefit from this (Bond et al. 1997; Crowther et al. 2001).

The importance of work for people with schizophrenia is an international experience (Priebe et al. 1998). Employment is associated with better subjective and objective quality of life, although this may be a result of self-selection. However, very low proportions of people with schizophrenia or other severe mental health problems are in employment, typically 10–20% in the USA and 30–40% in the UK (Bond et al. 1997; Crowther et al. 2001). Obstacles to employment are benefit disincentives, but also stigma and low self-esteem (Mowbray et al. 1997). When a group of people with severe mental illness was asked why they were not employed, the largest number of responses were related to their mental health (45%), including medication or admission, but many reasons were related to personal factors such as negative experiences or external reasons such as poor transport (Mowbray et al. 1997).

Many approaches have been developed to create employment opportunities, the emphasis shifting over time from protected and time-limited work experience to full competitive employment. An example of the former is the Clubhouse model, also known as the Fountain House, the name of the original Clubhouse (Beard et al. 1982). These offer transitional employment programmes (TEP), which are characterized by:
1 placements are identified by the Clubhouse;
2 the placement of a patient is for a limited period, typically 6 months;
3 the Clubhouse is responsible for filling the post even if the patient is absent; and
4 the employer pays the patient directly.
The limitation of TEPs is that most jobs are very basic, and that they only offer experience rather than stable employment. As a consequence, membership of a Clubhouse can become a career in itself.

Recently, supported employment has become very prominent in the USA, probably as a consequence of the Rehabilitation Act Amendments of 1986 (Bond et al. 1997), and the same commitment has been shown in the UK in the Disability Discrimination Act 1995. Supported employment aims to place people in regular competitive employment at prevailing wage rates while receiving ongoing support to sustain the position. Several principles emerge (Bond et al. 1997).
1 Patients only find and keep jobs if they receive specialist support focusing on competitive employment.
2 Supported employment is most effective if people are placed directly in jobs; prevocational training on its own is less effective.
3 Integration of vocational and clinical services, especially those following assertive community treatment principles, are more effective than brokerage programmes.

A good example of strengths and limitations of supported employment is a study conducted in New Hampshire (Drake et al. 1994). A rehabilitative day centre in one town was changed to a supported employment service, and compared with an unchanged day programme in another town. Competitive employment increased from 25% to 39% in the new service, but remained at 13% in the unchanged programme. The new service was particularly effective for those people who were unemployed at baseline. Clearly, not everyone could obtain employment, and many were not able to hold on to it. The average length of a job in the follow-up year was 5.5 months, and people worked on average 22 h/week. Most jobs were basic, such as ground keeper and sales clerk. There is no evidence that the stress related to employment negatively affects clinical variables or increases relapse (Drake et al. 1999). On the other hand, there is also little consistent evidence that the improved vocational functioning leads to benefits in other domains of outcome, and if so, may be a result of the comprehensive nature of programmes (Bond et al. 1997). A suggestion raised by one study (Bell et al. 1996) is that payment may be a powerful intermediate variable. Patients with schizophrenia or schizoaffective disorder randomly allocated to a payment group worked many more hours than the non-payment group with access to similar jobs in a supportive hospital environment. Those people working actively (most but not exclusively in the payment group) performed better clinically and suffered fewer relapses.

A degree of caution is warranted because, by their nature, competitive employment studies are only of assistance to people with the potential to work, even though more people fall within this category than was once thought. People are self-selected, and it is likely that the capable persons will succeed at competitive employment and benefit most. This is not an argument against intensive attempts to find employment for people with schizophrenia, because the reduction in stigma for the group of people with mental illness as a whole and benefits to individuals are very worthwhile. However, it does mean that this approach will not benefit all, and that in addition a diverse range of occupational and social services is necessary, not ignoring the needs of the most dependent. Much more research can be expected in this area.

Service integration

Despite the controversies addressed in this chapter, knowledge of effectiveness of mental health care has increased but so has the complexity of services and the challenges to researchers. No longer are research questions focused on a direct comparison of a community service and standard hospital care. Instead, questions are more sophisticated, hoping to clarify the advantages of specialized care for subgroups of patients. Frequently, several models emerge, each claiming to be effective, such as the ICM and ACT (Mueser et al. 1998). This has implications for planning because a number of questions have to be addressed before a service can be designed:

1 What is the evidence for an intervention?
2 How do different effective models compare?
3 How do models fit together into an effective service?
4 Can they be afforded?

It is hardly surprising that several countries have designed strategies based on evidence, most explicitly England with its National Service Framework and NHS Plan (Department of Health 1999, 2001). Other countries have also developed plans strongly influenced by the outcome of mental health services research, such as Canada, Australia and New Zealand (Goering 1997; Australian Health Ministers 1998; Mental Health Commission 1999).

Most plans propose a range of services, such as primary care, crisis teams, assertive outreach, long-term support and hospital care. Specific activities such as advocacy, day activity, employment and education are often stated, as are services for specific groups such as people with alcohol or substance misuse and mental illness (dual diagnosis). Emphasis tends to be placed on functions such as access and co-ordination. Monitoring, the identification of best practice and the development of standards are also often part of the process (Goering 1997). None of these plans, strategies and service frameworks describe a precise and integrated service model that can be replicated everywhere in its

jurisdiction, although policy guidance in England with its associated performance management apparatus is becoming increasingly prescriptive (Department of Health 2001).

Incidence, course and outcome of mental illness vary around the world (Jablensky et al. 1992) and differences in service configuration and capacity are also striking, even across the Western world (Goldberg & Thornicroft 1998). However, we know very little about the association between service configurations and outcome for specific patient groups. There are remarkably few controlled studies to assist this process. Nearly all studies evaluate single interventions. If interventions are combined, this is criticized as confounding the purity of the result of the single target intervention, e.g. in supported employment interventions combined with assertive outreach (Bond et al. 1997).

The reason for the absence of well-controlled whole service evaluations is that they are very difficult and costly and, if attempted, tend to raise further questions rather than provide authoritative answers. Context, services, patient characteristics and interventions need to be carefully standardized across sites for the results to be meaningful. This is obviously a major challenge, but a few attempts have been made.

At an organizational level, the Robert Wood Johnson Foundation Programme on chronic mental illness was evaluated for its 6-year duration (Goldman et al. 1994a,b). It promoted the concept of a local mental health authority responsible for the integration of all services for people with a long-term mental illness, including social care and housing in nine US cities. The outcome was a successful establishment of these authorities, achieving improved organizational centralization and reduced fragmentation of services (Morrissey et al. 1994). Client outcomes improved, but this did not coincide with system improvements. Reasons for improvement were speculative only, probably relating to the availability of housing and intensive case management (Ridgely et al. 1996). A subsequent demonstration programme, 'Access to Community Care and Effective Services', targeting homeless persons with severe mental illness, supports the benefits of assertive community treatment and the association of better service integration with the successful transfer of people into supported housing (Rosenheck et al. 1998).

The problems of an evaluation of different services, even if an attempt is made to control, is illustrated by an ambitious research project carried out in Inner London (Thornicroft et al. 1998). It studied the impact of the introduction of two contrasting models of community care on people with psychosis. One sector had a generic CMHT and the other sector had two teams offering acute treatment and continuing care (Becker et al. 1998). Despite striking differences in the level of community provision and costs between the sectors, differences in outcome were not marked, with outcome possibly marginally favouring the better-resourced two-team model (Thornicroft et al. 1998). However, there was some evidence that the more intensive service resulted in worse functional outcomes (Wykes et al. 1998). Both services, which in the UK context were relatively well resourced, were highly effective in maintaining contact with patients. The suggested conclusion that the structure of community services in themselves do not determine outcome is valuable, but not sufficient for planners to act on. The question relevant to researchers is how any positive or negative findings in such studies can be interpreted, because invariably baseline characteristics of population differ, drop-outs are high and precise interventions offered are unknown and often changing during a study. It is tempting to conclude that service research without randomization is a sophisticated form of audit, and that effectiveness of interventions can only be identified in well-conducted trials with precisely defined questions. This returns us to the problem that we have little understanding of interactions within a system.

This is possibly inevitable considering the challenge. If a typical service comprises seven service elements (e.g. primary care, crisis, early intervention, assertive outreach, hospital, occupation, housing), this produces $6 \times 5 \times 4 \times 3 \times 2 = 720$ interactions. A thorough system evaluation would have to take into account the effectiveness of each of these services and their various combinations, unless one is prepared to conceptualize the components of the system as a black box. Moreover, the system will interact with other systems, such as the quality of family and community support. It is therefore understandable that researchers limit themselves to single interventions. The reality is probably that we have to accept a need to extrapolate effectiveness of single interventions to effectiveness at a system level, and that we have to rely on audit to warn us about any negative interactions. The question of how policy can become evidence-based, having to design policies for whole systems, is a challenge service researchers will have to accept as much as politicians (Goldman *et al.* 2000).

Conclusions

Mental health care has changed profoundly over the past 50 years, and models of care have converged locally and internationally. Complex systems have emerged to replace the traditional mental hospital, comprising community services and hospital care, interacting with essentials of daily living such as housing and employment. Research faces a growing challenge on how to provide the evidence required by policy makers.

Currently, a number of unresolved questions are pressing:
1 What care is specifically beneficial for subgroups of patients (e.g. people with dual diagnosis of psychosis and substance misuse or mentally ill offenders)?
2 Should such care be provided as specialist services or integrated into generic services?
3 What is the most effective system of care?
4 How should such systems differ according to epidemiological variables?
5 What are the human resource implications?
None of these questions is simple to address, and we would be surprised if unequivocal answers to any of these questions become available quickly. However, answers do need to be found

as the alternative is a continuing fruitless debate. There is a risk that, in the face of uncertainty, funding may shift to areas of medicine easier to research and therefore less affected by controversy. Worse still, there is a potential for the implementation of ineffective policy that may set a pattern of care for the decades to come.

However, we tend to belittle how much we have learnt in the last few decades. Even though we may not be able to identify the finer details, we know that successful community care can be delivered and is popular with patients and staff. Maybe it is the opinion of the users, and the many who in the past would have refused to accept care, that should in the end carry most weight.

References

Anthony, W.A., Cohen, M.R. & Vitalo, R. (1978) The measurement of rehabilitation outcome. *Schizophrenia Bulletin* 4, 365–383.

Appleby, L., Luchins, D.J., Desai, P.N. *et al.* (1996) Length of inpatient stay and recidivism among patients with schizophrenia. *Psychiatric Services* 47, 985–990.

Australian Health Ministers (1998) *Second National Mental Health Plan, Mental Health Branch*. Commonwealth Department of Health and Family Services.

Bachrach, L. (1991) Community mental health centers in the USA. In: *Community Psychiatry* (eds D.H. Bennett & H.L. Freeman), pp. 543–569. Churchill Livingstone, Edinburgh.

Barnes, T.R.E., Hutton, S.B., Chapman, M.J. *et al.* (2000) West London first-episode study of schizophrenia: clinical correlates of duration of untreated psychosis. *British Journal of Psychiatry* 177, 207–211.

Bassuk, E.L. & Gerson, S. (1978) Deinstitutionalization and mental health services. *Scientific American* 238, 46–53.

Beard, J.H., Propst, R.N. & Malamud, T.J. (1982) The Fountain House model of psychiatric rehabilitation. *Psychosocial Rehabilitation Journal* 5, 47–53.

Beck, A., Croudace, T.J., Singh, S. & Harrison, G. (1997) The Nottingham acute bed study: alternatives to acute psychiatric care. *British Journal of Psychiatry* 170, 247–252.

Becker, T., Holloway, F., McCrone, P. *et al.* (1998) Evolving service interventions in Nunhead and Norwood: PRiSM Psychosis Study 2. *British Journal of Psychiatry* 173, 371–375.

Bell, M.D., Lysaker, P.H. & Milstein, R.M. (1996) Clinical benefits of paid work activity in schizophrenia. *Schizophrenia Bulletin* 22, 51–67.

Bezold, H.S., MacDowell, M. & Kunkel.R. (1996) Predicting psychiatric length of stay. *Administration and Policy in Mental Health* 23, 407–423.

Blom-Cooper, L., Hally, H. & Murphy, E. (1995) *The Falling Shadow*. Duckworth, London.

Bond, G.R. Drake, R.E., Mueser, K.T. & Becker, D.R. (1997) An update on supported employment for people with severe mental illness. *Psychiatric Services* 48, 335–346.

Brewin, C.R., Wing, J.K., Mangen, S.P. *et al.* (1989) Needs for care among the long-term mentally ill: a report from the Camberwell High Contact Survey. *Psychological Medicine* 18, 457–468.

Brown, G.W., Bone, M., Dalison, B. & Wing, J.K. (1966) *Schizophrenia Social Care*. Oxford University Press, London.

Burns, T., Beadsmoore, A., Bhat, A.V. *et al.* (1993) A controlled trial of home-based acute psychiatric services: clinical and social outcome. *British Journal of Psychiatry* 163, 49–54.

Burns, T., Creed, F., Fahy, T.*et al.* (1999) Intensive versus standard case management for severe psychotic illness: a randomised trial. *Lancet* **353**, 2185–2189.

Bynum, W.F. (1983) Psychiatry in its historical context. In: *Handbook of Psychiatry 1: General Psychopathology* (eds M. Shepherd & O.L. Zangwill), pp. 11–38. Cambridge University Press, Cambridge.

Chinman, M., Allende, M., Bailey, P. *et al.* (1999) Therapeutic agents of assertive community treatment. *Psychiatric Quarterly* **70**, 137–162.

Chinman, M.J., Rosenheck, R. & Lam, J.A. (2000) The case management relationship and outcomes of homeless persons with serious mental illness. *Psychiatric Services* **51**, 1142–1147.

Creed, F., Black, D., Anthony, P. *et al.* (1990) Randomised controlled trial of day patient versus inpatient psychiatric treatment. *British Medical Journal* **300**, 1033–1037.

Creed, F., Mbaya, P., Lancashire, S. *et al.* (1997) Cost effectiveness of day and inpatient psychiatric treatment: results of a randomised controlled trial. *British Medical Journal* **314**, 1381–1385.

Crowther, R.E., Marshall, M., Bond, G.R. & Huxley, P. (2001) Helping people with severe mental illness to obtain work. *British Medical Journal* **322**, 204–208.

Deci, P.A., Santos, A., Hiott, D.W. *et al.* (1995) Dissemination of assertive community treatment programs. *Psychiatric Services* **46**, 676–678.

Department of Health (1998) *Modernising Mental Health Services Safe, Sound and Supportive.* Department of Health, London.

Department of Health (1999) *National Service Frameworks, Mental Health.* Department of Health, London.

Department of Health (2001) *The Mental Health Policy Implementation Guide.* Department of Health, London.

Drake, R.E., Becker, D.R., Biesanz, J.C. *et al.* (1994) Rehabilitative day treatment vs. supported employment. I. Vocational outcomes. *Community Mental Health Journal* **30**, 519–532.

Drake, R.E., McHugo, G.J., Clark, R.E. *et al.* (1998) Assertive community treatment for patients with co-occurring severe mental illness and substance abuse disorder. *American Journal of Orthopsychiatry* **68**, 201–215.

Drake, R.E., McHugo, G.J., Bebout, D.R. *et al.* (1999) A randomised controlled trial of supported employment for inner-city patients with severe mental illness. *Archives of General Psychiatry* **56**, 627–633.

Erickson, R.C. (1975) Outcome studies in mental hospitals: a review. *Psychological Bulletin* **82**, 519–540.

Essock, S., Friedman, I.K., Kopntos, N.J. *et al.* (1998) Cost-effectiveness of assertive community treatment teams. *American Journal of Orthopsychiatry* **68**, 179–190.

Fenton, F.R., Tessier, L., Struening, E.L. *et al.* (1984) A two-year follow-up of a comparative trial of the cost-effectiveness of home and hospital psychiatric treatment. *Canadian Journal of Psychiatry* **29**, 205–211.

Ford, R., Durcan, G., Warner, L., Hardy, P. & Muijen, M. (1998) One day survey by the Mental Health Act Commission of acute adult psychiatric inpatient wards in England and Wales. *British Medical Journal* **317**, 1279–1283.

Frangou, S. & Byrne, P. (2000) How to manage the first episode of schizophrenia. *British Medical Journal* **321**, 522–523.

Freeman, H. (1999) Psychiatry in the National Health Service, 1948–98. *British Journal of Psychiatry* **175**, 3–11.

Garety, P. & Jolley, S. (2000) Early intervention in psychosis. *Psychiatric Bulletin* **24**, 321–323.

Gater, R., Amaddeo, F., Tansella, M., Jackson, G. & Goldberg, D. (1995) A comparison of community-based care for schizophrenia in South Verona and South Manchester. *British Journal of Psychiatry* **166**, 344–352.

Glick, I.D., Hargreaves, W.A., Drues, J. & Showstack, J.A. (1976) Short

versus long hospitalization: a prospective controlled study. IV. One year follow-up results for schizophrenic patients. *American Journal of Psychiatry* **133**, 509–514.

Goering, P. (1997) *Review of Best Practices in Mental Health Reform.* Health Canada, Ottawa.

Goldberg, D. & Thornicroft, G. eds. (1998) *Mental Health in Our Future Cities* (Maudsley Monographs No. 42). Psychology Press/Taylor & Francis, Philadelphia, PA.

Goldman, H.H. (1998) Deinstitutionalisation and community care: social welfare policy as mental health policy. *Harvard Review of Psychiatry* **6**, 219–222.

Goldman, H.H., Morrissey, J.P. & Ridgely, M.S. (1994a) Evaluating the Robert Wood Johnson Foundation Program on chronic mental illness. *Milbank Quarterly* **72**, 37–47.

Goldman, H.H., Morrissey, J.P. & Ridgely, M.S. (1994b) Evaluating the program on chronic mental illness (RWJ PCMI). *Milbank Quarterly* **72**, 48–56.

Goldman, H.H., Thelander, S. & Westrin, C.-G. (2000) Organizing mental health services: an evidence-based approach. *Journal of Mental Health Policy and Economics* **3**, 69–75.

Greengross, P., Hollander, D. & Stanton, R. (2000) Pressure on adult acute psychiatric beds: results of a national questionnaire survey. *Psychiatric Bulletin* **24**, 54–56.

Grob, G.N. (1994) *The Mad Among Us.* Free Press, New York.

Hansson, L., Muus, S., Saarento, O. *et al.* (1999) The Nordic comparative study on sectorized psychiatry: rates of compulsory care and use of compulsory admissions during a 1-year follow-up. *Social Psychiatry and Psychiatric Epidemiology* **34**, 99–104.

Hargreaves, W.A., Glick, I.D., Drues, J., Showstack, J.A. & Feigenbaum, E. (1977) Short versus long hospitalization: a prospective controlled study. VI. Two year follow-up results for schizophrenics. *Archives of General Psychiatry* **34**, 305–311.

Harrison, J. (2000) Prioritising referrals to a community mental health team. *British Journal of General Practice* **50**, 194–198.

Health Committee (2000) *Fourth Report of Session 1999–2000: Provision of NHS Mental Health Services*, Vol. 1. HMSO, London.

Herz, M.I., Endicott, J. & Spitzer, R.L. (1977) Brief hospitalization: a two-year follow-up. *American Journal of Psychiatry* **134**, 502–507.

Hirsch, S.R., Platt, S., Knights, A. & Weyman, A. (1979) Shortening hospital stay for psychiatric care: effect on patients and their families. *British Medical Journal* **1**, 442–446.

Hoge, M.A., Davidson, L., Hill, W.L., Turner, V.E. & Ameli, R. (1992) The promise of partial hospitalization: a reassessment. *Hospital and Community Psychiatry* **43**, 345–354.

Holloway, F. (1989) Psychiatric day care: the users' perspective. *International Journal of Social Psychiatry* **35**, 252–264.

Holloway, F. (2001) Balancing clinical values and finite resources. In: *Textbook of Community Psychiatry* (eds G. Thornicroft & G. Szmukler), pp. 179–192. Oxford University Press, Oxford.

Holloway, F. & Carson, J. (1998) Intensive case management for the severely mentally ill: controlled trial. *British Journal of Psychiatry* **172**, 19–22.

Holloway, F., Szmukler, G. & Carson, J. (2000) Support systems. I. Introduction. *Advances in Psychiatric Treatment* **6**, 226–237.

Hoult, J. & Reynolds, I. (1984) Schizophrenia: a comparative trial of community orientated and hospital orientated psychiatric care. *Acta Psychiatrica Scandinavica* **69**, 359–372.

Intagliata, J. (1982) Improving the quality of community care for the chronically mentally ill: the role of case management. *Schizophrenia Bulletin* **8**, 655–674.

Jablensky, A., Sartorius, N., Ernberg, E.*et al.* (1992) Schizophrenia: manifestations, incidence and course in different cultures. A World

Health Organisation 10-Country Study. *Psychological Medicine Monograph Supplement* 20, 1–97.

Jackson, G., Gater, R., Goldberg, D. *et al.* (1993) A new community mental health team based in primary care: a description of the service and its effect on service use in the first year. *British Journal of Psychiatry* 162, 375–384.

Jayaram, G., Tien, A.Y., Sullivan, P. & Gwon, H. (1996) Elements of a successful short-stay inpatient psychiatric service. *Psychiatric Services* 47, 407–412.

Johnson, S. & Thornicroft, G. (1993) The sectorisation of psychiatric services in England and Wales. *Social Psychiatry and Psychiatric Epidemiology* 28, 45–47.

Johnstone, P. & Zolese, G. (1999) Systematic review of the effectiveness of planned short hospital stays for mental health care. *British Medical Journal* 318, 1387–1390.

Joy, C.B., Adams, C.E. & Rice, K. (2000) *Crisis Intervention for People with Severe Mental Illness*. The Cochrane Library, 3. Update Software, Oxford.

Korkeila, J.A., Lehtinen, V., Tuori, T. & Helenius, H. (1998) Patterns of psychiatric hospital service use in Finland: a national register study of hospital discharges in the early 1990s. *Social Psychiatry and Psychiatric Epidemiology* 33, 218–223.

Kovess, V., Boisguérin, B., Antoine, D. & Reynauld, M. (1995) Has sectorization of psychiatric services in France really been effective? *Social Psychiatry and Psychiatric Epidemiology* 30, 132–138.

Kulkarni, J. & Power, P. (1999) Initial treatment of first-episode psychosis. In: *The Recognition and Management of Early Psychosis* (eds P.D. McGrorry & H.J. Jackson), pp. 184–205. Cambridge University Press, Cambridge.

Le Count, D. (1998) The Madison model: keeping the focus of treatment in the community. In: *Mental Health in Our Future Cities* (Maudsley Monographs No. 42) (eds D. Goldberg & G. Thornicroft), pp. 147–172. Psychology Press/Taylor & Francis, Philadelphia, PA.

Lehman, A.F. & Steinwachs, D.M. and the Co-Investigators of the PORT Project (1998) At issue: translating research into practice. The Schizophrenia Patient Outcomes Research Team (PORT) Treatment Recommendations. *Schizophrenia Bulletin* 24, 1–10.

Ley, A., Jeffrey, D.P., McLaren, S. & Siegfried, N. (2000) *Treatment Programmes for People with Both Severe Mental Illness and Substance Misuse*. The Cochrane Library, 3. Update Software, Oxford.

McGorry, P.D. & Jackson, H.J. (1999) *The Recognition and Management of Early Psychosis*. Cambridge University Press, Cambridge.

McGrew, J.H., Bond, G.R., Dietzen, L. & Saylers, M. (1994) Measuring the fidelity of implementation of a mental health program model. *Journal of Consulting and Clinical Psychology* 62, 670–678.

Mark, T., McKusick, D., King, E., Harwood, H. & Genuardi, J. (1998) *National Expenditures for Mental Health, Alcohol, and Other Drug Abuse Treatment, 1996*. Substance Abuse and Mental Health Admnistration, Rockville, MD.

Marks, I.M., Connolly, J., Muijen, M. *et al.* (1994) Home-based versus hospital-based care for people with serious mental illness. *British Journal of Psychiatry* 165, 179–194.

Marshall, M., Gray, A., Lockwood, A. *et al.* (2000a) *Case Management for Severe Mental Disorders*. The Cochrane Library, 3. Update Software, Oxford.

Marshall, M., Gray, A., Lockwood, A. *et al.* (2000b) *Assertive Community Treatment* The Cochrane Library, 3. Update Software, Oxford.

Mattes, J.A., Rosen, B., Klein, D.F. & Milan, D. (1977) Comparison of the clinical effectiveness of 'short' versus 'long' stay psychiatric hospitalisation. II. Results of a 3-year post hospital follow-up. *Journal of Nervous and Mental Disease* 165, 395–402.

Mellsop, G.W., Blair-West, G.W. & Duraiappah, V. (1997) The effect of a new integrated mental health service on hospitalization. *Australian and New Zealand Journal of Psychiatry* 31, 480–483.

Mental Health Commission (1999) *New Zealand's National Mental Health Strategy*. Mental Health Commission, Wellington.

Merson, S., Tyrer, P., Onyett, S. *et al.* (1992) Early intervention in psychiatric emergencies: a controlled clinical trial. *Lancet* 339, 1311–1314.

Mollica, R.F. (1983) From asylum to community: the threatened disintegration of public psychiatry. *New England Journal of Medicine* 308, 367–373.

Moore, C. (1998) Admission to an acute psychiatric ward. *Nursing Times* 94, 58–59.

Morrissey, Y., Calloway, M., Baztko, T. et al. (1994) Mental health authorities and service system changes from the RWY PCMY. *Milbank Quarterly* 72, 19–80.

Morse, G.A., Calsyn, R.J., Klinkenberg, W.D. *et al.* (1997) An experimental comparison of three types of case management for homeless mentally ill persons. *Psychiatric Services* 48, 497–503.

Mosher, L.R. (1999) Soteria and other alternatives to acute psychiatric hospitalization. *Journal of Nervous and Mental Disease* 187, 142–149.

Mowbray, C.T., Leff, S., Warren, R., McCrohan, N.M. & Bybee, D. (1997) Enhancing vocational outcomes for persons with psychiatric disabilities: a new paradigm. In: *Innovative Approaches for Difficult to Treat Populations* (eds S.W. Henggeler & A.B. Santos), pp. 311–350. American Psychiatric Press, Washington DC.

Mueser, K.T., Bond, G.R., Drake, R.E. *et al.* (1998) Models of community care for severe mental illness: an overview of research on case management. *Schizophrenia Bulletin* 24, 363–380.

Nienhuis, F.J., Giel, R., Kluiter, H., Ruphan, M. & Wiersma, D. (1994) Efficacy of psychiatric day treatment: course and outcome of psychiatric disorders in a randomised trial. *European Archives of Psychiatry and Clinical Neurosciences* 244, 73–80.

Oiesvold, T., Saarento, O., Sytema, S. *et al.* (1999) The Nordic Comparative Study on Sectorized Psychiatry: length of in-patient stay. *Acta Psychiatrica Scandinavica* 100, 220–228.

Oliver, N. & Kuipers, E. (1996) Stress and its relationship to expressed emotion in community mental health workers. *International Journal of Social Psychiatry* 42, 150–159.

Onyett, S., Heppleston, T. & Bushnell, D. (1994) A national survey of community mental health teams: team structure and process. *Journal of Mental Health* 3, 175–194.

Pelosi, A.J. & Jackson, G.A. (2000) Home treatment: enigmas and fantasies. *British Medical Journ* 320, 308–309.

Perring, C. (1992) The experience and perspectives of patients and care staff on the transition from hospital to community-based care. In: *Psychiatric Hospital Closure: Myths and Realities* (ed. S. Ramon), pp. 122–169. Chapman & Hall, London.

Pfeiffer, S.I., Malley, D.S. & Shott, S. (1996) Factors associated with outcome of adults treated in psychiatric hospitals: a synthesis of findings. *Psychiatric Services* 47, 263–269.

Polak, P.R. & Kirby, M.W. (1976) A model to replace psychiatric hospitals. *Journal of Nervous and Mental Disease* 162, 13–22.

Power, P. & McGorry, P.D. (1999) Initial assessment of first episode psychosis. In: *The Recognition and Management of Early Psychosis* (eds P.D. McGrorry & H.J. Jackson), pp. 155–183. Cambridge University Press, Cambridge.

Priebe, S., Warner, R., Hubschmid, T. & Eckle, I. (1998) Employment, attitudes towards work, and quality of life among people with schizophrenia in three countries. *Schizophrenia Bulletin* 24, 469–477.

Raftery, J. (1992) Mental health services in transition: the United States and the United Kingdom. *British Journal of Psychiatry* 161, 589–593.

Ramon, S. (1988) Community care in Britain. In: *Community Care in Practice* (eds A. Lavender & F. Holloway), pp. 9–26. John Wiley, Chichester.

Ramsay, R. & Holloway, F. (1998) Mental Health Services. In: *General Psychiatry College Seminars in Psychiatry* (eds G. Stein & G. Wilkinson), pp. 1274–1333. Gaskell, London.

Reding, G.R. & Raphelson, M. (1995) Around the clock mobile crisis intervention: another effective alternative to psychiatric hospitalization. *Community Mental Health Journal* 31, 179–190.

Reid, Y., Johnson, S., Morant, N. *et al.* (1999) Explanations for stress and satisfaction in mental health professionals: a qualitative study. *Social Psychiatry and Psychiatric Epidemiology* 34, 301–308.

Ridgely, M., Morrissey, J., Paulson, R., Goldman, H. & Calloway, M. (1996) Characteristics and activities of case managers in the RWJ Foundation program on chronic mental illness. *Psychiatric Services* 47, 737–743.

Rosenheck, R., Morrissey, J., Lan, J. *et al.* (1998) Service system integration, access to services, and housing outcomes in a programme for homeless persons with severe mental illness. *American Journal of Public Health* 88, 1610–1615.

Rosie, J.S., Hassan, F.A.A., Piper, W.E. & Joyce, A.S. (1995) Effective psychiatric day treatment: historical lessons. *Psychiatric Services* 47, 137–138.

Royal College of Psychiatrists (2000) *Good Psychiatric Practice 2000.* Council Report CR83. Royal College of Psychiatrists, London.

Sainsbury Centre for Mental Health (1998a) *Keys to Engagement.* Sainsbury Centre for Mental Health, London.

Sainsbury Centre for Mental Health (1998b) *Acute Problems.* Sainsbury Centre for Mental Health, London.

Sashidharan, S.P., Smyth, M. & Owen, A. (1999) PriSM Psychosis study. Thro' a glass darkly: a distorted appraisal of community care. *British Journal of Psychiatry* 175, 504–507.

Saylers, M.P., Masterton, T.W., Fekete, D.M. *et al.* (1998) Transferring clients from intensive case management: impact on client functioning. *American Journal of Orthopsychiatry* 68, 233–245.

Scull, A.T. (1977) *Decarceration.* Polity Press, Cambridge.

Scull, A.T. (1979) *Museums of Madness.* Penguin, Harmondsworth.

Sederer and Dickey (1995) Acute and chronic psychiatric care: establishing boundaries. *Psychiatric Quarterly* 66, 263–274.

Shepherd, G., Beadsmoore, A., Moore, C., Hardy, P. & Muijen, M. (1997) Relation between bed use, social deprivation, and overall bed availability in acute adult psychiatric units, and alternative residential options: a cross sectional survey, one day census data, and staff interviews. *British Medical Journal* 314, 262–266.

Shepherd, M., Gunnell, D., Maxwell, B. & Mumford, D. (1998) Development and evaluation of an inner city mental health team. *Social Psychiatry and Psychiatric Epidemiology* 33, 129–135.

Sledge, W.H., Tebes, J., Rakfeldt, J. *et al.* (1996) Day hospital/crisis respite care versus inpatient care. I. Clinical outcomes. *American Journal of Psychiatry* 153, 1065–1073.

Smyth, M.G. & Hoult, J. (2000) The home treatment enigma. *British Medical Journal* 320, 305–308.

Snowden, L.R. & Cheung, F.A. (1990) Use of inpatient mental health services by members of ethnic minority groups. *American Psychologist* 45, 347–355.

Solomon, P. & Draine, J. (1995) One year outcomes of a randomised trial of case management with seriously mentally ill clients leaving jail. *Evaluation Review* 19, 256–273.

Stein, L. & Santos, A. (1998) *Assertive Community Treatment of Persons with Severe Mental Illness.* Norton, New York.

Strathdee, G. & Thornicroft, G. (1996) Core components of a. comprehensive mental health service. In: *Commissioning Mental Health Services* (eds. G. Thornicroft & G. Strathdee), pp. 133–145. HMSO, London.

Surgeon General (1999) *Mental Health: A Report of the Surgeon General.* http://www.surgeongeneral.gov/library/mentalhealth/toc.html.

Sytema, S. & Burgess, P. (1999) Continuity of care and readmission in two service systems. a comparative Victorian and Groningen case-register study. *Acta Psychiatrica Scandinavica* 100, 212–219.

Sytema, S., Micciolo, R. & Tansella, M. (1996) Service utilisation by schizophrenic patients in Groningen and South Verona: an event history analysis. *Psychological Medicine* 26, 109–119.

Szmukler, G. & Holloway, F. (2001) Inpatient treatment. In: *Textbook of Community Psychiatry* (eds G. Thornicroft & G. Szmukler), pp. 321–338. Oxford University Press, Oxford.

Tansella, M. (1986) Community psychiatry without mental hospitals: the Italian experience – a review. *Journal of the Royal Society of Medicine* 79, 664–669.

Teague, G.B., Bond, G.R. & Drake, R.E. (1998) Program fidelity in assertive community treatment: development and use of a measure. *American Journal of Orthopsychiatry* 68, 216–232.

Thornicroft, G. & Goldberg, D. (1999) *Has Community Care Failed?* Maudsley Discussion Paper No 5. Institute of Psychiatry, London.

Thornicroft, G., Wykes, T., Holloway, F., Johnson, S. & Szmukler, G. (1998) From efficacy to effectiveness in community mental health services: PriSM Psychosis Study 10. *British Journal of Psychiatry* 173, 423–427.

Tyrer, P., Evans, K., Gandhi, N. *et al.* (1998) Randomised controlled trial of two models of care for discharged psychiatric patients. *British Medical Journal* 316, 106–109.

Tyrer, P., Coid, J., Simmonds, S., Joseph, P. & Marriott, S. (2000) Community mental health teams (CMHTs) for people with severe mental illnesses and disordered personality. *Cochrane Library* 3. Update Software, Oxford.

Vendsborg, P.B., Norentoft, M., Hvenegaard, A. & Sogaard, J. (1999) *Assertive Community Treatment.* Danish Institute for Health Services Research, Copenhagen.

Wasylenki, D., Gehrs, M., Goering, P. & Toner, B. (1997) A home based programme for the treatment of acute psychosis. *Community Mental Health Journal* 33, 151–165.

Weller, M.P.I. (1989) Mental illness: who cares? *Nature* 339, 249–252.

Wilder, J.F., Levin, G. & Zwerling, I. (1966) A two-year follow-up evaluation of acute psychotic patients treated in a day-hospital. *American Journal of Psychiatry* 122, 1095–1101.

Wykes, T. & Holloway, F. (2000) Community rehabilitation. past failures and future prospects. *International Review of Psychiatry* 12, 197–205.

Wykes, T., Stevens, W. & Everitt, B. (1997) Stress in community care teams: will it affect the sustainability of community care? *Social Psychiatry and Psychiatric Epidemiology* 32, 398–407.

Wykes, T., Leese, M., Taylor, R. & Phelan, M. (1998) Effects of community services on disability and symptoms: PRiSM Psychosis Study 4. *British Journal of Psychiatry* 173, 385–390.

Ziguras, S.J. & Stuart, G.W. (2000) A meta-analysis of the effectiveness of mental health case management over 20 years. *Psychiatric Services* 51, 1410–1421.

35 Psychosis and recovery: some patients' perspectives*

Peter Chadwick, Robert Lundin, Grace Brown,† Alison McPartlin, Claire Brookman and Janey Antoniou

Six stories, 701
  Peter, 701
  Robert, 702
  Grace, 702
  Alison, 702
  Claire, 703
  Janey, 703
Treatment experiences, 703
  Peter, 703
  Robert, 704
  Grace, 704
  Alison, 705
  Claire, 706
  Janey, 706

Living with the illness, 707
  Peter, 707
  Robert, 707
  Grace, 708
  Alison, 708
  Janey, 709
Reflections, 709
  Peter, 709
  Robert, 710
  Grace, 710
  Alison, 711
  Claire, 711
  Janey, 711
References, 712

Professionals in the field of psychiatry are becoming more aware than ever that there is a great amount of insight to be gleaned from the stories of people who have experienced serious psychiatric illnesses. There are many reasons. Patients can, and often do, have unique and powerful perspectives into the nature of their illnesses. Through intimate experiences, they subjectively understand manias, psychoses and other symptoms, therein reaching a depth of appreciation that an 'outsider' can scarcely match. Moreover, as recipients of treatment, patients know the success and shortcomings of mental health services from a user's perspective. Patients' roles as knowledgeable informants are being recognized throughout the mental health service industry.

Here are interwoven stories from six patients who have suffered mental illness. Peter discusses in detail his experiences with anger, anxiety, passion, psychosis, medications and their fascinating relationship to his sexuality. Robert also describes his experiences with mental illness, from its onset in his life in 1979 at the age of 23 to his current success in controlling his symptoms and living a productive life. Janey was ill for many years before she realized it in 1985 when working as a scientist and has also had to make many adjustments to accommodate her illness to her changing life. Grace and Alison experience mental illness each in their own way and Claire expresses triumph in her

account. All have had some misgivings about their treatment of which their psychiatrist has not been fully aware. While schizophrenia and schizoaffective disorder are terribly disabling, these authors cope well with their mental illnesses. Their stories are of triumph over adversity.

Six stories

Peter

I often was accused of being tactless, off-beat, cheeky, of getting the wrong end of the stick, of being tangential, of not getting things across first time, of being strange, different, maybe queer, and so it would go on. To say I did not 'mesh' with society would be an understatement. But in madness I did not retreat or run away from that society, rather, it was that I had never been at one with it in the first place.

In my emotional life it was as if the volume controls on my basic affects – anger, fear and sex – were turned up too high. The high level of anxiety and my extreme sensitivity to detail made me feel thin-skinned to the point of 'skinlessness'. I vacillated by the minute, sometimes by the second, between rage, terror and sensual passion.

My home environment had been one of extremely high expressed emotion in the sense of Vaughn and Leff (1976) and Bebbington and Kuipers (1994). There was totally conditional love – and emotional abuse – the latter repeated at school. By the time I was 21 I was an exceedingly nervous and insecure man prone to nervous sweating, insomnia and repeated flashbacks to bullying episodes at school (school was in many ways the

Editors' note: A book which summarizes our knowledge of schizophrenia would be incomplete without a first-hand expression of patients' experiences. Six have generously given their accounts and reflections. While this is different from the critical reductionist approach which characterizes most of the book, we think that practitioners and scientists will be better able to appreciate their tasks if they are in touch with the experience which patients can best describe themselves.
†Alias.

seedbed of my later paranoia). In short, I was basically a nervous wreck, with tobacco smoking being my only prop and palliative.

As a young man I was also a transvestite and lived in mortal terror of being discovered. I entered on the road to psychosis when I was discovered, in 1974, and outed by neighbours in Bristol, UK. What previously had been my one asset, my creative imagination, now became my deadliest enemy. The slightest evidence of my transvestism being discovered – such as a long stare from a passer-by, a lorry driver honking his horn as he sped past or somebody not answering the phone when I rang – I took as confirmation that my cross-dressing had been in some way broadcast far and wide.

When I was 33, this process, obviously fed by guilt and fear, had reached pandemonium proportions such that almost anything and everything happening around me I took as evidence that I was being tormented and mocked. This was by a collection of people I termed 'The Organization', who persecuted me for my decadent, sybaritic, satyriacal ways. Eventually, and by now thinking that I must be possessed by Satan, I was admitted to hospital after a suicide attempt (Chadwick 1992, 1993).

Robert

My history of mental illness began with a hospitalization after a suicide attempt in 1974, only a few days after my graduation from high school in the USA. It was a complete surprise to me. High school had been an unerring success; I valued my clean reputation among my peers and the school's faculty. For reasons of the school's strict drug policy, I had stayed away from the drug-using crowd. After graduation, however, with the authority of the school gone, I imbibed with a friend who offered me some potent marijuana. The resulting high flipped me into a drug-induced psychosis, one so powerful, frightening and confounding that it led to my making a violent suicide attempt that evening. I recovered rapidly after the drug wore off, but my reputation among many of my friends was seriously undermined. That summer of 1974 I was very confused, lonely and ashamed. I now had a terrible secret to hide.

I didn't remain depressed for long; by the fall there was college to look forward to. As I began my college career I once again immersed myself in school life. But there were many lonely evenings of pensive thoughts, trying to comprehend why I had attempted my own life. I knew very little about psychosis. At this point, mental illness was out of the question. Yet, in my senior year the telltale signs of intrusive thoughts crept in – I didn't recognize them at the time – they were so slight that they didn't spur me to seek help.

From 4 years of college, relying greatly on my sister's guidance, I moved onto graduate school in business administration. I was having a terrible time making decisions for my future. None the less, I was accepted to a graduate programme at Vanderbilt University in Nashville. By my third semester, psychosis visited me again with unfortunate vigour, this time without the catalyst of illegal drug use.

I remember the night I went mad. An acute psychotic episode can be a vivid experience. My thoughts became expansive, sweeping; one fantastic idea triggered another, then another. My mind was both exhilarated and terrified with frightful revelations about life and the universe. I was horrified to realize that nothing in the world existed outside my perception. Then, as I lay beneath the covers to my bed, perspiration beading on my brow, God was communicating to me through a light bulb from behind the louvered door to the closet in my bedroom. In reality, I was very ill. That night I drove to Vanderbilt University Medical Centre and demanded that I speak to the university's chancellor. The nurses led me to an examining room and summoned the psychiatry resident on call. She arrived in the brightly lighted room and spoke to me softly. I refused to talk. After several tense moments I opened up, and within an hour I was admitted to the adult psychiatric ward.

Grace

I was diagnosed as paranoid schizophrenic when I was 30 years old, 18 years ago. I had a happy protected childhood and knew I was loved by both parents. Following university, I got a good job in television, shared a flat with a friend and had a busy social life. A friend invited me to Tai Chi classes – an eastern form of meditation and martial arts. After a weekend session, with time spent examining people's auras, I started feeling spaced out and could not sleep. I lost my concentration and became deeply concerned about spiritual matters. I went to see a spiritualist who claimed he could heal people through listening to his spirit guides. For a period of time I would hear the central light bulb ticking loudly in my bedroom. Was it an evil spirit? Convinced of a supernatural world, I picked up a Bible I had had as a child and turned to the gospel of Luke. A bright light shone on significant passages to do with healing. I believe and still believe the light was from God. Consequently, I asked Jesus to come into my life and read most of the New Testament the following day. That night a voice in my head like my own convinced me that I must jump out of my bedroom window, so as not to disturb my parents, and get a message to television broadcasters that the world was coming to an end.

I was admitted to hospital by my anxious family. Since then I have had 15 short psychotic episodes, which have involved a deceptive voice leading me into situations where I have often been in danger.

Alison

I became aware I was special at the age of 15. Luminous spikes emerged from my head, an empowering sensation, which I enhanced by cropping my hair. At age 18, the spikes told me to discover my special purpose in life; in contrast, my parents insisted I go to university. I wound up miserable and isolated in halls of residence.

Meanwhile, the spikes were still radiating from my head like antennae; I felt solid and objects seemed extra real; I was bursting with LIFE and it clicked that what I had to do was study

LIFE. So I decided to make biochemistry my Alien Mission. As an Alien, I needed space, so I lived alone in a cheap flat and went for long cycle trips in my free time rather than socialize with the other students. This was a success: I graduated with a first class honours degree, a publication and an offer to do a PhD. My success reinforced my belief in my mission of research by indicating I had special abilities.

On the down side, I had been having trouble with my sleep. I put it down to species difference but, living alone with flexible working hours, I coped until, shortly after my finals, I had to vacate my flat and I decided to share. This was a big mistake as I felt suffocated. To make matters worse, the other students kept asking me out to parties, pubs, etc. and I felt pressured to go. I find such socializing horribly stressful and draining and, without space to recover at home, had difficulty coping with work. I complained of tiredness and was given clomipramine. This made me extremely groggy. I found it even harder to cope, started making mistakes in the lab and became so despondent that I begged to be admitted to hospital. The doctors asked me over and over if I heard voices or had any unusual thoughts and eventually I thought perhaps, perhaps my spikes and alienity might fall into that category, so they said that indeed was a problem but it would be cured by chlorpromazine.

Claire

Having depression when I was 16 and given antidepressants to cure the sadness and self-loathing, the thought of ever having to go into hospital never crossed my mind. Uncontrollable crying set in. The ability to concentrate, even for a minute, became more difficult. I couldn't watch a television programme and could not concentrate when listening to others. I suspected that everyone was out to kill me and that my parents were poisoning my food. I started to make myself sick. Then one morning my parents called the police and I was taken into hospital and sectioned.

I refused all medication and, when given any orally, I would go to my room and spit them out. Food also became my enemy, believing I could only be given food that was from a shop and sealed. I then started to become psychotic. My symptoms were thoughts of someone killing me. Still having no appetite and losing weight, I continued to have delusional thoughts and began to not communicate with anyone. I withdrew from a life I had loved. I didn't believe I had an illness. My symptoms worsened and eventually I had to have slow-release injections. My mind was muddled. I could not distinguish between the truth and lies.

My illness was beginning to get worse. The antidepressants had no effect. My job began to suffer. My till wouldn't balance, which in the past had been a simple task. My need for food became less and not being able to sit still began to annoy me.

Janey

I originally thought that I'd become ill at work in 1985, because that was when I was hospitalized for the first time. However, in retrospect I was ill for a while in the late 1970s at university and had seen a psychiatrist then, although I'd managed to persuade him I was okay. I also remember being on chlorpromazine after a suicide attempt when I was 14 and am vividly aware of being depressed when I was seven.

Both my parents had been London children who had been evacuated during World War II, an experience so traumatic my father still won't talk about it. This caused my childhood to be difficult in a family who came to the collective (unconscious) decision that emotions and all other problems should be sorted out quietly by the individual concerned. In addition, my parents found making friends difficult and had moved away from their parents so I had no other significant adults in my life.

I constantly hear voices: scary, horrible, horrible voices that do not stop. In a poem I once described them as 'red-hot voices howling in my mind' and I would go walking all night to attempt to get away from them. I also have horrendous delusions which I don't realize are not real until I become well again afterwards, like nightmares where the horror turns out to be real and had been lived. I always have to apologize to people when I recover because of the strange things I have done when I am ill. Trying to pretend I was 'normal' is always physically exhausting.

I had no official label or diagnosis until about 1988 when I asked my psychiatrist if he knew of a group I could join, whose members had been through hospital but still worked. He suggested contacting the National Schizophrenia Fellowship. I was shocked, I had never thought of schizophrenia in connection to myself.

Over the last 14 years I've had huge problems with illness, fights with doctors over medications and been sectioned a large number of times. I have wandered the streets in my dressing gown, jumped in the Thames and, on one occasion, was naked in public. The police have taken me back to the hospital when I went AWOL from the hospital, with all the neighbours watching me go. But, to a certain degree and with a lot of help, I have learned to live with the way things are for me.

Treatment experiences

Peter

When I received a diagnosis of schizophrenia/schizoaffective psychosis in 1979 it was a relief, not a death sentence. Accepting that I had a mental illness, and perhaps had had one to some degree all my life, made sense out of a lot of my past experiences, agonies and traumas. It also made me face my need for medication which, when my drug and dosage finally were agreed on, has since given me some 20 years of productive and essentially happy and normal life (Chadwick 1995).

Medication, when at last I received it, slowed down my racing thoughts, gave me control over my own mind and restored my metacognitive capacities: I could once again easily reflect on my own thoughts and perceptions. It calmed my emotions, widened my attentional beam, helped me to sleep at night and in some manner calmed me cognitively. In this sense it made my thinking clearer and less distractible and made me less likely to jump to conclusions or to the most dramatic interpretation of a situation.

I do not believe that all the conditions that psychiatry and clinical psychology have terms for are illnesses. But I have no doubt that psychosis is an illness, I do not believe, and few users do, that medication alone is sufficient to ameliorate our problems. Still, if it is adhered to it can form a powerful foundation to treatment.

No one can get out of hell on their own. They need help from other people. Just rearranging the way you think will not do it, nor will a pill, nor will kindness and acceptance. But put all three together and you start moving in the right direction. Help has to be tailored to the individual psychological needs of the service user.

Because of the religious nature of my delusions, talks with vicars and with the hospital chaplain were helpful. Because of my alternative sexual orientation, the acceptance of my transvestism by straight people in West London gave me much peace (Chadwick 1997b). Because of the abnormalities in my attentional style and emotional intensity, medication was a great source of support for me. Because my thinking had been so pervaded by confirmation-seeking, a deliberate shift to a more balanced use of evidence prevented a reactivation of the old style.

In addition to all of this, I had to attack my own guilty conscience and merciless 'internal critic' which was largely built up from internalized images of my mother, father and of bullies at school. I had, so to speak, to put my changed mentality on the road and get positive social feedback to gradually increase my self-esteem and dampen my self-abusing conscience. All of this took time, years in fact.

When I was psychotic my mind was out of control. I had no capacity for metacognition, in the sense that I could not think about my own thinking. Hence, I could not reflect on, reroute or stop what was happening within me. It was like being on a roller-coaster heading for a brick wall. The (very few) attempts I did make to think about my own thinking and perceiving actually caused distress as I noticed how bizarre and inaccurate – particularly my hearing of things said at a distance – they were proving to be.

The side-effects of medication, particularly restlessness and constipation, were at their worst when I was in hospital and on high dosages of haloperidol and pimozide (Chadwick 1997a, chapter 5). After discharge I was on oral administration, and restlessness and occasional sluggishness still troubled me. But the former was easily subdued by orphenadrine and the sluggishness I eased by taking the occasional drug holiday or by titrating (in the sense of self-adjusting) my dose. Although side-effects were irritating, I always felt that the medication was so helpful to my mental state that they never motivated me to cease taking it (I remain on 2.5 mg haloperidol nocte to this day).

Other patients I know complained of sluggishness and sleepiness on antipsychotic medication and that it affects their general level of motivation. They were particularly irritated by those psychiatrists who did not realize this. I was given the freedom to self-adjust my dose and this was very helpful but others were not (and indeed were actively dissuaded from doing so). I think this was a mistake and may have played a part in many people discontinuing medication and then relapsing.

Robert

When they placed me on medication in hospital at Vanderbilt, they chose a moderate dosage of Navane (tiotixene). There seemed to be some haste to get me back into classes at the graduate business school. The psychiatric unit summoned my parents while I was still an inpatient, but the doctors were unwilling to label my case schizophrenia. I was released to the university's student health service with the optimistic label of some kind of adjustment problem. While remaining on antipsychotic medication, with both my concentration and ability to cope with anxiety disturbed, within a few weeks I contacted my parents and told them it was impossible for me to continue school. Their disappointment was palatable. Both they and I realized that this marked a real blemish on my educational record, which, up to then, had been quite solid. But I would do anything to release myself from the stresses of school. I was continually racked with anxiety, my ability to concentrate was badly impeded, and the effects of medication were making me groggy.

Home again I was faced with the humiliation of failure. I came from a high-achieving family where a letdown like this was viewed with concern. I lapsed into a depression, one that was to last several months. Inexplicably I was given no drug therapy, rather, I was convinced that a regimen of exercise and a positive attitude would lift me from it. This I did, and in 4 months I was back on my feet again, symptom free. Like the remission of symptoms I experienced after the 1974 crisis, again I thought myself clear of any psychiatric problem. So my family hoped. That fall, of 1980, I began a career in college administration; I was now free of medications and their side-effects. I thought my problems were over.

Grace

Inpatient experiences over 18 years

I fought not to take medication because of the side-effects. My psychiatrist, family and later my church leaders were all adamant I had to take medication. I've been on at least nine different drugs, gained 4 stone in weight and have experienced a range of side-effects from incontinence, sleepiness and lethargy to such an inner restlessness that I couldn't relax enough to sit down. The drug haliperidol gave me hallucinations of snakes and greatly increased my state of anxiety. My psychiatrist has at last found a drug that suits me. I now take the minimum dose of 200 mg/day quetiapine. Last year I lost the weight I had gained. I am not aware of any side-effects.

My first admission was to a private hospital; the subsequent admissions were mainly to Charing Cross Hospital.

I remember thinking in 1985 that the care in the NHS was as good as I received in the pricey private hospital. Wards were generally quite peaceful. I remember the nurses as being caring and friendly, happy to spend time chatting. Nurses made the beds daily. Menus were delivered to each cubicle or room and meals served individually on trays, instead of the present system of queuing at a food trolley. Daily needs were attended to. As my admissions were generally the day before my monthly cycle, nurses were willing to even go off the ward to buy what I needed the several times when I was sectioned.

Although there was never much to do on the wards, there was a ping-pong table at one end and, at various times on different admissions, there was art therapy, aerobics to music, discussion around newspaper articles or a more nebulous 'group therapy'. My episodes of illness were characterized by anxious religious thoughts and delusions. I would arrive on the ward feeling spaced out and fearful. I became self-focused which I now realize to be destructive. Conversation with other people was key to recovery, whether with nurses, patients or communication with friends and family. Within 4 days I was often able to return to complete normality. The pay-box phone was a lifeline to the outside world and it was in constant use. My shortest hospital admission was 5 days, the longest 6 weeks. When I was at my worst and extremely anxious, believing God had forsaken Jesus on the cross, so everyone in the world was going to hell, a trainee Christian doctor came to my side and quoted scriptures. It had an immediate calming effect and I was soon off the ward.

Gradually life on the ward changed. With the closure of many long-term psychiatric hospitals, a significant percentage of the patients who were admitted were noticeably more disturbed. There was often a radio blaring loudly and it was difficult to find a quiet place when I wanted to read my Bible and pray. Physically there were improvements made on the ward but nursing care deteriorated. Most of the nurses I knew left.

On one admission about 2 years ago I became aware of the seclusion room being used as a punishment room as an easy option for nursing staff. A girl of about 20, who had suffered much abuse and neglect in her life, started screaming. I saw her bodily being carried by her hands and feet by two male nurses to the seclusion room. A few days later, some gunshots rang out at night – perhaps army practice fire. The woman in the room next to me started screaming. I heard a nurse outside her room say 'We'd better take her to the seclusion room'. Where were the compassionate nurses who would ask why the patients were distressed and give reassurance?

In September 2001 I was on the adjacent ward 3 West. Now the only activity on the ward was watching TV. Nursing care was at its lowest level. The patients were mostly left to make their own beds 'to encourage patients to take responsibility for everyday activities' (I quote from a reply to an official complaint I made). Nurses didn't check whether patients washed or ate. In the past a nurse would go to each cubicle to encourage the patients to come to meals. There was no towel offered or supplied on admission to me. One woman who was receiving treatment for cancer was in such fear that she wet herself very obviously.

(Her thin trousers were soaked half way down to her thigh.) She was wandering anxiously round the ward. I asked two different nurses to help the woman change, but it was over half an hour before someone went with her to her cubicle to help her. Her soaked sheets were left unchanged and I ended up making her bed myself. During the 3 weeks I was on the ward there were no plates or bowls for breakfast. I was told by a nurse to put my cereal in a plastic cup and I buttered my bread on the table. Breakfast was brought in a box and dumped on the table. There were no vases on the ward, no iron, no ashtrays and one evening there was only half a loo roll between the three loos I checked. There was only one bath on the ward, which always looked filthy. I spent about 10 minutes trying to clean the bath one evening but the bath was old and the dirt ingrained. I twice used the shower nearest to me. The curtain didn't meet the shower base and large quantities of water spread across the floor. Four times (directed by the nurses to do so and only assisted once), I used the mop and bucket and old towels to mop up the water. I did this twice for two unknown patients, who I'm sure were not as well as me, and if I hadn't there was no alternative but to wade through water to get to the loo. I've always had friends and family visiting. However, communication was made more difficult on my last admission with no pay phone. Calls had to be made in the staff office where there was no privacy.

Some of the homeless people on the ward had no one to call or perhaps just one person. For the homeless people and those in hostels daily interest and encouragement from a nurse could have made all the difference. But there was virtually no interaction between staff and patients. Surely a nurse could have had a 15-min daily conversation with each patient, relating purely on a human level. A revision of the nursing and management of inpatient services is now being undertaken.

Alison

For me, the treatment is far worse than the 'illness'. It did not stop me thinking I was special but I lost the ability to do my mission which led to a suicide attempt. I could not even do simple things like cook proper meals, let alone think clearly or develop other coping strategies. I was also unable to feel pleasure. The end result was paranoia and fear of psychiatrists, hospitals and drug companies, which persists to this day; and guilt for wasting so many years of my life.

The first antipsychotic I was given was chlorpromazine. A 'heavy squad' pinned me down and sat on my limbs and head and chest so I couldn't breathe and injected me. Next I was given a depot injection of Modecate. I lay in bed for a month feeling like cement. Over the next year, I tried a succession of antipsychotics, all of which made me sluggish, sleepy and unable to function. Yet I complied with treatment and accepted my diagnosis, and tried to get on with things. I returned to labwork – repetitive routine work was all I was capable of; I joined a roadrunners club and a badminton club; went to a drop-in centre where I made some friends, but there was no point to it. After some 6 months of Haldol I seized up, froze to my bed, panicked and ended up back in hospital. During 1992–93 I had frequent admissions to hospital. Without procyclidine my eyes rolled upwards in my blank deathlike face; restless legs prevented restful sleep but for years I was never truly awake.

By the end of 1993 I felt I couldn't take any more. I had already attempted suicide and, although it was dawning on me that my doctor did not care, I naively trusted her and thought we could talk about a new approach, but she refused to speak to me and suddenly I thought, 'it is time to make a stand for my life, I have nothing to lose'. I ran up to my doctor and hurled her to the ground.

This landed me in a maximum security hospital. Although I resented the loss of freedom, having staff present all the time made it possible to build up rapport. My new consultant, to whom I am deeply indebted, agreed to take me off Haldol. The fog lifted; I could smile again, and get up in the mornings.

I will note here that I have found the newer medications just as tortuous. As a prophylactic I was put on risperidone for a month but it made me groggy and irritable once more and the nursing staff agreed I was better without it. Later, when I took olanzapine for 2 years, it also sapped my energy and motivation, and stopped me breathing when I tried to sleep. At the end of 1999 I was persuaded to take clozapine but I soon changed my mind because the starting dose made me feel like I was about to die and I knew I wouldn't be able to go home and look after myself at the end of the week as planned. I think it is important for psychiatrists to realize that for some people medication side-effects are not just a minor discomfort but can leave the patient unable to shop, feed themselves or wash. The lesson I have learned is not to trust psychiatrists on this, because it is me who will end up in trouble.

Claire

Having a diagnosis of schizophrenia, manic depression and having had a psychotic episode the outlook was not great. A year in hospital and having been sectioned twice I wondered if I would ever get out of hospital. My family visited me every day, they cared for me as best they could even though my hatred for them was overwhelming. I cut myself off from all but one of my friends and I am pleased to say my grandmother never suffered the abuse I gave to my parents. The hospital days went so quick, a whole year of my life was spent sectioned and not knowing why I was hospitalized. The insight into my illness took a long time, I was convinced the doctors were wrong, and only now do I look back and realize they were trying to help someone with an acute mental illness.

Becoming acutely ill happened over night. Literally, well one minute then ill the next. I refused all medication so injections were the only way to stabilize this manic phase. Oral medication was then introduced and the side-effects were extremely frightening: milk from my breasts, a sense of tiredness and weight gain but most importantly a general sense of not being me. I would go to sleep asking my brain to get well so I could get out of this place, which was now my home.

I saw people come and go, but I remained in hospital. Why was I not allowed to go home? I never cut myself, I never tried suicide, I was just a bit high.

My constant rejection of medication forced the doctors to make a compulsory admission to hospital under Section 2 of the Mental Health Act. I fought the 'section' and won. However, I returned to hospital as soon as I returned home. The drugs I took made no difference until I decided to take part in a study. Wanting my life back I tried Clozaril. Within 2 months I was well, not completely but a sense of normality returned to my life. I could go home without being abusive to my family. I could do simple tasks, like making dinner and watching television without thinking it was about me. My thoughts were not so muddled and I could differentiate between the truth and lies, reality and fantasy. I talked in English, not the made-up language I had thought up. Most importantly, I realized I had a mental health problem and was going to beat it.

Janey

Over the last years I have been on: trazodone, amitriptyline, imipramine, chlorpromazine, lithium, pimozide, Depixol, haloperidol, chlordiazepoxide, diazepam, nitrazipam, Haldol, Stelazine, sulpiride, remoxipride, Melleril, flupentixol, risperidone, fluoxetine, lofepramine, citalopram, carbamazepine, lorazepam, quetiapine and sertraline. All of them have given me some side-effects. There is a myth that the symptoms have got to be worse than side-effects, they are not – just different. The side-effects can include impotence, weight gain, permanent drowsiness and a feeling that one is never going to enjoy anything again. It becomes an effort just to carry on with one's life, and can in itself lead to suicidal feelings.

One of the greatest fantasies I and the other patients in hospital shared was stirring a therapeutic dose of haloperidol or chlorpromazine into the psychiatrist's coffee to see if he could function normally for the rest of the day! Maybe all psychiatrists should try taking one of the older medications at a therapeutic dose for a couple of days before they start prescribing these things!

I have found in the past that doctors will maintain the status quo concerning drugs because it is easier, despite endless complaints from their patients, and that nothing will happen unless the patient takes the initiative and stops taking the medication. Of course, awkward patients (like me) start complaining the instant the side-effects start, so now I compromise with my GP over new treatments, I can try them but have to take them for 6 weeks before I change anything. Mostly though, through trial and error, I have found what drugs work best for me and will cooperate in taking them. Occasionally, however, I become ill and then stop taking my medication.

Living with the illness

Peter

Struggling on: I remained fragile for 5 or 6 years after my crisis in 1979. I could not withstand very much stress and certain things were particularly detrimental to my recovery. The highest in this league were verbally and/or physically abusive people that I might see in pubs, shops or hotels. I always avoided such people or indeed anyone who seemed loud and aggressive. Second came overtalkative people, people who did not listen and arrogant self-opinionated people. Thirdly, and not surprisingly in my case, came 'transvestophobic' people and men and women who were cynically sensitive to and intolerant of behaviour in a man that was not fully masculine and heterosexual. (I had had horrific experience of such people at school – I called them 'The Masculinity and Heterosexuality Thought Police'.) I learned to try to avoid all these categories of individual or to minimize contact with them as much as possible.

I also found it helpful to have gradual re-employment rather than being thrown in at the deep end to work full-time from day one. In the teaching work I eventually did, I gradually took on more courses each year from 1982 until I was able to work full time. But this took about 5 years and hence for a long time after the episode I was only able to work part-time. None the less, working was therapeutic and made me feel useful and at one with the world.

It also is difficult for me to overestimate the value of thousands of hours of everyday chat about nothing in particular in soothing my troubled mind. It is not always time spent examining one's deep motives and buried childhood and teenage experiences or time spent looking critically at one's habitual ways of thinking and interpreting that is the most therapeutic. Small talk enculturates a person back into everyday society, a society one has been divorced from when deluded and helps to rebuild the foundations of one's life. In this vein many chats I had with paraprofessionals and other public servants such as ward domestics, auxiliaries, trainee reflexologists, hairdressers and trainee counsellors had a significant part to play in rebuilding trust, feelings of self-worth and hope for the future. The fostering of hope was especially critical (Nunn 1996).

As part of my recovery I spent 18 months in a psychiatric aftercare hostel in Shepherd's Bush, London. In 1981, after I left, my future wife, Jill, and I moved into a flat. It was like a 'three-quarter way house' for other people we had known to drop in for chats, and visit when they were feeling very distressed. Socializing in this way gave me plenty of opportunity to talk with other patients and with residential social workers about my delusions, delusional perceptions, background and feelings. Sharing talk about such things also gave plenty of opportunities for sharing of insights and therapeutic strategies, reality testing and also for humour. Indeed, it was refreshing and therapeutic to find oneself laughing at experiences previously taken to be so portentous in quality.

My treatment team in hospital in 1979 had been headed by three psychiatrists but, in those days, no psychologists. In recent years, clinical psychologists have, of course, made extensive contributions to the treatment of psychosis (Fowler et al. 1995; Chadwick et al. 1996; Haddock & Slade 1996) and hence now have a significant part to play in such rehabilitation. In my case the actual psychological work was done not with a clinician but with other patients in the aftercare hostel and later at home in a kind of psychological cocounselling role. However, this produced many useful ideas about rehabilitation in psychosis (Chadwick 1992, chapter 12) and also revealed that the delusions many people had were not 'empty speech acts' (Berrios 1991) but intimately related to their personal concerns, life experiences and motives and were hence extremely meaningful. This was also the case in my own crisis (Chadwick 1992). Indeed, in 1979 the persecutors who populated my delusional system were similar in character and in intelligence to those people who had abused me in the past. Thoughts of my 'final punishment', death by crushing under the wheels of a double decker bus, were pretty well in ratio to the hatred that certain people had shown me in my formative years. In many ways my delusions were therefore 'existentially true'.

Robert

Despondence and depression

When I began a job as assistant director of admissions at the college where my father taught, many eyes were on me. For a young man, it was a good appointment. I was looked upon by many people in my small town as bound for success; my bouts with mental illness, to this time, had remained hidden.

About 2 months into the job I was actively having psychotic episodes. I remember I would think I was an angel given the mission to save the college from evil or incompetence of some sort. I could not be sure of reality. More debilitating were the bouts of anxiety that often accompanied delusions. While on my first recruiting trip to South Carolina, I became racked with anxiety. Following desperate telephone conversations with my parents and my psychiatrist, I cut short the recruiting trip and came home on the next available plane. Everyone knew this was the end of my job – and it was – but I could bear the stress no longer. When I returned I was sternly ordered to clear my desk by the next afternoon. Now there was no doubting or hiding that I had a mental illness. I was terribly upset, forlorn. I fell into a dogged depression that lasted for 9 months. In that time I moved to Tucson, Arizona to be with relatives and to find better treatment and a more accurate diagnosis. Although I showed every sign of a schizoaffective disorder, I was diagnosed as manic-depressive, and my treatment would depend upon that diagnosis for the next 12 years.

Recovery by chance

During the decade following the abrupt dismissal from my job with the college admissions department, I found and was fired from several jobs, mostly for behaviour stemming from one type of delusion or another. I frequently had delusions of reference, more occasionally delusions of grandeur (often thinking I was the reincarnation of Jesus Christ), paranoid delusions (thinking the Secret Service was following me), delusions of mission (thinking I was chosen to 'save' the US equestrian team), and occasionally visual hallucinations (seeing tiny spacecraft attacking me). These, in sum, and for that matter individually, made any long-term employment futile. Likewise, I was unable to develop meaningful personal relationships, except one brief affair with a volatile and well-known sculptress which ended when I was emotionally unable to carry it on.

At the inception of being diagnosed as manic-depressive, I was treated with lithium which seemed to do little other than protect me from future depressions. But in 1985 I was started on an anticonvulsant, Tegretol, which had very good results. My moods stabilized significantly and, better still, lost social skills returned, enough so that I attempted running my own business in the equestrian industry. Predictably, the business failed but I gained enough independence to leave my parents' home in Tennessee and move to Chicago.

At first, life in Chicago was difficult. I was unemployed, living in a run-down apartment building. Within a year I relapsed and had two hospitalizations. During the second hospitalization, where the police escorted me to hospital following a terrible psychotic break, the man who became my psychiatrist seemed to have insight into my disorder. He began me on the antipsychotic *tiotixene* that I had given up years before when they first diagnosed me manic-depressive. The combination of the mood stabilizers and the antipsychotic had tremendous efficacy for me. From that hospitalization forward I would begin to embark upon an editing and journalism career, I would become an award winning photographer and mental health advocate, and eventually I would be fully employed by the University of Chicago. I have not been in hospital since.

Grace

For the first 5 years of my 'schizophrenia' and despite five brief hospital admissions, I carried on working in television production. As I was perfectly well in between episodes, I was well able to do my job efficiently although I sometimes had to battle against the side-effects of the drugs.

When I became disillusioned with the content of the programmes I was working on, I left my job and applied to be a nurse. I was accepted, only to be refused after filling in my medical form. Instead, I worked as a home help for a year looking after the elderly. It was humbling after my academic achievements and successful career, but I thoroughly enjoyed it. Suddenly, I had a very bad attack. My thoughts became very confused and I became convinced in my mind that I had to take a lighted light bulb out of its socket. I pressed against the hot glass with all my strength until the bulb came out. For about the third time God saved my life because the bulb should have smashed under the pressure. I had third-degree burns and lost the top of

my index finger, but a skin graft saved the use of my hand. How was it that I, who in between episodes was well and happy, could be persuaded by a deceptive voice to do such a horrendous thing? At such times I had no discernment and it seemed to me that with a child-like trust I followed the voice that was intent on destroying me.

I found understanding through my Christian faith. Although the voice in my head sounded like my own, the source was demonic. I now realize Tai Chi and spiritualism can open us up to evil spirits. I confessed and turned away from what I now know to be ungodly.

I am now able to hear the voice of God in my heart along with thousands of other born-again Holy Spirit-filled Christians. Listening for God's voice is considered a normal part of daily Christian living – the voice of comfort, love and encouragement gently guiding us, which is such a different voice. The Bible says 'For God has not given us a spirit of fear but of power, of love and of a sound mind' (2 Timothy 1 verse 7 NKJV). I recognized in myself areas of pain, which only God has been able to heal through prayer and His healing voice and presence.

I have gained further qualifications and worked as a teacher for the past 8 years and have been in a position of leadership at my church for the past 4 years.

Alison

In spring of 1995, free of medication, I was accepted for a Masters in neuroscience in London. To my delight I found that my brain still worked and I completed the course with Distinction.

When results were announced the whole class went to a pub to celebrate. On the way home I became detached from the group and I was attacked by a man who stuck a knife in my neck and choked me to the point of losing consciousness. He sexually assaulted me, then abducted me and imprisoned me overnight in a room in a house where he did the same again. It felt like when the 'heavy squad' went for me in hospital, so I immediately suspected that he was a psychiatric hit-man.

In the following weeks I was so wound up that I would stay awake for 48 h and felt I was going to explode. I had phoned Dr C. and she suggested I try olanzapine and a psychologist – I thought I had been attacked because I had gone against the system and if I took treatment, then I would be safe. Olanzapine helped at first but several months later I was extremely hot and agitated, with sweat pouring out from me; I thought I was finally going mad, but it turned out to be an overactive thyroid.

In January 1998 I moved to a group home run by a mental health charity. A support worker visited the house a few times a week: we talked and went on outings to parks, cinema, etc. I learned how to dress normally, make small-talk, appreciate popular culture; I have the sneaking feeling that this is superficial and that being normal is a lot of work for little reward – for me at least – but at least I understand normal people better and can put on an act when I have to.

In the year 2000, Dr H. agreed to have me as his patient. I trusted him because he seemed open-minded and promised not to poison me. In April 2000 my thyroid became underactive so I now take thyroxine. In the past year I have moved out of London and into my own flat. Since moving to my own flat, I have managed to stop smoking; I cook proper food instead of ready meals; I have started going to yoga class; I sleep better; I have improved concentration and energy; and I do not have a crisis every other week. I still have slow days, but I think I am on the road to recovery.

Janey

Employment

Until January 1998 I was employed as a research scientist. I had managed to keep working all the way through the early years of being ill but, in the end, because of the pressure of the work, I was having to keep my medication very high to stay well enough. I should say this was not the fault of my colleagues; they were mostly wonderful and very supportive. In the late 1980s though, I was denied the chance to do a PhD and of promotion – specifically because of my health – something I have always regretted.

I had no choice about being 'out' about having schizophrenia in the workplace because I had been ill when I was at work. Some people were very nervous around me but in the end I learned to accept it philosophically. With new young PhD students at work who had come from a fairly sheltered background, I used to take them down the bar and pour a couple of beers into them and then let them ask any questions that they needed to. After that it was usually all right!

Now I work as a freelance training consultant and writer and have travelled around the country talking about my experiences to the police, social services, housing and the prison service. I have found this type of communication really helpful, both for them to learn from me and me from them.

Reflections

Peter

Psychosis is a terrible illness to have and patients should be told from the onset how hard the road to recovery is. A psychotic episode has an incredibly disruptive effect on a sufferer's life, and leaves one disorientated and dilapidated. Changes in a productive direction tend to be slow. But a good 40% in my group did make real progress even if they were not all relapse-free, and I found over the years that the material released to consciousness in the acute stage and later could be understood and used for genuine insight and growth. In this respect the psychotic experience was potentially positive and some of us are now not only well but better than we have ever been.

It has become evident in recent years that delusions and hallucinations are not the only problems that sufferers of psychosis face. They have difficulties with attention, perception, memory and thinking skills (Green 1996; Laws & McKennal 1997; Marland 2000). Outside of cognitive deficits they have prob-

lems with relationships and family, illicit drug use, work or the stresses of unemployment, accommodation, weight and, indeed, problems with their general attitude to life. Psychiatrists and clinical psychologists can no longer assume that the patient is a treatment success if he or she merely is delusion- and hallucination-free (Marland 2000).

Generally, among patients I know, a concatenation of influences came together to determine positive or negative outcome. Factors that many people found a help or a hindrance include: having a supportive social network; structure to one's day and week; and goals to aim for in the form of realistic ambitions, and dreams. Also having a clinician who was optimistic rather than pessimistic about one's chances of getting well again gave a positive ambience to patients' lives.

Reactions to medication and to the concept of illness were very individual. Although I found it extremely helpful to have seen myself as having had an illness and likely to benefit from medication, this was not the case with everybody. Others felt that it helped their self-esteem and motivation to change not to see themselves as having been ill but rather 'in crisis', and still others found medication to be of little help other than as a means of 'flattening' and numbing them against stress, but at the cost of decreased vitality for life. These reactions clearly have to be seen as something real rather than as signs of ignorance or 'lack of insight'. Many idiosyncratic factors also came to light over the years from the boost to self-confidence of a new wardrobe of clothes, or a new hairdo, to the value of the unconditional love of a pet, and the logical reliability of a computer.

Finding a partner or very close friend who was supportive and a good confidante was, not surprisingly, very important indeed. In fact, if one had just one person with whom one could talk about anything and everything, this was a tremendous buffer against stress.

Finding an outlet for creative self-expression (drama group, painting, poetry group, creative writing, etc.) was something many people highly valued, some more so than psychotherapy. The active wish on the part of the person to get better, and not to settle cosily into the mental health subculture of being looked after and state-assisted, was particularly critical.

The spiritual component of some psychoses was something we found that needed to be treated with respect rather than merely as a symptom of basic derangement. Such experiences can, of course, be very profound and moving (Chadwick 1992; Jackson 1997; Clarke 2000).

The two most widespread problems that sufferers I have been in contact with had to deal with were lack of motivation and lack of psychological insight – the latter particularly was the case in those of manic or hypomanic temperaments. Patients should be given an environment where they can fully express themselves. Generally, insight and understanding into the causes and meaning of one's distress did promote positive movement and those who gained more insight with time did seem to do better. My mind was psychologically clearer and less distracted by irrelevancies and overwhelming emotions if I maintained my usual, admittedly low, dosage of medication. I should also say that many insight sessions (with my journal/diary) terminated with me having to take extra medication for a day or two to deal with the terrible stress the insights had provoked. Particularly painful were recollections of the damaging effects of my mother's acrid cynicism about love and about the character of people in general. Also rerunning obnoxious experiences I had had at school and later at the hands of homophobes and transvestophobes helped me to see how I could have come to see myself as possessed by Satan but the experiences in themselves were still terribly distressing.

Over the years, work of this kind was cumulatively helpful. It did not result in my being able to take less medication, or in my becoming drug-free. It did, however, result in more happiness, richer experience, more self-acceptance and more peace of mind.

The motivational problem was eased in some people by their doing courses leading to a qualification. I embarked on a second doctorate, others studied for GCSEs or A levels, with success. These courses gave structure to the week, a goal to aim for, a sense of progression and an opportunity to mix with and bond with people outside the mental health subculture. They also acted as a distraction from mental health problems and induced a degree of mental self-discipline and attention control.

Developments over the past 20 years present a much improved scenario facing psychosis sufferers than the one I and my peers confronted in 1979. Many patients now actively want to be involved in research and in the evaluation of treatments and services (Rogers *et al.* 1993). They are also coming to be respected for the inside knowledge they have of the conditions from which they suffer. In addition, they have their own methods of coping and getting well, which valuably are shared with others (Sutherland 1976; Toates 1990; Jamison 1993, 1996; Mental Health Foundation 1997, 2000). Units are also increasingly hiring staff who have themselves been users in the past to swell the ranks of suffering healers. These initiatives, however, still have a long way to go (Campbell 2000).

Robert

Many patients who go through the mental health system, both in the USA and Britain, feel that they are powerless over an institution that has great control over their lives. In the worst case, this breeds contempt. In more benign cases, this spurs the mental health user to become involved in the system, both as an advocate and as a provider.

At the root of the conflict between users and providers are several conditions. The first is the fact that the treatment of patients is very expensive, so expensive that in the USA, at least, most patients are unable to afford it without some direct assistance by government agencies. A year's supply of medications, for instance, may easily top $8000 in the USA. For a patient disabled by schizophrenia, the private market purchase of services and medications is untenable – they find themselves dependent upon public assistance. However, with public assistance often comes a limitation of options. The patient may be assigned to a doctor, not of their choice, and allowed only a brief periodic visit. Physicians and other service providers, on their part, are loaded down with a great number of cases, more than they can realistically accommodate. Should the patient not like his or her treatment, there is little the patient can do. Subsequently, there is sometimes a feeling of being trapped within the system, or disempowered. Disempowerment is a leading cause of self-stigma.

Another condition ripe for conflict is the practice of involuntary commitment and involuntary outpatient commitment. In most states in the USA, a person may be involuntarily committed to a psychiatric hospital if they are determined to be a threat to themselves or others. There are movements in many states to loosen up these standards to make involuntary commitment easier. Proponents of this view often cite the grave situation of violent tendencies in the mentally ill or of homelessness. Opponents among patients cite involuntary commitment as an equally grave threat to their freedom of movement. Ditto with involuntary outpatient commitment.

There are more agitated patients, who prefer terms such as survivor or ex-patient, who believe the system is designed to muffle, coerce and control. They decry the use of injected tranquillizers, like Haldol or Prolixin, which are employed in some psychiatric hospitals to reduce a patient to a manageable stupor for weeks on end. There is a contingent of ex-patients who condemn the involuntary use of ECT, calling it, and its side-effects, inhumane. The use, or rather misuse, of constraints and isolation is also on their list of appalling practices.

Grace

Some Christian friends and fellow sufferers say they have been helped by drugs, although I personally feel they have often been a hindrance rather than a help. My psychiatrist did allow me once not to take any drugs during one hospitalization and I still came round within 4 days. Whether I was on drugs or had taken myself off drugs I still had psychotic episodes, so it is difficult to prove their usefulness to me.

I have learned a lot through what I have experienced. Contrary to what one might expect, I have grown in confidence because I have had to make a stand for what I believe. My greatest struggle has been with my own family who have found my Christian faith too radical, but have loved me through it all.

After a long search I found Christians who understood there was such a thing as spiritual warfare and supported me in prayer. The self-sacrificial Christ-like love I received through my pastors increased the desire in me to find the unconditional love of God.

There are many people on the wards searching for spiritual truth like myself. I would like doctors and psychiatrists to study the Christian faith ,and indeed other faiths, as part of their training. It was often difficult to find a common frame of reference. What seemed to be very significant spiritual experiences were considered to be 'just part of my illness' by my family, doctors and psychiatrists.

Over the years a mutual respect has developed between my psychiatrist and myself. I believe the Church and the medical profession can and should work together to bring hope and healing to those suffering from mental illness.

Alison

Here are some things I have found most useful for recovery:
• My own living space and financial support in the form of state benefits.
• Attention to medical problems, such as thyroid and sleep disorder; the latter was cured by a lightbox.
• Goals to work for that have personal significance (what I used to call my Mission) – this provides stimulation and motivation.
• A supportive psychiatrist and GP who allow me to be involved in my treatment and in research.
• Internet – I find others who share my experiences, and I can learn about things without having to go out and socialize.
• Friends and family – better than paid support because it is a two-way relationship and is not focused on illness-related topics
• Keeping a journal – to monitor effects of changes, and also to write down thoughts or weigh up pros and cons of things.
• Exercise – yoga, running, cycling, walking.
• Building on my strengths, while accepting differences and limitations, and not trying too hard to fit in or take on too much (imagining I am alien helps me do this but I have learnt that it is best kept to myself and not taken too seriously).
If I build on my strengths I think I can have a good life and eventually earn my own living.

Claire

Having a mental health problem can rule your life and can consume your whole well-being; fighting it is the only way to achieve success. I have met people who have beaten cancer. Beating a mental health problem has to be on a par.

I now make speeches to other mental health charities and educate people about the stigma surrounding mental health. I can now hold down a job, 5 days a week. I can socialize with friends; I can go to the cinema; I cook dinner without it being a task to achieve. I have made television and radio interviews and now live a normal life. People never know I have a mental illness unless I choose to tell them.

I know now I can conquer anything; to me nothing is as bad as a mental health problem.

So is success making money or having the strength to combat such a stigmatized relatively incurable illness?

So the story so far has progressed onto a life of well being and joy, but what will happen next. Will I be able to function without medication? Or is it the medication which is keeping me well? Will I be able to sustain a life of never having to go back into hospital. The questions I have asked are the ones that frighten me every day. Every day is a new start; every day is an achievement.

Janey

Personally, one of the biggest frustrations about having schizophrenia is losing control of one's thoughts. For me, the worse

thing about living with it afterwards is that control then seems to be taken from me by mental health professionals, who make decisions about the way I will live, often without discussing them with me. It is as if I am being perceived by some to be unable to make decisions about what is best for me and when I question a decision that has been made I am not listened to. While I personally can understand this when I have been very psychotic and deluded, I resent it in my day-to-day life. But I am very lucky in that I am both educated and articulate; some people are less able to ask for things or explain how they feel. A friend of mine complained that his medication gave him bad side-effects but was not listened to until he attempted suicide.

That one in 10 people with schizophrenia commit suicide (or die accidentally) is probably the saddest statistic concerned with mental illness. I have lost six friends and have, in the past, been depressed enough about my future and what was happening to me to make several serious attempts to end my life. Most suicide attempts by the mentally ill are during the first week after discharge, which suggests to me that people are taking a look at what is happening to them generally, after leaving psychiatric hospital, and saying 'no thanks'. The negative publicity and stigma surrounding mental illness may add to someone's isolation and make suicide more likely, as can rejection by one's friends and family.

There has been an increasing amount of publicity about the 'failure' of community care, mostly when someone who is ill has been violent. Myths have grown up around this and the degree to which failure to take medication is involved in it. In addition, people with a mental health problem always seem to be labelled collectively as 'the mentally ill' or 'these people', when in reality, like any other group in society, they are all different and include stubborn, nice, nasty, lazy, violent, timid and many other types of people.

I have a neighbour who used to run inside when she saw me but now ignores me. I guess she has read headlines like 'Nutter Kills Stranger', plus she has seen aspects of my personal drama that I have already mentioned, like me being taken to the hospital by the police when I have been very ill. I do not have a problem with her being scared of the unknown. The first time I went into psychiatric hospital I was terrified at what seemed like very strange people around me. But I was living with them so it only took me about 24 h to work out that they were okay really. Later a very good friend of mine told me that the person who scared her the most on her first admission was me.

As I see it, the reality of community care is that it is expensive; schizophrenia is difficult to live with; the medication is not perfect; the media and charities highlight the failures; the professionals get disillusioned with taking the blame; and the users/survivors get shunned by the community!

In the real world, good news does not sell newspapers. However, those with mental health problems having trouble with employment, housing and education could be written up alongside those of suicide and the image of the occasional violence that admittedly does happen. Some of us get by and for some community care is a success; it would be nice for the public to be able to read about this too! The tabloids have no right to be using words like 'nutter' and 'psycho' when they stopped using 'spastic' and 'nigger' years ago.

In the real world of community care, there is a shortage of money and the professionals in the field have to live with this. Therefore, it is unfortunate but not surprising that they attempt not to provide services for those who they regard as not from their 'patch'. It is also human nature to spend time with those who will accept help or who one finds more rewarding. In addition, those looking after someone who kills will receive some of the blame, no matter how hard they tried, which must be heartbreaking if they have made a huge effort.

In the real world, the pharmaceutical companies answer primarily to their Board and the shareholders. This means that the newer medications, which have fewer side-effects, are very expensive and are therefore rationed by most authorities and GP Trusts to a small percentage of the people who could benefit from them. Those who do not receive them have to put up with the older drugs, or just refuse to co-operate. I have learned to compromise with my GP over medication. I do not know what is the right answer for others, although I can see that *both* the good of the individual and that of the community have to be considered.

In the real world, there are a fairly large group of users who claim that psychiatry causes the problem of stigma by the labelling and diagnosis of mental health problems. But there are others who have told me that they have been relieved to know what is wrong with them. This whole labelling issue is a very emotive subject. The sufferer/patient/user/survivor population is a very heterogeneous one. A person who is, say, able to go on the train to the Survivors Speak Out AGM in Birmingham is going to have very different needs to someone who is scared to get on the bus to go to the local drop-in centre. Some people find the whole psychiatric experience something they just do not want, regardless of what others think that they need, while others see hospital as a safe place and it is, for them, part of their community. This means that user involvement in service provision can be difficult unless all the users involved are aware that other users may think differently from them.

Fifteen years on from getting schizophrenia I have sifted through the system and learnt coping skills. I cannot use television and radio as 'white noise' as most people do, nor can I go to loud pubs or nightclubs. I take medication at absolutely the smallest dose I can manage and am now not keen to try new things. I work in a carpentry workshop which also conditions tools for the developing world (a room littered with knives and axes), as well as helping with training when I can. I do not mind one-to-one counselling, hate group therapy and find aromatherapy and transcendental meditation really useful. I have both user and non-user friends and try to influence politicians' and professionals' thinking while keeping an open mind about conflicting user views. It is not a perfect world and it does go horribly wrong but I manage.

References

Bebbington, P.E. & Kuipers, L. (1994) The predictive utility of expressed emotion in schizophrenia: an aggregate analysis. *Psychological Medicine* **24**, 707–718.

Berrios, G. (1991) Delusions as 'wrong beliefs': a conceptual history. *British Journal of Psychiatry* **159**, 6–13.

Campbell, P. (2000) The consumer in mental health care. In: *Mental Health Nursing: an Evidence-based Approach* (ed. R. Newell & K. Gournay), pp. 11–26. Churchill-Livingstone, Edinburgh.

Chadwick, P.D.J., Birchwood, M. & Trower, P. (1996) *Cognitive Therapy for Delusions: Voices and Paranoia*. Wiley, Chichester.

Chadwick, P.K. (1992) *Borderline: a Psychological Study of Paranoia and Delusional Thinking*. Routledge, London and New York.

Chadwick, P.K. (1993) The stepladder to the impossible: a first hand phenomenological account of a schizoaffective psychotic crisis. *Journal of Mental Health* **2**, 239–250.

Chadwick, P.K. (1995) Learning from patients. *Clinical Psychology Forum* **82**, 30–34.

Chadwick, P.K. (1997a) *Schizophrenia: the Positive Perspective. In Search of Dignity for Schizophrenic People*. Routledge, London and New York.

Chadwick, P.K. (1997b) Recovery from psychosis: Learning more from patients. *Journal of Mental Health* **6** (6), 577–588.

Clarke, I. (2000) Psychosis and spirituality: finding a language. *Changes* **18**, 208–214.

Fowler, D., Garety, P. & Kuipers, E. (1995) *Cognitive Behaviour Therapy for Psychosis*. Wiley, Chichester.

Green, M. (1996) What are the functional consequences of neurocognitive deficits in schizophrenia? *American Journal of Psychiatry* **153**, 321–330.

Haddock, G. & Slade, P.D. (1996) *Cognitive–Behavioural Interventions with Psychotic Disorders*. Routledge, London and New York.

Jackson, M. (1997) Benign schizotypy? The case of spiritual experience. In: *Schizotypy: Implications for Illness and Health* (ed. G.S. Claridge), pp. 227–250. Oxford University Press, Oxford.

Jamison, K.R. (1993) *Touched with Fire: Manic-Depressive Illness and the Artistic Temperament*. Free Press, New York.

Jamison, K.R. (1996) *An Unquiet Mind: A Memoir of Moods and Madness*. Picador, London.

Laws, K. & McKennal, J. (1997) Psychotic symptoms and cognitive deficits: what relationship? *Neurocase* **3**, 41–49.

Marland, G. (2000) Cognitive deficits in schizophrenia. *Nursing Times* **96** (16), 43–44.

Mental Health Foundation (1997) *Knowing Our Own Minds*. Mental Health Foundation, London.

Mental Health Foundation (2000) *Strategies for Living*. Mental Health Foundation, London.

Nunn, K.P. (1996) Personal hopefulness: a conceptual review of the relevance of the perceived future to psychiatry. *British Journal of Medical Psychology* **69** (3, September), 227–245.

Rogers, A., Pilgrim, D. & Lacey, R. (1993) *Experiencing Psychiatry: Users' Views of Services*. Macmillan & Mind Publications, London.

Sutherland, N.S. (1976) *Breakdown: A Personal Crisis and a Medical Dilemma*. Weidenfeld & Nicolson, London.

Toates, F. (1990) *Obsessive–Compulsive Disorder: What it is, How to Deal with It*. Thorsons, London.

Vaughn, C.E. & Leff, J.P. (1976) The influence of family and social factors on the course of psychiatric illness: a comparison of schizophrenic and depressed neurotic patients. *British Journal of Psychiatry* **129**, 125–137.

36

Economics of the treatment of schizophrenia

S.M. Essock, L.K. Frisman and N.H. Covell

Economics of mental health and schizophrenia, 713
  Costs of schizophrenia, 713
  Cost perspective, 714
  Cost components, 714
Cost-effectiveness, 715
Cost of the newer antipsychotic medications, 717
  Clozapine cost-effectiveness studies as case
    examples, 717

Costs associated with risperidone, olanzapine and
  quetiapine, 719
Conclusions and additional resources, 719
Acknowledgements, 721
References, 721

Economics of mental health and schizophrenia

Until recently, the economics of mental illness were little understood. For most of the last century, economists paid scant attention to schizophrenia, or indeed to mental health in general (McGuire 1990). Yet today, with new and expensive medications arriving on the market, and conventional treatments under pressure to meet financial strictures, economic considerations in mental health policy are growing ever more important. This chapter focuses on two aspects of the economics of schizophrenia: the costs of the mental illness and the cost-effectiveness of treatment modalities.

Studies of the cost of mental illnesses appeared before other types of work in the economics of mental health. Early work in the 1980s considered the impact of organization and financing on system efficiency and addressed the supply of personnel in caring for persons with mental illness. One study reviewed the market for psychotherapy and the insurability of mental health care (McGuire 1981), and another examined the supply of psychiatrists (Frank 1983). The impact of cost sharing on demand for mental health care was analysed by researchers at the RAND corporation (RAND) (Manning *et al.* 1984). The use of diagnosis-related groupings to pay for care under prospective payment was considered (Taube *et al.* 1984). The impact of various funding mechanisms in public mental health was reviewed by Dickey and Goldman (1986).

More recently, economic analyses have contributed to a range of activities in the field of mental health economics, including the economics of schizophrenia. During the 1990s, studies continued with work on insurance, regulation and the organization of mental health services. Examination of insurance mandates for mental health care, such as simulation of mandates and related costs, provided valuable information to legislators in the USA considering such laws (Frank *et al.* 1991). Advocates for systems change considered major reorganizational efforts, such as those implemented through the Robert Wood Johnson Program on Chronic Mental Illness and other types of organizational reforms (Goldman *et al.* 1994, 1995; McGuire *et al.* 1995; Semke *et al.* 1995; Shepherd *et al.* 1996). The 1990s also brought analysis of the increasing implementation of managed care with behavioural health carve-outs (Mechanic 1998).

Cost studies lay the foundation for cost-effectiveness and cost–benefit studies because they identify the range of resources that are consumed as a result of an illness. Cost-effectiveness analyses of mental health programmes began to appear in the early 1980s with a hallmark study on the cost–benefit of assertive community treatment teams (Weisbrod *et al.* 1980). Together, studies of costs and cost-effectiveness are perhaps the most important measures of the economics of schizophrenia. First, the sizeable cost to society captures the attention of policymakers and taxpayers, and convinces them of the huge fiscal impact of schizophrenia. Secondly, decisions by clinicians, managers and policymakers that are informed by research on costs and cost-effectiveness lead to better distribution of the resources available for mental health care.

Costs of schizophrenia

Early studies of the costs of mental illness (Cruze *et al.* 1981; Harwood *et al.* 1984; Rice *et al.* 1990) did not distinguish between the costs of different diagnostic categories (McGuire 1991). Samples that were examined included bipolar disorder and major depression as well as schizophrenia. More recent studies have estimated specific costs for schizophrenia and other illnesses. Rice estimated the cost of schizophrenia in the USA at $32.5 billion in 1990 (Rice 1999a) and $44.9 billion in 1994 (Rice 1999b). In Canada, costs in 1996 were calculated to be approximately $2.35 billion (Goeree *et al.* 1999), while costs of schizophrenia in the UK were estimated to be £2.6 billion (Knapp 1997). Some schizophrenia cost studies focus only on service costs, such as Rund and Ruud's (1999) study of costs in Norway and Martin and Miller's (1998) study of Medicaid recipients in Georgia. In contrast, Rice's and Knapp's studies included both direct costs, such as treatment and other service costs, and indirect costs, such as lost income. However, no study of the cost of schizophrenia can claim to capture all costs. As noted by McGuire (1991), even comprehensive studies of the cost of schizophrenia often underestimate two types of costs: the costs to families and the costs of publicly owned capital.

Cost perspective

Cost-effectiveness and cost–benefit analysis should always state the perspective from which the study is undertaken. Cost-of-illness studies like Rice's and Knapp's, which consider economic costs, typically reflect the perspective of society in general (Knapp 1997; Rice 1999a,b). Economic, or social, costs are the costs of resources consumed because of an illness. Although a societal perspective presumably provides the balanced view of a neutral scientist, it is also helpful to examine costs from perspectives of particular stakeholders. In an analysis of the impact of Assertive Community Treatment in Connecticut, Essock *et al.* (1998) presented costs from the perspectives of society, the state and the Department of Mental Health. Comparison of the results from multiple perspectives may identify areas of cost-shifting that result from certain programmes and policies. For example, a treatment that reduces hospital days may shift costs from state-run inpatient facilities to private non-profit outpatient settings. These shifts in cost may mean that changes within treatment systems that are beneficial to patients and revenue-neutral from a societal perspective may still be more expensive from the vantage point of particular stakeholders. By identifying such stakeholders, policy-makers can identify important potential sticking points to implementing system changes and intervene (e.g. by creating fiscal incentives for the stakeholders who would otherwise be fiscal losers to co-operate).

Cost components

Costs of treatment and other services

The examples provided by Rice and Knapp are instructive for those conducting cost-of-illness studies and cost-effectiveness studies in the area of schizophrenia. They show that there are many ways in which the illness is associated with costs greater than those found with other illnesses. First are the costs of treatment, including medication. Treatment may be offered by public, private or voluntary sector settings, and many persons with schizophrenia receive care in multiple places. Besides treatment, services such as case management, vocational rehabilitation and psychosocial clubhouses generate significant costs. Medical and surgical costs also may be relevant in cost-effectiveness analyses, because utilization of these services may vary depending on the adequacy of mental health care (Mumford & Schlesinger 1987; Pallack & Cummings 1992).

Lost productivity and family burden

Mental illnesses, like other disorders, cause people to lose work days (Kessler & Frank 1997) and sometimes even to forfeit aspirations of having any career at all. Comprehensive studies of the costs of schizophrenia may address lost productivity, but because of the high rates of disability in this population many studies of interventions for persons with schizophrenia ignore productivity losses. However, new strategies for improving the employment outcomes for persons with serious mental illness, such as Individual Placement and Support (Drake *et al.* 1996), have made employment a realistic goal of rehabilitation. These new successes suggest that loss of productivity should be included when calculating the cost of interventions for persons with schizophrenia. In addition to the productivity losses of the individuals affected, cost studies should attend to the work losses of family members and others who contribute time and in-kind services (Clark 1994).

Capital costs

Economic cost studies appropriately study the opportunity costs of all resources, i.e. the value of resources in their best alternative use. In a cost-effectiveness study of a new residential model for persons with serious mental illness, Cannon *et al.* (1985) carefully considered the value of capital costs of a public hospital, which would have been underestimated if valued through traditional methods of depreciation. Capital costs can be large enough to change the most basic findings of a cost study, as shown by Rosenheck *et al.* (1994). Public administrators may not consider the value of buildings and property to be part of a cost equation because they are not always part of the operating costs, but the value of the property in alternative use may be considerable. For example, in the USA, for the past 20 years states have decreased their reliance on large state hospitals, leaving them with many-acre campuses, many of which are located in areas where the market rate for land is very high.

Other components

It is important to attend to criminal justice costs, especially when an intervention is expected to have an impact on co-occurring substance use disorders (Clark *et al.* 1999). Another neglected aspect of cost studies is the cost of administering transfer payments (such as social security). Although disability payments themselves do not represent the use of new resources, the cost of administering these payments should be counted, especially if the intervention could change the rate of receipt of disability payments or other public benefits (Frisman & Rosenheck 1996). An intervention that returns people to work will not only increase their productivity (a benefit), but also decrease disability payments (decrease a cost).

Whether a particular cost is included in a cost-effectiveness study is related to the potential impact of that type of cost on the study findings. The larger the cost per unit, or the more frequently it is used, the more carefully it should be assessed (Hargreaves *et al.* 1998). But should cost-effectiveness analyses always be conducted? Because of the wide range of costs and cost perspectives that might be included, these studies can be expensive to implement. This expense is further increased because, in order to be able to detect significant differences, a highly variable outcome such as cost may require many more study participants than would be needed for an effectiveness study alone. The usefulness of a cost study depends in large part on the likelihood that the treatment or intervention under study will have an effect on costs – either positive or negative. Cost studies are critical in the analysis of second-generation antipsychotic agents because of the relatively high purchase price of the drugs compared with first-generation (conventional) antipsychotic medications, and because of the potential that these drugs can reduce the number of days that people with schizophrenia are hospitalized (Byrom et al. 1998).

Cost-effectiveness

The success of interventions in schizophrenia, whether medications or psychosocial rehabilitation programmes, is reflected in multiple domains. An antipsychotic medication may have an impact on cognition, hallucinations, affect, disruptiveness, sexual functioning, extrapyramidal side-effects (EPS), weight and employment – the list goes on and on. Some of the measures of the effectiveness of the agent may be positive and some may be negative. Some domains, such as hallucinations and delusions, may be influenced much more directly by the medication than more distal outcomes, such as housing or employment. Different individuals value changes in the domains differently, e.g. eliminating voices that other people do not hear may be much more important to the person troubled by harassing voices than to the person whose voices are good company or connect him or her to an imagined network of internationally renowned researchers. Similarly, some people are very troubled by changes in weight or sexual functioning, while such changes may mean little to others.

Hence, much as we would like a composite measure across all effectiveness domains, this reductionistic approach is fraught with untenable compromises. Just as there is variation among different patients, so providers and payers may ascribe different values to the same outcome. Legislators who make funding allocations to public mental health systems may be more concerned about decreases in violence, while patients may be more concerned with increases in quality of life. How much is a symptom-free day worth? It depends on who is asking and who is paying.

Cost-effectiveness analyses have evolved to deal with the multiple domains touched by a single treatment. Such analyses report the change in a given effectiveness measure associated with a particular cost investment in treatment. A medication may be cost-effective with respect to certain outcomes, cost neutral for others and costly for yet others. Lehman (1999) reminds us that the current explosion of new knowledge about effective treatments and the advent of evidence-based quality standards for treating schizophrenia come at a time when cost containment is paramount on the health policy agenda. Policy-makers need to know the impact of dollars invested in treatment – but not just in a single domain such as reductions in hospital care. Those who make purchasing decisions for the public systems of care, which fund most treatment for schizophrenia, need information on multiple domains of effectiveness.

An alternative to cost-effectiveness analysis is cost–utility analysis, which calculates a comprehensive outcome indicator as a preference-weighted sum of the outcome measures. This tool is useful in cases as noted above, where different stakeholder groups value outcomes differently. An example of a cost–utility approach is the use of Quality-Adjusted Life Years (QALYs) (Gold et al. 1996; Drummond et al. 1997). This approach creates an effectiveness metric representative of one stakeholder group; at worst, the resulting metric is representative of no one. Although a QALY representation of different stakeholder groups is elegant, making it is like creating sausages – observing their manufacture may reduce enthusiasm for their use. One must find or create weights to apply to the various effectiveness measures and then choose a combination scheme, deciding, for example, what weight gain is the equivalent of what change in EPS and what change in psychotic symptoms. Typically, one does this either by interviewing individuals representative of the population under study (e.g. treatment-refractory patients with schizophrenia) or by adopting someone else's measures as 'close enough'. Because 'close enough' is a very subjective call, it is important for researchers to disclose the sources of the weighting estimates so that readers can make their own call. For example, in their report of changes in QALYs among mostly male veterans with schizophrenia, Rosenheck et al. (1999) used weights derived as part of a doctoral dissertation where the sample was mainly African American women (Kleinman 1995). Only about half of these women (55%) were diagnosed with schizophrenia, and the rest were diagnosed with major depression, bipolar and other affective disorders. The authors of this chapter are unwilling to take the leap of faith needed to generalize from groups this disparate when presenting cost-effectiveness results from our own work (Essock et al. 2000). Nevertheless, Rosenheck and colleagues are to be commended for providing the information necessary to follow back their methods to see what was used. This is not always the case.

Another type of utility analysis compares interventions with respect to the number of symptom-free days they produce. One such analysis followed the methodology of Lave et al. (1998) and credited a study participant with having 1 depression-free day if the study participant had 2 days with a depression score of 0.5 (Simon et al. 2000). Many people with depression, as well as many researchers, would take issue with saying that someone was symptom-free for half a year if they reported having 50% of full symptoms for each day of that year. Symptom-free days may be a poor measure within schizophrenia studies simply because, unlike depression, symptoms and functioning in schizophrenia are poorly correlated, and the likelihood of someone with schizophrenia having a completely symptom-free day may be small.

In a population where individuals may live for a long period of time with a relatively debilitating illness like schizophrenia, measures of mortality alone do not adequately capture the impact of the disability. Disability-Adjusted Life Years (DALYs) can be used to express years lost either to premature death or to disabilities associated with living with schizophrenia (Shore 1999). In contrast to QALYs, which estimate symptom-free days, 1 DALY equals 1 lost year of healthy life. DALYs are proxies for negative outcomes (Murray & Lopez 1997), and thus the calculation of cost-effectiveness centres on how many DALYs are saved by using a particular intervention. DALYs are calculated by adding together the number of years between mortality and life expectancy (years of life lost, YLL) and the number of years lived with a disability (YLDs).

Calculating YLDs requires making assumptions about the relative impact of illness onset, duration and severity on healthy living (e.g. making an assumption that a first psychotic episode at age 15 is worse than a first episode at age 25). As with QALYs, these metrics can be derived by surveying individuals with schizophrenia or their proxies, with the accompanying assumptions that how one weights hypothetical events is the same as the trade-offs one would make if one could trade fewer days of healthy life for more days of life with particular disabilities. Because such ratings are inherently untestable by rigorous methods, whether reliable or not, their validity remains suspect. Further, the calculation of DALYs 'presupposes that life years of disabled people are worth less than life years of people without disabilities' (Arneson & Nord 1999), and may even rank some individuals' lives as worse than death (Rock 2000). Schizophrenia does bring with it an increased risk of suicide (Radomsky *et al.* 1999), which is consistent with DALYs ranking some lives as worse than death. However, to assume that person A and person B would in fact make the same choices regarding what fates are worse than death presumes an ecological validity to DALY ratings that may be unwarranted.

Cost utility measures, such as QALYs, DALYs and measures like symptom-free days, have enormous appeal because of their ability to reduce multiple effectiveness domains to a single bullet measure. By deriving a single measure, one can compare any treatment approach to any other treatment approach. Where the measure is reduced to dollars (as in QALYs), one may even compare the values of interventions between different conditions, such as whether dollars expended on diabetes reap more benefits than dollars spent on schizophrenia (Drummond *et al.* 1997). However, the assumptions built into such bullet measures may have limited usefulness for informing decisions at the level of the individual patient, prescriber or health care payer. These individuals weigh their particular circumstances, and may be unwilling to have others' preferences serve as proxies for their own. Instead, these stakeholders ask more specific questions. The mental health commissioner may ask, 'If I put an extra three million dollars in the pharmacy budget for medication X, what can I expect this to buy me in terms of other programme costs? What is the downside risk? What will it buy me in terms of reductions in hospital use, improvements in vocational functioning, reductions in violent episodes and reductions in side-effects?' Similarly, patients and families paying for medica-

tions ask, 'If I increase or decrease my spending by changing to medication X, what changes may I realize in the voices I hear, in my employability, in my sexual functioning and in my body movements?' An alternative to composite measures is measures that contrast invested costs to a variety of outcome domains that are more important to some stakeholders than others. An analogy is a proposal for a city park to be funded from multiple sources. The park may or may not be a good idea depending on your perspective – whether you would use the park, and how the park would impact on the value of your property, your safety, your recreational options or what you are called on to invest. Depending on who is paying for what, and which outcome domains are most important to you, you will stand to get a lot or a little out of your dollars that pay for the park. The challenge in funding the park is to present the data on costs and effects in such a way that the various payers (the city, private foundations, neighbourhood organizations, individual contributors) can look from their different perspectives and identify the expected gains and losses in the outcome domains that are relevant to them. Each stakeholder can weigh factors such as less street noise, more open space, more dogs and more people drawn to the neighbourhood, and decide whether to support the park.

In contrast to cost–utility analysis, cost-effectiveness analysis does not reduce the impact of an intervention to one measure. Some outcomes, such as lower costs and higher effectiveness, may be clearly preferred or 'dominant choices'. Other outcomes, such as higher costs and higher effectiveness, are not as clearly dominant. In these cases, it may be useful to show the likely range of cost compared with multiple domains of effectiveness. One method of examining these ranges is to create sampling distributions for costs and effectiveness measures that show the precision of estimates as well as their mean. Bootstrap techniques, for example, create an empirical sampling distribution for every study participant's test data, using incremental cost-effectiveness ratios (ICERs) calculated by dividing the difference in cost (clozapine – usual care) by the difference in effectiveness (clozapine – usual care). We used 10 000 bootstrap replications to calculate the numerator and denominator of the ICER, and each of the 10 000 bootstrap replications was plotted as a point on the cost-effectiveness plane (Fig. 36.1). Cost data are often highly positively skewed, and ICERs can be used to provide less biased estimates of confidence intervals (Black 1990; Pollack *et al.* 1994; Chaudhary & Stearns 1996; Briggs & Fenn 1998; Lave *et al.* 1998).

Figure 36.1 shows the cost-effectiveness of clozapine compared with first-generation antipsychotic medications among long-stay state hospital patients (Essock *et al.* 2000). The cluster of points displays the sampling distribution of ICERs. Most of the points fall in the lower right quadrant, indicating that clozapine is most likely to be less costly and more effective than first-generation antipsychotic agents from the cost perspective (total societal cost) and for the effectiveness measure in question (reduction in EPS). Such displays of information give the reader/policymaker two important pieces of information at a glance:

1 a sense of the precision of the point estimate (a large cloud

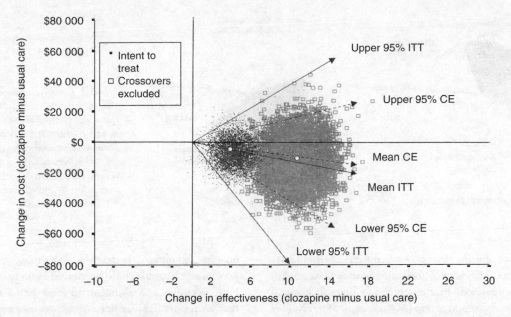

Fig 36.1 Cost-effectiveness plane: number of extrapyramidal side-effect (EPS)-free months. Difference in effectiveness (x-axis) compared with difference in cost (y-axis) for 10 000 bootstrap replications plotted in the cost-effectiveness plane. The x and y axes, respectively, show the difference between clozapine and usual-care groups in estimated number of EPS-free months and total cost during a 2-year period, with $n = 136$ clozapine, intent-to-treat (ITT), and $n = 87$ usual care, ITT, and with $n = 89$ clozapine, treatment crossovers excluded (CE) and $n = 30$

usual care, CE. The quadrant to the lower right of the origin (0,0) contains those estimates where clozapine was found to be less costly and more effective than usual care (80% of the estimates for the ITT analyses and 81% of the estimates when treatment crossovers are excluded). The cluster of points displays the sampling distribution of the incremental cost-effectiveness ratio (ICER). (Essock *et al.* 2000; used with permission of the American Medical Association, © 2000.)

around the central point indicates great variability in the estimate whereas a compact cloud means that the central point is a good estimate of what they might expect to see); and

2 the risk of falling into a quadrant other than the one indicating the intervention is dominant (less costly and more effective); the more points outside of the lower right quadrant, the more likely the intervention will be less effective or will be more costly in addition to being more effective.

It is incumbent on mental health services researchers to report their findings in ways that speak to funders and service system managers by providing estimates of the most likely outcome, as well as the likelihood of alternative outcomes. Saul Feldman, formerly head of the National Institute of Mental Health Staff College and chief executive officer of one of the largest managed behavioural health care organizations in the USA, has been in a position to make policy based on research, and to inform policy-makers with research. He poses the question, 'Is good research good if it does not inform policy and practice?' (Feldman 1999).

Cost of the newer antipsychotic medications

In general, the purchase price of the newer antipsychotic medications is greater than that of first-generation ones. These costs are reflected in formulary budgets. Once a relatively small component of treatment costs, formulary budgets in psychiatric settings have risen dramatically in the past decade, and the market

share of the newer agents has risen as they have replaced the less costly first-generation antipsychotic medications. Figure 36.2 shows the distribution of antipsychotic prescriptions paid for by Medicaid in 1998 (left) and the dollars that Medicaid paid for these prescriptions (right). These data show that the newer agents account for 58% of all antipsychotic prescriptions paid for by Medicaid, but they represent 90% of the $1.28 billion in Medicaid costs for antipsychotic prescriptions. These charts dramatically display the disparity in medication costs associated with the first- vs. second-generation agents.

In the USA, the price difference between the first- and second-generation antipsychotic medications can be 100-fold as, for example, when contrasting generic oral haloperidol with brand-name clozapine. This large price differential has prompted scores of studies that consider more than simply the cost of the medication when determining the cost impact of using the newer medications. For example, let us say that using new and expensive medication X results in fewer days hospitalized than a lower cost alternative. Using X will reduce overall costs as long as the cost savings associated with fewer days in the hospital are greater than the cost difference between medication X and the alternative – all else being equal.

Clozapine cost-effectiveness studies as case examples

The rub, of course, is that 'all else' is rarely equal in effectiveness or cost-effectiveness studies, and the early cost projections con-

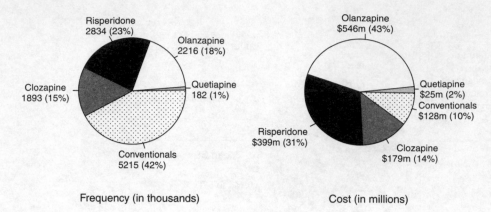

Fig 36.2 Antipsychotic prescriptions: 1998, United States Medicaid. Distribution of frequency prescribed (left circle) and total dollars paid (right circle) by Medicaid for antipsychotic medication prescriptions during 1998. Newer antipsychotic medications represented slightly over half of the total prescriptions and were responsible for 90% of the total cost.

cerning the impact of using clozapine often suffered from faulty assumptions about what was equivalent. Many of these studies were prepost comparisons that examined changes in hospital use but lacked a comparison group (Meltzer *et al.* 1993; Reid *et al.* 1994; Jonsson & Walinder 1995; Aitchison & Kerwin 1997; Blieden *et al.* 1998; Ghaemi *et al.* 1998; Luchins *et al.* 1998). The study by Meltzer *et al.* (1993) collected retrospective cost data for 2 years before and after 47 individuals began taking clozapine, and they concluded that clozapine was associated with a 23% drop in treatment costs. This conclusion generated a series of letters criticizing the study's methodology (Essock 1995; Rosenheck *et al.* 1995; Schiller & Hargreaves 1995; response by Meltzer & Cola 1995). Critics focused on the problem of regression toward the mean that can be expected whenever study participants are enrolled during a low point in their functioning (such as may have prompted the initiation of clozapine). They also noted that, unless there is random assignment to treatment conditions, studies comparing individuals who were and were not selected to begin a new medication are also open to case-mix confounds (differences in the characteristics of people who were and were not selected to receive the new medication).

Two randomized clinical trials of the cost-effectiveness of clozapine each showed much more modest benefits associated with clozapine than predicted by the mirror-image analyses. The first study was a 2-year open-label trial comparing clozapine to the usual care with a range of first-generation antipsychotics among long-term patients in state hospitals (Essock *et al.* 1996a,b, 2000). The second study was a 1-year, masked (blinded) trial comparing clozapine to haloperidol among veterans hospitalized for a year or less (Rosenheck *et al.* 1997). Each trial showed clozapine to be somewhat more effective than the comparison agents, and this increase in effectiveness came at no additional cost when costs were viewed from a societal perspective. Each study also showed that clozapine was more effective than usual care in minimizing days hospitalized, enough so that the reduction in hospital days more than covered the increased cost of the medication plus increased outpatient services.

If cost-effectiveness studies are to influence planning and policy-making, the perspectives of different payers need to be taken into account. From more narrow perspectives, such as the

hospital formulary budget or capitated outpatient service providers, clozapine could be viewed as increasing costs. These local incentives and disincentives must be addressed to be sure that fiscal incentives are lined up to promote good care. If a hospital has a fixed budget (the case with many state hospitals), it would have a great incentive to use clozapine for a heavy user of hospital services, but a hospital that is paid per diem would have no such incentive.

Lengthy randomized clinical trials in routine practice settings, such as the clozapine studies in Connecticut state hospitals and in Department of Veterans Affairs (VA) hospitals, suffer from treatment crossovers. By the end of 6 months in the Connecticut study, only 11% of the usual care patients had begun a trial on clozapine, but by the end of 24 months 66% had begun such a trial. In the VA clozapine study, 72% of the patients assigned to masked haloperidol had ceased taking that medication by the end of the 1-year study period, with 31% (49 of 157) switching to clozapine and the rest to first-generation antipsychotics, including unmasked haloperidol (Rosenheck *et al.* 1997). Because of the biases introduced by what is likely to be highly nonrandom discontinuation of the assigned treatment, the importance of intent-to-treat analyses, and the hazards of unspecified biases in crossover-excluded analyses, are well documented (Lavori 1992).

When crossovers are common, analyses excluding crossovers may offer a proxy for the best case scenarios for each treatment condition by comparing only those who do well enough on treatment A to stay on it with only those who do well enough on treatment B to stay on it. Figure 36.1 illustrates such an analysis using data from the Connecticut clozapine study. The exclusion of treatment crossovers increases the apparent effectiveness of clozapine because the crossovers-excluded cluster is shifted to the right of the intent-to-treat cluster in Fig. 36.1. Relative to the intent-to-treat analysis, the crossovers-excluded analysis has decreased the estimate of the relative costliness of clozapine because the crossover-excluded cluster is shifted lower by about $5500 (Essock *et al.* 2000). Clearly, individuals who leave their assigned treatment are different in terms of costs and outcomes from those who remain in their assigned treatment condition.

Another difficulty when trying to assess relative costs is the great variability in costs across patients. For example, in the VA study just cited, health care costs in the 6 months prior to randomization were approximately $27 000 with a standard deviation of about $17 000 (Rosenheck *et al.* 1997). For the Connecticut clozapine study, the 95% confidence interval for patients assigned to clozapine was $96 847–114 308 for year 2, vs. $103 665–121 144 for those assigned to usual care. With such variability, cost differences are very difficult to detect, even with the relatively large sample sizes of the VA and Connecticut trials (*n* = 423 and 227 respectively). Even for individuals who are heavy service users at study entry, mounting a trial powered to detect cost differences requires hundreds of individuals per treatment arm. If the trial were a study of outpatients who are infrequent users of expensive services like hospitals, it would require even larger samples to detect cost differences apart from medication.

From a public health perspective, an emphasis on point estimates of costs and effectiveness is misguided when the confidence intervals are so broad. Economists would call clozapine the dominant alternative in these randomized trials because most of the range spanned by the cost confidence intervals includes the values where clozapine costs less than or the same as usual care, and the effectiveness measures favour clozapine or are neutral. The reduction of data to such a point estimate belies the broad distribution of possible outcomes that are likely to occur across patients. Planners and policy-makers, as well as patients and their treating clinicians, need a sense of the range of possible outcomes, as well as the relative likelihood of these outcomes, to inform their decisions about what chances they want to take.

Costs associated with risperidone, olanzapine and quetiapine

Figure 36.3 shows the frequency of prescribing by type of antipsychotic in three large states in different parts of the USA among individuals whose medications are paid via Medicaid. Because Medicaid formularies allow unrestricted access to any of these medications, independent of location in the country, and because the same financial incentives apply, one would expect to see similar rates of prescribing these medications. Indeed, the distributions do appear quite similar to each other and to the national data (Fig. 36.2). That these distributions do not reflect what we know about the relative effectiveness of these agents suggests that other factors are strong influences on medication choice and that these influences combine to create similar patterns of antipsychotic prescribing under Medicaid nationwide. In addition to effectiveness, factors as disparate as patients' past histories of medication use, order of receiving Food and Drug Administration (FDA) approval, convenience of use, purchase price, relative marketing budgets, and side-effect profiles may be at play. These Figures serve as reminders that medications are started and discontinued for reasons other than effectiveness. (Data for these pie charts were extracted from the Health Care Financing Administration (HCFA)

website at http://medicare.hcfa.gov/medicaid/drug5.htm; as of March 2000, the website reports Medicaid expenditures in cents rather than dollars and does not label the cost units.)

Several studies of risperidone and olanzapine also suggest that the purchase prices of these medications may be offset by the reduction in use of more expensive health care services such as inpatient treatment. Many of these studies have methodological shortcomings similar to those of the earlier cost studies of clozapine described above. Another concern is that, because of industry sponsorship of many of these studies, they do not meet the criteria of lack of an incentive for bias set forth by the *New England Journal of Medicine* (Kassiter & Angell 1994). The editors of that journal noted that opportunities for introducing bias into economic studies are far greater than in studies of biological phenomena. The unusually discretionary nature of model building and data selection in such analyses allow the introduction of bias, and drug costs in particular can be quite arbitrary because they are prices (not costs) set by the manufacturer. Hence, additional work is needed in this area.

In general, studies by pharmaceutical companies show support for cost reductions favouring that manufacturer's medication, such as risperidone (Nightengale *et al.* 1998) or olanzapine (Hamilton *et al.* 1999; Tunis *et al.* 1999). Although such studies may form useful starting points for further investigation, they need follow-up by independent investigators to assess how the agents' cost-effectiveness plays out in broader settings with representative patients. Otherwise, best-case examples might be generalized to settings where they are not applicable and used to set policy there. For example, an important follow-up study found that, among 84 treatment-refractory patients randomly assigned to a double-blind 8-week fixed dose trial of either olanzapine or chlorpromazine, olanzapine appeared to have limited efficacy, showing only a 7% response (Conley *et al.* 1998). Hence, the reduction in treatment costs associated with olanzapine noted in the reviews of Palmer *et al.* (1998) and Foster and Goa (1999) would not be expected among treatment-refractory patients, even though these patients are heavy users of inpatient services. Under other scenarios, these patients are the very ones for whom new interventions produce cost savings because their higher initial rates of utilization allow the potential to show greater savings (Essock *et al.* 1998; Rosenheck *et al.* 1999). An independent study among outpatients with schizophrenia, using a matched comparison group, compared risperidone with first-generation antipsychotics and found no difference in total treatment costs or effectiveness measures. There was a trend for the risperidone-treated group to have higher costs, attributable to higher medication costs (Schiller *et al.* 1999).

Conclusions and additional resources

The economics of the treatment of mental illness introduces methodological complexities not always present when considering the economics of other medical conditions. We have illustrated the importance of estimating and eliminating bias when

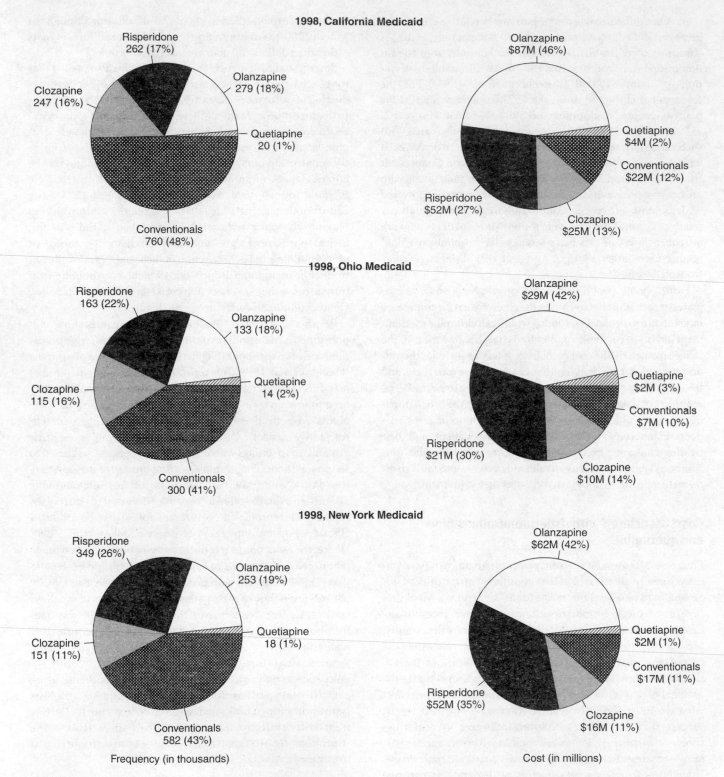

1998, California Medicaid

Risperidone 262 (17%)
Clozapine 247 (16%)
Olanzapine 279 (18%)
Quetiapine 20 (1%)
Conventionals 760 (48%)

Olanzapine $87M (46%)
Quetiapine $4M (2%)
Conventionals $22M (12%)
Risperidone $52M (27%)
Clozapine $25M (13%)

1998, Ohio Medicaid

Risperidone 163 (22%)
Olanzapine 133 (18%)
Clozapine 115 (16%)
Quetiapine 14 (2%)
Conventionals 300 (41%)

Olanzapine $29M (42%)
Quetiapine $2M (3%)
Conventionals $7M (10%)
Risperidone $21M (30%)
Clozapine $10M (14%)

1998, New York Medicaid

Risperidone 349 (26%)
Olanzapine 253 (19%)
Clozapine 151 (11%)
Quetiapine 18 (1%)
Conventionals 582 (43%)
Frequency (in thousands)

Olanzapine $62M (42%)
Quetiapine $2M (1%)
Conventionals $17M (11%)
Risperidone $52M (35%)
Clozapine $16M (11%)
Cost (in millions)

Fig 36.3 Antipsychotic prescriptions. Distribution of frequency prescribed (left circles) and total dollars paid (right circles) by Medicaid for antipsychotic medication prescriptions in California, Ohio and New York during 1998.

constructing studies and reporting results. We especially stress the importance of reporting results from the perspective of different payers and have described how to estimate the variability of any findings when reporting them as point estimates. These

factors should be acknowledged and accounted for when addressing treatment costs for schizophrenia. It is important to tell patients, prescribers and payers not just the best estimate of costs and effectiveness, but the likelihood that their costs and outcomes will fall within the acceptable ranges of what they are willing to pay or risk to achieve a given outcome.

Fortunately, the literature of the economics of schizophrenia is currently evolving. Many active champions in this field now publish widely and lead the way in documenting how fiscal incentives and disincentives, as well as overall societal costs, impact access to treatment, quality of care received and patient outcomes. Although all of this work cannot be summarized here, useful sourcebooks include those by Drummond *et al.* (1997), Frank and Manning (1992), Gold *et al.* (1996) and Hargreaves *et al.* (1998). The journal *Health Affairs* continues to be a particularly valuable resource for reports on mental health economics, and contains thoughtful analyses of economic influences on the treatment of individuals with schizophrenia.

Acknowledgements

The material in this chapter is based on a chapter in *Neuropsychopharmacology: The Fifth Generation of Progress*, 2002, edited by Kenneth L. Davis, Dennis Charney, Joseph T. Coyle and Charles Nemeroff, American College of Neuropsychopharmacology, Lipincott, Williams and Wilkins. This research is the product of the collaboration of many individuals, both within and outside the Connecticut Department of Mental Health and Addiction Services (DMHAS). In particular, we would like to thank Carlos Jackson, PhD, for his assistance with the data extraction and statistical analyses of the Medicaid prescription data and Linda Dunakin and Sally Clay for helpful comments on the manuscript. The research was funded in part by USPHS Grants R01 MH-48830 and R01 MH-52872 from the National Institute of Mental Health (NIMH) to Susan Essock, Principal Investigator, as well as by DMHAS. This publication does not express the views of the Department of Mental Health and Addiction Services or the State of Connecticut. The views and opinions expressed are those of the authors.

References

Aitchison, K.J. & Kerwin, R.W. (1997) Cost-effectiveness of clozapine: a UK clinic-based study. *British Journal of Psychiatry* 171, 125–130.

Arneson, T. & Nord, E. (1999) The value of DALY life: problems with ethics and validity of disability adjusted life years. *British Medical Journal* 319, 1423–1425.

Black, W.C. (1990) The CE plane: a graphic representation of cost-effectiveness. *Medical Decision Making* 10, 212–214.

Blieden, N., Flinders, S., Hawkins, K. *et al.* (1998) Health status and health care costs for publicly funded patients with schizophrenia started on clozapine. *Psychiatric Services* 49, 1590–1593.

Briggs, A. & Fenn, P. (1998) Confidence intervals or surfaces? Uncertainty on the cost-effectiveness plane. *Health Economics* 7, 723–740.

Byrom, B.D., Garratt, C.J. & Kilpatrick, A.T. (1998) Influence of antipsychotic profile on cost of treatment in schizophrenia: a decision analysis approach. *International Journal of Psychiatry in Clinical Practice* 2, 129–138.

Cannon, N.C., McGuire, T.G. & Dickey, B. (1985) Capital costs in economic program evaluation: the case of mental health services. In: *Economic Evaluation of Public Programs New Direction for Program Evaluation*, Vol. 26 (ed. J. Catterall), pp. 69–82. Jossey-Bass, San Francisco, CA.

Chaudhary, M.A. & Stearns, S.C. (1996) Estimating confidence intervals for cost-effectiveness ratios: an example from a randomized trial. *Statistics in Medicine* 15, 1447–1458.

Clark, R.E. (1994) Family costs associated with severe mental illness and substance use. *Hospital and Community Psychiatry* 45, 808–813.

Clark, R.E., Ricketts, S.K. & McHugo, G.J. (1999) Legal system involvement and costs for person in treatment for severe mental illness and substance use disorders. *Psychiatric Services* 50, 641–647.

Conley, R., Tamminga, C. & Group, M.S. (1998) Olanzapine compared with chlorpromazine in treatment-resistant schizophrenia. *American Journal of Psychiatry* 155, 914–920.

Cruze, A.M., Harwood, H.J., Kristiansen, P.L. *et al.* (1981) *Economic Costs to Society of Alcohol and Drug Abuse and Mental Illness, 1977.* Research Triangle Institute, Research Triangle Park, NC.

Dickey, B. & Goldman, H.H. (1986) Public health care for the chronically mentally ill: financing operating costs. *Administration in Mental Health* 14, 63–77.

Drake, R.E., McHugo, G.J., Becker, D.R. *et al.* (1996) The New Hampshire study of supported employment for people with severe mental illness. *Journal of Consulting and Clinical Psychology* 64, 391–399.

Drummond, M.F., O'Brien, B., Stoddart, G.L. *et al.* (1997) *Methods for the Economic Evaluation of Health Care Programs*, 2nd edn. Oxford University Press, New York.

Essock, S.M. (1995) Clozapine's cost effectiveness [letter]. *American Journal of Psychiatry* 152, 152.

Essock, S.M., Hargreaves, W.A., Covell, N.H. *et al.* (1996a) Clozapine's effectiveness for patients in state hospitals: results from a randomized trial. *Psychopharmacological Bulletin* 32, 683–697.

Essock, S.M., Hargreaves, W.A., Dohm, F.A. *et al.* (1996b) Clozapine eligibility among state hospital patients. *Schizophrenia Bulletin* 22, 15–25.

Essock, S.M., Frisman, L.K. & Kontos, N.J. (1998) Cost effectiveness of assertive community treatment teams. *American Journal of Orthopsychiatry* 68, 179–190.

Essock, S.M., Frisman, L.K., Covell, N.H. *et al.* (2000) Cost-effectiveness of clozapine compared to conventional antipsychotic medication for patients in state hospitals. *Archives of General Psychiatry* 57, 987–944.

Essock, S.M., Frisman, L.K. & Covell, N.H. (2002) The economics of the treatment of schizophrenia. In: *Neuropsychopharmacology: the Fifth Generation of Progress American College of Neuropsychopharmacology* (eds K.L. Davis, D. Charney, J.T. Coyle & C. Nemeroff), pp. 809–818. Lippincott, Williams & Wilkins, New York.

Feldman, S. (1999) Strangers in the night: research and managed mental health care. *Health Affairs* 18, 48–51.

Foster, R.H. & Goa, K.L. (1999) Olanzapine: a pharmacoeconomic review of its use in schizophrenia. *Pharmacoeconomics* 15, 611–640.

Frank, R.G. (1983) Is there a shortage of psychiatrists? *Community Mental Health Journal* 19, 42–53.

Frank, R.G. & Manning, W.G., eds. (1992) *Economics and Mental Health.* Johns Hopkins University Press, Baltimore, MA.

Frank, R.G., McGuire, T.G. & Salkever, D.S. (1991) Benefit flexibility, cost shifting, and mandated mental health coverage. *Journal of Mental Health Administration* 18, 264–271.

Frisman, L. & Rosenheck, R. (1996) How transfer payments are treated in cost-effectiveness and cost–benefit analyses. *Administration and Policy in Mental Health* 23, 533–545.

Ghaemi, S.N., Ziegler, D.M., Peachey, T.J. *et al.* (1998) Cost-effectiveness of clozapine therapy for severe psychosis. *Psychiatric Services* 49, 829–831.

Goeree, R., O'Brien, B.J., Goering, P. *et al.* (1999) The economic burden of schizophrenia in Canada. *Canadian Journal of Psychiatry* 44, 464–472.

Gold, M.R., Siegel, J.E., Russell, L.B. *et al.*, eds. (1996) *Cost-Effectiveness in Health and Mental Health*. Oxford University Press, New York.

Goldman, H.H., Morrissey, J.P. & Ridgely, M.S. (1994) Evaluating the Robert Wood Johnson Foundation program on chronic mental illness. *Millbank Quarterly* 72, 37–47.

Goldman, H.H., Frank, R.G. & Gaynor, M.S. (1995) What level of government? Balancing the interests of the state and the local community. *Administration and Policy in Mental Health* 23, 127–135.

Hamilton, S.H., Revicki, D.A., Edgell, E.T. *et al.* (1999) Clinical and economic outcomes of olanzapine compared with haloperidol for schizophrenia. *Pharmacoeconomics* 15, 469–480.

Hargreaves, W.A., Shumway, M., Hu, T. *et al.* (1998) *Cost–Outcome Methods for Mental Health*. Academic Press, New York.

Harwood, H.J., Napolitano, D.M., Kristiansen, P.L. *et al.* (1984) *Economic Costs to Society of Alcohol and Drug Abuse and Mental Illness, 1980*. Research Triangle Institute, Research Triangle Park, NC.

Jonsson, D. & Walinder, J. (1995) Cost-effectiveness of clozapine treatment in therapy-refractory schizophrenia. *Acta Psychiatrica Scandinavica* 92, 199–201.

Kassirer, J.P. & Angell, M. (1994) Journal's policy on cost-effectiveness analyses. *New England Journal of Medicine* 331, 669–670.

Kessler, R.C. & Frank, R.G. (1997) The impact of psychiatric disorders on work loss days. *Psychological Medicine* 27, 861–873.

Kleinmann, L.S. (1995) Preferences for outpatient mental health treatment. PhD dissertation. The Johns Hopkins University, Baltimore, MD.

Knapp, M. (1997) Costs of schizophrenia. *British Journal of Psychiatry* 171, 509–518.

Lave, J.R., Frank, R.G., Schulberg, H.C. *et al.* (1998) Cost-effectiveness of treatments for major depression in primary care practice. *Archives of General Psychiatry* 55, 645–651.

Lavori, P.W. (1992) Clinical trials in psychiatry: should protocol deviation censor patient data? *Neuropsychopharmacology* 6, 39–48.

Lehman, A.F. (1999) Quality of care in mental health: the case of schizophrenia. *Health Affairs* 18, 52–70.

Luchins, D.J., Hanrahan, P., Shinderman, M. *et al.* (1998) Initiating clozapine treatment in the outpatient clinic: service utilization and cost trends. *Psychiatric Services* 49, 1034–1038.

McGuire, T.G. (1981) *Financing Psychotherapy: Costs, Effects, and Public Policy*. Ballinger Books, Cambridge, MA.

McGuire, T.G. (1990) Growth of a field in policy research: the economics of mental health. *Administration and Policy in Mental Health* 17, 165–175.

McGuire, T.G. (1991) Measuring the economic costs of schizophrenia. *Schizophrenia Bulletin* 17, 375–388.

McGuire, T.G., Hodgkin, D. & Shumway, D. (1995) Managing Medicaid mental health costs: the case of New Hampshire. *Administration and Policy in Mental Health* 23, 97–117.

Manning, W.G., Wells, K.B., Duan, N. *et al.* (1984) Cost sharing and the use of ambulatory mental health services. *American Psychologist* 39, 1077–1089.

Martin, B.C. & Miller, L.S. (1998) Expenditures for treating schizophrenia: a population-based study of Georgia Medicaid recipients. *Schizophrenia Bulletin* 24, 479–488.

Mechanic, D., ed. (1998) Managed Behavioral Health Care: Current Realities and Future Potential. *New Directions for Mental Health Services*, no. 78. Jossey-Bass, San Francisco, CA.

Meltzer, H.Y. & Cola, P. (1995) Clozapine's cost effectiveness [reply]. *American Journal of Psychiatry* 152, 153–154.

Meltzer, H.Y., Cola, P., Way, L. *et al.* (1993) Cost effectiveness of clozapine in neuroleptic-resistant schizophrenia. *American Journal of Psychiatry* 150, 1630–1638.

Mumford, E. & Schlesinger, H.J. (1987) Assessing consumer benefit: cost offset as an incidental effect of psychotherapy. *General Hospital Psychiatry* 9, 360–363.

Murray, C.J.L. & Lopez, A.D. (1997) Alternative projections of mortality and disability by cause 1990–2020: global burden of disease study. *Lancet* 349, 1498–1504.

Nightengale, B.S., Crumly, J.M., Liao, J. *et al.* (1998) Current topics in clinical psychopharmacology. *Psychopharmacological Bulletin* 34, 373–382.

Pallack, M.S. & Cummings, N.A. (1992) Inpatient and outpatient psychiatric treatment: the effect of matching patients to appropriate level of treatment on psychiatric and medical–surgical hospital days. *Applied and Preventive Psychology* 1, 83–87.

Palmer, C.S., Revicki, D.A., Genduso, L.A. *et al.* (1998) A cost-effectiveness clinical decision analysis model for schizophrenia. *American Journal of Managment Care* 4, 345–355.

Pollack, S., Bruce, P., Borenstein, M. *et al.* (1994) The resampling method of statistical analysis. *Psychopharmacological Bulletin* 30, 227–234.

Radomsky, E.D., Haas, G.L., Mann, J.J. *et al.* (1999) Suicidal behavior in patients with schizophrenia and other psychotic disorders. *American Journal of Psychiatry* 156, 1590–1595.

Reid, W.H., Mason, M. & Toprac, M. (1994) Savings in hospital bed-days related to treatment with clozapine. *Hospital and Community Psychiatry* 45, 261–264.

Rice, D.P. (1999a) The economic impact of schizophrenia. *Journal of Clinical Psychiatry* 60 (Suppl. 1), 4–6.

Rice, D.P. (1999b) Economic burden of mental disorders in the United States. *Economics of Neuroscience* 1, 40–44.

Rice, D.P., Kelman, S., Miller, L.S. *et al.* (1990) *The Economic Costs of Alcohol and Drug Abuse and Mental Illness: 1985*. National Institute of Mental Health, DHHS Publications, (ADM) 90–1694, Rockville, MD.

Rock, M. (2000) Discounted lives? Weighing disability when measuring health and ruling on 'compassionate' murder. *Social Science and Medicine* 51, 407–417.

Rosenheck, R.A., Frisman, L.N. & Neale, M. (1994) Estimating the capital component of mental health care costs in the public sector. *Administration and Policy in Mental Health* 21, 493–509.

Rosenheck, R., Charney, D.S., Frisman, L.K. *et al.* (1995) Clozapine's cost effectiveness [letter]. *American Journal of Psychiatry* 152, 152–153.

Rosenheck, R.A., Cramer, J., Xu, W. *et al.* (1997) A comparison of clozapine and haloperidol in the treatment of hospitalized patients with refractory schizophrenia. *New England Journal of Medicine* 337, 451–458.

Rosenheck, R., Cramer, J., Allan, E. *et al.* (1999) Cost-effectiveness of clozapine in patients with high and low levels of hospital use. *Archives of General Psychiatry* 56, 565–572.

Rund, B.R. & Ruud, T. (1999) Costs of services for schizophrenic patients in Norway. *Acta Psychiatrica Scandinavica* 99, 120–125.

Schiller, M. & Hargreaves, W.A. (1995) Clozapine's cost effectiveness [letter]. *American Journal of Psychiatry* 152, 151–152.

Schiller, M.J., Shumway, M. & Hargreaves, W.A. (1999) Treatment costs and patient outcomes with use of risperidone in a public mental health setting. *Psychiatric Services* 50, 228–230.

Semke, J., Fisher, W.H., Goldman, H.H. *et al.* (1995) The evolving role of the state hospital in the care and treatment of older adults: state trends 1984–93. *Psychiatric Services* 47, 1082–1087.

Shepherd, G., Muijen, M., Hadley, T.R. *et al.* (1996) Effects of mental health services reform on clinical practice in the United Kingdom. *Psychiatric Services* 47, 1351–1355.

Shore, M.F. (1999) Replacing cost with value. *Harvard Review of Psychiatry* 6, 334–336.

Simon, G.E., VonKorff, M., Rutter, C. *et al.* (2000) Randomised trial of monitoring, feedback, and management of care by telephone to improve treatment of depression in primary care. *British Medical Journal* 320, 550–554.

Taube, C.A., Lee, E.S. & Forthofer, R.N. (1984) DRGs in psychiatry: an empirical evaluation. *Medical Care* 22, 597–610.

Tunis, S.L., Bryan, M.J., Gibson, J. *et al.* (1999) Changes in perceived health and functioning as a cost-effectiveness measure for olanzapine versus haloperidol treatment of schizophrenia. *Journal of Clinical Psychiatry* 60 (Suppl.), 38–45.

Weisbrod, B.A., Test, M.A. & Stein, L.I. (1980) Alternative to hospital treatment. II. Economic benefit–cost analysis. *Archives of General Psychiatry* 37, 400–405.

Index

All entries in the index refer to schizophrenia unless otherwise stated, cross-references in *italics* are for general references (*e.g. see also specific drugs*) and abbreviations used as subentries are defined in the main body of the index.

Abnormal Involuntary Movement Scale (AIMS)
  ECT combination therapy 527
  tardive dyskinesia 560
abulia 22
abuse/neglect
  disease development role 626–7, 661, 678
    patients' perspectives 701
  violence association 599, 603
accessory symptoms 22, 25–6
acetylcholine 356–7
  dopamine relationship 553–4
  extrapyramidal syndrome role 553–4
  muscarinic receptors 357
    agonists 452–3
    novel antipsychotics 434, 452–3
  nicotinic receptors 356–7
    linkage studies ($\alpha 7$) 265, 278, 287, 292, 357, 395
  psychopharmacological studies 357
  psychosis role 452
  tardive dyskinesia role 566
  see also anticholinergic drugs
acoustic startle reflex, personality disorders 85
actuarial assessment, violence 600–1
adenosine receptors, genetic models 395
adjunctive therapy 434, 448–50, 461, 521, 525–8
  drug-resistant schizophrenia 503–7
  see also specific drugs/treatments
adolescent onset *see* child/adolescent onset schizophrenia
adoptees family study 255
adoption studies 255–6
  cognitive deficits 280
  design 255
  environmental factors 256
    early effects 627
  need-adapted therapy 672
  schizophrenia spectrum disorder 255
  violence 595
adrenergic receptors
  α_1 antagonists 453
    sertindole (pseudo-irreversible) 432
  α_2 agonists 453
  α_2 antagonists 453
    clozapine 426
  adjunctive therapy 450
  β antagonists (β-blockers) 450
  genetic models 395

hypotension 578
adrenoleukodystrophy (ALD), schizophrenic symptoms 193
aetiology
  animal models 390–1
  child/adolescent onset 40–1
  late-onset schizophrenia 71–4
affect 21, 628
  blunted/flattened 21
  inappropriate (parathymia) 21
  judgement 619
affective disorders 21, 285
  bipolar *see* bipolar disorder
  comparative studies 172
  depression *see* depression
  late-onset schizophrenia 70–1
  misdiagnosis of child/adolescent onset schizophrenia 38
  psychotic 285
African-Caribbean immigrants 222–3
aftercare hostels 707
age as risk factor 215–16, 338
  extrapyramidal syndromes 555
  family studies 251, 255
  for suicide 123
  tardive dyskinesia (TD) 562, 563
aggression, treatment 443
  clozapine 500
  valproate 504–5
  see also violence
agitation, treatment of 443, 505
agranulocytosis 499, 580
  clozapine and 425, 444, 501
  combination therapy 499
akathisia
  antipsychotic-induced 150, 444, 552–3
  misdiagnosis 553
  reduced risk, clozapine 501
  serotonin role 554
  tardive 559
  treatment 556, 558
akinesia 553
  antipsychotic-induced 150, 444, 553
  depression and 483, 574
  negative symptoms *versus* 553
alcohol abuse 213
  depression induction 143
  pregnancy 329
  social course effects 127
Aldomet (methyldopa) 566

allele interactions 257
allelic heterogeneity 258
allergic reactions, antipsychotics 578
Alzheimer's disease
  antipsychotics and 311
  delusions and hallucinations 192
  genetics 257
  neuropathology 320
  P300 (P3) ERP component 300
  prevalence in schizophrenia 311
American Psychiatric Association (APA)
  Task Force on ECT 517, 535
  Task Force on Tardive Dyskinesia 565
amisulpride 428–30
  clinical effects 428
  dosage 446
  efficacy 429, 445–6, 447
  pharmacological profile 428
  side-effects 428–30
ampakines 455–7
AMPA receptors 350, 455
  antagonists 393
  decreases in schizophrenia 350–3
  therapeutic strategies 455–7
amphetamines
  dopaminergic response 376–7
    exaggerated 372
    neuroimaging studies 372, 373
  ketamine effects 377
  NMDA receptor role 376–7
  psychosis 372
  schizotypal personality studies 90, 92
amygdala 410, 411
  function 411
  volume reductions 42, 288, 410
amygdalo-hippocampal complex 410–12
anaesthesia, neuroleptic malignant syndrome 535
anastrophae 120–1
Andreasen classification system 114
anhedonia 21
  Physical Anhedonia Scale (PAS) 285
  schizotypy 285
  Social Anhedonia Scale (SAS) 285
animal models 388–402
  antipsychotics testing 393, 394, 427, 429
  clinical/behavioural aspects 389, 392
  controversy 388
  creating 389–90
  delayed onset 340

dopamine-based 388–9
genetic 389, 394–6
glutamatergic 389, 390, 394
goals 389
neurodevelopmental 389, 390–4
  aetiological 390–1
  disrupted neurogenesis 391–2
  neonatal lesion 390, 392–4, 396
  perinatal stress 392
  see also neurodevelopmental hypothesis
novel (heuristic) 389–90
transgenic 394, 396
'two hit' models 392
validity 388, 427
anomalous experiences 15, 16
antecedents 215–23
see also risk factors
anticholinergic drugs 461
  EPS treatment 444, 556, 558
  side-effects 444, 558, 564
    cognitive impairment 575
  tardive dyskinesia treatment 566
  see also acetylcholine
anticipatory saccades 281, 283
anticonvulsant drugs
  adjunctive therapy 448, 450, 504–5
  mood effects 483
  psychopharmacology 356
  see also individual drugs
antidepressant drugs
  antipsychotic adjuncts 159–60, 449–50
    drug-resistant schizophrenia 505–6
    negative symptom efficacy 449–50
  atypical antipsychotics as 445, 446–7, 483, 492
  depression management 156–60, 483, 505
    efficacy 449
    studies 157–9
  SSRIs *see* selective serotonin reuptake inhibitors (SSRIs)
  tricyclic 156, 449
  see also specific drugs
antipsychotic drugs 47–8, 421–41, 444
  acute treatment 444–56
  adjuncts 434, 448–50, 461, 503–7, 521, 525–8
    see also specific adjuncts/treatments
  Alzheimer's disease link 311
  'atypical' *see* atypical antipsychotic drugs
  'atypicality' controversy 428, 476
  background 421–2
  benefits and drawbacks 173
  chronic/residual disease treatment 460–2
  cognitive effects 461, 574–5
  combination therapy 498–9, 605
  comparisons 173–4
  compliance/adherence 443, 477
    cheeking/spitting 458
    continuum 477
    factors affecting 477
    relapse risk 476
    side-effects and 573
    strategies for improving 477
  depression management 155–6
    influence on antidepressants 159–60

see also depression
dopamine receptors and 268, 421, 422
  D_2 occupancy threshold 424–5, 459, 553, 555
  D_2 receptor hypothesis 422–5, 427
  side-effects and 424, 425, 553
  see also dopamine hypothesis; dopamine receptors
dose–response relationships 76, 458–9
  dose reduction 479–80
  effective doses 458–9
  EPS and 555
  guidance 459
  heterogeneity 489
  therapeutic window 424
  threshold hypothesis 459
ECT *versus* 521–5
eye tracking effects 282
first-episode treatment 456, 459–60
  early intervention 457
glutamatergic modulation 434
goals 428
late-onset schizophrenia treatment 72–7
limitations 119
maintenance treatment *see* maintenance treatment
modelling
  animal model testing 393, 394, 427, 429
  cellular/behavioural models 426–7
  see also animal models
molecular neurobiology 268
negative symptoms and 444
neurochemistry 304, 352, 375, 447, 494
neuropathology and 311, 315, 319
non-specificity problem 434
novel therapeutic targets 423–4
parenteral forms 447–8, 457
  depot preparations 76–7, 478
  depot *versus* oral 478
  pharmakokinetics 478
  prescription 478–9
patients' perspectives 703–6
pharmacogenomics 433, 496
positive symptoms and 376
prescribing practice 706, 712
  cost analysis 717, 718
  late-onset guidelines 76–7
  long-acting depot preparations 478–9
prophylaxis 443
refractoriness to *see* treatment-resistant schizophrenia
regimens
  determination 443
  drug choice 457–8, 478–9
  early intervention 457, 480–82
  emergency settings 457
  high-dose/megadose 498
  maintenance *see* maintenance treatment
  'rapid neuroleptization' 457, 458
  refractory disease 498–507
  targeted/intermittent strategy 456, 481
relapse prevention 380, 456, 474, 627
  see also maintenance treatment
response prediction 456, 492–6
  comorbid disorders 491–3
  neuroimaging studies 493–5

plasma levels 495–6
risk–benefit analysis 564
safety 444
schizotypal personality disorder treatment 91–2
second generation *see* atypical antipsychotic drugs
side-effects 47, 433, 474, 573–88
  cardiovascular 577–8
  cognitive 574–5
  cutaneous 578–9
  D_2 related 424, 425, 553, 573
  diabetes 563, 576–7
  dysphoria induction 143, 150, 573–4
  extrapyramidal *see* extrapyramidal syndromes (EPSs)
  gastrointestinal 579
  haematological 580
  hepatic 579–80
  hyperprolactinaemia 425, 428, 575–6, 577
  major effect 706
  management 443
  neuroleptic malignant syndrome 535–6, 581
  ocular 579
  orthostatic hypotension 578
  parenteral forms 478
  seizures 580–81
  sexual dysfunction 577
  thyroid toxicity 576
  weight gain 576
stress vulnerability effects 627
third-generation 433–4
see also dopamine receptors; serotonin receptors; *specific drugs*
antisocial behaviour, obstetric complications and 329
anxiety disorders 22, 483–4, 573
  management 484, 505
  patients' perspectives 704, 707
  relative's distress 598
  secondary *versus* primary 484
apathy 22
  cognitive adaptive therapy 650
apocalypse 121
apomorphine-induced stereotypic behaviour 395
apopheny 120
apoptosis 338
aripiprazole 433, 450–51
arrhythmias, fatal 577
art therapy 677
Asperger's syndrome 6
assertive community treatment (ACT) 604–5, 639, 640, 691–3, 714
associations, loosening of 20
association studies 260, 266–8
  case–control design 280
  classical markers 267
  contradictory results 266
  dopamine receptor genes 267
  family-based design 280–1
  intermediate phenotypes 280–1
  linkage disequilibrium 260, 262
  linkage studies *versus* 280

problems 266
quantitative traits 279
recruitment 281
serotonin receptor genes 267–8
transmission disequilibrium test 266, 267
see also DNA markers; linkage studies
asylums 688
asymmetrical abnormalities *see* brain
    asymmetry
atropine 357
attentional impairment 22, 28, 169–70, 290,
    291
    auditory ERPs 300
    cognitive disruption 169–70
    delusion formation 177–8
    eye tracking effects 282
    selective, cingulate cortex role 410
    spectrum personality disorder 87–8
atypical antipsychotic drugs 47–8, 267, 268,
    425–33, 444–7
    adjunctive therapy 434, 448–50, 503–7
    'atypicality' controversy 428, 476
    basal ganglia effects 494
    chronic/residual disease 460–1
    clinical profiles 446
    cognitive improvement 173–5, 446, 461–2,
        482, 492, 574
    combination therapy 498–9
    comparison between 447
    cost analysis 717–19
    depression and
        antidepressant effects 445, 446–7, 483
        treatment alteration in depressive patients
            155–6
        see also depression
    drug choice 458
    effective doses 459, 495
    efficacy 445–6
    ERP effects 304
    extrapyramidal symptoms and 174, 425,
        428
        EPS profiles 555–6
        mechanism of action 556
        see also extrapyramidal syndromes (EPSs);
            tardive dyskinesia (TD)
    first-episode treatment 460
    formulations 458
        parenteral forms 447–8
    goals 428
    impact 425–8
    late-onset schizophrenia treatment 76
    mechanistic issues 428
    negative symptom effect 429, 446, 460–1,
        482
        treatment-resistant schizophrenia 491
    neurochemistry 447
    pharmacogenomics 433, 496
    pharmacology 494–5
        'loose' binding 426, 427
        NMDA actions 304
        'tight' binding 431
    prototypical drug (clozapine) *see* clozapine
    psychosocial interactions 485
    side-effects 428–9, 433, 446, 573–88
        agranulocytosis 425, 444, 499, 501, 580
        cardiac conduction 430, 432, 433, 577–8

cataracts 430, 579
constipation 501
diabetes 577
extrapyramidal 555
hepatic/gastrointestinal 579–81
hyperprolactinaemia 428, 431, 530–76,
    577
leucopenia 580
ocular 579
orthostatic hypotension 578
seizures 501, 505, 532, 580–2
weight gain 429–30, 433, 579
    tardive dyskinesia and 564
    third-generation 433–4
    treatment-resistant schizophrenia 498–503
    typical drugs comparison 173–4, 479
    violence management 605
    see also dopamine receptors; serotonin
        receptors; *specific drugs*
atypical psychotic disorders 54–67
    DSM-IV classification 60–2
    historical background 54
    ICD-10 classification 62–4
    see also psychosis
auditory verbal hallucinations (AVHs) 16–17
    command 443
        violence and 597, 598
    neuropsychological investigations 175–7
        inner speech 176
        language and hallucinations 176
        reality/source monitoring 176–7
    post-traumatic stress disorder 626
autism 6–7
autistic spectrum disorders 6–7
    misdiagnosis 38–9
autoimmune disorders 193
avoidant personality disorder 81

Barker hypothesis 241
basal ganglia 412
    abnormalities 42, 412
        antipsychotic effects 319, 494
    cholinergic effects 553
    see also dopamine
behavioural abnormalities 331
    acute pharmacological treatment 443
    animal modelling 389
    token economy programmes 640
behavioural family management 650
benzamides 370, 371
benzodiazepines
    agitation management 504
    antipsychotic adjunct 448
        acute treatment 457–8
        treatment-resistant schizophrenia 505
    anxiety management 484, 505
    eye tracking effects 282
    psychopharmacology 356
    rapid actions 457
    side-effects 505
    tardive dyskinesia treatment 567
β-blockers 450
bipolar disorder
    chromosomal associations 265
    comparative studies 172
    eye tracking 282

life events 625
linkage studies 265
neuropathology 319
obstetric complications and 328
P300 (P3) ERP component 300
symptoms 122
birth
    place of 221, 236, 330
    season of 221–2, 236, 330
    trauma 254–5
    see also pregnancy and birth complications
        (PBCs)
birth cohort studies
    epidemiology findings 205
    Mannheim cohort 129
    violence 594, 608
blepharospasm–oromandibular dystonia 560
Bleuler, E. 4–5, 25–6, 657
blunted affect 21
BOLD fMRI 298, 405
bone density, hyperprolactinaemia effects 575
Bonn Scale for the Assessment of Basic
    Symptoms (BSABS) 121
borderline personality disorder 81
borderline schizophrenia 80
Borna disease virus (BDV) 219, 391
Borrelia encephalitis 194
botulinum toxin, tardive dyskinesia treatment
    567
Bouffées délirantes 55
bradykinesia *see* akinesia
brain
    imaging *see* neuroimaging studies
    lesions 196–7
        child/adolescent onset schizophrenia 41
        late-onset schizophrenia 72, 74
        laterality, locus and nature 189
        see also brain asymmetry
        neurodevelopment and 330
        occult 197
        pathophysiology 93
    mapping, depressive patients 153
    perfusion changes 332
    structural abnormalities 42, 255, 304, 310,
        406–11
        asymmetry *see* brain asymmetry
        cognitive impairment course 116–17
        CT studies 287–8
        developmental 240–1, 255, 319
        MRI studies 288
        obstetric complications 240
        progression 406, 493
        see also progressive brain changes
        refractory disease and 493
        ventricular *see* ventricular enlargement
        volumetric reductions 406
        see also neurodevelopmental hypothesis;
            neuropathology
    see also entries beginning cerebral/cortical;
        specific regions
brain asymmetry
    brain lesions 189
    hippocampal formation 336, 410
    lateralization 89
    neurodevelopmental hypothesis and 335–6
    neuropathology 317, 335–6

P300 (P3) ERP 304–5
planum temporale 289
positron emission tomography (PET) 335–6
superior temporal gyrus (STG) 304, 305
sylvian fissure 289
temporal cortex 289, 317
temporal sulci 336
twin studies 336
breast cancer, hyperprolactinaemia effect 574
Brief Psychiatric Rating Scale (BPRS) 490
brief psychotic disorders
diagnostic criteria 12
DSM-IV classification 61
brief reactive psychosis, DSM-IV classification 61
British National Schizophrenia Guideline Group 618
Brown–Peterson task deficits 170
BSF 190555 (BTS 79018) 452
BTS 79018 (BSF 190555) 452
buspirone 483
butyrophenones 370, 371, 444

California Verbal List Test (CVLT) 290
Camberwell Collaborative Psychosis Study 623
Camberwell Family Interview (CFI) 615
cAMP 350
Canadian Psychiatric Association, ECT recommendations 518
cancer
antipsychotics link 575
negative comorbidity 213
schizophrenia associations 196–7
candidate genes/loci 262, 267–8, 278, 390, 395
cannabinoid receptor abnormalities 214
cannabis
comorbidity 213–14
psychosis induction 39–40, 353, 702
Capgras syndrome (illusion des sosies) 59
carbamazepine 449, 483
adjunctive therapy 450, 483, 504–5
drug interactions 504
side-effects 450, 504
cardiovascular disease 577–8
see also QTc prolongation
Care Programme Approach 604
case management 691
social skills training 642
cataracts 430, 579
catastrophae 121
catatonia 18–19, 122
autism and 7
definition and classification 18–19, 534
ECT and 519, 534–5
incidence and variety 19
lethal 535, 581
symptoms 197
catch-up saccades 281
catechol-O-methyl transferase (COMT) 291, 408
fMRI studies 287, 289
gene location 263
genetic linkage 263, 278, 292, 341
categorical models 26–7

caudate nucleus, clozapine effects 494
cavum septum pellucidum, anomalies 91, 197
cerebellum 412
cerebral blood flow
functional imaging (regional; rCBF) 91, 401
perfusion changes 332
cerebral disconnectivity see under cortical connectivity
cerebral hemispheres
asymmetry see brain asymmetry
dysfunction 89
auditory hallucinations 175
cerebral tumours, schizophrenia association 196–7
cerebral ventricle enlargement see ventricular enlargement
cerebrospinal fluid (CSF)
glutamate levels 349
homovanillic acid (HVA) levels 90
cerebrovascular disease, schizophrenic symptoms 192
c-fos induction, antipsychotics drugs 426–7, 450
chandelier neurones 316–17, 355–6
checklists, cognitive adaptive therapy 650
'chemical restraint' 457, 605
Chestnut Lodge Follow-up Study 128
child/adolescent onset schizophrenia 34–53
aetiology and risk factors 40–1
pregnancy and birth complications (PBCs) 40
psychosocial risks 41
puberty 40–1
clinical features 35–6
premodal phase 36
premorbid impairments 35–6
psychotic symptoms 36
symptom dimensions 36
course 46
developmental issues in assessment 37–8
diagnosis 37–8
differential diagnosis 37, 38–40
affective/schizoaffective/atypical psychoses 38
autistic spectrum disorders 38–9
drug psychoses 39–40
epilepsy 39
multidimensionally impaired (MDI) syndrome 39
neurodegenerative disorders 39
schizotypal personality disorder 39
epidemiology 40
genetics 44
history 34–5
investigations 38, 39–40
mortality 46
neurobiology 41–4
absence of gliosis 41, 42
dendritic elimination 41, 42
excessive synaptic pruning 41, 42
functional imaging 43
lesion 41
neurodevelopmental hypothesis 41–2, 43–4
progressive brain changes 42–3
structural abnormalities 42

neuropsychology 44–6
course of cognitive defects 45–6
executive functions and onset 45
pattern of cognitive defects 44–5
outcome 46, 493
prognosis 46
refractoriness 47–8, 492–3
see also treatment-resistant schizophrenia
treatment 47–8
cognitive–behavioural therapy (CBT) 48
cognitive remediation 48
organization of services 48
pharmacological 47–8
primary prevention and early detection 47
psychosocial and family interventions 48
see also antipsychotic drugs; treatment
childhood encephalitis 194
childhood experiences, late-onset schizophrenia and 74
childhood Sydenham's chorea, secondary schizophrenia 193
chi-squared automatic interaction detector (CHAID) 602
chlorpromazine 349
cardiac conduction defects 577
cutaneous effects 578–9
dysphoric reactions 573
ECT combination therapy 527
ECT versus 521–5
first-episode patients 460
hepatotoxicity 579–80
ocular effects 579
seizure induction 580
choice reaction time 291
cholinergic receptors see under acetylcholine
chorea gravidum 561
chorea of pregnancy 561
chromosomes
bipolar disorder associations 265
cytogenetic abnormalities, child/adolescent onset 44
homologous 258
linkage associations 262–6
chromosome 1q 265
chromosome 2 266
chromosome 5 262–3, 266
chromosome 6 264, 268
chromosome 7 266
chromosome 8p 263–4
chromosome 9 266
chromosome 10p 264
chromosome 11 268
chromosome 13q 264–5
chromosome 15q 265, 287
chromosome 18 265
chromosome 22q 263
errors 263
X chromosome 265–6
see also linkage studies
recombination and crossover 258–9, 261
translocation 265
trisomy (chromosome 5) 262–3
chronic delusional states (délires chroniques) 58–9

CI-1007 451

cingulate cortex 409–10
  abnormal cingulate gyrification 409–10
  disconnection 413
  GABAergic reductions 354
  imaging difficulties 409
  selective attention/response competition 410
  symptom expression 410
  volume reductions 409
classification 3–14, 114
  categorical approach 26–7, 112
  dimensional approach 27
  empirical approaches 8–9
  ICD-10 *see* International Classification of Disease-10 (ICD-10)
  modern systems and limitations 9–10
  standards for symptom definition and combination 9
  testing clinical concepts 8–9
Clérambault syndrome 59–60
Client's Assessment of Strengths, Interests and Goals (CASIG) 638
clinical assessment, violence 600–1
clinical phenotypes, intermediate 285, 292
clinicopathological relationship 317–18
clonazepam 457
clozapine 47, 444, 499–501
  adjunctive therapy 498
    ECT 507, 532–3
    lamotrigine 505
    lithium 503
    safety issues 532
    SSRIs 506
    valproate 505
  advantages 479
  antidyskinetic effect 566
  blood testing 500, 501
  chronic disease 461
  cognitive functioning 461–2
  combination therapy 498
  cost-effectiveness 716, 717–18
    randomized trials 718
  effective dose 495
  efficacy 425, 445, 499–501
  extrapyramidal symptoms, reduction 425, 501, 555, 566
  first-episode patients 460
  functional imaging 427
  hostility/agression effects 500
  impact 425–7
  late-onset schizophrenia treatment 76
  maintenance treatment 500
  molecular neurobiology 268
  pharmacogenetics 496
  pharmacology
    dopamine receptor binding 425, 450
    kinetics 494
    'loose' binding 426, 427
    non-dopamine receptor binding 426
    pharmacological profile 425
    striatal D_2 *versus* $5-HT_2$ occupancy 427, 494
    variant D_2 occupancy 427
  refractory schizophrenia 499–501, 532–3
  side-effects 500–501
    agranulocytosis 425, 444, 499, 501

eye tracking effects 282
insulin sensitivity 577
obsessive–compulsive disorder 506
oesophageal epistasis 579
orthostatic hypotension 578
seizure-induction 501, 505, 532, 580
sialorrhoea 579
weight gain 576
structural effects, caudate nucleus 494
substance abuse and 484–5
suicide reduction 500
violence management 500, 605
clubhouse model 646, 695
Cochrane Collaboration Review 478, 500
cognitive adaptive therapy 649–50
cognitive–behavioural therapy (CBT) 48, 657, 667–9
  anxiety management 484
  assessment role 8
  'befriending' 48
  conceptualization 669
  drug-resistant schizophrenia 497
  efficacy 667–8
  focus 669
  late-onset schizophrenia treatment 75
  long-term goals 639
  non-specific effects 668–9
  outcome measures 669
  psychopathology and 669
  randomized controlled trials 668
  research evidence 667–8
    interpretation 668–9
  short-term goals 639
  strategies 639
  symptom reductions 668
  violence management 606
cognitive dysmetria 27–8
Cognitive Enhancement Therapy (CET) 676–7
cognitive impairment 30, 168–84, 289–91, 365, 381, 643, 662, 676
  adoption studies 280
  adrenergic receptor role 452
  brain anomalies 116–17
  child/adolescent onset 44–5
  clinicopathological relationship 318
  concurrent and predictive validity 172–3
  core deficits 169–71
  course 168–9
  deficit criteria 461
  differential deficits 171–2
  drug-induced 574–5
  ECT and 536, 538
  fundamental deficits 171
  genetics 280, 289
  historical aspects 168
  intermediate phenotype 179
  late-onset schizophrenia 71
  negative symptoms 30, 115–16
  neuropsychiatry comparative studies 171–2
  neuropsychology 289–91, 292
    behavioural abnormalities 289–90
    psychotic symptoms 175–9
    test performances 168–9, 171
    see also specific tests
  novel approaches 175–9

outcome prediction 279
patients' perspectives 704, 709
psychopharmacology 351
relative risk (RR) investigations 179, 280
  as risk factor 220
social course indicator 125
spectrum personality disorders 86–9
tardive dyskinesia effects 563, 574
treatment 173–5
  atypical antipsychotic drugs 446, 461–2, 482, 492, 574
  maintenance therapy and 482
  problems 662
  psychosocial 497–8
  see also cognitive remediation/rehabilitation
treatment-resistant schizophrenia 492
twin studies 179, 290–1
see also memory impairment
cognitive problem-solving model, social skills training 641, 676
cognitive remediation/rehabilitation 48, 628, 643–5, 676–7
  Cognitive Enhancement Therapy (CET) 676–7
  computer programmes 644
  individualized 643
  Integrated Psychological Therapy model 644–5, 676
  molecular approach 676
  psychosocial interventions 497–8, 628
  self-instruction 643
  see also social skills training
combat experience, stress and 626
communication deviance, families of patients 618
community-based child and adolescent mental health services (CAMHS) 48
community care 690–2
  assertive community treatment (USA) 604–5, 639, 640, 691–2
    cost analysis 714
    fidelity criteria 691
  case management (USA) 691
  child and adolescent mental health services (CAMHS) 48
  Community Mental Health Care Team (UK) 690–1
  community psychiatric nurse (CPN) 75, 690
  costs 691, 692, 711
  crisis intervention services 692
  early psychosis services 692
  efficacy 690–1
  'failure' 689
  home treatment team 692
  integration 696–7
  multidisciplinary approach 690
  structure 696–7
  violence and schizophrenia 594–5
Community Mental Health Care Team (CMHT) 690–1
Community Mental Health Centers (CMHC) Act (USA; 1979) 688–9
community psychiatric nurse (CPN) 75, 690
comorbidity 213–14
  cognitive impairment 482, 492

depression 482–3, 505
management
  during maintenance treatment 481–5
  refractory disease 491–2, 505–6
negative 213, 481–2
obsessive–compulsive disorder 484, 506
personality disorder 597
substance abuse 127, 213–14, 484–5
see also specific conditions
complexity science, risk assessment 600
compulsory treatment orders 607, 693, 706, 710
computerized tomography (CT) 29, 287–8
depressive patients 153
history 403
late-onset schizophrenia 72
neurodevelopmental hypothesis 331
secondary schizophrenias 188–9
spectrum personality disorders 90
computer programmes, cognitive remediation 644
concrete thinking 19
consciousness disorder 28
constipation, clozapine 500
content-related behaviour model, social skills training 641
Continuous Performance Test (CPT) 43, 290
errors 169
heritability 290
performance 220
spectrum personality disorder 87–8
conventional antipsychotic drugs see antipsychotic drugs
coping strategies
deficits 625
learning 661
older versus younger patients 660–1
coping style 620, 622
corpus callosum, abnormalities 91, 197
cortical connectivity 316–17
abnormal/disconnectivity 43, 340, 412–13
  dopamine role 376–8
  frontal–temporal 412–13
  functional 'dysconnection' 340–1
  see also neuropathology
adolescent changes 378
functional 316, 413
prefrontal cortex 335, 339–90, 376
structural imaging 317
twin studies 316, 412
cortical efferents, glutamatergic 349, 367
corticostriatal–thalamocortical loops 366–7, 411
cost-effectiveness analysis 716–17
costs 713–14
atypical antipsychotics 717–19
capital 714
community care 691, 692
components 714–15
family burden 714
hospitalization 692–3
legal 714
perspective 714
planning/policy-making effect 718
productivity loss 714
range of 714–15

schizophrenia-specifc 713–14
  direct versus indirect 713
treatment/services 714
see also economics
costs-of-illness studies 714
cost–utility analysis 715–16
Cotard syndrome 60
counterfactual theory 593
course of disease 11–12, 101–41
brain anomalies 116–17
cognitive impairment 116–17
comorbidity with substance abuse 127
description measures 112–13
early course 118–20
geographical variation 129–30
indicators 112, 118–19
long-term 127–30
  sociodemographic outcome indicators 129
  studies 104–10, 128–9
negative symptoms 28, 116
  cognitive impairment correlations 115–16
neurodegeneration and 337
positive symptoms 28
short-term, child/adolescent onset 46
social see social course
stages 120–1
symptom dimensions/clusters 117–18
symptom-related see symptom-related course
time trends 101–2
types 113
see also comorbidity; outcome; prognosis
craniofacial abnormalities 330
crisis intervention services 692
cross-fostering adoption studies 255
Crow classification system 114
crude mortality rate (CMR) 123
cultural issues
culture-specific psychoses 56, 57
life events 623
psychosocial interventions 659
violence studies 598
culture-specific psychoses 56, 57
cutaneous drug reactions 577–8
cyclic AMP (cAMP) 350
cycloid psychoses 56
in late-onset schizophrenia 70–1
D-cycloserine 454
cytogenic abnormalities 44

'dangerous severe personality disorder' 602
day care (partial hospitalization) 694–6
deafferentation 93
deafness, late-onset schizophrenia 73–4
declarative memory 290
deficit syndromes 115, 461, 482, 491
deinstitutionalization 688, 695
violence and schizophrenia 594, 599
délire de négation 60
délires chroniques 58–9
delusional disorders 56–60
chronic states 58–9
clinical outcome 532
diagnostic criteria 12

DSM-IV classification 61
ECT response 533
erotomanic type 59–60
ICD-10 classification 62–3, 69
induced 59
  diagnostic criteria 12
  ICD-10 classification 64
persistent 56–60
  diagnostic criteria 12
  ICD-10 classification 62–3
see also delusions
delusional jealousy 59
delusional memories, investigations 178
delusional mood 16
delusional speech, treatment 641
delusions 5–6, 17–18
Alzheimer's disease 192
definitions and classification 17, 18
formation theories 177–8
incidence and variety 17–18
late-onset schizophrenia 70
neuropsychological investigations 177–8
patients' perspectives 702, 703, 708
reality/source monitoring 176–7
religious 702, 704
violence association 596, 597
  content role 597
  hallucination role 597
see also delusional disorders
dementia 116, 311
Lewy body 356
dementia praecoccissima 34
dementia praecox 45, 54, 326
family study 251
demographic variables, treatment resistance 492–3
demoralization syndrome 151
demyelinating diseases, schizophrenic symptoms 192–3
dendritic abnormalities
delayed onset role 339
elimination 41, 42
hippocampal 312–13
prefrontal 316
depot preparations 76–7, 478–9
depression 21–2, 142–67, 504
antipsychotic-induced 573–4
bereavement relationship 625
biochemical measures 154
biological validation 152–5
brain structure and function 153–4
  brain mapping studies 153
  neuroimaging 153–4
  neuropsychology 154
clinical validation 152
differential diagnosis 143, 150–2
  akinesia and akathisia 150, 574
  antipsychotic-induced dysphoria 143, 150
  disappointment reactions 151
  independent diathesis 151–2
  negative symptoms 150–1
  organic factors 143
  prodrome of psychotic relapse 151
  schizoaffective disorder 151
dopamine role 153–4

endocrine measures 154
genetic studies 154–5
historical aspects 142
life events 152
misdiagnosis of child/adolescent onset
	schizophrenia 38
patients' perspectives 703, 707
postpsychotic 11–12, 142, 574
prevalence and incidence 122, 143
	studies 144–9
primary 483
prognosis 152
prognostic value 122
relative's distress 598
secondary 483
serotonin role 154
social factors 613
suicide 152
symptoms 121–2
treatment 504–5
	antidepressant medications 156–60, 449
	antipsychotic medications 155–6
	atypical antipsychotics 445, 446–7, 492
	ECT 517, 518, 534, 536, 538, 541
	implications 155–60
	lithium 160
	maintenance therapy and 482
	psychosocial interventions 160
	see also antidepressant drugs
treatment-resistant schizophrenia 492,
	505–6
see also suicide
derailment 20
dermatoglyphic abnormalities 330–1
	marker of disturbed development 233,
	235–6
desipramine 484
destructive phase 117
developing countries, course and outcome
	variations 129
development
	animal models 390–4
	dopaminergic systems 326–7, 340, 378
	hippocampal formation 318
		genetics 396–7
		lesion models 390, 392, 393, 395
		prefrontal cortex role 392, 393
	markers of disturbances 217, 232–6
		dermatoglyphic features 233, 235–6,
		330–1
		minor physical abnormalities (MPAs)
		232–3
	neurodevelopmental genes 395
	neuroimaging studies 327, 331–6
	prefrontal cortex (PFC) 318, 339–40
		hippocampus role 392, 393
	risk factors for schizophrenia 232–50
	structural abnormalities 240–1, 255, 319
	thalamus changes 318–19
	see also neurodevelopmental hypothesis;
		neuropathology; pregnancy and birth
		complications (PBCs)
dexamethasone suppression (DST), depressive
	patients 154
diabetes mellitus
	antipsychotic-induced 563, 576–7

tardive dyskinesia and 563
diagnosis 113–14, 205–6
	neuropathological 319–20
	time lag 213
Diagnostic and Statistical Manuals (DSM)
	DSM-III 26
	DSM-IIIR, delusion 17
	DSM-IV 9, 10–12
		atypical psychotic disorders 60–2
		brief psychotic disorders 61
		brief reactive psychosis 61
		delusional disorders 61
		diagnostic criteria 10–11
		late-onset schizophrenia 69–70
		schizoaffective disorder 62
		schizophreniform disorder 61–2
		schizotypal personality disorder 62
		shared psychotic disorders (folie à deux)
		62
diagnostic criteria 11–12, 206
	DSM see Diagnostic and Statistical Manuals
		(DSM)
	genetic studies and 252, 253, 277
	problems 206
	reactive psychosis 614
dialectic behaviour therapy 604
didactic training, violence management 604
diffusion tensor/weighted imaging (DTI/DWI)
	404–5
dimensional models 27
N,N-dimethyltryptamine (DMT) 353
direct interaction tasks 618
disabilities 113
Disability-Adjusted Life Years (DALYs)
	715–16
Disability Discrimination Act (UK; 1995) 695
disappointment reactions 151
disease course see course of disease
disinhibition 88
disorganization syndrome 22–3
	child/adolescent onset schizophrenia 36
	neuroimaging studies 43
		cingulate cortex 410
		parietal cortex 409
	neuropsychological tests 175
disulfiram 484
DMT (N,N-dimethyltryptamine) 353
DNA markers 260–1
	microsatellite 260–1
	RFLPs 260
	SNPs 261
	VAPSEs 267
	VNTR 260
DNA microarrays, prefrontal cortex profiling
	314
domestic violence 598
door-to-door case findings 204–5
dopamine 349
	acetylcholine relationship 552–3
	amphetamine-induced release 372, 374,
	376–7
	anatomy see dopaminergic systems
	dysfunction see dopaminergic dysfunction
	enhancing agents 92
	metabolism 286
	neuromodulatory role 367, 379

neuroplasticity 379
	receptors see dopamine receptors
	release 153
		tonic versus phasic 375
	sensitization 378, 379
	serotonin interactions 451
	suppression, tardive dyskinesia treatment
	566
	synaptic 374
	synthesis 153, 369
	tissue level studies 368–9
	transporter (DAT) 369
	see also dopamine hypothesis
dopamine-enhancing agents 92
dopamine hypothesis 89–90, 349, 365–87
	antipsychotics role 421
	classical versus revised 365
	evolution 422–3
	neurodevelopmental hypothesis and 376,
		379–80
		lesion models 393
	see also dopamine; dopaminergic
		dysfunction
'dopamine-in, dopamine-out' models 388–9
dopamine receptors 267, 368
	agonism 450–51, 461, 462
	antagonism 422–5
		subtype selective 423–4, 450
	autoreceptors 451
	D_1-like–D_2-like receptor interactions 423
	D_1-like receptors 422
	see also D_1 and D_5 (below)
	D_1 receptors 267, 368, 422
		agonists 451, 462
		D_5 receptors versus 423
		neuromodulation 367
		occupancy 553
		post-mortem studies 369
		premotor cortex 314, 365
		selective antagonists 423–4
	D_2-like receptors 422
	see also D_2, D_3 and D_4 (below)
	D_2 receptors 267, 365, 368, 422
		antipsychotic side-effects 424, 425
		'atypical' antipsychotic action 428, 429,
		430, 431, 432
		availability 412
		blockade hypothesis 173, 175, 381,
		422–5
		$D_{2longer}$ variant 422
		DRD2 gene 265
		imaging 370–2
		increase in depressive patients 153
		linkage studies 265
		neuromodulation 367
		occupancy 375, 424–5, 427, 459, 553
		olanzapine binding 430
		partial agonists 433, 450–1
		psychosis and 372
		sensitization and 378
		striatal increase 369
		unmasking 374
	D_3 receptors 267, 368, 422
		imaging 370
		increases 369
		knockouts 423

mRNA levels 268
  polymorphism 267
  selective antagonists 423
D_4 receptors 267, 368, 422
  clozapine 425
  imaging 370
  increases 369
  knockouts 426
  occupancy 553
  role in clozapine drug response 268
  selective antagonists 423, 450
D_5 receptors 267, 368, 422
  D_1 receptors versus 423
genes 268, 496
genetic models 395
imaging studies 370–2
  functional (PET/SPECT) 424–5
localization 368
typology 422–3
see also antipsychotic drugs
dopaminergic dysfunction 267, 365–6
  animal models 388–9
  cortical–subcortical interactions 376–8
  dysregulation of release 372, 376–7
  endogenous sensitization 378, 379
    hippocampal lesion effects 393
  extrapyramidal syndrome 553
  eye tracking effects 282
  imaging studies 370–6, 378
  neurochemical analysis 286, 368–9, 369–70
  neurodevelopmental hypothesis 326–7, 376, 379–80
  postmortem studies 368–70
  receptors/transporter changes 369
  stress effects 372, 374, 378, 625
  subcortical dysregulation 365–6, 376–8, 380, 393, 411
  synaptic depletion 374
  tardive dyskinesia
    hypersensitivity hypothesis 561
    suppression therapy 566
  see also dopamine hypothesis; dopamine receptors
dopaminergic systems 366–8
  baseline activity 374–6
  circuitry 367
  development 326–7, 340, 378
  direct pathways 367, 368
  dysfunction see dopaminergic dysfunction
  endogenous sensitization 378, 379, 393
  GABA role 367, 377
  glutamate role 367, 379
    NMDA receptors 376–7, 379
  indirect pathways 367, 368
  neuroimaging studies 370–6
  postmortem studies 368–70
  projections 366–7
    corticostriatal–thalamocortical loops 366–7, 411
    pFC 314, 365, 408
  subcortical 365–6, 380, 393, 411
    cortical regulation 376–8
  see also dopamine receptors; NMDA receptors
drug abuse see substance abuse

duration of untreated psychosis (DUP) 118–19
  outcome association 119, 692
  reduction 664
  symptom association 119
  treatment resistance 493
dyskinesias
  clozapine effects 566
  drug-induced (other than TD) 560
  hereditary 560–61
  spontaneous 560
  systemic 561
  tardive see tardive dyskinesia (TD)
dysmorphic features, comorbidity 213
dysphoria, antipsychotic-induced 143, 150, 573–4
dystonia
  acute drug-induced 553, 554, 556
  tardive 559

early onset schizophrenia see child/adolescent onset schizophrenia
early signs questionnaire 481
economics 713–23
  cost-effectiveness analysis 716–17
    atypical antipsychotics 717–19
    clinical trials 718–19
    crossovers effect 718
    incremental cost-effectiveness ratios (ICERs) 716
  cost–utility analysis 715–16
  display of information 716–17
  effectiveness of interventions 715–17
    clozapine 716, 717–19
    industrial sponsorship 719
    intent-to-treat (ITT) 717, 718
  mental illness 713
  methodological complexities 719–21
  stakeholders 714, 716
  see also costs
ECT see electroconclusive therapy (ECT)
education 661, 664
EEG see electroencephalography (EEG)
elation 22
elderly-onset see late-onset schizophrenia
electroconclusive therapy (ECT) 485, 517–51
  adjunctive/combination therapy 521, 538, 542
    clozapine and 532–3
    drug-resistant schizophrenia 506–7, 528–32, 541
    increased efficacy 521, 527, 528, 538
    monotherapy versus 525–7
  American Psychiatric Association (APA) Task Force 517
  antipsychotics versus 521–5, 542
  background 517
  catatonia 519, 534–5
  clinical trials (summaries)
    antipsychotics/insulin coma versus (prospective) 522–3
    combination versus monotherapy (prospective) 525–6
    drug-resistant patients 529–30
    sham versus real ECT (prospective) 520

unilateral versus bilateral (prospective) 537
  current practice/recommendations 517–18
  depressive disorders 517, 518, 534, 536, 538, 541
  early studies 518–19
  efficacy 517, 518–33
    as combination therapy 521, 527, 528, 538
  electrode placement 536
    left versus right 536
    modified bilateral 524, 531
    right unilateral 536
    unmodified bilateral 521, 523
  insulin coma versus 521, 522, 523
  lethal catatonia 535
  maintenance/continuation 538
  manic patients 538
  mechanism of action 434, 541–2
    antipsychotic concentration effect 541
    dopaminergic enhancement 542
    serotonergic enhancement 542
  'middle prognosis' patients 523, 527
  morbidity/mortality 538
  movement disorders 540–1
    antiparkinsonian effects 524, 543
    tardive dyskinesia treatment 541, 567
  neuroimaging 540
  neuroleptic malignant syndrome (NMS) 535–6
  outcome 519
    combination therapy 527
    drug-resistant patients 531
    duration of effects 506, 519, 520, 524
    positive predictors 533
    prediction 533–6
    sex differences 533, 534
    short- versus long-term 524, 525
  photoshock versus 519
  psychotic exacerbations 517, 532
  regressive 524, 537
  relapse rates 521, 528, 538
  remission 519
  schizoaffective disorder 530–1, 535
  schizophreniform patients 521
  sham versus real ECT 519–21, 534, 535
  side-effects 536, 538–41
    cognitive consequences 536, 539
    neuropathological 539–40
  stimulus intensity 536
  symptoms responsive to ECT 533–4, 538
  technique 536–8
  treatment duration/frequency 536–8
  variation in use 518
electroencephalography (EEG) 39, 298
  epochs 298
  event-related (evoked) potentials see event-related potentials (ERPs)
  historical aspects 298–300
  limitations 298
  mean power spectra 301
  MEG and 307
  quantitative (Q-EEG) 299
  resolution 299
  structural imaging and 299
  utility 298–9

electrophysiology 298–309
  intermediate phenotypes 286–7, 292
  see also electroencephalography (EEG);
    event-related potentials (ERPs)
emotional delusional states 58
emotional disturbance 21–2
empirical symptom dimensions and clusters,
    three-factor model 117–18
employment
  Clubhouse (Fountain House) model 647,
    695
  competitive studies 695–6
  costs of lost productivity 714
  day care (partial hospitalization) 695–6
  importance of 646, 695
  job-finding clubs 648
  mental health issues 646
  obstacles 695
  patients' perspectives 707, 709
  right to 646
  sheltered employment 647
  'social' firms 647
  supported employment 647–8, 695
  tardive dyskinesia effects 563
  unemployment rates in schizophrenia 646
  vocational rehabilitation 646–8, 695–6
empowerment (patients) 637, 661–2
encephalitis, schizophrenic symptoms 193–4
encephalopathies, paraneoplastic 193
endocrine dysfunction, antipsychotic-induced
    530–76
endophenotypes *see* intermediate phenotypes
entorhinal cortex
  neuronal disarray 312
  tyrosine hydroxylase decreases 369
environmental factors 219–20, 330
  adoption studies 256, 627
  early social 74, 626–7, 628, 701
  genetic factor interaction 279–80, 292, 627
  intrauterine 328
  lack of specific discovery 223, 279–80
  'microenvironment' 254
  nature *versus* nurture debate 252
  obstetric complications and 329
  psychological 256
  psychosocial therapy and 675
  relapse role 475
  stress *see* stress (psychosocial)
  twin studies 254
  see also families; genetic factors; life events
Epidemiologic Catchment Area (ECA) survey
    593–4
epidemiology 203–31, 331
  antecedents 215–23
    see also risk factors
  birth cohort studies 205
  case findings 204–5
  child/adolescent onset 40
  comorbidity *see* comorbidity
  door-to-door and sample surveys 204–5
  ethnicity *see* ethnicity
  extrapyramidal syndromes (EPSs) 554–6
  fertility 215
  first-reported cases 212
  geographic variation *see* geographical
    variations

instruments 206–7
  investigators 206
  morbidity measures 207
  morbid risk (disease expectancy) 211
  mortality 214
  neurodevelopmental hypothesis 327
  pregnancy and birth complications (PBCs)
    328
  prospects in search for causes 223
  season of birth 221–2, 236, 330
  secular trends 212–13
  sex differences *see* gender differences
  tardive dyskinesia (TD) 562
  urban birth 221, 236, 330
  variation sources related to investigation
    methods 203–7
  see also incidence; prevalence
epigenetic changes 335
epilepsy 580
  kindling 191
  lesions 191
  misdiagnosis of child/adolescent onset 39
  schizophrenic symptoms 190, 191
  see also seizures
episodic memory deficits 170
epistatic transmission 257
equivalent outcomes paradox 662
ergot alkaloids 370, 371
erotomania 59–60
ERPs *see* event-related potentials (ERPs)
errorless learning 645
ethnicity
  genetic markers 266
  risk factor 222–3
    tardive dyskinesia 564
event-related potentials (ERPs) 298, 299–306
  chronic schizophrenia 302, 303, 305, 306
  confounds 299
  first-episode schizophrenia 302, 303, 304,
    306
  functional imaging *versus* 299, 300
  gamma-band oscillations 299, 300–302
  historical aspects 299–300
  mismatch negativity *see* mismatch negativity
    (MMN)
  N2b component 302
  N100 component 286, 287, 299–300, 306
    attenuation, spectrum personality
      disorders 86
  N200 component 286, 306
  oddball paradigm 286, 300, 304
  p50 deficit *see* P50 sensory gating deficit
  p300 (P3) component *see* P300 (P3) ERP
    component
  prediction paradigm 300
  resolution 299, 307
  startle response 305
  utility 307
evoked potentials *see* event-related potentials
    (ERPs)
excitatory amino acid neurotransmission
  gamma-band oscillations 301
  neurodegeneration role 303–4
  see also glutamate
executive functions 45
  cognitive adaptive therapy 650

impairments 45, 170–1
  late-onset schizophrenia 71
  spectrum personality disorders 87
  risk model of deficit 45
'experimental' drug use 269
explanatory insight oriented therapy (EIO)
    671
explanatory theories 23
expressed emotion (EE) 497, 628, 701
  blood pressure analogy 620
  burden measure 621–2, 665
  CFI measures 615, 620
  changing 650
  construct validity (meaning) 618–20
  critical comments 615, 618, 619, 620
    'benign' 621
  distress level association 619
  emotional overinvolvement (EOI) 615, 619
  family intervention 617–18, 650, 664, 667
    number needed to treat (NNT) 618
    see also family interventions
  FMSS measures 615
  geographical differences 616
  high *versus* low 620
  hostility 615
  medication effect *versus* 616
  Negative Affective Style 618
  origins 620–1
  positive remarks 615
  in professional carers 621
  reactive nature 620
  reduction 48
  relapse 615–22
    high EE association 615–17
    prediction 615–18
    prospective studies 616
    rates 617
    social constraint 617
  risk factor in child/adolescent onset 41
  sex differences 616
  social outcome effect 617
  studies in high EE families 619
  warmth 615
extrapyramidal syndromes (EPSs) 552–8
  antipsychotic drug-induced 76, 150, 356,
    425, 444
  atypical antipsychotic reduction 174, 425,
    428, 555–6
  clinical manifestations 552–3
    acute dystonia 553
    akathisia *see* akathisia
    parkinsonism *see* parkinsonism
  combination therapy 499
  ECT protection against 524, 540–1, 543
  epidemiology 554–6
  management 556–8
    algorithm for 557
    anticholinergic treatment 444, 461, 556,
      558
    antihistaminergic treatment 556
    indications for anti-EPS drugs 558
    prophylaxis 556, 557
  pathophysiology 553–4
  psychological consequences 557
  spontaneous 456
  susceptibility 554

tardive dyskinesia risk factor 564
tardive dyskinesia *versus* 560
see also tardive dyskinesia
eye movement
  dysfunction 281–5, 291–2
    family studies 283–4
    genetic models 284
    inconsistencies 291
    intermediate phenotypes 279
    medication effects 282
    phenocopies 284
    schizophrenia spectrum disorders 283
    schizophrenic patients 281–2
    spectrum personality disorders 86
    tracking 281–5, 291–2
    twin studies 284
  fixation 281
  gain 281, 283
  saccades 281–2, 283
  smooth pursuit 281, 283
  see also eye tracking
eye tracking
  antisaccade task 281
  attention role 282
  confounds 282, 283
  gain 281, 283
  genetic component 284
  measures 281
  methodological problems 284
  neurobiology 21
  root mean square (RMS) error 281, 283
  saccades 281–2, 283
  see also eye movement

families 615
  bidirectional interactions 618–19
  communication deviance 618
  coping style 620, 622
  genetic studies *see* family studies
  interventions *see* family interventions
  personality studies 619
    see also expressed emotion (EE)
family burden 615, 620, 665
  costs 714
  measures 621–2
  violence and 598
  see also expressed emotion (EE)
family interventions 48, 444, 475, 481, 497,
    606, 650–1, 664–78
  advocacy/consumer movements 665
  benefits 650
  care, impact of 664–5
  efficacy 665
  expressed emotion (EE) 617–18, 650, 664,
    667
  'Falloon' style interventions 667
  future directions 667
  implementation 667
  long-term 665–6
  models 665
  need-adapted approach 673
  number needed to treat (NNT) 618
  relapse rates 666
  short-term 665
  strategies 665–6
  timing of 667

treatment strategies for schizophrenia (TSS)
    666–7
family studies 251–2
  depressive patients 154
  see also genetics; genetic studies
fananserin 423
feelings 21
  intensification of 21
  loss of *see* anhedonia
fertility 215
fetal hypoxia 240–1
first-episode psychosis 118–20, 210–11
  early detection 663–4, 678, 679
    services 692
  ERPs 302, 303, 304
  relapse/remission 459
  treatment 456, 459–60
    atypical drugs 460
    early intervention 457
    maintenance 477
    response rate 459
first-rank symptoms 5, 26
  see also positive symptoms
Fisher344 rats 395
Five Minute Speech Sample (FMSS) 615
flashbacks, psychosis *versus* 626
flattening of affect 21
flight of ideas 20
flunitrazepam 457
fluoxetine 483
flupenthixol 531
fluphenazine
  depot preparation 478
  dose reduction 480
folie à deux see shared psychotic disorders
    (*folie à deux*)
Foucault's concept of schizophrenia 3
Fountain House model 646, 695
free radicals
  photosensitivity 578
  reduction 567
  tardive dyskinesia 561, 567
frontal cortex 406–8
  dysfunction 87, 93
    eye tracking 282
    frontal–temporal disconnection 412–13
    see also cognitive impairment
  metabolism defects 494
  MRS studies 407
  neuropsychology 407–8
  prefrontal *see* prefrontal cortex (PFC)
  volume reduction 42, 91
    grey matter 406–7
    staging 407
fundamental symptoms 22, 25

GABA 354–6
  cognitive function 356
  membrane transporter (GAT) 316, 319,
    355–6
  neuropathology 316–17, 355–6
  psychopharmacological studies 356
  receptors 356
  serotonin and 354
  tardive dyskinesia hypothesis 561, 567
GABAergic interneurones 354–5

chandelier neurones 316–17, 355–6
  dopamine and 367, 368, 377
  dorsal prefrontal cortex pathology 315,
    316–17
  dysfunction 355–6
  gamma-band oscillations 301
  neurodevelopmental hypothesis 355
  NMDA antagonist effects 455
  reductions 354
GAD *see* glutamic acid decarboxylase (GAD)
galactorrhoea, hyperprolactinaemia effect 575
gamma-aminobutyric acid *see* GABA
GAP-43 reduction 337
gender differences
  age of onset 215
    child/adolescent onset 40
    late-onset 73
  expressed emotion (EE) 616
  extrapyramidal syndromes 555
  genetic studies 252
    X chromosome linkage 265–6
  marital status as risk factor 222
  mortality rate 214
  outcome prediction 533
  progression of brain changes in males 116
  refractoriness 493
  social course 124–5
  tardive dyskinesia 563
genetic counselling 268–9
genetic disorders
  complex traits 256–7, 266, 277, 279
  heterogeneity 257–8
  insulin-dependent diabetes 266
  minor physical abnormalities (MPAs)
    associations 233
  schizophrenia associations 194–6
  single *versus* multiple genes 256–7
  tardive dyskinesia *versus* 560–1
genetic factors 216–18, 269, 341
  environmental factor interaction 279–80,
    292, 627
  genotype relative risk (GRR) 262, 266
  high-risk child cases 217–18
  late-onset, aetiology 71–2
  liability curve 256
  lifetime risk 251, 252, 269
  markers 217
  neurodevelopmental hypothesis 329,
    341
  obstetric complication interaction 329
  pandysmaturation syndrome 217
  structural abnormalities 216–18, 288
  susceptibility genes 262, 267–8, 278, 390,
    395
  tardive dyskinesia 564
  ventricular enlargement 406
  violence 596
  see also environmental factors
genetic mapping 262
genetic markers
  classical 260, 262
  DNA *see* DNA markers
genetic models 389, 394–6
genetics 251–76, 341
  animal models 389, 394–6
  anticipation 258, 268

candidate genes/loci 262, 267–8, 278, 390, 395
child/adolescent onset 44
chromosomal loci implicated 262–6
cognitive impairment 280
eye tracking 284
heterogeneity 257–8, 277
intermediate phenotypes *see* intermediate phenotypes
molecular neurobiology 268
nature *versus* nurture debate 252
negative symptoms 30, 44, 285
neurodevelopmental genes 395
non-genetic components 254–5, 392
penetrance 256
phenocopies 255
phenotype misclassification 277
prenatal/presymptomatic testing 269
risk factors *see* genetic factors
schizophrenia spectrum personality disorders 84, 255
schizotypy 84, 285
studies *see* genetic studies
transmission mode 256–7, 269
    complexity 277
    dominance 257
    epistasis 257
    variance 279–80, 284
see also environmental factors
genetic studies 30
    adoption studies *see* adoption studies
    anomalies 251–2
    association studies *see* association studies
    Bezugsziffer (BZ) 251
    cognitive impairment 179
    controls 252
    depressive patients 154–5
    diagnostic criteria and 252, 253, 277
    family studies 251–2
        design 279–80
        eye tracking 283–4
    genome screens 262
    intermediate phenotypes 277–96
        design 280–1
    linkage *see* linkage studies
    'loaded' families 262, 269
        pedigree analysis 257–8
    loci identification attempts 216–17
    model fitting 253–4
    polydiagnostic approach 252
    quantitative measures 278–9
    repeat expansion analysis 268
    twin studies *see* twin studies
genetic variance 279–80, 284
genome, variation 260
genome screens 262
genotype relative risk (GRR) 262, 266
geographical variations 330, 696
    developing countries 129
    expressed emotion (EE) 616
    populations and groups 211–12
gliosis 310–11
    absence 41, 42, 310–11, 326
    reactive astrocytosis 310
    in utero timing 311
globus pallidum 366

glucose metabolism rate (GMR), functional imaging 91
glutamate
    animal models of schizophrenia 390, 394, 397, 454
        see also glutamate hypothesis
    cortical distribution 349
    dopamine and 367, 376–7, 379
    novel antipsychotics 434, 453–6
    psychopharmacological studies 351–2
    receptors 350–1
        AMPA *see* AMPA receptors
        kainate 350, 455
        metabotropic 350, 455
        NMDA *see* NMDA receptors
        sensitization 455
    release inhibiting drugs 455
    tardive dyskinesia role 561
glutamate hypothesis 349–52, 453–4
    animal models 389, 390, 394
glutamic acid decarboxylase (GAD) 315, 316, 355
glycine, NMDA receptor modulation
    glycine site agonists 454–5, 461
    glycine uptake inhibition 455
goal-directed behaviour 661
    personal therapy 677–8
goal-oriented therapeutic contracting 645–6
    stages 646
G-protein
    dopamine receptor linkage 368
    olfactory (GOLF) 265
grey matter volume reductions 42, 116, 288
    frontal cortex 406–7
Griesinger's concept of schizophrenia 3–4
guilt proneness, in relatives 619
gynaecomastia, hyperprolactinaemia effects 575

habituation, spectrum personality disorders 85–6
hallucinations 15–17
    Alzheimer's disease 192
    auditory *see* auditory verbal hallucinations (AVHs)
    clinical outcome 533
    definitions and classification 15–16
    ECT response 534
    hippocampus role 411
    incidence and variety 16–17
    neuroimaging 409, 411
    neuropsychological investigations 175–7
    patients' perspectives 708
    reality/source monitoring 176–7
    subtypes 16
    temporal cortex role 409
    visual 17
    voice 16–17, 176
        see also auditory verbal hallucinations (AVHs)
hallucinatory psychosis, chronic 58–9
hallucinogenic drugs 353–4
    psychosis induction 39–40, 353, 702
    see also specific drugs
haloperidol 47–8

atypical antipsychotics *versus* 445, 446, 447, 458, 501
cost-effectiveness, clozapine *versus* 717
depot preparation 478
dysphoria induction 574
ECT and 527
extrapyramidal symptoms 555
first-episode patients 460
late-onset schizophrenia treatment 76
schizotypal personality disorder treatment 91
side-effects
    hyperprolactinaemia 575
    QTc prolongation 578
    SIADH 576
    thyroid toxicity 576
    weight gain 576
working memory deficits 574
Hamilton Depression Rating Scale (HAM-D) 143
handedness studies 335–6
    inconsistency 89
'hard-wiring' symptoms, dopamine role 379
HCR-20 risk assessment 601
head injury, schizophrenic symptoms 190, 191–2
health belief model 599
hepatic toxicity, antipsychotics 579–80
Heschl's gyrus 304
hippocampal formation 410–11
    asymmetry 336, 410
    development 318
        genetics 395–6
        lesion models 390, 392, 393, 395
        prefrontal cortex role 392, 393
    hippocampal–prefrontal relationship 317, 392, 393, 412
        delayed onset role 339, 392
    neuropathological findings 311–13, 336
        functional imaging 311–12, 411
        morphometric 312, 333
        structural imaging 410–11
        synaptic/dendritic 312–13
    obstetric complications and 410
    symptom expression 411
    volume reductions 42, 288, 311, 410–11
        inconsistencies 332, 410
        neuronal loss 312
        progression 410
        twin studies 410
HLA antigens *see* human leucocyte antigens (HLA)
homeobox genes 395–6
home treatment 692
homicide 592–3
homocystinuria 195
homovanillic acid (HVA)
    cerebrospinal fluid levels 90
    decreases in first-degree relatives 286
    postmortem studies 368–9
    relation to drug resistance 496
hospitalization 692–4
    acute pharmacological treatment 443–4
    availability 692
    beds 692–3
    costs 692–3

discharge from 694
duration 693
outcome studies 103–4, 693, 694
partial (day care) 694–6
pressure on 693
rates 693
  decline in 212
role 692–3
therapeutic environment 693–4
violence management 603–4
voluntary *versus* compulsory admission 693
see also inpatients; mental health services
hospital samples, case findings 204
hostility, treatment 443
  clozapine 500
  valproate 505
5-HT (5-hydroxytryptamine) *see* serotonin
human leucocyte antigens (HLA) 260, 262
  association studies 267
  ethnicity 266
  HLA 9 267
  HLA-A9 linkage 264
  HLA BW16 266
Huntington's disease
  antipsychotic treatment 565
  schizophrenia associations 194
  tardive dyskinesia *versus* 560–1
HVA *see* homovanillic acid (HVA)
5-hydroxytryptamine (5-HT) *see* serotonin
hyperprolactinaemia 575–6
  amisulpride 428
  clinical side-effects 575, 577
  D_2 blockade and 425
  haloperidol 575
  olanzapine 575–6
  risperidone 431, 575
hypofrontality 43
hypogonadism, hyperprolactinaemia effect 575
hypomanic symptoms 122
hypoxia, fetal 240–1

idiopathic focal dystonias 560
IEPA (International Early Psychosis Association) 678
illogicality 20
illusion des sosies 59
illusions 15, 17
image analysis 312
imaginative psychosis, chronic 59
immune disorders, tardive dyskinesia *versus* 561
inappropriate affect (parathymia) 21
incidence 209–11
  broad and narrow cases 209, 211
  catatonia 19
  child/adolescent onset 40
  delusions 17–18
  depression 122, 143, 144–9
  disturbance of emotion 21–2
  extrapyramidal syndromes 554–5
  first-episode psychosis 210–11
  hallucinations 16–17
  problems with definition 209
  secular trends 212–13
  studies 210

thought disorder 20–1
incoherence 20
inconsistent handedness 89
incremental cost-effectiveness ratios (ICERs) 716
industrialized countries, course and outcome variations 129
infection as risk factor
  postnatal infections 219
  prenatal infections 219, 241, 242–4, 255
    animal models 390–1
    neurodevelopmental hypothesis 329–30, 390–1
    second trimester 329
  respiratory 219
  schizophrenic symptoms 193–4
influenza, *in utero* exposure 219, 241, 242–4, 329
  animal model 390–1
information-processing deficits 28
  spectrum personality disorders 84–6, 86–9
inner speech, neuropsychology 176
inpatients
  patients' perspectives 704–5
  skills training 643
  token economy/social learning 640–1
  violence management 603–4
  see also hospitalization
insulin coma 521, 522, 523
Integrated Psychological Therapy (IPT) model 644–5, 676
intellectual decline 22
intellectual delusional states 58
intelligence quotient (IQ) 220
  reduction in child/adolescent onset 35, 44, 45–6
intent-to-treat (ITT) 717, 718
intermediate phenotypes 277–96
  assumptions 278
  characteristics 278–9
  clinical phenotypes 285, 292
  cognitive phenotypes 289–91
  concept 278
  controls 280, 283
  electrophysiological phenotypes 286–7
  eye tracking dysfunction (ETD) 281–5, 291–2
  genetic variance 279–80
    environment 279–80, 292
    epidemiological approach 279
  identification 277
  inconsistencies 291
  methodological issues 278–81, 292
  neurochemical phenotypes 286
  neuroimaging 287–9
    see also neuroimaging studies
    see also event-related potentials (ERPs)
International Classification of Disease-10 (ICD-10) 9, 10–12
  acute and transient psychotic disorders 63–4
  atypical psychotic disorders 62–4
  delusional disorders 62–3, 69
  diagnostic criteria 10–11
  induced delusional disorder 64
  late-onset schizophrenia 69–70

schizoaffective disorder 64
schizotypal personality disorder 64
International Early Psychosis Association (IEPA) 678
International Pilot Study of Schizophrenia (IPSS) 205
International Study of Schizophrenia 128
interneurones
  GABAergic *see* GABAergic interneurones
  prefrontal cortex 316–17
interpretive psychosis, chronic 58
interviews 206
intraclass correlation coefficient (ICC) 280
intracranial volume (ICV) 406
intradimensional and extradimensional set shifting (ID/ED) deficits 170–1
intrauterine environment 328
  insults 255, 280
  see also infection as risk factor; neurodevelopmental hypothesis
investigator allegiance 662–3
ion channels 268, 350
  see also specific types
isolation role 629

jealousy 59
jimson weed 357
jobs *see* employment

kainate receptors 350, 455
  reduction in schizophrenia 351
Kallman's syndrome 196
Kennard principle 339
ketamine 351, 379
  amphetamine-induced dopamine release 377
  animal models of schizophrenia 394
  psychopharmacological studies 351–2
  psychosis 351, 452
Klinefelter's syndrome 194
knight's move thinking 20
Kraepelin, E. 657
  classification of psychoses 54
  concept of schizophrenia 4, 25, 326

lack of will 22
lamotrigine, clozapine adjunct 505
language development disorders 35, 38–9
latent inhibition 88
latent schizophrenia 4, 80
late-onset schizophrenia 68–79
  aetiology 71–4
    brain abnormalities, imaging 72–3
    gender 73
    genetic factors 71–2
    premorbid personality and other factors 74
    sensory deficits 73–4
  clinical features 70–1
  diagnostic guidelines 69–70
  historical development 68–70
  management and treatment 74–7
    cognitive and behavioural interventions 75
    medication *see* antipsychotic drugs
    rehousing 75

paraphrenia *see* paraphrenia
terminology and future classification 70
lateralization 89
Law 180 (Italy; 1978) 688
legal issues
    coercion/security 607
    Community Mental Health Centers
        (CMHC) Act (USA; 1979) 688–9
    compulsory treatment orders 607, 706
    criminal justice costs 714
    Disability Discrimination Act (UK; 1995)
        695
    Law 180 (Italy; 1978) 688
    Mental Health Act 607, 706
    mental health legislation reform 591–2
    Mental Health Treatment Act (UK; 1930)
        688
    Rehabilitation Act Amendments (USA;
        1996) 695
    *Tarasoff vs Regents of University of
        California*; duty to warn 592
    violence 591–2
    vulnerability of patients 600
lesion models 390, 392–4
lethal catatonia 535, 581
leucopenia 580
leucoplakia 580
Lewis–Murray scale 236
Lewy body dementia 356
Lhx5 homeobox genes 395–6
life events 622–5, 628–9
    bipolar disorder 625
    cultural setting 623
    dating events 622
    depression 152
    increased sensitivity to 625
    'inventory' approach 622
    LEDS 622
    priming event 629
    range of events reaction 622
    relapse relationship 627
    single event reaction 622
    studies 623–4
        prospective 622–3
        retrospective 622
    survival function 625
    triggering concept 623, 629
Life Events and Inventory Schedule (LEDS)
    622
lifetime prevalence 207
limbic encephalitis 193
limbic system 366
    amygdalo-hippocampal complex 410–11
    encephalitis 193
    see also amygdala; hippocampal formation
linkage disequilibrium 260, 262, 281
linkage studies 262–6
    association studies *versus* 280
    complex traits 259–60
        problems 261
    correlated phenotypes 217
    eye tracking dysfunction 284–5
    genotype relative risk (GRR) 262, 266
    heterogeneity 259
    identical by descent 259
    identical by state 259

independent assortment 258
intermediate phenotypes 280
LOD scores 259, 261
markers 259
    chromosomal linkages 262–6, 287
    classical 260, 262
    DNA 260–1
    NMDA receptors 351
    non-parametric linkage (NPL) 259
        problems 262
    principles 258–62
    problems 261–2, 280
    recombination and crossover 258–9, 261
    Schizophrenia Linkage Collaborative Group
        263–4
    see also association studies
lithium 483
    adjunctive therapy 448, 483, 503–4
        drug interactions 504
    depression management in patients 160
    eye tracking effects 282
liver toxicity, antipsychotics 579–80
Locke, John 3
locus heterogeneity 258
long-term depression (LTD) 379
long-term potentiation (LTP) 379
loosening of associations 20
lorazepam 457
low birth weight (LBW) 240
LSD (lysergic acid diethylamide) 379
    psychopharmacology 353
    serotonin receptor binding 352, 353
lung cancer, negative comorbidity 213
LY-354740 455
lymphocytic choriomeningitis virus (LCMV)
    391
lysergic acid diethylamide *see* LSD (lysergic
    acid diethylamide)

M-100907 (formerly MDL-100,907) 451
'MacArthur' violence risk assessment study
    592, 597, 598, 600, 601–2
Magical Ideation Scale (MIS) 285
magnetic resonance imaging (MRI) 29, 335,
    404–5
    depressive patients 153
    functional (fMRI) 287, 289, 404, 405
        BOLD fMRI 299, 405
        ERPs *versus* 300
        treatment response 494
    inconsistencies 332
    interpretation 332
    late-onset schizophrenia 72
    neurodevelopmental hypothesis and 331–2,
        335, 337
        inconsistencies 332
        twin studies 335
    principles 404
    resolution 299
    secondary schizophrenias 189
    spectrum personality disorders 91
    structural abnormalities 288
    T2-relaxometry 404
    volumetric/morphologic measurement
        404
    white matter analysis (DTI/DWI) 404–5

magnetic resonance spectroscopy (MRS) 43,
    404
    frontal cortex 407
    glutamate abnormalities 350
    hippocampus 411
magnetization transfer imaging (MTI) 405
magnetoencephalography (MEG) 302, 306–7
    M100 component 307
magnocellular system, spectrum personality
    disorders 86–7
maintenance treatment 443, 474–88
    adherence 477
    clinical trials 476
    comorbid condition management 481–5
        anxiety disorders 483–4
        cognitive deficits 482
        depression 482–3
        mood effects 483
        negative symptoms 481–2
        substance abuse 484–5
        see also individual conditions
    drug selection 478–9
    duration 477
    early intervention 457, 480–1
    ECT 538
    effectiveness of long-term therapy 476–7
    effect on functional outcome 481
    first-episode patients 477
    guidelines 477
    long-acting depot preparations 478–9
        bioavailability 479
        oral drugs *versus* 478
        side-effects 478
    multiepisode patients 477
    need for 637
    pharmacological–psychosocial interactions
        485
    side-effects 476
        adherence factor 477
    strategies 380, 479–81
        continuous use 456
        dose reduction 479–80
        prodromal monitoring 480–1
    typical *versus* atypical drugs 479
        clozapine 500
    see also relapses
malnutrition 219, 329, 390
    neurological consequences for fetus 241,
        244
mania
    ECT and 538
    misdiagnosis of child/adolescent onset 38
    symptoms 122
Mannheim cohort 129
Marfan's syndrome 195
marital status
    risk factor 222
    role in social course 123
marker genes, linkage studies 259
masking deficit, spectrum personality disorders
    87
maternal effects
    influenza as risk factor 219, 241, 242–4
    stress as risk factor 219, 244, 330
    see also infection as risk factor; pregnancy
        and birth complications (PBCs)

Maudsley Assessment of Delusions Schedule
  (MADS) 597
Maudsley Child and Adolescent Psychosis
  Follow-up Study 37
mazindol 433
m-chlorophenylpiperazine (mCPP) 354
media coverage 591, 592–3, 711–12
Medicaid fomularies 719
medication see antipsychotic drugs; specific
  drugs
MEG see magnetoencephalography (MEG)
meiotic recombination 258–9
memory impairment 22, 88–9, 290–1
  child/adolescent onset disease 44–5
  declarative memory 290
  episodic memory 170
  hippocampus role 411
  positron emission tomography (PET) 411
  schizotypal personality disorder 88–9
  sensory memory 304
  verbal 290
  working memory see working memory
  see also cognitive impairment
menstruation, hyperprolactinaemia effect 575
Mental Health Act 607, 706
mental health legislation see legal issues
mental health policy
  psychosocial interventions and 676
  service integration 697
mental health problems
  changing perspectives 688
  disabilities 638, 689
  economics 713
  employment issues 646
  handicaps 638
  humanist approach to 658–9
  impairments 638
mental health services 688–700
  acute hospital care 692–4
    see also hospitalization
  asylums 688
  availability 692
  child/adolescent onset treatment 48
  community see community care
  components 689–90
  consumer movement 665, 678
  core elements 689–90
  day care/partial hospitalization 694–6
    admission alternative 694–5
    drop-out rate 694
    employment services 695–6
      see also employment
  evaluation 696–7
  evidence-based strategies 696
  exclusion from, substance abusers 484
  history 688
  integration 696–7
  international challenges 689
  Israel 676
  organization/delivery 48, 639–41, 696
  patients' perspectives 701–12
  policy issues 676
  principles 689
  reform movement 688
  state of 637
  see also legal issues; rehabilitation

Mental Health Treatment Act (UK; 1930) 688
mental retardation association 220
mescaline 353
mesocortical system 366
  glutamate role 394
mesolimbic system 366
  dopamine sensitization 378
  glutamate role 394
metabolic disorders 193
  tardive dyskinesia and 563
  tardive dyskinesia versus 561
  see also specific disorders
metabotropic receptors
  dopamine see dopamine receptors
  glutamate (mGluRs) 350
    agonists 455
metachromatic leucodystrophy (MLD) 193
  functional 'dysconnection' 340–1
  misdiagnosis of child/adolescent onset 39
  schizophrenic symptoms 193
metacognition 704
methylazoxymethanol acetate (MAM),
  neurogenesis disruption 391
methyldopa (Aldomet) 566
microsatellite DNA (simple sequence repeats;
  SSR) 260–1
microtubule-associated protein-2 (MAP-2)
  313
midazolam 457
migrant status, as risk factor 222–3
MIND (National Association for Mental
  Health) 665, 678
minor physical abnormalities (MPAs) 232
  comorbidity 213
  craniofacial 330
  dermatoglyphic see dermatoglyphic
    abnormalities
  disturbed development 232–3, 330–1
  genetic disorder associations 233
  interpretation limitations 331
  late-onset schizophrenia 74
  medication effects 331
  studies 233, 234
mismatch negativity (MMN) 299, 300, 302–4
  bilateral generation 302
  negative symptom correlation 302
  neurodegeneration link 303–4
  NMDA receptor activity 302, 303, 304
  pitch 302, 303
  progressive reduction 303
  sensory memory 304
models 26–8
  type I/type II 491, 493
molecular neurobiology 268, 337
monoamine oxidase (MAO) inhibitors,
  depression management 156
mood
  delusional 16
  disorders see affective disorders
  drug effects 573–4
  instability 483
  stabilization 483, 503–5
morbidity
  chronic schizophrenia 460
  electroconculsive therapy (ECT) 538
  measures 207

morbid jealousy 59
morbid risk (disease expectancy) 211
mortality 214
  in child/adolescent onset 46
  crude mortality rate (CMR) 123
  electroconvulsive therapy (ECT) 538
  neuroleptic malignant syndrome 581
  standard mortality rate (SMR) 123, 214
motion sensitivity, magnocellular deficits 87
motivation 21, 709, 710
motor disorders
  child/adolescent onset 35
  extrapyramidal see extrapyramidal
    syndromes (EPSs)
  schizophrenic phenomena 6
  tardive dyskinesia see tardive dyskinesia
    (TD)
MRI see magnetic resonance imaging (MRI)
MRS see magnetic resonance spectroscopy
  (MRS)
multidimensionally impaired syndrome (MDI),
  misdiagnosis 39
multidisciplinary approach, community care
  690
multiepisode patient, treatment 456
  maintenance 477
multifactorial threshold model (MFT) 256–7
multiple sclerosis, secondary schizophrenia
  192
muscarinic receptors see under acetylcholine
music therapy 677
mutism 20

N2b ERP component 302
N100 ERP component 86, 286, 287,
  299–300, 306
N200 component 286, 306
N-acetylaspartate (NAA) signal 43
  dorsal prefrontal cortex 313, 376, 407
  hippocampus 311
N-acetylaspartyl glutamate (NAAG) 351
naltrexone 484
NAMI (National Alliance for the Mentally Ill)
  665, 678
National Alliance for the Mentally Ill (NAMI)
  665, 678
National Association for Mental Health
  (MIND) 665, 678
National Confidential Inquiry (NCI)
  homicide rates 593
  violence prevention 602
National Institute of Mental Health
  millennium schizophrenia genome screen
    264
  treatment strategies for schizophrenia (TSS)
    666–7
  Treatment Strategies in Schizophrenia study
    481
National Institutes of Health Consensus
  Development Panel on ECT use 518
National Schizophrenia Fellowship (NSF)
  665, 703
nature versus nurture debate 252
need-adapted approach 658, 671–4
  case study 672–3
  evidence for 671–2

hermeneutic basis 673
medication role 673
outcome studies 673–4
Negative Affective Style, expressed emotion 618
negative symptoms 6, 15, 114–15
  akinesia differentiation 553
  assessment difficulties 27
  associated conditions 30
  child/adolescent onset 36
  correlations
    cognitive impairment 30, 115–16
    functional outcome 173, 491–2
  course 28, 116
  depression resemblance 150–1
  fluctuation 492
  genetics 30, 44, 285
  history 25–6
  intermediate phenotypes 285
  late-onset schizophrenia 70
  management 481–2, 605
    antidepressant effects 449–50, 506
    atypical antipsychotic effect 429, 446, 460–1, 482, 491
    ECT 538
    NMDA receptor modulation 482
  mismatch negativity and 302
  neuroimaging studies 43
  neuropsychological tests 175
  premorbid behaviours 83
  primary/deficit syndromes 115, 482, 491
  prognostic significance 28–9
    social course indicator 125
    symptom-related course indicator 126
    treatment-resistant schizophrenia 491–2
  secondary/non-deficit syndromes 115, 481, 482, 491, 661
  social factors association 125, 614
  stability 28
  violence association 605
neologisms 20
neural cell adhesion molecules (NCAMs) 395
  PSA-NCAM reduction 337, 395
neural circuitry-based model 317–18
neurobiological correlates 29–30
  cerebral ventricles 255
  molecular 268
  neural systems, late-maturing 339
  see also brain; specific regions
neurochemistry 286, 349–64
  antipsychotic drugs 304, 352, 375, 447, 494
    resistance to 496
  cholinergic hypothesis 356–7
  dopamine hypothesis see dopamine hypothesis
  GABA hypothesis 354–6
  glutamate hypothesis 349–52
  imaging in depressive patients 153
  serotonin hypothesis 352–4
  see also specific neurotransmitters
neurocognitive deficits see cognitive impairment
neurocysticercosis 194
neurodegeneration 310–11, 443, 457, 494
  Alzheimer's disease link 311
  evidence against 326, 332, 337–8

see also neurodevelopmental hypothesis
excitatory amino acid role 303–4
gliosis 310–11
mismatch negativity and 302
progressive 302, 304
tardive dyskinesia 561
see also neuropathology; progressive brain changes
neurodegenerative disorders 116
  schizophrenia, misdiagnosis 39
neurodevelopmental hypothesis 28, 232, 326–48
  adult changes 327
  asymmetry and 335–6
  cortical gyral development 335
  dopaminergic involvement 326–7, 376, 379–80
  epidemiological studies 327
  functional 'dysconnection' 340–1
    see also cortical connectivity
  GABAergic interneurones and 355
  intrauterine infection 329–30, 390–1
  malnutrition 329, 390
  minor physical abnormalities (MPAs) 232–3, 330–1
  models 41–2, 389, 390–4
    aetiological 390–1
    candidate processes 341
    delayed onset 338–41
    early onset schizophrenia 41–2, 43–4
    implications 43–4
    late-onset schizophrenia 74
    neonatal lesion 390, 392–4, 396
    neurogenesis 391–2
    perinatal stress 392
    risk model 42
    weaknesses 41
  neurodegeneration versus 332, 337–8
  neuroimaging studies 327, 331–6
    CT analysis 331
    MRI challenge 332, 335
    PET scans 335–6
  neuronal migration disturbance 312, 318
    GABAergic 355
  neuropathological evidence 318–19, 326, 327–37, 414
    gliosis findings 311, 326
    neuronal disarray 312, 335, 390
    postmortem studies 336–7
    see also neuropathology
  obstetric abnormalities 327–9
    see also pregnancy and birth complications (PBCs)
  Occam's razor approach 339
  plausibility 393
  premorbid neurological/behavioural abnormalities 331
  public health implications 341–2
  relation to other developmental diseases 319
  second trimester importance 329, 330, 335
  strengths/weaknesses 342
  synaptic abnormalities 41, 337, 338, 339, 341
  twin studies 255, 335
  ventricular size and 327, 331–2

see also development; genetics
neurogenesis
  animal models of disruption 391–2
  cytoarchitectonic neuropathology 335–6
neuroimaging studies 29, 43, 403–17
  depressive patients 153–4
  developmental disease 327, 331–6
  disorganization syndrome 43
  dopaminergic systems 370–6, 424–5
    amphetamine-induced changes 372, 374
    baseline activity 374–6
    receptors 370–2
    striatal presynaptic DA 373
  functional 298–9, 405
    D_2 receptor blockade 424–5
    hippocampal dysfunction 311–12
    treatment response 494
  history 403–4
  intermediate phenotypes 287–9
  late-onset schizophrenia 72–3
  negative symptoms 43
  positive symptoms 43, 409
  resolution 299
  secondary schizophrenias 188–9
  spectrum personality disorders 90–1
  structural 90–1, 287–8, 404–5
    connectivity assessment 416
    depression 153
    ECT effects 540
    tardive dyskinesia 562
  techniques 404–5
  treatment-resistant schizophrenia 493–5
  twins 255, 288–9
  volumetric studies 406
  see also specific regions; specific techniques
neuroleptic malignant syndrome (NMS) 535–6, 581
neuroleptics see antipsychotic drugs
neurological disorders
  neurodevelopmental hypothesis and 331, 340
  neuropsychiatry comparative studies 171–2
  see also specific disorders
neurological signs, refractoriness 493
neuronal metabolism, investigations 43
neuronal migration, disturbance 312, 318, 355
neuropathology 310–25
  antipsychotic drugs and 311, 316, 319, 494
  asymmetry 317, 335–6
  child/adolescent onset schizophrenia 41–4
  clinicopathological relationship 317–18
  connectivity 316–17, 412–13
    prefrontal cortex 314–16, 335, 376
    see also cortical connectivity
  cytoarchitectonics 335–6, 391
  dementia correlates 311
  dendritic see dendritic abnormalities
  developmental disease evidence 311, 312, 318–19, 326, 327–37
  ECT and 539–40
  entorhinal cortex 336
  gliosis see gliosis
  hippocampus see hippocampal formation
  image analysis 312
  interpretation 317–20

key findings 317
molecular biology 336
morphometric findings 332, 333–4
  hippocampal 312
  prefrontal 313–14
neuroimaging *see* neuroimaging studies
prefrontal cortex *see* prefrontal cortex
specificity 319
synaptic *see* synaptic abnormalities
tardive dyskinesia 562
see also neurodegeneration;
    neurodevelopmental hypothesis;
    specific regions
neurophysiological abnormalities, drug
  resistance 496
neuroplasticity 332, 341
  positive symptoms 379
neuropsychiatry comparative studies 171–2
neuropsychology 30, 168, 289–91
  behavioural abnormalities 289–90
  child/adolescent onset schizophrenia 44–6
  cognitive impairment 168–9, 171, 289–91,
    292
  delusions 177–8
  depression 154
  disorganization syndrome 175
  drug-resistant disease 497–8
  following ECT 539
  frontal cortex abnormality 407–8
  hallucinations 175–7
  negative symptoms 175
  prefrontal cortex (PFC) 407–8
  psychomotor poverty syndrome 175
  psychotic symptoms 175–9
  reality monitoring 176–7
  reasoning 177–8
  risk factor markers 220
  source monitoring 176–7
  thought disorder 178–9
  twin studies 172–3
  validity of impairments 172–3
  see also specific tests
neurotoxicity 337
nicotine, eye tracking effects 282
nicotinic receptors *see under* acetylcholine
Niemann–Pick type C disease 195
nigrostriatal system 366, 367, 554
  see also striatum
nitric oxide synthase inhibition 391
NMDA receptors 349–50
  5-HT_{2A} antagonist modulation 452
  animal models of schizophrenia 390, 394,
    395, 397, 454
  antagonist effects 455
  antipsychotic drugs 434, 482
    atypical 304
  cognitive role 352
  dopamine and 368, 376–7, 379
  event-related potentials 302, 303, 306
  genes 350
  glycine site agonists 454–5, 461
  hypofunction hypothesis 453–4
  ketamine binding 351–2, 394, 453
  linkage studies 351
  MK801 binding 350
  neurodegeneration role 304, 443

tradive dyskinesia 561
phencyclidine (PCP) binding 306, 349–50,
  394, 453
  sensory gating role 302
  subunit alterations 350
NNC01-1689 423
Noonan's syndrome 194
NOTCH4 gene 268
novel antipsychotics *see* atypical antipsychotic
  drugs
nucleus accumbens, dopamine release 452
nutrition, prenatal 241, 244
  see also malnutrition

obsessive–compulsive disorder 484, 506
obstetric complications *see* pregnancy and
  birth complications (PBCs)
occupancy (receptor)
  $5\text{-HT}_{2A/C}$ receptors 424, 427
  D_2 receptor 375, 424–5, 459
    amisulpride 428
    clozapine 427
    extrastriatal occupancy *versus* 424–5
    side-effects and 424, 425, 553, 556
  D_2 receptor *versus* 5-HT receptors 424–5,
    430
  D_4 receptors 553
  treatment resistance 494
occupational therapy, cognitive remediation
  versus 644
oculocutaneous albinism 195
oculography 281
oestrogen
  protective effect 215
  replacement therapy 575
olanzapine 429–30, 502–3
  advantages 479
  chronic disease 460–1
  clinical trials 429, 445, 447, 458, 502–3
  cognitive benefits 174, 461–2
  costs 719, 720
  depression treatment 445
  dose range 429, 503
  drug-resistant disease 502–3
  efficacy 445
  EPS profile 555
  first-episode patients 460
  formulations 458
  high-dose treatments 502
  late-onset schizophrenia treatment 76
  pharmacological profile 429
  preclinical testing 429
  side-effects 429–30
    diabetes 577
    hyperprolactinaemia 575–6
    QTc prolongation 578
    weight gain 429–30, 576
  violence treatment 605
Olsen's classification system 114
onset 45
  age of 338, 492–3
    juvenile *see* child/adolescent onset
     schizophrenia
    late *see* late-onset schizophrenia
  delayed
    animal models 392

mechanisms 74, 338–41
difficulties in identification 209
gender differences 215
indicator studies 119–20
violence association 595
operant conditioning, token economy 640
orbitofrontal cortex 406
organic delusional syndrome 187
organic disease 187–8
  classification problems 187–8
  co-occurence of schizophrenia-like
    symptoms 190–1
organic hallucinosis 187
organic mental disorders 187
orgasm, antipsychotic effects 577
Orientation–Remedial Module 644
orofacial dyskinesia, spontaneous 560
orthostatic hypotension 578
Othello syndrome 59
outcome 101–41
  catch-up prospective studies 111
  child/adolescent onset 46
  description measures 112–13
  domains 112
  DUP association 119, 692
  ECT effects 519
  follow-up studies 103–4
  functional
    drug-resistant patients 489
    inpatients 694
    maintenance therapy effect 481
  geographical variation 129–30
  indicators 101, 279, 533
  longitudinal studies 326
  long-term studies 104–10
  methodological aspects 102–13
    assessment scales 112
    requirements for studies 102–3
  need-adapted approaches 673–4
  patients' perspectives 709
  quality of life 130
  real-time studies 111
  social, EE effect 617
  vocational rehabilitation 647–8
  see also course of disease
outpatient populations, case findings 204
overinclusion 19–20
oxidative stress, tardive dyskinesia 561
oxypertine 566

P50 sensory gating deficit 174
  linkage studies 265, 278, 280, 287, 292,
    306, 395
  spectrum personality disorders 85
P300 (P3) ERP component 286, 292, 299,
  300, 304–5
  amplitude reduction 300, 304, 305
  asymmetry 304–5
  atypical antipsychotics and 304
  cognitive function 304
  latency 300, 304
  scalp distribution 306
  spectrum personality disorders 86
PABS (Perceptual Aberration Scale) 285
pandysmaturation syndrome 217
panic disorder 484

parachute study 674
parahippocampal gyrus 408
paraneoplastic encephalopathies,
    schizophrenic symptoms 193
paranoia 54, 56–7
    patients' perspectives 702
    psychoses in late-onset schizophrenia 73, 74
paranoid disorders 56–7
    diagnostic criteria 81
    overlap in clinical studies 81
paraphrenia 54, 57–8
    cognitive deficits 71
    diagnostic guidelines 69
    European use 68–9
    late 58
    misconceptions of term 69
    subtypes 69
parathymia 21
parental loss, disease development role 626
parenteral formulations see under
    antipsychotic drugs
parietal cortex 409
parkinsonism
    akinesia see akinesia
    antipsychotic-induced 444, 540, 553
    clozapine reduction 501
    ECT, antiparkinsonian effects 524, 540–1,
        543
    management 556, 558
    mechanisms 554
    rigidity 553
    serotonin role 554
    tremor 553
Parkinson's disease
    ECT effects 540
    subclinical in schizophrenia 554
partial hospitalization (day care) 694–6
partnerships, role in social course 123
'partners in autonomous living' 643
parvocellular system, spectrum personality
    disorders 87
PAS (Physical Anhedonia Scale) 285
pathological jealousy 59
pathophysiology 389
patient individuality 709
patients' perspectives 701–12
PCP see phencyclidine (PCP)
PCR (polymerase chain reaction) 260–1
penile dysfunction, antipsychotic-induced 577
Perceptual Aberration Scale (PABS) 285
perceptual impoverishment 22
periventricular leucomalacia 240–1
perphenazine, thyroid toxicity 576
personality disorder see schizotypal personality
    disorder
personal space
    importance 703, 711
    violence relationship 604
pharmaceutical companies, cost-effectiveness
    studies 719
pharmacogenomics 433, 496
phencyclidine (PCP) 306
    animal models of schizophrenia 394
    ketamine analogue see ketamine
    NMDA receptor binding 306, 349–50, 351,
        394

psychopharmacological studies 351–2
    schizophrenomimetic drug 349, 351, 453
phenocopies
    eye tracking dysfunction 284
    schizophrenia 255
phenomena 5–7
phenomenology, primary versus secondary
    cases 197–8
phenothiazines 444
phenotypes, intermediate see intermediate
    phenotypes
phenylketonuria, tardive dyskinesia and 563
'philosophy of care' 673
phobias 484
phosphodiester (PDE) investigations 43, 289
phospholipase A2 (PLA2) 268
phosphomonoester (PME) investigations 43,
    407
photosensitivity, drug-induced 578–9
photoshock, ECT versus 519
Physical Anhedonia Scale (PAS) 285
physical anomalies, minor see minor physical
    abnormalities (MPAs)
physical illness, treatment-resistant
    schizophrenia 492
pigmentation changes, drug-induced 578–9
place of birth 221, 236, 330
planum temporale 408
    asymmetry studies 289
plasma drug levels, treatment resistance 495–6
pneumoencephalography 403
point prevalence 207
polymerase chain reaction (PCR) 260–1
polymorphic syndrome 64
porphobilinogen deaminase (PBGD) 268
porphyria, acute intermittent 194–5
positive symptoms 5–6, 15, 114–15
    child/adolescent onset 36
    course 28
    dopamine role 375, 379
        amphetamine-induced psychosis 372,
            374
        'hard-wiring' 379
        subcortical systems 365–6, 376–8, 380
        see also antipsychotic drugs
    ECT response 534
    genetic studies 285
    history 25–6
    intermediate phenotypes 285
    late-onset schizophrenia 70
    neural circuitry 375
    neuroimaging studies 43
    premorbid behaviours 83
    prognostic significance 28–9
        symptom-related course indicator 126
    stability 28
positron emission tomography (PET) 29, 299,
    405
    atypical antipsychotics 427, 428
    brain asymmetry 335–6
    D_2 receptor bockade 424–5, 555
        5-HT$_2$ versus 427
    dopamine receptors 370, 372
    ERPs versus 300
    history 403
    memory 411

neural stimulation 405
neurodevelopmental hypothesis 335–6
regional cerebral blood flow (rCBF) imaging
    91, 405
resolution 299, 375
resting state 405
superior temporal gyrus 409
postmortem studies 336–7
    dopamine 368–70
    see also neuropathology
postnatal infections, as risk factor 219
postpsychotic depression 11–12, 142, 574
postsynaptic potential (PSP) 298, 299
post-traumatic stress disorder (PTSD) 625–6,
    661, 664
poverty of content of speech 20
poverty of speech 20
pre-eclampsia 328
prefrontal cortex (PFC)
    animal studies 340
        lesion 393
    antipsychotic drugs 426
    development 318, 339–40
        hippocampus role 392
    dopamine receptors 365, 368
    dorsal (DPFC) 313–17
    dysfunction 28, 365, 376
        deficits 290, 291
        specificity of alterations 319
    functions 407–8
        cognitive 313
        modulatory role 376, 377
    hippocampal–prefrontal relationship 317,
        392, 412
        delayed onset role 339
    interneurones 316–17
    neuropathology 313–17, 335, 376, 412
        disconnectivity 413
        GABAergic reductions 354
        grey matter decrease 314, 406
        synaptic abnormalities 313–14
        tyrosine hydroxylase decreases 369
        volumetric changes 313
    neuropsychology 407–8
    subcortical inputs
        adrenergic 453
        dopaminergic 314, 365, 376, 408, 451
        targets 316
        thalamic 314–16, 318–19
    temporal–prefrontal relationship 340
    thalamic projections 317
pregnancy and birth complications (PBCs) 40,
    218, 236–41
    animal models 391
    caesarean section 391
    child/adolescent onset schizophrenia 40
    demographic and clinical correlates 240
    determining exposure status 236, 239
    disease associations 328–9
    epidemiology 328
    frequency 327
    genetic factor interaction 238
    hippocampal anomalies 410
    inconsistencies 328–9
    intrauterine environment 328
    malnutrition 329, 390

neurodevelopmental hypothesis 327–9
pre-eclampsia 328
prematurity (extreme) 328
putative mechanism of action 240–1
schizophrenic mothers and 329
specific types 239–40
timing 329
type 328
ventricular enlargement 406
see also neurodevelopmental hypothesis
prejudice 678
see also stigma
prematurity, extreme 328
premodal phase, child/adolescent onset 36
premorbid personality 82–4
investigations 83
late-onset schizophrenia 74
schizoid 220
premorbid personality disorder 597
prenatal risk factors 219
infections *see* infection as risk factor
maternal stress 219, 244, 330
nutritional 219, 241, 244, 329, 390
obstetric *see* pregnancy and birth
complications (PBCs)
see also epidemiology; neurodevelopmental
hypothesis
pre-pulse inhibition, dysfunction 84–5
preschizophrenia
early developmental peculiarities 220
gender traits 83
schizoid personality disorder 83–4
schizotypal personality disorder 83–4
spectrum personality disorders 82–4
Present State Examination (PSE) 26
symptom definition 9
test performance comparisons 197–8
pressure of speech 20
prevalence 207
child/adolescent onset 40
depression 122, 143
extrapyramidal syndromes 554–5
secondary schizophrenias 188–9
secular trends 212–13
studies 208
tardive dyskinesia 562
prevention 47
procreational habits hypothesis 222
prodromal stage 118–20, 168, 663, 675, 678
monitoring 480–1
social course 123
violence in 595
professional carers, expressed emotion 621
prognosis
child/adolescent onset 46
depression 152
improvement in 710
indicators
negative symptoms 28–9, 125, 126
positive symptoms 28–9
symptom-related course 126–7
'middle prognosis' patients 523, 527
treatment-resistant schizophrenia 491–2
programmed cell death 318
progressive brain changes 406, 493–4
child/adolescent onset 42–3

gender differences 116
hippocampal volume reductions 410
mismatch negativity (MMN) reduction 303
neurodegeneration 302, 304
see also neurodegeneration; neuropathology
proportion of survivors affected (PSA) 207
protection motivation theory 599
proton resonance spectroscopy *see N*-
acetylaspartate (NAA) signal
PSA-NCAM reduction 337, 395
pseudohallucination 16
psychiatric disorders
classification 613
hierarchy 7–8
psychogenic elements 613–14
rehabilitation *see* rehabilitation
Psychiatric Epidemiology Interview Schedule
(PERI) 596
psychoanalysis 657–8
explanatory insight-oriented therapy (EIO)
671
psychodynamic theories/therapies 670–1
reality adaptive supportive therapy (RAS)
671
psychodynamic theories/therapies 670–1
psychogenic (reactive) psychoses 55, 614
psychological impairments 22, 113
psychomotor poverty syndrome 22
neuropsychological test performance 175
parietal cortex role 409
psychopathology 15–24
cognitive–behavioural therapy 669
descriptive 15–24
genetics role 595
pathological jealousy 59
rating scales 669
refractory schizophrenia 489–90
see also violence
psychopathy, violence link 595–8
Psychopathy Check List-Revised (PCL-R) 601
psychopharmacological studies
acetylcholine 357
ethical concerns 352
GABA 356
glutamate 351–2
serotonin 353–4
psychosis
abuse role 626, 661
acetylcholine role 452
acute 702
diagnostic criteria 12
ICD-10 classification 63–4
symptom-related course indicator 126
treatment 442–73
atypical *see* atypical psychotic disorders
chronic
hallucinatory 58–9
imaginative 59
interpretive 58
classification problems 188
culture-specific 56, 57
cycloid 56, 70–1
delusional/persistent *see* delusional disorders
drug-induced
amphetamine 372
hallucinogens 354

ketamine 351
misdiagnosis 39–40
patients' perspectives 702
phencyclidine (PCP) 349, 351, 453
stimulant 39–40, 378
early investigation/intervention 663–4, 678,
679
services 692
first episode *see* first-episode psychosis
flashbacks *versus* 626
frequency in 'normal' population 626
Lewy body dementia 356
neurotoxicity 337
normalization of concept 628
patients' perspectives 701–12
post-traumatic stress disorder 626
prepsychotic state 663, 675, 678
see also prodromal stage
problems associated 661
psychodynamic theories/therapies 670–1
psychogenic (reactive) 55, 61, 614
remission 121
social factors 614
symbolic expression 677
vulnerability to 152
see also individual psychotic disorders
psychosocial interventions 48, 485, 498,
657–87
adherence and 485
aims 663–4
art/music therapy 677
cognitive–behavioural *see*
cognitive–behavioural therapy (CBT)
cognitive functioning and 660
problems arising from 662
see also cognitive impairment; cognitive
remediation/rehabilitation
cultural issues 659
depression management in patients 160
drug-resistant schizophrenia 496–8
duration of treatment 660, 670
early interventions 663–4, 678, 679
future direction 678–9
goals 658, 659
group therapy 675–6, 705
small groups 675
therapeutic community 675–6
history 657–8
medication *versus* 658
mental health policy and 676
need-adapted therapy *see* need-adapted
approach
patients' perspectives 704
personal therapies 677–8
pharmacological interactions 485
principles 658–64
psychodynamic theories/therapies 670–1
psychoeducation therapy *see* family
interventions
psychosis and 658–9, 663–4
relevance 659
social skills *see* social skills training
special needs/considerations 659–63
cognitive limitations 662
individual differences 660–1
patient's role 661–2

therapist variables 662–3
substance abuse 606–7, 678–9
therapeutic milieu treatments 675–6
violence management 606–7
see also environmental factors;
    rehabilitation; social factors; *specific interventions*
psychosocial risks
child/adolescent onset schizophrenia 41
expressed emotion *see* expressed emotion (EE)
relapse 443–4, 475, 615–22
stress *see* stress (psychosocial)
see also social factors
psychosocial stress *see* stress (psychosocial)
psychostimulants, dopamine sensitization 378, 393
psychotherapy 485
PTAC 452
puberty, risk factor 40–1
public health 341
pulvinar reduction 91
putamen reduction, schizotypal personality disorder 91
pyramidal neurones
hippocampal disarray 312
prefrontal thalamic targets 316

QTc prolongation 433
atypical antipsychotics 430, 432, 578
typical antipsychotics 577, 578
Quality-Adjusted Life Years (QALYs) 715, 716
quality of life 130
quetiapine 430, 503
controlled trials 430, 445, 458, 503
costs 719, 720
drug-resistant disease 503
efficacy 445
EPS profile 555–6
late-onset schizophrenia treatment 76
pharmacological profile 430
side-effects 430
orthostatic hypotension 578
QTc prolongation 430, 578

'rapid neuroleptization' 457, 458
reaction time, impairment 169, 291
reactive (psychogenic) psychoses 55, 61, 614
reality adaptive supportive therapy (RAS) 671
reality distortion syndrome 23
hippocampus role 411
reality monitoring 176–7
reasoning 177–8
recombination, meiotic 258–9
recovery rate, outcome indicator 101, 103
reduction in child/adolescent onset 35, 44, 45–6
reelin expression 391, 396
refractoriness to antipsychotics *see* treatment-resistant schizophrenia
regional cerebral blood flow (rCBF)
functional imaging 91, 405
perfusion changes 332

rehabilitation 637–56, 688
assertive community treatment (ACT) 604–5, 639, 640, 691–2, 714
assessment and 638
conceptual framework 638
enhancing skills 641–6
cognitive 48, 497–8, 643–5, 649–50, 676–7
goal-oriented contracts 645–6
social 641–3
general principles 638–9
innovations 651
modifying environments 646–51
family 650
housing 75, 648–9, 707
vocational 646–8, 695–6
need for continuous management 637
patients' perspectives 707–9
programme strategies 639
task *versus* social performance 639
token economy/social learning programme 639, 640–1
see also mental health services; treatment; *specific interventions*
Rehabilitation Act Amendments (USA; 1996) 695
rehousing 75
relapses 125, 474–6
chronic exacerbation 460
drug effects on severity 476, 480
factors affecting 474–6, 484
following ECT 521, 528, 538
following first episode 459
impact 476
minor exacerbation 480
prevention strategies 380, 479–81, 664
depot *versus* oral drugs 478
targeted/intermittent strategy 456, 481
see also maintenance treatment; remission
prodrome 151, 480–1
rates 617, 666
risk 456, 474–6
stress role 475, 628, 637
expressed emotion 615–22, 664
life events 627
relationships 603, 606, 709
patient–carer 658
need-adapted approach 673
poor 706
relative risk (RR) investigations 179, 220, 280
religion and spirituality 705, 710
delusions and 702, 704, 709
respect for 709
remission 121
ECT effects 519
following first episode 459
psychoses 121
therapeutic goal 443–4
without medication 456
see also relapses
repeat expansion detection (RED) 268
Research Diagnostic Criteria 26
reserpine 349, 565
respiratory infections, risk factors 219
response topography model 641
restriction endonucleases 260

restriction fragment length polymorphism (RFLP) 260
retardation 20
retinal pigmentation 579
retinopathy 579
rewards, goal-oriented therapeutic contracting 645–6
RFLP (restriction fragment length polymorphism) 260
rheumatoid arthritis, negative comorbidity 213
rigidity 553
risk factors 215–23, 232–50
age *see* age as risk factor
definition 232
environmental *see* environmental factors
genetic *see* genetic factors
infections *see* infection as risk factor
malnutrition *see* malnutrition
marital status 222
maternal stress 219, 244, 330
migrant status and ethnic minorities 222–3
neurocognitive/neuropsychological markers 220
neuroleptic malignant syndrome 581
obstetric complications *see* pregnancy and birth complications (PBCs)
premorbid traits 74, 82–4
intelligence (IQ) 220
social impairments 220
prenatal exposures *see* prenatal risk factors
search for candidate exposure 236
season of birth 221–2, 236, 330
sex 215–16
tardive dyskinesia 563
see also gender differences
social *see* social factors
tardive dyskinesia 563–4
urban birth 221, 236, 330
see also life events; stress (psychosocial)
risperidone 430–1, 502
advantages 479
chronic disease 460–1
clinical trials 431, 445, 447, 458, 501
cognitive functioning 461–2
combination therapy 499
costs 719, 720
drug-resistant disease 501
effective dose 459
efficacy 431, 445
EPS profile 555
formulations 458
late-onset schizophrenia treatment 76
pharmacological profile 430
preclinical testing 431
psychosis treatment 431
schizotypal personality disorder treatment 91
side-effects 431, 499
hyperprolactinaemia 575
weight gain 576
violence treatment 605
Robert Wood Johnson Program on Chronic Mental Illness 713
root mean square (RMS) error 281, 283

Royal College of Psychiatrists, violence
    management 602–5
rubella, risk factor 219

S-16944 452
saccades 281–2, 283
sample surveys 204–5
SANE (Schizophrenia – A National
    Emergency) 665
SAS (Social Anhedonia Scale) 285
Scale for the Assessment of Negative Symptoms
    (SANS) 26, 285
Scale for the Assessment of Positive Symptoms
    (SAPS) 26, 285
Schedule for Affective Disorders and
    Schizophrenia 26
Schedule for the Deficit Syndrome (SDS) 115
Schedules for Clinical Assessment in
    Neuropsychiatry (SCAN) 9
Schilder's disease 193
schizoaffective disorder
    diagnostic criteria 12
    differential diagnosis from depression 151
    DSM-IV classification 62
    ECT and 530–1, 535
    GABA neurone reductions 355
    ICD-10 classification 64
    late-onset schizophrenia 70–1
    misdiagnosis of child/adolescent onset 38
    outcome 531
schizoid personality disorder 81
    overlap in clinical studies 81
    preschizophrenia 83–4
schizophrenia
    chronic disease
        delusional disorders 58–9
        event-related potentials (ERPs) 302, 303,
            305, 306
        exacerbations 460
        morbidity 460
        treatment 460–2
    concepts of 3–14
        Bleuler 4–5, 25–6, 657
        early concepts 3–5
        evolution in child and adolescent onset
            cases 34–5
        Griesinger 3–4
        historical views 3
        Kraepelin 4, 25
    dementia 116, 311
    first episode see first-episode psychosis
    secondary 187–202
        categories 188
        cause–effect relationship 189–90
        co-occurence with organic brain disease
            190–1
        criteria to support causal relationships
            190
        imaging studies 188
        phenomenology comparison with primary
            cases 197–8
        physical screening procedures 198
        prevalence 188–9
        problems with definition 188
        terminology and classification 187–8
    simple 4, 11–12

stages of development 120–1
subgroups 26
subtypes 11–12, 113–14
    see also individual disorders
Schizophrenia – A National Emergency
    (SANE) 665
Schizophrenia Linkage Collaborative Group
    263–4
Schizophrenia Patient Outcomes Research
    Team (PORT) 605
schizophrenia spectrum personality disorders
    80–100
    attentional performance 87–8
    clinical overlap 81–2
        personality disorder 81
    cognitive function 86–9
        Continuous Performance Test (CPT)
            87–8
        frontal executive functions 87
        lateralization 89
        memory 88–9
        thought disorder and disinhibition 88
        visual processing 86–7
    definition 255
    genetics 84, 255
    imaging studies 90–1
        CT scans 288
    neurochemistry 89–90
    outcome 92
    pathophysiology integration 92–3
    phenomenology 80–2
    preschizophrenia 82–4
    psychometric assessment 82
    psychophysiology 84–6
        eye movement disorders 86, 283
        habituation 85–6
        N100 and P300 attenuation 86
        P50 suppression 85
        pre-pulse inhibition 84–5
    treatment studies 91–2
schizophreniform disorder 55
    diagnostic criteria 12
    DSM-IV classification 61–2
    ECT and 521
schizotaxia 82
schizotypal personality disorder 60, 80
    amphetamine studies 90
    anhedonia 285
    cognitive disorganization 82
    continuous performance test (CPT) 87–8
    deficits
        executive function 87
        frontal lobe dysfunction 87, 93
        memory impairments 88–9
        thought disorder and disinhibition 88
        ventricle/brain ratio (VBR) 91
    diagnostic criteria 12, 80, 81
        DSM-III classification 285
        DSM-IV classification 62
    dopaminergic function 90
    evoked potentials 86
    eye movement abnormalities 86
    genetics 84, 285
    habituation anomalies 85–6
    ICD-10 classification 64
    imaging studies 90–1

misdiagnosis of child/adolescent onset 39
negative schizotypy 82, 285
non-conformity 82
outcome 92
overlap in clinical studies 81
positive schizotypy 82, 285
premorbid studies 82–4
preschizophrenia 83–4
psychotic-like symptoms 92
self-report scales 82, 285
treatment studies 91–2
schizotypal premorbid traits 220
Schneider's concept of schizophrenia 26
scopolamine 357
screening procedures 198, 206
seasonal ovopathy 222
season of birth 221–2, 236, 330
second-generation antipsychotics see atypical
    antipsychotic drugs
seizures
    cell death 540
    deliberate induction 517
        ECT see electroconvulsive therapy (ECT)
        photoconvulsive 519
    drug-induced 580–1
        chlorpromazine 580
        clozapine 501, 505, 532, 580
    grand mal 532
    kindling 191
    management 505
        see also anticonvulsant drugs
    status epilepticus 532
    threshold alteration 580
    see also epilepsy
selective serotonin reuptake inhibitors
    (SSRIs)
    adjunctive therapy 461, 505, 506
        drug-resistant schizophrenia 506
        negative symptoms 449–50, 506
    anxiety management 484
    depression management 156, 483
    drug abuse management 506
self-absorption 670, 705
self-awareness impairment 28
self-blame, high EE relatives 621
self-control
    strategies 677
    violence and 599
self-instruction, cognitive remediation 643
senile dyskinesia 560
sensitiver Beziehungswahn 60
sensitization to dopamine 378, 379, 393
sensory deficits
    acetylcholine role 265, 278, 287, 292, 357,
        395
    late-onset schizophrenia 73–4
    NMDA receptor role 302
    P50 deficit see P50 sensory gating deficit
    spectrum personality disorders 84–6
D-serine 454
serotonergic dysfunction
    extrapyramidal syndromes 554
    hallucinations 353
    investigations in depressive patients 154
    schizophrenia 286
    tardive dyskinesia 566

serotonin 352–4
  dopamine interactions 451
  dysfunction *see* serotonergic dysfunction
  GABA and 354
  neural architecture 352
  projections 352
  psychopharmacological studies 353–4
  receptors *see* serotonin receptors
  selective depletion model 393
  transporter 353
    see also selective serotonin reuptake
      inhibitors (SSRIs)
serotonin receptors 352–3
  5-HT1$_A$ receptors 352
    agonists 452
    autoreceptors 452
    clozapine partial agonism 426, 452
    upregulation 352
  5-HT1$_B$ receptors 352, 354
  5-HT$_{2A/C}$ receptors 352, 353
    5-HT$_{2A}$ antagonists 451–2, 461
    association studies 267–8
    'atypical' antipsychotics 267, 268, 353,
      354, 426, 427, 429, 430, 431, 432, 433
    chromosome 13q location 264
    decrease in depressive patients 154
    dopamine interaction 451
    hallucinogenic drugs 353–4
    occupancy threshold 424, 427
    polymorphism 268
  antipsychotics and 267, 268, 352, 353, 354,
    451–2
  genes
    expression studies 353
    pharmacogenetics 496
  LSD binding 352, 353
  occupancy, D$_2$ receptors *versus* 424–5, 430
  polymorphism 352, 353
  see also atypical antipsychotic drugs
sertindole 431–2
  clinical trials 431–2
  pharmacological profile 431
  preclinical testing 431
  side-effects 432
severity–liability model 114
sex chromosome abnormalities 194
sex differences *see* gender differences
sex hormones, development of schizophrenia
  73
sex ratio, child/adolescent onset schizophrenia
  40
sexual dysfunction 575
shared psychotic disorders (*folie à deux*) 59
  DSM-IV classification 62
sheltered employment 647
SIADH (syndrome of inappropriate
  antidiuretic hormone secretion) 576
sialorrhoea, drug-induced 579
simple sequence repeats (SSR; microsatellite
  DNA) 260–1
single major locus models (SML) 256
single nucleotide polymorphism (SNP) 261
single photon emission computerized
  tomography (SPECT) 29, 289, 405
  atypical antipsychotic pharmacology 426,
    428, 431, 433

dopamine receptors 370
  5-HT$_2$ *versus* D$_2$ receptor bockade 427
  D$_2$ receptor bockade 424–5
  regional cerebral blood flow (rCBF) imaging
    91
  resolution 299, 375
  resting *versus* haemodynamic state 405
  serotonin transporter studies 353
sleep disturbance 703
smooth pursuit eye movements (SPEM)
    abnormalities 45
  spectrum personality disorders 86
SNP (single nucleotide polymorphism) 261
Social Anhedonia Scale (SAS) 285
social class, risk factor 221
social constraint 617
social course 123–5
  alcohol and drug abuse effects 127
  developmental impairments 35
  first admission 123
  gender differences 124–5
  indicators 123, 125
  outcome 5 years after first admission 126
social factors 638
  child/adolescent onset schizophrenia 41
  depression 613
  employment/unemployment 646
  historical background 614–15
  negative symptom association 614
  relapse 443–4, 475, 615–22
  social class as risk factor 221
  stress *see* stress (psychosocial)
  violence 598–9, 608
  see also expressed emotion (EE);
    psychosocial risks
'social' firms 647
social impairment 637, 674
  child/adolescent onset schizophrenia 35
  neurodevelopment and 326
  patients' perspectives 701, 703
  phobias 484
  presychotic state 675
  rehabilitation *see* social skills training
  tardive dyskinesia effect 563
social learning programmes 639, 640–1
social phobias 484
social reactivity 614, 628
social security costs 714
social skills training 641–3, 660, 674–5, 677
  'booster' sessions 643
  clinical trials 642, 643
  formats 642
  models 641, 676
  supported employment and 648
  see also cognitive remediation/rehabilitation
social stigma 678, 711, 712
sodium valproate *see* valproate (valproic acid)
source monitoring 176–7
speech deficits 20
SSR (simple sequence repeats; microsatellite
  DNA) 260–1
SSRIs *see* selective serotonin reuptake
  inhibitors (SSRIs)
standard mortality rate (SMR) 123, 214
starvation, as risk factor 219, 241, 244
status epilepticus 532

stereotypic behaviour
  apomorphine-induced 395
  tardive dyskinesia *versus* 560
stigma 678, 711, 712
stimulant-induced psychosis 39–40, 378
stress (psychosocial) 613–36, 638, 661, 678
  coping/responses to 628
    family style 620, 622
    patient deficits 625
  debate 613
  domains 613–14
  dopamine dysfunction and 372, 374, 378,
    379, 393, 625
  early social environment 626–7, 628
  EE measures *see* expressed emotion (EE)
  Fisher344 rats 395
  genetics role 627
  historical background 614–15
  isolation role 629
  life events *see* life events
  maternal, as risk factor 219, 244, 330
  medication effects 627
  perinatal 392
  post-traumatic stress disorder 625–6, 661
    definition 625
    treatment 664
  pre-existing schemata 628
  relapse role 475, 615–22, 627, 637
  social-buffering 625
  vulnerability threshold 627
  see also psychosocial interventions
stress–vulnerability paradigm 626, 638
striatum 366, 367
  D$_2$ receptor blockade hypothesis 424–5
  dopamine hypothesis 374
  extrapyramidal symptoms correlate 427
  imaging 373
subacute sclerosing panencephalitis (SSPE)
  193–4
substance abuse 492, 506
  alcohol *see* alcohol abuse
  antidepressant drug effects 506
  antipsychotic drug effects 484–5
  comorbidity 127, 213–14, 484–5
  depression induction 143
  exclusion from services 484
  motivational treatment model 484
  pharmacotherapy 484
  pregnancy 329
  psychosocial intervention 606–7, 678–9
  relapse risk 476, 484, 492
  social course effects 127
  tardive dyskinesia and 563
  treatment-resistant schizophrenia 492
  violence risk 593, 594, 606–7
substantia nigra 366, 367
sudden unexplained death 214
suicide 122, 214
  depressive patients 152, 446
  indicators 123
  patients' perspectives 702, 703, 711
  prevention 442, 443
  reduction with clozapine 500
  risk factors 214
    age 123
  see also depression

sulpiride 428
  combination therapy 499
superior temporal gyrus (STG) 408–9
  asymmetry 304, 305
  functional disconnection 412–13
  P300 ERP 304
  symptom expression 409
  see also planum temporale
supernatural delusions 702
supported employment 647–8, 695
supported housing 648–9, 707
sylvian fissure, asymmetry 289
symptom-related course 125–7
  prognostic indicators 126–7
symptoms 25–33
  accessory 22
  arrangement in time matrix 120
  assessment 638
  child/adolescent onset 36
  clinicopathological relationship 317–18
  clustering of 22–3, 27
    investigations 29
  definitions, standards for 9
  DUP association 119
  empirical symptom dimensions and clusters
    117–18
  frequency, WHO study 111
  fundamental 22
  negative see negative symptoms
  neurobiological correlates 409, 410, 411
  outcome prediction 533
  positive see positive symptoms
  prodromal see prodromal stage
  psychotic see psychosis
  suppression of 442–3
  violence associations 595–6
    causal links 597–8
    evidence 596–7
    see also delusional disorders
  see also individual symptoms
synaptic abnormalities 337, 393
  excessive pruning 41, 42, 338, 339
  hippocampal 312–13
  prefrontal cortex 313–14
synaptic reorganization 338
synaptophysin 313, 314
syndrome of inappropriate antidiuretic
    hormone secretion (SIADH) 576
systemic illness, tardive dyskinesia versus
    560–1
systemic lupus erythematosus (SLE) 193

T2-relaxometry 404
tangentiality 20
Tarasoff vs Regents of University of California,
    duty to warn 592
tardive akathisia 559
tardive dyskinesia (TD) 76, 558–67
  antipsychotics and 76, 444, 456, 540, 562,
    563–4
    atypical 564
  atypical forms 559
  characteristics 558
  clinical manifestations 559
  cognitive functioning 461

complications 563
differential diagnosis 560–1
ECT protection 540–1, 543
epidemiology 562
neuroimaging/neuropathology 562
outcome, long-term 562
pathophysiology 561–2
prevention 564
risk factors 563–4
terminology 559–60
treatment 565–7
  alternate therapies 566
  anticholinergics see anticholinergic drugs
  botulinum toxin 567
  dopamine suppression 566
  ECT 541, 567
  free radical reduction 567
  GABAergic drugs 567
  management algorithm 564–5
  serotonin suppression 566
  typical abnormal movements (Marsalek)
    559
  withdrawal TD 559
see also extrapyramidal syndromes (EPSs)
tardive dystonia 559
task versus social performance 639
temporal cortex 408–9
  asymmetry 289, 317
  demyelination 192
  epilepsy 191
  ERPs 304, 306
  eye tracking 282
  frontal–temporal disconnection 412–13
  parahippocampal gyri 408
  superior temporal gyri see superior temporal
    gyrus (STG)
  symptom expression 409
  tumours 196
  volume reduction 42, 91, 408
    investigations 29
    schizotypal personality disorder 91
temporal sulci, asymmetry 336
tetrabenazine 566
thalamus 412
  animal lesion models 393
  imaging 412
  mediodorsal nucleus (MDN)
    developmental changes 318–19
    MDN–DPFC reductions 315–16
  prefrontal inputs 317
  prefrontal projections 314–16, 366, 367
  size alterations 91, 315, 412
    late-onset schizophrenia 72–3
therapeutic community approach 675–6
thioridazine, side-effects 575, 577, 578, 579
thioxanthenes 444
  schizotypal personality disorder treatment
    91
thought disorder 19–21, 88
  components 19
  definitions and classification 19–20
  disordered content 19
  disordered form 19
  incidence and variety 20–1
  late-onset schizophrenia 70

neuropsychological investigations 178–9
priming changes 178–9
schizotypal personality disorder 88
spreading activation 178
superior temporal gyrus 409
threat, perception of 596
three-factor model 117–18
thyroid toxicity, antipsychotics 576
token economy 639, 640–1
Tourette's syndrome
  antipsychotic treatment 565, 574
  tardive dyskinesia versus 560
Tower of London test deficits 171
trail making tests 290, 291
trait markers, fronto-temporal disconnection
    413
transgenic models 394, 396
transient psychotic disorders 54–6
  diagnostic criteria 12
  ICD-10 classification 63–4
  symptom-related course indicator 126
trans-institutional residential models 649, 689
transmission disequilibrium test (TDT) 266,
    267
transporters
  dopamine 369
  GABA 316, 319, 355–6
  glycine 455
  serotonin 353
    see also selective serotonin reuptake
      inhibitors (SSRIs)
treatment
  acute pharmacological 442–73
    hospital care 692–4
    see also hospitalization
  child/adolescent onset schizophrenia 47–8
  clinical issues 456–9
    dose–response relationship 458–9
    early intervention 457, 480–1, 662–4
    emergencies, drug choice 457–8
    predictors of response 456
    who to treat 456
  compliance 443
  cost-effectiveness 715–17
  at different stages 459–62
    chronic exacerbations 460
    chronic/residual 460–2
    first episode 459–60
  early phase 474
  maintenance see maintenance treatment
  outcome domains 485
  patient choice 443
  patients' perspectives 703–6
  pharmacological agents 444–56, 498–507
    adjunctive therapies 448–50, 503–6, 521,
      525–8
    adrenergic agents 453
    antipsychotics see antipsychotic drugs;
      atypical antipsychotic drugs
    dopamine agonists 450–1
    experimental 434, 450–6
    glutamatergic agents 434, 453–6
    muscarinic agents 434, 452–3
    psychosocial therapy interactions 485
    selective dopamine antagonists 450

serotonergic agents 451–2
violence remediation 443, 500, 505, 605–6
see also dopamine receptors; serotonin receptors; *specific drugs/treaments*
psychosocial *see* psychosocial interventions
resistance to *see* treatment-resistant schizophrenia
response to 30, 460, 492–6
services *see* mental health services
somatic
  ECT *see* electroconvulsive therapy (ECT)
  insulin coma 521
stabilization phase 474
stable phase 474
therapeutic goals 442–4, 658
  behavioural improvement 443
  regimen determination 443
  remission 443–4
  symptom suppression 442–3
violence 602–8
see also rehabilitation
treatment-resistant schizophrenia 425, 489–516
characteristics 491–6, 530–1
  age of onset 492–3
  brain metabolism 494
  cognitive function 492
  demographic/clinical variables 492–3
  depression 492
  gender 493
  negative symptoms 491–2
  neurochemical/neurophysiological 496
  neurological signs 493
  physical illness 492
  plasma drug levels 495–6
  substance abuse 492
child/adolescent onset schizophrenia 48, 492–3
continuum of response 490
definitions 489–91
  clinical criteria 489–90, 528
  concept change 507
  research criteria 490–1
endogenous trait 489
neuroimaging 493–5
'partial responders' 490
pharmacogenetics 496
pharmacological approach 498–507
  adjunctive therapies 503–7, 528–32
  antipsychotic drugs 498–503, 507
  see also antipsychotic drugs; *specific drugs/treatments*
poor functional outcome 489
psychopathology scores 489–90, 502
psychosocial approach 496–8
  see also psychosocial interventions
receptor occupancy 494
see also prognosis
treatment strategies for schizophrenia (TSS) 666–7
trema 120
tremor 553
tricyclic antidepressants (TCAs) 156, 449
trisomy (chromosome 5) 262–3

tuberous sclerosis 196
tumour associations 196–7
see also cancer
Turner's syndrome 194
twin studies 252–5
biases 253
cognitive impairment 179, 290–1
concordance rates 252–3
  proband-wise 254
criticism 254–5
  diagnostic criteria 253
  'microenvironment' 254
discordant pairs 255
environmental factors 254
eye tracking dysfunction 284
model fitting 253–4
monozygotic reared apart (MZA) 254
monozygotic *versus* dizygotic 252–3
MZ/DZ ratio 253
neuropathology/neuroimaging 288–9, 335, 410
  brain asymmetry 336
  brain volume 406
  cortical connectivity 316, 412
neuropsychological impairments 172–3
penetrance 256
polydiagnostic approach 253
positive *versus* negative symptoms 285
pregnancy and birth complications (PBCs) 218
  birth trauma 254–5
registers 253
typical antipsychotic drugs *see* antipsychotic drugs
tyrosine hydroxylase, immunolabelling studies 369–70

unemployment rates in schizophrenia 646
unitary models 27–8
child/adolescent onset schizophrenia 35
Universal Declaration of Human Rights, right to employment 646
urban risk factor 221, 236, 330
Usher's syndrome 195

valproate (valproic acid)
adjunctive therapy 450, 483, 504–5
  clozapine 505
  mood stabilization 483
aggression control 504–5
VAPSEs (variations affecting protein structure or expression) 267
variable number tandem repeat (VNTR) 260
variations affecting protein structure or expression (VAPSEs) 267
velocardiofacial syndrome (VCFS) 44, 196, 340
chromosome 22q 263
MPAs association 233
neuronal migration 355
schizophrenia associations 196, 198
ventral tegmental area (VTA) 366, 367
PFC modulation 377
ventricle/brain ratio (VBR) 91
schizotypal personality disorder 91

ventricular enlargement 42, 255, 326
birth/obstetric complications 406
ECT effects 540
genetic factors 406
lack of correlation with duration 331
late-onset schizophrenia 72–3
neuroimaging 29, 331–2, 406, 540
  CT studies 287–8, 331
  inconsistencies 332, 335
  MRI studies 331–2, 335, 337
  pneumoencephalography 403
treatment-resistant schizophrenia 493
variation with time 332
Vermont Longitudinal Study 128
violence 591–612
birth cohort studies 594, 608
'chemical restraint' 457, 605
community-based studies 593–4, 608
crime rate relationship 592
cross-cultural studies 598
early *versus* late starters 595–6
Epidemiologic Catchment Area (ECA) survey 593–4
factors affecting 596
  comorbid personality disorder 597
  cultural influence 598
  genetics role 595
  parental abuse/neglect 599, 603
  personal space 604
  social network influence 598–9
  substance misuse 593, 594, 606–7
is there a schizophrenia–violence association? 592–5
  community care 594–5
  homicide 592–3
  non-fatal violence 593–5
  public inquiries 592–3
legal aspects 591–2, 600, 607
management/prevention 602–8
  assertive community treatment (ACT) 604–5
  basic principles 602–3
  behaviour therapy 604
  Care Programme Approach 604
  coercion/security 607–8
  community patients 604–5
  compulsory treatment orders 607
  containment/restraint 604
  didactic training 604
  drug treatment 443, 500, 505, 605–6
  environment change 603
  inpatients 603–4
  psychological therapy 606
  Royal College of Psychiatrists guidelines 602–3
  social support/therapy 606–7
media coverage 591, 592–3, 711–12
National Confidential Inquiry (NCI) 593, 602
psychopathy and 595–8
  hypothesis of common causation 595
reoffending 607–8
risk assessment 599–602
  acceptability of risk 599–600
  appropriateness of setting 603

assessment tools 601–2
clinical *versus* actuarial judgment 600–1
'MacArthur' study 592, 597, 598, 600, 601–2
redistribution of risk 599
statistics 601
self-control and 599
social attitudes/climate 591–2
in social context 598–9, 608
staff attitudes 604
symptom associations 595–6, 596–7
causal links 597–8
delusions 596, 597
hallucinations 596, 597
negative symptoms 605
threat/control override 597
targets of 598
see also psychopathology
Violence Risk Appraisal Guide (VRAG) 601
visual hallucinations 17
visual impairments
late-onset schizophrenia 74
processing deficits in spectrum personality disorders 86–7
visual pathway 282
vitamin B_{12} deficiency, psychotic symptoms 193
VNTR (variable number tandem repeat) 260

vocational rehabilitation 646–8, 695–6
see also employment
voice hallucinations 16–17, 176
see also auditory verbal hallucinations (AVHs)
volitional saccade 281–2
vulnerability of patients, legal issues 600

Waldrop scale 233
ward functioning 694
Washington International Pilot Study 128
Wechsler Adult Intelligence Scale–Revised (WAIS-R) deficits 170, 290
weight gain 433, 576
atypical antipsychotics 429–30, 433, 576
conventional antipsychotics 576
white matter lesions (WMLs)
DTI/DWI 404–5
late-onset schizophrenia 72
whole brain volume (WBV) 406
will, lack of 22
Wilson's disease 195
misdiagnosis of child/adolescent onset 39
schizophrenia associations 195
Wisconsin Card Sorting Test 45, 290, 291
performance deficits 170
imaging 403
withdrawal, in depression 143

Wolfram syndrome 195–6
working memory 28
deficits 28, 88–9, 170–1
haloperidol-induced deficits 574
neurobiology 291
tests 290, 291
Workplace Fundamentals Module 648
World Health Organization (WHO)
10-country investigation 209
life event study 623
symptom frequency 111

xanomeline 452–3
X chromosome, linkage studies 265–6
xerostomia, drug-induced 579
X-ray irradiation, neurogenesis disruption 391

years of life lost (YLL) 716

ziprasidone 432
efficacy 445
EPS profile 556
parenteral administration 447
pharmacological profile 432
zotepine 432–3
pharmacological profile 433
side-effects 433
zuclopentixol, depot preparation 478